Procedures

P9-BJT-892

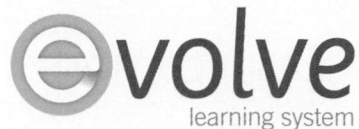
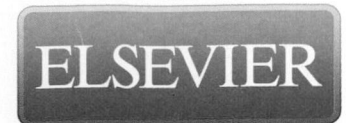
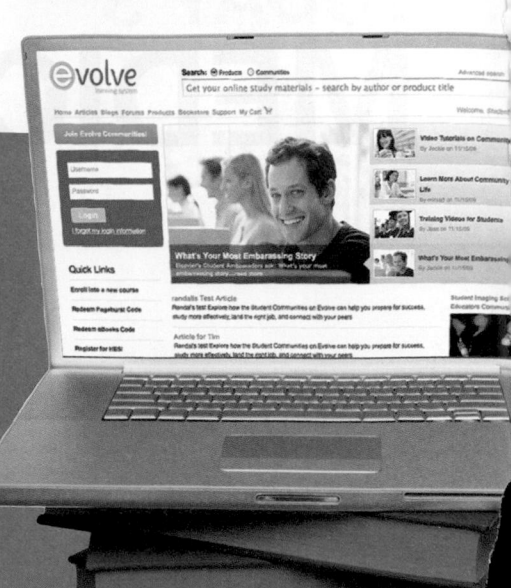

TODAY'S
MEDICAL ASSISTANT
Clinical & Administrative Procedures

2ND EDITION

TODAY'S
MEDICAL ASSISTANT
Clinical & Administrative Procedures

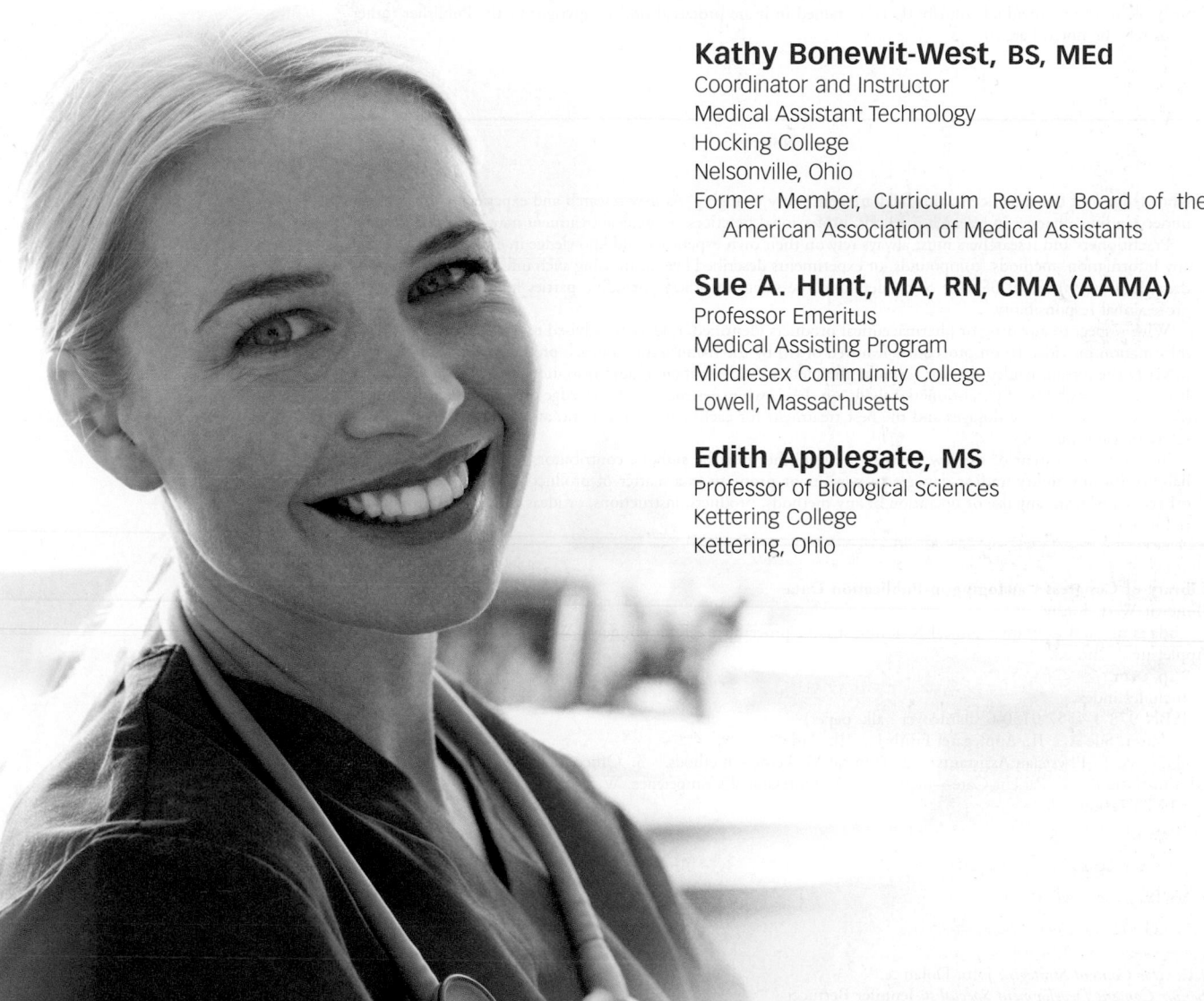

Kathy Bonewit-West, BS, MEd
Coordinator and Instructor
Medical Assistant Technology
Hocking College
Nelsonville, Ohio
Former Member, Curriculum Review Board of the
American Association of Medical Assistants

Sue A. Hunt, MA, RN, CMA (AAMA)
Professor Emeritus
Medical Assisting Program
Middlesex Community College
Lowell, Massachusetts

Edith Applegate, MS
Professor of Biological Sciences
Kettering College
Kettering, Ohio

ELSEVIER

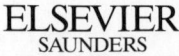

ELSEVIER
SAUNDERS

3251 Riverport Lane
St. Louis, Missouri 63043

Notices

Knowledge and best practice in this field are constantly changing. As new research and experience broaden our
understanding, changes in research methods, professional practices, or medical treatment may become necessary.

Practitioners and researchers must always rely on their own experience and knowledge in evaluating and using
any information, methods, compounds, or experiments described herein. In using such information or methods
they should be mindful of their own safety and the safety of others, including parties for whom they have a
professional responsibility.

With respect to any drug or pharmaceutical products identified, readers are advised to check the most current
information provided (i) on procedures featured or (ii) by the manufacturer of each product to be administered,
to verify the recommended dose or formula, the method and duration of administration, and contraindications.
It is the responsibility of practitioners, relying on their own experience and knowledge of their patients, to make
diagnoses, to determine dosages and the best treatment for each individual patient, and to take all appropriate
safety precautions.

To the fullest extent of the law, neither the Publisher nor the authors, contributors, or editors, assume any
liability for any injury and/or damage to persons or property as a matter of products liability, negligence or
otherwise, or from any use or operation of any methods, products, instructions, or ideas contained in the material herein.

Library of Congress Cataloging-in-Publication Data
Bonewit-West, Kathy.
    Today's medical assistant : clinical & administrative procedures / Kathy Bonewit-West, Sue A. Hunt, Edith
Applegate.—2nd ed.
      p. ; cm.
    Includes index.
    ISBN 978-1-4557-0150-6 (hardcover : alk. paper)
    I. Hunt, Sue A.   II. Applegate, Edith J.   III. Title.
    [DNLM: 1. Physician Assistants.   2. Clinical Medicine—methods.   3. Office Management—organization &
administration.   4. Patient Care—methods.   5. Professional Competence. W 21.5]
    610.73′72069—dc23
                                                                          2012025089

Executive Content Strategist: John Dolan
Senior Content Development Specialist: Jennifer Bertucci
Publishing Services Manager: Julie Eddy
Senior Project Manager: Celeste Clingan
Design Direction: Jessica Williams

Printed in China
Last digit is the print number: 9 8 7 6 5 4 3 2 1

Your laughter is contagious;
Your determination never swayed;
Your quest for knowledge is heart-warming;
Your generous spirit runs deep;
Your ability to overcome any obstacle is unmatched;
You are the medical assisting students of today and the future of health care of tomorrow.

KBW

For Melissa
Thank you for your support

SH

For Stan—my best friend and husband for over 50 years
You are the GPS in my life

EA

Reviewers

Virgie Allen, MBA
Medical Assistant Instructor/Academic Coordinator
American Career College
Ontario, California

Jodi Anderson, LVN
Campus Chair—MA Program
UEI College
San Diego, California

Patrick R. Callico, AS
Instructor
San Joaquin Valley College
Bakersfield, California

Jane Moore Crawford, MS, RD, SNS
Education Consultant
Tennessee Department of Education, School Nutrition
Program
Nashville, Tennessee

Christine Cusano, CMA (AAMA), CPhT
Senior Regional Director of Education
Lincoln Technical Institute
Lincoln, Rhode Island

Patricia DeBenedetto, CMA (AAMA), CHI
Medical Assistant Program Instructor
Medical Career Institute
Ocean Township, New Jersey

Brian Dickens, MBA, RMA, CHI
Medical Assistant Program Director
Keiser Career College/Southeastern Institute
Greenacres, Florida

Debra Downs, LPN, AAS, RMA (AMT)
Medical Assisting Program
Director/Instructor
Okefenokee Technical College
Waycross, Georgia

Ekbal Fakhoury, MD, DTMH, MS
Instructor
Heald College
Concord, California

Tracie Fuqua, BS, CMA (AAMA)
Program Director
Medical Assistant Program
Wallace State Community College
Hanceville, Alabama

Terri-Lee Hall, AAS
Instructor
YTI Career Institute
Mechanicsburg, Pennsylvania

Glenda H. Hatcher, BSN, RN, CMA (AAMA)
Medical Assisting Faculty
Southwest Georgia Technical College
Thomasville, Georgia

Shirley A. Jelmo, BS, CMA (AAMA), RMA
Medical Assisting Instructor
Pima Medical Institute
Colorado Springs, Colorado

Amy M. Link, BS, LPN, AHI, CIC
Lead Medical Assisting Instructor
Pima Medical Institute
Tucson, Arizona

Tabitha Lyons, NCMA
Corporate Program Manager for the Medical Assisting
Program
Anthem Education Group
Phoenix, Arizona

Kristin M. Maguire, NCMA, NCPT, NCET, MOS
Medical Assisting Instructor
Anthem Institute
Cherry Hill, New Jersey

Tracy L. Martin, RN, MSN, Ed.
Instructor
YTI Career Institute
Mechanicsburg, Pennsylvania

Laura Melendez, BS, RMA, RT BMO
Medical Assistant Instructor
Keiser Career College
Greenacres, Florida

Melody A. Miller
Medical Assisting Instructor
Lancaster County Career and Technology Center
Willow Street, Pennsylvania

Octavio M. Miranda
Medical Assistant Program Director
UEI College
Chula Vista, California

Marjorie A. Nibert, LPN
Education Supervisor
Lincoln College of Technology
Melrose, Illinois

Mary S. Nichols, RMA (AMT)
Medical Assisting Instructor
Heald College
Roseville, California

Brigitte M. Niedzwiecki, RN, MSN
Medical Assisting Program Director
Chippewa Valley Technical College
Eau Claire, Wisconsin

Julie Pepper, CMA (AAMA)
Instructor, Medical Assistant Program
Chippewa Valley Technical College
Eau Claire, Wisconsin

Carol Qare, DPM, CPT, RMA
Director of Healthcare
Heald College
San Francisco, California

Diana J. Richards, CPT, CMA (AAMA)
Medical Assisting Instructor
UEI College
Huntington Park, California

Theresa Rieger, CMA (AAMA), CPC
Manager
Mercy Health Northwest Family Clinic
Oklahoma City, Oklahoma

Dawn M. Szczesny, MA
Allied Health Instructor
Tri-State Business Institute
Erie, Pennsylvania

Charles W. Taber, Jr., AAS, NREMT-B, RMA (AMT)
Medical Assisting Instructor
High Tech Institute
St. Louis Park, Minnesota

Sandra Moaney Wright, M.Ed, Ph.D
Former Campus President
Atlanta Medical Academy
Atlanta, Georgia

Preface

Medical assistants, for many years an integral part of most physicians' staff, now fulfill an ever-expanding and varied role in the medical office, both clinically and administratively. With increased responsibilities, however, comes a greater need for professional knowledge and skills. This text has been designed to provide the basics of administrative and clinical competency combined with background knowledge of anatomy and physiology.

The underlying principle of this book is to provide a format for the achievement of professional competency in skills performed in the medical office, and the understanding of their application to real-life or on-the-job situations. When professional competency is achieved in the classroom, less of a gap should exist between the academic world and the real world, and thus the transition from student to practicing medical assistant is made more easily.

Although the book's usefulness to students in medical assisting educational programs has been emphasized, the practicing medical assistant will also find this text helpful as a learning and reference source. The organization of the text lends itself well to individualized instruction and convenient reference use.

FEATURES IN THIS TEXTBOOK

This second edition provides up-to-date information in both the administrative and clinical areas, and it incorporates current trends in technology.

Important Features Include the Following:

- Information about compliance to all aspects of HIPAA in the medical office
- Introduction to anatomy and physiology by body system
- Current information on the OSHA Bloodborne Pathogens Standard (including a new video)
- The theory and step-by-step procedure for measuring temperature using a temporal artery thermometer
- The theory and step-by-step procedure for performing pulse oximetry
- The theory and step-by-step procedure for proper body mechanics and wheelchair transfer of a patient (including a new wheelchair transfer video)
- Automated blood pressure cuffs information
- Latex glove allergy information
- The theory of intravenous therapy

- The A_{1c} blood glucose test
- Comprehensive updated pharmacology drug table of medications commonly administered and prescribed in the medical office
- Expanded information on the Electronic Medical Record (EMR)
- Prescriptions and the EMR
- Laboratory documents and the EMR
- The PT/INR laboratory test and the PT/INR home testing
- The theory and assistance required for mole removal
- The theory of home oxygen therapy
- Expanded information on CLIA-waived testing kids and CLIA-waived automated analyzers
- Information about obtaining an entry-level position as a medical assistant after graduation
- Up-to-date information on ICD-10 coding
- Brand new chapter on Emergency preparedness and Disaster planning

STANDARD PEDAGOGICAL FEATURES IN THIS TEXTBOOK

Other very important features include valuable learning aids:

- **On the Web Resources** allow students to access websites containing additional information relating to the chapter.

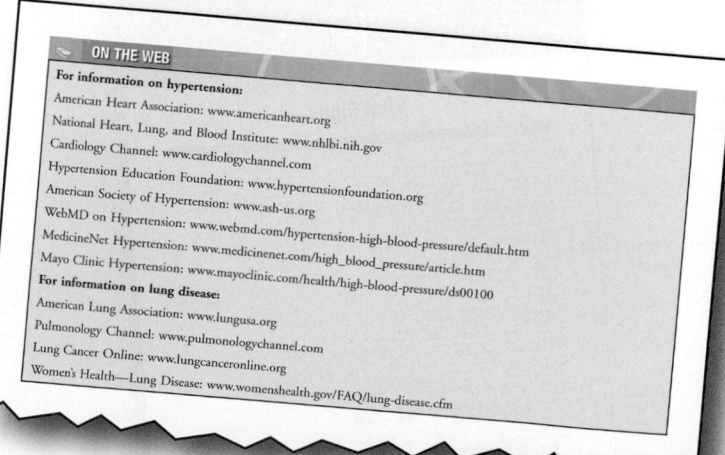

• The organizational format of this textbook facilitates the learning process by providing students and educators with detailed objectives and an in-depth study of the most current and up-to-date administrative and clinical procedures performed in the medical office. Presented at the beginning of each chapter are **Learning Objectives** and related **Procedures,** a **Chapter Outline,** and **Key Terms.** The learning objectives address the cognitive knowledge required to perform the procedures. Procedures coincide with the objectives to delineate the task or skill to be mastered by the student. (In the student Study Guide, most procedures are expanded into detailed performance objectives, including outcomes, and conditions and standards of acceptable performance.) The chapter outline provides a quick reference of the cognitive knowledge included in that chapter. The Key Terms list designates the terms and definitions that should be mastered for each chapter.

• The **knowledge** or **theory** that the student must acquire to perform each skill is presented in a clear and concise manner. **Numerous illustrations** accompany the theory section to aid the student in acquiring the knowledge relating to each skill.

• **Procedures** for each skill follow the theory section and are designed to help the student perform the skill with the level of competency required on the job. Each procedure is presented in an organized step-by-step format, with underlying principles and illustrations accompanying the techniques. A charting example follows each clinical procedure to provide the student with a guide for charting his or her own procedure. Students should find it much easier to acquire competency in charting with these examples.

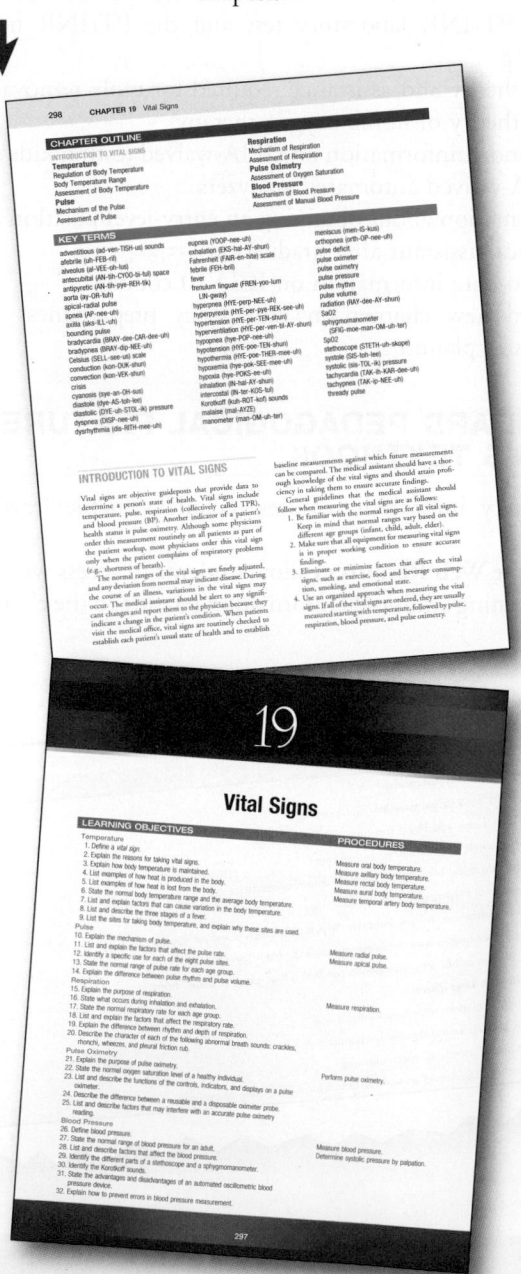

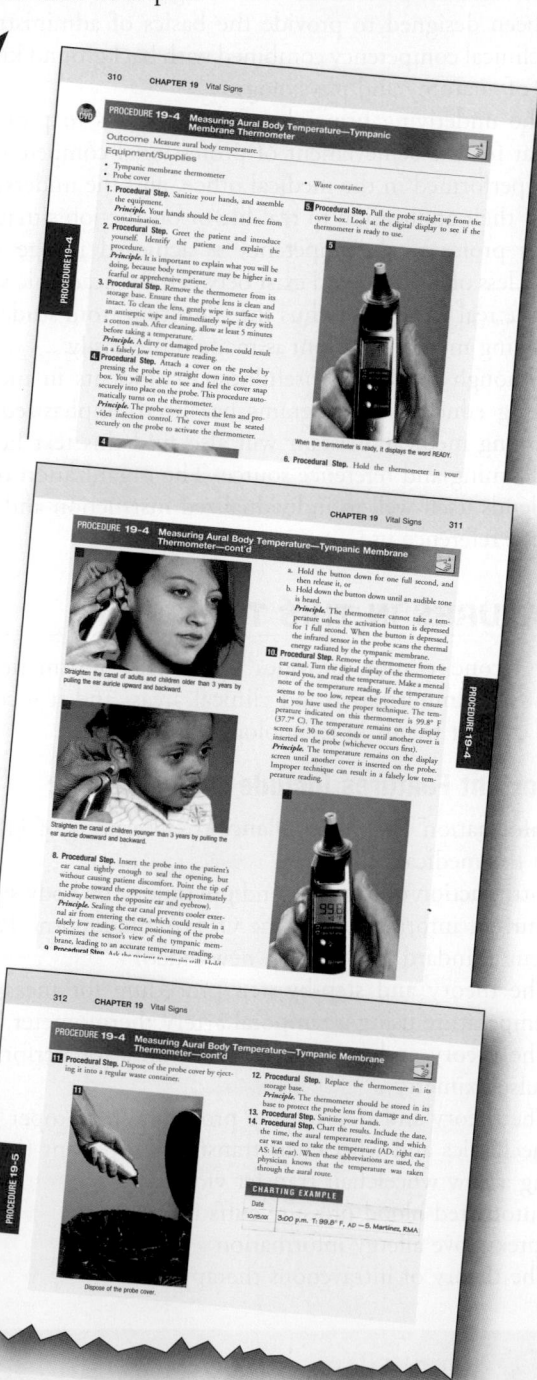

- The unique and memorable medical assistant biographical profiles (**Memories from Externship** and **Putting It All into Practice**) help students "connect" with their future beyond the classroom. The medical assistants featured are real people sharing their fears, likes, hopes, and aspirations, providing a "real-world" feel to the book and an inspiration for the student.

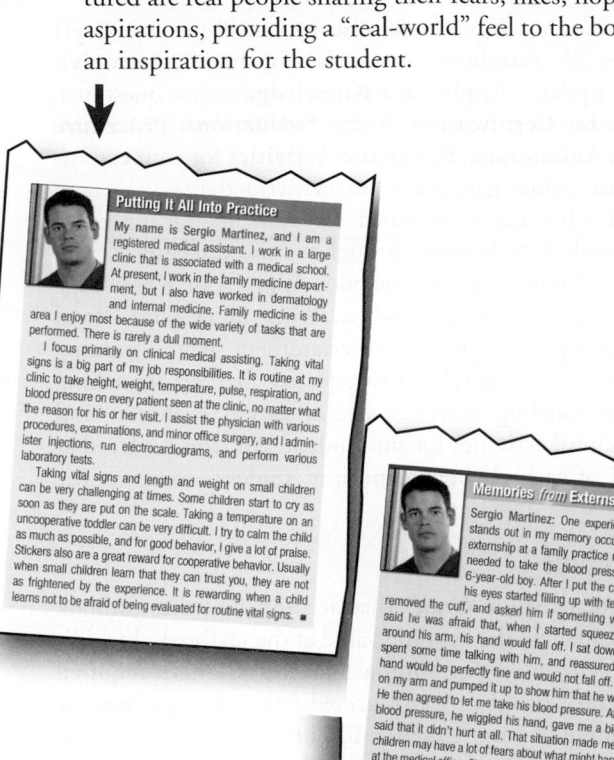

Putting It All Into Practice

My name is Sergio Martinez, and I am a registered medical assistant. I work in a large clinic that is associated with a medical school. At present, I work in the family medicine department, but I also have worked in dermatology and internal medicine. Family medicine is the area I enjoy most because of the wide variety of tasks that are performed. There is rarely a dull moment.

I focus primarily on clinical medical assisting. Taking vital signs is a big part of my job responsibilities. It is routine at my clinic to take height, weight, temperature, pulse, respiration, and blood pressure on every patient seen at the clinic, no matter what the reason for his or her visit. I assist the physician with various procedures, examinations, and minor office surgery, and I administer injections, run electrocardiograms, and perform various laboratory tests.

Taking vital signs and length and weight on small children can be very challenging at times. Some children start to cry as soon as they are put on the scale. Taking a temperature on an uncooperative toddler can be very difficult. I try to calm the child as much as possible, and for good behavior, I give a lot of praise. Stickers also are a great reward for cooperative behavior. Usually when small children learn that they can trust you, they are not as frightened by the experience. It is rewarding when a child learns not to be afraid of being evaluated for routine vital signs. ∎

Memories *from* Externship

Sergio Martinez: One experience that really stands out in my memory occurred during my externship at a family practice medical office. I needed to take the blood pressure of a small 6-year-old boy. After I put the cuff on his arm, his eyes started filling up with tears. I stopped, removed the cuff, and asked him if something was wrong. He said he was afraid that, when I started squeezing that thing around his arm, his hand would fall off. I sat down next to him, spent some time talking with him, and reassured him that his hand would be perfectly fine and would not fall off. I put the cuff on my arm and pumped it up to show him that he would be safe. He then agreed to let me take his blood pressure. After I took his blood pressure, he wiggled his hand, gave me a big smile, and said that it didn't hurt at all. That situation made me realize that children may have a lot of fears about what might happen to them at the medical office. Since that experience, I always take the time to explain procedures to children before I perform them. ∎

- **Patient Teaching** boxes emphasize this important aspect of the medical assistant's job and present it in context to make it more relevant, thereby making it more memorable.

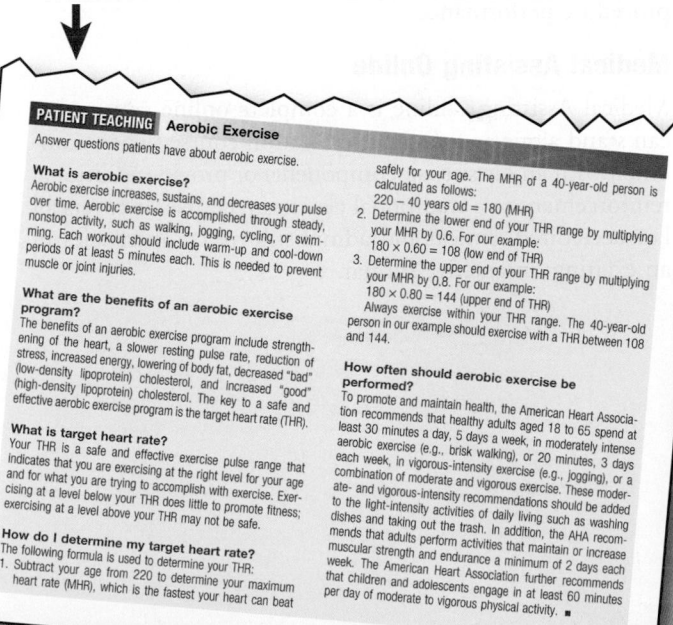

PATIENT TEACHING   Aerobic Exercise

Answer questions patients have about aerobic exercise.

What is aerobic exercise?
Aerobic exercise increases, sustains, and decreases your pulse over time. Aerobic exercise is accomplished through steady, nonstop activity, such as walking, jogging, cycling, or swimming. Each workout should include warm-up and cool-down periods of at least 5 minutes each. This is needed to prevent muscle or joint injuries.

What are the benefits of an aerobic exercise program?
The benefits of an aerobic exercise program include strengthening of the heart, a slower resting pulse rate, reduction of stress, increased energy, lowering of body fat, decreased "bad" (low-density lipoprotein) cholesterol, and increased "good" (high-density lipoprotein) cholesterol. The key to a safe and effective aerobic exercise program is the target heart rate (THR).

What is target heart rate?
Your THR is a safe and effective exercise pulse range that indicates that you are exercising at the right level for your age and for what you are trying to accomplish with exercise. Exercising at a level below your THR does little to promote fitness; exercising at a level above your THR may not be safe.

How do I determine my target heart rate?
The following formula is used to determine your THR:
1. Subtract your age from 220 to determine your maximum heart rate (MHR), which is the fastest your heart can beat safely for your age. The MHR of a 40-year-old person is calculated as follows:
   220 − 40 years old = 180 (MHR)
2. Determine the lower end of your THR range by multiplying your MHR by 0.6. For our example:
   180 × 0.60 = 108 (low end of THR)
3. Determine the upper end of your THR range by multiplying your MHR by 0.8. For our example:
   180 × 0.80 = 144 (upper end of THR)
   Always exercise within your THR range. The 40-year-old person in our example should exercise with a THR between 108 and 144.

How often should aerobic exercise be performed?
To promote and maintain health, the American Heart Association recommends that healthy adults aged 18 to 65 spend at least 30 minutes a day, 5 days a week, in moderately intense aerobic exercise (e.g., brisk walking), or 20 minutes, 3 days each week, in vigorous-intensity exercise (e.g., jogging), or a combination of moderate and vigorous exercise. These moderate- and vigorous-intensity recommendations should be added to the light-intensity activities of daily living such as washing dishes and taking out the trash. In addition, the AHA recommends that adults perform activities that maintain or increase muscular strength and endurance a minimum of 2 days each week. The American Heart Association further recommends that children and adolescents engage in at least 60 minutes per day of moderate to vigorous physical activity. ∎

- **Case Studies** are designed to assist the student in responding to "real-life" situations that occur in the medical office. A practitioner's response is given for each case study too, as a means of comparison for the student.

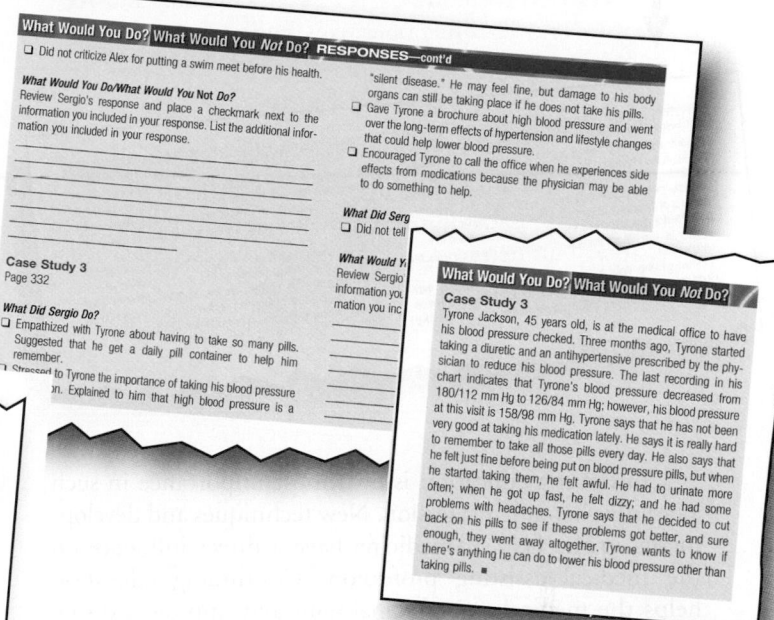

What Would You Do? What Would You *Not* Do? RESPONSES—cont'd

☐ Did not criticize Alex for putting a swim meet before his health.

What Would You Do/What Would You Not Do?
Review Sergio's response and place a checkmark next to the information you included in your response. List the additional information you included in your response.

"silent disease." He may feel fine, but damage to his body organs can still be taking place if he does not take his pills.
☐ Gave Tyrone a brochure about high blood pressure and went over the long-term effects of hypertension and lifestyle changes that could help lower blood pressure.
☐ Encouraged Tyrone to call the office when he experiences side effects from medications because the physician may be able to do something to help.

What Did Sergio
☐ Did not tell

Case Study 3
Page 332

What Would Y
Review Sergio
information you
mation you inc

What Did Sergio Do?
☐ Empathized with Tyrone about having to take so many pills. Suggested that he get a daily pill container to help him remember.
☐ Stressed to Tyrone the importance of taking his blood pressure

What Would You Do? What Would You *Not* Do?

Case Study 3
Tyrone Jackson, 45 years old, is at the medical office to have his blood pressure checked. Three months ago, Tyrone started taking a diuretic and an antihypertensive prescribed by the physician to reduce his blood pressure. The last recording in his chart indicates that Tyrone's blood pressure decreased from 180/112 mm Hg to 126/84 mm Hg; however, his blood pressure at this visit is 158/98 mm Hg. Tyrone says that he has not been very good at taking his medication lately. He says it is really hard to remember to take all those pills every day. He also says that he felt just fine before being put on blood pressure pills, but when he started taking them, he felt awful. He had to urinate more often; when he got up fast, he felt dizzy; and he had some problems with headaches. Tyrone says that he decided to cut back on his pills to see if these problems got better, and sure enough, they went away altogether. Tyrone wants to know if there's anything he can do to lower his blood pressure other than taking pills. ∎

- **Key Terms** identified at the beginning of the chapter are defined at the end of the chapter in the **Terminology Review**, providing students with a valuable terminology overview for each chapter. The Terminology Review now contains a helpful "Word Parts" column for key terms that are easily broken down into meaningful word portions.

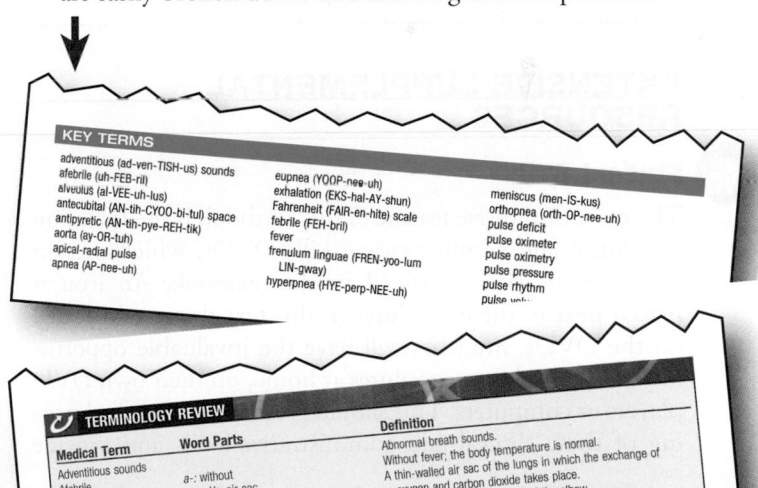

KEY TERMS

adventitious (ad-ven-TISH-us) sounds
afebrile (uh-FEB-ril)
alveolus (al-VEE-uh-lus)
antecubital (AN-tih-CYOO-bi-tul) space
antipyretic (AN-tih-pye-REH-tik)
aorta (ay-OR-tuh)
apical-radial pulse
apnea (AP-nee-uh)

eupnea (YOOP-nee-uh)
exhalation (EKS-hal-AY-shun)
Fahrenheit (FAIR-en-hite) scale
febrile (FEH-bril)
fever
frenulum linguae (FREN-yoo-lum LIN-gway)
hyperpnea (HYE-perp-NEE-uh)

meniscus (men-IS-kus)
orthopnea (orth-OP-nee-uh)
pulse deficit
pulse oximeter
pulse oximetry
pulse pressure
pulse rhythm
pulse vol—

TERMINOLOGY REVIEW

Medical Term	Word Parts	Definition
Adventitious sounds		Abnormal breath sounds.
Afebrile	a-: without	Without fever; the body temperature is normal.
Alveolus	alveol/o: air sac	A thin-walled air sac of the lungs in which the exchange of oxygen and carbon dioxide takes place.
Antecubital space	ante-: before cubitum: elbow	The space located at the front of the elbow.
Antipyretic	anti-: against pyr/o: fever -ic: pertaining to	An agent that reduces fever.
Aorta		The major trunk of the arterial system of the body. The aorta arises from the upper surface of the left ventricle.
Apnea	a-: without or absence of -pnea: breathing	The temporary cessation of breathing.
Axilla		The armpit.
Bounding pulse		A pulse with an increased volume that feels very strong and full.
Bradycardia	brady-: slow cardi/o: heart -ia: condition of diseased or abnormal state	An abnormally slow heart rate (less than 60 beats per minute).
Bradypnea	brady-: slow -pnea: breathing	An abnormal decrease in the respiratory rate of less than 10 respirations per minute.

- Legal issues are important for medical assisting students to understand; it is damage control for the medical practice for which they will eventually work. **Medical Practice and the Law** boxes at the end of each chapter provide the student with current legal information pertaining to the chapter.

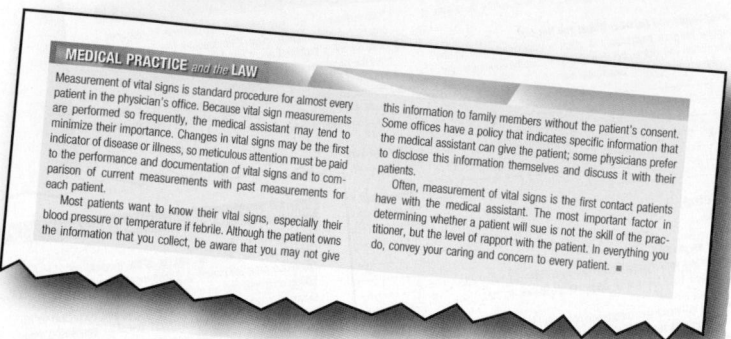

MEDICAL PRACTICE *and the* **LAW**

Measurement of vital signs is standard procedure for almost every patient in the physician's office. Because vital sign measurements are performed so frequently, the medical assistant may tend to minimize their importance. Changes in vital signs may be the first indicator of disease or illness, so meticulous attention must be paid to the performance and documentation of vital signs and to comparison of current measurements with past measurements for each patient.

Most patients want to know their vital signs, especially their blood pressure or temperature if febrile. Although the patient owns the information that you collect, be aware that you may not give this information to family members without the patient's consent. Some offices have a policy that indicates specific information that the medical assistant can give the patient; some physicians prefer to disclose this information themselves and discuss it with their patients.

Often, measurement of vital signs is the first contact patients have with the medical assistant. The most important factor in determining whether a patient will sue is not the skill of the practitioner, but the level of rapport with the patient. In everything you do, convey your caring and concern to every patient. ∎

Continuing education is of utmost importance in such a rapidly changing profession. New techniques and developments in the field of medicine have a direct influence on the medical assisting profession. Continuing education helps the medical assistant maintain and improve existing skills and learn new skills. A list of helpful community resources for the medical assistant is found in Appendix C on the Evolve site.

The authors hope that individuals who use this approach to medical assisting will view this text not as a stopping place but as a means of opening doors to new paths to be explored in the medical assisting profession.

EXTENSIVE SUPPLEMENTAL RESOURCES

Student DVDs

The most impressive feature of this textbook is the inclusion of clinical and administrative skills DVDs, which present many of the skills outlined in the textbook. An icon is placed next to the procedures in this text that are included on the DVDs. Students will have the invaluable opportunity to watch these procedures at home, on their own DVD players or computers. This should greatly enhance the learning of these clinical and administrative skills and provide the medical assistant graduate with competence and confidence to perform clinical and administrative skills in the medical office.

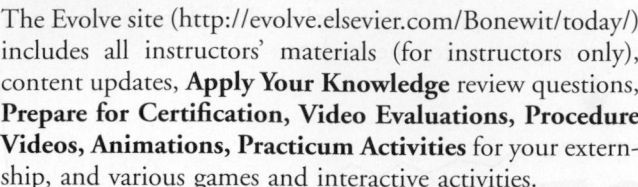

Evolve Resources

The Evolve site (http://evolve.elsevier.com/Bonewit/today/) includes all instructors' materials (for instructors only), content updates, **Apply Your Knowledge** review questions, **Prepare for Certification, Video Evaluations, Procedure Videos, Animations, Practicum Activities** for your externship, and various games and interactive activities.

An Evolve site is designed for students to apply the theory and skills learned throughout the textbook. Organized by chapter, the site includes Apply Your Knowledge questions and several games (i.e., "Quiz Show" and "Road to Recovery") to provide entertainment while learning important concepts related to selected chapters, matching exercises, labeling exercises, identification exercises, and other helpful activities for the student. An icon is placed at the end of each chapter to prompt students to access the site.

Study Guide

The student *Study Guide* that accompanies the textbook greatly enhances the learning value of the textbook. In addition, its outcome-based approach meets the criteria required for outcome-based program accreditation as stipulated by the Commission on Accreditation of Allied Health Educational Programs (CAAHEP) and the Curriculum Review Board of the American Association of Medical Assistants (AAMA). Included are extensive exercises for each chapter, as well as performance checklists. The study guide includes pretests and posttests, which help better prepare students for chapter tests, a textbook and student Study Guide assignment sheet for documenting completion of assignments and calculating points earned for each assignment, and a laboratory assignment sheet to keep track of student procedure performance.

Medical Assisting Online

Medical Assisting Online is a complete online course that can stand alone as a distance education course (when combined with an on-site lab component) or provide additional reinforcement to a traditional classroom course. It covers all key accredited clinical and administrative competencies in an exciting, interactive format.

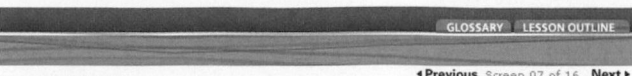

Body Temperature

Methods for Measuring Body Temperature

There are different methods for taking a person's temperature. The three most-used methods—oral, **aural**, and rectal—all have similar considerations:

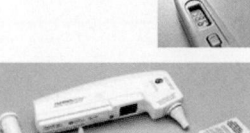

- Type of equipment used
- Placement of the thermometer tip
- Length of time needed to reach temperature
- Normal temperature range
- Contraindications, or when not to use a method

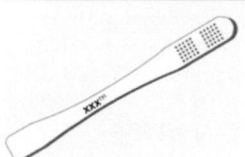

We'll look at oral, tympanic, and rectal methods and the considerations for each.

Click **Next** to continue.

◀ **Previous**   **Next** ▶

Body Temperature

Oral Method of Measuring Body Temperature: Procedure

Follow these guidelines for measuring the body temperature orally.

Placement: The tip is placed under the tongue.

Length of time needed to reach temperature: Approximately 1 minute is required for an accurate reading. Wait until the temperature is displayed or the unit beeps.

Contraindications: Do not use the oral method if the patient is not able to hold the tip under the tongue for the required time period. It is not acceptable for children under the age of 2 years old.

View the following for details about taking and documenting an oral temperature.

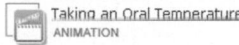 Taking an Oral Temperature
ANIMATION

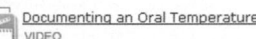 Documenting an Oral Temperature
VIDEO

Click **Next** to continue.

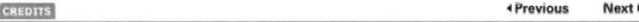

CREDITS   ◀ **Previous**   **Next** ▶

Acknowledgments

The completion of the second edition of this text permits the opportunity to relay appreciation to the medical assisting educators who so eagerly and enthusiastically use and enjoy this text. To them the authors are also indebted for their helpful assistance and suggestions for this new text.

The photographs in the textbook were taken by Brian Blauser and Jack Foley, professional photographers. We are indebted to them for their careful precision and patience in taking and editing the photographs, thus greatly enhancing the learning value of this text.

We would like to gratefully acknowledge the following practicing medical assistants for contributing many hours to be photographed for demonstration of the clinical procedures in the text: Megan Baer, Dawn Bennett, Trudy Browning, Janet Canterbury, Theresa Cline, Marlyne Cooper, Hope Fauber, Dori Glover, Jennifer Hawk, Kevin Hickey, Cammie Lindner, Judy Markins, Korey McGrew, Natalie Morehead, Traci Powell, Linda Proffitt, Latisha Sharpe, Michelle Shockey, Kara Van Dyke, Michelle Villers, and Huang Ying.

We would also like to acknowledge the following individuals who portrayed patients in the text: Brian Adevc, Travis Allman, Jessica Bennett, Kim Bingham, Pamela Bitting, Caitlin Brennan, David Brennan, Hollie Bonewit, Phillip Carr, Chloe Cline, Angie Coffin, Chad Cron, Dawn Decaminada, Aja Fox, Markly Georges, Connie Hazlett, Gary Hazlett, Isabella Ipacs, Joey Ipacs, Susan Ipacs, Charles Larimer, Pam Larimer, Christopher Mace, Deborah Murray, Delaney Murray, Michael Nkrumah, Heather Pike, Jan Six, Megan Skidmore, Colton Smith, Sydney Smith, Clinton Swart, Tristen West, and Lynn Witkowski.

We would like to extend our appreciation to the authors, publishers, and equipment companies who have granted us permission to use their illustrations.

The publication of this text was accomplished through the capable guidance of many talented individuals at Elsevier. Many thanks to Senior Project Manager, Celeste Clingan, for her outstanding production work. This book could not have attained this level of excellence without the exceptional capabilities of Jennifer Bertucci, Senior Content Development Specialist. Jessica Williams created these beautiful interior and cover designs. And, finally, we want to relay a very special thank you to John Dolan, Executive Content Strategist, for his dedication to quality medical assisting education and his encouragement in helping us achieve our very best in this edition.

With warm regard, we would like to recognize those very important individuals—the medical assisting students, graduates, and practicing medical assistants—who continually strive for excellence in meeting the demands and ever-increasing requirements of such a challenging profession. A quote by an unknown author really says it better: "Celebrate your talents, for they are what make you unique."

Kathy Bonewit-West, BS, MEd
Sue A. Hunt, MA, RN, CMA (AAMA)
Edith Applegate, MS

Clinical Procedure Icons

The OSHA Bloodborne Pathogens Standard must be followed when performing many of the clinical procedures presented in this text. To assist the student in following the OSHA Standard, icons have been incorporated into the procedures. An illustration of each icon along with its description is outlined below.

 HAND HYGIENE is an important medical aseptic practice and is crucial in preventing the transmission of pathogens in the medical office. The medical assistant should sanitize the hands frequently, using proper technique. When performing clinical procedures, the hands should always be sanitized before and after patient contact, before applying gloves and after removing gloves, and after contact with blood or other potentially infectious materials.

 CLEAN DISPOSABLE GLOVES should be worn when it is reasonably anticipated that you will have hand contact with the following: blood and other potentially infectious materials, mucous membranes, nonintact skin, and contaminated articles or surfaces.

 BIOHAZARD CONTAINERS are closable, leakproof, and suitably constructed to contain the contents during handling, storage, transport, or shipping. The containers must be labeled or color coded and closed before removal to prevent the contents from spilling.

 APPROPRIATE PROTECTIVE CLOTHING such as gowns, aprons, and laboratory coats should be worn when gross contamination can reasonably be anticipated during performance of a task or procedure.

 **FACE SHIELDS OR MASKS IN COMBINATION WITH EYE-PROTECTION DEVICES** must be worn whenever splashes, spray, spatter, or droplets of blood or other potentially infectious materials may be generated, posing a hazard through contact with your eyes, nose, or mouth.

Contents

1

The Health Care System

1. Describe the role of medical office care in the health care system.
2. Describe the historical development of managed care.
3. Identify the flow of activity in ambulatory care.
4. Identify the various types of health care professionals, and describe the job responsibilities of each professional.
5. State the educational requirements for physicians.
6. List and describe the parts of the medical office.
7. Identify and describe the various types of medical specialties.
8. Identify three medical practice types.
9. Compare and contrast various complementary and traditional medical treatments.

CHAPTER OUTLINE

KEY TERMS

ambulatory (AM-byoo-la-toe-ree) care
capitation (cap-ih-TAY-shun)
curative (KYUR-a-tive) treatment
empirical (em-PEER-ih-cle)
fee for service

formulary (FORM-you-lay-ree)
health insurance
holistic (hole-IH-stick)
managed care
palliative (PAL-ee-a-tive) treatment

residency (RES-ih-dense-ee)
symptomatic (simp-toe-MA-tick) treatment
utilization review

INTRODUCTION TO HEALTH AND THE HEALTH CARE SYSTEM

The World Health Organization (WHO) defines *health* as the absence of illness or disease and a state of being in which the individual feels well and is able to carry out the daily functions of life with no difficulties and no pain. In reality, no one reaches this optimum level of health. Everyone has aches and pains, psychological if not physical.

In our health care system, the physician's responsibility is to examine hundreds of people in the course of a week and try to focus on medical problems that meet the following criteria: The problem is causing or can cause severe difficulties in carrying out the daily functions of life, and the problem can be treated either by reducing the effects of the symptoms or by eradicating the problem altogether.

Each individual the physician sees has a different group of presenting physical symptoms as well as a different set of social circumstances and emotional issues. The physician listens to the patient's description of his or her life, performs objective laboratory and diagnostic tests, identifies medical problems, and assesses the nature of each problem.

Physicians know that the vast majority of medical problems do not pose a long-term threat to health. Most medical conditions get better over time. Effective treatments are available to cure many conditions **(curative treatment).** In other cases the physician can reduce the symptoms even if the underlying medical condition is not significantly affected. This type of treatment is called **symptomatic treatment** (responding to symptoms) or **palliative treatment** (seeking to reduce the effects of a disease or condition without curing the underlying disease). For example, a patient with a urinary tract infection who is given a prescription for antibiotics receives curative treatment, whereas a patient who has diabetes mellitus receives palliative treatment. The patient is prescribed insulin, which alleviates the symptoms of the diabetes; however, the treatment does not cure the diabetes.

Most treatments are based on scientific study. In Western scientific medicine, as in no other medical tradition, approaches to diagnosis and treatment have been studied and tested over hundreds of years. As long ago as the fourth century BC, a physician named Hippocrates in Greece believed that disease was not a punishment for transgressions against the gods, but rather the result of physiologic and environmental factors that could be studied. Since the time of Hippocrates, the practice of medicine has changed considerably in response to scientific discoveries (Table 1-1).

SHIFT FROM HOSPITAL-BASED TO COMMUNITY-BASED HEALTH CARE

Three trends running in parallel through modern medicine have led to an increasingly important role for office-based health care.

The first trend is the desire by those who pay the bills—employers, the federal and state governments, and insurance companies—to reduce the costs of health care whenever and wherever possible.

A second trend is the pressure for medical offices and clinics to provide a broad range of diagnostic and treatment services to avoid having to admit patients to the hospital. The increased cost of hospitalization has provided this pressure. Developments in diagnostic equipment, increased availability of home health care, and less invasive surgical procedures have facilitated the process.

The third trend is an increased understanding, through **empirical** evidence (information learned from experimental research), that people *feel better* the less they must be confined to a hospital or go to a hospital for treatment. Being able to be diagnosed and treated in an outpatient setting with follow-up at home allows people to feel more in control of their lives as medical patients. This is especially important for people who have frequent contact with the medical system, such as the parents of infants and children, the elderly, and those with chronic illnesses. Many people who would have been hospitalized for long periods or possibly even institutionalized 50, 25, or even 10 years ago are currently living independently in the community.

Today the hospital's role is primarily to provide acute care and diagnostic services. In order for a patient to be hospitalized, his or her condition must be unstable or necessitate constant regulation of therapy. If the patient does not meet these strict criteria, he or she goes home to be followed as an outpatient; is transferred to a rehabilitation facility for intense, regular rehabilitative treatment; or is sent to a nursing home for long-term maintenance care.

MANAGED CARE VERSUS PATIENT CARE: COMPETING FORCES FACING THE MEDICAL OFFICE IN THE TWENTY-FIRST CENTURY

Fee-for-Service Insurance Plans

Traditionally, medical care in the United States was paid for on a **fee-for-service** basis. Each service was billed and paid for as a separate charge: so much for the office visit, so much for the electrocardiogram, so much for the urinalysis, and so on. Fee-for-service payments can be thought of as ordering food at a restaurant à la carte: so much for the main course, so much for a salad, so much for coffee.

During the first part of the twentieth century, health insurance (if the patient had any) paid only for hospitalization, and usually the patient completed most of the paperwork. **Health insurance** is a system by which a person or the person's employer pays an insurance company a yearly amount of money, and the insurance company pays some or most of the person's medical expenses for that year. The theory behind insurance is that, although a few people will have large medical bills over the course of the year, most people will have small bills. By setting the fee for everyone

Table 1-1	Milestones in the History of Medicine
3000 BC	Writings about the circulation of blood in China.
c. 460 BC	Birth of Hippocrates (called the "Father of Medicine") in Greece—based medical care on observation and believed that illness was a natural biologic event.
1514-1564	Andreas Vesalius—wrote the first relatively correct anatomy textbook.
1578-1657	William Harvey—discovered circulation of blood (England).
1632-1723	Antony van Leeuwenhoek—discovered the microscope (Holland).
1728-1793	John Hunter—developed surgical techniques used in surgery.
1749-1823	Edward Jenner—first vaccine for smallpox (England).
1818-1865	Ignaz Semmelweis—theorized that handwashing prevents childbirth fever (Austria); his theories were rejected during his lifetime and not accepted until the work of Pasteur and Lister.
1820-1910	Florence Nightingale—began training for nurses; established first nursing school; before this time nurses received no training and the profession had little status (England).
1821-1910	Elizabeth Blackwell—first woman to complete medical school in the United States; established a medical school in Europe for women only.
1821-1912	Clara Barton—acted as a nurse on the battlefields of the Civil War; was a civil rights activist and suffragette; organized the American Red Cross.
1822-1895	Louis Pasteur—developed pasteurization of wine, beer, and milk to prevent growth of microorganisms; microbiology (France).
1827-1912	Joseph Lister—demonstrated that microorganisms cause illness; his experiments with phenol, carbolic acid, and other antiseptics laid the groundwork for modern surgery (England).
Mid-1800s	First large hospitals, such as Bellevue, Johns Hopkins, and Massachusetts General, established in U.S. cities. Discovery of anesthesia in the United States is credited to a Southern physician named Crawford Williamson Long.
1843-1910	Robert Koch—isolated the bacteria that cause anthrax and cholera; established principles to determine that a specific type of bacteria causes a specific disease (Germany).
1845-1923	Wilhelm Roentgen—discovered x-rays (Germany) based on the discovery of radium and radioactivity by Marie Curie (1867-1934) and Pierre Curie (1859-1906).
1851-1902	Walter Reed—proved that yellow fever is transmitted by mosquitoes, not direct contact, while working as a U. S. army physician in Cuba. An aggressive spraying program made it possible to complete the Panama Canal.
1854-1915	Paul Ehrlich—coined the term *chemotherapy;* predicted autoimmunity; developed Salvarsan (arsphenamine), an effective treatment for syphilis, in 1909. This led to the development of sulfa drugs and other antibiotics (Germany).
1881-1955	Alexander Fleming—discovered penicillin (England); identified it in 1929, but an efficient method of producing large amounts was not developed until needed in World War II. Other antibiotic medications such as sulfa were soon discovered.
1891-1941	Frederick Banting—co-discoverer of insulin with Charles Best and John Macleod in 1922 (Canada).
1906-1993	Albert Sabin—developed oral polio vaccine.
1914-1995	Jonas Salk—developed parenteral polio vaccine.
1922-2001	Christiaan Neethling Barnard—South African surgeon who is remembered for succeeding at the first human-to-human heart transplant in 1967.
1978	Birth of Louise Joy Brown, the first child born by in vitro fertilization, in Great Britain.

at a level above the actual cost of care for most people, the insurance company can pay for the care of the well, the occasionally ill, and the often ill and still make a profit.

This system encouraged health care providers to provide a high level of care for everyone with health insurance because the insurance paid for every test and every procedure. Physicians' incomes soared between the end of World War II and the early 1980s. With the increasing costs of laboratory and diagnostic testing, hospital services, and office visits, the cost of medical care increased far more rapidly than the cost of other goods and services in the U.S. economy. (In economic terms, health care inflation increased much more rapidly than the general rate of inflation.)

During this time, ever-better health insurance became a standard employee benefit at many companies. The first kind of health insurance offered, in the 1950s and 1960s, was coverage for hospital care. Coverage for office visits became standard in the 1970s.

Government Insurance Plans

Recognizing that there were large segments of the population without insurance because they are not employed, the federal government began to provide health insurance to large segments of the population starting in the 1960s. Medicaid began to provide health insurance for low-income children without parental support and later expanded to cover all low-income people. Medicare initiated health insurance for the elderly, the disabled, and those with end-stage kidney disease. The Civilian Health and Medical Program of the Uniformed Services (CHAMPUS; now called *TRICARE*) provided health insurance for dependents of active-duty military personnel. With these programs, the

Highlight on the History of Medical Treatment of Infectious Disease

Historians generally place the beginning of Western medicine with Hippocrates, an ancient Greek physician who saw medicine as an independent discipline based on clinical practice rather than prayer and ritual. For several centuries there were few treatment methods other than rest, exercise, diet, and a few medications derived from plants. The intensive study of the human body in the 1500s fostered a better understanding of physiologic processes. For example, the English scientist William Harvey, who rejected the traditional belief that blood was made up of "spirits" and that body fluids were "humors," developed a theory, later proved true, that blood flows from the heart to the lungs, throughout the body via arteries, and back to the heart via veins.

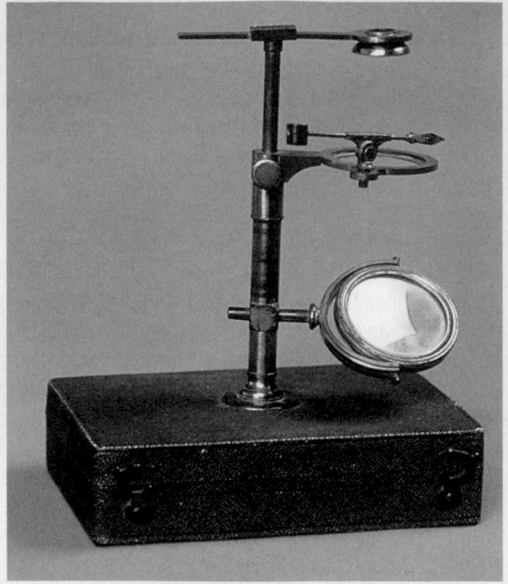

Early microscope, about 1765.

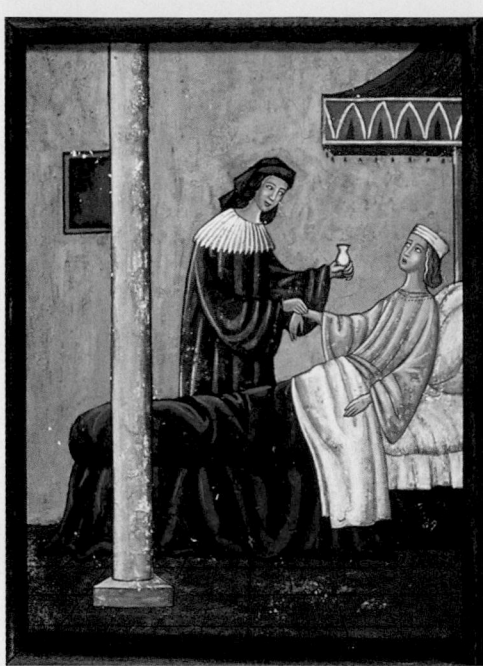

Physician in the Middle Ages taking a patient's pulse and holding a flask of urine.

The first microscopic lens was invented in 1677 by Antony van Leeuwenhoek. Through his microscope van Leeuwenhoek saw yeasts, molds, and algae, adding evidence to the theory that diseases could be caused by particles too small to be seen with the eyes. He also identified red blood cells passing through capillaries.

Throughout the nineteenth century, other scientists and physicians advanced the understanding of the cause of disease. Some found ways to combat disease without understanding the mechanism by which the disease acted; others determined the actual cause of a particular disease.

In the 1840s the Viennese obstetric assistant Ignaz Semmelweis discovered that puerperal fever, or so-called "childbed fever," a fatal illness of women who had just given birth, could be reduced if physicians washed their hands. He came to believe that physicians were infecting women by transferring disease-causing substances from one woman to another.

Semmelweis conducted what today would be called an *epidemiologic study*. He studied the records of women who had died and determined which physicians and medical students had attended which birth. His study of the records led him to conclude that most of the women who died had been attended to by

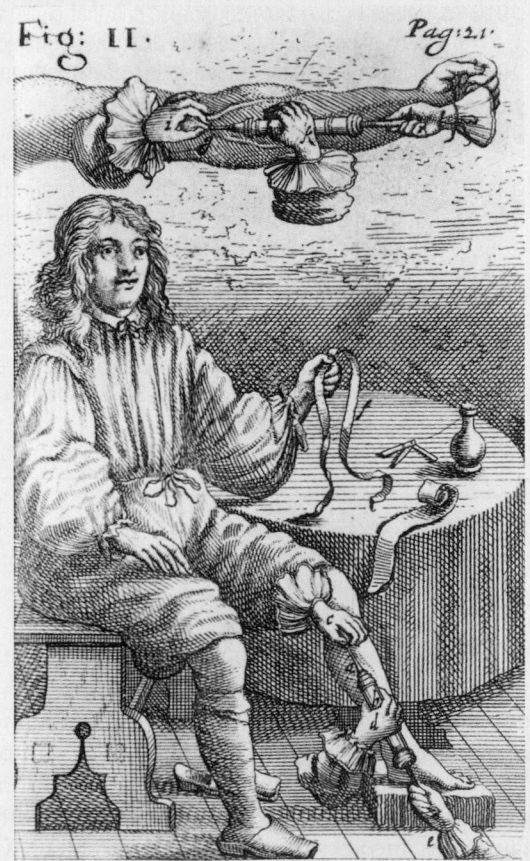

Extracting blood for a transfusion, eighteenth century.

physicians and medical students who had come into the birthing room directly from the anatomy laboratory, where they had worked with cadavers, without first washing their hands. Most of Semmelweis's colleagues dismissed his notion that simple handwashing could reduce childbirth deaths as nonsense, and during his lifetime, Semmelweis was ridiculed. It was not until decades later that physicians regularly began washing their hands.

The Scottish surgeon Joseph Lister worked on similar ideas to develop the first practice of antisepsis (cleaning areas where germs may be) and later asepsis (creating a germ-free environment). Lister started by pouring carbolic acid on the wounds of those who had just had surgery. Over time, he found milder substances. Lister found that far fewer patients who were treated with these substances died from gangrene that developed in the open wounds.

Semmelweis, Lister, and others worked empirically, which means they sought results through experiments that could be repeated with the same results. Although they were able to decrease infection rates, they never completely understood what caused infectious diseases. Other scientists sought to determine that bacteria caused specific diseases.

The German physician Robert Koch is called the "Father of Microbiology" because of his work with specific bacteria such as *Mycobacterium tuberculosis,* the bacterial agent that causes tuberculosis. Koch also isolated the bacterial agent that causes anthrax. Koch grew the anthrax bacillus in a number of different liquid media in his laboratory, used the microscope to identify it, injected the organism into a healthy animal, waited for the animal to become sick, and then recovered the same organism from the sick animal. This proved that one specific type of bacteria causes one specific disease. Today we know that it is possible to break the chain of illness by keeping those who are contagious away from those who are vulnerable to disease.

The work of Louis Pasteur and Koch, among others, helped set the stage for the understanding of infectious disease and for worldwide vaccination programs to eradicate smallpox and to try to eradicate the "childhood illnesses" of mumps, measles, and rubella (German measles).

The first vaccination actually had been performed a century earlier. Edward Jenner , an English physician in the farming country of Gloucestershire, used the pus from one person's cowpox lesion to vaccinate another individual against smallpox in 1796.

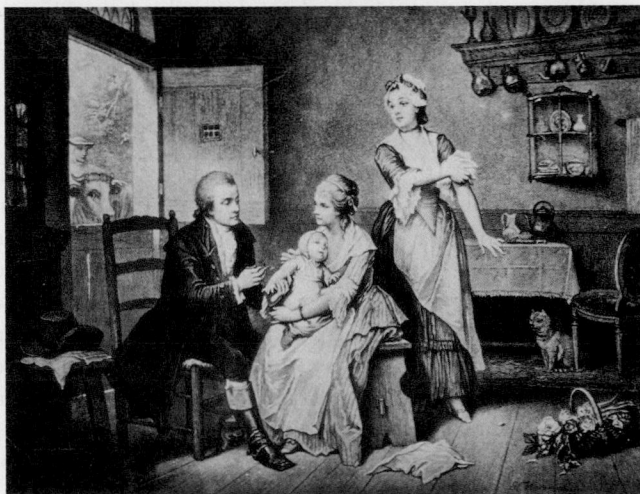

Edward Jenner vaccinating an infant.

Cowpox is a variant of smallpox. It is lethal to animals but relatively harmless to humans. For centuries, people had realized that people who had been infected with cowpox did not develop smallpox. Today, we understand what had happened—their immune systems had developed antibodies to cowpox that also prevented smallpox infection by attacking the smallpox virus.

Jenner used "humanized cowpox" to establish immunity by taking pus from a lesion on a human infected with cowpox and rubbing it into an open wound on another human. A couple of weeks later, he inoculated the second person with smallpox. Not only did the individual not become ill, but he also was not contagious. A century later Pasteur would discover fully the mechanism by which vaccination works. Vaccines were discovered for many diseases. By the beginning of the twentieth century, vaccines had been developed for diphtheria and tetanus, and most children received these vaccines as infants by the middle of the twentieth century. New immunizations continue to be developed not only for infants but also for adolescents, adults, and the elderly.

Medications to kill bacteria were another important tool in the fight against infectious disease. Paul Ehrlich is credited with the development of the first medication to kill bacteria. In 1909 he developed a drug called *Salvarsan* (arsphenamine), which could be used to effectively treat syphilis. Unfortunately the medication itself was extremely toxic. The first of the sulfanilamide drugs, Prontosil, was developed in 1932 in Germany. It was effective against infections caused by streptococci and some other types of bacteria. The sulfanilamides became popular before and during World War II because they were the only antiinfective agents widely available. Penicillin, a mold that kills bacteria, had been discovered in 1922 by Alexander Fleming in London after it attacked bacteria that he was growing on agar plates. Initially the scientific community did not believe that it would be effective inside the body, and little follow-up research was done. During World War II, two medical researchers, Howard Florey and Ernst Chain, took up the research on penicillin and managed to prove that the medication was effective. The first human was treated in 1941, and within a few years mass production had been established and penicillin was in widespread use.

Discovery of the first virus is credited to Dimitri Ivanowski, a Russian botanist, in 1892. He discovered that a substance could pass through a ceramic filter that trapped all known bacteria and still cause a disease of tobacco called *mosaic tobacco disease.* We now know that the culprit is the tobacco mosaic virus. Yellow fever was the first viral disease of humans to be identified. During construction of the Panama Canal, workers were devastated by this disease. Research done by Walter Reed established that the disease was caused by a virus transmitted by mosquitoes and not direct contact. Controlling mosquitoes facilitated the work on the canal. The development of the electron microscope in 1930 allowed viruses to be seen, but progress to control viral diseases was slow. For most viruses the body has adequate defenses to overcome the infection, but there are some significant exceptions. The retroviruses, such as human immunodeficiency virus (HIV), are notable because they are able to overcome the body's immune system. In the 1970s the first deaths from acquired immunodeficiency syndrome (AIDS) were reported in the United States. Within the next 20 years, a worldwide epidemic occurred. By 1997 more than 6 million deaths worldwide had been caused by the AIDS virus. Treatments have been developed to slow the progression of the disease, but to date there is no effective immunization or cure for this disease. The ability of viruses to mutate rapidly has resulted in recent viral pandemics from diseases such as severe acute respiratory syndrome (SARS) in 2004 and H1N1 influenza in 2009. ∎

federal government has become the primary insurer for more than 50 million Americans. These plans, which included payments for office visits for illness, greatly increased the number of Americans who had medical insurance. There was little incentive for the consumer (the patient) to control costs because insurance was covering those costs, and care in most cases was "free" to the consumer.

Although most Americans who were insured did not feel that they were "paying" for their medical care, they were, indirectly. The huge increases in health care costs were one of the major sources of the generally high rates of inflation in the 1970s. Employers, who paid for the insurance, had to pay ever-rising premiums and offset these large premium increases with small increases in cash wages, which did not keep up with inflation. So American workers did, in fact, pay for health insurance and health care costs in lower purchasing power for the cash they received as salary.

Managed Care

Health maintenance organizations (HMOs) were originally formed with a belief that consistent, routine care would help prevent later expensive care. The expansion of health insurance to cover office visits originally covered only visits for illness or injury and did not cover so-called "routine care" (well-child visits, immunizations, regular checkups, or physical examinations). Managed care was based on the belief that increasing prevention and promoting early detection and diagnosis of chronic and life-threatening medical conditions would reduce costs. The HMO movement, which gained acceptance in the 1970s, pushed traditional health insurance companies to begin providing coverage for routine care.

In the late 1970s, insurance companies began to respond to escalating health care costs by reviewing care to find out if it was medically necessary. This process, called **utilization review**, identifies patients who, according to the insurance companies, no longer need to be hospitalized. Originally, utilization review was used by Medicare and Medicaid. Other insurance companies soon realized that shortening hospital stays was an important way of reducing overall health care costs. The combination of HMO insurance plans and strict utilization review for hospitalized patients is the basis of what we call **managed care.**

The original HMO model had two components: insurance and services including diagnostic tests and pharmacy. HMO plans set up full-service medical clinics. Physicians were employees. The HMO established a contractual relationship with a hospital for inpatient services, and patients had to go to the specific hospital with which the HMO had a contract.

In the late 1980s HMO services began to separate from HMO insurance. A second type of HMO model based on networks of physicians who agreed to provide care for HMO patients came into being. Some of these networks operated under the old fee-for-service plans but agreed to discounted fees from the HMOs in exchange for access to the rapidly growing patient populations enrolled in HMOs. In an effort to reduce payments, HMOs tried to have physicians accept a flat monthly fee for each subscriber in their practice and agree to provide all necessary primary care for that fee. This type of payment is called **capitation.** This reduces the incentive to provide extra services because their cost will not be reimbursed separately.

The managed care movement in general, as well as the trend to decrease reimbursement for primary care in particular, put the burden on physicians to compete with one another to provide the most care for the least money. As a result, physicians often feel pressure to limit diagnostic tests, reduce hospitalizations and the number of days patients stay in the hospital, and use generic instead of brand-name drugs. (Generics are identical in chemical formulation to brand-name drugs and can be manufactured only after the brand-name drug's patent protection has expired.)

Managed care also puts pressure on physicians to see more patients, spend less time with each patient, and justify all services including diagnostic tests and referrals. The expense of handling sicker patients is expected to be balanced by those patients who use less than the average amount of medical services.

In addition, insurance plans have tried to reduce their costs for prescription medications by restricting drug coverage to lists of approved drugs. Such a list, called a **formulary,** usually includes one or two of the less expensive drugs for each possible medical condition. Exceptions are made if the physician can show that the less expensive drugs have been ineffective for his or her patient and that a more expensive drug is necessary. In some plans the patient can receive a more expensive medication by paying more of the cost.

Health Care Reform

Despite these measures, however, beginning in the late 1990s, both insurance premiums and health care costs began to increase at more than double and even triple the underlying rate of inflation. There has also been an increase in the number of individuals and families who do not qualify for government insurance plans, and also do not have health insurance through their employers. This may be because they work part-time or are self-employed. The Patient Protection and Affordable Care Act, which became law in March 2010, expands insurance coverage to an estimated 32 million Americans who were previously uninsured. Among the provisions that went into effect in September 2010, insurance companies are no longer allowed to exclude children with preexisting health conditions or to drop customers after discovering technical mistakes on applications. By 2014 this law will require all individuals to purchase health insurance or pay an annual fine. Even though this law has been challenged in the courts, a strong belief persists that society has an obligation to make appropriate health care accessible to all citizens.

AMBULATORY CARE

There is no such thing as a "typical" medical office. The style of any particular medical office depends on the personality of the physician or physicians who practice there, as well as the general population of patients who come there. Regardless of the physician's personality and the patients' personal background, the same kinds of activities occur in any physician's office setting.

Today, the trend in medical care is toward an increasing amount of **ambulatory care**—defined as the patient coming to the care rather than the patient receiving care in a home or hospital setting (Figure 1-1). To take advantage of ambulatory care, the patient must be able to walk into the physician's office or at least be brought to the office in a wheelchair.

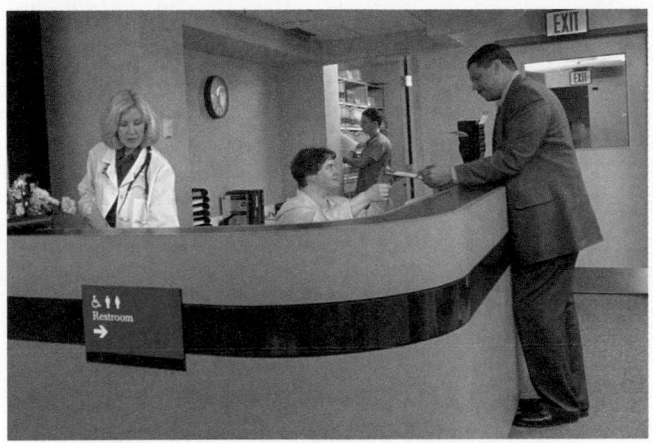

Figure 1-1 The patient check-in area in a clinic.

In addition to private physicians' offices, offices of physicians who make up a staff model HMO, community health centers, multispecialty clinics, and hospitals are increasingly making more space available for outpatient care.

Flow of Activity in Ambulatory Care

The flow of activities for each patient in an outpatient setting is similar. The patient will do the following:
- Enter the office
- Approach the reception desk, identify the physician and time of appointment, provide the office staff with personal and payment information, and make a copayment (if necessary)
- Be seen by a physician (or by a nurse practitioner [NP] or physician assistant [PA] if the practice uses such personnel)
- Undergo diagnostic or laboratory tests in the office
- Receive a diagnosis, treatment, or a referral to another health care provider
- Receive instruction for follow-up care and any diagnostic tests to be done elsewhere before leaving the medical office; if seriously ill, the patient may be admitted to the hospital

Figure 1-2 is a flowchart of how a patient moves through the medical office.

Once a patient has been seen in the medical office, the office begins the process of obtaining payment for its services. The medical payment may come from a private

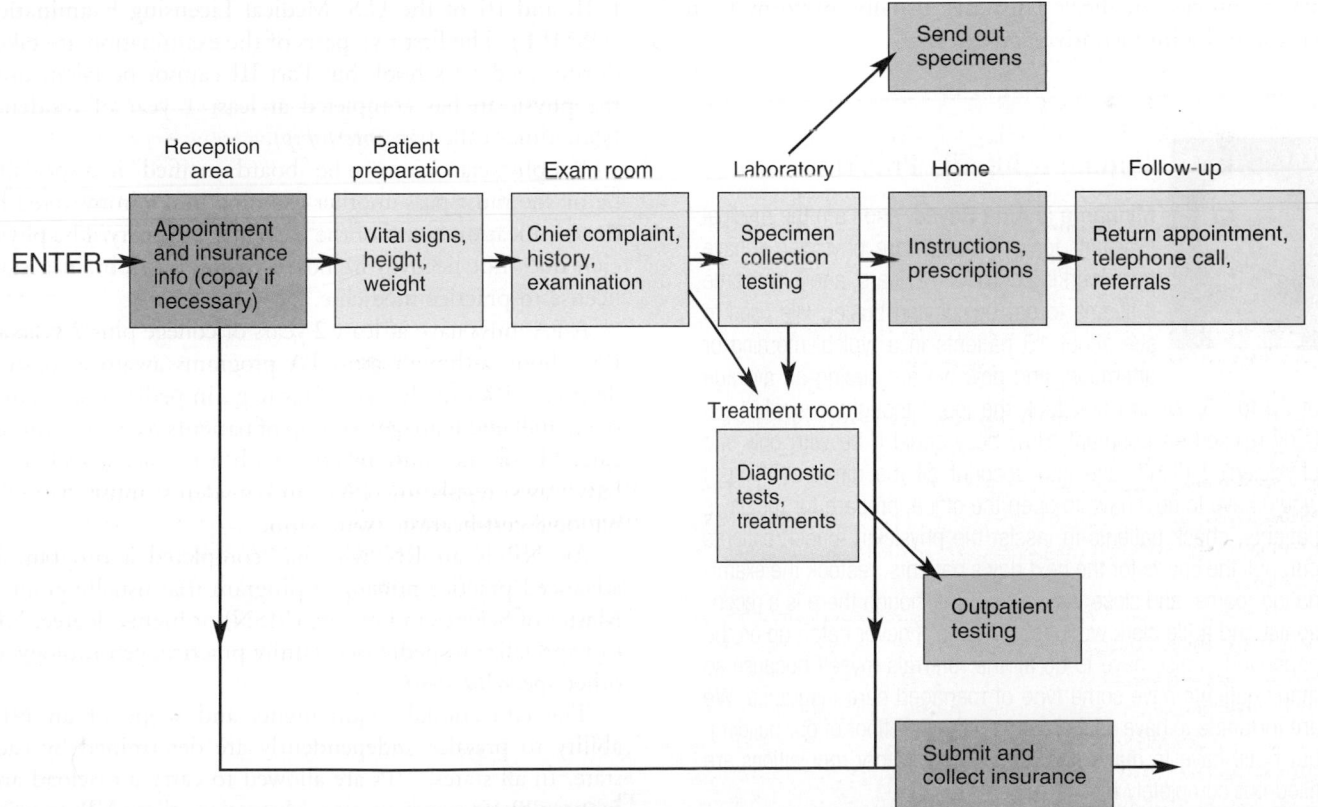

Figure 1-2 Patient progress through a medical office.

insurance plan, a government-funded insurance program, and/or from the patient. The patient may be responsible for a percentage of the charges or the entire bill if he or she does not have insurance.

After the examination the patient receives instructions to prepare for a test or procedure to be performed or information about medication that has been prescribed. Patients who are seen regularly because of a chronic illness may spend time with a physician or medical assistant reviewing the patient's individual treatment plan. A follow-up appointment is made if necessary.

Most medical offices provide health education materials in the waiting room. These materials may consist of pamphlets, article reprints, health education videos, or health news reports specially prepared for viewing in the medical office.

The Health Care Team

A medical assistant works as a member of a dedicated health care team. The physician or group of physicians expects each medical assistant to fill a slightly different role within the office team. This role will depend on the style of the practice, the region of the country where the practice is located, and what types of medical professionals make up the team.

As the operations of a medical practice become more complex, physicians may employ individuals with more specialized medical business and medical management experience to run the business side of the office. In these offices, medical assistants play more of a clinical role. In smaller offices, medical assistants usually perform both clinical and administrative activities.

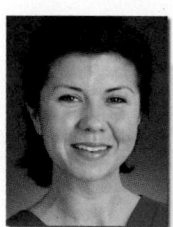

Putting It All Into Practice

My name is Aida Reyes, and I am the medical assistant for a primary care physician. I have been working here for 12 years, and in that time it seems to get busier and busier. We used to see about 15 patients in a typical morning or afternoon, and now we are seeing an average of 20 to 25. When I first took the job, I thought it would be a fairly relaxed environment. How busy could it be with only one physician? I didn't take into account all the different things I would have to do. I have to open the office, prepare for the day's patients, check patients in, assist the physician, check patients out, pull the charts for the next day's patients, restock the examination rooms, and close the office. Even though there is a receptionist and a file clerk working part time, I never catch up on the paperwork. I also have to do all the referrals myself because so many patients have some type of managed care insurance. We are fortunate to have a laboratory on the first floor of our building, but I still have to make sure that all laboratory requisitions are filled out completely for our patients. ∎

Members of the Health Care Team

The members of the medical team who typically work in ambulatory care, be it a private practice, a community or public health clinic, or a hospital clinic, include physicians, NPs, PAs, medical assistants, registered nurses (RNs) or licensed practical nurses, a business manager, a receptionist, a medical secretary, file clerks, and one or more insurance specialists. Medical transcription is occasionally done in the medical office, but increasingly it is outsourced or replaced by the electronic medical record or voice recognition software. If the office performs moderate- or high-complexity laboratory tests, a certified medical technologist may also be on the staff or serve as a consultant.

Hospital or community-based clinics will possibly also have a staff of social workers, outreach workers, and case managers to provide social services to patients. Practices specializing in women's health (obstetrics and gynecology) may also have certified nurse-midwives.

Table 1-2 lists various nurses and allied health professionals and describes their roles.

Physicians and Other Health Care Providers

Physicians have either an MD (medical doctor) or DO (doctor of osteopathy) degree, either of which is awarded after 4 years of college, then 4 years of medical or osteopathic school. In addition, they complete a hospital-based, intensive postgraduate training period, traditionally called a **residency,** which lasts from 2 to 7 years, depending on the specialty. To receive a medical license from the state where he or she will practice, the physician must pass Parts I, II, and III of the U.S. Medical Licensing Examination (USMLE). The first two parts of the examination are taken during medical school, but Part III cannot be taken until the physician has completed at least 1 year of residency (sometimes called an *internship*).

If a physician wants to be "board certified" in a specialty, he or she must pass another examination, administered by the certification board of the particular specialty. The physician does not need to be board certified to obtain a state license to practice medicine.

A PA must have at least 2 years of college plus 2 years of PA school, although most PA programs award a master's degree. A PA usually specializes (e.g., in pediatrics, in adult medicine) and manages a group of patients receiving routine care. He or she must practice with a physician. All states have laws regulating PAs, and students must pass the national certification examination.

An NP is an RN who has completed a program in advanced practice nursing, a program that usually grants a Master of Science in Nursing (MSN) or higher degree. NPs can specialize in pediatrics, family practice, gerontology, or other specialty areas.

The educational requirements and scope of an NP's ability to practice independently are determined by each state. In all states, NPs are allowed to carry a caseload and manage routine patient care. Most states allow NPs to write

Table 1-2   Nurses and Allied Health Professionals

Occupation	Credentials	Responsibilities
Certified Professional Coder Certified Coding Associate	CPC CCA	Assigns codes to patient charges and diagnoses for insurance billing. There are many coding certifications depending on knowledge and specialty.
Diagnostic Medical Sonographer	DMS	Performs ultrasound scans in hospitals and ambulatory care facilities. Ultrasound uses high-frequency sound waves to produce images. A sonographer may specialize in ultrasound of the heart (echocardiography).
Emergency Medical Technician Paramedic	EMT; paramedic	Provides emergency services and life support in the community. Several levels of emergency service personnel exist, depending on training and experience.
Health Information Specialist	RHIA; RHIT	Works with patient medical records; may provide assistance in planning, managing information, gathering data for medical research, and policy making.
Medical Assistant	CMA (AAMA); RMA	Performs administrative and clinical tasks in ambulatory care.
Medical (Clinical) Technologist	MT; MLT	Performs laboratory tests in the clinical laboratory and may supervise laboratory operations or provide consulting services.
Medical Secretary	CMS	Secretary who specializes in administrative procedures in a health care setting.
Nuclear Medicine Technologist	CNMT	Operates devices that detect and map absorption of radioactive substances given by injection to create diagnostic images.
Nurse, Practical	LPN; LVN	Performs direct patient care and clinical procedures. May work in hospitals, nursing homes, and ambulatory care settings.
Nurse Practitioner	NP	Specializes in a specific area such as internal medicine, pediatrics, and women's health and often manages routine patient care in ambulatory care settings.
Nurse, Registered	RN	Plans and provides nursing care in inpatient settings. Provides supervision for caregivers in both inpatient and outpatient settings.
Occupational Therapist Occupational Therapy Assistant	OT; OTA	Plans therapeutic activities for rehabilitation, especially for activities of daily living (ADLs). Implements treatment plans.
Physical Therapist Physical Therapy Assistant	PT; PTA	Plans exercises for large muscle groups for rehabilitation and implements treatment plans.
Physician Assistant	PA	Manages routine patient care under the supervision of a physician. Usually works in ambulatory care.
Radiologic Technologist	RT	Takes radiographs and assists with special radiographic examinations. After completing education, may specialize in computed tomography, mammography, or therapeutic radiation.
Registered Dietician	RD	Assists with nutrition of patients in hospitals and ambulatory care. Performs nutrition screening and counseling. Coordinates all aspects of food service in many settings.
Respiratory Therapist	RRT	Provides respiratory treatments and manages patients on ventilators.
Surgical Technologist	CST	Assists during surgery in hospital and day surgery centers by setting up operating rooms, preparing instruments and equipment, and passing instruments during surgery.

What Would You Do? What Would You *Not* Do?

Case Study 1

In the examination room, Alicia Darwin, a new patient, tells Aida that she has switched physicians because she had often been seen by a nurse practitioner in the medical office where she used to go. "I don't think a nurse practitioner has as much experience as a doctor," she said, "and besides, the nurse practitioner can't give me medication if I need it." She asked Aida to confirm that she would always be seen by the physician in this office. She added, "I don't have anything against nurses like you; I just want to have a real doctor take care of me." ■

prescriptions; in other states a physician must cosign the order. In some states, NPs are allowed to practice independently, but in most they must practice in an office with supervision by a physician. In a few states, NPs are allowed to admit patients to hospitals.

Effective Teamwork

Working as an effective health care team does not just happen. To be effective, team members work together to provide appropriate care for each patient. The more people involved, the more crucial this teamwork is. Each member of the team must be committed to problem solving, communicating, and coordinating effective care.

Teamwork is reinforced at regular staff meetings, which can be directed by either the medical or the business director of the office, depending on the particular topics of the meeting. But the true test of teamwork occurs on a daily basis as health care is provided.

Each health care team member has a certain responsibility and restrictions on activities and areas about which he or she is allowed to make decisions. Sometimes this scope is defined by federal or state law. For example, medical assistants are allowed to administer injections in some states, but in others they cannot. The medical assistant must learn what areas fall within the proper scope of decision-making responsibility in his or her state.

The specific education and role of the medical assistant is discussed in Chapter 2. The medical assistant plays an important role by keeping the work of the office flowing smoothly. He or she must communicate well with other health team members. Because a patient will not always repeat all information to the physician, the medical assistant must communicate anything related to the patient's health verbally or through the medical record. At the same time, the medical assistant must be careful to avoid using diagnostic terminology in the medical record or giving medical advice to the patient (unless following specific guidelines established by the physician).

Teamwork is enhanced when each team member helps and supports other members and avoids blaming or criticizing others. Because the number of employees in a medical office is often small, it is important for everyone to do his or her best to get along and deal with conflict. When a problem arises, it is important to try to find solutions to the problem rather than focusing on who caused the problem or whose fault it is. It is also helpful to maintain perspective and accept that things do go wrong, and most problems can be dealt with. In any conflict situation, it is important to listen to the point of view of others and validate their feelings. Effective communication techniques are discussed in more detail in Chapter 4.

PARTS OF THE MEDICAL OFFICE

A physician's office has a number of different physical spaces in it. Each space has a particular purpose. Every physician's office has three basic areas: a reception area and waiting room, examination and treatment rooms, and an area for other activities. This may include medical records storage, if the office uses paper medical records; storage for supplies; and staff offices or cubicles.

In most offices, physicians also have their own offices, separate from examination rooms, but some physicians have examination tables in their offices, combining the two spaces in one room.

Larger offices may have several additional areas such as an office laboratory; separate treatment rooms or special procedure rooms; a business office, which is separate from the front office (reception, telephones, appointments); and a lunch or break room for the staff.

All physicians' offices must meet a number of specifications laid out by regulatory agencies. These include the federal Occupational Safety and Health Administration (OSHA), which regulates workplace health and safety. They also must meet the specifications of the Americans with Disabilities Act, which requires that doorways be at least 3 feet wide and hallways at least 5 feet wide. Restroom facilities must be available for both patients and staff. Office laboratories are regulated by the Clinical Laboratory Improvement Amendments of 1988 (CLIA'88). Local boards of health also inspect and regulate hospitals and clinics.

Figure 1-3 shows the layout of a small physician office.

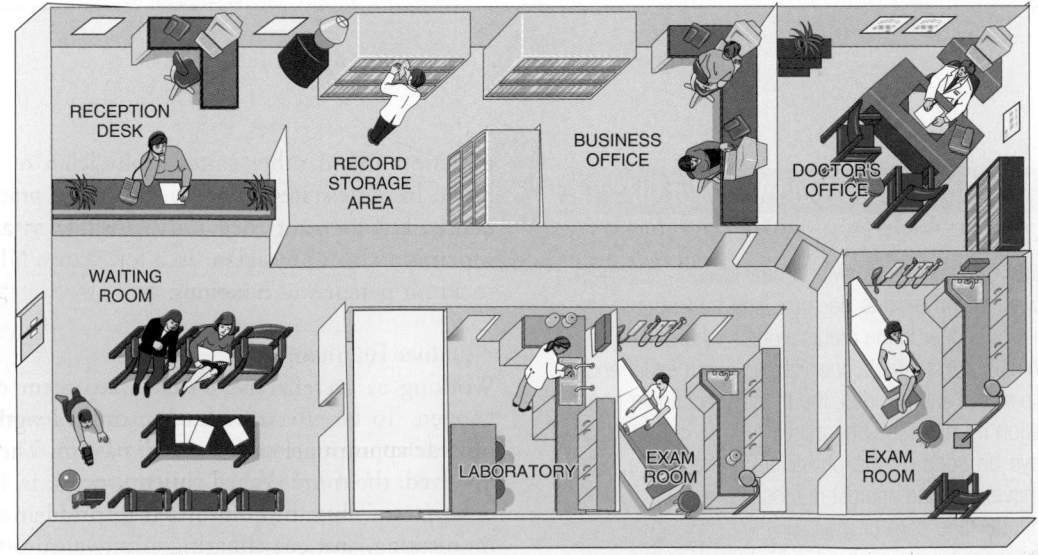

Figure 1-3 Layout of a small medical office.

Reception Area and Waiting Room

The reception area and waiting room are the first place any new or prospective patient will see. First impressions are important. The waiting room should be clean and well lit. Furniture should be arranged and not haphazardly placed. Up-to-date, general-interest reading material should be available; many physicians also have patient education materials available in the waiting room. Waiting rooms in pediatric and family practice offices also have toys available for children. Large pediatric practices may have a separate waiting room for sick children or for adolescents.

The waiting room should have enough chairs for two people per patient visit, multiplied by the number of patients seen in 2 hours. It needs to present a calm atmosphere and look professional. Usually the waiting area is carpeted. It should have comfortable chairs, grouped in blocks if possible rather than just lined up around the walls. Colors should be muted, and music should be soft. Red, yellow, and orange are typically avoided; today, physician's office decor often uses shades of green, dusty pink, or salmon. Music is usually a tape or radio station of the "easy listening" variety.

The reception area adjoins the waiting room. The medical assistant at the reception desk should greet each patient as he or she enters the waiting room. Most reception areas have a counter so that the patient can fill out or sign forms, and many have a sliding window so that patients cannot hear the conversations occurring behind the receptionist.

Patients check in here when they enter the office. New patient forms are received here, and health insurance cards are copied. Copayments are taken from patients whose insurance is provided through HMOs. Appointments may be made by the receptionist or in a separate area of the office.

Examination Rooms and Laboratory

Examination rooms are designed for the convenience of the physician and assisting personnel who will work there. However, they also need to be as comfortable and calming to the patient as possible. Reading material should be available in each examination room. Although good scheduling will ensure that patients will not wait too long in these rooms for a physician, most physicians do see patients in at least two examination rooms. Additional delays may occur if the physician has to respond to urgent telephone calls or office emergencies (Figure 1-4).

Many physicians perform treatments or diagnostic procedures in examination rooms, but complex procedures (such as suturing a laceration) are often performed in larger rooms with extra equipment and/or supplies. These are called *treatment rooms.*

If laboratory tests are performed in the medical office, there is a special room or area set aside for this. CLIA '88 regulates laboratory testing. Medical assistants are trained to perform low-complexity tests (CLIA-waived tests) and

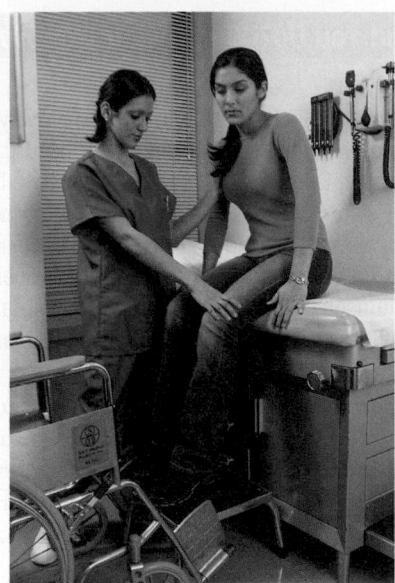

Figure 1-4 Examination rooms are usually compact, but each should be large enough to accommodate a wheelchair.

may also perform more complex texts with special training.

CLIA '88 specifies who can supervise laboratories and lays out the process for inspection and accreditation. It sets strict guidelines for quality control, quality assurance, handling of hazardous materials, documentation, and proficiency training. Offices that perform only CLIA-waived laboratory tests may perform laboratory testing in the patient preparation area. Ideally the bathroom is adjacent to this area, with an opening in the wall so that urine samples can be passed directly into the laboratory area.

Medical Records Storage and Business Office

If the office uses paper records, the medical records may be stored near the reception area, in the business areas, adjacent to the patient preparation area, or in a separate room. Charts of active patients—those who have been seen within the past 2 to 3 years—are kept in the records storage area in the office. Inactive charts are removed regularly and stored in a less accessible location such as the basement of the building or off-site in a facility that maintains records in storage. Charts needed for patients who will be coming in during a specified period—morning, afternoon, or an entire day—are removed from the storage area and prepared for use.

Some practices are moving away from paper records to computerized medical records. In this case, patient records are stored on a computer's hard disk and are simply pulled up from the database as needed. The process of placing old records into the computerized record is lengthy, and many offices that use an electronic medical record store the former paper record of established patients in an accessible area and make it available to the provider during patient visits.

Posting of patient charges, billing, and computer operations may be performed in an area behind the reception

Case Study 2

The physician complains to Aida that there are always dishes in the sink in the break room and crumbs and used paper coffee cups on the table. Even though the area is not seen by patients, the physician is concerned that an insect or rodent problem could develop. Aida knows that the part-time file clerk and the part-time receptionist have a tendency to leave dirty dishes and trash after their afternoon break. She herself is so busy that she rarely has time to either clean or sit down in the break room. ∎

desk or in a separate business office. If the practice has one or more satellite locations, the billing and insurance tasks are usually done in the practice's main office for all locations. Some offices contract billing and insurance claim processing to an outside company, which may even be located in another state.

Additional Areas Found in Many Offices

Physicians' private offices are often a reflection of their personal tastes. This room is where a physician meets privately with patients, patients' families, and other visitors. He or she usually displays degrees and certificates of membership in professional organizations on the walls of the office. Even if the practice has a small library for the use of all staff, physicians will usually have at least a few important references in this office. Art and memorabilia that show the physician's personal taste also help to make the private office a pleasant place for the physician to do quiet work and hold meetings.

Recognizing the needs of staff for a quiet place to take their breaks and eat their lunch, newer offices often include a staff break or lunch room. This room may have a refrigerator and microwave for staff to prepare lunches they bring from home. There should be at least one table and chairs. The lunch or break room should not double as a storage area, and staff should avoid using the room for meetings that deprive others of use of the room. Depending on the type of medical practice, particular rooms may be set aside for specific treatments or diagnostic procedures. Types of special rooms include the following:

- A pediatrics examination or treatment room in a family practice group's office
- A surgical procedure room in a general surgery group's office
- A room for more complex testing such as colposcopy and pelvic ultrasounds in a group practice specializing in obstetrics and gynecology
- A trauma room in a large clinic or community health center

MEDICAL SPECIALTIES

Since the middle of the twentieth century, the practice of medicine has been broken down into fields of specialty and

Aida Reyes: The clinic where I did my externship was so large that at first I kept getting lost. Another thing that confused me was the doors that the staff used to get from one part of the clinic to another. It was arranged by department, but the layout of rooms in each department was different. I spent the majority of my time in internal medicine working with one medical assistant and one physician, but my preceptor arranged for me to spend time in other departments like medical records, billing, and pediatrics and with the referral coordinator. In addition to the full-time physicians, there were some specialists who came in once or twice a week, including a neurologist, an orthopedic surgeon, and an ophthalmologist. The clinic also employed a social worker and a dietician. In each department there was a nurse and there were at least two medical assistants in addition to the receptionist. The amazing thing was how quickly I adapted and became comfortable finding my way around. After only a few weeks, it felt like I belonged there. I was so proud when my preceptor said, "Aida, you have become one of the team. I don't know how we ever got along without you." ∎

subspecialty. In 1950 most Americans received their medical care from a general practitioner, who took care of adults and children, often delivered babies, and performed many general surgical procedures.

Today, Americans may see two, three, or more physicians routinely. Box 1-1 describes the medical specialties recognized by the American Board of Medical Specialties. In many areas, there are several subspecialties. If the physician wants to work in a subspecialty, after the residency training he or she participates in additional training called a *fellowship* for 2 to 3 years. It is not possible to be board certified in any specialty or subspecialty without completing a residency.

Primary Care

Primary care physicians specialize in internal medicine (treatment of the internal organs of adults by other than surgical means), pediatrics (general medical care of children and adolescents), or family medicine (general medical care of children, adolescents, and adults—today's equivalent of general practice).

Over the course of time, the activities of different types of physicians have shifted. For instance, fewer family practitioners deliver babies today than did general practitioners in the 1950s and 1960s, preferring to leave that task to obstetricians owing to the cost of malpractice insurance. Although some women continue to see a gynecologist for an annual pelvic examination and Pap test, the primary care provider performs these activities more often today than in the past.

Because of the requirements for a primary care provider in managed care plans, some specialists, especially

BOX 1-1 Medical Specialties

Allergy and Immunology (Allergist, Immunologist): Treats adults and/or children with allergies and problems of the immune system. Many individuals experience allergies and/or asthma in the presence of allergens. The immune system can also malfunction either through inherited or acquired diseases. Allergists and immunologists diagnose, manage, and treat allergic diseases, immunodeficiency conditions, and autoimmune diseases.

Anesthesiology (Anesthesiologist): Provides anesthesia during surgery and other procedures, as well as medical care to patients before, during, and after surgery. The anesthesiologist also supervises other anesthesia personnel in the operating room such as nurse anesthetists and anesthesia residents.

Colon and Rectal Surgery: Performs surgical treatment on the large intestine and rectum. These surgeons specialize in the diagnosis and treatment of diseases of the colon and rectum in addition to full training in general surgery. They perform diagnostic and screening procedures and perform surgery when necessary.

Dermatology (Dermatologist): Specializes in conditions of the skin. Dermatologists diagnose skin diseases and also perform surgery on the skin. Laser treatments are commonly used for skin conditions in addition to medication, cryotherapy, and surgery.

Emergency Medicine: Treats patients for emergency conditions, usually in the emergency department of a hospital. Emergency medicine focuses treatment of acute illnesses and injuries that require immediate care. The physician is often an employee of a hospital emergency department or other urgent care center.

Family Medicine (Family Practitioner): Treats adults and children for routine care and complaints; often the primary care physician for all family members. The family practitioner is concerned with the total health of the individual and the family. Specialized training is available for the subspecialties of geriatric medicine and sports medicine.

Internal Medicine (Internist): Provides medical treatment for conditions of various body systems. The internist may be the primary care provider for adults. Within the discipline of internal medicine are several subspecialties such as adolescent medicine, cardiovascular disease, critical care medicine, endocrinology, gastroenterology, geriatric medicine, hematology, medical oncology, nephrology, pulmonary disease, rheumatology, and sports medicine.

Medical Genetics: Provides diagnostic procedures and treatment for individuals with genetically linked diseases. Also provides genetic counseling and prenatal diagnosis. May specialize in laboratory testing or in research related to genetic diseases.

Neurological Surgery (Neurosurgeon): Performs prevention, diagnosis, surgical and nonsurgical treatment, and rehabilitation for conditions of the brain, spine, and nervous system. Also provides surgical and nonsurgical treatment of pain. Subspecialties include vascular neurosurgery and pediatric neurosurgery.

Nuclear Medicine: Specializes in diagnosis using radionuclides, atoms that give off electromagnetic radiation. Nuclear physicians are usually employed by a hospital or university (or both) and have little direct patient care. They are responsible for diagnosis and recommending treatment of abnormalities detected by the various imaging modalities used in the nuclear medicine department.

Obstetrics (Obstetrician) and Gynecology (Gynecologist): Specializes in care during pregnancy and delivery (obstetrician); specializes in other care and surgery of the female reproductive system (gynecologist). The gynecologist is responsible for screening procedures, diagnostic procedures, and both medical and surgical treatments. He or she also frequently uses hormone-modulating treatments.

Ophthalmology (Ophthalmologist): Specializes in the care of the eye. The ophthalmologist manages diseases and conditions of the eye with both medical and surgical treatment including laser treatments. May also manage errors of refraction and prescribe corrective lenses, although this is often delegated to an optometrist. Several subspecialties deal with specific eye diseases or parts of the eye.

Orthopedic Surgery (Orthopedic Surgeon): Specializes in diagnosis and treatment of acute and traumatic injuries of the musculoskeletal system, as well as diseases of the muscular or skeletal system. Both surgical and nonsurgical treatments are used. Some orthopedic surgeons specialize in specific joints, specific age groups, orthopedic sports medicine, or orthopedic oncology.

Otolaryngology (Otolaryngologist or ENT): Specializes in the care of the ear, nose, throat, head, and neck. The ENT is responsible for the diagnosis and surgical or nonsurgical treatment of a variety of disorders. Many physicians specialize in the care of only one organ or area and may focus on either reconstruction or diseases of that organ.

Pathology (Pathologist): Examines cells, tissues, and other specimens to determine whether their structure is normal or abnormal; attempts to determine the nature or cause of disease. Pathologists examine tissue biopsies and other specimens to identify abnormal cells. They also perform autopsies. They may be trained within two primary specialty areas: clinical pathology and/or anatomic pathology.

Pediatrics (Pediatrician): Specializes in the care of children from birth through adolescence. In the United States, pediatricians are considered to be primary care practitioners. However, many pediatricians specialize, and almost every specialty for adult medicine is represented as a pediatric subspecialty.

Physical Medicine and Rehabilitation (Physiatrist): Specializes in the treatment and rehabilitation of patients with disabling conditions such as spinal cord injury and stroke. A physiatrist sees patients across several age groups and specialty areas and focuses on restoring maximal function to patients. He or she may specialize in specific age groups or types of injury such as spinal cord injury.

Plastic Surgery: Specializes in surgical and nonsurgical treatment of physical defects of various areas of the body. The plastic surgeon performs procedures for cosmetic enhancement or reconstruction of various parts of the body. Cosmetic surgery has become popular in the past 2 decades. Reconstructive surgery includes craniofacial surgery, hand surgery, and maxillofacial surgery to repair congenital defects and problems that result from injury or disease.

Preventative Medicine: Includes aerospace medicine, occupational medicine, and public health. In this medical specialty, physicians practice in one of the specialty areas or one of the subspecialties (medical toxicology or undersea and hyperbaric medicine).

Psychiatry (Psychiatrist) and Neurology (Neurologist): Specializes in preventing, diagnosing, and treating mental illness and conditions of the nervous system. Psychiatrists have completed the same general training as any other physician, and they are able to prescribe medication for mental illness and monitor the effects of medication therapy. Like other mental health professionals, they usually also have training in psychotherapy, psychoanalysis, and/or cognitive behavioral therapy.

Radiology (Radiologist): Specializes in the use of x-ray and other ionizing radiation for diagnosis (diagnostic radiology) and treatment (radiation oncology). A radiologist has the training to manage several types of diagnostic imaging including x-ray, computed tomography (CT) scan, and magnetic resonance imaging (MRI).

Surgery (General Surgeon or Vascular Surgeon): Performs general surgical procedures or vascular surgical procedures. A general surgeon performs primarily abdominal surgery using traditional methods or laparoscopic methods. A vascular surgeon manages diseases or conditions of the arteries and veins, except for the blood vessels of the heart and brain. Cardiothoracic surgeons manage conditions of the heart including the blood vessels, and neurosurgeons manage all conditions of the brain.

Thoracic Surgery (Thoracic Surgeon): Performs surgery of the chest including cardiac surgery, although thoracic surgeons usually specialize in surgery of the chest or cardiac surgery. Because cardiac surgery requires a high degree of skill, preparation for this specialty requires long and intensive training. Thoracic surgeons may limit their practice by age group served or by type of condition (such as congenital heart disease or heart transplantation).

Urology (Urologist): Specializes in the care of the urinary system in males and females and the reproductive tract in males; also specializes in surgery of the urinary tract and male reproductive tract. The urologist may provide medical conditions as for infections or surgical repair for abnormal growths or correction of congenital malformations.

obstetrician/gynecologists, also provide general care for some patients in their practice.

Osteopathy

Osteopathy is a mix of traditional scientific medicine and **holistic** medicine which focuses more on healing the entire person than a specific disease or condition. This branch of medical practice seeks to balance the structure and function of the body through manipulation of muscles and joints. Osteopathy was started in the late 1800s by Andrew Taylor Still (1828-1917). Osteopaths see disease as the result of dysfunction in the skeletal and muscular systems. Pain,

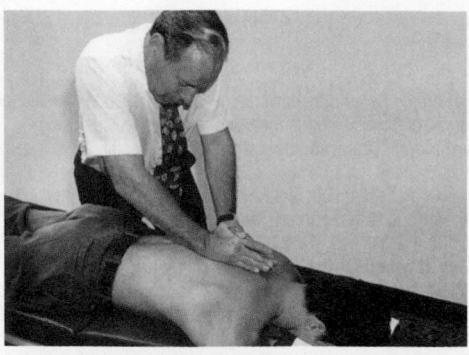

Figure 1-5 Spinal adjustment with patient in prone position.

"asymmetry" (the difference in anatomy or joint movement between one side of the body and the other), and tissue tenderness are used to gauge symptoms. Osteopaths, who hold DO degrees, today are given all the privileges of those with MD degrees. The majority of osteopaths practice as primary care doctors, where they believe their holistic and structural approach can be most effective.

Podiatry

Podiatrists use traditional medical and surgical techniques but are limited in their practice to treatment of disorders of the feet and ankles. Since the 1970s, podiatry has worked to enlarge its area of practice by focusing on surgery of the foot to alleviate such problems as bone spurs and bunions. Podiatrists work closely with primary care doctors in the management of diabetic patients and the elderly, who often require specialized foot care.

Chiropractic

Chiropractic is the technique of spinal manipulation. Chiropractors believe that vertebral subluxations (partially dislocated spinal joints) cause nerve blockages, which in turn lead to pain in the back, neck, shoulders, and legs. Begun in 1895 by Daniel David Palmer (1845-1913), chiropractic holds that the body has its own ability to heal and maintain balance. According to chiropractic theory, the nervous system is the center of all disease and healing. Some chiropractors believe that subluxation is the reason for all disease. Today's chiropractors, who are licensed by the state in which they practice, limit their treatment to discomfort clearly associated with the spine and integrate their practices into standard Western medical practice.

Figure 1-5 demonstrates a chiropractic adjustment.

PRACTICE TYPES

Fifty years ago most physicians who were not full-time members of hospital staffs worked by themselves in an office, either in their home or in an office building. They paid their office expenses, taxes, and liability insurance out of their income, and the difference was considered their "net income" from their practice. As their practice got busier, their income increased. Today many physicians work with other physicians. Some of them have an ownership position

in the practice or facility in which they work, but others are employees and receive a salary from their employer. The following categories refer to the way the office is structured, not the business arrangement or ownership.

Solo Practice

It is still possible for a physician to work in a solo practice. But to do so, he or she must make a number of trade-offs. Solo practices are limited in their size by the number of patients one physician can manage. When a physician practices alone, the medical assistant is usually responsible for aspects of both administrative and clinical support.

Even if a solo practitioner employs an NP or PA to see additional patients, the physician still must factor into his or her workday some time to oversee the work of these nonphysician professionals. In addition, the physician, as the employer, is usually responsible for paying the malpractice insurance premiums for all of the licensed professionals in his or her office. Physicians in solo practice are also completely responsible for their patients. Usually they make arrangements with other physicians to share after-hours and weekend call responsibilities and to cover for vacations.

Group Practice

Many physicians today participate in a group practice. The most common type of group practice includes three or four physicians of the same medical specialty who band together to share resources such as office space and personnel. In these groups, medical assistants usually specialize in either clinical or administrative work, although they expect to help out in other areas.

Depending on the business form used, patients are the responsibility of either one physician or "the group." In either case, if a patient's regular physician is not available, another physician in the office can see the patient. In addition, physicians who work in group practices usually share after-hours and weekend call responsibilities. They usually split the cost of malpractice insurance, and the policy is written for the group rather than for each individual.

Large medical groups with physicians who provide primary care, as well as physicians with other medical specialties, are becoming increasingly common throughout the country. Their names often include the words "associates" or "medical associates." This organizational form allows a sharing of resources that, in turn, allows each physician in the group to provide a broader range of services. In the past, these groups have been more common in particular regions and in rural areas, where a single group of physicians has the responsibility of being both the physicians in town and the staff of a small, rural hospital. HMOs that provide all services in one building, so-called "closed-panel HMOs," also operate as multispecialty groups.

These practices often have separate administrative departments for billing, appointment scheduling, and referrals and separate clinical departments for phlebotomy, electrocardiography, laboratory work, and radiography. In such practices, medical assisting jobs can be limited in scope, and specific responsibilities depend on the department where the medical assistant works.

Clinic

Traditionally a clinic was connected to a hospital and provided ambulatory care, often to patients with limited financial resources. Patients were either seen at no charge or billed by the clinic, and physicians were paid a salary for their services and/or saw patients as part of their residency program. Today a *clinic* usually refers to a public or nonprofit facility that provides outpatient public health services, although multispecialty group practices may use the word "clinic" in their name. Community health centers, established by the federal government in the late 1960s, operate as clinics and have physicians as well as NPs, PAs, and nurse-midwives all on salary. In many states separate laws apply to clinics related to licensing and supervision by public health agencies.

COMPLEMENTARY AND ALTERNATIVE MEDICINE

Numerous other practices are used for the treatment of illness, some of which have a long tradition and some of which have developed more recently. Studies from the early 1990s found that Americans annually spend literally millions of dollars on therapies that are not part of their physician's standard approach. Patients often do not even tell their physicians about these other treatments. When practices have been used for extended periods in specific cultures, they may be called *traditional medicine.* The term *complementary medicine* is usually used for medical treatments that patients use in addition to standard medical treatments. The term *alternative medicine* refers to practices that are used instead of standard medical treatment. For many patients, these may overlap. Acupuncture, for example, has been a definitive method of treatment in traditional Chinese medicine for centuries (Figure 1-6). In the United States it has become a popular treatment method used in addition to standard treatment. It has become so popular that there are many schools to train practitioners, and the practice of acupuncture requires a license in about 40 states.

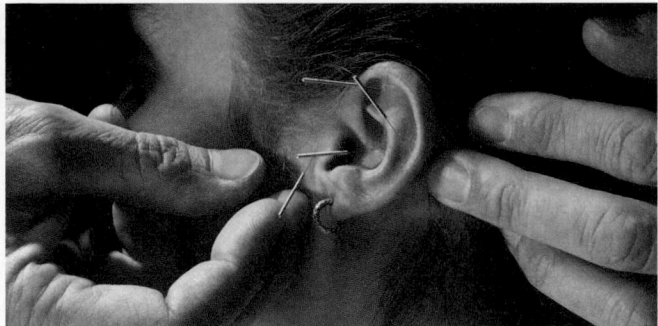

Figure 1-6 Acupuncture involves the placement of several extremely thin needles in various parts of the body.

Since the early 1990s, scholars of medicine have begun to take an interest in studying complementary and alternative practices scientifically. The federal government has since established the National Center for Complementary and Alternative Medicine within the National Institutes of Health. This agency coordinates and funds scientific research to study the effectiveness of these health practices. The most well respected medical journals such as the *New England Journal of Medicine* and *JAMA* have published a number of studies about the effectiveness of various nonstandard therapies, and numerous specialized journals have also been established to publish research about such therapies. When research demonstrates that practice is effective, physicians trained in the classical Western medical tradition are more accepting and may even incorporate some of these practices or refer patients to practitioners.

What Would You Do? What Would You *Not* Do?

Case Study 3
While Aida is taking John Carter's medical history, he mentions that he has been getting acupuncture and taking several herbal preparations that he buys at a health food store. He also says that he wears shoe insoles with magnets in them because he has had heel pain for several months. He says, "You should try them. They have really helped my heel pain." ∎

MEDICAL PRACTICE *and the* LAW

Although all states require a physician to have a license to practice medicine, it does not always have to be from the state in which the physician is working. Although individual state laws vary, in the following cases a physician is usually exempt:

1. A physician who is licensed in another state or country who is meeting with a physician of the state in question for the purposes of consultation.
2. A physician who is licensed in another state or country who is visiting a medical school or teaching hospital to receive instruction or to provide instruction, as long as it is under the supervision of a licensed physician.
3. A physician who is authorized by a foreign government may usually practice medicine in relation to that government's diplomatic, consular, or maritime staff.
4. Any commissioned medical officer serving in the U.S. Armed Forces or Public Health Service or any physician employed by the U.S. Department of Veterans Affairs.

In addition, medical students and interns or residents in postgraduate programs who are under the supervision of a licensed physician may practice medicine in the institutions with which their training programs are affiliated. ∎

What Would You Do? What Would You *Not* Do? RESPONSES

Case Study 1
Page 9

What Did Aida Do?

❑ Accepted Alicia Darwin's reason for changing medical offices without making a judgment.

❑ Stated that she hoped Alicia would feel comfortable as a patient in their practice.

❑ Stated that she was a medical assistant, not a nurse, and explained the difference briefly.

❑ Clarified the legal position of a nurse practitioner in her state related to prescribing medications.

What Did Aida Not Do?

❑ Did not agree verbally or by implication that she is a nurse.

❑ Did not ask for additional information about Alicia's previous physician or medical office.

❑ Did not make any critical remarks about nurse practitioners or Alicia's previous physician.

❑ Did not make any statement that could be interpreted as a guarantee that Alicia would like this physician better.

What Would You Do/What Would You Not *Do?*

Review Aida's response and place a checkmark next to the information you included in your response. List the additional information you included in your response.

_____

_____

_____

_____

_____

_____

_____

Case Study 2
Page 12

What Did Aida Do?

❑ Agreed that the condition of the break room could be improved.

❑ Promised to talk to all staff members about keeping the break room clean.

❑ Arranged time to speak to staff members either individually or as a group to discuss ways to keep the break room clean and make a plan.

❑ Encouraged all staff members to take an active part in developing a plan to keep the break room clean.

❑ Followed up to be sure that any plan made was implemented and was effective.

What Did Aida Not Do?

❑ Did not focus on identifying who was responsible when talking to either the physician or other staff members.

❑ Did not become defensive when talking to the physician or other staff members.

❑ Did not single out any staff member(s) as responsible for the problem.

❑ Did not complain about one staff member's behavior to any other staff member.

What Would You Do/What Would You Not *Do?*

Review Aida's response and place a checkmark next to the information you included in your response. List the additional information you included in your response.

_____

_____

_____

_____

_____

_____

_____

Case Study 3
Page 15

What Did Aida Do?

❑ Accepted John Carter's description of his complementary and alternative medical practices.

❑ Documented all practices in the medical record.

❑ Asked questions to explore the underlying problems such as heel pain or the reason for acupuncture.

What Did Aida Not Do?

❑ Did not tell John that he might be endangering his health because of his use of complementary or alternative medical practices.

❑ Did not tell John that acupuncture, magnets, or herbs would not help him.

❑ Did not ask John where to buy foot insoles with magnets.

❑ Did not dismiss John's practices as insignificant and fail to document them.

What Would You Do/What Would You Not *Do?*

Review Aida's response and place a checkmark next to the information you included in your response. List the additional information you included in your response.

_____

_____

_____

_____

_____

_____

_____

TERMINOLOGY REVIEW

Medical Term	Word Parts	Definition
Ambulatory Care	*ambulare:* to walk *-ory:* pertaining to	Medical care that is provided on an outpatient basis. The patient is able to come to the facility providing care and return home after receiving services.
Capitation		A set payment provided by managed care insurance per patient per month regardless of the amount of service the patient receives.
Curative Treatment		Treatment that cures disease.
Empirical	*empiricus:* experienced *-al:* pertaining to	Learned from observation or experiment.
Fee for service		A means of payment for health care in which the cost for each service provided is reimbursed in full or in part.
Formulary		A list of prescription drugs covered or preferred by a managed care insurance company.
Health Insurance		Purchase of protection for covered services related to health care.
Holistic	*holos:* whole *-ic:* pertaining to	Considering the whole; in medicine, considering the entire person when providing health care.
Managed Care		A system that manages the delivery of health care with the intention of controlling costs.
Palliative Treatment		Therapy that reduces the effects of a disease or condition but does not remove the disease itself.
Residency		A program to provide training in a medical specialty to a physician who has finished medical school.
Symptomatic Treatment		Therapy for symptoms of a disease or condition that does not remove the disease itself.
Utilization Review		Assessing medical services to determine whether they are appropriate, necessary, and of high quality.

ON THE WEB

For information on health:

- World Health Organization: www.who.int/en

- National Institutes of Health: www.nih.gov

For information on physicians and osteopathic physicians:

- American Medical Association: www.ama-assn.org

- American Osteopathic Association: www.osteopathic.org

For information on medical specialties:

- American Board of Medical Specialties (ABMS): www.abms.org

For information on complementary and alternative medicine:

- National Center for Complementary and Alternative Medicine (NCCAM), National Institutes of Health: www.nccam.nih.gov

Check out the Evolve site at http://evolve.elsevier.com/Bonewit/today/ to actively Prepare for your Certification, and to access additional interactive activities and exercises to help you study and prepare for success.

2

The Professional Medical Assistant

INTRODUCTION TO PROFESSIONAL MEDICAL ASSISTING

Medical assisting came into existence as a career during the second half of the twentieth century. As recently as 1950, most physicians established their own practice when they completed their medical education and hospital training. A physician (almost always a man) usually saw patients and had no assistance, except possibly from his wife who answered the telephone and often did the billing.

The physician spent a large portion of each day making house calls. During a house call the physician would examine a patient with only the equipment he could carry in his medical bag. The physician's office was often located in a room in his house or the first floor of a building, with the physician living in an apartment above. Patients who went to the physician's office may or may not have had an appointment. They expected to wait to be seen.

In the first 20 years after World War II (before the increasing use of technology caused medical costs to skyrocket), a physician usually charged $2 to $5, possibly $10, for an office visit, a sum that seems small today. For some patients, however, even this small charge was more than a day's pay. For physicians the low fee was enough because the expenses of the practice were also low. In fact, physicians rarely pressed poor patients for full payment. They always had many patients who owed them money, and it was not uncommon for patients to pay small amounts on a weekly basis for many months or even years, especially the parents of young children. Sometimes physicians would even barter by exchanging medical care for goods or services provided by the patient. For example, a patient might pay for his medical care by bringing the physician fresh produce from his farm.

In the past 60 years, the practice of medicine has changed dramatically. This, in turn, has changed the way in which physicians operate their medical practice. With the advent of government insurance programs, not only were office visits covered by insurance, but the medical office was also expected to complete and submit the insurance forms to receive payment. Physicians soon discovered that the cost of employing a person to complete these forms was offset by improved collections and cash flow. Gradually almost all insurance billing shifted to the health care provider.

Advances in medical science made many more diagnostic tests, laboratory tests, and treatments available and even necessary for good medical care. It made sense to have an assistant in the office to perform these tests and allow the physician to concentrate on seeing patients.

Even as laboratory and diagnostic testing has increased in amount and in complexity, so too have the administrative equipment and technology used in a physician's office. Today there are computers, wireless electronic devices, printers, fax machines, photocopiers, intercoms, and voice-mail systems.

Physicians send claims to a number of different insurance companies. Many insurance plans require prior approval for certain medical procedures, referrals to specialists, or surgical procedures. Insurance companies and government programs prefer electronic claims filing and often make electronic payments directly into physicians' office accounts at banks. This creates a need not only for more staff, but also for more highly trained staff.

Physicians have also almost completely stopped making house calls. Because of this, physicians need more office space. In addition, patients with more complex needs are seen in physicians' offices, rather than the hospital emergency department or outpatient department. Sometimes a patient must occupy an examination or treatment room for an extended period of time, such as when an individual with asthma is receiving an inhalation treatment.

Another change that has had an impact on the medical practice involves the increase in medical litigation. Since the 1970s, physicians have practiced what has come to be called "defensive medicine." Because of the fear of a malpractice lawsuit and the high cost of malpractice insurance, physicians began to perform more laboratory and diagnostic tests to rule out even the most unlikely cause of an illness.

As services expanded, physicians employed nurses to help them in their offices. This helped ease their burden of performing procedures and caring for patients, but nurses were often unable and unwilling to assist with the administrative aspects of the practice. As a result, many physicians found a willing candidate and trained that person to assist first with administrative duties and then with both patient care and administrative duties. This evolved over time into what today is the medical assistant position.

In 1956, medical assistants from 15 states organized to form the American Association of Medical Assistants (AAMA). In 1978 the profession was recognized by the U.S. Department of Education. The AAMA and other organizations, especially the American Medical Technologists (AMT), have worked to define professional training for the medical assistant and to provide certification for medical assistants through national examinations.

EDUCATIONAL PROGRAMS FOR MEDICAL ASSISTANTS

Initially, medical assistants received on-the-job training, but as the profession grew, formal educational programs were established. These programs vary in length from 6 months to 2 years. Medical assisting programs include theoretical and practical preparation in all aspects of the medical assisting profession. To maintain quality, many of these programs seek **accreditation,** credit, or recognition for maintaining certain standards from a regional or national organization. The two recognized accrediting agencies for medical assisting programs are the Commission on Accreditation of Allied Health Education Programs (CAAHEP) in collaboration with the AAMA and the Accrediting Bureau of Health Education Schools (ABHES).

A medical assisting program seeking accreditation from one of these agencies must prepare a written report showing how the educational standards of the agency are being met. After the report has been submitted, an accreditation visit is made to validate the information presented in the report. Once accreditation has been granted, graduates of the program are eligible to take either the certified medical assistant (CMA) (AAMA) or registered medical assistant (RMA) certification examination. Accredited programs must include at least 160 hours of practical work experience in a medical office or clinic, known as an **externship** or **practicum.**

CHARACTERISTICS OF MEDICAL ASSISTANTS

Medical assistants possess or develop a number of characteristics that make them effective in their work. Although a person's character and personality have been shaped by heredity and environment, a medical assisting student can work to enhance the traits that are important for health care delivery. Appearance and behavior are important means of projecting competence in the medical office (Figure 2-1).

Character Traits

The most important character traits of a competent medical assistant are dependability, honesty, and tolerance. The medical assistant is an integral part of the office practice and must arrive at work on time and not take days off, except when ill or if a family emergency arises. A medical assistant must be reliable enough to organize the day's work and be prepared for each patient interaction.

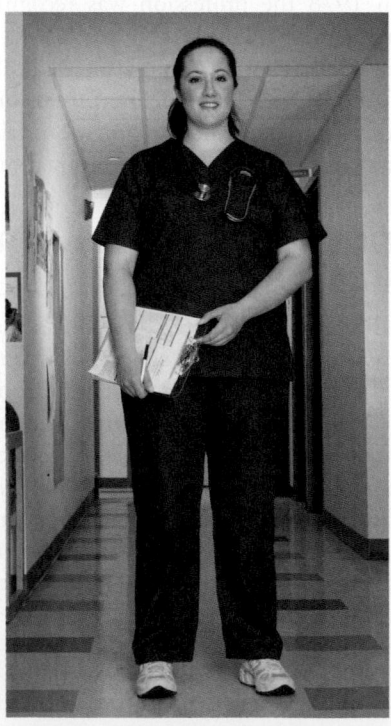

Figure 2-1 A professional appearance projects competence and increases the patient's confidence in the medical assistant.

A medical assistant projects honesty by working within his or her "scope of practice"—that is, doing only what he or she is trained to do and being comfortable in saying "I don't know" or "I don't know how to" when appropriate. The medical assistant must always maintain confidentiality and behave ethically. The medical assistant must recognize that a high level of trust is an important component of high-quality patient care. Tolerance or a willingness to accept the beliefs and practices of others is an important character trait. Tolerance allows the medical assistant to work effectively with co-workers and patients from a variety of religious, ethnic, and cultural backgrounds.

Personality Traits

Certain personality traits are essential to being a successful medical assistant. A medical assistant needs to be genuinely interested in helping people. The medical assistant must be outgoing, warm and caring, and able to put the needs of others first. The ability to remain calm in challenging or difficult situations is also important.

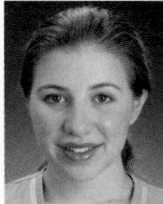

Putting It All into Practice

My name is Beth Ann Wilson, and I am a certified medical assistant. I attended a medical assisting training program at the community college near my home. I was the first person in my family to go to college, and my family was very proud of me. After the first year (two semesters), I received a certificate in medical assisting, and I found a job in our town at a group practice specializing in obstetrics and gynecology. My instructor encouraged me to take the CMA (AAMA) examination, and I was glad when I found out that I had passed it. I continued to take night classes so that I could get my associate's degree. I also attend the state and local chapter meetings of the AAMA so that I can get the contact hours I need to renew my CMA (AAMA) certification.

When I started working, I spent most of my time at the front desk answering the telephone, checking patients in, and filing, but after about 8 months I began to escort patients back to the examination rooms, prepare them for examinations, perform laboratory tests, and assist during examinations. We do some specialized tests in our office, including colposcopy, and I was trained to set up for the test and assist the physicians. Janice, our office manager who is also a CMA (AAMA), has asked me to be responsible for ordering all the supplies for the office and taking inventory. She has also encouraged me to take business courses and attend seminars related to changes in insurance billing. Not too long ago, Janice told me that she is planning to cut back her hours in the spring, and she hopes that I will be able to take over some of her duties in running the practice. That will be a big challenge, but I think I am ready for it. I have a few ideas of my own, and I will be glad for an opportunity to try them out. ■

The practice of medicine is one of the "caring professions." Each professional in the medical office needs to have a serious interest in helping people. Although the medical assistant must know how to perform the necessary administrative activities effectively and efficiently, the first priority is the care of patients who visit the office.

The concepts of warmth and caring are discussed in more detail in Chapter 4, in the section on communication. For now, it is important to say that caring is a key personality trait. Some aspects of caring can be learned and practiced. If an individual does not have a naturally caring personality, he or she will find it much harder to learn the communication skills needed to express caring.

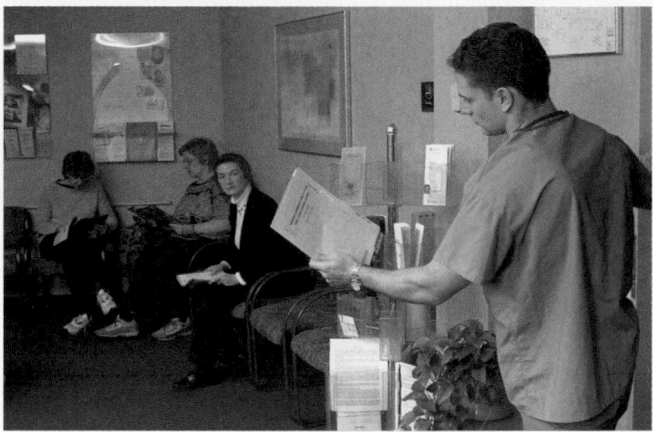

Figure 2-2 The patient judges the medical assistant's professionalism when called from the waiting room.

What Would You Do? What Would You *Not* Do?

Case Study 1

It is a busy Monday and Beth Ann is getting ready to leave the office for her lunch break at 1:30 PM when a male physician steps out of an examination room and asks her to assist him with a Pap test and pelvic examination. Beth Ann knows that it is office policy to always have a female staff member in the examination room when a pelvic examination is done. She tells the physician that she is about to go for lunch, but she will find someone to assist him. She goes to the front and finds the receptionist at the desk checking in patients, but neither of the two other medical assistants working that day is in sight. ■

The ability to put the needs of others first is important. The medical assistant must not allow personal circumstances to interfere with interactions with patients, colleagues, or physicians. Remaining objective and concentrating on the situation at hand is important. The patient's needs take precedence over the needs of the medical assistant.

The atmosphere in a medical office may change quickly from calm and orderly to rushed and somewhat disorganized. The medical assistant who can remain calm when things do not go as planned will be more successful than one who is thrown completely off balance by sudden changes in schedule or plans and who becomes emotionally unable to respond effectively.

Appearance

Personal appearance influences both the feelings and the behavior of the medical assistant. It also influences the way in which the patients respond to the medical assistant. Psychologists have long recognized the importance of physical appearance. Important judgments are made within seconds of meeting a stranger on the basis of appearance and body language.

When the medical assistant calls a patient to come from the waiting room to the examination or treatment room, the patient immediately forms an impression of the quality of care the medical assistant—and the physician—are going

to provide (Figure 2-2). A medical assistant who is neat, clean, and well groomed projects a sense of professionalism, authority, and competence. When medical assistants are courteous, they project respect for a person's dignity. This is important because many patients feel awkward, especially when dressed in underwear and an examination gown. In the same way, anything that the patient experiences as negative can result in an instant feeling of doubt in the medical assistant's ability. This may be generalized to a general feeling of doubt about all office staff. Patients often react negatively to rumpled clothing, dirty or worn shoes, unpleasant body odor, strong scent from perfume or personal products, piercings, tattoos, or an appearance that seems too "dressed up" because of jewelry, false nails, heavy makeup, and/or elaborate hairstyle.

Most medical offices require that medical assistants wear a uniform when performing clinical tasks. The uniform worn by most medical assistants consists of scrub pants with a scrub top or short-sleeved shirt; clean, white, soft-soled shoes; and a laboratory coat or jacket as needed. The top and/or jacket may be patterned, especially in a pediatric practice. Both top and bottom should fit well without being too tight. Pants should be hemmed neatly so that they do not drag on the ground (Figure 2-3). In some practices all staff wear coordinated uniforms. When performing administrative tasks, the medical assistant wears scrubs or street clothes. If street clothes are worn, they should project a businesslike appearance (Figure 2-4). Jeans, for example, are always unacceptable attire in the medical office.

Neatness and good grooming are also important for health and safety reasons. Hair carries bacteria, even if regularly washed. Medical assistants who perform clinical activities should pull their hair back and tie it, usually in a ponytail. A little bit of makeup can enhance a female medical assistant's professional image, but too much is not appropriate for a work environment. Both female and male medical assistants should always present a businesslike appearance.

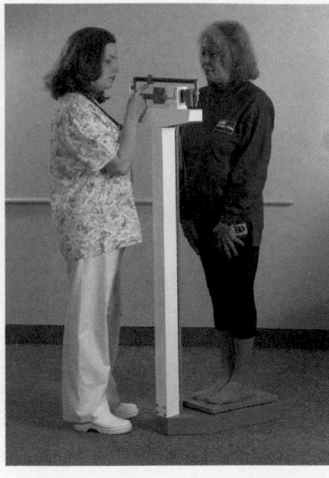

Figure 2-3 Scrub tops and pants should fit well and look professional.

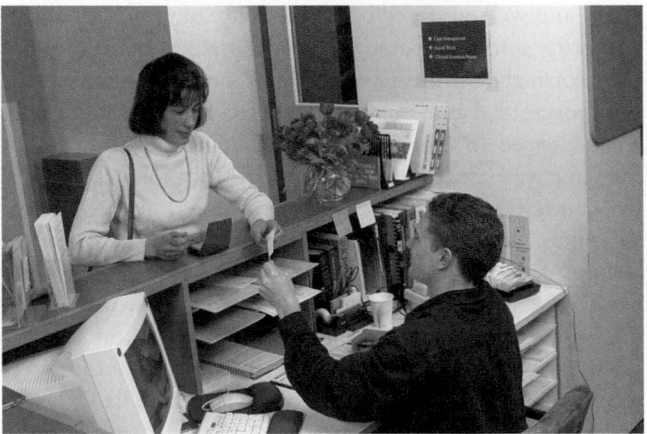

Figure 2-4 Street clothes may be worn for administrative tasks in some offices.

Medical assistants should maintain scrupulous personal hygiene and avoid perfume or scented personal care products. Many patients have allergies or respiratory problems that can be aggravated by perfumes, colognes, and scented hairspray or deodorants.

Nails should be kept relatively short and should not be polished. Long nails are not functional for keyboard work, patient care, or laboratory procedures. The Centers for Disease Control and Prevention (CDC) recommends that artificial nails not be worn and fingernails be kept ¼ inch or shorter when caring for patients at high risk of acquiring infections.

Traditionally, health professionals were allowed to wear only "functional" jewelry—a wristwatch and a plain wedding band—because jewelry is not regularly washed and can become tangled in equipment. Today, most medical offices allow staff to wear small earrings that do not dangle below the earlobe and necklaces that can be tucked into the

shirtfront. Wearing rings other than a wedding band is not a good idea. Rings can cut through protective gloves or scrape a patient. Also, they need to be taken off frequently for handwashing. Most medical offices do not allow visible piercings, except for the ears. It may also be a policy of the medical office that visible tattoos must be covered. Tattoos on the arms can be covered with a long-sleeved jersey worn under the scrub top or special sleeves designed specifically to cover tattoos.

Initiative and Behavioral Skills

Initiative is the ability to begin or follow through on a plan without being supervised. Initiative is an important quality for a medical assistant. The willingness to take initiative and perform tasks that need to be done without being specifically instructed to do so improves the functioning of the office as a whole.

Initiative, however, does not mean taking over. The office is the physician's place of business, and the physician expects to run it. Initiative does not mean redecorating the waiting room without asking the physician. It does mean doing things that need to be done without being asked, keeping up with current issues in practice without being told, and identifying helpful educational opportunities and asking permission to attend. It also means finding useful things to do when the office is slow, such as restocking supplies, ordering supplies, and cleaning out cabinets and cupboards.

Office managers who supervise medical assisting students during externships relay that some medical assisting students do not take enough initiative. Taking appropriate initiative is an important skill to develop. While in school, students learn to wait for someone to tell them exactly what to do and how to do it. In the workplace the opposite quality is valued. A medical assistant is expected to figure out what needs to be done and how to help out—even during a practicum or externship.

When a medical assistant begins a practicum or a new position, he or she must learn when to jump in and perform a task without being asked. The task that is most comfortable for the medical assistant to perform may not be the one that shows the most initiative. Medical assisting students often work on filing during slack periods because they are comfortable with the task, but it might be more important to restock examination rooms or make telephone calls to remind patients about appointments.

Initiative is a quality that employers look for in new medical assistants. An employer may even test a new employee's initiative by showing them how to do something, such as restocking an examination room at the end of the day, and then watching to see if the new medical assistant restocks the examination room without being told.

Managing activities, tasks, and schedules efficiently requires attention and effort first as a student and later as a professional medical assistant. This concept of **time**

management goes beyond day-to-day use of time to include planning, setting goals, prioritizing, and analyzing the effectiveness of how time has been used.

Getting organized requires a method to keep track of personal, class, and/or work schedules. An effective schedule includes classes, work schedules, meetings, and/or other regular activities, but it can also be helpful to schedule time for specific tasks such as homework (for a student) or preparing an inventory (for a working medical assistant). There is a tendency to put off tasks that seem difficult or unappealing. Scheduling specific times to work on these types of tasks increases the likelihood of completing them so that they are done well and on time.

For class and work activities, it may be helpful to create and update a task list. In its simplest form, this is created daily as a list of tasks to be done; each task is checked off or crossed off when it is completed. Task lists do not have to be limited to a single day, and they can be prioritized with the tasks placed in order from most important to least important. In analyzing a schedule, some unimportant activities may stand out as items that can be eliminated or reduced in frequency. It may provide a psychological boost to limit the task list to tasks that can really be completed within the allotted time span.

In order to perform many tasks efficiently, it is important to have easy access to information including names, addresses, and telephone numbers of friends, classmates, or business contacts. Reference materials needed for the job or for schoolwork should also be easily accessible.

There are many tools to facilitate effective use of time, including a personal organizer, or personal planning book, or scheduling and information management software on a smartphone or computer. Address books and reference materials can also be in book or index card format or electronic format.

The willingness to adapt to change is important for medical assistants, as well as all health care workers. The pace of change within ambulatory care is fairly rapid, so it is unwise to become attached to one way of doing things. Changes in equipment, procedure, staff, and setting can occur quite frequently, but patient care needs to remain excellent. When the medical assistant approaches changes with tolerance and even enthusiasm, the office runs more smoothly. The medical assistant needs to adapt to the office setting rather than expecting the office to adapt to his or her preferences.

Finally, it is important for the medical assistant to work well with others and be a team player. Behavior that enhances patient care includes helping others, maintaining a positive attitude and not complaining, avoiding gossip, working within the established chain of command, and handling stress without losing emotional control or creating emotional scenes. Keeping perspective, accepting corrections or criticism without becoming defensive, and learning from mistakes are important. These behaviors facilitate working with others over the long term with a minimum of discord.

What Would You Do? What Would You *Not* Do?

Case Study 2

Dawn Elliot, a 48-year-old woman, brings her mother, Ruth Mitchell, who is 70 years old, to the office with complaints of vaginal bleeding. The physician asks for blood to be drawn in the office to determine if Mrs. Mitchell has anemia from blood loss. Diane, a medical assisting externship student who has been working with Mrs. Mitchell, comes to Beth Ann and says, "Can you draw the blood from my patient? She says she doesn't want a student to draw her blood." ■

PROFESSIONALISM

Professionalism is behavior based on a body of knowledge and ethical standards to serve the public. The particular body of knowledge is different for each profession, but ethical standards for professionals are similar.

Professionalism for Physicians

For physicians, *professionalism* means treating patients based on the body of scientific knowledge the physicians have accumulated, and continue to accumulate, over their working lifetime. In addition, physicians are bound by both ethical standards and legal regulations.

One source of guidance for physicians is the American Medical Association's (AMA's) *Principles of Medical Ethics.* The AMA code of ethics is reviewed and updated periodically by that organization.

Other sources of professional guidance for physicians include the following:

- State and federal regulations
- Regulations of the hospital(s) to which the physicians admit patients
- Any open-panel health maintenance organizations or preferred provider organizations in which the physicians participate
- The national medical board of their specialty or subspecialty

Physicians may have traditionally taken guidance from Hippocrates (c. 460-377 BC). Hippocrates was an ancient Greek physician who wrote the Hippocratic Oath. The Hippocratic Oath served as a guide to good conduct for ancient physicians, and parts of it are still applicable today. Its philosophic underpinnings are still taught in medical school and adhered to by physicians, especially the key concept: "First, do no harm."

For more information on unprofessional activities of physicians, and by extension all office staff, see *Highlight on Unprofessional Conduct for a Physician*.

Professionalism for Medical Assistants

The AAMA maintains a code of ethics that is similar to the AMA principles for physicians. The AMT also maintains a set of standards that define professional practice. These codes of ethics can be viewed at the websites of each organization.

Highlight on Unprofessional Conduct for a Physician

Even if they are not illegal, many activities are considered unprofessional for physicians, and by extension for their employees, including the following:

- Receiving payment for referrals to other physicians, laboratories, treatment centers, or pharmacies. Although physicians often make specific referrals, it is unethical for them to have arrangements to receive payments for those referrals, and especially to refuse to refer a patient unless a payment is made. This practice is sometimes called **fee splitting**. It is also unethical to charge a patient simply for being admitted to a hospital, without any other service being provided.
- Prescribing medication or diagnostic tests for financial gain rather than because of the patient's need for the test.
- Pressuring patients to use pharmacies or laboratories in which the physician has a financial interest. It is also unethical to prescribe medication, tests, or procedures that are not medically necessary. Billing an insurance company for unnecessary procedures is illegal.
- Accepting gifts from pharmaceutical companies or medical equipment manufacturers or suppliers in return for promoting the company's product or prescribing only the company's drug. Physicians may accept inexpensive or educational gifts with the understanding that they have no obligation to promote the product.
- Allowing another physician or surgeon to perform surgery without informing the patient. The patient has the right to know who is performing a procedure.
- Failing to disclose the source of sperm used for artificial insemination (e.g., husband, sperm bank, paid donor). The physician may not substitute sperm without informing the patient.

- Failing to practice medicine appropriately.
- Practicing medicine under the influence of mind-altering drugs, alcohol, or any prescription medication that may impair mental function, alertness, or physical performance.
- Allowing an unlicensed person to practice medicine.
- Failing to order a consultation for any medical problem that is beyond a physician's personal experience and expertise. For example, a gynecologist should not treat a patient for renal failure.
- Withholding information about a patient's medical care from another medical facility just because the patient has an outstanding bill.
- Putting a patient at risk of human immunodeficiency virus (HIV) infection, or refusing to treat a patient who is HIV positive. It is considered ethical for physicians to limit their practice to certain medical specialties and to refuse to accept specific types of insurance.
- Performing a procedure that might transmit the HIV virus to a patient if a physician or any other health care worker is HIV positive.
- Engaging in a sexual relationship with a patient. Something inherent in the relationship between two individuals in which one is perceived to be more influential than the other puts pressure on the "weaker" party to please the more powerful party. Because this makes it difficult to determine if consent is freely given, such a relationship should never be sexual in nature. Sexual relationships between professionals and the people they serve (e.g., physician-patient, attorney-client, teacher-student) are thus considered unethical and unprofessional. ∎

The medical assistant's ethical responsibilities are to admit mistakes, stay within the personal limits of his or her training, maintain confidentiality, stay current, and uphold the honor of the profession. This may mean having to confront a co-worker who is not adhering to such principles.

Dealing with a co-worker's inappropriate conduct is difficult, especially for a new employee or if the co-worker is higher in the organizational hierarchy. We live in a society that does not like "tattletales." On the other hand, unprofessional behavior in a medical office is disruptive to the concept of teamwork. Even if the unprofessional behavior does not pose an immediate threat to a patient, any behavior that results in people not working well together can lead to an uncomfortable or dangerous situation. The medical assistant should first discuss the situation with the co-worker by calmly and objectively describing the actions or behavior that he or she considers unprofessional. If the person does not correct the situation, it is appropriate to report the behavior to the office manager.

What Would You Do? What Would You *Not* Do?

Case Study 3

Before examining Ruth Mitchell, the physician asked Beth Ann to recheck her blood pressure. It was 190/100 in the right arm and 186/98 in the right arm. Beth Ann noticed that the blood pressure had been taken that day by Diane, a medical assisting externship student, who had recorded it as 130/80. Beth Ann asked Diane if she was confident about the blood pressure reading she obtained from Mrs. Mitchell. Diane said, "It was really faint, and I didn't hear it that well, so I wrote down the same blood pressure as she had the last time she was here. I didn't want to look incompetent. Besides, I was afraid it might affect my grade if you thought I was having trouble hearing the blood pressure." ∎

CREDENTIALS OF MEDICAL ASSISTANTS

Medical assistants usually graduate from an educational program that may vary in length from 6 months to 2 years. If the medical assistant graduates from a program accredited by CAAHEP or ABHES, he or she is eligible to take a national certification examination. Certification is a process by which an organization, often a national body, validates the credentials of an individual or a program. Certification is important for health care professionals. Certification is also important for medical assistants who live in a state that does not regulate unlicensed health professionals. When an unbiased national organization validates knowledge and skills, the employer can be sure that the medical assistant has excellent qualifications.

Two organizations provide nationally accepted certification for medical assistants: the AAMA and the AMT. In many areas, employers hire only medical assistants who have passed a certification examination. As medical assistants perform more specialized clinical tasks, employers have become increasingly concerned about validating skills and knowledge before hiring them.

Certified Medical Assistant

A CMA (AAMA) has passed the certification examination administered by the AAMA. In order to take the examination, the individual must have graduated from a medical assisting program accredited by CAAHEP or ABHES or be a CMA (AAMA) recertificant.

The examination is computer-based and is administered online at testing centers. Most states have several testing locations.

Application material can be obtained from the AAMA Certification Department, 20 North Wacker Dr., Suite 1565, Chicago IL 60606-2903; from the director of accreditation at the medical assisting program attended; or from the AAMA website (www.aama-ntl.org).

Passing this examination allows a medical assistant to use the title CMA (AAMA) after his or her name on all official documents, including patient records and business cards.

Registered Medical Assistant

An RMA has passed the examination administered by the AMT. The AMT is an organization that certifies medical assistants, medical technologists, medical laboratory technicians, phlebotomists, and other health professionals.

In order to take the RMA examination, an individual must have (1) graduated from a medical assisting program accredited by CAAHEP or ABHES; (2) graduated from a medical assisting program that includes at least 720 hours of training in an institution that is accredited by an organization approved by the U.S. Department of Education; (3) graduated from a formal medical services program of the U.S. Armed Forces; or (4) been employed full-time in the profession of medical assisting for 5 years. The AMT may also grant the credential of RMA to an applicant who has passed another approved medical assisting certification examination.

Applications for the RMA examination can be obtained from the Registrar's Office, American Medical Technologists, 10700 W. Higgins, Suite 150, Rosemont, IL 60018. Information about the examination can be obtained from the AMT website (www.americanmedtech.org). The RMA examination may be given at a student's school, or an applicant may take the test online at testing centers located throughout the country.

Passing this examination entitles the medical assistant to use the initials RMA after his or her name on all official documents.

Obtaining Additional Credentials

A medical assistant may need to validate other skills as a condition of employment.

Training in cardiopulmonary resuscitation (CPR) is offered directly through the American Red Cross (ARC) and the American Heart Association (AHA) and by hospitals and other health care agencies. Like other health professionals, medical assistants recertify at the health care provider level every 2 years to be sure their skills are current as required by their professional organization and/or employer. Most health care facilities require current CPR credentials.

Medical assistants may also take courses in performing first aid, hearing tests, limited x-ray examinations, or other specialized tests, depending on state law and the needs of the medical practice. In many areas, medical assisting certification or registration is a valid qualification to perform phlebotomy, but some states and/or institutions require separate certification in phlebotomy. This can be obtained through the AMT, the American Society for Clinical Pathology (ASCP), or the American Society of Phlebotomy Technicians. The websites of these organizations are listed at the end of the chapter.

A medical assistant who obtains experience working for a podiatrist or ophthalmologist may obtain certification as a podiatric medical assistant, certified (PMAC) or a certified ophthalmic assistant (COA).

If the medical assistant has specialized in the administrative area, additional credentials can be obtained, such as the certified medical administrative specialist (CMAS) from the AMT or one of the various certifications in medical coding, such as a certified coding associate (CCA), a certified coding specialist (CCS), or a certified coding specialist–physician-based (CCS-P) from the American Health Information Management Association (AHIMA). The CCS-P is a coding practitioner who specializes in coding for physicians in settings such as physician offices, group practices, multispecialty clinics, or specialty centers. Additional education may be required to obtain these credentials.

PROFESSIONAL ORGANIZATIONS

The AAMA and the AMT are professional organizations for medical assistants. For an annual membership fee, many benefits are available. Medical assisting students can join either the AAMA or the AMT for a reduced annual rate and receive member services. Membership information is available at the website for each organization.

Peer Support

Through local and national meetings and workshops, medical assistants are able to enter a network of peers with whom they can share and from whom they can learn. They can also obtain insurance at reasonable cost, professional journals, and access to other sources of information important to the profession.

Continuing Education

With the constant change in the medical field, it is not merely important but necessary to keep skills up to date, attain new skills, and obtain new information about professional practices. Most health professions require a certain amount of continuing education for licensure or certification renewal. These are designed either as contact hours or **continuing education units (CEUs)**. A CEU is a unit of participation in professional continuing education.

Medical assisting contact hours and CEUs can be obtained from educational programs that have been approved by the particular certifying agency. The AAMA validates continuing education programs given through the state and national organization. Attending meetings of professional organizations is the best way to find educational programs specifically for the needs of professional medical assistants. Home study programs are also available to obtain continuing education credit.

An individual must be recertified as a CMA (AAMA) every 5 years. This can be accomplished by retaking the certification examination or by successfully completing the required continuing education programs. Sixty points must be accumulated during the 5-year period: 10 in the administrative area, 10 in the clinical area, and 10 in the general area, with 30 additional hours in any of the three categories. Of these, 30 points must be CEUs (one contact hour each) from AAMA-approved programs.

If certified after January 2006, RMAs must accumulate 30 points of continuing education every 3 years. (One contact hour is equivalent to one point.) Those who were certified before this date are expected to keep up to date with current practice, but there are no specific continuing education requirements.

Legislative Advocacy

One of the tasks of professional organizations is to monitor legislative initiatives at the state and national level that may affect the profession. In many states the profession of medical assisting is defined in state law, whereas in other states it is not. The state professional organization provides a forum to push for legislation that will advance the medical assisting profession.

Publications, Newsletters, and Websites

Both the national and state organizations provide a means for communication among professional medical assistants, including *CMA Today,* published by the AAMA, and the *Journal of Continuing Education Topics and Issues,* published by the AMT. The national organizations have state associations, often with several chapters within the state. The state organizations may produce newsletters and maintain websites. Conferences are held annually both nationally and at the state level to enhance communication and contact among members of the profession.

ROLE OF THE MEDICAL ASSISTANT

Administrative Responsibilities

Various administrative responsibilities must be performed on a daily basis in a medical office. We like to think of a physician's office as a place where patients receive medical treatment, but in reality much of the activity in a physician's office involves managing the logistics of scheduling patients, preparing to provide services, and receiving payment for services. The medical assistant may be responsible for a number of these activities, although larger offices may employ specialists to perform these tasks.

1. Scheduling appointments, both over the telephone and in person, is a primary responsibility of the medical assistant. A patient may also need to have appointments made with other medical facilities; examples include a consultation with a specialist, a diagnostic procedure, outpatient surgery, continuing therapy or rehabilitation, and a hospital admission. Some patients may need to schedule multiple appointments with other facilities as the result of a single office visit. The medical assistant must learn the procedure for making and documenting each type of appointment.

2. Maintaining the medical record and filing records and reports has traditionally been one of the medical assistant's roles. With the increasing use of electronic medical records, there is less actual filing in many offices, but it still may be necessary to scan paper reports and keep track of laboratory and diagnostic test results. Each patient encounter with a clinician—physician, nurse practitioner (NP), or physician assistant (PA)—is followed by documentation of the patient's visit. Clinicians create handwritten or dictated patient notes, or they may enter information directly into an electronic medical record. If the dictation method is used, it may be transcribed using voice recognition software or it may be sent to an outside service electronically. In this case the medical assistant prints the reports after they have been returned and files them after the physician has approved them. The medical assistant may prepare letters and other documents for the physician.

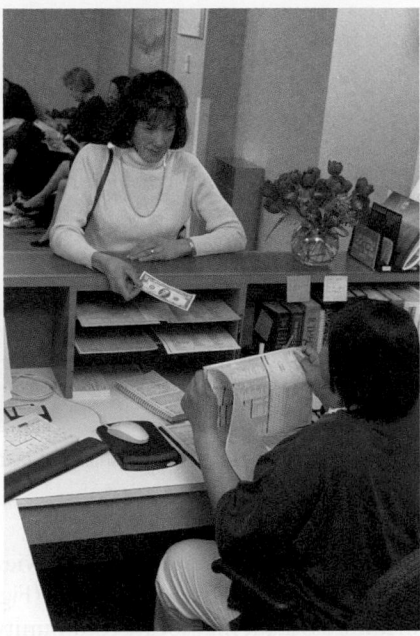

Figure 2-5 Medical assistant taking a payment.

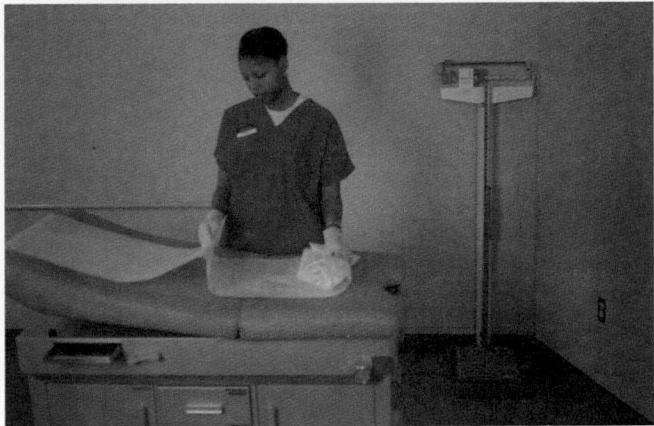

Figure 2-6   Medical assistant preparing an examination room.

Clinical Responsibilities

Depending on the type of medical office, clinical activities may make up the bulk of the medical assistant's responsibilities. The medical assistant prepares patients for examination, performs diagnostic tests, performs treatments, and assists the physician with examination and treatment.

1. Medical assistants are often asked to collect and process specimens. Some specimens are tested in the office, and others are sent to an outside laboratory.
2. Medical assistants perform several diagnostic tests, such as electrocardiograms and respiratory testing.
3. Medical assistants prepare patients for examination, including taking medical histories, weighing the patient, measuring vital signs, and obtaining information about the chief complaint. Having this done by a medical assistant may allow the physician to see at least one extra patient per hour.
4. After each patient appointment, the medical assistant prepares the examination and/or treatment room for the next patient (Figure 2-6). This involves making sure there is fresh paper on the table, that the proper instruments and supplies are available for the next examination or procedure, and that the necessary equipment is available and in working order.
5. Medical assistants help the physician with examinations and procedures. The medical assistant settles a patient into an examination room and positions and drapes the patient for portions of the examination. Another duty is to pass instruments and supplies to the physician during procedures. The medical assistant may also remove sutures and change sterile dressings. If minor surgery or sterile procedures are performed in the office, the medical assistant sets up the equipment and supplies and then assists the physician as needed.
6. Medical assistants perform treatments, including nebulizer treatments or application of hot and cold packs or compresses.
7. Medical assistants prepare and administer medications and immunizations. The administration of

3. Every patient visit generates activities that are necessary for the physician to be paid for the services provided. The medical assistant must know how to accept and document payments (Figure 2-5), total and enter charges, code the procedures and/or diagnostic tests performed, and enter payments received. These charges and payments are entered into the office computer and sometimes into various paper records, such as the day sheet, to keep track of money owed to and received by the practice. In turn, the charges are used to generate insurance claims and patient bills. In larger offices and clinics, a separate business office usually handles financial matters. Small offices often send billing information to an outside billing service. If billing is performed in the office, the medical assistant must be able to create patient bills and submit insurance claims.
4. On a regular basis, checks and cash need to be deposited into the office's bank account. Preparing bank deposits and recording the deposits in the office's checkbook are activities that medical assistants often perform.
5. Every business has bills to pay. These include rent (or mortgage, if the office is owned), electricity, lease payments on equipment, staff salaries, and a number of other regular payments, such as liability and malpractice insurance. Medical assistants, or business office personnel, usually pay these bills and maintain records of these and other bills owed by the office. (Some offices have an outside bookkeeping service perform these tasks. Even in many offices that pay their own regular bills, salary is handled by an outside payroll service.)

medication requires concentration and precision. All medications must be documented according to office procedure.

8. Sometimes a medical assistant also has to perform emergency care and administer first aid or assist with an office emergency. This does not happen often, but every medical assistant must be prepared.

Managing the Medical Office

The medical assistant may have many responsibilities to keep the medical office running smoothly.

1. Operational activities involve maintaining the inventory of supplies. This can include everything from purchasing tongue blades and gauze to contracting with a uniform service to launder the staff's laboratory coats or patient gowns. It may also involve evaluating and recommending changes in the supplies purchased and evaluating new equipment for potential purchase or lease.

2. A second group of activities involves personnel policy and procedures. Businesses are always reviewing their policies and procedures and updating and revising them as needed. As offices move from one or two physicians and a small staff to a larger organization, policies and procedures become more important to standardize the way all employees are dealt with.

3. **Risk management** is the development of policies and procedures that minimize the chances of the practice being sued by a patient or disciplined by a regulatory agency. Every physician's office needs to have one person responsible for risk management, which involves, among other areas, the promotion of health and safety for office personnel and patients, implementation of a quality control program, maintenance of proper infection control measures, fire prevention, and the proper disposal of hazardous waste and controlled substances.

4. Record keeping is an important activity for the individual who manages a medical office. In addition to patient records, many other kinds of records must be kept, including office insurance records, quality control records, maintenance contracts, personnel records, and financial records.

Patient Education

Instructing patients is an important role for medical assistants because the medical assistant actually conveys information to the patient from the physician.

1. The medical assistant is often responsible for educating the patient about office procedures, including giving information to a new patient who is making the first appointment, as well as instructing an established patient whose circumstances have changed.

2. The medical assistant may provide information about maintaining health to patients directly as directed by the physician or by making educational materials

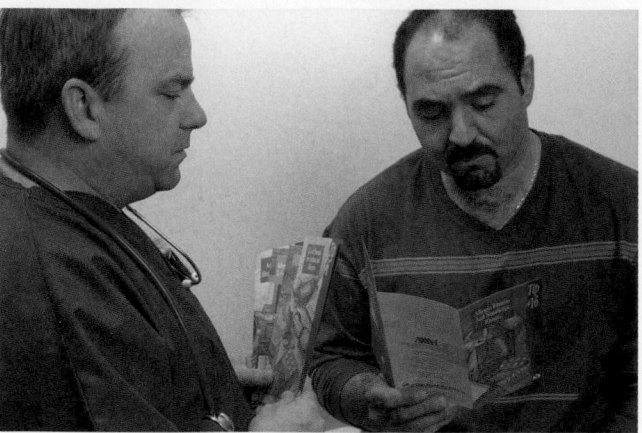

Figure 2-7   The medical assistant uses brochures to teach a patient.

available in the office. These are always reviewed by the physician before being given to patients (Figure 2-7).

3. The medical assistant may locate community resources for a patient or provide brochures from community agencies in order to improve follow-up care for a patient.

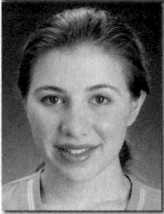

Memories *from* Externship

Beth Ann Wilson: I could not believe how nervous I was before I went to my externship the first day. I had worked at several jobs and even done filing at a medical office during the summer when I was in high school, but it felt totally different to know that I would be responsible to act like a "real" medical assistant. Fortunately, the staff members at my placement were wonderful. They let me shadow one of the medical assistants until I felt comfortable to work with patients on my own. They were also careful to expose me gradually to each part of the medical office, so it didn't get overwhelming. The person who helped me the most was Cheryl, the office manager. Every day she sought me out and asked how it was going. There was one time when a physician asked me to take out a patient's sutures, and I hadn't even seen someone perform that procedure. I didn't know what to say, but I told him I would find another medical assistant to help him. Then I went to Cheryl. She found someone else to perform the procedure and made sure that I had an opportunity to observe. I never could decide whether I liked checking patients in up front or assisting the physicians better, as long as I had a chance to interact with patients. It has always made me feel good to know that I am helping others. ■

EMPLOYMENT OPPORTUNITIES

According to the U.S. Department of Labor Bureau of Labor Statistics, medical assisting is projected to be one of the fastest-growing occupations in the period between 2008 and 2018. Job prospects are expected to be excellent, especially for medical assistants who have completed a formal educational program. Certification may help to distinguish a medical assistant who meets recognized standards from an entry-level assistant.

The majority of medical assistants work in physician's offices. Other common places of employment include hospitals and offices of other health practitioners, such as chiropractors, podiatrists, or optometrists. Medical assistants also work in outpatient care centers, schools or other educational facilities, medical laboratories, government agencies, employment services, and nursing care facilities.

The median annual income reported by medical assistants in May 2010 was $28,860, but salaries varied greatly depending on geographic location, skill level, and type of facility in which the medical assistant was employed.

The Bureau of Labor Statistics reported median annual income for medical assistants in May 2010 as follows:

Offices of physicians	$30,110
General medical and surgical hospitals	$30,770
Offices of other health practitioners	$26,820
Outpatient care centers	$30,490

The most direct route for career advancement is probably to become an office, practice, or department manager. This may require additional education, especially in business administration, but often management skills can be learned mainly on the job. In order to become a medical assisting instructor, it is necessary to have an Associate in Science degree or a higher degree in a related field and to be either a CMA (AAMA) or an RMA (for an accredited medical assisting program). Clinical advancement usually requires additional training in a formal educational program preparing for a health career, such as dental hygiene, laboratory technology, nursing, radiologic technology, or respiratory therapy.

MEDICAL PRACTICE *and the* LAW

Medical assistants are not licensed, and in most states their role is not clearly defined in the law. State medical practice laws usually allow physicians to delegate clinical tasks to qualified medical assistants under their supervision, provided that the task is not prohibited by another law. Some states do define the role of a medical assistant, sometimes related to general duties and sometimes related to specific tasks that the medical assistant is allowed to perform. In some states, medical assistants are required to register with the state before practicing as a medical assistant. Because state laws vary so greatly, a medical assisting student should always find out the legal status of a medical assistant in his or her own state or the state in which he or she intends to work after graduation. ■

What Would You Do? What Would You *Not* Do? RESPONSES

Case Study 1
Page 21

What Did Beth Ann Do?

❑ Looked in the back part of the office for an available staff member.

❑ Asked the receptionist if she knew where one of the other medical assistants was.

❑ Used the intercom to locate a medical assistant.

❑ Checked the examination rooms with open doors to see if a medical assistant might be almost finished checking in a patient.

❑ Assisted the physician if she was unable to find another medical assistant to do it.

What Did Beth Ann Not Do?

❑ Did not leave for lunch without finding someone to assist the physician.

❑ Did not tell the physician that she was sorry she could not assist him at this time.

❑ Did not knock on closed examination room doors.

What Would You Do/What Would You Not Do?

Review Beth Ann's response and place a checkmark next to the information you included in your response. List the additional information you included in your response.

_____
_____
_____
_____
_____
_____
_____

Case Study 2
Page 23

What Did Beth Ann Do?

❑ Agreed to draw the blood without complaining.

❑ Tried to make the patient feel comfortable and confident.

❑ Explained to Diane later that some patients do not want students to perform certain procedures.

❑ Told Diane that she was glad she had called her to help.

What Would You Do? What Would You *Not* Do? RESPONSES—cont'd

❑ Reinforced that even if Diane's pride was slightly hurt, Diane did the correct thing by not showing this to the patient.

What Did Beth Ann Not Do?
❑ Did not make the patient feel as if she were asking for special treatment.
❑ Did not tell Diane that she looked very young or unprofessional.
❑ Did not talk about the incident as a funny story in the break room to other staff.

What Would You Do/What Would You Not Do?
Review Beth Ann's response and place a checkmark next to the information you included in your response. List the additional information you included in your response.

_____
_____
_____
_____
_____
_____
_____

Case Study 3
Page 24

What Did Beth Ann Do?
❑ Told the patient that the physician asked her to recheck the blood pressure because it sometimes changes when patients sit in a quiet examination room.

❑ Found a private place to speak to Diane and agreed with her that sometimes it is really hard to hear the blood pressure.
❑ Explained to Diane that it is important to take and record the blood pressure correctly even if she has to ask for assistance.
❑ Reminded Diane that the staff understands she is a student and will not be able to perform every procedure perfectly.
❑ Offered to work with Diane to improve her technique.

What Did Beth Ann Not Do?
❑ Did not talk down to Diane or try to make her feel bad.
❑ Did not tell others in the office not to rely on Diane's blood pressure measurements.
❑ Did not tell the patient that Diane had not been sure of her measurement.

What Would You Do/What Would You Not Do?
Review Beth Ann's response and place a checkmark next to the information you included in your response. List the additional information you included in your response.

_____
_____
_____
_____
_____
_____
_____

TERMINOLOGY REVIEW

Medical Term	Word Parts	Definition
Accreditation		Credit or recognition from a regional or national organization for maintaining certain standards.
Continuing education unit (CEU)		A standard unit of measure of continuing education for professionals, defined as 1 contact hour by the AAMA, but also commonly 10 contact hours of participation.
Externship		A supervised work experience that is required in an educational program and usually unpaid. Sometimes called a *practicum*.
Fee splitting		The practice of sharing fees with colleagues, especially for making referrals.
Initiative		The ability to begin or carry through on a plan of action independently.
Practicum		A supervised work experience that is required in an educational program and usually unpaid. Sometimes called an *externship*.
Risk management		Processes to protect a health care facility from the risk of legal action.
Time management		Skills and techniques used to manage time in order to accomplish tasks and meet goals.

ON THE WEB

For information on professional organizations:

Accrediting Bureau of Health Education Schools: www.abhes.org

American Association of Medical Assistants: www.aama-ntl.org

American Health Information Management Association: www.ahima.org

American Medical Association: www.ama-assn.org

American Medical Technologists: www.americanmedtech.org

American Society for Clinical Pathology: www.ascp.org

American Society of Phlebotomy Technicians: www.aspt.org

American Society of Podiatric Medical Assistants: www.aspma.org

Commission on Accreditation of Allied Health Education Programs: www.caahep.org

Joint Commission on Allied Health Personnel in Ophthalmology: www.jcahpo.org

For information on occupational outlook for medical assistants:

U.S. Department of Labor Bureau of Labor Statistics: www.bls.gov

 Check out the Evolve site at http://evolve.elsevier.com/Bonewit/today/ to actively Prepare for your Certification, and to access additional interactive activities and exercises to help you study and prepare for success.

3

Ethics and Law for the Medical Office

LEARNING OBJECTIVES

Ethics and Health Care

1. Identify key differences between law and ethics.
2. List reasons for medical assistants to study ethics.
3. Identify specific rights that patients have in relation to health care.
4. Correlate the concept of duties to the actions expected of health professionals.
5. Be a patient advocate.
6. Report illegal and/or unsafe activities and behaviors affecting patient care to proper authorities.
7. Describe how certain ethical issues generate ethical conflict in society.
8. Describe ways to separate and prioritize personal and professional ethics.
9. Describe six steps that may be used to make ethical decisions.

Law and Professional Liability

10. Identify similarities and differences between public law and private law.
11. Identify the process through which laws are created on the federal and state level.
12. Differentiate between types of crimes, such as felonies and misdemeanors, as well as between violent and nonviolent crimes.
13. Differentiate between criminal law and civil law.
14. List and explain the elements of a valid contract.
15. State the rights and duties of each party in the physician-patient relationship.
16. Incorporate the Patient's Bill of Rights into personal practice.
17. Define "standard of care," and describe how this concept affects the behavior of health professionals.
18. Describe the medical assistant's role in obtaining informed consent.
19. Explain the principles of negligence and professional negligence as they apply to the behavior of health professionals.
20. Explain the purpose and need for professional liability insurance.
21. Describe the process of malpractice litigation.
22. List and explain specific defenses to intentional and unintentional torts.

Federal and State Laws Affecting the Medical Office

23. Describe and explain the laws regulating controlled substances and prescription medications.
24. List and explain several laws that protect employees of medical offices.
25. Describe how the provisions of the Health Insurance Portability and Accountability Act (HIPAA) affect the medical office.
26. List and explain the situations where mandatory reporting is required by the medical office.
27. Describe how states regulate the practice of medicine and health occupations.
28. Differentiate between licensing and voluntary accreditation for health care facilities.

CHAPTER OUTLINE

KEY TERMS

abandonment
act
advocate (ADD-va-kit)
arbitration
assumption of risk
autonomy (ah-TAH-noe-mee)
beneficence (ben-IH-fih-sens)
bill
case law
civil law
cloning (KLOH-ning)
common law
comparative negligence (NEG-lih-jhens)
contingency (kon-TIN-jhen-see)
contributory negligence
controlled substance
crime
criminal law
defendant
do-not-resuscitate (DNR) orders
Drug Enforcement Administration (DEA)

duty
emancipated minor
embezzlement (em-BEZ-el-ment)
etiquette
felony
fidelity
fraud
gene therapy
genetic engineering
health care proxy (PROX-ee)
informed consent
larceny
liability
license
licensure (LI-sen-sur)
litigation (lih-tih-GAY-shun)
living will
malfeasance (mal-FEE-suns)
malpractice
mediation
misdemeanor (mis-de-MEAN-or)

misfeasance (mis-FEE-suns)
negligence (NEG-lih-jhens)
nonfeasance (non-FEE-suns)
nonmalfeasance (non-mal-FEE-suns)
plaintiff (PLANE-tiff)
prescription
privilege
prudent
reciprocity (re-sip-RAW-city)
respondeat superior (ray-SPON-day-at sue-PEER-ee-or)
right
standard of care
statute (STA-chewt) of limitations
statutory (STA-chew-toe-ree) law
stem cells
subpoena (su-PEE-na)
subpoena *duces tecum* (su-PEE-na DEW-chess TAY-come)
tort
veracity (ver-ASS-ih-tee)

INTRODUCTION TO MEDICAL ETHICS

Within a democracy, society tolerates a wide range of beliefs about what is moral or right and uses the democratic process to create rules and laws that regulate public behavior. This process allows for change and flexibility because laws are continually reviewed through the judiciary process.

It is important to remember that society's beliefs about right and wrong precede laws and also influence their interpretation. Currently the rapid pace of technologic innovation and changing beliefs places considerable stress on the social structure.

There is also a wide diversity of expectations about normal, acceptable behavior, sometimes called **etiquette,** or manners. Breaches of etiquette pose no true threat to the integrity of an individual or society. However, individuals may have just as strong an emotional reaction to what they see as bad manners as they would have to a true ethical breach.

In the context of the medical office, a patient may feel that being rushed by the physician and treated "as a number, not a name" by the front-office staff is being treated without dignity. The patient's emotional response to how he or she is treated may seem more important than the actual quality of care.

REASONS TO STUDY ETHICS

Although ethics is an abstract discipline and medical assisting is firmly grounded in practice and procedure, medical assistants should study ethics for a number of reasons.

First, it is an important part of an individual's education to develop the intellectual skills to analyze complex problems and justify the choices made in particular situations. In the case of ethics, the choice is between alternative courses of action that have moral and social consequences.

Second, as society has become increasingly complex, average citizens are more aware that choices affect not only people living now, but those who will live in the future. People hesitate to allow only elected and appointed officials to deal with these choices. Learning about ethics and social issues encourages ordinary people to have input into social beliefs and expectations. There is also a greater sense of interconnections involving the whole world, sometimes called *globalism.* Many individuals feel some level of responsibility for all human beings, and indeed for all living beings on the earth.

Third, in the specific realm of medicine and science, more sophisticated medical treatment and new technologies are constantly becoming available. However, society does not have unlimited resources to provide everything to everyone, even in the developed world. There is a need to make informed choices about what care will be provided to whom, and when, rather than simply responding to special interests.

Fourth, every year new biomedical research makes it possible to do more things with which the world has no previous experience. Society must have informed citizens who can analyze issues and guide the future. Within the health care system, health professionals, including medical assistants, need skills in considering ethical questions in order to improve health care for individuals and society.

ETHICS AND HEALTH CARE

Ethical Concepts

Current thinking about biomedical ethics identifies several rights (very strong claims) for patients and duties (requirements) for the institutions and individuals who provide health care. Sources for these ideas include religious traditions, social belief systems, and political documents such as the Declaration of Independence and the U.S. Constitution and the Bill of Rights, as well as ethical theories developed by individual philosophers.

Rights

A **right** is a claim that is expected to be honored. It is stronger than a wish or a need.

The early leaders of the American government believed in natural rights and the duty of any government to preserve them. Natural rights were considered to exist through the natural order or to be granted by God. These include the following:

1. Right to life
2. Right to privacy
3. Right to autonomy
4. Right to the means to sustain life

Right to Life

One of the rights mentioned in the Declaration of Independence is the right to life.

Since the 1970s the term "right to life" has come to be associated with the movement against abortion. But in a broader context, it reflects the belief that human beings may not kill others. The belief in the right to life is found in all major religions and traditions.

The right to life has many implications for medicine. Historically, physicians and other health care workers may not harm patients because this may threaten their lives. They may not assist with suicide; this is expressly stated in the Hippocratic Oath. In the United States today, however, many individuals want some control over death, including the choice of suicide assisted by their physician.

Two important areas of conflict appeared in the middle of the twentieth century. First, advances in medical care made it possible to keep people alive who could not recover their health. Sometimes this sustaining of life came at the cost of prolonged suffering.

Second, the absolute right to life of an unborn fetus conflicts with the right of a woman to control her own reproductive capacity. Birth-control methods, artificial conception methods, and abortion, if necessary, are measures to control the size of a woman's family. Many women and their physicians have come to believe they have a right to make decisions related to reproduction, including using available technology, as they see fit.

Right to Privacy

The Supreme Court has ruled that there is an implicit right to privacy in the Bill of Rights, specifically in the Fourth Amendment. A series of court decisions affirming a woman's right to use mechanical birth control and to have an abortion hinged on justices' perceiving this right to privacy.

Patient confidentiality, which has been upheld by courts, is another manifestation of the right to privacy. Patient confidentiality is discussed in detail later in this chapter.

Right to Autonomy

Currently, medical ethics takes the position that an individual has the right to **autonomy,** which means the right to make independent decisions about his or her health care according to individual values and concerns, without constraint or coercion by others. This right is preserved even when the individual's decisions do not match the values of the medical community or the individual physician. The right of autonomy is the basis for **informed consent.** Informed consent is consent based on understanding of a medical procedure and its possible outcomes. Health care professionals must provide complete information in order for patients to make informed decisions. The patient must have the mental capacity to reason and consider alternatives. Because of this, the law limits the autonomy of children or individuals with decreased mental capacity such as the mentally retarded or individuals whose mental capacity has been impaired by illness, those acting under the influence of drugs or alcohol, and those experiencing mental illness.

Respect for autonomy does not derive from the Hippocratic Oath. Rather, it comes from the thinking of European philosophers such as Immanuel Kant and John Locke.

Right to the Means to Sustain Life

Every society must grapple with the problem of equitable distribution of goods and services to its citizens and how to regulate that distribution over time.

This is not a problem when the supply is adequate, or when supply is greater than demand. For instance, in ordinary circumstances the supply of oxygen is more than adequate to meet the needs of the entire population.

It is when the amount of a particular resource is less than the desire for that resource that problems develop. In this case, resources are said to be *scarce,* and the society's government must determine who will have access to the scarce resources.

At a minimum, every individual should have access to what is necessary to sustain life and preserve human dignity. Consideration of justice in distribution and access is especially important in social and political movements. Any society must find ways to respond to need while also rewarding contribution and providing for stability within the social system.

Duties

A **duty** is a commitment to act in a certain way on the basis of religious beliefs, moral principles, or a particular professional code of conduct. Traditionally five main duties of a health care professional have been identified.

Do No Harm

The concept of **nonmalfeasance** means, first of all, doing no harm in any treatment given. This duty is found in the Hippocratic Oath. It is not taken in a literal sense because many treatments can have adverse effects. Rather, it is taken to mean that medical benefits should outweigh adverse effects.

This concept applies especially to scientific research. Guidelines for ethical research not only require informed consent but also restrict research with possible harmful effects to those patients whose conditions are so serious that doing nothing is likely to be as dangerous as the treatment or procedure being studied.

Do the Best Possible

The concept of **beneficence,** doing the best possible, is seen in some systems of ethics as a separate duty, whereas in

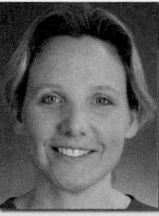

Putting It All into Practice

My name is Vicki Edmonds, and I have worked in a family practice for about 6 years. There are two physicians and two nurse practitioners in my practice, and I usually assist one of the physicians. Of course, if it is busy or one of the other medical assistants is ill, we all pitch in and help out. Neither of the physicians in my practice has ever been sued, and we all work together to be sure it stays that way. We do everything we can so that our patients not only receive great care but are also satisfied with their treatment. We also document everything carefully because our physicians are aware that it is hard to prove that you gave good care if you don't write it down. Every once in a while we have a patient who constantly breaks appointments or doesn't take his or her medication, and if the physician thinks that it is harmful to the patient's health, sometimes he will instruct the patient to find another practitioner to care for him or her. I remember one time when the patient lived far away, and she said that it was difficult for her to make the trip to our office. After she missed three appointments in a row, the physician had me write a letter suggesting that she find another physician nearer to her home. He explained that he couldn't be responsible for her if she was unable to keep appointments. In the letter he gave her a month to find another physician, and he offered to help her if she was having difficulty. We sent that letter by certified mail and obtained a return receipt. Then we documented everything in the patient's medical record. The patient sent a letter back saying that she was going to an office much closer to home, and she thought that would work out better for her. ■

others it is considered an extension of doing no harm. It is often difficult to pinpoint exactly what harm and good are; they may vary with a particular individual's viewpoint.

Be Faithful to Reasonable Expectations

The concept of **fidelity,** being faithful, comes from the Latin term *fides,* which means faith. In the case of medical practice, fidelity is usually interpreted as meaning faithful to reasonable expectations. Although patient expectations vary, there is general agreement that a patient can reasonably expect to be treated with dignity, treated by individuals who honor their agreements, and treated by competent providers. Patients can also expect that they will be cared for by individuals who adhere to the ethical standards of their profession, to statutory law, and to accepted medical and scientific practice.

Be a Patient Advocate

The concept of fidelity includes the expectation that patient needs come first. An **advocate** is a person who intercedes on behalf of another person. A medical assistant functions as an advocate for patients by suggesting appropriate community referrals to the physician, by making sure that all insurance claims are complete, by following up to help patients receive insurance coverage if additional information will make that possible, and generally by working to protect patients' rights (see Highlight on Patient's Bill of Rights later in this chapter).

In order to protect patient safety, it may even be necessary for a medical assistant to report unsafe or illegal behavior to proper authorities. The first step is always to follow up within the organization by reporting to the supervisor any incident or situation that could cause potential harm. If no action is taken after a reasonable amount of time, the situation should be documented in writing (as a memory aid) and reported to the next person in the chain of command. If a medical assistant has followed up within the organization without resolution of an unsafe or illegal situation, he or she should report the incident to the appropriate government agency. For example, if unsafe or illegal behavior is being exhibited by a physician or nurse, the medical assistant should report the behavior to the state authority that licenses that individual. These agencies have different names in different states—for example, Board of Registration (Massachusetts), Board of Medical Practice (Minnesota, Delaware, and Vermont), or Board of Medical Examiners (Oregon, Louisiana, New Jersey, Nevada, and others). Any type of report must be based on firsthand evidence. In most states, reports can be made online, and these reports can usually be made anonymously. Information about professionals whose licenses have been revoked or suspended is also available online in many states.

Tell the Truth

The concept of **veracity** has increased in importance since the nineteenth century. Veracity is not found in the Hippocratic Oath. It has developed with the evolution of the scientific tradition. Today it is seen as a proactive duty—physicians and other health care professionals must provide truthful information without having to be asked. It is a tenet of modern science that scientific knowledge belongs to all. Results of experiments must be accurate and reviewed by other scientists to see if the results can be replicated, then published for the benefit of all.

Give Each Person a Fair Share

The concept of justice requires that each individual be given his or her due and implies that he or she deserves a fair share of resources. However, there is often an underlying belief that an individual must contribute or bear a portion of the burden before being allowed to get certain resources. Justice in the context of medical practice appears not only in terms of distribution of medical resources, but also in the belief in the right to compensation if a mistake is made.

Deciding what is "fair" is difficult because different situations may require different guidelines. In the United States, the tendency is to believe in "first come, first served." But in an emergency department, serious conditions must take precedence.

What Would You Do? What Would *Not* Do?

Case Study 1

Denise Fitzgerald is a 16-year-old girl who has come to the office with complaints of a sore throat and fever. While Vicki is taking vital signs, she notices a circular wound on Denise's arm that looks like a cigarette burn. It is red and has some crusted areas. When she asks Denise about it, the patient blushes and says in a low voice that her boyfriend burned her a few days ago to teach her a lesson. Then Denise says, "Please don't tell the doctor because he will tell my mother, and I'm afraid she will make me break up with my boyfriend." ■

Ethical Conflict

Many issues become controversial when there is a disagreement within society about the relative hierarchy of certain rights and duties.

Reproductive Issues

Conflict surrounds the issues of contraception, abortion, and other issues related to reproduction. With regard to pregnancy, some people feel that the duty to follow divine law or natural measures takes precedence over an individual's right to autonomy. This results in differing beliefs about how appropriate it is to use contraception and artificial measures to become pregnant. There has been controversy about the "morning-after pill" (marketed under the name *Plan B*). Because it has been found to be relatively safe, it was approved as an over-the-counter medication for women older than age 18 by the Food and Drug Administration (FDA) in 2006.

Another controversial issue is abortion. Some argue that the fetus's right to life outweighs the woman's right to privacy in determining—with her physician—the proper course of her medical care. Since the original U.S. Supreme Court decision in 1973 upholding a woman's right to obtain an abortion in any state *(Roe v Wade)*, the Court has been called on to rule many times on various state laws that seek to limit this right. The Partial-Birth Abortion Ban Act of 2003, which prohibits a specific abortion procedure that can be done in the second trimester of pregnancy, is an example of a federal law that restricts a woman's right to abortion in some cases. It was upheld in the Supreme Court case of *Gonzales v Carhart* in 2007.

Stem Cell Research

A promising area of research for medical treatment involves the use of embryonic **stem cells.** These cells, taken from fetal tissue, are able to mature into different types of tissue. Embryonic cells may be found to be able to reduce, or possibly even reverse, the symptoms of Parkinson disease and other diseases.

The ethical conflict arises because the cells of live human embryos may be killed during research activities. In addition, a possible source of embryonic cell tissue is from aborted fetuses or fertilized ova not used for in vitro fertilization. Researchers who use fetal tissue stress that they use only tissue from spontaneous abortions (miscarriages). Antiabortion advocates argue that if there is an increased need for fetal tissue, a time may come when women might be influenced in their decision whether or not to have an abortion if they could sell their fetus's tissue for research and/or treatment. In 2001 the federal government introduced a policy that federal funding would be available only for research using the 64 then-existing stem cell lines. This policy was reversed in 2009, and federal funding is now available for additional stem cell lines.

Genetic Engineering and Cloning

A number of ethical issues surround the practices of **genetic engineering** (making, altering, or repairing genetic material) and **cloning** (reproducing genetically identical cells or individuals).

One is the issue of genetically engineered crops and other food products. This encompasses practices as diverse as injecting milk cows with growth hormones in order to get them to produce more milk to incorporating material from bacteria into plant seeds. Opponents argue that we cannot predict all of the possible effects of manipulating genetic material and are likely to see unexpected and unwanted consequences to ourselves or other species.

Gene therapy is a term used for experimental treatments that attempt to treat or cure disease by giving patients new genes or parts of genes that may have been synthesized in the laboratory, taken from human tissue, or engineered from genetic material of animals or other species. Research efforts are overseen by the Recombinant DNA Advisory Committee of the National Institutes of Health (NIH). A clinical study of a gene therapy treatment for arthritis was suspended in July 2007 after the death of a patient.

Human cloning is prohibited by several states, but efforts to pass legislation on the federal level have not succeeded to date. Experiments in animal cloning continue, although critics claim that it results in unhealthy animals and needless suffering. There are serious concerns about safety and health if cloned animals were introduced into the food supply chain.

Refusing or Withholding Treatment and Physician-Assisted Suicide

The right to refuse treatment is well established for adults. The 1990 Patient Self-Determination Act establishes the duty of hospitals, nursing homes, and health maintenance organizations (HMOs) to inform patients or new subscribers of their right to express their wishes related to health care and to refuse treatment. The act also establishes the right of an individual to prepare an advance directive that specifies what treatments he or she would like to receive, and what ones he or she would not wish to receive, if the individual were to become incapable of making those decisions at a later time. Courts have held an individual's right to refuse treatment in such high regard that they have allowed mentally ill patients to refuse treatments for their mental illness.

When an individual requires resuscitation or life support to stay alive, there may come a point where it seems that the treatment is resulting in more suffering (harm) than benefit. This is especially true if it is unlikely that the person can recover his or her health or normal function. If there is a written document expressing the person's wishes, life support may be removed or discontinued. In the absence of an advance directive, an individual's family may bring to court a petition to remove life support. Such a petition must be supported by witnesses other than those who file the petition, stating that the incompetent individual expressed a desire to avoid being kept alive by artificial means. Life support has been interpreted to include ventilators, antibiotics, and even tube feedings.

Physician-assisted suicide and euthanasia (literally, "good death"), sometimes called *mercy killing,* evoke fears that the power to take life will be abused—that it will be used more for the convenience of others than for the well-being of those who are dying. Advocates for the disabled have argued that allowing physician-assisted suicide or euthanasia could be the first step in society's determining that the severely disabled are too much of a financial and physical burden and having them euthanized.

Throughout the 1990s, an individual physician named Jack Kevorkian provided patients with degenerative, terminal illness a machine that provided an injection of lethal drugs. He was sentenced to 10 to 25 years in prison in 1999 and was released after 8 years in 2007 after he promised not to assist in any additional deaths.

In 1997, Oregon became the first state to legalize physician-assisted suicide, allowing physicians to write a prescription for a patient of a lethal dose of pain killer or other medication. The physician is not allowed to administer the medication. The U.S. Supreme Court upheld a challenge to the Oregon law in 2006. The discussion about physician-assisted suicide occurs in every state, but to date similar legislation has failed to pass in any other state.

Terminally ill patients and their families are often looking for a trusted advisor with whom they can discuss their fears and concerns. Even when a physician is not morally willing or legally able to provide a means for a patient to end his or her life, there is increasing recognition of the value of frank discussion and reassurance that patients will not be left to cope alone.

Advance Directives

On the basis of personal beliefs, patients can formalize their decisions about treatment in terminal or end-of-life situations in a number of ways. These include **do-not-resuscitate (DNR) orders,** living wills, health care proxies, and organ donor cards, all of which fall under the heading of "advance directives" (Box 3-1). An advance directive may specify care to be given or avoided and name a person to make medical decisions for the individual should he or she become incompetent. This is usually a spouse, child older than age 18, member of the clergy, or close friend. Medical advance directives should always name a single individual

BOX 3-1 Advance Directives

DO-Not-Resuscitate (DNR) Order

Requested by either patient or health care agent. A written order from the physician in the patient's medical record that allows medical staff to not resuscitate in the event of cardiac or respiratory arrest.

Living Will

Executed by an individual before or during illness. Identifies the patient's wishes about which life-prolonging actions should or should not be taken. In states that accept it, it provides instructions to health professionals about treatment to be provided and may include instructions to a health care agent as to which treatments he or she should authorize. Provisions for organ donation, autopsy, or donation of remains to a medical school are also usually included in a living will.

Health Care Proxy

Executed by an individual before or during illness. Names a health care agent who has the ability to make decisions about care, including signing a DNR order. It may also outline the types of care that the individual does or does not wish to receive. It becomes effective only when the individual becomes incapable of making his or her own decisions.

Durable Power of Attorney

A written authorization to act on the behalf of another, especially in business affairs. An ordinary power of attorney expires when a person becomes incapacitated, but a *durable power of attorney* remains in effect, even if the grantor does become incapacitated. An authorization limited to health care decisions only is called a *durable power of attorney for health care decisions* or a *medical durable power of attorney*.

Organ Donor Card

A card stating that an individual wishes to donate organs. Many states have done away with a separate organ donor card, preferring to place the organ-donor designation on an individual's driver's license.

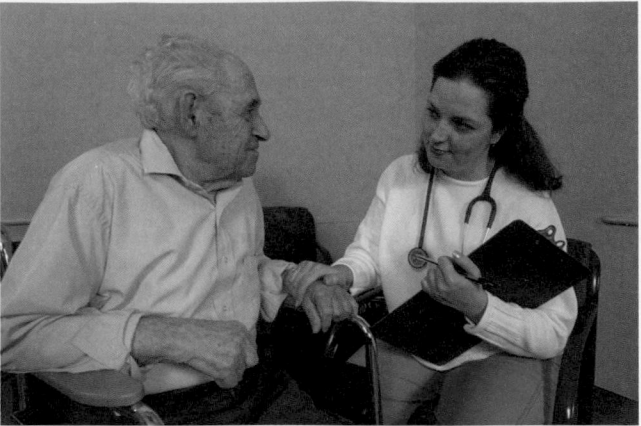

Figure 3-1 Elderly patients are grateful when office staff respond to their fears and concerns.

DNR orders should be in the medical record, and the staff should be informed of the patient's wishes. If the patient is at home, the family must have a copy of the DNR order to show emergency personnel, who otherwise will be legally obligated to resuscitate the patient.

Removal of life support means that no form of support, including mechanical breathing, feeding, or medications to prolong life, should be given. Pain medication and sedation are continued if necessary after removal of life support.

A **living will** is a document executed by an individual that gives medical professionals instructions about how that person wishes to be treated in the event he or she becomes incompetent. A living will may also give instructions regarding organ donation, autopsy, or donation of the remains to a medical school for anatomy dissection. Many states allow an individual's wishes to donate organs to be noted on his or her driver's license or on an organ donor card that can be carried in the wallet. In the event of a fatal auto accident, the police—who usually use the license or other documents to make identification—can notify ambulance personnel that the deceased is an organ donor.

A person usually names an agent to carry out his or her wishes if he or she is unable to do so. A **health care proxy** names the person who is charged with this responsibility and may also give specific instructions to the designated person concerning medical issues. Laws regulating living wills and health care proxies vary from state to state, and it is important for patients to use forms that will be valid where they live. This may require the assistance of an attorney.

Personal and Professional Ethics

It is important to distinguish between personal and professional ethics. In the work situation, professional ethics usually takes precedence over personal beliefs and morals. For example, a medical assistant may believe that a parent who is paying the medical bill should be given the results of laboratory tests done on his or her child. Legally, however, after age 18, information about a patient can be given only with the patient's consent. In this case, professional ethics

to make decisions, with an alternate if possible. This is often a difficult choice, especially for an elderly person with several children (Figure 3-1). In addition, the patient may want to provide for donation of any organs that are useful. Organ donation (or donation of one's entire body) and procedures for determining who may give permission if the patient has not left a directive are outlined in the Uniform Anatomical Gift Act.

Signed originals rather than photocopies of the advance directives should be held by the named surrogate, and the patient should keep copies with his or her important papers. It should also be noted in the primary care physician's records with a copy if possible so that the surrogate can be contacted if necessary.

requires that the medical assistant follow the law, no matter what he or she believes personally, and maintain the patient's confidentiality.

Acting according to professional ethics means that the medical assistant cannot ethically withhold from the physician information given by the patient related to the medical condition. Even if the medical assistant does not agree with how the physician is managing a patient's care, the medical assistant cannot ethically (or legally) suggest another treatment plan for the patient.

It is important to clarify one's personal set of moral values and beliefs and identify areas where there may be potential conflict with professional ethics to avoid having to make a difficult decision on the spot. Using the process outlined in the following section, the medical assisting student should determine his or her own personal beliefs related to issues of potential ethical conflict. Then he or she should decide what professional ethics requires in those situations.

An individual or medical practice can look to a professional organization for guidance related to ethical questions. Medical associations publish guidelines related to medical ethics. Professional associations for medical assistants can be a source of information and guidelines. For problems affecting the medical office, a discussion by all office staff may assist in decision making (Figure 3-2).

Process Used to Make Ethical Decisions

Making ethical decisions involves measures to respond to conflict between different values and their relative importance. In order to decide on a course of action, it is helpful to clarify the conflict and make a thoughtful choice. A six-step process can be used to make these decisions. Actions should be well considered and in accordance with beliefs about what is right and wrong, rather than simply impulse reactions.

Gathering Information

Information that needs to be gathered includes (1) background about the situation; (2) facts related to the specific

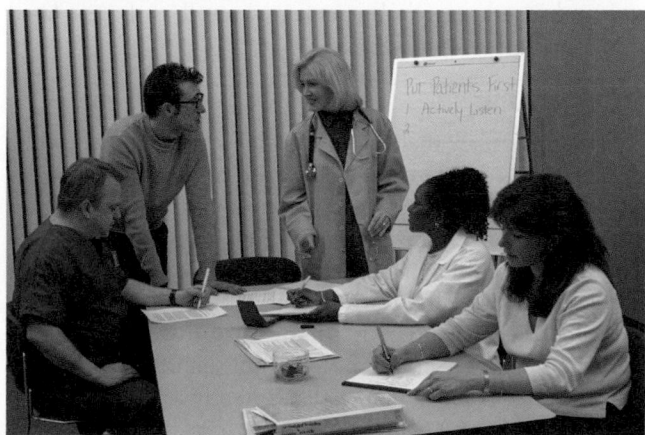

Figure 3-2 A staff meeting may be helpful to discuss problems affecting the medical office.

problem; (3) information about the people involved, such as their knowledge of the situation or their mental capacity; and (4) the laws or institutional policies that relate to the situation.

Identifying Conflicting Values

A conflict does not always involve lofty values. It may be as simple as one person's wish to not cause problems, to save time, or to avoid a hassle. However, this desire may conflict with professional duties or with another individual's right.

If a medical assistant is working in a facility where individual staff members do not always follow established procedures (e.g., do not always run controls for laboratory tests), the desire to go along with co-workers and avoid conflict may be strong; however, the duty to act with fidelity is not being met. The medical assistant may be personally performing the needed controls, but the knowledge that others are not doing so creates a conflict between personal reluctance to violate the autonomy of a co-worker and the professional duty of fidelity to patients.

Determining Relative Importance of Conflicting Claims

To determine the relative importance of conflicting claims, an individual needs to clarify his or her goals and weigh the conflicting values. It is important to remember that when values conflict, an individual or group makes a decision about importance that is valid within its own context but may not conform to the values of other individuals or groups.

For example, in the case of abortion, some people believe that the right of a fetus to life outweighs all other rights. Others believe that a woman's right to autonomy in medical decisions about her body, and the consequences to a child of being unwanted, diminish or outweigh the absolute right to life in the early stages of a pregnancy.

Exploring Alternatives

Once it has been established which values are more important, it is important to consider the possible outcomes of possible actions. It is helpful to identify as many courses of action as possible, predict the consequences of each action, and project how different goals would be met or not met by following each possible course of action.

Choosing and Justifying One Alternative

Conflicting claims require choices. By analyzing hypothetic situations in detail, a person can construct some sort of personal framework for ethical decisions; once on the job, there is often little time to analyze each situation individually.

In the end, there are four ways to justify a decision:
1. By presenting logical arguments—deductions based on facts
2. By social justification—consideration of the larger consequences to society
3. By projection of consequences—imagining what might happen if a given alternative is chosen

4. By refuting alternative claims—stating explicitly why alternative choices have less merit than the one chosen

If it is impossible to select any alternative that seems comfortable, or "right," the choice to do nothing becomes a chosen alternative rather than simply the avoidance of a decision.

Implementing the Decision

The final step in this process is to put the ethical decision into action. This does not have to be a permanent solution. The decision can be reconsidered and another solution can be tried, or the question can be reconsidered at intervals to see if circumstances, beliefs, or knowledge has changed.

INTRODUCTION TO LAW

Difference between Public Law and Private Law

The legal system in the United States is primarily divided into two parts, public law and private law. *Public law* refers to laws that define the relationship between the individual and society as a whole. The term **criminal law** is used to refer to the set of laws that protect society. Examples include laws against robbery, rape, and operating a motor vehicle while under the influence of alcohol or a controlled drug. Private law, also called **civil law,** is the set of laws that deals with disputes between individuals and/or groups of people. This may involve two individuals or groups of people; individuals and corporations, government, or other organizations; or one corporate, government, or organizational entity and another such entity. Contracts are considered a part of civil law, and disputes about contracts that go to court are tried as part of the civil court system.

Lawsuits

Both civil and criminal action disputes can lead to lawsuits that are tried in the court system. In any court proceeding, there is a **plaintiff,** the person or entity that makes the complaint, and a **defendant,** the person or entity against whom a lawsuit is brought. In a criminal lawsuit, the plaintiff is the district or state's attorney, a representative of the government. In a civil lawsuit, the plaintiff is the injured party.

In criminal law the criminal activity itself is held to be harmful or potentially harmful to society or individual members of society. The act itself is punishable, regardless of whether anyone was actually harmed by the act. In civil law, an injury or damage must result because of someone's wrongful act for **liability** (legal responsibility) to arise. The same misdeed can provoke both a criminal charge and a civil lawsuit. The criminal suit will determine if the person is guilty of committing a crime punishable by an imprisonment or fine paid to the government. The civil suit will determine what liability the person has to the injured party, if any.

A well known example of this dual legal picture is the O. J. Simpson case. Simpson was found not guilty by a jury of the murder of his ex-wife, Nicole, and her friend, Ronald Goldman. However, her estate filed a civil suit against him on the grounds of "wrongful death." In the civil case, he was found liable for their deaths, and more than 30 million dollars was awarded in damages. In a criminal case the charge must be proven "beyond a reasonable doubt," but in a civil case the burden of proof is only to a level at which the supporting evidence is more convincing than the opposing evidence ("a preponderance of the evidence").

Specialized Areas of Public Law

Specialized areas of public law include constitutional law, international law, and administrative law. Constitutional law is the study of law of countries and other political organizations. International law concerns the relationships among countries and includes maritime law and regulations applying to ocean-going vessels. Administrative law arises from the actions of federal government agencies, such as the Social Security Administration and the Internal Revenue Service.

Creation of Laws

Law was created by tradition through accepted social practices and decisions of the courts. This type of law is called **common law** or **case law.** Today most laws are created through a vote by a legislative body. The term for this is **statutory law.** Legislators are elected by popular vote to serve either in the state or federal legislature. One of their important duties is to draft new legislation, which is called a **bill** while it is under consideration. Once passed by either the House of Representatives or the Senate, a bill that contains several parts becomes an **act.** Once passed by both houses, the act is signed into law by the President (for a federal law) or a state governor (for law applicable to one state). Cities and towns can also enact laws, called *ordinances;* these usually have to do with local issues, such as smoking in public places, parking, leash laws for pets, and curfews at parks.

All employees of the medical office must be aware of the federal and state laws that regulate the provision of health care and insurance reimbursement, as well as those related to the operation of a business.

Criminal Law

The branch of law that describes offenses against the public welfare is called *criminal law.* A **crime** is an offense in violation of a law that prohibits or requires certain behavior. When a person is convicted of a crime (or pleads guilty to a crime), punishment is imposed. A **felony** is a serious crime, punishable by death or imprisonment in a state or federal penal institution for more than 1 year. A **misdemeanor** is a less serious crime, punishable by a fine or imprisonment for less than 1 year, often in a local or county penal institution. Another term sometimes used to describe a criminal act is **malfeasance**—a wrongdoing that is illegal or contrary to official obligation.

Nonviolent Crimes

Occasionally a physician is charged with manslaughter or criminal negligence if a patient dies or sustains serious injury as a result of incorrect or negligent treatment. This is usually in addition to a civil lawsuit brought by the patient or family for wrongful death (see the discussion of professional malpractice later in this chapter). Euthanasia and assisted suicide (except for physician-assisted suicide in Oregon) are usually considered murder whether performed by a health professional or family member.

Two or more people who have joined together to commit an unlawful act may be accused of conspiracy; this may be applied to actions that are illegal in and of themselves, or actions to prevent detection of a prior crime.

Stealing another person's property (without violence) is called **larceny.** In the medical office, this may take the form of **embezzlement**—appropriating funds from a client, customer, or employer.

A growing problem in the health care industry is **fraud**—deliberate deception carried out to secure unfair or unlawful gain. Billing for services not provided, billing for services provided to imaginary patients, performing unneeded services, and even deliberately using codes from a higher level of service than that provided are all forms of insurance fraud. Every instance of such a billing can be considered a separate act. If the fraud involves the use of mail (mail fraud) or electronic resources (wire fraud), it becomes a federal offense.

In the mind of an office employee, there may be a difference between billing an insurance company using a code for more complex service than was actually provided, "because they pay us so little anyway," and billing for procedures that were never performed. But from a legal perspective, both are considered fraud and, if proved, both carry serious penalties.

Insurance companies and agencies of the federal and state government are victims of billions of dollars in fraudulent claims each year. They have increasing incentives to investigate health care facilities they suspect of fraudulent billing.

Civil Law

The branch of law that regulates interactions among individuals, groups, organizations, and the government is civil law. Disputes arise when one individual or group believes that the actions of another individual or group have caused personal injury or damage to property. In medical offices these usually relate to the actual care received by the patient and/or the relationship between the patient and the physician or office staff. Two types of obligations that may give rise to civil lawsuits are contracts and torts.

Contracts involve agreements between two or more parties and are discussed in detail later. If a contract exists, failure to meet the terms of the contract by either party is called a *breach of contract.* A **tort** is an injury or wrong against a person or property that does not involve breach of contract. If a person knows, or should know, the

---

BOX 3-2 Intentional and Unintentional Torts

Intentional Torts

Abandonment Failure to continue to provide medical care to a patient without proper notification.

Assault Threat to touch another person or his or her property without permission in a way that will cause pain, injury, or damage or is offensive.

Battery Touching of another person or his or her property without permission in a way that will cause pain, injury, or damage or is offensive.

Defamation Making a false claim that may harm a person's reputation, business, or group. If the claim is made verbally, it is called *slander.* If the claim is made in writing, it is called *libel.*

False imprisonment Confining a person without legal authority, such as using restraints without a proper physician order.

Invasion of privacy Public disclosure of private information, such as releasing medical information or photographs without consent of the patient.

Misrepresentation Providing information with knowledge that it is incorrect or reckless disregard for the truth.

Unintentional Torts

Negligence Failure to act with reasonable prudence in a situation. Negligence by a professional is also called *malpractice.*

Strict liability Responsibility for injury, even if there was no negligence. This is often applied when individuals are injured by products or equipment.

---

consequences of his or her action, the wrong is called an *intentional tort.* If the action is a mistake or has unintended consequences, it is called an *unintentional tort.* See Box 3-2 for a list of torts. Keep in mind that intentional torts may also be prosecuted as criminal acts if they are performed with specific intent to cause injury.

Two other terms may be used for acts that can result in civil lawsuits. The term **misfeasance** refers to a legal act performed in an improper way, especially if it causes injury or damage. The term **nonfeasance** means failing to perform an act that should have been performed to prevent injury or damage.

LAW AND PROFESSIONAL LIABILITY

Physician-Patient Relationship

The physician-patient relationship is a contractual relationship. Each party has certain rights and responsibilities under the relationship.

Several elements must be present in order for there to be a contract:

1. There must be a mutual agreement.
2. There must be intent to do (or not do) something that is legal.

3. The action must occur in exchange for service (called *consideration*) or for payment.
4. The parties must be legally able to enter into a contract.

A contract does not have to be written or sometimes even discussed in detail. When clothes are left for dry cleaning, it is assumed that there will be an obligation to pay for the service. The same is true if a patient makes a visit to a medical office. Written contracts are used when there is a considerable amount of money at stake (such as a car loan or mortgage), and in the medical office a patient may be asked to sign a statement confirming that payment will be made for any charges not covered by insurance.

Certain groups of people are not legally able to be a party to contracts, including most medical care contracts. These people are also not able to give informed consent. Such groups include the following:

1. Children younger than the age of 18
2. Mentally ill adults or adults with severe intellectual disabilities
3. Individuals who are temporarily mentally incapacitated (including those who have received narcotic analgesics or other mind-altering medications)
4. Individuals who are under threat or duress (fear of a threat)
5. Individuals who have been found incompetent to handle their affairs

All consent forms should be signed and all implied contracts made with a competent party acting as a willing health care decision maker for the child or incompetent person. In some circumstances, adult rights, including the right to consent to medical treatment, are given to individuals younger than the age of 18. Such an individual is called an **emancipated minor.** In most states, an individual between 14 and 18 years old can obtain a court order from a judge to become free of control of a parent or guardian after proving the ability to be financially independent.

The Physician

Within the physician-patient relationship, the physician provides skillful care to the patient and continues to treat the patient unless he or she informs the patient that the relationship will be terminated. In this case the physician must give the patient time to make other arrangements for care. The physician arranges for someone else to treat the patient if the physician is unavailable (such as on nights, on weekends, and during vacations). The physician informs the patient about treatments or procedures and carries out only those treatments and procedures to which the patient consents. The physician informs the patient of test results, diagnoses, and medical conditions and gives the patient instructions for follow-up care and procedures to follow at home.

A physician has the following rights:
- To accept or decline to treat a patient
- To choose to limit the medical practice to a particular size or certain specialty
- To decide where to practice

Decisions not to treat particular patients must be based on general principles (such as limiting a practice to urology) rather than arbitrary decisions (based on a whim or subjective judgment).

The Patient

The patient agrees to keep appointments, give accurate information about his or her medical condition, provide an accurate medical history, follow directions, and pay for service.

The patient has the following rights:
- To refuse treatment
- To receive complete information about procedures
- To select a physician
- To expect continuity of care
- To expect confidentiality of verbal and written communication with the physician and the physician's agents
- To be treated with respect and dignity
- To receive complete information about the treatment suggested, alternatives, and possible consequences of alternatives or no treatment

Patients' rights may be legally defined by the state or an institution. The *Patient's Bill of Rights* is a name that is often used to refer to the Consumer Bill of Rights and Responsibilities, which was adopted by the Presidential Advisory Commission on Consumer Protection and Quality in the Health Care Industry in 1998 (see Highlight on the Patient's Bill of Rights). This document was created to improve consumer trust in the health care system by defining the rights and responsibilities of consumers, health care professionals, health care institutions, and insurance plans. The Bipartisan Patient Protection Act (also known as the *McCain-Edwards-Kennedy Patients' Bill of Rights*) was an attempt to enact the findings of this commission into federal law. It failed in the U.S. House of Representatives in 2002. In the next decade, most individual states did pass legislation defining what was commonly called a "patient's bill of rights," although the focus varies from state to state. Some concentrate primarily on rights of patients in residential facilities, whereas others have a broader scope. The federal Patient Protection and Affordable Care Act, which became law in March 2010, has shifted focus somewhat from merely defining patients' rights to ensuring that all Americans will have access to affordable, high-quality health care and preventative care.

Terminating the Physician-Patient Relationship

To end a relationship with a patient, a physician must notify the patient in writing. It is recommended that such a letter be sent using certified mail with return receipt requested. The letter needs to be dated, must state the reasons for termination of care, and should describe how medical records will be made available. Copies of any correspondence regarding termination and receipts should be kept in the medical record. If the patient notifies the physician by telephone that he or she wishes to terminate the

Highlight on the Patient's Bill of Rights

Eight areas of consumer rights and responsibilities were emphasized in the Consumer Bill of Rights and Responsibilities that was adopted by the President's Advisory Commission on Consumer Protection and Quality in the Health Care Industry in 1998.

1. Consumers have the right to receive accurate, easy-to-understand information about their health plans, professionals, and facilities. Some patients require assistance to make informed health care decisions and should receive that assistance.
2. Consumers have the right to enough choices about health care providers (including individuals and institutions) to be sure that they have access to appropriate high-quality health care.
3. Consumers have the right to access emergency health care services when and where they need them without having to obtain prior authorization or risk financial penalty.
4. Consumers should receive easy-to-understand information so that they can fully participate in all decisions related to

their health care. If they cannot make their own decisions, they have a right to be represented by parents, guardians, family members, or others.
5. Consumers always have a right to respectful care from all health care providers and health care institutions.
6. Consumers always have a right to have the confidentiality of their individually identifiable health care information protected. In addition, they have a right to review and copy their medical records and request corrections to their medical information.
7. Consumers have a right to an appeal system that allows for resolution of differences with their health plans, health providers, and health care institutions. Systems should be in place for internal and external review.
8. Consumers should take responsibility for greater involvement in their care in order to achieve the best outcomes and support a quality improvement, cost-conscious environment. ∎

relationship, the physician should send a similar letter as documentation.

Common reasons for a physician terminating care of a patient include the following:

- The physician moves.
- The physician retires.
- The physician dies.
- The physician closes the practice for other reasons.
- The patient regularly and continually breaks appointments.
- The patient regularly and continually refuses to follow medical advice.

If a patient can convince a court that he or she was under the belief that a physician-patient relationship still existed and because of such belief did not seek out another practitioner, and sustained injury, a successful case can be made for **abandonment.** This is rare and should never happen if the physician keeps good written records about any termination notification.

Personal and Professional Liability

A person is responsible for his or her actions and may be held liable if those actions injure another person. In daily life we are required to act as a reasonable person would act in the same circumstances. The failure to act—or refrain from acting—as a reasonable person would act in similar circumstances is called **negligence.**

A common example of negligence relates to a wet floor. If someone washes the floor or spills water on the floor and does not wipe it up, the floor becomes slippery. When an unsuspecting person comes along and is not aware that the floor is wet, that person could slip and be injured. The person responsible for making the floor wet would be

expected to know that the wet floor would be slippery and could cause someone to fall. A person who notices the spill would also be expected to know that the wet floor could cause a fall.

If a person falls, is injured, and files a lawsuit, the person who washed the floor, or another person with responsibility for public safety who noticed the spill, could be found to be negligent and be responsible (liable) to pay for the injured person's medical care, lost wages, and any other costs caused by the fall on the wet floor.

Standard of Care

A person without any special training is held only to the standard of a "reasonably prudent person." The term **prudent** means careful or using common sense. For instance, any reasonably prudent person is expected to realize that an infant or unconscious person will not be able to remove a heating pad that is too hot. If an infant or unconscious person is burned by a heating pad, the person who placed it will be considered liable and will be responsible for medical bills as well as compensation for pain and suffering.

A medical assistant is generally held to a professional standard, especially when performing procedures that are often done by a licensed health professional. The medical assistant must be especially careful to avoid offering advice or making decisions that may be interpreted as diagnosing illness or prescribing treatment.

If the medical assistant administers medication, he or she must do so correctly and must follow proper procedures and precautions to protect the patient from injury. A physician must be on the premises (not necessarily in the room) any time medication is given by a medical assistant, because in most states the medical assistant can perform the procedure only under the authority and supervision of a physician. It is important for medical assistants to find out what they are legally allowed to do in the state where they work.

In emergency situations, when no qualified professional is available, health care practitioners are expected to give care for which they have been trained but at which they may not be proficient. For instance, any physician would be expected to initiate emergency care for a patient who suddenly goes into cardiac arrest, even a specialist such as an ophthalmologist. Patients make an assumption that in a medical office they will receive medical treatment, even in the event of an emergency. All medical office personnel are expected to be able to give advice in an emergency or to activate the local emergency medical system if they cannot handle the situation.

Many, if not most, medical offices train all of their personnel in cardiopulmonary resuscitation (CPR) and first aid. If a medical assistant, secretary, or receptionist tells any patient that a problem is not serious, and it is, then he or she may be liable if there is injury to the patient caused by delay of treatment. Failure to respond correctly to an emergency can be considered a "breach of contract" because there is an implied contract between a patient and a medical office that any emergency will be handled by competent staff.

Health professionals are generally held to a high standard of care. For physicians and other health professionals, the term **standard of care** defines the level of appropriate care legally required of any other practitioner with the same education and training providing the same care in the same geographic region. In general, if a legal question arises, a medical assistant will be held to the standard of care of the professional who would normally perform the care in question.

For example, if a family practice physician prescribes blood pressure medication, he or she has to do it as competently as another family practice physician in the same area. If a nurse practitioner prescribes blood pressure medication, he or she has to meet the same standard as the family

practice physician. If a patient sustains injury from taking the medication, in either case, the court would look at the appropriateness of the medication for the particular patient, the dose, and the follow-up to see whether either practitioner has acted at an acceptable level.

Informed Consent

Consent can be implied by a patient's actions. If a medical assistant says, "Would you please roll up your sleeve so that I can give you an injection?" and the patient does so, the patient has given implied consent to the medical assistant to administer the injection. Even though the patient has not verbally agreed, the act of preparing for the injection suggests that the patient is willing to undergo the procedure.

Expressed consent can be verbal or written. We know, however, that simply expressing consent does not always represent understanding. Patients today have the legal right to completely understand what will be done to them or for them. For this reason, many medical offices now use written consent forms to obtain informed consent.

Written consent forms are now always used for surgery, for procedures involving entry into a sterile body cavity, for procedures that carry a risk to the patient's health, and for testing for human immunodeficiency virus (HIV), the virus that causes acquired immunodeficiency syndrome (AIDS). Written consent forms are increasingly being used as well for immunizations; treatment with birth control pills; transfusions of blood or blood products, such as plasma; and other treatments and procedures.

Legally, it is not the form, but the understanding by the person on whom the treatment or procedure will be performed, that truly represents consent. It is the responsibility of the person performing the procedure, prescribing the medication, or performing the test or examination to inform the patient about the potential risks of the action, the discomfort it may cause, the common side effects, the importance of the procedure, and the probable results if the test or procedure is not done (Figure 3-3).

Often the medical assistant is asked to obtain the signature on the consent form and witness that signature. If the

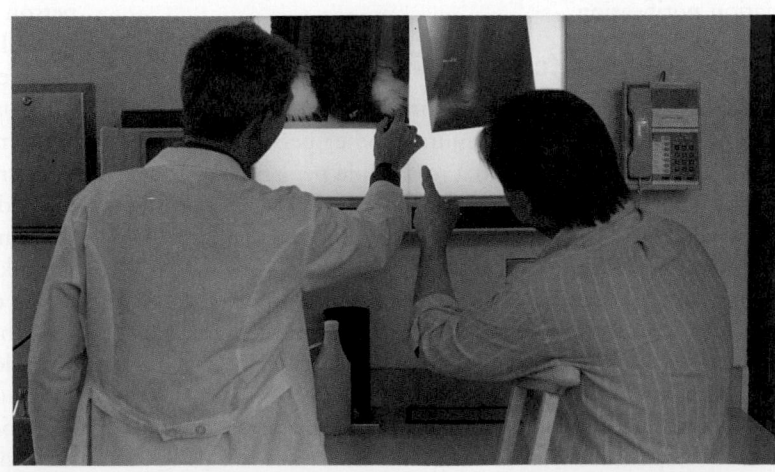

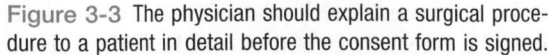
Figure 3-3 The physician should explain a surgical procedure to a patient in detail before the consent form is signed.

medical assistant believes that the patient does not fully understand what he or she is consenting to, the matter should be referred back to the physician. This is a good example of the medical assistant acting as a liaison between the patient and the physician and being an advocate for the patient.

Depending on state law, there may be special consent forms for the release of information about HIV test results and/or treatment, drug and alcohol rehabilitation, services for mental health, or other health-related information.

A patient can rescind (withdraw) the authorization to release information at any time by notifying the medical office in writing.

What Would You Do? What Would You *Not* Do?

Case Study 2

Howard Morton is a 72-year-old patient who has come to the office for an office visit for severe back pain. After examining him, the physician referred him to an orthopedic surgeon for evaluation. While Vicki is preparing the referral form for Mr. Morton, he says, "If I see an orthopedic surgeon, he is probably going to want to do surgery. Do you think surgery is the best treatment for my kind of problem? What else could I try? Should I see a chiropractor? Or do you think acupuncture might help?" ■

Professional Negligence

Professional negligence is often called **malpractice.** To avoid lawsuits for malpractice, a health professional must be sure that he or she is acting within the limits of his or her profession and must act (or refrain from acting) in a given situation as a reasonable and prudent person of the same profession would. When the medical assistant performs procedures that are usually performed by other professionals, such as nurses, the medical assistant will be held to the same standard as the professional who usually performs the procedure. No one always does everything perfectly, and both negligence and malpractice are assumed to be mistakes and unintentional.

Requirements to Prove Professional Negligence

To prove that a professional is guilty of professional negligence and liable for the outcome, four things must be proved by a preponderance of the evidence. This means that they are more likely than not. Sometimes these things are called the *4 Ds of malpractice:*

1. The person who caused the injury has a *duty* to the person who was injured.
2. The person was *derelict* (neglectful) in performing that duty.
3. The failure to perform the duty was the *direct cause* of the injury and nothing could have intervened.
4. The failure to perform the duty caused *damage* or injury.

In some instances the plaintiff has no direct knowledge of the incident (e.g., if the plaintiff is under general anesthesia). In such a case a lawsuit may be allowed under the doctrine of *res ipsa loquitur,* whereby the court assumes that negligence must have occurred because of the type of injury. An example would be if the gallbladder was removed when the patient was scheduled for a hysterectomy.

A physician who gives casual medical advice at a party may not consider the person a patient he or she has a duty to take care of. But if the person fails to seek medical treatment on the basis of the physician's casual words, a court may have to decide if the physician owed a duty to the person.

If a professional does exactly what any other professional would have done and the patient has a poor outcome, the physician is not necessarily negligent. For example, even with the best sterile technique it is possible to get a wound infection. A person with a wound infection must show that proper technique was not used. If the injured person does not follow directions to keep the wound dry and the wound gets infected, the infection might have occurred because the patient did not follow directions.

If someone makes a mistake but there is no injury, the person who makes the mistake will not be liable and will not have to pay any damages. Many mistakes can be corrected if they are reported promptly.

Professional Liability Insurance

To protect against financial loss if the patient sues, physicians usually have professional liability insurance (also called *malpractice insurance*). This is for two reasons. One is to protect physicians for their own negligent actions. The second is to protect physicians if they are sued for the negligent actions of their employees while on the job.

If an injury occurs, the law allows the injured person to sue both the person responsible for causing the injury *and that person's employer,* provided that the incident occurred at work. This occurs under what is known as the doctrine of **respondeat superior.** The English translation of this Latin term is literally "let the master answer," meaning let the person at the head of the organization answer for the injuries caused by his or her employees.

This legal doctrine provides an incentive for employers to be sure that their employees are careful and gives the injured person a better chance of collecting damages for any injury. Even if the employee does not have insurance to cover such an incident or enough money to pay the amount received in judgment, the employer ought to have liability insurance. As the number of lawsuits for outpatient care increases, it is recommended that medical assistants carry their own malpractice insurance.

Laws that protect health professionals from being sued for giving emergency care at the scene of an accident are called *Good Samaritan Acts.* They vary from state to state and may cover physicians, nurses, emergency medical technicians, anyone certified to perform CPR, and other professionals.

Malpractice Litigation

Litigation (the process of taking a lawsuit or criminal case through the courts) is complex. Having a general understanding of the process is important, even though less than 5% of all lawsuits brought against medical professionals or medical institutions ever reach the stage of going to trial.

Initiating a Lawsuit

A person who believes he or she has received inappropriate medical care consults an attorney, who obtains information from the patient and usually tries to obtain copies of the relevant medical records. A letter containing a patient's authorization to send a copy of medical records to a lawyer may be the first indication to the medical office that the patient is actively contemplating a lawsuit.

After receiving written authorization from the patient, the medical office provides a copy of the record to a lawyer. Under the Health Insurance Portability and Accountability Act of 1996 (HIPAA), health care facilities, including physicians' offices, are allowed to charge a reasonable copying fee for records sent to an attorney or requested by a patient.

At the time a lawsuit is actually filed, the patient signs a document releasing the physician from the requirements of patient confidentiality. This is necessary because information about the patient's medical record becomes part of the public record in the litigation process.

When he or she obtains the patient's medical records, the attorney has them reviewed by physicians or other health professionals uninvolved in the patient's treatment to determine if a case can clearly be made for malpractice. Appropriateness of care is clearly the major issue in a suit for malpractice. However, incomplete, illegible, or altered records decrease the medical record's credibility, even if the care actually given was appropriate.

Most malpractice suits are accepted by attorneys on a **contingency** basis. In such a case the individual filing the lawsuit pays for the attorney's time and effort only if he or she collects an award from the party being sued. This is usually a percentage of the settlement or judgment amount. Contingency payments to the attorney are usually from 20% to 40% of the amount collected.

Response to a Possible Lawsuit

The first thing a physician should do on receiving a request for patient records by an attorney or on being served with notice of a lawsuit is to inform the company that provides his or her professional liability insurance. If a suit is filed, the malpractice insurance provider will appoint an attorney to represent the physician as a policyholder. The physician may also wish to hire an independent attorney because the physician's interests are not always the same as the malpractice insurance carrier's. If other staff members are named in the lawsuit, it may be in their best interest to hire their own attorneys as well.

As the legal process continues, the attorneys usually negotiate a settlement in order to avoid the time and expense of going to court, as well as the possibility of a large damage award. Because juries are unpredictable, the attorneys appointed by the insurance provider will hesitate to risk a jury trial, even if there does not appear to be any negligence in the care provided to the plaintiff. If there is a lawsuit, the court may issue a **subpoena,** a court order that requires an individual to be present to testify during some part of the trial process. In order to require that the original medical record is present, the court will issue a **subpoena** *duces tecum,* a court order requiring that documents (or other material evidence) be made available. An employee of the health care facility should bring the original medical record to court each day that it is required and be present wherever the medical record is at all times.

Alternative Dispute Resolution

Instead of a trial, both parties may agree to have their dispute decided by a neutral third party. This process can reduce time, expense, and publicity of a dispute. Such a process may take the form of mediation or arbitration.

Mediation uses a facilitator to help two parties in conflict settle their differences. This can be done in different ways, and if no settlement is reached, either party may find recourse in the court system.

Arbitration is a process whereby a neutral party settles the dispute. The arbitration can be either binding or nonbinding.

In nonbinding arbitration, the parties do not have to accept the decision and one party can proceed with a court case. In binding arbitration, the parties agree at the beginning to be bound by the decision of the arbitrator(s).

Various organizations provide lists of arbitrators, and depending on the circumstances and applicable state law, the parties in arbitration either select a mutually acceptable arbitrator or are assigned one from a list prepared during the arbitration process.

Arbitration is not common in malpractice cases; it is far more common in commercial contract and labor contract disputes.

Tort Defenses

Privilege

Privilege is a special right or permission granted to a certain group of individuals. For example, a health care facility's policy and procedure manual may give physicians the power to order soft restraints or leather restraints for a patient in certain circumstances. With such an order, other health professionals may legally apply the restraints. A patient who is placed in restraints according to established procedures could not make a case for false imprisonment, an intentional tort.

Consent

Consent has been already discussed in detail. A patient may be asked to sign a consent form allowing photographs to be taken and published in a medical journal or textbook, or used as a slide in a lecture (without personal identifying information) for the purpose of providing education. If informed consent was obtained, especially if it is in writing, the patient cannot make a case for invasion of privacy.

Self-Defense or the Defense of Others

Self-defense or the defense of others is another defense against intentional tort. When physical contact occurs, a person accused of assault and/or battery may assert that he or she was defending against contact initiated by another person.

Expiration of the Statute of Limitations

Several defenses can be used against a charge of negligence or malpractice. The **statute of limitations** is the law that limits the time period during which a person can sue. The period varies from 1 to 3 years, depending on the laws of the particular state and whether the suit is for negligence or malpractice (negligence usually has a shorter statute of limitations than malpractice).

Although state law can vary slightly, the statute of limitations usually begins at one of three points:

1. When the injury occurs
2. When the individual first realizes that an injury has occurred; for instance, if a hemostat is left in the body during surgery, the statute of limitations begins to run when the instrument is discovered by a radiograph taken at a later date for another reason
3. When a minor reaches the age of majority or some other specific age (such as 21)

Contributory or Comparative Negligence

If the injured person has played a part in causing the injury, some states regard this as a complete defense (**contributory negligence**). Other states determine **comparative negligence**—how much of the negligence was caused by the professional and how much was caused by the injured individual. Judges and juries are asked to assess damages to the injured party depending on the percentage of the injury caused by the health care professional.

For example, after minor surgery a patient developed a wound infection that required additional surgery and resulted in an unsightly scar. The physician's attorney brought out that the patient had failed to seek medical attention for several days after noting swelling, drainage from the wound, and a fever of 102° F. Prompt medical attention, the attorney argued, would have prevented the second surgery and minimized scarring.

In a state using contributory negligence, establishing that the patient contributed to the injury would be a complete defense and the patient would not collect any damages. In a state using comparative negligence, the judge or jury would determine a percentage for the amount of negligence on the part of the physician and award the patient that percentage of the total damages established by the court.

Assumption of Risk

A patient who does not follow medical advice becomes responsible for any problems that occur as a result of his or her decision. This is called **assumption of risk.** This is easier to establish if the patient has signed a waiver, such as a form acknowledging that a patient is leaving the hospital against medical advice. In the medical office, there is usually no form for the patient to sign, so a complete note should be written in the patient's medical record if he or she refuses to follow medical advice. This note should include the patient's exact words if possible, and the name of any staff or family member who was present during the discussion. If a patient frequently misses appointments, it is also an example of disregarding medical advice. By documenting all missed appointments, the medical assistant can provide evidence that the patient, not the physician, is responsible for any problem that may arise.

What Would You Do? What Would You *Not* Do?

Case Study 3

While walking down the hall to call the next patient, Vicki notices a large wet area on the linoleum floor of the hall. She gets several dry paper towels and goes to clean up the spill. Just as she bends over to wipe up the water, the physician comes out of examination room 4. He looks at the open door of his other examination room, and noticing that it is empty, he says, "Where's my next patient? And can you take an ECG on the patient in room 4 right away?" ∎

FEDERAL AND STATE LAWS AFFECTING THE MEDICAL OFFICE

Controlled Substances and Prescriptions

Controlled Substances

The **Drug Enforcement Administration (DEA)** enforces the Controlled Substances Act of 1970. A **controlled substance** is a drug that has a potential for addiction and/or abuse. Physicians who prescribe controlled substances must register with the DEA and renew their registration every year, but the physician's DEA number should not be preprinted on prescription forms. The DEA updates the five schedules of controlled substances annually. Schedule I controlled substances have the highest potential for abuse and currently have no accepted medical use in the United States, whereas Schedule V controlled substances have the lowest potential for abuse. The specific medications are discussed in more detail in Chapter 26.

Federal law requires that controlled substances be stored away from other medications, in a sturdy, locked cabinet. It is recommended to use a double-locked box or drawer—a box or drawer with an outer lock or key and an inner compartment that also has a lock or key. A physician may not legally obtain Schedule I controlled substances unless participating in an authorized experiment. Schedule II controlled substances are ordered from a manufacturer or a distributor using federal triplicate order form DEA Form 222. Schedule III through V controlled substances do not require the special triplicate form; however, they do require that invoices and packing slips be kept for 2 years.

If controlled substances are kept in a medical office, an inventory sheet must be maintained. The controlled substance stock should be counted daily and verified by a second person. The two people must sign the inventory sheet. Every 2 years, a record of daily inventory of controlled substances must be submitted to the DEA. If controlled substances need to be wasted or destroyed, two witnesses must sign the inventory sheet. If any controlled substances are stolen, local police must be alerted immediately.

Prescribing, dispensing, and/or administering controlled substances also requires documentation. States vary on what paperwork is necessary; some require a special narcotic prescription form for Schedule II prescriptions. Any physician copies of controlled substance prescription forms should be kept in a secure, fireproof safe or other storage. If controlled substances are administered or dispensed only rarely, records can be kept in the patients' records and made available to DEA investigation.

A medical assistant must know the legal requirements regarding controlled substances that have been set by the DEA and the state in which he or she works. A medical assistant will often be responsible for flagging the physician's DEA registration renewal date, as well as for providing security and inventory record keeping for all controlled substances. A medical assistant may also be responsible for properly disposing of expired controlled substances and keeping records. In some states medical assistants are not permitted to administer controlled substances, although they are allowed to administer other medications.

Prescriptions

Federal law also identifies drugs that require a prescription. A **prescription** is an order from a physician or other licensed health care provider to a pharmacist to dispense a supply of medication. Individual states have different regulations within a set of federal guidelines. The medical assistant must know the laws of the state in which he or she works.

In order to prevent theft or alteration of prescriptions, it is recommended that physicians adhere to the following recommendations:

1. Store all prescription blanks in a safe place where they cannot be stolen, and keep the number of prescription pads in use to a minimum.
2. Write out the actual amount prescribed in words in addition to the number. This makes it more difficult to alter the amount.
3. Use prescription blanks only for writing prescriptions and not for notes.
4. Do not sign prescription blanks in advance.
5. Use tamper-resistant prescription pads.

The physician may also write on the prescription whether a generic substitute may be provided. Different states have different laws regarding substitution of a generic preparation for a brand-name drug.

Federal and State Laws Protecting Employees

Hiring and Firing

A person who works for an organization that has more than 15 employees is protected by federal Equal Opportunity Employment laws (Title VII of the Civil Rights Act of 1964) and the federal Age Discrimination in Employment Act of 1967. These laws make it illegal for a company to discriminate in hiring practices on the basis of race, sex, religion, national origin, or age. Some states also have legislation making it illegal to discriminate on the basis of sexual orientation. Complaints about discrimination in hiring are submitted to the federal Equal Employment Opportunity Commission (EEOC).

Employment policies must treat employees equally and cannot discriminate against any category of employees by paying one group (such as men) more than another group for the same duties.

Preemployment Testing

Preemployment testing is allowed only to determine if the potential employee has the skills and abilities to perform a specific job. If keyboarding is included in the job description, the employer may administer a keyboarding test to test a candidate's qualifications for the position. This also applies to any testing done before an individual with a disability is hired.

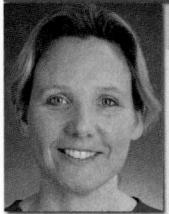

Memories *from* Externship

Vicki Edmonds: When I was at my externship at a clinic affiliated with a community hospital, the employees were implementing a plan for the physicians to discuss advance directives with all patients. They hoped to have each patient prepare a written health care proxy and provide the office with a copy. When we pulled each patient's medical record for the visit, we checked the record to see if there was already a complete form. If not, we placed a blank health care proxy form loosely in the front of the folder for the physician to give to the patient. Then when patients checked out, we would remind them to return the completed form. At first I found this embarrassing because it seemed like such a private thing. Then one of our elderly patients told me that she was so grateful that her husband had signed a health care proxy before he had a stroke, which left him completely paralyzed and unable to speak. She said that the discussions they had had when he was preparing the form had helped her understand exactly what his wishes were. On the basis of those discussions, she had asked the hospital staff not to resuscitate him if he stopped breathing or his heart stopped. She told me that before they talked about it, she would not have been comfortable making that decision. I was impressed by this patient's ability to talk frankly about her family's preparations to face serious illness, and I was grateful because it helped me become more comfortable with the subject. ■

The Americans with Disabilities Act (ADA) discusses the need for employers to make "reasonable accommodations" for any individual with a physical or mental disability who is otherwise qualified to perform the tasks necessary in the job. The law also deals with the necessity of making public accommodations accessible to disabled individuals. The EEOC also hears complaints about possible failure to comply with the workplace portions of the ADA.

Preemployment drug tests have been ruled legal for any position. However, random drug tests while on the job are usually legal only if the demands of public safety outweigh the employee's right to privacy. Some health care facilities perform drug tests on all new employees.

Occupational Safety and Health Act of 1970

The Occupational Safety and Health Administration (OSHA) was created in 1970 to be the federal agency responsible for the physical protection of employees in the workplace. OSHA regulates all workplace environments but has two specific functions related to the medical office. The Bloodborne Pathogens Standard relates to preventing exposure to pathogens that cause disease. This standard is discussed in detail in Chapter 17. OSHA also regulates the exposure of employees to hazardous chemicals in the workplace and requires employers to inform employees of the hazards of any chemicals used. See Chapter 18 for a discussion of the Hazard Communication Standard. The 1988 Clinical Laboratory Improvement Amendments, which regulate office laboratories, are discussed in detail in Chapter 29.

Family and Medical Leave Act

The Family and Medical Leave Act of 1993 (FMLA) applies to employers with 50 or more employees. Under FMLA, employees are entitled to up to 12 weeks of unpaid leave to accommodate a serious health crisis of any family member or the birth or adoption of a child. The employee must notify the employer before the beginning of the leave how much of the leave he or she intends to take. After the employee returns, he or she must be given former job and seniority status.

Sexual Harassment

Sexual harassment is defined as any unwanted physical or verbal sexual attention from anyone an individual interacts with on the job that causes that individual to fear reprisal if the attention is refused. Sexual harassment is not flirting. Flirting occurs when both parties engage in actions or verbal exchanges intended to attract or compliment the other. Harassment occurs when one party (most often a man) engages another party (most often a woman) in unwanted comments or physical contact of a sexual nature. If a comment or attention is unwanted, it should be clearly stated to the offending party. Sometimes individuals hesitate to "hurt the other person's feelings" or are uncomfortable speaking out, and communication is unclear.

Minimum Wage and Overtime

The federal Fair Labor Standards Act regulates the minimum wage, although some states have a higher minimum wage than that set under federal law. The Fair Labor Standards Act also requires overtime pay of one-and-one-half the employee's regular rate of pay for time worked beyond 40 hours in 1 week. Professional and supervisory employees are exempt from the law. Registered nurses and office managers are considered professional employees, but medical assistants are not and are covered by the overtime rules.

Employee Retirement Income Security Act

The Employee Retirement Income Security Act of 1974 (ERISA) regulates employee benefit plans, including managed care health plans, pension plans, and other employee benefits. ERISA sets minimum standards for pension plans to prevent unfair denial of pension rights. Under ERISA, employee health plans cannot use health status or medical condition to deny certain employees the right to insurance.

Health Insurance Portability and Accountability Act of 1996

HIPAA provides legislation related to several aspects of health insurance, privacy of patient information, and standards for filing health insurance claims electronically. This act has several sections.

Health Insurance Availability and Coverage

The first part deals with health insurance availability and coverage. It provides specific regulations for group health insurance plans to prevent eligibility rules that exclude patients with certain diagnoses or genetic conditions or require them to pay higher premiums. It also regulates the length of time that group health plans can refuse to pay for preexisting conditions, especially if the new subscriber had other health insurance before enrolling in the group insurance plan.

Privacy Rule

The HIPAA Privacy Rule (one part of the law) went into effect in 2003. This rule provides patients with control over the use and disclosure of their health information. The Privacy Rule contains provisions that describe how personal health information may be used, stored, maintained, or transmitted electronically. In addition, it describes how patients must be informed of their right to control their health information.

1. The medical office must inform patients in writing how their protected health information (PHI) will be used by the medical office. This document is called a *Notice of Privacy Practices* (NPP). Protected health information includes written, oral, and electronic health information that contains data through which the patient can be identified, such as the Social Security number, name, and telephone number. Patients

must sign a document indicating that they have received a notice regarding privacy protection.

2. A patient's written consent is not required for the use of or disclosure of PHI if the purpose of disclosure is medical treatment, payment, or health care operations. Therefore individuals who are involved in caring for the patient (including medical assistants and medical assisting students) may have access to PHI.

3. Patients have the right to access their medical records and to request changes to the records if they believe they are inaccurate.

4. The medical office must have procedures in place to prevent unnecessary or inappropriate access to PHI, including request forms for information; procedures to prevent unauthorized individuals from viewing records, appointment books, computer screens, or other material that might contain PHI; and procedures for storing and destroying records containing PHI so that no unauthorized access occurs.

5. Patients have a right to request an accounting of the transfer of their information for purposes other than treatment, payment, or health care operations.

6. The medical office must have written agreements with each outside agency that handles PHI, such as medical laboratories, transcription services, law and accounting firms, software and hardware consultants, and billing services, to ensure that these other agencies handle PHI in accordance with the HIPAA Privacy Rule.

7. All employees must be trained in privacy and security of PHI.

Transaction and Code Set Rule

The Transaction and Code Set Rule prescribes electronic data interchange standards for structuring information that must be used for Medicare and Medicaid insurance claims. As of July 1, 2005, almost all providers that file Medicare claims electronically must adhere to these electronic data interchange standards.

Security Rule

The Security Rule complements the Privacy Rule by setting standards to maintain security of personal health information that is transmitted electronically. It identifies administrative, physical, and technical security safeguards for electronic protected health information (EPHI). The final compliance date was April 21, 2006.

Other Provisions

The Unique Identifiers Rule established a new provider identification number called the *National Provider Identifier* (NPI), a 10-digit identification number issued to each provider by the Centers for Medicare and Medicaid Services (CMS). The NPI replaces other physician insurance identification numbers but not the DEA number or state physician license number.

The final part of HIPAA is the Enforcement Rule, which describes penalties for violating HIPAA rules.

Health Information Technology for Economic and Clinical Health Act

The Health Information Technology for Economic and Clinical Health (HITECH) Act, part of the American Recovery and Reinvestment Act of 2009, includes incentives to encourage adoption of electronic medical records by physicians and health care facilities and to create a national health care infrastructure. This act also includes a 1% reduction in the Medicare fee schedule if an electronic medical record has not been adopted by 2015.

In order to continue to protect the individual's right to privacy in the face of increased sharing of health care data, this act also increases the security provisions of HIPAA and adds increased financial penalties for privacy violations. It requires notification of patients for unauthorized use and unencrypted disclosure of PHI; breaches involving more than 500 patients must be reported to federal agencies and sometimes local media. Privacy requirements are imposed directly on business associates, whereas formerly, health care providers were required to have contracts with business associates. Business associates also become liable for financial penalties for privacy violation.

Mandatory Reporting

For public health reasons and the good of society as a whole, physicians are required to make certain reports, usually to a state or local agency. Some are required by law and cannot be refused because the patient does not want the information released.

1. Records of births, stillbirths, and deaths.

2. Reports must be made to the medical examiner or coroner (the name depends on the state) for certain types of deaths that may indicate suspicious circumstances or may be a result of a crime. The medical examiner then decides whether to investigate.

3. Infectious disease cases have to be reported to the local board of health. Each state has a list of reportable diseases, which include diseases that pose a public health risk, such as rabies, measles, and AIDS. Dog bites and human bites must usually also be reported.

4. Injuries that may have occurred as a result of violence must be reported to the police. Sometimes a patient asks that the report not be made. Even if the injured person does not intend to press charges, the injury still must be reported. If there is a likely need for evidence to be collected from the injured person (e.g., in the case of a rape), the person should be directed to an emergency department, which has personnel trained in the procedure.

5. Possible abuse or neglect must be reported to the police or a particular state agency, depending on state law. Suspicion does not have to be backed up with evidence. Certain professions are mandated (legally required) to report, especially child abuse or elder

abuse. Physicians and nurses are always required to make such reports, and in some states medical assistants, as allied health care professionals, are also included in the list of those required to make reports.

6. Various other reports are mandated by the states. Some states require reports of seizures (a symptom of epilepsy) to the department of motor vehicles, and some states require that all cancer cases treated by health professionals be reported to a state cancer registry.

Failure to make a mandated report is a crime. When a report is required by law, the patient should be informed why the report is required and to whom the report will be made.

State Regulation of Health Occupations

The laws that regulate the practice of medicine are called *medical practice acts,* and they generally contain the following two elements:

- Definition of the practice of medicine.
- Limitation to qualified practitioners by **licensure**—the process by which the state examines a person's qualifications and issues a **license** to practice medicine. All states require a license to practice medicine, although a physician may practice in certain federal facilities and agencies with a license from a different state than the one in which the facility is located. Practicing medicine without a license is a criminal act.

Physicians can also be licensed in most states if they have held a medical license in another state for more than 5 to 10 years. This is called **reciprocity** or *reciprocal licensing.* Usually this is simply a matter of requesting a license if a physician is moving from one state to another. In states with many physicians, reciprocal licensing is more difficult to obtain. Florida severely limits reciprocal licensing in an effort to keep older physicians from "retiring" to Florida and then opening practices or taking hospital or clinic jobs.

The physician licensing board approves the original application for a license then renews the license yearly or biannually (every 2 years).

Revoking or Suspending a Physician's License

A physician licensing board can revoke or suspend a physician's license for conviction of a crime, unprofessional activity, and physical or mental incapacity, including alcoholism, drug abuse, and senility. If the physician is convicted of a crime, the seriousness and nature of the crime will influence the physician licensing board's decision about the length of time a person's license may be suspended.

Similar laws govern the licensure and revocation of licenses for such professionals as registered nurses, nurse practitioners, and physician assistants. These laws clarify what the member of the profession can and cannot do.

BOX 3-3 List of Health Care Facilities That May Be Licensed by the State

- Ambulatory surgical centers
- Blood banks
- Clinics or community clinics
- Commercial independent laboratories
- Substance abuse treatment facilities
- End-stage renal disease centers
- Health departments
- Home health agencies
- Hospices
- Hospitals
- Intermediate care facilities
- Nursing homes
- Physician office laboratories
- Pregnancy counseling centers

Facility Licensing and Accreditation

State Requirements

Each state requires certain types of health care facilities to obtain a license. This gives the state oversight into the activities of the facility and allows for on-site surveys to maintain quality standards. A list of these types of facilities can be found in Box 3-3. Physician offices are usually not included, but if laboratory testing is done in the office, it may be necessary to get a license or certificate of waiver for the laboratory depending on the type of testing being done. Health insurance companies and HMOs are also licensed by the state, which sets certain requirements for their business operations.

Federal Requirements

In addition to state licensure, health care facilities that bill Medicare and Medicaid for services fall under CMS oversight and are responsible for meeting all regulatory standards.

The CMS also participates with state and private agencies to regulate clinical laboratories and determine compliance with regulations for quality assurance. This is discussed in more detail in Chapter 29.

Voluntary Accreditation

Many health care facilities, including hospitals, ambulatory surgical centers, clinical laboratories, health clinics, and physician offices, seek accreditation by independent accrediting agencies as a means to improve health care and maintain high standards. Accreditation may also be a means to comply with regulations for state licensure and regulations of the CMS.

The Joint Commission (formerly the Joint Commission on Accreditation of Healthcare Organizations [JCAHO]) was originally established in 1951 to accredit hospitals, rehabilitation centers, and nursing homes. In recent years it has expanded its activities to accredit almost all kinds of health care facilities, including clinics and physician offices. In order to become accredited, the health care facility must prepare a report demonstrating compliance with all standards of the Joint Commission. This is followed by a survey visit with follow-up to improve in any areas of weakness that might be found during that visit.

The Accreditation Association for Ambulatory Health Care (AAAHC) performs a similar type of accreditation for most types of ambulatory health care facilities.

MEDICAL PRACTICE and the LAW

Two elements are important to avoid malpractice suits. The first is to implement proper procedures to prevent mistakes. These procedures are part of the overall process of *risk management,* a term that is usually applied to measures taken to reduce risk of injury and lawsuits within the medical office.

Safety plans, chemical hygiene plans, evacuation plans, and standard precautions are all part of risk management, as are measures to avoid theft by patients or staff or fraud by financial staff. In addition, education and training of all staff help each staff member provide proper care to patients.

A second element of risk management is to prevent patients from becoming angry about the care (or lack of care) they receive. This requires all staff to be courteous, give complete explanations, and treat patients and their families with respect and dignity. If the office maintains good relations with patients, patients will be more likely to understand when there is a poor outcome or a mistake is made. Demonstrating respect and concern for patients at all times is one of the most important ways to prevent malpractice lawsuits.

Although the owners of the practice are ultimately responsible, the job of developing and implementing risk management plans usually falls to the office manager and, in a small office, to the head medical assistant. The best way to protect against malpractice lawsuits is to use the following procedures to prevent mistakes:

1. Make sure all equipment is in good working order and that staff have been properly trained to use it.
2. Make sure all staff members know how to do procedures and can review them in an up-to-date procedure manual.
3. Be sure that patients understand the nature of procedures and surgery and sign written consent forms for surgery and invasive procedures.
4. Always document accurately and completely. Promptly report any problems, and document your report.
5. Protect patients from injury by the proper use of equipment and safe transfers to and from wheelchairs.
6. Be sure that patients are not left alone if there is any question of their balance or mental status, if hot packs are used, or where hot water or hot pipes are present. Children should never be left unattended in an examination room or the waiting room.
7. Identify all patients using two identifiers before providing care, administering medications, or obtaining laboratory specimens.
8. Label all specimens in the presence of the patient. Log and track all results so that none slip through the cracks.
9. Wipe up all liquid spills promptly and use signs if floors are wet.
10. Do not make promises about outcomes.
11. Notify the physician of any patient complaints and/or requests for patient records from an attorney. ∎

What Would You Do? What Would You *Not* Do? RESPONSES

Case Study 1
Page 36

What Did Vicki Do?
❑ Told Denise that she would have to point out the burn to the physician because he needed to be sure it was healing properly.
❑ Told Denise that she would have to tell the physician what Denise had said about the burn.
❑ Explained that burning someone with a cigarette is not acceptable behavior and encouraged Denise to discuss the incident with the physician or another adult.

❑ Asked Denise if her boyfriend had hurt her any other time.

What Did Vicki Not Do?
❑ Did not tell Denise that she needed to break up with her boyfriend immediately.
❑ Did not agree to hide the information about the burn from the physician.
❑ Did not promise that the physician would not tell her parents.
❑ Did not discuss Denise's burn or explanation for it with anyone other than the physician.

What Would You Do? What Would You *Not* Do? RESPONSES—cont'd

What Would You Do/What Would You Not *Do?*
Review Vicki's response and place a checkmark next to the information you included in your response. List the additional information you included in your response.

_____
_____
_____
_____
_____

What Would You Do/What Would You Not *Do?*
Review Vicki's response and place a checkmark next to the information you included in your response. List the additional information you included in your response.

_____
_____
_____
_____
_____

Case Study 2
Page 45

What Did Vicki Do?
❏ Told Mr. Morton that the orthopedic surgeon specialized in musculoskeletal conditions and would not always recommend surgery.
❏ Asked Mr. Morton if he had asked the physician about other kinds of treatments.
❏ Asked Mr. Morton if he wanted her to complete the referral and make a new appointment.
❏ Asked Mr. Morton if he needed more time to speak to the physician.

What Did Vicki Not Do?
❏ Did not make recommendations about other types of treatment for back pain.
❏ Did not give an opinion about the benefits of one type of procedure compared with another.
❏ Did not promise that the orthopedic surgeon would not want to do surgery.
❏ Did not tell Mr. Morton that the physician should have done a better job explaining possible treatments.

Case Study 3
Page 47

What Did Vicki Do?
❏ Told the physician politely that she has to finish cleaning up the spill in the hall because someone might slip and fall.
❏ Worked as quickly as possible to dry the floor of the hall and then called the next patient.
❏ Asked the physician if he wanted to talk to the next patient before she took the vital signs.
❏ Obtained the electrocardiogram (ECG) for the patient in room 4 after calling and preparing the physician's next patient.

What Did Vicki Not Do?
❏ Did not leave the spilled water on the floor while she called the next patient and took the ECG.
❏ Did not ask if the physician thought she could do two things at once.
❏ Did not go around the office later trying to find out who had spilled water without cleaning it up.

What Would You Do/What Would You Not Do?
Review Vicki's response and place a checkmark next to the information you included in your response. List the additional information you included in your response.

_____
_____
_____
_____
_____
_____

↻ TERMINOLOGY REVIEW

Medical Term	Word Parts	Definition
Abandonment		Failure to continue to provide medical care to a patient without proper notification.
Act		A bill or measure that has become law. Often refers to legislation with several parts.
Advocate		A person who intercedes on another person's behalf.
Arbitration		A formal process whereby the parties to a dispute agree to submit to the decision of a neutral party.
Assumption of risk		A defense to a lawsuit that establishes that the plaintiff assumed the risk of whatever caused the injury.

Continued

TERMINOLOGY REVIEW—cont'd

Medical Term	Word Parts	Definition
Autonomy		Ability to make independent decisions without constraint or coercion by others.
Beneficence		Acting in the best possible way; performing good deeds.
Bill		A law proposed by a legislative body.
Case law		Law established by decisions of previous court cases.
Civil law		Law that regulates relationships and interactions between individuals and groups.
Cloning		Producing genetically identical cells or individuals artificially.
Common law		Unwritten body of law based on general custom.
Comparative negligence		A defense to a lawsuit that establishes a percentage of responsibility for injury on the part of the plaintiff.
Contingency		A condition that must be met before a contract is binding.
Contributory negligence		A defense to a lawsuit that establishes any responsibility for injury on the part of the plaintiff.
Controlled substance		A drug that has the potential for addiction or abuse.
Crime		An offense in violation of a law that prohibits or requires certain behavior.
Criminal law		Law that regulates offenses against the public welfare.
Defendant		The person or group against which an action is brought in a court of law.
Do-not-resuscitate (DNR) order		A medical order signed by a physician that relieves health care personnel from the obligation to resuscitate a patient who stops breathing or whose heart stops.
Drug Enforcement Administration (DEA)		The federal agency that enforces the Controlled Substances Act of 1970.
Duty		Commitment to act in a certain way.
Emancipated minor		A person younger than the age of 18 with the rights of an adult including the ability to consent to medical care.
Embezzlement		Fraudulent appropriation of funds or property of an employer or client.
Etiquette		Rules of socially acceptable behavior; manners.
Felony		A serious crime punishable by death or imprisonment.
Fidelity		Faithfulness.
Fraud		Intentional deception resulting in injury or loss.
Gene therapy		Giving patients new genes or parts of genes to treat a disease or condition.
Genetic engineering		Making, altering, or repairing genetic material.
Health care proxy		A legal document that names an agent to make decisions about a person's medical care if he or she becomes unable to make wishes known.
Informed consent		Agreement to a medical procedure based on understanding of the procedure and its possible consequences and effects.
Larceny		Stealing another person's property or money without violence.
Liability		Legal responsibility.
License		Official permission to perform an activity or practice a profession.
Licensure		The process by which the state examines qualifications and gives permission to an individual or organization to engage in a profession or business.
Litigation		The process of taking a lawsuit through the courts.
Living will		A legal document that specifies the kind of medical treatment a patient wants or does not want if he or she becomes incapacitated.
Malfeasance		A crime or wrongdoing that is illegal or contrary to official obligation.
Malpractice		Negligence by a professional.
Mediation		Negotiation by a third party to help two parties resolve a dispute.
Misdemeanor		A less serious crime, punishable by a fine or imprisonment for less than 1 year.
Misfeasance		Performing a legal act in an improper way.
Negligence		Failure to act (or to refrain from acting) as a reasonably prudent person would in similar circumstances.
Nonfeasance		Failing to perform an act that should have been performed, resulting in injury.
Nonmalfeasance		Ethical concept requiring that an action do no harm, or do less harm than good.
Plaintiff		The person or group that makes the complaint in a lawsuit.
Prescription		An order to a pharmacist to dispense a supply of a medication.

TERMINOLOGY REVIEW—cont'd

Medical Term	Word Parts	Definition
Privilege		A special immunity that protects against legal liability.
Prudent		Using care or common sense.
Reciprocity		Automatic issuing of a license in one state to the holder of a license in another state.
Respondeat superior		A legal doctrine making an employer liable for the negligent acts of employees.
Right		A claim that is expected to be honored.
Standard of care		Level of appropriate care required of a health professional.
Statute of limitations		A law limiting the time period for beginning a lawsuit.
Statutory law		Law enacted by a legislative body.
Stem cells		Cells that have the capacity to develop into various types of body tissue.
Subpoena		A court order for a witness to appear and give testimony.
Subpoena duces tecum		A court order to produce documents or records.
Tort		An injury or wrong against a person or property that does not involve breach of contract.
Veracity		Truthfulness.

ON THE WEB

For information on accreditation of ambulatory care facilities:

Accreditation Association for Ambulatory Health Care (AAAHC): www.aaahc.org/eweb/StartPage.aspx

The Joint Commission: www.jointcommission.org

For information on federal supervision of laboratories and ambulatory surgery centers:

U.S. Department of Health and Human Services, Centers for Medicare and Medicaid Services: www.cms.hhs.gov

For information on genetic engineering:

Office of Biotechnology Activities, National Institutes of Health: http://oba.od.nih.gov

For information on organ and tissue donation:

U.S. Department of Health and Human Services, Information on Organ and Tissue Donation and Transplantation: www.organdonor.gov

For information on National Provider Identifier (NPI) numbers:

NPI Registry Search: https://nppes.cms.hhs.gov/NPPES/NPIRegistryHome.do

For Information on the Patient's Bill of Rights:

Executive Summary of the Consumer Bill of Rights and Responsibilities from the *Report of the President's Advisory Commission on Consumer Protection and Quality in the Health Care Industry* : www.hcqualitycommission.gov

 Check out the Evolve site at http://evolve.elsevier.com/Bonewit/today/ to actively Prepare for your Certification, and to access additional interactive activities and exercises to help you study and prepare for success.

4

Interacting with Patients

KEY TERMS

active listening	hierarchy (HIGH-er-ark-ee)	projection
anxiety	hospice	reflecting
body language	judgmental	self-actualization
chronic	nonverbal	summarizing
closed questions	open questions	sympathy
denial	oral	terminal phase
ego defense mechanism	paraphrasing	verbal
empathy	physiologic	webcam

INTRODUCTION TO COMMUNICATION

In order to respond to a patient effectively, the medical assistant must be able to communicate effectively. Major components of health care include reducing a patient's fear and anxiety and helping the patient understand how to promote health and manage illness. To assess a patient's perception of his or her health status, the medical assistant must be effective at both sending and receiving messages.

COMMUNICATING WITH PATIENTS

Figure 4-1 outlines the basic model of communication. A sender sends a message to a receiver. The message can be **verbal,** meaning that spoken or written words are used to send the message. It can also be **nonverbal,** meaning the message is expressed without words through body language, facial expression, and other means. Most messages are sent using a combination of verbal and nonverbal communication. The *feedback* from the receiver to the sender, also verbal or nonverbal, helps the sender decide whether to initiate a new message, expand on the original message, or clarify the message.

Verbal and Nonverbal Communication

Verbal communication is either **oral** (spoken) or written. Written communication has traditionally been thought of as more formal than oral conversation—a letter rather than a phone call. Today, however, with the increasing use of e-mail, written communication may be as informal as oral communication.

Nonverbal communication refers to information that is received from body language. **Body language** is the way a person's body signals feelings or emotions. For example, hands folded across the chest and a rigid posture may signal anger. Nonverbal communication also includes the secondary communication that occurs during oral conversation. Secondary communication consists of tone of voice, voice pitch, voice volume, and voice quality. Nonverbal communication often provides more information than the words themselves (Figure 4-2).

The response to a simple question such as "How are you feeling today, Mr. Jackson?" may consist only of the words "All right." The quality of the voice—pinched, pained, flat,

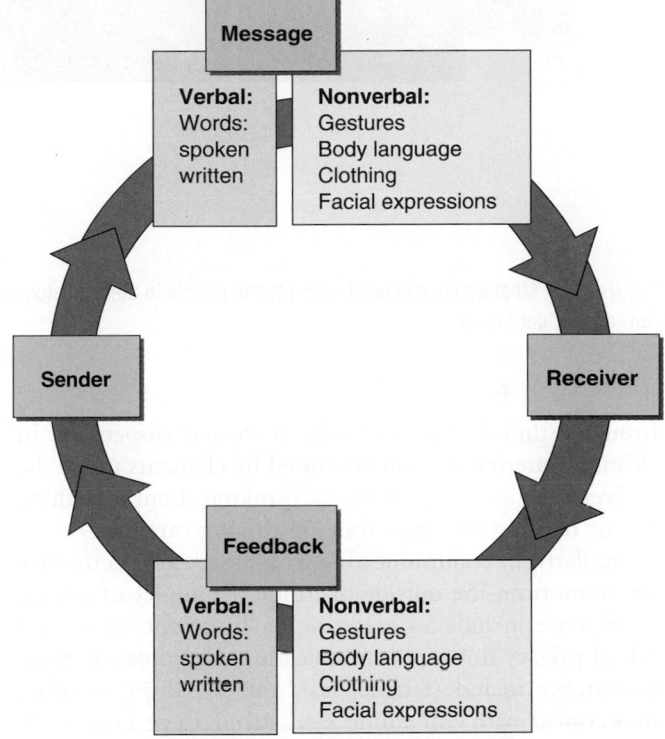

Figure 4-1 Model of communication.

excited, spoken with a deep sigh—gives more information than the words about Mr. Jackson's physical condition and his state of mind.

Other types of nonverbal communication include facial expression, body position, and gestures used while speaking. These are known as *nonverbal cues.*

Interference with Communication

Numerous elements can interfere with communication between the sender and receiver. An analogy for interference is listening to the radio. The radio station can be thought of as the sender of a message. The message is sent through radio signals. Any number of outside elements can interfere with the radio station's signal to the receiver, such as a storm that causes electrical interference in the atmosphere, air traffic controllers switching to a radio frequency that interferes with the broadcast frequency, or the receiver driving

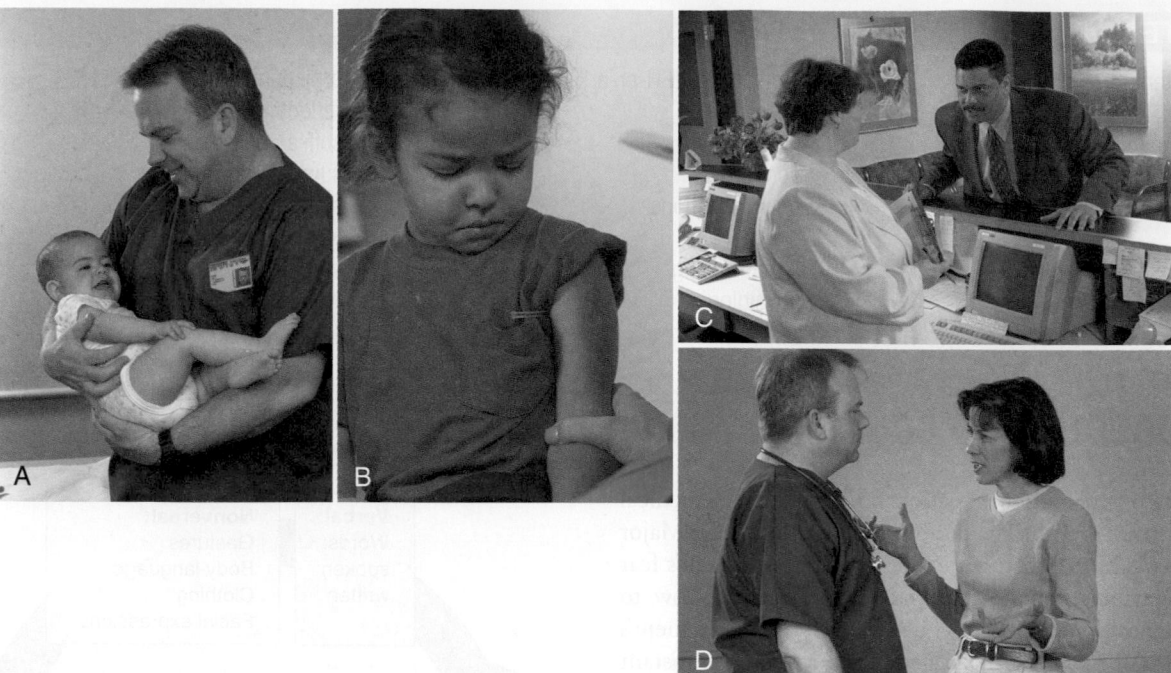

Figure 4-2 Most adults can easily identify the people in these photographs as expressing **A,** pleasure; **B,** uncertainty or lack of confidence; **C,** aggression; and **D,** confusion.

through a tunnel or over a bridge with steel suspension. In addition, interference can be caused by elements inside the receiver, such as strong emotions, thinking about something else, or needing to concentrate on driving carefully.

Similarly, in communicating with a patient, interference can come from the outside or inside. Examples of outside interference include a distracting environment, noise, and lack of privacy during communication. Examples of inside interference include fatigue, fear, anxiety, anger, or being preoccupied with something else. All of these factors can cause the message to be diluted, changed, or not completely understood by the receiver. Other barriers arise because understanding or senses are impaired.

The ability to identify a patient's strong emotions or feelings from the nonverbal cues exhibited by the patient may cross cultural boundaries. For example, infants and children from all cultures cry when they receive immunizations. The ability for the medical assistant or a patient to interpret subtle feelings or gestures, however, does not typically cross cultural boundaries. For example, shaking the head from side to side does not always mean "no." In some cultures it may mean "yes," or it may be used to express other meanings such as an acknowledgement that the listener has heard what was said.

Individuals who come from different cultures also have a different idea of personal space and may interpret physical touch in a different way. Cultural sensitivity is especially important for communication to be effective. Nonverbal communication that is accepted in the sender's culture, such as smiling, looking straight into the speaker's eyes, or lightly touching someone's shoulder to show concern, may create

interference if the gesture has a different significance in the listener's culture.

First impressions based on personal appearance may influence the way an individual is addressed. For example, it is easy to assume that an individual who looks homeless, who is dressed in dirty clothing, or who has a strong body odor is also uneducated. In the same way, individuals who are dressed in expensive suits often are treated with great respect. It is important to be aware of this tendency and respond to each patient as an individual.

Listening Skills

Good listening skills are major components of good communication. Some health professionals are naturally better listeners than others, but listening skills can be learned and practiced.

The most important listening skill is known as *active listening*. **Active listening** means being "in the moment" and paying close attention to what is being said without thinking about anything else. Focusing all the attention on the sender of the message is important. To receive a message clearly, the listener cannot allow emotions or thoughts to interfere with the sender's message.

What a sender says will naturally trigger a response. Letting go of the urge to respond verbally, take over the conversation, and air one's own views is important. By focusing on the sender, the medical assistant will not be tempted to let his or her own mental responses become spoken responses. It will also prevent the medical assistant from focusing on his or her mental responses, thereby preventing messages from the sender from being received clearly.

Additional guidelines for the medical assistant to demonstrate good listening techniques include the following:

1. Checking to make sure the patient's interpretation of a message is correct. This may involve asking the patient to repeat what has been said by rephrasing a question.
2. Listening for feelings. Medical assistants should be alert for key words or themes the patient uses frequently to describe his or her medical condition. These can be important clues as to the patient's emotional state. The medical assistant should also be aware of changes in his or her own feelings. The medical assistant's emotions may mirror the emotions of patients. For example, if the medical assistant begins to get impatient or aggravated with a patient, it may be a clue that the patient is upset or angry.
3. Being observant while listening. The patient's facial expressions, body language, tone of voice, and other nonverbal cues can tell a lot about what the patient is feeling.
4. Being patient and listening completely. Patients should be allowed to "tell their story" in their own time and in their own way. Interruption interferes with this process. Although there are questions that need to be asked, the medical assistant should introduce questions in a way that interferes as little as possible with the patient's natural storytelling flow.

Nonverbal Measures to Facilitate Communication

In the United States, eye contact is important (Figure 4-3). Maintaining eye contact is a sign of interest and involvement. However, being aware that in many cultures it is not respectful to look directly at older people is important. This is especially true in Asian and Native American cultures. Many Latinos also do not look directly at a person they respect, such as a teacher or a physician.

If the patient looks away and the medical assistant continues to seek eye contact, the patient may perceive this as aggression. Maintaining eye contact with someone who is culturally uncomfortable with that nonverbal communication creates a barrier between the two individuals.

For the most part, control of body language is unconscious. Therefore it is important for the medical assistant to be aware of the patient's nonverbal messages. Being alert to the patient's body language allows the medical assistant to notice when a patient feels uncomfortable or anxious. When a patient's words and body language do not match, the body language is usually a more genuine reflection of the patient's feelings.

Touching a person, even gently, can also be interpreted in many different ways. Moving closer can indicate interest, but it may also be viewed as aggressive. Many adults do not like to be touched by people they do not know well.

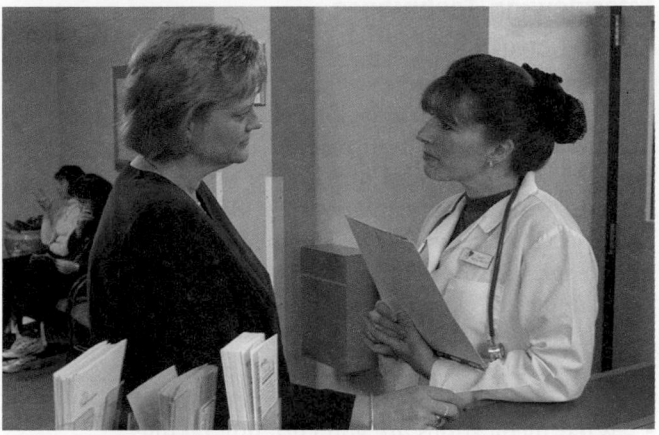

Figure 4-3 Photograph showing a comfortable talking distance and eye contact that is typical for the United States.

Cultural sensitivity is extremely important. For example, some Asians do not like to have their heads or their children's heads touched. This may present a problem when the medical assistant must measure the head circumference of an Asian infant. If this occurs, the medical assistant should stress to the infant's parent in a reassuring tone of voice that measuring head circumference is an important health assessment procedure and that there is no disrespect intended in the action.

A gentle pat on the shoulder can be reassuring to a patient, but it is important to notice if the patient becomes tense or appears uncomfortable when touched. If the medical assistant steps back, the patient will usually relax. In the United States, people normally maintain a distance of about 3 to 4 feet for conversation with others, but in other cultures this comfort zone varies.

If the medical assistant must penetrate the patient's personal comfort zone for a procedure, it may help to make a statement that prepares the patient for movement into the patient's personal space. For example, when applying a sterile dressing to a wound, the medical assistant might say, "I'm going to have to move in now so I have a better view of the area."

What Would You Do? What Would You *Not* Do?

Case Study 1
Nancy Walker, CMA (AAMA), has called Jennifer Boland, a 32-year-old married mother of three, from the waiting room. Nancy notices that Jennifer is not looking at her, but the patient cooperates with getting her weight and vital signs. When Nancy asks the reason for today's visit, it seems to take Jennifer a long time to answer. She picks at the sleeve of her jersey and finally says in a low voice that she is afraid she might be pregnant. Her voice cracks a little, and then she wipes one of her eyes. ■

Interviewing Techniques

Closed Questions

Two types of questions can be used when conducting a patient interview. These include closed questions and open questions. **Closed questions** are questions that can be answered with one word (e.g., yes or no) or a short answer (e.g., I was born on January 16, 1985). Closed questions are especially effective when the medical assistant needs to obtain specific information.

Examples of closed questions include the following:
- What is your date of birth?
- Who referred you to our office?
- Have you taken any medication for your pain?
- What medications are you currently taking?

Open Questions

Open questions consist of questions that encourage the patient to open up and talk. Examples of open questions include the following:
- What brings you to see the doctor today?
- What is your pain like?
- What has been going on with you since you were last here?
- How has your appetite changed over the past few months?

Open questions help the patient do the following:
- Identify what is important
- Express feelings
- Relay perceptions

Open questions are particularly effective in allowing the patient to describe a problem in his or her own words and explain how the patient feels about the problem. Because of this, open questions should be used to obtain a patient's chief complaint and conduct a patient interview. When using open questions, it is important for the medical assistant to employ active listening techniques.

If the medical assistant asks primarily closed questions, the patient may fail to give important details or mention other problems. If the medical assistant asks directly if the patient has been following a special diet or taking prescribed medication, the patient may feel pressure to agree, even if this has not always been the case. When a patient is encouraged to talk freely, a more realistic picture may emerge.

Keeping the Conversation Going

On occasion the medical assistant will need to employ techniques to keep a conversation going with a patient. For example, the medical assistant may need additional information from a patient, but the patient stops talking. When this occurs, the medical assistant should employ techniques that encourage the patient to continue speaking without steering the conversation in a particular direction. A useful technique in such a situation is to ask the patient an open question; however, "why" questions should not be used. Examples of "why" questions include the following:
- Why aren't you taking your medication?
- Why aren't you following your diet?

"Why" questions tend to make people defensive. Rather than having the patient justify his or her actions, it is important to identify the underlying reasons as to why the patient did not take the medication or stay on the diet. Effective questions that keep the conversation flowing without making a patient defensive include the following:
- How do you set up your meals and snacks?
- What problems are you having taking your medication?
- What do you think about having to take medication at school?

In answering these questions, the patient may provide clues as to the underlying reasons for not staying with the prescribed treatment plan.

Drawing Patients Out

Active listening includes techniques to draw a patient out and/or clarify what a patient is saying. This is especially important when the patient is trying to cope with strong feelings about his or her medical problems. Refer to Table 4-1 for a full listing of communication techniques that demonstrate active listening.

Avoiding Responses That Inhibit Communication

The medical assistant should avoid communication techniques that exhibit disapproval or blame as well as statements that are challenging or not genuine. If a patient feels that the medical assistant is not really listening, does not understand his or her point of view, or does not validate emotions, the patient may become defensive or stop speaking altogether. The medical assistant's ability to demonstrate acceptance of strong emotions experienced by the patient is especially important.

When a patient expresses concerns, it is tempting to try to reassure the patient. For example, a patient might express anxiety about the results of a diagnostic test. If the medical assistant reassures the patient that the results will probably be normal, the fact that the patient is worried is not validated and the reassurance implies that the patient's worry is unreasonable or unacceptable. If the medical assistant confirms that it is difficult to wait for test results, the patient is more likely to feel that his or her feelings have been accepted.

Because the medical assistant's job is to make the person feel comfortable, it is important to avoid being too casual or familiar with a patient. If a subject is sensitive, but it is important to ask about it, the medical assistant can do so in a somewhat tentative way to make it easier for the patient to reply. The medical assistant can identify what the patient might be feeling, but the patient will not always agree. Many people are not always aware of their feelings and may deny feelings that they are communicating nonverbally. This should be respected. Others are only too glad to have their feelings recognized.

Medical assistants should express themselves honestly, without being **judgmental,** which means critical or negative. They can disagree with what a patient is saying,

Table 4-1 Communication Techniques That Demonstrate Active Listening

Technique	Description	Example
Using open questions	Asking questions that do not expect a particular answer, especially a yes or no answer.	"What's been going on lately?" "How would you describe your stomach pain?"
Repeating or rephrasing	Saying the same thing as the patient either as a statement or a question to encourage agreement, disagreement, or clarification.	*Patient:* " It feels like someone is stabbing me in the side." *Medical assistant:* "Like a knife in your side…"
Translating a nonverbal message into words	Translating the patient's nonverbal expression of emotion into a verbal expression.	*Patient:* "All the doctor visits, the medication, the pain—it's really too much." *Medical assistant:* "You sound like you feel overwhelmed."
Reflecting	**Reflecting** is turning a question or statement around to reflect back to the patient; this gives the patient confidence to continue.	*Patient:* "Would you have this surgery if you were me?" *Medical assistant:* "What do you think about having the surgery?"
Paraphrasing and summarizing	**Paraphrasing** puts the patient's statement into the medical assistant's own words; **summarizing** restates the meaning but may leave out some of the details. The purposes are to validate that the medical assistant has understood and to encourage clarification.	*Medical assistant:* "So for the past week the pain has been getting steadily more intense and more frequent, and since this morning it hasn't let up at all."
Providing silence	Simply waiting for the patient to continue; allows the patient to choose whether to continue or choose a new topic.	(Silence)
Verbalizing the implied	Saying what the patient seems to mean but has not expressed.	*Patient:* "Usually I don't mind coming to see Dr. Hughes." *Medical assistant:* "But you didn't want to come today…"
Asking for clarification	Asking for more detail or a clearer statement; lets the patient know that the medical assistant has not understood and may show the patient how to make the message clearer.	*Medical assistant:* "It's not clear to me how often you have been taking this medication. Do you take it before every meal, or just when you are at home?"

especially if that disagreement will get the patient to elaborate on what is being said. But they should not argue because arguing sets up a competitive situation. Because the medical assistant represents medical authority, the patient can easily feel threatened and unworthy.

The responses that should be avoided are summarized in Table 4-2.

Barriers to Effective Communication

Impaired Level of Understanding

Occasionally, a patient with an impaired level of understanding visits the medical office. When this occurs, the medical assistant needs to simplify his or her method of speaking. The medical assistant should use short sentences and simple words. Speaking slowly in a normal speaking tone is important. Raising one's voice does not help in this situation. The tone of voice should express concern and empathy without being condescending or implying that the patient is not intelligent. Strong and constant eye contact also helps the patient to focus.

It may be necessary to say the same thing more than once, either by repeating it or saying the same thing in a different way. In addition, gestures and demonstration help to reinforce the information.

Those with limited understanding of medical information—children, the elderly (especially those with some degree of dementia), and those who are mentally disabled—need constant reassurance. Giving a direct and complete explanation at the patient's level of understanding is important. Even young children need to be informed about what is going to be done to them. For instance, if the medical assistant is going to draw blood, it is not enough to say, "I'm going to draw your blood. It's going to hurt for just a moment."

It may be necessary to say something like, "I'm going to use this needle to take some blood from your arm. I'm going to put it through the skin, into where your blood is. It will feel kind of like someone is pinching you, but only for a second. Then I'll put a Band-Aid on it, and it will stop bleeding."

After an explanation to an individual with impaired understanding, the medical assistant should ask the patient to repeat the explanation back in his or her own words. If the patient simply repeats a small part of the explanation, communication may have been ineffective. If the medical assistant explains a procedure such as a colonoscopy, for example, he or she should then ask the patient, "Can you tell me what a colonoscopy is?" An answer that may indicate

Table 4-2   Responses That Inhibit Communication

Technique	Description	Example
Offering false reassurance	Telling the patient that everything will be all right; implies that the patient should not feel anxiety or concern. Especially inappropriate when the medical assistant does not know what will happen.	"Don't worry; your husband will come through this with flying colors."
Disapproving, blaming	Making a negative value judgment about the patient's thinking or behavior; by implying or stating that a patient is responsible for his or her health problem, the medical assistant encourages the patient to defend against attack rather than establishing trust.	"You shouldn't be smoking, you know. No wonder you have trouble breathing."
Challenging	Insisting that the patient prove a statement or belief.	"Just show me something in writing that says people should never take a bath."
Defending	Protecting oneself or someone else from criticism, which implies that the patient does not have a right to have a different opinion.	"Dr. Lawler's patients never have to wait very long."
Asking for explanations of feelings or behavior	Because patients often don't know why they feel or act as they do, asking why may be frustrating and cause them to become defensive.	"Why don't you stick to your diet?" "Why are you angry?"
Belittling or negating feelings	Acting as if feelings are less intense than they are or not even present; this implies that the patient's feelings are not real or not justified	"You are really making a big deal out of a little cut."

lack of understanding is, "It's when they do a colonoscopy." The medical assistant can then make another attempt to provide a simple explanation.

A young child or an individual with an impaired level of understanding cannot give informed consent. This must be obtained from an individual who can legally give informed consent for the impaired patient before the medical assistant can proceed.

Sight Impaired

Many degrees of vision loss exist. Total blindness is the complete inability to perceive light and form. *Legally blind* is a term used to describe individuals whose vision cannot be corrected beyond 20/200 in the better eye. This means that with glasses, at 20 feet the person sees the same as or less than a person with normal vision sees at 200 feet. A person may be called *sight impaired* if his or her vision is better than 20/200 but he or she still has low vision or a decreased field of vision.

It is important for the medical assistant to be verbally descriptive when working with a patient with impaired vision. The medical assistant should use touch and guidance when escorting patients who cannot see to walk safely from the waiting room to the examination room and also when helping them around the examination room. Patients with impaired vision usually prefer to take the medical assistant's arm and follow his or her movements rather than vice versa. To explain exactly where things are, a clock image sometimes helps. Saying that the examination table is at three o'clock tells a blind patient that the examination table is on the right directly to the side.

Hearing Impaired

The term *deaf* is usually used when individuals cannot hear well enough to use the sense of hearing to process information. However, there are many more individuals whose hearing is impaired than those who are deaf, especially in certain tone ranges or when sound is not loud enough.

Special techniques should be used with patients who are hearing impaired. The medical assistant should speak clearly, slowly, and in short sentences. The medical assistant's voice should be slightly louder than normal but not so loud that it loses clarity or sounds like shouting. Eye contact is also important when communicating with a hearing-impaired patient. Even if the hearing-impaired patient does not lip-read, most people who lose their hearing learn how to associate facial expression and mouth shape with words they know and recognize.

When beginning a conversation with a hearing-impaired patient, it may be necessary to touch the person gently to get his or her attention. If the patient is wearing a hearing aid, it may be helpful to ask if the hearing aid has been working well for him or her.

Sign language is often used to communicate with the deaf. Hand and finger positions represent letters or words. Several different systems exist, but American Sign Language is the recognized language in the United States.

Because each sign can represent an entire word, a person who uses sign language may be able to communicate as fast as, or faster than, a person who is speaking. Sign language has its own structure and grammar system, so it takes considerable practice to become fluent. A patient who uses sign language to communicate is usually accompanied by an interpreter. If the patient does not have an interpreter, the law requires the office to provide one. Sign language interpretation can be provided by an interpreter. It can also be provided by setting up a video relay service account. Video service links the deaf patient with a sign language interpreter. When a sign language interpreter's services are being used, it is important that the medical assistant maintain eye contact with the patient. Hearing-impaired and deaf patients are able to obtain information from facial expressions and body language. They may also be able to read lips.

Language Barriers

A language barrier interferes with communication when two people speak different languages. Depending on the patient's facility with English, this interference may vary from slight to severe.

The best way to work around language barriers is with translation assistance. It is preferred to use trained medical interpreters or translators whenever possible. When scheduling an appointment for a patient with a language barrier, the medical assistant should arrange translation assistance at the same time. Sometimes a patient with a language barrier brings a child to translate. The medical assistant should be aware that children are the least reliable interpreters because they have a tendency to skip over medical words they do not understand or cannot translate without realizing that important information may be lost. It may also be embarrassing for a patient to discuss certain medical problems if a child is translating for him or her.

When conversing with a patient through an interpreter, the medical assistant should speak to the patient and not to the interpreter. The medical assistant should allow the interpreter to translate a sentence before going on to the next sentence. The medical assistant should speak slowly and carefully, using simple terms and short sentences. Many people who do not feel comfortable speaking English can still understand much of what is said to them in English.

At times the medical assistant may need to improvise when working with a patient with a language barrier. This may be required during the following circumstances: the office does not have translation services, the interpreter is busy, or the patient's family member is translating but the patient wants to converse with the medical assistant in private. In these situations the medical assistant should use gestures and pantomime to convey his or her ideas.

Translation assistance is required before a patient with a language barrier gives written consent to an invasive procedure or minor office surgery. The law states that a patient must be fully informed as to the nature of his or her surgery or procedure. Consent forms are usually written in English, but the verbal explanation of the procedure needs to be in a language the patient understands well. If a practice has a large number of non–English-speaking patients, it is a good idea to have routine consent forms and instructional materials translated and available.

Telephone and video translation services can be purchased from several companies. Telephone translation assistance allows the patient, medical assistant, and/or physician to speak to the interpreter using a speakerphone. A video translation service requires a computer, a **webcam** (small video camera attached to the computer), and a speakerphone and allows all parties to see one another during the conversation.

What Would You Do? What Would You *Not* Do?

Case Study 2

When Nancy calls Harold Underwood, a 67-year-old man, from the waiting room, he does not answer until she has repeated his name three times. Because he is a new patient, Nancy introduces herself. He says that he has moved into senior housing nearby so that he can be close to his daughter. Nancy finds that she has to repeat all instructions, and she notices that Harold is wearing a hearing aid in his left ear. When she asks him if he needs help to step up to sit on the examination table, he looks at her blankly. ∎

UNDERSTANDING AND MEETING THE NEEDS OF PATIENTS

Patient Expectations of Health Care

Patient expectations depend on many factors including unmet needs and experiences the person has had in the past. Previous interactions with health care facilities also shape a patient's expectations. For example, if there is a long waiting time, a patient who has always had to spend 30 to 40 minutes in the waiting room will be less upset than a patient who is used to being seen within 10 minutes.

Patients usually want to be seen by a physician in a reasonable amount of time, and they hope that the physician will "fix" whatever is wrong. Patients do not expect to have long-term problems. They want to be treated as if they were cars and physicians were mechanics—"fix what's broken and get me back on the road of life!"

In addition, people expect physicians to take care of them when they are really sick and not fuss too much over them when they are generally well. People certainly do not want physicians to nag them about changing their lifestyle to improve their health. But physicians are much more likely today to bring up lifestyle issues, such as eating healthy foods in reasonable portions, not smoking, reducing alcohol intake, exercising, and using seat belts. Physicians are well aware that a healthy lifestyle can reduce the amount and intensity of medical care a person needs in the future.

Patients are sometimes so wrapped up in their primary concern—to get relief from pain or other symptoms—that they have difficulty accepting that physicians are often looking for the cause of their illness, not just to alleviate symptoms. This can cause a lot of frustration for patients, especially if no significant relief can be given or if the physician does not seem to think that alleviating the symptoms would be appropriate.

A common example of this is a viral illness such as the common cold. A patient may have a fever, muscle aches, weakness, vomiting, and diarrhea. Once the physician establishes that the patient does not have a more serious condition, the physician may recommend only rest, fluids, and over-the-counter medications (e.g., acetaminophen or ibuprofen for fever reduction and relief of soreness). This

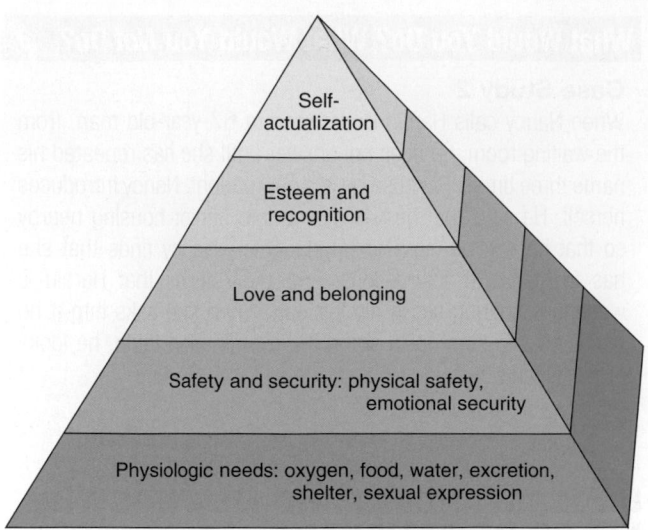

Figure 4-4 Maslow's hierarchy of needs.

plan of treatment can be frustrating for a patient who wants to feel better and have a speedy recovery.

How Basic Needs Affect the Behavior of Patients

Maslow's Hierarchy of Needs

Abraham Maslow was an American psychiatrist. In his book titled *Motivation and Personality*, he defined what has come to be known as "Maslow's hierarchy of needs." A **hierarchy** is an arrangement in order of importance. Maslow describes human needs as a hierarchy with the most important needs at the lowest level. The image of a pyramid is often used to depict this visually, as shown in Figure 4-4. On the bottom of the pyramid (Level 1) are the **physiologic** needs. These are the basic biologic needs for survival, which include oxygen, water, food, excretion, sleep, shelter, and sexual expression.

On the next level of the pyramid (Level 2) are the needs for safety and security. Level 2 needs include avoiding harm, attaining physical safety, and the emotional security that comes with freedom from fear and anxiety.

On the middle level of the pyramid (Level 3) are the needs for love and belonging. Level 3 needs include both receiving and giving personal affection, companionship with another individual, and identification with a group.

On the fourth level of the pyramid (Level 4) are the needs for esteem and recognition. Level 4 needs include self-esteem, the respect of others in one's peer group, success in work, and prestige in the community.

Finally, at the pyramid's pinnacle (Level 5) is the need for **self-actualization.** This is the fulfillment of each individual's potential.

Effects of Unmet Needs during Illness

Understanding that an individual cannot step up to the next level on Maslow's pyramid until his or her needs have been fully met at the current level is important. An individual's current level may shift several times, even in the course of a day, as different needs are experienced. An individual moves up or down the pyramid depending on what needs are currently unmet. Only when lower-level needs are met will the person be able to devote a significant amount of energy or concern to needs that are higher on the pyramid. In fact, a person has all the needs (outlined on the pyramid) all the time but becomes aware of higher-level needs only once the lower-level needs are met.

This has a number of implications for how patients relate to the medical care they receive.

Many patients who come to the medical office are struggling to meet basic needs because they are ill. Health care professionals must recognize any difficulties in that area.

Health and happiness require more than just meeting basic needs, however. Part of the role of health professionals is to foster the meeting of needs beyond physiologic needs. For example, intervening for an abused child or battered woman helps meet needs for safety and security, as well as some sense of love and belonging, by knowing someone cares. Teaching patients how to manage a **chronic** disease—one that continues to exist over time—helps a person's self-esteem by making the person feel competent in self-care.

Another area where understanding the hierarchy of needs helps in the health care setting includes learning to recognize situations when attention-getting behavior by patients might be an attempt to satisfy needs for love and belonging, or for esteem and recognition. When people are ill, their usual means for meeting their attention needs (both for love and belonging, as well as esteem and recognition) may be interrupted.

Medical assistants must be able to recognize that they cannot meet all of a patient's needs. For example, the medical assistant is not a close friend and should not attempt to be one, but recognizing when a patient feels a loss in this area, the medical assistant helps the person to identify his or her feelings and to cope with whatever need is not being met.

Establishing Caring Relationships

A patient who visits the medical office is often fragile, emotionally as well as physically. Illness interrupts an individual's daily routine and threatens self-concept and self-esteem. A patient who is ill often has a difficult time meeting his or her physiologic needs. One of the primary roles of a medical assistant is to create and maintain a caring relationship with the patient. The medical assistant is often the patient's earliest, most frequent, and most consistent point of contact with the medical office.

Empathy

In order to meet a patient's needs, the medical assistant must first be able to identify the patient's feelings. In addition, the medical assistant must be able to understand those feelings, not in an intellectual way but in an emotional way. This understanding is called *empathy*. **Empathy** is the capacity to make an emotional connection with another person's feelings without allowing the emotional connection to become overpowering. Empathy is often contrasted with sympathy. **Sympathy** is defined as experiencing the same emotions as another. Sympathy is often accompanied by a feeling of pity.

Empathy is more objective than sympathy. Experiencing empathy requires a person to retain perspective and have confidence that strong emotions are not dangerous. The medical assistant must be sensitive to the feelings patients have when they go through the medical office routine. It is important for the medical assistant to be constantly aware that strong emotions may arise when individuals experience a threat such as an illness. By showing empathy to patients, a medical assistant can support them more effectively.

Expression of Caring

Caring can be expressed through words and body language. The medical assistant expresses caring through words, by drawing patients out and letting them tell their story in their own way, in their own time. This was described earlier in this chapter in the section on interviewing techniques. The medical assistant should accept and validate a patient's feelings. Patients benefit by being acknowledged and having someone else accept them.

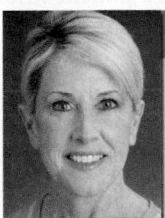

Putting It All into Practice

My name is Nancy Walker, and I have been working for an oncologist for the past 5 years. Our patients have many different types of cancer and are at many different stages of their diseases. One thing that they all have in common is that they need a lot of emotional support. We provide this primarily by keeping the lines of communication open. We try to create an atmosphere where patients feel able to discuss whatever is on their minds. Some patients never say the word "cancer," and they talk about future plans as if they will be in the peak of health. Other patients are amazingly open and frank, even if they have not responded well to treatment. One patient told me that this is the only place she can talk about dying because her husband and her daughter become so emotional that she feels she has to spare them. We do not push patients to talk about anything they are uncomfortable with, but we do make time if patients want to talk about their feelings. The physicians also refer our patients to support groups or counselors because they believe that it is equally important to manage a patient's emotions and physical symptoms. ■

Caring can also be expressed nonverbally through body language and through the way a medical assistant positions himself or herself during conversations with patients (Figure 4-5). The medical assistant should be positioned at the patient's eye level and at a distance of no more than 3 to 4 feet. If the medical assistant stands while the patient sits at a lower level, the patient may feel intimidated or inferior.

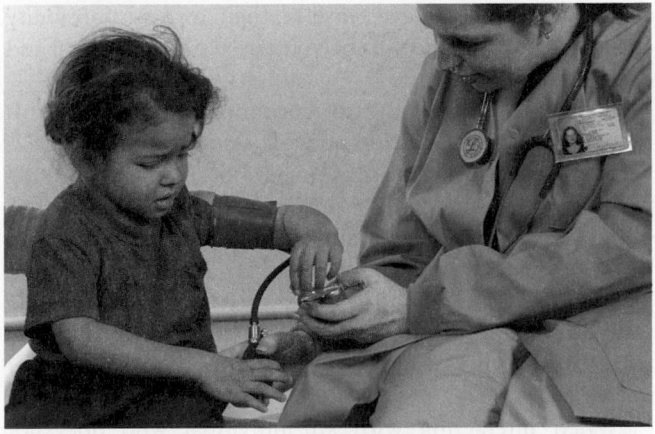

Figure 4-5   Allowing a preschool child to handle and use the blood pressure cuff may prevent anxiety by giving the child a sense of control.

Typically, the patient sits on the examining table while the medical assistant stands, which has both at almost equal height. If the patient is more comfortable sitting in the examining room chair, the medical assistant can sit on the physician's stool, which again puts both at about equal height. This is much more friendly than if the medical assistant stands while the patient sits in the chair.

Maintaining eye contact and lightly touching the patient, if it seems appropriate, also communicate interest and caring.

Value of Effective Relationships with Patients

The medical assistant is often the patient's most frequent, and long-term, point of contact with the medical office. A medical assistant who gets to know a patient well can be of invaluable assistance to both the patient and the physician, through trust established over time.

The experience of being understood and cared for is one of the most important steps in beginning to heal or cope effectively with illness, especially if the patient has a chronic illness. Ideally, each professional the patient comes in contact with at the office will convey this sense, but it is most important for those who are performing procedures. If the patient feels understood, he or she will also develop trust and be able to relax during procedures. This makes the procedure easier and less painful for the patient. It also makes it easier for the medical assistant to perform the procedure.

Personal Boundaries

Personal boundaries or self-boundaries include physical, mental, and spiritual guidelines or limits that a person uses to define how close other people can come without posing a threat to personal integrity. They indicate a sense of being separate from others instead of defined and controlled by others. The medical assistant and other health professionals allow others to maintain the personal physical space that is necessary for them to feel comfortable, and they do not allow others to intrude into their own physical space. They should also have a clear sense of their own responsibility and right to decide how to behave based on clear moral and ethical principles.

It is not uncommon to encounter individuals with mental boundaries that are too weak or too strong. A person who is very unsure about his or her boundaries goes along with his or her companions and is easily manipulated. The opposite type of person maintains rigid control, refuses to be influenced, and usually keeps others at a distance so that no one can get close. Either of these types may be totally self-absorbed, seeing themselves as the center of the universe and treating others as if their only function is to meet their needs.

When interacting with an individual who does not respect physical or emotional boundaries, it is important for the medical assistant to recognize what is happening and take appropriate steps to maintain personal boundaries. If possible, this should be done in a straightforward way without acting upset or angry. For example, a patient may act as if he or she is a good friend of the medical assistant and ask for a cell phone number or may ask the medical assistant to meet him or her for lunch. Initially most medical assistants would offer excuses not to comply. If the patient continues to ask for a telephone number, for example, the medical assistant may state calmly that he or she does not give his or her cell phone number to patients.

Emotional Responses to Illness

Guilt

Patients may feel guilt about their illness. The amount of guilt they feel varies from one patient to another. The amount of guilt that a patient is willing to express, as opposed to the amount that is repressed, varies from one patient to the next.

Some individuals engage in behaviors that are known to be risky to health, such as cigarette smoking, drinking, and drug abuse. These patients sometimes feel guilty about a respiratory disease, but others may display a devil-may-care attitude about their disease. People often know intellectually that their high-calorie, high-fat diet or sedentary lifestyle predisposes them to certain illnesses or conditions. Smokers, for example, have been bombarded with scientifically valid information for almost 40 years about the link between smoking and heart disease, lung cancer, and chronic obstructive pulmonary disease. Yet many of these individuals continue established habits without an outward sense of guilt. It seems as though they have convinced themselves that their risky behavior is not the cause of their disease or that they are somehow immune to the consequences of their behavior.

On the other hand, patients with conditions totally out of their control may experience guilt. For example, someone with pancreatic cancer might say that he could have avoided the disease if he had taken better care of himself, eaten a healthy diet, or gotten more exercise.

As with other emotions, the medical assistant should accept and validate a patient's description of his or her feelings. If the patient's previous behavior is partially responsible for current medical problems, the patient requires support and acceptance. If it is unlikely that previous behavior is related to the medical problem, the medical assistant can encourage the patient to discuss the causes of his or her condition with the physician.

Loss of Control

When people are ill, they often have a feeling of a loss of control. This is especially true if they have sought medical care for their condition. In addition to physiologic changes that may be unwelcome, they feel unable to control their schedule and/or environment. Some decisions are made for them. They have to take off their clothes. People get physically close to them and sometimes even touch them. People tell them to do things they do not want to do. They are anxious and become defensive. The medical assistant should respond to the patient's irritation with patience and kindness. It is important to give the patient choices and make every effort to accommodate the patient's wishes.

Anxiety

Anxiety is a response to a perceived threat. A person who is moderately to severely anxious is not able to converse coherently and will not pick up nonverbal cues that he or she would normally notice. When working with a patient who is anxious, the medical assistant must first get the person's attention, slow down the conversation, and then help the person to focus on the conversation. It is important to validate the patient's concern, which reduces his or her anxiety level. This allows the patient's energy to be channeled in a more productive way. When patients are anxious, they may not remember what they are told. The medical assistant can help the patient by creating memory aids. For example, the medical assistant can prompt the patient to record a follow-up appointment in his or her appointment calendar. It is also a good idea to write the instructions down or provide the patient with a preprinted instruction sheet.

Severe anxiety can be medically problematic. Physical symptoms occur with a full-blown anxiety attack, often termed a *panic attack*. An overly anxious person hyperventilates, has an extremely rapid heart rate, and becomes unresponsive. Some people experience numbness in their fingers and toes; others feel a sensation of fluid in their ears. Some people become intensely fearful and have an overpowering sense of dread.

An anxiety attack must be dealt with as a medical issue first. Helping the patient acknowledge the anxiety is important. Acknowledging the anxiety helps a person gain control. In addition, having strong emotions accepted by another person decreases the sense of fear that many people have about their emotions.

If the patient is breathing rapidly, the medical assistant should encourage the patient to take slow, deep breaths. Experts no longer recommend having a patient breathe into a brown paper bag because this may cause blood oxygen levels to fall dangerously low.

If possible, the medical assistant should encourage the patient to validate that anxiety is present without minimizing its significance. If the patient has not experienced severe anxiety before, he or she may not realize the effects it can cause. The medical assistant can explain that any physical symptoms are the result of anxiety and stay with the patient until the symptoms begin to subside. With most patients, the symptoms begin to diminish after 1 or 2 minutes. After the person has returned to a level of relative calm, it may be possible to discuss how the person handles anxiety. The physician may also refer the patient to a counselor to work on strategies to manage it.

What Would You Do? What Would You *Not* Do?

Case Study 3

Julie Ann Reynolds is a 20-year-old patient who comes to the office and describes four or five recent episodes of shortness of breath, palpitations, feeling faint, sweating, and nausea. She states that she has just started taking classes at a local university after transferring from a community college. The episodes have occurred mainly in the car on the way to school or shortly after she arrives. She says that on one occasion her heart was beating so fast that she had to pull her car over and wait for about 10 minutes before she felt well enough to drive. She says that she has never had a heart problem, but now she is afraid that there is something wrong with her heart. She also says that her mother is worried about her and has suggested that she get an electrocardiogram and other tests because she might have a serious medical condition. ■

Anger

Anger is a natural response to a perceived threat. Anger is often a subconscious response, which means that the patient is unaware of its cause, its intensity, or even its presence. A patient may express anger at a target that did not actually cause the angry feeling. Anger can also escalate quickly if it triggers an angry response from another individual. When dealing with an angry patient, the medical assistant needs to identify the emotion without feeling attacked. If possible, the medical assistant should help the angry person identify the true source of the anger.

Anger is one of the more difficult of the incapacitating emotions to deal with. Anger tests a medical assistant's empathy and ability to put aside private issues to help patients. The first instinct is to defend oneself against a perceived attack by the angry patient, but this is counterproductive. It is more effective to respond with calmness and control using a quiet voice. Accepting that a patient is angry is not the same as allowing the patient to threaten office staff or other patients. It is perfectly acceptable to set personal boundaries by telling the patient that he or she is acting inappropriately, that he or she is making it difficult for other patients, or that shouting will not be tolerated. To protect the confidentiality of the patient who is temporarily out of control, the medical assistant should escort the patient to a private area. It is also appropriate for the medical assistant to request assistance from the office manager in dealing with an angry patient. Sometimes anger, like electricity, loses intensity when the connection is broken.

The Grieving Process

Any time a disease causes actual or potential loss including loss of function as well as loss of life, both the patient and family go through a fairly predictable sequence of stages called the *grieving process.* This process was described in detail by the spiritual author Elisabeth Kübler-Ross in relation to individuals with a terminal illness. The **terminal phase** is defined as when the patient is not expected to live more than 6 months. People go through this sequence over varying lengths of time, and may move from one stage to another out of the order presented here. Although the process is individual, it is important to know that even a dying person can come to a type of acceptance, and after death has occurred there is a time when the grieving relatives and friends will again be able to engage in loving and fulfilling relationships.

The following five steps are those described by Kübler-Ross for the patient with a terminal illness:

1. Denial. This is the initial response to knowledge that one has a terminal illness. It is a state of shock and disbelief. Most people simply deny the idea. Denial can be useful; it can provide a period of time to find a way to deal with death or disability. If a patient is using denial, the medical assistant should remember that this is a defense against unmanageable anxiety.

The medical assistant should listen to the patient actively, without confronting unrealistic statements. Acceptance of the patient's need to deny reality provides support for a patient to accept at his or her own pace. The patient and family will start to accept reality when they are ready to handle the strong emotions.

2. Anger. Frustration and anger usually follow denial. The patient is in the "why me?" mode. The illness seems unfair, and the patient may respond by being belligerent, uncooperative, and critical of those around him or her. Health care providers may become targets of this anger and criticism. The medical assistant must keep in mind that any such display of anger is not directed at him or her personally but toward the situation and circumstances over which the patient has no control.

3. Bargaining. In this stage, which usually follows anger closely, the patient may try to give something up to gain more time. Most bargaining is done between the patient and his or her personal concept of God. If bargaining is verbalized, the medical assistant should be accepting of the patient's wish to make a bargain that will reverse his or her condition or prolong his or her life.

4. Depression. The patient recognizes the facts that cannot be denied and becomes depressed. Most people become silent in this stage and prefer to be

Highlight on Ego Defense Mechanisms

Ego defense mechanisms are unconscious mental processes that offer psychological protection. Everyone uses defense mechanisms at some time or another to protect against being overwhelmed by painful feelings. Although people are sometimes aware of using these mechanisms, usually they operate on an unconscious level—that is, people are not aware that they are disguising or blocking emotions or impulses.

Everyone tends to use defense mechanisms that have been effective in the past to reduce stress or anxiety. When a person first encounters a situation, such as a diagnosis of serious illness, that would provoke strong feelings, a defense mechanism like denial helps him or her avoid feeling overwhelmed and unable to cope. (**Denial** is unconsciously refusing to acknowledge something that is difficult to accept.) People say things like, "It doesn't seem real to me" or "This must be a mistake."

Denial allows the truth to penetrate gradually so the person has a chance to get used to the threat, to seek privacy to experience intense emotion, and to avoid total disorientation. However, if a person continues to use denial without attempting to accept the situation, negative consequences may occur.

The person may not take appropriate actions to respond to illness. Friends and family may respond negatively to the person's perceived lack of responsibility. And the person may miss the opportunity to grow and strengthen his or her sense of self-worth and ability to cope with adversity.

If a medical assistant can identify a patient's defense mechanisms and coping patterns, he or she can gain a better understanding of the patient's underlying fears and concerns. The medical assistant can try to respond to these concerns but should not directly challenge the defenses or label them.

When defense mechanisms are attacked, it takes more energy to defend against threatening emotions. On the other hand, accepting defenses tends to promote a feeling of being understood and may decrease the need for rigidity in the defenses.

Example

Mr. Sykes has had to wait for about 45 minutes past his appointment time to see Dr. Lopez. When Kathy, the medical assistant, takes him back to the examination room, he says, "I think you should know that some of the people in the waiting room are really upset about how long they have been waiting."

Kathy may suspect that this is an example of **projection**—unconsciously identifying thoughts or feelings as originating in someone else when they really are one's own thoughts and feelings. She can be helpful to Mr. Sykes by responding in a way that reassures him that it is understandable for a person to be upset when there is an unusually long wait. Responses that are not helpful (because they reinforce Mr. Sykes's fear that it would be dangerous to express a negative emotion directly) are as follows:

1. Making it seem as though Mr. Sykes is overreacting and should not feel upset ("Oh, it hasn't been that long.")
2. Labeling or challenging the defense mechanism ("Do you always project your own feelings on people around you?")
3. Defending the physician or office staff ("Dr. Lopez has been very busy with several sick patients.")
4. Talking negatively about the patients in the waiting room ("Some people are never happy, no matter how quickly they are seen.")

Following is a list of several other ego defense mechanisms, with examples that might occur in a medical office. Remember that using defense mechanisms usually helps people adapt to stressful situations. ■

Other Ego Defense Mechanisms

Selective inattention	Failing to hear or pay attention to information that may provoke anxiety	A patient expresses the belief that his cancer will definitely be cured if he has the primary tumor removed.
Regression	Returning to the emotional adjustment of an earlier stage of growth and development	An ill person who could be independent asks for assistance with personal hygiene.
Depersonalization	Removing feeling from something that is perceived as stressful	A medical assistant who is assisting with a lumbar puncture on a young child experiences the child as looking like a toy or doll.
Rationalization	Assigning logical reasons or excuses for actions that may have been motivated by self-interest or other emotions the person does not wish to acknowledge	A patient might justify not telling the physician that he smokes by saying to himself, "The doctor isn't interested because he didn't ask about it."
Repression	Unconsciously excluding unacceptable ideas, impulses, or emotions from awareness	A diabetic patient who hates finger sticks often forgets to test her blood sugar.
Suppression	Deciding to put uncomfortable or painful thoughts out of awareness	A patient says, "I don't want to think about my surgery until the day before."
Displacement	Shifting an emotion or behavior from the original object to a more acceptable substitute	A medical assistant who has just been given a poor evaluation is extremely rude to the next person she talks to on the telephone.
Undoing	An attempt to make amends for a feeling or behavior that makes a person feel guilty	A patient notices that she hates the medical assistant's hairstyle and hair color. Immediately she tells the medical assistant that she has beautiful eyes.
Compensation	Attempting to overcome a real or perceived handicap by developing some other ability or trait	A person who thinks that she isn't very intelligent in school always offers to help the teacher.

alone. The patient who is withdrawn is more difficult to deal with than the person who is openly angry. In this situation, a medical assistant needs to be available and present with the patient for companionship and to provide a nonjudgmental listening ear. The medical assistant should always strive to maintain communication with a patient in the depression stage. Counseling and support groups may be appropriate referrals for both patients and family members in this stage.

5. Acceptance. Some people find a degree of peace within themselves when they accept their imminent death. They willingly stop resisting death and rest quietly. This is seldom seen by professionals who work in medical offices, because those who reach this stage may be in a hospital, in a hospice center, or at home. The dying person may want loved ones present at death and may not interact with others at all. Most people fear dying alone and want the comfort of having someone, preferably a loved one, present in the final moments.

A dying person has a number of fears, such as fear of the unknown, fear of pain, and fear of helplessness. It is a challenge for all health care professionals to accept the difficult feelings of fear.

Listening closely to the patient allows the medical assistant to help the patient respond to all hints of deterioration, as well as actual problems, as soon as they become apparent. The patient may need to be seen by several health care professionals while receiving additional care at home. The medical assistant can be helpful by being aware of community resources and by communicating the needs of the patient and his or her family to the doctor. This requires knowledge of insurance benefits and of the types of insurance the office accepts, as well as other sources of funding assistance the patient may be able to obtain.

A patient whose condition has stabilized or whose active treatment has ended but who still requires pain relief, nursing care, and/or comfort measures must receive them at home, in a nursing home, in a rehabilitation center, or in a hospice center. A **hospice** is an organization that provides comfort, pain relief, and personal care for dying patients.

Most hospices provide nursing care, nursing assistants, and volunteers to visit terminal patients in their homes, working with the families to increase the individual's comfort once active treatment is no longer effective or desired. There are also some hospice centers, which provide centralized care. In some areas a patient can receive similar services from home health care agencies and visiting nurse associations.

The medical assistant may serve as a liaison to obtain appropriate referrals from the doctor and assist the patient and/or family to locate providers of needed services. Communication on this level must be two-way; if a patient is being seen by visiting nurses, hospice, or other health professionals, the medical assistant may be the person who facilitates communication between the doctor and these other parties.

Cultural Influences Affecting Health Care

Patients often come from cultures that have some level of distrust of Western scientific medicine and/or strong belief in their own medical traditions. In addition to seeking care from a physician, these patients may complement their care by visiting traditional practitioners. In many traditional practices, religion and medicine are tightly interwoven. Both patients and practitioners hope to affect health by influencing spirits or gods in the unseen world. People from many cultures believe in the effectiveness of sacred words, tattoos, or amulets (objects worn to prevent injury or evil), as well as specific rituals that may involve chanting, fire, or even animal sacrifice.

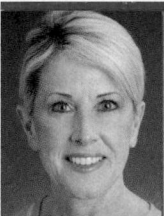

Memories *from* Externship

Nancy Walker: I did my externship in the adult medicine area of a clinic in a large metropolitan area. We had several African patients who came to our area as refugees from Somalia. If they were recent immigrants, we had to explain many things about our clinic to them because they were not familiar with preventative care from their own country. The female patients were modest; they did not shake hands with male physicians and avoided undressing for examinations. We tried to assign them to female practitioners, if possible, and everyone in the office learned to adapt procedures by having the patient remove the minimum possible amount of clothing. For example, the physicians usually listened to a female patient's heart and respirations just by placing the stethoscope under her clothing. One of these patients told me that some offices were not as accepting of their customs as we were. She said that it is considered immodest for a woman to remove clothing in front of any male, even a physician. She told me that if she had to do it, she would just stay sick. ∎

Causes of Illness

Many cultures distinguish between illness caused by bad spirits or evil people and illness with physiologic origins. It is important to not ridicule these theories if patients believe them. When patients feel that health professionals do not respect their beliefs, they may not follow recommendations or return for follow-up care. An open attitude and the willingness to listen to the patient's beliefs are required in order to establish a relationship of trust with the patient.

Fundamentals of scientific medical practice—such as frequent handwashing to remove invisible organisms, taking medicine when one does not feel ill, and causing pain to healthy children by giving them immunizations—may be foreign to certain traditional practices.

Treatments and Traditional Practices

When patients have different beliefs, it is important for all members of the health care team to keep the lines of communication open. Patients need to be able to discuss other treatments that are being used. They also need to understand the importance of the treatments being offered by scientific medicine so that they can comply with standard medical treatment regimens in addition to their traditional practices.

As a general rule, the medical assistant should accept any traditional practice that is not dangerous. For example, some patients from Cambodia and other parts of Southeast Asia believe that rubbing the skin with the side of a coin dipped in a camphor preparation is a treatment for colds and headaches. This treatment leaves bruises on the skin but does not cause breaks in the skin. A child with bruises from this type of treatment is not a victim of child abuse, but the bruises might look like abuse. The medical assistant should learn about traditional treatments used by patients in the practice where he or she works.

One area in which family and cultural traditions may be strong relates to diet and herbal preparations. In many traditions, certain diseases and conditions are considered "hot" and others are considered "cold." The patient may be advised to either eat or avoid certain foods or to take certain herbal preparations in order to restore balance. If the patient can describe traditional treatments, it will be easier for the physician to identify any practices that might be harmful or that might interfere with prescribed medical treatments.

Behavioral Requirements

In some cultures there are specific behavioral requirements for women and men. There may be cultural norms requiring women to have a male escort when they leave their homes. In some cultures the oldest male in the family must make important decisions. For some individuals there are also cultural requirements prohibiting the removal of clothing, jewelry, and head coverings, even for medical examinations. Medical assistants must learn about cultural norms and respond with acceptance and sensitivity. If necessary, adaptations must be made so that the patient is not forced to violate personal standards.

MEDICAL PRACTICE and the LAW

The Civil Rights Act of 1964 and its amendments require access to federally funded health programs and services for individuals with limited English proficiency (LEP). State laws require similar access for state programs and services. This has been interpreted as a requirement for some translation services to be provided by all government-funded health care providers. These services include consent forms in the languages of the service population and access to qualified medical interpreters either in person or by telephone. Health care providers are also required to provide sign language interpreters if necessary under the provisions of the Americans with Disabilities Act.

The U.S. Department of Health and Human Services also requires translation services before informed consent can be given for medical research. Before enrolling a subject in a medical research program, it is necessary to provide written consent forms in the language that the subject understands and a translator fluent in English. ■

What Would You Do? What Would You *Not* Do? RESPONSES

Case Study 1
Page 59

What Did Nancy Do?
❑ Maintained a warm and accepting posture and a friendly tone of voice.
❑ Used an open response to encourage Jennifer to say more about how she felt about possibly being pregnant.
❑ Identified verbally that Jennifer seemed a little upset.

What Did Nancy Not Do?
❑ Did not immediately congratulate Jennifer or respond as if this was good news.
❑ Did not immediately assume a businesslike tone of voice and ask closed questions to obtain information.
❑ Did not imply that Jennifer was experiencing a different emotion.
❑ Did not act as if the patient had nothing on her mind.
❑ Did not appear to be in a hurry to finish the interview.

What Would You Do/What Would You Not Do?
Review Nancy's response and place a checkmark next to the information you included in your response. List the additional information you included in your response.

_____
_____
_____
_____
_____
_____
_____

Case Study 2
Page 63

What Did Nancy Do?
❑ Made sure that Harold was looking at her when she spoke to him.

What Would You Do? What Would You *Not* Do? RESPONSES—cont'd

❏ Spoke clearly and a little more slowly than usual, using a strong voice.

❏ Asked Harold if his hearing aid was working well for him.

❏ Used gestures to reinforce her directions.

❏ Used short sentences.

❏ Repeated instructions or questions as needed.

What Did Nancy Not Do?

❏ Did not speak so loudly that she was shouting.

❏ Did not express impatience in her tone of voice or body language.

❏ Did not speak in long, complicated sentences.

❏ Did not turn away from the patient and keep talking.

❏ Did not drop her voice at the end of sentences.

What Would You Do/What Would You Not Do?

Review Nancy's response and place a checkmark next to the information you included in your response. List the additional information you included in your response.

_____

_____

_____

_____

_____

_____

Case Study 3
Page 67

What Did Nancy Do?

❏ Expressed to Julie Ann that these symptoms are upsetting.

❏ Agreed that it is a good decision to see the doctor.

❏ Asked Julie Ann to describe the emotions she was experiencing during these episodes.

❏ Maintained an open, friendly, and calm demeanor during the interview.

What Did Nancy Not Do?

❏ Did not try to identify the cause of the episodes for Julie Ann.

❏ Did not rush through the interview so that the patient would be ready for the physician quickly.

❏ Did not say, "It's probably just anxiety."

❏ Did not say that there was probably nothing seriously the matter with Julie Ann.

What Would You Do/What Would You Not Do?

Review Nancy's response and place a checkmark next to the information you included in your response. List the additional information you included in your response.

_____

_____

_____

_____

_____

↻ TERMINOLOGY REVIEW

Medical Term	Word Parts	Definition
Active listening		Paying close attention to a speaker without thinking of anything else.
Anxiety		A vague, unpleasant emotion of fear or dread often accompanied by restlessness or nervousness.
Body language		Communication that is expressed through facial expressions, body position, muscle activity, and other nonverbal means.
Chronic		Existing over a long period of time.
Closed questions		Questions that anticipate a yes or no or a short answer.
Denial		Failure to acknowledge the reality of a situation.
Ego defense mechanism		Unconscious mental process that offers psychological protection.
Empathy		Objective awareness and sensitivity to the feelings and emotions of others.
Hierarchy		Classified according to rank or importance.
Hospice		An organization that manages care for dying patients including comfort, pain relief, and personal care.
Judgmental		Critical or negative; making judgments about what is good or bad based on personal opinion.
Nonverbal	*non-*: not *verbum*: word *-al*: pertaining to	Communication that occurs without words, such as through body posture or facial expression.

Continued

TERMINOLOGY REVIEW—cont'd

Medical Term	Word Parts	Definition
Open questions		Questions that could have a variety of answers and encourage a personal response.
Oral	*os (gen. oris):* mouth *-al:* pertaining to	Spoken; pertaining to the mouth.
Paraphrasing		A restatement of the words of another, often to clarify meaning.
Physiologic	*physis:* nature *logia:* study *-ic:* pertaining to	Pertaining to body processes.
Projection		Experiencing one's own emotions as those of another.
Reflecting		Expressing the meaning and emotion of another's words back to the person.
Self-actualization		The fulfillment of each individual's potential.
Summarizing		Expressing the most important points of a conversation or written document.
Sympathy		Feeling the same emotions as another.
Terminal phase		The last stage of illness, usually used when death is expected to occur within 6 months.
Verbal	*verbum:* word *-al:* pertaining to	Using words to communicate.
Webcam		Small video camera attached to a computer that allows video to be transmitted on the Internet.

ON THE WEB

For information on multicultural resources:

U.S. National Library of Medicine—Multi-Cultural Resources for Health Information: sis.nlm.nih.gov/outreach/multicultural.html

For information on hearing impairment:

National Association of the Deaf: www.nad.org

For information on limited English proficiency:

Department of Health and Human Services Office for Civil Rights: Limited English Proficiency (LEP): http://www.hhs.gov/ocr/civilrights/resources/specialtopics/lep

For information on psychology:

American Psychological Association: www.apa.org

Social Psychology Network: www.socialpsychology.org

For information on vision impairment:

American Foundation for the Blind: www.afb.org

The Blind Reader's Page: blindreaders.info

 Check out the Evolve site at http://evolve.elsevier.com/Bonewit/today/ to actively Prepare for your Certification, and to access additional interactive activities and exercises to help you study and prepare for success.

5

Introduction to Anatomy and Physiology

LEARNING OBJECTIVES

1. Explain why it is important for the medical assistant to be knowledgeable about anatomy and physiology.
2. Explain the relationship between anatomy and physiology.
3. State the six levels of organization within the human body.
4. List the 11 organ systems of the body, and describe the function of each.
5. Describe homeostasis and its importance to the human body.
6. Explain how the body maintains homeostasis using a negative feedback system.
7. List the four criteria used to describe the anatomic position.
8. Identify body planes, body regions, and relative positions using anatomic terms.
9. Distinguish between the dorsal body cavity and the ventral body cavity, and list the subdivisions of each cavity.
10. Describe the cell membrane.
11. Describe the composition of the cytoplasm.
12. Describe the components of the nucleus, and state the function of each component.
13. Identify and describe each of the cytoplasmic organelles, and state the function of each organelle.
14. Explain how the cell membrane regulates the composition of the cytoplasm.
15. Describe the various mechanisms that result in the transport of substances across the cell membrane.
16. List the phases of a cell cycle, and describe the events that occur in each phase.
17. Explain the difference between mitosis and meiosis.
18. List the four main types of tissues found in the body.
19. Describe the various types of epithelial tissues in terms of structure, location, and function.
20. Describe the general characteristics of connective tissue.
21. List three types of connective tissue cells, and state the function of each.
22. Describe the features and location of the various types of connective tissue.
23. Explain the differences among skeletal muscle, smooth muscle, and cardiac muscle in terms of structure, location, and control.
24. State the two categories of cells in nerve tissue, and explain their function.

CHAPTER OUTLINE

A Brief Summary of Medical History
THE HUMAN BODY
Anatomy and Physiology
Levels of Organization
Organ Systems
Homeostasis
Anatomic Terms

Cell Structure and Function
Structure of the Generalized Cell
Cell Functions
Tissues and Membranes
Body Tissues
Body Membranes

KEY TERMS

active transport (AK-tiv TRANS-port)

anatomic position (an-ah-TOM-ik poh-ZIH-shun)

chondrocyte (KON-droh-syte)

collagenous fiber (koh-LAJ-eh-nuss FYE-bur)

cytokinesis (sye-toh-kih-NEE-sis)

diffusion (dif-YOO-zhun)

elastic fiber (ee-LAS-tick FYE-bur)

fibroblast (FYE-broh-blast)

histology (hiss-TAHL-oh-jee)

homeostasis (hoh-mee-oh-STAY-sis)

human anatomy (ah-NAT-o-mee)

human physiology (fiz-ee-AHL-oh-jee)

macrophage (MAK-roh-fayj)

mast cell (MAST SELL)

meiosis (mye-OH-sis)

metabolism (meh-TAB-oh-lizm)

mitosis (mye-TOH-sis)

negative feedback (NEG-ah-tiv FEED-bak)

neuroglia (noo-ROG-lee-ah)

neuron (NOO-ron)

osmosis (os-MOH-sis)

osteocyte (AH-stee-oh-syte)

passive transport (PASS-iv TRANS-port)

phagocytosis (fag-oh-sye-TOH-sis)

pinocytosis (pin-oh-sye-TOH-sis)

tissue (TISH-yoo)

A BRIEF SUMMARY OF MEDICAL HISTORY

Studies of illness and aging of the human body are major components in the field of medicine. The study of "modern" medicine began in the fifth century BC.

Hippocrates, who was born in approximately 460 BC on the island of Cos, Greece, is recognized as the "Father of Medicine." After his death, all the existing writings on medicine were gathered into a work called the *Hippocratic Collection* and attributed to him whether he wrote them or not. The Hippocratic Oath, which is still in use today, is from the *Collection*. Hippocrates concluded that illness had rational explanations instead of being caused by evil spirits or disfavor of the gods. This freed medicine from superstition and allowed for scientific study.

In 1249, Roger Bacon invented eyeglasses, bringing better vision to many. Leonardo da Vinci advanced the understanding of human anatomy by carefully dissecting corpses and making detailed anatomic drawings during the fifteenth century. William Harvey published *An Anatomical Essay on the Motion of the Heart and Blood in Animals* in 1628, detailing how blood was pumped from the heart throughout the body and then returned to the heart and recirculated. This work showed that food was not converted into blood by the liver and then consumed as fuel by the body, as was widely alleged at that time.

A Dutch cloth merchant, Antony van Leeuwenhoek discovered blood cells in 1670. This discovery was made possible by his microscope. Although the microscope had been invented by Robert Hooke a few years earlier, van Leeuwenhoek, by grinding his own glass lenses, greatly improved the microscope's design and achieved magnifications of greater than 270 diameters. He also observed bacteria, yeast cells, spermatozoa, and protozoa. In addition, his microscope allowed capillaries to be observed, thus showing the link between arteries and veins and confirming Harvey's theory of blood circulation.

Edward Jenner, an English microbiologist, is known as the "Father of Immunology." He observed that people who had contracted cowpox seemed immune to the deadly smallpox. He theorized that deliberately infecting people with cowpox would protect them from smallpox. He tested his theory on a young boy in 1796 and then demonstrated that the lad was indeed immune to smallpox.

William Beaumont, while serving as an army post surgeon, treated a patient who had been blasted by a musket at close range. The resulting large wound affected part of his lung, two ribs, and his stomach. Beaumont treated the wounds but was unable to get the hole in the stomach to completely close; repeated bandaging was required to prevent food and drink from coming out. He quickly realized this was an opportunity to study the digestion process. He tied small pieces of food with silk string and dangled them through the hole in the patient's stomach, removing the items at 1-hour intervals. He published his observations in 1833.

Medicine truly came of age during the second half of the nineteenth century. Louis Pasteur and Robert Koch established the germ theory of disease. Florence Nightingale showed the importance of hygiene and sanitation to reduce hospital infections. Sir Humphry Davy discovered the anesthetic properties of nitrous oxide, and Joseph Lister pioneered the use of carbolic acid as an antiseptic to clean wounds and surgical instruments. His antiseptic technique reduced deaths from infection after surgery from about 60% to under 4%. Then in 1895 a German scientist named Wilhelm Roentgen discovered the x-ray. Medicine has never been the same since.

The twentieth century continued to build on all these discoveries. The pharmaceutical industry mushroomed with the development of thousands of new medicines. Vaccines were developed to prevent polio, measles, mumps, and many other diseases. Cardiac pacemakers and defibrillators were invented. Medical imaging advanced with the development of computed tomography (CT), magnetic resonance imaging (MRI), positron emission tomography (PET), ultrasound, and many other techniques. Numerous advances occurred in surgery, including open-heart surgery and organ transplants. Radiation therapy and chemotherapy for the treatment of cancer were developed. Kidney dialysis machines were invented, and hospital intensive care units (ICUs) were established to better treat very sick patients. The list of medical advances goes on and on and is added to every year.

THE HUMAN BODY

The human body is an awesome masterpiece. Imagine billions of microscopic parts, each with its own identity, working together in an organized manner for the benefit of the total being. The human body is more complex than the greatest computer, yet it is personal. The study of the human body is as old as history itself because people have always had an interest in how the body is put together, how it works, why it becomes defective (illness), and why it wears out (aging).

The study of the human body is essential for those planning a career in health sciences, just as knowledge about automobiles is necessary for those planning to repair them. How can you fix an automobile if you do not know how it is put together or how it works? How can you help fix a human body if you do not know how it is put together or how it works?

Anatomy and Physiology

Human anatomy is the study of the shape and structure of the human body and its parts. It encompasses a wide range of study, including the development and microscopic organization of structures, the relationship between structures, and the interrelationship between structure and function. **Gross human anatomy** deals with the large structures of the human body that can be seen through normal dissection. **Microscopic anatomy** deals with the smaller structures and fine detail that can be seen only with the aid of a microscope.

Human physiology is the scientific study of the functions or processes of the human body. It answers how, what, and why anatomic parts work. Anatomy and physiology are interrelated because structure and function are always closely associated. The function of an organ, or how it works, depends on how it is put together. Conversely, the anatomy or structure provides clues to understanding how it works. The structure of the hand, with its long, jointed fingers, is related to its function of grasping things. The heart is designed as a muscular pump that can contract to force blood into the blood vessels. By contrast, lungs are made of a thin tissue and function to exchange oxygen and carbon dioxide between the outside environment and the blood. Imagine what would happen if the heart were made of thin tissue and the lungs were made of thick muscle. Structure and function are always related.

Levels of Organization

Among the most outstanding features of the complex human body are its order and organization—how all the parts, from tiny cells to visible organs, work together to make a functioning whole. The organizational scheme of the body has six levels (Figure 5-1).

Starting with the simplest and proceeding to the most complex, the six levels of organization are chemical, cellular, tissue, organ, body system, and total organism. The structural and functional characteristics of all organisms are determined by their chemical makeup.

Chemical Level The *chemical level* deals with the interactions of atoms, such as hydrogen and oxygen, and their combinations into molecules, such as water. Molecules contribute to the makeup of a cell, which is the basic unit of life.

Cells *Cells*, discussed later in this chapter, are the basic living units of all organisms. Estimates indicate that there are about 75 trillion dynamic, living cells in the human body. These cells represent a variety of sizes, shapes, and structures and provide a vast array of functions.

Tissues Cells with similar structure and function are grouped together as *tissues*. All of the tissues of the body are grouped into four main types: epithelial, connective, muscle, and nervous. The tissue level of organization is discussed later in this chapter.

Organs Two or more tissue types that form a more complex structure and work together to perform one or more functions make up *organs*, the next higher level of organization. Examples of organs include the skin, heart, ear, stomach, and liver.

Body Systems A *body system* consists of several organs that work together to accomplish a set of functions. Some examples of body systems include the nervous system, the digestive system, and the respiratory system.

Total Organism Finally, the most complex of all the levels is the *total organism,* which is made up of several systems that work together to maintain life.

Organ Systems

The human body has 11 major organ systems, each with specific functions, yet all are interrelated and work together to sustain life. Each system is described briefly here and then in more detail in later chapters. The organ systems are illustrated and summarized in Table 5-1.

Integumentary System *Integument* means skin. The integumentary (in-teg-yoo-MEN-tar-ee) system consists of the skin and the various accessory organs associated with it. These accessories include hair, nails, sweat glands, and sebaceous (oil) glands. The components of the integumentary system protect the underlying tissues from injury, protect against water loss, contain sense receptors, help in temperature regulation, and synthesize chemicals to be used in other parts of the body.

Skeletal System The skeletal (SKEL-eh-tull) system forms the framework of the body and protects underlying organs, such as the brain, lungs, and heart. It consists of the

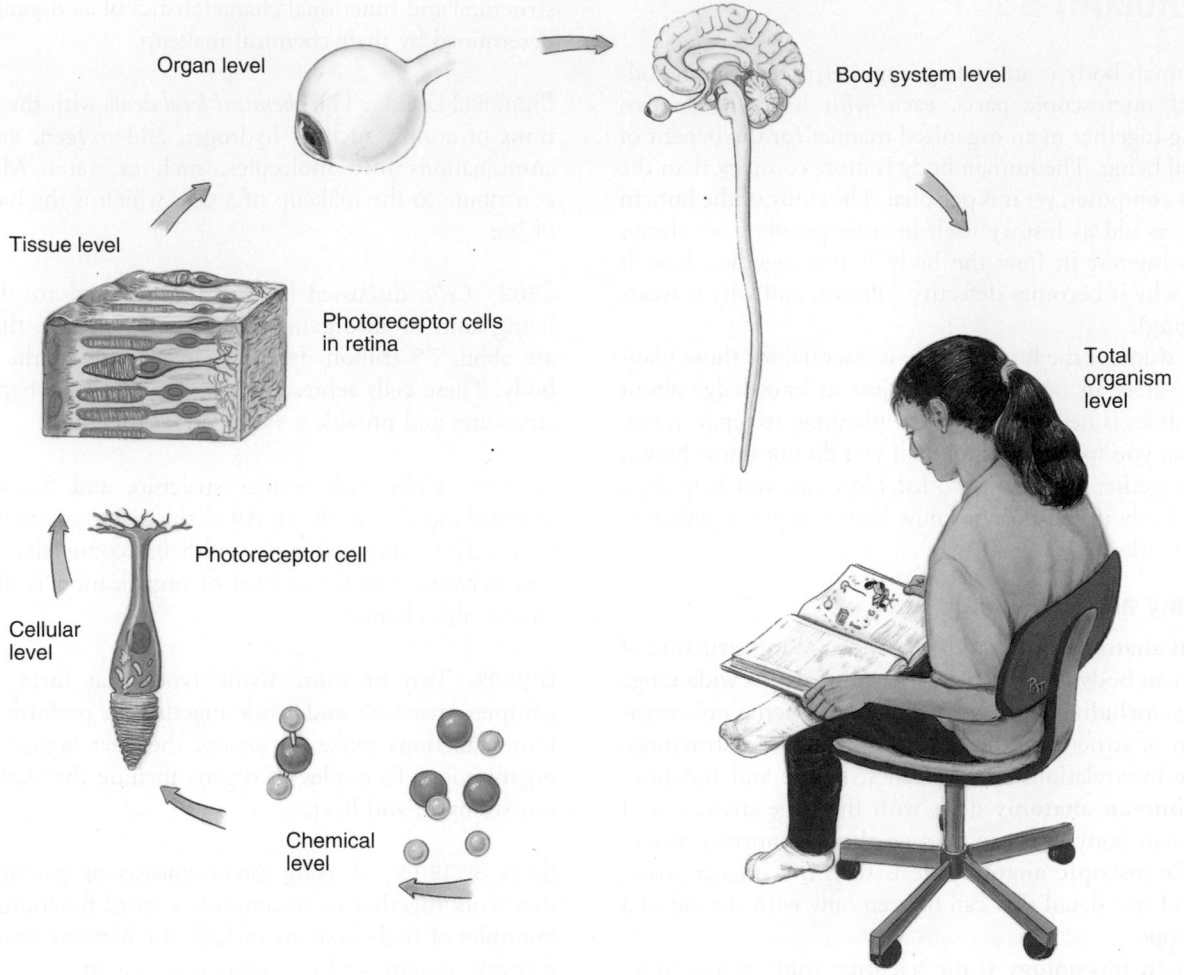

Organ level

Tissue level

Photoreceptor cells
in retina

Body system level

Total
organism
level

Photoreceptor cell

Cellular
level

Chemical
level

Figure 5-1 Organizational scheme of the body. From simple to complex, the levels are chemical, cellular, tissue, organ, body system, and total organism.

bones and joints along with ligaments and cartilage that bind the bones together. Bones serve as attachments for muscles and act with the muscles to produce movement. Tissues within bones produce blood cells and store inorganic salts containing calcium and phosphorus.

Muscular System   Muscles are the organs of the muscular (MUS-kyoo-lar) system. As muscles contract, they create the forces that produce movement and maintain posture. Muscles can store energy in the form of glycogen and are the primary source of heat within the body.

Nervous System   The nervous (NER-vus) system consists of the brain, spinal cord, and associated nerves. These organs work together to coordinate body activities. Nerve cells, or neurons, are specialized to transmit impulses from one point to another. In this way, body parts can communicate with each other and with the outside environment. Some nerve cells have special endings called *sense receptors* that detect changes in the environment.

Endocrine System   The endocrine (EN-doh-krin) system includes all the glands that secrete chemicals called *hormones*. These hormones travel through the blood and act as messengers to regulate cellular activities. The endocrine and nervous systems work together to coordinate and regulate body activities to maintain a proper balance. The nervous system typically acts quickly, whereas the endocrine system acts slowly but with a more sustained effect. The endocrine system also regulates reproductive functions in both males and females.

Cardiovascular System   The cardiovascular (kar-dee-oh-VAS-kyoo-lar) system consists of the blood, heart, and blood vessels. The blood transports nutrients, hormones, and oxygen to tissue cells and removes waste products such as carbon dioxide. Certain cells within the blood known as *white blood cells* defend the body against disease. The heart acts as a pump to create the forces necessary to maintain blood pressure and to circulate the blood. The blood vessels serve as pipes or conduits for the flow of blood.

Table 5-1 Organ Systems of the Body

Integumentary System	Skeletal System	Muscular System
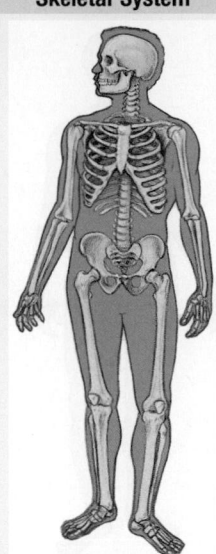		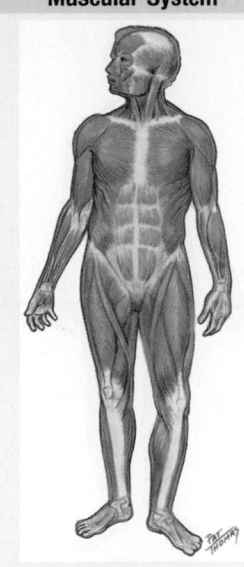
COMPONENTS: Skin, hair, nails, sweat, sebaceous glands	COMPONENTS: Bones, cartilage, ligaments	COMPONENTS: Muscles
FUNCTIONS: Covers and protects body; regulates temperature	FUNCTIONS: Provides body framework and support; protects; attaches muscles to bones; provides calcium storage	FUNCTIONS: Produces movement; maintains posture; provides heat

Nervous System	Endocrine System	Cardiovascular System
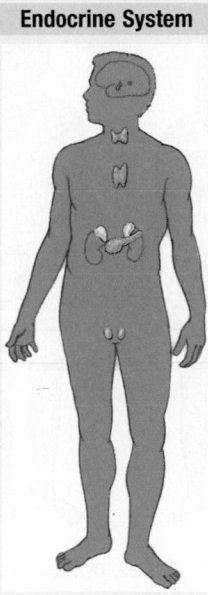		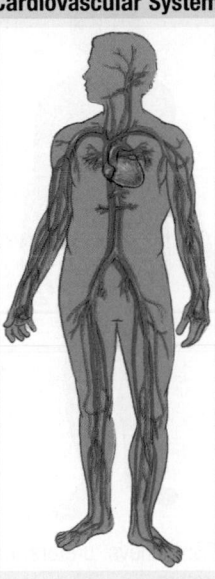
COMPONENTS: Brain, spinal cord, nerves, sense receptors	COMPONENTS: Pituitary, adrenal, thyroid, other ductless glands	COMPONENTS: Heart, blood vessels, blood
FUNCTIONS: Coordinates body activities; receives and transmits stimuli	FUNCTIONS: Regulates metabolic activities and body chemistry	FUNCTIONS: Transports material from one part of the body to another; defends against disease

Continued

Lymphatic System The lymphatic (lim-FAT-ik) system consists of a series of vessels that transport a fluid called *lymph* from the tissues back into the blood. In addition to lymph, the system includes lymph nodes and lymphoid organs, such as the tonsils, spleen, and thymus, that filter the lymph to remove foreign particles as a protection against disease. Lymphoid organs also function in the body's defense mechanism by enhancing the activities of cells that inactivate specific pathogenic agents. The lymphatic system is sometimes considered to be a part of the cardiovascular system.

Table 5-1   Organ Systems of the Body—cont'd

Lymphatic System	Digestive System	Respiratory System
COMPONENTS: Lymph, lymph vessels, lymphoid organs	COMPONENTS: Mouth, esophagus, stomach, intestines, liver, pancreas	COMPONENTS: Air passageways, lungs
FUNCTIONS: Returns tissue fluid to the blood; defends against disease	FUNCTIONS: Ingests and digests food; absorbs nutrients into blood	FUNCTIONS: Exchanges gases between blood and external environment

Urinary System	Reproductive System
COMPONENTS: Kidneys, ureters, urinary bladder, urethra	COMPONENTS: Testes, ovaries, accessory structures
FUNCTIONS: Excretes metabolic wastes; regulates fluid balance and acid-base balance	FUNCTIONS: Forms new individuals to provide continuation of the human species

From Applegate E: *The anatomy and physiology learning system,* ed 4, St Louis, 2011, Saunders.

Digestive System   The organs of the digestive (dye-JES-tiv) system include the mouth, pharynx, esophagus, stomach, small intestine, and large intestine (colon), which make up the digestive tract. Accessory organs of this system include the teeth, tongue, salivary glands, liver, gallbladder, and pancreas. The functions of this system are to ingest

food, process it into molecules that can be used by the body, and then eliminate the residue.

Respiratory System   The respiratory (reh-SPY-rah-tor-ee or res-per-ah-TOR-ee) system brings oxygen, in the form of air, into the lungs; removes the carbon dioxide; and provides a membrane for the exchange of these gases between the blood and lungs. The system consists of the nasal cavities, pharynx, larynx, trachea, bronchi, and lungs.

Urinary System The kidneys, ureters, urinary bladder, and urethra make up the urinary (YOO-rin-air-ee) system. The kidneys remove various waste materials, especially nitrogenous wastes, from the blood and help to regulate the fluid level and chemical content of the body. The product of kidney function is urine, which is transported through the ureters and urethra. The urinary bladder serves as a reservoir or storage area for the urine.

Reproductive System The purpose of the reproductive (ree-pro-DUK-tiv) system is the production of new individuals. The primary organs of the system are the gonads, which produce the reproductive cells. These are the ovaries in the female and testes in the male. In addition to gonads, there are accessory glands, supporting structures, and duct systems for the transport of the reproductive cells. In the female the reproductive system produces ova or eggs, receives sperm from the male, and provides for the support and development of the embryo and fetus. The male reproductive system is concerned with the production and maintenance of sperm and the transfer of these cells to the female.

Homeostasis

Homeostasis refers to the constant internal environment that must be maintained for the cells of the body. The word is derived from two Greek words: *homeo,* which means "alike" or "the same," and *stasis,* which means "always" or "staying." Putting these together, the word *homeostasis* means "staying the same." When the body is healthy, the internal environment always stays the same. It remains stable within limited normal ranges.

Everyone is familiar with aspects of the external environment—whether it is cold or hot, humid or dry, smoggy or clear. The internal environment is not quite as obvious. It involves the tissue fluid that surrounds and bathes every cell of the body. Normal functional activities of the cell depend on the internal environment being maintained within limited normal ranges. The chemical content, volume, temperature, and pressure of the fluid must stay the same (homeostasis), regardless of external conditions, so that the cell can function properly. If the conditions in the tissue fluid deviate from normal, mechanisms respond that try to restore conditions to normal. If the mechanisms are unsuccessful, the cell malfunctions and dies. This leads to illness and disease. Ultimately the goal of medical treatment is to restore homeostasis.

Negative and Positive Feedback

Any condition or stimulus that disrupts the homeostatic balance in the body is a *stressor.* When a stressor causes internal conditions to deviate from normal, all the body systems work to bring conditions back to the normal range.

This is usually accomplished by a **negative feedback** mechanism in which a stimulus initiates reactions that reduce the stimulus. This mechanism works similarly to a thermostat connected to a furnace and an air conditioner. When the temperature in the room decreases (stressor) below the thermostat setting (normal), the sensing device in the thermostat detects the change and causes the furnace to add heat to the room. When the room becomes too warm, the furnace stops and the air conditioner begins to cool the room. Negative feedback mechanisms do not prevent variation, but they keep variation within a normal range.

An example of a physiologic negative feedback mechanism in the human body involves blood pressure. When blood pressure decreases below normal, body sensors detect the deviation and initiate changes that bring the pressure back within the normal range. When the pressure increases above normal, changes occur to decrease the pressure to normal. Variations in blood pressure occur, but homeostatic mechanisms keep them within the limits of a normal range.

The nervous and endocrine systems work together to control homeostasis, but all the organ systems in the body help maintain the normal conditions of the internal environment. The brain contains centers that monitor temperature, pressure, volume, and the chemical conditions of body fluids. Endocrine glands secrete hormones in response to deviations from normal conditions, and these hormones affect other organs. The changes required to bring conditions back to the normal range are mediated by various organ systems. Good health depends on homeostasis. Illness results when the negative feedback mechanisms that maintain homeostasis are disrupted. Medical therapy attempts to assist the negative feedback process to restore balance, or homeostasis.

Anatomic Terms

Certain basic terms need to be understood to communicate effectively in the health care profession. In other words, you have to speak the language. This section explains some basic terms that relate to the anatomy of the body. They are used to describe directions and regions of the body.

Anatomic Position

If directional terms are to be meaningful, there must be some knowledge of the beginning position. If you give a person directions to go somewhere, you must have a starting reference point. When using directions in anatomy and physiology, it is assumed that the body is in **anatomic position.** In this position, the body is standing erect, the face is forward, and the arms are at the sides with the palms and toes directed forward. Figure 5-2 illustrates the body in anatomic position.

Directions in the Body

Directional terms are used to describe the relative position of one part to another. Note that in the following list of directional terms, the two items in each pair of terms are opposites.

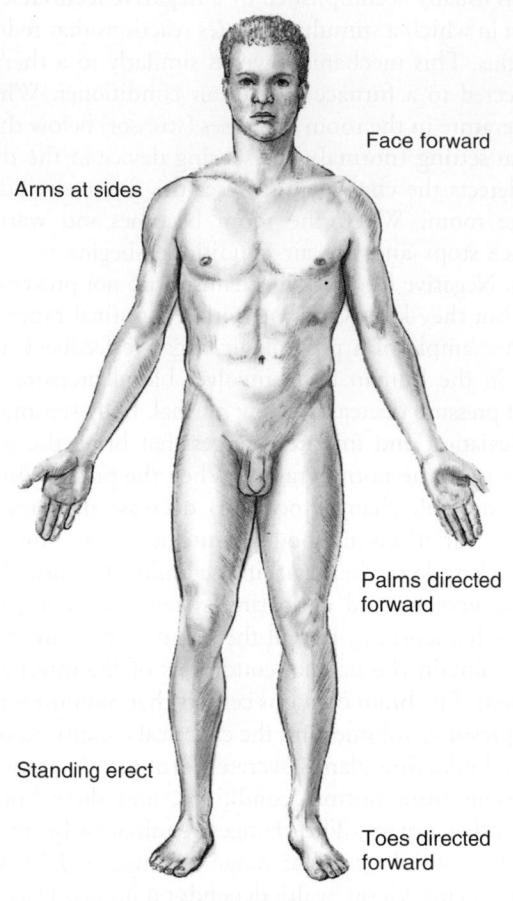

Face forward

Arms at sides

Palms directed
forward

Standing erect

Toes directed
forward

Figure 5-2 The body in anatomic position.

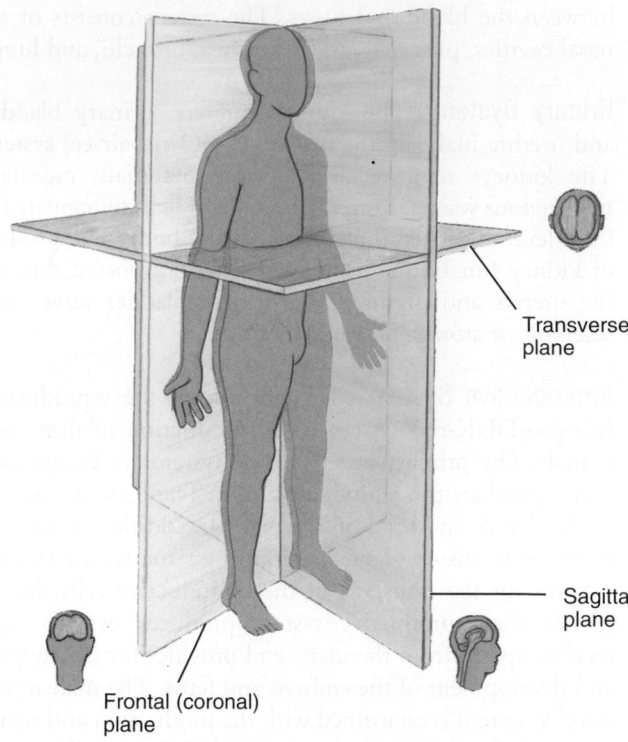

Transverse
plane

Sagittal
plane

Frontal (coronal)
plane

Figure 5-3 Transverse, sagittal, and frontal planes of the body.

Superior means that a part is above another part, or closer to the head. The nose is superior to the mouth. *Inferior* means that a part is below another part, or closer to the feet. The heart is inferior to the neck.

Anterior (or ventral) means toward the front surface. The heart is anterior to the vertebral column. *Posterior* means that a part is toward the back. The heart is posterior to the sternum.

Medial means toward, or nearer, the midline of the body. The nose is medial to the ears. *Lateral* means toward, or nearer, the side, away from the midline. The ears are lateral to the eyes.

Proximal means that a part is closer to a point of attachment, or closer to the trunk of the body, than another part. The elbow is proximal to the wrist. The opposite of proximal is *distal*, which means that a part is farther away from a point of attachment than is another part. The fingers are distal to the wrist.

Superficial means that a part is located on or near the surface. The superficial (or outermost) layer of the skin is the epidermis. The opposite of superficial is *deep*, which means that a part is away from the surface. Muscles are deep to the skin.

Visceral pertains to internal organs or the covering of the organs. The visceral pericardium covers the heart. *Parietal* refers to the wall of a body cavity. The parietal peritoneum lines the wall of the abdominal cavity.

Planes and Sections of the Body

To aid in visualizing the spatial relationships of internal body parts, anatomists use three imaginary planes, each of which is cut through the body in a different direction. Figure 5-3 illustrates these three planes.

The *sagittal* plane refers to a lengthwise cut that divides the body into right and left portions. This is sometimes called a *longitudinal section*. If the cut passes through the midline of the body, it is called a *midsagittal plane,* and it divides the body into right and left halves.

The *transverse plane* or horizontal plane is perpendicular to the sagittal plane and cuts across the body horizontally to divide it into superior and inferior portions. Sections cut this way are sometimes called *cross sections*.

The *frontal plane* divides the body into anterior and posterior portions. It is perpendicular to both the sagittal plane and the transverse plane. This is sometimes called a *coronal plane*.

Body Cavities

Spaces within the body that contain the internal organs or viscera are called *body cavities*. The two main cavities are the *dorsal cavity* and the larger *ventral cavity,* which are

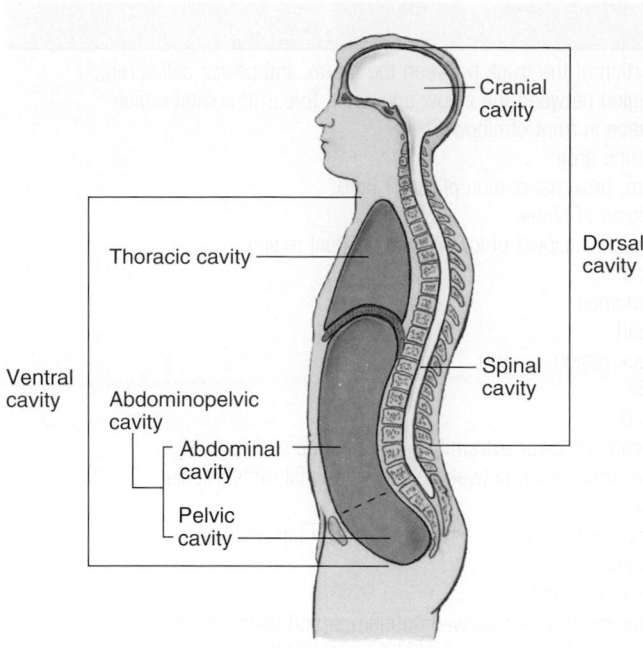

Figure 5-4 The two major cavities in the body and their subdivisions.

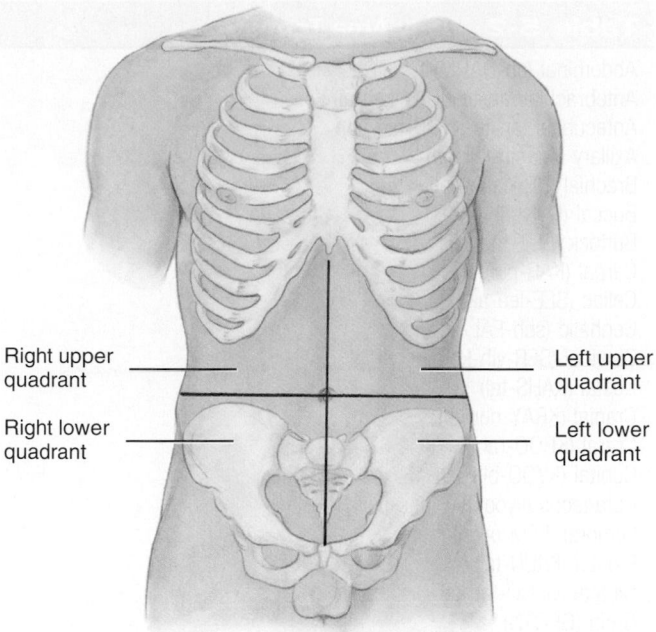

Figure 5-5 Abdominopelvic quadrants that are formed by a midsagittal plane and a transverse plane through the umbilicus.

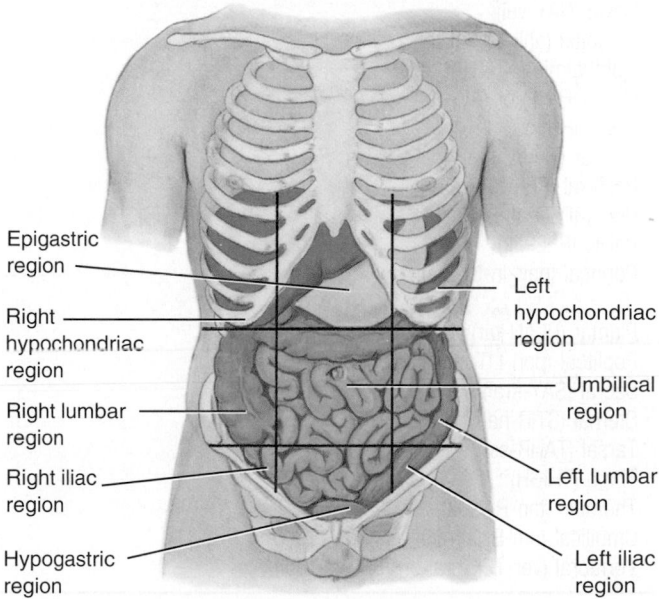

Figure 5-6 Nine abdominopelvic regions formed by two sagittal planes and two transverse planes.

illustrated in Figure 5-4. The dorsal cavity is divided into the *cranial cavity,* which contains the brain, and the *spinal cavity,* which contains the spinal cord. The cranial and spinal cavities join with each other to form a continuous space.

The ventral cavity is much larger than the dorsal cavity and is subdivided into the *thoracic* (tho-RAS-ik) *cavity* and the *abdominopelvic* (ab-dahm-ih-noh-PEL-vik) *cavity.* The thoracic cavity is superior to the abdominopelvic cavity and contains the heart, lungs, esophagus, and trachea. It is separated from the abdominopelvic cavity by the muscular diaphragm. Although there is no clear-cut partition to divide it, the abdominopelvic cavity is separated into the *superior abdominal cavity* and the *inferior pelvic cavity.* The stomach, liver, gallbladder, spleen, and most of the intestines are in the abdominal cavity. The pelvic cavity contains portions of the small and large intestines, the rectum, the urinary bladder, and the internal reproductive organs.

To help describe the location of body organs or pain, health care professionals frequently divide the abdominopelvic cavity into regions using imaginary lines. One such method uses the midsagittal plane and a transverse plane that passes through the umbilicus. This divides the abdominopelvic area into four quadrants, illustrated in Figure 5-5. Another system uses two sagittal planes and two transverse planes to divide the abdominopelvic area into the nine regions illustrated in Figure 5-6. The three central regions are, from superior to inferior, the *epigastric* (ep-ih-GAS-trik), *umbilical* (um-BIL-ih-kal), and *hypogastric* (hye-poh-GAS-trik) regions. Lateral to these, from superior to inferior, are the right and left *hypochondriac* (hye-poh-KAHN-dree-

ak), right and left *lumbar,* and right and left *iliac* (ILL-ee-ak) or *inguinal* (IN-gwih-nal) regions.

Regions of the Body

The body may be divided into the *axial* (AK-see-al) portion, which consists of the head, neck, and trunk, and the *appendicular* (ap-pen-DIK-yoo-lar) portion, which consists of the limbs. The trunk, or *torso,* includes the thorax, abdomen,

Table 5-2   Body Area Terms

Abdominal (ab-DAHM-ih-nal)	Portion of the trunk between the thorax and pelvis; celiac region
Antebrachial (an-te-BRAY-kee-al)	Region between the elbow and wrist; forearm; cubital region
Antecubital (an-te-KYOO-bih-tal)	Space in front of elbow
Axillary (AK-sih-lair-ee)	Armpit area
Brachial (BRAY-kee-al)	Arm; proximal portion of upper limb
Buccal (BUK-al)	Region of cheek
Buttock (BUT-tuck)	Posterior aspect of lower trunk; gluteal region
Carpal (KAR-pal)	Wrist
Celiac (SEE-lee-ak)	Abdomen
Cephalic (seh-FAL-ik)	Head
Cervical (SER-vih-kal)	Neck region
Costal (KAHS-tal)	Ribs
Cranial (KRAY-nee-al)	Skull
Crural (KROO-rahl)	Portion of lower extremity between knee and foot; leg
Cubital (KYOO-bih-tal)	Forearm; region between elbow and wrist; antebrachial
Cutaneous (kyoo-TAY-nee-us)	Skin
Femoral (FEM-or-al)	Thigh; part of lower extremity between hip and knee
Frontal (FRUN-tal)	Forehead
Gluteal (GLOO-tee-al)	Buttock region
Groin (GROYN)	Depressed region between abdomen and thigh; inguinal
Inguinal (IN-gwih-nal)	Depressed region between abdomen and thigh; groin
Leg (LEG)	Portion of lower extremity between knee and foot; also called *crural* region
Lumbar (LUM-bar)	Region of lower back and side between lowest rib and pelvis
Mammary (MAM-ah-ree)	Pertaining to the breast
Navel (NAY-vel)	Middle region of abdomen; umbilical region
Occipital (ahk-SIP-ih-tal)	Lower portion of the back of the head
Ophthalmic (off-THAL-mik)	Pertaining to the eyes
Oral (OH-ral) or (AW-ral)	Pertaining to the mouth
Otic (OH-tik)	Ears
Palmar (PAWL-mar)	Palm of hand
Pectoral (PEK-toh-ral)	Chest region
Pedal (PED-al)	Foot
Pelvic (PEL-vik)	Inferior region of abdominopelvic cavity
Perineal (pair-ih-NEE-al)	Region between anus and pubic symphysis; includes region of external reproductive organs
Plantar (PLAN-tar)	Sole of foot
Popliteal (pop-LIT-ee-al or pop-lih-TEE-al)	Area behind knee
Sacral (SAY-kral)	Posterior region between hip bones
Sternal (STIR-nal)	Anterior midline of the thorax
Tarsal (TAHR-sal)	Ankle and instep of foot
Thigh (THIGH)	Part of lower extremity between hip and knee; femoral region
Thoracic (tho-RAS-ik)	Chest; part of trunk inferior to neck and superior to diaphragm
Umbilical (um-BIL-ih-kal)	Navel; middle region of abdomen
Vertebral (ver-TEE-bral or VER-teh-bral)	Pertaining to spinal column; backbone

From Applegate E: *The anatomy and physiology learning system,* ed 4, St Louis, 2011, Saunders.

and pelvis. In addition to these terms and the nine abdominopelvic regions identified in the previous section, there are numerous other terms that apply to specific body areas. Some of these are listed in Table 5-2 and are identified in Figure 5-7.

CELL STRUCTURE AND FUNCTION

Structure of the Generalized Cell

Every individual begins life as a single cell, a fertilized egg. This single cell divides into two cells, then four, eight, 16,

and on and on, until the adult human body has an estimated 75 trillion cells. Cells are the structural and functional units of the human body. Homeostasis depends on the interaction between the cell and its environment.

During development, cells become specialized in size, shape, characteristics, and function, resulting in a large variety of cells in the body. For descriptive purposes it is convenient to imagine a typical, generalized cell that contains the components of all the different cell types. Not all the components of a "generalized" cell are present in every cell type, but each component is present in some cells and has its particular function to maintain life. A generalized

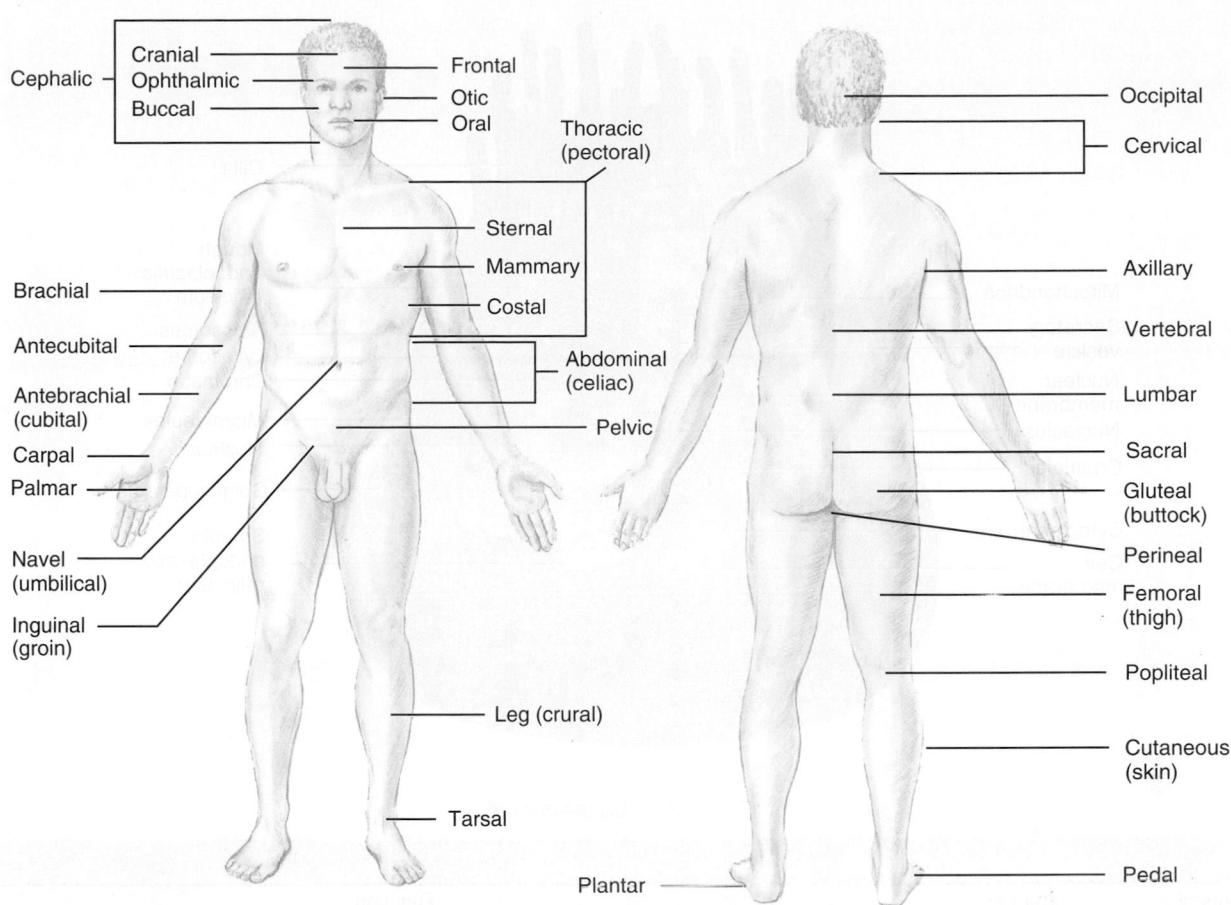

Figure 5-7 Terms for selected regions of the body.

cell is illustrated in Figure 5-8, and the structure and functions of the cellular components are summarized in Table 5-3.

Plasma Membrane

Every cell in the body is enclosed by a *plasma (cell) membrane*. The plasma membrane separates the material outside the cell (extracellular) from the material inside the cell (intracellular). If the membrane breaks, the cell dies. The plasma membrane determines what can go into, or out of, the cell. It is ***selectively permeable***, which means that some substances can pass through the membrane but others cannot. The main structural components of the plasma membrane are *phospholipids* and *proteins.*

Cytoplasm

The *cytoplasm* (SYE-toh-plazm) is the gel-like fluid inside the cell. The cytoplasm has numerous small structures, called *organelles,* suspended in it. These organelles (or-guh-NELZ), or "little organs," are the functional machinery of the cell, and each organelle type has a specific role in the metabolic reactions that take place in the cytoplasm.

The cytoplasm is primarily water known as the **intracellular fluid**. About two thirds of the water in the body is in the cytoplasm of cells. The intracellular fluid contains dissolved electrolytes, metabolic waste products, and nutrients such as amino acids and simple sugars.

Nucleus

The *nucleus* (NOO-klee-us) is the control center that directs the activities of the cell. All cells have at least one nucleus at some time during their existence; some, however, such as red blood cells, lose their nucleus as they mature. Other cells, such as skeletal muscle cells, have multiple nuclei.

The nucleus is a relatively large, spheric body that is usually located near the center of the cell (see Figure 5-8). It is enclosed by a double-layered **nuclear membrane** that separates the cytoplasm of the cell from the **nucleoplasm**, the fluid portion inside the nucleus.

The nucleus contains the genetic material of the cell. In the nondividing cell, the genetic material, deoxyribonucleic acid (DNA), is present as long, slender, filamentous threads called **chromatin** (see Figure 5-8). When the cell starts to divide or replicate, the chromatin condenses and becomes tightly coiled to form short, rodlike **chromosomes**. Each chromosome, composed of DNA with some protein, contains several hundred genes arranged in a specific linear order. Human cells have 23 pairs of chromosomes that

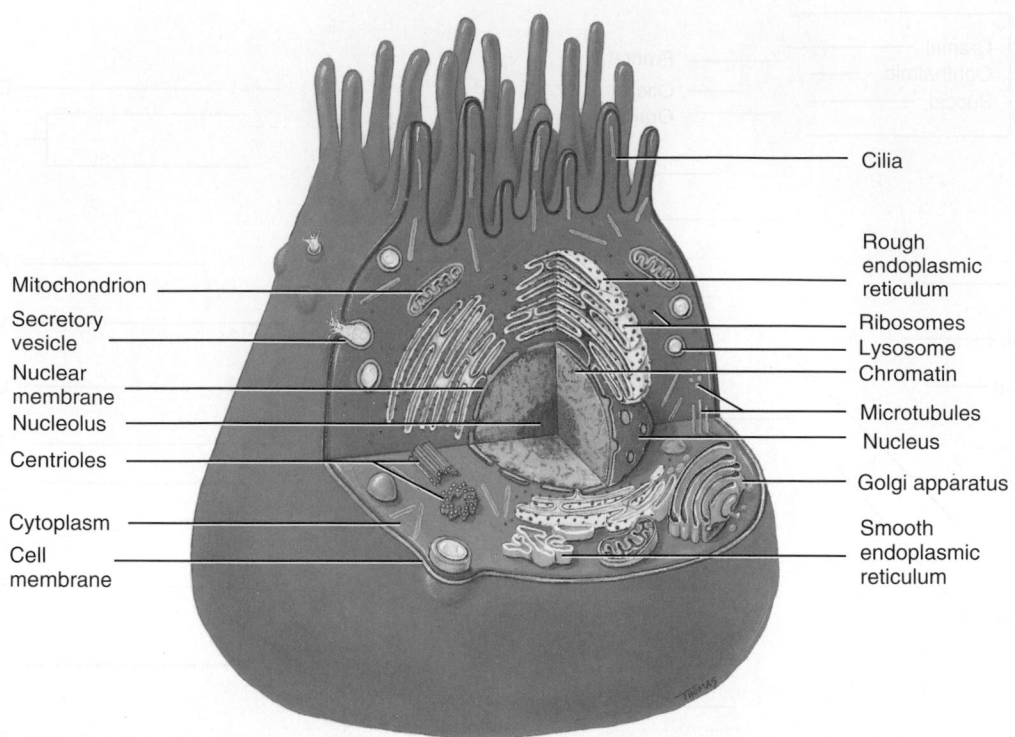

Figure 5-8 Generalized cell.

Table 5-3   Structure and Function of Cellular Components

Component	Structure	Function
Plasma membrane	Bilayer of phospholipid and protein molecules	Maintains integrity of cell; controls passage of materials into and out of cell
Cytoplasm	Water; dissolved ions and nutrients; suspended colloids	Medium for chemical reactions; suspending medium for organelles
Nucleus	Spheric body near center of cell; enclosed in a membrane	Contains genetic material; regulates activities of cell
Nuclear membrane	Double-layered membrane around nucleus; has pores	Separates cytoplasm from nucleoplasm; pores allow passage of material as needed
Chromatin	Strands of DNA in nucleus	Genetic material of cell; becomes chromosomes during cell division
Nucleolus	Dense, nonmembranous body in nucleus; composed of RNA and protein molecules	Forms ribosomes
Mitochondria	Rod-shaped bodies enclosed by a double-layered membrane in cytoplasm; folds of inner membrane form cristae	Major site of adenosine triphosphate synthesis; convert energy from nutrients into a form that is usable by body
Ribosomes	Granules of RNA in cytoplasm	Protein synthesis
Endoplasmic reticulum	Interconnected membranous channels and sacs in cytoplasm	Transports material through cytoplasm; rough endoplasmic reticulum aids in synthesis of protein; smooth endoplasmic reticulum involved in lipid synthesis
Golgi apparatus	Group of flattened membranous sacs usually near nucleus	Packages products for secretion; forms lysosomes
Lysosomes	Membranous sacs of digestive enzymes in cytoplasm	Digest material taken into cell, debris from damaged cells, worn-out cell components
Cytoskeleton	Protein microfilaments and microtubules in cytoplasm	Provides support for cytoplasm; helps in movement of organelles
Centrioles	Pair of rod-shaped bodies composed of microtubules; located near nucleus at right angles to each other	Distribute chromosomes to daughter cells during cell division
Cilia	Membrane-enclosed bundles of microtubules that extend outward from cell membrane; short and numerous	Move substances across surface of cell
Flagella	Similar to cilia, except usually long and single	Cell locomotion

From Applegate E: *The anatomy and physiology learning system,* ed 4, St Louis, 2011, Saunders.

together contain all the information necessary to direct the synthesis of more than 100,000 different proteins.

The **nucleolus** (noo-KLEE-oh-lus) ("little nucleus") appears as a dark-staining, discrete, dense body within the nucleus (see Figure 5-1). It has no enclosing membrane, and the number of nucleoli may vary from one to four in any given cell. The function of the nucleolus is to produce ribonucleic acid (RNA) and combine it with protein to form ribosomes. Ribosomes function in protein synthesis, as described later in this section. In growing cells and other cells that are making large amounts of protein, the nucleoli are large and distinct.

Cytoplasmic Organelles

Cytoplasmic organelles are "little organs" that are suspended in the cytoplasm of the cell. Each type of organelle has a definite structure and a specific role in the function of the cell.

Mitochondria

Mitochondria (mye-toh-KON-dree-ah) are elongated, oval, fluid-filled sacs in the cytoplasm that contain their own DNA and can reproduce themselves (see Figure 5-8). Enzymes necessary for the production of adenosine triphosphate (ATP) are located inside the mitochondria. ATP is a chemical that stores chemical energy within the cell and provides energy for use by the body cells. Mitochondria could be called the "power plant" of the cell because they convert energy from nutrients into ATP.

Ribosomes

Ribosomes (RYE-boh-sohmz) consist of small granules of RNA located in the cytoplasm. The RNA in the ribosomes is from the nucleolus, and when fully assembled, ribosomes function in protein synthesis. Some ribosomes are found free in the cytoplasm. These ribosomes function in the synthesis of proteins for use within that same cell. Other ribosomes are attached to the membranes of the endoplasmic reticulum (ER) and function in the synthesis of proteins that are exported from the cell and used elsewhere.

Endoplasmic Reticulum

The *endoplasmic reticulum* (ER) (end-oh-PLAZ-mik reh-TICK-yoo-lum) is a complex series of membranous channels extending throughout the cytoplasm. The interconnected membranes form fluid-filled flattened sacs and tubular canals. The membranes are connected to the outer layer of the nuclear membrane, to the inner layer of the cell membrane, and to certain other organelles. The ER provides a path to transport materials from one part of the cell to another.

Some of the membranes of the ER have granular ribosomes attached to the outer surface (see Figure 5-8). This is called **rough endoplasmic reticulum** (RER) and, because of the ribosomes, it functions in the synthesis and transport of protein molecules. Other portions of the ER lack the ribosomes and appear smooth. This is the **smooth**

endoplasmic reticulum (SER), which functions in the synthesis of certain lipid molecules, such as steroids.

Golgi Apparatus

The *Golgi apparatus* (GOL-jee ap-ah-RAT-us) is a series of four to six flattened membranous sacs, usually located near the nucleus, and is connected to the ER (see Figure 5-8). It is the "packaging and shipping plant" of the cell.

Proteins and lipids are carried through the channels of the ER to the Golgi apparatus. Within the Golgi apparatus, the proteins become surrounded by a piece of the Golgi membrane. Then they are pinched off the end of the apparatus to become a **secretory vesicle**, a temporary inclusion in the cytoplasm. The secretory vesicles move to the cell membrane and release their contents to the exterior of the cell.

The Golgi apparatus are especially abundant and well developed in glandular cells that secrete a product, but they also function in nonsecretory cells. In these cells they appear to package intracellular enzymes in the form of lysosomes. Because of the vesicles pinching off the ends of the flattened membranous sacs, the Golgi apparatus is sometimes described as looking like a stack of pancakes with syrup dripping off the edge.

Lysosomes

Lysosomes (LYE-soh-sohmz) are membrane-enclosed sacs of various enzymes that have been packaged by the Golgi apparatus. When cells are damaged, these enzymes destroy the cellular debris. They also function in the destruction of worn-out cell parts. The enzymes break down particles, such as bacteria, that have been taken into the cell. When a white blood cell phagocytizes or engulfs bacteria, the enzymes from the lysosomes destroy the bacteria. Lysosomal activity also seems to be responsible for decreasing the size of some body organs at certain periods. Atrophy of muscle because of lack of use, reduction in breast size after breastfeeding, and decrease in the size of the uterus after parturition all seem to be caused by lysosomal function.

Filamentous Protein Organelles

Several types of protein filaments are considered to be cellular organelles. The cytoskeleton and centrioles are in the cytoplasm, but the cilia and flagella project outward, away from the cell surface.

Cytoskeleton

The *cytoskeleton* helps to maintain the shape of the cell. At times it anchors certain organelles in position, but it may also move organelles from one position to another. Some parts of the cytoskeleton may move a portion of the cell membrane, whereas others may move the entire cell. The cytoskeleton also plays a role in muscle contraction.

The cytoskeleton is made up of protein **microfilaments** and **microtubules**. Microfilaments are long, slender rods of protein that support small projections of the cell membrane called *microvilli*. Microtubules are thin cylinders, larger than the microfilaments. In addition to their role as part of the cytoskeleton, microtubules are also found in centrioles, cilia, and flagella.

Centrioles

A dense area called the *centrosome* (SEN-troh-sohm), located near the nucleus, contains a pair of *centrioles* (SEN-tree-ohlz) (see Figure 5-8). Each centriole is a nonmembranous rod-shaped structure composed of microtubules. The two members of the pair are at right angles to each other. Centrioles function in cell reproduction by aiding in the distribution of chromosomes to the new daughter cells.

Cilia

Cilia (SIL-ee-ah) are short, cylindric, hairlike processes that project outward from the cell membrane. Each cilium consists of specialized microtubules surrounded by a membrane and anchored under the cell membrane. Cilia have an organized pattern of movement that creates a wavelike motion to move substances across the surface of the cell. They are found in large quantities on the surfaces of cells that line the respiratory tract. Their motion moves mucus, in which particles of dust are embedded, upward and away from the lungs.

Flagella

Similar in structure to cilia, *flagella* (fluh-JELL-ah) are much longer and fewer. In contrast to cilia, which move substances across the surface of the cell, flagella beat with a whiplike motion to move the cell itself. In the human, the tail of the spermatozoon, or sperm cell, is a single flagellum that causes the swimming motion of the cell.

Cell Functions

The structural and functional characteristics of different types of cells are determined by the nature of the proteins present. Cells of various types have different functions because cell structure and function are closely related. A very thin cell is not well suited for a protective function. Bone cells do not have an appropriate structure for nerve impulse conduction. Just as there are many cell types, there are varied cell functions. The specific functions of cells will become more apparent as the tissues, organs, and systems are studied. This section deals with the more generalized cell functions—the functions that relate to the sustained viability and continuation of the cell itself. These functions include movement of substances across the cell membrane, cell division to make new cells, and protein synthesis.

Movement of Substances across the Cell Membrane

The cell membrane provides a surface through which substances enter and leave the cell. The cell membrane controls the composition of the cell's cytoplasm by regulating the passage of substances through the membrane. If the membrane breaks, this control is removed and the cell dies. The survival of the cell depends on maintaining the difference between extracellular and intracellular material.

Table 5-4	Summary of Membrane Transport Mechanisms
Mechanism	**Description**
Passive	
Simple diffusion	Molecular movement down a concentration gradient
Osmosis	Movement of solvent toward high solute (low solvent) concentration; requires membrane
Filtration	Movement of solvent using hydrostatic pressure; requires membrane filter
Active	
Active transport	Movement of ions or molecules against a concentration gradient; requires carrier molecule and ATP
Phagocytosis	Ingestion of solid particles by creating vesicles; requires ATP
Pinocytosis	Ingestion of fluid by creating vesicles; requires ATP
Exocytosis	Secretion of cellular products by creating vesicles, then liberating contents to outside of cell; requires ATP

From Applegate E: *The anatomy and physiology learning system*, ed 4, St Louis, 2011, Saunders.

Mechanisms of movement across the cell membrane include **diffusion**, osmosis, filtration, active transport, endocytosis, and exocytosis. These are summarized in Table 5-4.

Diffusion

Simple diffusion is the movement of substances from a region of high concentration to a region of low concentration. Odors permeate a room because the aromatic molecules diffuse through the air. A crystal of dye will color a whole beaker of water because the dye particles diffuse from the region of high concentration in the dye crystal to regions of low concentration in the water (Figure 5-9).

In the examples of diffusion cited, there has been no membrane involved. Diffusion can also occur across a membrane as long as the membrane is permeable to the substances involved. For example, oxygen and carbon dioxide are able to diffuse through the cell membrane. When carbon dioxide builds up in the capillaries to a concentration that is higher than in the lungs, the carbon dioxide diffuses into the lungs to be exhaled. Similarly, when the level of oxygen in the capillaries is lower than the level of oxygen in the lungs, oxygen diffuses into the capillaries for distribution to the body cells. In this way, the gases are exchanged between the air and the blood in the lungs, and between the blood and the cells of the various tissues (Figure 5-10).

Osmosis

Osmosis (os-MOH-sis) involves the movement of **solvent** (water) molecules through a **selectively permeable** membrane from a region of higher concentration of water molecules (where the **solute** concentration is lower) to a region of lower concentration of water molecules (where the solute

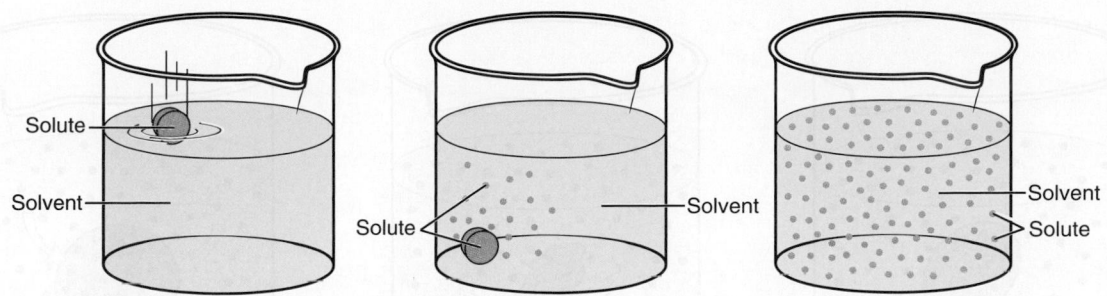

Figure 5-9 Simple diffusion. Molecules of solute diffuse throughout the solvent until equilibrium exists.

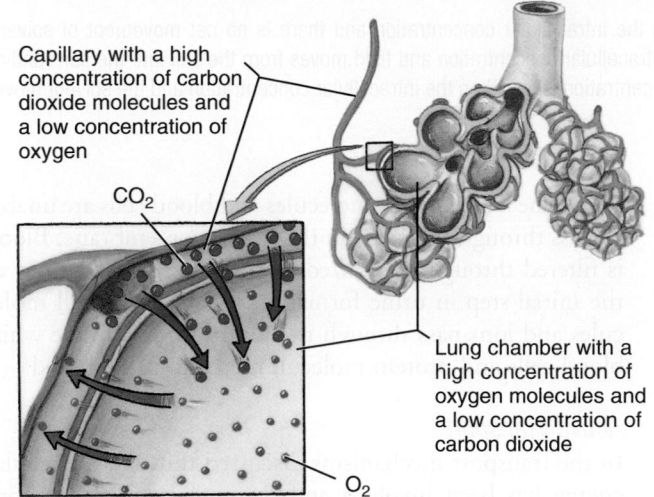

Figure 5-10 Diffusion of oxygen and carbon dioxide in the lungs. Oxygen moves from the higher concentration in the lung into the lower concentration in the capillary. Carbon dioxide moves in the opposite direction.

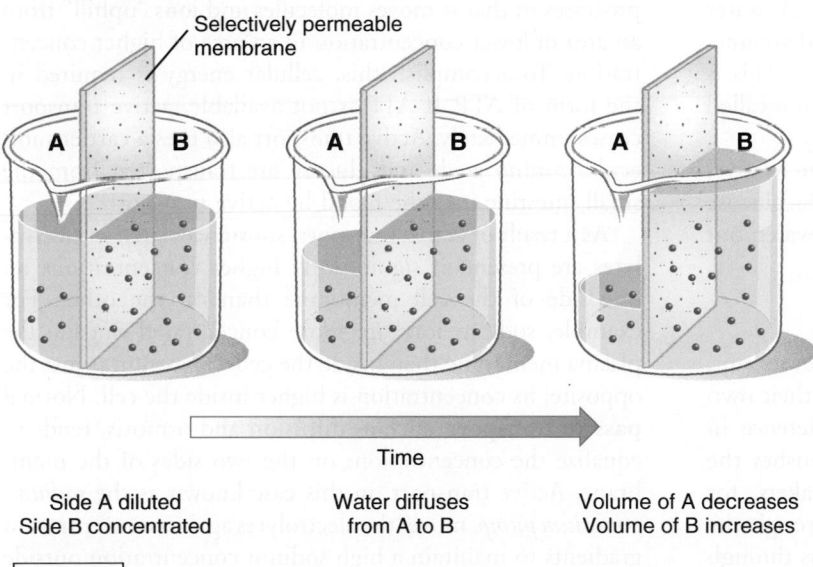

Figure 5-11 Osmosis. Solvent molecules move across the membrane but solute molecules do not because the membrane is selectively permeable.

concentration is higher). Figure 5-11 illustrates osmosis. When equilibrium is reached, the solutions on both sides of the membrane have the same concentration but the solution that was more concentrated at the start (had more solute) will now have a greater volume. Water molecules continue to pass through the membrane after equilibrium,

but because they move in both directions at the same rate there is no change in concentration or volume.

If a red blood cell, which contains 5% glucose, is placed in a container of 5% glucose solution, water will move in both directions at the same rate because the glucose concentrations inside and outside the cell are the same.

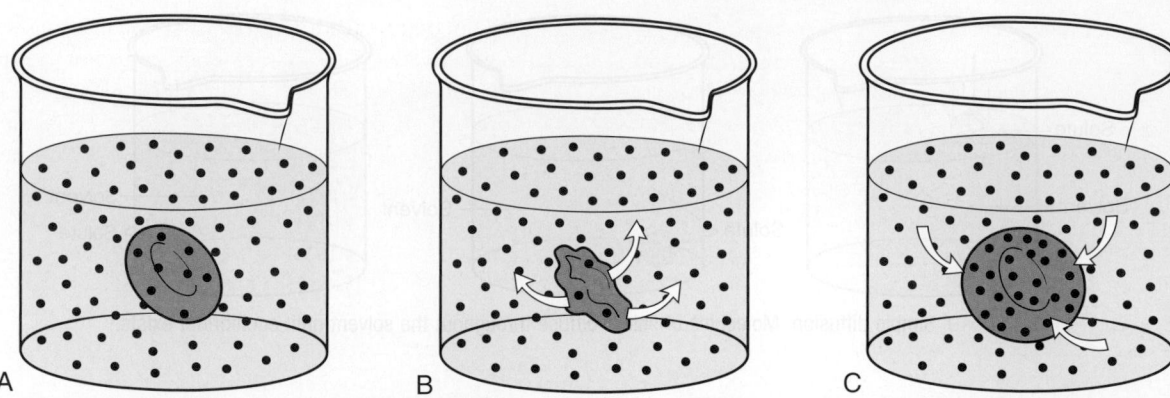

Figure 5-12 **A,** Isotonic solution. The extracellular concentration equals the intracellular concentration and there is no net movement of solvent. **B,** Hypertonic solution. The extracellular concentration is greater than the intracellular concentration and fluid moves from the cell into the surrounding fluid. The cell shrinks (crenates). **C,** Hypotonic solution. The extracellular concentration is less than the intracellular concentration and the solvent moves into the cell. The cell expands.

Solutions that have the same solute concentration are **iso-tonic** (Figure 5-12, *A*).

When a red blood cell is placed in a 10% glucose solution, water will leave the cell (where there are more water molecules) and enter the surrounding fluid (where there are fewer water molecules). When fluid leaves the cells, they will shrink or *crenate.* The 10% glucose solution is **hypertonic** (greater solute concentration) in relation to the cell (Figure 5-12, *B*).

When a red blood cell is placed in distilled water, water will enter the cell because there are more water molecules outside the cell than inside. The distilled water is **hypotonic** (lower solute concentration) in relation to the cell. As water enters the cell, it will swell because of the increased volume. If enough water goes into the cell, it may rupture. This is called *lysis.* When this happens to a red blood cell, it is called *hemolysis* (hee-MAHL-ih-sis) (Figure 5-12, *C*).

The terms *isotonic, hypotonic,* and *hypertonic* are relative. They are used to compare two solutions. A 5% glucose solution is hypertonic in relation to distilled water but hypotonic in relation to a 10% glucose solution.

Filtration

In diffusion and osmosis, particles (whether solute, solvent, or both) pass through a membrane by virtue of their own random movement, which is directed by a difference in concentration. In *filtration,* however, pressure pushes the particles through a membrane. Drip coffee makers, for example, use this principle. Water drips first through the coffee and then the water, and small particles pass through a filter. The large granules of coffee are too big to go through the pores in the filter. The size of the pores determines the size of the particles that can pass through the filter. The pressure is created by the weight of the water on the paper filter.

Contraction of the heart creates pressure in the blood. This fluid pressure or *hydrostatic pressure,* which is greater inside the blood vessels, pushes fluid, dissolved nutrients, and small ions through the capillary walls to form tissue fluid. The large protein molecules and blood cells are unable to pass through the pores in the capillary membrane. Blood is filtered through specialized membranes in the kidney as the initial step in urine formation. Water and small molecules and ions pass through the filtration membrane while blood cells and protein molecules remain in the blood.

Active Transport

In the transport mechanisms discussed thus far, no cellular energy has been involved and the molecules and/or ions have moved from a region of high concentration to one of low concentration. **Active transport** differs from these processes in that it moves molecules and ions "uphill" from an area of lower concentration to an area of higher concentration. To accomplish this, cellular energy is required in the form of ATP. If ATP is not available, active transport ceases immediately. Active transport also uses a carrier molecule. Amino acids and glucose are transported from the small intestine into the blood by active transport.

As a result of active transport, substances such as electrolytes are present in significantly higher concentrations on one side of the cell membrane than on the other. For example, sodium ions are more concentrated outside the plasma membrane than inside the cell. Potassium is just the opposite; its concentration is higher inside the cell. Normal **passive transport,** such as diffusion and osmosis, tends to equalize the concentrations on the two sides of the membrane. Active transport, in this case known as the *sodium-potassium pump,* moves the electrolytes against concentration gradients to maintain a high sodium concentration outside the cell and a high potassium concentration inside the cell. The process requires ATP and a protein carrier molecule.

Endocytosis

Endocytosis (en-doh-sye-TOH-sis) refers to the formation of vesicles to transfer particles and droplets from outside to inside the cell. In this case, the material is too large to enter the cell by diffusion or active transport. The process requires energy in the form of ATP. **Phagocytosis,** which means "cell eating," is a form of endocytosis that involves solid material. The cell membrane engulfs a particle to form a vesicle in the cytoplasm. Lysosomes fuse with the vesicle and the enzymes digest the particle. Certain white blood cells are called *phagocytes* because they engulf and destroy bacteria in this manner. Another form of endocytosis is **pinocytosis** or "cell drinking." It differs from phagocytosis in that the vesicles that are formed are much smaller and their contents are fluids. Pinocytosis is important in cells that function in absorption.

Exocytosis

In certain cells, secretory products are packaged into vesicles by the Golgi apparatus and are then released from the cell by a process called *exocytosis* (eck-soh-sye-TOH-sis). The secretory vesicle moves to the cell membrane, where the vesicle membrane fuses with the cell membrane and the contents are discharged to the outside of the cell. Secretion of digestive enzymes from the pancreas and secretion of milk from the mammary glands are examples of exocytosis. Exocytosis and endocytosis are similar except for working in opposite directions. They are both active processes that require cellular energy (ATP). Exocytosis releases substances to the outside of the cell, and endocytosis transports substances to the inside of the cell.

Cell Division

Cell division is the process by which new cells are formed for growth, repair, and replacement in the body. This process includes division of the nuclear material and division of the cytoplasm. Periods of growth and repair are special periods in the life of an individual when it is obvious that new cells are needed either to increase the number of

cells or to repair tissues after an injury. General maintenance and replacement needs of the body may not be quite as obvious. More than 2 million red blood cells are worn out and replaced in the body every second of every day. Skin cells are continually sloughed off the body's surface and must be replaced. The lining of the stomach is replaced every few days. All cells in the body (somatic cells), except those that give rise to the eggs and sperm (gametes), reproduce by **mitosis**. Egg and sperm cells are produced by a special type of nuclear division called **meiosis,** in which the number of chromosomes is halved. Division of the cytoplasm is called **cytokinesis.**

Mitosis

All somatic cells reproduce by mitosis, in which a single cell divides to form two new "daughter cells," each identical to the parent cell. Humans have 23 pairs of chromosomes (or 46 chromosomes) in their cells. Each new cell that forms must also have that same number. For this to occur, events must proceed in an organized manner, chromosome material must replicate exactly, and then the chromosomes must separate precisely so that each new cell receives a set of chromosomes that is a carbon copy of the parent cells. For descriptive purposes, it is convenient to divide the events of mitosis into stages, as illustrated in Figure 5-13. It is important to remember that the process is a continual one and that there are no starting and stopping points along the way.

Interphase

The period between active cell divisions is called *interphase*. This is a time of growth and **metabolism** and is usually the longest period of the cell cycle. In cells that are rapidly dividing it may last for as little as a few hours, but in other cells it may take days, weeks, or even months. Some highly

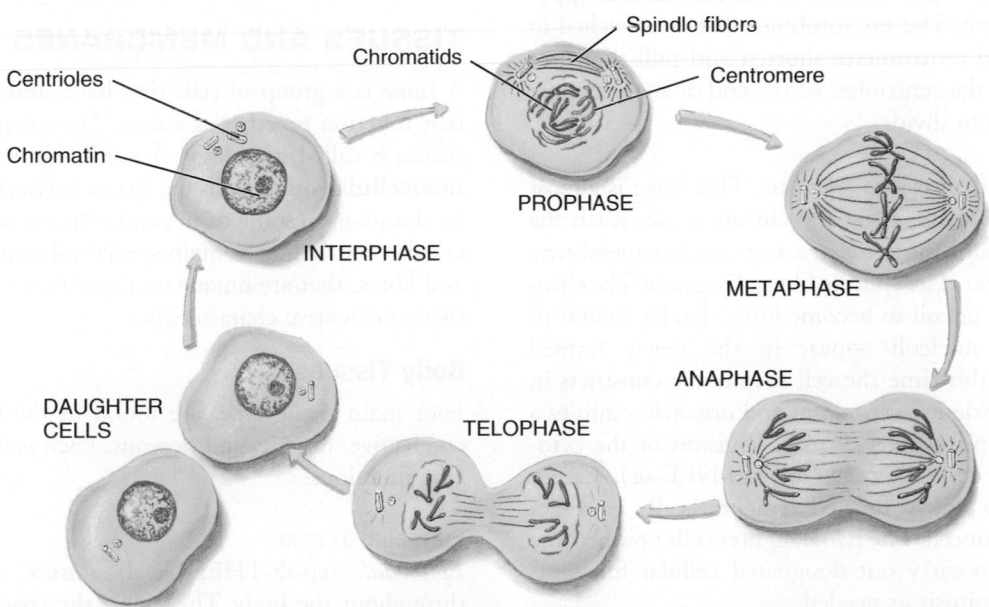

Figure 5-13 Mitosis. Interphase is the period between active cell divisions. Prophase is the first stage of mitosis. The process continues through metaphase, anaphase, and telophase. Cytokinesis occurs in telophase. With the division of nuclear material and cytoplasm, two exact copies of the parent cell are produced.

specialized cells, such as nerve and muscle cells, may never divide and spend their whole life in interphase.

During interphase the cell increases in size and synthesizes an exact copy of the DNA in its nucleus so that when the cell begins to divide it has identical sets of genetic information. In addition, just before division the cell synthesizes an additional pair of centrioles and some new mitochondria. In addition to these synthetic activities, which are a preparation for division, normal cellular function takes place during interphase.

Prophase

After interphase, the cell begins mitosis. The first stage of mitosis is *prophase.* During prophase, the chromatin shortens, thickens, and becomes tightly coiled to form chromosomes. As a result of the replication in interphase, each chromosome has two identical parts, called *chromatids,* that are joined by a special region on each called the *centromere.* The two pairs of centrioles separate and go to opposite ends of the cytoplasm. Microtubules called *spindle fibers* form and extend from the centromeres to the centrioles. The nucleolus and nuclear membrane disappear during the latter part of prophase.

Metaphase

Prophase ends when the nuclear membrane disintegrates, and this signals the beginning of the next stage, *metaphase.* The chromosomes align themselves along the center of the cell during metaphase. This is the time when the chromosomes are most clearly visible and distinguishable.

Anaphase

The third stage of mitosis is *anaphase.* After the chromosomes are aligned along the center of the cell, the centromeres separate so that each chromatid now becomes a chromosome. At this time, there are actually two sets of chromosomes in the cell. The two chromatids (now chromosomes) from each pair migrate to the centrioles at opposite ends of the cell. The microtubules that are attached to the centrioles and centromeres shorten and pull the chromosomes toward the centrioles. At the end of anaphase, the cytoplasm begins to divide.

Telophase

The final stage of mitosis is *telophase.* This stage is almost the reverse of prophase. After the chromosomes reach the centrioles at the ends of the cell, a new nuclear membrane forms around them. The spindle fibers disappear. The chromosomes start to uncoil to become long, slender strands of chromatin, and nucleoli appear in the newly formed nucleus. During this time the cell membrane constricts in the middle to divide the cytoplasm and organelles into two parts that are approximately equal. Division of the cytoplasm is called cytokinesis (sye-toh-kih-NEE-sis). Except for size, the two newly formed daughter cells are exact copies of the parent cell. The two daughter cells now become interphase cells to carry out designated cellular functions and to undergo mitosis as needed.

Normally, body cells divide at a rate required to replace the dying ones. Normal cells are subject to control mechanisms that prevent overpopulation and competition for nutrients and space. Occasionally, a series of events occurs that alters some cells, so they lack the control mechanisms that tell them when to stop dividing. When the cells do not stop their mitotic activity, they form an abnormal growth called a *tumor,* or neoplasm.

Meiosis

Meiosis is a special type of cell division that occurs in the production of the gametes, or eggs and sperm. These cells have only 23 chromosomes, one half the number found in somatic cells, so that when fertilization takes place the resulting cell will again have 46 chromosomes, 23 from the egg and 23 from the sperm. Meiosis is discussed in greater detail in Chapter 16. In brief, meiosis consists of two divisions, but DNA is replicated only once. The result is four cells, but each one has only 23 chromosomes. Figure 5-14 compares mitosis and meiosis.

DNA Replication and Protein Synthesis

Proteins that are synthesized in the cytoplasm function as structural materials, enzymes that regulate chemical reactions, hormones, and other vital substances. Because DNA in the nucleus directs the synthesis of the proteins in the cytoplasm, it ultimately determines the structural and functional characteristics of an individual. Whether a person has blue or brown eyes, brown or blond hair, or light or dark skin is determined by the types of proteins synthesized in response to the genetic information contained in the DNA in the nucleus. The portion of a DNA molecule that contains the genetic information for making one particular protein molecule is called a *gene.* If a cell produced for replacement or repair is to function exactly as its predecessor, then it must have the same genes, a carbon copy of the DNA. This is the purpose of DNA replication in cell division.

TISSUES AND MEMBRANES

A *tissue* is a group of cells that have similar structure and that function together as a unit. The microscopic study of tissues is called **histology**. A nonliving material called the **intercellular matrix** fills the spaces between cells. This may be abundant in some tissues and scarce in others. The intercellular matrix may contain special substances, such as salts and fibers, that are unique to a specific tissue and give that tissue distinctive characteristics.

Body Tissues

Four main tissue types are found in the body: epithelial, connective, muscle, and nervous. Each is designed for specific functions.

Epithelial Tissue

Epithelial (ep-ih-THEE-lee-al) *tissues* are widespread throughout the body. They form the covering of all body surfaces, line body cavities and hollow organs, and are the major tissue in glands. They perform a variety of functions that include protection, secretion, absorption, excretion, filtration, diffusion, and sensory reception.

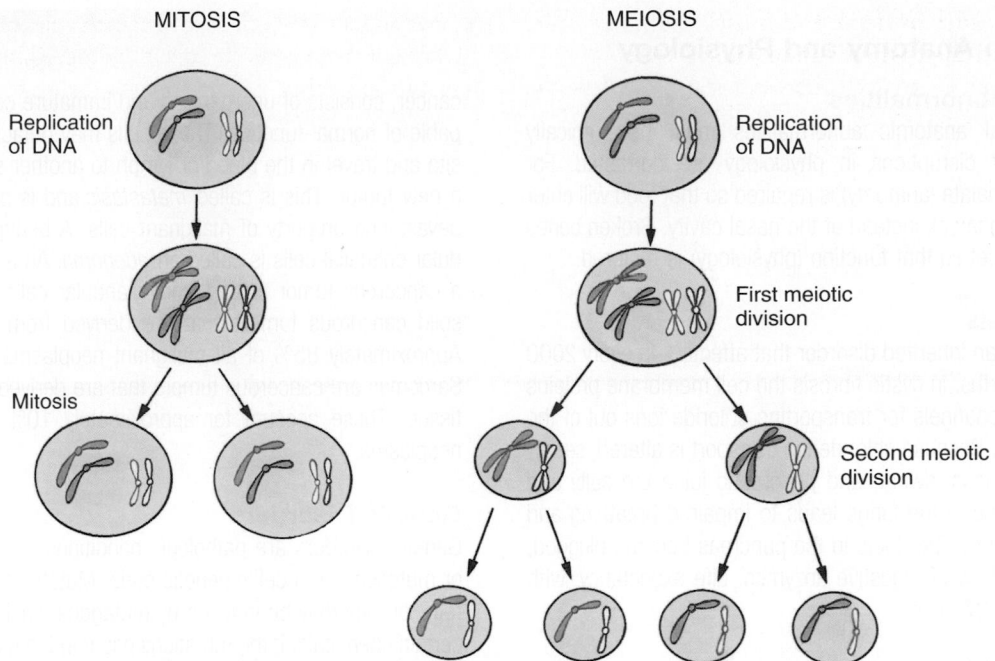

Figure 5-14 Comparison of mitosis and meiosis. The result of mitosis in humans is two cells, each with 46 chromosomes (23 pairs). Meiosis results in four cells, each with 23 chromosomes.

The cells in epithelial tissue are tightly packed with little intercellular matrix. Because the tissues form coverings and linings, the cells have one free surface that is not in contact with other cells. Opposite the free surface, the cells are attached to underlying connective tissue by a noncellular *basement membrane.* Because epithelial tissues are typically *avascular* (without blood vessels), they must receive their nutrients and oxygen supply by diffusion from the blood vessels in the underlying tissues. Another characteristic of epithelial tissues is that they regenerate, or reproduce, quickly. For example, the cells of the skin and stomach are continually damaged and replaced, and skin abrasions heal quite rapidly.

Epithelia are classified according to cell shape and the number of layers in the tissue. Classified according to shape, the cells are squamous, cuboidal, or columnar, and the shape of the nucleus corresponds to the cell shape. **Squamous** cells are flat and the nuclei are usually broad and thin. **Cuboidal** cells are cubelike, as tall as they are wide, and the nuclei are spheric and centrally located. **Columnar** cells are tall and narrow, resembling columns, and the nuclei are usually in the lower portion of the cell near the basement membrane. According to the number of layers, epithelia are **simple** if they have only one layer of cells and **stratified** if they have multiple layers. Stratified epithelia are named according to the type of cells at the free surface of the tissue.

Simple Squamous Epithelium
Simple squamous epithelium (Figure 5-15) consists of a single layer of thin, flat cells that fit closely together with little intercellular matrix. Because it is so thin, simple squamous epithelium is well suited for areas in which diffusion and filtration take place. The alveoli or air sacs of the lungs, where diffusion of oxygen and carbon dioxide gases occurs, are made of simple squamous epithelium. This tissue is also found in the kidney, where the blood is filtered. Capillary walls, where oxygen and carbon dioxide diffuse between the blood and tissues, are made of simple squamous epithelium. Because it is so thin and delicate, this tissue is damaged easily and offers little protective function.

Simple Cuboidal Epithelium
Simple cuboidal epithelium (Figure 5-16) consists of a single layer of cube-shaped cells. These cells have more volume than squamous cells and also have more organelles. Simple cuboidal epithelium is found as a covering of the ovary, as a lining of kidney tubules, and in many glands, such as the thyroid, pancreas, and salivary glands. In the kidney tubules, the tissue functions in absorption and secretion. In glands, simple cuboidal cells form the secretory portions and the ducts that deliver the products to their destination.

Simple Columnar Epithelium
A single layer of cells that are taller than they are wide makes up *simple columnar epithelium* (Figure 5-17). The nuclei are in the bottom portion of the cell near the basement membrane. Simple columnar epithelium is found lining the stomach and intestines, where it secretes digestive enzymes and absorbs nutrients. Because the cells are taller (or thicker) than either squamous or cuboidal cells, this tissue offers some protection to underlying tissues.

In regions where absorption is of primary importance, such as in parts of the digestive tract, the cell membrane on the free surface has numerous small projections called *microvilli.* Microvilli increase the surface area that is

Highlight on Anatomy and Physiology

Congenital Abnormalities

Often, congenital anatomic abnormalities must be surgically repaired so that disruptions in physiology are corrected. For example, a cleft palate (anatomy) is repaired so that food will enter (physiology) the pharynx instead of the nasal cavity. Broken bones (anatomy) are reset so that function (physiology) is restored.

Cystic Fibrosis

Cystic fibrosis is an inherited disorder that affects 1 in every 2000 Caucasian live births. In cystic fibrosis the cell membrane proteins that function as channels for transporting chloride ions out of the cell are defective. Because chloride ion transport is altered, secretions such as mucus, sweat, and pancreatic juice are salty and thick. Thick mucus in the lungs leads to impaired breathing and increased infections. The ducts in the pancreas become plugged, which stops the flow of digestive enzymes. Life expectancy, with therapy, is about 27 years.

Kidney Dialysis

Normally functioning kidneys remove waste products from the blood. When the kidneys do not function properly, waste molecules can be removed from the blood artificially by a process called *dialysis.* Dialysis is a form of diffusion in which the size of the pores in a selectively permeable membrane separates smaller solute particles from larger solutes. In kidney dialysis, small waste molecules pass through the membrane and are removed from the blood. The protein molecules, which are needed in the blood, are too large to pass through the pores and thus are retained.

Neoplasms

A benign neoplasm consists of highly organized cells that closely resemble normal tissue. In contrast, a malignant neoplasm, or cancer, consists of unorganized and immature cells that are incapable of normal function. These cells may detach from the tumor site and travel in the blood or lymph to another site and establish a new tumor. This is called *metastasis* and is probably the most devastating property of malignant cells. A benign tumor of glandular epithelial cells is called an *adenoma.* An adenocarcinoma is a cancerous tumor arising from glandular cells. Carcinomas are solid cancerous tumors that are derived from epithelial tissue. Approximately 85% of all malignant neoplasms are carcinomas. Sarcomas are cancerous tumors that are derived from connective tissue. These account for approximately 10% of all malignant neoplasms.

Genetic Disorders

Genetic disorders are pathologic conditions caused by mistakes, or mutations, in a cell's genetic code. Mutations may occur naturally, or they may be induced by mutagens, such as radiation and certain chemicals. If the mutations occur in the gametes, the faulty code is passed from one generation to the next. Errors in the genes (DNA) cause the production of abnormal proteins, which result in abnormal cellular function. For example, in sickle cell anemia, a genetic blood disorder, red blood cells have abnormal hemoglobin because there is an "error" in the gene that directs hemoglobin synthesis.

Peritonitis

An inflammation of the serous membranes in the abdominal cavity is called *peritonitis.* This is sometimes a serious complication of an infected appendix. ∎

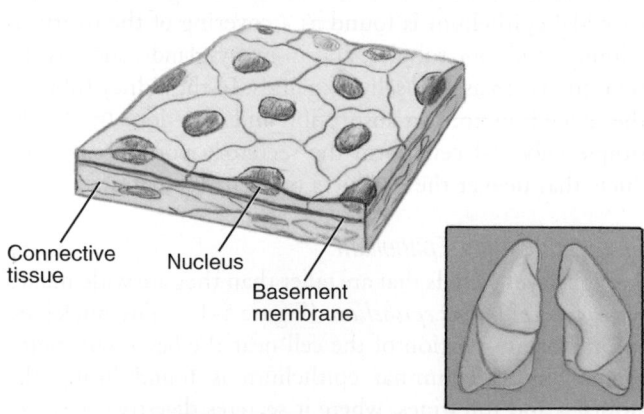

Connective tissue
Nucleus
Basement membrane

Figure 5-15 Simple squamous epithelium in the alveoli of the lungs. It is also found in capillary walls and in renal corpuscles of the kidney.

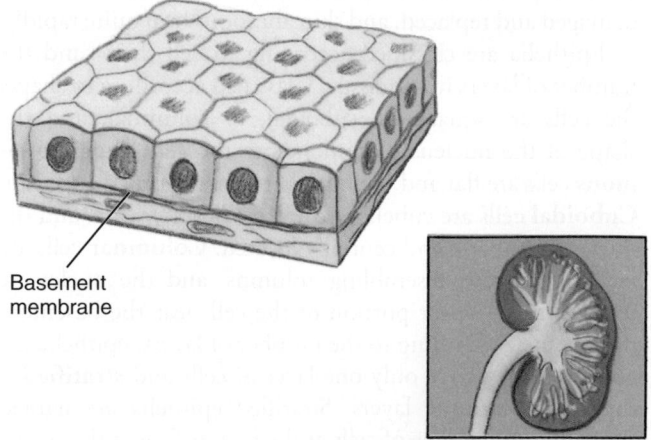

Basement membrane

Figure 5-16 Simple cuboidal epithelium in the kidney tubules. It is also found in many glands and as a covering of the ovary.

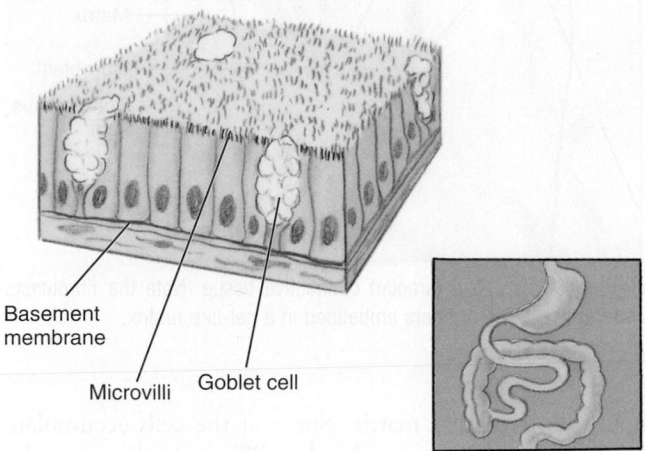

Figure 5-17 Simple columnar epithelium in the lining of the stomach and intestines.

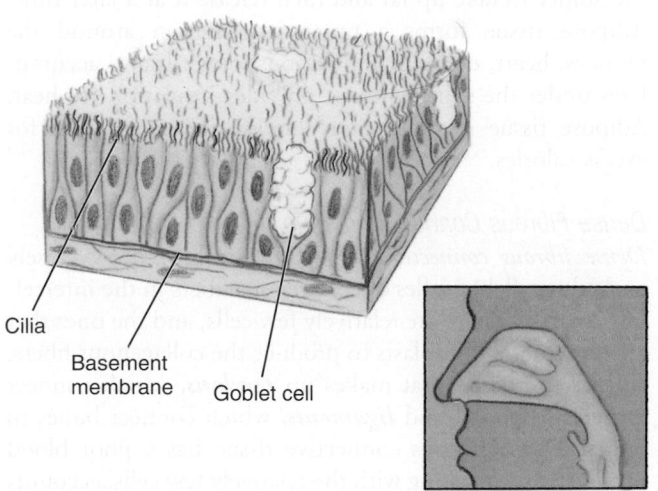

Figure 5-18 Pseudostratified columnar epithelium in the respiratory tract. It also lines some of the male reproductive system.

available for absorption of nutrients. **Goblet cells** are frequently interspersed among the simple columnar cells. Goblet cells are flask- or goblet-shaped cells that secrete mucus onto the free surface of the tissue. Cilia may be present to move secretions along the surface.

Pseudostratified Columnar Epithelium

Pseudostratified columnar epithelium (Figure 5-18) appears to have multiple layers (stratified), but it really does not. This is because the cells are not all the same height. Some cells are short and some are tall, and the nuclei are at different levels. Close examination reveals that all the cells are attached to the basement membrane but that not all cells reach the free surface of the tissue. Cilia and goblet cells are often associated with pseudostratified columnar epithelium. This tissue lines portions of the respiratory tract in which the mucus, produced by the goblet cells, traps dust particles and is then moved upward by the cilia. Pseudostratified columnar epithelium also lines some of the tubes of the male reproductive system. Here the cilia help propel the sperm from one region to another.

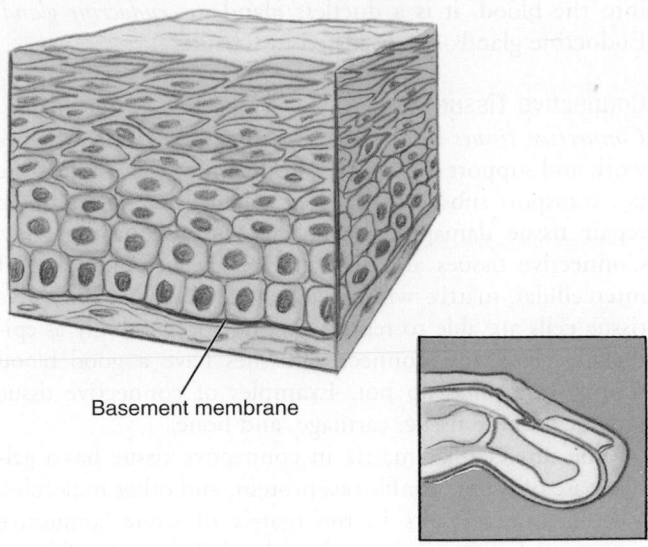

Figure 5-19 Stratified squamous epithelium from the outer layer of the skin. Note the numerous cell layers and the flattened cells at the surface.

Stratified Squamous Epithelium

Stratified squamous epithelium, the most widespread stratified epithelium, is thick because it consists of many layers of cells (Figure 5-19). The cells on the bottom layer, next to the basement membrane, are usually cuboidal or columnar, and these are the cells that undergo mitosis. As the cells are pushed toward the surface, they become thinner, so the surface cells are squamous. As the cells are pushed farther away from the basement membrane, it is more difficult for them to receive oxygen and nutrients from underlying connective tissue, and the cells die. As cells on the surface are damaged and die, they are sloughed off and replaced by cells from the deeper layers. Because this tissue is thick, it is found in areas in which protection is a primary function. Stratified squamous epithelium forms the outer layer of the skin and extends a short distance into every body opening that is continuous with the skin.

Transitional Epithelium

Transitional epithelium is a specialized type of tissue that has several layers but can be stretched in response to tension. The lining of the urinary bladder is a good example of this type of tissue. When the bladder is empty and contracted, the epithelial lining has several layers of cuboidal cells. As the bladder fills and is distended or stretched, the cells become thinner and the number of layers decreases.

Glandular Epithelium

Glandular epithelium consists of cells that are specialized to produce and secrete substances. Glandular epithelium normally lies deep to the epithelia that cover and line parts of the body. If the gland secretes its product onto a free surface via a duct, it is called an *exocrine gland*. Examples of exocrine glands include sebaceous glands, mammary glands, and salivary glands. If the gland secretes its product directly into the blood, it is a ductless gland, or *endocrine gland.* Endocrine glands are discussed in Chapter 11.

Connective Tissue

Connective tissues bind structures together, form a framework and support for organs and the body as a whole, store fat, transport substances, protect against disease, and help repair tissue damage. They occur throughout the body. Connective tissues are characterized by an abundance of intercellular matrix with relatively few cells. Connective tissue cells are able to reproduce but not as rapidly as epithelial cells. Most connective tissues have a good blood supply, but some do not. Examples of connective tissue include adipose tissue, cartilage, and bone.

The intercellular matrix in connective tissue has a gel-like base of water, nonfibrous protein, and other molecules. Various mineral salts in the matrix of some connective tissues, such as bone, make them hard. Two types of fibers, collagenous and elastic, are frequently embedded in the matrix. **Collagenous fibers,** composed of the protein collagen, are strong and flexible but are only slightly elastic. They are able to withstand considerable pulling force and are found in areas in which this is important, such as in tendons and ligaments. When collagenous fibers are grouped together in parallel bundles, the tissue appears white, so they are sometimes called *white fibers.* **Elastic fibers,** composed of the protein elastin, are not very strong, but they are elastic. They can be stretched and will return to their original shape and length when released. Elastic fibers, also called *yellow fibers,* are located where structures are stretched and released, such as the vocal cords.

Numerous cell types are found in connective tissue. Three of the most common are the **fibroblast, macrophage,** and **mast cell.** As the name implies, fibroblasts produce the fibers that are in the intercellular matrix. Macrophages are large phagocytic cells that are able to move about and clean up cellular debris and foreign particles from the tissues. Mast cells contain heparin, an anticoagulant, and histamine, a substance that promotes inflammation and that is active in allergies.

Loose Connective Tissue

Loose connective tissue, also called *areolar* (ah-REE-oh-lar) *connective tissue,* is one of the most widely distributed tissues in the body. It is the packing material in the body. It attaches the skin to the underlying tissues and fills the spaces between muscles. Most epithelial tissue is anchored to this tissue by the basement membrane, and the blood vessels in the loose connective tissue supply nutrients to the epithelium above. The matrix is characterized by a loose network of collagenous and elastic fibers. The predominant cell is the fibroblast, but other connective tissue cells are also present (Figure 5-20).

Adipose Tissue

Commonly called *fat, adipose* (ADD-ih-pose) *tissue* is really a specialized form of loose connective tissue in which there

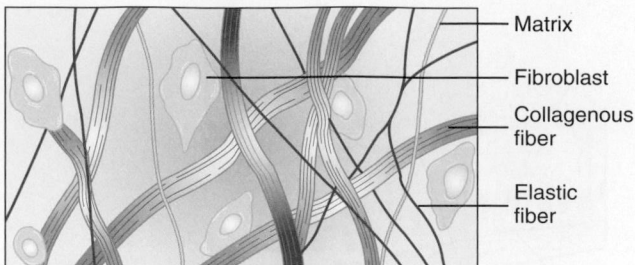

Figure 5-20 Loose (areolar) connective tissue. Note the fibroblasts and the two types of fibers embedded in a gel-like matrix.

is little intercellular matrix. Some of the cells accumulate liquid triglyceride, or fat, droplets. When this happens, the cytoplasm and nucleus are pushed off to one side, and the cells swell and become closely packed together. Fat cells have the ability to take up fat and then release it at a later time. Adipose tissue forms a protective cushion around the kidneys, heart, eyeballs, and various joints. It also accumulates under the skin, where it provides insulation for heat. Adipose tissue is an efficient energy storage material for excess calories.

Dense Fibrous Connective Tissue

Dense fibrous connective tissue is characterized by closely packed parallel bundles of collagenous fibers in the intercellular matrix. There are relatively few cells, and the ones that are present are fibroblasts to produce the collagenous fibers. This is the tissue that makes up *tendons,* which connect muscles to bones, and *ligaments,* which connect bones to bones. Dense fibrous connective tissue has a poor blood supply, and this, along with the relatively few cells, accounts for the slow healing of this tissue.

Elastic Connective Tissue

Elastic connective tissue has closely packed elastic fibers in the intercellular matrix. This type of tissue yields easily to a pulling force and then returns to its original length as soon as the force is released. The vocal cords and the ligaments that connect adjacent vertebrae are composed of elastic connective tissue.

Cartilage

Cartilage has an abundant matrix that is solid, yet flexible, with fibers embedded in it. The matrix contains the protein *chondrin* (KON-drihn). Cartilage cells, or **chondrocytes,** are located in spaces called *lacunae* (lah-KOO-nee) that are scattered throughout the matrix. Typically, cartilage is surrounded by a dense fibrous connective tissue covering called the *perichondrium.* The perichondrium has blood vessels, but they do not penetrate the cartilage itself, and the cells obtain their nutrients by diffusion through the solid matrix. Cartilage heals slowly because there is no direct blood supply, and this also contributes to slow cellular reproduction. Cartilage protects underlying tissues, supports other structures, and provides a framework for attachments.

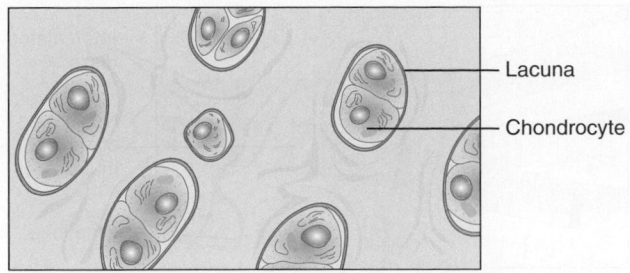

Figure 5-21 Hyaline cartilage. Note the chondrocytes within the lacunae.

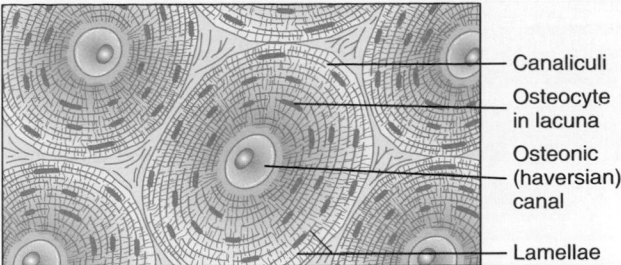

Figure 5-22 Compact bone (osseous tissue). Note the osteons with a central haversian canal and concentric lamellae of matrix. Canaliculi extend from the osteocytes, which are located within lacunae.

Hyaline cartilage (Figure 5-21) is the most common type of cartilage. It has fine collagenous fibers in the matrix and a shiny, white, opaque appearance. It is found at the ends of long bones, in the costal cartilage that connects the ribs to the sternum, and in the supporting rings of the trachea. Most of the fetal skeleton is formed of hyaline cartilage before it is replaced by bone.

Fibrocartilage has an abundance of strong collagenous fibers embedded in the matrix. This allows it to withstand compression, act as a shock absorber, and resist pulling forces. It is found in the intervertebral discs, or pads between the vertebrae; in the symphysis pubis, or pad between the two pubic bones; and between the bones in the knee joint.

Elastic cartilage has numerous yellow elastic fibers embedded in the matrix, which makes it more flexible than hyaline cartilage or fibrocartilage. It is found in the framework of the external ear, the epiglottis, and the auditory tubes.

Bone

Osseous tissue or *bone* is the most rigid of all the connective tissues. Collagenous fibers in the matrix give strength to bone, and its hardness is derived from the mineral salts, particularly calcium, that are deposited around the fibers. Bones form the framework for the body and help protect underlying tissues. They serve as attachments for muscles and act as mechanical levers in producing movement. Bone also contributes to the formation of blood cells and functions as a storage area for mineral salts.

Cylindric structural units, called *osteons* or *haversian* (hah-VER-shun) *systems,* are packed together to form the substance of compact bone (Figure 5-22). The center or hub of the osteon is a tubular *osteonic* or *haversian canal* that contains a blood vessel. The matrix is deposited in concentric rings called *lamellae* (lah-MEL-ee) around the canal. **Osteocytes,** or bone cells, are located in lacunae between the lamellae so that they are also arranged in concentric rings. Slender processes from the bone cells extend through tiny tubes in the matrix called *canaliculi* (kan-ah-LIK-yoo-lye) to other cells or to the osteonic canals. This provides a readily available blood supply for the bone cells, which allows a faster repair process for bone than for cartilage.

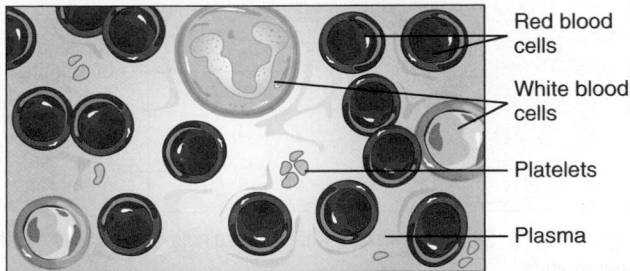

Figure 5-23 Blood. Note the blood cells and platelets, which are suspended in a liquid plasma.

Blood

Blood is a unique connective tissue because it is the only one that has a liquid matrix. It is a vehicle for transport of substances throughout the body. **Erythrocytes,** or red blood cells, and **leukocytes,** or white blood cells, are suspended in a liquid matrix called *plasma* (Figure 5-23). The red blood cells transport oxygen from the lungs to the tissues. White blood cells are important in fighting disease. Another formed element in the blood is the *platelet,* or **thrombocyte,** which is not actually a cell but a fragment of a giant cell in the bone marrow. Platelets are important in initiating the blood clotting process. Blood is discussed in more detail in Chapter 12.

Muscle Tissue

Muscle tissue is composed of cells that have the special ability to shorten or contract in order to produce movement of body parts. The tissue is highly cellular and is well supplied with blood vessels. The cells are long and slender, so they are sometimes called *muscle fibers,* and these are usually arranged in bundles or layers that are surrounded by connective tissue. Muscle tissue is of three types: skeletal muscle, smooth muscle, and cardiac muscle.

Skeletal Muscle

Skeletal muscle tissue (Figure 5-24) is what is commonly thought of as "muscle." It is the meat of animals, and it constitutes about 40% of an individual's body weight. Skeletal muscle cells (fibers) are long and cylindric with many nuclei (multinucleated) peripherally located next to the cell membrane. The cells have alternating light and dark bands

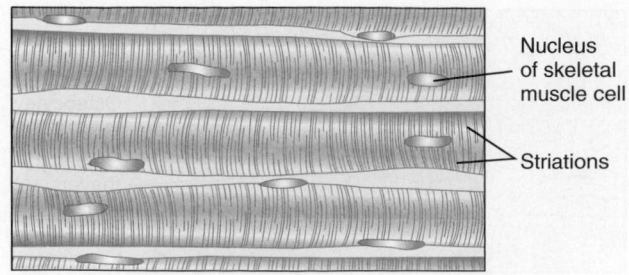

Figure 5-24 Skeletal muscle. Note the long cylindric fibers with striations.

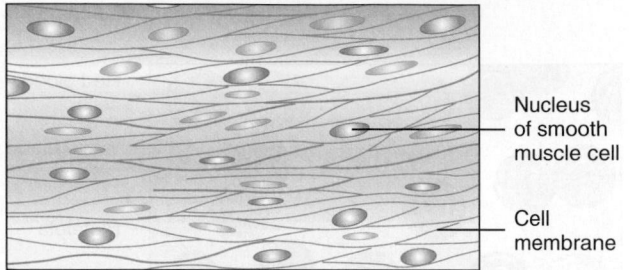

Figure 5-25 Smooth muscle. Note the spindle-shaped cells with tapered ends.

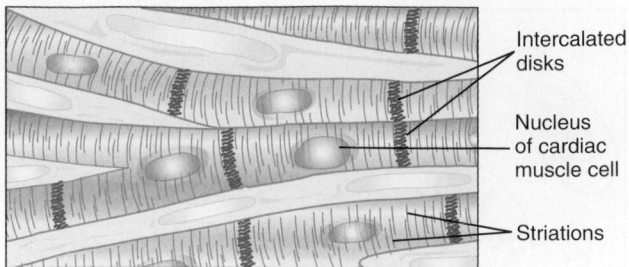

Figure 5-26 Cardiac muscle. Note the branching striated cells and intercalated disks.

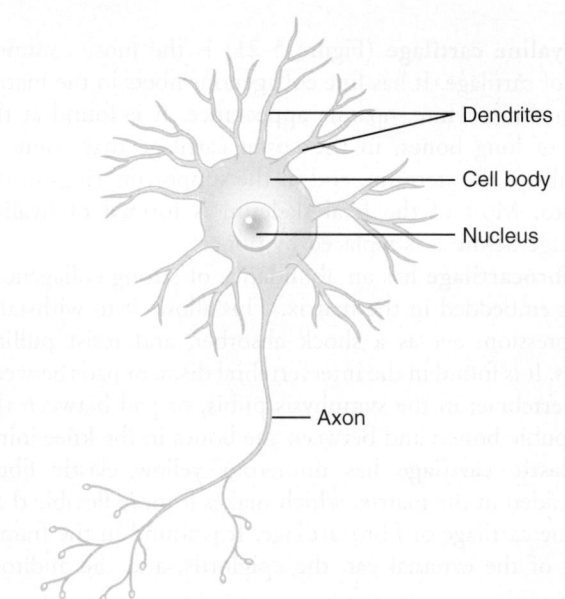

Figure 5-27 Neuron (nervous tissue). Note the dendrites, axon, and cell body.

that are perpendicular to the long axis of the cell. These bands are a result of the organized arrangement of the contractile proteins in the cytoplasm and give the cell a *striated* appearance. Skeletal muscle fibers are collected into bundles and wrapped in connective tissue to form the muscles, which are attached to the skeleton and which cause body movements when they contract in response to nerve stimulation. Skeletal muscle action is under conscious or voluntary control. Chapter 8 describes skeletal muscles in more detail.

Smooth Muscle

Smooth muscle tissue (Figure 5-25) is found in the walls of hollow body organs, such as the stomach, intestines, urinary bladder, uterus, and blood vessels. It normally acts to propel substances through the organ by contracting and relaxing. It is called *smooth muscle* because it lacks the striations evident in skeletal muscle. Because it is found in the viscera or body organs, it is sometimes called *visceral muscle*. Smooth muscle cells are shorter than skeletal muscle cells, are spindle-shaped and tapered at the ends, and have a single, centrally located nucleus. Smooth muscle usually cannot be stimulated to contract by conscious or voluntary effort, so it is called *involuntary muscle*.

Cardiac Muscle

Cardiac muscle tissue (Figure 5-26) is found only in the wall of the heart. The cardiac muscle cells are cylindric and appear striated, similar to skeletal muscle cells. Cardiac muscle cells are shorter than skeletal muscle cells and have only one nucleus per cell. The cells branch and interconnect to form complex networks. At the point where one cell attaches to another, there is a specialized intercellular connection called an **intercalated** (in-TER-kuh-lay-ted) *disc*.

Cardiac muscle appears striated like skeletal muscle, but its contraction is involuntary. It is responsible for pumping the blood through the heart and into the blood vessels.

Nervous Tissue

Nervous tissue is found in the brain, spinal cord, and nerves. It is responsible for coordinating and controlling many body activities. It stimulates muscle contraction, creates an awareness of the environment, and plays a major role in emotions, memory, and reasoning. To do all of these things, cells in nervous tissue need to be able to communicate with each other by way of electrical nerve impulses.

The cells in nervous tissue that generate and conduct impulses are called **neurons** or *nerve cells*. These cells have three principal parts: the dendrites, the cell body, and one axon (Figure 5-27). The main part of the cell, the part that carries on the general functions, is the **neuron cell body**. **Dendrites** are extensions, or processes, of the cytoplasm that carry impulses to the cell body. An extension or process called an **axon** carries impulses away from the cell body.

Nervous tissue also includes cells that do not transmit impulses but instead support the activities of the neurons. These are the *glial* (GLEE-al) *cells* (or neuroglial cells),

Highlight on Conditions Affecting Tissues

Adhesion (add-HEE-shun) Abnormal joining of tissues by fibrous scar tissue

Carcinoma (kar-sih-NOH-mah) A malignant growth derived from epithelial cells

Lipoma (lih-POH-mah) Benign tumor derived from fat cells

Marfan syndrome (mahr-FAHN SIN-drohm) A congenital disorder of connective tissue characterized by abnormal length of the extremities and cardiovascular abnormalities

Myoma (mye-OH-mah) Benign tumor formed of muscle tissue

Papilloma (pap-ih-LOH-mah) Benign epithelial tumor; may occur on any epithelial surface or lining

Sarcoma (sar-KOH-mah) A malignant growth derived from connective tissue cells

Scurvy (SKUR-vee) A condition caused by a deficiency of vitamin C in the diet, which results in abnormal collagen synthesis

Systemic lupus erythematosus (sih-STEM-ik LOO-pus air-ith-eh-mah-TOH-sis) Chronic autoimmune connective tissue disease characterized by injury to the skin, joints, kidneys, nervous system, and mucous membranes, but can affect any organ of the body ■

together termed the **neuroglia.** Supporting, or glial, cells bind neurons together and insulate the neurons. Some are phagocytic and protect against bacterial invasion, whereas others provide nutrients by binding blood vessels to the neurons. Further detail on nerve tissue is presented in Chapter 9.

Body Membranes

Body membranes are thin sheets of tissue that cover the body, line body cavities, cover organs within the cavities, and line the cavities in hollow organs. By this definition, the skin is a membrane because it covers the body, and indeed, the skin, or integument, is sometimes called the *cutaneous membrane.* This membrane is discussed in Chapter 6. This section examines two epithelial membranes and two connective tissue membranes. Epithelial membranes consist of epithelial tissue and the connective tissue to which it is attached. The two main types of epithelial membranes are the mucous membranes and serous membranes. Connective tissue membranes contain only connective tissue. Synovial membranes and meninges belong to this category.

Mucous Membranes

Mucous membranes are epithelial membranes that consist of epithelial tissue attached to underlying loose connective tissue. These membranes (sometimes called *mucosae*) line the body cavities that open to the outside. The entire digestive tract is lined with mucous membranes. Other examples include the respiratory, urinary, and reproductive tracts. The type of epithelium varies depending on its function. In the mouth, the epithelium is stratified squamous for its protection function, but the stomach and intestines are lined with simple columnar epithelium for absorption and secretion. The mucosa of the urinary bladder is transitional epithelium so that it can expand. Mucous membranes get their name from the fact that the epithelial cells secrete mucus for lubrication and protection.

Serous Membranes

Serous membranes line body cavities that do not open directly to the outside, and they cover the organs located in those

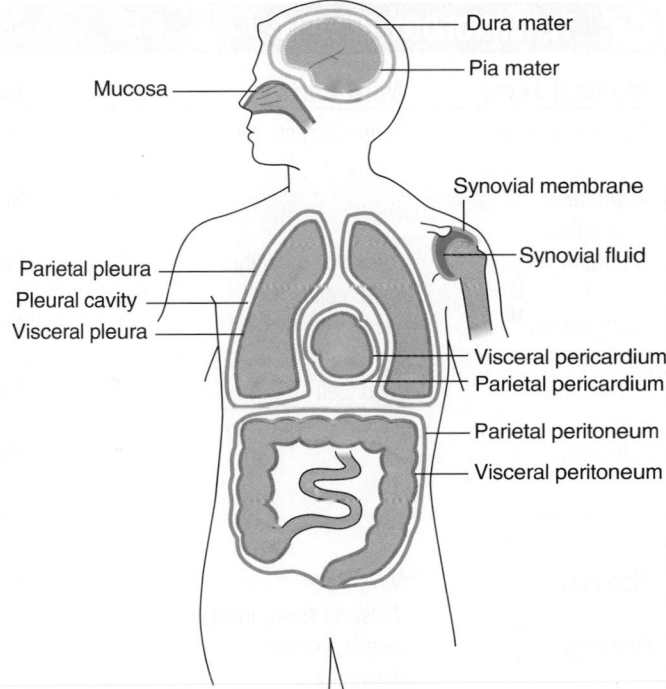

Figure 5-28 Body membranes.

cavities. A serous membrane, or *serosa,* consists of a thin layer of loose connective tissue covered by a layer of simple squamous epithelium called *mesothelium.* These membranes always have two parts. The part that lines a cavity wall is the *parietal* layer, and the part that covers the organs in the cavity is the *visceral* layer (Figure 5-28). Serous membranes are covered by a thin layer of *serous fluid* that is secreted by the epithelium. Serous fluid lubricates the membrane and reduces friction and abrasion when organs in the thoracic or abdominopelvic cavity move against one another or the cavity wall.

Serous membranes have special names according to their location. The serous membrane that lines the thoracic cavity and covers the lungs is the *pleura,* with the parietal pleura lining the cavity and the visceral pleura covering the lungs. The *pericardium* (pair-ih-KAR-dee-um) lines the pericardial cavity and covers the heart. The serous membrane in the abdominopelvic cavity is the *peritoneum* (pair-ih-toh-NEE-um).

Synovial Membranes

Synovial (sih-NOH-vee-al) *membranes* are connective tissue membranes that line the cavities of the freely movable joints such as the shoulder, elbow, and knee. Similar to serous membranes, they line cavities that do not open to the outside. Unlike serous membranes, they do not have a layer of epithelium. Synovial membranes secrete *synovial fluid* into the joint cavity, and this lubricates the cartilage on the ends of the bones so that they can move freely and without friction. In certain types of arthritis, these membranes become inflamed and the fluid becomes viscous. This

reduces lubrication and increases friction, and movement becomes difficult and painful.

Meninges

The connective tissue coverings around the brain and spinal cord, within the dorsal cavity, are called *meninges* (meh-NIN-jeez). They provide protection for these vital structures. The outermost layer of the meninges is the toughest and is called the **dura mater** (DOO-rah MAY-ter). The middle layer, the **arachnoid** (ah-RAK-noyd), is quite fragile. The **pia mater** (PEE-ah MAY-ter), the innermost layer, is delicate and closely adherent to the surface of the brain and spinal cord. Inflammation of the meninges is *meningitis*. Further discussion of the meninges appears in Chapter 9.

↻ TERMINOLOGY REVIEW

Medical Term	Word Parts	Definition
Active transport	*trans-:* across, through	Process that moves substances across or through a membrane and requires cellular energy.
Anatomic position		Standard reference position for the body.
Chondrocyte	*chondr/o:* cartilage *-cyte:* cell	Cartilage cell.
Collagenous fibers	*-ous:* pertaining to	Strong and flexible connective tissue fibers that contain the protein collagen.
Cytokinesis	*cyt/o:* cell *-kinesis:* movement	Division of the cell at the end of mitosis to form two separate daughter cells.
Diffusion		Movement of substances from a region of high concentration to a region of low concentration.
Elastic fibers		Yellow connective tissue fibers that are not particularly strong but can be stretched and will return to their normal shape when released.
Fibroblast	*fibr/o:* fiber *-blast:* to form, immature cell	Connective tissue cell that produces fibers.
Histology	*-hist/o:* tissues *-logy:* study	Branch of microscopic anatomy that studies tissues.
Homeostasis	*home/o:* sameness, unchanging, constant *-stasis:* to stop, control, place	A normal stable condition in which the body's internal environment remains the same; constant internal environment.
Human anatomy	*anatomy:* structure	Study of human body shape and structure and the relationships of its parts.
Human physiology	*physi/o:* nature, function *-logy:* study	Study of the functions of humans and their separate parts.
Macrophage	*macro-:* large *-phage:* eat, swallow	Large phagocytic connective tissue cell that functions in the immune response.
Mast cell		A connective tissue cell that produces heparin and histamine.
Meiosis		Type of nuclear division in which the number of chromosomes is reduced to one half the number found in a body cell; results in the formation of egg or sperm.
Metabolism		The total of all biochemical reactions that take place in the body; includes anabolism and catabolism.
Mitosis		Process by which the nucleus of a body cell divides to form two new cells, each identical to the parent cell.
Negative feedback		A mechanism of response in which a stimulus initiates reactions that reduce the stimulus.

↻ TERMINOLOGY REVIEW—cont'd

Medical Term	Word Parts	Definition
Neuroglia	*neur/o:* nerve *-glia:* glue	Supporting cells of nervous tissue; cells in nervous tissue that do not conduct impulses; nerve glue.
Neuron	*neur/o:* nerve	Nerve cell, including its processes; conducting cell of nervous tissue.
Osmosis		Diffusion of water through a selectively permeable membrane.
Osteocyte	*oste/o:* bone *-cyte:* cell	Mature bone cell.
Passive transport	*trans-:*	Process that moves substances across or through a membrane and does not require cellular energy.
Phagocytosis	*phag/o:* eat, swallow *-cyt-:* cell *-osis:* condition	Condition of cell eating; a form of endocytosis in which solid particles are taken into the cell.
Pinocytosis	*pin/o:* to drink *-cyt-:* cell *-osis:* condition	Condition of cell drinking; a form of endocytosis in which fluid droplets are taken into the cell.
Tissue		Group of similar cells specialized to perform a certain function.

🖎 ON THE WEB

For information on the human body:

American Medical Association: www.ama-assn.org

Cell Biology: www.cytochemistry.net/cell-biology

Cells Alive: www.cellsalive.com

Healthfinder: www.healthfinder.gov

Inner Body: Human Anatomy Online: www.innerbody.com

Loyola University Medical Education Network: www.lumen.luc.edu/lumen/meded/histo/frames/histo_framcs.html

MadSci Network: www.madsci.org

MedlinePlus Tutorials: www.nlm.nih.gov/medlineplus/tutorials

Medscape: www.medscape.com

Medtropolis: The Virtual Body: www.medtropolis.com

The Virtual Cell Web Page: www.ibiblio.org/virtualcell

The Visible Human Project: www.nlm.nih.gov/research/visible

University of Utah Health Sciences Center: library.med.utah.edu

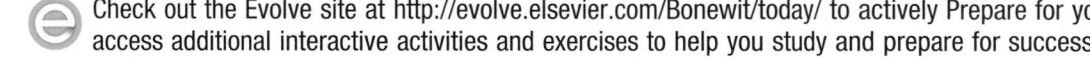

⊖ Check out the Evolve site at http://evolve.elsevier.com/Bonewit/today/ to actively Prepare for your Certification, and to access additional interactive activities and exercises to help you study and prepare for success.

6

Integumentary System

KEY TERMS

arrector pili (ah-REK-tor PY-lee)
ceruminous gland (see-ROOM-in-us GLAND)
dermis (DER-mis)

epidermis (ep-ih-DER-mis)
keratinization (ker-ah-tin-ih-ZAY-shun)
melanin (MEL-ah-nin)
sebaceous gland (see-BAY-shus GLAND)

subcutaneous layer (sub-kyoo-TAY-nee-us LAY-ER)
sudoriferous gland (soo-door-IF-er-us GLAND)

INTRODUCTION TO THE INTEGUMENTARY SYSTEM

The skin and the glands, hair, nails, and other structures that are derived from it make up the *integumentary* (in-teg-yoo-MEN-tar-ee) *system*. Because it is on the outside of the body, this organ system is our contact with the external environment and is subjected to continual abuse from the environment. However, the skin is resilient and versatile. Generally, it quickly repairs itself and continues to perform its many functions year after year.

STRUCTURE OF THE SKIN

The skin (sometimes called the *cutaneous* [kyoo-TAY-nee-us] *membrane*) consists of two distinct layers of tissues. The outer layer is the **epidermis,** and the inner layer is the **dermis.** These are anchored to underlying structures by a third layer, the *hypodermis* or *subcutaneous tissue*.

The structure of the skin is illustrated in Figure 6-1.

Epidermis

The outer layer of the skin is the *epidermis*. This layer consists of stratified squamous epithelium (see Figure 6-1). There are no blood vessels present in the epidermis, and the cells receive their nutrients by diffusion from vessels in the underlying tissue. The bottom row of cells in the epidermis is called the *stratum basale*. It consists of actively dividing (mitotic) columnar cells and melanocytes. This is the layer next to the basement membrane and closest to the blood supply. As older cells are pushed upward toward the surface by the growing cells next to the basement membrane, they receive fewer nutrients. They also undergo a process called **keratinization** (ker-ah-tin-ih-ZAY-shun). During keratinization, a protein called *keratin* is deposited in the cell. This causes the chemical composition of the cell to change, and the cell changes shape. By the time the cells reach the surface, they are flat or squamous. They are also dead from

lack of nutrients and are sloughed off. They are replaced by other cells that are pushed upward from the stratum basale. About one fourth of the cells in the stratum basale are melanocytes (meh-LAN-oh-sytes). Melanocytes are specialized epithelial cells that produce a dark pigment called **melanin** (MEL-ah-nin), which is primarily responsible for skin color.

The outermost or surface region of the epidermis is the stratum corneum (KOR-nee-um). It makes up about three fourths of the epidermal thickness and consists of 20 to 30 layers of flattened, dead, completely keratinized cells. The cells in the stratum corneum are continually shed and replaced. About 5 weeks after a cell has been produced in the stratum basale, it is sloughed off the surface of the stratum corneum. The keratin that is present is a tough, water-repellent protein, and its inclusion in the stratum corneum provides protection against water loss from the body.

Dermis

The *dermis,* or *stratum corium* (KOR-ee-um), is dense connective tissue that is deeper and usually thicker than the epidermis (see Figure 6-1). Hair, nails, and certain glands (although derived from the stratum basale of the epidermis) are embedded in the dermis. The dermis contains both collagenous and elastic fibers to give it strength and elasticity. If the skin is overstretched, the dermis may be damaged, leaving white scars called *striae* (STRY-ee), commonly called "stretch marks." Fibers also form a framework for the numerous blood vessels and nerves that are present in the dermis but generally absent in the epidermis. Many of the nerves in the dermis have specialized endings called *sensory receptors* that detect changes in the environment, such as heat, cold, pain, pressure, and touch. Because there are no nerves in the epidermis, these receptors are the body's contact with the environment.

The upper region of the dermis has numerous *papillae,* or projections, that extend into the epidermis. Blood vessels, nerve endings, and sensory receptors extend

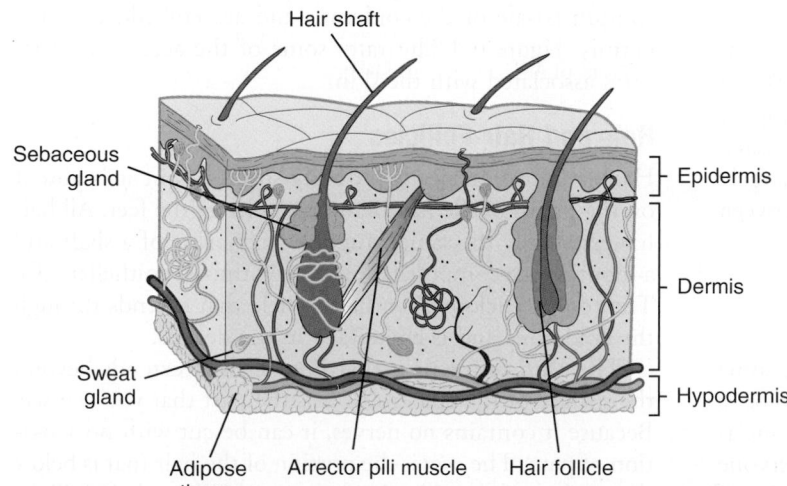

Figure 6-1 Structure of the skin. Note the epidermis, dermis, and hypodermis.

Highlight on the Integumentary System

Skin: For an "average" person, the skin weighs about 5 kg (11 lb), has a surface area of approximately 2 m² (21 ft²), and varies in thickness from 0.05 to 0.4 cm (0.02 to 0.16 inch).

Neoplasms: Cancerous neoplasms composed of melanocytes, called *malignant melanomas,* account for 3% of all cancers, and the incidence is rising at a rate of 4.5% annually. Exposure to sunlight is the major risk factor for the development of malignant melanoma, and individuals with fair skin and light hair are at greatest risk. Melanomas often metastasize to the lung, liver, and brain.

Dermis: The dermis is the portion of an animal's skin that is used to make leather because the collagen in the dermis becomes tough when treated with tannic acid.

Blister: A blister is a fluid-filled pocket between the dermis and the epidermis. When the skin is burned or irritated, some plasma escapes from the blood vessels in the dermis and accumulates between the two layers, where it forms the blister.

Dermal blood vessels: In people with light skin, when dermal blood vessels dilate and blood flow increases (e.g., during blushing and increased temperature), the skin may be quite red. If the vessels constrict and blood flow decreases, the individual is pale or "white as a sheet."

Hair type: The shape of the hair shaft determines whether hair is straight or curly. If the shaft is round, the hair is straight. If it is oval, the hair is wavy. If it is flat, the hair is curly or kinky. To make their hair curly, individuals often get a "permanent," which flattens the hair.

Acne: Acne is a problem that plagues many teenagers. Increased hormone activity at puberty causes an increase in sebaceous gland activity. Sebum and dead cells may block the hair follicle and form blackheads. Bacteria infect the blocked follicle, and the sebum–dead cell mixture accumulates until the follicle ruptures. This initiates an inflammatory response that soon appears on the surface as a pus-filled pimple.

Adipose tissue: People who lose weight rapidly may feel cold because they have reduced their adipose insulation. ∎

---

into the papillae to bring them into closer proximity to the epidermis and the surface. On the palms, the fingertips, and the soles of the feet, the papillae form distinct patterns or ridges that provide friction for grasping objects. The patterns are genetically determined and are unique for each individual. These are the basis of fingerprints and footprints.

Subcutaneous Layer

The **subcutaneous layer** (see Figure 6-1) is not actually a part of the skin, but it loosely anchors the skin to underlying organs. Because it is beneath the dermis, it is sometimes called the *hypodermis.* It is also referred to as *superficial fascia.* The subcutaneous layer consists largely of loose connective tissue and adipose tissue. The fibers in the loose connective tissue are continuous with those in the dermis, and as a result there is no distinct boundary between the dermis and the subcutaneous tissue.

The adipose tissue in the subcutaneous layer cushions the underlying organs from mechanical shock and acts as a heat insulator in temperature regulation. Fat in the adipose tissue can be mobilized and used for energy when necessary. The distribution of subcutaneous adipose tissue is largely responsible for the differences in body contours between men and women.

SKIN COLOR

Skin color is a result of many factors: some genetic, some physiologic, and some environmental. Basic skin color is caused by the dark pigment *melanin* produced by the melanocytes in the stratum basale of the epidermis. Everyone has about the same number of melanocytes. The activity of the melanocytes, however, is genetically controlled. Although many genes are responsible for skin color, a single mutation can result in an inability to produce melanin. This results in a condition called *albinism* (AL-bih-nizm) in which individuals have light skin, white hair, and unpigmented irises in the eyes.

Some people have the yellowish pigment *carotene* (KAIR-oh-teen) in addition to melanin. This gives a yellow tint to the skin. A pinkish tint in the skin is attributable to the blood vessels in the dermis. Ultraviolet light increases melanocyte activity so that more melanin is produced and the skin becomes darker or tanned.

EPIDERMAL DERIVATIVES

Accessory structures of the skin include hair, nails, sweat glands, and sebaceous glands. They are derived from the stratum basale of the epidermis and are embedded in the dermis. Figure 6-1 illustrates some of the accessory structures associated with the skin.

Hair and Hair Follicles

Hair is found on nearly all body surfaces, but it is absent on the palms of the hands and the soles of the feet. All hair has essentially the same structure. It consists of a shaft and a root that are composed of dead, keratinized epithelial cells. The root is enclosed in a hair follicle that extends through the epidermis and is embedded in the dermis.

The *shaft* of a hair is that portion that extends beyond the surface of the epidermis. It is the part that you can see. Because it contains no nerves, it can be cut with no sensation of pain. The *root* is the portion of the hair that is below the surface of the skin. It is surrounded by a hair follicle.

The shaft and root are continuous and together make up the hair, which is produced by the hair follicle. The outermost covering on a hair is a single layer of overlapping, keratinized cells called the *cuticle.* On the shaft of the hair, the cuticle is exposed to the environment and subjected to abrasion. It tends to wear away at the tip of the shaft. When this happens, the inner portion projects from the tip of the shaft, resulting in "split ends."

The root of a hair is enclosed in a tubular *hair follicle* that is embedded in the dermis. Blood vessels in the dermis provide the blood supply for the epithelial cells of the hair follicle. Stratum basale cells, like those in the skin, provide the mitotic cells that divide and undergo keratinization to produce the hair.

Hair color is determined by the type of melanin produced by the melanocytes in the stratum basale. Yellow, brown, and black pigments are present in varying proportions to produce different hair colors. With age, the melanocytes become less active. Hair in which melanin is replaced with air bubbles is white.

A bundle of smooth muscle cells, called the **arrector pili** muscle, is associated with each hair follicle. Most hair follicles are at a slight angle to the surface of the skin. The arrector pili muscles are attached to the hair follicles in such a way that contraction pulls the hair follicles into an upright position or causes the hair to "stand on end." Contraction of the arrector pili muscles also causes raised areas on the skin, or "goose bumps." Action of the arrector pili muscles is controlled by the nervous system in response to cold and fright.

Nails

Nails are thin plates of dead stratum corneum that contain a very hard type of keratin and cover the dorsal surfaces of the distal ends of the fingers and toes. Each nail has a *free edge;* a *nail body,* which is the visible portion; and a *nail root,* which is covered with skin. The *eponychium* (ch-poh-NICK-ee-um) or *cuticle* is a fold of stratum corneum that grows onto the proximal portion of the nail body. Stratum basale from the epidermis grows under the nail body and is responsible for nail growth. The portion of the body over the growth area appears as a whitish, crescent-shaped area called the *lunula* (LOO-nyoo-lah). Nails appear pink because of the rich supply of blood vessels in the underlying dermis.

Glands

The two major glands associated with the skin are the **sebaceous glands** and the *sweat glands.* A third type, the **ceruminous glands,** are modified sweat glands.

Sebaceous Glands

Generally, sebaceous glands are associated with hair follicles and are found in all areas of the body that have hair (see Figure 6-1). Those not associated with hair follicles open directly onto the surface of the skin. The oily secretion, called *sebum,* is transported by a duct into a hair follicle,

and from there it reaches the surface of the skin. Sebum functions to keep hair and skin soft and pliable. It also inhibits growth of bacteria on the skin and helps to prevent water loss. Secretory activity of the sebaceous glands is stimulated by sex hormones; consequently, the glands are relatively inactive in childhood, become highly active during puberty, and decrease in activity during old age. Decreased sebum, in part, accounts for the dry skin and brittle hair that are common in older people.

Sweat (Sudoriferous) Glands

Sweat glands (also called **sudoriferous glands**) are widely distributed over the body. They are most numerous in the palms and soles. The glandular portion of a sweat gland is a coiled tube that is embedded in the dermis of the skin, and the duct opens onto the surface of the skin through a *sweat pore* (see Figure 6-1). The secretion of these glands is primarily water with a few salts. When the body's temperature increases, the glands are stimulated to produce sweat, which evaporates and has a cooling effect. Sweat, or *perspiration,* is also produced in response to nerve stimulation as a result of emotional stress.

Ceruminous Glands

Ceruminous glands are modified sweat glands that are found in the external auditory (ear) canal. They secrete an oily, sticky substance called *cerumen* (see-ROOM-men), or earwax, that is thought to repel insects and trap foreign material.

FUNCTIONS OF THE SKIN

Protection

The skin forms a protective covering over the entire body. The keratin in the cells waterproofs the cells and helps prevent fluid loss from the body. This waterproofing also prevents too much water from entering the body during swimming and bathing. Unbroken skin forms the first line of defense against bacteria and other invading organisms. The oily secretions of the sebaceous glands are acidic and inhibit bacterial growth on the skin. Melanin pigment absorbs light and helps protect underlying tissues from the damaging effects of ultraviolet light. Skin also protects underlying tissues from mechanical, chemical, and thermal injury.

Sensory Reception

The dermis contains numerous sensory receptors for heat, cold, pain, touch, and pressure. Even though hair itself has no sensory receptors, the movement of hair can be detected by receptors clustered around a hair follicle. The sensory receptors in the dermis relay information about the environment to the brain so that changes can be made to prevent or minimize injury. The sensory receptors are also a means of communication between individuals.

Regulation of Body Temperature

Normally, body temperature is maintained at 37° C (98.6° F). It is important that body temperature be regulated because changes in temperature alter the speed of chemical reactions in the body. The skin helps to regulate body temperature in two ways: by dilation and constriction of blood vessels, and by activity or inactivity of the sweat glands. Both of these mechanisms are examples of negative feedback in maintaining homeostasis. Blood vessels dilate and sweat glands become active in response to an increase in body temperature. Both mechanisms tend to remove heat from the body. In response to cold, blood vessels constrict and sweat glands are inactive to conserve body heat. The adipose tissue in the subcutaneous layer also helps by acting as an insulator.

Synthesis of Vitamin D

Vitamin D is required for calcium and phosphorus absorption in the small intestine. The calcium and phosphorus are essential for normal bone metabolism and muscle function. Skin cells contain a precursor molecule that is converted to vitamin D when the precursor is exposed to ultraviolet rays in sunlight. It takes only a small amount of ultraviolet light to stimulate vitamin D production, so this should not be used as an excuse to expose the skin to sun unnecessarily and to risk the damage that may result.

AGING OF THE INTEGUMENTARY SYSTEM

As the skin ages, the number of elastic fibers decreases and adipose tissue is lost from the dermis and subcutaneous layer. This causes the skin to wrinkle and sag. Loss of collagen fibers in the dermis makes the skin more fragile and makes it heal more slowly. Mitotic activity in the stratum basale slows so that the skin becomes thinner and appears more transparent. Reduced sebaceous gland activity causes dry, itchy skin. Loss of adipose tissue in the subcutaneous layer and reduced sweat gland activity lead to an intolerance to cold and susceptibility to heat. The ability of the skin to regulate temperature is reduced. There is a general reduction in melanocyte activity, which decreases protection from ultraviolet light, resulting in increased susceptibility to sunburn and skin cancer. Some melanocytes, however, may increase melanin production, resulting in "age spots."

Despite all the creams and "miracle" lotions, there is no known way to prevent skin from aging. Good nutrition and cleanliness may slow the aging process. Because skin that is exposed to sunlight ages more rapidly than unexposed skin, one of the best ways to slow the aging process is to avoid exposure by wearing protective clothing and by using sunblock whenever possible.

Highlight on Conditions Affecting the Integumentary System

Alopecia (al-oh-PEE-shee-ah) Absence of hair from skin areas where it normally grows; baldness; may be hereditary or caused by disease, injury, or chemotherapy or may occur as part of aging

Basal cell carcinoma (BAY-sal SELL kar-sih-NOH-mah) Malignant tumor of the basal cell layer of the epidermis; most common form of skin cancer and usually grows slowly

Cellulitis (sell-yoo-LYE-tis) Infection of connective tissue with severe inflammation of the dermis and subcutaneous layers of the skin

Dermatitis (der-mah-TYE-tis) Inflammation of the skin

Eczema (ECK-zeh-mah) An inflammatory skin disease with red, itching, vesicular lesions that may crust over; common allergic reaction, but may occur without any obvious cause

Eschar (ESS-kar) A slough produced by a burn or gangrene

Impetigo (im-peh-TYE-go) Superficial skin infection caused by staphylococcal or streptococcal bacteria and characterized by vesicles, pustules, and crusted-over lesions; most common in children

Malignant melanoma (mah-LIG-nant mel-ah-NOH-mah) Cancerous growth composed of melanocytes; often arises in a preexisting mole; an alarming increase in the prevalence of malignant melanoma is attributed to excessive exposure to sunlight

Nevus (NEE-vus) An elevated, pigmented lesion on the skin; commonly called a *mole;* a dysplastic nevus is a mole that does not form properly and may progress to a type of skin cancer; plural, *nevi*

Pruritus (proo-RYE-tus) Severe itching; one of the most common problems in dermatology; arises as a result of stimulation of nerves in the skin by enzymes released in allergic reactions or by other irritating substances

Urticaria (ur-tih-KAIR-ee-ah) Allergic transient skin eruptions characterized by elevated lesions, called *wheals,* and often accompanied by severe itching and burning; also called *hives*

Wart (WORT) Epidermal growth on the skin caused by a virus; plantar warts occur on the soles of the feet, juvenile warts occur on the hands and face of children, and venereal warts occur in the genital area

Xeroderma pigmentosum (zee-roh-DER-mah pig-men-TOH-sum) A pigmentary and atrophic inherited disease of the skin and eyes that is characterized by vascular lesions, excessive freckling, keratinous growths, carcinoma, photophobia, ocular opacities, and tumors; involves defect in the enzymes active in the repair of DNA damaged by ultraviolet light ■

TERMINOLOGY REVIEW

Medical Term	Word Parts	Definition
Arrector pili	*pil/o:* hair	Muscle associated with hair follicles.
Ceruminous gland	*cerumin/o:* cerumen	A gland in the ear canal that produces cerumen or ear wax.
Dermis	*derm/o:* skin	Inner layer of the skin that contains the blood vessels, nerves, glands, and hair follicles.
Epidermis	*epi-:* above, upon *-derma:* skin	Outermost layer of the skin.
Keratinization	*kerat/o:* hard, horny tissue *-ation:* process, condition	Process by which the cells of the epidermis become filled with keratin and move to the surface where they are sloughed off.
Melanin	*melan/o:* black	A dark brown or black pigment found in parts of the body, especially skin and hair.
Sebaceous gland	*seb/o:* sebum *-ous:* pertaining to	An oil gland of the skin that produces sebum or body oil.
Subcutaneous layer	*sub-:* under, below *cutane/o:* skin *-ous:* pertaining to	Below the skin; a sheet of areolar connective tissue and adipose tissue beneath the dermis of the skin; also called *hypodermis* or *superficial fascia*.
Sudoriferous gland	*sud-:* sweat *-ous:* pertaining to	A gland in the skin that produces perspiration; also called *sweat gland*.

ON THE WEB

For information on the integumentary system:

British Medical Journal: Dermatology: www.bmj.com/cgi/collection/dermatology

Loyola University Medication Education Network: Dermatology Atlas: www.meddean.luc.edu/lumen/MedEd/medicine/dermatology/melton/title.htm

Merck Manual—Dermatologic Disorders: www.merck.com/mmpe *(Click on "Dermatologic Disorders")*

Skin Cancer Risk Analyzer: www.telemedicine.org/melanoma.htm

University of Delaware—Integumentary System: www.udel.edu/biology/Wags/histopage/colorpage/cin/cin.htm

 Check out the Evolve site at http://evolve.elsevier.com/Bonewit/today/ to actively Prepare for your Certification, and to access additional interactive activities and exercises to help you study and prepare for success.

7

Skeletal System

LEARNING OBJECTIVES

1. List and describe five functions of the skeletal system.
2. Explain the difference between compact and spongy bone.
3. Classify bones according to size and shape.
4. Identify the general features of a long bone.
5. Explain the process by which long bones grow in length.
6. Explain the difference between the axial and appendicular skeletons.
7. Identify the bones of the skull.
8. Identify the structural features of vertebrae.
9. List and describe the divisions of the vertebral column.
10. Describe the structural features of the sternum and ribs.
11. Identify the parts of the pectoral girdle.
12. Identify the bones of the upper extremities.
13. Identify the parts of the pelvic girdle.
14. Identify the bones of the lower extremities.
15. List and describe the different types of joints.
16. Describe ways in which the aging of an individual affects the skeletal system.
17. Identify pathology related to the skeletal system.

CHAPTER OUTLINE

INTRODUCTION TO THE SKELETAL SYSTEM
Overview of the Skeletal System
Functions of the Skeletal System
Structure of Bone Tissue
Classification of Bones
General Features of a Long Bone
Bone Development and Growth
Bone Growth in Length
Divisions of the Skeleton
Bones of the Axial Skeleton
Skull
Hyoid Bone

Vertebral Column
Thoracic Cage
Bones of the Appendicular Skeleton
Pectoral Girdle
Upper Extremity
Pelvic Girdle
Lower Extremity
Articulations
Synarthroses
Amphiarthroses
Diarthroses
Aging of the Skeletal System

INTRODUCTION TO THE SKELETAL SYSTEM

The skeletal system consists of the bones and the cartilage, ligaments, and tendons associated with the bones. It accounts for about 20% of the body weight. Bones are rigid structures that form the framework for the body. People often think of bones as dead, dry, inert pipes and plates because that is how they are seen in the laboratory. In reality, the living bones in our bodies contain active tissues that consume nutrients, require a blood supply, use oxygen and discharge waste products in metabolism, and change shape or remodel in response to variations in mechanical stress. The skeletal system is strong but lightweight. It is well adapted for the functions it must perform. It is a masterpiece of design.

OVERVIEW OF THE SKELETAL SYSTEM

Functions of the Skeletal System

The skeletal system gives form and shape to the body. Without the skeletal components, we would appear as big "blobs" inefficiently "oozing" around on the ground. Besides contributing to shape and form, our bones perform several other functions and play an important role in homeostasis.

Support
Bones provide a rigid framework that supports the soft organs of the body. Bones support the body against the pull of gravity, and the large bones of the lower limbs support the trunk when standing.

Protection
The skeleton protects the soft body parts. The fused bones of the cranium surround the brain to make it less vulnerable to injury. The vertebrae surround and protect the spinal cord. The bones of the rib cage help protect the heart and lungs in the thorax.

Movement
Bones provide sites for muscle attachment. Bones and muscles work together as simple mechanical lever systems to produce body movement.

Storage
The intercellular matrix of bone contains large amounts of calcium salts, the most important being calcium phosphate.

Calcium is necessary for vital metabolic processes. When blood calcium levels decrease below normal, calcium is released from the bones so that there will be an adequate supply for metabolic needs. When blood calcium levels are increased, the excess calcium is stored in the bone matrix. Storage and release are dynamic processes that go on almost continually.

Blood Cell Formation
Blood cell formation, called *hematopoiesis* (hee-mat-oh-poy-EE-sis), takes place mostly in the red marrow of bones. Red marrow is found in the cavities of most bones in an infant. With age, it is largely replaced by yellow marrow for fat storage. In the adult, red marrow is limited to the spongy bone in the skull, ribs, sternum, clavicles, vertebrae, and pelvis. Red marrow functions in the formation of red blood cells, white blood cells, and blood platelets.

Structure of Bone Tissue

There are two types of bone tissue: compact and spongy. As the names imply, the two types differ in density, or how tightly the tissue is packed together. Three types of cells contribute to bone homeostasis: osteoblasts, osteoclasts, and osteocytes. Osteoblasts are bone-forming cells, osteoclasts resorb or break down bone, and osteocytes are mature bone cells. An equilibrium between osteoblasts and osteoclasts maintains bone tissue.

Compact Bone
The microscopic unit of compact bone is known as the **osteon** (haversian system). The osteon consists of a central canal called the *osteonic* (haversian) *canal,* which is surrounded by concentric rings (lamellae) of hard, calcified matrix. Between the rings of matrix, the bone cells (osteocytes) are located in spaces called *lacunae.* Small channels (canaliculi) radiate from the lacunae to the osteonic (haversian) canal to provide passageways through the hard matrix. In compact bone the haversian systems are packed tightly together to form what appears to be a solid mass. The osteonic canals contain blood vessels that are parallel to the long axis of the bone. These blood vessels interconnect, by way of perforating (Volkmann) canals, with vessels on the surface of the bone. The microscopic structure of compact bone is illustrated in Figure 7-1.

Spongy (Cancellous) Bone
Spongy (cancellous) bone is lighter and less dense than compact bone (see Figure 7-1). Spongy bone consists of plates and bars of bone adjacent to small, irregular cavities

Highlight on the Skeletal System

Osteoporosis: Osteoporosis is a bone disorder caused by decreased osteoblast activity. It is characterized by loss of the organic matrix, collagenous fibers, and minerals in the bone tissue. People with osteoporosis are susceptible to deformities of the vertebral column and fractures because the bones are too weak to support the weight of the body. Osteoporosis occurs most frequently in postmenopausal Caucasian women. Factors that influence its occurrence are aging, malnutrition, lack of exercise, and hormone imbalance. Supplemental estrogen after menopause may be of benefit, and exercise is always important in maintaining bone strength.

Epiphyseal plate: The epiphyseal plates of specific long bones ossify at predictable times. Radiologists frequently can determine a young person's age by examining the epiphyseal plates to see whether they have ossified. A difference between bone age and chronologic age may indicate some type of metabolic dysfunction.

Mastoiditis: The mastoid air cells are separated from the cranial cavity by only a thin partition of bone. A middle ear infection that spreads to the mastoid air cells (mastoiditis) is serious because there is danger that the infection will spread from the air cells to the membranes around the brain.

Sinus problems: The bones with paranasal sinuses are the frontal, the sphenoid, the ethmoid, and the two maxillae. The sinuses are lined with mucous membranes that are continuous with the nasal cavity. Allergies and infections cause inflammation of the membranes, which results in sinusitis. The swollen membranes may reduce drainage from the sinuses so that pressure within the cavities increases, resulting in sinus headaches.

Soft spots: The bones in the skull of a newborn are not completely joined together but are separated by fibrous membranes. The six large areas of membranes are called *fontanels*, or soft spots. The anterior fontanel is on the top of the head, at the junction of the frontal and parietal bones. The posterior fontanel is at the junction of the occipital and parietal bones. On each side of the head there is a mastoid (posterolateral) fontanel near the mastoid region of the temporal bone and a sphenoid (anterolateral) fontanel just superior to the sphenoid bone.

Abnormal spinal curvatures: An abnormally exaggerated lumbar curvature is called *lordosis,* or swayback. This is often seen in pregnant women as they adjust to their changing center of gravity. An increased roundness of the thoracic curvature is kyphosis, or hunchback. This is frequently seen in elderly people. Abnormal side-to-side curvature is scoliosis. Abnormal curvatures may interfere with breathing and other vital functions.

Yes and no: The atlas holds up the skull and permits you to nod "yes." The axis allows you to rotate your head from side to side to indicate "no."

Marrow biopsy: The sternum is frequently used for a red marrow biopsy because it is accessible. The sample for biopsy is obtained by performing a sternal puncture, in which a large needle is inserted into the sternum to remove a sample of red bone marrow.

Fractured clavicle: The clavicle is the most frequently fractured bone in the body because it transmits forces from the arm to the trunk. The force from falling on the shoulder or outstretched arm is often sufficient to fracture the clavicle.

Tennis elbow: Tennis elbow is an inflammation of the tissues surrounding the lateral epicondyle of the humerus. Six muscles that control movement of the hand attach in this region, and repeated contraction of these muscles irritates the attachments. The medical term for tennis elbow is *lateral epicondylitis.*

Pelvic outlet and childbirth: The female pelvis is shaped to accommodate childbearing. Because the fetus must pass through the pelvic outlet, the physician carefully measures this opening to make sure there is enough room. The distance between the two ischial spines is a good indication of the size of the pelvic outlet. If the opening is too small, a cesarean delivery is indicated.

Broken hip: Elderly people, particularly those with osteoporosis, are susceptible to "breaking a hip." The femur is a weight-bearing bone, and when it is weakened, it cannot support the weight of the body and the neck of the femur fractures under the stress. Instead of saying, "Grandma fell and broke her hip," often it is more appropriate to say, "Grandma broke her hip, then fell."

Bunion: Poorly fitted shoes may compress the toes so that there is a lateral deviation of the big toe toward the second toe. When this occurs, a bursa and callus form at the joint between the first metatarsal and proximal phalanx. This creates a bunion.

Gout: Gout was commonly known as the disease of the kings because it was believed to be caused by a rich diet and fine wines. Gout is an equal-opportunity disease, however, and occurs across the entire population. A rich diet and fine wines may contribute to the disease, but they are not the definitive cause. Gout is caused by the excessive accumulation of uric acid that forms needle-like crystals within the joint, producing pain and inflammation. The great toe is the most commonly affected joint. The disorder is diagnosed by aspirating joint fluid and observing the crystals under the microscope. Although there is no cure for gout, it can be effectively controlled with antiinflammatory drugs and dietary measures.

Knee problems: The term *torn cartilage* refers to a damaged meniscus, usually the medial, in the knee. Frequently this can be repaired with relatively minor arthroscopic surgery. A torn ligament in the knee usually involves one of the cruciate ligaments. The surgical procedure to repair this damage is quite involved, and recovery of function may require months of rehabilitative therapy. ■

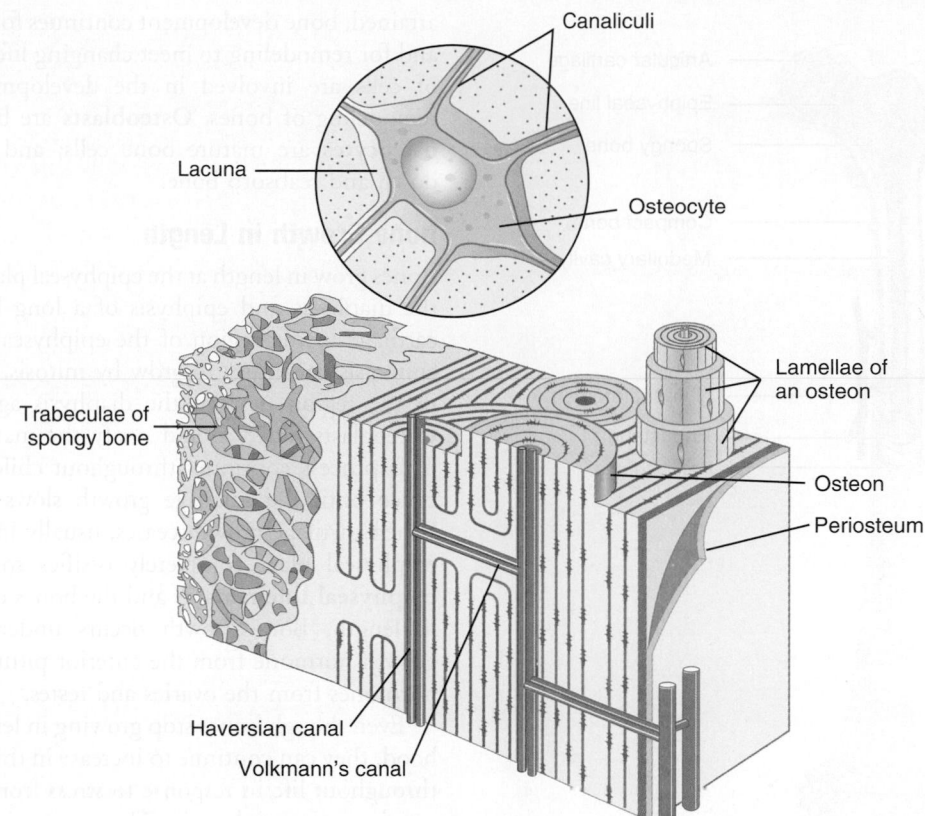

Figure 7-1 Structure of compact and spongy bone. Note the osteons packed together for compact bone and trabeculae of spongy bone.

that contain red bone marrow. The plates of bone are called *trabeculae* (trah-BEK-yoo-lee). The canaliculi, instead of connecting to a central haversian canal, connect to the adjacent cavities to receive their blood supply. It may appear that the trabeculae are arranged in a haphazard manner, but they are organized to provide maximum strength in the same way that braces are used to support a building. The trabeculae of spongy bone follow the lines of stress and can realign if the direction of stress changes.

Classification of Bones

Bones come in a variety of sizes and shapes. Bones that are longer than they are wide are called *long bones*. They consist of a long shaft with two bulky ends or extremities. They are primarily compact bone but may have a large amount of spongy bone at the ends. Examples of long bones are those in the thigh, leg, arm, and forearm.

Short bones are roughly cube-shaped with vertical and horizontal dimensions approximately equal. They consist primarily of spongy bone, which is covered by a thin layer of compact bone. Examples of short bones include the bones of the wrist and ankle.

Flat bones are thin, flattened, and often curved. They are usually arranged like a sandwich with a middle layer of spongy bone called the *diploë* (DIP-loh-ee). The diploë is covered on each side by a layer of compact bone; these layers are called the *inner* and *outer tables*. Most of the bones of the cranium are flat bones.

Bones that are not in any of the previously mentioned three categories are classified as *irregular bones*. They are primarily spongy bone that is covered with a thin layer of compact bone. The vertebrae and some of the bones in the skull are irregular bones.

General Features of a Long Bone

Most long bones have the same general features, which are illustrated in Figure 7-2.

Diaphysis: The shaft of a long bone is called the **diaphysis** (dye-AF-ih-sis). It is formed from relatively thick compact bone that surrounds a hollow space called the *medullary* (MED-yoo-lair-ee) *cavity.*

Medullary cavity: In adults the medullary cavity contains yellow bone marrow, so it is sometimes called the *yellow marrow cavity.*

Epiphysis: At each end of the diaphysis, there is an expanded portion called the **epiphysis** (ee-PIF-ih-sis). The epiphysis is spongy bone covered by a thin layer of compact bone. The end of the epiphysis, where it meets another bone, is covered by hyaline cartilage, called the *articular cartilage.* This provides smooth surfaces for movement in the joints. In growing bones, there is an **epiphyseal** (ep-ih-FIZ-ee-al) **plate** of hyaline cartilage between the diaphysis and epiphysis. Bones grow in length at the epiphyseal plate. Growth ceases when the cartilaginous epiphyseal plate is replaced by a bony epiphyseal line.

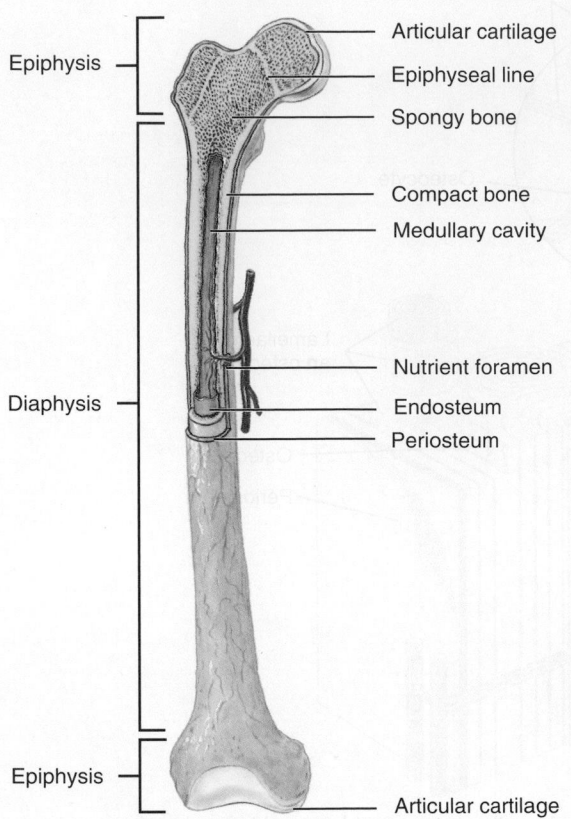

Figure 7-2 General features of long bones.

Periosteum: Except in the region of the articular cartilage, the outer surface of long bones is covered by a tough, fibrous connective tissue called the *periosteum.* The periosteum is richly supplied with nerve fibers, lymphatic vessels, blood vessels, and osteoblasts.

Nutrient foramina: Blood vessels enter the diaphysis of the bone through small openings called *nutrient foramina.*

Endosteum: The surface of the medullary cavity is lined with a thinner connective tissue membrane, the endosteum, which contains osteoclasts.

In addition to the general features that are present in most long bones, all bones have surface markings and characteristics that make a specific bone unique. Bones have holes, depressions, smooth facets, lines, projections, and other markings. These usually represent passageways for vessels and nerves, points of articulation with other bones, or points of attachment for tendons and ligaments.

Bone Development and Growth

The terms *osteogenesis* and *ossification* are often used synonymously to indicate the process of bone formation. Parts of the skeleton form during the first few weeks after conception. By the end of the eighth week after conception, the skeletal pattern is formed in cartilage and connective tissue membranes and ossification begins. Bone development continues throughout adulthood. Even after adult stature is attained, bone development continues for repair of fractures and for remodeling to meet changing lifestyles. Three types of cells are involved in the development, growth, and remodeling of bones. **Osteoblasts** are bone-forming cells; **osteocytes** are mature bone cells; and **osteoclasts** break down and reabsorb bone.

Bone Growth in Length

Bones grow in length at the epiphyseal plate located between the diaphysis and epiphysis of a long bone. The hyaline cartilage in the region of the epiphyseal plate next to the epiphysis continues to grow by mitosis. The chondrocytes in the region next to the diaphysis age and degenerate. Osteoblasts move in and ossify the matrix to form bone. This process continues throughout childhood and adolescence until the cartilage growth slows and finally stops. When cartilage growth ceases, usually in the early 20s, the epiphyseal plate completely ossifies so that only a thin **epiphyseal line** remains and the bones can no longer grow in length. Bone growth occurs under the influence of growth hormone from the anterior pituitary gland and sex hormones from the ovaries and testes.

Even though bones stop growing in length in early adulthood, they can continue to increase in thickness or diameter throughout life in response to stress from increased muscle activity or to weight gain. The increase in diameter is called *appositional* (ap-poh-ZISH-un-al) *growth.* Osteoblasts in the periosteum form compact bone around the external bone surface. At the same time, osteoclasts in the endosteum break down bone on the internal bone surface, around the medullary cavity. These two processes together increase the diameter of the bone and at the same time keep the bone from becoming excessively heavy and bulky.

Divisions of the Skeleton

The typical adult human skeleton consists of 206 named bones. For convenience, the bones of the skeleton are grouped in two divisions, as illustrated in Figure 7-3. The 80 bones of the *axial skeleton* form the vertical axis of the body. They include the bones of the head, vertebral column, ribs, and breastbone or sternum. The *appendicular skeleton* consists of 126 bones and includes the free appendages and their attachments to the axial skeleton. The free appendages are the upper and lower extremities, or limbs, and their attachments are called *girdles.* Table 7-1 lists the named bones of the body by category.

BONES OF THE AXIAL SKELETON

The axial skeleton, with 80 bones, is divided into the skull, hyoid, vertebral column, and rib cage.

Skull

The skull has 28 bones, as illustrated in Figures 7-4 and 7-5. The eight bones of the *cranium* are interlocked to enclose the brain. The anterior aspect of the skull, the *face,* consists of 14 bones. The remaining six bones are the

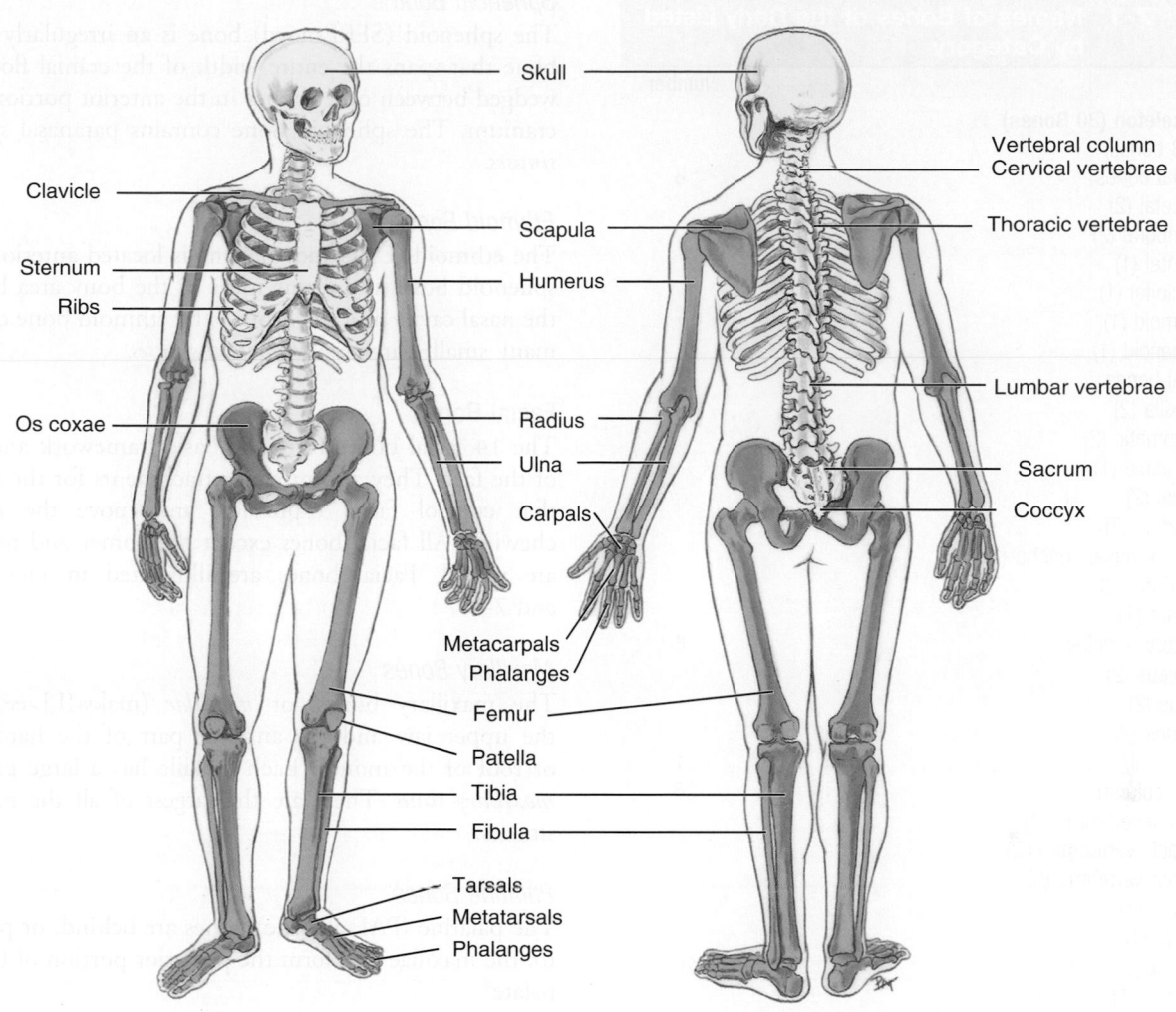

Figure 7-3 Divisions of the skeleton with major bones identified. Yellow = axial skeleton. Blue = appendicular skeleton.

auditory ossicles, tiny bones in the middle ear cavity. With the exception of the lower jaw, or mandible, and the auditory ossicles, the bones in the skull are tightly interlocked along irregular lines called *sutures.* Some of the bones in the skull contain *sinuses,* which are air-filled cavities lined with mucous membranes. The sinuses help to reduce the weight of the skull. The paranasal sinuses are arranged around the nasal cavity and drain into it.

Cranium

Frontal Bone
The frontal bone forms the anterior portion of the skull above the eyes (forehead). The paranasal *frontal sinuses* are cavities in the frontal bone.

Parietal Bones
The two parietal (pah-RYE-eh-tal) bones form most of the superolateral aspect of the skull.

Occipital Bone
The single occipital (ahk-SIP-ih-tal) bone forms most of the posterior part of the skull. The *foramen magnum* is a large opening on the lower surface of the occipital bone. The spinal cord passes through this opening. *Occipital condyles* are rounded processes on each side of the foramen magnum. They articulate with the first cervical vertebra.

Temporal Bones
The two temporal bones, one on each side of the head, form parts of the sides and base of the cranium. Near the inferior margin of the temporal bone, there is an opening, the *external auditory meatus,* which is a canal that leads to the middle ear. Just anterior to the external auditory meatus, the temporal bone articulates with the mandible to form the *temporomandibular joint* (TMJ). Posterior and inferior to each external auditory meatus, there is a rough protuberance, the *mastoid process.* The mastoid process contains air cells that drain into the middle ear cavity.

Table 7-1 Names of Bones of the Body Listed by Category	
Bones	**Number**
Axial Skeleton (80 Bones)	
Skull (28 bones)	
Cranial bones	8
Parietal (2)	
Temporal (2)	
Frontal (1)	
Occipital (1)	
Ethmoid (1)	
Sphenoid (1)	
Facial bones	14
Maxilla (2)	
Zygomatic (2)	
Mandible (1)	
Nasal (2)	
Palatine (2)	
Inferior nasal concha (2)	
Lacrimal (2)	
Vomer (1)	
Auditory ossicles	6
Malleus (2)	
Incus (2)	
Stapes (2)	
Hyoid	1
Vertebral column	26
Cervical vertebrae (7)	
Thoracic vertebrae (12)	
Lumbar vertebrae (5)	
Sacrum (1)	
Coccyx (1)	
Thoracic cage	25
Sternum (1)	
Ribs (24)	
Appendicular Skeleton (126 Bones)	
Pectoral girdles	4
Clavicle (2)	
Scapula (2)	
Upper extremity	60
Humerus (2)	
Radius (2)	
Ulna (2)	
Carpals (16)	
Metacarpals (10)	
Phalanges (28)	
Pelvic girdle	2
Coxal, innominate, or hip bones (2)	
Lower extremity	60
Femur (2)	
Tibia (2)	
Fibula (2)	
Patella (2)	
Tarsals (14)	
Metatarsals (10)	
Phalanges (28)	

From Applegate E: *The anatomy and physiology learning system*, ed 4, St Louis, 2011, Saunders.

Sphenoid Bone

The sphenoid (SFEE-noyd) bone is an irregularly shaped bone that spans the entire width of the cranial floor. It is wedged between other bones in the anterior portion of the cranium. The sphenoid bone contains paranasal *sphenoid sinuses.*

Ethmoid Bone

The ethmoid (ETH-moyd) bone is located anterior to the sphenoid bone and forms most of the bony area between the nasal cavity and the orbits. The ethmoid bone contains many small, paranasal *ethmoidal sinuses.*

Facial Bones

The 14 facial bones form the basic framework and shape of the face. They also provide attachments for the muscles that control facial expression and move the jaw for chewing. All facial bones except the vomer and mandible are paired. Facial bones are illustrated in Figures 7-4 and 7-5.

Maxillary Bones

The maxillary bones, or *maxillae* (maks-ILL-ee), form the upper jaw and the anterior part of the hard palate or roof of the mouth. Each maxilla has a large paranasal *maxillary sinus.* These are the largest of all the paranasal sinuses.

Palatine Bones

The palatine (PAL-ah-tyne) bones are behind, or posterior to, the maxillae and form the posterior portion of the hard palate.

Nasal Bones

The two nasal bones are small rectangular bones that form the bridge of the nose.

Lacrimal Bones

The small, thin lacrimal (LACK-rih-mal) bones are located in the medial walls of the orbits, between the ethmoid bone and the maxilla. Each one has a small *lacrimal groove* that is a pathway for a tube that carries tears from the eyes to the nasal cavity.

Zygomatic Bones

The zygomatic (zye-goh-MAT-ik) bones, also called *malar* bones, form the prominences of the cheeks.

Inferior Nasal Conchae

The inferior nasal conchae (KONG-kee) are thin, curved bones that are attached to the lateral walls of the nasal cavity and project into the nasal cavity.

Vomer

The thin, flat vomer (VOH-mer) is in the inferior portion of the midline in the nasal cavity. It forms part of the *nasal septum.*

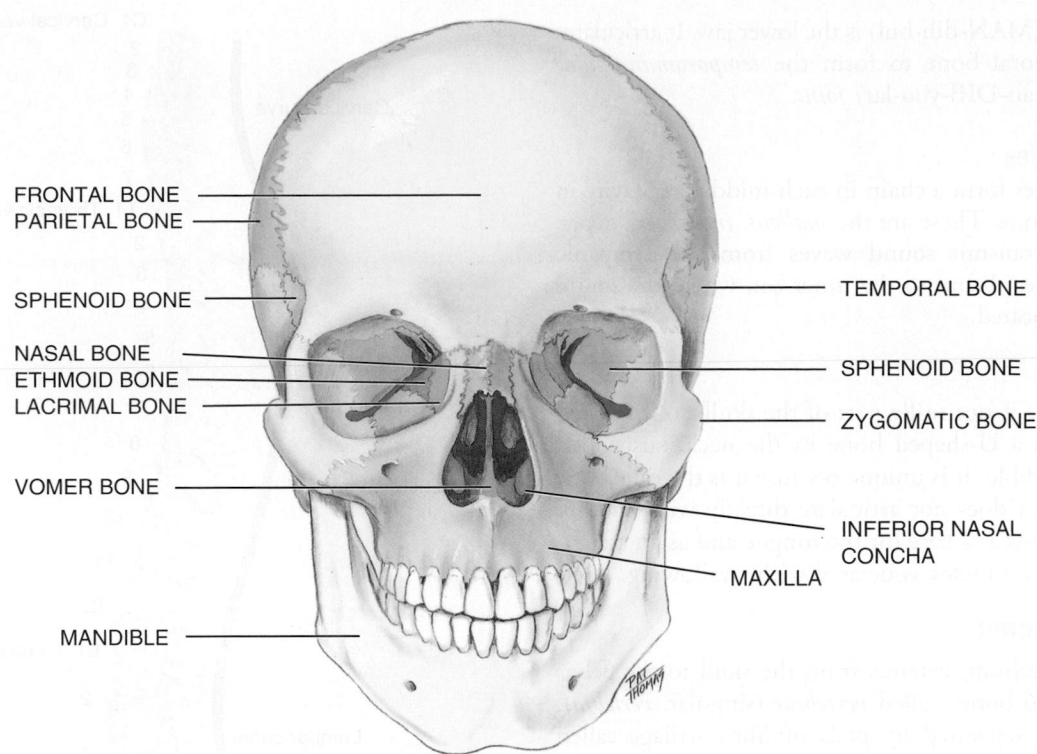

FRONTAL BONE
PARIETAL BONE
SPHENOID BONE
NASAL BONE
ETHMOID BONE
LACRIMAL BONE
VOMER BONE

TEMPORAL BONE
SPHENOID BONE
ZYGOMATIC BONE
INFERIOR NASAL CONCHA
MAXILLA
MANDIBLE

Figure 7-4 Skull, anterior view.

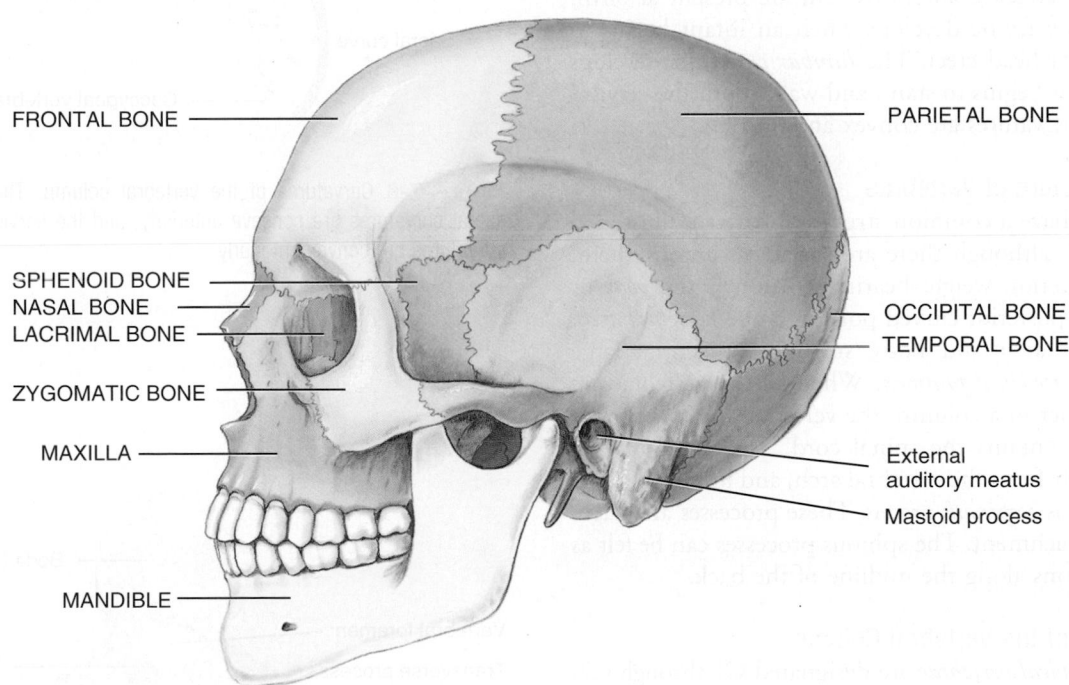

FRONTAL BONE
SPHENOID BONE
NASAL BONE
LACRIMAL BONE
ZYGOMATIC BONE
MAXILLA
MANDIBLE

PARIETAL BONE
OCCIPITAL BONE
TEMPORAL BONE
External auditory meatus
Mastoid process

Figure 7-5 Skull, lateral view.

Mandible

The mandible (MAN-dih-bul) is the lower jaw. It articulates with the temporal bone to form the *temporomandibular* (tem-por-oh-man-DIB-yoo-lar) *joint.*

Auditory Ossicles

Three tiny bones form a chain in each middle ear cavity in the temporal bone. These are the *malleus, incus,* and *stapes.* These bones transmit sound waves from the tympanic membrane, or eardrum, to the inner ear, where the sound receptors are located.

Hyoid Bone

The hyoid bone is not really part of the skull, so it is listed separately. It is a U-shaped bone in the neck, suspended under the mandible. It is unique because it is the only bone in the body that does not articulate directly with another bone. It functions as a base for the tongue and as an attachment for several muscles associated with swallowing.

Vertebral Column

The vertebral column extends from the skull to the pelvis and contains 26 bones called *vertebrae* (singular, *vertebra*). The bones are separated by pads of fibrocartilage called *intervertebral discs.* The discs act as shock absorbers and allow the column to bend. Normally there are four curvatures, illustrated in Figure 7-6, that increase the strength and resilience of the column. They are named according to the region in which they are located. The *thoracic* and *sacral curvatures* are concave anteriorly and are present at birth. The *cervical curvature* develops when an infant begins to hold his or her head erect. The *lumbar curvature* develops when an infant begins to stand and walk. Both the cervical and lumbar curvatures are convex anteriorly.

General Structure of Vertebrae

All vertebrae have a common structural pattern, illustrated in Figure 7-7, although there are variations among them. The thick anterior, weight-bearing portion is the *body* or *centrum.* The posterior curved portion is the *vertebral arch.* The vertebral arch and body surround a central large opening, the *vertebral foramen.* When all the vertebrae are stacked together in a column, the vertebral foramina make a canal that contains the spinal cord. *Transverse processes* project laterally from the vertebral arch, and in the posterior midline there is a *spinous process.* These processes are places for muscle attachment. The spinous processes can be felt as bony projections along the midline of the back.

Composition of the Vertebral Column

The seven *cervical vertebrae* are designated C1 through C7. The 12 *thoracic vertebrae* are designated T1 through T12. Five *lumbar vertebrae,* designated L1 through L5, make up the part of the vertebral column in the small of the back. The lumbar vertebrae have large, heavy bodies because they support most of the body weight and have many back muscles attached to them.

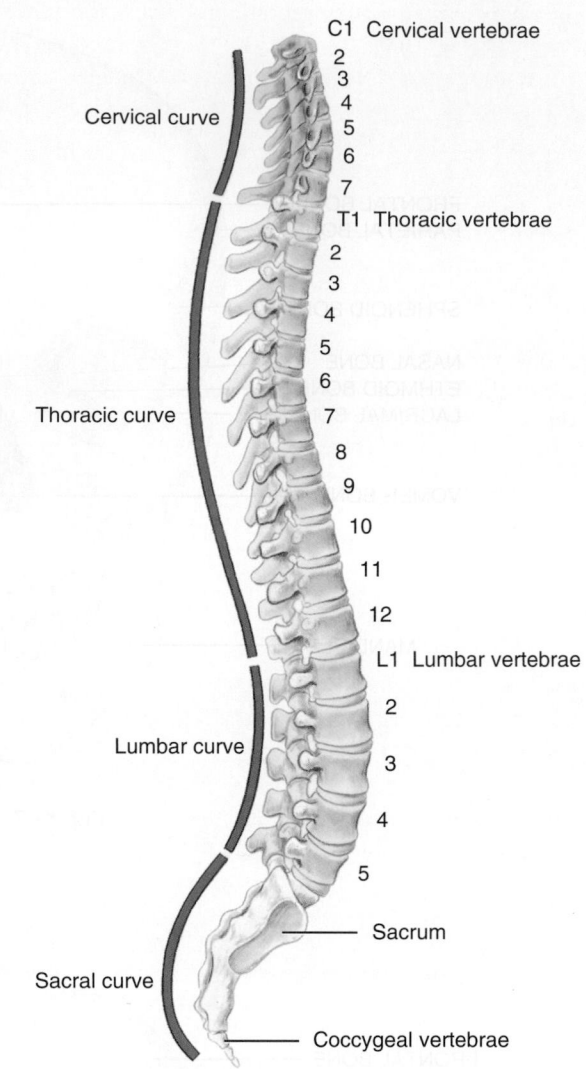

Figure 7-6 Curvatures of the vertebral column. The thoracic and sacral curvatures are concave anteriorly, and the cervical and lumbar curvatures are convex anteriorly.

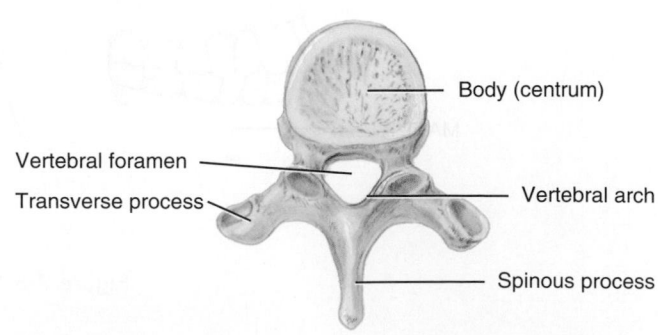

Figure 7-7 General features of vertebrae, viewed from above.

The *sacrum* is a triangular bone just below the lumbar vertebrae. In the child there are five separate bones, but these fuse to form a single bone in the adult. The sacrum articulates with the pelvic girdle laterally, at the *sacroiliac (say-kro-ILL-ee-ak) joint,* and forms the posterior wall of the pelvic cavity.

The *coccyx* (KOK-siks), or tailbone, is the last part of the vertebral column (see Figure 7-8). A child has four (the number varies from three to five) separate small bones, but these fuse to form a single bone in the adult.

Thoracic Cage

The thoracic cage, or bony thorax, protects the heart, lungs, and great vessels. It also supports the bones of the shoulder girdle and plays a role in breathing. The components of the thoracic cage are the thoracic vertebrae dorsally, the ribs laterally, and the sternum and costal cartilage anteriorly.

Sternum

The *sternum,* or breastbone, is in the anterior midline (Figure 7-8). An important anatomic landmark, the *jugular (suprasternal) notch* is an easily palpable, central indentation in the superior margin of the sternum. The superior portion of the sternum articulates with the clavicles and the first two pairs of ribs. The body of the sternum has notches along the sides where it attaches to the cartilage of the third through seventh ribs.

Ribs

Twelve pairs of *ribs,* illustrated in Figure 7-8, form the curved, lateral margins of the thoracic cage. One pair is attached to each of the 12 thoracic vertebrae. The upper seven pairs of ribs are called *true,* or *vertebrosternal* (ver-TEE-broh-stir-nal), *ribs* because they attach to the sternum directly by their individual *costal cartilage.* The lower five pairs of ribs are called *false ribs* because their costal cartilage does not reach the sternum directly. The first three pairs of false ribs reach the sternum indirectly by joining with the cartilage of the ribs above. These are called *vertebrochondral* (ver-TEE-broh-kahn-dral) *ribs.* The bottom two rib pairs have no anterior attachment and are called *vertebral ribs* or *floating ribs.*

BONES OF THE APPENDICULAR SKELETON

The 126 bones of the appendicular skeleton are suspended from two yokes or girdles that are anchored to the axial skeleton. They are additions or appendages to the axis of the body. The appendicular skeleton is designed for movement. If a portion is immobilized for a period of time, life without appendicular movement can be awkward.

Pectoral Girdle

Each half of the *pectoral girdle,* or *shoulder girdle,* consists of two bones: an anterior *clavicle* (KLAV-ih-kul) and a posterior *scapula* (SKAP-yoo-lah). The bones of the pectoral girdle, illustrated in Figure 7-9, form the connection between the upper extremities and the axial skeleton. The clavicles and scapulae, with their associated muscles, also form the shoulder.

The *clavicle* is commonly called the *collarbone.* It is an elongated, S-shaped bone that articulates proximally with the manubrium of the sternum. The distal end articulates with the scapula.

The *scapula,* commonly called the *shoulder blade,* is a thin, flat triangular bone on the posterior surface of the thoracic wall. It articulates with the clavicle and the humerus. The acromion process of the scapula forms the point of the shoulder. On the lateral margin of the scapula there is a

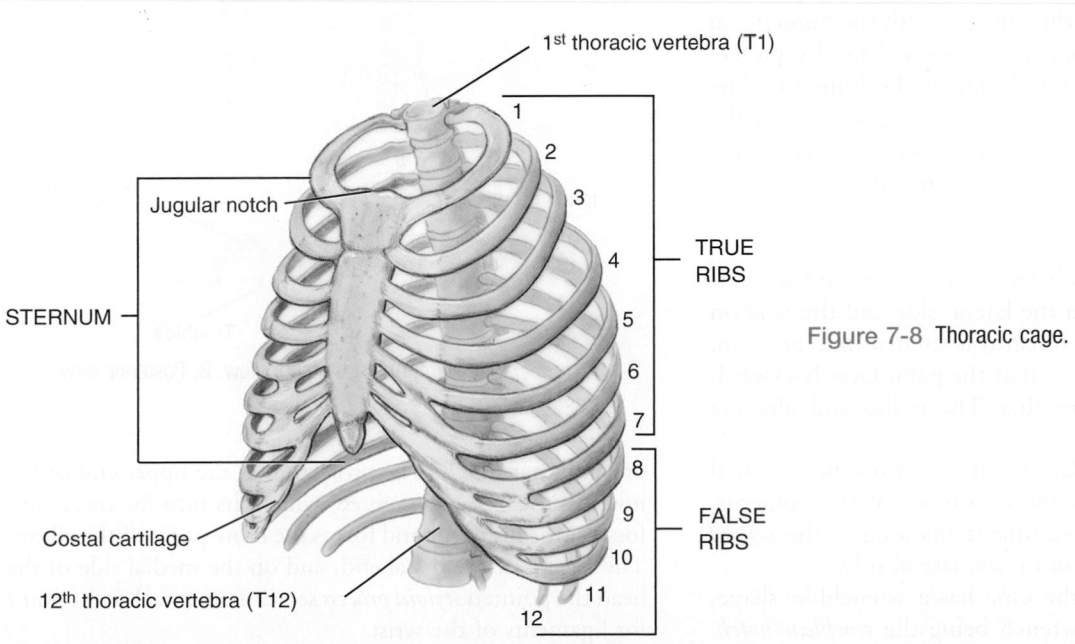

1st thoracic vertebra (T1)

Jugular notch

STERNUM

Costal cartilage

12th thoracic vertebra (T12)

1
2
3
4
5
6
7
8
9
10
11
12

TRUE RIBS

FALSE RIBS

Figure 7-8 Thoracic cage.

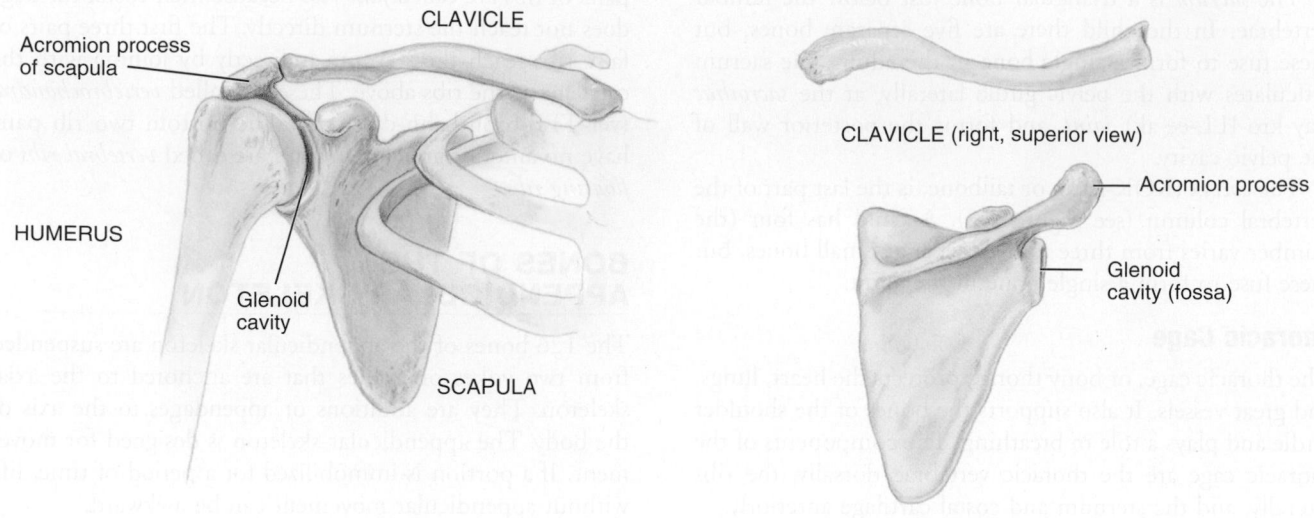

CLAVICLE

Acromion process of scapula

HUMERUS

Glenoid cavity

SCAPULA

CLAVICLE (right, superior view)

Acromion process

Glenoid cavity (fossa)

SCAPULA (right, posterior view)

Figure 7-9 Components of the pectoral girdle: clavicle and scapula.

shallow depression, the *glenoid cavity* (fossa), where the head of the humerus connects to the scapula. The clavicle and scapula provide attachments for numerous muscles.

Upper Extremity

The upper extremity (limb) consists of the bones of the arm, forearm, and hand.

Arm

The arm, or *brachium,* is the region between the shoulder and the elbow. It contains a single long bone, the *humerus,* illustrated in Figure 7-10. The *head* is the large, smooth, rounded end that fits into the scapula. The deltoid muscle attaches to the humerus along the shaft of the humerus. At the distal end, on the posterior surface, there is a depression, the *olecranon fossa,* where the ulna fits with the humerus to form the hinged elbow joint. Two smooth, rounded projections are evident on the distal end of the humerus. The capitulum is on the lateral side and articulates with the radius of the forearm. The trochlea is on the medial side and articulates with the ulna of the forearm.

Forearm

The forearm is the region between the elbow and wrist. It is formed by the *radius* on the lateral side and the *ulna* on the medial side when the forearm is in anatomic position. When the hand is turned so that the palm faces backward, the radius crosses over the ulna. The radius and ulna are illustrated in Figure 7-11.

The radius has a circular, disclike *head* on the proximal end. This articulates with the capitulum of the humerus. On the distal end, the prominent marking is the *styloid process,* a pointed projection on the lateral side.

The proximal end of the ulna has a wrenchlike shape, with the opening of the wrench being the *trochlear notch,*

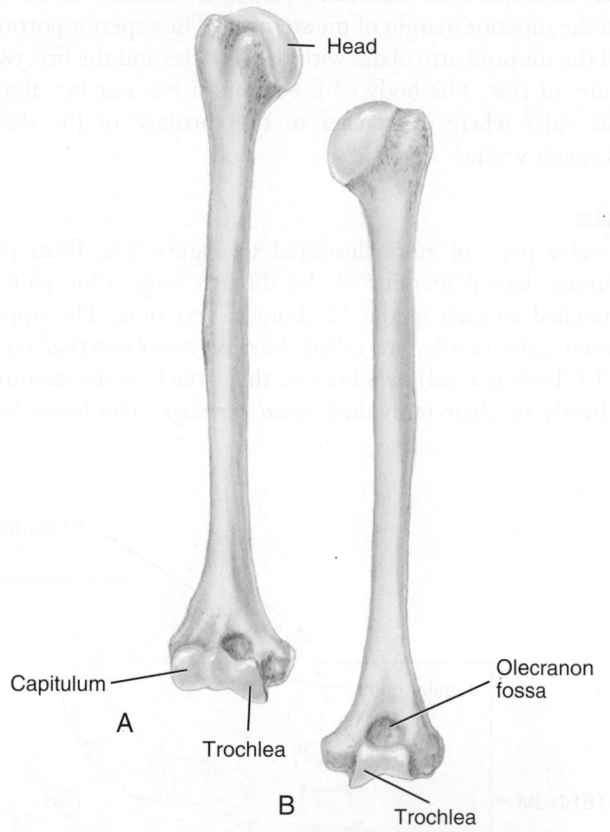

Head

Capitulum

A

Trochlea

Olecranon fossa

B

Trochlea

Figure 7-10 Humerus. **A,** Anterior view. **B,** Posterior view.

or semilunar notch. The projection at the upper end of the notch is the *olecranon process,* which fits into the olecranon fossa of the humerus and forms the bony point of the elbow. The *head* is at the distal end, and on the medial side of the head the pointed *styloid process* serves as an attachment point for ligaments of the wrist.

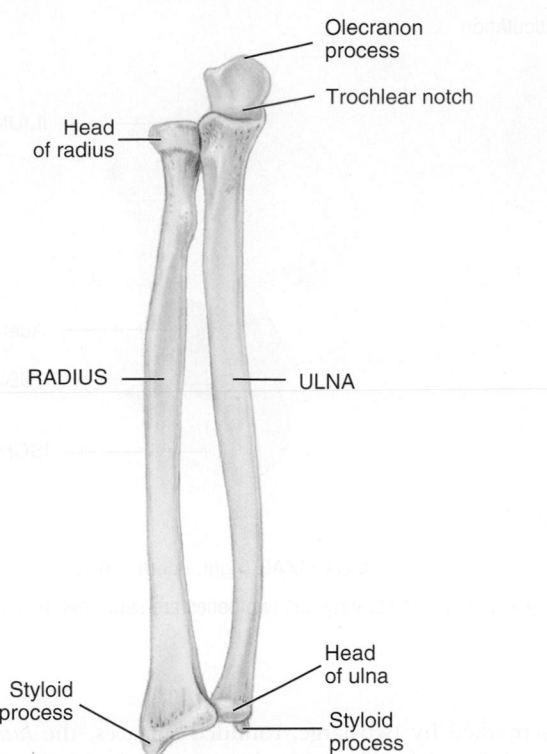

Figure 7-11 Radius and ulna, anterior view. The radius is on the lateral side, and the ulna is the medial bone.

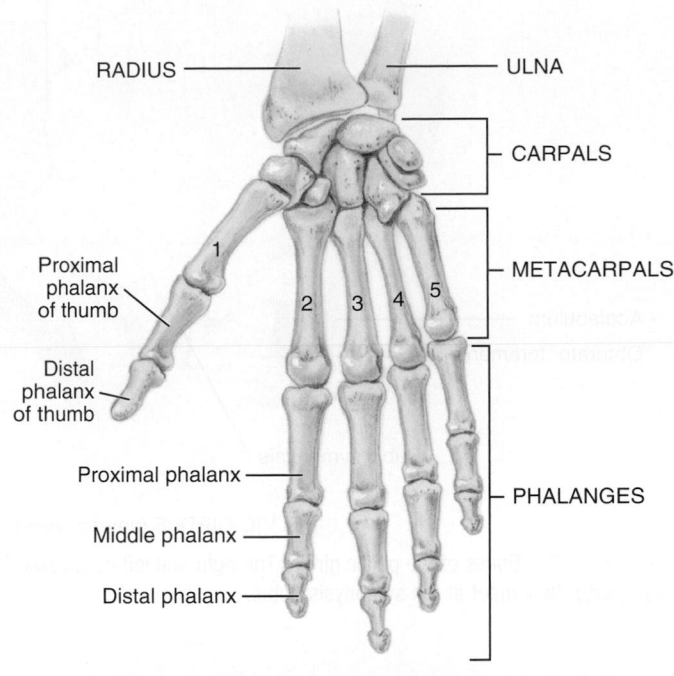

Hand (right, palmar aspect)

Figure 7-12 Hand. The carpals form the wrist, the metacarpals form the palm, and the phalanges form the fingers.

Hand

The hand, illustrated in Figure 7-12, is composed of the wrist, palm, and five fingers. The wrist, or *carpus,* contains eight small *carpal bones,* tightly bound by ligaments. The palm of the hand, or *metacarpus,* contains five *metacarpal bones,* one in line with each finger. These bones are not named but are numbered one through five starting on the thumb side. The 14 bones of the fingers are called *phalanges* (fah-LAN-jeez). Some people refer to these as *digits.* Three phalanges are in each finger (a proximal, middle, and distal phalanx) except the thumb, or *pollex,* which has two. The thumb lacks a middle phalanx. The proximal phalanges articulate with the metacarpals.

Pelvic Girdle

The *pelvic girdle,* or *hip girdle,* attaches the lower extremities to the axial skeleton and provides a strong support for the weight of the body. It also provides support and protection for the urinary bladder, a portion of the large intestine, and the internal reproductive organs, which are located in the pelvic cavity.

The pelvic girdle consists of two *coxal* (hip) *bones,* illustrated in Figure 7-13. The coxal bones are also called the *ossa coxae,* or *innominate bones.* Anteriorly, the two bones articulate with each other at the *symphysis pubis;* posteriorly, they articulate with the sacrum at the *iliosacral joints.* During childhood, each coxal bone consists of three separate parts: the *ilium, ischium,* and *pubis.* In the adult, these

bones are firmly fused to form a single bone. Where the three bones meet, there is a large depression, the *acetabulum* (as-seh-TAB-yoo-lum), which holds the head of the femur. The *obturator foramen* is a large opening between the pubis and ischium that functions as a passageway for blood vessels, nerves, and muscle tendons.

Together, the sacrum, coccyx, and pelvic girdle form the basin-shaped pelvis. The *false pelvis* (greater pelvis) is surrounded by the flared portions of the ilium bones and the lumbar vertebrae. The *true pelvis* (lesser pelvis) is smaller and inferior to the false pelvis. It is the region below the *pelvic brim,* or *pelvic inlet,* and it is encircled by bone. The large opening at the bottom of this region is the *pelvic outlet.* The dimensions of the true pelvis are especially important in childbirth.

Lower Extremity

The lower extremity (limb) consists of the bones of the thigh, leg, foot, and patella, or kneecap. The lower extremities support the entire weight of the body when we are erect, and they are exposed to tremendous forces when we walk, run, and jump. With this in mind, it is not surprising that the bones of the lower extremity are larger and stronger than those in the upper extremity.

Thigh

The *thigh* is the region from the hip to the knee. It contains a single long bone, the *femur,* illustrated in Figure 7-14. It is the largest, longest, and strongest bone in the body.

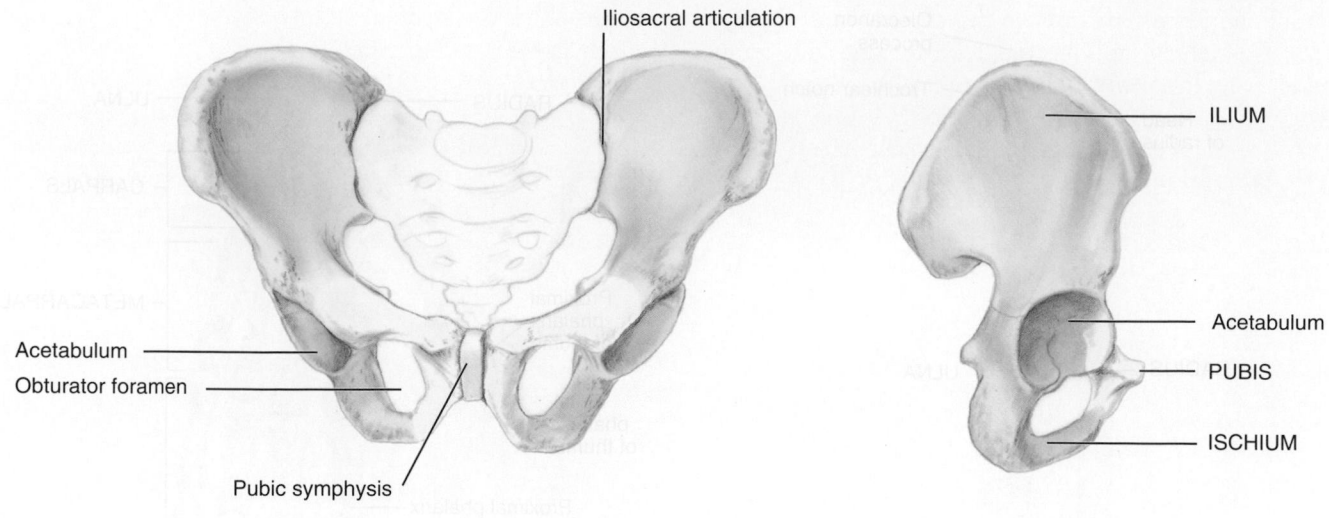

PELVIC GIRDLE (anterior view)

OS COXAE (right, lateral view)

Figure 7-13 Bones of the pelvic girdle. The right and left ossa coxae form the pelvic girdle. Posteriorly, the two bones are separated by the sacrum. Anteriorly, they meet at the symphysis pubis.

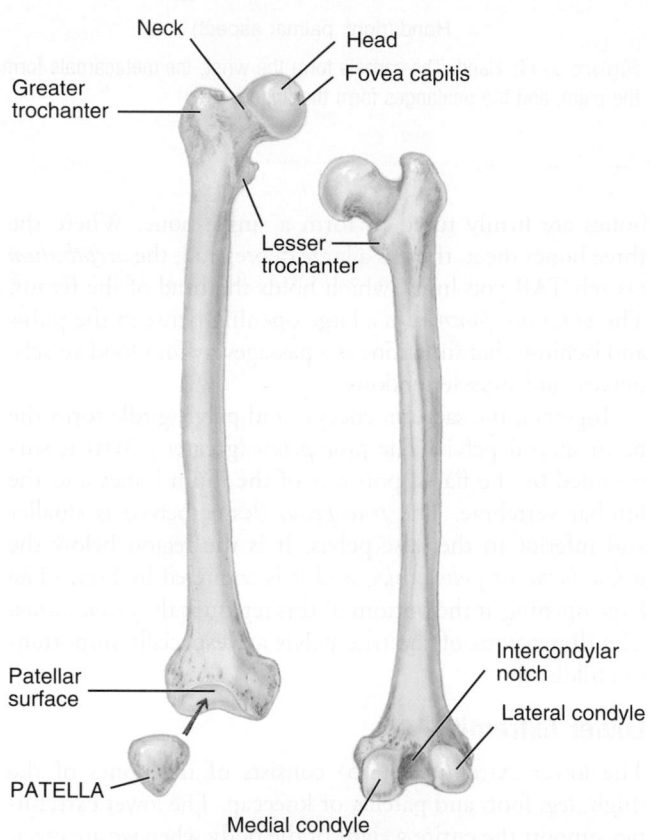

FEMUR and PATELLA (right)

Figure 7-14 Femur and patella *(right)*. **A,** Anterior view. **B,** Posterior view.

The large, smooth, ball-like *head* of the femur has a small depression called the *fovea capitis.* A ligament attaches here. Prominent projections at the proximal end, the *greater* and *lesser trochanters,* are major sites for muscle attachment. The *neck* is between the head and the trochanters. The distal end is marked by two large, rounded surfaces, the *lateral* and *medial condyles.* These form joints with the bones of the leg. The *intercondylar notch* is a depression between the condyles that contains ligaments associated with the knee joint. On the anterior surface, between the condyles, a smooth *patellar surface* marks the area for the kneecap.

Leg

The *leg* is the region between the knee and the ankle. It is formed by the slender *fibula* (FIB-yoo-lah) on the lateral side and the larger, weight-bearing *tibia* (TIB-ee-ah), or shin bone, on the medial side. The tibia articulates with the femur to form the knee joint and with the *talus* (one of the foot bones) to allow flexion and extension at the ankle.

The proximal end of the fibula is the *head,* and the projection at the distal end is the *lateral malleolus,* which forms the lateral bulge of the ankle. The superior surface of the tibia is flattened and smooth, with two slightly concave regions called the *lateral* and *medial condyles.* The condyles of the femur fit into these regions. The *anterior crest* is a sharp ridge on the anterior surface and forms the shin. On the medial side of the distal end, the *medial malleolus* forms the medial bulge of the ankle. Figure 7-15 illustrates the tibia and fibula.

Foot

The *foot,* illustrated in Figure 7-16, is composed of the ankle, instep, and five toes. The ankle, or *tarsus,* contains seven *tarsal bones.* These correspond to the carpals in the wrist. The largest tarsal bone is the *calcaneus* (kal-KAY-nee-us), or heel bone. The *talus,* another tarsal bone, rests on top of the calcaneus and articulates with the tibia. The instep of the foot, or *metatarsus,* contains five *metatarsal bones,* one in line with each toe. The distal ends of these bones form the ball of the foot. These bones are not named but are numbered one through five starting on the medial side. The tarsals and metatarsals, together with strong tendons and ligaments, form the arches of the foot. The 14 bones of the toes are called *phalanges.* Three phalanges are in each toe (a proximal, middle, and distal phalanx), except in the great (or big) toe, or hallux, which has only two. The

great toe lacks a middle phalanx. The proximal phalanges articulate with the metatarsals.

Patella

The *patella,* or *kneecap,* is a flat, triangular bone enclosed within the major tendon that anchors the anterior thigh muscle to the tibia. It provides a smooth surface for the tendon as it turns the corner between the thigh and leg when the knee is flexed. It also protects the knee joint anteriorly.

ARTICULATIONS

An *articulation* (ahr-tik-yoo-LAY-shun), or joint, is where two bones come together. In terms of the amount of movement they allow, there are three types of joints: immovable, slightly movable, and freely movable.

Synarthroses

Synarthroses (sin-ahr-THROH-seez) are immovable joints. The singular form is *synarthrosis.* In these joints, the bones come in close contact and are separated by only a thin layer of fibrous connective tissue. The *sutures* in the skull are examples of immovable joints.

Amphiarthroses

Slightly movable joints are called **amphiarthroses** (am-fee-ahr-THROH-seez). The singular form is amphiarthrosis. In this type of joint, the bones are connected by hyaline cartilage or fibrocartilage. The ribs connected to the sternum by costal cartilage are slightly movable joints connected by hyaline cartilage. The symphysis pubis is a slightly movable joint in which there is a fibrocartilage pad between the two bones. The joints between the vertebrae, the intervertebral discs, are also of this type.

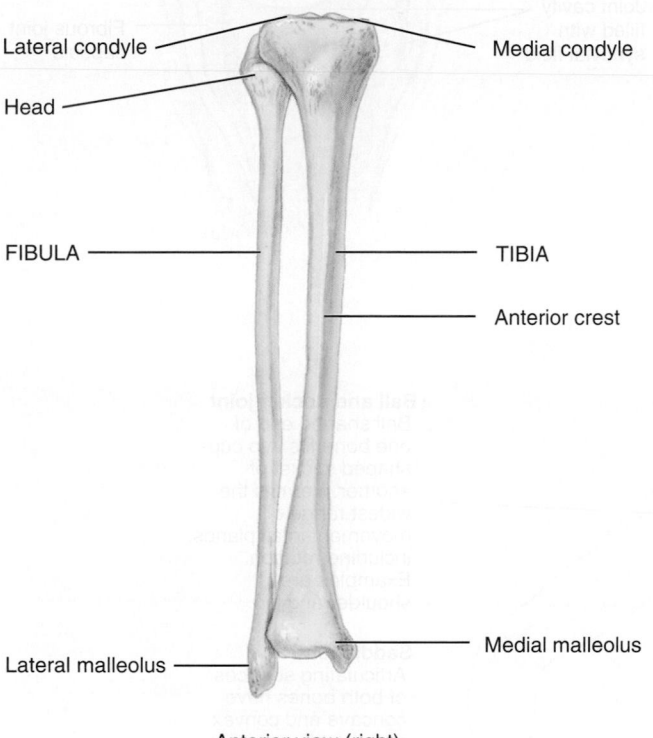

Figure 7-15 Tibia and fibula, anterior view *(right).* The fibula is on the lateral side of the leg, and the tibia is on the medial side.

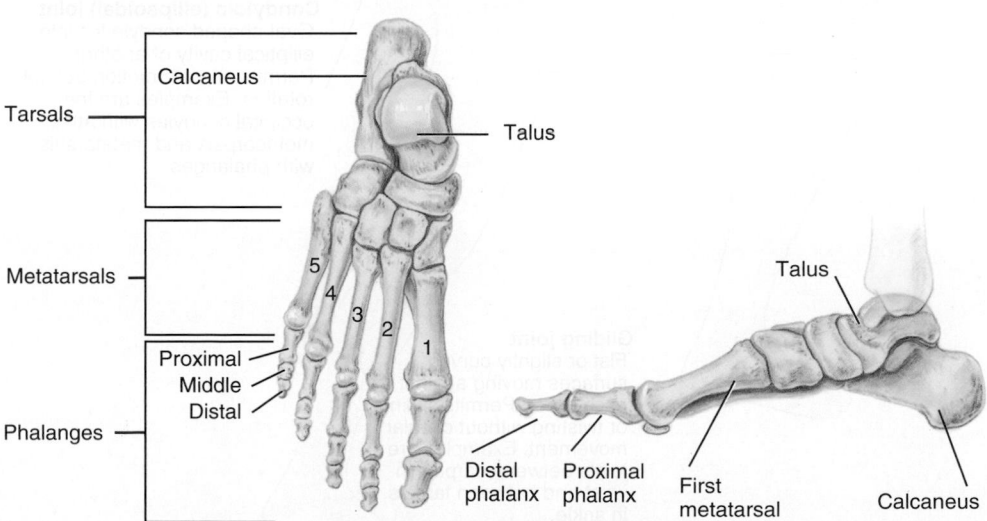

Figure 7-16 Bones of the foot. **A,** Superior view. **B,** Lateral view.

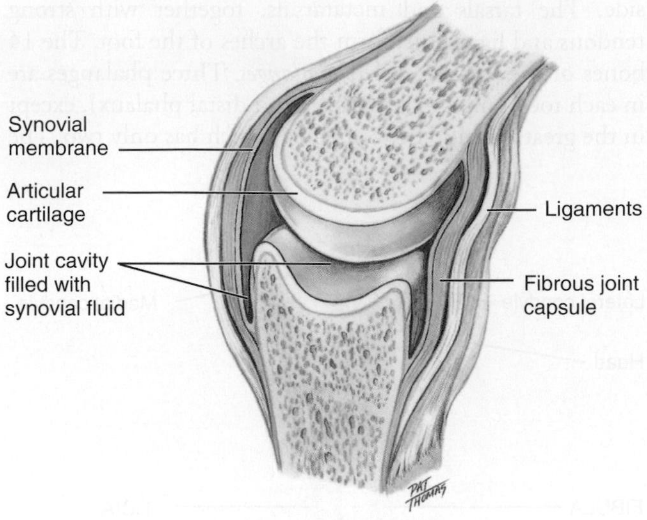

Figure 7-17 Generalized structure of a synovial joint.

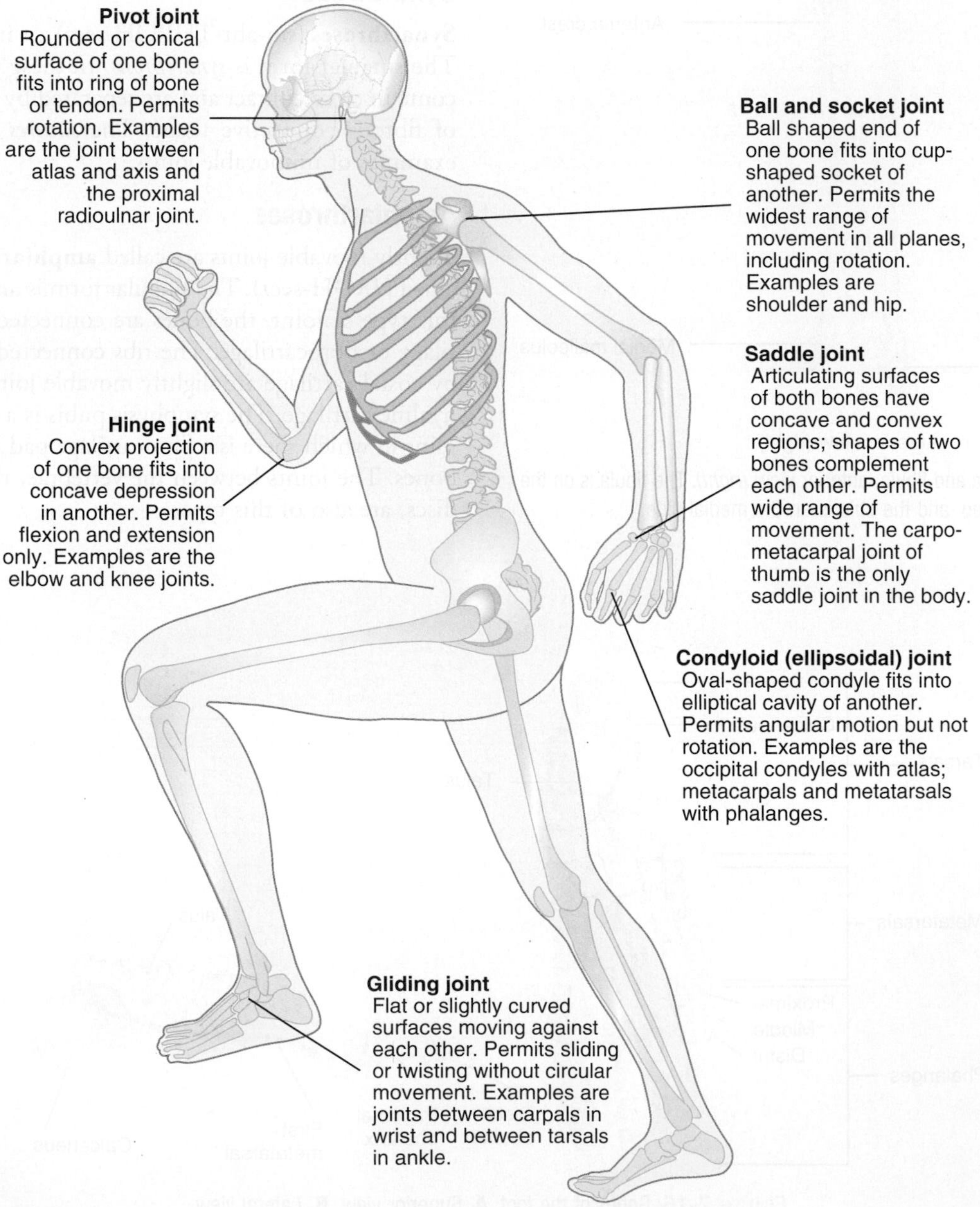

Synovial membrane

Articular cartilage

Joint cavity filled with synovial fluid

Ligaments

Fibrous joint capsule

Pivot joint
Rounded or conical surface of one bone fits into ring of bone or tendon. Permits rotation. Examples are the joint between atlas and axis and the proximal radioulnar joint.

Ball and socket joint
Ball shaped end of one bone fits into cup-shaped socket of another. Permits the widest range of movement in all planes, including rotation. Examples are shoulder and hip.

Saddle joint
Articulating surfaces of both bones have concave and convex regions; shapes of two bones complement each other. Permits wide range of movement. The carpo-metacarpal joint of thumb is the only saddle joint in the body.

Hinge joint
Convex projection of one bone fits into concave depression in another. Permits flexion and extension only. Examples are the elbow and knee joints.

Condyloid (ellipsoidal) joint
Oval-shaped condyle fits into elliptical cavity of another. Permits angular motion but not rotation. Examples are the occipital condyles with atlas; metacarpals and metatarsals with phalanges.

Gliding joint
Flat or slightly curved surfaces moving against each other. Permits sliding or twisting without circular movement. Examples are joints between carpals in wrist and between tarsals in ankle.

Figure 7-18 Types of freely movable joints.

Diarthroses

Most joints in the adult body are **diarthroses** (dye-ahr-THROH-seez) or freely movable joints. The singular form is diarthrosis. In this type of joint, the ends of the opposing bones are covered with hyaline cartilage, the *articular cartilage,* and they are separated by a space called the *joint cavity.* The components of the joints are enclosed in a dense fibrous *joint capsule* (Figure 7-17).

The outer layer of the capsule consists of the ligaments that hold the bones together. The inner layer is the *synovial membrane,* which secretes *synovial fluid* into the joint cavity for lubrication. Because all of these joints have a synovial membrane, they are sometimes called *synovial joints.*

Some diarthroses have pads and cushions associated with them. The knee has fibrocartilaginous pads, called *semilunar cartilages* or the *lateral meniscus* (meh-NIS-kus) and *medial meniscus,* which rest on the lateral and medial condyles of the tibia. The pads help stabilize the joint and act as shock absorbers. *Bursae* are fluid-filled sacs that act as cushions and help reduce friction. Bursae are lined with a synovial membrane that secretes synovial fluid into the sac. They are commonly located between the skin and underlying bone or between tendons and ligaments. Inflammation of a bursa is called *bursitis.*

There are six types of diarthrotic or freely movable joints based on the shapes of their parts and the types of movement they allow. These are described and illustrated in Figure 7-18.

AGING OF THE SKELETAL SYSTEM

The major age-related change in the skeletal system is the loss of calcium from the bones. Calcium loss occurs in both men and women, but it starts at an earlier age and is more severe in women. The exact reasons for the loss are unknown and possibly involve a combination of several factors. These may include an imbalance between osteoblast and osteoclast activity, imbalance between calcitonin and parathormone levels, reduced absorption of calcium and/or vitamin D from the digestive tract, poor diet, and lack of exercise. Whatever the cause, there is no sure way of preventing the loss, but adequate calcium and vitamin D in the diet may help reduce the effects.

Another change with age is a decrease in the rate of collagen synthesis. This means that the bones have less strength and are more brittle. Bones fracture more readily in elderly individuals, and the healing process may be slow or incomplete. Tendons and ligaments become less flexible because of the changes in collagen.

The articular cartilage at the ends of bones tends to become thinner and deteriorates with age. This causes joint disorders that are commonly found in older individuals. People also appear to get shorter as they get older. This is caused partially by loss of bone mass and partially by compression of the intervertebral discs.

Age-related changes in the skeletal system cannot be prevented. An active and healthy lifestyle with appropriate exercise and an adequate diet help reduce the effect of the changes in the skeletal system.

Highlight on Conditions Affecting the Skeletal System

Ankylosing spondylitis (ANG-kih-loh-sing spahn-dih-LYE-tis) Inflammation of the spine that is characterized by stiffening of the spinal joints and ligaments so that movement becomes increasingly painful and difficult; also called *rheumatoid spondylitis*

Arthritis (ahr-THRYE-tis) Inflammation of a joint

Bunion (BUN-yun) Abnormal swelling of the joint between the big toe and the first metatarsal bone, resulting from a buildup of soft tissues and bone caused by chronic irritation from ill-fitting shoes

Carpal tunnel syndrome (KAHR-pull TUH-nul SIN-drohm) Condition characterized by pain and burning sensations in the fingers and hand, caused by compression of the median nerve as it passes between a wrist ligament and the bones and tendons of the wrist

Dislocation (dis-loh-KAY-shun) Displacement of a bone from its joint with tearing of ligaments, tendons, and articular capsule; also called *luxation*

Gout (GOWT) A form of acute arthritis in which uric acid crystals develop within a joint and irritate the cartilage, causing acute inflammation, swelling, and pain; most commonly occurs in middle-aged and older men

Lyme disease (LYME dih-ZEEZ) A bacterial disease transmitted to humans by deer ticks; characterized by joint stiffness, headache, fever and chills, nausea, and back pain; complications include severe arthritis and cardiac problems; early stages of the disease respond well to antibiotics

Osteoarthritis (ahs-tee-oh-ahr-THRYE-tis) A noninflammatory disease of the joints that is characterized by degeneration of the articular cartilage and changes in the synovial membrane; also called *degenerative joint disease* (DJD)

Osteomalacia (ahs-tee-oh-mah-LAY-shee-ah) Softening of bone because of inadequate amounts of calcium and phosphorus; bones bend easily and become deformed; in childhood this is called *rickets*

Continued

Highlight on Conditions Affecting the Skeletal System—cont'd

Osteomyelitis (ahs-tee-oh-my-eh-LYE-tis) Inflammation of the bone marrow caused by bacteria

Osteoporosis (ahs-tee-oh-por-OH-sis) Decrease in bone density and mass; commonly occurs in postmenopausal women as a result of increased osteoclast activity caused by diminished estrogen levels; bones fracture easily

Osteosarcoma (ahs-tee-oh-sahr-KOH-mah) Malignant tumor derived from bone; also called *osteogenic sarcoma;* osteoblasts multiply without control and form large tumors in bone

Rheumatoid arthritis (ROO-mah-toyd ahr-THRYE-tis) A chronic systemic disease with changes occurring in the connective tissues of the body, especially the joints; in contrast to osteoarthritis, the symptoms are usually more generalized

and severe; evidence indicates it may be an autoimmune disease

Spina bifida (SPY-nah BIFF-ih-dah) A developmental anomaly in which the vertebral laminae do not close around the spinal cord, leaving an opening through which the cord and meninges may or may not protrude

Sprain (SPRAYN) Twisting of a joint with pain, swelling, and injury to ligaments, tendons, muscles, blood vessels, and nerves; most often occurs in the ankle; more serious than a strain, which is the overstretching of the muscles associated with a joint

Talipes (TAL-ih-peez) Congenital deformity of the foot in which the patient cannot stand with the sole of the foot flat on the ground; also called *clubfoot* ■

TERMINOLOGY REVIEW

Medical Term	Word Parts	Definition
Amphiarthrosis	*arthr/o:* joint *-osis:* condition of	A slightly movable joint; plural, amphiarthroses.
Diaphysis	*dia-:* through	The long straight shaft of a long bone.
Diarthrosis	*arthr/o:* joint *-osis:* condition of	Freely movable joint characterized by a joint cavity; also called a *synovial joint;* plural, *diarthroses.*
Epiphyseal plate	*epi-:* above, upon, on *-phys:* to grow	The cartilaginous plate between the epiphysis and diaphysis of a bone; responsible for the lengthwise growth of a long bone.
Epiphysis	*epi-:* above, upon, on	The end of a long bone.
Osteoblast	*oste/o:* bone *-blast:* immature cell	Bone-forming cell; immature bone cell.
Osteoclast	*oste/o:* bone *-clast:* to break	Cell that destroys, breaks down, or resorbs bone tissue.
Osteocyte	*oste/o:* bone *-cyte:* cell	Mature bone cell.
Osteon	*oste/o:* bone	Structural unit of bone; haversian system.
Synarthrosis	*syn-:* together *arthr-:* joint *-osis:* condition of	An immovable joint; plural, *synarthroses.*

ON THE WEB

For information on the skeletal system:

Loyola University Medical Education Network: Pick a Bone: www.meddean.luc.edu/lumen/MedEd/GrossAnatomy/learnem/bones/main_bone.htm

Merck Manual: Bone, Joint, and Muscle Disorders: www.merck.com/mmhe *(Click on "Bone, Joint, and Muscle Disorders")*

National Osteoporosis Foundation: www.nof.org

 Check out the Evolve site at http://evolve.elsevier.com/Bonewit/today/ to actively Prepare for your Certification, and to access additional interactive activities and exercises to help you study and prepare for success.

8

Muscular System

KEY TERMS

antagonist (an-TAG-oh-nist)
insertion (in-SIR-shun)
motor unit (MOH-toar YOO-nit)

neuromuscular junction (noo-roe-MUSK-yoo-lar JUNK-shun)
neurotransmitter (noo-roh-TRANS-mit-ter)

origin (OR-ih-jin)
prime mover (PRYM MOO-ver)
synergist (SIN-er-gist)

INTRODUCTION TO THE MUSCULAR SYSTEM

As described in Chapter 5, there are three types of muscle tissue: skeletal, visceral, and cardiac. These are reviewed in Table 8-1. This chapter takes a closer look at skeletal muscle, which makes up about 40% of an individual's body weight. It forms more than 600 muscles that are attached to the bones of the skeleton. Skeletal muscles are under conscious control, and when they contract they move the bones. Skeletal muscles also allow us to smile, frown, pout, show surprise, and exhibit other forms of facial expression.

CHARACTERISTICS AND FUNCTIONS OF THE MUSCULAR SYSTEM

Skeletal muscle has four primary characteristics that relate to its functions:

Excitability: Excitability (eks-eye-tah-BILL-ih-tee) is the ability to receive and respond to a stimulus. To function properly, muscles have to respond to a stimulus from the nervous system.

Contractility: Contractility (kon-track-TILL-ih-tee) is the ability to shorten or contract. When a muscle responds to a stimulus, it shortens to produce movement.

Extensibility: Extensibility (eks-ten-sih-BILL-ih-tee) means that a muscle can be stretched or extended. Skeletal muscles are often arranged in opposing pairs. When one muscle contracts, the other muscle is relaxed and stretched.

Elasticity: Elasticity (ee-lass-TISS-ih-tee) is the capacity to recoil or return to the original shape and length after contraction or extension.

Muscle contraction fulfills four important functions in the body:

- Movement
- Posture
- Joint stability
- Heat production

Nearly all *movement* in the body is the result of muscle contraction. Some exceptions to this are the action of cilia, the motility of the flagella on sperm cells, and the ameboid movement of some white blood cells. The integrated action of joints, bones, and skeletal muscles produces obvious movements such as walking and running. Skeletal muscles also produce more subtle movements that result in various facial expressions, eye movements, and respiration. *Posture,* such as sitting and standing, is maintained as a result of muscle contraction. The skeletal muscles are continually making fine adjustments that hold the body in stationary positions. Skeletal muscles contribute to *joint stability.* The tendons of many muscles extend over joints and in this way contribute to joint stability. This is particularly evident in the knee and shoulder joints, where muscle tendons are a major factor in stabilizing the joint. *Heat production,* to maintain body temperature, is an important by-product of muscle metabolism. Nearly 85% of the heat produced in the body is the result of muscle contraction.

STRUCTURE OF SKELETAL MUSCLE

A whole skeletal muscle is considered an organ of the muscular system. For example, the biceps muscle is an organ of the muscular system. Each organ or muscle consists of skeletal muscle tissue, connective tissue, nerve tissue, and blood or vascular tissue.

Whole Skeletal Muscle

An individual skeletal muscle such as the biceps muscle may consist of hundreds, or even thousands, of muscle fibers bundled together and wrapped in a connective tissue covering. Each muscle is surrounded by a connective tissue sheath called the *epimysium* (ep-ih-MYE-see-um). Fascia consists of connective tissue located outside the epimysium. Fascia surrounds and separates the muscles. Skeletal muscle cells (fibers), like other body cells, are soft and fragile. The connective tissue coverings furnish support and protection for the delicate cells and allow them to withstand the forces of contraction. The coverings also provide pathways for the passage of blood vessels and nerves.

Skeletal Muscle Fibers

Each individual skeletal muscle fiber consists of a single cylindric muscle cell. The cell membrane is called the *sarcolemma* (sar-koh-LEM-mah), and the cytoplasm is the *sarcoplasm* (SAR-koh-plazm). Multiple nuclei are next to the sarcolemma at the periphery of the cell. Because the muscle

Table 8-1	Summary of Muscle Tissue		
Feature	**Skeletal**	**Visceral**	**Cardiac**
Location	Attached to bones	Walls of internal organs and blood vessels	Heart
Function	Produce body movement	Contraction of viscera and blood vessels	Pump blood through heart and blood vessels
Cell shape	Cylindric	Spindle-shaped; tapered ends	Cylindric, branching
Number of nuclei	Many	One	One
Striations	Present	Absent	Present
Type of control	Voluntary	Involuntary	Involuntary

From Applegate E: *The anatomy and physiology learning system,* ed 4, St Louis, 2011, Saunders.

Highlight on the Muscular System

Rigor mortis: The term *rigor mortis* means the "stiffness of death." Within a short time of death, the adenosine triphosphate in muscles breaks down. This causes the myofilaments to remain locked in a contracted position and the body becomes rigid. A day or so later, muscle proteins begin to deteriorate and the rigor mortis disappears.

Tetanus: The word *tetanus* is often confusing because it means different things to different people. In reference to muscle contraction, the term denotes a steady contraction of a muscle fiber, without a relaxation phase. The word also refers to a disease, commonly called "lockjaw," that is caused by the bacterium *Clostridium tetani.* The toxin from the bacteria causes nerves to be highly excitable, which, in turn, causes uncontrollable muscle contractions, or spasms. A third use of the word is to denote a condition caused by a deficiency of calcium ions in the extracellular fluid. The lack of calcium increases nerve excitability with resulting muscle spasms, particularly of the extremities. The word *tetany* is also sometimes used to mean tetanus.

Cramps: Cramps are painful, spastic contractions of muscles. They are usually caused by an irritation within the muscles that results in reflex contractions. Local inflammation from the accumulation of lactic acid is one source of irritation.

Wryneck: Injury to one of the sternocleidomastoid muscles may result in torticollis, or wryneck. This is characterized by a twisting of the neck and an unnatural position of the head.

Diaphragm: Voluntary forceful contractions of the diaphragm increase intraabdominal pressure to assist in urination, defecation, and childbirth.

Electrical shock: The muscles that flex the fingers and hand are stronger than the extensor muscles. In a normal relaxed position the fingers are slightly flexed because the normal muscle tone is greater in the flexors. Persons who receive a high-voltage electrical shock through the arms flex their hands tightly and "can't let go." All of the flexors and extensors receive the electrical stimulus, but because the flexor muscles are stronger, they contract more forcefully.

Intramuscular injections: The gluteus medius is a common site for intramuscular injections. Generally, the injection is given in the center of the upper outer quadrant of the buttock, or gluteal, area. The gluteus medius, rather than the gluteus maximus, is used to avoid damaging the sciatic nerve.

Horseback riding: The adductor muscles in the medial compartment are the horse rider's muscles. These muscles adduct, or press, the thighs together to keep a person on a horse.

Quads: The quadriceps femoris group is a powerful knee extensor that is used in climbing, running, and rising from a chair. ■

---

cell needs energy for contraction, there are numerous mitochondria.

Nerve and Blood Supply

Skeletal muscles have an abundant supply of blood vessels and nerves. This is directly related to the primary function of skeletal muscle contraction. Before a skeletal muscle fiber can contract, it must receive an impulse from a nerve cell. Muscle contraction requires adenosine triphosphate (ATP), and blood vessels deliver the necessary nutrients and oxygen to produce it. Blood vessels also remove the waste products that are produced as a result of muscle contraction.

In general, an artery and at least one vein accompany each nerve that penetrates the epimysium of a skeletal muscle. Branches of the nerve and blood vessels follow the connective tissue components of the muscle so that each muscle fiber is in contact with a branch of a nerve cell and with one or more minute blood vessels called *capillaries.*

Skeletal Muscle Attachments

In some instances, fibers of the epimysium fuse directly with the periosteum of a bone to form a *direct* attachment. The fleshy part of the muscle is known as the *belly* or *gaster.* More commonly, the connective tissue coverings extend beyond the belly of the muscle to form a thick, ropelike *tendon* or a broad, flat, sheetlike *aponeurosis* (ah-pah-noo-ROE-sis). The tendons or aponeuroses form *indirect* attachments from muscles to the periosteum of bones or to the connective tissue of other muscles. Typically, a muscle spans a joint and is attached to bones by tendons at both ends. One of the bones remains relatively fixed or stable while the other end moves as a result of muscle contraction. The fixed or stable end is called the **origin** of the muscle, and the more movable attachment is called the **insertion.**

CONTRACTION OF SKELETAL MUSCLE

Skeletal muscle contraction is the result of a complex series of events based on chemical reactions at the cellular (muscle fiber) level. This chain of reactions begins with stimulation by a nerve cell and ends when the muscle fiber is again relaxed. Contraction of a whole muscle is the result of the simultaneous contraction of many muscle fibers.

Stimulus for Contraction

Skeletal muscles are stimulated to contract by special nerve cells called *motor neurons.* As the axon of the motor neuron penetrates the muscle, the axon branches, so there is an axon terminal for each muscle fiber. A single motor neuron and all the muscle fibers it stimulates make up a **motor unit.** Some motor units include several hundred individual fibers; others contain fewer than 10. Because all the muscle fibers in a motor unit receive a nerve impulse at the same time, all the fibers contract at the same time.

The region in which an axon terminal meets a muscle fiber is called a **neuromuscular junction** or myoneural

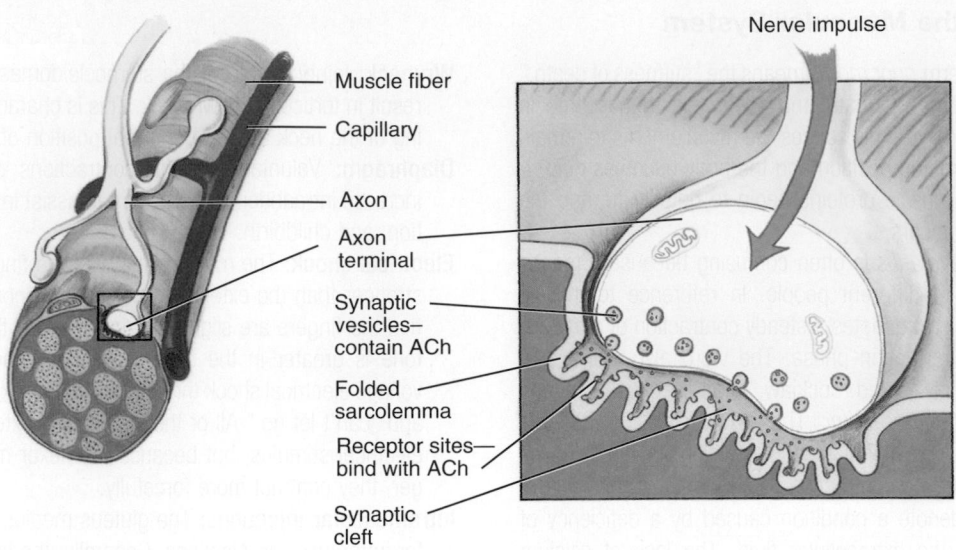

Figure 8-1 Neuromuscular junction. The axon terminal fits into a depression on the sarcolemma. A nerve impulse travels down the axon to the axon terminal. The impulse causes the synaptic vesicles to release acetylcholine, which diffuses across the synaptic cleft and binds with receptors on the sarcolemma.

junction, which is illustrated in Figure 8-1. The axon terminal does not actually touch the sarcolemma of the muscle cell but fits into a shallow depression in the cell membrane. The fluid-filled space between the axon terminal and sarcolemma is called a *synaptic cleft* (gap). *Acetylcholine (ACh)* (ah-see-till-KOH-leen), a **neurotransmitter,** is contained within synaptic vesicles in the axon terminal. Receptor sites for the ACh are located on the sarcolemma.

When a nerve impulse reaches the axon terminal, ACh is released. The ACh diffuses across the synaptic cleft and binds with the receptor sites on the sarcolemma. This reaction is the stimulus for contraction.

The ACh is rapidly inactivated by the enzyme *acetylcholinesterase* (ah-see-till-koh-lin-ES-ter-ase). This ensures that one nerve impulse will result in only one contraction of the muscle fiber. Anything that interferes with the production, release, or inactivation of ACh, or its ability to bind with the receptor sites on the sarcolemma, will have an effect on muscle contraction. Muscle relaxant drugs work in this manner.

Energy Sources and Oxygen Debt

The immediate or initial source of energy for muscle contraction is ATP. Surprisingly, muscles have limited storage facilities for ATP. In working muscles the stored ATP is depleted in about 6 seconds, and new ATP must be regenerated if muscle contraction is to continue.

Creatine phosphate (KREE-ah-tin FOS-fate) is a unique high-energy compound that is stored in muscles This compound provides almost instantaneous regeneration of ATP.

This reaction is so effective that there is little change in ATP levels during the initial stages of muscle contraction. Muscles store enough creatine phosphate to regenerate sufficient ATP to sustain contraction for about 10 seconds.

When muscles are actively contracting for extended periods of time, *fatty acids* and *glucose* become the primary energy sources. As ATP and creatine phosphate stores are being used, more ATP is produced from the metabolism of glucose and fatty acids.

If adequate oxygen is available, fatty acids and glucose are broken down in the mitochondria by a process called *aerobic respiration.* The products are carbon dioxide, water, and large amounts of ATP.

When muscles are contracting vigorously for long periods of time, the circulatory system is unable to deliver oxygen fast enough to maintain the aerobic pathways. Processes that do not require oxygen are necessary. Under these conditions, glucose is the primary energy source. If adequate oxygen is not available, glucose is broken down by a process called *anaerobic respiration.* The products of the anaerobic pathway are lactic acid and a small amount of ATP.

Some of the lactic acid accumulates in the muscle and causes a burning sensation. Most of it diffuses out of the muscle and into the bloodstream, which takes it to the liver. Later, when sufficient oxygen is available, the liver converts the lactic acid back to glycogen, the storage form of glucose.

The aerobic pathway produces about 20 times more ATP than the anaerobic pathway. However, the anaerobic pathway provides ATP about two and one-half times faster than the aerobic pathway. Most of the energy for vigorous activity over a moderate period of time comes from anaerobic respiration. Prolonged activities requiring endurance depend on aerobic mechanisms.

Periods of strenuous exercise that require anaerobic mechanisms to regenerate ATP create an *oxygen debt* that must be repaid before equilibrium can be restored. There is an accumulation of lactic acid in the muscle that may cause

Highlight on Conditions and Procedures Related to the Muscular System Conditions

Conditions

Cramp (KRAMP) Painful involuntary muscle spasm; often caused by myositis but can be a symptom of any irritation or ion imbalance

Muscular dystrophy (MUSS-kyoo-lar DIS-troh-fee) An inherited, chronic, progressive wasting and weakening of muscles without involvement of the nervous system

Myasthenia gravis (mye-as-THEE-nee-ah GRAY-vis) An autoimmune disease, more common in females, that is characterized by weakness of skeletal muscles caused by an abnormality at the neuromuscular junction

Myoparesis (mye-oh-pah-REE-sis) Weakness or slight paralysis of a muscle

Myopathy (mye-AHP-ah-thee) Muscle disease

Myorrhexis (mye-oh-REK-sis) Rupture of a muscle

Myositis (mye-oh-SYE-tis) Inflammation of muscle tissue

Repetitive stress disorder (ree-PET-ah-tiv STRESS dis-OAR-der) Condition with symptoms caused by repetitive motions that involve muscles, tendons, nerves, and joints; most commonly occur as work-related or sports injuries

Shin splint (SHIN SPLINT) Strain of the long flexor muscle of the toes resulting in pain along the tibia (shinbone); usually caused by repeated stress to the lower leg

Tic (TIK) A spasmodic involuntary twitching of a muscle that is normally under voluntary control

Procedures

Electromyography (ee-lek-troh-mye-AHG-rah-fee) The process of recording the strength of muscle contraction as a result of electrical stimulation

Muscle biopsy (MUSS-uhl BYE-ahp-see) Removal of muscle tissue for microscopic examination

Tenomyoplasty (ten-oh-MY-oh-plas-tee) Surgical repair of a tendon and muscle; applied especially to an operation for inguinal hernia

Tenoplasty (TEN-oh-plas-tee) Surgical repair of a tendon

Tenorrhaphy (ten-OAR-ah-fee) Suture of a tendon ■

temporary muscular pain and cramping. The ATP and creatine phosphate in the muscle are depleted and need to be replenished. This additional oxygen is necessary to convert the lactic acid into glycogen, a process that occurs in the liver. Oxygen is also necessary to replenish the ATP and the creatine phosphate in the muscle. Oxygen debt is defined as the additional oxygen that is required after physical activity to restore resting conditions. The debt is paid back by labored breathing that continues after the activity has stopped.

Movements

Most intact skeletal muscles are attached to bones by tendons that span joints. When the muscle contracts, one bone (the insertion) moves relative to the other bone (the origin). Frequently muscles work in groups to perform a particular movement. If one muscle has a primary role in providing a movement, it is called a **prime mover.** Muscles that work with, or assist, the prime mover to cause a movement are called **synergists** (SIN-er-jists). Often muscles span more than one joint, and a synergist will stabilize one joint while the prime mover acts on the other joint. For example, the fingers can be flexed to make a fist without bending the wrist because certain muscles fix the wrist in a stabilized position. **Antagonists** are muscles that oppose, or reverse, a particular movement. The biceps brachii muscle on the anterior arm flexes the forearm at the elbow. The triceps brachii muscle on the posterior arm extends the forearm at the elbow. The two muscles are on opposite sides of the humerus and have opposite functions. They are antagonists.

Bones and muscles work together to perform different types of movement at the various joints. Describing muscular action or movement at joints requires a frame of reference and descriptive terminology with definite meaning. Some commonly used terms that are used to describe particular movements are defined and illustrated in Figure 8-2.

SKELETAL MUSCLE GROUPS

The body is composed of more than 600 skeletal muscles. A discussion of each muscle is certainly beyond the scope of this book. Only the more significant and obvious muscles are identified and described here. These are arranged in groups according to location and/or function. If you identify and learn the muscles as group associations, it will make them easier to remember. If you can locate a muscle on your own body, you will be able to contract the muscle and describe its action. Learning anatomy in this manner makes it more meaningful.

Naming Muscles

Most skeletal muscles have names that describe some feature of the muscle. Often several criteria are combined into one name. Associating the muscles' characteristics with their names will help you learn and remember them. The following are some terms relating to muscle features that are used in naming muscles:

- *Size:* vastus (huge); maximus (large); longus (long); minimus (small); brevis (short)
- *Shape:* deltoid (triangular); rhomboid (like a rhombus with equal and parallel sides); latissimus (wide); teres (round); trapezius (like a trapezoid, a four-sided figure with two sides parallel)

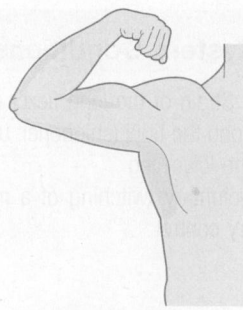

Flexion (FLEK-shun)
Means to bend. Flexion usually brings two
bones closer together and decreases the
angle between them. Example: bending
the elbow or the knee.

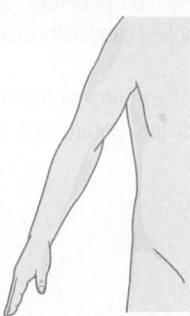

Extension (ek-STEN-shun)
Means to straighten. Extension is the opposite
of flexion. It increases the angle between two
bones. Example: straightening the elbow or the
knee after it has been flexed.

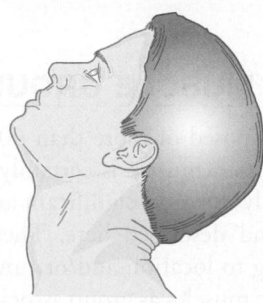

Hyperextension (hye-perk-ek-STEN-shun)
Hyperextension occurs when a part of the body
is extended beyond the anatomical position. The
joint angle becomes greater than 180°.
Example: moving the head backward.

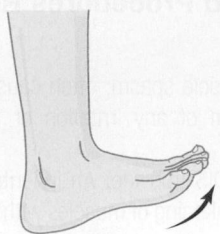

Dorsiflexion (dor-sih-FLEK-shun)
Flexion of the ankle in which the dorsum
or top of the foot is lifted upward, decreasing
the angle between the foot and leg.
Example: standing on your heels.

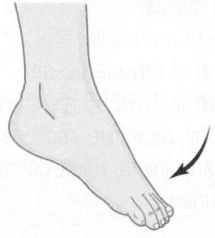

Plantar flexion (PLAN-tar FLEK-shun)
Plantar flexion is movement at the ankle that
increases the angle between the foot and leg.
Example: standing on your toes.

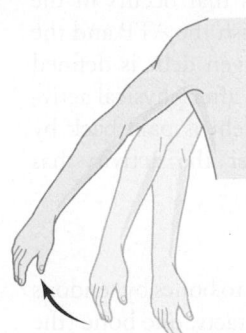

Abduction (ab-DUCK-shun)
Means to take away. Abduction moves a bone or limb away
from the midline or axis of the body. Examples: the outward
movement of the legs in "jumping jacks," moving the arms
away from the body, or spreading the fingers apart.

Figure 8-2 Types of body movements.

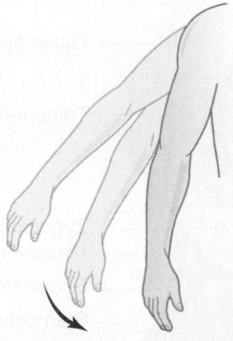

Adduction (ad-DUCK-shun)
Means to bring together. Adduction is the opposite of abduction. It moves a bone or limb toward the midline of the body. Examples: bringing the arms back to the sides of the body after they have been abducted or moving the legs back to anatomical position after abduction.

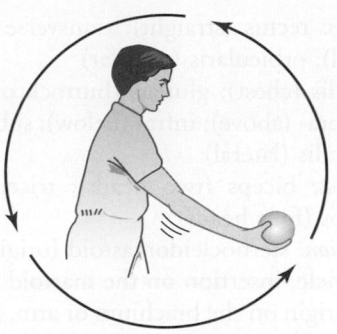

Circumduction (sir-kum-DUCK-shun)
Circumduction is the conelike, circular movement of a body segment. The proximal end of the segment remains relatively stationary while the distal end outlines a large circle. Example: the movement of the arm at the shoulder joint, with the elbow extended, so that the tips of the fingers move in a large circle.

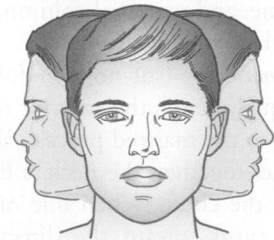

Rotation (roh-TAY-shun)
Rotation is the movement of a bone around its own axis in a pivot joint. Example: shaking your head "no".

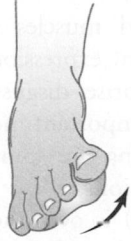

Inversion (in-VER-zhun)
Inversion is the movement of the sole of the foot inward or medially.

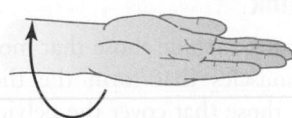

Supination (soo-pih-NAY-shun)
Supination is a specialized rotation of the forearm that turns the palm of the hand forward or anteriorly. If the elbow is flexed, supination turns the palm of the hand upward or superiorly.

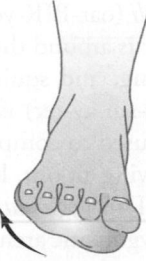

Eversion (ee-VER-zhun)
Eversion is the opposite of inversion. It is the movement of the sole of the foot outward or laterally.

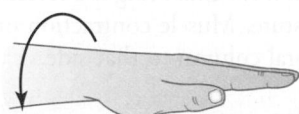

Pronation (proh-NAY-shun)
Pronation is the opposite of supination. It is a specialized rotation of the forearm that turns the palm of the hand backward or posteriorly. If the elbow is flexed, pronation turns the palm of the hand downward or inferiorly.

Figure 8-2, cont'd

- *Direction of fibers:* rectus (straight); transverse (across); oblique (diagonal); orbicularis (circular)
- *Location:* pectoralis (chest); gluteus (buttock or rump); brachii (arm); supra- (above); infra- (below); sub- (under or beneath); lateralis (lateral)
- *Number of origins:* biceps (two heads); triceps (three heads); quadriceps (four heads)
- *Origin and insertion:* sternocleidomastoid (origin on the sternum and clavicle, insertion on the mastoid process); brachioradialis (origin on the brachium or arm, insertion on the radius)
- *Action:* abductor (to abduct a structure); adductor (to adduct a structure); flexor (to flex a structure); extensor (to extend a structure); levator (to lift or elevate a structure); masseter (to chew)

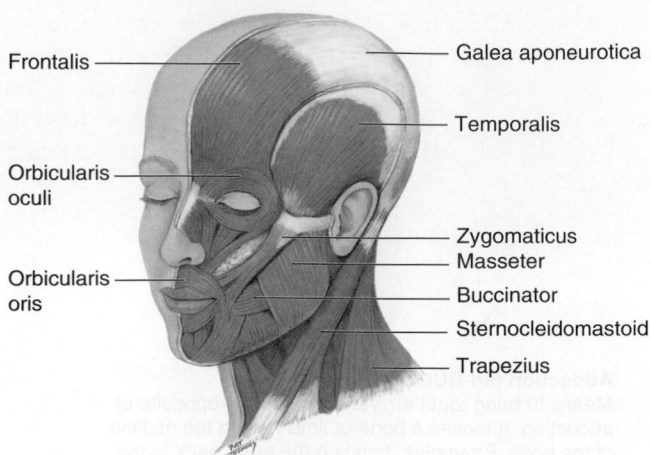

Figure 8-3 Muscles of the head and neck.

Muscles of the Head and Neck

Muscles of Facial Expression

Humans have well-developed muscles in the face that permit a large variety of facial expressions. Because these muscles are used to show surprise, disgust, anger, fear, and other emotions, they are an important means of nonverbal communication. The following are some of the muscles used to produce facial expressions.

The *frontalis* (frun-TAL-is) is over the frontal bone of the forehead. It is attached to the soft tissue of the eyebrow; when it contracts, it raises the eyebrows and wrinkles the forehead. The *orbicularis oris* (oar-BIK-yoo-lair-is OAR-is) is a sphincter that encircles the mouth. This muscle is used to close the mouth, to form words, and to pucker the lips as in kissing. The *orbicularis oculi* (oar-BIK-yoo-lair-is OK-yoo-lye) is another sphincter but is around the eye (oculus). The actions of winking, blinking, and squinting use this muscle. The *buccinator* (BUCK-sin-ay-ter) is the principal muscle in the cheek area and is used to compress the cheek when whistling, sucking, or blowing air out. It is sometimes called the *trumpeter's muscle.* The *zygomaticus* (zye-goh-MAT-ih-kus) extends from the zygomatic arch to the corners of the mouth. It contracts to raise the corner of the mouth when we smile.

Muscles of Mastication

Four pairs of muscles are responsible for chewing movements or mastication. All of these muscles insert on the mandible, and they are some of the strongest muscles in the body. Two of the muscles, the *temporalis* (tem-poar-AL-is) and *masseter* (MASS-eh-ter), are superficial and are identified in Figure 8-3. The others, the lateral and medial pterygoids, are deep to the mandible and are not shown in the figure. The *temporalis* is the largest of the mastication muscles. As the name implies, it has its origin on the temporal bone. The *masseter* is located along the ramus of the mandible and is a synergist of the temporalis.

Neck Muscles

Only two of the more obvious and superficial neck muscles are considered here. Numerous muscles are associated with the throat, hyoid bone, and vertebral column, a discussion of which is beyond the scope of this text.

The *sternocleidomastoid* (stir-no-klye-doh-MAS-toyd) muscles ascend obliquely across the anterior neck from the sternum and clavicle to the mastoid process. When both of these muscles contract together, the neck is flexed and the head is bent toward the chest. When one of the muscles contracts, the head turns toward the direction opposite the side that is contracting. When the left muscle contracts, the head turns to the right. A portion of the *trapezius* (trah-PEEZ-ee-us) muscle is in the neck region and moves the head. Each trapezius muscle extends from the occipital bone at the base of the skull to the end of the thoracic vertebrae and also inserts on the scapula laterally. A portion of this muscle extends the head and is antagonistic to the sternocleidomastoid.

Muscles of the Trunk

The muscles of the trunk include those that move the vertebral column, the muscles that form the thoracic and abdominal walls, and those that cover the pelvic outlet.

Vertebral Column Muscles

The *erector spinae* (ee-REK-ter SPY-nee) group of muscles on each side of the vertebral column is a large muscle mass that extends from the sacrum to the skull. These muscles are primarily responsible for extending the vertebral column to maintain erect posture. Muscle contraction on only one side bends the vertebral column to that side.

Thoracic Wall Muscles

The muscles of the thoracic wall are involved primarily in the process of breathing. The intercostal muscles are located in spaces between the ribs. The *external intercostal muscles* contract to elevate the ribs during the inspiration phase of breathing. The *internal intercostals* contract during forced expiration.

The *diaphragm* is a dome-shaped muscle that forms a partition between the thorax and the abdomen. It has three openings in it for structures that have to pass from the thorax to the abdomen. The diaphragm is responsible for the major movement in the thoracic cavity during quiet, relaxed breathing. When the diaphragm contracts, the dome is flattened. This increases the volume of the thoracic cavity and results in inspiration. When the muscle relaxes, it again resumes its dome shape and decreases the volume of the thoracic cavity, which forces air out during expiration.

Abdominal Wall Muscles

The abdomen, unlike the thorax and pelvis, has no bony reinforcements or protection. The wall consists entirely of four muscle pairs, arranged in layers, and the fascia that envelops them (Figure 8-4). The aponeuroses of the muscles on opposite sides meet in the anterior midline to form the *linea alba* ("white line"), a band of connective tissue that extends from the sternum to the pubic symphysis. The outer muscle layer is the *external oblique.* The *internal oblique* lies just underneath it, and the deepest layer of muscle is the *transversus abdominis.* The arrangement of the muscle layers with the fibers in each layer going in different directions is similar to the type of construction found in plywood and adds strength to the anterolateral abdominal wall. The fascia of these muscles extends anteriorly to form a broad aponeurosis along much of the anterior aspect of the abdomen. The fascia also envelops the *rectus abdominis* muscle, which runs vertically from the pubic bones to the ribs and the sternum on each side of the midline. All of these muscles compress the abdominal wall and increase intraabdominal pressure. The rectus abdominis also flexes the vertebral column.

Pelvic Floor Muscles

The *pelvic diaphragm* forms the floor of the pelvic cavity. Most of the pelvic diaphragm is formed by the two *levator ani* muscles, which support the pelvic viscera. They resist increased pressure in the abdominopelvic cavity and thus play a role in the control of the urinary bladder and rectum.

Muscles of the Upper Extremity

The muscles of the upper extremity include those that attach the scapula to the thorax and generally move the scapula, those that attach the humerus to the scapula and generally move the arm, and those that are located in the arm or forearm and move the forearm, wrist, and hand. Figure 8-5 illustrates the anterior view of body musculature and Figure 8-6 illustrates the posterior view.

Muscles That Move the Shoulder and Arm

The *trapezius* attaches the scapula to the axial skeleton. It is a large superficial triangular muscle of the back. When the trapezius contracts, it adducts and elevates the scapula, as in shrugging the shoulders.

Both the *pectoralis major* (pek-tor-AL-iss MAY-jer) and the *latissimus dorsi* (lah-TISS-ih-mus DOR-sye) muscles attach the humerus to the axial skeleton. The pectoralis major is a superficial muscle on the anterior chest. It has a broad origin on the sternum, costal cartilages, and clavicle, but then the fibers converge to insert on the humerus by way of a short tendon. The primary function of the pectoralis major is to adduct and rotate the arm medially across the chest. The latissimus dorsi is a large, superficial muscle located in the lower back region. It has an extensive origin from the spines of the thoracic vertebrae, ilium, and ribs and then extends upward to insert on the humerus. The latissimus dorsi adducts and rotates the arm medially and lowers the shoulder. It is an important muscle in swimming and rowing motions.

The *deltoid* is a large, fleshy muscle that covers the shoulder and attaches the humerus to the scapula. This muscle

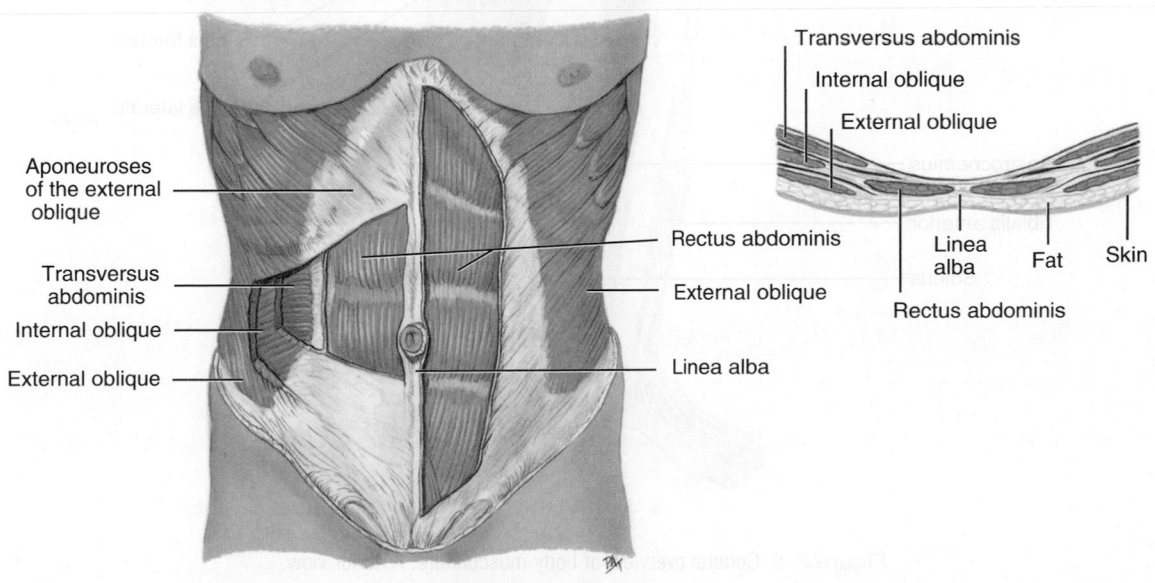

Figure 8-4 Abdominal wall muscles.

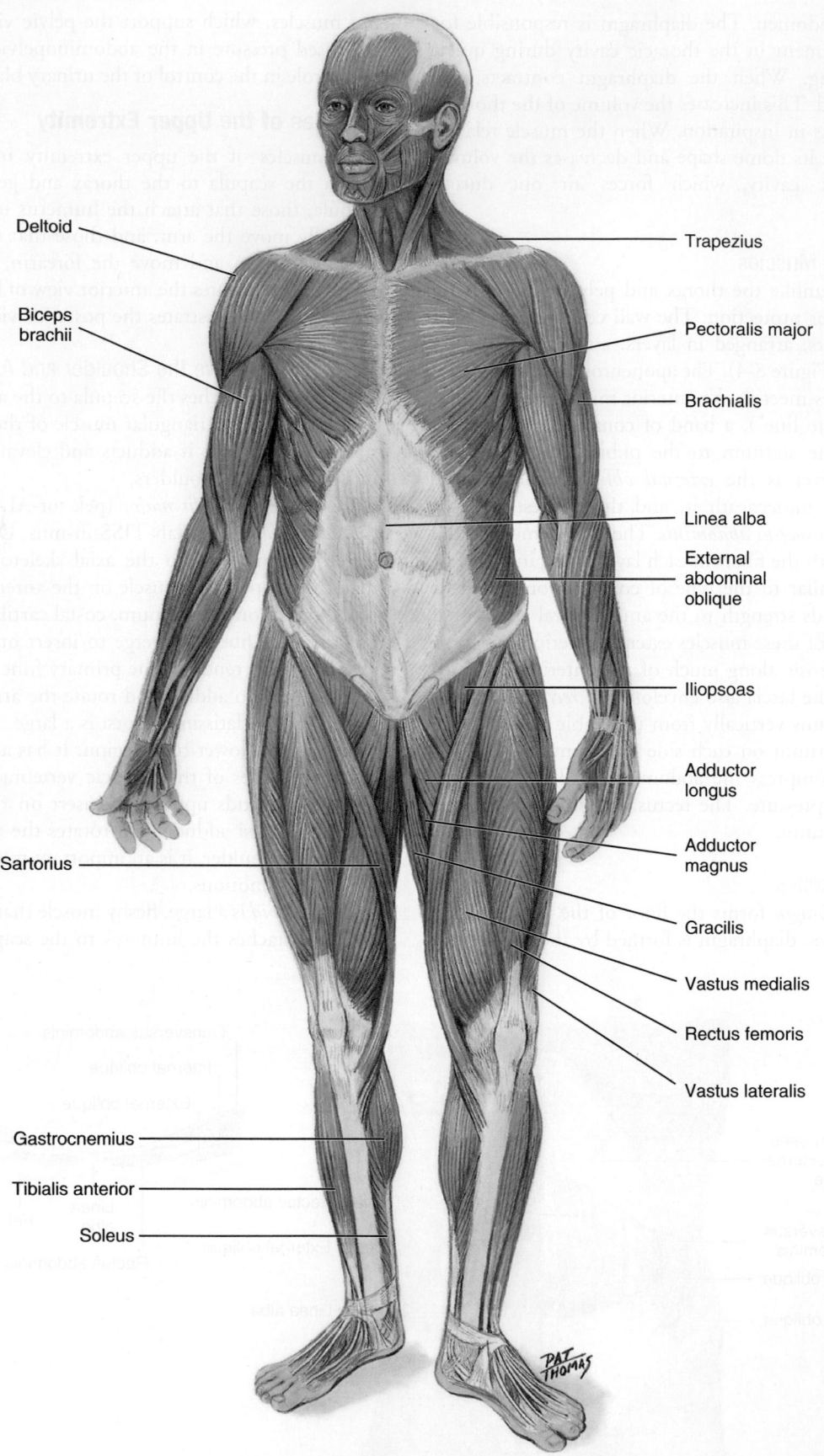

Deltoid

Biceps
brachii

Trapezius

Pectoralis major

Brachialis

Linea alba

External
abdominal
oblique

Iliopsoas

Adductor
longus

Adductor
magnus

Sartorius

Gracilis

Vastus medialis

Rectus femoris

Vastus lateralis

Gastrocnemius

Tibialis anterior

Soleus

PAT
THOMAS

Figure 8-5 General overview of body musculature. Anterior view.

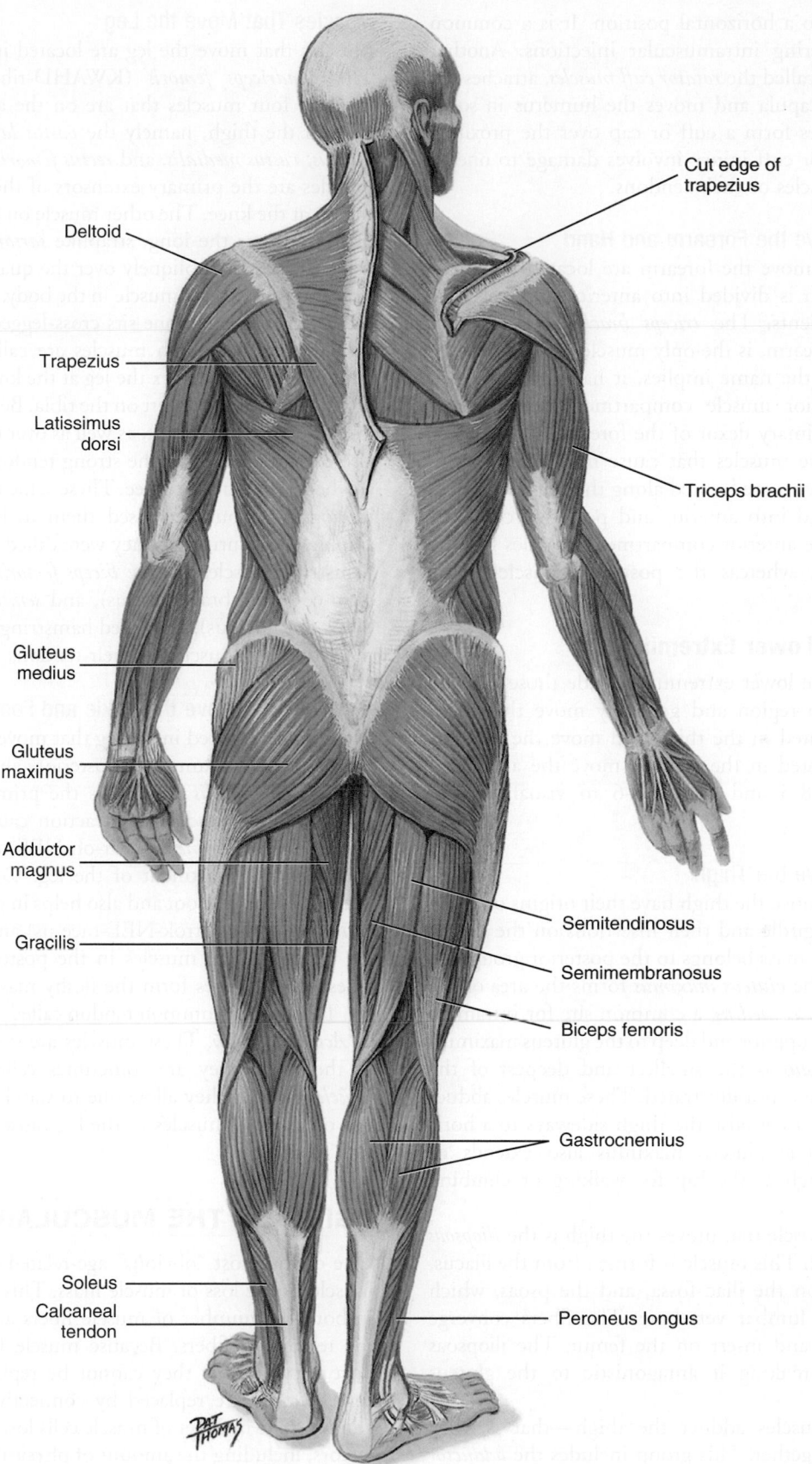

Cut edge of trapezius

Deltoid

Trapezius

Latissimus dorsi

Triceps brachii

Gluteus medius

Gluteus maximus

Adductor magnus

Gracilis

Semitendinosus

Semimembranosus

Biceps femoris

Gastrocnemius

Soleus

Calcaneal tendon

Peroneus longus

PAT THOMAS

Figure 8-6 General overview of body musculature. Posterior view.

abducts the arm to a horizontal position. It is a common site for administering intramuscular injections. Another group of muscles, called the *rotator cuff muscles,* attaches the humerus to the scapula and moves the humerus in some way. These muscles form a cuff or cap over the proximal humerus. A rotator cuff injury involves damage to one or more of these muscles or their tendons.

Muscles That Move the Forearm and Hand
The muscles that move the forearm are located along the humerus. The arm is divided into anterior and posterior muscle compartments. The *triceps brachii,* the primary extensor of the forearm, is the only muscle in the posterior compartment. As the name implies, it has three heads of origin. The anterior muscle compartment contains the *biceps brachii,* a primary flexor of the forearm.

The 20 or more muscles that cause most wrist, hand, and finger movements are located along the forearm. These muscles are divided into anterior and posterior compartments. Most of the anterior compartment muscles flex the wrist and fingers, whereas the posterior muscles cause extension.

Muscles of the Lower Extremity
The muscles of the lower extremity include those that are located in the hip region and generally move the thigh, those that are located in the thigh and move the leg, and those that are located in the leg and move the ankle and foot. See Figure 8-5 and Figure 8-6 to visualize these muscles.

Muscles That Move the Thigh
The muscles that move the thigh have their origins on some part of the pelvic girdle and their insertions on the femur. The largest muscle mass belongs to the posterior group, the gluteal muscles. The *gluteus maximus* forms the area of the buttocks. The *gluteus medius,* a common site for intramuscular injections, is superior and deep to the gluteus maximus. The *gluteus minimus* is the smallest and deepest of the gluteal muscles and is not illustrated. These muscles abduct the thigh—that is, they raise the thigh sideways to a horizontal position. The gluteus maximus also extends or straightens the thigh at the hip for walking or climbing stairs.

The anterior muscle that moves the thigh is the *iliopsoas* (ill-ee-oh-SOH-as). This muscle is formed from the iliacus, which originates on the iliac fossa, and the psoas, which originates on the lumbar vertebrae. The fibers converge into the iliopsoas and insert on the femur. The iliopsoas flexes the thigh, making it antagonistic to the gluteus maximus.

The medial muscles adduct the thigh—that is, they press the thighs together. This group includes the *adductor longus, adductor brevis, adductor magnus,* and *gracilis* (grah-SILL-is) muscles. These muscles are often called the *horse rider's muscles* because their action keeps the rider on the horse.

Muscles That Move the Leg
Muscles that move the leg are located in the thigh region. The *quadriceps femoris* (KWAHD-rih-seps FEM-oar-is) includes four muscles that are on the anterior and lateral sides of the thigh, namely the *vastus lateralis, vastus intermedius, vastus medialis,* and *rectus femoris.* As a group, these muscles are the primary extensors of the leg, straightening the leg at the knee. The other muscle on the anterior surface of the thigh is the long, straplike *sartorius* (sar-TOAR-ee-us), which passes obliquely over the quadriceps group. The sartorius, the longest muscle in the body, flexes and medially rotates the leg when one sits cross-legged.

The posterior thigh muscles are called the *hamstrings,* and they are used to flex the leg at the knee. All have origins on the ischium and insert on the tibia. Because these muscles extend over the hip joint, as well as over the knee joint, they also extend the thigh. The strong tendons of these muscles can be felt behind the knee. These same tendons are present in hogs, and butchers used them to hang the hams for smoking and curing, so they were called "ham strings." The hamstring muscles are the *biceps femoris, semimembranosus* (sem-ee-MEM-brah-noh-sus), and *semitendinosus* (sem-ee-TEN-dih-noh-sus). A "pulled hamstring" is a tear in one or more of these muscles or their tendons.

Muscles That Move the Ankle and Foot
The muscles located in the leg that move the ankle and foot are divided into anterior, posterior, and lateral compartments. The *tibialis anterior* is the primary muscle in the anterior group, and its contraction causes dorsiflexion of the foot. The *peroneus* (pear-oh-NEE-us) muscles occupy the lateral compartment of the leg. Contraction of these muscles everts the foot and also helps in plantar flexion. The *gastrocnemius* (gas-trok-NEE-mee-us) and *soleus* (SOH-lee-us) are the major muscles in the posterior compartment. These two muscles form the fleshy mass in the calf of the leg. They have a common tendon called the *calcaneal tendon* or *Achilles tendon.* These muscles are strong plantar flexors of the foot. They are sometimes called the *toe dancer's muscles* because they allow one to stand on tiptoe. Numerous other deep muscles in the leg cause flexion and extension of the toes.

AGING OF THE MUSCULAR SYSTEM
One of the most "obvious" age-related changes in skeletal muscles is the loss of muscle mass. This involves a decrease in both the number of muscle fibers and the diameter of the remaining fibers. Because muscle fibers are amitotic, once they are lost they cannot be replaced by new ones. Instead, they are replaced by connective tissue, primarily adipose. The number of muscle cells lost depends on several factors, including the amount of physical activity, the nutritional state of the individual, heredity, and the condition of the motor neurons that supply the muscle tissue. There is an age-related loss of motor neurons to skeletal muscle cells, and this is considered an important cause of muscle atrophy.

It is probable that exercise enhances the ability of nerves to stimulate muscle fibers and to reduce atrophy.

As muscle mass decreases, there is a corresponding reduction in muscle strength. The amount of strength loss differs, depending to a large extent on the amount of physical activity. There is evidence that the mitochondria function less effectively in nonexercised muscle cells than in exercised cells. When mitochondria are inefficient, lactic acid accumulates, which contributes to muscle weakness.

There is a tendency for the skeletal muscles of older people to be less responsive, or to respond more slowly, than those of younger people. This is because the latent, contraction, and relaxation phases of muscle action all increase in duration. The increase in response time is less in muscles that are used regularly. Continued physical activity and good nutrition are probably the best deterrents to loss of muscle mass and muscle strength and to increased muscle response time.

TERMINOLOGY REVIEW

Medical Term	Word Parts	Definition
Antagonist	*anti-:* against	A muscle that has an action opposite to that of the prime mover.
Insertion		The end of a muscle that is attached to a relatively movable part; the end opposite the origin.
Motor unit		A single neuron and all the muscle fibers it stimulates.
Neuromuscular junction	*neur/o:* nerve	The area of communication between the axon terminal of a motor neuron and the sarcolemma of a muscle fiber; also called a *myoneural junction.*
Neurotransmitter	*neur/o:* nerve *trans-:* across	A chemical substance that is released at the axon terminals to stimulate a muscle fiber contraction or an impulse in another neuron.
Origin		The end of a muscle that is attached to a relatively immovable part; the end opposite the insertion.
Prime mover		The muscle that is mainly responsible for a particular body movement; also called *agonist.*
Synergist	*syn-:* together *erg/o:* work	A muscle that assists a prime mover but is not capable of producing the movement by itself; two or more muscles work together to produce a movement.

ON THE WEB

For information on muscles and joints:

Gateway Community College: Muscles Tutorial: www.gwc.maricopa.edu/class/bio201/muscle/mustut.htm

Loyola University Medical Education Network: Master Muscle List: www.meddean.luc.edu/lumen/meded/grossanatomy/dissector/mml/index.htm

Merck Manual—Musculoskeletal Disorders: www.merck.com/mmpe/sec04.html *(Click on "Musculoskeletal Disorders")*

San Diego State University College of Sciences: Actin Myosin Crossbridges: www.sci.sdsu.edu/movies/actin_myosin_gif.html

Science Animations: science.nhmccd.edu/biol/animatio.htm

Skeletal Muscles of the Human Body: ptcentral.com/muscles

Skeleton: The Joints: www.zoology.ubc.ca/%7Ebiomania/tutorial/bonejt/outline.htm

University of Washington: Lower Extremity Muscle Atlas: www.rad.washington.edu/atlas2

University of Washington: Upper Extremity Muscle Atlas: www.rad.washington.edu/atlas

University of Wisconsin Medical School: Anatomy Dissections: www.anatomy.wisc.edu/courses/gross/index.html

 Check out the Evolve site at http://evolve.elsevier.com/Bonewit/today/ to actively Prepare for your Certification, and to access additional interactive activities and exercises to help you study and prepare for success.

9

Nervous System

LEARNING OBJECTIVES

1. Describe the organization and functions of the nervous system.
2. Describe the structure and functions of neurons and neuroglia.
3. Explain how an impulse is conducted along the length of a neuron.
4. List and describe the three layers of meninges around the central nervous system.
5. Describe the location, components, and functional areas of the cerebrum, diencephalon, brain stem, and cerebellum.
6. Compare the composition of gray matter and white matter.
7. Explain the function of cerebrospinal fluid.
8. Describe the structure and functions of the spinal cord.
9. Explain the difference in composition of sensory, motor, and mixed nerves.
10. List the 12 cranial nerves, and state the function of each.
11. Identify the region of the body that is innervated by each of the following spinal nerve plexuses: cervical, brachial, lumbosacral.
12. Explain the difference between the sympathetic and parasympathetic divisions of the autonomic nervous system.
13. Describe ways in which the aging of an individual affects the nervous system.
14. Identify pathology related to the nervous system.

CHAPTER OUTLINE

INTRODUCTION TO THE NERVOUS SYSTEM

The nervous system is the major controlling, regulatory, and communicating system in the body. It is the center of all mental activity, including thought, learning, and memory. Together with the endocrine system, the nervous system is responsible for regulating and maintaining homeostasis. Through its receptors, the nervous system keeps us in touch with our environment, both external and internal.

Like other systems in the body, the nervous system is composed of organs, principally the brain, spinal cord, nerves, and ganglia. These, in turn, consist of various tissues, including nerve, blood, and connective tissues. Together these carry out the complex activities of the nervous system.

FUNCTIONS OF THE NERVOUS SYSTEM

The various activities of the nervous system can be grouped together as three general functions:
- Sensory functions
- Integrative functions
- Motor functions

Together these functions keep us in touch with our environments, maintain homeostasis, and account for thought, learning, and memory.

Millions of sensory receptors detect changes, called *stimuli,* that occur inside and outside the body. They monitor such things as temperature, light, and sound from the external environment. Inside the body, the internal environment, receptors detect variations in pressure, pH, carbon dioxide concentration, and the levels of various electrolytes. All of this gathered information is called *sensory input.*

Sensory input is converted into electrical signals called *nerve impulses* that are transmitted to the brain. In the brain the signals are brought together to create sensations, produce thoughts, or add to memory. Decisions are made each moment on the basis of sensory input. This is called *integration.*

Based on the sensory input and integration, the nervous system responds by sending signals to muscles, causing them to contract, or to glands, causing them to produce secretions. Muscles and glands are called *effectors* because they cause an effect in response to directions from the nervous system. This is the *motor output* or *motor function.*

ORGANIZATION OF THE NERVOUS SYSTEM

There is really only one nervous system in the body, although terminology seems to indicate otherwise. Although each subdivision of the system is also called a "nervous system," all of these smaller systems belong to the single, highly integrated nervous system. Each subdivision has structural and functional characteristics that distinguish it from the others. The nervous system as a whole is divided into two subdivisions: the *central nervous system* (CNS) and the *peripheral nervous system* (PNS) (Figure 9-1).

Central Nervous System

The *brain* and *spinal cord* are the organs of the CNS. Because they are so vitally important, the brain and spinal cord, located in the dorsal body cavity, are encased in bone for protection. The brain is in the cranial vault, and the spinal cord is in the vertebral canal of the vertebral column. Although considered to be two separate organs, the brain and spinal cord are continuous at the foramen magnum.

Peripheral Nervous System

The organs of the PNS are the *nerves* and *ganglia.* Nerves are bundles of nerve fibers, much as muscles are bundles of muscle fibers. Cranial nerves (12 pairs) and spinal nerves (31 pairs) extend from the CNS to peripheral organs, such as muscles and glands. Ganglia are collections, or small knots, of nerve cell bodies outside the CNS.

The PNS is further subdivided into an *afferent (sensory) division* and an *efferent (motor) division.* The afferent or sensory division transmits impulses from peripheral organs to the CNS. The efferent or motor division transmits impulses from the CNS out to the peripheral organs to cause an effect or action.

Finally, the efferent or motor division is again subdivided into the *somatic nervous system* and the *autonomic nervous system* (ANS). The somatic nervous system, also called the *somatomotor* or *somatic efferent* nervous system, supplies motor impulses to the skeletal muscles. Because these nerves permit conscious control of the skeletal muscles, the somatic nervous system is sometimes called the *voluntary nervous system.* The ANS, also called the *visceral efferent* nervous system, supplies motor impulses to cardiac muscle, smooth muscle, and glandular epithelium. It is further subdivided into *sympathetic* and *parasympathetic* divisions. Because the ANS regulates involuntary or automatic functions, it is sometimes called the *involuntary nervous system.*

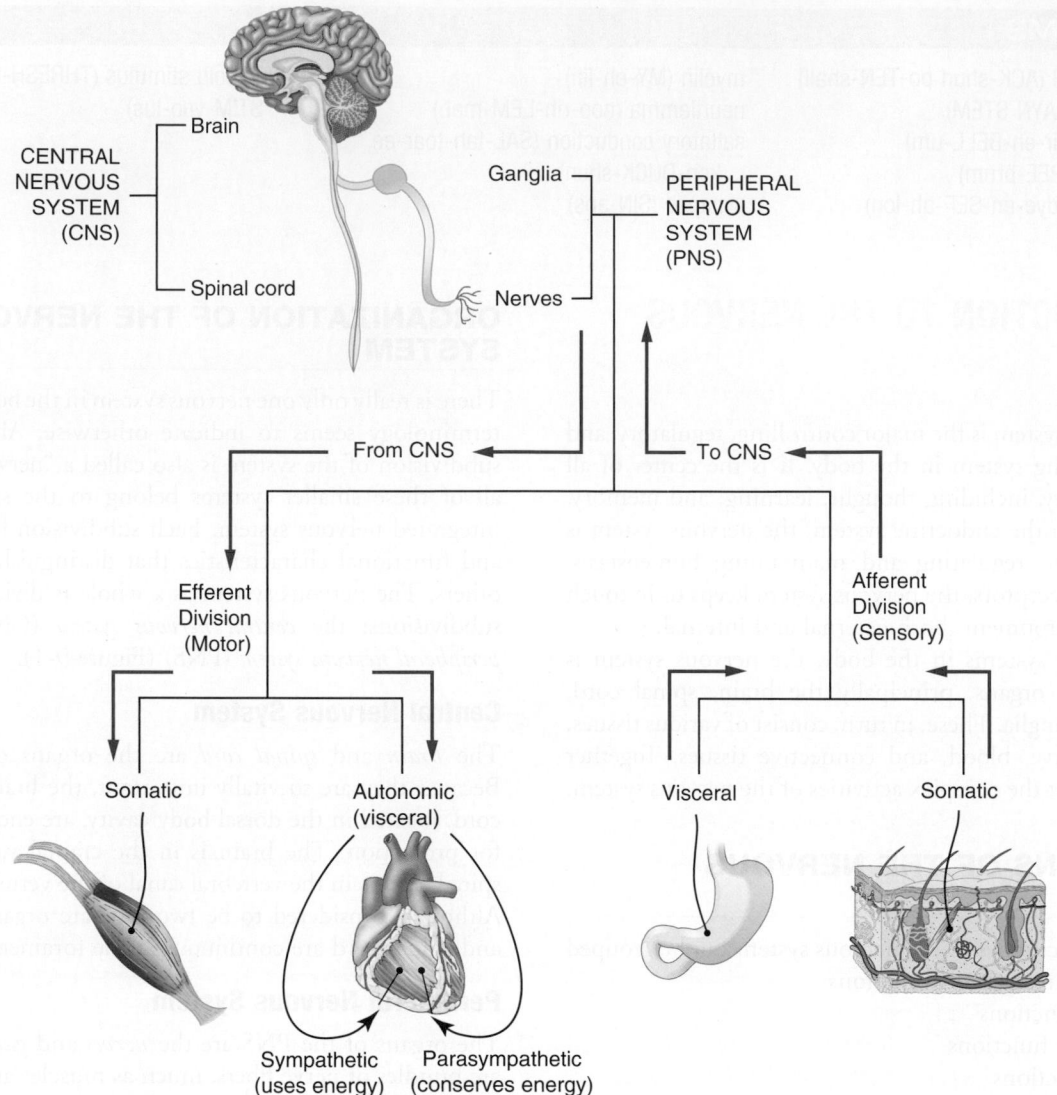

Figure 9-1 Organization of the nervous system.

Highlight on Conditions Affecting the Nervous System

Amyotrophic lateral sclerosis (a-my-oh-TROF-ick LAT-er-al sclair-OH-sis) A neurologic disease caused by degeneration of motor neurons of the spinal cord, medulla, and cortex; marked by progressive muscular weakness and atrophy with spasticity and exaggerated reflexes; mental capabilities are not impaired; also called *Lou Gehrig disease* or *motor neuron disease*

Bell palsy (BELL PAUL-zee) Neuropathy of the seventh cranial nerve (facial) that causes paralysis of the muscles on one side of the face with sagging of the mouth on the affected side of the face

Cerebral concussion (seh-REE-brull kon-KUSH-un) Loss of consciousness as the result of a blow to the head; usually clears within 24 hours; no evidence of permanent structural damage to the brain tissue

Cerebral contusion (seh-REE-brull kon-TOO-shun) Bruising of brain tissue as a result of direct trauma to the head; neurologic problems persist longer than 24 hours

Cerebral palsy (seh-REE-brull PAWL-zee) Partial paralysis and lack of muscular coordination caused by damage to the cerebrum during fetal life, birth, or infancy

Cerebrovascular accident (CVA) (seh-ree-broh-VAS-kyoo-lar AK-sih-dent) Most common brain disorder; may be caused by decreased blood supply to the brain or rupture of a blood vessel in the brain; commonly called a *stroke*

Multiple sclerosis (MS) (MULL-tih-pull skler-OH-sis) A disorder in which there is progressive destruction of the myelin sheaths of central nervous system neurons, interfering with their ability to transmit impulses; characterized by progressive loss of function interspersed with periods of remission; cause is unknown and there is no satisfactory treatment

Reye syndrome (RS) (RYE SIN-drohm) Brain dysfunction that occurs primarily in children and teenagers and is characterized by edema of the brain that leads to disorientation, lethargy, and personality changes and may progress to a coma; seems to

NERVE TISSUE

Although the nervous system is complex, there are only two main types of cells in nerve tissue. The actual nerve cell is the *neuron*. It is the "conducting" cell that transmits impulses. It is the structural unit of the nervous system. The other type of cell is the *neuroglia* or *glial cell*. The word *neuroglia* means "nerve glue." These cells are nonconductive and provide a support system for the neurons. They are a special type of "connective tissue" for the nervous system.

Neurons

Neurons, or nerve cells, carry out the functions of the nervous system by conducting nerve impulses. They are highly specialized and amitotic. This means that if a neuron is destroyed, it cannot be replaced because neurons do not undergo mitosis.

Each neuron has three basic parts:
- Cell body
- One or more dendrites
- A single axon

Figure 9-2 illustrates a typical neuron. The main part of the neuron is the *cell body* or *soma*. In many ways the cell body is similar to other types of cells. It has a nucleus with at least one nucleolus and contains many of the typical cytoplasmic organelles. It lacks centrioles, however. Because centrioles function in cell division, the fact that neurons lack these organelles is consistent with the amitotic nature of the cell.

Dendrites and *axons* are cytoplasmic extensions, or processes, that project from the cell body. They are sometimes referred to as *fibers*. Dendrites are usually, but not always, short and branching, which increases their surface area to receive signals from other neurons. The number of dendrites on a neuron varies. They are called *afferent processes* because they transmit impulses to the neuron cell body. Only one axon projects from each cell body. It is usually elongated, and because it carries impulses away from the cell body, it is called an *efferent process*.

An axon may have infrequent branches called *axon collaterals*. Axons and axon collaterals terminate in many short branches or *telodendria* (tell-oh-DEN-dree-ah). The distal ends of the telodendria are slightly enlarged to form *synaptic bulbs*. Many axons are surrounded by a segmented, white, fatty substance called **myelin** (MY-eh-lin) or the *myelin sheath*. Myelinated fibers make up the white matter in the CNS, whereas cell bodies and unmyelinated fibers make up the gray matter. The unmyelinated regions between the myelin segments are called the *nodes of Ranvier* (nodes of ron-vee-AY). In the PNS the myelin is produced by Schwann cells. The cytoplasm, nucleus, and outer cell membrane of the Schwann cell form a tight covering around the myelin and around the axon itself at the nodes of Ranvier. This covering is the **neurilemma** (noo-rih-LEM-mah), which plays an important role in the regeneration of nerve fibers. In the CNS, *oligodendrocytes* (ah-lee-go-DEN-droh-sites) produce myelin, but there is no neurilemma, which is why fibers within the CNS do not regenerate. The structure of an axon and its coverings is illustrated in Figure 9-2.

Functionally, neurons are classified as afferent, efferent, or interneurons (association neurons) according to the direction in which they transmit impulses relative to the CNS (Table 9-1). *Afferent*, or *sensory*, *neurons* carry impulses from peripheral sense receptors to the CNS. They usually have long dendrites and relatively short axons. *Efferent*, or *motor*, *neurons* transmit impulses from the CNS to effector organs, such as muscles and glands. Efferent neurons usually have short dendrites and long axons. *Interneurons*, or *association neurons*, are located entirely within the CNS, where they form the connecting link between the afferent and efferent neurons. They have short dendrites and may have either a short or a long axon.

Neuroglia

Neuroglia cells do not conduct nerve impulses; instead, they support, nourish, and protect the neurons. They are far more numerous than neurons and, unlike neurons, are capable of mitosis.

NERVE IMPULSES

The functional characteristics of neurons are *excitability* and *conductivity*. Excitability is the ability to respond to a stimulus; conductivity is the ability to transmit an impulse from one point to another. All the functions associated with the nervous system, including thought, learning, and memory, are based on these two characteristics. These functional characteristics are the result of structural features of the cell membrane.

Highlight on the Nervous System

Brain tumors: Because neurons are not capable of mitosis, primary malignant tumors of the brain are tumors of the glial cells rather than of the neurons themselves. These tumors, called *gliomas,* have extensive roots, making them extremely difficult to remove.

Blood-brain barrier: Neuroglia, particularly astrocytes, form a wall around the outside of the blood vessels in the nervous system. This astrocyte wall plus the blood vessel wall form the blood-brain barrier. Water, oxygen, carbon dioxide, alcohol, and a few other substances are able to pass through this barrier and move between the blood and brain tissue. Other substances, such as toxins, pathogens, and certain drugs, cannot pass through this barrier. This is a protective mechanism to keep harmful substances out of the brain. It has clinical significance because drugs such as penicillin that may be used to treat disorders in other parts of the body have no effect on the brain because they do not cross the blood-brain barrier.

Anesthetics: Some anesthetics produce their effects by inhibiting the diffusion of sodium through the cell membrane and thus blocking the initiation and conduction of nerve impulses.

Meningitis: Meningitis is an acute inflammation of the pia mater and the arachnoid. It is most commonly caused by bacteria. However, viral infections, fungal infections, and tumors may also cause inflammation of the meninges. Depending on the primary cause, meningitis may be mild or it may progress to a severe and life-threatening condition.

Left and right brain: In most people (approximately 90%), the left cerebral hemisphere dominates for language and mathematic abilities. It is the reasoning and analytic side of the brain. The right cerebral hemisphere is involved with motor skills, intuition, emotion, art, and music appreciation. It is the poetic and creative side of the brain. These people are generally right-handed. In about 10% of the people, these sides are reversed. In some cases, neither hemisphere dominates. This may result in "confusion" and learning disabilities.

Parkinson disease: Parkinson disease is a condition in which the basal ganglia do not produce enough of the inhibitory transmitter dopamine. Without dopamine, there is an excess of excitatory signals that affect certain voluntary muscles, producing rigidity and tremors.

Emotions: The *limbic system* consists of scattered but interconnected regions of gray matter in the cerebral hemispheres and diencephalon. The limbic system is involved in memory and in emotions such as sadness, happiness, anger, and fear. It is our emotional brain.

Hydrocephalus: In hydrocephalus, an obstruction in the normal flow of cerebrospinal fluid (CSF) causes the fluid to accumulate in the ventricles. The obstruction may be a congenital defect or an acquired lesion such as a tumor. As the fluid accumulates, it causes the ventricles to enlarge and CSF pressure to increase. When this happens in an infant, before the cranial bones ossify, the cranium enlarges. In an older child or adult, the pressure damages the soft brain tissue.

Lumbar puncture: A lumbar puncture is the withdrawal of some CSF from the subarachnoid space in the lumbar region of the spinal cord. The extension of the meninges beyond the end of the cord makes it possible to do this without injury to the spinal cord. The needle is usually inserted just above or just below the fourth lumbar vertebra, and the spinal cord ends at the first lumbar vertebra. The CSF that is removed can be tested for abnormal characteristics that may indicate an injury or infection.

Carpal tunnel syndrome: Carpal tunnel syndrome is a common occupational injury to the hand and wrist that is associated with repetitive hand motions. It is also associated with several diseases, including arthritis, diabetes, and gout. Symptoms, which include tingling of the thumb and fingers, result from the compression of the median nerve because of inflammation and swelling of the tendons within the carpal tunnel. ■

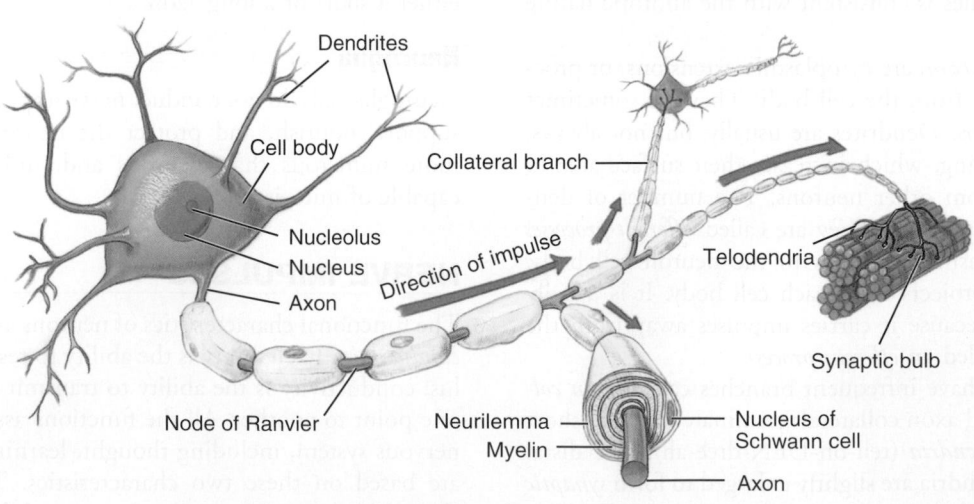

Figure 9-2 Structure of a typical neuron.

Table 9-1	Types of Neurons Classified According to Function	
Type of Neuron	**Structure**	**Function**
Afferent (sensory)	Long dendrites and short axon; cell body located in ganglia in PNS; dendrites in PNS; axon extends into CNS	Transmits impulses from peripheral sense receptors to CNS
Efferent (motor)	Short dendrites and long axon; dendrites and cell body located within CNS; axons extend to PNS	Transmits impulses from CNS to effectors, such as muscles and glands in periphery
Association (interneurons)	Short dendrites; axon may be short or long; located entirely within CNS	Transmits impulses from afferent neurons to efferent neurons

From Applegate E: *The anatomy and physiology learning system*, ed 4, St Louis, 2011, Saunders.
CNS, Central nervous system; *PNS*, peripheral nervous system.

Resting Membrane

A *resting membrane* is the cell membrane of a nonconducting, or resting, neuron. The membrane is impermeable to the passive diffusion of sodium (Na$^+$) and potassium (K$^+$) ions. An active transport mechanism, the sodium-potassium pump, maintains a difference in concentration of these ions on the two sides of the membrane. Sodium ions are concentrated in the extracellular fluid, whereas the potassium ions are inside the cell. The intracellular fluid also contains proteins and other negatively charged ions. The result is a polarized membrane with more positive charges outside the cell and more negative charges inside the cell. This difference in charges on the two sides of the resting membrane is the *resting membrane potential.* Electrical measurements show the resting membrane potential to be about −70 millivolts (mV), which means that the inside of the membrane is 70 mV less positive (more negative) than the outside.

Stimulation of a Neuron

A stimulus is a physical, chemical, or electrical event that alters the permeability of the neuron cell membrane. This allows sodium ions to move inside the cell, then potassium ions move to the outside. This ionic movement briefly changes the polarization of the membrane.

This response to a stimulus—namely, depolarization, reverse polarization, and repolarization—is called the **action potential.** Electrical measurements show the action potential to peak at approximately +30 mV (Figure 9-3). At the conclusion of the action potential, the sodium-potassium pump actively transports sodium ions out of the cell and

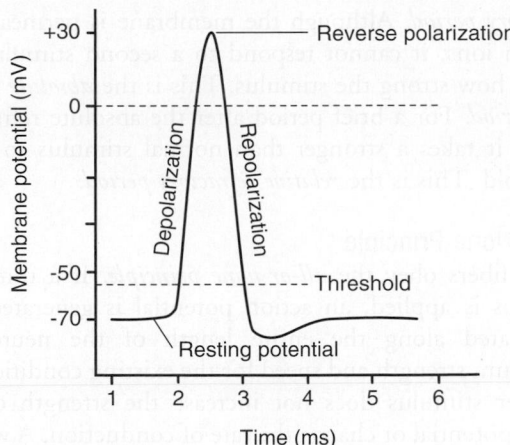

Figure 9-3 Recording of an action potential. The resting potential is −70 mV and the peak action potential is +30 mV.

potassium ions into the cell to completely restore resting conditions.

The minimum stimulus necessary to initiate an action potential is called a **threshold stimulus** or liminal stimulus. A weaker stimulus, called a *subthreshold (subliminal) stimulus,* does not cause sufficient depolarization to elicit an action potential.

Conduction along a Neuron

Once a threshold stimulus has been applied and an action potential generated, it must be conducted along the total length of the neuron either to an effector or to another neuron.

The threshold stimulus causes a localized area of reverse polarization on the membrane. In that one area, the membrane is negative on the outside and positive on the inside. The rest of the membrane is in the resting condition. When a given area reverses its polarity, the difference in potential between that area and the adjacent area creates a current flow that depolarizes the second point. When the second point reverses its polarity, current flow between the second point and the third point depolarizes the third point. This continues point by point, in domino fashion, along the entire length of the neuron, creating a *propagated action potential,* or *nerve impulse.*

Saltatory Conduction

The conduction described in the previous paragraph is representative of an unmyelinated axon. Because myelin is an insulating substance, it inhibits the flow of current from one point to another. In myelinated fibers, depolarization occurs only at the places where there is no myelin, at the nodes of Ranvier. The action potential "jumps" from node to node. This "jumping" is **saltatory conduction,** which is faster than conduction in unmyelinated fibers.

Refractory Period

The period of time during which a point on the cell membrane is "recovering" from depolarization is called the *refractory period.* Although the membrane is permeable to sodium ions, it cannot respond to a second stimulus, no matter how strong the stimulus. This is the *absolute refractory period.* For a brief period after the absolute refractory period it takes a stronger than normal stimulus to reach threshold. This is the *relative refractory period.*

All-or-None Principle

Nerve fibers obey the *all-or-none principle.* If a threshold stimulus is applied, an action potential is generated and propagated along the entire length of the neuron at maximum strength and speed for the existing conditions. A stronger stimulus does not increase the strength of the action potential or change the rate of conduction. A weaker stimulus is subthreshold and does not evoke an action potential. If a stimulus is threshold or greater, an impulse is conducted. If the stimulus is subthreshold, there is no conduction.

Conduction across a Synapse

A nerve impulse, or propagated action potential, travels along a nerve fiber until it reaches the end of the axon; then it must be transmitted to the next neuron. The region of communication between two neurons is called a **synapse** (SIN-aps). This is similar to the neuromuscular junction described in Chapter 8. A synapse has three parts (Figure 9-4):

• Synaptic knob
• Synaptic cleft
• Postsynaptic membrane

The first neuron, the one preceding the synapse, is called the *presynaptic neuron;* the second neuron, the one following the synapse, is called the *postsynaptic neuron.* Synaptic knobs are tiny bulges at the end of the telodendria on the presynaptic neuron. Small sacs within the synaptic knobs, called *synaptic vesicles,* contain chemicals known as *neurotransmitters* (noo-roh-TRANS-mitters).

When a nerve impulse reaches the synaptic knob, a series of reactions releases neurotransmitters into the synaptic cleft. The neurotransmitters diffuse across the synaptic cleft and react with receptors on the postsynaptic cell membrane. This is synaptic transmission. To prevent prolonged reactions with the postsynaptic receptors, the transmitters are quickly inactivated by enzymes. One of the best known neurotransmitters is *acetylcholine* (ah-see-till-KOH-leen), which is inactivated by the enzyme *cholinesterase* (koh-lin-ES-ter-ase). Table 9-2 lists some of the common neurotransmitters.

In *excitatory transmission,* the neurotransmitter-receptor reaction on the postsynaptic membrane depolarizes the membrane and initiates an action potential. This is excitation or stimulation. Acetylcholine is typically an excitatory neurotransmitter. Some neurotransmitters result in *inhibitory transmission.* In this case, the reaction between the neurotransmitter and the receptor makes it more difficult to generate an action potential. This is inhibition. Gamma-aminobutyric acid (GABA) is an inhibitory neurotransmitter in the CNS.

The billions of neurons in the CNS are organized into functional groups called *neuronal pools.* The neuronal pools

Figure 9-4 Components of a synapse. The impulse travels from the presynaptic neuron to the postsynaptic neuron.

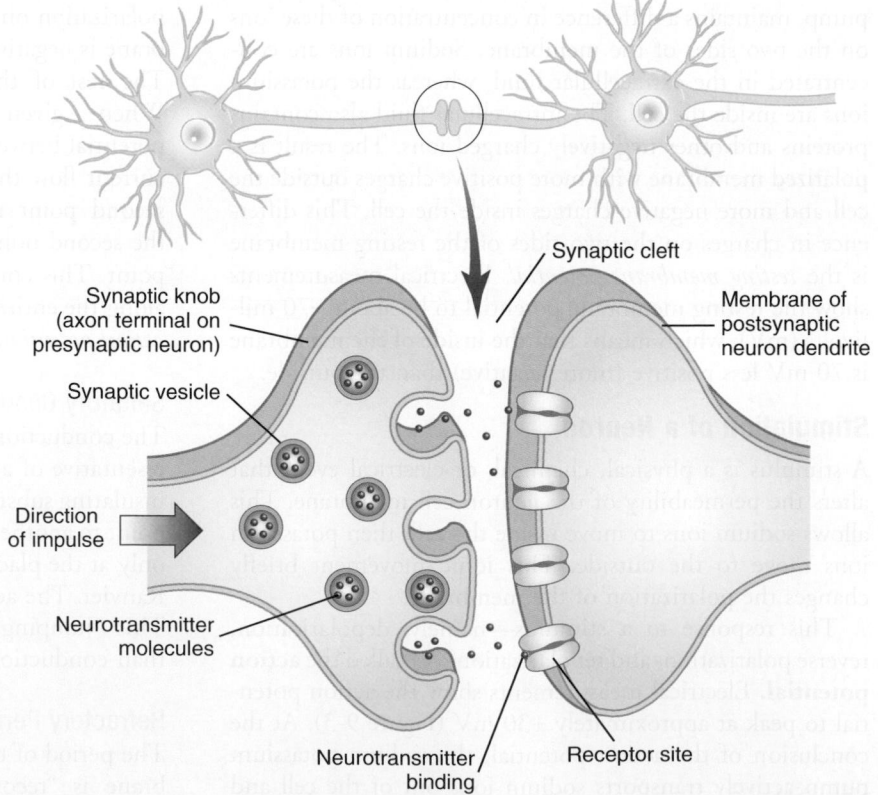

Synaptic knob
(axon terminal on
presynaptic neuron)

Synaptic vesicle

Direction
of impulse

Neurotransmitter
molecules

Neurotransmitter
binding

Synaptic cleft

Membrane of
postsynaptic
neuron dendrite

Receptor site

Table 9-2   Some Common Neurotransmitters

Neurotransmitter	Location	Function	Comments
Acetylcholine	CNS and PNS	Generally excitatory but inhibitory to some visceral effectors	Found in skeletal neuromuscular junctions and in many ANS synapses
Norepinephrine	CNS and PNS	May be excitatory or inhibitory depending on receptors	Found in visceral and cardiac muscle neuromuscular junctions; cocaine and amphetamines exaggerate effects
Epinephrine	CNS and PNS	May be excitatory or inhibitory depending on receptors	Found in pathways concerned with behavior and mood
Dopamine	CNS and PNS	Generally excitatory	Found in pathways that regulate emotional responses; decreased levels in Parkinson disease
Serotonin	CNS	Generally inhibitory	Found in pathways that regulate temperature, sensory perception, mood, onset of sleep
Gamma-aminobutyric acid (GABA)	CNS	Generally inhibitory	Inhibits excessive discharge of neurons
Endorphins and enkephalins	CNS	Generally inhibitory	Inhibit release of sensory pain neurotransmitters; opiates mimic effects of these peptides

From Applegate E: *The anatomy and physiology learning system*, ed 4, St Louis, 2011, Saunders.
ANS, Autonomic nervous system; *CNS*, central nervous system; *PNS*, peripheral nervous system.

receive information, process and integrate that information, and then transmit it to some other destination. Neuronal pools are arranged in pathways, or circuits, over which the nerve impulses are transmitted. The simplest pathway is the *simple series circuit* (Figure 9-5, *A*) in which a single neuron synapses with another neuron, which in turn synapses with another, and so on. Most pathways are more complex. In a *divergence circuit* (Figure 9-5, *B*), a single neuron synapses with multiple neurons within the pool. This permits the same information to diverge or go along different pathways at the same time. This type of pathway is important in muscle contraction when many muscle fibers, or even several muscles, must contract at the same time. Another type of pathway is the *convergence circuit* (Figure 9-5, *C*). In this case, several presynaptic neurons synapse with a single postsynaptic neuron. This accounts for the fact that many different stimuli may have the same ultimate effect. For example, thinking about food, smelling food, and seeing food all have the same effect—the flow of saliva.

Reflex Arcs

The neuron is the structural unit of the nervous system; the *reflex arc* is the functional unit. The reflex arc is a type of conduction pathway. It is similar to a one-way street because it allows impulses to travel in only one direction. The simplest reflex arc consists of two neurons, but most have three or more neurons in the conduction pathway. Figure 9-6 illustrates a three-neuron reflex arc. There are five basic components in a reflex arc (Table 9-3):

- Receptor
- Sensory neuron
- Integration center
- Motor neuron
- Effector

A *reflex* is an automatic, involuntary response to some change, either inside or outside the body. Reflexes are important in maintaining homeostasis by making adjustments to

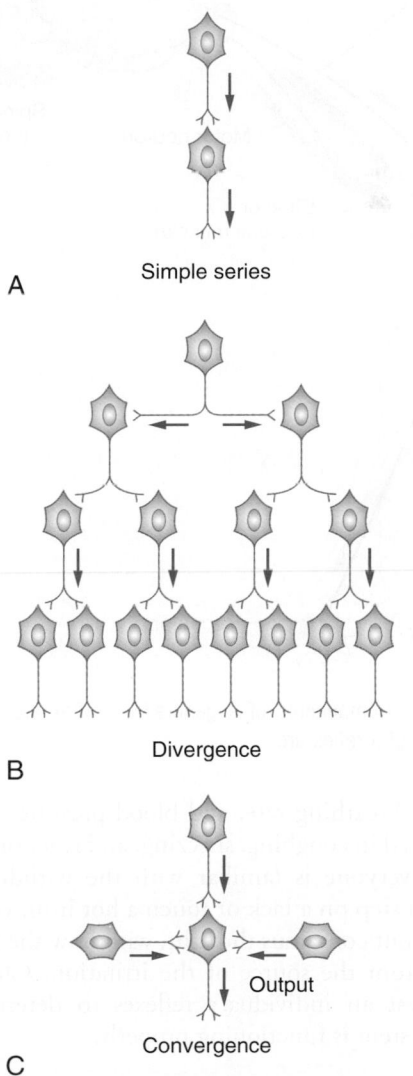

Figure 9-5 Neuronal pools. **A,** Simple series circuit: one neuron synapses with another. **B,** Divergence circuit: a single neuron synapses with multiple neurons. **C,** Convergence circuit: several neurons synapse with a single postsynaptic neuron.

Table 9-3   Components of a Reflex Arc

Component	Description	Function
Receptor	Site of stimulus action; receptor end of dendrite or special cell in receptor organ	Responds to some change in internal or external environment
Sensory neuron	Afferent neuron; cell body is in ganglion outside CNS; axon extends into CNS	Transmits nerve impulses from receptor to CNS
Integration center	Always within CNS; in simplest reflexes, it consists of synapse between sensory and motor neurons; more commonly one or more interneurons are involved	Processing center; region in CNS where incoming sensory impulses generate appropriate outgoing motor impulses
Motor neuron	Efferent neuron; dendrites and cell body are in CNS; axon extends to periphery	Transmits nerve impulses from integration center in CNS to effector organ
Effector	Muscle or gland outside CNS	Responds to impulses from motor neuron to produce an action, such as contraction or secretion

From Applegate E: *The anatomy and physiology learning system,* ed 4, St Louis, 2011, Saunders.
CNS, Central nervous system.

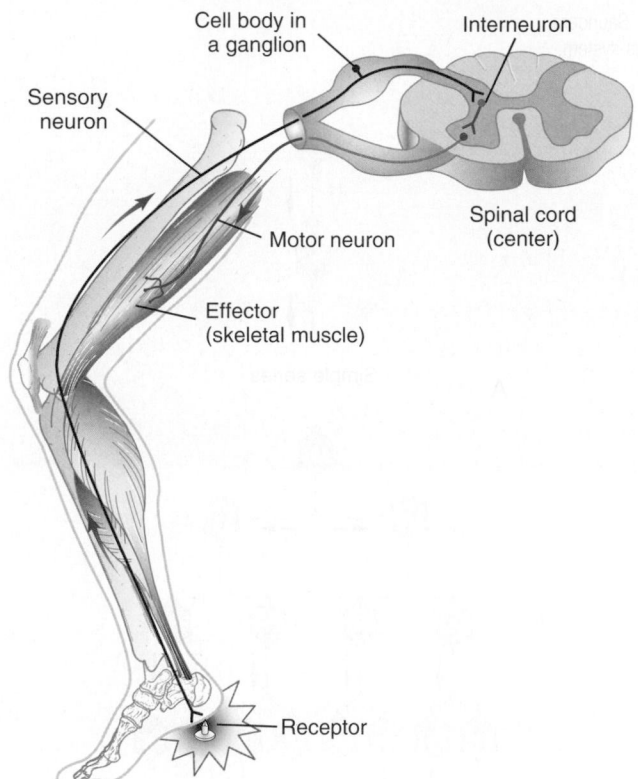

Figure 9-6 Components of a generalized reflex arc. Note the five components of a reflex arc.

heart rate, breathing rate, and blood pressure. Reflexes are also involved in coughing, sneezing, and reactions to painful stimuli. Everyone is familiar with the withdrawal reflex. When you step on a tack or touch a hot iron, you immediately, without conscious thought, withdraw the injured foot or hand from the source of the irritation. Clinicians frequently test an individual's reflexes to determine if the nervous system is functioning properly.

CENTRAL NERVOUS SYSTEM

The CNS consists of the brain and spinal cord, which are located in the dorsal body cavity. These are vital to our well-being and are enclosed in bone for protection. The brain is surrounded by the cranium, and the spinal cord is protected by the vertebrae. The brain is continuous with the spinal cord at the foramen magnum in the occipital bone. In addition to bone, the CNS is surrounded by connective tissue membranes, called *meninges,* and by *cerebrospinal fluid* (CSF).

Meninges

Three layers of meninges (men-IN-jeez) surround the brain and spinal cord (Figure 9-7). The outer layer, the *dura mater* (DOO-rah MAY-ter), is tough, white fibrous connective tissue. It is just inside the cranial bones and lines the vertebral canal. The dura mater contains channels, called *dural sinuses,* that collect venous blood to return it to the cardiovascular system.

The middle layer of meninges is the *arachnoid* (ah-RAK-noyd). The arachnoid, which resembles a cobweb in appearance, is a thin layer with numerous threadlike strands that attach it to the innermost layer. The space under the arachnoid, the *subarachnoid space,* is filled with CSF and contains blood vessels.

The *pia mater* (PEE-ah MAY-ter) is the innermost layer of meninges. This thin, delicate membrane is tightly bound to the surface of the brain and spinal cord and cannot be dissected away without damaging the surface. It closely follows all surface contours.

Brain

The brain is divided into the cerebrum, diencephalon, brain stem, and cerebellum.

Cerebrum

The largest and most obvious portion of the brain is the **cerebrum** (seh-REE-brum), which is divided by a deep *longitudinal fissure* (FISH-ur) into two *cerebral hemispheres.* The two hemispheres are two separate entities but are connected by an arching band of white fibers, called the *corpus callosum* (KOR-pus kah-LOH-sum), that provides a communication pathway between the two halves. The surface of the cerebrum is marked by convolutions, or *gyri* (JYE-rye), separated by grooves, or *sulci* (SULL-see). The pia mater closely follows the convolutions and goes deep into the sulci, and then up and over the gyri.

Each cerebral hemisphere is divided into five lobes, as illustrated in Figure 9-8. Four of the lobes have the same name as the bone over them. The *frontal lobe,* under the frontal bone, is the most anterior portion of each hemisphere. The posterior boundary of the frontal lobe is the *central sulcus.* The *parietal lobe* is immediately posterior to the central sulcus, under the parietal bone. The *occipital lobe,* under the occipital bone, is the most posterior portion of the cerebral hemisphere. Laterally, the *temporal lobe* is inferior to the frontal and parietal lobes. The *lateral sulcus* (fissure) separates the temporal lobe from the two lobes that

are superior to it. A fifth lobe, the *insula* (IN-sull-ah) or *island of Reil,* lies deep within the lateral sulcus. It is covered by parts of the frontal, parietal, and temporal lobes.

The cerebral hemispheres consist of gray matter and white matter. A thin layer of *gray matter,* the *cerebral cortex,* forms the outermost portion of the cerebrum. Gray matter consists of neuron cell bodies and unmyelinated fibers. The *white matter,* which makes up the bulk of the cerebrum, is just beneath the cerebral cortex. White matter is myelinated nerve fibers that form communication pathways in the cerebrum.

The cerebral cortex is the neural basis of what makes us "human." It is the center for sensory and motor functions. It is concerned with memory, language, reasoning, intelligence, personality, and all the other factors that we associate with human life. Even though the two cerebral hemispheres are nearly symmetric in structure, they are not always equal in function; instead, there are areas of specialization. However, there is considerable overlap in these regions and no area really works alone; all the areas are dependent on one another for mental "consciousness"—those abilities that involve higher mental processing, such as memory, reasoning, logic, and judgment.

It is possible to identify regions of the cerebral cortex that have specific functions. *Sensory areas* receive information from the various sense organs and receptors throughout the body. The primary sensory area, the *somatosensory* (soh-mat-oh-SEN-soar-ee) *cortex,* is located in the *postcentral gyrus* of the parietal lobe, immediately posterior to the central sulcus. This region receives sensory input from sensory receptors in the skin and skeletal muscles. The right

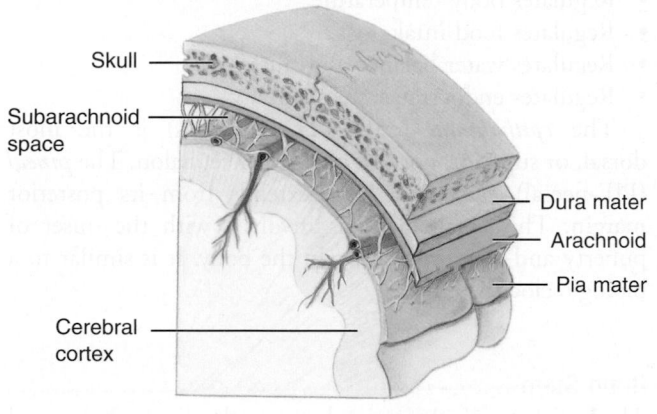

Figure 9-7 Meninges of the central nervous system.

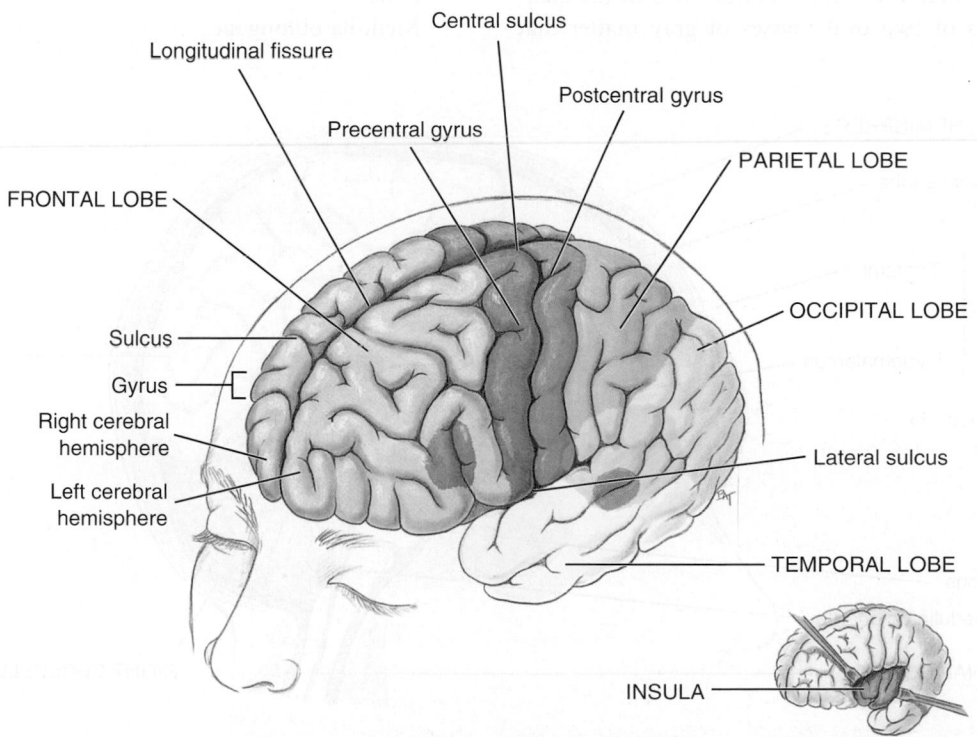

Figure 9-8 Lobes and landmarks of the cerebrum.

side of the somatosensory cortex receives input from the left side of the body and vice versa. *Motor areas* responsible for muscle contraction are located in the frontal lobe. The primary motor area, the *somatomotor* (soh-mat-oh-MOH-ter) *cortex,* is in the *precentral gyrus,* immediately anterior to the central sulcus. Neurons in this area allow us to consciously control our skeletal muscles. The right primary motor gyrus controls muscles on the left side of the body and vice versa. The primary motor cortex is also highly organized in a manner similar to the primary sensory cortex, with neurons in a specific region responsible for controlling movement in a specific part of the body.

Association areas of the cerebral cortex are involved in the process of recognition. They analyze and interpret sensory information, and based on previous experiences they integrate appropriate responses through the motor areas. Table 9-4 describes some of the specific functional areas of the cerebral cortex.

The *basal ganglia* are functionally related regions of gray matter that are scattered throughout the white matter of the cerebral hemispheres. These regions function as relay stations, or areas of synapse, in pathways going to and from the cortex. The major effects of the basal ganglia are to decrease muscle tone and inhibit muscular activity. Because of these effects, they play an important role in posture and coordinating motor movements. Also, nearly all the inhibitory neurotransmitter dopamine is produced in the basal ganglia.

Diencephalon

The **diencephalon** (dye-en-SEF-ah-lon) is centrally located and is nearly surrounded by the cerebral hemispheres. Regions of the diencephalon are illustrated in Figure 9-9.

The *thalamus* (THAL-ah-mus), about 80% of the diencephalon, consists of two oval masses of gray matter that serve as relay stations for sensory impulses, except for the sense of smell, going to the cerebral cortex. The thalamus channels the impulses to the appropriate region of the cortex for discrimination, localization, and interpretation.

The *hypothalamus* (HYE-poh-thal-ah-mus) is a small region below the thalamus. It plays a key role in maintaining homeostasis because it regulates many visceral activities. The hypothalamus also serves as a link between the nervous and endocrine systems because it regulates secretion of hormones from the pituitary gland. A slender stalk, the *infundibulum,* extends from the floor of the hypothalamus to the pituitary gland and acts as a connector between the two structures. Functions of the hypothalamus include the following:

- Regulates and integrates the ANS
- Regulates emotional responses and behavior
- Regulates body temperature
- Regulates food intake
- Regulates water balance and thirst
- Regulates endocrine system activity

The *epithalamus* (ep-ih-THAL-ah-mus) is the most dorsal, or superior, portion of the diencephalon. The *pineal* (PIE-nee-al) *gland,* or *body,* extends from its posterior margin. This small gland is involved with the onset of puberty and rhythmic cycles in the body. It is similar to a biologic clock.

Brain Stem

The **brain stem** is the region between the diencephalon and the spinal cord. It consists of three regions:
- Midbrain
- Pons
- Medulla oblongata

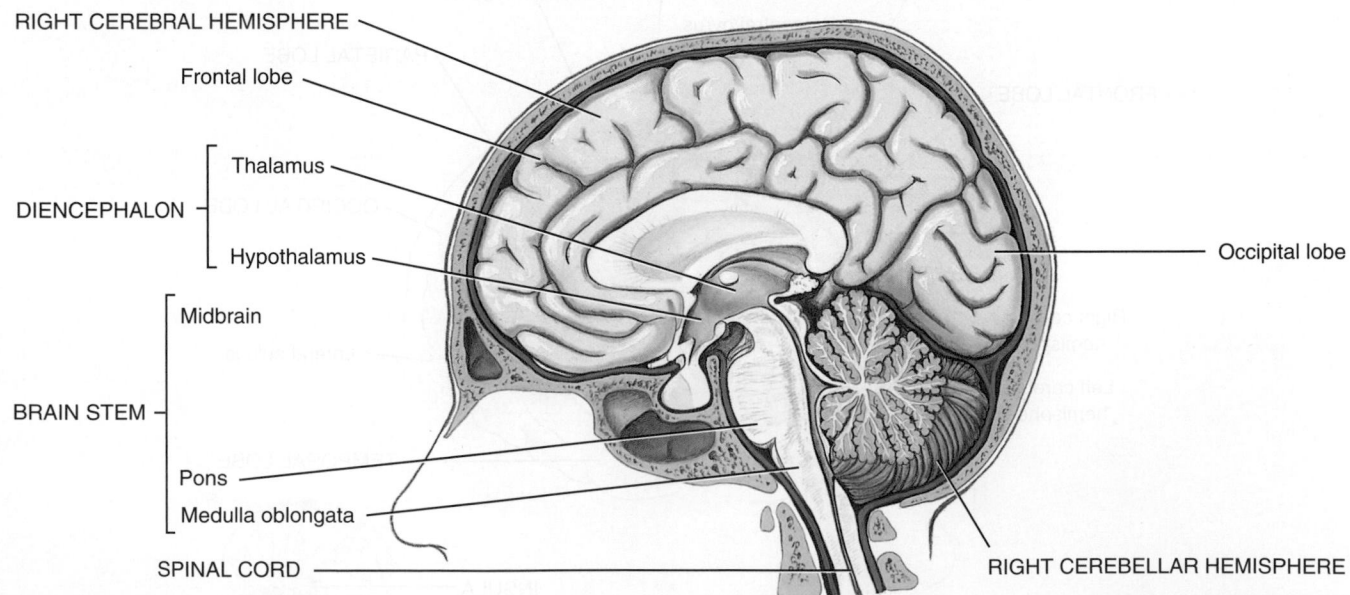

Figure 9-9 Midsagittal section of the brain showing the major portions of the diencephalon, brain stem, and cerebellum.

Table 9-4   Functional Regions of the Cerebral Cortex

Functional Region	Location	Description	Comments
Primary sensory cortex (somatosensory cortex)	Postcentral gyrus in parietal lobe	Receives sensory input from receptors in skin and skeletal muscles	Functions in sensations of temperature, touch, pressure, pain
Primary visual cortex	Posterior region of occipital lobe	Receives sensory input from retina of eye	Perceives current visual image
Auditory cortex	Superior margin of temporal lobe, along lateral sulcus	Receives auditory impulses related to pitch, rhythm, and loudness from inner ear	Allows the hearing of "sounds"
Olfactory cortex	Medial aspect of temporal lobe	Receives input from olfactory (smell) receptors in nasal cavity	Permits perception of different odors
Gustatory cortex	Parietal lobe where it is overlapped by temporal lobe	Receives input from taste buds on tongue	Permits perception of different tastes
Primary motor cortex (somatomotor cortex)	Precentral gyrus in frontal lobe	Initiates efferent action potentials that control voluntary movements	Permits skeletal muscle contraction
Premotor cortex	Anterior to primary motor cortex in frontal lobe	Controls learned motor skills that involve skeletal muscles, either simultaneously or sequentially	Examples of learned motor skills are playing piano, typing, writing
Broca area (motor speech area)	Inferior portion of frontal lobe in one hemisphere, usually the left	Programs and coordinates muscular movements necessary to articulate words	Person with injury in this area is able to understand words but is unable to speak because of inability to coordinate muscles necessary to form words
Prefrontal cortex	Anterior portion of frontal lobes	Involved with thought, reasoning, intelligence, judgment, planning, conscience	This area is well developed only in humans
Gnostic area (general interpretation area)	Region where parietal, temporal, and occipital lobes meet; found in one hemisphere (usually the left)	Integrates sensory interpretations from adjacent association areas to form thoughts; then transmits signals for appropriate responses	Stores complex memory patterns; allows person to recognize words and arrange them appropriately to express thoughts or to read and understand written ideas

From Applegate E: *The anatomy and physiology learning system,* ed 4, St Louis, 2011, Saunders.

Regions of the brain stem are illustrated in Figure 9-9.

The *midbrain* is the most superior portion of the brain stem, the region next to the diencephalon. It consists of bundles of myelinated fibers that contain the voluntary motor tracts descending from the cerebral cortex. The *pons* is the bulging middle portion of the brain stem. This region primarily consists of nerve fibers that form conduction tracts between the higher brain centers and the spinal cord. Four cranial nerves originate in the pons. It also contains the *pneumotaxic* (noo-moh-TACK-sik) and *apneustic* (ap-NOO-stick) *areas,* which help regulate breathing movements.

The *medulla oblongata* (meh-DULL-ah ahb-long-GAH-tah), or simply *medulla,* extends inferiorly from the pons. It is continuous with the spinal cord at the foramen magnum. All the ascending (sensory) and descending (motor) nerve fibers connecting the brain and spinal cord pass through the medulla. Most of the descending fibers cross over from one side to the other. In other words, fibers descending on the left side cross over to the right and vice versa. This is called *decussation* (dee-kuh-SAY-shun). Because the fibers decussate, or cross over, the brain controls motor functions on the opposite side of the body. The medulla contains three vital centers that control visceral activities. The *cardiac center* adjusts the heart rate and contraction strength to meet body needs. The *vasomotor center* regulates blood pressure by effecting changes in blood vessel diameter. The *respiratory center* acts with the centers in the pons to regulate the rate, rhythm, and depth of breathing. Other centers are involved in coughing, sneezing, swallowing, and vomiting.

Cerebellum

The **cerebellum** (sair-eh-BELL-um), the second largest portion of the brain, is located below the occipital lobes of the cerebrum. It consists of two *cerebellar hemispheres* connected in the middle by a structure called the *vermis.*

Like the cerebrum, the cerebellum consists of white matter surrounded by a thin layer of gray matter, the *cerebellar cortex.* Because the surface convolutions are less prominent in the cerebellum than in the cerebrum, the cerebellum has proportionately less gray matter.

Bundles of myelinated nerve fibers form communication pathways between the cerebellum and other parts of the CNS.

The cerebellum functions as a motor area of the brain that mediates subconscious contractions of skeletal muscles necessary for *coordination, posture,* and *balance.* The cerebellum coordinates skeletal muscles to produce smooth muscle movement rather than jerky, trembling motion. When the cerebellum is damaged, movements such as running, walking, and writing become uncoordinated. Posture is dependent on muscle tone, which is mediated by the cerebellum. Impulses from the inner ear concerning position and equilibrium are directed to the cerebellum, which uses that information to maintain balance.

Ventricles and Cerebrospinal Fluid

A series of interconnected, fluid-filled cavities is found within the brain. These cavities are the *ventricles* of the brain, and the fluid is *cerebrospinal* (seh-ree-broh-SPY-null) *fluid* (CSF). The *lateral ventricles* in the cerebrum are the largest of these cavities. One lateral ventricle exists in each cerebral hemisphere. The CSF is a clear fluid that forms as a filtrate from the blood in specialized capillary networks, the *choroid plexus* (KOR-oyd PLEKS-us), within the ventricles of the brain. It circulates through the ventricles and the central canal of the spinal cord and surrounds the brain in the subarachnoid space. From the subarachnoid space, CSF carrying waste products is returned to the blood. In addition to providing support and protection for the CNS, the CSF helps to nourish the brain and maintain constant ionic conditions for the brain and spinal cord and provides a pathway for removal of waste products.

Spinal Cord

The *spinal cord,* illustrated in Figure 9-10, extends from the foramen magnum at the base of the skull to the level of the first lumbar vertebra, a distance of about 43 to 46 cm (approximately 17 to 18 inches). The cord is continuous with the medulla oblongata at the foramen magnum. Distally, it terminates in the *conus medullaris* (KOH-nus med-yoo-LAIR-is). Like the brain, the spinal cord is surrounded by bone, meninges, and CSF. The spinal dura is separated from the vertebral bones by an *epidural space.* The meninges extend beyond the end of the spinal cord, down to the upper part of the sacrum. From there, a fibrous cord of pia mater, the *filum terminale* (FYE-lum term-ih-NAL-ee), extends down to the coccyx, where it is anchored.

The spinal cord is divided into 31 segments, with each segment giving rise to a pair of spinal nerves. At the distal end of the cord, many spinal nerves extend beyond the conus medullaris to form a collection that resembles a horse's tail. This is the *cauda equina* (KAW-dah ee-KWYNE-ah). There are two enlargements in the cord, one in the cervical region and one in the lumbar region. The *cervical enlargement* gives rise to the nerves that supply the upper extremity. Nerves from the *lumbar enlargement* supply the lower extremity.

In cross section, the spinal cord appears oval (Figure 9-11). Peripheral white matter surrounds a core of gray matter that resembles a butterfly or the letter *H.* The gray

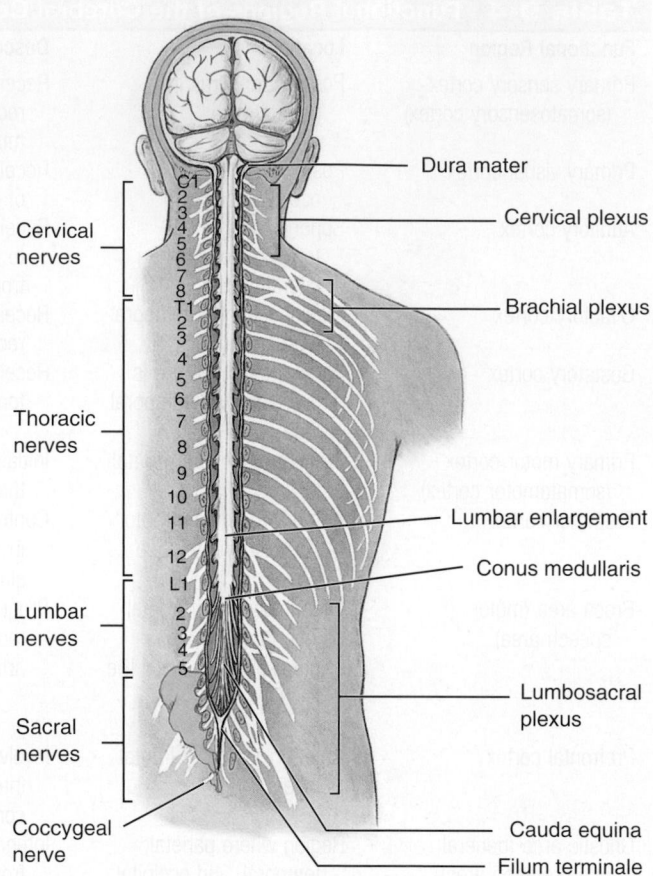

Figure 9-10 Gross anatomy of the spinal cord.

matter contains the terminal portions of sensory neuron axons, entire interneurons, and the dendrites and cell bodies of motor neurons. The central connecting bar between the two large areas of gray matter is the *gray commissure* (KOM-ih-shur). This surrounds the *central canal,* which contains CSF. The white matter that surrounds the gray matter contains longitudinal bundles of myelinated nerve fibers, called *nerve tracts.*

The spinal cord has two main functions. It is a conduction pathway for impulses going to and from the brain, and it serves as a reflex center. The conduction pathways that carry sensory impulses from body parts to the brain are called *ascending tracts.* Pathways that carry motor impulses from the brain to muscles and glands are *descending tracts.*

In addition to serving as a conduction pathway, the spinal cord functions as a center for spinal reflexes. The reflex arc, described earlier in this chapter and illustrated in Figure 9-6, is the functional unit of the nervous system. Reflexes are responses to stimuli that do not require conscious thought, and consequently they occur more quickly than reactions that require thought processes. For example, with the withdrawal reflex, the reflex action withdraws the affected part before one is aware of the pain. Many reflexes are mediated in the spinal cord without going to the higher brain centers. Table 9-5 describes some clinically significant reflexes.

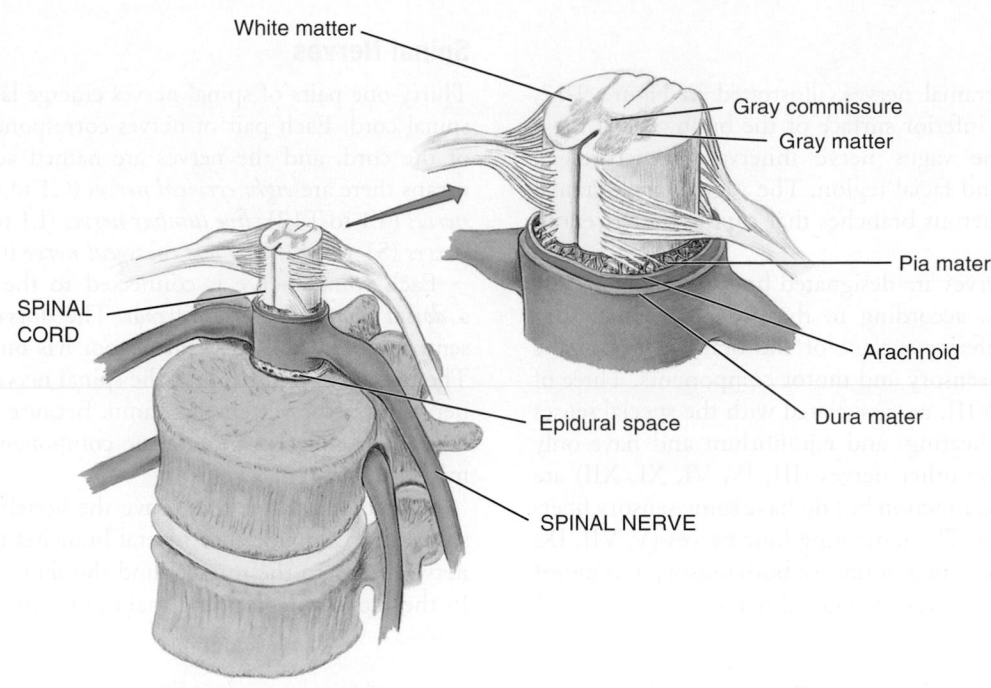

Figure 9-11 Cross section of the spinal cord.

Table 9-5	Some Clinically Significant Reflexes	
Reflex	**Description**	**Indications**
Patellar (knee-jerk reflex)	Stretch reflex; two-neuron path; reflex hammer strikes patellar tendon just below knee; receptors in quadriceps femoris muscle are stretched; reflex results in immediate "kick"	Reflex is blocked by damage to nerves involved and by damage to lumbar segments of spinal cord; also absent in people with chronic diabetes mellitus and neurosyphilis
Achilles tendon (ankle-jerk reflex)	Stretch reflex; two-neuron path; reflex hammer strikes Achilles tendon just above heel; gastrocnemius and soleus muscles contract to plantarflex foot	Weak or no reflex action indicates damage to nerves involved or to L5-S2 segments of spinal cord; also absent in chronic diabetes, neurosyphilis, and alcoholism
Abdominal	Stroking lateral abdominal wall produces reflex action that compresses abdominal wall and moves umbilicus toward stimulus	Absent in lesions of peripheral nerves, in lesions in thoracic segments of spinal cord, and in multiple sclerosis
Babinski	Lateral sole of foot is stroked from heel to toe; positive sign results in dorsiflexion of big toe and spreading of other toes; negative sign results in toes curling under with a light inversion of foot	Positive Babinski sign is normal in children younger than 18 months of age; negative sign is normal after 18 months of age; if motor tracts in spinal cord are damaged, positive Babinski sign reappears

From Applegate E: *The anatomy and physiology learning system,* ed 4, St Louis, 2011, Saunders.

PERIPHERAL NERVOUS SYSTEM

The PNS consists of the nerves that branch out from the brain and spinal cord. These nerves form the communication network between the CNS and the remainder of the body. The PNS is further subdivided into the *somatic nervous system* and the *autonomic nervous system.* The somatic nervous system consists of nerves that go to the skin and muscles and is involved in conscious activities. The ANS consists of nerves that connect the CNS to the visceral organs such as the heart, stomach, and intestines. It mediates unconscious activities.

Structure of a Nerve

A nerve contains bundles of nerve fibers, either axons or dendrites, surrounded by connective tissue. *Sensory nerves* contain only afferent fibers—long dendrites of sensory neurons. *Motor nerves* have only efferent fibers—long axons of motor neurons. *Mixed nerves* contain both types of fibers.

Cranial Nerves

Twelve pairs of cranial nerves, illustrated in Figure 9-12, emerge from the inferior surface of the brain. All of these nerves except the vagus nerve innervate structures in the head, neck, and facial region. The vagus nerve, cranial nerve X, has numerous branches that supply the viscera in the body.

The cranial nerves are designated both by name and by Roman numerals, according to the order in which they appear on the inferior surface of the brain. Most of the nerves have both sensory and motor components. Three of the nerves (I, II, VIII) are associated with the special senses of smell, vision, hearing, and equilibrium and have only sensory fibers. Five other nerves (III, IV, VI, XI, XII) are primarily motor in function but do have some sensory fibers for proprioception. The remaining four nerves (V, VII, IX, X) consist of significant amounts of both sensory and motor fibers. Table 9-6 itemizes the cranial nerves.

Spinal Nerves

Thirty-one pairs of spinal nerves emerge laterally from the spinal cord. Each pair of nerves corresponds to a segment of the cord, and the nerves are named accordingly. This means there are *eight cervical nerves* (C1 to C8), *12 thoracic nerves* (T1 to T12), *five lumbar nerves* (L1 to L5), *five sacral nerves* (S1 to S5), and *one coccygeal nerve* (Co).

Each spinal nerve is connected to the spinal cord by a *dorsal root* and a *ventral root*. The dorsal root has only sensory fibers, and the ventral root has only motor fibers. The two roots join to form the spinal nerve just before the nerve leaves the vertebral column. Because all spinal nerves have both sensory and motor components, they are all mixed nerves.

Immediately after they leave the vertebral column, the spinal nerves divide into several branches that provide the nerve supply to the muscles and the skin of the body wall. In the thoracic region, the main portions of the nerves go

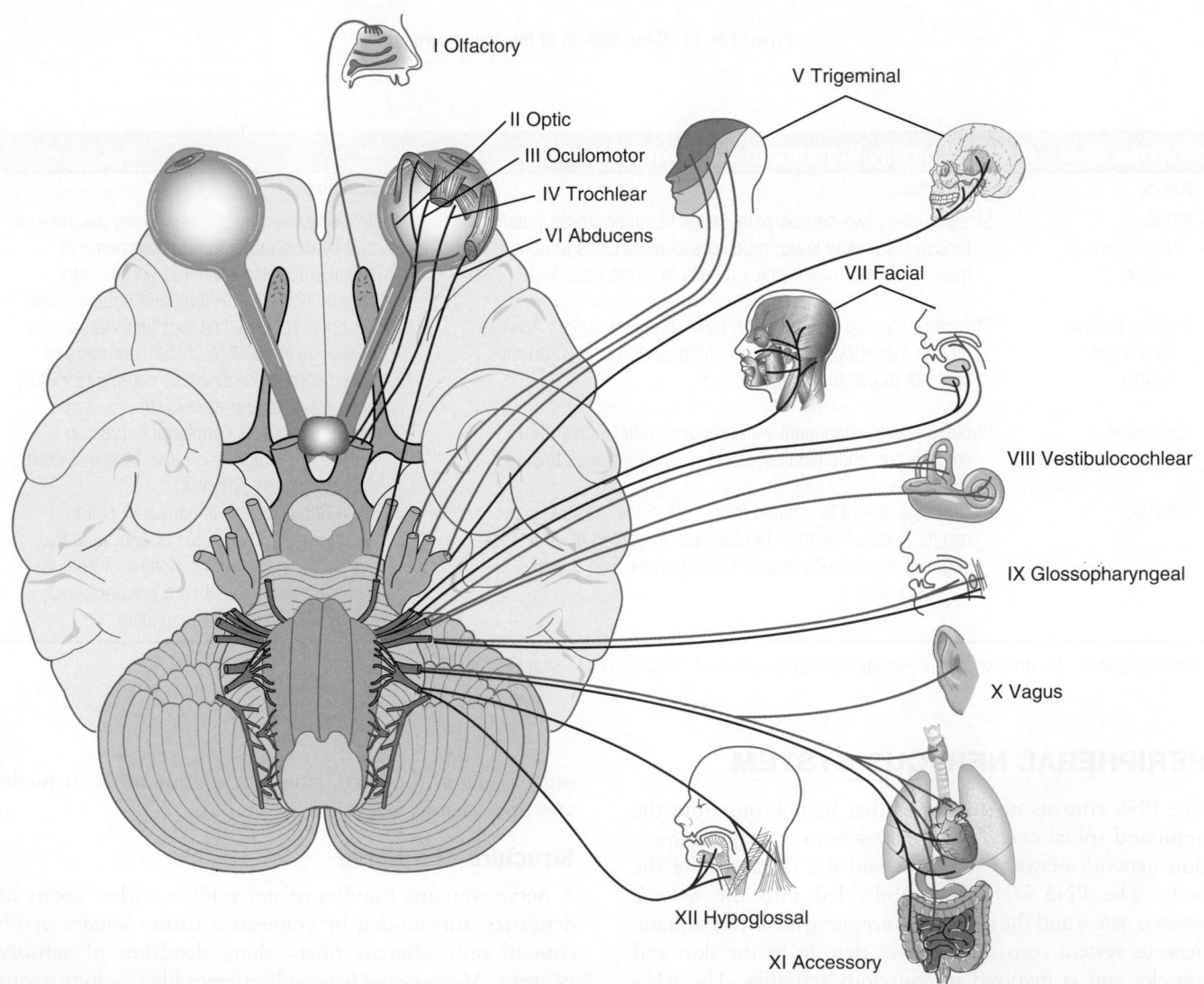

I Olfactory

II Optic

III Oculomotor

IV Trochlear

VI Abducens

V Trigeminal

VII Facial

VIII Vestibulocochlear

IX Glossopharyngeal

X Vagus

XII Hypoglossal

XI Accessory

Figure 9-12 Cranial nerves. The red lines indicate motor function, and the blue lines indicate sensory function.

Table 9-6   Summary of Cranial Nerves

Number	Name	Type	Function
I	Olfactory	Sensory	Sense of smell
II	Optic	Sensory	Vision
III	Oculomotor	Primarily motor	Movement of eyes and eyelids
IV	Trochlear	Primarily motor	Movement of eyes
V	Trigeminal	Mixed	
	Ophthalmic branch		Sensory fibers from cornea, skin of nose, forehead, and scalp
	Maxillary branch		Sensory fibers from cheek, nose, upper lip, and teeth
	Mandibular branch		Sensory fibers from skin over mandible, lower lip, and teeth
			Motor fibers to muscles of mastication
VI	Abducens	Primarily motor	Eye movement
VII	Facial	Mixed	Sensory fibers from taste receptors on anterior two thirds of tongue
			Motor fibers to muscles of facial expression, lacrimal glands, and salivary glands
VIII	Vestibulocochlear	Sensory	Hearing and equilibrium
IX	Glossopharyngeal	Mixed	Sensory fibers from taste receptors on posterior one third of tongue
			Motor fibers to muscles used in swallowing and to salivary glands
X	Vagus	Mixed	Sensory fibers from pharynx, larynx, esophagus, and visceral organs
			Somatic motor fibers to muscles of pharynx and larynx
			Autonomic motor fibers to heart, smooth muscles, and glands to alter gastric motility, heart rate, respiration, and blood pressure
XI	Accessory	Primarily motor	Contraction of trapezius and sternocleidomastoid muscles
XII	Hypoglossal	Primarily motor	Contraction of muscles of tongue

From Applegate E: *The anatomy and physiology learning system,* ed 4, St Louis, 2011, Saunders.

directly to the thoracic wall, where they are called *intercostal nerves.* In other regions, the main portions of the nerves form complex networks called *plexuses* (see Figure 9-10). In the plexus the fibers are sorted and recombined so that the fibers associated with a particular body part are together even though they may originate from different regions of the cord. The *cervical plexus* is located in the neck and sends nerves to the skin and muscles of the neck, shoulder, and diaphragm. The *brachial plexus* is deep to the clavicle and innervates the skin and muscles of the upper extremities. The *lumbosacral plexus* is in the lumbar region of the back. Nerves from this plexus go to the skin and muscles of the lower abdominal wall, the lower extremities, the buttocks, and the external genitalia.

Autonomic Nervous System

General Features

The ANS is a visceral efferent system, which means it sends motor impulses to the visceral organs. It functions automatically and continuously, without conscious effort, to innervate smooth muscle, cardiac muscle, and glands. It is concerned with heart rate, breathing rate, blood pressure, body temperature, and other visceral activities that work together to maintain homeostasis.

The ANS has two parts: the *sympathetic division* and the *parasympathetic division* (Table 9-7). Many visceral organs are supplied with fibers from both divisions *(dual innervation).* In this case, one stimulates and the other inhibits. This antagonistic functional relationship serves as a balance to help maintain homeostasis.

Sympathetic Division

The sympathetic division, illustrated in Figure 9-13, is concerned primarily with preparing the body for stressful or emergency situations. Sometimes called the *fight-or-flight system,* it is an energy-expending system. It stimulates the responses that are necessary to meet the emergency and inhibits the visceral activities that can be delayed momentarily. For example, during an emergency, the sympathetic system increases breathing rate, heart rate, and blood flow to skeletal muscles. At the same time, it decreases activity in the digestive tract because that is not necessary to meet the emergency.

The sympathetic preganglionic fibers arise from the thoracic and lumbar regions of the spinal cord; thus the sympathetic division is sometimes called the *thoracolumbar* (thoar-ah-koh-LUM-bar) *division.*

Parasympathetic Division

The parasympathetic division is most active under ordinary, relaxed conditions (see Figure 9-13). It also brings the body's systems back to a normal state after an emergency by slowing the heart rate and breathing rate, decreasing blood pressure, decreasing blood flow to skeletal muscles, and increasing digestive tract activity. Sometimes called the *rest-and-repose system,* it is an energy-conserving system.

The parasympathetic preganglionic fibers arise from the brain stem and sacral region of the spinal cord; thus the parasympathetic division is sometimes called the *craniosacral* (kray-nee-oh-SAY-kral) *division.*

Table 9-7 Comparison of Sympathetic and Parasympathetic Actions on Selected Visceral Effectors

Visceral Effectors	Sympathetic Action	Parasympathetic Action
Pupil of eye	Dilates	Constricts
Lens of eye	Lens flattens for distance vision	Lens bulges for near vision
Sweat glands	Stimulates	No innervation
Arrector pili muscles of hair	Stimulates contraction; goose bumps	No innervation
Heart	Increases heart rate	Decreases heart rate
Bronchi	Dilates	Constricts
Digestive glands	Decreases secretion of digestive enzymes	Increases secretion of digestive enzymes
Digestive tract	Decreases peristalsis	Increases peristalsis
Digestive tract sphincters	Stimulates—closes sphincters	Inhibits—opens sphincters
Blood vessels to digestive organs	Constricts	No innervation
Blood vessels to skeletal muscles	Dilates	No innervation
Blood vessels to skin	Constricts	No innervation
Adrenal medulla	Stimulates secretion of epinephrine	No innervation
Liver	Increases release of glucose	No innervation
Urinary bladder	Relaxes bladder and closes sphincter	Contracts bladder and opens sphincter

From Applegate E: *The anatomy and physiology learning system,* ed 4, St Louis, 2011, Saunders.

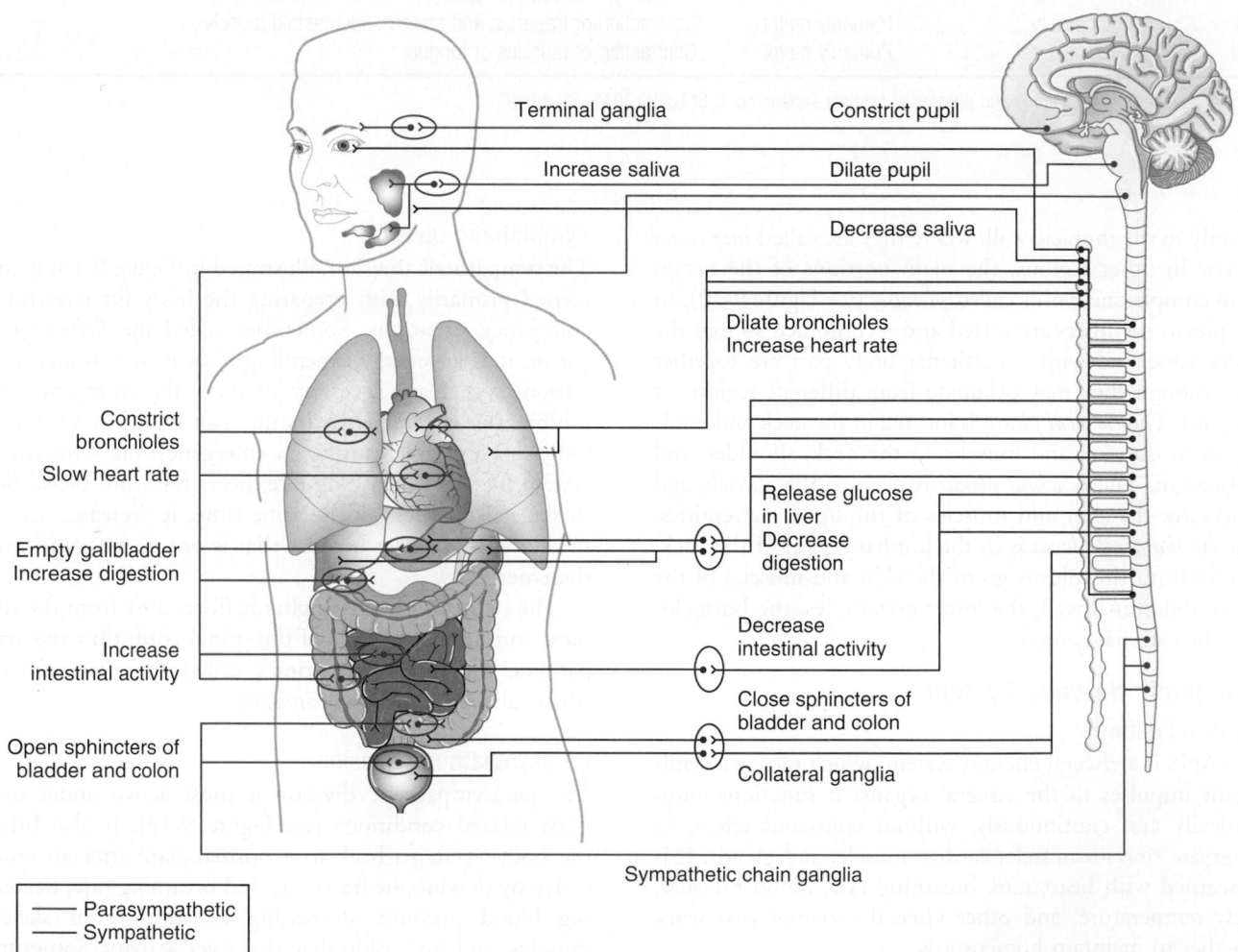

Figure 9-13 Structure and function of autonomic nervous system. The red lines indicate the sympathetic division, and the blue lines indicate parasympathetic innervations. Note the location of the ganglia for each division.

AGING OF THE NERVOUS SYSTEM

Aging of the nervous system is of major importance because changes in this system affect organs in other systems and can cause disturbances of many bodily functions. For example, changes in nerves decrease stimulation of skeletal muscle, which contributes to muscle atrophy with age. Because of its widespread consequences, aging of the nervous system is one of the most distressing aspects of growing old.

Like other cells, nerve cells are lost as a person ages, even in the absence of disease processes. Because neurons are amitotic, those that are lost are not replaced. Loss of neurons is largely responsible for the decrease in brain mass that occurs with aging. Fortunately, the brain has a large reserve supply of neurons, many more than are necessary to carry out its functions, so the decrease in neuron number alone is not devastating. The loss of neurons is not constant in all areas of the brain. For example, about 25% of the specialized cells in the cerebellum, which are responsible for coordinated movements, are lost during aging. This may affect balance and cause difficulty in coordinating fine movements. In other areas of the brain, the number of neurons remains essentially constant throughout life.

It is generally accepted that there is a decline in intelligence with aging, and this is thought to be associated with the loss of neurons. However, it is important to remember that there are wide variations in individuals regarding changes in intellect with age. Because a person is old does not mean that person is "dumb." Many elderly people retain a keen intellect until death. Along with the decline in intelligence, there is a general decline in memory. Again, this varies from person to person. In general, short-term memory seems to be affected more than long-term memory. Intellect and memory appear to be retained better in people who remain mentally and physically active.

Another change observed in older people is a decrease in the rate of impulse conduction along an axon and across a synapse. A reduction in the amount of myelin around the axon probably accounts for the diminished conduction rate along the axon. Decreases in the quantity of neurotransmitter and in the number of receptor sites cause slower conduction across the synapses. These factors contribute to the slower reflexes and the longer time required to process information that are observed in many elderly people.

TERMINOLOGY REVIEW

Medical Term	Word Parts	Definition
Action potential	*act-:* motion	A nerve impulse; a rapid change in membrane potential that involves depolarization and repolarization.
Brain stem		The portion of the brain, between the diencephalon and spinal cord, that contains the midbrain, pons, and medulla oblongata.
Cerebellum	*cerebell/o:* cerebellum	Second largest part of the human brain, located posterior to the pons and medulla oblongata and involved in the coordination of muscular movements.
Cerebrum	*cerebr/o:* cerebrum	The largest and uppermost part of the human brain; concerned with consciousness, learning, memory, sensations, and voluntary movements.
Diencephalon	*cephal/o:* head	Part of the brain between the cerebral hemispheres and the midbrain; includes the thalamus, and hypothalamus.
Myelin		White, fatty substance that surrounds many nerve fibers.
Neurilemma	*neur/o:* nerve *-lemma:* sheath, covering	The layer of cells that surrounds a nerve fiber in the peripheral nervous system and in some cases produces myelin; also called *Schwann sheath.*
Saltatory conduction	*-tion:* process of	Process in which a nerve impulse travels along a myelinated nerve fiber by jumping from one node of Ranvier to the next.
Synapse	*syn-:* together, with	The region of communication between two neurons.
Threshold stimulus		Minimum level of stimulation that is required to start a nerve impulse or muscle contraction; also called *liminal stimulus.*

Check out the Evolve site at http://evolve.elsevier.com/Bonewit/today/ to actively Prepare for your Certification, and to access additional interactive activities and exercises to help you study and prepare for success.

10

The Senses

1. Explain the difference between general senses and special senses, and state examples of each.
2. List and describe the five groups of sense receptors.
3. Identify the sense receptors for touch, pressure, proprioception, temperature, and pain.
4. List and identify the location of the four different taste sensations.
5. Locate the sense receptors for smell, and trace the impulse pathway to the cerebral cortex.
6. Describe the structure of the eye, and explain the function of each structure.
7. Explain how light is focused on the retina.
8. Explain the function of the following photoreceptor cells in the retina: rods and cones.
9. Explain how nerve impulses for sight are initiated in response to light.
10. Describe the structure of the ear, and explain the function of each structure.
11. Explain how nerve impulses for hearing are initiated in response to sound waves.
12. Explain the difference between static equilibrium and dynamic equilibrium.
13. Explain how impulses for static equilibrium and dynamic equilibrium are initiated.
14. Describe ways in which the aging of an individual affects the senses.
15. Identify pathology related to the senses.

CHAPTER OUTLINE

KEY TERMS

accommodation (ah-kahm-oh-DAY-shun)
chemoreceptor (kee-moh-ree-SEP-tor)
mechanoreceptor
   (mek-ah-noh-ree-SEP-tor)

nociceptor (noh-see-SEP-tor)
photoreceptor (foh-toh-ree-SEP-tor)
proprioception (proh-pree-oh-SEP-shun)

sensory adaptation (SEN-soh-ree
   add-dap-TAY-shun)
thermoreceptor (ther-moh-ree-SEP-tor)

INTRODUCTION TO THE SENSES

Sensory perception depends on receptors that respond to various stimuli. When a stimulus triggers an impulse in a receptor, the action potentials travel to the cerebral cortex, where they are processed and interpreted. Only after this occurs is a particular sensation perceived. Some senses, such as pain, touch, pressure, and proprioception, are widely distributed in the body. These are called **general senses.** Other senses, such as taste, smell, hearing, and sight, are called **special senses** because their receptors are localized in a particular area.

RECEPTORS AND SENSATIONS

Although there are many different kinds of sense receptors, they can be grouped into five types. The basis for these receptor types is the kind of stimulus to which they are sensitive or have a low threshold. The five types of receptors are chemoreceptors, mechanoreceptors, nociceptors, thermoreceptors, and photoreceptors (Table 10-1).

Perceived sensation occurs only after impulses have been interpreted by the brain. Steps involved in sensory perception include the following:

1. There must be a **stimulus.**
2. A **receptor** must detect the stimulus and create an action potential.
3. The action potential (impulse) must be **conducted** to the central nervous system (CNS).
4. Within the CNS, the impulse must be **translated** into information.
5. Information must be **interpreted** in the CNS into an awareness or perception of the stimulus.

The impulses from all the receptors are alike. The difference in perception is where they are interpreted in the brain. For example, all impulses going to one particular region are interpreted as sound, whereas those going to another region are interpreted as taste. As the brain interprets a sensation,

it projects that sense back to its original source so that the "feeling" seems to come from the receptors that are stimulated. This projection allows us to locate the source of the stimulus.

Some sense receptors, when they are continually stimulated, undergo **sensory adaptation.** They have a decreased sensitivity to a continued stimulus and trigger impulses only if the strength of the stimulus is increased.

GENERAL SENSES

General senses, or **somatic senses,** are those that are found throughout the body. They are associated with the visceral organs, as well as the skin, muscles, and joints, and include the following:

* Touch
* Pressure
* Proprioception
* Temperature
* Pain

Touch and Pressure

As a group, the receptors for touch and pressure are **mechanoreceptors** that are sensitive to forces that deform or displace tissues. They are widely distributed in the skin. Three of the mechanoreceptors involved in touch and pressure are free nerve endings, Meissner corpuscles, and pacinian corpuscles.

Free nerve endings are the dendritic ends of sensory neurons that are interspersed between the cells in epithelial tissue. They do not have a connective tissue covering. They are important in sensing objects, such as clothing, that are in continuous contact with the skin. **Meissner corpuscles** (MYZE-ner KOAR-pus-als) consist of the ends of sensory nerve fibers surrounded by connective tissue and are specific in localizing tactile sensations. They are located in the dermal papillae, just beneath the epidermis, where they are important in sensing light-discriminative touch stimuli. **Pacinian corpuscles** (pah-SIN-ee-an KOAR-pus-als) are called *lamellated corpuscles* because several layers of connective tissue surround the nerve endings. These are common in deeper dermis and subcutaneous tissues, tendons, and ligaments. They are stimulated by heavy pressure.

Proprioception

Proprioception (proh-pree-oh-SEP-shun) is the sense of position or orientation. It allows us to sense the location and rate of movement of one body part relative to another. **Golgi tendon organs,** found at the junction of a tendon with a muscle, and **muscle spindles,** located in skeletal muscles, are important mechanoreceptors for proprioception.

Temperature

Thermoreceptors are located immediately under the skin and are widely distributed throughout the body. They are most numerous on the lips and are least numerous on some

Table 10-1	Types of Sense Receptors	
Receptor	**Stimulus**	**Example**
Chemoreceptors	Changes in chemical concentration of substances	Taste and smell
Mechanoreceptors	Changes in pressure or movement in fluids	Proprioceptors in joints, receptors for hearing and equilibrium
Nociceptors	Tissue damage	Pain receptors
Thermoreceptors	Changes in temperature	Heat and cold
Photoreceptors	Light energy	Vision

From Applegate E: *The anatomy and physiology learning system,* ed 4, St Louis, 2011, Saunders.

of the broad surfaces of the trunk. Thermoreceptors include at least two types of free nerve endings that are sensitive to temperature changes. In general, there are up to 10 times more **cold receptors** in a given area than **heat receptors.** Extremes in temperature stimulate pain receptors. A person determines gradations in temperatures by the degree of stimulation of each type of receptor. Extreme cold and extreme heat feel almost the same—both are painful—because the pain receptors are being stimulated. Thermoreceptors are strongly stimulated by abrupt changes in temperature and then fade after a few seconds or minutes. In other words, thermoreceptors show rapid **sensory adaptation.**

Pain

The sense of pain is initiated by **nociceptors** (noh-see-SEP-tors), which are free nerve endings that are stimulated by tissue damage. They are widely distributed throughout the skin and in the tissues of the internal organs. The nervous tissue of the brain has no pain receptors; however, other tissues in the head, including the meninges and blood vessels, have an abundant supply. Pain receptors have a protective function because pain is usually perceived as unpleasant and is a signal to locate and remove the source of the tissue damage. Nociceptors usually do not adapt and may continue to send signals after the stimulus is removed.

GUSTATORY SENSE

The **gustatory sense,** or **taste,** is one of the special senses. As previously explained, the senses of taste, smell, hearing, and sight are called *special senses* because their receptors are localized in a particular area.

The organs of taste, the **taste buds,** are localized in the mouth region, primarily on the surface of the tongue, where they lie along the walls of projections called **papillae** (Figure 10-1).

Highlight on the Senses

Odors: Nearly everyone is familiar with sensory adaptation in the sense of smell. A particular odor becomes unnoticed after a short time, even though the odor molecules are still present in the air, because the system quickly adapts to the continued stimulation. Odors have the quality of being interpreted as pleasant or unpleasant. Because of this, the sense of smell is as important as taste in the selection of food. For example, a person who has became sick after eating a certain type of food is often nauseated by the smell of that same food at a later occasion.

Cold adaptation: When a person first enters a cool swimming pool on a hot day, there is an abrupt change in temperature; therefore the cold receptors are strongly stimulated and there is a feeling of discomfort. After a brief time, the receptors adapt, the stimulation fades, and the cool water feels comfortable.

Headache: If there are no pain receptors in the nervous tissue of the brain, what are headaches? Headaches are a type of referred pain, pain that is referred to the surface of the head from deeper structures. The pain stimuli may originate in the meninges or blood vessels within the cranium. Other pain stimuli may originate outside the cranium from muscular spasms, the nasal sinuses, or the eyes.

Bitter taste: The taste receptors with the highest degree of sensitivity are those that are stimulated by bitter substances, and a highly intense bitter taste usually causes a person to reject that substance. This is probably an important protective mechanism because many of the deadly toxins found in poisonous plants have an intensely bitter taste.

Blinking: The eye blinks six to 30 times a minute. Blinking stimulates the lacrimal glands to secrete a sterile fluid, or "tears," and helps move the fluid across the eyes.

Corneal transplant: The cornea was one of the first organs transplanted. Surgical removal of deteriorating corneas and replacement with donor corneas is a common medical procedure for several reasons. The cornea is readily accessible and relatively easy to remove. The tissue is avascular, so there is no bleeding problem or difficulty in establishing circulatory pathways. Corneas are less active than other tissues immunologically and are less likely to be rejected. Long-term success after corneal implant surgery is excellent.

Pupil size: In addition to regulating the amount of light that enters the eye, pupillary reflexes may also reflect interest or emotional state. For example, frequently the pupils dilate during problem solving or when the subject is appealing. If the subject is boring or repulsive, the pupils constrict.

Detached retina: Sometimes the sensory portion of the retina breaks away from the pigmented layer, resulting in a **detached retina.** This may be caused by trauma, such as a blow to the head, or by certain eye disorders. If allowed to progress, the result is distorted vision and eventually blindness. In many cases the retina can be reattached by laser surgery.

Color blindness: Color blindness occurs because there is an absence or deficiency of one or more of the visual pigments in the cones, and the person cannot distinguish certain colors. In the most common form, red-green color blindness, the cones lack the red pigment and the person is unable to distinguish red from green. Most color blindness is inherited and occurs more frequently in males.

Ruptured eardrum: The eardrum is sometimes ruptured, or perforated, by shock waves from an explosion, scuba diving, trauma, or acute middle ear infections. A perforated eardrum is characterized first by acute pain, then by noise in the affected ear, and then by hearing impairment.

Motion sickness: Motion sickness is nausea and vomiting resulting from repetitive and excessive stimulation of the equilibrium receptors. Some people are more susceptible than others. ∎

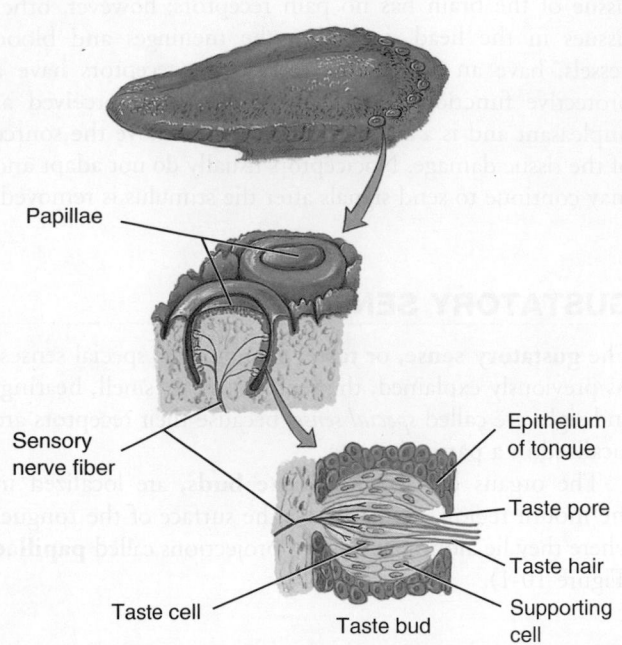

Papillae

Sensory
nerve fiber

Epithelium
of tongue

Taste pore

Taste hair

Supporting
cell

Taste cell

Taste bud

Figure 10-1 Taste buds on the papillae of the tongue. The taste hairs on taste (gustatory) cells are the receptors for taste.

The receptors belong to the **chemoreceptor** (kee-moh-ree-SEP-tor) category because they are sensitive to chemicals in the food we eat. In order for these chemicals to be detected by a chemoreceptor, they must be dissolved in water.

Within the taste bud, specialized epithelial cells called **taste cells** or **gustatory cells** are interspersed with supporting cells and nerve fibers (see Figure 10-1). The entire taste bud opens to the surface through a **taste pore.** Tiny **taste hairs** (microvilli) project from the taste cells through the taste pore, and it is these hairs on the taste cells that function as the receptors.

Although all the taste receptors appear to be alike, there are at least four different types, each one sensitive to a particular kind of stimulus. Consequently, there are four different taste sensations:

- Salty
- Sweet
- Sour
- Bitter

When the microvilli, or taste hairs, are stimulated, an impulse is triggered on a nearby nerve fiber. Impulses from the anterior two thirds of the tongue travel along the **facial nerve,** and those from the posterior one third travel along the **glossopharyngeal** (glos-so-fah-RIN-jee-al) **nerve.** The impulses are interpreted in the sensory cortex on the parietal lobe of the cerebrum, near the lateral sulcus.

OLFACTORY SENSE

The receptors for **olfaction** (sense of smell) are neurons in the **olfactory epithelium** of the nasal cavity. The **olfactory** neurons are concentrated in the superior region of the cavity. These neurons have long cilia that extend to the surface and project into the nasal cavity. The cilia are believed to be the sensitive receptors of the neuron.

Like those for taste, the olfactory receptors are **chemoreceptors.** They are stimulated by chemicals dissolved in liquids. In this case, airborne molecules responsible for odors dissolve in the fluid on the surface of the olfactory epithelium and then bind to the receptors and trigger impulses. Axons from the olfactory neurons pass through foramina in the ethmoid bone and enter the **olfactory bulb** of the olfactory nerve (cranial nerve I). Here they synapse with association neurons that conduct the impulses to the **olfactory cortex** in the temporal lobe, where they are interpreted.

The senses of taste and smell are closely related and complement each other. They often have a combined effect when they are interpreted in the cerebral cortex. This implies that part of what we "taste" is really smell. Also, part of what we "smell" is taste because some airborne molecules move from the nose down to the mouth and stimulate taste buds.

VISUAL SENSE

Most of us consider vision to be one of the most important senses we have. The eyes, which contain the photoreceptors, are the organs of vision. They are protected by a bony socket and are assisted in their function of vision by accessory structures that protect and move them.

Protective Features and Accessory Structures of the Eye

Only a small portion of the eye is visible from the exterior. Most of it is surrounded by a protective bony **orbit,** or socket, that is formed by portions of seven cranial bones: frontal, lacrimal, ethmoid, maxilla, zygomatic, sphenoid, and palatine. It also contains fat, various connective tissues, blood vessels, and nerves.

Eyebrows help to keep perspiration, which can be an irritant, out of the eyes. **Eyelids** function to open and close the eye and to keep foreign objects from entering the eye. The muscles associated with the eyelids are the **orbicularis oculi,** which is a sphincter that closes the eye, and the **levator palpebrae superioris,** which elevates the eyelid to open the eye. The conjunctiva, a thin mucous membrane, lines the eyelid and then folds back to cover the anterior portion of the eyeball, except for the central portion, which is the cornea. Mucus from the conjunctiva helps keep the eye from drying out. **Eyelashes** line the margin of the eyelid and help trap foreign particles. **Sebaceous glands** associated with the eyelashes secrete an oily fluid that helps lubricate the region. Inflammation of the sebaceous glands is called a **stye.**

The **lacrimal** (LACK-rih-mal) **apparatus,** shown in Figure 10-2, consists of the lacrimal gland and various ducts. The **lacrimal gland** is located in the superior and lateral region of the orbit. Tears produced by the lacrimal gland flow through **lacrimal ducts** and across the surface of the eye to the medial side, where they drain into two small **lacrimal canals** (canaliculi). From the lacrimal canals, the tears flow into the **lacrimal sac,** and then into the **nasolacrimal duct,** which opens into the nasal cavity. Tears moisten, lubricate, and cleanse the anterior surface of the eye. Tears also contain an enzyme (lysozyme) that helps destroy bacteria and prevent infections.

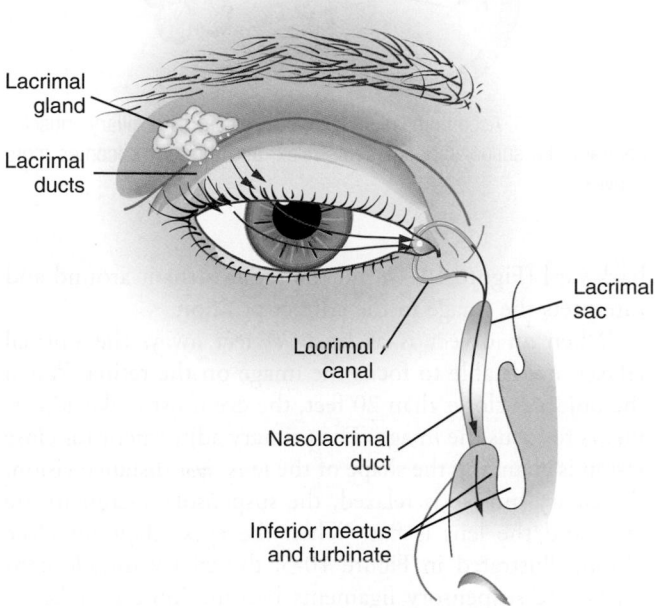

Figure 10-2 Lacrimal apparatus of the eye.

Structure of the Eyeball

The eyeball, or **bulbus oculi** (BUL-bus AHK-yoo-lye), is somewhat spheric, is 2 to 3 cm in diameter, and has an anterior bulge. It is surrounded by orbital fat within the orbital cavity. Figure 10-3 illustrates the structure of the bulbus oculi.

The wall of the eyeball is made up of three concentric layers or coats called tunics. The outermost layer is the **fibrous tunic.** It consists of the white, opaque **sclera** (SKLEE-rah) and the transparent **cornea.** The sclera, the white part of the eye, covers the posterior five sixths of the eyeball, and the muscles that move the eye are attached to it. The transparent cornea, which covers the anterior one sixth of the eyeball, is the "window" of the eye. It helps focus light rays entering the eye.

The middle layer of the eyeball is the **vascular tunic.** It consists of the **choroid** (KOAR-oyd), **ciliary body,** and **iris.** The **choroid** is a highly vascular, brown-pigmented layer located between the sclera and the retina in the posterior portion of the eye. It is the largest part of the middle tunic and lines most of the sclera, although it is only loosely connected to the fibrous coat and can be stripped away easily. The choroid is, however, firmly attached to the retina. The brown pigment in the choroid absorbs excess light rays that might interfere with vision. The blood vessels nourish the interior of the eye. Anteriorly, the choroid is continuous with the **ciliary body.** Numerous finger-like **ciliary processes** within the ciliary body secrete aqueous humor, a fluid in the anterior portion of the eye. The ciliary body also contains the **ciliary muscle. Suspensory ligaments** connect the ciliary body to the transparent, biconvex **lens** of the eye. When the ciliary muscle contracts, the suspensory ligaments relax and the lens bulges to allow focusing for close vision. The **iris** is the conspicuous, colored portion of the

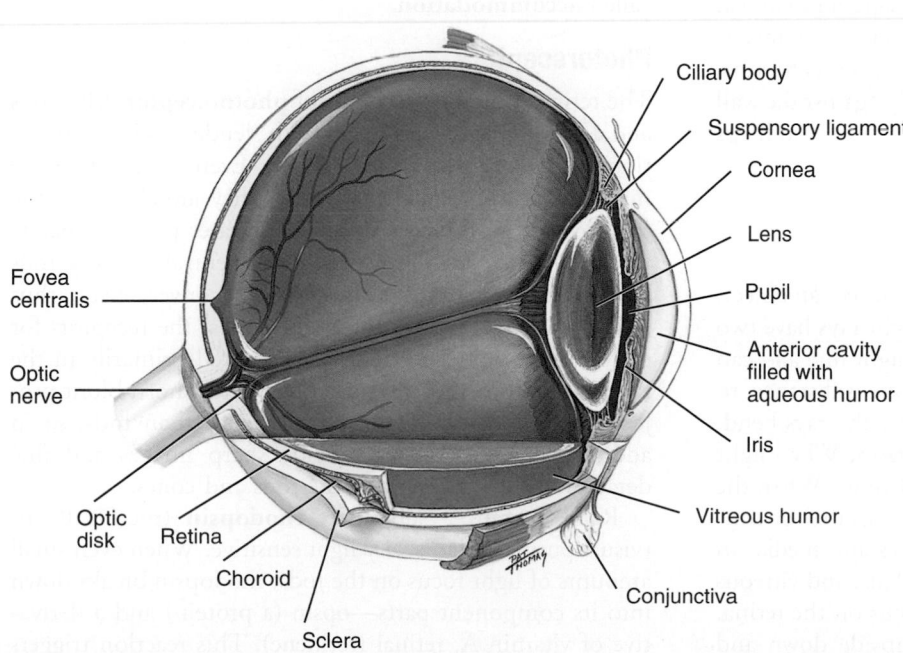

Figure 10-3 Anatomy of bulbus oculi or eyeball.

eye. It is a doughnut-shaped diaphragm with a central aperture, called the **pupil.** The iris contains two groups of smooth muscles, a radial group and a circular group. When the radial muscles contract, the pupil dilates; when the circular group contracts, the pupil gets smaller. These muscles of the iris continually contract and relax to change the size of the pupil, which regulates the amount of light entering the eye.

The innermost coat of the eyeball is the **nervous tunic,** or **retina** (RET-ih-nah), which is found only in the posterior portion of the eye. It ends at the posterior margin of the ciliary body. The retina contains several layers. The outer layer is deeply pigmented and firmly attached to the choroid. The layer next to the pigmented layer contains the **rods and cones,** which are the receptor (photoreceptor) cells. Other layers consist of bipolar neurons and ganglion cells. The axons of the ganglion cells converge to form the **optic nerve,** which penetrates the tunics at the **optic disk** and passes through the apex of the orbital cavity to reach the brain. Because there are no photoreceptor cells in the optic disk, it is commonly referred to as the "blind spot" of the eye. Just lateral to the optic disk, near the center of the retina, there is a yellow spot called the **macula lutea** (MACK-yoo-lah LOO-tee-ah). The region of the retina that produces the sharpest image is a depression, the **fovea centralis** (FOE-vee-ah sen-TRAL-is), in the center of the macula lutea.

The lens, suspensory ligaments, and ciliary body form a partition that divides the interior of the eyeball into two cavities. The space anterior to the lens, between the cornea and the lens, is the anterior cavity and is filled with **aqueous humor** secreted by the ciliary body. Aqueous humor helps maintain the shape of the anterior part of the eye and nourishes the structures in that region. It is largely responsible for the internal pressure of the eye. The aqueous humor circulates through the anterior cavity and then is reabsorbed into blood vessels at the junction of the sclera and cornea. The posterior cavity, between the lens and the retina, is filled with a colorless, transparent, gel-like **vitreous humor.** The vitreous humor presses the retina firmly against the wall of the eye, supports the internal parts of the eye, and helps maintain the eye's shape.

Pathway of Light and Refraction

Vision depends on light rays. When a person sees an object, light rays from the object enter the eye. Light rays have two important properties—they travel in a straight line and can be bent. When light rays travel from one substance to another that has a different optical density, the rays bend. The bending of light rays is called **refraction.** When light rays hit a concave surface, they scatter or diverge. When the rays meet a convex surface, they get closer together or converge. The eyes have four refractive surfaces and media. In a normal eye, the cornea, aqueous humor, lens, and vitreous humor bend the light rays so that they focus on the retina. The image that forms on the retina is upside down and

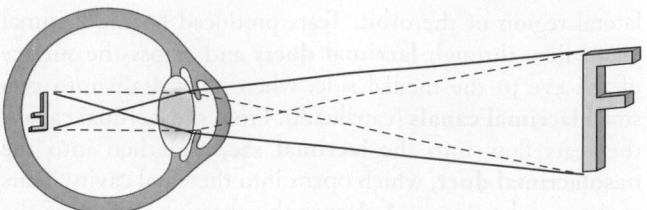

Figure 10-4 Formation of images on the retina. The image on the retina is upside down and backward.

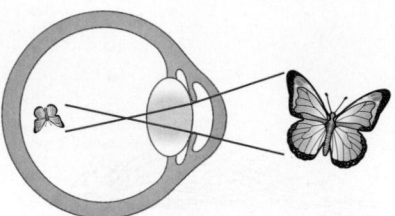

Figure 10-5 Accommodation for close vision. The ciliary muscles contract, the suspensory ligaments relax, and the lens becomes more convex.

backward (Figure 10-4), but the brain turns it around and interprets the image in the correct position.

When an object is at least 20 feet away, the normal relaxed eye is able to focus the image on the retina. When the object is closer than 20 feet, the eye must make adjustments to focus the image. The primary adjustment for close vision is changing the shape of the lens. For distance vision, the ciliary muscle is relaxed, the suspensory ligaments are taut, and the lens is flat. When the eyes adapt for close vision, illustrated in Figure 10-5, the ciliary muscle contracts, the suspensory ligaments become loose or relaxed, and the lens bulges or becomes more convex. The closer the object, the more the light rays have to bend to focus and the greater the curvature of the lens. These adjustments are called **accommodation.**

Photoreceptors

The retina contains two kinds of **photoreceptor** cells: rods and cones. **Rods** are thin cells with slender, rodlike projections and are sensitive to dim light. Even though rods are much more numerous than cones, they are absent in the fovea centralis and their number increases proportionately to the distance away from the fovea centralis. Many rods synapse with a single sensory fiber (convergence); thus vision with rods lacks fine detail. **Cones,** the receptors for color vision and visual acuity, are located primarily in the fovea centralis. They are thicker cells with short, blunt projections. Cones exhibit less convergence than rods, so in addition to color, cones provide sharp images and fine detail. Table 10-2 compares the rods and cones.

Rods contain a substance, **rhodopsin** (roe-DOP-sin) (visual purple), that is very light sensitive. When even small amounts of light focus on the rods, rhodopsin breaks down into its component parts—opsin (a protein) and a derivative of vitamin A, retinal (retinene). This reaction triggers

Table 10-2 Comparison of Rods and Cones

Feature	Rods	Cones
Shape	Long, slender projections	Short, thick projections
Location	None in fovea centralis; increase in density away from fovea centralis	Concentrated in fovea centralis; decrease in density away from fovea centralis
Quantity	More numerous than cones	Less numerous than rods
Convergence	High degree of convergence	Less convergence
Pigments	Single pigment, rhodopsin	Three pigments, one each for red, green, blue
Functions	Black and white vision; dim light; night vision; lacks detail	Color vision; bright light; precise vision with fine detail

From Applegate E: *The anatomy and physiology learning system,* ed 4, St Louis, 2011, Saunders.

a nerve impulse. Rhodopsin is resynthesized from opsin and retinal to prepare the rods for receiving subsequent stimuli. The more rhodopsin there is in the rods, the greater the sensitivity to light. In bright light, nearly all the rhodopsin in the rods is decomposed. After entering a dimly lit area, it takes some time for the eyes to adapt to the dim light. During this period, rhodopsin is regenerated in the rods so that they become more sensitive.

Cones function similarly to rods. Light-sensitive pigments break down into component parts, and the reaction triggers nerve impulses. Three different types of cones exist, each with a different visual pigment. All the pigments contain retinal, but the protein portion is different. One type responds best to green light, another responds best to blue light, and a third type responds best to red light. The perceived color of an object depends on the quantity and combination of cones that are stimulated. If all the pigments are stimulated, the person senses white. If none are stimulated, the person senses black.

Visual Pathway

Visual impulses generated in the rods and cones of the retina leave the eyes in the axons that form the **optic nerves.** Just anterior to the pituitary gland, these nerves form an X-shaped structure, the **optic chiasma** (OP-tik kye-AZ-mah). Within the optic chiasma, the axons from the medial portion of each retina cross over to enter the **optic tract** on the opposite side (Figure 10-6). The right optic tract contains the fibers from the lateral portion of the right eye and the medial portion of the left eye. The left optic tract contains the fibers from the lateral portion of the left eye and the medial portion of the right eye. The optic tracts lead to the **thalamus,** where they synapse with neurons that carry the impulses in the **optic radiations** to the visual cortex of the occipital lobes. Because some of the fibers cross

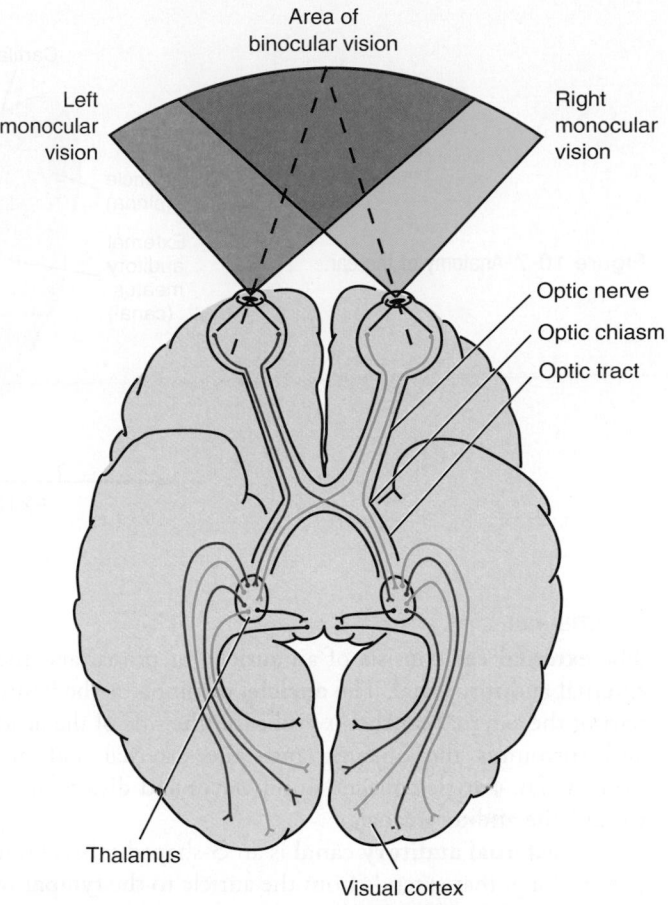

Figure 10-6 Visual pathway. The optic nerves converge at the optic chiasma, where some axons cross to the opposite side. Impulses then travel to the thalamus, then to the visual cortex of the occipital lobe, where they are interpreted.

over to the other side in the optic chiasma, each occipital lobe receives an image of the entire object from each eye but from slightly different perspectives. This enables vision in three dimensions.

AUDITORY SENSE

The **ear** is the organ of hearing (auditory or acoustic organ). It is also the organ for the sense of equilibrium, which is covered later in this chapter. The receptors for hearing, located within the ear, are mechanoreceptors (mek-ah-noh-ree-SEP-tors). Physical forces, in the form of sound vibrations, are responsible for initiating impulses that are interpreted as sound.

Structure of the Ear

The "ears" on the sides of the head are only a portion of the actual organ of hearing. A large part of the organ, actually the most important part, lies hidden from view in the temporal bone. Anatomically, the organ of hearing is divided into the external ear, middle ear, and inner ear. The anatomy of the ear is illustrated in Figure 10-7.

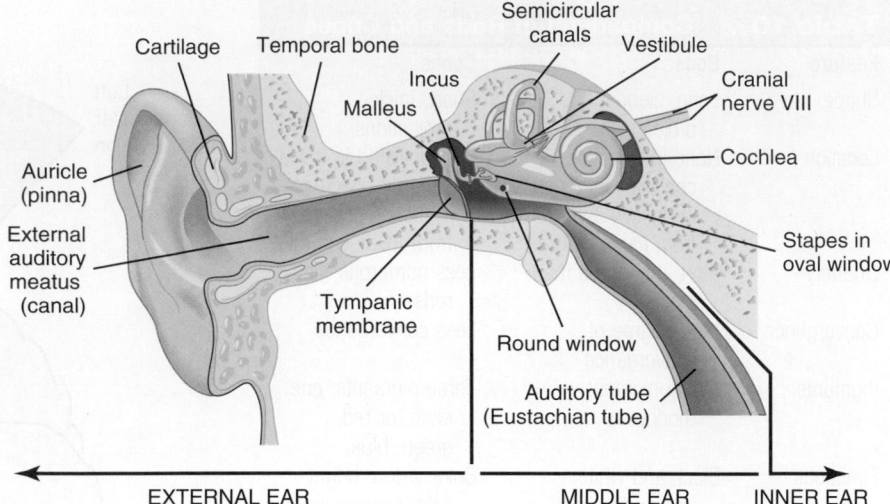

Figure 10-7 Anatomy of the ear.

External Ear

The **external ear** consists of an auricle, or pinna, and the external auditory canal. The **auricle,** or pinna, is the fleshy part of the external ear that is visible on the side of the head and surrounds the opening into the external auditory meatus. The auricle collects sound waves and directs them toward the auditory canal.

The **external auditory canal** is an S-shaped tube, about 2.5 cm long, that extends from the auricle to the **tympanic membrane.** The skin that lines the external auditory canal has numerous hairs and **ceruminous glands,** which secrete a waxy substance called **cerumen.** The hairs and cerumen help prevent foreign objects from reaching the eardrum. The external ear ends at the tympanic membrane.

Middle Ear

The **middle ear** is an air-filled cavity, called the **tympanic cavity,** in the temporal bone. It begins at the tympanic membrane, contains the auditory ossicles, and has an opening into the eustachian tube. The **oval window** and the **round window** in the medial wall of the middle ear connect the middle ear with the inner ear. The oval window is closed by the stapes, one of the bones in the middle ear. The round window is closed by a membrane.

The **tympanic membrane,** or eardrum, is a thin membrane that separates the external ear from the middle ear. Sound waves cause the tympanic membrane to vibrate.

An **auditory tube** (eustachian tube) connects each middle ear with the throat. Its purpose is to equalize the pressure between the outside air and the middle ear cavity, a condition necessary for normal hearing. Throat infections may spread to the middle ear through the auditory tube.

The **auditory ossicles** are three tiny bones: the **malleus** (hammer), **incus** (anvil), and **stapes** (stirrup). These bones are linked together by tiny ligaments and form a bridge across the space of the tympanic cavity. The malleus is attached to the tympanic membrane, and the stapes is attached to the oval window between the middle ear and

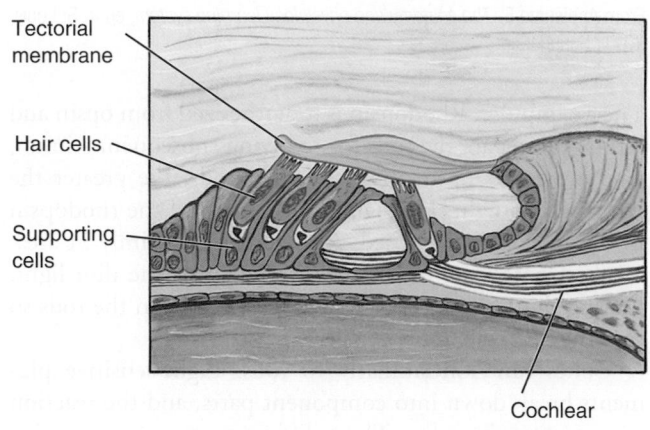

Figure 10-8 Organ of Corti enlarged to show the hair cells and tectorial membrane.

the inner ear. The incus is between the malleus and stapes. When the tympanic membrane vibrates, the ossicles transmit the vibrations across the cavity to the oval window, which transfers the motion to the fluids in the inner ear. This fluid motion excites the receptors for hearing.

Inner Ear

The **inner ear** consists of a series of interconnecting chambers in the temporal bone. It is divided into the vestibule, semicircular canals, and cochlea. The vestibule and semicircular canals function in the sense of equilibrium. The cochlea functions in the sense of hearing.

The **cochlea** (KOK-lee-ah) is the coiled portion of the inner ear. It encloses the **organ of Corti** (KOAR-tee), which contains the receptors for sound. The organ of Corti consists of **supporting cells** and **hair cells** (Figure 10-8). The hair cells are specialized sensory cells that have hairlike projections (microvilli) extending from their free surface. The tips of the projections contact a gelatinous **tectorial** (tek-TOE-ree-al) **membrane** that extends over them. Hair cells have no axons, but they are surrounded by sensory nerve fibers that form the **cochlear branch** of the **vestibulocochlear nerve** (cranial nerve VIII).

Physiology of Hearing

Sound travels through the atmosphere in waves of alternating compressions and decompressions of molecules. Low-pitched tones create low-frequency sound waves; high-pitched tones create high-frequency sound waves. An individual with normal hearing should be able to hear the frequencies of normal speech, which range from 300 to 4000 vibrations per second. Hearing is most acute with frequencies between 2000 and 3000 vibrations per second.

Initiation of Impulses

The process of hearing begins when sound waves enter the external auditory canal. As the waves travel through the external ear, they hit the tympanic membrane and cause it to vibrate. Because the malleus is attached to the membrane, the vibrations are transferred from the tympanic membrane to the malleus, then to the incus, and then to the stapes, which creates vibrations in the membrane of the oval window. Movement of the oval window passes the vibrations to the inner ear.

The vibrations cause the organ of Corti to move and the hairs on the hair cells rub against the tectorial membrane. As the hairs contact the membrane, they bend, and this mechanical deformation initiates the nerve impulses that result in hearing. The following list summarizes the sequence of events in the initiation of auditory impulses:

1. The tympanic membrane vibrates in response to sound waves.
2. The malleus, incus, and stapes transfer vibrations to the oval window membrane.
3. Movement from the oval window starts oscillations within the cochlea.
4. As the cochlea moves, the hairs on the hair cells in the organ of Corti rub against the tectorial membrane and bend.
5. Bending of the hairs on the hair cells stimulates the formation of impulses.
6. Impulses are transmitted to the auditory cortex of the temporal lobe by the cochlear branch of cranial nerve VIII, the vestibulocochlear nerve.

Pitch and Loudness

Hair cells in the organ of Corti have varying sensitivities to different frequencies. Pitch is detected by the portion of the organ of Corti that vibrates in response to the sound and the sensitivity of the hair cells.

Loudness is determined by the intensity of the sound waves. Loud sounds create a greater magnitude of oscillation than low-level sounds. This means that more hair cells are stimulated and more impulses travel to the auditory cortex.

SENSE OF EQUILIBRIUM

The sense of equilibrium is a combination of two different senses: the sense of **static equilibrium** and the sense of **dynamic equilibrium.** Static equilibrium is involved in evaluating the position of the head relative to gravity. It occurs when the head is motionless or moving in a straight line. Dynamic equilibrium occurs when the head is moving in a rotational or angular direction.

Static Equilibrium

The organs of static equilibrium are located in the **vestibule** portion of the inner ear. The vestibule is divided into two portions, the **utricle** (YOO-trih-kull) and the **saccule** (SACK-yool). Each of these contains a small structure called a **macula** (MACK-yoo-lah), which is the organ of static equilibrium. The macula consists of sensory hair cells, similar to those in the organ of Corti, and supporting cells. The projections, or hairs, of the hair cells are embedded in a gelatinous mass that covers the macula. Grains of calcium carbonate, called **otoliths** (OH-toe-liths), are embedded on the surface of the gelatinous mass.

When the head is in an upright position, the hairs are straight. When the head tilts or bends forward, the otoliths and the gelatinous mass move in response to gravity. As the gelatinous mass moves, it bends some of the hairs on the receptor cells. This action initiates an impulse that travels to the CNS by way of the vestibular branch of the vestibulocochlear nerve. The CNS interprets the information and sends motor impulses out to appropriate muscles to maintain balance.

Dynamic Equilibrium

The sense organs for dynamic equilibrium, the equilibrium of rotational or angular movements, are located in the **semicircular canals.** Three semicircular canals, positioned at right angles to one another, exist in three different planes (see Figure 10-7). At the base of each canal, near where it attaches to the utricle, there is a swelling called the **ampulla.** The sensory organs of the semicircular canals are located within the ampullae. Each of these organs, called a **crista ampullaris** (KRIS-tah amp-yoo-LAIR-is), contains sensory hair cells and supporting cells. The crista ampullaris is covered by a dome-shaped gelatinous mass called the **cupula** (KEW-pew-lah). The hairs of the hair cells are embedded in the cupula.

When the head turns rapidly, the semicircular canals move with the head but the cupula tilts to one side. As the cupula tilts, it bends some of the hairs on the hair cells, which triggers a sensory impulse. Because the three canals are in different planes, their cristae are stimulated differently by the same motion. This creates a mosaic of impulses that are transmitted to the CNS on the **vestibular branch** of the **vestibulocochlear nerve.** The CNS interprets the information and initiates appropriate responses to maintain balance. The cerebellum is particularly important in mediating the sense of balance and equilibrium.

Highlight on Conditions Affecting the Senses

Astigmatism (ah-STIG-mah-tizm) Defective curvature of the cornea or lens of the eye resulting in a distorted image on the retina

Blepharitis (bleff-ahr-EYE-tis) Inflammation of the edges of the eyelid

Glaucoma (glaw-KOH-mah) Disease of the eye characterized by increased intraocular pressure from an accumulation of aqueous humor caused by either increased production or decreased drainage; the increased pressure causes pathologic changes in the optic disk and typical defects in the field of vision; if untreated, glaucoma leads to blindness

Macular degeneration (MACK-yoo-lahr dee-jen-er-AY-shun) A gradually progressive condition that results in the loss of central vision because of the breakdown of cells in the macula lutea; frequently affects older people

Meniere disease (men-ih-ARZ dih-ZEEZ) A chronic disease of the inner ear characterized by recurring attacks of dizziness, tinnitus, and fluctuating hearing loss; attacks vary in duration and frequency

Nyctalopia (nick-tah-LOH-pee-ah) A condition in which the individual has difficulty seeing at night; night blindness

Otosclerosis (oh-toe-sklee-ROH-sis) Progressive formation of bony tissue around the oval window, immobilizing the stapes; results in conduction deafness

Presbycusis (prez-bih-KUS-is) Impairment of hearing resulting from aging

Presbyopia (prez-bih-OH-pee-ah) Impairment of vision caused by aging

Sensorineural deafness (sen-soh-ree NEW-rahl DEFF-nis) Hearing loss as a result of damage along any part of the auditory pathway from the receptor cells in the cochlea to the auditory cortex of the cerebrum; noise-related damage to the receptor cells in the cochlea is this type of deafness

Tinnitus (tin-EYE-tus) A ringing or buzzing sound in the ears

Tympanitis (tim-pan-EYE-tis) Inflammation of the tympanic membrane

Vertigo (VER-tih-goh) A feeling of dizziness, loss of balance, and lightheadedness caused by a disturbance of the semicircular canals, utricle, saccule, or vestibular nerve ∎

AGING OF THE SENSES

As the body ages, a general decline in all of the special senses occurs. The most significant changes in the eye occur in the lens. It tends to become thicker and less elastic, which makes it less able to change shape to accommodate for near vision. This condition, called **presbyopia** or farsightedness of aging, probably is the most common age-related dysfunction of the eye. The lens also tends to become cloudy or opaque, forming cataracts. About 90% of people older than age 70 have some degree of cataract formation; however, it is not always significant enough to affect vision. The cornea tends to become more translucent and less spheric, which contributes to an increase in astigmatism in older people. Older people require more light to see well because atrophy of the muscles in the iris reduces the ability of the pupil to dilate and decreases the amount of light that reaches the retina. The chemical processes that rebuild the visual pigment, rhodopsin, are slower in older people, so dark adaptation takes longer and is not as complete as in young people. These changes in the eye may make it more difficult for older people to read and fill out forms correctly, especially if the forms are printed in small type and the individual is reading in dim light.

Most age-related changes in the external ear and middle ear have little effect on hearing. A buildup of cerumen, or earwax, in the external ear may contribute to hearing loss in the low-frequency range. The joints between the auditory ossicles in the middle ear may become less movable, which interferes with the transmission of sound waves to the inner ear, but generally it is not clinically significant. Most of the gradual loss of hearing that usually begins by the age of 40 is a result of degeneration of the receptor cells in the spiral organ of Corti in the inner ear. Another factor is the decrease in the number of nerve fibers in the vestibulocochlear nerve. The reduction in fibers in the cochlear branch contributes to hearing loss. A decrease in vestibular fibers affects balance and equilibrium. Age-related changes in the ear may make it more difficult for individuals to hear verbal instructions and other communication correctly.

Taste and smell, both chemical senses, show a decline with age; however, the mechanism is unclear. Diminished perception may be caused by degeneration of the receptor cells, by changes in the way the impulses are processed in the brain, or by other factors. It is likely that decreases in sensory perception result from a combination of several factors. Whatever the cause, deterioration in the sense of taste may make food unappetizing. Loss in the sense of smell may lead to an inability to detect harmful odors such as smoke and gas.

TERMINOLOGY REVIEW

Medical Term	Word Parts	Definition
Accommodation		Mechanism that allows the eye to focus at various distances, primarily achieved by changing the curvature of the lens.
Chemoreceptor	*chem/o:* chemical	A sensory receptor that detects the presence of chemicals; responsible for taste, smell, and monitoring of the concentration of certain chemicals in body fluids.
Mechanoreceptor	*mechan/o:* mechanical	A sensory receptor that responds to a bending or deformation of the cell; examples include receptors for touch, pressure, hearing, and equilibrium.
Nociceptor	*noci:* causing harm or damage *-ceptor:* receptor	A sensory receptor that responds to tissue damage; pain receptor.
Photoreceptor	*phot/o:* light	A sensory receptor that detects light; located in the retina of the eye.
Proprioception	*propri/o:* one's own *-ceptor:* receptor	The sense of body position and movements; responds to stimuli originating within an organism or muscle.
Sensory adaptation		Phenomenon in which some receptors respond when a stimulus is first applied but decrease their response if the stimulus is maintained; receptor sensitivity decreases with prolonged stimulation.
Thermoreceptor	*therm/o:* heat	A sensory receptor that detects changes in temperature.

ON THE WEB

For information on the senses:

Ear Nose & Throat: www.entusa.com

National Eye Institute: www.nei.nih.gov

National Institute on Deafness: www.nidcd.nih.gov

The Inner Ear: oto.wustl.edu/cochlea

The Joy of Visual Perception: A Web Book: www.yorku.ca/eye

Vestibular Disorders Association: www.vestibular.org

Check out the Evolve site at http://evolve.elsevier.com/Bonewit/today/ to actively Prepare for your Certification, and to access additional interactive activities and exercises to help you study and prepare for success.

11

Endocrine System

KEY TERMS

adenohypophysis
 (add-eh-noe-hye-PAH-fih-sis)
endocrine gland (EN-doh-krin GLAND)

exocrine gland (EKS-oh-krin GLAND)
hormone (HOAR-mohn)

neurohypophysis
 (noo-roh-hye-PAH-fih-sis)
target tissue (TAR-get TISH-yoo)

INTRODUCTION TO THE ENDOCRINE SYSTEM

The endocrine system is composed of the endocrine glands, which secrete hormones into the blood. Unlike the organs in other systems, endocrine glands are scattered throughout the body. In addition, they are small and unimpressive; however, as you study this chapter, you will discover that they are extremely important. The study of endocrine glands and hormones is called *endocrinology.*

COMPARISON OF THE ENDOCRINE AND NERVOUS SYSTEMS

The endocrine system, along with the nervous system, functions in the regulation of body activities. The nervous system acts through electrical impulses and neurotransmitters to cause muscle contraction and glandular secretion. The effect is of short duration, measured in seconds, and localized. The endocrine system acts through chemical messengers called *hormones* that influence growth, development, and metabolic activities. The action of the endocrine system is measured in minutes, hours, or weeks and is more generalized than the action of the nervous system.

COMPARISON OF EXOCRINE AND ENDOCRINE GLANDS

The two major categories of glands in the body are exocrine and endocrine. **Exocrine glands** have ducts that carry their secretory product to a surface. These have a variety of functions and include the sweat, sebaceous, and mammary glands and the glands that secrete digestive enzymes. The **endocrine glands** do not have ducts to carry their product to a surface. They are called *ductless glands.* The word "endocrine" is derived from the Greek terms *endo,* meaning "within," and *krine,* meaning "to separate or secrete." The secretory products of endocrine glands are called **hormones** and are secreted directly into the blood and then carried throughout the body where they influence only those cells that have receptor sites for that hormone. Other cells are not affected. Endocrine glands have an extensive network of blood vessels, and organs with the richest blood supply include some of the endocrine glands, such as the thyroid and adrenal glands.

CHARACTERISTICS OF HORMONES

Each hormone produced in the body is unique. Each one is different in its chemical composition, structure, and action. In spite of the differences, there are similarities in these molecules.

Chemical Nature of Hormones

Chemically, hormones may be classified as either **proteins** or **steroids.** All of the hormones in the human body, except the sex hormones and those from the adrenal cortex, are proteins or protein derivatives. This means that their fundamental building blocks are **amino acids.** Protein hormones are difficult to administer orally because they are quickly inactivated by the acid and pepsin in the stomach. These hormones must be administered by injection. Sex hormones and those from the adrenal cortex are steroids, which are lipid derivatives. These lipid-soluble hormones may be taken orally.

Mechanism of Hormone Action

Hormones are potent substances. This means that small amounts of a hormone may have profound effects on metabolic processes. Hormones are carried by the blood throughout the entire body, yet they affect only certain cells. The specific cells that respond to a given hormone have **receptor sites** for that hormone. This is sort of a lock and key mechanism. If the key fits the lock, then the door will open. If a hormone fits the receptor site, then there will be an effect (Figure 11-1). If a hormone and a receptor site do not match, then there is no reaction. All the cells that have receptor sites for a given hormone make up the **target tissue** for that hormone. In some cases the target tissue is localized in a single gland or organ. In other cases, the target tissue is diffuse and scattered throughout the body so that many areas are affected. Hormones bring about their characteristic effects on target cells by modifying cellular activity.

ENDOCRINE GLANDS AND THEIR HORMONES

The organs of the endocrine system are the glands that secrete hormones. Figure 11-2 illustrates that the eight major endocrine glands are scattered throughout the body; however, they are still considered to be one system because they have similar functions, similar mechanisms of influence, and many important interrelationships.

Some glands also have nonendocrine regions that have functions other than hormone secretion. The pancreas is one of these glands. It has a major exocrine portion that secretes digestive enzymes and an endocrine portion that secretes hormones. The ovaries and testes secrete hormones and also produce the ova and sperm. Some organs, such as the stomach, intestines, and heart, produce hormones, but their primary function is not hormone secretion. These organs are discussed in more detail in the chapters dealing with their predominant function. Table 11-1 summarizes the major endocrine glands and their hormones.

Pituitary Gland

The **pituitary gland** or **hypophysis** is a small gland about 1 cm in diameter, or about the size of a pea. The gland is connected to the hypothalamus of the brain by a slender stalk called the *infundibulum.* The gland has two distinct regions. The anterior portion is called the **adenohypophysis** (add-eh-noe-hye-PAH-fih-sis). The posterior region is called the **neurohypophysis** (noo-roh-hye-PAH-fih-sis).

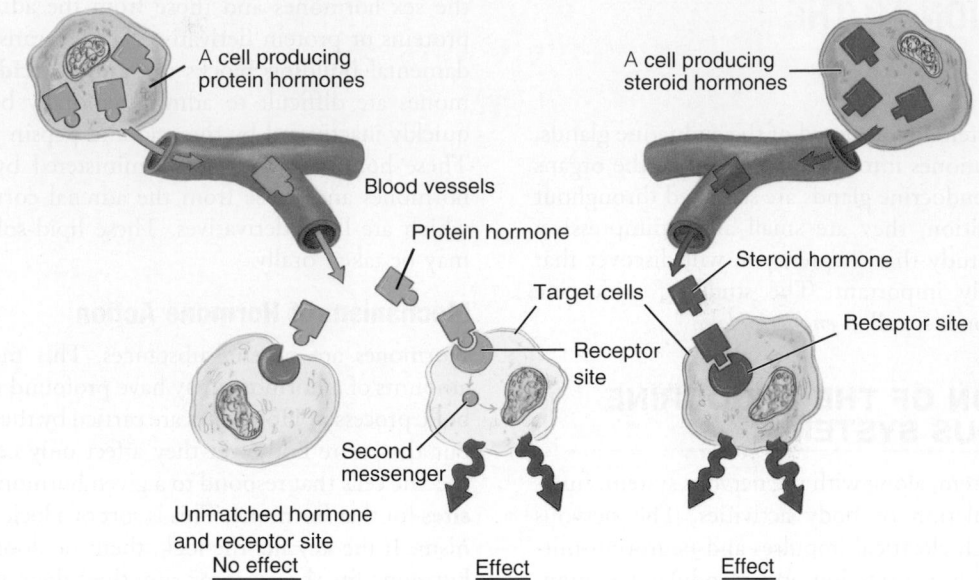

Figure 11-1 Hormone-receptor action. There must be a match between hormone and receptor. Receptors for protein hormones are on the cell surface. Receptors for steroid hormones are inside the cell.

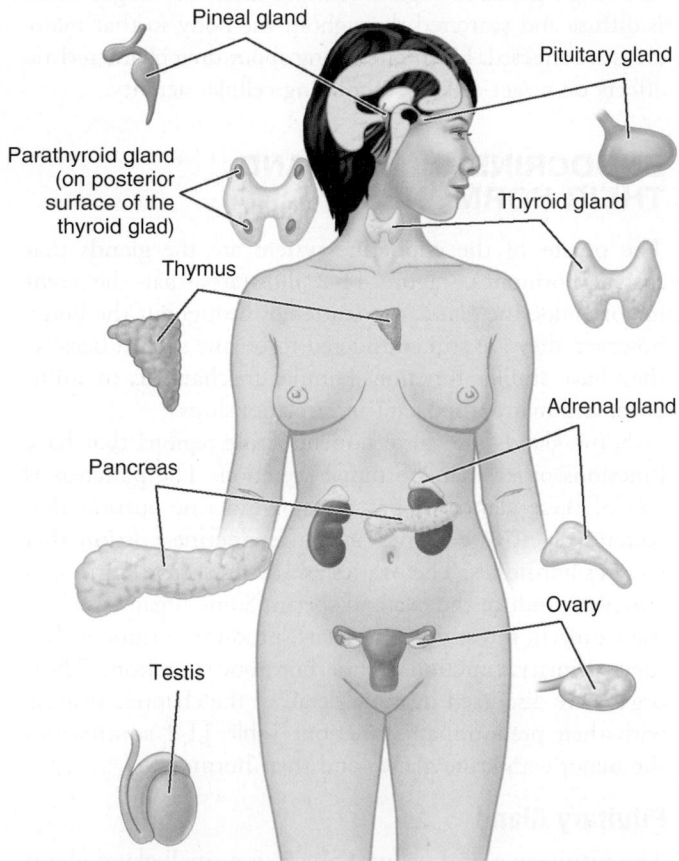

Figure 11-2 Major endocrine glands.

Table 11-1 and Figure 11-3 summarize the hormones from the pituitary gland.

Hormones of the Anterior Lobe (Adenohypophysis)
Growth Hormone

Growth hormone (GH) stimulates the growth of bones, muscles, and other organs by promoting protein synthesis. This hormone dramatically affects the appearance of an individual because it influences height. If there is too little of the hormone in a child, that person may become a pituitary dwarf of normal proportions but small stature. An excess of the hormone in a child results in exaggerated bone growth, and the individual becomes exceptionally tall or a giant. After ossification is complete and an increase in bone length is no longer possible, excess GH causes an enlargement in the diameter of the bones. The result is a condition called *acromegaly* (ack-roh-MEG-ah-lee), in which the bones of the hands and face become abnormally large.

Thyroid-Stimulating Hormone

Thyroid-stimulating hormone (TSH), or thyrotropin (thye-roh-TROH-pin), causes the glandular cells of the thyroid to secrete thyroid hormone. When there is a hypersecretion of TSH, the thyroid gland enlarges and secretes too much thyroid hormone. Hyposecretion of TSH results in atrophy of the thyroid gland and too little hormone.

Adrenocorticotropic Hormone

Adrenocorticotropic (ah-dree-noh-kor-tih-koh-TROH-pik) hormone (ACTH) reacts with receptor sites in the cortex of the adrenal gland to stimulate the secretion of cortical hormones, particularly cortisol. ACTH also affects the melanocytes in the skin and increases pigmentation.

Table 11-1 Principal Endocrine Glands and Their Hormones

Gland	Hormone	Target Tissue	Principal Actions
Anterior lobe of pituitary	Growth hormone (GH)	Most tissues in body	Stimulates growth by promoting protein synthesis
	Thyroid-stimulating hormone (TSH)	Thyroid gland	Increases secretion of thyroid hormone; increases size of thyroid gland
	Adrenocorticotropic hormone (ACTH)	Adrenal cortex	Increases secretion of adrenocortical hormones, especially glucocorticoids, such as cortisol
	Follicle-stimulating hormone (FSH)	Ovarian follicles in females; seminiferous tubules of testis in males	Follicle maturation and estrogen secretion in females; spermatogenesis in males
	Luteinizing hormone (LH); also called *interstitial cell–stimulating hormone* (ICSH) in males	Ovary in females, testis in males	Ovulation; progesterone production in females; testosterone production in males
	Prolactin	Mammary gland	Stimulates milk production
Posterior lobe of pituitary	Antidiuretic hormone (ADH)	Kidney	Increases water reabsorption (decreases water lost in urine)
	Oxytocin	Uterus; mammary gland	Increases uterine contractions; stimulates ejection of milk from mammary gland
Thyroid gland	Thyroxine and triiodothyronine	Most body cells	Increases metabolic rate; essential for normal growth and development
	Calcitonin	Primarily bone	Decreases blood calcium by inhibiting bone breakdown and release of calcium; antagonistic to parathyroid hormone
Parathyroid gland	Parathyroid hormone (PTH) or parathormone	Bone, kidney, digestive tract	Increases blood calcium by stimulating bone breakdown and release of calcium; increases calcium absorption in digestive tract; decreases calcium lost in urine
Adrenal cortex	Mineralocorticoids (aldosterone)	Kidney	Increases sodium reabsorption and potassium excretion in kidney tubules; secondarily increases water retention
	Glucocorticoids (cortisol)	Most body tissues	Increases blood glucose levels; inhibits inflammation and immune response
	Androgens and estrogens	Most body tissues	Secreted in small amounts so that effect is generally masked by hormones from ovaries and testes
Adrenal medulla	Epinephrine, norepinephrine	Heart, blood vessels, liver, adipose	Helps cope with stress; increases heart rate and blood pressure; increases blood flow to skeletal muscle; increases blood glucose level
Pancreas (islets of Langerhans)	Glucagon	Liver	Increases breakdown of glycogen to increase blood glucose levels
	Insulin	General, but especially liver, skeletal muscle, adipose	Decreases blood glucose levels by facilitating uptake and use of glucose by cells; stimulates glucose storage as glycogen and production of adipose
Testes	Testosterone	Most body cells	Maturation and maintenance of male reproductive organs and secondary sex characteristics
Ovaries	Estrogens	Most body cells	Maturation and maintenance of female reproductive organs and secondary sex characteristics; menstrual cycle
	Progesterone	Uterus and breast	Prepares uterus for pregnancy; stimulates development of mammary gland; menstrual cycle
Pineal gland	Melatonin	Hypothalamus	Inhibits gonadotropin-releasing hormone, which consequently inhibits reproductive functions; regulates daily rhythms, such as sleep and wakefulness

From Applegate E: *The anatomy and physiology learning system,* ed 4, St Louis, 2011, Saunders.

Highlight on the Endocrine System

Insulin: Insulin is a small protein molecule. It cannot be taken by mouth because it is rapidly inactivated by digestive enzymes.

Growth hormone (GH): Excessive secretion of a hormone is called *hypersecretion*. A deficiency of a hormone is called hyposecretion. Usually hyposecretion of GH in the adult poses no problems. However, in rare instances the deficiency may be so drastic that body tissues atrophy and premature aging occurs.

Antidiuretic hormone (ADH): Ingestion of alcoholic beverages inhibits ADH secretion and results in increased urine output. Certain drugs, called *diuretics,* counteract the effects of ADH and result in fluid loss. These drugs are sometimes prescribed for patients with high blood pressure or those with edema caused by congestive heart failure because the drugs have the effect of removing fluid from the body.

Oxytocin: Oxytocin, or similar synthetic drugs, may be used to hasten the delivery of the placenta, control bleeding after delivery, or stimulate milk ejection.

Thyroid function: When thyroxine and triiodothyronine, with their incorporated iodine, are released into the blood, more than 99% combines with plasma proteins. This iodine is called protein-bound iodine (PBI). The amount of PBI can be measured by a laboratory procedure and is widely used as a test of thyroid function.

Cortisone: Persons with inflamed joints often receive injections of a pharmaceutic glucocorticoid, cortisone, to relieve the pain and inflammation. Over-the-counter creams and ointments containing hydrocortisone are available to relieve the itching and inflammation of rashes.

Gonadocorticoids: Tumors that result in hypersecretion of gonadocorticoids may have dramatic effects in prepubertal boys and girls. There is a rapid onset of puberty and sex drive in males. Females develop the masculine distribution of body hair, including a beard, and the clitoris enlarges to become more like a penis.

Hypoglycemia: Hyperinsulinism is usually caused by an overdose of insulin. The result is hypoglycemia, or low blood sugar level. The low blood sugar stimulates the secretion of glucagon, epinephrine, and GH, which causes anxiety, nervousness, tremors, and a feeling of weakness. Insufficient glucose levels in the brain lead to disorientation, convulsions, and unconsciousness. Death can occur quickly unless the blood glucose level is raised. The early symptoms can be treated easily by eating sugar.

Melatonin: Melatonin production appears to be related to the amount of light that enters through the eye. People who work at night and sleep during the day have a reversed cycle of melatonin production. The high melatonin levels occur during the day while they are asleep and the low levels are at night when they are working and light is entering the eye. ■

Highlight on Conditions Affecting the Endocrine System

Acromegaly (ack-roh-MEG-ah-lee) Enlargement of the extremities caused by excessive growth hormone in the adult

Adenoma (add-eh-NOH-mah) A tumor of a gland

Cretinism (KREE-tin-izm) Dwarfism caused by a deficiency of thyroid hormone in childhood and usually accompanied by mental retardation

Cushing syndrome (KOOSH-ing SIN-drohm) A group of symptoms caused by prolonged exposure to high levels of cortisol; characterized by excessive deposition of fat in the subscapular area and in the face (moon face), high blood pressure, generalized weakness, and loss of muscle mass because of excessive protein catabolism; may be caused by overproduction of cortisol or by taking glucocorticoid hormone medications to treat inflammatory diseases, such as asthma and rheumatoid arthritis

Diabetes insipidus (di-ah-BEE-teez in-SIP-ih-dus) A metabolic disorder caused by a deficient quantity of antidiuretic hormone, resulting in a large quantity of dilute urine (polyuria) and great thirst (polydipsia)

Diabetes mellitus (di-ah-BEE-teez mell-EYE-tus) Disorder caused by a deficiency of insulin from the beta cells of the pancreatic islets; characterized by a disturbance in the metabolism of blood glucose and manifested by polyuria, polyphagia, and polydipsia

Myxedema (miks-eh-DEE-mah) A condition of swelling attributable to an accumulation of mucus in the skin; results from deficiency of thyroid hormone in the adult

Progeria (pro-JEER-ih-ah) A condition of premature old age occurring in childhood; may be caused by hormone dysfunction ■

Hypersecretion and hyposecretion of ACTH are reflected in the activity of the adrenal cortex.

Gonadotropic Hormones

Gonadotropic (go-nad-oh-TROH-pik) hormones react with receptor sites in the gonads—ovaries and testes—to regulate the development, growth, and function of these organs. Follicle-stimulating hormone (FSH) stimulates the development of eggs or ova in the ovaries and of sperm in the testes. In addition, it stimulates estrogen production in the female. Luteinizing hormone (LH) causes ovulation and the production and secretion of progesterone and estrogen. In the male, LH is sometimes called *interstitial cell–stimulating hormone* (ICSH) because it stimulates the interstitial cells of the testes to produce and secrete the male sex hormone testosterone. Without FSH and LH, the ovaries and testes decrease in size, ova and sperm are not produced, and sex hormones are not secreted.

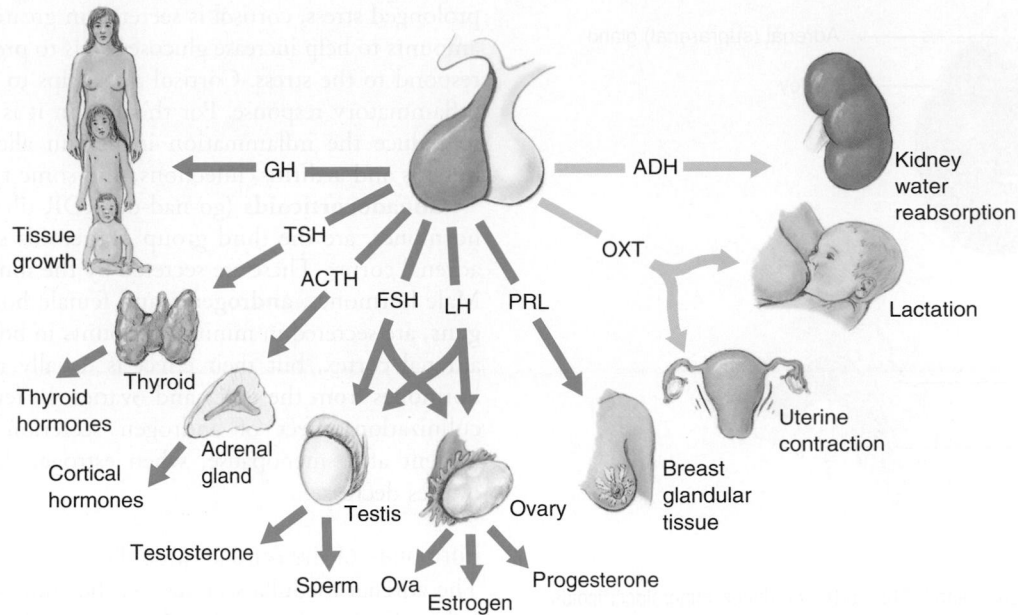

Figure 11-3 Effects of hormones from the pituitary gland.

Prolactin

Prolactin (PRL), or lactogenic hormone, promotes the development of glandular tissue in the female breast during pregnancy and stimulates milk production after the birth of the infant. This hormone does not cause the milk to be ejected from the breast. A hormone from the posterior pituitary and other neural influences are responsible for the ejection of the milk.

Hormones of the Posterior Lobe (Neurohypophysis)

Antidiuretic Hormone

Antidiuretic (ant-eye-dye-yoo-RET-ik) hormone (ADH) promotes the reabsorption of water by the kidney tubules, with the result that less water is lost as urine. This mechanism conserves water for the body. Insufficient amounts of ADH cause excessive water loss in the urine. Large amounts of a dilute urine are produced. This condition is called *diabetes insipidus*. ADH, especially in large amounts, also causes blood vessels to constrict, which increases blood pressure. For this reason, ADH is sometimes called *vasopressin*.

Oxytocin

Oxytocin (ahk-see-TOH-sin) (OXY) causes contraction of the smooth muscle in the wall of the uterus. It also stimulates the ejection of milk from the lactating breast. A commercial preparation of this hormone, *Pitocin,* is sometimes used to induce labor.

Thyroid Gland

The thyroid (THYE-royd) gland is a vascular organ that is located in the neck (see Figure 11-2). It consists of two lobes, one on each side of the trachea, just below the larynx or voice box. The two lobes are connected by a narrow band of tissue called the *isthmus.*

Thyroxine and Triiodothyronine

About 95% of the active thyroid hormone is thyroxine, and the remaining 5% is triiodothyronine. Both of these require iodine for their synthesis. The iodine is actively transported into the thyroid gland, and then it is incorporated into the hormone molecules.

If there is an iodine deficiency, the thyroid cannot make sufficient hormone. This stimulates the thyroid gland to increase in size in a vain attempt to produce more hormone. However, it cannot produce more hormone because it does not have the necessary raw materials, namely, iodine. This type of thyroid enlargement is called *simple goiter* or *iodine deficiency goiter.* The use of iodized salt has reduced the incidence of simple goiter.

Thyroxine and triiodothyronine help to regulate the metabolism of carbohydrates, proteins, and lipids in the body. They do not have a single target organ; instead, they affect most of the cells in the body. Thyroid hormones increase the rate at which cells release energy from carbohydrates, enhance protein synthesis, are necessary for normal growth and development, and stimulate the nervous system.

Calcitonin

Calcitonin is secreted by the thyroid gland and reduces the calcium level in the blood. If the blood calcium level becomes too high, calcitonin is secreted until the calcium ion level decreases to normal.

Parathyroid Glands

Four small masses of epithelial tissue are embedded in the connective tissue capsule on the posterior surface of the thyroid glands. These are the parathyroid glands, and they secrete **parathyroid hormone** (PTH), or parathormone. PTH is the most important regulator of blood calcium

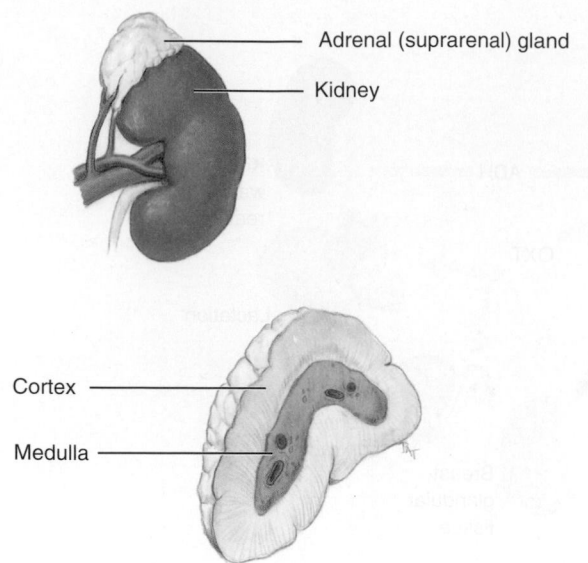

Figure 11-4 Adrenal gland. The cortex produces mineralocorticoids, glucocorticoids, and gonadocorticoids. The medulla produces epinephrine and norepinephrine.

levels. The hormone is secreted in response to low blood calcium levels, and its effect is to increase those levels. PTH is antagonistic to calcitonin from the thyroid gland. Calcitonin reduces blood calcium levels, and PTH increases blood calcium. The two hormones work together to maintain homeostasis.

Adrenal (Suprarenal) Glands

The adrenal, or suprarenal (soo-prah-REE-null), glands are paired with one gland located near the upper portion of each kidney. The glands are embedded in the fat that surrounds the kidneys. Each gland is divided into an outer region—the adrenal cortex—and an inner region—the adrenal medulla (Figure 11-4).

Hormones of the Adrenal Cortex

The adrenal cortex consists of three different regions, with each region producing a different group or type of hormones. Chemically, all the cortical hormones are steroids.

Mineralocorticoids (min-er-al-oh-KOR-tih-koyds) are secreted by the outermost region of the adrenal cortex. As a group, these hormones help regulate blood volume and the concentration of mineral electrolytes in the blood. The principal mineralocorticoid is **aldosterone** (al-DAHS-ter-ohn), which primarily affects the kidneys. In general, the primary effect of aldosterone is to conserve sodium ions and water in the body and to eliminate potassium ions. The levels of sodium and potassium ions are important in maintaining blood pressure, nerve impulse conduction, and muscle contraction. **Glucocorticoids** (gloo-koh-KOR-tih-koyds) are secreted by the middle region of the adrenal cortex. The principal glucocorticoid is **cortisol,** also called *hydrocortisone.* The overall effect of the glucocorticoids is to increase blood glucose levels. This helps to maintain appropriate blood glucose levels between meals. In times of

prolonged stress, cortisol is secreted in greater than normal amounts to help increase glucose levels to provide energy to respond to the stress. Cortisol also helps to counteract the inflammatory response. For this reason it is used clinically to reduce the inflammation in certain allergic reactions, bursitis and arthritis, infections, and some types of cancer.

Gonadocorticoids (go-nad-oh-KOR-tih-koyds), or sex hormones, are the third group of steroids secreted by the adrenal cortex. These are secreted by the innermost region. Male hormones, **androgens,** and female hormones, **estrogens,** are secreted in minimal amounts in both sexes by the adrenal cortex, but their effect is usually masked by the hormones from the testes and ovaries. In females the masculinization effect of androgen secretion may become evident after menopause, when estrogen levels from the ovaries decrease.

Hormones of the Adrenal Medulla

The adrenal medulla secretes two hormones: **epinephrine** (adrenaline) and **norepinephrine** (noradrenaline). About 80% of the medullary secretion is epinephrine. These two hormones are secreted in response to stimulation by sympathetic nerves, particularly during stressful situations. Epinephrine, a cardiac stimulator, and norepinephrine, a vasoconstrictor, together cause increases in heart rate, the force of cardiac muscle contraction, and blood pressure. They divert blood supply to the skeletal muscles and decrease the activity of the digestive tract, dilate the bronchioles and increase the breathing rate, and increase the rate of metabolism to provide energy. They prepare the body for strenuous activity and are sometimes called the *fight-or-flight hormones.* Their effect on the body is similar to effects of the sympathetic nervous system but lasts up to 10 times longer because the hormones are removed from the tissues slowly. The effects of epinephrine are summarized in Figure 11-5.

Pancreas—Islets of Langerhans

The pancreas is a long, soft organ that lies transversely along the posterior abdominal wall, posterior to the stomach, and extends from the region of the duodenum to the spleen. This gland has an exocrine portion that secretes digestive enzymes that are carried through a duct to the duodenum and an endocrine portion that secretes hormones into the blood. The endocrine portion consists of more than 1 million small groups of cells, called *pancreatic islets* or *islets of Langerhans,* which are interspersed throughout the exocrine tissue. The pancreatic islets contain alpha cells that secrete the hormone **glucagon** and beta cells that secrete the hormone **insulin.** Both of these hormones have a role in regulating blood glucose levels. Maintaining blood glucose levels within a normal range is important because this is the primary source of energy for the nervous system. If blood glucose levels fall too low, the nervous system does not function properly. If blood glucose levels become too high, the kidneys produce large quantities of urine, and dehydration may result.

mellitus, which is characterized by abnormally high blood glucose levels.

Gonads (Test+12es and Ovaries)

The gonads, the primary reproductive organs, are the testes in the male and ovaries in the female. These organs are responsible for producing the sperm and ova, but they also secrete hormones and are considered to be endocrine glands. A brief description of their endocrine functions is given here. Information regarding reproductive functions and a more thorough discussion of the hormones appear in Chapter 16.

Testes

Male sex hormones, as a group, are called **androgens** (AN-droh-jenz). The principal androgen is **testosterone** (tess-TAHS-ter-ohn), which is secreted by the testes. A small amount is also produced by the adrenal cortex. Production of testosterone begins during fetal development, continues for a short time after birth, nearly ceases during childhood, and then resumes at puberty. This steroid hormone is responsible for the following:

- Growth and development of the male reproductive structures
- Increased skeletal and muscular growth
- Enlargement of the larynx accompanied by voice changes
- Growth and distribution of body hair
- Increased male sexual drive

Ovaries

Two groups of female sex hormones are produced in the ovaries: the **estrogens** (ESS-troh-jenz) and **progesterone** (proh-JESS-ter-ohn). These steroid hormones contribute to the development and function of the female reproductive organs and sex characteristics. At the onset of puberty, estrogens promote the following:

- Development of the breasts
- Distribution of fat evidenced in the hips, legs, and breasts
- Maturation of reproductive organs, such as the uterus and vagina

Progesterone causes the uterine lining to thicken in preparation for pregnancy. Together, progesterone and estrogens are responsible for the changes that occur in the uterus during the female menstrual cycle.

Pineal Gland

The **pineal** (PIE-nee-al) gland, also called *pineal body* or **epiphysis cerebri,** is a small cone-shaped structure that extends posteriorly from the third ventricle of the brain.

The pineal gland consists of portions of neurons, neuroglial cells, and specialized secretory cells called **pinealocytes** (PIE-nee-al-oh-cytes). The pinealocytes synthesize the hormone **melatonin** (mell-ah-TOH-nihn) and secrete it directly into the cerebrospinal fluid, which takes it into the blood. Melatonin secretion is rhythmic in nature, with high levels secreted at night and low levels secreted during the day.

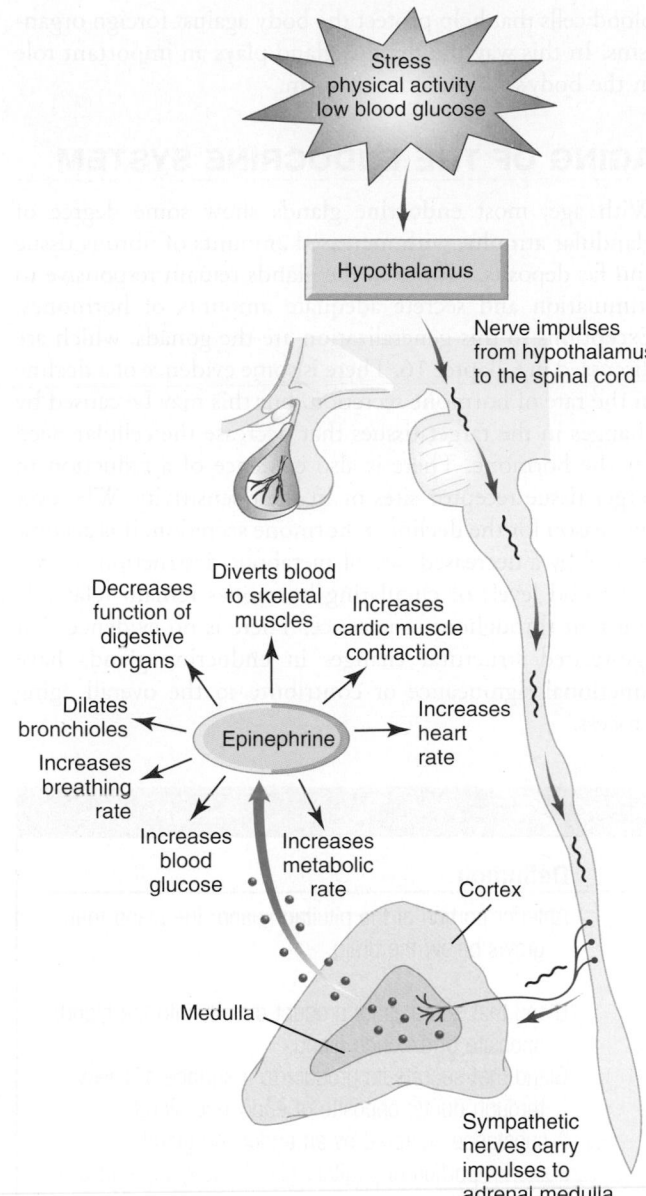

Figure 11-5 Epinephrine—its effects and control of its secretion.

Glucagon

Alpha cells in the pancreatic islets secrete the hormone glucagon in response to a low concentration of glucose in the blood. Glucagon's principal action is to raise blood glucose levels to prevent hypoglycemia from occurring between meals or when glucose is being used rapidly.

Insulin

Beta cells in the pancreatic islets secrete the hormone insulin in response to a high concentration of glucose in the blood. The action of insulin is the opposite of or antagonistic to the action of glucagon. Insulin decreases the blood glucose concentration. Hypoactivity of insulin may be caused by insufficient insulin secretion, insufficient receptor sites on target cell membranes, or defective receptor sites that do not recognize insulin. These dysfunctions lead to diabetes

The function of the pineal gland and melatonin in humans has been the subject of controversy and speculation for centuries. Even the ancient Greeks wrote about it. Evidence accumulated during the 1980s indicates that melatonin has a regulatory role in sexual and reproductive development. Melatonin acts on the hypothalamus to inhibit gonadotropin-releasing hormone (GnRH), which then inhibits gonadal development.

Another function of melatonin involves the organization and regulation of circadian rhythms, or daily changes in physiologic processes that follow a regular pattern. An example of this is the sleepiness-wakefulness cycle. Increased plasma melatonin levels, which occur at night, are associated with sleepiness. The hormone also seems to play a role in hunger-satiety cycles, mood changes, and jet lag. The high nighttime level of melatonin seems to be a mechanism to "reset" the biologic clock daily.

Thymus Gland

The thymus gland is located near the midline, posterior to the sternum and slightly superior to the heart. Through the production of the hormone **thymosin** (THYE-moh-sin), the thymus gland assists in the development of certain blood cells that help protect the body against foreign organisms. In this way the thymus gland plays an important role in the body's immune mechanism.

AGING OF THE ENDOCRINE SYSTEM

With age, most endocrine glands show some degree of glandular atrophy, with increased amounts of fibrous tissue and fat deposits. However, the glands remain responsive to stimulation and secrete adequate amounts of hormones. Exceptions to this generalization are the gonads, which are discussed in Chapter 16. There is some evidence of a decline in the rate of hormone secretion, but this may be caused by changes in the target tissues that decrease the cellular need for the hormone. There is also evidence of a reduction in target-tissue receptor sites or in their sensitivity. Whatever the reason for the decline in hormone secretion, it is accompanied by a decreased rate of metabolic destruction so that the blood levels of circulating hormones remain relatively constant throughout senescence. There is no evidence that age-related structural changes in endocrine glands have functional significance or contribute to the overall aging process.

TERMINOLOGY REVIEW

Medical Term	Word Parts	Definition
Adenohypophysis	*aden/o:* gland *hypo-:* beneath, below *-physis:* to grow	Anterior portion of the pituitary gland; the gland that grows below the brain.
Endocrine gland	*endo-:* in, within *-crine:* to secrete	Gland that secretes its product directly into the blood; opposite of exocrine gland.
Exocrine gland	*exo-:* out, away from *-crine:* to secrete	Gland that secrets its product to a surface or cavity through ducts; opposite of endocrine gland.
Hormone	*hormon/o:* hormone	A substance secreted by an endocrine gland.
Neurohypophysis	*neur/o:* nerve *hypo-:* beneath, below *-physis:* to grow	Posterior portion of pituitary gland; the gland that grows beneath the brain and contains axons of neurons.
Target tissue		A tissue (cells) that responds to a particular hormone because it has receptor sites for that hormone.

ON THE WEB

For information on the endocrine system:

Endocrine Diseases: www.mic.ki.se/diseases/C19.html

Endocrine System: www.emc.maricopa.edu/faculty/farabee/BIOBK/BiobookENDOCR.html

Endocrine Web: www.endocrineweb.com

Inner Body: www.innerbody.com

 Check out the Evolve site at http://evolve.elsevier.com/Bonewit/today/ to actively Prepare for your Certification, and to access additional interactive activities and exercises to help you study and prepare for success.

12

Circulatory System

LEARNING OBJECTIVES

1. Describe the size and location of the heart.
2. Identify the layers of the heart wall, and state the type of tissue in each layer.
3. Label a diagram of the heart, including the chambers, valves, and associated vessels.
4. Trace the pathway of blood flow through the heart.
5. Describe the components and function of the conduction system of the heart.
6. Summarize the events of a cardiac cycle, and correlate the heart sounds heard with these events.
7. Describe the physical characteristics and functions of blood.
8. Identify the composition of blood plasma.
9. Identify the formed elements of the blood.
10. State the function of each formed element in blood.
11. Describe the life cycle of an erythrocyte.
12. List and describe the five types of leukocytes.
13. Explain the blood clotting mechanism of the body.
14. Explain the basis of blood types.
15. Describe the structure and function of arteries.
16. Describe the structure and function of capillaries.
17. Describe the structure and function of veins.
18. Describe ways in which the aging of an individual affects the circulatory system.
19. Identify pathology related to the circulatory system.

CHAPTER OUTLINE

INTRODUCTION TO THE CIRCULATORY SYSTEM
Heart
Overview of the Heart
Structure of the Heart
Physiology of the Heart
Blood
Functions and Characteristics of Blood

Composition of Blood
Hemostasis
Blood Types
Blood Vessels
Classification and Structure of Blood Vessels
Circulatory Pathways
Aging of the Circulatory System

KEY TERMS

atrioventricular valve (ay-tree-oh-ven-TRIK-yoo-lar VALVE)
cardiac cycle (KAR-dee-ak SYE-kul)
coagulation (koh-ag-yoo-LAY-shun)
conduction myofibers (kon-DUCK-shun my-o-FYE-bers)

diapedesis (dye-ah-peh-DEE-sis)
diastole (dye-AS-toh-lee)
erythrocyte (ee-RITH-roh-syte)
erythropoiesis (ee-rith-roh-POY-ee-sis)
erythropoietin (ee-rith-roh-POY-ee-tin)
hematopoiesis (hee-ma-to-poy-EE-sis)

hemocytoblast (hee-moh-SYTE-oh-blast)
leukocyte (LOO-koh-syte)
semilunar valve (seh-mee-LOO-nar VALVE)
systole (SIS-toh-lee)
thrombocyte (THROM-boh-syte)

INTRODUCTION TO THE CIRCULATORY SYSTEM

The circulatory system is made up of the heart, blood, and blood vessels. A central pump, the heart, provides the force to move the blood through a system of blood vessels that extend throughout the body. Blood is the primary transport medium that is responsible for meeting the demands of the cells. This chapter focuses on the three components making up the circulatory system: heart, blood, and blood vessels.

HEART

The heart is a muscular pump that provides the force necessary to circulate the blood to all the tissues in the body. Its function is vital because, to survive, the tissues need a continuous supply of oxygen and nutrients, and metabolic waste products must be removed from them. Deprived of these necessities, cells soon undergo irreversible changes that lead to death. Although blood is the transport medium, the heart is the organ that keeps the blood moving through the vessels. The normal adult heart pumps about 5 L of blood every minute throughout life. If it loses its pumping effectiveness for even a few minutes, the individual's life is jeopardized.

Overview of the Heart

Form, Size, and Location of the Heart

Knowledge of the heart's position in the thoracic cavity is important in hearing heart sounds, obtaining electrocardiograms (ECGs), and performing cardiopulmonary resuscitation (CPR). The heart, illustrated in Figure 12-1, is located in the thoracic cavity between the two lungs. It is posterior to the sternum and anterior to the vertebral column, and it rests on the diaphragm. About two thirds of the heart mass is to the left of the body's midline, and one third is to the right. The **apex,** or pointed end of the heart, extends downward to the level of the fifth intercostal space. The opposite end, the **base,** is larger and less pointed than the apex and has several large vessels attached to it. Its most superior portion is at the level of the second rib. The size of the heart varies with the size of the individual. On average, it is about 9 cm wide and 12 cm long, which is about the size of a closed fist.

Coverings of the Heart

The heart is enclosed by a loose-fitting, double-layered sac called the **pericardium** (pair-ih-KAR-dee-um) or *pericardial sac.* The outer layer of the pericardium consists of tough, white fibrous connective tissue and is called the **fibrous pericardium.** The fibrous pericardium is lined with a serous membrane called the **parietal pericardium.** Where the pericardium is attached to the vessels at the base of the heart, the parietal pericardium reflects onto the surface of the heart to form the **visceral pericardium,** or **epicardium.** The small space between the parietal and visceral layers of the pericardium is the **pericardial cavity.** It contains a thin layer of serous fluid that reduces friction between the membranes as they rub against each other during heart contractions.

Structure of the Heart

Layers of the Heart Wall

The heart wall is formed by three layers of tissue: an outer epicardium, a middle myocardium, and an inner endocardium. The **epicardium** (eh-pih-KAR-dee-um) (which is the same as the visceral pericardium) consists of a serous membrane. It is a thin protective layer that is firmly anchored to the underlying muscle. Blood vessels that nourish the heart wall are located in the epicardium.

The thick middle layer is the **myocardium** (my-oh-KAR-dee-um). It forms the bulk of the heart wall and is

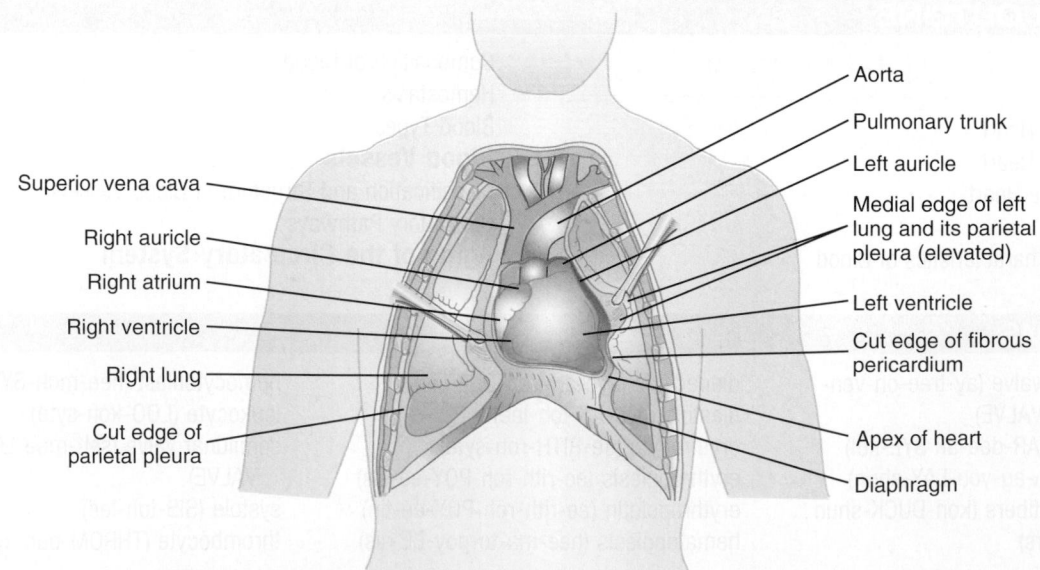

Figure 12-1 Frontal view of the mediastinum, showing the position of the heart.

composed of cardiac muscle tissue. Refer to Chapter 5 for a review of the different types of muscle tissue. Contractions of the myocardium provide the force that ejects blood from the heart and moves it through the vessels.

The smooth inner lining of the heart wall is the **endocardium** (en-doh-KAR-dee-um). Its smooth surface permits blood to move easily through the heart. The endocardium also forms the valves of the heart and is continuous with the lining of the blood vessels. Figure 12-2 illustrates the layers of the heart wall.

Chambers of the Heart

The internal cavity of the heart is divided into four chambers (Figure 12-3):

- Right atrium
- Right ventricle
- Left atrium
- Left ventricle

The two atria are thin-walled chambers that receive blood from the veins. The two ventricles are thick-walled chambers that forcefully pump blood out of the heart. Differences in thickness of the heart chamber walls are caused by variations in the amount of myocardium present, which reflects the amount of force each chamber is required to generate.

The **right atrium** (AY-tree-um) receives deoxygenated blood from the superior vena cava and the inferior vena cava. The superior vena cava returns blood to the heart from the head, neck, and upper extremities. The inferior vena cava returns blood to the heart from the thorax, abdomen, pelvis, and lower extremities. The **left atrium** receives oxygenated blood from the lungs through four pulmonary

veins, two on the right and two on the left. Because the atria are "receiving" chambers rather than "pumping" chambers, their myocardium is relatively thin. The right and left atria are separated by a partition called the **interatrial septum.** A thin region, the **fossa ovalis,** is found in the

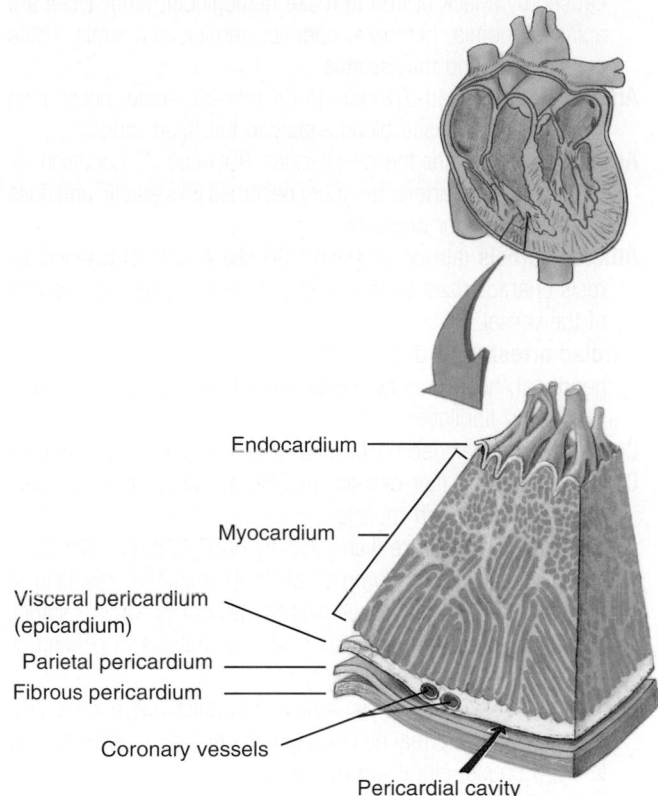

Endocardium

Myocardium

Visceral pericardium
(epicardium)

Parietal pericardium

Fibrous pericardium

Coronary vessels

Pericardial cavity

Figure 12-2 Layers of the heart wall.

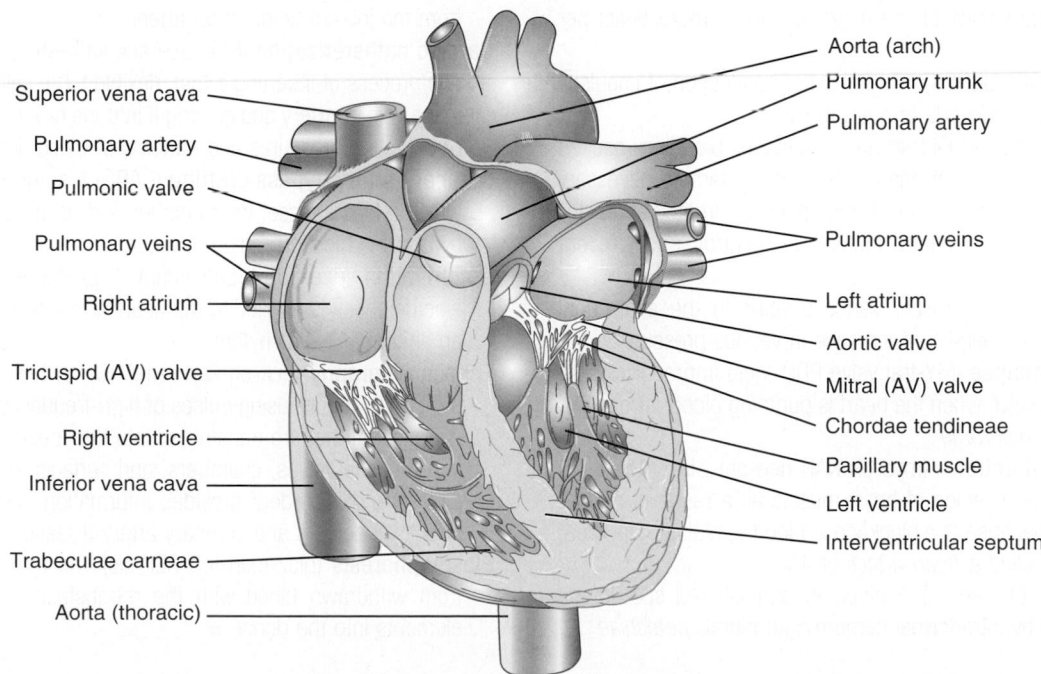

Superior vena cava

Pulmonary artery

Pulmonic valve

Pulmonary veins

Right atrium

Tricuspid (AV) valve

Right ventricle

Inferior vena cava

Trabeculae carneae

Aorta (thoracic)

Aorta (arch)

Pulmonary trunk

Pulmonary artery

Pulmonary veins

Left atrium

Aortic valve

Mitral (AV) valve

Chordae tendineae

Papillary muscle

Left ventricle

Interventricular septum

Figure 12-3 Internal view of the heart showing the chambers and valves.

Highlight on Conditions and Procedures Affecting the Circulatory System

Conditions

Anemia (ah-NEE-mee-ah) Deficiency in red blood cells (RBCs) or hemoglobin; most common form is iron deficiency anemia caused by a lack of iron to make hemoglobin; other types are aplastic anemia, hemolytic anemia, pernicious anemia, sickle cell anemia, and thalassemia

Angina pectoris (an-JYE-nah PECK-tohr-is) Acute chest pain caused by decreased blood supply to the heart muscle

Arteriosclerosis (ahr-tee-rih-oh-skleh-ROH-sis) A condition of hardening of an artery; an artery becomes less elastic and does not expand under pressure

Atherosclerosis (ath-er-oh-skleh-ROH-sis) A form of arteriosclerosis characterized by the buildup of fatty plaques in the wall of the vessel

Cardiac arrest (KAR-dee-ack ah-REST) Cessation of an effective heartbeat; heart may be completely stopped or quivering ineffectively in fibrillation

Cardiomegaly (kar-dee-oh-MEG-ah-lee) Enlargement of the heart

Cardiomyopathy (kar-dee-oh-my-AHP-ah-thee) Any primary disease of the heart muscle

Congestive heart failure (kahn-JES-tiv HART FAIL-yer) Condition in which the heart's pumping ability is impaired, resulting in fluid accumulation in vessels and tissue spaces; various stages of difficult breathing occur as fluid accumulates in pulmonary vessels and lung tissue

Ecchymosis (eck-ih-MOH-sis) A blue or purplish patch in the skin caused by intradermal hemorrhage; larger than a petechia (see later); a bruise; plural, *ecchymoses*

Embolus (EMM-boh-lus) A moving clot or other plug; an object, often a blood clot, that moves in the blood until it obstructs a small vessel and blocks circulation

Fibrillation (fib-rih-LAY-shun) Rapid, random, ineffectual, and irregular contractions of the heart at 350 or more beats per minute

Heart block (HART BLOCK) Impairment of conduction of impulses from the sinoatrial node to heart muscle

Hemophilia (hee-moh-FILL-ih-ah) Excessive bleeding caused by a congenital lack of one or more of the factors necessary for blood clotting; treatment of hemophilia is directed at replacing the missing clotting factors to control and prevent bleeding

Hemorrhoids (HEM-oh-royds) Varicose veins in the anal canal resulting from a persistent increase in venous pressure

Mitral valve prolapse (MY-tral valve PRO-laps) Improper closure of the mitral valve when the heart is pumping blood; also called *floppy valve syndrome*

Myocardial infarction (mye-oh-KAR-dee-ahl in-FARK-shun) Destruction of a region of heart muscle as a result of oxygen deprivation because of a blockage in blood vessels to that area; sometimes called a *heart attack* or *MI*

Petechia (pee-TEE-kee-ah) A pinpoint, purplish red spot in the skin caused by intradermal hemorrhage; plural, *petechiae*

Phlebitis (fleh-BYE-tis) Inflammation of veins, which may be caused by pooling and stagnation of blood; often leads to the formation of blood clots within the vessel

Polycythemia (pahl-ee-sye-THEE-mee-ah) Any type of increase in the number of RBCs

Purpura (PER-pyoo-rah) A group of disorders characterized by multiple pinpoint hemorrhages and accumulation of blood under the skin

Thrombus (THRAHM-bus) A blood clot

Valvular heart disease (VAL-vyoo-lar HART dih-ZEEZ) Any disorder of the heart valves including insufficiency, stenosis, and prolapse

Varicose veins (VAIR-ih-kohs VANES) Abnormally swollen, distended, and knotted veins, usually in the subcutaneous tissues of the leg

Vasculitis (vas-kew-LYE-tis) Inflammation of a vessel; also called *angiitis*

Venous insufficiency (VANE-us in-suh-FISH-en-see) Condition in which damaged or missing valves, especially in the deep veins of the leg, interfere with the return of blood to the heart and the blood collects in the legs and feet; often results in the formation of blood clots

Procedures

Angioplasty (AN-jih-oh-plas-tee) Surgical repair of a blood vessel or vessels

Arterectomy (ahr-teh-RECK-toh-mee) Surgical removal of an artery

Artificial pacemaker (ahr-tih-FISH-al PAYSE-may-ker) An electronic device that stimulates the initiation of an impulse within the heart

Atherectomy (ath-er-ECK-toh-mee) Surgical removal of plaque from the interior lining of an artery

Cardiac catheterization (KAR-dee-ack kath-eh-ter-ih-ZAY-shun) The process of inserting a thin, flexible tube, called a *catheter,* into a vein or artery and guiding it into the heart for the purpose of detecting pressures and patterns of blood flow

Coronary artery bypass grafting (CABG) A surgical procedure in which a blood vessel from another part of the body is used to bypass the blocked region of a coronary artery

Defibrillation (dee-fib-rih-LAY-shun) A procedure in which an electric shock is applied to the heart with a defibrillator to stop an abnormal heart rhythm

Echocardiography (eck-oh-kar-dee-AHG-rah-fee) A noninvasive clinical procedure using pulses of high-frequency sound waves (ultrasound) that are transmitted into the chest; echoes returning from the valves, chambers, and surfaces of the heart are plotted and recorded; provides information about valvular or structural defects and coronary artery disease

Plasmapheresis (plaz-mah-feh-REE-sis) The removal of plasma from withdrawn blood with the retransfusion of the formed elements into the donor ∎

interatrial septum. This represents an opening, the foramen ovale, that is present between the atria in the fetal heart.

The **right ventricle** (VEN-trih-kull) receives blood from the right atrium and pumps it out to the lungs, where it picks up a new supply of oxygen. The **left ventricle** receives blood from the left atrium and pumps it out to the tissues of the whole body. The ventricles are "pumping" chambers, and this is reflected by a thick myocardium. Because the left ventricle pumps blood to the whole body and the right ventricle sends blood only to the lungs, the left ventricle has to generate a lot more pumping force than the right ventricle. This is reflected in the fact that the left ventricular wall has a thicker myocardium than the right. Both ventricles hold about the same volume of blood. The thick, muscular partition between the right and left ventricles is the **interventricular septum.**

Highlight on the Circulatory System

Blood doping: Blood doping is a practice reportedly used by some athletes to improve their endurance for aerobic activities such as running, swimming, and cycling. A few weeks before a competition, blood is drawn from the athlete and the red blood cells (RBCs) are separated and frozen. Normal hematopoiesis replaces the lost RBCs and brings the blood cell count back to normal. Then, just before the competition, the frozen RBCs are thawed and injected into the athlete. This creates an artificial polycythemia. The idea is that the additional RBCs are able to deliver more oxygen to the muscles and improve aerobic endurance. Whether this occurs is questionable, and the practice is not without danger. All blood transfusions carry some risk. Furthermore, the additional cells increase the viscosity or thickness of the blood and put a strain on the heart.

Pericarditis: Pericarditis is an inflammation of the pericardium. This may interfere with production of the serous fluid that lubricates the surfaces of the parietal and visceral layers. Painful adhesions may form and interfere with contraction of the heart.

Damaged heart valves: Sometimes disease processes damage the heart valves so that they are unable to function properly. Incompetent valves permit a "backflow" of blood, and the heart has to pump the same blood over and over to get it into the vessels. In valvular stenosis, the valves are stiff and have narrow openings. The heart has to work harder to pump blood out through the small opening. Defective heart valves may result in abnormal heart sounds. For example, if the atrioventricular valves are faulty, a hissing sound may be heard between the first and second heart sounds.

Angina pectoris: Angina pectoris is chest pain that results when the heart muscle's demand for oxygen exceeds the oxygen supply. Nitroglycerin is sometimes used in the treatment of angina pectoris because it dilates blood vessels, so the patient is less likely to develop a myocardial oxygen deficit.

Coronary artery blockage: If a branch of a coronary artery becomes blocked, blood supply to that region of the heart is cut off and the muscle cells in that area die because of lack of oxygen. This is a myocardial infarction (MI), also called a *coronary* or a *heart attack.* The extent of the damage and chances of recovery depend on the location of the blockage and the length of time that elapses before medical intervention occurs.

Heart enzymes: When heart muscle is damaged, the dying cells release enzymes into the bloodstream. These enzymes can be measured and are useful in confirming an MI. The enzymes assayed are creatine kinase (CK) and lactate dehydrogenase (LDH).

Dysrhythmias: Variations in normal contraction patterns are called *dysrhythmias* (arrhythmias). One type of dysrhythmia occurs when a conduction myofiber or heart muscle cell independently depolarizes to threshold and triggers a premature heart contraction. The cell responsible for the premature contraction is called an *ectopic focus.* Sometimes ectopic foci form feedback loops within the conduction system, causing myocardial contractions to occur at a rapid rate. If not treated properly, this often leads to ventricular tachycardia, fibrillation, and death.

Red bone marrow: By the age of 25 years, a person's red bone marrow for hematopoiesis is limited to the flat bones of the skull, iliac crests, ribs, sternum, vertebrae, and proximal ends of the humerus and femur.

Smoking: About 20% of a cigarette smoker's hemoglobin is nonfunctional for transporting oxygen because it is bound to carbon monoxide from the cigarette smoke.

Reticulocytes: The reticulocyte count in circulating blood gives information about the rate of hematopoiesis. Normally 0.5% to 1.5% of the RBCs in normal blood are reticulocytes. A number below 0.5% indicates a slowdown in production. Values above 1.5% indicate a greater-than-normal rate of RBC formation.

Vitamin K: The *K* in vitamin K is for *koagulation,* the German word for clotting. In other words, vitamin K is the "koagulation" vitamin. Although this vitamin is necessary in the diet, it is also produced by bacteria in the large intestine and absorbed into the blood.

Aneurysm: An aneurysm is a bulge, or bubble, that develops at a weakened region in the wall of an artery. This is especially dangerous if it is in the aorta or arteries of the brain. If diagnosed soon enough, the aneurysm sometimes may be removed and the vessel surgically repaired. Because the wall is weakened, an aneurysm is subject to rupture. Little can be done when this happens because the massive bleeding usually leads to death before medical care can be obtained.

Continued

Highlight on the Circulatory System—cont'd

Blood vessels: It is estimated that if all the capillaries in the body were placed end to end, they would encircle the earth at the equator two and one-half times! The difference in blood pressure between arteries and veins is obvious when the vessels are cut. Blood flows smoothly and freely from a vein, but it spurts forcefully from an artery.

Varicose veins: Varicose veins are veins that are twisted and dilated with accumulated blood. These frequently occur in the legs. Conditions that hinder venous return, such as pregnancy, obesity, and standing for long periods of time, allow blood to accumulate in the veins of the extremities. This stretches the veins, so the valve flaps no longer overlap and they permit the backflow of blood. Superficial veins are more susceptible because they receive less support from surrounding tissue.

Sunbathing: When you are in the sun for an extended period, the cutaneous blood vessels dilate to bring more blood to the skin's surface, which helps keep the body cool. This action decreases the amount of blood in other parts of the body and may diminish the blood supply to the brain. If you are sunbathing and stand up abruptly, you may feel dizzy. This is because the blood momentarily remains in the dilated cutaneous vessels instead of returning to the heart. This causes a decrease in blood pressure. The dizziness is a signal that the brain is not receiving enough oxygen.

Rising rapidly and dizziness: Sometimes there is a feeling of dizziness when rising rapidly from lying down to a standing position. This is because the body has not had time to respond to the decrease in blood pressure caused by the downward pull of gravity on the blood. The dizziness is a signal that the brain is not receiving enough blood.

Hole in the heart: When the foramen ovale between the two atria fails to close after birth, the result is an interatrial septal defect. Because pressure in the right atrium is lower than in the left, blood flows from the left atrium back into the right atrium without going through the systemic circulation. This defect overloads the pulmonary circulation and puts a strain on the heart as it attempts to pump enough blood to maintain adequate supplies to the body tissues. ∎

Valves of the Heart

Pumps need a set of valves to keep the fluid flowing in one direction, and the heart is no exception. The heart has two types of valves that keep the blood flowing in the correct direction. The valves between the atria and ventricles are called **atrioventricular** (ay-tree-oh-ven-TRIK-yoo-lar) **(AV) valves.** The valves at the base of the large vessels leaving the ventricles are called **semilunar** (seh-mee-LOO-nar) **(SL) valves**.

Atrioventricular Valves

The AV valves permit the flow of blood from the atria into the corresponding ventricle. They also prevent the backflow of blood from the ventricles into the atria. Each valve consists of a fibrous connective tissue ring and double folds of endocardium that form the **cusps** of the valve. The valve cusps are attached to the ventricles by connective tissue strings called **chordae tendineae** (KOR-dee ten-DIN-ee) (see Figure 12-3). As blood returns to the atria, it pushes the valve cusps open and the blood flows into the ventricles. When the ventricles contract, the force of the blood against the cusps causes them to close and prevents the backward flow of blood into the atria.

The AV valve between the right atrium and right ventricle has three cusps and is called the **tricuspid valve.** The valve between the left atrium and left ventricle has only two cusps and is called the **bicuspid,** or **mitral, valve** (see Figure 12-3).

Semilunar Valves

The **SL valves** are located at the bases of the large vessels that carry blood from the ventricles (see Figure 12-3). Each valve consists of three cuplike cusps. Contraction of the ventricles increases the pressure of the blood so that it pushes the valves open and the blood leaves the heart. As the ventricles relax and pressure decreases, the blood starts to flow back down the large vessels toward the ventricles. When the blood flows toward the ventricles, it enters the "cups" of the valve cusps. This closes the opening of the valves and prevents the flow of blood back into the ventricles.

The valve at the exit of the right ventricle is in the base of the pulmonary trunk and is called the **pulmonary SL valve.** The valve at the exit of the left ventricle is in the base of the ascending aorta. It is called the **aortic SL valve** (see Figure 12-3).

Pathway of Blood through the Heart

Although it is convenient to describe the flow of blood through the right side of the heart and then through the left side, it is important to realize that both atria contract at the same time and that both ventricles contract at the same time. The heart functions as two pumps, one on the right and one on the left, that work simultaneously. The "right pump" pumps the blood to the lungs (**pulmonary circulation**) at the same time that the "left pump" pumps blood to the rest of the body (**systemic circulation**). The sequence in which the chambers contract is described in more detail with the cardiac cycle.

The arrows in Figure 12-4 depict the direction in which blood flows through the heart. Venous blood from the systemic circulation is relatively low in oxygen and high in carbon dioxide content. This blood enters the **right atrium** through the superior vena cava and inferior vena cava. It

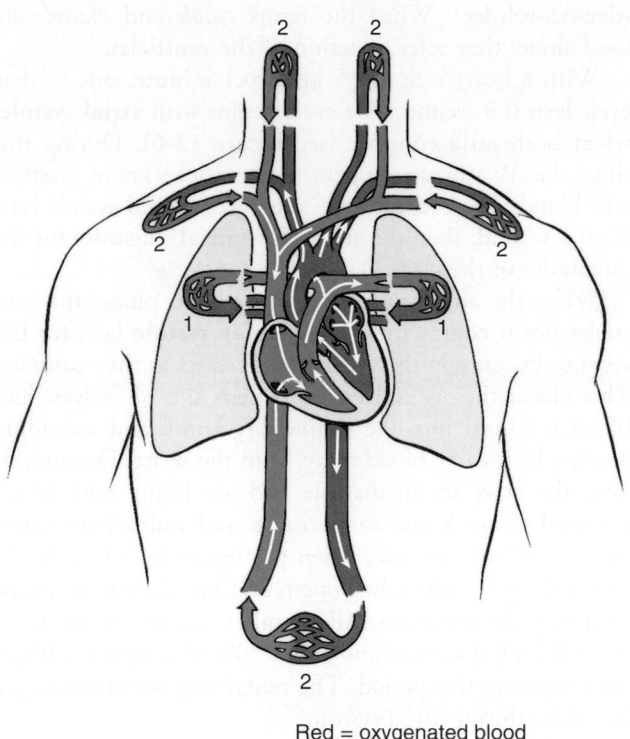

Red = oxygenated blood

Blue = deoxygenated blood

1 = capillary beds of lungs
where gas exchange occurs

2 = capillary beds of body tissues
where gas exchange occurs

Figure 12-4 Pathway of the blood through the heart: Superior vena cava (SVC) and inferior vena cava (IVC) → Right atrium → Tricuspid valve → Right ventricle → Pulmonary semilunar (SL) valve → Pulmonary trunk → Pulmonary arteries → Capillaries of lungs → Pulmonary veins → Left atrium → Bicuspid valve → Left ventricle → Aortic SL valve → Ascending aorta → Systemic circulation.

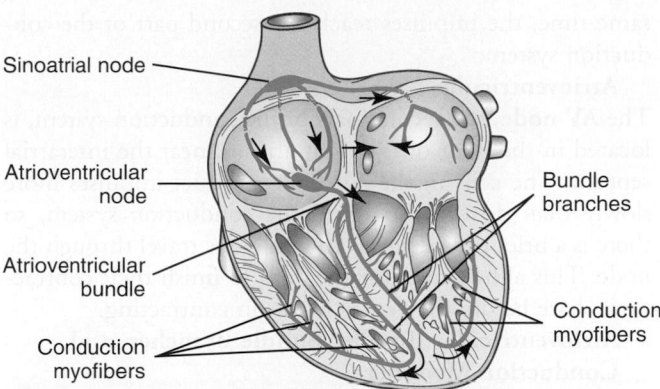

Figure 12-5 Conduction system of the heart. Impulses travel from the sinoatrial (SA) node (pacemaker) → Atrioventricular (AV) node → AV bundle → Right and left bundle branches → Conduction myofibers → Myocardium.

then flows through the **tricuspid valve** into the **right ventricle.** From the right ventricle, it passes through the **pulmonary SL valve** into the **pulmonary trunk** and then into the **pulmonary arteries.** The **pulmonary arteries** carry the blood to the **lungs.** In the lungs the blood releases carbon dioxide and picks up a new supply of oxygen. **Pulmonary veins** then carry the blood to the **left atrium.** From the left atrium, the blood flows through the **bicuspid valve** into the **left ventricle.** The blood then flows through the **aortic SL valve** into the **ascending aorta.** Oxygen-rich blood flowing into the aorta is distributed to all parts of the body through the systemic circulation.

Blood Supply to the Myocardium

The myocardium of the heart wall is working muscle that needs a continuous supply of oxygen and nutrients to function with efficiency. Unlike skeletal muscle, cardiac muscle cannot build up an oxygen debt to be repaid at a later time. It needs a continuous oxygen supply or it dies. For this reason, cardiac muscle has an extensive network of blood vessels to bring oxygen to the contracting cells and to remove waste products.

Two main coronary arteries branch from the ascending aorta just distal to the aortic SL valve. They are the **right and left coronary arteries.** The right and left coronary arteries have numerous branches. Blood flow through the coronary arteries is greatest when the myocardium is relaxed. When the ventricles contract, they compress the arteries, which reduces the flow.

Physiology of the Heart

The work of the heart is to pump blood to the lungs through the pulmonary circulation and to the rest of the body through the systemic circulation. This is accomplished by contraction and relaxation of the cardiac muscle in the myocardium.

Conduction System

An effective cycle for productive pumping of blood requires that the heart be synchronized accurately. Both atria need to contract simultaneously, followed by contraction of both ventricles. Contraction of the chambers is coordinated by specialized cardiac muscle cells that make up the **conduction system** of the heart.

Components of the Conduction System

Sinoatrial Node

The conduction system includes several components (Figure 12-5). The first part of the conduction system is the **sinoatrial (SA) node** (sye-noh-AY-tree-al node), which is located in the right atrium, near the entrance of the superior vena cava. Without any neural stimulation, the SA node rhythmically initiates impulses 70 to 80 times per minute. Because it establishes the basic rhythm of the heartbeat, it is called the **pacemaker** of the heart. The impulses from the SA node rapidly travel throughout the atrial myocardium and cause the two atria to contract simultaneously. At the same time, the impulses reach the second part of the conduction system.

Atrioventricular Node

The **AV node,** the second part of the conduction system, is located in the floor of the right atrium, near the interatrial septum. The cells in the AV node conduct impulses more slowly than do other parts of the conduction system, so there is a brief time delay as the impulses travel through the node. This allows time for the atria to finish their contraction phase before the ventricles begin contracting.

Atrioventricular Bundle, Bundle Branches, and Conduction Myofibers

From the AV node, the impulses rapidly travel through the **AV bundle** (bundle of His) to the **right** and **left bundle branches.** The bundle branches extend along the right and left sides of the interventricular septum to the apex. These branch profusely to form **conduction myofibers** (Purkinje fibers), which transmit the impulses to the myocardium. The AV bundle, bundle branches, and conduction myofibers rapidly transmit impulses throughout all the ventricular myocardium so that both ventricles contract at the same time. As the ventricles contract, blood is forced out through the SL valves into the pulmonary trunk and the ascending aorta. After the ventricles complete their contraction phase, they relax and the SA node initiates another impulse to start another cardiac cycle.

Cardiac Cycle

The **cardiac cycle** refers to the alternating contraction and relaxation of the heart chambers during one heartbeat (Figure 12-6). The two atria contract at the same time; then they relax while the two ventricles simultaneously contract. The contraction phase of the chambers is called **systole** (SIS-toh-lee); the relaxation phase is called **diastole** (dye-AS-toh-lee). When the terms *systole* and *diastole* are used alone, they refer to action of the ventricles.

With a heart rate of 75 beats per minute, one cardiac cycle lasts 0.8 second. The cycle begins with **atrial systole,** when both atria contract (see Figure 12-6). During this time, the AV valves are open, the ventricles are in diastole, and blood is forced into the ventricles. Atrial systole lasts for 0.1 second; then the atria relax **(atrial diastole)** for the remainder of the cycle, 0.7 second.

When the atria finish their contraction phase, the ventricles begin contracting. **Ventricular systole** lasts for 0.3 second. Pressure in the ventricles increases as they contract. This closes the AV valves and opens the SL valves, and blood is forced into the pulmonary trunk and ascending aorta, which carry blood away from the heart. During this time the atria are in diastole and are filling with blood returned through the venae cavae and pulmonary veins. After ventricular systole, when the ventricles relax, the SL valves close, the AV valves open, and blood flows from the atria into the ventricles. All chambers are in simultaneous diastole for 0.4 second, and about 70% of ventricular filling occurs during this period. The remaining blood enters the ventricles during atrial systole.

Heart Sounds

The sounds associated with the heartbeat are caused by the closure of the valves of the heart. A **stethoscope** is used to listen to these sounds, usually described as *lubb-dupp.* The **first heart sound,** the lubb, is caused by closure of the AV valves. The **second heart sound,** the dupp, is caused by closure of the SL valves. It has a higher pitch than the first heart sound. There is a pause between the dupp of the first beat and the lubb of the second beat when the entire heart is resting. Therefore the sequence is lubb-dupp, pause,

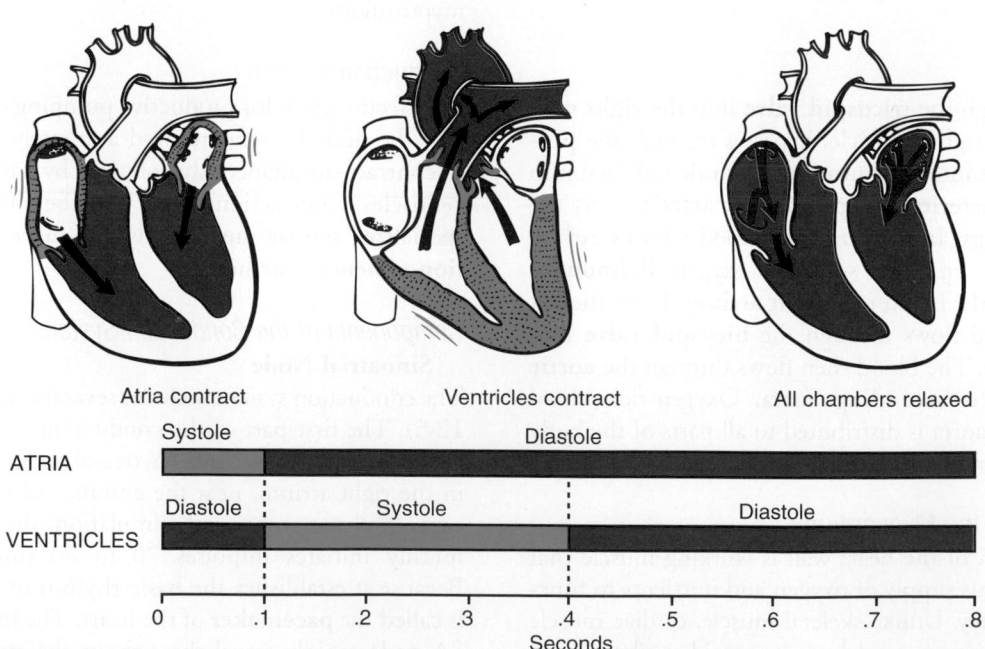

Figure 12-6 Cardiac cycle. Atrial systole is followed by ventricular systole. All chambers are simultaneously in diastole for one half of the cycle.

lubb-dupp, pause, lubb-dupp, pause, and so on. Abnormal heart sounds, called **murmurs,** are caused by faulty valves.

BLOOD

The body consists of active cells that need a continuous supply of nutrients and oxygen. Metabolic waste products need to be removed from the cells for maintenance of a stable cellular environment. Blood is the primary transport medium responsible for meeting these cellular demands. The heart provides the force to move the blood through a system of vessels that extend throughout the body.

Functions and Characteristics of Blood

Blood is one of the connective tissues. As a connective tissue, it consists of cells and cell fragments (**formed elements**) suspended in an intercellular matrix (**plasma**). Blood is the only liquid tissue in the body. The total blood volume in an average adult is 4 to 5 L in women and 5 to 6 L in men. It accounts for approximately 8% of the total body weight. Blood is slightly heavier and four to five times more viscous than water. It is slightly alkaline, with a normal pH range of 7.35 to 7.45.

The activities of the blood may be categorized as **transportation, regulation,** and **protection.** These functional categories overlap and interact as the blood carries out its role in providing suitable conditions for cellular functions. The following activities of blood are transport functions:

- It carries oxygen and nutrients to the cells of the body.
- It transports carbon dioxide and nitrogenous wastes from the tissues to the lungs and kidneys, where these wastes can be removed from the body.
- It carries hormones from the endocrine glands to the target tissues.

The following activities of blood are in the regulation category:

- It helps regulate body temperature by removing heat from active areas, such as skeletal muscles, and transporting it to other regions or to the skin, where it can be dissipated.
- It plays a significant role in fluid and electrolyte balance because the salts and plasma proteins contribute to the osmotic pressure.
- It functions in pH regulation through the action of buffers in the blood.

Functions of the blood that are in the protection category include the following:

- Its clotting mechanisms prevent fluid loss through hemorrhage when blood vessels are damaged.
- Certain cells in the blood, the phagocytic white blood cells (WBCs), help to protect the body against microorganisms that cause disease by engulfing and destroying the agent.
- Antibodies in the plasma help protect against disease by their reactions with offending agents.

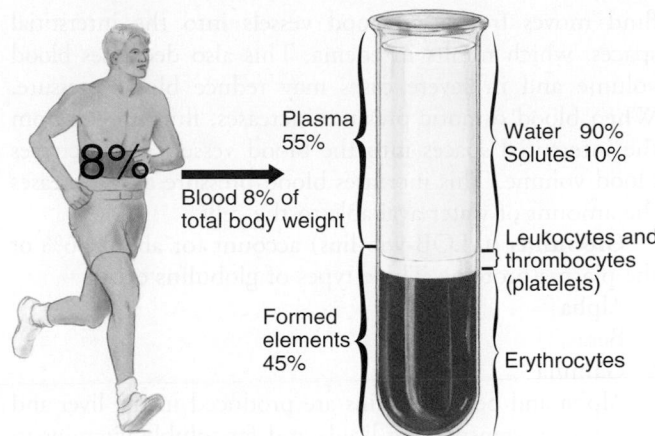
Figure 12-7 Composition of the blood.

Composition of Blood

When a sample of blood is spun in a centrifuge, the cells and cell fragments are separated from the liquid part of the blood (Figure 12-7). Because the **formed elements** are heavier than the liquid, they are packed in the bottom of the tube by the centrifugal force. The straw-colored liquid on the top is the **plasma.** Figure 12-7 illustrates that the plasma accounts for about 55% of the blood volume and red blood cells (RBCs) make up the remaining 45% of the volume. The WBCs and platelets form a thin white layer, called the "buffy coat," between the plasma and RBCs.

Plasma

Plasma, the liquid portion of the blood, is about 90% water. The remaining portion consists of more than 100 different organic and inorganic solutes dissolved in the water. Because plasma is a transport medium, its solutes are continuously changing as substances are added or removed by the cells. With a healthy diet, the plasma is normally in a state of dynamic balance that is maintained by various homeostatic mechanisms.

Plasma Proteins

Plasma proteins are the most abundant of the solutes in the plasma. These proteins normally remain in the blood and interstitial fluid and are not used for energy. The three major classes of plasma proteins are as follows:

- Albumins
- Globulins
- Fibrinogen

Many of the plasma proteins are synthesized in the liver, and each one has a different function. Liver damage or dysfunction affects the synthesis of plasma proteins.

Albumins (al-BYOO-mins) account for about 60% of the plasma proteins. Albumin molecules are produced in the liver and are the smallest of the plasma protein molecules. Because they are so abundant, they contribute to the osmotic pressure of the blood and play an important role in maintaining fluid balance between the blood and interstitial fluid. If the osmotic pressure of the blood decreases, fluid moves from the blood vessels into the interstitial spaces, which results in edema. This also decreases blood volume and in severe cases may reduce blood pressure. When blood osmotic pressure increases, fluid moves from the interstitial spaces into the blood vessels and increases blood volume. This increases blood pressure and decreases the amount of water available to the cells.

Globulins (GLOB-yoo-lins) account for about 36% of the plasma proteins. Three types of globulins exist:

- Alpha
- Beta
- Gamma

Alpha and beta globulins are produced in the liver and function in transporting lipids and fat-soluble vitamins in the blood. Gamma globulins are the antibodies that function in immunity. These are produced in lymphoid tissue.

The remaining 4% of the plasma proteins consists of **fibrinogen** (fye-BRIN-oh-jen), which is the largest of the plasma protein molecules. It is produced in the liver and functions in blood clotting. During the clotting process, a series of reactions converts the soluble fibrinogen into insoluble fibrin, which forms the foundation of a blood clot. When blood clots in a test tube, the liquid that remains is called **serum.** It is similar to plasma but has no fibrinogen because the fibrinogen is converted to fibrin.

Other Solutes

Although protein molecules are the most abundant of the solutes in the plasma, there are additional solutes that play a significant role in homeostasis. Urea and uric acid are waste products of protein metabolism and may become toxic if allowed to accumulate. They are transported, as solutes in plasma, to the kidneys for excretion. The simple molecules that are the end products of digestion are transported as solutes in the plasma. Other plasma solutes include the respiratory gases, oxygen and carbon dioxide, and electrolytes that are important in muscle contraction, nerve impulse conduction, and pH of body fluids.

Formed Elements

The formed elements are cells and cell fragments suspended in the plasma. The three classes of formed elements are the **erythrocytes** (ee-RITH-roh-sytes), or RBCs; the **leukocytes** (LOO-koh-sytes), or WBCs; and the **thrombocytes** (THROM-boh-sytes), or platelets.

The production of these formed elements, or blood cells, is called **hematopoiesis** (hemopoiesis). Before birth, hematopoiesis (hee-ma-to-poy-EE-sis) occurs primarily in the liver and spleen. After birth, most production is limited to the red bone marrow in specific regions of the body, but some WBCs are produced in lymphoid tissue. All types of formed elements develop from a single cell type. The precursor cell, or stem cell, is called a **hemocytoblast** (hee-moh-SYTE-oh-blast). Seven different cell lines develop from the hemocytoblast. Figure 12-8 illustrates the formed elements.

Erythrocytes

Characteristics and Functions

Erythrocytes (ee-RITH-roh-sytes), or RBCs, are the most numerous of the formed elements. The normal RBC range for a woman is 4 to 5.5 million RBCs per cubic millimeter (mm^3) of blood. The normal RBC range for a man is 4.5 to 6.2 million RBCs per cubic millimeter of blood.

Erythrocytes are tiny **biconcave discs** about 7.5 micrometers (μm) in diameter. They are thin in the middle and thicker around the periphery. The shape of the RBC provides a combination of flexibility for moving through tiny capillaries along with a maximum surface area for the diffusion of gases. Mature RBCs are **anucleate,** meaning they do not have a nucleus. During development the nucleus is lost from the cell, presumably to give the cell more room for hemoglobin. Because the mature cells are anucleate, they cannot undergo mitosis, which means that replacement cells have to develop from the stem cells. The primary function of erythrocytes is to transport oxygen and, to a lesser extent, carbon dioxide. This function is directly related to the **hemoglobin** (hee-moh-GLOH-bin) within the RBC.

Production of Erythrocytes

Erythrocyte production, specifically called **erythropoiesis,** is regulated by a negative feedback mechanism that uses the hormone **erythropoietin** (ee-rith-roh-POY-ee-tin) to stimulate erythrocyte production (Figure 12-9). The liver produces erythropoietin in an inactive form and secretes it into the blood. The kidneys produce **renal erythropoietic factor** (REF), which activates the erythropoietin. When blood oxygen concentration is low, the kidneys release REF into the blood, which activates the erythropoietin, which then stimulates the red bone marrow to produce RBCs. The additional RBCs combine with oxygen to increase the blood oxygen concentration. As blood oxygen concentration increases, levels of REF and active erythropoietin decrease and RBC production decreases.

Iron, vitamin B$_{12}$, and folic acid are essential to normal RBC production. The iron is necessary for the synthesis of normal hemoglobin. Iron deficiency anemia results when there is a lack of iron in the diet. This results in a reduced amount of hemoglobin, which decreases the blood's oxygen-carrying capacity. All cells in the body require vitamins B$_{12}$ and folic acid for normal formation. This is especially significant in erythrocytes because of the large numbers produced every day. Certain cells in the stomach produce **intrinsic factor,** a factor necessary for the absorption of vitamin B$_{12}$ in the intestines. Without intrinsic factor, vitamin B$_{12}$ (even though present in the diet) cannot be absorbed. This results in a condition known as **pernicious anemia.**

Destruction of Erythrocytes

Normal erythrocytes live for approximately 120 days. During this time they travel thousands of miles as they circulate throughout the body. Normally the erythrocytes have a flexible cell membrane that allows them to bend and squeeze through the capillaries. As they age, however, their membrane loses its elasticity and becomes fragile. When they are defective or worn out, macrophages, which are

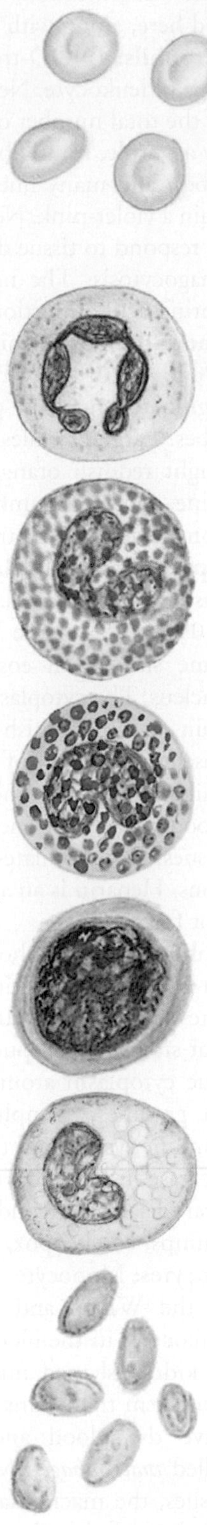

Erythrocytes

Biconcave disks; no nucleus; 7 to 8 μm in diameter; 4.5 to 6.0 million/mm^3
Function to transport oxygen and carbon dioxide

Leukocytes

Nucleated cells; 5000 to 9000/mm^3
Function as part of body's defense against disease

Neutrophils

Nucleus with 2 to 5 lobes; indistinct granules in cytoplasm; 12 to 15 μm in diameter 60% to 70% of total WBCs
Function in phagocytosis

Eosinophils

Bilobed nucleus; red-staining granules in cytoplasm; 10 to 12 μm in diameter 2% to 4% of total WBCs
Function to counteract histamine in allergic reactions; destroy parasitic worms

Basophils

U-shaped or bilobed nucleus; granules in cytoplasm stain blue; 10 to 12 μm in diameter
Less than 1% of total WBCs
Function to release histamine and the anticoagulant heparin; called *mast cells*, in the tissues

Lymphocytes

Agranulocyte; small cell with large round nucleus; 6 to 8 μm in diameter
20% to 25% of total WBCs
Function in immunity; produce antibodies

Monocytes

Agranulocyte; large cells with bean-shaped nucleus; may be 20 μm in diameter
3% to 8% of total WBCs
Function in phagocytosis; engulf relatively large particles; called *macrophages* in tissues

Thrombocytes

Cell fragments of megakaryocytes; 2 to 5 μm in diameter
250,000 to 500,000/mm^3
Function in hemostasis by forming platelet plug and releasing factors necessary for blood clotting

Figure 12-8 **Formed elements in the blood.**

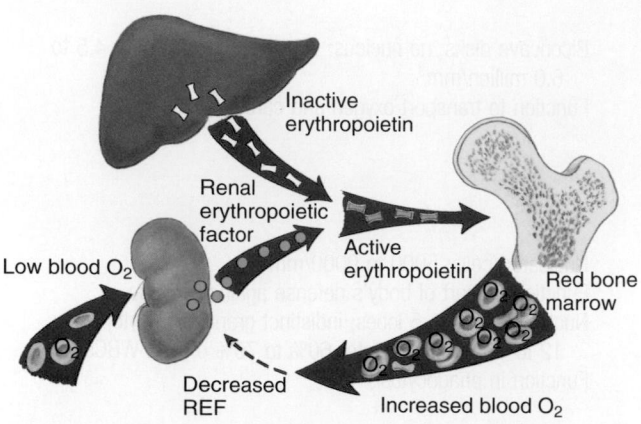

Inactive
erythropoietin

Renal
erythropoietic
factor

Low blood O$_2$

Active
erythropoietin

Red bone
marrow

Decreased
REF

Increased blood O$_2$

Figure 12-9 Regulation of erythrocyte production. The liver secretes inactive erythropoietin into the blood. In response to low blood O$_2$, the kidneys release renal erythropoietic factor (REF) into the blood. This activates the erythropoietin, which stimulates the bone marrow to produce RBCs.

phagocytic cells in the spleen and liver, remove them from circulation, and they are replaced by an equal number of new cells. Under typical conditions, more than 2 million erythrocytes are destroyed and replaced every second. Bilirubin, a yellow pigment, is a by-product of RBC destruction. It becomes a part of bile and is secreted by the liver.

Leukocytes

Characteristics and Functions

Leukocytes (WBCs) are generally larger than erythrocytes, but they are fewer in number. A normal WBC count ranges from 4500 to 11,000/mm^3. All leukocytes are derived from hemocytoblast stem cells (see Figure 12-8), but they do not lose their nuclei or accumulate hemoglobin during development. The lack of hemoglobin makes them appear whitish.

Even though they are considered to be blood cells, leukocytes do most of their work in the tissues. They use the blood as a transport medium. Some are phagocytic, others produce antibodies, some secrete histamine and heparin, and others neutralize histamine. Leukocytes are able to move through the capillary walls into the tissue spaces, a process called **diapedesis** (dye-ah-peh-DEE-sis). In the tissue spaces they provide a defense against organisms that cause disease.

Types of Leukocytes

Blood contains two main groups of leukocytes. The cells that develop granules in the cytoplasm are called **granular leukocytes (granulocytes),** and those that do not have granules are called **nongranular leukocytes (agranulocytes). Neutrophils, eosinophils,** and **basophils** are granular leukocytes. **Monocytes** and **lymphocytes** are nongranular leukocytes. Because WBCs are clear and colorless, they must be stained first with an appropriate dye (usually Wright stain) before they can be identified under the microscope. The nucleus, cytoplasm, and any granules in the cytoplasm take on the characteristic color of their cell type, which aids

in proper identification. The five types of WBCs are described here, along with their reactions to Wright stain.

Neutrophils: (NOO-troh-fills) are the most common type of leukocyte. Neutrophils make up 50% to 70% of the total number of WBCs. They are characterized by a purple, multilobed nucleus (usually three to five lobes) and many fine granules in the cytoplasm that stain a violet-pink. Neutrophils are the first leukocytes to respond to tissue damage, by engulfing bacteria by phagocytosis. The number of neutrophils increases during acute infections.

Eosinophils: Eosinophils (ee-oh-SIN-oh-fills) make up 1% to 4% of the WBCs. They are characterized by a segmented nucleus, generally of no more than two lobes. Large granules found in the cytoplasm stain a bright reddish orange. Eosinophils neutralize histamine, and their number increases during allergic reactions. They also destroy parasitic worms.

Basophils: Basophils (BAY-soh-fills) are the least numerous of the leukocytes. The normal range for basophils is 0% to 1% of the WBCs. A basophil is about the same size as an eosinophil and has an S-shaped nucleus. The cytoplasm has large, coarse granules that stain a dark bluish-black and almost completely obscure the details of the nucleus. In the tissues, basophils secrete histamine and heparin. Histamine dilates blood vessels to increase blood flow to damaged tissues. It also dilates blood vessels in allergic reactions. Heparin is an anticoagulant that inhibits blood clot formation.

Lymphocytes: Lymphocytes (LIM-foh-sytes) account for 20% to 35% of the WBCs in the blood. Lymphocytes have a large round or slightly indented nucleus that stains a deep purplish-blue. A small rim of sky-blue cytoplasm around the nucleus contains few or no granules. Lymphocytes are involved with the immune system and the production of antibodies. An increase in lymphocytes generally occurs with certain viral diseases, including infectious mononucleosis, mumps, chickenpox, rubella, and viral hepatitis.

Monocytes: Monocytes (MON-oh-sytes) are the largest of the WBCs and make up 3% to 8% of the leukocytes in the blood. Monocytes have a U-shaped or kidney-shaped nucleus surrounded by abundant cytoplasm that stains grayish-blue. When monocytes leave the blood and enter the tissues, they are called *macrophages* (MACK-roh-fayj-es). In damaged tissues, the macrophages engulf bacteria and cellular debris to finish the cleanup process started by the neutrophils.

Thrombocytes

Thrombocytes, or **platelets,** are not complete cells but small fragments of large cells called **megakaryocytes.** Megakaryocytes (meg-ah-KAIR-ee-oh-sytes) develop from hemocytoblasts in the red bone marrow. Platelets are one third to one half the size of an erythrocyte, and an average platelet count ranges from 150,000 to 500,000 platelets/mm³ of blood.

Thrombocytes become sticky and clump together to form platelet plugs that close breaks and tears in blood vessels. They also initiate the formation of blood clots.

Hemostasis

Blood vessels that are torn or cut permit blood to escape into the surrounding tissues or to the outside of the body. This has damaging effects on the tissues and, in cases of excessive blood loss, may result in death. Whenever blood vessels are injured, several reactions occur that attempt to minimize blood loss and tissue damage. The stoppage of bleeding is called **hemostasis** (hee-moh-STAY-sis). It includes three separate but interrelated processes:

- Vascular constriction
- Platelet plug formation
- Coagulation

Vascular Constriction

The first response to blood vessel injury is contraction of the smooth muscle in the vessel walls. This creates a **vascular constriction** that restricts the flow of blood through the opening in the vessel. The initial constriction lasts for only a few minutes but allows enough time for the other aspects of hemostasis to begin. As platelets accumulate at the site of the injury, they secrete **serotonin,** a chemical that stimulates smooth muscle contraction and prolongs the vascular constriction.

Platelet Plug Formation

Normally platelets do not stick to one another or to the lining of blood vessel walls. When the lining of the blood vessel breaks, the underlying connective tissue is exposed. The connective tissue attracts platelets and they accumulate in the damaged region, where they adhere to the connective tissue and to one another. This creates a mass of platelets, a **platelet plug,** that obstructs the tear in the vessel. Normal daily activities create numerous tears in minute blood vessels, and these are closed by platelet plugs so that there is no blood loss or damage to surrounding tissues.

Coagulation

The third and most effective mechanism in hemostasis is the formation of a blood clot, or **coagulation** (koh-ag-yoo-LAY-shun). The blood contains factors called **procoagulants** that promote clotting. It also contains **anticoagulants,** which inhibit clotting. Normally the anticoagulants predominate and override the procoagulants so that the blood remains fluid and does not clot. When vessels are damaged, the procoagulants increase their activity, which results in the formation of a clot.

The formation of a blood clot involves a complex series of chemical reactions and includes numerous clotting factors that are present in the plasma. Even though it is a complex process, it can be summarized in three main steps, as illustrated in Figure 12-10.

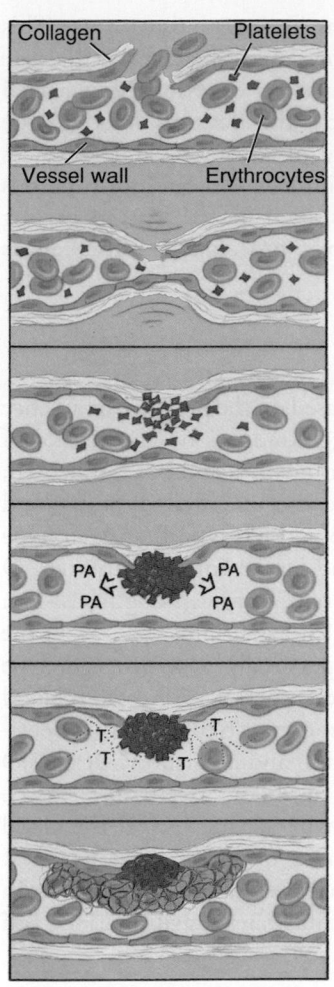

Figure 12-10 Hemostasis. The first response to vessel injury is a vascular spasm. This is followed by platelet plug formation. The third and most effective mechanism of hemostasis is the formation of a blood clot.

1. Platelets and damaged tissues release chemicals that initiate a series of reactions that result in the formation of **prothrombin activator.**
2. In the presence of calcium ions and prothrombin activator, **prothrombin** (pro-THROM-bin) in the plasma is converted from an inactive form to active **thrombin.**
3. Thrombin, in the presence of calcium ions, acts as an enzyme to convert inactive and soluble **fibrinogen** (fye-BRIN-oh-jen) into active and insoluble **fibrin.** The fibrin threads form a mesh that adheres to the damaged tissue and traps blood cells and platelets to form the clot.

Platelets and all the necessary clotting factors must be available for successful clot formation. The liver produces most of the clotting factors, and many of them require vitamin K for their synthesis. Numerous reactions in the clotting process also require calcium ions. A low platelet count (thrombocytopenia), deficiency of vitamin K or calcium, and liver dysfunction can impair the clotting process.

After a clot has formed, the fibrin strands contract. This process, called **clot retraction,** causes the clot to condense or shrink. Clot retraction pulls the edges of the damaged tissue closer together, reduces the flow of blood to the area, reduces the probability of infection, and enhances healing. Fibroblasts migrate into the clot and form fibrous connective tissue that repairs the damaged area. As healing occurs, the clot is dissolved by a process called **fibrinolysis** (fye-brin-AHL-ih-sis).

Blood Types

ABO Blood Groups

The ABO blood groups are based on the presence or absence of certain antigens called agglutinogens on the surface of the RBC membrane. These antigens, A and B, are inherited; consequently, blood types are also inherited. Type A blood has type A antigen; type B blood has type B antigen; type AB blood has both type A and type B antigens; and type O blood has neither type A nor type B antigen (Figure 12-11). Certain blood antibodies called agglutinins develop in the plasma shortly after birth. Specifically, a person with type A blood develops B antibodies; a person with type B blood develops A antibodies; a person with type AB blood develops neither A nor B antibodies; and a person with type O blood develops both A and B antibodies (see Figure 12-11).

Blood types are important in transfusions. If the blood types are different, the antibodies of the recipient may react with the antigens of the donor and cause hemolysis in the blood. Figure 12-12 illustrates agglutination and hemolysis.

Rh Blood Groups

Even after the ABO blood groups were well established and accurate blood typing procedures had been developed, there were still unexplained cases of transfusion reactions. This led to more research, which led to the discovery of the *Rh factor,* so named because it was first studied in the rhesus monkey.

People are Rh positive (Rh+) if they have Rh antigens on the surface of their RBCs. About 85% of people are Rh+. The other 15% do not have the Rh antigens and are Rh negative (Rh−). The presence or absence of Rh antigens is an inherited trait. Normally, neither Rh+ nor Rh− individuals have Rh antibodies. If an Rh− person is exposed to Rh+ blood, either through a blood transfusion or by transfer of blood between a mother and fetus, the Rh− individual develops Rh antibodies. If that individual is exposed to Rh+ blood a second time, a transfusion reaction results. When transfusions are given, it is necessary to match both the Rh type and the ABO type.

BLOOD VESSELS

Blood vessels are the channels through which blood is distributed to body tissues. The vessels make up two closed systems of tubes that begin and end at the heart (Figure 12-13). One system, the **pulmonary vessels,** transports

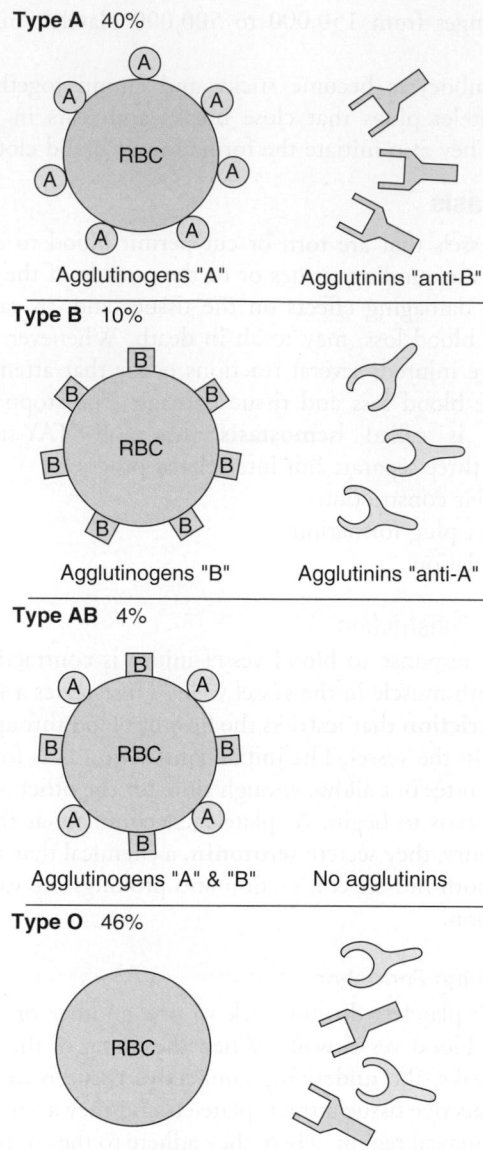

Figure 12-11 Agglutinogens (antigens) and agglutinins (antibodies) involved in the ABO blood groups.

blood from the right ventricle to the lungs and back to the left atrium. The other system, the **systemic vessels,** carries blood from the left ventricle to the tissues in all parts of the body and then returns the blood to the right atrium. Based on their structure and function, blood vessels are classified as arteries, capillaries, or veins.

Classification and Structure of Blood Vessels

Arteries

Arteries carry blood away from the heart. Pulmonary arteries transport blood that has a low oxygen content from the right ventricle to the lungs. Systemic arteries transport oxygenated blood from the left ventricle to the body tissues. Blood is pumped from the ventricles into large elastic arteries that branch repeatedly into smaller and smaller arteries until the branching results in microscopic arteries called

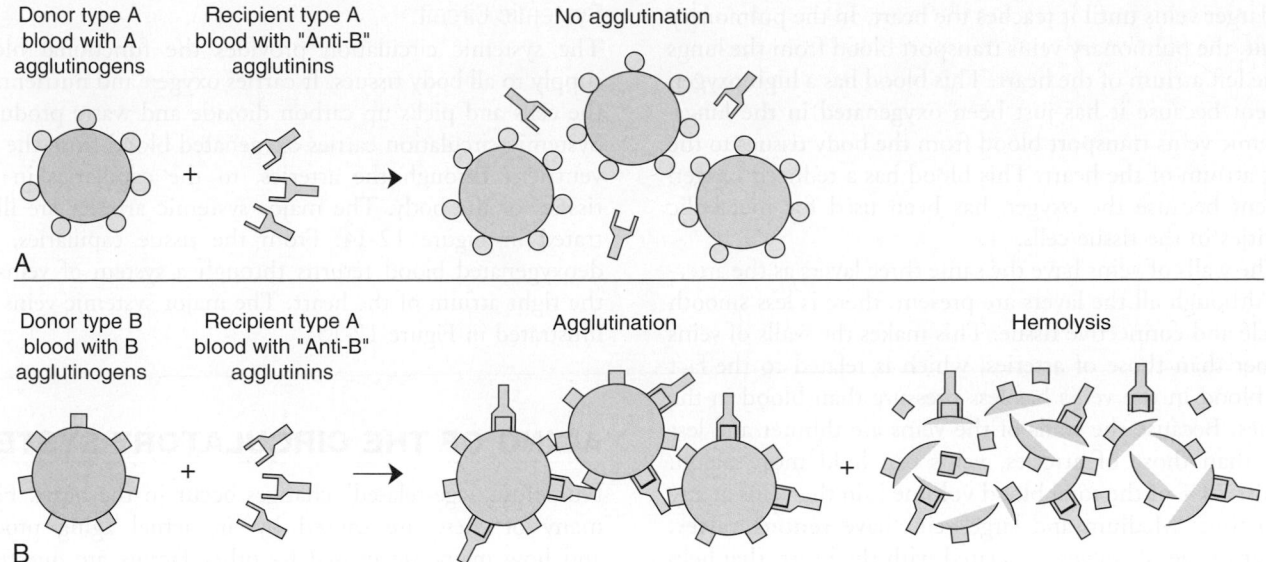

Donor type A
blood with A
agglutinogens

Recipient type A
blood with "Anti-B"
agglutinins

No agglutination

A

Donor type B
blood with B
agglutinogens

Recipient type A
blood with "Anti-B"
agglutinins

Agglutination

Hemolysis

B

Figure 12-12 Agglutination reactions. **A,** Type A donor and type A recipient results in no agglutination. **B,** Type B donor and type A recipient results in agglutination and hemolysis.

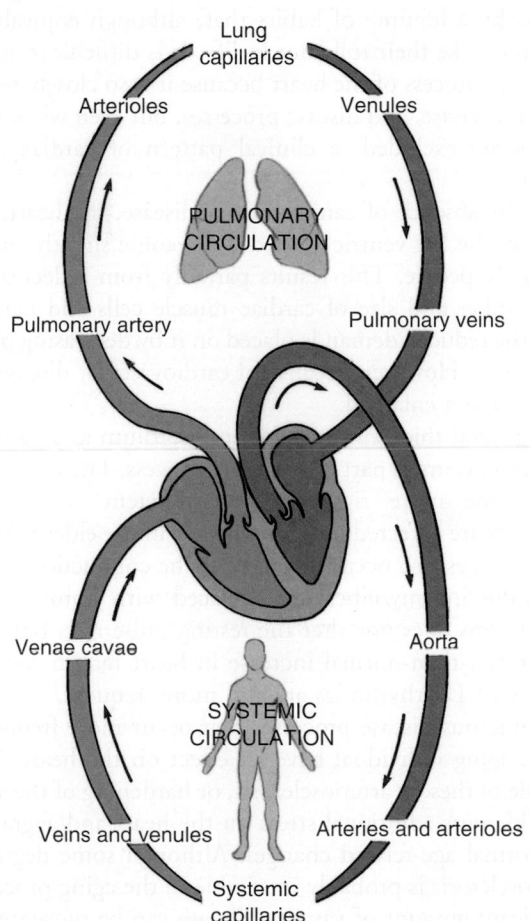

Figure 12-13 Scheme of circulation. In pulmonary circulation, arteries take blood from the right ventricle to the lungs, and veins return the blood to the left atrium. In systemic circulation, arteries take blood from the left ventricle to the body tissues, and veins return the blood to the right atrium.

arterioles (ar-TEER-ee-ohlz). The arterioles play a key role in regulating blood flow into the tissue capillaries. About 10% of the total blood volume is in the systemic arterial system at any given time.

The wall of an artery consists of three layers. The innermost layer is the **tunica intima** (also called **tunica interna**). The middle layer is the **tunica media,** which consists of smooth muscle and is usually the thickest layer. It not only provides support for the vessel but also changes vessel diameter to regulate blood flow and blood pressure. The outermost layer is the **tunica externa** or **tunica adventitia.**

Capillaries

Capillaries are the smallest and most numerous of the blood vessels. They form the connection between the vessels that carry blood away from the heart (arteries) and the vessels that return blood to the heart (veins). They are the continuation of the smallest arterioles. Arterioles are the smallest vessels that have three distinguishable layers in their wall. When the arterioles branch into capillaries, the middle and outer layers of the wall disappear so that the capillary wall is only a thin endothelium. This thin wall permits the exchange of materials between the blood in the capillary and the adjacent tissue cells. This exchange is the primary function of capillaries.

The diameter of a capillary is so small that erythrocytes must pass through them in single file. This slows the blood flow to allow ample time for the transport of substances across the capillary endothelium.

Veins

Veins carry blood toward the heart. After blood passes through the capillaries, it enters the smallest veins, called **venules.** From the venules, it flows into progressively larger and larger veins until it reaches the heart. In the pulmonary circuit, the pulmonary veins transport blood from the lungs to the left atrium of the heart. This blood has a high oxygen content because it has just been oxygenated in the lungs. Systemic veins transport blood from the body tissues to the right atrium of the heart. This blood has a reduced oxygen content because the oxygen has been used for metabolic activities in the tissue cells.

The walls of veins have the same three layers as the arteries. Although all the layers are present, there is less smooth muscle and connective tissue. This makes the walls of veins thinner than those of arteries, which is related to the fact that blood in the veins has less pressure than blood in the arteries. Because the walls of the veins are thinner and less rigid than those of arteries, veins can hold more blood. Almost 70% of the total blood volume is in the veins at any given time. Medium and large veins have **venous valves,** similar to the SL valves associated with the heart, that help keep the blood flowing toward the heart. Venous valves are especially important in the arms and legs, where they prevent the backflow of blood in response to the pull of gravity.

Circulatory Pathways

The blood vessels of the body are functionally divided into two distinct circuits:
- Pulmonary circuit
- Systemic circuit

The pump for the pulmonary circuit, which circulates blood through the lungs, is the right ventricle. The left ventricle is the pump for the systemic circuit, which provides the blood supply for the tissue cells of the body.

Pulmonary Circuit

The pulmonary circuit takes blood from the right side of the heart to the lungs and then returns it to the left side of the heart (see Figures 12-4 and 12-13). Oxygen-poor blood, which has increased levels of carbon dioxide, is returned to the **right atrium** from the tissue cells of the body. It passes through the **tricuspid valve** into the **right ventricle.** During ventricular systole, the blood is ejected through the **pulmonary SL valve** into the **pulmonary trunk,** which divides into the right and left **pulmonary arteries.** Each pulmonary artery enters a lung and repeatedly divides into smaller and smaller vessels until they become capillaries. The **capillaries of the lungs** form networks that surround the air sacs, or alveoli, of the lungs. Here CO_2 diffuses from the capillary blood into the alveoli of the lungs, and O_2 diffuses from the alveoli into the blood. The newly oxygenated blood enters pulmonary venules, which form progressively larger veins, until two **pulmonary veins** emerge from each lung and carry the blood to the **left atrium.** In the pulmonary circuit, the arteries carry deoxygenated blood away from the heart and the veins carry oxygenated blood to the heart.

Systemic Circuit

The systemic circulation provides the functional blood supply to all body tissues. It carries oxygen and nutrients to the cells and picks up carbon dioxide and waste products. Systemic circulation carries oxygenated blood from the left ventricle, through the arteries, to the capillaries in the tissues of the body. The major systemic arteries are illustrated in Figure 12-14. From the tissue capillaries, the deoxygenated blood returns through a system of veins to the right atrium of the heart. The major systemic veins are illustrated in Figure 12-15.

AGING OF THE CIRCULATORY SYSTEM

Numerous "age-related" changes occur in the heart. How many of these are caused by an actual aging process and how many are caused by other factors are questions worth considering. Is it possible to lessen the effects of aging by adjusting lifestyle? Cardiac changes that were once thought to be the result of aging are now believed to be the consequence of a sedentary lifestyle that many consider their "reward" after retirement. Other cardiac changes are caused by a lifetime of habits that, although enjoyable at the time, take their toll later in life. It is difficult to isolate the aging process of the heart because it is so closely related to diet, exercise, and disease processes, but even when these factors are excluded, a clinical pattern of cardiac aging emerges.

In the absence of cardiovascular disease, the heart, particularly the left ventricle, tends to become slightly smaller in elderly people. This results partially from a decrease in the number and size of cardiac muscle cells and partially from the reduced demands placed on it by decreasing physical activity. However, because of cardiovascular disease, the heart is often enlarged.

A general thickening of the endocardium and valves of the heart occurs as part of the aging process. The valves tend to become more rigid and incompetent. Thus heart murmurs are detected more frequently in the elderly. Structural changes also occur throughout the conduction system as conducting myofibers are replaced with fibrous tissue. Usually this does not alter the resting pulse rate, but there is a greater-than-normal increase in heart rate in response to activity. Dysrhythmias are also more frequent.

Numerous disease processes that occur more frequently in the aging individual have an effect on the heart. Most notable of these is arteriosclerosis, or hardening of the arteries. This puts additional stress on the heart and aggravates the normal age-related changes. Although some degree of arteriosclerosis is probably inevitable in the aging process, a significant amount of vascular disease can be prevented by a proper diet, regular walking or other aerobic exercise, and the elimination of cigarette smoking. In other words, lifestyle probably has more effect on the cardiovascular system than aging.

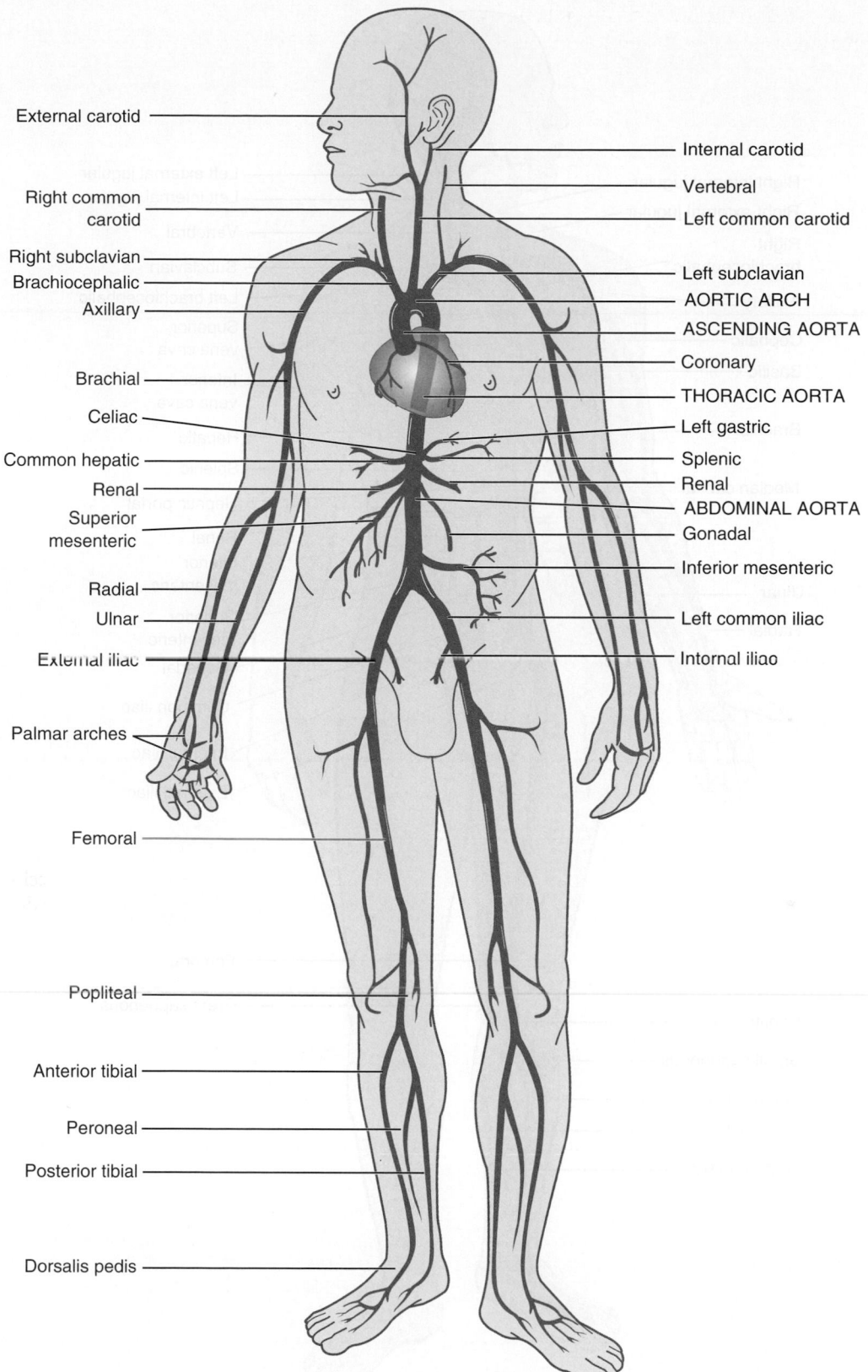

External carotid

Right common carotid

Right subclavian
Brachiocephalic
Axillary

Brachial

Celiac

Common hepatic
Renal
Superior mesenteric

Radial
Ulnar

External iliac

Palmar arches

Femoral

Popliteal

Anterior tibial

Peroneal

Posterior tibial

Dorsalis pedis

Internal carotid
Vertebral
Left common carotid

Left subclavian
AORTIC ARCH
ASCENDING AORTA
Coronary
THORACIC AORTA
Left gastric
Splenic
Renal
ABDOMINAL AORTA
Gonadal
Inferior mesenteric
Left common iliac
Internal iliac

Figure 12-14 Major systemic arteries.

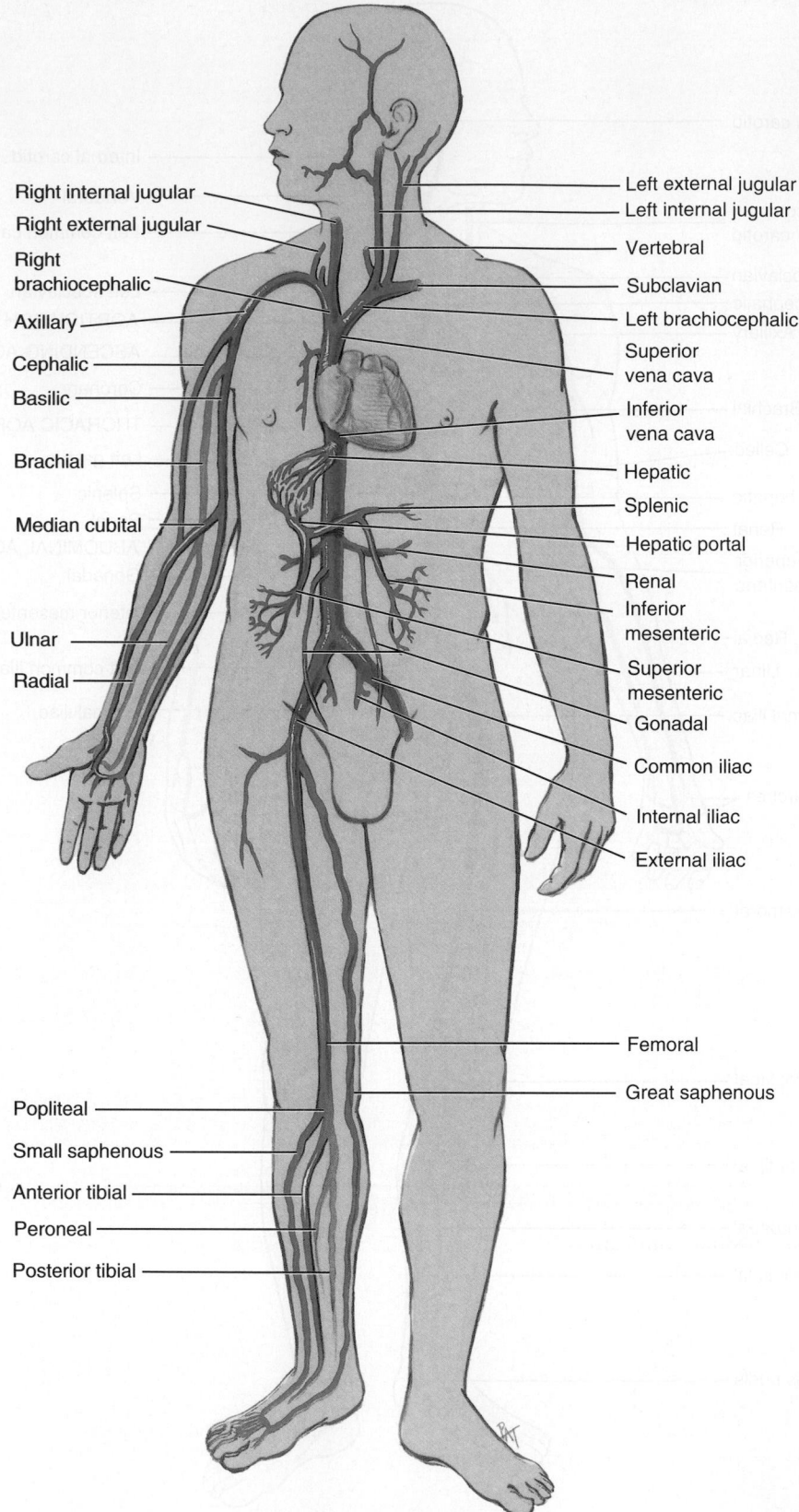

Right internal jugular

Right external jugular

Right brachiocephalic

Axillary

Cephalic

Basilic

Brachial

Median cubital

Ulnar

Radial

Left external jugular

Left internal jugular

Vertebral

Subclavian

Left brachiocephalic

Superior vena cava

Inferior vena cava

Hepatic

Splenic

Hepatic portal

Renal

Inferior mesenteric

Superior mesenteric

Gonadal

Common iliac

Internal iliac

External iliac

Femoral

Great saphenous

Popliteal

Small saphenous

Anterior tibial

Peroneal

Posterior tibial

Figure 12-15 Major systemic veins.

TERMINOLOGY REVIEW

Medical Term	Word Parts	Definition
Atrioventricular valve	*atri/o:* atrium *ventricul/o:* ventricle	Valve between an atrium and a ventricle in the heart.
Cardiac cycle		A complete heartbeat consisting of contraction and relaxation of both atria and both ventricles.
Coagulation	*coagul/o:* clotting *-tion:* process	The process of blood clotting.
Conduction myofibers		Cardiac muscle cells specialized for conducting action potentials to the myocardium; part of the conduction system of the heart; also called *Purkinje fibers.*
Diapedesis	*dia-:* through	The process by which white blood cells squeeze between the cells in a vessel wall to enter the tissue spaces outside the blood vessel.
Diastole		Relaxation phase of the cardiac cycle; opposite of systole.
Erythrocyte	*erythr/o:* red *-cyte:* cell	Red blood cell.
Erythropoiesis	*erythr/o:* red *-poieses:* formation	The process of red blood cell formation.
Erythropoietin	*erythr/o:* red *-poietin:* substance that forms	A hormone released by the kidneys that stimulates red blood cell production.
Hemocytoblast	*hem/o:* blood *-cyt-:* cell *-blast:* to form	A stem cell in the bone marrow from which the blood cells arise.
Hematopoiesis	*hemat/o:* blood *-poieses:* formation	Blood cell production, which occurs in the red bone marrow; also called *hemopoiesis.*
Leukocyte	*leuk/o:* white *-cyt-:* cell	White blood cell.
Semilunar valve		Valve between a ventricle of the heart and the vessel that carries blood away from the ventricle; also pertains to the valves in veins.
Systole		Contraction phase of the cardiac cycle; opposite of diastole.
Thrombocyte	*thromb/o:* clot *-cyte:* cell	One of the formed elements of the blood; functions in blood clotting; also called *platelet.*

ON THE WEB

For information on the circulatory system:

America's Blood Centers: www.americasblood.org

Cardio Guide: www.mymedline.com/cardio

The Franklin Institute—Blood: www.fi.edu/learn/heart/blood/blood.html

The Franklin Institute—The Human Heart: www.fi.edu/learn/heart

Heart Point: www.heartpoint.com

Human Blood: anthro.palomar.edu/blood

Inner Body: www.innerbody.com/html/body.html

The Internet Pathology Laboratory for Medical Education—Hematopathology: library.med.utah.edu/WebPath/ ORGAN.html *(Click on "Hematopathology")*

 Check out the Evolve site at http://evolve.elsevier.com/Bonewit/today/ to actively Prepare for your Certification, and to access additional interactive activities and exercises to help you study and prepare for success.

13

Respiratory System

KEY TERMS

alveoli (al-VEE-oh-ly)
bronchial tree (BRONG-kee-al TREE)
external respiration (eks-TER-nal
  res-per-RAY-shun)

internal respiration (in-TER-nal
  res-per-RAY-shun)
respiratory membrane (RES-per-ah-tor-ee
  MEM-brayn)

surfactant (sir-FAK-tant)
ventilation (ven-tih-LAY-shun)

INTRODUCTION TO THE RESPIRATORY SYSTEM

When the respiratory system is mentioned, people generally think of breathing, but this is only one of the activities of the respiratory system. The cells in the body need a continuous supply of oxygen for the metabolic processes that are necessary to maintain life. The respiratory system works with the circulatory system to provide this oxygen and to remove the waste products of metabolism. The respiratory system also helps to regulate the pH of the blood.

FUNCTIONS AND OVERVIEW OF RESPIRATION

Respiration is the sequence of events that results in the exchange of oxygen and carbon dioxide between the atmosphere and the body cells. Every 3 to 5 seconds nerve impulses stimulate the breathing process, or **ventilation,** which moves air through a series of passages into and out of the lungs. After this there is an exchange of gases between the lungs and the blood. This is called **external respiration.** The blood transports the gases to and from the tissue cells. The exchange of gases between the blood and tissue cells is known as **internal respiration.**

VENTILATION

Ventilation, or breathing, is the movement of air through the conducting passages between the atmosphere and the lungs.

Conducting Passages

The conducting passages are divided into the upper respiratory tract and the lower respiratory tract (Figure 13-1). The **upper respiratory tract** includes the nose, pharynx, and larynx. The **lower respiratory tract** consists of the trachea, bronchial tree, and lungs. These passageways open to the outside and are lined with mucous membrane. In some regions the membrane has hairs that help filter the air. Other regions have cilia to propel mucus.

Nose and Nasal Cavities

The framework of the **nose** consists of bone and cartilage. Two small nasal bones and extensions of the maxillae form the bridge of the nose, which is the bony portion. The remainder of the framework is cartilage. This is the flexible portion. Connective tissue and skin cover the framework.

The interior chamber of the nose is the **nasal cavity** (Figure 13-2). It is divided into two parts by the **nasal septum.** Air enters the nasal cavity from the outside through two openings—the **nostrils,** or **external nares** (NAY-reez). The openings from the nasal cavity into the pharynx are the **internal nares.** The **palate** forms the floor of the nasal cavity and separates the nasal cavity from the oral cavity. The anterior portion of the palate is called the **hard palate**

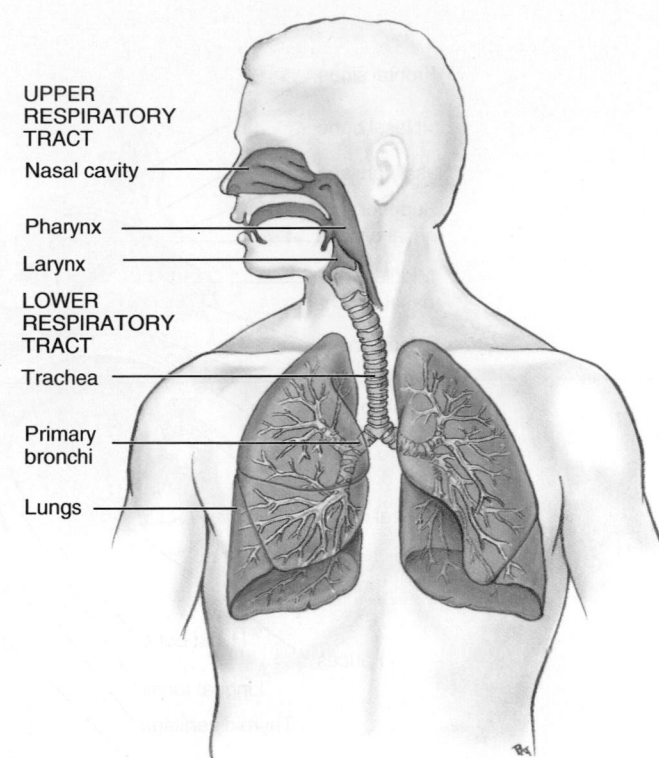

UPPER RESPIRATORY TRACT
Nasal cavity
Pharynx
Larynx
LOWER RESPIRATORY TRACT
Trachea
Primary bronchi
Lungs

Figure 13-1 Conducting passages of the respiratory system. The upper respiratory tract includes the nose, pharynx, and larynx. The lower respiratory tract consists of the trachea, bronchial tree, and lungs.

because it is supported by bone. The posterior portion has no bony support, so it is called the **soft palate.** The soft palate terminates in a projection called the **uvula** (YOO-vyoo-lah), which helps direct food into the oropharynx.

Nasal conchae (KONG-kee) are bony ridges that project into the nasal cavity (see Figure 13-2). The three nasal conchae increase the surface area of the nasal cavity to warm and moisten the air. They also help direct air flow through the nasal cavity. Dust and other particles in the air tend to become trapped in the mucous membrane around the nasal conchae.

Paranasal sinuses are air-filled cavities in the frontal, maxillae, ethmoid, and sphenoid bones. These sinuses surround the nasal cavity and open into it. They reduce the weight of the skull, produce mucus, and influence voice quality by acting as resonating chambers. The sinuses are lined with mucous membrane that produces mucus, which drains into the nasal cavity. During infections and allergies, the membranes in the passages that drain the sinuses become inflamed and swollen. The swelling may block the passages and cause the mucus to accumulate in the sinuses. As the mucus accumulates, pressure within the sinuses increases, resulting in a sinus headache.

As air passes through the nasal cavity, it is filtered, warmed, and moistened. Goblet cells in the mucous membrane produce mucus, which traps microorganisms, dust, and other foreign particles. **Cilia** attached to the epithelium

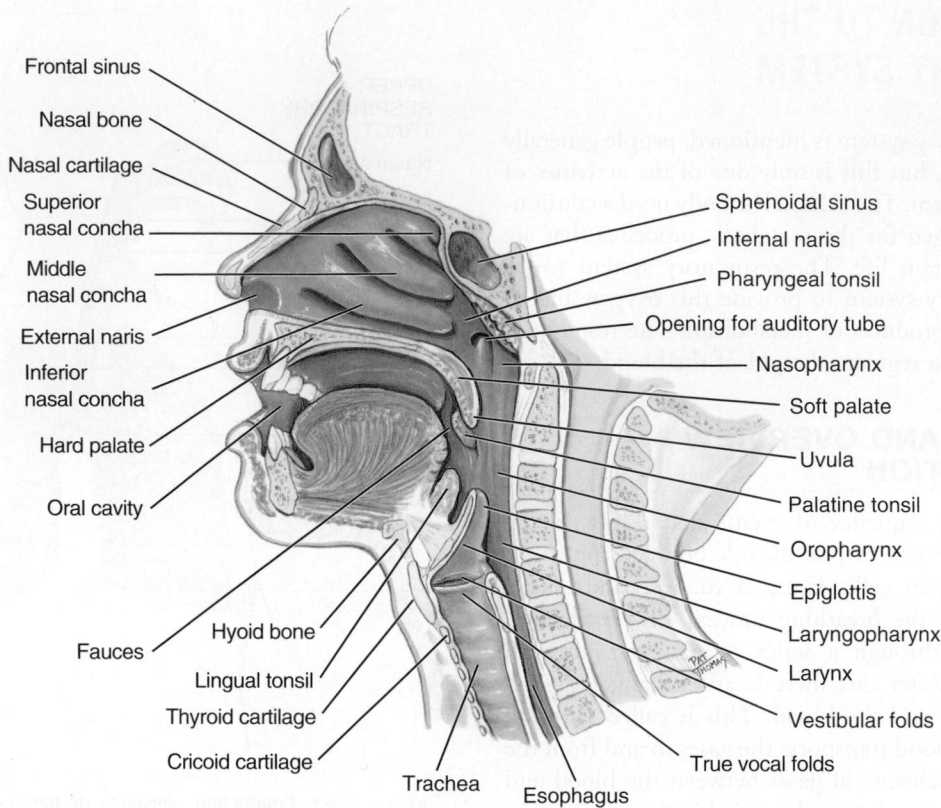

Figure 13-2 Features of the upper respiratory tract. The upper respiratory tract includes the nose, pharynx, and larynx.

propel the mucus with the trapped particles toward the pharynx, where it is swallowed. Acid in the gastric juice destroys most of the microorganisms that are swallowed. An extensive capillary network under the mucous membrane warms and moistens the air before it reaches the rest of the respiratory tract.

Pharynx

The **pharynx** (FAIR-inks), commonly called the *throat,* is a passageway about 13 cm long. It serves both the respiratory and digestive systems by receiving air from the nasal cavity and air, food, and water from the oral cavity. Inferiorly, it opens into the larynx and esophagus. The pharynx is divided into three regions according to location: nasopharynx, oropharynx, and laryngopharynx (see Figure 13-2).

The **nasopharynx** (nay-zoh-FAIR-inks) is the portion of the pharynx that is posterior to the nasal cavity and extends to the uvula. Air enters this region from the nasal cavity through the internal nares. The mucous membrane in the nasopharynx is similar to the lining of the nasal cavity. The **auditory** (eustachian) **tubes** from the two middle ear cavities open into the nasopharynx. The auditory tubes help to equalize the air pressure on both sides of the tympanic membrane. Collections of lymphoid tissue, called **pharyngeal tonsils** (or **adenoids**), are located in the posterior wall of the nasopharynx.

The **oropharynx** (ohr-oh-FAIR-inks) is the portion of the pharynx that is posterior to the oral cavity. It receives air, food, and water from the oral cavity. During swallowing, the soft palate and uvula move upward to prevent the material from going into the nasopharynx. The opening between the oral cavity and oropharynx is called the **fauces** (FAW-seez). The fauces is bordered by masses of lymphoid tissue called **tonsils.** The **palatine tonsils** are in the lateral walls of the oropharynx, adjacent to the fauces. The **lingual tonsils** are located on the surface of the posterior portion of the tongue, also in the region of the fauces. The tonsils in the pharynx function in immune responses and help prevent infections.

The most inferior portion of the pharynx is the **laryngopharynx** (lah-ring-goh-FAIR-inks) (see Figure 13-2). It is posterior to the larynx and is continuous with the esophagus.

Larynx

The **larynx** (LAIR-inks), commonly called the *voice box,* is the passageway for air between the pharynx and the trachea. It is about 5 cm long and formed by nine pieces of cartilage that are connected to one another by muscles and ligaments.

The three largest cartilaginous portions of the larynx are the thyroid cartilage, cricoid cartilage, and epiglottis (see Figure 13-2). The **thyroid cartilage** forms a projection in

Highlight on the Respiratory System

Rhinitis: Rhinitis is an inflammation of the nasal mucosa accompanied by excessive production of mucus. It can be caused by cold viruses, certain bacteria, and allergens.

Pharyngitis and laryngitis: Inflammation of the pharynx, or a sore throat, is pharyngitis. Inflammation of the vocal cords is laryngitis. The inflammation may be caused by overuse of the voice, infection with bacteria or viruses, or inhalation of irritating particles. Laryngitis results in hoarseness or an inability to speak above a whisper.

Tracheotomy: A tracheotomy is the creation of an opening into the trachea through the neck and insertion of a tube to facilitate passage of air or removal of secretions.

Respiratory obstruction: Foreign objects that become lodged in the larynx or trachea are usually expelled by coughing. If a person cannot speak or make a sound because of the obstruction, it means that the airway is completely blocked. This is a life-threatening situation. The Heimlich maneuver is a procedure in which the air in the person's own lungs is used to forcefully expel the object.

Bronchoscopy: Bronchoscopy is a procedure in which a fiberoptic bundle is inserted into the trachea and directed along the conducting passageways to the smaller bronchi. This allows direct visualization of the inside of the bronchi and collection of specimens for cytologic and bacterial studies.

Asthma: Several different forms of asthma exist, all of which have sensitive conducting passages. In many cases the agent that triggers the attack is an allergen in the air. The most obvious and dangerous symptom involves the constriction of the smooth muscle around the bronchial tree. The airways become narrow and breathing is difficult. Treatment includes the use of bronchodilators to dilate the respiratory passages to permit airflow.

Pleurisy: Pleuritis, or pleurisy, is an inflammation of the pleura and is often painful because the sensory nerves in the parietal pleura are irritated. As the condition progresses, the permeability of the membrane changes, which results in an accumulation of fluid in the pleural cavity, making breathing difficult.

Pneumothorax: The accumulation of air in the pleural cavity is called *pneumothorax*. This condition can occur in pulmonary disease, such as emphysema, carcinoma, tuberculosis, or lung abscesses, when rupture of a lesion allows air to escape from the alveoli into the pleural cavity. It also may follow trauma in which the chest wall is perforated and atmospheric air enters the cavity.

Surfactant: Surfactant is not produced until the late stages of fetal life. Newborns who are born prematurely may not have enough surfactant, and the forces of surface tension collapse the alveoli. The newborn must reinflate the alveoli with each breath, which requires tremendous energy. The lack of surfactant accounts for many of the signs and symptoms of infant respiratory distress syndrome (IRDS). The condition is treated by using positive-pressure respirators that maintain pressure within the alveoli to keep them inflated. ■

Highlight on Conditions Affecting the Respiratory System

Atelectasis (at-eh-LECK-tah-sis) Collapse of the alveoli; the lung is airless

Bronchogenic carcinoma (brong-koh-JEN-ik kar-sin-OH-mah) Cancerous tumors arising from a bronchus; lung cancer; smoking is the primary etiologic agent; spreads readily to the liver, brain, and bones

Chronic obstructive pulmonary disease (COPD) (KRAHN-ik ob-STRUCK-tiv PULL-mon-air-ee dih-ZEEZ) A chronic condition of obstructed airflow through the bronchial tubes and lungs, usually accompanied by dyspnea; includes emphysema and chronic bronchitis

Coryza (koh-RYE-zah) The common cold, characterized by sneezing, nasal discharge, coughing, and malaise; caused by a rhinovirus

Croup (KROOP) Acute respiratory syndrome in infants and children, characterized by obstruction of the larynx, barking cough, and strained, high-pitched, noisy breathing

Hemoptysis (hee-MAHP-tih-sis) Spitting of blood as a result of bleeding from any part of the respiratory tract

Pertussis (per-TUSS-is) Whooping cough; a highly contagious bacterial infection of the pharynx, larynx, and trachea; characterized by explosive coughing spasms ending in a "whooping" sound

Pneumoconiosis (new-moh-koh-nee-OH-sis) General term for lung pathology that occurs after long-term inhalation of pollutants such as coal dust or asbestos, characterized by chronic inflammation, infection, and bronchitis

Pneumothorax (new-moh-THOH-raks) Accumulation of air or gas in the pleural space, resulting in collapse of the lung on the affected side

Pulmonary edema (PULL-mon-air-ee eh-DEE-mah) Swelling and fluid in the air sacs and bronchioles; often caused by inability of the heart to pump blood; the blood then backs up in the pulmonary blood vessels and fluid seeps into the alveoli and bronchioles

Smoker's respiratory syndrome (SMOH-kers reh-SPY-rah-tor-ee SIN-drohm) A group of respiratory symptoms seen in smokers; includes coughing, wheezing, vocal hoarseness, pharyngitis, dyspnea, and susceptibility to respiratory infections ■

the neck called the *Adam's apple.* The projection is more pronounced in males than in females. The **cricoid** (KRY-koyd) **cartilage** forms the base of the larynx and is attached to the trachea. The **epiglottis** (eh-pih-GLOT-is) is a long, leaf-shaped structure. During swallowing, the epiglottis covers the opening into the larynx to prevent food and water from entering the trachea.

The larynx houses two pairs of ligaments. The upper pair are the **vestibular folds,** or **false vocal cords.** They work with the epiglottis to prevent particles from entering the lower respiratory tract. The lower pair are the **true vocal cords,** which function in sound production. Muscles control the length and tension of the true vocal cords. They are relaxed during normal breathing. When the vocal cords are under tension, exhaled air moving by them causes them to vibrate and produce sound. The length of the vocal cords determines the pitch of the sound, and the force of the moving air regulates the loudness. The opening between the true vocal cords is the **glottis,** which leads to the trachea.

Trachea

The **trachea** is commonly called the *windpipe.* The trachea consists of a tube that extends from the larynx and into the mediastinum, where it divides into the right and left bronchi (Figure 13-3). It is about 12 to 15 cm long. The walls of the trachea are supported by 15 to 20 C-shaped pieces of hyaline cartilage that hold the trachea open despite the pressure changes that occur during breathing. The posterior open part of the C-shaped cartilage is closed by smooth muscle and connective tissue and is next to the esophagus. During swallowing, the esophagus bulges into the soft part of the trachea.

The mucous membrane that lines the trachea is ciliated epithelium similar to that in the nasal cavity and nasopharynx. Goblet cells located in the mucous membrane produce mucus that traps airborne particles and microorganisms. The cilia propel the mucus upward, where it is either swallowed or expelled. Continued irritation from cigarette smoke and other air pollutants damages the cilia, and the mucus with the trapped particles is not removed. Microorganisms thrive in the accumulated mucus, which results in respiratory infections. Irritation and inflammation of the mucous membrane stimulate the cough reflex.

Bronchi and Bronchial Tree

In the mediastinum, the trachea divides into the **right** and **left primary bronchi.** After the bronchi enter the lungs, they branch several times into smaller and smaller passages to form the **bronchial tree** (see Figure 13-3). The primary bronchi divide to form **secondary (lobar) bronchi.** The branching continues until the pathway terminates in clusters of tiny air sacs called **alveoli.**

The alveoli consist primarily of **simple squamous epithelium,** which permits rapid diffusion of oxygen and carbon dioxide. Exchange of gases between the air in the lungs and the blood in the capillaries occurs across the walls of the alveoli.

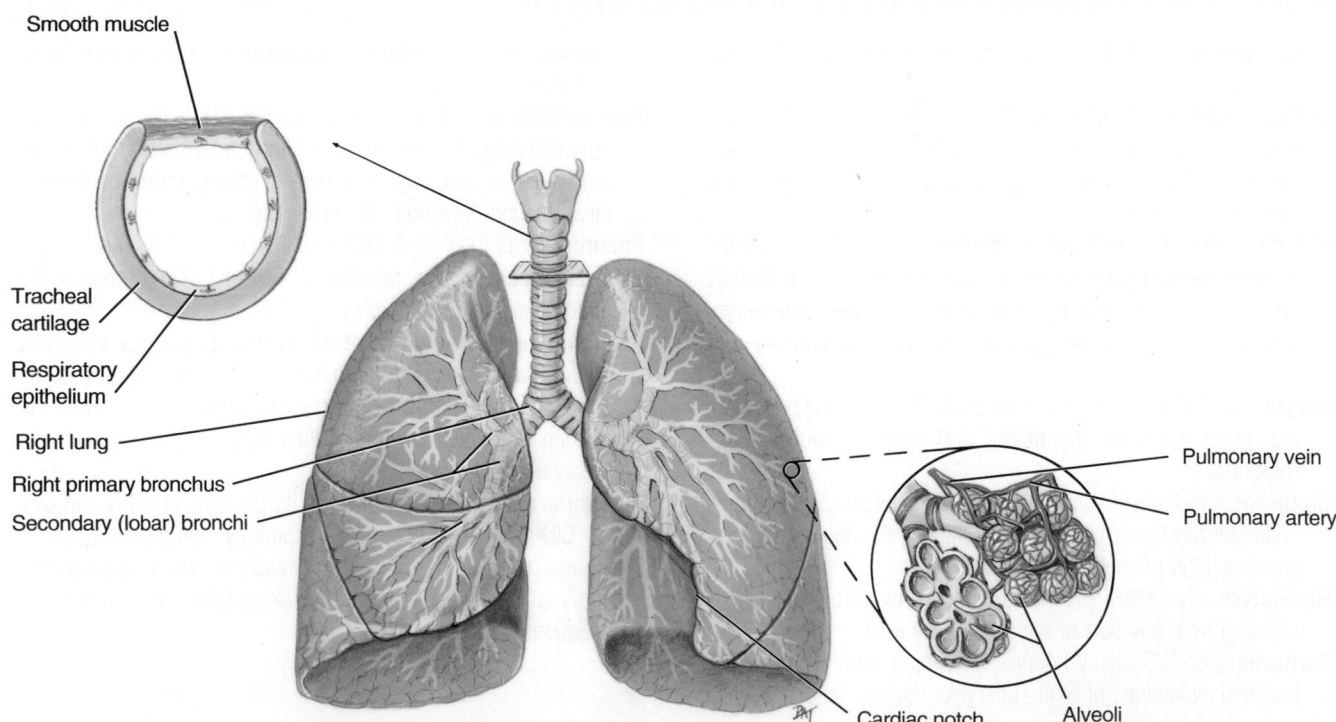

Figure 13-3 Features of the lower respiratory tract. The lower respiratory tract includes the trachea, bronchial tree, and lungs. Note the C-shaped cartilage ring of the trachea at the upper left and the clusters of alveoli in the lower right.

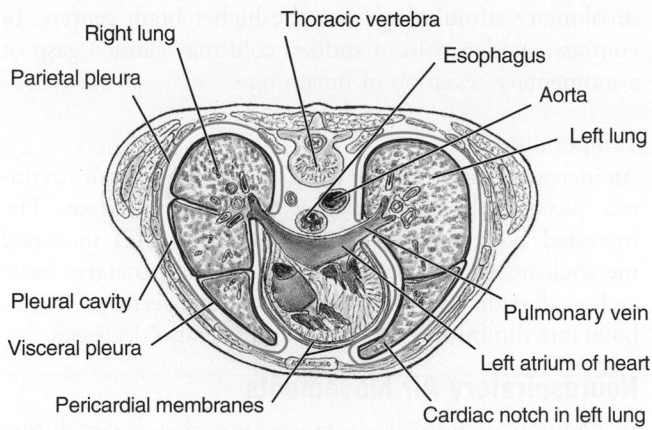

Figure 13-4 Features of the lungs and pleura. Note the three lobes in the right lung and two lobes in the left lung. Red indicates visceral pleura, and blue indicates parietal pleura.

Lungs

The two **lungs** occupy most of the space in the thoracic cavity (Figure 13-4). The lungs are soft and spongy because they are mostly air spaces surrounded by the alveolar cells and elastic connective tissue. They are separated from each other by the mediastinum, which contains the heart. Each lung is roughly cone-shaped, rests on the diaphragm, and extends upward just above the midpoint of the clavicle.

The **right lung** is shorter, is broader, and has a greater volume than the left lung. It is divided into three lobes (superior, middle, and inferior) by two fissures. The **left lung** is longer and narrower than the right lung. It has an indentation, called the **cardiac notch,** on its medial surface for the apex of the heart. The left lung is divided into two lobes by a single fissure.

Each lung is enclosed by a double-layered **serous membrane** called the **pleura** (see Figure 13-4). The **visceral pleura** is firmly attached to the surface of the lung. The visceral pleura is continuous with the **parietal pleura,** which lines the wall of the thorax. The small space between the visceral and parietal pleurae is the **pleural cavity.** It contains a thin film of serous fluid that is produced by the pleura. The fluid acts as a lubricant to reduce friction as the two layers slide against each other.

Mechanics of Ventilation

Pulmonary ventilation is commonly referred to as *breathing*. It is the process of air flowing into the lungs during inhalation and out of the lungs during exhalation. Air flows because of pressure differences between the atmosphere and the gases inside the lungs. Under normal conditions, the average adult takes 12 to 20 breaths per minute. A breath is one complete respiratory cycle that consists of one inhalation and one exhalation. The amount of air that is exchanged during one cycle varies with age, sex, size, and physical condition.

Inhalation

Inhalation (or **inspiration**) is the process of taking air into the lungs. It is the active phase of ventilation because it is the result of muscle contraction. In normal, quiet breathing, the primary muscle involved in inhalation is the dome-shaped diaphragm. When the diaphragm contracts, it drops, or becomes flatter. This increases the size (volume) of the thoracic cavity. When the thoracic volume increases, the pressure within the lungs decreases below atmospheric pressure. This causes air to flow from the region of higher atmospheric pressure outside the body into the region of lower pressure within the lungs. Air continues to flow into the lungs until the pressure equals atmospheric pressure.

Exhalation

Exhalation (or **expiration**) is the process of letting air out of the lungs during the breathing cycle. When the diaphragm relaxes, the volume of the thoracic cavity decreases to its normal resting size. This decrease in lung volume causes an increase in the pressure of the lungs. Air now flows from the region of higher pressure within the lungs to the region of lower atmospheric pressure outside the body until the two pressures are equal.

As air leaves the lungs during exhalation, the alveoli become smaller. The interior surfaces of the alveoli are coated with a thin layer of fluid. The fluid molecules are attracted to one another, which tends to cause the surfaces to adhere to each other. This makes it harder to inflate the lungs during inhalation and creates a tendency for the lungs to collapse. Normally this is prevented by a substance called **surfactant** (sir-FAK-tant). Surfactant is a substance that is produced by certain cells within the lung tissue and reduces the attraction between the fluid molecules. Without surfactant, the alveoli collapse and become nonfunctional.

RESPIRATION

External Respiration

External respiration is the exchange of oxygen and carbon dioxide between the lungs and the blood in the surrounding capillaries. Oxygen diffuses from the alveoli of the lungs into the blood, and carbon dioxide diffuses from the blood into the air in the alveoli. The surfaces in the lungs where diffusion occurs constitute the **respiratory membrane.** The rate of gaseous exchange across the respiratory membrane depends on the surface area of the membrane, thickness of the membrane, solubility of the gas, and difference in pressure of the gas on the two sides of the membrane.

Internal Respiration

Internal respiration is the exchange of gases between the tissue cells and the blood in the tissue capillaries. After the blood picks up oxygen in the lungs, the blood returns to the left side of the heart, which pumps it to the tissue capillaries. The oxygen is given off to the tissue cells, and the carbon dioxide is picked up by the blood to be transported as a waste product to the lungs.

REGULATION OF RESPIRATION

The normal breathing rate in adults averages 12 to 20 breaths per minute. The rate is higher, up to 40 breaths per minute, in children. The basic rate is established by the respiratory center in the brain stem, but environmental conditions and emotions influence variations in the rate.

Respiratory Center

Groups of neurons in the **pons** and **medulla oblongata** (regions of the brain stem) make up the **respiratory center.** This center controls the rate and depth of breathing and contains both inhalation and exhalation areas. The inhalation area sends impulses along the **phrenic nerve** to the diaphragm. This causes the diaphragm to contract, and inhalation results. The inhalation neurons fatigue quickly and quit sending impulses to the diaphragm. When the impulses cease, the muscles of the diaphragm relax and exhalation occurs. When forceful exhalation is needed, the exhalation area of the brain sends impulses to the intercostal muscles. If the respiratory center in the brain stem is damaged, the impulses cease and breathing stops. Death will occur within a few minutes unless artificial breathing mechanisms are applied.

Factors That Influence Breathing

Even though the respiratory center establishes the basic rhythm of breathing, it is influenced by factors that cause variations in the rate and depth of breathing.

Chemoreceptors

Chemoreceptors in the medulla are sensitive to changes in carbon dioxide concentrations in the blood and cerebrospinal fluid. They are not sensitive to changes in oxygen levels. If carbon dioxide concentrations increase, the receptors stimulate the respiratory center to increase the rate and depth of breathing. This decreases the concentrations back to normal levels. In contrast, low carbon dioxide levels decrease the rate and depth of breathing. Breathing may even stop for brief periods of time until concentrations increase to normal levels.

Stimulus from Higher Brain Centers

Impulses from higher brain centers may override the respiratory center temporarily. These impulses may be either voluntary or involuntary; however, the voluntary controls are limited. For example, if you try to voluntarily hold your breath, you can do so for only a limited time. When carbon dioxide levels reach a certain critical point, the impulses from the higher brain centers are ignored and the respiratory center resumes regular breathing.

Involuntary impulses from higher brain centers may stimulate rapid breathing in response to emotions, such as anxiety or excitement. Chronic pain also may result in

involuntary stimulation from the higher brain centers. In contrast, sudden pain or sudden cold may cause a gasp or a momentary cessation of breathing.

Temperature

An increase in body temperature caused by a fever or strenuous physical exercise increases the breathing rate. The increased body temperature is associated with increased metabolism, which uses more oxygen and generates more carbon dioxide. When body temperature decreases, metabolic rate diminishes and breathing rate also decreases.

Nonrespiratory Air Movements

In addition to normal air movements that occur during breathing and result in pulmonary ventilation, there are a number of modifications called **nonrespiratory air movements.** Some of these are reflexes that clear air passages, others are voluntary, and some express emotions. These nonrespiratory air movements are outlined in Table 13-1.

AGING OF THE RESPIRATORY SYSTEM

Various harmful substances, including cigarette smoke, air pollution, and pathogens, continually bombard the respiratory system and take their toll. There is no way to avoid all of these irritants except to stop breathing! Some irritants, such as cigarette smoke, can be decreased, but others are inescapable.

Because of the continual contact between the respiratory system and the environment, it is difficult to distinguish between the changes in the tissues of the breathing apparatus, including the lungs, that are the result of aging and

Table 13-1	Nonrespiratory Air Movements
Movement	**Description**
Sneezing	Spasmodic contraction of exhalation muscles that forces air through nose and mouth
Coughing	Long inhalation followed by closure of glottis; then a strong exhalation forces glottis open and sends a blast of air through upper respiratory tract
Sighing	Long inhalation followed by a shorter but forceful exhalation
Hiccupping	Spasmodic contraction of diaphragm followed by sudden closure of glottis to produce a sharp sound
Crying	An inhalation followed by many short exhalations; glottis remains open and vocal cords vibrate; usually accompanied by tears and characteristic facial expressions
Laughing	Same basic movements as crying but facial expressions differ; may be indistinguishable from crying
Yawning	A deep inhalation through a widely opened mouth

From Applegate E: *The anatomy and physiology learning system,* ed 4, St Louis, 2011, Saunders.

those that are the result of disease or other factors outside the body. Modifications in the lining of the respiratory tract probably are caused by environmental rather than solely aging-related factors. Long-term exposure to irritants results in deterioration of the cilia, which hinders their cleansing action and movement of mucus. As a consequence, the occurrence of emphysema and chronic bronchitis increases with age. Diminishing effectiveness of the immune system makes the elderly more susceptible to pneumonia and other microbial diseases. However, excluding external influences, there are changes that take place as a result of "normal" aging.

One of the most common signs of respiratory aging, in general, is when a person is unable to maintain the same level of physical activity that was experienced in younger years. This is a gradual decline and may not be noticeable until phrases such as, "I used to be able to…" become part of the conversation. The cardiovascular and muscular systems have an effect on endurance, and the skeletal system has an effect on thoracic volume, but the major change is a decreased ability of the respiratory system to acquire and deliver oxygen to the blood.

The impairment in oxygen delivery is the result of structural changes that take place in the respiratory tissues. One type of change is a loss of elasticity in the tissues of the respiratory system. The cartilage in the walls of the trachea and bronchi undergoes a progressive calcification. Smooth muscle fibers in the bronchioles are replaced by fibrous tissue, so they are less able to stretch and contract. Modifications in lung tissue cause the alveoli to lose some of their elastic recoil. The cumulative effect of these changes is a gradual decrease in respiratory volume and capacity and an increase in the volume of residual air in the lungs. Another change is deterioration of the walls between adjacent alveoli. This increases the size of each individual alveolus but reduces the total surface area of the respiratory membrane for diffusion of gases. A lower percentage of the oxygen in alveolar air is able to diffuse into the lung capillaries. These changes result in a decreased ability to acquire and deliver oxygen to the blood, which reduces the capacity for physical activity.

TERMINOLOGY REVIEW

Medical Term	Word Parts	Definition
Alveoli		Microscopic dilations of terminal bronchioles in the lungs, where diffusion of gases occurs; air sacs in the lungs.
Bronchial tree		The bronchi and all their branches that function as passageways between the trachea and the alveoli.
External respiration		Exchange of gases between the lungs and the blood.
Internal respiration		Exchange of gases between the blood and tissue cells.
Respiratory membrane		Any surface in the lungs where diffusion occurs; consists of the layers that the gases must pass through to get into or out of the alveoli.
Surfactant		A substance, produced by certain cells in lung tissue, that reduces surface tension between fluid molecules that line the respiratory membrane and helps keep the alveolus from collapsing.
Ventilation		Movement of air into and out of the lungs; breathing.

ON THE WEB

For information on the respiratory system:

Chronic Obstructive Pulmonary Diseases: www.priory.com/cmol/copd.htm

The Internet Pathology Laboratory for Medical Education—Gastrointestinal Pathology: library.med.utah.edu/WebPath/ORGAN.html *(Click on "Pulmonary Pathology")*

 Check out the Evolve site at http://evolve.elsevier.com/Bonewit/today/ to actively Prepare for your Certification, and to access additional interactive activities and exercises to help you study and prepare for success.

14

Digestive System

LEARNING OBJECTIVES

1. Identify the components of the digestive tract and the accessory organs.
2. List six functions of the digestive system.
3. Describe the general histology of the four layers in the digestive tract wall.
4. Describe the features and function of the oral cavity, teeth, pharynx, and esophagus.
5. List and describe the location of the three salivary glands.
6. Explain the function of saliva.
7. Describe the structure and features of the stomach and its role in digestion.
8. Describe the structure and features of the small intestine and its role in digestion and absorption.
9. Describe the structure, features, and function of the large intestine.
10. Describe the structure and function of the liver, gallbladder, and pancreas.
11. Explain how substances are absorbed into the body through the small intestine.
12. Describe ways in which the aging of an individual affects the digestive system.
13. Identify pathology related to the digestive system.

CHAPTER OUTLINE

INTRODUCTION TO THE DIGESTIVE SYSTEM
Functions of the Digestive System
General Structure of the Digestive Tract
Mucosa
Submucosa
Muscular Layer
Serosa or Adventitia
Components of the Digestive Tract
Mouth
Pharynx
Esophagus
Stomach

Small Intestine
Large Intestine
Accessory Organs of Digestion
Liver
Gallbladder
Pancreas
Chemical Digestion
Carbohydrate Digestion
Protein Digestion
Lipid Digestion
Absorption
Aging of the Digestive System

KEY TERMS

absorption (ab-SOARP-shun)
chyme (KYME)
mesentery (MEZ-en-tair-ee)

peristalsis (pair-ih-STALL-sis)
plicae circulares (PLY-kee
  sir-kyoo-LAIR-eez)

rugae (ROO-jee)

INTRODUCTION TO THE DIGESTIVE SYSTEM

The digestive system includes the **digestive tract** and its **accessory organs** (Figure 14-1). The function of the digestive system is to process food into molecules that can be absorbed and used by the cells of the body. Food is broken down, bit by bit, until the molecules are small enough to be absorbed and the waste products are eliminated. The digestive tract (also called the **alimentary canal** or **gastrointestinal [GI] tract**) consists of a long, continuous tube that extends from the mouth to the anus. It includes the mouth, pharynx, esophagus, stomach, small intestine, and large intestine. The tongue and teeth are accessory structures located in the mouth. The salivary glands, liver, gallbladder, and pancreas are not part of the digestive tract but are major accessory organs that have a role in digestion. These secrete fluids into the digestive tract.

FUNCTIONS OF THE DIGESTIVE SYSTEM

Food undergoes three types of processes in the body:
- Digestion
- Absorption
- Metabolism

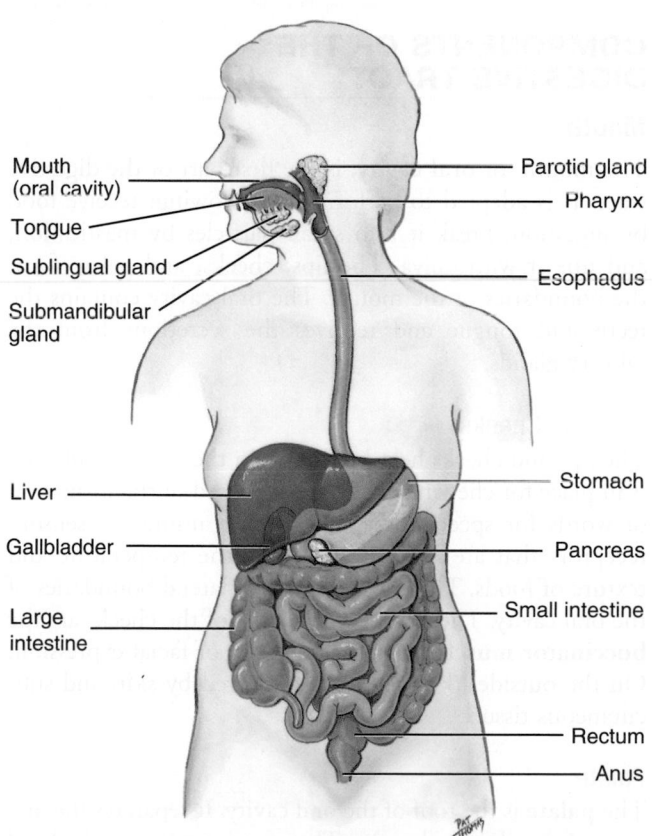

Figure 14-1 Organs of the digestive system.

Mouth (oral cavity)
Tongue
Sublingual gland
Submandibular gland
Liver
Gallbladder
Large intestine

Parotid gland
Pharynx
Esophagus
Stomach
Pancreas
Small intestine
Rectum
Anus

Digestion and absorption occur in the digestive tract. After the nutrients are absorbed, they are available to all cells in the body and are used by the cells in metabolism.

The digestive system prepares nutrients for use by the body's cells through the following six activities:
- **Ingestion**—The first activity of the digestive system is to take in food. This process is called *ingestion.* Ingestion has to take place before anything else can happen.
- **Mechanical digestion**—The large pieces of food that are ingested have to be broken into smaller particles that can be acted on by various enzymes. This is called *mechanical digestion.* Mechanical digestion begins in the mouth with chewing, or **mastication** (mas-tih-KAY-shun), and continues with churning and mixing actions in the stomach.
- **Chemical digestion**—The complex molecules of carbohydrates, proteins, and fats are transformed by chemical digestion into smaller molecules that can be absorbed and used by the cells. Chemical digestion uses water to break down the complex molecules. This process is known as **hydrolysis. Digestive enzymes** speed up the hydrolysis process, which is otherwise slow.
- **Movements**—After ingestion and mastication, the food particles move from the mouth into the pharynx, and then into the esophagus. This movement is called **deglutition** (dee-gloo-TISH-un), or swallowing. **Mixing movements** occur in the stomach as a result of smooth muscle contraction. These repetitive contractions mix the food particles with enzymes and other fluids. The movements that propel the food particles through the digestive tract are called **peristalsis.** These are rhythmic waves of contractions that move the food particles through the various regions in which mechanical and chemical digestion takes place.
- **Absorption**—The simple molecules that are produced from chemical digestion pass through the lining of the small intestine into the blood. This process is called *absorption.*
- **Elimination**—The food molecules that cannot be digested need to be eliminated from the body. The removal of indigestible wastes through the anus, in the form of feces, is **defecation** (def-eh-KAY-shun).

GENERAL STRUCTURE OF THE DIGESTIVE TRACT

The **digestive tract** is a long, continuous tube that is about 9 m (30 ft) in length. It opens to the outside at both ends, through the mouth at one end and through the anus at the other. Although there are variations in each region, the basic structure of the wall is the same throughout the entire length of the tube.

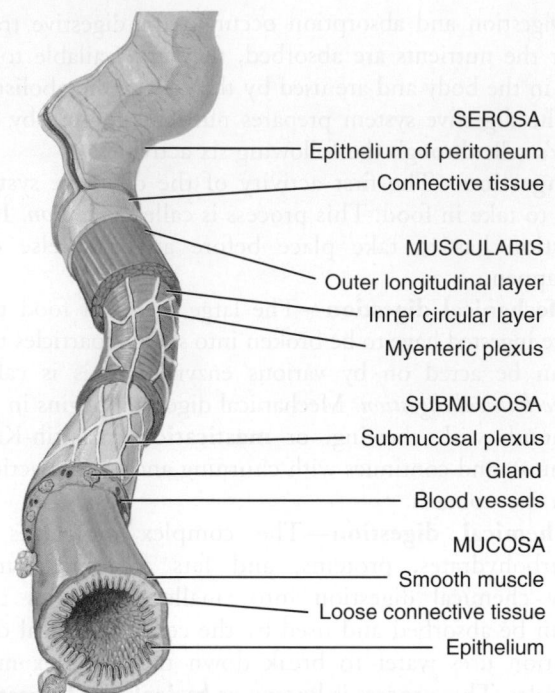

SEROSA
— Epithelium of peritoneum
— Connective tissue

MUSCULARIS
— Outer longitudinal layer
— Inner circular layer
— Myenteric plexus

SUBMUCOSA
— Submucosal plexus
— Gland
— Blood vessels

MUCOSA
— Smooth muscle
— Loose connective tissue
— Epithelium

Figure 14-2 Basic histology of the digestive tract. Progressing from the inner to outer, the tissue layers of the digestive tract are the mucosa, submucosa, muscularis, and serosa (adventitia if above the diaphragm).

The wall of the digestive tract has four layers or **tunics** (Figure 14-2):

- Mucosa
- Submucosa
- Muscular layer (muscularis)
- Serous layer or serosa

Mucosa

The mucosa, or mucous membrane layer, is the innermost tunic of the wall. It lines the lumen of the digestive tract. The mucosa consists of epithelium, an underlying loose connective tissue layer, and a thin layer of smooth muscle. In certain regions the mucosa develops folds that increase the surface area. Certain cells in the mucosa secrete mucus, digestive enzymes, and hormones. Ducts from other glands pass through the mucosa to the lumen of the digestive tract.

Submucosa

The submucosa is a thick layer of loose connective tissue that surrounds the mucosa. This layer also contains blood and lymphatic vessels, nerves, and some glands. Abundant blood vessels supply necessary nourishment to the surrounding tissues. Blood and lymph carry away absorbed nutrients that are the end products of digestion. The nerves in the submucosa form a network called the *submucosal plexus* that provides autonomic nerve impulses to the muscle layers of the digestive tract.

Muscular Layer

The muscular layer (labeled *muscularis* in Figure 14-2) consists of two layers of smooth muscle. The inner circular layer has fibers arranged in a circular manner around the circumference of the tube. When these muscles contract, the diameter of the tube is decreased. In the outer longitudinal layer the fibers run lengthwise along the long axis of the tube. When these fibers contract, their length decreases and the tube shortens. A network of autonomic nerve fibers, called the *myenteric* (mye-en-TAIR-ik) *plexus,* exists between the circular and longitudinal muscle layers. The myenteric plexus, along with the submucosal plexus, is important for controlling the movements and secretions of the digestive tract. In general, parasympathetic impulses stimulate movement and secretion in the GI tract and sympathetic impulses inhibit these activities.

Serosa or Adventitia

The fourth and outermost layer in the wall of the digestive tract is called the *adventitia* if it is above the diaphragm and the *serosa* if it is below the diaphragm. The adventitia is composed of connective tissue. The serosa, which is below the diaphragm, has a layer of epithelium covering the connective tissue. It is actually the visceral peritoneum and secretes serous fluid for lubrication. The serous fluid allows the abdominal organs to move smoothly against one another without friction.

COMPONENTS OF THE DIGESTIVE TRACT

Mouth

The mouth, or **oral cavity,** is the first part of the digestive tract. It is adapted to perform the following: receive food by ingestion, break it into small particles by mastication, and mix it with saliva. The lips, cheeks, and palate form the boundaries of the mouth. The oral cavity contains the teeth and tongue and receives the secretions from the salivary glands.

Lips and Cheeks

The lips and cheeks help hold food in the mouth and keep it in place for chewing. They are also used in the formation of words for speech. The lips contain numerous sensory receptors that are useful for judging the temperature and texture of foods. The cheeks form the lateral boundaries of the oral cavity. The main components of the cheeks are the **buccinator muscle** and other muscles of facial expression. On the outside, the muscles are covered by skin and subcutaneous tissue.

Palate

The **palate** is the roof of the oral cavity. It separates the oral cavity from the nasal cavity. The anterior portion, the **hard palate,** is supported by bone. The posterior portion, the **soft palate,** is skeletal muscle and connective tissue. The

Highlight on the Digestive System

Cold sores: Cold sores, or fever blisters, are small fluid-filled blisters that itch and are painful, usually appearing around the lips and in the mouth. They are caused by recurring infections with the herpes simplex virus. After the initial infection, the virus remains dormant in a cutaneous nerve until it is activated by stress, fever, or ultraviolet radiation.

Cleft palate: Cleft palate is a condition in which the bones in the hard palate do not fuse completely during prenatal development. This leaves an opening between the nasal and oral cavities. An infant with this problem has difficulty creating enough suction for proper feeding. Cleft palate can usually be corrected surgically.

Tongue-tied: A person with a short lingual frenulum is said to be "tongue-tied." The movement of the tongue is abnormally limited, which causes difficulties in speech. Surgically cutting the frenulum corrects this problem.

Wisdom teeth: The third molars are the last teeth to erupt. These are sometimes called "wisdom teeth" because they usually erupt between the ages of 17 and 25 years, when one is supposed to be wise. These teeth may remain embedded in the jawbone. If this happens, they are said to be impacted. In some cases, wisdom teeth are absent altogether.

Gingivitis: Gingivitis is an inflammation of the gingiva, or gum. The gums become sore and red and may bleed. This condition is reversible if it is not neglected and if corrective action is taken. Periodontal disease results when gingivitis is neglected and bacteria invade the bone around the tooth. This is a major cause of tooth loss in adults.

Cavities: Caries, or dental cavities, are caused by the demineralization of the teeth resulting from the action of bacteria that live in the mouth. The bacteria metabolize sugars in the mouth, producing acids that dissolve the calcium salts of the tooth. If the bacteria reach the pulp cavity, it is necessary to perform a root canal procedure. In this procedure, the pulp cavity with its nerve is destroyed, and the cavity is completely filled with a solid filling material.

Mumps: Mumps is a viral infection of the parotid glands. The infection causes inflammation in the gland, which makes opening the mouth and chewing difficult. If the disease occurs in postadolescent males, the infection may spread to the testes, which in severe cases may result in sterility.

Bad breath: Halitosis, commonly called "bad breath," results from an overabundance of bacteria in the mouth. In some cases it may be caused by poor oral hygiene. In others, it may be caused by a disease process that reduces the secretion of saliva for cleansing the mouth and moving food particles to the pharynx for swallowing. As a result, some food particles remain in the mouth and decompose, which provides a growth medium for the bacteria.

Hiatal hernia: A hiatal hernia occurs when a portion of the stomach protrudes into the thoracic cavity through a weakened area of the diaphragm. Frequently it develops when a small region of the fundus balloons backward through the esophageal hiatus. Symptoms of this condition include pain in the upper abdomen and "heartburn" caused by the reflux of stomach acid into the esophagus, especially when the person is lying down.

Vomiting: Vomiting is the forceful ejection of the stomach contents through the mouth. It can be initiated by extreme stretching of the stomach or by the presence of irritants such as bacterial toxins, alcohol, spicy foods, and certain drugs. The vomiting action is a coordinated reflex controlled by the vomiting center of the medulla oblongata.

Lactose intolerance: Lactose intolerance is caused by a deficiency of the intestinal enzyme lactase, which acts on lactose, a sugar found in milk. When people with lactose intolerance drink milk, this sugar is not digested properly. Bacterial action on the undigested sugar causes gas and a bloated feeling. The undigested lactose also prevents absorption of water from the small intestine, which leads to diarrhea. The solution to this problem is to avoid milk and milk products.

Appendicitis: Appendicitis is an inflammation that sometimes occurs when infectious material becomes trapped inside the appendix. If the inflamed appendix ruptures and releases the infectious contents into the abdominal cavity, the peritoneum may become involved, resulting in a potentially life-threatening inflammation of the peritoneum, called *peritonitis.* Treatment for appendicitis is usually the surgical removal of the appendix.

Cirrhosis: Cirrhosis is a chronic liver disease that may develop as a result of chronic alcoholism or severe hepatitis. The hepatic cells of the liver are destroyed and replaced with fibrous connective tissue such that the liver no longer functions properly. One consequence of cirrhosis is the buildup of bilirubin in the blood because it is not properly incorporated into the bile and excreted. The word *cirrhosis* means "orange-colored condition," which refers to the discoloration of the liver in this disease.

Gallstones: Gallstones are formed in the gallbladder when cholesterol precipitates from the bile and hardens into stones because there is a lack of bile salts. Problems develop when the stones leave the gallbladder and lodge in the bile duct. This obstructs the flow of bile into the small intestine and interferes with fat absorption. Surgery may be required to remove the gallstones. ■

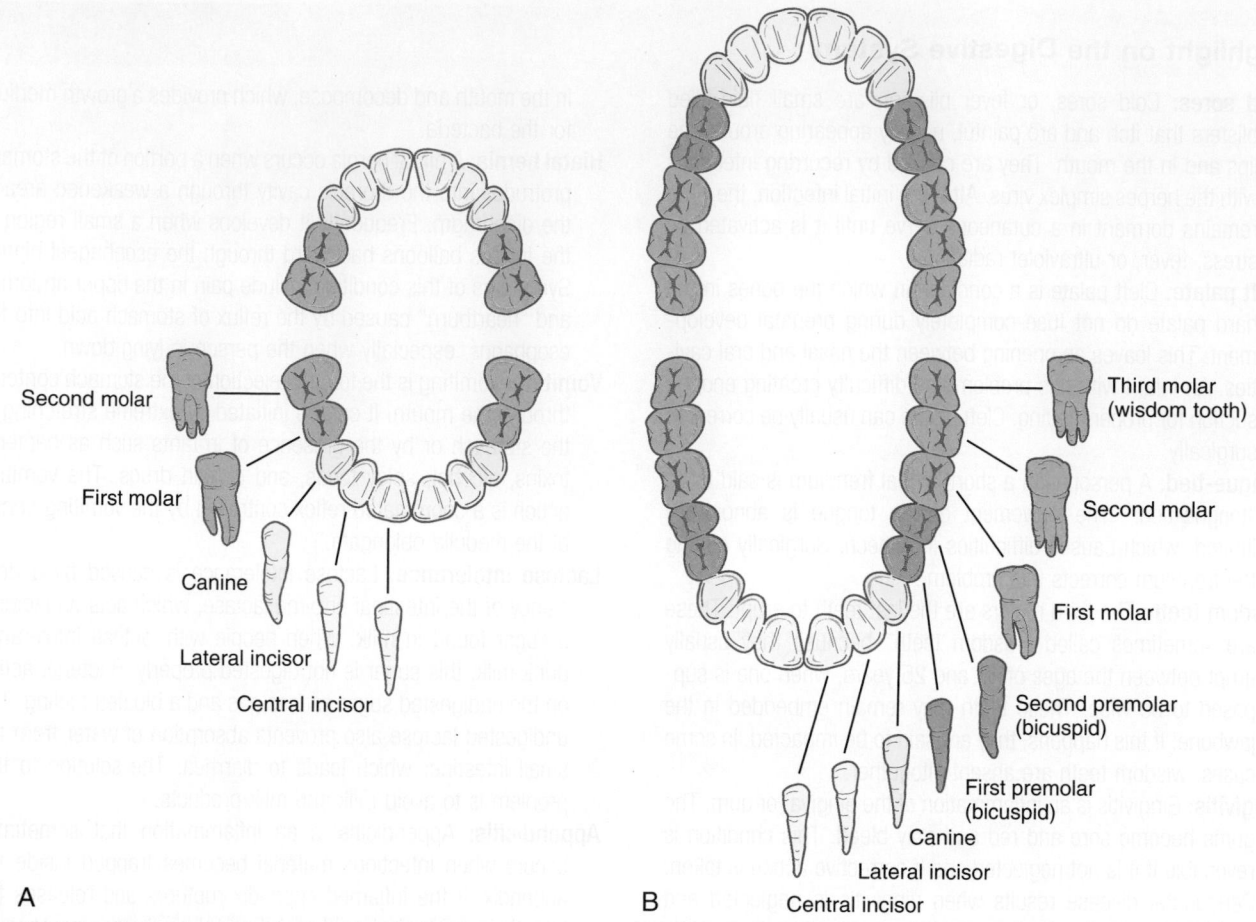

Figure 14-3 Deciduous **(A)** and permanent **(B)** teeth. The deciduous dentition on the left has 20 teeth. The permanent dentition on the right contains 32 teeth.

soft palate ends in a projection called the **uvula.** During swallowing, the soft palate and uvula move upward to direct food away from the nasal cavity and into the oropharynx.

Tongue

The largest and most movable organ in the oral cavity is the **tongue.** Most of the tongue consists of skeletal muscle. The major attachment for the tongue is the posterior region, or **root,** which is anchored to the hyoid bone. The anterior portion is relatively free but is connected to the floor of the mouth, in the midline, by a membranous fold of tissue called the **lingual frenulum.** The dorsal surface of the tongue is covered by tiny projections called **papillae.** The papillae provide friction for manipulating food in the mouth, and they also contain the taste buds (see Chapter 10). The **lingual tonsils** are embedded in the posterior surface of the tongue. The lingual tonsils provide defense against bacteria that enter the mouth.

The muscles in the tongue allow the tongue to perform the following: manipulate the food in the mouth for mastication, move the food around to mix it with saliva, shape it into a ball-like mass called a *bolus,* and direct it toward the pharynx for swallowing. It is a major sensory organ for taste and is one of the major organs used in speech.

Teeth

Two different sets of teeth develop in the mouth. The first set begins to appear at approximately 6 months of age and continues to develop until about 2½ years of age. This set is known as the **primary** or **deciduous teeth.** The primary teeth contain 10 teeth in each jaw for a total of 20 teeth. Figure 14-3, *A* illustrates the types of primary teeth. Starting at 6 years of age, the primary teeth begin to fall out and are replaced by the **secondary** or **permanent teeth.** This set contains 16 teeth in each jaw for a total of 32 teeth. These teeth are illustrated in Figure 14-3, *B.*

Different teeth are shaped to handle food in different ways. The **incisors** are chisel-shaped and have sharp edges for biting food. **Cuspids (canines)** are cone-shaped and have points for grasping and tearing food. **Bicuspids (premolars)** and **molars** have flat surfaces with rounded projections for crushing and grinding. Note the location of each type of tooth in Figure 14-3.

Although the different types of teeth have different shapes, each tooth has three parts:
- A crown
- A neck
- A root

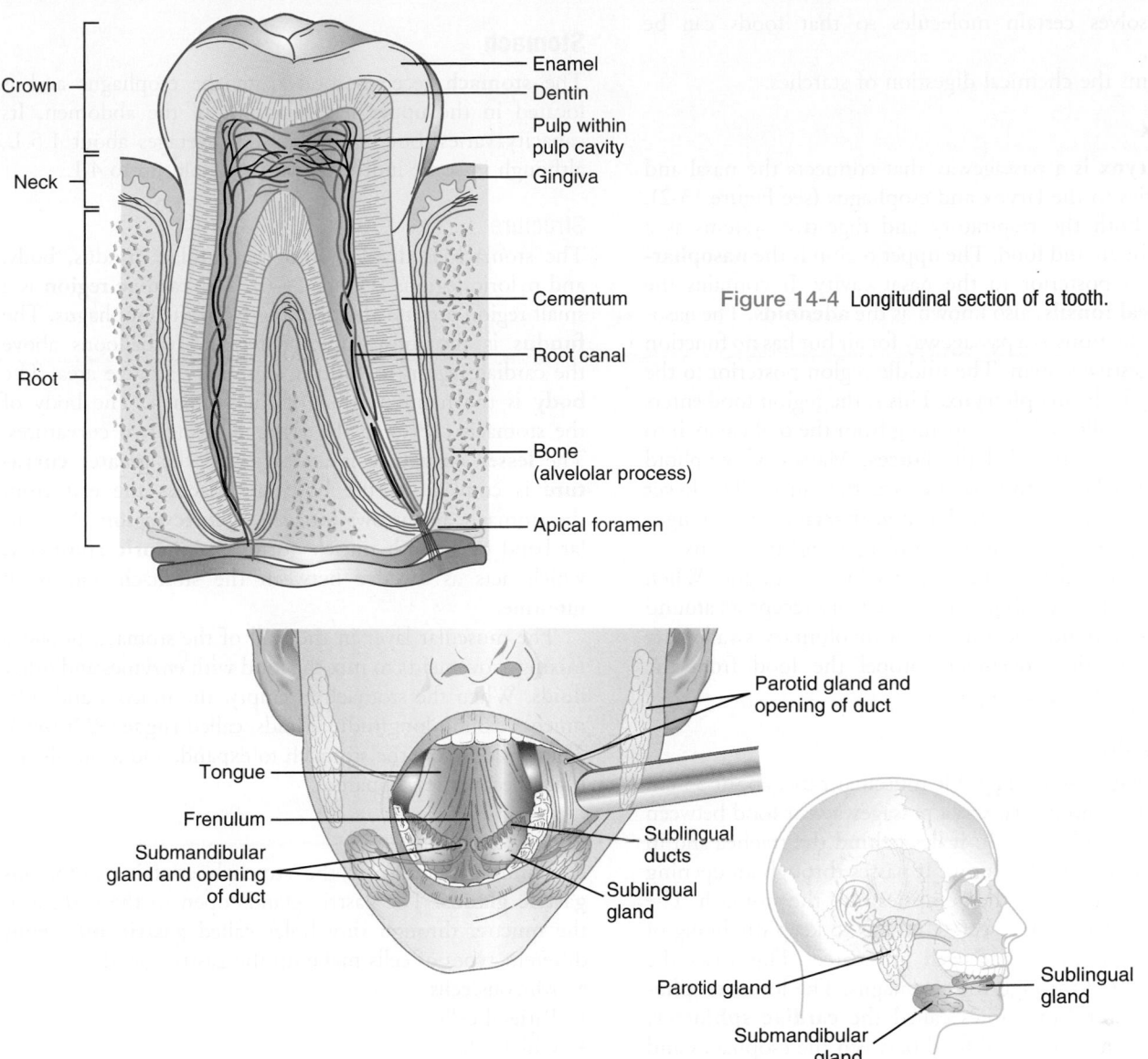

Figure 14-4 Longitudinal section of a tooth.

Figure 14-5 Locations of the salivary glands.

The **crown** is the visible portion of the tooth, covered by **enamel.** The **root** is the portion that is embedded in the sockets (alveolar processes) of the mandible and maxilla. The **neck** is a small region in which the crown and root meet and is adjacent to the **gingiva,** or **gum.**

The central core of a tooth is the **pulp cavity.** It contains the **pulp,** which consists of connective tissue, blood vessels, and nerves. In the root, the pulp cavity is called the **root canal.** Nerves and blood vessels enter the root through an **apical foramen.** The pulp cavity is surrounded by **dentin,** which forms the bulk of the tooth. Dentin is a living cellular substance similar to bone. In the root, the dentin is surrounded by a thin layer of calcified connective tissue called **cementum,** which attaches the root to the **periodontal ligaments.** The ligaments have fibers that firmly anchor the root in the alveolar process. **Enamel** surrounds the dentin in the crown of the tooth. Enamel is the hardest substance in the body. Figure 14-4 shows a longitudinal section of a tooth and illustrates the major features.

Salivary Glands

Three pairs of **salivary glands** secrete saliva into the oral cavity. The saliva is mixed with food during mastication (Figure 14-5). The **parotid glands** are the largest of the salivary glands. One gland is located on each side of the head just in front of the ear. **Submandibular glands** are located on the floor of the mouth. Small **sublingual glands** are also located in the floor of the mouth, anterior to the submandibular glands, and under the tongue.

Saliva contains water, mucus, and the enzyme **amylase.** Functions of saliva include the following:
- It has a cleansing action on the teeth.
- It moistens and lubricates food during mastication and swallowing.

- It dissolves certain molecules so that foods can be tasted.
- It begins the chemical digestion of starches.

Pharynx

The **pharynx** is a passageway that connects the nasal and oral cavities to the larynx and esophagus (see Figure 13-2). It serves both the respiratory and digestive systems as a channel for air and food. The upper region is the **nasopharynx** and is posterior to the nasal cavity. It contains the **pharyngeal tonsils,** also known as the **adenoids.** The nasopharynx functions as a passageway for air but has no function in the digestive system. The middle region posterior to the oral cavity is the **oropharynx.** This is the region food enters when it is swallowed. The opening from the oral cavity into the oropharynx is called the **fauces.** Masses of lymphoid tissue, the **palatine tonsils,** are near the fauces. The lower region of the pharynx is the **laryngopharynx.** The laryngopharynx opens into both the esophagus and the larynx.

Food is forced into the pharynx by the tongue. When food reaches the opening (fauces), sensory receptors around the fauces respond and initiate an involuntary swallowing reflex. Peristaltic movements propel the food from the pharynx into the esophagus.

Esophagus

The **esophagus** is a collapsible muscular tube, about 25 cm (10 in) long, and it serves as a passageway for food between the pharynx and stomach. It lies behind the trachea and in front of the vertebral column. It passes through an opening in the diaphragm and then empties into the stomach. The mucosa has glands that secrete mucus to keep the lining of the esophagus moist and well lubricated. This eases the passage of food through the esophagus. The lower **esophageal sphincter** (sometimes called the **cardiac sphincter**) controls the movement of food between the esophagus and the stomach.

Stomach

The **stomach** receives food from the esophagus and is located in the upper left quadrant of the abdomen. Its capacity varies, but in the adult it averages about 1.5 L, although in some individuals it may hold up to 4 L.

Structure

The stomach is divided into the cardiac, fundus, body, and pyloric regions (Figure 14-6). The **cardiac region** is a small region around the opening from the esophagus. The **fundus** is the most superior region. It balloons above the cardiac region to form a temporary storage area. The **body** is the main portion of the stomach. The body of the stomach curves to the right, creating two curvatures. The **lesser curvature** is concave and the **greater curvature** is convex. As the body approaches the exit from the stomach, it narrows into the **pyloric region.** A circular band of smooth muscle forms the **pyloric sphincter,** which acts as a valve between the stomach and small intestine.

The muscular layer in the wall of the stomach provides mixing movements to mix the food with enzymes and other fluids. When the stomach is empty, the mucosa and submucosa exhibit longitudinal folds, called **rugae** (ROO-jee). These folds allow the stomach to expand, and as it fills the rugae become less apparent.

Gastric Secretions

The mucosal lining of the stomach contains numerous **gastric glands.** The gastric glands open to the surface of the mucosa through tiny holes called **gastric pits.** Four different types of cells make up the gastric glands:
- Mucous cells
- Parietal cells
- Chief cells
- Endocrine cells

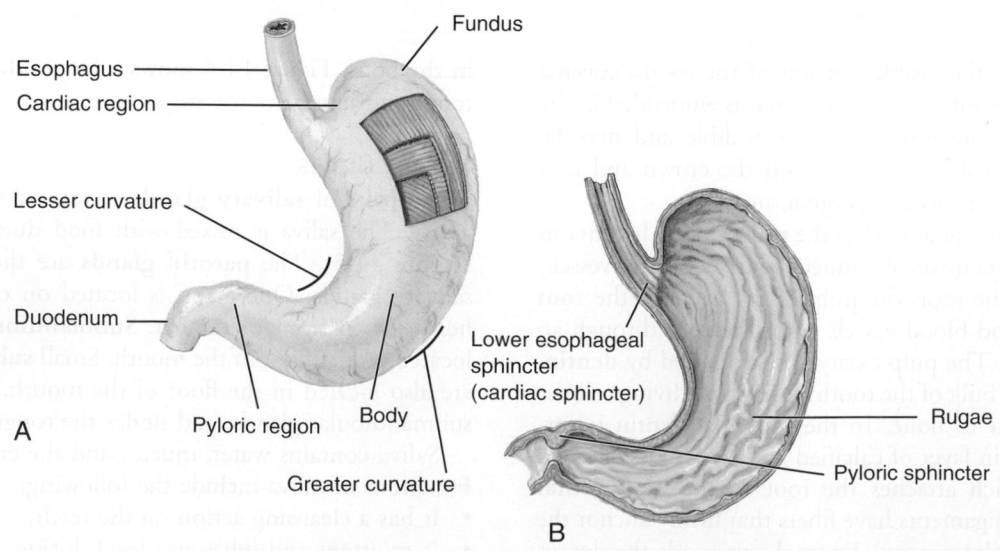

Figure 14-6 Features of the stomach. **A,** External view. **B,** Internal view. Note the rugae.

Exocrine gastric glands are composed of mucous cells, parietal cells, and chief cells. The secretions of the exocrine gastric glands make up the **gastric juice.** Approximately 2 to 3 L of gastric juice are produced every day. The products of the endocrine cells are secreted directly into the bloodstream and are not a part of the gastric juice.

Mucous cells produce two types of **mucus** in the stomach. One type is thick and alkaline and forms a protective coating for the stomach lining. The other type is thin and watery. It mixes with the food and creates a fluid medium for chemical reactions. **Parietal cells** secrete **hydrochloric acid** and **intrinsic factor.** The hydrochloric acid kills bacteria and provides an acidic environment for the action of enzymes in the stomach. Intrinsic factor aids in the absorption of vitamin B_{12}. **Chief cells** secrete **pepsinogen.** Pepsinogen is an inactive form of the enzyme pepsin. Hydrochloric acid converts the inactive pepsinogen into the active enzyme pepsin, which begins the chemical digestion of proteins.

The **endocrine cells** secrete the hormone **gastrin,** which functions in the regulation of gastric activity. Table 14-1 summarizes the various cells and secretions of the gastric glands.

The churning action of the muscles in the stomach wall breaks the food particles of the bolus that was swallowed into smaller sizes and mixes them with the gastric juice. This produces a semifluid mixture called **chyme** (KYME), which leaves the stomach through the pyloric sphincter and enters the small intestine.

Regulation of Gastric Secretions

The regulation of gastric secretions is accomplished through neural and hormonal mechanisms. Gastric juice is produced all the time, but the amount varies based on certain factors. Regulation of gastric secretions may be divided into cephalic, gastric, and intestinal phases.

The **cephalic phase** begins when an individual thinks pleasant thoughts about food or sees, smells, or tastes food. This phase anticipates food and prepares the stomach to receive it by increasing the secretion of gastric juice. The **gastric phase** accounts for more than two thirds of the gastric juice secretion. The gastric phase begins when food reaches the stomach. The presence of food in the stomach and the distention of the stomach wall stimulate reflexes that result in gastrin secretion. Gastrin, in turn, stimulates the secretion of gastric juice, which contains hydrochloric acid and pepsinogen. The hydrochloric acid acidifies the stomach contents and activates the pepsinogen into pepsin, which breaks down proteins.

The passage of chyme through the pyloric sphincter into the first part (duodenum) of the small intestine triggers the **intestinal phase** of regulation. Distention and the presence of acid chyme in the duodenum stimulate the secretion of intestinal hormones, which in turn inhibit gastric secretions. These inhibitory responses help prevent excess acid chyme from entering the small intestine. The intestinal phase regulates the entry of chyme into the small intestine.

Stomach Emptying

Peristalsis in the stomach pushes chyme toward the pyloric region. As the chyme accumulates, the pyloric sphincter relaxes and a small amount of chyme is pumped into the small intestine. The rate at which the stomach empties depends on the nature of the contents and the receptivity of the small intestine. The stomach is usually empty within 4 hours after a meal. Liquids tend to pass through the stomach quickly. Solids stay in the stomach until they are well mixed with gastric juice. Carbohydrates move through rather quickly, proteins take a little longer, and fatty foods may stay in the stomach as long as 4 to 6 hours.

Small Intestine

The small intestine is about 2.5 cm (1 in) in diameter and 6 m (20 ft) long. It extends from the pyloric sphincter to the ileocecal valve, where it empties into the large intestine. The function of the small intestine includes the following: finishing the process of digestion, absorbing the nutrients, and passing the residue on to the large intestine. The liver, gallbladder, and pancreas are accessory organs of the digestive system that are closely associated with the small intestine. These are described later in this chapter.

Structure

The small intestine follows the general structure of the digestive tract in that the wall has four layers: mucosa, submucosa, smooth muscle, and serosa. The mucosa and submucosa have circular folds, called **plicae circulares** (PLY-kee sir-kyoo-LAIR-eez), which increase the surface area for absorption (Figure 14-7). Finger-like extensions of the mucosa, called **villi,** project from the circular folds, and this further increases the surface area. Each villus surrounds a blood capillary network and a lymph capillary, or **lacteal.** These function in the absorption of nutrients. **Intestinal glands** extend downward between adjacent villi. The surface epithelium on the villi has tiny hairlike cytoplasmic extensions, called **microvilli,** that form a **brush border,** which again increases surface area.

Table 14-1	Secretions of Gastric Glands	
Cell Type	Secretion	Function
Mucous cells	Mucus (thick, alkaline)	Protects stomach lining
	Mucus (thin, watery)	Medium for chemical reactions
Parietal cells	Hydrochloric acid	Kills bacteria; activates pepsinogen
	Intrinsic factor	Absorption of vitamin B_{12}
Chief cells	Pepsinogen (active form is pepsin)	Begins digestion of proteins into polypeptides
Endocrine cells	Gastrin (a hormone)	Stimulates gastric gland secretion

From Applegate E: *The anatomy and physiology learning system,* ed 4, St Louis, 2011, Saunders.

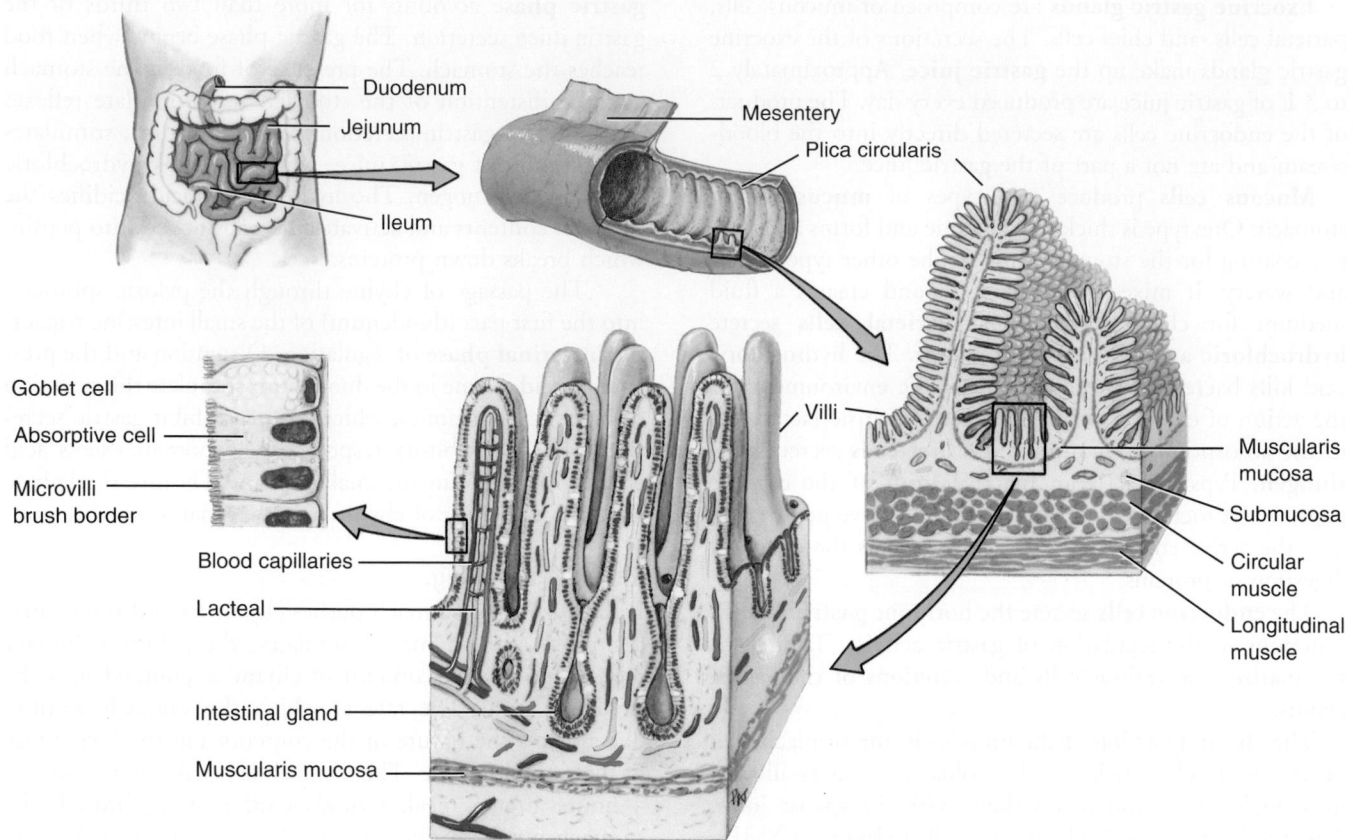

Figure 14-7 Wall of the small intestine.

Although the structure is similar throughout, the length of the small intestine is divided into three regions:

- Duodenum
- Jejunum
- Ileum

The **duodenum** is the first part and is about 25 cm (10 inches) long. It begins at the pyloric sphincter and continues in a C-shaped curve to the jejunum. The duodenum receives the chyme from the stomach and secretions from the liver and pancreas.

The second portion of the small intestine is the **jejunum,** which is about 2.5 m (8 ft) long. This is continuous with the third portion, the **ileum,** which is about 3.5 m (11.5 ft) long. No distinct separation exists between the jejunum and ileum. They are similar in structure and are suspended from the abdominal wall by a fold of peritoneum, called **mesentery.** There is a gradual decrease in the number and length of the villi and an increase in the number of goblet cells in the mucosa from the beginning of the jejunum to the terminal portion of the ileum.

Secretions of the Small Intestine

Intestinal glands secrete large amounts of watery fluid that is neutral or slightly alkaline in pH. It keeps the chyme in a liquid form and provides both an appropriate environment for the many chemical reactions of digestion and a fluid medium for the absorption of nutrients. The fluid is readily reabsorbed by the capillaries in the microvilli.

Mucus is secreted by the wall of the small intestine. The alkaline mucus protects the intestinal wall from the acid chyme and digestive enzymes.

Digestive enzymes are located in the microvilli of the mucosal epithelial cells. These enzymes include the following: **peptidase,** which acts on segments of proteins called *peptides;* **maltase, sucrase,** and **lactase,** which act on disaccharides (double sugars); and an **intestinal lipase,** which acts on neutral fats. **Enterokinase** (en-ter-oh-KYE-nayz), although not actually a digestive enzyme, is produced by the mucosal epithelial cells. This enzyme activates a protein-splitting enzyme from the pancreas.

In addition to mucus and digestive enzymes, intestinal cells secrete at least two hormones—secretin and cholecystokinin. **Secretin** (see-KREE-tin) stimulates the pancreas to secrete a fluid that has a high bicarbonate ion concentration. This fluid helps to neutralize chyme so that the intestinal enzymes can function. **Cholecystokinin** (koh-lee-sis-toh-KYE-nin) stimulates the release of bile from the gallbladder and the secretion of digestive enzymes from the pancreas. It also inhibits gastric motility and secretions.

The most important factor for regulating secretions in the small intestine is the presence of chyme. This is largely a local reflex action in response to chemical and mechanical

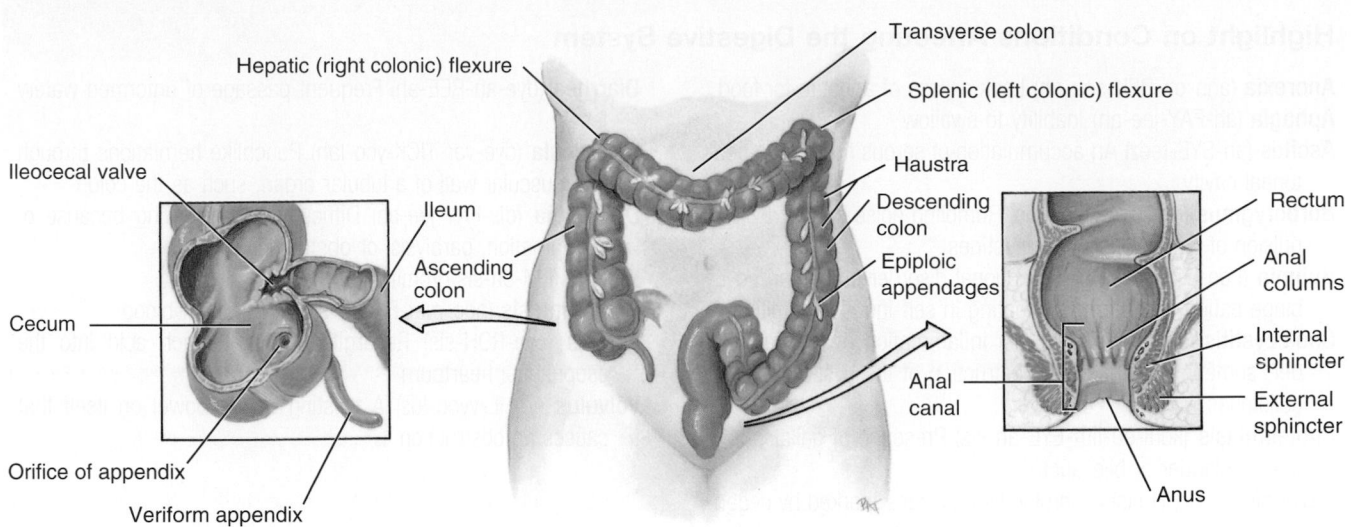

Figure 14-8 Features of the large intestine.

irritation from the chyme and in response to distention of the intestinal wall. This is a direct reflex action; thus the greater the amount of chyme, the greater the secretion.

Large Intestine

The **large intestine** is larger in diameter (6.25 cm or 2.5 inches) than the small intestine but is only about 1.5 m (5 ft) long (Figure 14-8). It begins at the **ileocecal** (ill-ee-oh-SEE-kul) **junction,** where the ileum enters the large intestine, and ends at the anus. The ileocecal junction has a circular band of smooth muscle fibers—the **ileocecal sphincter**—and a valve—the **ileocecal valve.**

Characteristics

The wall of the large intestine has the same types of tissue that are found in other parts of the digestive tract, but there are some distinguishing characteristics. The mucosa has large numbers of goblet cells but does not have any villi. The longitudinal muscle layer, although present, is incomplete. The longitudinal muscle is limited to three distinct bands, called **teniae coli** (TEE-nee-aye KOH-lye), that run the entire length of the colon. Contraction of the teniae coli exerts pressure on the wall and creates a series of pouches, called **haustra** (HAWS-trah), along the colon. **Epiploic** (ep-ih-PLOH-ik) **appendages,** pieces of fat-filled connective tissue, are attached to the outer surface of the colon.

Regions of the Large Intestine

The large intestine consists of the cecum, colon, rectum, and anal canal (see Figure 14-8).

Cecum: The cecum is the proximal portion of the large intestine. It is a blind pouch that extends from the ileocecal junction. The vermiform appendix is attached to the cecum. In humans the appendix has no function in digestion but does contain some lymphatic tissue.

Colon: The colon is the longest portion of the large intestine and is divided into ascending, transverse, descending, and sigmoid portions. The ascending colon begins at the ileocecal junction and travels upward on the right side, until it reaches the liver. Here it turns to the left, becomes the transverse colon, and continues across the abdomen toward the spleen on the left side. Here the colon turns sharply downward and travels along the posterior abdominal wall as the descending colon. The descending colon makes an S-shaped curve, called the *sigmoid colon,* and then becomes the rectum. The curve between the ascending and transverse portions is the hepatic flexure. The curve between the transverse and descending portions is the splenic flexure.

Rectum: The rectum continues from the sigmoid colon to the anal canal and has a thick muscular layer.

Anal canal: The last 2 to 3 cm (1 inch) of the digestive tract make up the anal canal, which opens to the outside at the anus. The mucosa of the anal canal is folded to form longitudinal anal columns. The smooth muscle layer is thick and forms the internal anal sphincter at the superior end of the anal canal. This sphincter is under involuntary control. At the inferior end of the anal canal is the external anal sphincter. This sphincter is composed of skeletal muscle and is under voluntary control.

Functions of the Large Intestine

The large intestine produces no digestive enzymes. Chemical digestion is completed in the small intestine before the chyme reaches the large intestine. There are no villi for the absorption of nutrients. This process is also accomplished in the small intestine. The primary functions of the large intestine are the absorption of fluid and electrolytes and the elimination of waste products.

Highlight on Conditions Affecting the Digestive System

Anorexia (ann-oh-REK-see-ah) Lack or loss of appetite for food

Aphagia (ah-FAY-jee-ah) Inability to swallow

Ascites (ah-SYE-teez) An accumulation of serous fluid in the peritoneal cavity

Borborygmus (bor-boh-RIG-mus) Rumbling noise caused by propulsion of gas through the intestines

Bulimia (boo-LIM-ee-ah) An emotional disorder characterized by binge eating and often terminating in self-induced vomiting

Cholecystitis (kohl-ee-sis-TYE-tis) Inflammation of the gallbladder; sometimes caused by obstruction of the cystic duct with gallstones

Cholelithiasis (kohl-ee-lith-EYE-ah-sis) Presence of gallstones in the gallbladder or bile duct

Cirrhosis (sih-ROH-sis) A chronic liver disease marked by degeneration of liver cells with eventual resistance to blood flow through the organ

Diarrhea (dye-ah-REE-ah) Frequent passage of unformed watery feces

Diverticula (dye-ver-TICK-yoo-lah) Pouchlike herniations through the muscular wall of a tubular organ, such as the colon

Dysphagia (dis-FAY-jee-ah) Difficulty in swallowing because of inflammation, paralysis, or obstruction

Emesis (EM-eh-sis) Vomiting

Hematemesis (hee-mat-EM-eh-sis) Vomiting of blood

Pyrosis (pye-ROH-sis) Regurgitation of stomach acid into the esophagus; heartburn

Volvulus (VAHL-vyoo-lus) A twisting of the bowel on itself that causes an obstruction ∎

The chyme that enters the large intestine contains materials that were not digested or absorbed in the small intestine—water, electrolytes, and bacteria. Some of the water and electrolytes are absorbed in the cecum and ascending colon. Although the quantity is relatively small, this absorptive function of the large intestine is important in maintaining fluid balance in the body. The residue that remains from the chyme becomes the feces.

The large intestine has the same types of mixing and peristaltic movements as occur in other parts of the digestive tract, but they are more sluggish and occur less frequently. They are more likely to occur after a meal as a result of reflexes initiated in the small intestine. As the rectum fills with feces, the defecation reflex is triggered and the waste products are eliminated.

The only secretory product in the large intestine is mucus from the numerous goblet cells. The mucus protects the intestinal wall against abrasion and irritation from the chyme. It also helps hold the particles of fecal matter together.

ACCESSORY ORGANS OF DIGESTION

The salivary glands, liver, gallbladder, and pancreas are not part of the digestive tract, but they have a role in digestive activities and are considered accessory organs. Because the salivary glands are so closely associated with the mouth and their primary function is performed in the mouth, they are considered part of the oral cavity. The liver and pancreas have functions in addition to digestion, and the gallbladder is closely related to the liver; thus these three organs are described as separate accessory organs in this section.

Liver

The liver is a large, reddish-brown organ. It is the largest gland in the body and is located in the right hypochondriac and epigastric regions of the abdomen, just beneath the diaphragm.

Structure of the Liver

The liver is divided into two major lobes and two minor lobes. The **falciform** (FALL-sih-form) **ligament** attaches the liver to the abdominal wall and separates the **right lobe** from the **left lobe.** Two additional small lobes are evident on the visceral surface: the **caudate lobe** and the **quadrate lobe** (Figure 14-9). The **porta** is also on the visceral surface. The porta is where the **hepatic artery** and **hepatic portal vein** enter the liver and where the **hepatic ducts** exit.

The substance of the liver is divided into functional units called **liver lobules.** A liver lobule consists of **hepatocytes** (liver cells) that radiate outward from the **central vein** like spokes of a wheel. Tiny channels, called **bile canaliculi,** are interwoven with the liver cells and carry the bile that is produced by the hepatocytes toward the periphery of the lobule. Bile canaliculi merge to form larger **right** and **left hepatic ducts.** These two ducts combine to form the common hepatic duct, which transports bile out of the liver. The plates of hepatocytes are separated from one another by venous channels, called **sinusoids,** which carry blood from the periphery of the lobule toward the central vein. The sinusoids are lined with special phagocytic cells, called *Kupffer cells,* that remove foreign particles from the blood as it flows through the sinusoids. **Portal triads,** which consist of a branch of the hepatic portal vein, a branch of the hepatic artery, and a branch of a hepatic duct, are located around the periphery of the lobule.

Blood Supply to the Liver

The liver receives blood from two sources. Freshly oxygenated blood is brought to the liver by the **common hepatic artery.** Blood that is rich in nutrients from the digestive tract is carried to the liver by the **hepatic portal vein.**

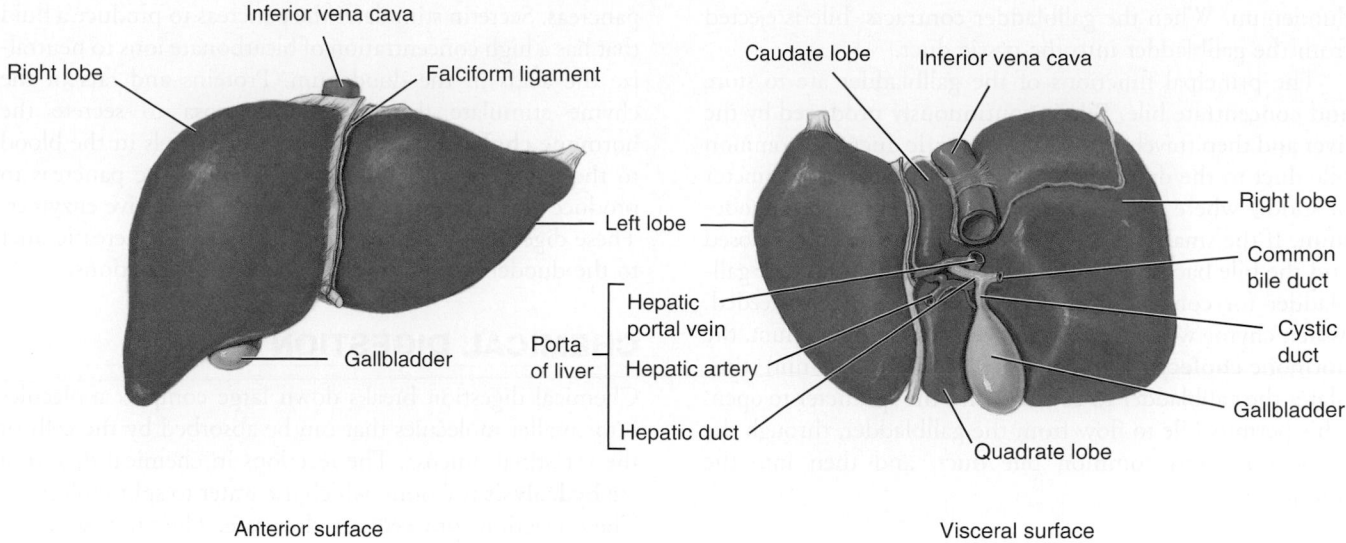

Figure 14-9 Features of the liver.

Venous blood from the hepatic portal vein and arterial blood from the hepatic arteries mix together as the blood flows through the sinusoids toward the **central vein.** The central veins of the liver lobules merge to form larger **hepatic veins** that drain into the inferior vena cava.

Functions of the Liver

The liver has a wide variety of functions, many of which are vital to life. Hepatocytes (liver cells) perform most of the functions attributed to the liver, but the phagocytic Kupffer cells that line the sinusoids are responsible for cleansing the blood. Liver functions include the following:

Secretion: The liver produces and secretes bile.

Synthesis of bile salts: Bile salts are produced in the liver and facilitate fat digestion and the absorption of fats and fat-soluble vitamins.

Synthesis of plasma proteins: The liver synthesizes albumin, fibrinogen, globulins, and clotting factors.

Storage: The liver stores glucose in the form of glycogen and also stores iron and vitamins A, B_{12}, D, E, and K.

Detoxification: The liver alters the chemical composition of toxic compounds to make them less harmful. It also changes the configuration of certain drugs, such as penicillin, and excretes them in the bile to remove them from the body.

Excretion: Hormones, drugs, cholesterol, and bile pigments from the breakdown of hemoglobin are excreted in the bile.

Carbohydrate metabolism: The liver has a major role in maintaining blood glucose levels. It removes excess glucose from the blood and converts it to glycogen for storage; it breaks down glycogen into glucose when more is necessary; and it converts noncarbohydrate molecules into glucose.

Lipid metabolism: The liver functions in the breakdown of fatty acids, in the synthesis of cholesterol and phospholipids, and in the conversion of excess carbohydrates and proteins into fats.

Protein metabolism: The liver converts certain amino acids into different amino acids as needed for protein synthesis. It also converts ammonia, produced in the breakdown of proteins, into urea, which is less toxic and can be excreted in the bile.

Filtering: The phagocytic Kupffer cells that line the sinusoids remove bacteria, damaged red blood cells, and other particles from the blood.

Bile

About 1 L of bile, a yellowish-green fluid, is produced by liver cells each day. Bile is slightly alkaline, with a pH of 7.6 to 8.6, so it helps neutralize the acid chyme. The main components of bile are water, bile salts, bile pigments, and cholesterol. The bile salts are useful secretory products of the liver, but the bile pigments and cholesterol are waste products excreted in the bile and eliminated from the body.

Bile salts function in the digestion of fats. Bile salts act as **emulsifying agents** that break large fat globules into tiny fat droplets. This increases the surface area of the fat and allows for more efficient enzyme action in fat digestion. Bile salts also facilitate the absorption of fat-soluble vitamins and the end products of fat digestion.

Bile pigments are produced in the breakdown of hemoglobin from damaged red blood cells. They are responsible for the color of the urine and feces. The principal bile pigment is **bilirubin** (bill-ih-ROO-bin). Cholesterol is a product of lipid metabolism. Bile salts act on cholesterol to make it soluble; then it is excreted in the bile.

Gallbladder

The **gallbladder** is a pear-shaped sac that is attached to the liver by the **cystic duct** (see Figure 14-9). The cystic duct joins the **hepatic duct** from the liver to form the **common bile duct.** The common bile duct empties into the duodenum. When the gallbladder contracts, bile is ejected from the gallbladder into the cystic duct.

The principal functions of the gallbladder are to store and concentrate bile. Bile is continuously produced by the liver and then travels through the hepatic duct and common bile duct to the duodenum. There is a sphincter (sphincter of Oddi) where the common bile duct enters the duodenum. If the small intestine is empty, the sphincter is closed and the bile backs up through the cystic duct into the gallbladder for concentration and storage until it is needed. When chyme with fatty contents enters the duodenum, the hormone **cholecystokinin** (koh-lee-sis-toh-KYE-nin) stimulates the gallbladder to contract and the sphincter to open. This permits bile to flow from the gallbladder, through the cystic duct and common bile duct, and then into the duodenum.

Pancreas

The **pancreas** is an elongated and flattened organ that is located along the posterior abdominal wall. One end of the pancreas, the **head,** is on the right side within the curve of the duodenum; the other end, the **tail,** is on the left side next to the spleen.

The pancreas has both endocrine and exocrine functions. The endocrine portion consists of the scattered **islets of Langerhans,** which secrete the hormones insulin and glucagon into the blood. These hormones and their functions are discussed in Chapter 11. The exocrine portion is the major part of the gland. It consists of **pancreatic acinar** (AS-ih-nar) **cells,** which secrete digestive enzymes into tiny ducts interwoven between the cells. These tiny ducts merge to form the main **pancreatic duct,** which extends the full length of the pancreas and empties into the duodenum. The pancreatic duct usually joins the common bile duct to form a single point of entry into the duodenum. Both ducts are controlled by the hepatopancreatic sphincter (sphincter of Oddi).

Pancreatic juice has a high concentration of bicarbonate ions and contains digestive enzymes that act on carbohydrates, proteins, and lipids. **Pancreatic amylase** acts on starch and other complex carbohydrates to break them into simpler sugars called *disaccharides.* Protein-splitting enzymes from the pancreas include trypsin. **Trypsin** breaks the proteins into shorter chains of amino acids, called *peptides.* Like other enzymes that act on proteins, trypsin is secreted in an inactive form, **trypsinogen.** Trypsinogen is activated by enterokinase when it reaches the duodenum. The pancreas also secretes peptidase enzymes that break peptides into amino acids. **Pancreatic lipase** breaks fats into fatty acids and monoglycerides.

Pancreatic secretion of digestive juice is regulated by the nervous system and by hormones. When parasympathetic impulses from the nervous system stimulate secretion of gastric juice, some impulses go to the pancreas and stimulate the secretion of pancreatic juice. When acid chyme enters the duodenum, the intestinal mucosa produces the hormone **secretin,** which travels in the blood to the pancreas. Secretin stimulates the pancreas to produce a fluid that has a high concentration of bicarbonate ions to neutralize the acids in the duodenum. Proteins and fats in the chyme stimulate the intestinal mucosa to secrete the hormone **cholecystokinin,** which also travels in the blood to the pancreas. This hormone stimulates the pancreas to produce a pancreatic juice that is rich in digestive enzymes. These digestive enzymes travel through the pancreatic duct to the duodenum, where they perform their actions.

CHEMICAL DIGESTION

Chemical digestion breaks down large complex molecules into smaller molecules that can be absorbed by the cells of the intestinal mucosa. The reactions in chemical digestion are **hydrolysis** reactions, which use water to split molecules. These reactions proceed at a slow rate. The purpose of the various digestive enzymes is to speed up the hydrolysis reactions of chemical digestion. The enzymes do not alter the reactions; they just make them occur more rapidly. Table 14-2 reviews the hormones and digestive enzymes that are discussed in previous sections of this chapter.

Carbohydrate Digestion

Starches and other complex carbohydrates are first broken down into disaccharides, or double sugars, by the action of salivary amylase and pancreatic amylase. The disaccharides **sucrose, maltose,** and **lactose** are the result of this stage of digestion. Sucrase, maltase, and lactase—enzymes from the small intestine—act on the disaccharides to convert them to monosaccharides, or simple sugars, that can be absorbed. The digestion of maltose yields two molecules of glucose; sucrose produces one molecule of glucose and one of fructose; lactose yields one molecule each of glucose and galactose. The end products of complete carbohydrate digestion are the monosaccharides **glucose, fructose,** and **galactose.**

Protein Digestion

The first digestive enzyme to act on proteins is pepsin in the stomach. Pepsin is secreted by the gastric glands in an inactive form, pepsinogen, which is activated by hydrochloric acid. When chyme reaches the duodenum, trypsin from the pancreas acts on the proteins. Trypsin is secreted in the inactive form, trypsinogen, which is activated by enterokinase in the small intestine. Pepsin and trypsin break down proteins into shorter chains of amino acids called **peptides.** Peptidase enzymes from the small intestine and pancreas break the peptide bonds to produce **amino acids.** The amino acids are the absorbable end products of protein digestion.

Lipid Digestion

The small intestine is the only place in which lipid (fat) digestion occurs because the necessary enzymes are produced by the pancreas and enter the small intestine through the pancreatic duct. Triglycerides are the most abundant

Table 14-2	Enzymes and Hormones of the Digestive System	
Secretion	Source	Action
Enzymes		
Amylase	Salivary glands Pancreas	Digestion of complex carbohydrates into disaccharides
Pepsin	Stomach	Digestion of proteins into polypeptides
Sucrase Maltase Lactase	Small intestine	Digestion of disaccharides into glucose, fructose, and galactose
Peptidase	Small intestine Pancreas	Digestion of peptides into amino acids
Lipase	Small intestine Pancreas	Digestion of fats into monoglycerides and fatty acids
Enterokinase	Small intestine	Activates trypsinogen
Hormones		
Gastrin	Stomach	Stimulates activity of gastric glands
Secretin	Small intestine	Stimulates pancreas to secrete bicarbonate ions to neutralize acid chyme
Cholecystokinin	Small intestine	Stimulates gallbladder to contract and release bile; stimulates pancreas to secrete digestive enzymes

From Applegate E: *The anatomy and physiology learning system,* ed 4, St Louis, 2011, Saunders.

dietary fats. Fat molecules tend to attract one another to form large globules, which reduces the surface area for enzyme action. After the fats enter the duodenum, they are **emulsified** by bile. Emulsification does not break any chemical bonds, but it reduces the attraction between molecules so that they disperse. Pancreatic lipases act on the surfaces of the emulsified fat droplets. Lipase action breaks two fatty acid chains from the triglyceride molecules, yielding **monoglycerides** and **free fatty acids.**

ABSORPTION

Approximately 10 L of food, beverage, and secretions enter the digestive tract every day. Usually less than 1 L enters the large intestine. The other 9 L or more are absorbed in the small intestine. Absorption takes place along the entire length of the small intestine, but most of it occurs in the jejunum. By the time the chyme reaches the distal part of the ileum and large intestine, all that remains are some water, indigestible materials, and bacteria.

AGING OF THE DIGESTIVE SYSTEM

Throughout life the digestive system normally functions day after day with relatively few problems. There may be an occasional episode of GI tract inflammation, called *gastroenteritis,* caused by eating something that "doesn't agree," by irritation from excessively spicy foods, or by eating food that is contaminated by bacteria or toxins. Appendicitis tends to be fairly common in teenagers, but the prevalence decreases with age because the opening into the appendix tends to become smaller and possibly eventually closes. Ulcers and gallbladder problems are associated with middle age, often considered to be the high-stress time of life. Most of the difficulties in the digestive system before "old age" are caused by external problems rather than to structural changes within the system itself.

Structural changes in the digestive system occur as part of the normal aging process. These changes affect the overall operation of the system and may influence the nutritional state of the aging individual. In the mouth, teeth may become loose as a result of periodontal disease and have to be extracted. Because of dental problems, chewing may be uncomfortable. Salivary glands decrease their production of saliva, which reduces the salivary cleansing action and leads to a dry mouth (xerostomia). Thus food is not adequately moistened for chewing and swallowing. Taste sensations diminish, partially because there is less saliva to dissolve the taste particles and partially because there are fewer taste receptors. Loneliness and the problems in the oral cavity associated with aging may make eating a chore rather than a pleasure.

The mucosa in the stomach and intestines undergoes some atrophy with advancing age. In the stomach this may lead to a deficiency in hydrochloric acid and gastric juice for digestion. Pernicious anemia may develop because there is a lack of intrinsic factor from the gastric mucosa. In the small intestine, mucosal atrophy may lead to fewer enzymes and shorter villi; however, this does not appear to impair digestion and absorption in normal healthy people. The wall of the large intestine becomes thinner and weakens. This makes older people more susceptible to diverticulosis, in which the wall bulges outward to form balloon-like pockets. Constipation is a common complaint in the elderly; statistically, however, there seems to be no basis for it. This is more likely caused by lifestyle and habits rather than by structural changes in the digestive system.

Although structural and functional changes take place in the digestive system as part of the aging process, digestion and absorption are not altered noticeably in healthy older persons. A balanced diet, exercise, and a positive outlook on life will keep the digestive system in good working order for a long time.

TERMINOLOGY REVIEW

Medical Term	Word Parts	Definition
Absorption		The passage of digestive end products from the gastrointestinal tract into the blood or lymph.
Chyme		The semifluid mixture of food and gastric juice that leaves the stomach through the pyloric sphincter.
Mesentery		Extensions of peritoneum that are associated with the intestine.
Peristalsis		Rhythmic contractions of the intestine that move food along the digestive tract.
Plicae circulares		Circular folds in the mucosa and submucosa of the small intestine.
Rugae		Longitudinal folds in the mucosa of the stomach.

ON THE WEB

For information on the digestive system:

American Dietetic Association: www.eatright.org

Atlas of Gastrointestinal Endoscopy: www.endoatlas.com

Inner Body: www.innerbody.com/html/body.html

National Institute of Health Digestive Diseases: digestive.niddk.nih.gov

National Institute of Health—Office of Dietary Supplements: dietary-supplements.info.nih.gov

Pathophysiology of the Digestive System: arbl.cvmbs.colostate.edu/hbooks/pathphys/digestion/

The Helicobacter Foundation: www.helico.com

The Internet Pathology Laboratory for Medical Education—Gastrointestinal Pathology: library.med.utah.edu/WebPath/ORGAN.html *(Click on "Gastrointestinal Pathology")*

The Internet Pathology Laboratory for Medical Education—Hepatic Pathology: library.med.utah.edu/WebPath/ORGAN.html *(Click on "Hepatic Pathology")*

 Check out the Evolve site at http://evolve.elsevier.com/Bonewit/today/ to actively Prepare for your Certification, and to access additional interactive activities and exercises to help you study and prepare for success.

15

Urinary System

LEARNING OBJECTIVES

1. State six functions of the urinary system.
2. Describe the location and structural features of the kidneys.
3. Draw and label the parts of a nephron.
4. State the two parts of the juxtaglomerular apparatus.
5. Describe the location, structure, and function of the ureters, urinary bladder, and urethra.
6. List and describe the three steps in urine formation.
7. Identify the hormones that affect kidney function, and explain how they do so.
8. Explain the function of renin.
9. Describe ways in which the aging of an individual affects the urinary system.
10. Identify pathology related to the urinary system.

CHAPTER OUTLINE

INTRODUCTION TO THE URINARY SYSTEM
Components of the Urinary System
Kidneys
Ureters
Urinary Bladder
Urethra
Urine Formation

Glomerular Filtration
Tubular Reabsorption
Tubular Secretion
Regulation of Urine Concentration and Volume
Micturition
Aging of the Urinary System

KEY TERMS

glomerular capsule (gloh-MER-yoo-lar
  KAP-sool)

juxtaglomerular apparatus (juks-tah-gloh-
  MER-yoo-lar ap-pah-RAT-us)

nephron (NEFF-rahn)
renal tubule (REE-nal TOOB-yool)

INTRODUCTION TO THE URINARY SYSTEM

The overall function of the **urinary system** is to maintain the volume and composition of body fluids within normal limits. The urinary system accomplishes this by excreting the waste products that accumulate as a result of cellular metabolism. Because of this, the urinary system is sometimes referred to as the *excretory system.* Although the urinary system has a major role in excretion, other organs contribute to the excretory function. Some waste products, such as carbon dioxide and water, are excreted by the lungs through the respiratory system. The skin excretes wastes through the sweat glands. The liver and intestines excrete bile pigments that result from the destruction of hemoglobin. The major task of excretion, however, still belongs to the urinary system. If the urinary system fails, the other organs cannot take over and compensate adequately. In addition to eliminating waste products, the urinary system maintains an appropriate fluid volume. It does this by regulating the amount of water that is excreted in the urine. Other functions of the urinary system include regulating the concentrations of various electrolytes in the body fluids and maintaining normal pH of the blood.

In addition to maintaining fluid balance in the body, the urinary system controls red blood cell production by secreting the hormone **erythropoietin** (ee-rith-roh-poy-EE-tin). The urinary system also plays a role in maintaining normal blood pressure by secreting the enzyme **renin.**

COMPONENTS OF THE URINARY SYSTEM

The **urinary system** consists of the kidneys, ureters, urinary bladder, and urethra. The kidneys produce the urine. The ureters transport the urine away from the kidneys to the urinary bladder. The urinary bladder stores the urine until it is excreted from the body. The urethra is a tubular structure that carries the urine from the urinary bladder to the outside of the body. The components of the urinary system are illustrated in Figure 15-1.

Kidneys

The **kidneys** are the primary organs of the urinary system. They are the organs that filter the blood, remove the wastes, and excrete the wastes into the urine. They are the organs that perform the functions of the urinary system. The other components of the urinary system are accessory structures to help eliminate the urine from the body.

Location

The kidneys are located between the twelfth thoracic and third lumbar vertebrae, one on each side of the vertebral column. The right kidney is usually slightly lower than the left because the liver displaces it downward. The kidneys are partially protected by the lower ribs and lie in shallow

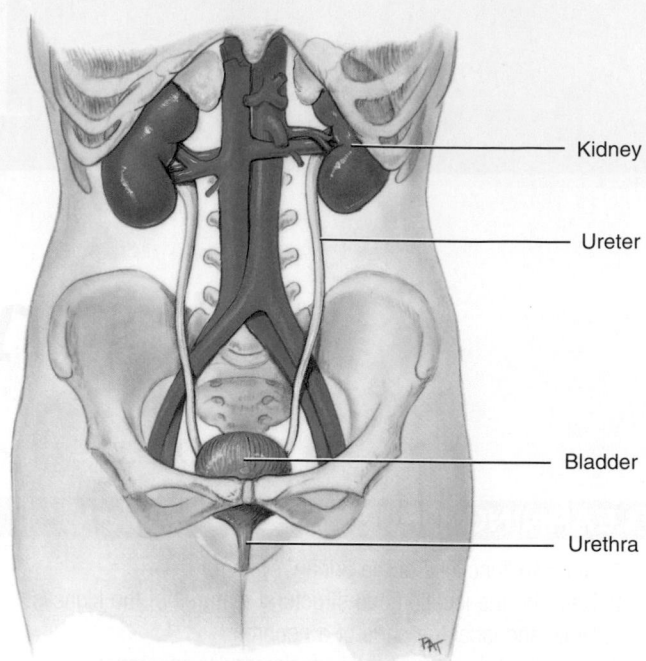

Figure 15-1 Components of the urinary system.

depressions against the posterior abdominal wall behind the peritoneum (retroperitoneal). Each kidney is held in place by connective tissue, called **renal fascia.**

A thick layer of adipose tissue surrounds each kidney. This is called *perirenal fat,* and it helps to protect the kidney. A tough, fibrous connective tissue encases each kidney and is called the *renal capsule.* The renal capsule provides support for the soft tissue that is inside.

Macroscopic Structure

In the adult, each kidney is approximately 3 cm thick, 6 cm wide, and 12 cm long (1.2 × 2.5 × 5 inches). The kidney is bean-shaped with an indentation, called the **hilum.** The hilum leads to a large cavity within the kidney called the **renal sinus.** The **ureter** and **renal vein** leave the kidney at the hilum, and the **renal artery** enters the kidney at the hilum.

The macroscopic internal structure of the kidney is illustrated in Figure 15-2. The outer, reddish region is the **renal cortex.** The renal cortex surrounds a darker reddish-brown region called the **renal medulla.** The renal medulla consists of a series of **renal pyramids.** The renal pyramids appear striated because they contain straight tubular structures and blood vessels. The wide bases of the pyramids are adjacent to the cortex. The pointed ends of the pyramids, called **renal papillae,** are directed toward the center of the kidney. Portions of the renal cortex extend into the spaces between adjacent pyramids to form **renal columns.** The cortex and medulla make up the functional tissue of the kidney.

The central region of the kidney contains the **renal pelvis,** a large cavity that collects the urine as it is produced.

Highlight on the Urinary System

Hangover: Alcohol inhibits the secretion of antidiuretic hormone, so when people drink alcohol, they experience diuresis, or excessive urination. Experts believe that the dehydration caused by diuresis contributes to "hangover" symptoms.

Kidney stones: Kidney stones develop when uric acid or calcium salts precipitate instead of remaining dissolved in the urine. The stones usually form in the renal pelvis, but they may also develop in the urinary bladder. If small enough, they may pass naturally with urine flow but usually cause a lot of discomfort. If kidney stones cause a serious obstruction, they may need to be surgically removed. A newer method of treatment called *lithotripsy* uses high-frequency sound waves to break the stone into small pieces so that it may pass naturally. The formation of stones in the urine is called **urolithiasis.**

Nephrons: The number of nephrons does not increase after birth. Growth of the kidney occurs from enlargement of the individual nephrons. When nephrons are damaged they are not replaced.

Nephroptosis: Nephroptosis, commonly referred to as a *floating kidney,* occurs when the kidney is no longer held in place by the renal fascia and it drops out of its normal position. This may make the kidney more vulnerable to injury if it is no longer protected by the ribs. Another danger is that the ureter may become twisted and block the flow of urine. Nephroptosis occurs more frequently in horseback riders, truck drivers, and people who ride motorcycles.

Polycystic kidney disease: This inherited condition affects the tubular portion of the nephrons. Swelling or cysts develop along the tubules, and as the cysts enlarge they displace and damage functional kidney tissue. This eventually leads to a total loss of kidney function. When this occurs in both kidneys, a transplant is necessary.

Uremia: When the kidneys do not function properly and fail to remove the waste products from the blood, uremia may result. Uremia is a condition in which there is a toxic level of urea in the blood.

Urinary incontinence: Urinary incontinence is the inability to control urination and to retain urine in the bladder. Temporary incontinence may result when the muscles around the bladder and urethra become weakened and lose muscle tone. This is sometimes caused by stretching of the muscles during childbirth. Because these muscles help restrict the outlet of the bladder, their weakness contributes to a leakage of urine. A cough or sneeze may increase pressure within the bladder sufficiently to force urine to escape. Permanent incontinence is usually caused by damage to the central nervous system or by extensive damage to the bladder or urethra.

Urinary tract infection (UTI): UTIs occur more frequently in women than in men because of differences in the urethra. In females the urethral opening is in close proximity to the anal opening, which gives intestinal bacteria easier access to the urethra. The female urethra is short, which allows any infection to spread to the urinary bladder. An infection of the urethra is called *urethritis,* and one of the urinary bladders is called *cystitis.* ∎

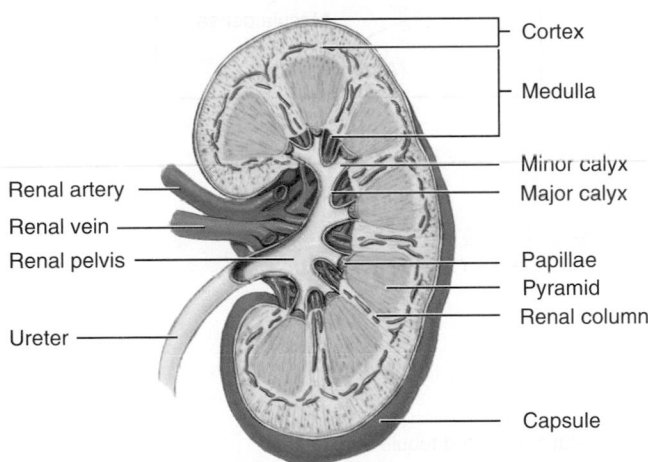

Figure 15-2 Coronal (frontal) section through the kidney.

The periphery of the renal pelvis is interrupted by cuplike projections called **calyces.** A **minor calyx** surrounds the renal papillae of each pyramid and collects urine from that pyramid. Several minor calyces converge to form a **major calyx.** From the major calyces the urine flows into the renal pelvis and from there into the ureter.

Nephrons

Each kidney contains more than 1 million functional units, called **nephrons,** located in the cortex and medulla. The nephron is where the blood is filtered and urine is formed. A nephron consists of a renal corpuscle and a renal tubule (Figure 15-3).

The **renal corpuscle** consists of the **glomerulus** (gloh-MER-yoo-lus) and the **glomerular capsule (Bowman capsule).** The glomerulus is a cluster of capillaries. Blood enters the glomerulus through an **afferent arteriole** and is filtered. The blood then leaves the glomerulus through an **efferent arteriole** (Figure 15-4). As the blood is filtered, the filtrate enters the glomerular capsule, which continues as the renal tubule. Renal corpuscles are located in the cortex of the kidney and give it a granular appearance.

The **renal tubule,** which carries fluid away from the glomerular capsule, consists of a proximal convoluted tubule, a nephron loop (Henle loop), and a distal convoluted tubule.

The first portion of the tubule, located in the cortex, is highly coiled and is known as the **proximal convoluted tubule.** Next the tubule straightens and dips into the medulla, makes a U-turn, and ascends back toward the cortex. This forms the **nephron loop** (Henle loop). The portion of the loop that descends from the proximal convoluted tubule into the medulla is the **descending limb,**

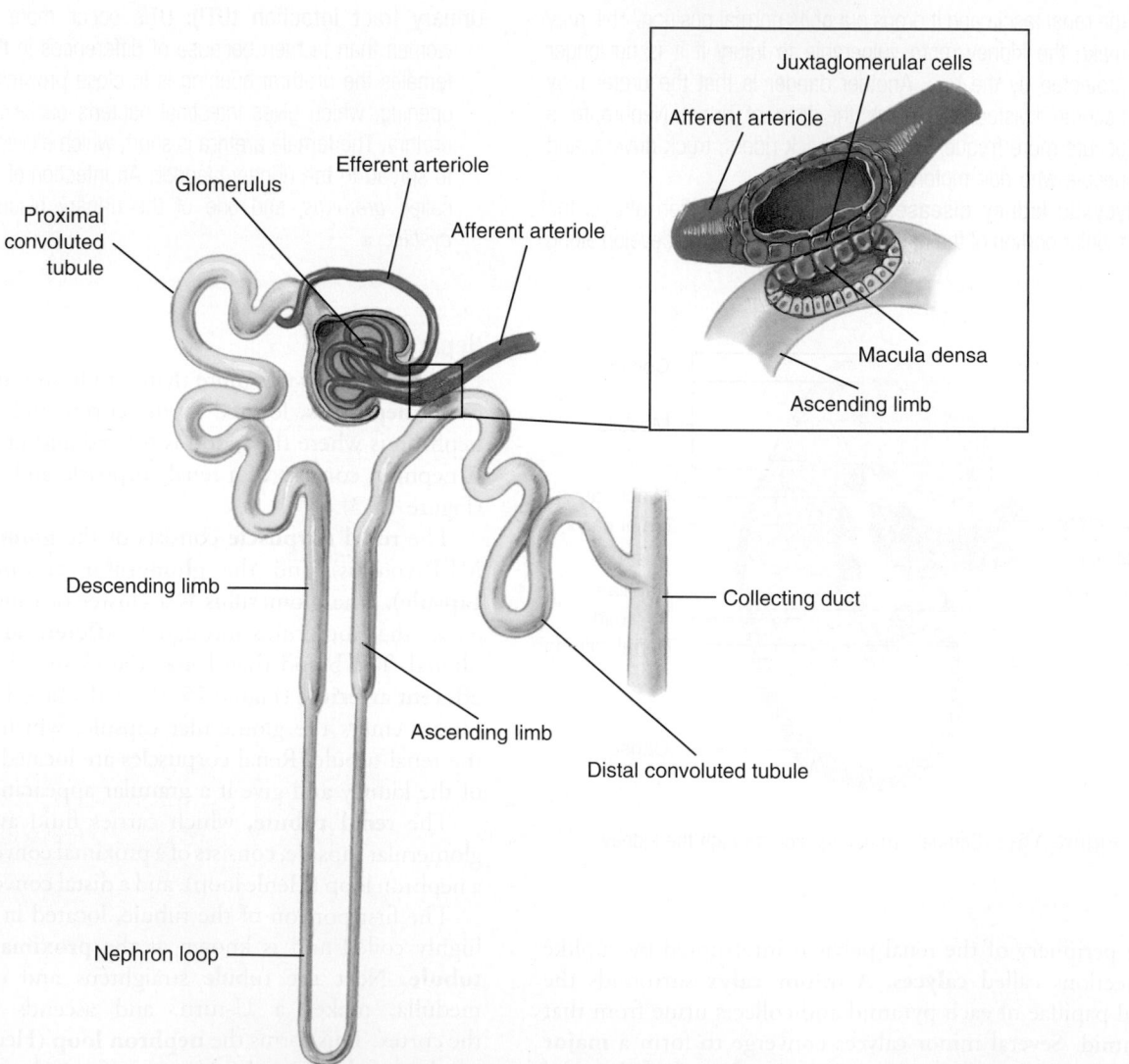

Figure 15-3 A section of a kidney showing the structures in the cortex and those in the medulla. The renal pyramids in the medulla contain the nephron loops and collecting ducts.

Figure 15-4 Juxtaglomerular apparatus and its relationship to the nephron. The juxtaglomerular apparatus is in the boxes. In the region of contact, the cells of the ascending limb are modified to form the macula densa, and the cells of the afferent arteriole are modified to form the juxtaglomerular cells. Together, these modified regions are the juxtaglomerular apparatus.

and the part that ascends back toward the cortex is the **ascending limb.** The final region of the tubule, which is also coiled and found in the cortex, is known as the **distal convoluted tubule** (see Figure 15-4).

Collecting Ducts

Urine passes from the distal convoluted tubules of the nephrons into **collecting ducts.** These straight tubules, with the nephron loops and blood vessels, give the medulla its striated appearance. Fluid flows from the collecting ducts into the minor calyces that surround the renal papillae.

Juxtaglomerular Apparatus

The ascending limb of the nephron loop, in the region where it continues into the distal convoluted tubule, comes into contact with the glomerular afferent arteriole of the same nephron (Figure 15-4). In the region of contact, the cells of the ascending limb are modified to form the **macula densa,** and those in the afferent arteriole are modified to form the **juxtaglomerular** (juks-tah-gloh-MER-yoo-lar) **cells.** The macula densa monitors sodium chloride concentration in the urine and also influences the juxtaglomerular cells. In the afferent arteriole, the juxtaglomerular cells produce the enzyme **renin,** which has a role in the regulation of blood pressure. Together, the macula densa and juxtaglomerular cells make up the **juxtaglomerular apparatus.**

Blood Flow through the Kidney

Blood flows through the kidneys at an approximate rate of 1200 mL/min. This is about one fourth of the total cardiac output. Blood is brought to the kidneys by the renal arteries, which are branches from the abdominal aorta. The blood flows through the arteries of the kidney until it enters the afferent arterioles. Each of these tiny vessels continues into a glomerulus, where the blood is filtered. The blood leaves the glomerulus through an efferent arteriole and enters a series of veins. The renal vein exits the kidney and takes blood to the inferior vena cava.

Ureters

Each **ureter** is a small tube, about 25 cm (10 inches) long, that carries urine from the renal pelvis to the urinary bladder. It descends from the renal pelvis and enters the urinary bladder on the posterior inferior surface.

The wall of the ureter consists of three layers (Figure 15-5). The outer layer is a supporting layer of fibrous connective tissue known as the **fibrous coat.** The middle layer is known as the **muscular coat.** It consists of smooth muscle. The main function of this layer is peristalsis to propel the urine through the ureter. The inner layer is the **mucosa.** This layer secretes mucus, which coats and protects the surface of the cells.

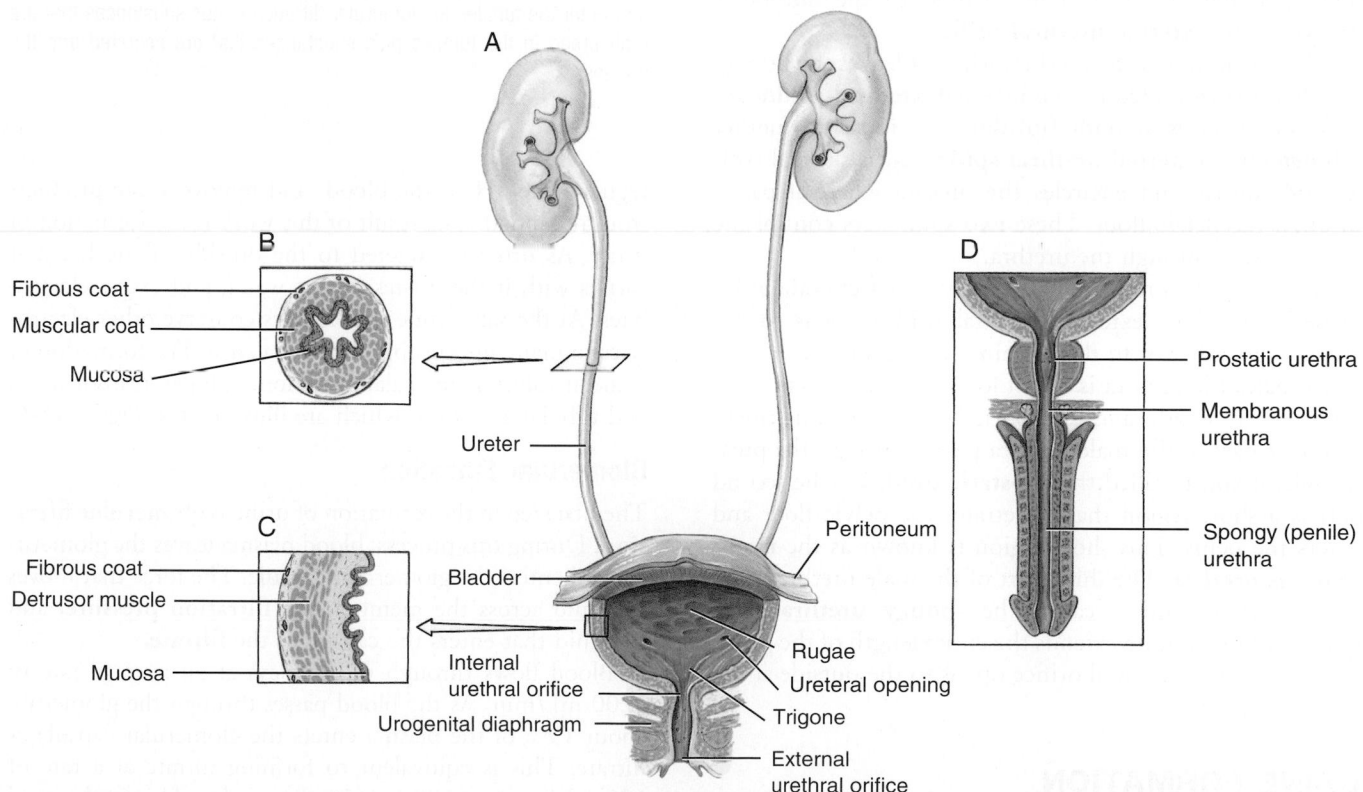

Figure 15-5 Ureter, urinary bladder, and urethra. **A,** Urinary tract. **B,** Cross section through the ureter. **C,** Cross section of the bladder wall. **D,** Regions of the male urethra.

Urinary Bladder

The **urinary bladder** is located in the pelvic cavity and is a temporary storage reservoir for urine (see Figure 15-5). The size and shape of the urinary bladder vary with the amount of urine it contains and with the pressure from surrounding organs.

The inner lining of the urinary bladder consists of a **mucous membrane.** When the bladder is empty, the mucosa has numerous folds called **rugae.** The rugae allow the bladder to expand as it fills. The next layer is the **muscularis,** which is composed of smooth muscle. The smooth muscle fibers in the muscular layer are interwoven in all directions, and collectively these are called the **detrusor** (dee-TROO-sor) **muscle.** Contraction of this muscle expels urine from the bladder.

A triangular area, called the **trigone,** is formed by three openings in the floor of the urinary bladder. Two of the openings are from the ureters and form the base of the trigone. Small flaps of mucosa cover these openings and act as valves that allow urine to enter the bladder but prevent it from backing up from the bladder into the ureters. The third opening, at the apex of the trigone, is the opening into the urethra. A band of the detrusor muscle encircles this opening to form the **internal urethral sphincter.**

Urethra

The final passageway for the flow of urine is the **urethra.** The urethra consists of a thin-walled tube that conveys urine from the floor of the urinary bladder to outside of the body (see Figure 15-5). The opening to the outside is known as the **external urethral orifice.**

The beginning of the urethra, where it leaves the urinary bladder, is surrounded by the **internal urethral sphincter.** This sphincter is smooth (involuntary) muscle. Another sphincter, the **external urethral sphincter,** is skeletal (voluntary) muscle and encircles the urethra where it passes through the pelvic floor. These two sphincters control the flow of urine through the urethra.

In females the urethra is short, only 3 to 4 cm (about 1½ inches) long. The external urethral orifice opens to the outside just anterior to the opening for the vagina.

In males the urethra is much longer, about 20 cm (7 to 8 inches) in length, and transports both urine and semen. The first part of the male urethra passes through the prostate gland and is called the **prostatic urethra.** The second part is a short region that penetrates the pelvic floor and enters the penis. This short region is known as the **membranous urethra.** The third part of the male urethra is the longest region and is called the **spongy urethra.** This portion of the urethra extends the entire length of the penis, and the external urethral orifice opens to the outside at the tip of the penis.

URINE FORMATION

The work of the kidneys, performed by the nephrons, is to maintain the volume and composition of body fluids,

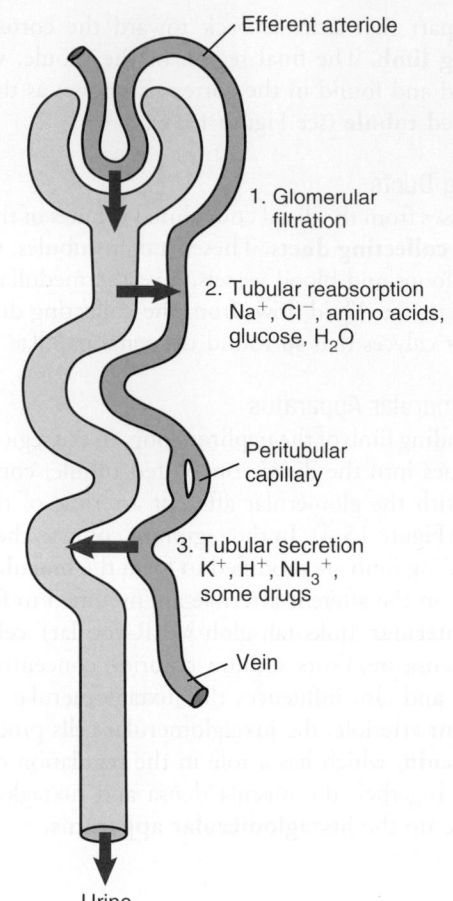

Figure 15-6 Steps in urine formation. Urine consists of the substances that enter the tubules in glomerular filtration minus substances that are reabsorbed in the tubules plus substances that are secreted into the tubules.

regulate the pH of the blood, and remove waste products from the blood. The result of this work is the formation of urine. As urine is excreted to the outside of the body, it carries with it the wastes, excess water, and excess electrolytes. At the same time the kidneys conserve other electrolytes to maintain the appropriate balance. The formation of urine involves glomerular filtration, tubular reabsorption, and tubular secretion, which are illustrated in Figure 15-6.

Glomerular Filtration

The first step in the formation of urine is **glomerular filtration.** During this process, blood plasma leaves the glomerulus and enters the glomerular capsule. The force that moves the fluid across the membrane is **filtration pressure,** and the fluid that enters the capsule is the **filtrate.**

Blood flows through the kidneys at an average rate of 1200 mL/min. As the blood passes through the glomeruli, about 19% of the plasma enters the glomerular capsule as filtrate. This is equivalent to forming filtrate at a rate of 125 mL/min, or 180 L (45 gal) per day. This is the total value for all the nephrons in both kidneys. The filtration membrane acts as a barrier that prevents blood cells and protein molecules from entering the capsule; therefore they are absent from the filtrate.

Tubular Reabsorption

If the volume and composition of the filtrate in the glomerular capsule are compared with the volume and composition of urine, it is obvious that changes occur after filtration. First of all, about 180 L (45 gal) of filtrate are formed in a 24-hour period. This volume is reduced to 1 to 2 L of urine. Glucose is present in the filtrate but normally absent in the urine. Urea and uric acid are present in higher concentrations in the urine than in the filtrate.

Tubular reabsorption is the first process that changes the volume and composition of the filtrate. Tubular reabsorption is the movement of substances from the filtrate in the kidney tubules into the blood. Only about 1% of the filtrate remains in the tubules and becomes urine. In general, water and other substances that are useful to the body are reabsorbed. Wastes remain in the filtrate and are excreted in the urine.

Tubular Secretion

The final process in the formation of urine is the transport of molecules and ions into the filtrate. This is called **tubular secretion.** Most of these substances are waste products of cellular metabolism that become toxic if allowed to accumulate in the body. Tubular secretion is the method by which some drugs, such as penicillin, are removed from the body. The tubular secretion of hydrogen ions plays an important role in regulating the pH of the blood. Other molecules and ions that may enter the filtrate by tubular secretion include potassium ions, creatinine, and histamine.

The final product, urine, produced by the nephrons of the kidney consists of the substances that are filtered, minus the substances that are reabsorbed in the tubules, plus the substances that are added by tubular secretion. If kidney function is impaired by disease or injury, dialysis may be necessary to maintain body fluid composition. Dialysis is a procedure used to separate waste material from the blood and to maintain fluid, electrolyte, and acid-base balance in the body.

Regulation of Urine Concentration and Volume

The concentration and volume of urine depend on conditions in the internal environment of the body. Cells in the hypothalamus are sensitive to changes in the composition of the blood and initiate appropriate responses that affect the kidneys. If the concentration of solutes in the blood increases above normal, the kidneys excrete a small volume of concentrated urine. This conserves water in the body and gets rid of solutes to restore the blood to normal. If the blood solute concentration decreases below normal, the kidneys conserve solutes and get rid of water by producing large quantities of dilute urine. Urine production plays an important role in maintaining homeostasis of blood concentration and volume. By regulating blood volume, the kidneys also play a role in regulating blood pressure because volume is directly related to pressure.

Under average conditions, the kidneys produce about 1500 mL of urine in a 24-hour period, but the volume may vary from 1 to 2 L. The pH may vary from 4.6 to 8, with an average of about 6. This means that urine is usually slightly acidic but may become alkaline under certain conditions such as vegetarian diets.

Three hormones—**aldosterone, antidiuretic hormone (ADH),** and **atrial natriuretic hormone**—influence urine concentration and volume. Aldosterone, secreted by cells of the adrenal cortex, acts on the kidney tubules to increase the reabsorption of sodium. When sodium is reabsorbed, water follows by osmosis. This reduces urine output.

Antidiuretic hormone (ADH) is produced by cells in the hypothalamus and is released from the posterior lobe of the pituitary gland. ADH makes the kidney tubules more permeable to water. When ADH is present, more water is reabsorbed, which reduces the volume of urine and makes it more concentrated. Water is conserved in the body. In the absence of ADH, the tubules are less permeable to water and there is less reabsorption. This results in large quantities of dilute urine, and water is lost from the body.

Special cells in the heart produce a hormone called *atrial natriuretic hormone,* or *atriopeptin,* which is secreted when the atrial cells are stretched. This hormone promotes the excretion of sodium and water by acting directly on the kidney tubules and by inhibiting the secretion of ADH, renin, and aldosterone. The result of atrial natriuretic hormone is a decrease in both blood volume and blood pressure.

Renin is an enzyme that is produced by the juxtaglomerular cells in the kidney in response to low blood pressure or decreased blood sodium concentration. Renin promotes the production of **angiotensin II** in the blood. Angiotensin II is a powerful vasoconstrictor, a substance that increases the blood pressure. Angiotensin II also stimulates the adrenal gland to secrete aldosterone, which acts on the kidney tubules to conserve sodium and water. This increases blood volume and consequently increases blood pressure.

Micturition

Micturition (mik-too-RISH-un), commonly called *urination* or *voiding,* is the act of expelling urine from the bladder. The bladder can hold up to a liter of urine, but normally when it contains 200 to 400 mL, stretch receptors in the bladder wall trigger impulses that initiate the **micturition reflex.** This is an automatic and involuntary response that is coordinated in the spinal cord. Impulses are transmitted along parasympathetic nerves to the detrusor muscle. Even though the micturition reflex is involuntary, it can be inhibited or stimulated by higher brain centers.

It is desirable to completely empty the bladder when urinating. Residual urine is what remains in the bladder if an individual is unable to completely empty the bladder. This may be indicative of a pathologic condition such as a urinary tract infection or, in males, an enlarged prostate.

AGING OF THE URINARY SYSTEM

Some of the more obvious and familiar aging changes occur in the urinary bladder and urethra. Muscles in the walls of these structures tend to weaken and become less elastic with age. As a person ages, the bladder is unable to expand or contract as much as in younger people. This reduces the capacity of the bladder and makes it more difficult to completely empty it during urination. Awareness of the need to urinate, which usually occurs when the bladder is half full in younger people, may be delayed in the elderly until the bladder is nearly full. Thus urgency accompanies awareness. The external urethral sphincter also weakens, which adds to the problems.

Several anatomic changes occur in the kidneys as a person ages, and these changes are reflected in their related functions. There is a general atrophy of nephrons so that by the age of 80, the kidney is about 80% of its young, but mature, size. Some of the remaining glomeruli are modified, and this, along with the decrease in number, results in a decreased glomerular filtration rate so that the blood is not filtered as quickly as before.

The tubules also undergo changes as a person ages. In general, the tubule walls thicken, which makes them less able to reabsorb water to form concentrated urine. The collecting ducts are less responsive to ADH, and this, along with a diminished thirst mechanism, may result in dehydration. The ability to reabsorb glucose and sodium is also diminished. The tubules become less efficient in the secretion of ions and drugs. They have a diminished ability to compensate for drastic changes in acid-base balance. Drugs that are normally eliminated from the body by tubular secretion may accumulate to toxic levels because they are not cleared from the blood as quickly as they are in younger people.

Amazingly, even with the changes caused by aging, the kidneys of elderly persons are capable of maintaining relatively stable balances in the blood and body fluids under normal conditions. However, their ability to compensate for drastic changes and abnormal conditions is diminished.

TERMINOLOGY REVIEW

Medical Term	Word Parts	Definition
Glomerular capsule		Double-layered epithelial cup that surrounds the glomerulus in a nephron; also called *Bowman capsule*.
Juxtaglomerular apparatus	*juxta-:* near to	Complex of modified cells in the afferent arteriole and the ascending limb and distal tubule in the kidney; helps regulate blood pressure by secreting renin; consists of the macula densa and juxtaglomerular cells.
Nephron	*nephr/o:* kidney	Functional unit of the kidney consisting of a renal corpuscle and a renal tubule.
Renal tubule	*ren/o:* kidney	Tubular portion of the nephron that carries the filtrate away from the glomerular capsule; site where tubular reabsorption and secretion occur.

ON THE WEB

For information on the urinary system:

Inner Body: www.innerbody.com/html/body.html

The Internet Pathology Laboratory for Medical Education—Renal Pathology: library.med.utah.edu/WebPath/ORGAN. html *(Click on "Renal Pathology")*

Urinary Incontinence: www.seekwellness.com/incontinence

 Check out the Evolve site at http://evolve.elsevier.com/Bonewit/today/ to actively Prepare for your Certification, and to access additional interactive activities and exercises to help you study and prepare for success.

16

Reproductive System

KEY TERMS

gametes (GAM-eets)
gonads (GO-nads)
oogenesis (oh-oh-JEN-eh-sis)
ovarian cycle (oh-VAIR-ee-an SYE-kul)

ovarian follicle (oh-VAIR-ee-an
    FAHL-ih-kul)
spermatogenesis
    (spur-mat-oh-JEN-eh-sis)

spermiogenesis (spur-mee-oh-JEN-eh-sis)
uterine cycle (YOO-ter-in SYE-kul)

INTRODUCTION TO THE REPRODUCTIVE SYSTEM

The major function of the reproductive system is to produce offspring. The reproductive system is responsible for the following four functions:

- To produce egg and sperm cells
- To transport and sustain these cells
- To nurture the developing offspring
- To produce hormones

These functions are divided between the **primary reproductive organs** and the **secondary** (or **accessory**) **reproductive organs.** The primary reproductive organs are called **gonads.** They include the ovaries and testes. These gonads are responsible for producing the egg and sperm cells, known as **gametes.** They are also responsible for producing hormones that function in the maturation of the reproductive system and the development of sexual characteristics. The hormones also play important roles in regulating the normal physiology of the reproductive system. All other organs, ducts, and glands in the reproductive system are considered secondary, or accessory, reproductive organs. These structures transport and sustain the gametes and nurture the developing offspring.

MALE REPRODUCTIVE SYSTEM

The male reproductive system produces, sustains, and transports sperm; introduces the sperm into the female vagina; and produces hormones. Figure 16-1 illustrates the organs of the male reproductive system.

Testes

The **testes** (or **testicles**) are the male gonads. The testes begin their development high in the abdominal cavity, near the kidneys. During the last 2 months before birth, or shortly after birth, the testes descend into the **scrotum.** The scrotum is a pouch that extends below the abdomen and behind the penis. The location of the testes outside the abdominal cavity may make them vulnerable to injury. However, this location provides a temperature about 3° C below normal body temperature. This lower temperature is necessary for the production of viable sperm. The scrotum consists of skin and subcutaneous tissue. A vertical septum, or partition, of subcutaneous tissue in the center of the scrotum divides it into two parts, each containing one testis. Smooth muscle fibers, called the **dartos muscle,** are located in the subcutaneous tissue. The dartos muscle contracts to give the scrotum its wrinkled appearance. When this muscle is relaxed, the scrotum is smooth. Another muscle known as the **cremaster muscle** is located in the spermatic cord. The cremaster controls the position of the scrotum and testes. When it is cold or a man is sexually aroused, this muscle contracts to pull the testes closer to the body for warmth.

Structure

Each testis is an oval structure about 5 cm long and 3 cm in diameter (Figure 16-2). A tough, white fibrous connective tissue capsule, known as the **tunica albuginea** (TOO-nik-ah al-byoo-JIN-ee-ah), surrounds each testis. The tunica albuginea extends inward to form **septa** that partition the testis into **lobules.** Each testis contains about 250 lobules. Each lobule contains one to four highly coiled **seminiferous** (seh-mye-NIFF-er-us) **tubules** that converge into a series of duets that exit the testes and enter the epididymis. **Interstitial cells** (cells of Leydig) are located between the seminiferous tubules within a lobule. Interstitial cells produce male sex hormones.

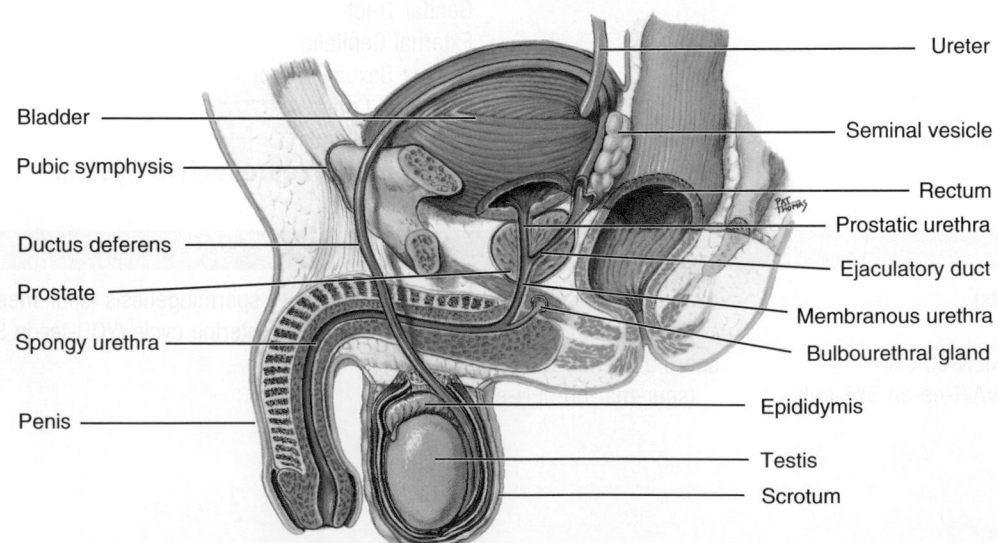

Figure 16-1 Structures in the male reproductive system. The testes are the primary reproductive organs in the male. The ducts and glands are accessory organs.

Spermatogenesis

Sperm are produced within the seminiferous tubules. The process of sperm formation is known as **spermatogenesis** (spur-mat-oh-JEN-eh-sis), which is a form of meiosis. The seminiferous tubules are packed with cells in various stages of spermatogenesis (Figure 16-3). Interspersed with these cells are large cells that extend from the periphery of the tubule to the lumen. These large cells are the **supporting cells** (Sertoli cells), which support and nourish the other cells.

Early in embryonic development, **primordial germ cells** enter the testes and differentiate into **spermatogonia**

(spur-mat-oh-GOH-nee-ah). Spermatogonia are immature cells that remain dormant until puberty. Spermatogonia are located around the periphery of the seminiferous tubules. They are diploid cells, meaning that they contain 46 chromosomes (23 pairs). At puberty, hormones stimulate these cells to begin dividing by mitosis. Some of the daughter cells produced by mitosis remain at the periphery as spermatogonia. Others are pushed toward the lumen and undergo some changes to become **primary spermatocytes.** Because they are produced by mitosis, primary spermatocytes are diploid and have 46 chromosomes.

Each primary spermatocyte goes through the first meiotic division (meiosis I) to produce two **secondary spermatocytes.** In the second meiotic division (meiosis II), each secondary spermatocyte divides to produce two **spermatids.** As a result of the two meiotic divisions, each primary spermatocyte produces four spermatids (Figure 16-4). During spermatogenesis there are two cellular divisions but only one replication of DNA, so each spermatid has 23 chromosomes (haploid), one from each pair in the original primary spermatocyte. Each successive stage in spermatogenesis is pushed toward the center of the tubule. This results in the more immature cells being at the periphery, and the more differentiated cells are nearer the center (see Figure 16-3).

Spermatogenesis (and oogenesis in the female) differs from mitosis (review Chapter 5) because the resulting cells have only half the number of chromosomes as the original cell. When the sperm cell nucleus unites with an egg cell

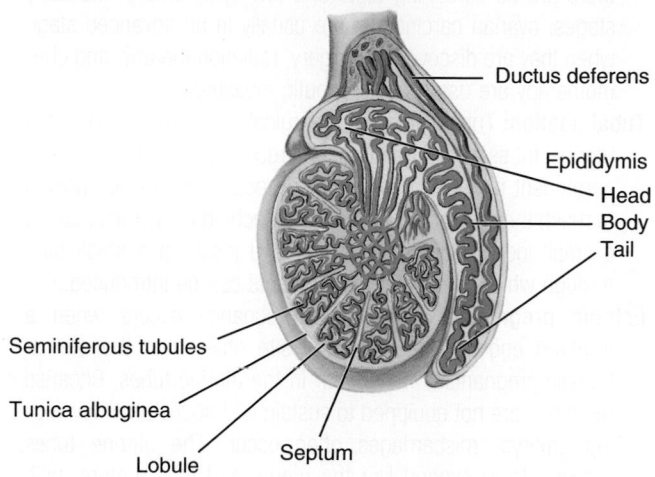

- Ductus deferens
- Epididymis
  - Head
  - Body
  - Tail
- Seminiferous tubules
- Tunica albuginea
- Lobule
- Septum

Figure 16-2 Sagittal section of a testis.

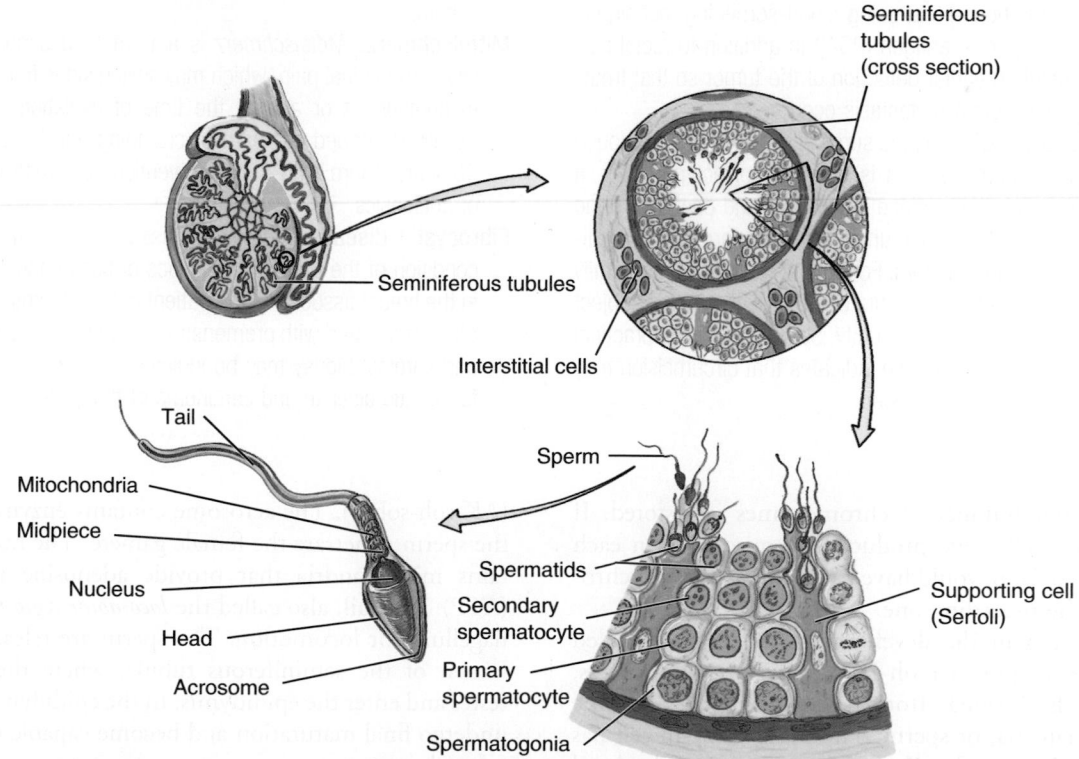

- Seminiferous tubules (cross section)
- Seminiferous tubules
- Interstitial cells
- Tail
- Mitochondria
- Midpiece
- Nucleus
- Head
- Acrosome
- Sperm
- Spermatids
- Secondary spermatocyte
- Primary spermatocyte
- Spermatogonia
- Supporting cell (Sertoli)

Figure 16-3 Cross section of a seminiferous tubule showing the different cell types. Interstitial cells that produce testosterone are between the seminiferous tubules. Spermatids in the lumen become sperm by a process called *spermiogenesis*.

Highlight on the Reproductive System

Inguinal hernia: The inguinal canal is a weak area in the abdominal wall that may rip open, resulting in an inguinal hernia. A portion of the intestine may pass through the opening into the scrotum. This is painful and potentially dangerous if the blood supply to the intestine is constricted. This condition is more common in men than in women. Inguinal hernias are frequently repaired by surgery.

Undescended testicles: The condition in which the testes do not descend into the scrotum is called **cryptorchidism**. *Crypt* means "hidden" and *orchid* refers to the testis, so the term means "hidden testis." Cryptorchidism results in sterility if it is not corrected before puberty because the cooler temperature of the scrotum is necessary for sperm production.

Vasectomy: A vasectomy is a surgical procedure, usually accomplished through a tiny incision in the scrotum, that severs the vas deferens. A bilateral vasectomy results in sterility because it interrupts the pathway of the sperm to the outside of the body.

Enlarged prostate gland: Benign prostatic hyperplasia is a common condition in older men. In this condition, the prostate enlarges and compresses the urethra, making urination difficult. This situation results in urine retention in the bladder, which makes the individual more susceptible to urinary tract infections.

Prostate cancer: Cancer of the prostate is a common cancer in men. It usually starts in one of the secretory glands, and as it continues it produces a lump on the surface of the prostate. In many cases by the time the lump can be palpated through the wall of the rectum, the cancer has metastasized to other areas of the body. It is hoped that using blood-screening techniques (e.g., prostate-specific antigen [PSA]) in addition to rectal palpation will result in earlier detection of the tumor so that treatment can begin before metastasis occurs.

Circumcision: Circumcision is the surgical removal of the prepuce of the penis. Sometimes this is done to correct phimosis, a condition in which the prepuce is too tight and obstructs urine flow. In certain cultures, circumcision is performed as a religious rite or an ethnic custom. For others, it is a matter of family preference. The medical benefits of circumcision are a subject of debate in the medical community. Some believe it is practical for hygienic reasons. Evidence indicates that circumcision may reduce the risk of penile cancer.

Impotence: Impotence is the inability to achieve an erection. Psychological stresses are often blamed for impotence, but other causes can lead to the difficulty. Impotence may result from an abnormality of the erectile tissue or failure of the parasympathetic reflexes that produce an erection. Drugs and alcohol may cause temporary impotence because they can interfere with the nerve and blood vessel actions that are necessary for an erection.

Ovarian cancer: Carcinomas of the ovary account for more deaths than those of cervical and uterine cancers together. Because there are no screening tests and few symptoms in the early stages, ovarian carcinomas are usually in an advanced stage when they are discovered. Surgery, radiation therapy, and chemotherapy are used as therapeutic measures.

Tubal ligation: Tubal ligation is a surgical procedure in which the uterine tubes are burned or severed and tied off. This is a permanent method of birth control because sperm are unable to reach the egg for fertilization. The technique involves making a small incision in the abdomen and inserting a small tube through which the ligation instruments can be introduced.

Ectopic pregnancy: An ectopic pregnancy occurs when a fertilized egg implants in some site other than the uterus. Ectopic pregnancies may occur in the uterine tubes. Because the tubes are not equipped to sustain and nourish the developing embryo, miscarriages often occur. The uterine tubes are unable to expand like the uterus and may rupture, with subsequent hemorrhage. Surgery may be indicated to remove the implant and to preserve the uterine tube before rupture occurs.

Mittelschmerz: *Mittelschmerz* is a term to describe one-sided lower abdominal pain, which may switch sides from one month to another, at or around the time of ovulation. The pain is usually described as sharp or cramping and lasts from 24 to 48 hours. There is no known prevention, and treatment consists of analgesics.

Fibrocystic disease: Fibrocystic disease is a common benign condition of the breast. Small sacs of tissue and fluid develop in the breast tissue, and the patient notices lumps in the breast often associated with premenstrual tenderness. Mammography and surgical biopsy may be indicated to differentiate between fibrocystic disease and carcinoma of the breast. ∎

---

nucleus, the full number of chromosomes is restored. If sperm and egg cells were produced by mitosis, then each successive generation would have twice the number of chromosomes as the preceding one.

The final step in the development of sperm is called **spermiogenesis** (spur-mee-oh-JEN-eh-sis). In this process, the spermatids formed from spermatogenesis become mature spermatozoa, or sperm. The mature sperm cell has a **head, midpiece,** and **tail** (see Figure 16-3). The head contains the 23 chromosomes surrounded by a nuclear membrane. The tip of the head is covered by an **acrosome** (AK-roh-sohm). The acrosome contains enzymes that help the sperm penetrate the female gamete. The midpiece contains mitochondria that provide adenosine triphosphate (ATP). The tail, also called the *locomotor region,* is a typical flagellum for locomotion. The sperm are released into the lumen of the seminiferous tubule, where they leave the testes and enter the epididymis. In the epididymis the sperm undergo final maturation and become capable of fertilizing a female gamete.

Sperm production begins at puberty and continues throughout the life of a male. The entire process, beginning

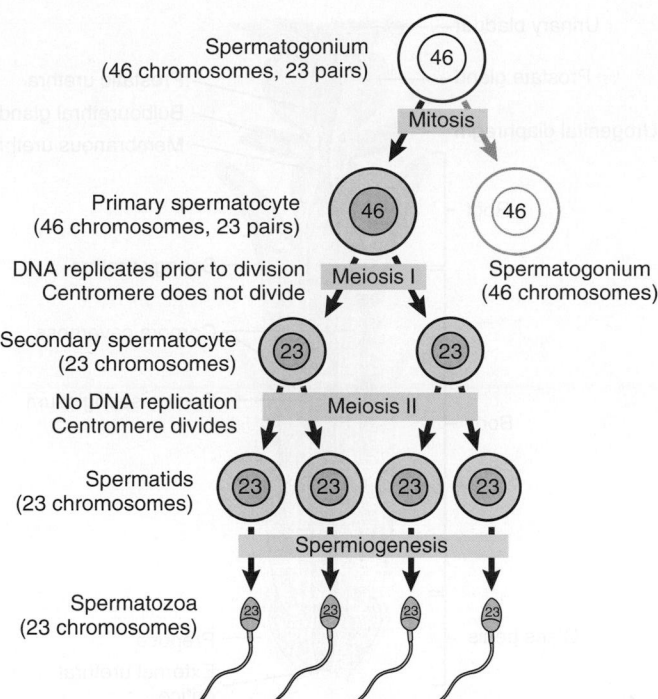

Spermatogonium
(46 chromosomes, 23 pairs)

Mitosis

Primary spermatocyte
(46 chromosomes, 23 pairs)

Spermatogonium
(46 chromosomes)

DNA replicates prior to division
Centromere does not divide

Meiosis I

Secondary spermatocyte
(23 chromosomes)

No DNA replication
Centromere divides

Meiosis II

Spermatids
(23 chromosomes)

Spermiogenesis

Spermatozoa
(23 chromosomes)

Figure 16-4 Spermatogenesis. Each primary spermatocyte yields four spermatids by meiosis.

with a primary spermatocyte, takes about 74 days. After ejaculation, the sperm can live for about 48 hours in the female reproductive tract.

Duct System

Sperm cells pass through a series of ducts to reach the outside of the body. After they leave the testes, the sperm pass through the epididymis, ductus deferens, ejaculatory duct, and urethra.

Epididymis

Sperm leave the testes through a series of ducts that enter the **epididymis** (ep-ih-DID-ih-mis) (see Figure 16-2). The epididymis is a long tube that is tightly coiled to form a comma-shaped organ. When the sperm leave the testes, they are immature and incapable of fertilizing ova. They complete their maturation process and become fertile as they move through the epididymis. Mature sperm are stored in the lower portion of the epididymis.

Ductus Deferens

The **ductus deferens** (also called **vas deferens**) is a tube that is continuous with the epididymis (see Figure 16-2). The ductus deferens enters the abdominopelvic cavity, then descends along the posterior wall of the bladder toward the prostate gland (see Figure 16-1). Sperm are stored in the ductus deferens, near the epididymis, and peristaltic movements propel the sperm through the tube.

The proximal portion of the ductus deferens is a component of the **spermatic cord,** which contains vascular and neural structures that supply the testes. The spermatic cord

contains the ductus deferens, testicular artery and veins, lymph vessels, testicular nerve, cremaster muscle (which elevates the testes for warmth and at times of sexual stimulation), and a connective tissue covering.

Ejaculatory Duct

Each ductus deferens joins the duct from the adjacent seminal vesicle to form a short **ejaculatory** (ee-JAK-yoo-lah-to-ree) **duct** (see Figure 16-1). Each ejaculatory duct passes through the prostate gland and empties into the urethra.

Urethra

The **urethra** (yoo-REE-thrah) extends from the urinary bladder to the external urethral orifice at the tip of the penis. It is a passageway for sperm and fluids from the reproductive system and for urine from the urinary system. While reproductive fluids are passing through the urethra, sphincters contract tightly to keep urine from entering the urethra.

The male urethra is divided into three regions (see Figure 16-1). The **prostatic urethra** is the portion that passes through the prostate gland. It receives the ejaculatory duct and numerous ducts from the prostate gland. The next portion, the **membranous urethra,** is a short region that passes through the pelvic floor. The longest portion is the **penile urethra** (also called *spongy urethra*), which extends the length of the penis and opens to the outside at the external urethral orifice. The ducts from the bulbourethral glands open into the penile urethra.

Accessory Glands

The accessory glands of the male reproductive system include the seminal vesicles, prostate gland, and bulbourethral glands. These glands secrete fluids that enter the urethra.

Seminal Vesicles

The paired **seminal vesicles** are saclike glands located between the urinary bladder and the rectum (see Figure 16-1). Each gland has a short duct that joins with the ductus deferens to form an ejaculatory duct. The ejaculatory ducts empty into the urethra. The seminal vesicles secrete a fluid that is viscous and contains fructose. The fructose provides an energy source for the spermatozoa.

Prostate

The **prostate gland** is a firm, dense structure that is located just inferior to the urinary bladder (see Figure 16-1). It is about the size of a walnut and encircles the urethra as it leaves the urinary bladder. Numerous short ducts from the prostate gland empty into the prostatic urethra. The secretions of the prostate are thin, milky colored, and alkaline. They enhance the motility of the sperm.

Bulbourethral Glands

The paired **bulbourethral (Cowper) glands** (see Figure 16-1) are small, about the size of a pea, and are located near the base of the penis. A short duct from each gland enters the penile urethra. In response to sexual stimulation, the bulbourethral glands secrete an alkaline, mucus-like fluid. This fluid performs the following functions: neutralizes the acidity of the urine residue in the urethra, helps to neutralize the acidity of the vagina, and provides some lubrication for the tip of the penis during intercourse.

Seminal Fluid

Seminal fluid (or **semen**) consists of a slightly alkaline (pH 7.5) mixture of sperm cells and secretions from the accessory glands. Secretions from the seminal vesicles make up about 60% of the **semen.** Most of the remaining semen consists of secretions from the prostate gland. Spermatozoa and secretions from the bulbourethral glands contribute only a small volume to the semen.

The volume of semen in a single ejaculation varies from 1.5 to 6 mL. There are usually between 50 and 150 million sperm per milliliter of semen. Sperm counts below 10 to 20 million per milliliter usually cause fertility problems. Although only one spermatozoon actually penetrates and fertilizes an ovum, it takes several million spermatozoa in an ejaculation to ensure that fertilization will take place.

Penis

The **penis** is the male copulatory organ located in front of the scrotum. The penis functions in transferring sperm to the vagina. It consists of three columns of erectile tissue that are wrapped in connective tissue and covered with skin (Figure 16-5). There are two dorsal columns known as the **corpora cavernosa** (KOR-por-ah kav-er-NOH-sah). A single, midline ventral column surrounds the urethra and is called the **corpus spongiosum** (KOR-pus spun-jee-OH-sum).

The penis has a root, body, and glans penis. The **root** of the penis attaches it to the pubic arch. The **body** (or **shaft**) of the penis is the visible, pendant portion. The corpus spongiosum expands at the end of the penis to form the **glans penis.** The urethra opens through the external urethral orifice at the tip of the glans penis. A loose fold of skin, called the **prepuce** (PREE-pyoos), or **foreskin,** covers the glans penis.

Male Sexual Response

In the absence of sexual arousal, the erectile tissue of the penis contains only a small volume of blood, causing the penis to be flaccid. During sexual excitement, arterioles that supply blood to the erectile tissue dilate. As a result, the spaces in the erectile tissue become engorged with blood, causing the penis to enlarge and become rigid. This is called **erection** and is necessary to allow the penis to enter the vagina. The erection reflex may be initiated by stimuli such as anticipation, memory, and visual sensations. It may also be the result of stimulation of touch receptors on the glans penis and skin of the genital area. Emotions and thoughts can inhibit erection.

Continued sexual stimulation causes the reflexes that promote an erection to become more and more intense

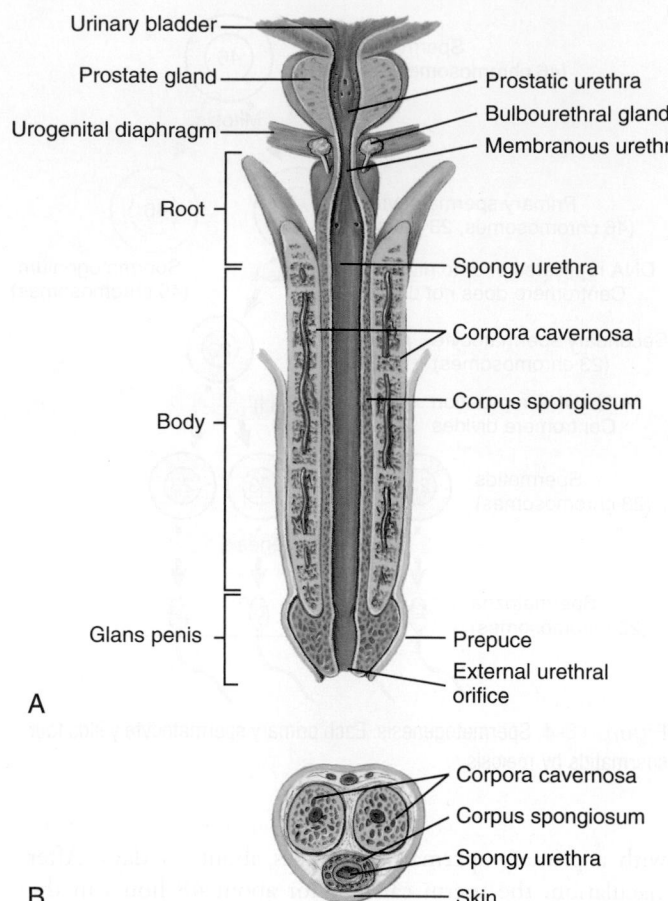

Figure 16-5 Structure of the penis. **A,** Longitudinal section. **B,** Cross section. Note that the penis has three regions: root, body, and glans penis. There are two dorsal columns of corpora cavernosum and a ventral column of corpus spongiosum.

until a level is reached that prompts a surge of impulses to the genital organs. These impulses stimulate rhythmic contractions of the epididymides, vasa deferentia, and ejaculatory ducts. The impulses also cause contractions of the accessory glands. This results in **emission,** which is the forceful discharge of semen into the urethra. **Ejaculation** immediately follows emission and is the forceful expulsion of semen from the urethra to the exterior. Concurrently with emission and ejaculation, the sphincters of the urinary bladder constrict to prevent semen from entering the bladder and to inhibit the flow of urine from the bladder.

The rhythmic muscle contractions of ejaculation are accompanied by feelings of intense pleasure, increased heart rate, elevated blood pressure, and increased respiration. Together, these physiologic activities are referred to as **climax,** or **orgasm.** This is quickly followed by relaxation, and blood leaves the penis so that it becomes flaccid. After orgasm, there is a latent period, lasting from several minutes to several hours, during which another erection is impossible.

Hormonal Control

The hypothalamus, anterior pituitary, and testes have significant roles in the hormonal control of male reproductive functions. Puberty in males usually begins at ages 10 to 12 and continues until ages 16 to 18. During this period the male reproductive organs become sexually mature. The sequence of events that triggers the onset of puberty is unknown. It begins when certain unknown stimuli cause the hypothalamus to start secreting **gonadotropin-releasing hormone** (GnRH), which enters the blood and goes to the anterior pituitary gland.

In response to GnRH, the anterior pituitary secretes luteinizing hormone and follicle-stimulating hormone (FSH). **Luteinizing hormone** (LH) promotes the growth of the interstitial cells in the testes and stimulates the cells to secrete **testosterone. Follicle-stimulating hormone** acts with testosterone to stimulate spermatogenesis in the seminiferous tubules. Figure 16-6 summarizes the hormonal control of testicular functions.

Male sex hormones are collectively called **androgens.** The most abundant androgen is testosterone. Before birth, testosterone from the adrenal cortex stimulates the development of the male reproductive organs. Between birth and puberty, testosterone levels are low. Then at puberty, under the influence of LH, the interstitial cells begin secreting high levels of testosterone. The adrenal cortex continues to secrete small amounts of androgens. The increase in testosterone levels at puberty promotes the maturation of the

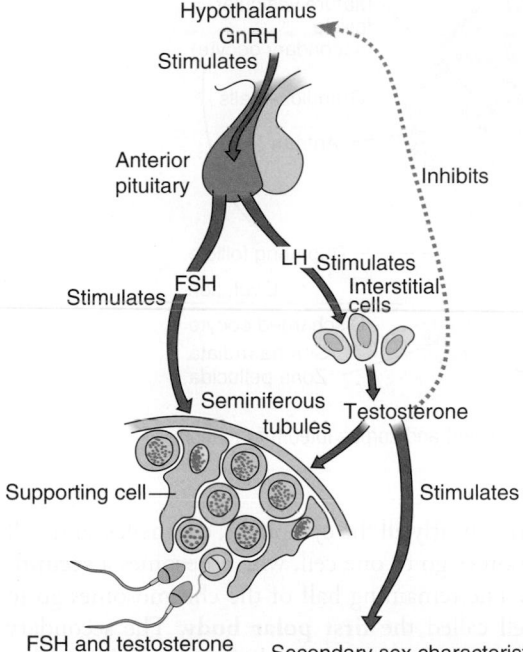

Figure 16-6 Hormonal regulation of testicular function.

male reproductive organs, stimulates spermatogenesis, and promotes the development of the male secondary sex characteristics.

After puberty, testosterone production is controlled by a negative feedback mechanism that involves the hypothalamus (see Figure 16-6). High blood testosterone levels inhibit GnRH. This removes the stimulus for LH, which reduces the testosterone level back to normal. Testosterone production continues from puberty throughout the rest of a man's life, although there is some decline in quantity in old age.

FEMALE REPRODUCTIVE SYSTEM

The organs of the female reproductive system perform the following functions: produce and sustain the female sex cells (egg cells, or ova), transport these cells to a site where they may be fertilized by sperm, provide a favorable environment for the developing offspring, move the offspring to the outside at the end of the development period, and produce the female sex hormones. The female reproductive system includes the ovaries, uterine tubes, uterus, vagina, accessory glands, and external genital organs (Figure 16-7).

Ovaries

The primary reproductive organs in the female are the paired **ovaries.** Each ovary is a solid, ovoid structure about the size and shape of an almond (approximately 3.5 cm long, 2 cm wide, and 1 cm thick). The ovaries are located in shallow depressions, called **ovarian fossae,** one on each side of the uterus. They are held loosely in place by peritoneal ligaments.

Structure

The ovaries are covered on the outside by a layer of epithelium called **germinal (ovarian) epithelium** (Figure 16-8) and a dense connective tissue capsule known as the **tunica albuginea.** The substance of the ovaries is indistinctly divided into an outer **cortex** and an inner **medulla.** The cortex appears more dense and granular because of the presence of numerous **ovarian follicles** in various stages of development. Each of the follicles contains a female germ cell known as an **oocyte.** The medulla consists of loose connective tissue with abundant blood vessels, lymphatic vessels, and nerve fibers.

Oogenesis

Female sex cells (or gametes) develop in the ovaries by a form of meiosis called **oogenesis** (oh-oh-JEN-eh-sis). The sequence of events in oogenesis is similar to the sequence in spermatogenesis, but the timing and final result are different (Figure 16-9). Early in fetal development, primitive germ cells in the ovaries differentiate into **oogonia** (oh-oh-GO-nee-ah). The oogonia divide rapidly to form thousands of cells that have a full complement of 46 chromosomes (23 pairs). Oogonia then enter a growth phase, enlarge, and become **primary oocytes.** The primary oocytes (with 46 chromosomes) replicate their DNA and begin the first

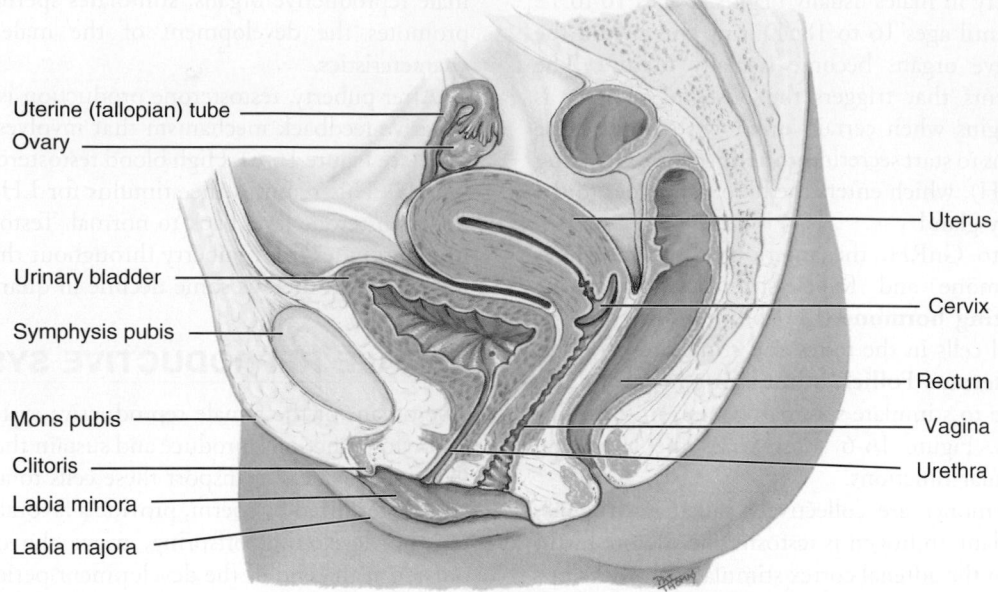

Figure 16-7 Organs of the female reproductive system.

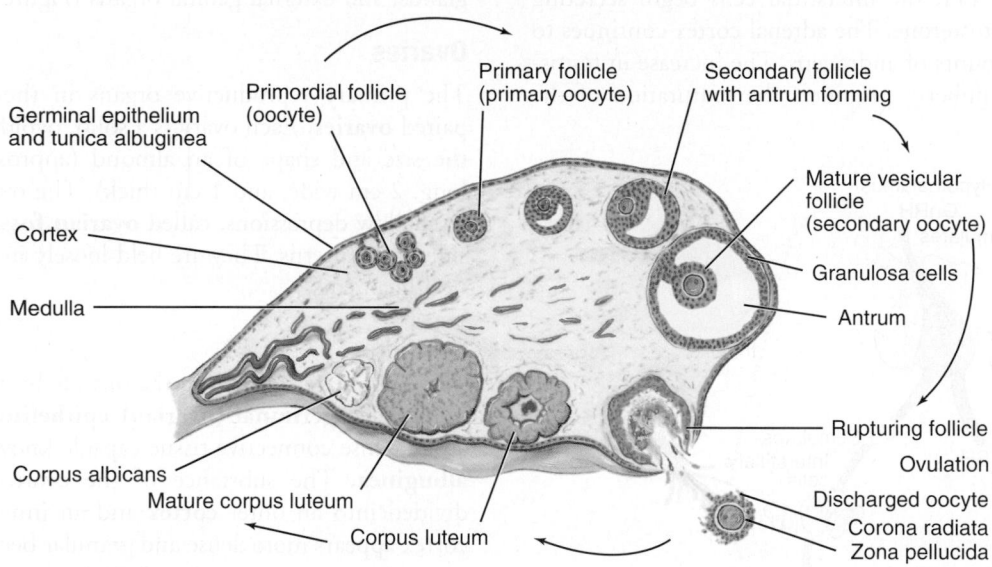

Figure 16-8 Structure of an ovary illustrating the stages in follicle development and corpus luteum formation.

meiotic division. This process stops in prophase, and the cells remain in this suspended state until puberty. Many of the primary oocytes degenerate before birth. Even with this decline, the two ovaries together contain approximately 700,000 oocytes at birth. This is the lifetime supply, and no more will develop. This is quite different than in the male, in whom spermatogonia and primary spermatocytes continue to be produced throughout the reproductive lifetime. By puberty the number of primary oocytes has further declined to about 400,000.

Beginning at puberty, several primary oocytes start to grow again each month. One of the primary oocytes seems to outgrow the others, and it resumes meiosis I. The other cells degenerate. The large cell undergoes an unequal

division so that nearly all the cytoplasm, organelles, and half the chromosomes go to one cell, which becomes a **secondary oocyte.** The remaining half of the chromosomes go to a smaller cell called the **first polar body.** The secondary oocyte begins the second meiotic division, but the process stops in metaphase. At this point, ovulation occurs. If fertilization occurs, meiosis II continues. Again, this is an unequal division, with all of the cytoplasm going to the ovum, which has 23 single-stranded chromosomes. The smaller cell from this division is a **second polar body.** The first polar body also usually divides in meiosis II to produce two even smaller polar bodies. If fertilization does not occur, the second meiotic division is never completed and the secondary oocyte degenerates. Here again there are

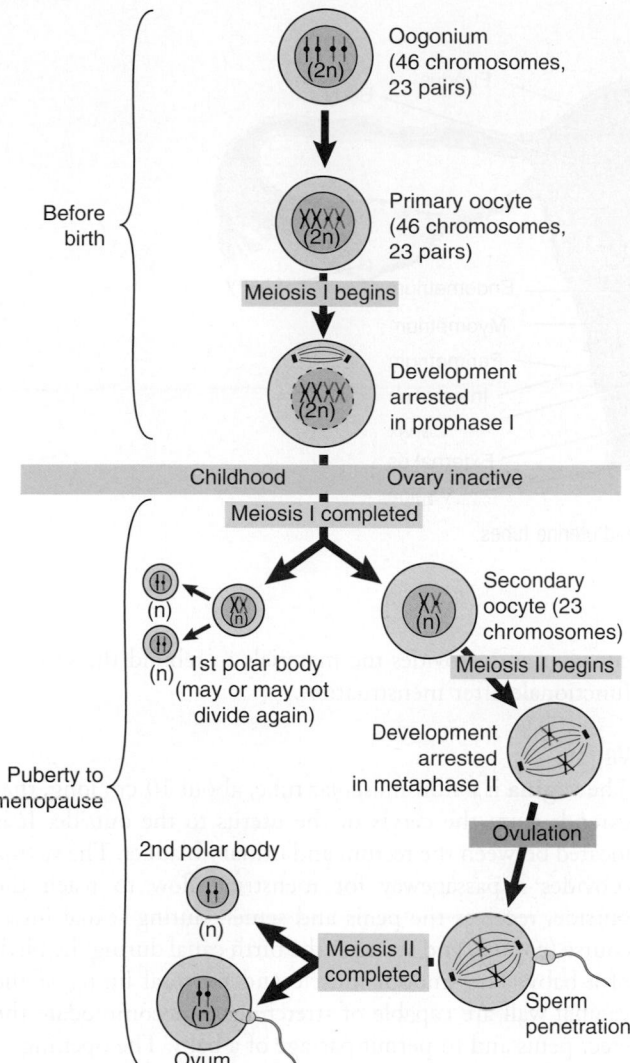

Figure 16-9 Oogenesis. The first meiotic division is interrupted in prophase before birth and does not resume until after puberty. The second meiotic division is interrupted in metaphase and does not resume unless a sperm penetrates the cell.

(Figure labels) Oogonium (46 chromosomes, 23 pairs); Before birth; Primary oocyte (46 chromosomes, 23 pairs); Meiosis I begins; Development arrested in prophase I; Childhood / Ovary inactive; Meiosis I completed; 1st polar body (may or may not divide again); Secondary oocyte (23 chromosomes); Meiosis II begins; Development arrested in metaphase II; Ovulation; Puberty to menopause; 2nd polar body; Meiosis II completed; Sperm penetration; Ovum

obvious differences between the male and female. In spermatogenesis, four functional spermatozoa develop from each primary spermatocyte. In oogenesis, only one functional fertilizable cell develops from a primary oocyte. The other three cells are polar bodies and they degenerate.

Ovarian Follicle Development

An ovarian follicle consists of a developing oocyte surrounded by one or more layers of cells called **follicular cells.** While the oocyte is progressing through meiosis, corresponding changes are taking place in the follicular cells (see Figure 16-8). **Primordial follicles,** which consist of a primary oocyte surrounded by a single layer of flattened cells, develop in the fetus and are the stage that is present in the ovaries at birth and throughout childhood.

Beginning at puberty FSH stimulates changes in the primordial follicles. The follicular cells become cuboidal, the primary oocyte enlarges, and a **primary follicle** is

created. The follicles continue to grow under the influence of FSH, and the follicular cells proliferate to form several layers of **granulosa cells** around the primary oocyte. Most of these primary follicles degenerate along with the primary oocytes within them, but usually one continues to develop each month. The granulosa cells start secreting estrogen. In addition, a cavity known as the *antrum* forms within the follicle. When the antrum starts to develop, the follicle becomes a **secondary follicle.** The granulosa cells also secrete a substance that forms a clear membrane, known as the **zona pellucida** (ZOH-nah peh-LOO-sih-dah), around the oocyte. After about 10 days of growth the follicle is a mature vesicular (graafian) follicle, which forms a "blister" on the surface of the ovary. It contains a secondary oocyte ready for ovulation.

Ovulation

Ovulation occurs when the mature follicle at the surface of the ovary ruptures and releases the secondary oocyte into the peritoneal cavity. The ovulated secondary oocyte is ready for fertilization. It is still surrounded by the zona pellucida and a few layers of cells called the **corona radiata** (koh-ROH-nah ray-dee-AH-tah). If it is not fertilized, the secondary oocyte degenerates in a couple of days. If a spermatozoon passes through the corona radiata and zona pellucida and enters the cytoplasm of the secondary oocyte, the second meiotic division resumes to form a polar body and a mature ovum.

After ovulation, the portion of the follicle that remains in the ovary enlarges and is transformed into a **corpus luteum** (see Figure 16-8). The corpus luteum is a glandular structure that secretes progesterone and some estrogens. Its fate depends on whether fertilization occurs. If fertilization does not take place, the corpus luteum remains functional for about 10 days and then begins to degenerate into a **corpus albicans.** This structure is primarily scar tissue, and its hormone output ceases. If fertilization occurs, the corpus luteum persists. The corpus luteum continues its hormone functions until the placenta develops sufficiently to secrete the necessary hormones. Again, the corpus luteum ultimately degenerates into a corpus albicans; it just remains functional for a longer period of time.

Genital Tract

Uterine Tubes

There are two **uterine tubes** (also called **fallopian** [fah-LOH-pee-an] **tubes**). Each tube is about 4 cm long and about 1 cm in diameter and extends laterally from the upper portion of the uterus to the region of the ovary on that side (Figure 16-10). One tube is associated with each ovary. The end of the tube near the ovary expands to form a funnel-shaped **infundibulum,** which is surrounded by finger-like extensions called **fimbriae.** Because there is no direct connection between the infundibulum and the ovary, the oocyte enters the peritoneal cavity before it enters the uterine tube. At the time of ovulation, the fimbriae increase their activity and create currents in the peritoneal fluid that

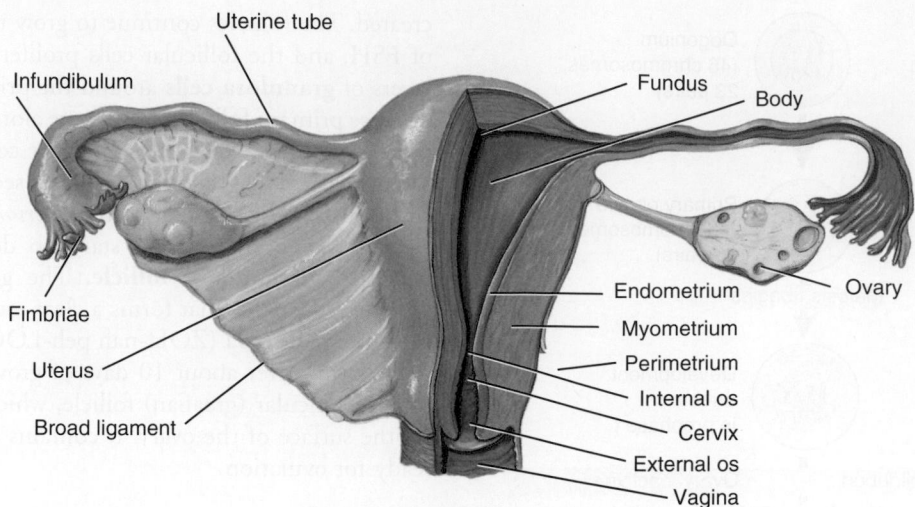

Figure 16-10 Uterus and uterine tubes.

help propel the oocyte into the uterine tube. Once inside the uterine tube, the oocyte is moved along by the rhythmic beating of cilia on the epithelial lining and by the peristaltic action of the smooth muscle in the wall of the tube. The journey through the uterine tube takes about 7 days. Because the oocyte is fertile for only 24 to 48 hours, fertilization usually occurs in the uterine tube.

Uterus

The **uterus** is a muscular organ that receives the fertilized oocyte and provides an appropriate environment for the developing offspring. It is located in the pelvic cavity, between the rectum and urinary bladder (see Figure 16-7). Before the first pregnancy, the uterus is about the size and shape of a pear, with the narrow portion directed inferiorly. After childbirth the uterus is usually larger, and then it regresses after menopause.

The upper, bulging surface of the uterus, above the entrance of the uterine tubes, is known as the **fundus** (see Figure 16-10). The large main portion of the uterus is the **body.** The narrow region of the uterus that is directed into the vagina is the **cervix.** The opening between the body and cervix is known as the **internal os,** and the opening from the cervix into the vagina is the **external os.** Several ligaments hold the uterus in place. The largest of these is the **broad ligament,** which drapes over the uterus like a sheet and extends laterally to the lateral pelvic wall. The broad ligament also encloses the uterine tubes.

The wall of the uterus consists of perimetrium, myometrium, and endometrium. The outer serous layer is known as the **perimetrium.** The thick middle layer is known as the **myometrium.** The myometrium consists of smooth muscle and makes up the bulk of the uterine wall. The inner layer is called the **endometrium.** It is a mucous membrane that is subdivided into two regions. The **stratum functionale** of the endometrium is the portion that is sloughed off during menstruation. The deeper, thinner **stratum basale** is more

constant and provides the materials to rebuild the stratum functionale after menstruation.

Vagina

The **vagina** is a fibromuscular tube, about 10 cm long, that extends from the cervix of the uterus to the outside. It is located between the rectum and urinary bladder. The vagina provides a passageway for menstrual flow to reach the outside, receives the penis and semen during sexual intercourse (coitus), and serves as the birth canal during the birth of a baby. The smooth muscle and mucosal lining of the vaginal wall are capable of stretching to accommodate the erect penis and to permit passage of a baby. The opening of the vagina to the outside is known as the **vaginal orifice.** The vaginal orifice may be incompletely covered by a thin fold of mucous membrane called the **hymen.**

External Genitalia

The external genitalia are accessory structures of the female reproductive system that are outside the vagina. They are also referred to as the **vulva.** The external genitalia include the labia majora, mons pubis, labia minora, clitoris, and glands within the vestibule (Figure 16-11).

The **labia majora** are two large fat-filled folds of skin that enclose the other external genitalia. Anteriorly the labia majora merge to form the **mons pubis.** The mons pubis is a rounded elevation of fat that overlies the pubic symphysis. After puberty the mons pubis and labia majora are covered with coarse pubic hair. The **labia minora** are two smaller folds of skin medial to the labia majora.

The area between the two labia minora is called the **vestibule.** At the anterior end of the vestibule (where the two labia minora meet), there is a small mass of erectile tissue called the **clitoris** (KLY-toh-ris). The clitoris becomes erect in response to sexual stimulation. The labia minora merge and form a hood over the clitoris, known as the **prepuce.** Posterior to the clitoris, the urethra and vagina

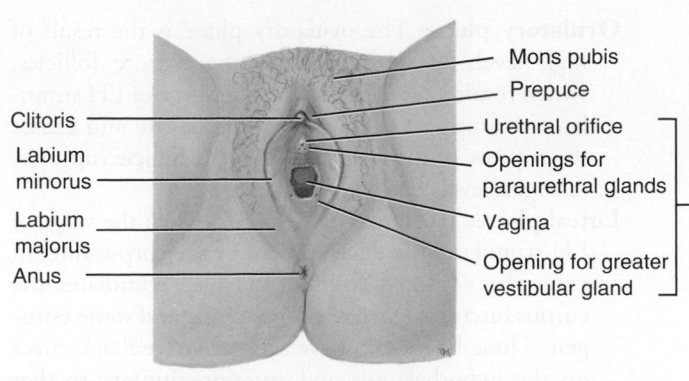

Mons pubis
Prepuce
Clitoris
Urethral orifice
Labium minorus
Openings for paraurethral glands
Labium majorus
Vagina
Anus
Opening for greater vestibular gland
Vestibule

Figure 16-11 Female external genitalia. The area between the two labia minora is the vestibule.

open into the vestibule. **Paraurethral glands** open into the vestibule on each side of the urethral orifice. These glands secrete mucus. The **greater vestibular glands** (Bartholin glands) open into the vestibule next to the vaginal orifice. These glands produce a mucus-like secretion for lubrication during sexual intercourse.

Female Sexual Response

The female sexual response is similar to that of the male and consists of erection and orgasm. The body's responses to sexual stimuli produce increased blood flow to the erectile tissue in the clitoris, the vaginal mucosa, breasts, and nipples. The clitoris and nipples become rigid and erect. The breasts and vaginal mucosa enlarge. Glands in the cervix and the vestibular glands secrete fluids that lubricate the vaginal mucosa and aid the entry of the penis.

With continued stimulation, the female response culminates in orgasm. This is accompanied by rhythmic contractions of the uterus and muscles of the pelvic floor. This helps the movement of sperm through the uterus toward the uterine tubes. The rhythmic muscle contractions are accompanied by feelings of intense pleasure, increased heart rate, elevated blood pressure, and increased respiration rate. This is followed by a general relaxation and feeling of warmth throughout the body.

Hormonal Control

As in the male, the hypothalamus, anterior pituitary, and gonads secrete hormones that have significant roles in the control of reproductive functions (Figure 16-12). The hypothalamus secretes GnRH, the anterior pituitary secretes FSH and LH, and the ovaries secrete the sex hormones **estrogen** and **progesterone.** Unlike in the male, the secretion of these hormones follows monthly cyclic patterns that affect the ovaries and uterus. These cycles, referred to as the **ovarian cycle** and the **menstrual** (uterine) **cycle,** begin at puberty and continue for about 40 years.

At puberty certain stimuli cause the hypothalamus to start secreting GnRH. This hormone enters the blood and goes to the anterior pituitary gland, where it stimulates the secretion of FSH and LH. These hormones, in turn, affect the ovaries and uterus, and the monthly cycles begin. In females the beginning of puberty is marked by the first

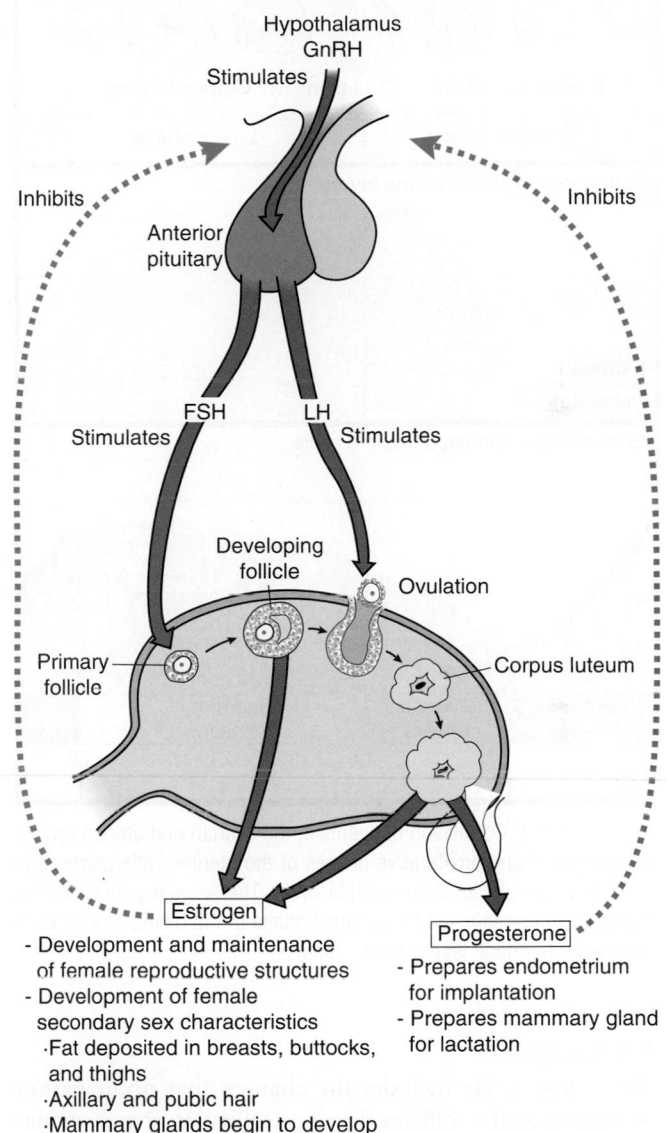

Hypothalamus GnRH
Stimulates
Inhibits
Inhibits
Anterior pituitary
FSH
LH
Stimulates
Stimulates
Developing follicle
Ovulation
Primary follicle
Corpus luteum

Estrogen
- Development and maintenance of female reproductive structures
- Development of female secondary sex characteristics
  - Fat deposited in breasts, buttocks, and thighs
  - Axillary and pubic hair
  - Mammary glands begin to develop in breasts
  - Pelvis broadens

Progesterone
- Prepares endometrium for implantation
- Prepares mammary gland for lactation

Figure 16-12 Hormonal regulation of ovarian functions.

period of menstrual bleeding, called **menarche** (meh-NAHR-kee). After this the cycles continue, more or less regularly, until the late 40s or early 50s. At this time the cycles become increasingly irregular until they finally stop. **Menopause** is the cessation of the reproductive cycles.

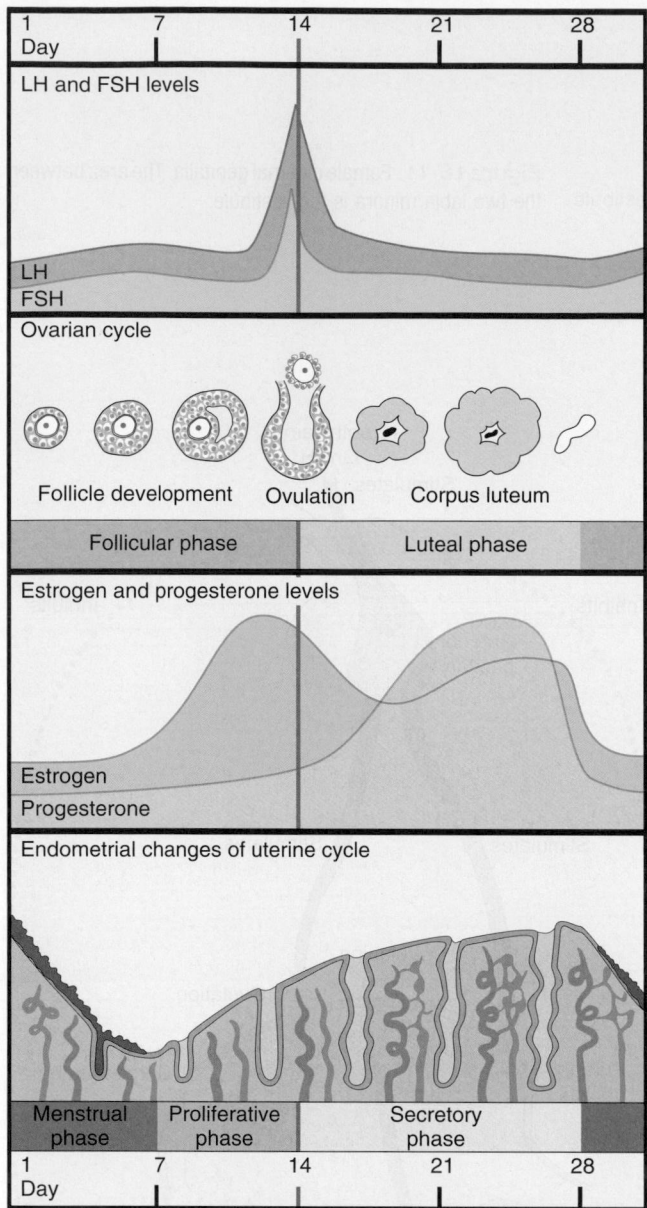

Figure 16-13 Correlation of events in the ovarian and uterine cycles. The menstrual and proliferative phases of the uterine cycle correspond to the follicular phase of the ovarian cycle. The secretory phase of the uterine cycle corresponds to the luteal phase of the ovarian cycle. Note the relative hormone levels in each phase.

Ovarian Cycle

The ovarian cycle includes the changes that occur within the ovaries as the follicles develop (follicular phase), ovulation occurs (ovulatory phase), and the corpus luteum develops (luteal phase) (Figure 16-13).

Follicular phase: The follicular phase of the cycle begins when GnRH from the hypothalamus stimulates increased secretion of FSH from the anterior pituitary. FSH stimulates growth of the ovarian follicles. As the follicles enlarge, estrogen secretion increases. The follicle continues to grow and mature until the middle of the cycle.

Ovulatory phase: The ovulatory phase is the result of high levels of estrogen from the mature follicles, which result in a surge of LH. The surge of LH stimulates resumption of meiosis in the oocyte and causes the rupture of the follicle. When the follicle ruptures, estrogen levels decline.

Luteal phase: The luteal phase occurs when the surge of LH stimulates the development of the corpus luteum from the ruptured follicle. LH also stimulates the corpus luteum to secrete progesterone and some estrogen. These hormones have a negative feedback effect on the hypothalamus and anterior pituitary so that FSH and LH levels decline. As the LH level declines, corpus luteum activity declines, the inhibitory effect is removed, and the cycle starts over.

Uterine (Menstrual) Cycle

The uterine (menstrual) cycle reflects changes in the endometrium of the uterus. These changes occur to the thick outer layer of the endometrium, known as the *stratum functionale*. Changes in estrogen and progesterone levels are responsible for the changes in the uterus. The **uterine cycle** is divided into the menstrual phase, proliferative phase, and secretory phase (see Figure 16-13).

Menstrual phase: The menstrual phase begins on the first day of the cycle and continues for 3 to 5 days. The thick stratum functionale detaches from the uterine wall and passes through the vagina as the menstrual flow. During this time, follicles are growing in the ovary.

Proliferative phase: The proliferative phase begins with the end of the menstrual phase and lasts for about 8 days. The growing follicles in the ovary secrete increasing levels of estrogen. The estrogen stimulates repair of the endometrium in the uterus. The endometrium thickens, glands develop, and blood vessels grow in the new tissue. Ovulation in the ovary occurs at the end of this uterine phase.

Secretory phase: During the secretory phase, the corpus luteum secretes progesterone, which stimulates continued growth and thickening of the endometrium. Arteries and glands grow and enlarge. The glands secrete glycogen, which will nourish a developing embryo if fertilization occurs. If fertilization does not occur, the corpus luteum in the ovary begins to degenerate. This leads to menstruation, and the cycle starts over again.

Menopause

Menopause is the cessation of the female reproductive cycles. Even though menopause is marked by the lack of menstrual cycles, the first changes occur in the ovary. By the age of 45 or 50, ovarian follicles cease responding to FSH and LH from the pituitary gland. As a result, the follicle cells do not produce estrogen and there is no ovulation, no corpus luteum, and no progesterone. Without estrogen and progesterone, the cyclic changes in the uterus stop and menstruation ceases. This is the visible evidence of meno-pause. As estrogen and progesterone levels decline, FSH and LH increase because of the lack of ovarian hormone feed-back. These high levels of pituitary hormones with the low levels of ovarian hormones are believed to be responsible for a variety of effects associated with the onset of menopause. Some women experience hot flashes, sweating, depression, headaches, irritability, and insomnia. However, many women experience few, if any, of these.

Mammary Glands

The mammary glands are the organs of milk production. Mammary glands are located in the breast, overlying the pectoralis major muscles. They are present in both sexes but usually functional only in the female.

Each breast has a raised **nipple,** which is surrounded by a circular pigmented area called the **areola** (ah-REE-oh-lah). The nipples are sensitive to touch, and they contain smooth muscle that contracts and causes them to become erect in response to stimulation.

The adult female breast contains 15 to 20 lobes of glandular tissue that radiate around the nipple (Figure 16-14). The **lobes** are separated by connective tissue and adipose. The connective tissue helps support the breast. Some bands of connective tissue, called **suspensory** (Cooper) **ligaments,** extend through the breast from the skin to the underlying muscles. The amount and distribu-tion of the adipose tissue determines the size and shape of

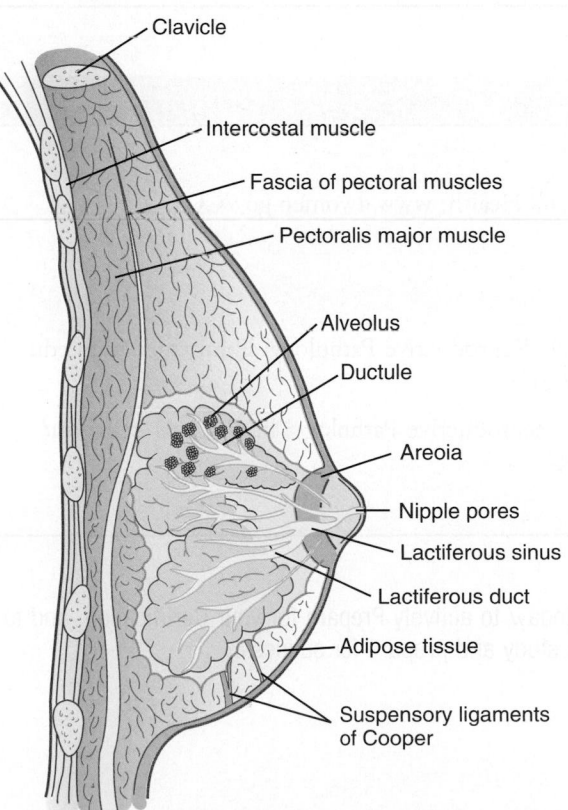

Figure 16-14 Breast and mammary glands.

- Clavicle
- Intercostal muscle
- Fascia of pectoral muscles
- Pectoralis major muscle
- Alveolus
- Ductule
- Areoia
- Nipple pores
- Lactiferous sinus
- Lactiferous duct
- Adipose tissue
- Suspensory ligaments of Cooper

the breast. Each lobe consists of **lobules** that contain the glandular units. A **lactiferous** (lak-TIFF-er-us) **duct** col-lects the milk from the lobules within each lobe and carries it to the nipple. Just before the nipple, the lactiferous duct enlarges to form a **lactiferous sinus (ampulla),** which serves as a reservoir for milk. After the sinus, the duct again narrows and each duct opens independently on the surface of the nipple.

Mammary gland function is regulated by hormones. At puberty, increasing levels of estrogen stimulate the develop-ment of glandular tissue in the female breast. Estrogen also causes the breasts to increase in size through the accumula-tion of adipose tissue. Progesterone stimulates the develop-ment of the duct system. During pregnancy these hormones further enhance development of the mammary glands. Pro-lactin from the anterior pituitary stimulates the production of milk within the glandular tissue, and oxytocin causes the ejection of milk from the glands.

AGING OF THE REPRODUCTIVE SYSTEM

Men normally do not experience a sudden decline in repro-ductive function comparable to menopause in women. Instead, they experience a gradual and subtle decline over many years. After age 50, men have some testicular atrophy, partially caused by a decrease in the size of the seminiferous tubules and partially a result of a reduction in the number of interstitial cells. These changes are accompanied by a decline in sperm and testosterone production. Both the seminal vesicles and the prostate show a decrease in secre-tory activity, which results in a reduction in the volume of semen. The portion of the prostate gland that surrounds the urethra often enlarges and may constrict the urethra, making urination difficult. The penis may undergo some atrophy and become smaller with age. The blood vessels and erectile tissue in the penis become less elastic, which hinders the ability to attain an erection. Although there is a general decline in the aging male reproductive system, many men are capable of achieving erection and ejaculation into old age.

After menopause, there is a gradual decline in the female reproductive system. Most of the changes are believed to be caused by the reduction in estrogen. The ovaries undergo progressive atrophy. The uterus becomes smaller, and fibrous connective tissue replaces much of the myometrium. The vagina becomes narrower and shorter, and its walls become thin and less elastic. Glands that lubricate the vagina reduce their secretory activity, and the vagina becomes dry. The vaginal secretions that remain are less acidic, which makes older women more susceptible to vaginal infections. The external genitalia and mammary glands undergo atrophic changes. The lack of estrogen also affects nonreproductive organs. This is particularly true in the case of bone metabo-lism, which is indicated by the increased prevalence of osteoporosis in postmenopausal women. There is also increased cardiovascular disease.

Estrogen replacement therapy is prescribed for many women to combat osteoporosis and other effects of menopause. However, there is controversy about the risks involved with this treatment, particularly the risks of uterine and breast cancer. Consideration should be given to the risks and benefits before beginning estrogen replacement therapy. Current practice often involves prescription of progesterone in conjunction with estrogen, which seems to reduce some of the risks.

There is a growing awareness that elderly people have sexual needs and enjoy sexual relations. Although age-related physical and hormonal changes that take place in the reproductive system may alter these needs and sexual functioning, studies demonstrate that sexuality remains important to many older people.

TERMINOLOGY REVIEW

Medical Term	Word Parts	Definition
Gametes		Sex cells: sperm and ova.
Gonads		Primary reproductive organs; organs that produce the gametes: testes in the male and ovaries in the female.
Oogenesis	*oo-:* egg, ovum *-genesis:* producing, forming	Process of meiosis in the female in which one ovum and three polar bodies are produced from one primary oocyte.
Ovarian cycle	*ovary/o:* ovary	Monthly cycle of events that occur in the ovary from puberty to menopause; occurs concurrently with the uterine cycle.
Ovarian follicle	*ovary/o:* ovary	An oocyte surrounded by one or more layers of cells within the ovaries.
Spermatogenesis	*spermat/o:* spermatozoa, sperm cells	Process of meiosis in the male in which four spermatids are produced from one primary spermatocyte.
Spermiogenesis	*spermi/o:* spermatozoa, sperm cells *-genesis:* producing, forming	Morphologic changes that transform a spermatid into a mature sperm.
Uterine cycle	*uter/o:* uterus, womb	Monthly cycle of events that occur in the uterus from puberty to menopause; also called the *menstrual cycle;* occurs concurrently with the ovarian cycle.

ON THE WEB

For information on the reproductive system:

Department of Health and Human Services, The Office of Women's Health: www.4women.gov/COE

Gene School: library.thinkquest.org/28599/index.htm

Inner Body: www.innerbody.com/html/body.html

The Internet Pathology Laboratory for Medical Education—Female Reproductive Pathology: library.med.utah.edu/WebPath/ORGAN.html *(Click on "Female Genital Tract Pathology")*

The Internet Pathology Laboratory for Medical Education—Male Reproductive Pathology: library.med.utah.edu/WebPath/ORGAN.html *(Click on "Male Reproductive Pathology")*

The Visible Embryo: visembryo.com

 Check out the Evolve site at http://evolve.elsevier.com/Bonewit/today/ to actively Prepare for your Certification, and to access additional interactive activities and exercises to help you study and prepare for success.

17

Medical Asepsis and the OSHA Standard

LEARNING OBJECTIVES	PROCEDURES
Microorganisms and Medical Asepsis	
1. Define a microorganism and give examples of types of microorganisms.	Handwashing.
2. Explain the difference between a nonpathogen and a pathogen.	
3. Define medical asepsis.	
4. List the six basic requirements for growth and multiplication of microorganisms.	
5. Outline the infection process and cycle, including the following:	
Give examples of the means of entry of microorganisms into the body.	
Give examples of the means of transmission of microorganisms from one person to another.	
Give examples of the means of exit of microorganisms from the body.	
List and explain the protective mechanisms the body uses to prevent the entrance of microorganisms.	
6. Explain the difference between resident flora and transient flora.	
7. State when each of the following is performed: handwashing, antiseptic handwashing, and alcohol-based hand rub.	Applying an alcohol-based hand rub.
8. Identify medical aseptic practices that should be followed in the medical office.	
9. Explain how proper handwashing helps prevent the transmission of microorganisms.	
10. List examples of when to wear clean disposable gloves.	Application and removal of clean disposable gloves.
OSHA Bloodborne Pathogens Standard	
11. Explain the purpose of OSHA.	Adhere to the OSHA Bloodborne Pathogens Standard.
12. Describe the purpose of the Needlestick Safety and Prevention Act.	
13. List and describe the elements that must be included in the OSHA exposure control plan.	
14. Explain the purpose of each of the following OSHA requirements: labeling requirements and sharps injury log.	
15. Define and give examples of each of the following: engineering controls, work practice controls, personal protective equipment, and housekeeping procedures.	
16. Identify the guidelines for use of personal protective equipment.	
Regulated Medical Waste	
17. List examples of medical waste and explain how to discard each type of waste.	Prepare regulated waste for pickup by an infectious waste service.
18. Explain how to handle and dispose of regulated medical waste.	
Bloodborne Diseases	
19. Explain how hepatitis B and C are transmitted in the health care setting.	
20. Describe postexposure prophylaxis for hepatitis B.	
21. Explain what occurs when HIV gains entrance into the body.	

KEY TERMS

aerobe (AIR-obe)
anaerobe (AN-er-obe)
antiseptic
asepsis (ay-SEP-sis)
cilia (SIL-ee-ah)
contaminated (kon-TAM-in-ated)
decontamination
  (DEE-kon-tam-in-AY-shun)
hand hygiene
infection

medical asepsis
microorganism (MYE-kroe-OR-gan-iz-um)
nonintact (NON-in-takt) skin
nonpathogen (non-PATH-oh-jen)
opportunistic (OP-pore-tune-IS-tik)
  infection
optimum (OP-tuh-mum) growth
  temperature
parenteral (pare-EN-ter-al)
pathogen (PATH-oh-jen)

perinatal (pare-ee-NAY-tul)
pH (PEE-AYCH)
postexposure prophylaxis (proe-fil-
  ACKS-is) (PEP)
regulated medical waste (RMW)
reservoir (REZ-er-vwar) host
resident flora (FLOE-ruh)
susceptible (sus-SEP-tih-bul)
transient (TRAN-zee-ent) flora

INTRODUCTION TO MEDICAL ASEPSIS AND THE OSHA STANDARD

Medical **asepsis** and **infection** control are crucial in preventing the spread of disease. The medical assistant should always practice good medical aseptic techniques to provide a safe and healthy environment in the medical office. The Occupational Safety and Health Administration (OSHA) Bloodborne Pathogens Standard is important for infection control. This standard is required by the federal government to reduce the exposure of health care employees to infectious diseases. This chapter presents a thorough discussion of medical asepsis, infection control, and the OSHA Bloodborne Pathogens Standard.

MICROORGANISMS AND MEDICAL ASEPSIS

Microorganisms are tiny living plants or animals that cannot be seen with the naked eye, but instead must be viewed with the aid of a microscope. Common types of microorganisms include bacteria, viruses, protozoa, fungi, and animal parasites. Most microorganisms are harmless and do not cause disease. They are termed **nonpathogens**. Other microorganisms, known as **pathogens**, are harmful to the body and can cause disease.

In the medical office, practices must be employed to reduce the number and hinder the transmission of pathogenic microorganisms. These practices are known as *medical asepsis*. **Medical asepsis** means that an object or area is clean and free from infection. Nonpathogens would still be present on a clean or medically aseptic substance or surface, but all the pathogens would have been eliminated.

Growth Requirements for Microorganisms

For microorganisms to survive, certain growth requirements must be present in the environment, as follows:

1. **Proper nutrition.** Microorganisms that use inorganic or nonliving substances as sources of food are known as *autotrophs*. Microorganisms that use organic or living substances for food are known as *heterotrophs*.
2. **Oxygen.** Most microorganisms need oxygen to grow and multiply and are termed **aerobes**. Other microorganisms, known as **anaerobes**, grow best in the absence of oxygen.
3. **Temperature.** Each microorganism has a temperature at which it grows best, known as the **optimum growth temperature**. Most microorganisms grow best at 98.6° F (37° C), the human body temperature.
4. **Darkness.** Microorganisms grow best in darkness.
5. **Moisture.** Microorganisms need moisture for cell metabolism and to carry away wastes.
6. **pH.** Most microorganisms prefer a neutral pH. If the environment of the microorganisms becomes too acidic or too basic, they die.

If growth requirements are taken away from the environment of microorganisms, they are unable to survive. Eliminating these conditions is one way to reduce the

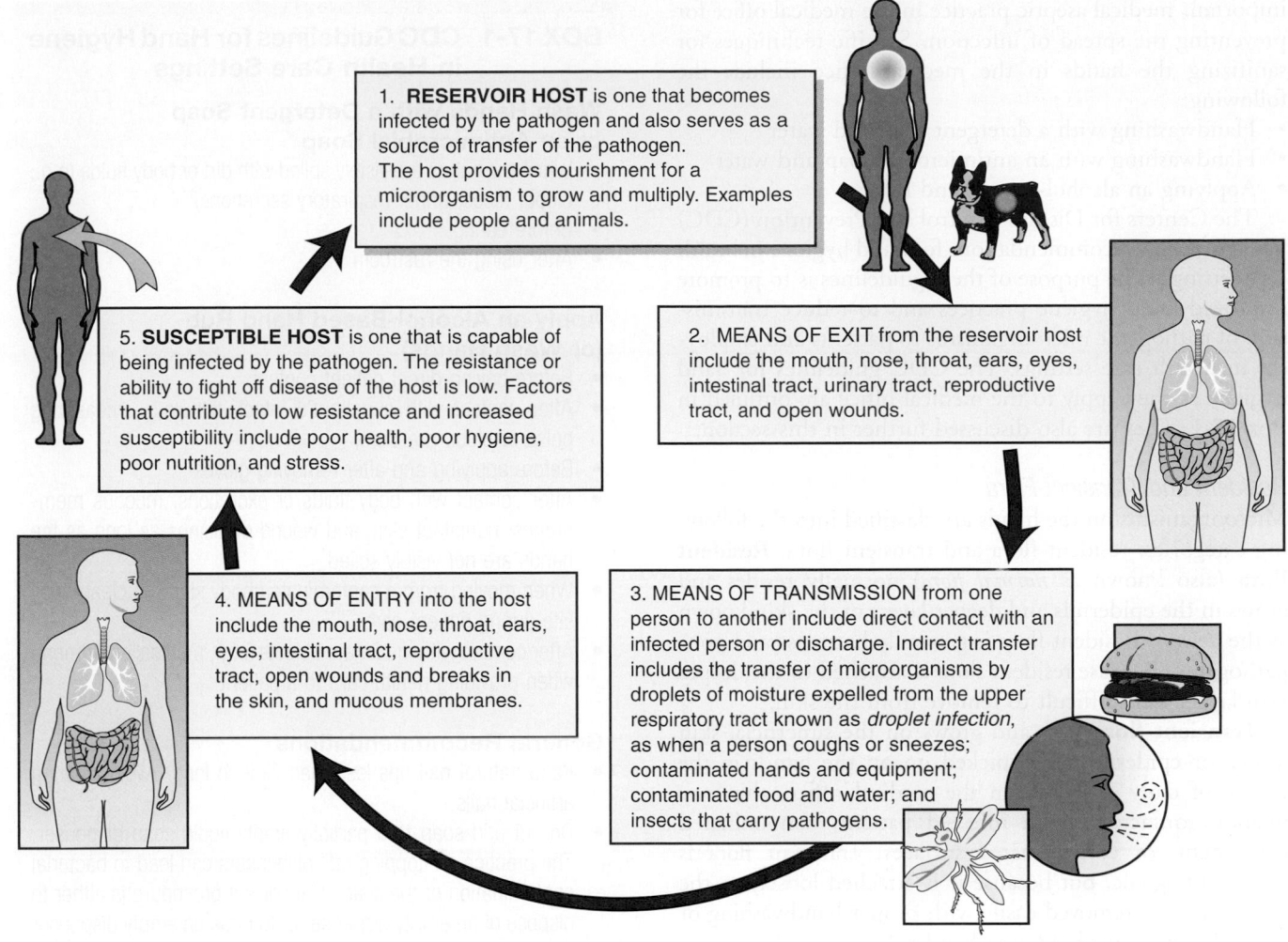

1. **RESERVOIR HOST** is one that becomes infected by the pathogen and also serves as a source of transfer of the pathogen. The host provides nourishment for a microorganism to grow and multiply. Examples include people and animals.

5. **SUSCEPTIBLE HOST** is one that is capable of being infected by the pathogen. The resistance or ability to fight off disease of the host is low. Factors that contribute to low resistance and increased susceptibility include poor health, poor hygiene, poor nutrition, and stress.

2. **MEANS OF EXIT** from the reservoir host include the mouth, nose, throat, ears, eyes, intestinal tract, urinary tract, reproductive tract, and open wounds.

4. **MEANS OF ENTRY** into the host include the mouth, nose, throat, ears, eyes, intestinal tract, reproductive tract, open wounds and breaks in the skin, and mucous membranes.

3. **MEANS OF TRANSMISSION** from one person to another include direct contact with an infected person or discharge. Indirect transfer includes the transfer of microorganisms by droplets of moisture expelled from the upper respiratory tract known as *droplet infection*, as when a person coughs or sneezes; contaminated hands and equipment; contaminated food and water; and insects that carry pathogens.

Figure 17-1 The infection process cycle.

growth and transmission of pathogens in the medical office.

Infection Process Cycle

For a pathogen to survive and produce disease, a continuous cycle must be followed; this is known as the *infection process cycle* (Figure 17-1). If the cycle is broken at any point, the pathogen dies. The medical assistant has a responsibility to help break this cycle in the medical office by practicing good techniques of medical asepsis. These techniques are discussed in the next section.

Protective Mechanisms of the Body

The body has protective mechanisms to help prevent the entrance of pathogens, and these help break the infection process cycle. Protective mechanisms of the body are as follows:

1. The skin is the body's most important defense mechanism; it serves as a protective barrier against the entrance of microorganisms.
2. The mucous membranes of the body, which line the nose and throat and respiratory, gastrointestinal, and genital tracts, help protect the body from invasion by microorganisms.
3. Mucus and cilia in the nose and respiratory tract fight off pathogens. Mucus traps the smaller microorganisms that enter the body, and the hairlike **cilia** constantly beat toward the outside to remove them from the body.
4. Coughing and sneezing help force pathogens from the body.
5. Tears and sweat are secretions that aid in the removal of pathogens from the body.
6. Urine and vaginal secretions are acidic. Pathogens cannot grow in an acidic environment.
7. The stomach secretes hydrochloric acid, which helps in the process of digestion. This acidic environment discourages the growth of pathogens that enter the stomach.

Medical Asepsis in the Medical Office

Hand Hygiene

Hand hygiene refers to the process of cleansing or sanitizing the hands. Hand hygiene is considered the most important medical aseptic practice in the medical office for preventing the spread of infection. Specific techniques for sanitizing the hands in the medical office include the following:

- Handwashing with a detergent soap and water
- Handwashing with an antimicrobial soap and water
- Applying an alcohol-based hand rub

The Centers for Disease Control and Prevention (CDC) has issued new recommendations for hand hygiene in health care settings. The purpose of these guidelines is to promote improved hand hygiene practices and to reduce transmission of pathogenic microorganisms to patients and employees in health care settings. The CDC guidelines for hand hygiene as they apply to the medical office are outlined in Box 17-1. They are also discussed further in this section.

Resident and Transient Flora

Microorganisms on the hands are classified into the following categories: resident flora and transient flora. **Resident flora** (also known as *normal flora*) normally resides and grows in the epidermis and deeper layers of the skin known as the *dermis*. Resident flora is generally harmless and nonpathogenic. Because resident flora is attached to the deeper skin layers, it is difficult to remove from the skin.

Transient flora lives and grows on the superficial skin layers, or epidermis. It is picked up on the hands in the course of daily activities. In the medical office, this may include contact with an infected patient, contaminated equipment, or contaminated surfaces. Transient flora is often pathogenic, but because it is attached loosely to the skin, it can be removed easily with proper handwashing or by applying an alcohol-based hand rub.

Handwashing

Handwashing refers to washing the hands with a detergent soap and water. Detergent soap (commonly known as *plain*

BOX 17-1   CDC Guidelines for Hand Hygiene in Health Care Settings

Wash Hands with a Detergent Soap or an Antimicrobial Soap

- When the hands are visibly soiled with dirt or body fluids (e.g., blood, feces, urine, respiratory secretions)
- Before eating
- After using the restroom

Apply an Alcohol-Based Hand Rub (or Wash Hands)

- Before having direct patient contact
- After contact with a patient's intact skin (e.g., measuring pulse or blood pressure)
- Before applying and after removing gloves
- After contact with body fluids or excretions, mucous membranes, nonintact skin, and wound dressings as long as the hands are not visibly soiled
- When moving from a contaminated body site to a clean body site during patient care
- After contact with inanimate objects (e.g., medical equipment) when providing health care to a patient

General Recommendations

- Keep natural nail tips less than $\frac{1}{4}$ inch long. Avoid wearing artificial nails.
- Do not add soap to a partially empty liquid soap dispenser. The practice of "topping off" dispensers can lead to bacterial contamination of the soap. The correct procedure is either to dispose of an empty dispenser or to rinse an empty dispenser thoroughly and then refill it.
- Multiple-use cloth towels of the hanging or roll type are not recommended.
- Use hand lotions or creams to minimize the occurrence of dermatitis associated with frequent handwashing.
- Wear gloves if contact with blood or other potentially infectious materials, mucous membranes, and nonintact skin could occur.
- Change gloves during patient care if moving from a contaminated body site to a clean body site.
- Remove gloves after caring for a patient. Do not wear the same pair of gloves for the care of more than one patient.

From Bonewit-West K: *Clinical procedures for medical assistants*, ed 8, St Louis, 2011, Saunders.

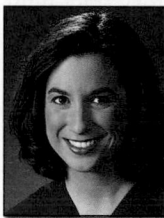

Putting It All Into Practice

My Name is Jennifer Hawk, and I work for a large group of physicians in a multispecialty clinic. I work in both the front and back areas of the office. I really enjoy experiencing all of these areas of the office, and I definitely never get bored.

The most interesting experience I have had as a practicing medical assistant is seeing the impact that I make in patients' lives. They rely on you and look to you first for help in their health care situation. You are most often the first person they come into contact with in the office, and they look to you for understanding and empathy. Especially patients who come to your office on a regular basis see you as a kind of family member. They appreciate a familiar face and a smile. Most often, you are the individual giving patients instructions concerning testing they will be having done or medication they will be taking. Patients truly do count on your knowledge and assistance throughout their course of care. I was genuinely surprised at what an impact I could have on others. ■

---

soap) contains agents that help break down and emulsify dirt and oil present on the skin. Soap is used to sanitize the hands through the physical removal of dirt and transient flora. It is important to use adequate friction during handwashing to ensure the removal of all transient flora. The CDC recommends that the hands be rubbed together for at least 15 seconds, making sure to cover all surfaces and to focus on the fingertips and fingernails. Procedure 17-1 outlines the handwashing procedure.

The CDC hand hygiene guidelines recommend that handwashing be performed when the hands are visibly

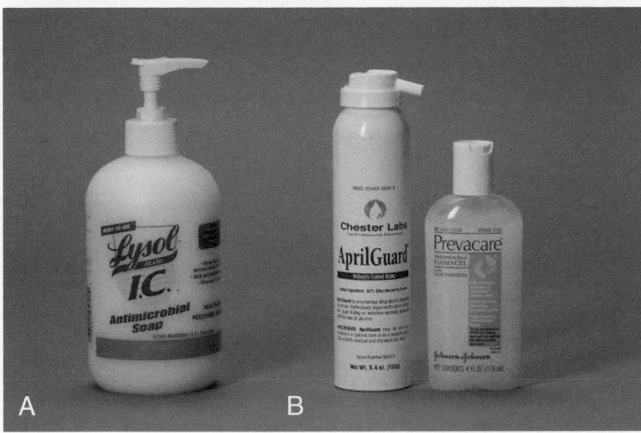

Figure 17-2 **A,** Antimicrobial soap. **B,** Alcohol-based hand rubs.

soiled with dirt or body fluids, before eating, and after using the restroom (see Box 17-1). If the hands are not visibly soiled, the CDC recommends that an alcohol-based hand rub, rather than handwashing, be used to sanitize the hands. This is because repeated handwashing tends to dry out the hands, leading to irritation, chapping, and dermatitis.

Antiseptic Handwashing

Washing the hands with an antimicrobial soap is termed *antiseptic handwashing*. Antimicrobial soaps contain an **antiseptic**, which is an agent that functions to kill or inhibit the growth of microorganisms (Figure 17-2, *A*). Antiseptic handwashing sanitizes the hands through the mechanical scrubbing action and through the action of the antiseptic. Proper handwashing with an antimicrobial soap removes all soil and transient flora from the hands. Most antimicrobial soaps also deposit an antibacterial film on the skin that discourages bacterial growth. Antiseptic handwashing should be performed by the medical assistant before assisting with minor office surgery. Examples of antiseptics contained in antimicrobial soaps include triclosan, chlorhexidine, hexachlorophene, iodine, and chloroxylenol.

Alcohol-Based Hand Rubs

CDC guidelines recommend the use of an alcohol-based hand rub for sanitizing the hands when they are not visibly soiled (see Box 17-1). Alcohol-based hand rubs, also known as *hand sanitizers,* consist of 60% to 90% alcohol (ethanol or isopropanol) and come in the forms of gels, lotions, and foams (Figure 17-2, *B*). Studies have shown that hand rubs are more effective than traditional soap and water handwashing in removing transient flora and reducing bacterial counts on the hands. The advantages that alcohol-based hand rubs offer over traditional handwashing are as follows:
- Alcohol-based hand rubs are usually more accessible than sinks.
- They do not require rinsing; water or hand drying with a towel is not needed.
- Less time is required to perform hand hygiene. It takes 20 to 30 seconds to sanitize the hands with an alcohol-

based hand rub compared with 1 to 2 minutes to perform proper handwashing.
- They are less damaging to the skin, resulting in less dryness and irritation. Most alcohol-based hand rubs contain emollients, which help prevent the skin of the hands from overdrying. As the alcohol dries, protective fats and oils remain on the hands.

Alcohol-based hand rubs have disadvantages. They are more expensive than plain soap. They also cause a brief stinging sensation if they are applied to broken skin, such as a cut or abrasion on the hand. Procedure 17-2 describes the proper steps for performing an alcohol-based hand rub.

Infection Control

In addition to hand hygiene, other good aseptic practices in the medical office include the following:
1. Follow the OSHA Bloodborne Pathogens Standard (presented in this chapter).
2. Keep the medical office free from dirt and dust, which can collect and carry microorganisms.
3. Ensure that the reception area and examining rooms are well ventilated. Stuffy rooms encourage microorganisms to settle on objects.
4. Keep the reception area and examining rooms bright and airy. Light discourages the growth of microorganisms.
5. Eliminate insects by the use of insecticides or window screens. Insects are a means of transmission of microorganisms.
6. Carefully dispose of wastes, such as urine, feces, and respiratory secretions; all wastes should be handled as though they contained pathogens.
7. Do not let soiled items touch clothing.
8. Avoid coughs and sneezes of patients. Moisture droplets expelled from the lungs with coughing and sneezing may contain pathogens.
9. Use discretion in the amount of jewelry worn; wear minimal jewelry or no jewelry at all. Microorganisms can become lodged in the grooves and crevices of jewelry and serve as a means of transmission of pathogens.
10. Teach patients aseptic practices to control the spread of infection at home.

Gloves

Gloves reduce hand contamination by 70% to 80%, reduce cross-contamination between patients, and protect patients and health care workers from infection. The CDC recommends that clean disposable gloves be worn when the medical assistant is likely to come in contact with any body substance, such as blood, urine, feces, mucous membranes, and nonintact skin. Clean disposable gloves should be worn when administering an injection, performing a venipuncture, or performing a urinalysis. Clean disposable gloves come in the following sizes: small, medium, large, and extra large, and sometimes extra small. Procedure 17-3 presents the proper method for applying and removing clean disposable gloves.

Text continued on p. 248

PROCEDURE 17-1   Handwashing

Outcome Perform handwashing.

Equipment/Supplies

- Liquid soap
- Paper towels
- Waste container

1. **Procedural Step.** Remove your watch or push it up on the forearm so that the wrist is clear. Avoid wearing rings. If you wear rings, remove all except a plain wedding band and put them in a safe place.
   Principle. Microorganisms can lodge in the crevices and grooves of rings.

2. **Procedural Step.** Stand at the sink, making sure clothing does not touch the sink.
   Principle. The sink is considered contaminated, and if the uniform touches the sink, it may pick up microorganisms and transfer them.

3. **Procedural Step.** Turn on the faucets, using a paper towel.
   Principle. The faucets are considered contaminated because they harbor microorganisms.

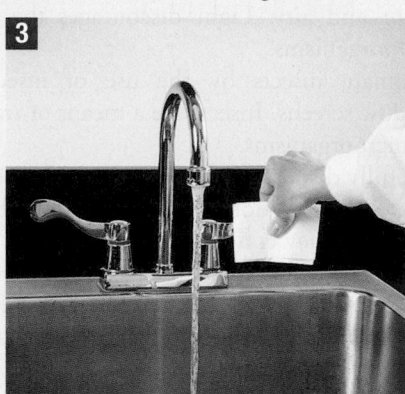

Turn on the faucet using a paper towel.

4. **Procedural Step.** Adjust the water temperature. The water should be warm to make the best suds.
   Principle. Water that is too hot or too cold tends to dry the skin, causing chapping and cracking and making it easy for pathogens to enter the body or be transferred to patients.

5. **Procedural Step.** Discard the paper towel in the waste container.
   Principle. The paper towel is considered contaminated after touching the faucets.

6. **Procedural Step.** Wet the hands and forearms thoroughly with water. The hands should be held lower than the elbows at all times. Do not touch the inside of the sink because it is also contaminated.
   Principle. When you hold the hands lower than the elbows, bacteria and debris are carried away from the arms and body and into the sink.

7. **Procedural Step.** Apply soap to the hands. Apply 1 teaspoon of liquid soap (approximately the size of a nickel) to the palm of one hand.

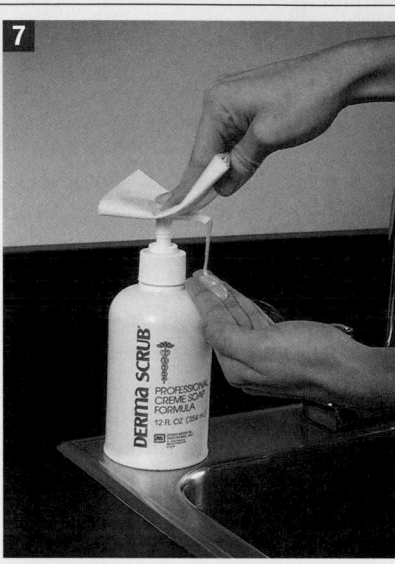

Apply soap to the hands.

8. **Procedural Step.** Wash the palms and backs of the hands with 10 circular motions. Use friction along with the circular motions to wash the palm and back of each hand.
   Principle. Friction helps to dislodge and remove microorganisms from the hands.

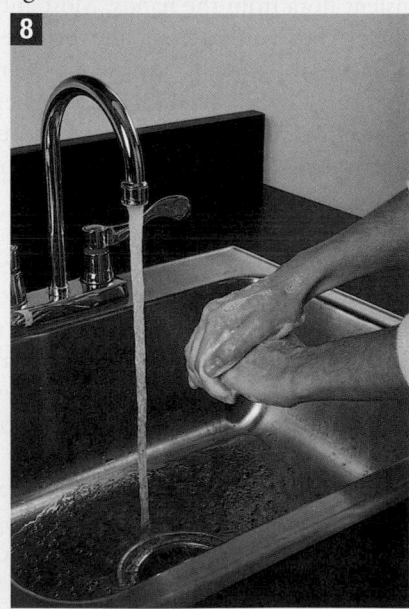

Wash the palms and backs of the hands.

9. **Procedural Step.** Wash the fingers with 10 circular motions while focusing on the fingertips and fingernails. Interlace the fingers and thumbs, and use friction and circular motions while rubbing the fingers back and forth.

Principle. This kind of movement helps remove microorganisms and debris that have accumulated between the fingers.

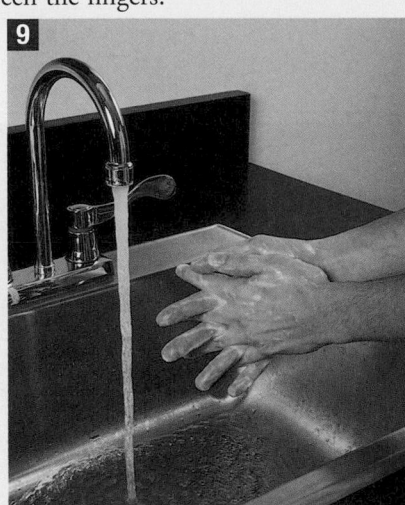

Interlace the fingers and thumbs, and use friction.

10. **Procedural Step.** Rinse well, making sure to hold the hands lower than the elbows.
Principle. Running water helps to rinse away dirt and microorganisms.

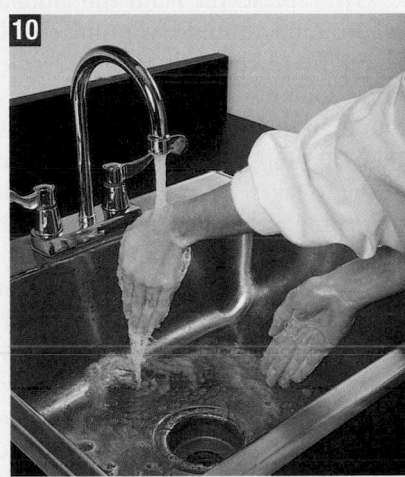

Rinse well, holding the hands lower than the elbows.

11. **Procedural Step.** Wash the wrists and forearms, using friction along with circular motions.

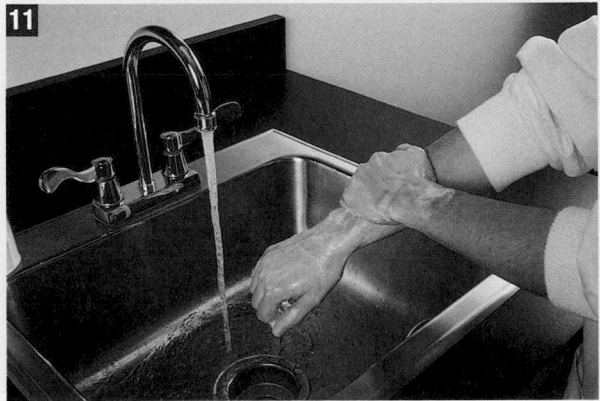

Wash wrists and forearms using friction.

(*NOTE:* The hands are washed first because they are the most contaminated; microorganisms and dirt are washed away and do not spread to the wrists and forearms.)

12. **Procedural Step.** Clean the fingernails with a manicure stick. The fingernails should be cleaned at least once daily, preferably during initial handwashing (i.e., handwashing performed just after arriving at the medical office to begin your day).
Principle. Dirt and microorganisms collect underneath the fingernails.

13. **Procedural Step.** Rinse the arms and hands.
Principle. The running water rinses away the dirt and microorganisms.

14. **Procedural Step.** Repeat the handwashing procedure. For initial handwashing or when the hands come into contact with blood or other potentially infectious materials, the handwashing procedure should be repeated to ensure removal of all pathogens.

15. **Procedural Step.** Dry the hands gently and thoroughly, and discard the paper towel.
Principle. Gently drying the hands prevents them from becoming chapped. Microorganisms can lodge in the crevices of chapped hands. Ensure that the hands are dried completely, because wet skin also may cause chapping.

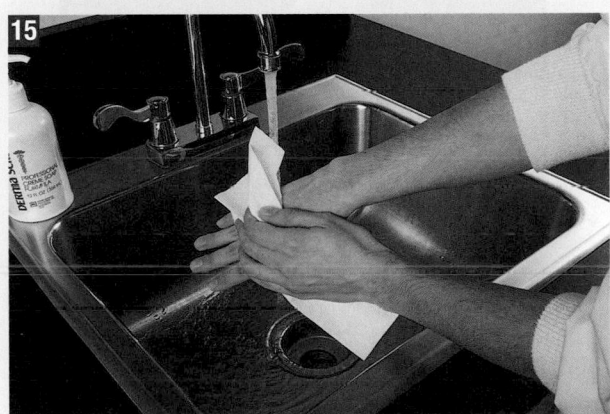

Dry the hands gently and thoroughly.

16. **Procedural Step.** Turn off the water, using a paper towel, and discard the paper towel in a waste container.
Principle. The faucet is considered contaminated, whereas the hands are medically aseptic or clean.

17. **Procedural Step.** Do not touch the sink with the bare hands.
Principle. The hands are now medically aseptic, and the sink is considered contaminated.

PROCEDURE 17-2 Applying an Alcohol-Based Hand Rub

Outcome Apply an alcohol-based hand rub.

Equipment/Supplies

- Alcohol-based hand rub

1. Procedural Step. Inspect the hands to ensure that they are not visibly soiled. Hands that are visibly soiled must be washed with soap and water.
Principle. Alcohol-based hand rubs are not intended for the removal of visible soil.

2. Procedural Step. Remove your watch or push it up on the forearm. Avoid wearing rings. If you wear rings, remove all except a plain wedding band and put them in a safe place.
Principle. Microorganisms can lodge in the crevices and grooves of rings.

3. Procedural Step. Apply the alcohol-based hand rub to the palm of one hand as follows:
Gel or Lotion. Apply approximately 1 mL of the gel or lotion to the palm of one hand; this amount is approximately equal to the size of a dime.

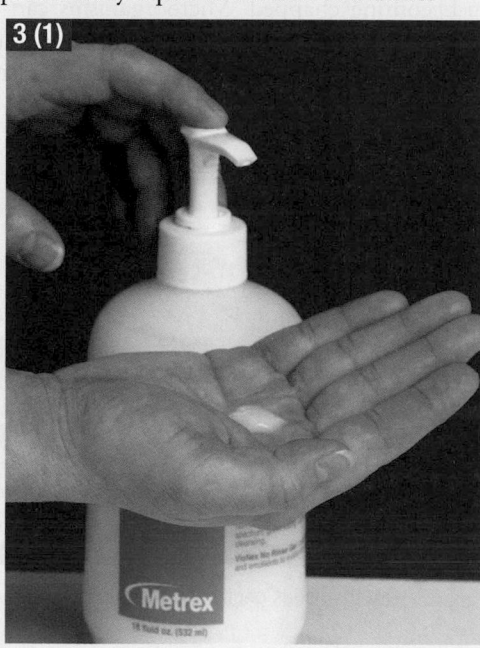

Apply lotion equal to the size of a dime.

Foam. Apply 3 grams of foam to the palm of one hand; this amount is approximately equal to the size of a walnut.
Principle. Using more than the recommended amount results in a prolonged (and unnecessary) period of time for your hands to dry.

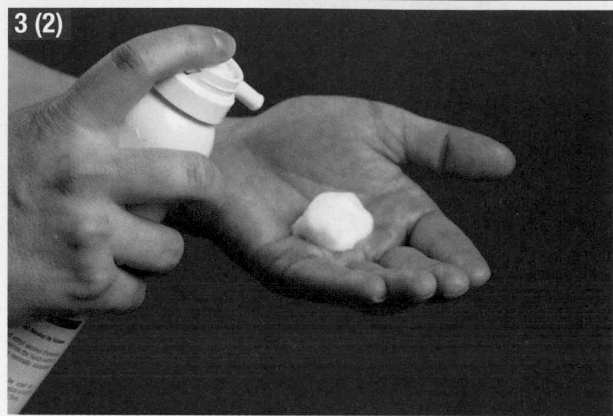

Apply foam equal to the size of a walnut.

4. Procedural Step. Thoroughly spread the hand rub over all surfaces of both hands (and fingers) up to ½ inch above the wrist. Spread the hand rub around the fingertips and around and under your fingernails.
Principle. Failure to cover all surfaces can leave areas of the hands contaminated. Microorganisms tend to collect around and underneath the fingernails.

5. Procedural Step. Rub the hands together until they are dry; this usually takes 10 to 30 seconds. Allow your hands to dry completely before touching anything. The hands are now medically aseptic.
Note: After cleaning your hands 5 to 10 times with a hand rub, a buildup of emollients may occur on your hands. The emollients can be easily removed by washing your hands with soap and water.
Principle. If you have applied a sufficient amount of hand rub, it should take at least 10 to 30 seconds for your hands to feel dry. Your hands will still feel a little wet at first. Let them dry completely before touching anything.

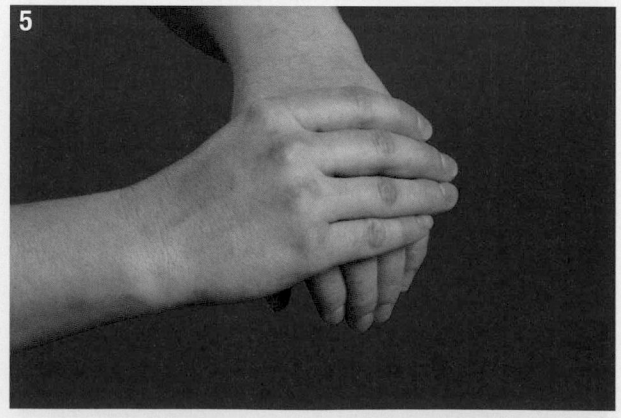

Rub the hands together until they are dry.

PROCEDURE **17-3** Application and Removal of Clean Disposable Gloves

Outcome Apply and remove clean disposable gloves.

Equipment/Supplies

• Clean disposable gloves

Applying Clean Disposable Gloves

No special technique is required when clean disposable gloves are applied. This is because the hands are clean and the gloves are clean; the medical assistant can touch any part of the gloves during application without contaminating them.

1. Procedural Step. Remove all rings, and sanitize your hands. Handwashing should be performed if the hands are visibly soiled. If this is not the case, use an alcohol-based hand rub to sanitize the hands. Ensure that your hands are completely dry.

Principle. Rings may cause the gloves to tear. The warm, moist environment inside gloves provides ideal growing conditions for the multiplication of transient microorganisms present on the hands. Sanitizing the hands removes these microorganisms and prevents the transmission of pathogens. Moisture encourages the growth of microorganisms.

2. Procedural Step. Choose the appropriate size of gloves; they should not be too small or too large. The gloves should fit snugly but not be too tight. Apply the gloves, and adjust them so they fit comfortably.

Principle. If your gloves are too small, they may rip as you are applying them or may become uncomfortable to wear. If they are too large, you may find it difficult to perform your tasks.

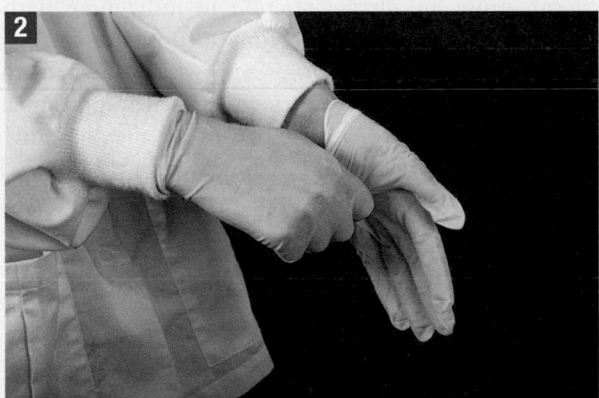
Apply the gloves.

3. Procedural Step. Inspect the gloves for tears. If a tear is present, a new pair of gloves must be applied.

Removing Clean Disposable Gloves

Gloves must be removed in a manner that protects the medical assistant from contaminating his or her clean hands with pathogens that may be present on the outsides of the gloves. This is accomplished by not allowing the bare hands to come in contact with the outsides of the gloves.

1. Procedural Step. Grasp the outside of the left glove 1 to 2 inches from the top with your gloved right hand. (*NOTE:* It does not matter which glove is removed first. You may start with the right glove if you prefer.)

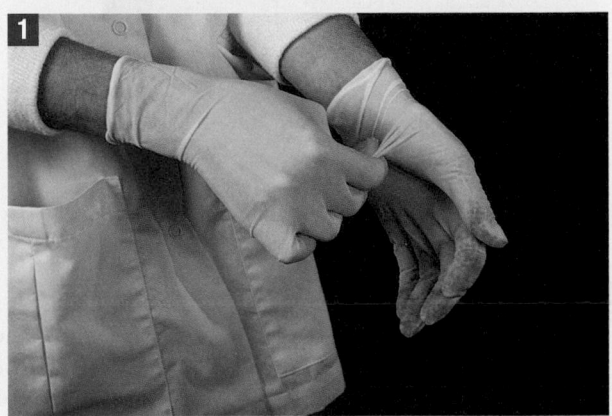
Grasp the glove 1 to 2 inches from the top of the glove.

2. Procedural Step. Slowly pull the left glove off the hand. It will turn inside out as it is removed from your hand.

3. Procedural Step. Pull the left glove free, and scrunch it into a ball with your gloved right hand.

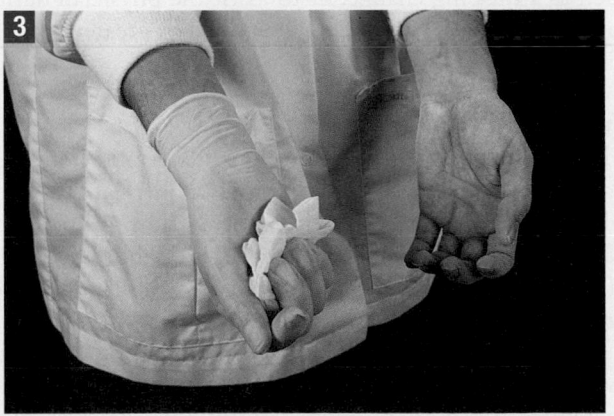
Scrunch the glove into a ball.

4. Procedural Step. Place the index and middle fingers of the left hand on the inside of the right glove. Do not allow your clean hand to touch the outside of the glove.

Continued

PROCEDURE 17-3   Application and Removal of Clean Disposable Gloves—cont'd

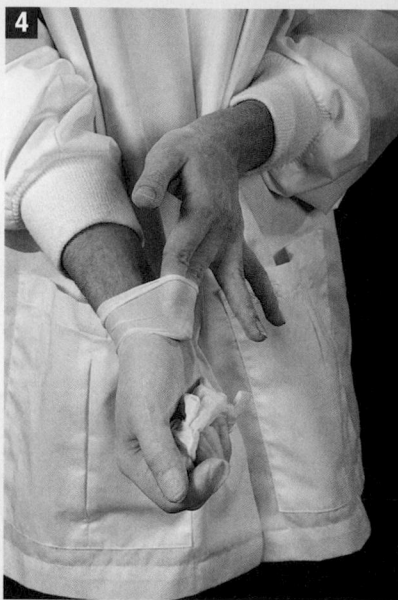

Place the index and middle fingers inside the glove.

5. Procedural Step. Pull the glove off the right hand. It will turn inside out as it is removed from your hand, enclosing the balled-up left glove. Discard both gloves in an appropriate container. If your gloves are visibly contaminated with blood or other potentially infectious materials, discard them in a biohazard waste

container. Otherwise, they can be discarded in a regular waste container.

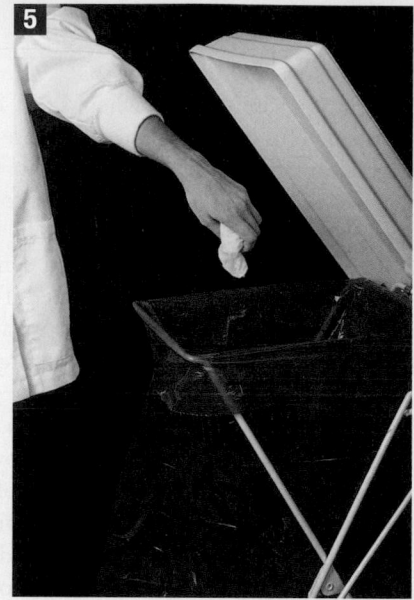

Discard both gloves in an appropriate container.

6. Procedural Step. Sanitize your hands to remove any microorganisms or other contaminants that may have come in contact with your hands during glove removal.

Sterile gloves are used to perform sterile procedures, such as a dressing change, or to assist the physician during minor office surgery, which is described in greater detail in Chapter 25.

Types of Gloves

There are two general types of gloves: latex and non-latex. Latex gloves are made from natural rubber latex (NRL), which is a milky liquid that is extracted from rubber trees. Non-latex gloves are made from synthetic rubber. Examples of non-latex gloves include nitrile, vinyl, and polychloroprene (neoprene) gloves.

Natural rubber latex gloves have a number of advantages over non-latex gloves. Latex gloves are soft and elastic and therefore stretch to fit more comfortably, whereas some non-latex gloves (e.g., vinyl gloves) are stiffer and are not as comfortable to wear. Latex gloves are thin, which allows the health care worker better feel, dexterity, and grip, and they are lower in cost than most non-latex gloves. In addition, latex has been in use for more than 100 years and has proven barrier protective capability, whereas the barrier effectiveness of non-latex gloves is not as well established at this time. The primary disadvantage of latex gloves is that

they can cause an allergic reaction in individuals with a hypersensitivity to latex. The primary substance causing a latex glove allergy is a protein present within the latex that enters the body through direct contact or through inhalation. When latex gloves are donned by an allergic individual, the protein comes in direct contact with the skin. The protein is absorbed into the skin, which then triggers an allergic reaction (Figure 17-3).

Glove Guidelines

The medical assistant should adhere to the following glove guidelines:

1. Keep fingernails trimmed short (less than ¼ inch long) to reduce the risk of tearing the gloves during application and use.
2. Wear the correct size glove. Gloves that are too small may rip as they are applied or may become uncomfortable to wear. Gloves that are too large may make it difficult to perform tasks.
3. Do not use oil-based hand lotions or creams because they can damage and deteriorate natural rubber latex gloves.

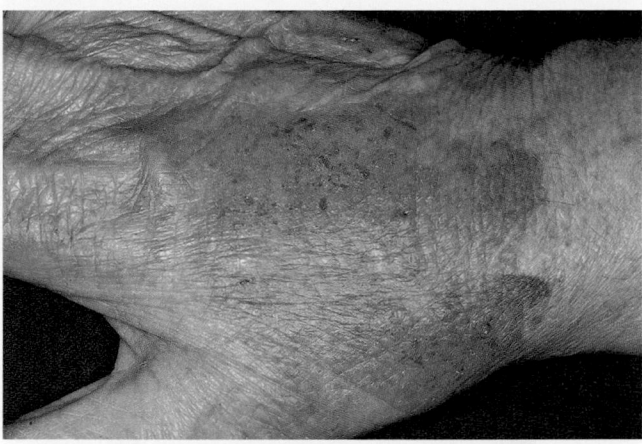

Figure 17-3 Latex glove allergy.

4. Do not store gloves in areas where there are extremes in temperatures (e.g., near a heater or air conditioner). These conditions can cause deterioration of the gloves.

OSHA BLOODBORNE PATHOGENS STANDARD

Purpose of the Standard

The federal government established OSHA (Occupational Safety and Health Administration) to assist employers in providing a safe and healthy working environment for their employees. To provide a safe working environment for health care workers, OSHA developed a comprehensive set of regulations known as the *OSHA Occupational Exposure to Bloodborne Pathogens Standard.*

These regulations went into effect in 1992 and are designed to reduce the risk to employees of exposure to infectious diseases.

The OSHA Bloodborne Pathogens Standard must be followed by any employee with occupational exposure to pathogens, regardless of the place of employment. In addition to medical assistants, employees with occupational exposure include physicians, nurses, dentists, dental hygienists, medical laboratory personnel, and emergency medical technicians. Employees who may have less obvious occupational exposure are correctional and law enforcement officers, firefighters, hospital laundry workers, morticians, and custodians.

Failure by employers to comply with the OSHA standard could result in a citation carrying a maximum penalty of $7000 for each violation and a maximum penalty of $70,000 for repeat violations.

Needlestick Safety and Prevention Act

Since the adoption of the OSHA Bloodborne Pathogens Standard, needlestick injuries among health care workers have continued to be a problem because of their high frequency of occurrence and the severity of the health effects associated with exposure to bloodborne pathogens.

To address this problem, Congress passed the Needlestick Safety and Prevention Act (NSPA). The NSPA directed OSHA to revise the Bloodborne Pathogens Standard to incorporate stronger measures to reduce needlesticks and other sharps injuries among health care workers. In response to this mandate, the primary measure instituted by OSHA was to establish detailed requirements that employers identify and make use of safer medical devices. This revised OSHA Bloodborne Pathogens Standard went into effect in 2001 and is described in detail in this chapter.

What Would You Do? What Would You *Not* Do?

Case Study 1
Petra Meyer has come in for her annual gynecologic examination. She notices that alcohol-based hand rubs are being used in the medical office. Petra wants to know if they are as good as regular soap and water for washing hands. Petra says she likes to garden and wants to know if hand rubs are effective in removing ground-in soil from the hands. Petra also is curious to know why they are now being used so much in health care settings. ∎

OSHA Terminology

The following definitions help clarify terms related to the OSHA Bloodborne Pathogens Standard.

Occupational exposure: *Occupational exposure* is reasonably anticipated skin, eye, mucous membrane, or parenteral contact with blood or other potentially infectious materials that may result from the performance of an employee's duties.

Parenteral: *Parenteral* refers to the piercing of the skin barrier or mucous membranes, such as through needlesticks, human bites, cuts, and abrasions.

Blood: *Blood* means human blood, human blood components, and products made from blood. Blood components include plasma, serum, platelets, and serosanguineous fluid (e.g., exudates from wounds). An example of a blood product is a medication derived from blood, such as immune globulins.

Bloodborne pathogens: *Bloodborne pathogens* are pathogenic microorganisms in human blood that can cause disease in humans. Bloodborne pathogens include, but are not limited to, hepatitis B virus (HBV), hepatitis C virus (HCV), and human immunodeficiency virus (HIV).

Other potentially infectious materials: *Other potentially infectious materials* (OPIM) include the following:
* Semen and vaginal secretions
* Cerebrospinal, synovial, pleural, pericardial, peritoneal, and amniotic fluids
* Any body fluid that is visibly contaminated with blood
* Any body fluid that has not been identified
* Saliva in dental procedures

- Any unfixed human tissue
- Any tissue culture, cells, or fluid known to be HIV infected

Contaminated: *Contaminated* is defined as the presence or reasonably anticipated presence of blood or other potentially infected materials on an item or surface.

Decontamination: *Decontamination* is the use of physical or chemical means to remove, inactivate, or destroy pathogens on a surface or item to the point where they are no longer capable of transmitting infectious particles, and the surface or item is rendered safe for handling, use, or disposal.

Nonintact skin: *Nonintact skin* is skin that has a break in the surface. It includes, but is not limited to, skin with dermatitis, abrasions, cuts, burns, hangnails, chapping, and acne.

Exposure incident: *Exposure incident* is defined as a specific eye, nose, mouth, or other mucous membrane, nonintact skin, or parenteral contact with blood or other potentially infectious materials that results from an employee's duties.

Components of the OSHA Standard

The OSHA Bloodborne Pathogens Standard is presented on the following pages as it pertains to the medical office and includes the following categories:
- Exposure control plan
- Safer medical devices
- Labeling requirements
- Communication of hazards to employees
- Record-keeping

Exposure Control Plan

The OSHA standard requires that the medical office develop an exposure control plan (ECP) (Figure 17-4). The ECP is a written document stipulating the protective measures that must be followed in that medical office to eliminate or minimize employee exposure to bloodborne pathogens and other potentially infectious materials. The ECP must be made available for review by all medical office staff. The ECP must include the following elements:

1. **An exposure determination.** The purpose of this section of the ECP is to identify employees who must receive training, protective equipment, hepatitis vaccination, and other protections required by the OSHA Bloodborne Pathogens Standard. The exposure determination must include (1) a list of all job classifications in which *all* employees are likely to have occupational exposure, such as physicians, medical assistants, and laboratory technicians, and (2) a list of job classifications in which only *some* employees have occupational exposure, such as custodians. For the second classification of jobs, the determination must include a list of tasks in which occupational exposure may occur, such as emptying the trash.

2. **The method of compliance.** The method of compliance section of the ECP must document the specific

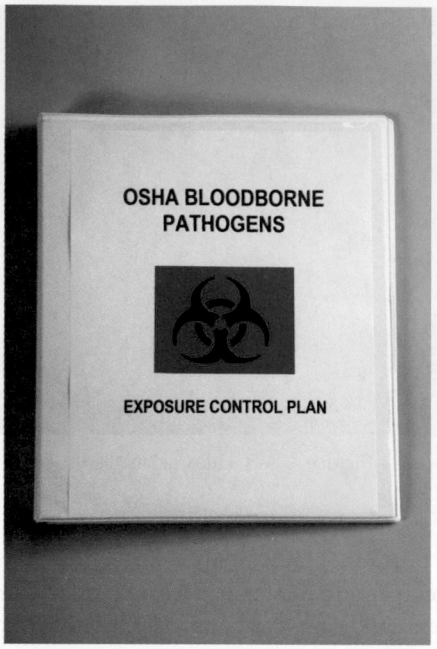

Figure 17-4 Example of an exposure control plan.

health and safety control measures that are taken in the medical office to eliminate or minimize the risk of occupational exposure. These measures are extremely important in reducing the risk of infectious disease for the medical assistant and are discussed in greater detail later in this section (see *Control Measures*).

3. **Postexposure evaluation and follow-up procedures.** Postexposure evaluation and follow-up must specify the procedures to follow in the event of an exposure incident in the medical office, including the method of documenting and investigating an exposure incident and the postexposure evaluation, medical treatment, and follow-up that would be made available to the employee. (Refer to the *OSHA Postexposure Evaluation and Follow-Up Procedures* box.)

OSHA requires employers to review and update their ECP at least annually to ensure that the plan remains current with the latest information on eliminating or reducing exposure to bloodborne pathogens. The ECP also must be updated whenever necessary to reflect new or modified tasks and procedures that affect occupational exposure.

Labeling Requirements

The OSHA Bloodborne Pathogens Standard requires that containers and appliances containing biohazardous materials be labeled with a *biohazard warning label*. The biohazard warning label must be fluorescent orange or orange-red and must contain the biohazard symbol and the word BIOHAZARD in a contrasting color (Figure 17-5, *A*).

A warning label must be attached to the following: (1) containers of regulated waste; (2) refrigerators and freezers

OSHA Postexposure Evaluation and Follow-Up Procedures

An exposure incident is a specific eye, nose, mouth, or other mucous membrane, nonintact skin, or parenteral contact with blood or other potentially infectious materials that results from an employee's duties. In the event of an exposure incident to bloodborne pathogens or other potentially infectious materials, OSHA requires the following steps to be performed:

1. Perform initial first aid measures immediately (e.g., wash a needlestick injury thoroughly with soap and water).

2. Document the route of exposure and the conditions and circumstances of the exposure incident. This includes such information as the engineering controls, the work practice controls, and personal protective equipment being used at the time of the incident.

3. Identify and document the source individual (unless the employer can establish that identification is not feasible or is prohibited by state or local law). A source individual is any person, living or dead, whose blood or OPIM may be a source of occupational exposure to the health care worker.

4. Obtain consent to test the source individual's blood. Test it as soon as possible to determine HBV, HCV, and HIV infectivity. The following guidelines apply to this requirement:
   - If consent is not obtained, the employer must document that legally required consent cannot be obtained.
   - If the source individual's consent is not required by law, the source individual's blood (if available) must be tested and the results documented.
   - If the source individual is already known to be infected with HBV, HCV, or HIV, testing does not need to be repeated.

5. Provide the exposed employee with the source individual's test results. Inform the employee of applicable laws and regulations concerning disclosure of the identity and infectious status of the source individual.

6. Obtain consent to test the employee's blood. Collect and test the blood of the employee as soon as possible for HBV, HCV, and HIV serologic status. If the employee does not give consent for HIV serologic testing, the baseline blood sample must be preserved for at least 90 days. If the employee elects to have the baseline sample tested during the 90-day waiting period, such testing must be done as soon as feasible.

7. When medically indicated, provide the employee with appropriate postexposure prophylaxis, as recommended by the U.S. Public Health Service.

used to store blood and other potentially infectious materials; and (3) containers and bags used to store, transport, or ship blood or other potentially infectious materials (Figure 17-5, *B*). Red bags or red containers may be substituted for biohazard warning labels. The labeling requirement is

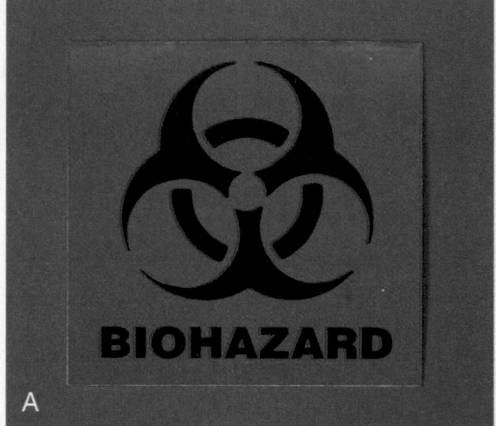

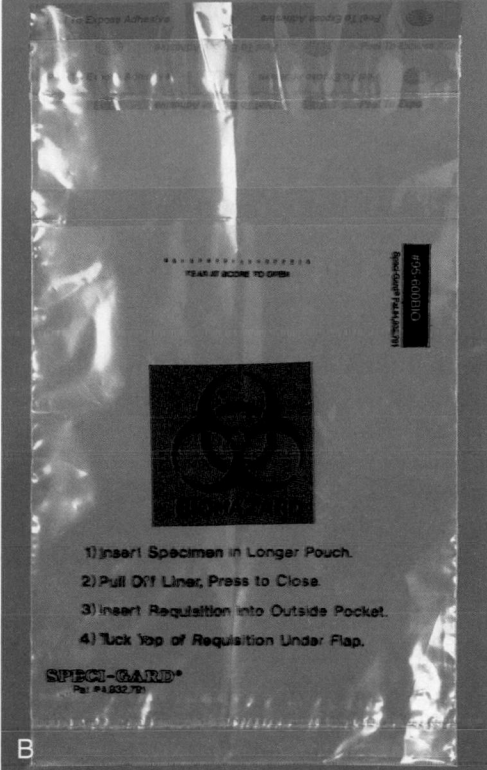

Figure 17-5 **A,** Biohazard warning label. **B,** Biohazard bag used to hold and transport blood or other potentially infectious materials.

designed to alert employees to possible exposure, particularly in situations in which the nature of the material or contents is not readily identifiable as blood or other potentially infectious materials.

Communicating Hazards to Employees

According to the OSHA standard, employers must ensure that all medical office employees with risk of occupational exposure participate in a training program. This program must present the ECP for the medical office, while focusing on the measures that employees are to take for their safety. Training must be provided at the time an employee is initially assigned to tasks in which occupational exposure may occur and at least annually thereafter.

The employer must maintain records of the training sessions, which must include presentation dates, content of the sessions, names and qualifications of the trainers, and names and job titles of employees who attended. These records must be maintained for 3 years from the date of the training session.

Record-Keeping

The OSHA Bloodborne Pathogens Standard requires that the following records be maintained:

1. **OSHA medical record.** The OSHA standard requires that the employer maintain an accurate OSHA record of every medical office employee at risk for occupational exposure. These records must be kept confidential except for review by OSHA officials and as required by law. The record must include the following: employee's name; social security number; hepatitis B vaccination status, including dates of vaccination; results of any postexposure examinations, medical testing, and follow-up procedures; and a written evaluation of any exposure incident along with a copy of the exposure incident report. The employer is required to maintain records for the duration of employment plus 30 years.
2. **Sharps injury log.** Employers with more than 10 employees at risk for occupational exposure are required to maintain a log of injuries from contaminated sharps. The log must be maintained in a way that protects the confidentiality of injured employees (e.g., removal of personal identification). The purpose of the log is to help employers and employees keep track of all needlestick injuries. This tracking helps in identifying problem areas that need attention and ineffective devices that need to be replaced. The sharps injury log must contain the following information:
   • Type and brand of device involved in the injury
   • Location of the incident (i.e., work area)
   • Explanation of how the incident occurred

Control Measures

Specific health and safety control measures are required by OSHA to eliminate or minimize the risk of occupational exposure in the medical office. These measures are divided into six categories: engineering controls, work practice controls, personal protective equipment, housekeeping, hepatitis B vaccination, and universal precautions.

Engineering Controls

The medical office must use engineering controls to eliminate or minimize the risk of occupational exposure. *Engineering controls* include all control measures that isolate or remove health hazards from the workplace. Engineering controls must be examined and maintained or replaced as required to ensure their effectiveness. Examples of engineering controls include the following:
• Readily accessible handwashing facilities
• Safer medical devices
• Biohazard sharps containers and biohazard bags
• Autoclaves

Safer Medical Devices

Safer medical devices are one example of an engineering control. A *safer medical device* is a device that, based on reasonable judgment, would make an exposure incident involving a contaminated sharp less likely. *Reasonable judgment* refers to the judgment of the health care worker who would be using the device.

Safer medical devices include sharps with engineered sharps injury protection and needleless systems. A *sharp with engineered sharps injury protection (SESIP)* is a non-needle sharp or a needle device with a built-in safety feature used for procedures that involve the risk of sharps injury. Examples of SESIPs include safety-engineered syringes and phlebotomy devices (Figure 17-6).

A *needleless system* is a device that does not use a needle for (1) the administration of medication or other fluids, (2) the collection or withdrawal of body fluids after initial access to a vein or artery is established, or (3) any other procedure involving the potential for occupational exposure to bloodborne pathogens as a result of percutaneous injuries from contaminated sharps. An example of a needleless system is a jet injection syringe, which uses compressed air to administer an injection rather than a needle.

Employers are required to evaluate and implement commercially available safer medical devices and other engineering controls that eliminate occupational exposure to the lowest extent feasible. Input from employees involved in direct patient care must be taken into consideration in making this determination. This helps to ensure that the individuals who are using the devices have the opportunity for input. As part of the annual review of the exposure control plan, the following information must be documented: (1) safer medical devices that reflect changes in technology are being evaluated and implemented in the workplace, and (2) input was obtained from employees in selecting safer medical devices.

Work Practice Controls

Work practice controls reduce the likelihood of exposure by altering the manner in which the technique is performed. It is important that the medical assistant consistently adhere to these safety rules, which include the following:

1. Perform all procedures involving blood or other potentially infectious materials in a manner that minimizes splashing, spraying, spattering, and generation of droplets of these substances.
2. Observe warning labels on biohazard containers and appliances. Bags or containers that bear a biohazard

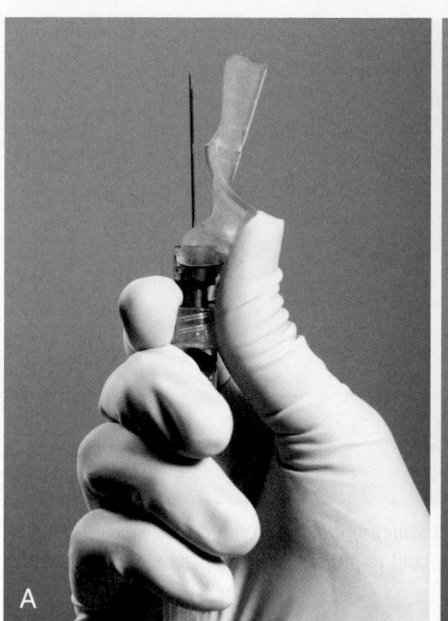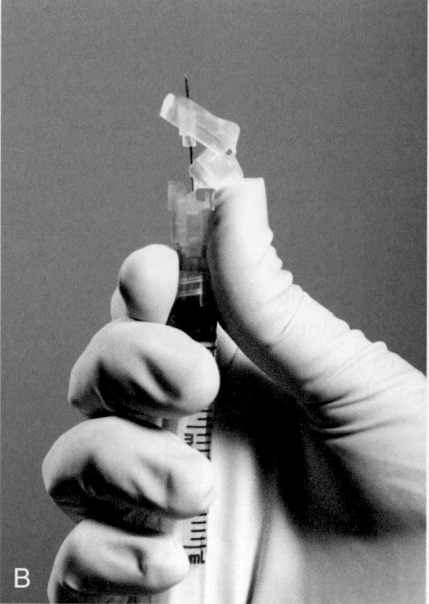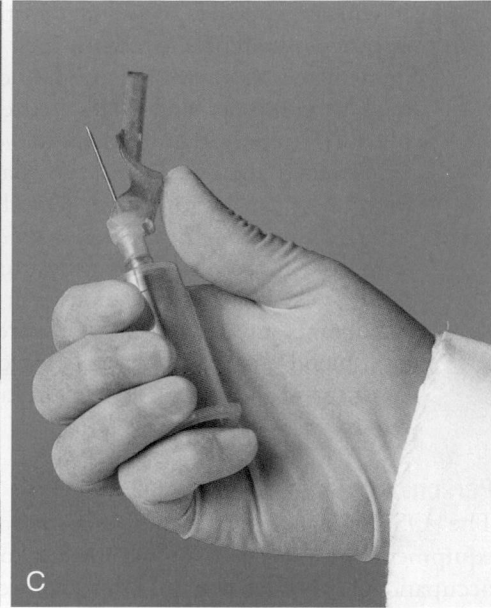

Figure 17-6 **A** and **B**, Safety-engineered syringes. **C**, Safety-engineered phlebotomy device.

warning label or are color-coded red indicate that they hold blood or other potentially infectious materials. Refrigerators, freezers, and other appliances that contain hazardous materials also must bear a biohazard warning label.

3. Bandage cuts and other lesions on the hands before gloving.
4. Sanitize the hands after removing gloves, regardless of whether or not the gloves are visibly contaminated.
5. If your hands or other skin surfaces come in contact with blood or other potentially infectious materials, thoroughly wash the area as soon as possible with soap and water.
6. If your mucous membranes (e.g., eyes, mouth, nose) come in contact with blood or other potentially infectious materials, flush them with water as soon as possible.
7. Do not break or shear contaminated needles.
8. Do not remove, recap, or bend a contaminated needle except in unusual circumstances when no other alternative is possible, or when this is required by a specific medical procedure. Such actions must be performed by a method other than the traditional two-handed procedure. Needle removal can be accomplished with a one-handed technique using a sharps container with a well-designed unwinder. Recapping must be performed through the use of a one-handed technique; using a two-handed technique is strictly prohibited. The one-handed recapping technique involves holding the syringe in the dominant hand and picking up the needle with the cap, using a scooping motion. The cap is secured

onto the needle by pushing it against a hard surface. (*Note:* Sterile needles may be recapped, such as after the withdrawal of medication from a vial or ampule.)

9. Immediately after use, place contaminated sharps in a puncture-resistant, leakproof container that is appropriately labeled or color-coded. *Contaminated sharps* are contaminated objects that can penetrate the skin, including (but not limited to) needles, lancets, scalpels, broken glass, and capillary tubes.
10. Do not eat, drink, smoke, apply cosmetics or lip balm, or handle contact lenses in areas where you may be exposed to blood or other potentially infectious materials.
11. Do not store food or drink in refrigerators, freezers, or cabinets or on shelves or countertops where blood or other potentially infectious materials are present.
12. Place blood specimens or other potentially infectious materials in containers that prevent leakage during collection, handling, processing, storage, transport, or shipping. Ensure that the containers are closed before they are stored, transported, or shipped, and are labeled or color-coded for easy identification.
13. Before any equipment that might be contaminated is serviced or shipped for repair or cleaning, such as a centrifuge, it must be inspected for blood or other potentially infectious materials. If such material is present, the equipment must be decontaminated. If it cannot be decontaminated, it must be appropriately labeled to indicate clearly the contamination site, to enable those coming into contact with the equipment to take appropriate precautions.

14. If you are exposed to blood or other potentially infectious materials, perform first aid measures immediately (e.g., wash a needlestick injury thoroughly with soap and water). After taking these measures, report the incident to your physician-employer as soon as possible so that postexposure procedures can be instituted. (See the box entitled *OSHA Postexposure Evaluation and Follow-Up Procedures.*) The most obvious exposure incident is a needlestick, but any eye, mouth, or other mucous membrane, nonintact skin, or parenteral contact with blood or other potentially infectious materials constitutes an exposure incident and should be reported.

Personal Protective Equipment

The OSHA standard specifies that personal protective equipment must be used in the medical office whenever occupational exposure remains after engineering and work practice controls are instituted. *Personal protective equipment* is clothing or equipment that protects an individual from contact with blood or other potentially infectious materials; examples include gloves, chin-length face shields, masks, protective eyewear, laboratory coats, and gowns. The type of protective equipment appropriate for a given task depends on the degree of exposure that is anticipated, as outlined here:

1. Wear gloves when it is reasonably anticipated that your hands will have contact with blood and other potentially infectious materials, mucous membranes, or nonintact skin; when performing vascular access procedures; and when handling or touching contaminated surfaces or items. Gloves cannot prevent a needlestick or other sharps injury, but they can prevent a pathogen from entering the body through a break in the skin, such as a cut, abrasion, burn, or rash.
2. Wear chin-length face shields or masks in combination with eye-protection devices whenever splashes, spray, spatter, or droplets of blood or other potentially infectious materials may be generated, posing a hazard through contact with the eyes, nose, or mouth (e.g., removing a stopper from a tube of blood, transferring serum from whole blood) (Figure 17-7).
3. Wear appropriate protective clothing, such as gowns, aprons, and laboratory coats, when gross contamination can reasonably be anticipated during performance of a task or procedure (e.g., laboratory testing procedure). The type of protective clothing needed depends on the task and degree of exposure anticipated.

Personal Protective Equipment Guidelines
Certain guidelines must be followed when using protective equipment:
1. Protective equipment must not allow blood or other potentially infectious materials to pass through or

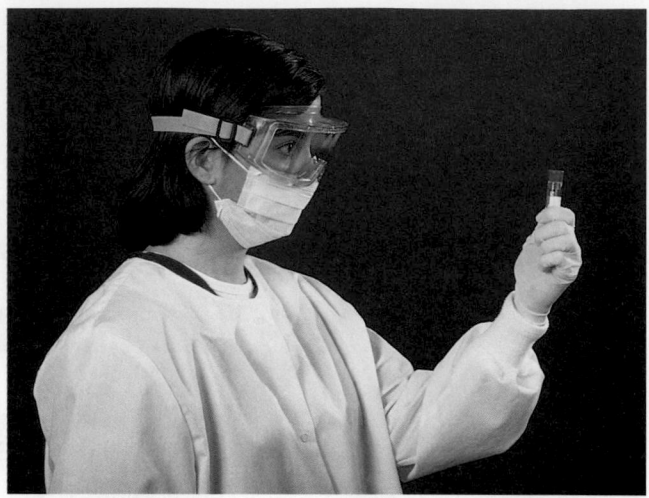

Figure 17-7 Jennifer wears a combination mask and eye-protection device and a laboratory coat to protect against splashes, spray, spatter, and droplets of blood.

reach the skin, underlying garments (e.g., scrubs, street clothes, undergarments), eyes, mouth, or other mucous membranes under normal conditions of use and for the duration of time the protective equipment is used.
2. The employer must provide appropriate personal protective equipment at no cost to you. The employer is responsible for ensuring that the equipment is available in appropriate sizes, is readily accessible, and is used correctly. In addition, the employer must ensure that the equipment is cleaned, laundered, repaired, replaced, or disposed of as necessary to ensure its effectiveness.
3. Alternatives must be provided for employees who are allergic to latex gloves. Examples of alternatives include non-latex gloves and powderless gloves.
4. If gloves become contaminated, torn, or punctured, replace them as soon as practical.
5. All eye-protection devices must have solid side shields; chin-length face shields, goggles, and glasses with solid side shields are acceptable (Figure 17-8); standard prescription eyeglasses are unacceptable as eye protection.
6. If a garment is penetrated by blood or other potentially infectious materials, it must be removed as soon as possible and placed in an appropriately designated container for washing.
7. All personal protective equipment must be removed before leaving the medical office.
8. When protective equipment is removed, it must be placed in an appropriately designated area or container for storage, washing, decontamination, or disposal.
9. Utility gloves may be decontaminated and reused unless they are cracked, peeling, torn, punctured, or no longer provide barrier protection.

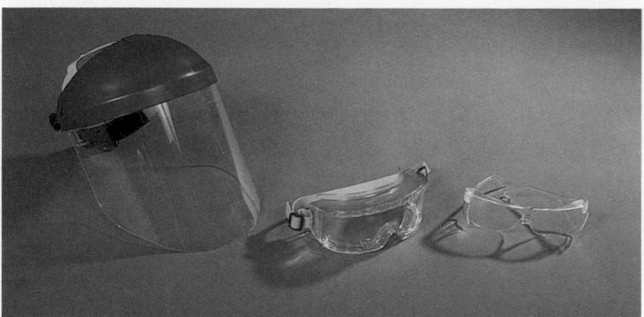

Figure 17-8 Examples of eye-protection devices. *Left,* Face shield; *center,* goggles; *right,* glasses with solid side shields.

10. If you believe that using protective equipment would prevent proper delivery of health care or would pose an increased hazard to your safety or that of a coworker, in extenuating circumstances you may temporarily and briefly decline its use. After such an incident, the circumstances must be investigated to determine whether the situation could be prevented in the future.

Housekeeping

The OSHA standard requires that specific housekeeping procedures be followed to ensure that the work site is maintained in a clean and sanitary condition. The medical office must develop and implement a written schedule for cleaning and decontaminating each area where exposure occurs. The cleaning and decontamination method must be specified for each task and should be based on the type of surface to be cleaned, the type of soil present, and the tasks or procedures being performed in that area. Housekeeping procedures include the following:

1. Clean and decontaminate equipment and work surfaces after completing procedures that involve blood or other potentially infectious materials. Cleaning is accomplished using a detergent soap, and decontamination is performed using an appropriate disinfectant (Figure 17-9).
2. Clean and decontaminate all equipment and work surfaces as soon as possible after exposure to blood or other potentially infectious materials. For decontamination of blood spills, OSHA recommends the use of a 10% solution of sodium hypochlorite (household bleach) in water (1 part bleach to 10 parts water).
3. Inspect and decontaminate all reusable receptacles, such as bins, pails, and cans, on a regular basis. If contamination is visible, the item must be cleaned and decontaminated as soon as possible.
4. Do not pick up broken, contaminated glassware with the hands, even if gloves are worn. Use mechanical means, such as a brush and dustpan, tongs, and forceps (Figure 17-10).
5. Protective coverings, such as plastic wrap and aluminum foil, may be used to cover work surfaces or

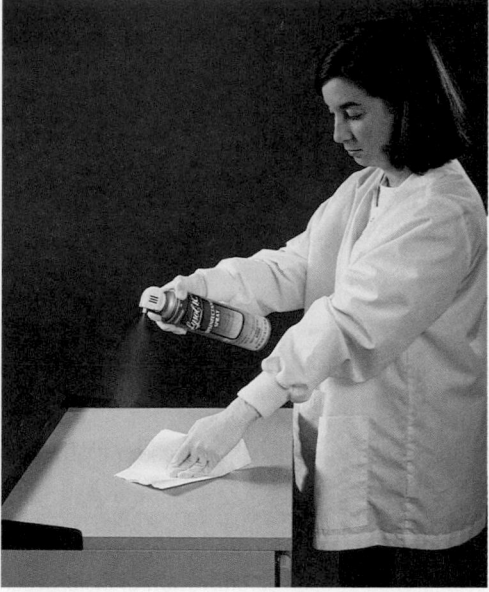

Figure 17-9 Clean and decontaminate work surfaces with an appropriate disinfectant after completing procedures involving blood and other potentially infectious materials.

equipment, but they must be removed or replaced if contamination occurs.
6. Handle contaminated laundry as little as possible and with appropriate personal protective equipment. Place all contaminated laundry in leakproof bags that are properly labeled or color-coded. Contaminated laundry must not be sorted or rinsed at the medical office.
7. If the outside of a biohazard container becomes contaminated, it must be placed in a second suitable container.
8. Biohazard sharps containers (Figure 17-11) must be closable, puncture-resistant, and leakproof. They must bear a biohazard warning label and must be color-coded red to ensure identification of the contents as hazardous. To ensure effectiveness, the following guidelines must be observed:
   • Locate the sharps container as close as possible to the area of use to avoid the hazard of transporting a contaminated needle through the workplace.
   • Maintain sharps containers in an upright position to keep liquid and sharps inside.
   • Do not reach into the sharps container with your hand.
   • Replace sharps containers on a regular basis, and do not allow them to overfill. (It is recommended that sharps containers be replaced when they are three-quarters full.)

Hepatitis B Vaccination

The OSHA standard requires employers to offer the hepatitis B vaccination series free of charge to all medical office

What Would You Do? What Would You *Not* Do?

Case Study 2

Tracy Smith is pregnant and is at the medical office to have her blood drawn for a prenatal profile. Tracy says she does not understand why gloves have to be worn when her blood is drawn. She says that it makes her feel like a leper, and she is absolutely sure that she doesn't have any diseases. Tracy says she has been reading information about the hepatitis B vaccine because she knows her baby will be given this vaccine soon after birth. She wants to know why it is recommended that an infant be immunized for hepatitis B. Tracy says that infants are not at risk for contracting hepatitis B because the way it is transmitted is mostly through sexual contact and illegal drug use. ■

Highlight on OSHA Bloodborne Pathogens Standard

General information

The exposure control plan must be made available to OSHA on request.

OSHA inspectors are responsible for determining whether the medical office meets the Bloodborne Pathogens Standard. This is accomplished through careful review of the exposure control plan, interviews with the medical office employer and employees, and observation of work activities.

Feces, nasal secretions, saliva, sputum, sweat, tears, urine, and vomitus are not considered by OSHA to be potentially infectious materials unless they contain blood.

Control measures

Employees must be trained in proper use of the following: engineering controls (including safer medical devices), work practice controls, and personal protective equipment.

General work clothes, such as scrubs, uniforms, pants, shirts, and blouses, are not intended to function as protection against a hazard and are not considered personal protective equipment.

Employees are not permitted to launder contaminated clothing at home; it is the employer's responsibility to have contaminated clothing laundered.

If an employee is allergic to standard latex gloves, the employer must provide a suitable non-latex alternative.

Needlestick injuries

The CDC estimates that every year, 600,000 to 800,000 health care workers in the United States experience needlestick and other sharps injuries, and 1000 of these individuals contract serious infections as a result of these injuries. The CDC estimates that 62% to 88% of sharps injuries can be prevented by the use of safer medical devices.

A wide variety of commercially available safer medical devices has been developed to reduce the risk of needlestick and other sharps injuries.

Safer medical devices that eliminate exposure to the lowest extent feasible must be evaluated and implemented in the health care setting. Lack of injuries on the sharps injury log does *not* exempt the employer from this provision. ■

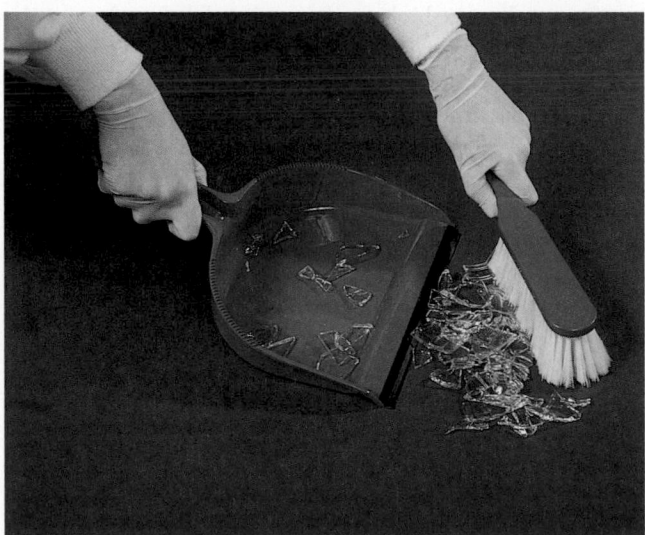

Figure 17-10 Use mechanical means to pick up broken contaminated glass.

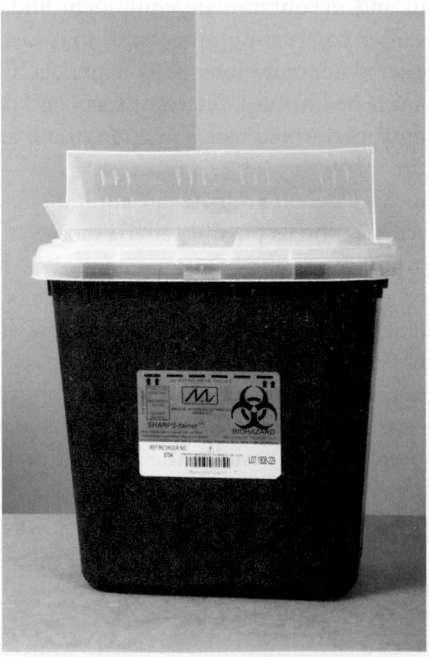

Figure 17-11 Biohazard sharps container.

HEPATITIS B VACCINE REFUSAL

I understand that due to my occupational exposure to blood or other potentially infectious materials, I may be at risk of acquiring hepatitis B virus (HBV) infection. I have been given the opportunity to be vaccinated with hepatitis B vaccine at no charge to myself. However, I decline hepatitis B vaccination at this time. I understand that by declining this vaccine I continue to be at risk of acquiring hepatitis B, a serious disease. If in the future I continue to have occupational exposure to blood or to other potentially infectious materials and I want to be vaccinated with hepatitis B vaccine, I can receive the vaccination series at no charge to me.

_____
Employee Name (printed)

_____   _____
Employee Signature   Date

_____   _____
Witness Signature   Date

Figure 17-12 Hepatitis B declination form. This form must be signed by an employee with occupational exposure who declines hepatitis B vaccination.

personnel who have occupational exposure. The vaccination must be offered within 10 working days of initial assignment to a position with occupational exposure, unless the following factors exist: (1) the individual has previously received the hepatitis B vaccination series, (2) antibody testing has revealed that the individual is immune to hepatitis B, or (3) the vaccine is contraindicated for medical reasons.

Medical office personnel who decline vaccination must sign a hepatitis B waiver form documenting refusal. This form must be filed in the employee's OSHA record (Figure 17-12). Employees who decline vaccination may request the vaccination later; the employer must then provide it, according to the aforementioned criteria.

Universal Precautions

Before the release of the OSHA standard, the CDC issued recommendations for health care workers known as the *Universal Precautions.* According to the concept of Universal Precautions, all human blood and certain human body fluids are treated as though they are known to be infectious for HIV, HBV, HCV, and other bloodborne pathogens. The OSHA standard states that the Universal Precautions must be observed; these precautions form the heart of the OSHA standard itself.

REGULATED MEDICAL WASTE

Medical waste is generated in the medical office through the diagnosis, treatment, and immunization of patients. Some of this waste poses a threat to health and safety and is known as **regulated medical waste (RMW)**. The OSHA Bloodborne Pathogens Standard defines RMW as follows:

- Any liquid or semiliquid blood or OPIM
- Items contaminated with blood or OPIM that would release these substances in a liquid or semiliquid state if compressed
- Items that are caked with dried blood or OPIM and are capable of releasing these materials during handling
- Contaminated sharps
- Pathologic and microbiologic wastes that contain blood or OPIM

Regulated medical waste must be discarded properly so as not to become a source of transfer of disease. According to the OSHA definition, a dressing saturated with blood is considered RMW and must be discarded in a biohazard bag. A bandage with a spot of blood on it is not considered RMW and can be discarded in a regular waste container. Box 17-2 gives the guidelines for discarding medical waste in the medical office.

Handling Regulated Medical Waste

Regulated medical waste must be handled carefully to prevent an exposure incident. The OSHA Bloodborne Pathogens Standard outlines specific actions to take when handling regulated medical waste, as follows:

1. Separate regulated waste from the general refuse at its point of origin. Disposable items containing regulated medical waste should be placed directly into biohazard containers and should not be mixed with the regular trash.
2. Ensure that biohazard containers are closable, leakproof, and suitably constructed to contain the contents during handling, storage, and transport. These containers include biohazard bags and sharps containers.

BOX 17-2 Guidelines for Discarding Medical Waste in the Medical Office

Regular Waste Container

The following items that have been used for health care *are not* considered regulated medical waste and can be discarded in a covered waste container lined with a regular trash bag.

- Disposable drapes
- Disposable patient gowns
- Examining table paper
- Disposable clean or sterile gloves
- Gauze tinged with blood or other body fluids
- Disposable probe covers for thermometers
- Tongue depressors
- Tissues with respiratory secretions
- Disposable ear speculums
- Empty urine containers
- Urine testing strips
- Disposable diapers
- Feminine hygiene products

Biohazard Sharps Container

The following items are sharps. They *are* considered regulated medical waste and must be discarded in a biohazard sharps container.

- Hypodermic syringes and needles
- Venipuncture needles
- Lancets
- Razor blades
- Scalpel blades
- Suture needles
- Blood tubes
- Capillary pipets
- Microscope slides and coverslips

- Broken glassware

Biohazard Bag Waste Container

The following items *are* considered regulated medical waste. They are not sharps and can be discarded in a covered waste container lined with a biohazard bag.

- Any item saturated or dripping with blood or OPIM (e.g., dressings, gauze, cotton balls, paper towels, tissues that are saturated or dripping with blood)
- Any item caked with dried blood or OPIM, such as dressings and sutures
- Disposable clean or sterile gloves contaminated with blood or OPIM
- Disposable vaginal speculums and collection devices (e.g., swabs, spatulas, brushes)
- Tissue or fluid removed during minor office surgery
- Microbiologic waste, such as specimen cultures and collection devices
- Discarded live and attenuated vaccines

Sanitary Sewer

Disposal of small quantities of blood and other body fluids to the sanitary sewer is considered a safe method of disposing of these waste materials. The following fluids can be carefully poured down a utility sink, drain, or toilet. (*NOTE:* State regulations may dictate the maximum volume allowable for discharge of blood or body fluids into the sanitary sewer.)

- Blood
- Body excretions such as urine
- Body secretions such as sputum

From Bonewit-West K: *Clinical procedures for medical assistants*, ed 8, St Louis, 2011, Saunders.

Highlight on Hepatitis B Vaccine

The hepatitis B vaccine became available in 1982 and is 95% effective in providing immunity. The hepatitis B vaccine is administered intramuscularly in a series of three doses. The hepatitis B vaccine is well tolerated by most patients. The most common side effect is soreness at the injection site, including induration, erythema, and swelling. Occasionally, a low-grade fever, headache, and dizziness occur.

Approximately 5% of the population does not form antibodies to the hepatitis B vaccine. Because of this, the CDC recommends that an antibody titer test be performed on all health care workers between 1 and 2 months after the last dose of the hepatitis B vaccine. The titer test is performed to determine if the health care worker has developed protective antibodies to hepatitis B and has immunity to HBV infection. Health care workers who do not respond to the primary vaccination series, as indicated by a negative titer test, must be revaccinated with a second three-dose vaccination series and then have a repeat titer test. If the titer test is still negative, this means that the health care worker probably lacks immunity to HBV infection.

Current data show that vaccine-induced antibodies may decline over time, but the immune system memory that programs the body to produce these antibodies remains intact indefinitely. Because of this, an individual with declining antibodies is still protected against hepatitis B. At present, the CDC does not recommend a booster dose once an individual has received the initial (three-dose) vaccine series.

The hepatitis B vaccine is recommended for all infants and children, and for adolescents who are 18 years old or younger. It also is recommended for adults older than 18 years who are at increased risk for developing hepatitis B. This population includes employees with occupational exposure (e.g., health care workers), hemodialysis patients, hemophiliacs, individuals with multiple sex partners, homosexually active men, injection drug users, individuals with HIV infection, household and sexual contacts of individuals infected with HBV, individuals with chronic liver or kidney disease, residents and staff in institutions for the developmentally disabled, and people who travel to countries where hepatitis B is common.

The number of individuals contracting hepatitis B has decreased sharply since the development of the hepatitis B vaccine. As more people become immune to hepatitis B through the immunization of infants, the goal of eliminating hepatitis B in the United States may be realized. ■

3. To prevent spillage or protrusion of the contents, close the lid of a sharps container before removing it from an examining room. Never open, empty, or clean a contaminated sharps container. If there is a chance of leakage from the sharps container, the medical assistant should place it in a second container that is closable, leakproof, and appropriately labeled or color-coded.

4. Securely close biohazard bags before removing them from an examining room. To provide additional protection, some medical offices double-bag by placing the primary bag inside a second biohazard bag.

5. Transport full biohazard containers to a secured area away from the general public, using personal protective equipment (e.g., gloves).

Disposal of Regulated Medical Waste

Each state is responsible for developing policies for disposal of regulated medical waste. To avoid noncompliance, it is important for the medical assistant to know and understand the specific regulated waste policies and guidelines set forth in his or her state. Regulated waste policies and guidelines for each state can be found at the following website: www.envcap.org/statetools/rmw/rmwlocator.html.

Most medical offices use a commercial medical waste service to dispose of regulated medical waste. This service is responsible for picking up and transporting the medical waste to a treatment facility for incineration to destroy pathogens and render them harmless. The waste can then be safely disposed of in a sanitary landfill. Regulated waste treatment facilities must be licensed and hold permits issued by the Environmental Protection Agency (EPA), allowing them to dispose of regulated medical waste.

A series of steps must be followed for preparing and storing regulated medical waste for pickup by the service. Although these steps may vary slightly from state to state, general measures required by most states include the following:

1. Place biohazard bags and sharps containers into a receptacle provided by the medical waste service. The receptacle is usually a cardboard box (Figure 17-13). The box should be securely sealed with packing tape, and a biohazard warning label must appear on two opposite sides of the box.

2. Store the biohazard boxes in a locked room inside the facility or in a locked collection container outside for pickup by the medical waste service. This step is aimed at preventing unauthorized access to items such as needles and syringes. The regulated waste storage area should be labeled with one of the following:
   • "Authorized Personnel Only" sign
   • International biohazard symbol

3. Many states require that a tracking record be completed when the waste is picked up by the medical waste service. This form includes such information as the type and quantity of waste (weighed in pounds) and where it is being sent. The form must be signed

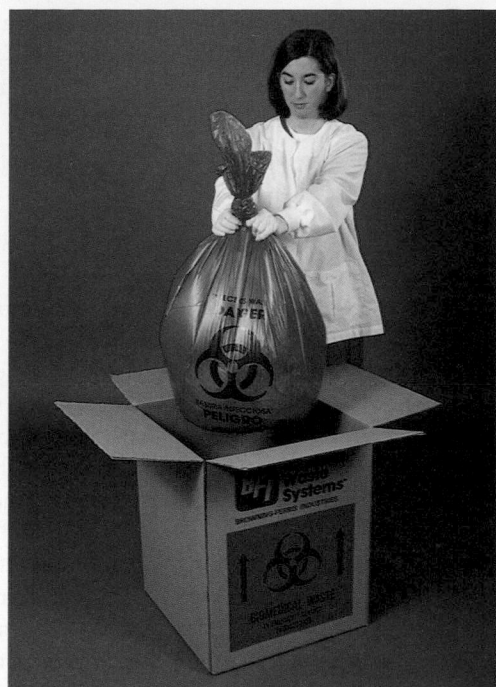

Figure 17-13 Jennifer places a biohazard bag inside a cardboard box in preparation for pickup by the medical waste service.

by a representative of the medical waste service and the medical office. After the waste has been destroyed at the regulated waste treatment facility, a record documenting its disposal is mailed to the medical office.

What Would You Do? What Would You *Not* Do?

Case Study 3

Giles Lee is 45 years old and is at the medical office. Twenty-five years ago, he was in a serious car accident and had to have a blood transfusion. He says that he donated blood for the first time 2 months ago. Last week he received a letter saying that his blood tested positive for hepatitis C and that he should see his physician. Giles says that he must have gotten hepatitis C from the blood transfusion he received when he was 20. He does not understand how that could have happened because the blood supply is tested for these types of diseases. Giles wants to know why he has not had any symptoms. He also wants to know if he can give hepatitis C to his wife and teenage children. ■

BLOODBORNE DISEASES

The biggest threats to health care workers from occupational exposure are HBV, HCV, and HIV. Hepatitis is much easier to transmit than HIV. After a needlestick exposure to blood infected with HBV, health care workers who are not immune to hepatitis B have a 6% to 30% chance of developing the disease. The risk of infection after a needlestick exposure to blood infected with HCV is approximately 2%.

After a needlestick exposure to HIV-infected blood, a health care worker has a 0.3% chance of developing HIV; he or she has a 0.1% chance of developing HIV after a mucous membrane exposure of the eyes, nose, or mouth.

Hepatitis B

Hepatitis B is an infection of the liver caused by HBV. The most common means of transmitting hepatitis B in the health care setting are blood and blood components, such as serum and plasma.

Health care workers are most likely to contract hepatitis B through needlesticks and cuts with contaminated sharps. The virus also is spread in the health care setting, but less effectively, through blood splashes to the eyes, mouth, and nonintact skin and through body fluids such as semen and vaginal secretions.

The number of health care workers who contract hepatitis B in the workplace has declined dramatically since the development of the OSHA standard and the hepatitis B vaccine. Statistics show that in 1983 there were more than 10,000 health care workers who contracted hepatitis B in the workplace, but by 2001, that number had decreased to fewer than 400 health care workers. Preventive treatment is available for individuals exposed to hepatitis B who have not been vaccinated.

Postexposure Prophylaxis

Postexposure prophylaxis (PEP) refers to treatment administered to an individual after exposure to an infectious disease, to prevent the disease. PEP for unvaccinated individuals exposed to hepatitis B involves the administration of a passive and an active immunizing agent. It is important to administer both of these agents as soon as possible after an exposure incident—preferably within 24 hours, but no later than 7 days.

The passive immunizing agent provides temporary immunity to hepatitis B, giving the active agent a chance to take effect. The passive agent is hepatitis B immune globulin (HBIG), which contains antibodies that provide immunity to hepatitis B for 1 to 3 months.

The active immunizing agent in the hepatitis B vaccine (Figure 17-14) is produced from genetically altered yeast cells; brand names are Recombivax HB and Engerix-B. The hepatitis B vaccine is administered intramuscularly in a series of three doses. The second dose is given 1 month after the first dose, and the third dose is administered 6 months after the first dose (i.e., 0, 1 month, and 6 months). Mild side effects, such as soreness at the injection site, may occur, but serious reactions to the vaccine are extremely rare.

As previously discussed, the OSHA standard recommends that all health care workers receive the hepatitis B vaccine (an active immunizing agent) as a preventive measure against hepatitis B. After an exposure incident, a medical assistant who has previously been vaccinated probably would not require further treatment.

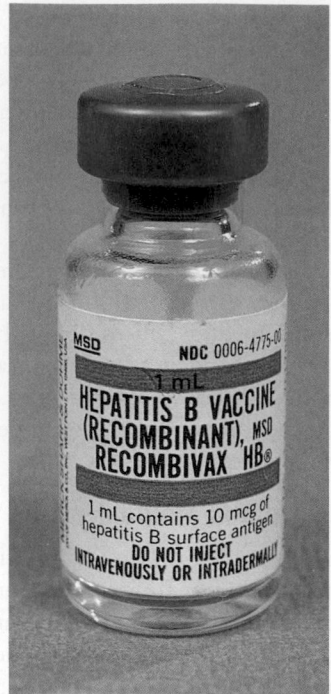

Figure 17-14 Hepatitis B vaccine.

Hepatitis C

Hepatitis C is an infection of the liver caused by HCV. Currently, no vaccine is available for the prevention of hepatitis C. In the medical office, the most likely means of contracting hepatitis C is through parenteral exposure to contaminated blood such as through needlesticks and other sharps injuries. The chance of contracting hepatitis C in the health care setting is much lower than that of contracting hepatitis B.

Most individuals with acute hepatitis C have no symptoms; if symptoms do occur, they are mild and flulike. Approximately 55% to 85% of individuals with acute hepatitis C develop chronic hepatitis C. After 10 to 30 years, about 20% of these individuals develop serious liver disease, including cirrhosis of the liver and cancer of the liver. Ultimately, 1% to 5% of individuals with chronic hepatitis C die from liver failure (see the *Highlight on Viral Hepatitis*). Antiviral drugs have been developed to treat chronic hepatitis C and are effective in 40% of cases.

Acquired Immune Deficiency Syndrome

Acquired immune deficiency syndrome (AIDS) is a chronic disorder of the immune system that eventually destroys the body's ability to fight off infection. AIDS is caused by a retrovirus known as *human immunodeficiency virus (HIV)*. The following description helps to clarify the difference between these two terms. The virus and the infection itself are known as *HIV*, whereas the term *AIDS* is used to refer to the last stage of HIV infection. Simply put, the terms *HIV infection* and *AIDS* refer to different stages of the same disease.

When HIV gains entrance into the body, it begins to attack and destroy certain white blood cells known as *CD4+*

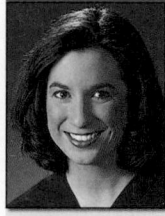

Memories *from* Externship

Jennifer Hawk: As a student, I was extremely nervous to go out on externship. I was so scared to think that I was actually going to be in a medical office setting and would have to put everything I had learned into practice. Would I remember everything? Would I do something wrong and hurt the patient? It was such an overwhelming feeling! But to my relief, I had a very good experience. The office staff was so friendly and helpful to me, and I surprised myself at how easily everything I had learned stayed with me. It was so exciting to see that I was actually functioning as a team member in the health care field. I could not have had better training. ■

T cells, which are involved in protecting the body against viral, fungal, and protozoal infections. As more and more CD4+ T cells are destroyed, the immune system is gradually weakened. After a period of time, which may last 10 years or longer, the body's immune system becomes so ravaged by the attack that it succumbs to the diseases associated with AIDS.

AIDS is characterized by the presence of severe and life-threatening opportunistic infections and unusual cancers that rarely affect individuals with healthy immune systems. An **opportunistic infection** is an infection that results from a defective immune system that cannot defend itself from pathogens normally found in the environment. Opportunistic infections are extremely difficult to treat because the infection tends to recur quickly after a course of therapy is completed.

Highlight on Viral Hepatitis

In 2007, there were an estimated 85,000 new cases of viral hepatitis in the United States. Approximately 51% of these infections were caused by the hepatitis B virus, 29% were caused by the hepatitis A virus, and 20% were caused by the hepatitis C virus.

Symptoms common to all types of hepatitis include fatigue, nausea, loss of appetite, abdominal pain, and jaundice.

Hepatitis A, B, and C are designated by the CDC as nationally notifiable diseases. When the physician diagnoses a case of hepatitis A, B, or C, a reportable disease form must be completed and filed with the local public health department.

In recent years, antiviral drugs have been developed to treat chronic forms of hepatitis B and C; however, not all infected individuals are candidates for treatment. These drugs, which must be taken for a prolonged time, are effective in removing the virus from approximately 40% of chronically infected patients.

Hepatitis B
The virus that causes hepatitis B is found in the blood and in certain body fluids (e.g., semen, vaginal secretions) of HBV-infected individuals. The most common means of transmission of hepatitis B is through sexual contact with an infected individual, by sharing needles for injection drug use with an infected individual, and perinatally from an infected mother to her infant during birth. Other modes of transmission include contact with blood or open sores of an infected individual and sharing of items such as razors or toothbrushes with an infected individual. Hepatitis B is not spread by sneezing, coughing, hugging, kissing, casual contact, breast-feeding, food, water, or sharing eating utensils or drinking glasses.

The highest rate of new hepatitis B infection occurs in adults, particularly among males between 25 and 44 years of age. The greatest decline has occurred among children and adolescents as a result of routine hepatitis B immunization.

It is estimated that more than 1.25 million people in the United States are infected with chronic hepatitis B; this means that these individuals are carriers of hepatitis B and are capable of

transmitting the disease to others. Many of these individuals do not know that they are carriers.

Every year, approximately 3000 Americans die as a result of the long-term consequences of chronic hepatitis B, such as cirrhosis and liver cancer.

Whether or not an HBV-infected individual goes on to develop chronic hepatitis B depends primarily on age. After infection with acute viral hepatitis B occurs, chronic infection develops in 90% of infants infected by their mothers at birth, 30% of children infected between ages 1 and 5 years, and 6% of individuals infected after age 5 years.

Hepatitis B can survive outside the body in a dried state for at least 1 week and still can be capable of causing infection. Examples of surfaces that could harbor dried blood or body fluids infected with HBV include contaminated worktables, equipment, and instruments.

Hepatitis C
Chronic hepatitis C is the most common chronic viral infection in the United States. Approximately 4 million Americans have been diagnosed with chronic hepatitis C, and each year it causes an estimated 12,000 deaths resulting from cirrhosis and liver cancer.

The most common means of transmission of hepatitis C is by sharing needles for injection drug use with an infected individual. Hepatitis C is not spread by casual contact, such as sneezing, coughing, hugging, sharing food or water, or sharing eating utensils or drinking glasses. It is rarely transmitted through sexual contact.

Individuals infected with hepatitis C should not share with other members of the household personal items that may have blood on them (e.g., toothbrushes, nail-grooming equipment, razors).

Chronic hepatitis C is known as "an epidemic that occurred in the past." Numerous individuals became infected with hepatitis C more than 30 years ago and are now being diagnosed with it. This is because the symptoms of chronic hepatitis C often do not appear until 10 to 30 years after infection, and many times the first

Continued

Highlight on Viral Hepatitis—cont'd

symptoms come only with advanced liver disease. Chronic hepatitis C surpasses alcoholism as the leading cause of liver cirrhosis and liver transplantation in the United States.

Before 1992, a blood test to determine the presence of hepatitis C did not exist. Because of this, a significant number of people contracted hepatitis C from HCV-infected blood transfusions. The CDC encourages people who received blood transfusions before July 1992 to ask their physicians if they should be tested for hepatitis C.

Postexposure prophylaxis with immune globulin is not effective in preventing hepatitis C, and no vaccine exists yet to prevent hepatitis C. Vaccines for hepatitis C are difficult to develop because the virus mutates so frequently. The only way to control the disease is by preventing exposure to the hepatitis C virus. ∎

Highlight on AIDS

Prevalence

AIDS was first reported in the United States in 1981, but most likely it existed here and in other parts of the world for many years before that. Since 1981, more than 1 million cases of AIDS have been reported in the United States, and every year approximately 40,000 people in the United States are newly infected with HIV. Since 1981, there have been an estimated 550,000 deaths from AIDS in the United States.

Currently, almost 75% of those individuals newly diagnosed with HIV are adolescent and adult males, and the largest proportions of these are men who have sex with men, followed by individuals infected through high-risk heterosexual contact. Individuals between the ages of 25 and 44 account for the largest proportion of newly diagnosed HIV cases.

Transmission

HIV is spread primarily through sexual contact with an infected individual and by sharing drug injection needles with infected individuals. Scientific evidence shows that HIV is not spread through casual, everyday contact. There is no evidence that HIV is spread by sharing facilities or equipment, such as telephones, computers, food utensils, bedding, doorknobs, and bathrooms. Because HIV is not passed through the air, it is not spread through coughing and sneezing. HIV also is not spread through tears or sweat, or by shaking hands, hugging, or donating blood.

Most individuals infected with HIV show no symptoms and may not develop full-blown AIDS for 10 years or longer. After infection with HIV, the individual is infected for life.

Women can transmit HIV to their fetuses during pregnancy or birth. Approximately one quarter to one third of pregnant women infected with HIV who are not being treated with antiretroviral drugs pass the infection to their infants. HIV also can be spread to infants through the breast milk of mothers infected with the virus. Because of this, the CDC recommends that testing for HIV be included in the routine panel of prenatal screening tests for all pregnant women, and that separate written consent not be required. The CDC further recommends that the patient should be notified that HIV testing will be performed, unless the patient declines the test (known as *opt-out screening*). The CDC recommends that repeat HIV screening be performed in the third trimester in areas that have elevated rates of HIV infection among pregnant women.

Worldwide, more than 700,000 infants are infected with HIV each year. If antiretroviral drugs are taken during pregnancy and the infant is delivered by cesarean section, the chance of transmitting HIV to the infant is reduced significantly. In developing countries, such as sub-Saharan Africa, women seldom know their HIV status, and treatment is often unavailable.

HIV testing

The CDC recommends HIV screening for patients in all health care settings after the patient is notified that the testing will be performed, and separate written consent is not required. HIV screening should be performed unless the patient declines (known as *opt-out screening*). The CDC further recommends that individuals at high risk for HIV infection undergo HIV screening at least annually.

The enzyme immune assay (EIA) test and the enzyme-linked immunosorbent assay (ELISA) test are used as screening tests for the presence of HIV. Newer rapid HIV testing kits are also commercially available; brand names include Uni-Gold Recombigen HIV (Trinity Biotech, County Wicklow, Ireland), Clearview HIV (Inverness Medical, Princeton, New Jersey), and OraQuick Rapid HIV test (OraSure Technologies, Bethlehem, Pennsylvania). Because of the possibility of a false-positive result, a second screening test is always performed if a blood specimen tests positive. If the second test also is positive, a more specific test, such as the Western blot test, is performed to confirm the test results. An individual who tests positive for HIV is seropositive.

A negative HIV test is not conclusive for the absence of HIV infection. If an individual has recently been infected with HIV, the antibodies may not have had time to develop. It generally takes 2 to 12 weeks (but possibly as long as 6 months) for the HIV antibodies to appear in the blood.

CDC definition of AIDS

As scientists have learned more about the disease, the CDC's definition of AIDS has changed several times since the beginning

Highlight on AIDS—cont'd

of the AIDS epidemic. The current AIDS definition includes the presence of one or both of the following conditions:

1. HIV positive and a CD4$^+$ T-cell count below 200 cells/μL (normal CD4$^+$ T-cell count for a healthy individual ranges from 500 to 1500 cells/μL)
2. Presence of one or more AIDS-defining conditions

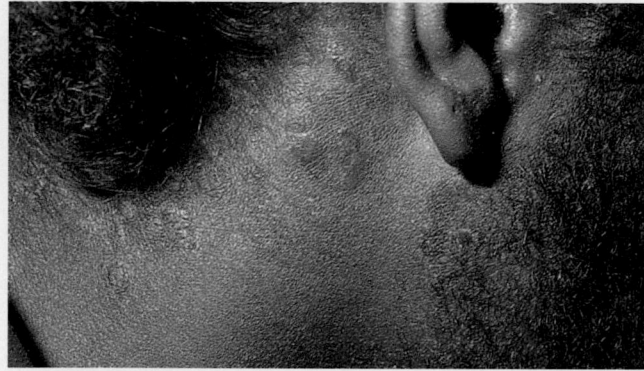

Kaposi sarcoma is an example of an AIDS-defining condition.

Treatment

There is no known cure for AIDS; there is no vaccine to prevent it. Powerful antiviral drugs have been developed that slow the reproduction of the virus and reduce the viral load in the body. In many patients, these drugs have dramatically delayed HIV from progressing to full-blown AIDS, thereby allowing them to live longer. These drugs can have serious side effects, and they do not prevent the spread of the disease to someone else. Numerous drugs also are available to treat the opportunistic infections and cancers that occur with AIDS. ■

MEDICAL PRACTICE and the LAW

There are three behaviors that are crucial in protecting yourself from a lawsuit:

1. Establish a rapport. If patients believe that you truly care about them and have their best interests at heart, they rarely sue, even if you make a mistake.
2. Follow all procedures according to your procedures manual. If you do everything right and the patient has an adverse outcome, you will not likely be found liable.
3. Document everything you do objectively. Lawsuits often come to court years after the incident, and nobody's memory is as good as written documentation. Document only the facts, not your opinion. Document the patient's reactions to treatments.

Ethics and law

Ethics is the highest standard of behavior and is loosely based on the Golden Rule. No law can force you to behave ethically, but most major professions, including the American Association of Medical Assistants (AAMA), have a written code of ethics. Ethics uses words such as *should* and *may*. If you are angry with someone, ethically, you should not yell at him or her. This is not against the law, but it is unethical.

Law is the lowest standard of behavior and is enforced by federal, state, and local law enforcement personnel. Laws use words such as *must* and *shall*. If you are angry with someone, legally, you must not hit him or her. This behavior is illegal, and you could be charged with assault and battery.

Regarding medical asepsis and infection control, you have a duty and a responsibility to protect yourself, your co-workers, and, most important, your patients. Follow specific guidelines established by OSHA and the CDC to prevent the transmission of pathogens. ■

What Would You Do? What Would You *Not* Do?   RESPONSES

Case Study 1
Page 249

What Did Jennifer Do?
❑ Told Petra that the hand sanitizers (alcohol-based hand rubs) are as good as, if not better than, soap and water for removing germs from the hands.
❑ Stressed to Petra that hand sanitizers are not designed to remove soil from the hands and that she should wash her hands with soap and water when they are visibly soiled.
❑ Explained that the Centers for Disease Control and Prevention now recommends that hand sanitizers be used in health care settings to help prevent the spread of disease.

What Did Jennifer Not Do?
❑ Did not tell Petra that she should switch from soap and water to hand sanitizers.

What Would You Do/What Would You Not Do?
Review Jennifer's response and place a checkmark next to the information you included in your response. List additional information you included in your response.

_____
_____
_____
_____
_____
_____

Case Study 2
Page 256

What Did Jennifer Do?
❑ Explained to Tracy that a federal agency known as the Occupational Safety and Health Administration (OSHA) requires that gloves be worn when drawing a patient's blood in the office. Told her that the office could be fined if they were not worn.
❑ Told Tracy that having her infant immunized for hepatitis B is an investment in her child's future. Explained that her child could come into contact with the virus anytime in his or her life. Stressed that if a young child becomes infected with hepatitis B, the child has a higher risk of developing chronic hepatitis, which can cause serious liver problems later in life.
❑ Gave Tracy a brochure on hepatitis B to take home.

What Did Jennifer Not Do?
❑ Did not discourage Tracy from having her baby immunized for hepatitis B.

What Would You Do/What Would You Not Do?
Review Jennifer's response and place a checkmark next to the information you included in your response. List additional information you included in your response.

_____
_____
_____
_____
_____
_____

Case Study 3
Page 259

What Did Jennifer Do?
❑ Explained to Giles that the blood supply was not tested for hepatitis C until 1992 because a test to detect the presence of hepatitis C was not developed until then.
❑ Told Giles that it is possible for someone to have hepatitis C and not exhibit any symptoms.
❑ Told Giles that he should ask the physician his question about giving hepatitis C to others.

What Did Jennifer Not Do?
❑ Did not automatically assume that Giles had hepatitis C because he had not yet been seen by the physician. It would be up to the physician to make a diagnosis of hepatitis C.
❑ Did not tell Giles about the serious complications of hepatitis C. If Giles is diagnosed with hepatitis C, it would be the physician's responsibility to relay this information.

What Would You Do/What Would You Not Do?
Review Jennifer's response and place a checkmark next to the information you included in your response. List additional information you included in your response.

_____
_____
_____
_____
_____
_____

TERMINOLOGY REVIEW

Medical Term	Word Parts	Definition
Aerobe	*aer/o:* air	A microorganism that needs oxygen to live and grow.
Anaerobe	*an-:* without *aer/o:* air	A microorganism that grows best in the absence of oxygen.
Antiseptic	*anti-:* against *septic:* infection	An agent that inhibits the growth of or kills microorganisms.
Asepsis	*a-:* without *sepsis:* infection	Free from infection or pathogens; the actions practiced to make and maintain an area or object free from infection or pathogens.
Cilia		Slender, hairlike projections that constantly beat toward the outside to remove microorganisms from the body.
Contaminate		To soil or to make impure. An aseptic object is contaminated when it touches something that is not clean.
Decontamination		The use of physical or chemical means to remove, inactivate, or destroy pathogens on a surface or item to the point where they are no longer capable of transmitting infectious particles; the surface or item is rendered safe for handling, use, or disposal.
Hand hygiene		The process of cleansing or sanitizing the hands.
Infection		The condition in which the body, or part of it, is invaded by a pathogen.
Medical asepsis	*a-:* without *sepsis:* infection	Practices that are employed to reduce the number and hinder the transmission of pathogens.
Microorganism	*micro-:* small *organism:* organism	A microscopic plant or animal.
Nonintact skin	*non-:* not	Skin that has a break in the surface. It includes, but is not limited to, abrasions, cuts, hangnails, paper cuts, and burns.
Nonpathogen	*non-:* not *path/o:* disease *-gen:* producing	A microorganism that does not normally produce disease.
Opportunistic infection		An infection that results from a defective immune system that cannot defend the body from pathogens normally found in the environment.
Optimum growth temperature		The temperature at which an organism grows best.
Parenteral	*para-:* apart from *enter/o:* intestine *-al:* pertaining to	Taken into the body through piercing of the skin barrier or mucous membranes, such as through needlesticks, human bites, cuts, and abrasions.
Pathogen	*path/o:* disease *-gen:* producing	A disease-producing microorganism.
Perinatal	*peri-:* surrounding *natal:* pertaining to birth	Relating to the period shortly before and after birth.
pH		The degree to which a solution is acidic or basic.
Postexposure prophylaxis (PEP)	*post-:* after *pro:* before *phylaxis:* prevention of disease	Treatment administered to an individual after exposure to an infectious disease to prevent the disease.
Regulated medical waste (RMW)		Medical waste that poses a threat to health and safety.
Reservoir host		The organism that becomes infected by a pathogen and serves as a source of transfer of the pathogen to others.
Resident flora		Harmless, nonpathogenic microorganisms that normally reside on the skin and usually do not cause disease. Also known as *normal flora.*
Susceptible		Easily affected; lacking resistance.
Transient flora		Microorganisms that reside on the superficial skin layers and are picked up in the course of daily activities. They are often pathogenic but can be removed easily from the skin by sanitizing the hands.

ON THE WEB

For information on federal regulations and recommendations for infection control:

Occupational Safety and Health Administration (OSHA): www.osha.gov

Centers for Disease Control and Prevention (CDC): www.cdc.gov

National Institute for Occupational Safety and Health (NIOSH): www.cdc.gov/niosh

CDC Recommendations for Hand Hygiene in the Healthcare Setting: www.cdc.gov/handhygiene

Food and Drug Administration (FDA): www.fda.gov

Environmental Protection Agency: www.epa.gov

Association for the Advancement of Medical Instrumentation (AAMI): www.aami.org

Division of Healthcare Quality Promotion (DHQP): www.cdc.gov/ncidod/dhqp

Epidemiology Program Office: www.cdc.gov/epo

Morbidity and Mortality Weekly Report: www.cdc.gov/mmwr

For information on hepatitis:

CDC National Center for Infectious Diseases: www.cdc.gov/hepatitis

Hepatitis Foundation International: www.hepfi.org

Hepatitis B Foundation: www.hepb.org

National Institute of Allergy and Infectious Diseases: www.niaid.nih.gov

HealthTalk: www.healthtalk.com

For information on AIDS:

CDC National Center for Infectious Diseases: www.cdc.gov/ncidod/diseases

AIDS Education Global Information System: www.aegis.com

AIDS Information: www.aidsinfo.nih.gov

The Body—AIDS and HIV Information Resource: www.thebody.com

About AIDS: aids.about.com

HIV Positive.Com: www.hivpositive.com

Mayo Clinic: www.mayoclinic.com

 Check out the Evolve site at http://evolve.elsevier.com/Bonewit/today/ to actively Prepare for your Certification, and to access additional interactive activities and exercises to help you study and prepare for success.

18

Sterilization and Disinfection

LEARNING OBJECTIVES

Hazard Communication Standard

1. Explain the purpose of the Hazard Communication Standard.
2. List and describe the information that must be included on the label of a hazardous chemical.
3. List and describe the information that must be included in a material safety data sheet (MSDS).

Sanitization

4. State the purpose of sanitization.
5. State the advantages of using an ultrasonic cleaner to clean instruments.
6. List and describe the guidelines that should be followed when sanitizing instruments.

Disinfection

7. State the uses of the three levels of disinfection: high, intermediate, and low.
8. Explain the differences among the following: critical item, semicritical item, and noncritical item.
9. List and describe the primary use of disinfectants in the medical office.

Sterilization

10. Explain how the autoclave functions to sterilize articles.
11. List the components of a sterilization monitoring program.
12. List and describe types of sterilization indicators.
13. Identify the advantages and disadvantages of each of the following types of wraps: sterilization paper, sterilization pouches, and muslin.
14. List the guidelines that should be followed when the autoclave is loaded.
15. Identify the sterilization times for each of the following categories: unwrapped articles, wrapped articles, liquids, and large wrapped packs.
16. Describe the method for storing wrapped articles.
17. Describe the daily, weekly, and monthly maintenance of the autoclave.

Other Sterilization Methods

18. State the primary use of each of the following types of sterilization methods: dry heat, ethylene oxide gas, chemicals, and radiation.

PROCEDURES

Read and interpret an MSDS.

Sanitize Instruments.

Wrap articles to be autoclaved.
Sterilize articles in the autoclave.
Maintain the autoclave.

KEY TERMS

antiseptic (an-tih-SEP-tik)
autoclave (AU-toh-klave)
contaminate (kon-TAM-in-ate)
critical item
decontamination
   (DEE-kon-tam-in-AY-shun)
detergent
disinfectant (dis-in-FEK-tant)
hazardous chemical
incubate (IN-kyoo-bate)
load
material safety data sheet (MSDS)
noncritical item
sanitization (san-ih-tih-ZAY-shun)
semicritical item
spore
sterilization (stare-ill-ih-ZAY-shun)
thermolabile (ther-moh-LAH-bul)

INTRODUCTION TO STERILIZATION AND DISINFECTION

The air and all objects around us contain microorganisms. The medical assistant is responsible for helping to reduce and eliminate microorganisms to prevent the spread of disease. This can be accomplished by practicing good techniques of medical and surgical asepsis (see Chapters 17 and 25).

Physical and chemical agents are used to destroy microorganisms in the medical office. The agent selected depends on the intended use of the article. Articles that penetrate sterile tissue or the vascular system, such as surgical instruments, must be sterilized. Articles that come in contact with the skin, such as stethoscopes, blood pressure cuffs, and percussion hammers, should be disinfected.

Sanitization, disinfection, and sterilization involve hazardous chemicals. It is essential for the medical assistant to know the precautions that are required when working with hazardous chemicals.

DEFINITIONS OF TERMS

Terms that aid in understanding this chapter are listed and defined here.

Sanitization Sanitization is a process that removes organic material and reduces the number of microorganisms to a safe level as determined by public health requirements. Sanitization removes all organic material, such as blood, body fluids, and tissue, from an article. For articles that are used in examinations, treatments, and office surgery to be properly sterilized or disinfected, they must first be sanitized.

Decontamination Decontamination refers to the use of physical or chemical means to remove or destroy pathogens on an item so that it is no longer capable of transmitting disease; this makes the item safe to handle.

Detergent A detergent is an agent that cleanses by emulsifying dirt and oil.

Disinfectant A disinfectant is an agent used to destroy pathogenic microorganisms; however, it does not kill the resistant bacterial spores. Disinfectants are generally applied to inanimate objects.

Spore A spore is a hard, thick-walled capsule that some bacteria form by losing moisture and condensing their contents to contain only the essential parts of the protoplasm of the cell. Spores represent a resting and protective stage of the bacterial cell and are more resistant to drying, sunlight, heat, and disinfectants than is the vegetative form of the bacterium. Favorable conditions cause the spore to germinate into a vegetative bacterium again that is capable of reproducing. Two examples of species of bacteria that form spores are *Clostridium botulinum*, which causes botulism, and *Clostridium tetani*, which causes tetanus.

Sterilization Sterilization is the process of destroying all forms of microbial life, including bacterial spores. An object that is *sterile* is free of all living microorganisms and spores. There can be no relative degrees of sterility—an object is either sterile or not sterile. The device most commonly used to sterilize articles in the medical office is the autoclave.

HAZARD COMMUNICATION STANDARD

The Hazard Communication Standard (HCS) is a requirement of the Occupational Safety and Health Administration (OSHA). The purpose of the HCS is to ensure that employees are informed of the hazards associated with chemicals in their workplaces. Chemicals can be in the form of a liquid, a solid, or a gas. A **hazardous chemical** is any chemical that presents a threat to the health and safety of an individual coming into contact with it. Hazardous chemicals are those that are corrosive, toxic, irritating, carcinogenic, flammable, or reactive.

The HCS is based on the concept that employees have a right to know about the hazardous chemicals in their workplace and the precautions to take to protect themselves when working with hazardous chemicals. In the medical office, sanitization, disinfection, and sterilization procedures involve the use of hazardous chemicals; the medical assistant must have a thorough knowledge of the HCS.

The HCS consists of the following components:
- Development of a hazard communication program
- Inventory of hazardous chemicals
- Labeling requirements
- Material safety data sheet requirements
- Employee information and training

Hazard Communication Program

As part of the HCS, employers are required to develop a hazard communication program. The hazard communication program consists of a written plan that describes what the facility is doing to meet the requirements of the HCS.

The information in the plan must be made available and communicated to all employees who work with hazardous chemicals.

Inventory of Hazardous Chemicals

The employer must develop and maintain a list of hazardous chemicals that are used and stored in the workplace. This list must include the name of the chemical, the name of the manufacturer, the hazardous ingredients, and the health and safety ratings of the chemical. The list must be updated as new chemicals are introduced into the workplace. In the medical office, hazardous chemicals often include the following:
- Products used for sanitization, disinfection, and sterilization(e.g.,chemicaldisinfectants,autoclave cleaners)
- Chemicals used for laboratory testing (e.g., laboratory testing reagents, developing solutions, controls)
- Pharmaceutical products such as local anesthetics (e.g., lidocaine [Xylocaine])
- Front office products (e.g., toner for copying machine and laser printer)
- Cleaning products (e.g., drain cleaner)

Labeling of Hazardous Chemicals

The HCS requires that each container of a hazardous chemical be labeled by the manufacturer with a warning to alert the user that the chemical is dangerous (Figure 18-1). This label must include the possible hazards of the chemical and the steps that can be taken to protect against those risks. Hazard warnings can use words, pictures, or symbols to provide the user with an understanding of the physical and

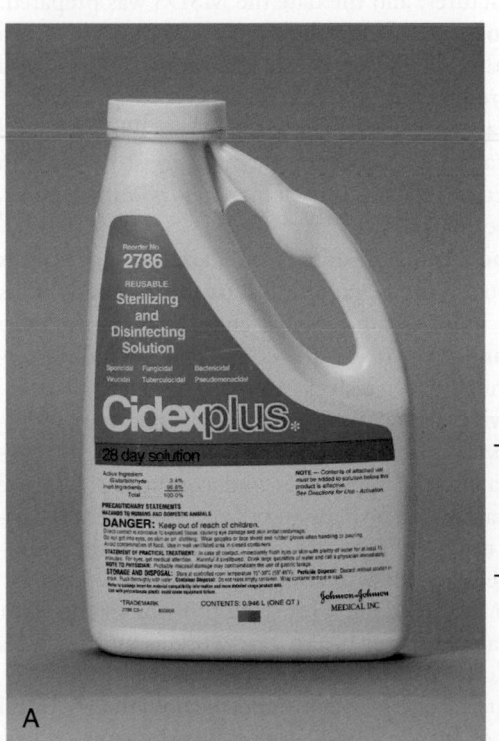

PRECAUTIONARY STATEMENTS
HAZARDS TO HUMANS AND DOMESTIC ANIMALS
DANGER: Keep out of reach of children.
Direct contact is corrosive to exposed tissue, causing eye damage and skin irritation/damage. Do not get into eyes, on skin or on clothing. Wear goggles or face shield and rubber gloves when handling or pouring. Avoid contamination of food. Use in well ventilated area in closed containers.
STATEMENT OF PRACTICAL TREATMENT: In case of contact, immediately flush eyes or skin with plenty of water for at least 15 minutes. For eyes, get medical attention. Harmful if swallowed. Drink large quantities of water and call a physician immediately.
NOTE TO PHYSICIAN: Probable mucosal damage may contraindicate the use of gastric lavage.
STORAGE AND DISPOSAL: Store at controlled room temperature 15°-30°C (59°-86°F).
Disposal: Discard residual solution in drain. Flush thoroughly with water.
Container disposal: Do not reuse empty container. Wrap container and put in trash.
Refer to package insert for material compatibility information and more detailed usage/product data.
Use with polycarbonate plastic could cause equipment failure.

*TRADEMARK   CONTENTS: 0.946 L (ONE QT.)
2786 C2-1   830006

Figure 18-1 A, Hazardous chemical container label. **B,** The label must indicate the possible hazards of the chemical.

health hazards of the chemical. If a label falls off a product or is damaged or obscured, a replacement label must be applied. If a chemical is transferred to a new container, a label with all the required information must be attached to the new container.

Container Label Requirements

The HCS requires that manufacturers label the containers of hazardous chemicals they produce with specific information. This information allows the user of the chemical to tell at a glance the hazards of using the chemical and the basic steps to take to protect oneself. Information required by the HCS includes the following:

1. **Name of the chemical.** The name of the chemical must be clearly indicated on the label.
2. **Manufacturer information.** The name, address, and emergency phone number of the company that manufactures the chemical must be stated on the label.
3. **Physical hazards of the chemical.** Physical hazards that must be stated include the potential of the chemical to catch fire, explode, or react with other chemicals or materials.
4. **Health hazards of the chemical.** Health hazards include the potential of the chemical to cause irritation to tissue, cancer, a sensitivity reaction, or a toxic or corrosive reaction.
5. **Safety precautions.** The protective clothing, equipment, and procedures that are recommended when working with the chemical must be stated on the label. Examples include gloves, protective eyewear, and working with the chemical in a well-ventilated area.
6. **Storing, handling, and disposal of the chemical.** Information on how the chemical should be stored, handled, and disposed of must be stated on the label.

Material Safety Data Sheets

A **material safety data sheet (MSDS)** provides more detailed information than the container label regarding the chemical, its hazards, and measures to take to prevent injury and illness when handling the chemical (Figure 18-2). The HCS requires that a current MSDS be kept on file for each hazardous chemical used or stored in the workplace. MSDSs must be readily accessible to employees and provided to them on request. It is important that the medical assistant review the MSDS before working with a hazardous chemical.

Companies that manufacture and distribute hazardous chemicals must provide an MSDS with every product. A hazardous chemical should never be used unless an MSDS is available. In the event of an accidental exposure, information on the MSDS must be readily available as a reference for emergency treatment. If an MSDS is missing, it must be replaced. This can be accomplished by contacting the supplier or the manufacturer of that chemical for a replacement or by going to the manufacturer's website; most manufacturers post their MSDSs on their websites for easy access.

An MSDS does not have to be kept on file for a hazardous chemical that is used in the workplace in the same way that a household consumer would use it. For example, correction fluids, such as Wite-Out and Liquid Paper, contain a hazardous chemical. If the medical assistant uses it in the same way, however, that a household consumer would use it (i.e., to correct errors on a document), an MSDS does not need to be kept on file. If household bleach (sodium hypochlorite) is used to decontaminate blood spills in the medical office, an MSDS would need to be kept on file because the bleach is not being used in the same way that a household consumer would use it.

What Would You Do? What Would You *Not* Do?

Case Study 1

Elba Cordera has brought her daughter Maria in for a well-baby visit. Maria is 9 months old and is just starting to crawl. Mrs. Cordera is taking precautions to baby-proof her house to protect Maria from accidents. Mrs. Cordera wants to know how to tell whether a cleaning product is poisonous. She also wants to know what she should do if Maria gets into a cleaning product and spills it on herself or swallows it. ∎

Material Safety Data Sheet Requirements

The HCS requires that manufacturers of hazardous chemicals include the following information on the MSDS (see Figure 18-2):

1. **Identification.** This section provides information used to identify the chemical and must include the chemical's generic name and its brand name; the name, address, and emergency phone number of the manufacturer; and the date the MSDS was prepared.
2. **Composition of ingredients.** This section provides a list of the ingredients in the hazardous chemical and exposure limits of each chemical.
3. **Physical and chemical properties.** Physical and chemical properties of the chemical must be listed in this section, such as appearance, odor, boiling point, and freezing point.
4. **Fire and explosion data.** Some hazardous chemicals may cause a fire or explosion if used improperly. This section indicates under what circumstances this may occur and what to do if it does occur, including recommended extinguishing agents.
5. **Reactivity data.** Some chemicals react when combined with other chemicals or materials. The reactivity data list the substances and conditions that the chemical should be kept away from to prevent a dangerous reaction. This information helps in determining where and how to store the chemical.
6. **Health hazard data.** This section is one of the most important areas for health care workers and includes the following information:
   • Route of entry, which indicates how the chemical can enter the body, including skin contact, eye contact, inhalation, and ingestion

MATERIAL SAFETY DATA SHEET (MSDS)

Date of Issue: 4/28/04　　　　　　　　　　　　　　　　　　Date of Revision: 8/8/12

SECTION 1　IDENTIFICATION

GENERIC NAME: Glutaraldehyde	INFORMATION TELEPHONE NUMBER: 1 (800) 733-8690
BRAND NAME: Aldecide	EMERGENCY TELEPHONE NUMBER:
MANUFACTURER'S NAME: Brennan Corporation	1 (800) 331-0766
MFG. ADDRESS: P.O. Box 93	
CITY: Camden　　STATE: NJ　　ZIP: 08106	

SECTION 2　COMPOSITION OF INGREDIENTS

CAS NUMBER	CHEMICAL NAME OF INGREDIENTS	PERCENT	PEL	TLV
111-30-8	Glutaraldehyde	2.5	0.2 ppm	0.2 ppm
7732-18-5	Water	97.4	None	None
7632-00-0	Sodium Nitrite	<1	None	None

SECTION 3　PHYSICAL AND CHEMICAL PROPERTIES

BOILING POINT: 212° F	SPECIFIC GRAVITY (H_2O = 1): 1.004
VAPOR PRESSURE (mm Hg): 0.20 at 20° C	VAPOR DENSITY (AIR = 1): 1.1
ODOR: Sharp odor	pH: 7.5-8.5
SOLUBILITY IN WATER: Complete (100%)	MELTING POINT: n/a
APPEARANCE: Bluish-green liquid	FREEZING POINT: 32° F
EVAPORATION RATE: 0.98　(Water = 1)	ODOR THRESHOLD: 0.04 ppm

SECTION 4　FIRE AND EXPLOSION HAZARD DATA

FLASH POINT: Not flammable (aqueous solution)	NFPA Rating:
FLAMMABILITY LIMITS:　　　　　LEL: n/a	Health: 2
EXTINGUISHING MEDIA: n/a (aqueous solution)	Flammability: 0
SPECIAL FIRE FIGHTING PROCEDURES: n/a	Reactivity: 0
UNUSUAL FIRE/EXPL HAZARDS: None	

SECTION 5　REACTIVITY DATA

STABILITY: Stable under recommended storage conditions.

CONDITIONS TO AVOID: Avoid direct sunlight and temperatures above 104° F (40° C).

INCOMPATIBILITY (MATERIAL TO AVOID): Strong acids and alkalines will neutralize active ingredient.

HAZARDOUS DECOMPOSITION BYPRODUCTS: None

HAZARDOUS POLYMERIZATION: Will not occur

Figure 18-2 Material safety data sheet (MSDS).

Continued

- Signs and symptoms of overexposure (e.g., burning eyes, nausea, dizziness, difficulty in breathing)
- Medical conditions that are aggravated by exposure to the chemical (e.g., asthma, dermatitis)
- Acute and chronic health hazards that could result from overexposure (e.g., skin irritation, eye damage, lung damage)

This section also indicates whether the hazardous chemical has been identified as a potential carcinogen by the National Toxicology Program (NTP), the International Agency for Research on Cancer (IARC), and OSHA.

7. **Emergency first-aid procedures.** This section identifies the first-aid measures to take if exposed to the chemical (e.g., in case of eye contact, immediately flush eyes with water for 15 minutes).

8. **Precautions for safe handling and use.** This section tells what to do for a spill or leak, the method of

MATERIAL SAFETY DATA SHEET

SECTION 6   HEALTH HAZARD DATA

ROUTE OF ENTRY: SKIN: yes   EYES: yes   INHALATION: yes   INGESTION: yes

SIGNS AND SYMPTOMS OF OVEREXPOSURE:

SKIN: Moderate irritation. May aggravate existing dermatitis.

EYES: Serious eye irritant. May cause irreversible damage which could permanently impair vision.

INHALATION: Vapors may be severely irritating and cause stinging sensations in the eyes, nose, throat, and lungs. May aggravate pre-existing asthma.

INGESTION: May cause irritation or chemical burns of the mouth, throat, esophagus, and stomach. May cause vomiting, diarrhea, epigastric distress, headache, dizziness, faintness, mental confusion, and general systemic illness.

CARCINOGENICITY DATA: NTP: No   AIRC: No   OSHA: No

SECTION 7   EMERGENCY FIRST AID PROCEDURES

SKIN: Wash skin with soap and water for 15 minutes. If skin redness or irritation persists, seek medical attention. Remove contaminated clothing and wash before reuse.

EYES: Immediately flush with water for 15 minutes. Seek medical attention.

INHALATION: Remove to fresh air. If irritation persists, seek medical attention.

INGESTION: Do not induce vomiting. Seek medical attention immediately. Call a physician or Poison Control Center.

SECTION 8   PRECAUTIONS FOR SAFE HANDLING AND USE

SPILL PROCEDURES: Ventilate area, wear protective gloves and eye gear. Wipe with sponge, mop, or towel. Flush with large quantities of water. Collect liquid and discard it.

WASTE DISPOSAL METHOD: Container must be triple rinsed and disposed of in accordance with federal, state, and/or local regulations. Used solution should be flushed thoroughly with water into sewage disposal system in accordance with federal, state, and/or local regulations.

PRECAUTIONS IN HANDLING AND STORAGE: Store in a cool, dry place (59-86° F) away from direct sunlight or sources of intense heat. Keep container tightly closed when not in use.

SECTION 9   CONTROL MEASURES

VENTILATION: Ensure adequate ventilation to maintain recommended exposed limit.

RESPIRATORY PROTECTION: None normally required for routine use.

SKIN PROTECTION: Wear chemical resistant protective gloves. Butyl rubber, nitrile rubber, polyethylene, or double-gloved latex.

EYE PROTECTION: Safety goggles or safety glasses

WORK/HYGIENE PRACTICES: Prompt rinsing of hands after contact. Handle in accordance with good personal hygiene and safety practices. These practices include avoiding unnecessary exposure.

Figure 18-2, cont'd

disposal of the chemical, and how to handle and store the chemical.

9. **Control measures.** This section lists engineering controls, work practice controls, and personal protective equipment that should be used to protect oneself from the hazardous chemical. Examples of these measures include using chemical-resistant gloves and eye protection and working in a well ventilated area.

Employee Information and Training

The HCS requires that employees be provided with information and training regarding hazardous chemicals in the workplace. The training session must be offered at the time of an employee's initial assignment to a work area where hazardous chemicals are present, and whenever a new chemical hazard is introduced into the work area. The training program must be an ongoing activity, and each training session must be documented. The HCS requires that the following information be relayed to employees who work with hazardous chemicals:

1. Requirements making up the HCS.
2. Physical and health hazards associated with exposure to chemicals in the workplace.
3. Measures employees can take to protect themselves from injury or illness from hazardous chemicals.

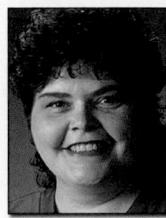
4. Emergency procedures to carry out in the event of exposure to a hazardous chemical or a chemical spill.
5. The meaning of the information on container labels and how to use that information.
6. The meaning of the information on the MSDS and how to use that information.
7. The location of the following: hazard communication program plan, list of hazardous chemicals in the workplace, and MSDS for each chemical in the workplace.

SANITIZATION

Sanitization involves a series of steps designed to remove organic material from an article and to reduce to a safe level the number of microorganisms on the article (Procedure 18-1). Organic material on an article may result in incomplete sterilization or disinfection. This is because the organic material acts as a physical barrier preventing the physical or chemical agent from reaching the surface of the article to kill microorganisms.

Sanitizing Instruments

Items most frequently sanitized in the medical office are medical and surgical instruments. This section focuses on the theory and procedure for sanitizing instruments. The general steps in the sanitization procedure of instruments are as follows:

1. *Rinse* the instruments to prevent organic material from drying on the instruments.
2. *Decontaminate* the instruments with a chemical disinfectant to remove pathogenic microorganisms, making the instrument safe to handle.

3. *Clean* the instruments to remove all organic matter.
4. *Thoroughly rinse* the instruments to remove all detergent residue.
5. *Dry* the instruments to prevent stains on the instruments.
6. *Check the instruments* for defects and working condition.
7. *Lubricate* hinged instruments to make the instruments function well and last longer.

Cleaning Instruments

Two methods can be used to perform the cleaning step (step 3 in the preceding list) of the sanitization procedure: the manual method and the ultrasound method.

Manual Method

The manual method is used most often in the medical office. It involves the manual cleaning of instruments using a cleaning solution and a brush. Manual cleaning is recommended for delicate instruments because vibrations that occur with the ultrasound method may damage these instruments.

Ultrasound Method

The ultrasound method uses a machine known as an *ultrasonic cleaner* (Figure 18-3). The ultrasound method offers a safety advantage in that instruments do not have to be handled during the cleaning process. This decreases the incidence of an accidental puncture or cut from a sharp instrument. An ultrasonic cleaner works by converting sound waves into mechanical energy, which creates small bubbles all over the instruments. When the bubbles burst, vibrations occur that loosen and remove debris from the instruments. Ultrasonic cleaners are especially good at removing debris from hard-to-reach areas, such as box locks of hemostats and screw locks of scissors.

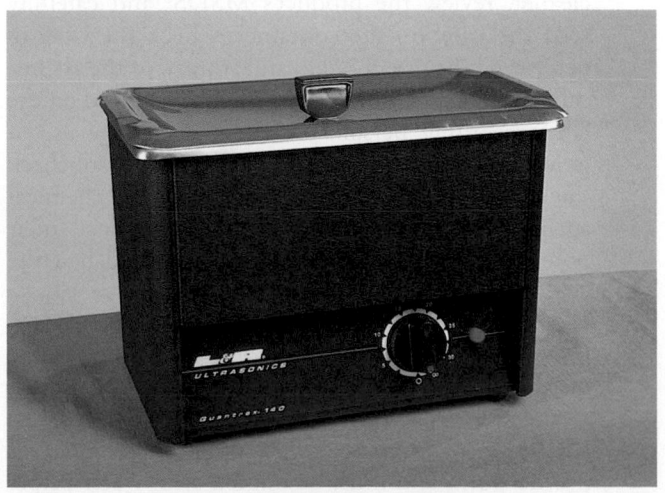

Figure 18-3 Ultrasonic cleaner.

Before the instruments are placed in the ultrasonic cleaner, they should be separated according to the type of metal (e.g., stainless steel, aluminum, brass). Instruments made of dissimilar metals should not be cleaned together in the ultrasonic cleaner. When different metals are in close contact, the ions from one metal can flow to another. This may result in a permanent blue-black stain on an instrument, which can be removed only by having the instrument refinished.

Guidelines for Sanitizing Instruments

The following guidelines should be followed when sanitizing surgical instruments:

1. **Wear gloves during the sanitization process.** While following the OSHA Bloodborne Pathogens Standard, the medical assistant should wear disposable gloves during the entire sanitization procedure. This protects the medical assistant from bloodborne pathogens and other potentially infectious materials. The medical assistant should be especially careful when working with hazardous chemicals and when handling sharp instruments. Heavy-duty utility gloves should be worn over the disposable gloves to provide protection from the irritating effects of chemical agents and accidental punctures or cuts from sharp instruments.

2. **Handle instruments carefully.** Instruments are expensive and delicate, yet durable. They can last for many years if handled and maintained properly. Dropping an instrument on the floor or throwing an instrument into a basin may damage it. Instruments should never be piled in a heap because they become entangled and may be damaged when separated. Keep sharp instruments separate from other instruments to prevent damaging or dulling the cutting edge. Also, keep delicate instruments separate to protect them from damage.

3. **Follow instructions on labels of chemical agents.** Before using a chemical agent such as a chemical disinfectant, an instrument cleaner, or an autoclave cleaner, review the product's MSDS, and carefully read the label on the container. Check the label to determine the use, mixing, and storage of the chemical agent. Read and observe precautions listed on the label regarding personal safety, such as the use of gloves and eye protection (Figure 18-4). Also, check the expiration date on the label of the chemical agent. Chemicals have a tendency to lose their potency over time and should not be used past the expiration date.

4. **Use a proper cleaning agent.** A low-sudsing detergent with a neutral pH should be used to clean the instruments. Commercially available instrument cleaners meet these criteria (Figure 18-5). These cleaners usually come in a concentrated liquid or powder form and must be diluted with water before use. Never substitute any other type of detergent, such

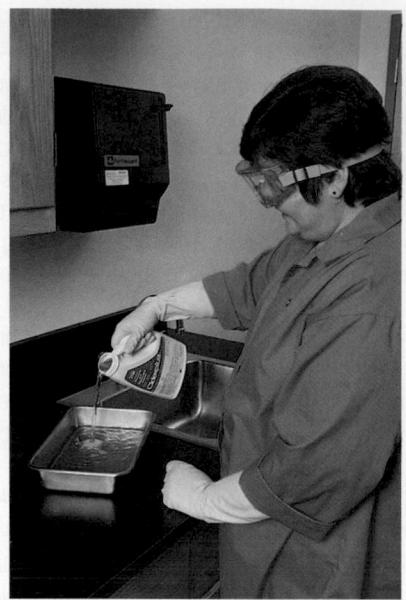

Figure 18-4 Kara wears utility gloves and safety goggles to protect herself from the irritating effects of glutaraldehyde.

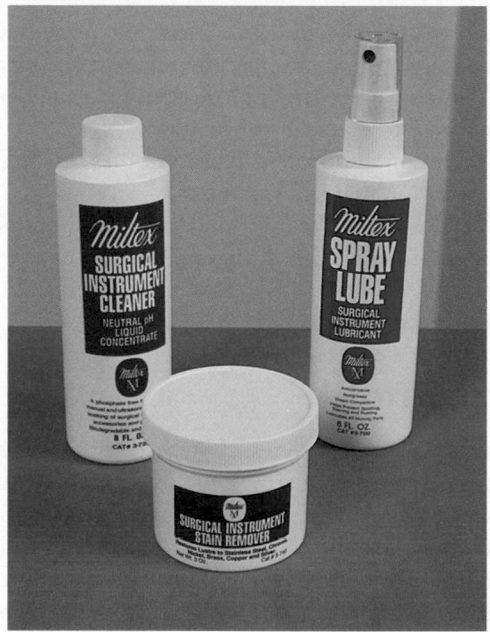

Figure 18-5 Commercially available surgical instrument cleaners. *Left,* Instrument cleaner; *center,* stain remover; *right,* spray lubricant.

as dishwasher detergent or laundry detergent; these detergents may not be low-sudsing or may not have the proper pH for sanitizing instruments. If a detergent with an alkaline pH is used and is not completely rinsed off, it could leave a residue on the instrument. This could result in an orange-brown stain on the instrument that resembles rust. Using an acid detergent also can cause staining and permanent corrosion.

5. **Use proper cleaning devices.** Proper cleaning devices should be used for the manual cleaning of surgical instruments. A stiff nylon brush should be used to clean the surface of the instrument. A stainless steel wire brush can be used to clean grooves, crevices, or serrations. A stain on an instrument often can be removed by using a commercial instrument stain remover (see Figure 18-5). Never use steel wool or other abrasives to remove stains because damage to the instrument could occur.

6. **Carefully inspect each instrument for defects and proper working condition.** After cleaning, rinsing, and drying the instrument, it is important to check it for defects and proper working condition as follows:
   - The blades of an instrument should be straight and not bent.
   - The tips of an instrument should approximate tightly and evenly when the instrument is closed.
   - An instrument with a box lock (e.g., hemostatic forceps, needle holders) should move freely but must not be too loose. The pin that holds the box lock together should be flush against the instrument.
   - An instrument with a spring handle (e.g., thumb and tissue forceps) should have sufficient tension to grasp objects tightly.
   - The cutting edge of a sharp instrument should be smooth and devoid of nicks.
   - Scissors should cut cleanly and smoothly. To test for this, the medical assistant should cut into a thin piece of gauze. The scissors are in proper working condition if they cut all the way to the end of the blade without catching on the gauze.

7. **Lubricate hinged instruments.** Lubricate box locks, screw locks, scissor blades, and any other moving part of each instrument. The lubricant makes the instrument function better and last longer. Use a lubricant that can be penetrated by steam, such as a commercial spray lubricant or a lubricant bath (see Figure 18-5). Lubricate after performing the final rinse (and drying of the instrument); otherwise, the lubricant would be rinsed off the instrument. Never use industrial oils or silicon sprays. These substances are not steam penetrable and can build up on the instrument, affecting its working condition.

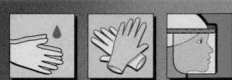

PROCEDURE 18-1 Sanitization of Instruments

Outcome Sanitize instruments.

Equipment/Supplies

- Sink
- Disposable gloves
- Heavy-duty utility gloves
- Contaminated instruments
- EPA-approved chemical disinfectant and MSDS
- Disinfectant container
- Cleaning solution and MSDS

- Basin
- Stiff nylon brush
- Stainless-steel wire brush
- Paper towels
- Cloth towel
- Instrument lubricant

---

1. **Procedural Step.** Review the MSDS for the hazardous chemicals you will be using in the sanitization process.
   Principle. The MSDS provides information regarding the chemical, its hazards, and measures to take to prevent injury and illness when handling the disinfectant.

2. **Procedural Step.** Apply disposable gloves. Transport the contaminated instruments to the cleaning area as soon as possible after use. The instruments should be carried in a covered basin from the examining room to the cleaning area.
   Principle. Disposable gloves act as a barrier to protect the medical assistant from infectious materials. Transporting contaminated instruments in a covered basin promotes infection control.

3. **Procedural Step.** Apply heavy-duty utility gloves over the disposable gloves.

Principle. Utility gloves help protect the hands from the irritating effects of chemical solutions.

4. **Procedural Step.** Separate sharp instruments and delicate instruments from other instruments.
   Principle. Separating sharp instruments from others prevents damage to or dulling of the cutting edge of these instruments. Delicate instruments should be separated to protect them from damage.

5. **Procedural Step.** Immediately rinse the instruments thoroughly under warm, not hot, running water (approximately 110° F [44° C]) to remove organic material, such as blood, body fluids, tissue, and other debris.
   Principle. Rinsing the instruments as soon as possible prevents organic material from drying on the instruments, making it difficult to remove later. Hot water may cause coagulation of organic material, making it more difficult to remove.

Continued

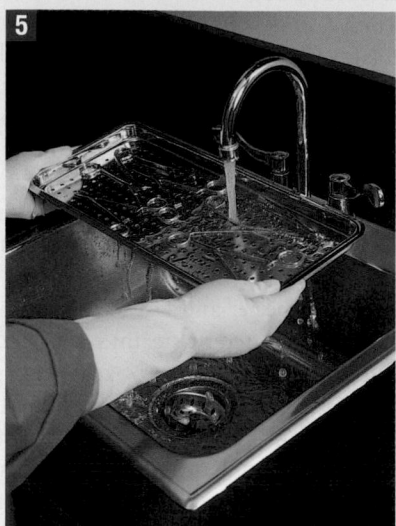

Rinse instruments under warm water to remove organic matter.

6. **Procedural Step.** Decontaminate the instruments by disinfecting them in an EPA-approved chemical disinfectant as follows:

a. Select the proper chemical disinfectant; check the expiration date on the container label.

b. Observe all personal safety precautions listed on the label of the disinfectant (e.g., wearing safety goggles).

c. Follow the manufacturer's directions on the label for proper mixing and use of the disinfectant.

d. Label the plastic or stainless steel disinfecting container with the name of the disinfectant and the date when the disinfectant is no longer effective and must be discarded (reuse life).

e. Pour the disinfectant into the labeled container and immerse the articles into the disinfectant. Ensure the articles are completely submerged in the disinfectant.

f. Cover the container that holds the chemical disinfectant.

g. Disinfect the articles for 10 minutes.

   Principle. Decontaminating the instruments removes pathogenic microorganisms from them, making them safe to handle. A disinfectant past its expiration date loses its potency and should not be used. An EPA-approved disinfectant has been determined by the U.S. Environmental Protection Agency to be effective when used as directed, without causing an unreasonable risk to the public or the environment. The container must be kept covered to prevent the escape of toxic fumes and to prevent evaporation of the disinfectant, which could change its potency.

7. **Procedural Step.** Clean the instruments. The instruments can be cleaned using the manual method or the ultrasound method as follows.

Manual Method for Cleaning Instruments

a. Obtain the instrument cleaning solution; check its expiration date.

b. Observe all personal safety precautions listed on the label of the cleaning agent.

c. Follow the directions on the manufacturer's label for proper mixing and use of the cleaning agent. The detergent may need to be diluted with water.

d. Remove the articles from the chemical disinfectant and place them in the basin containing the cleaning solution.

e. Use a stiff nylon brush to clean the surface of each instrument. Scrub all parts of the instrument thoroughly. Brush delicate instruments carefully to prevent damaging them.

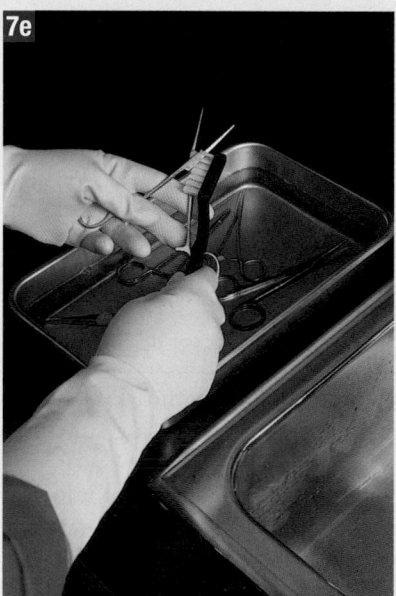

Clean the surface of the instrument with a stiff nylon brush.

f. Use a stainless-steel wire brush to clean grooves, crevices, or serrations where contaminants such as blood and tissue may collect.

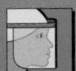
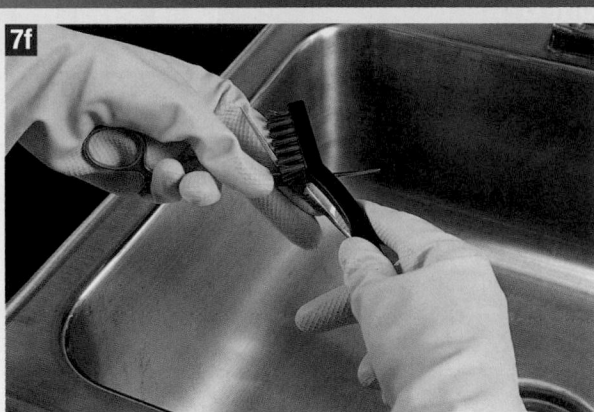

Clean grooves, crevices, or serrations with a wire brush.

g. If there is a stain on the instrument, attempt to remove it using a damp cloth or sponge to which a commercial stain remover has been applied.

h. Scrub each instrument until it is visibly clean and free from organic material and stains.

   Principle. A cleaning agent past its expiration date loses its potency and should not be used. Taking appropriate precautions with cleaning agents prevents harm to the medical assistant from hazardous chemicals. All organic material must be removed from the instruments to ensure complete sterilization in the autoclave.

Ultrasound Method for Cleaning Instruments

a. Using a cleaning agent recommended by the manufacturer, prepare the cleaning solution in the ultrasonic cleaner. Observe all personal safety precautions listed on the label.

b. Remove the articles from the chemical disinfectant, and separate instruments made of dissimilar metals, such as stainless steel, aluminum, and bronze.

c. Place the instruments in the ultrasonic cleaner with hinged instruments in an open position.

d. Ensure that sharp instruments do not touch other instruments.

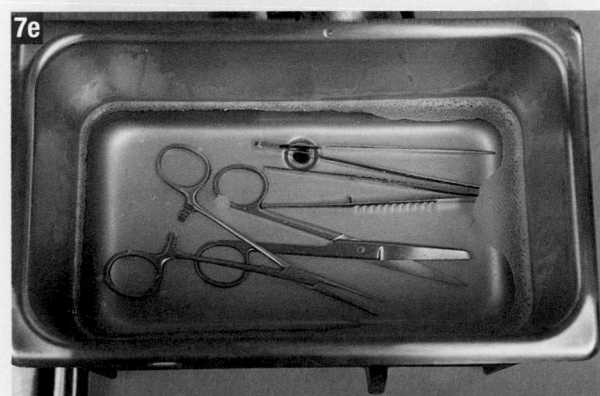

Completely submerge instruments in the cleaning solution.

e. Ensure that all instruments are fully submerged in the cleaning solution.

f. Place the lid on the ultrasonic cleaner.

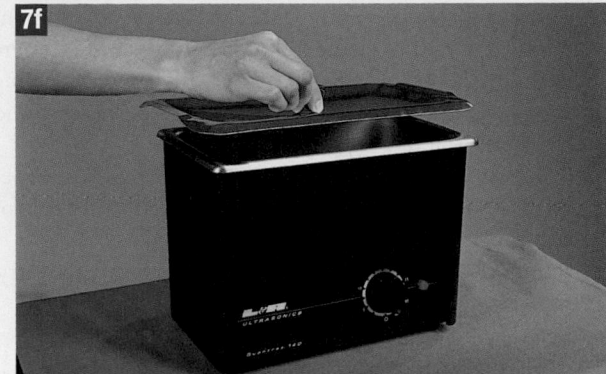

Place the lid on the ultrasonic cleaner.

h. Turn on the ultrasonic cleaner, and clean the instruments for the length of time recommended by the manufacturer.

i. After completion of the cleaning cycle, remove the instruments from the machine.

   Principle. Taking appropriate precautions with chemical agents prevents harm to the medical assistant from hazardous chemicals. Mixing dissimilar metals together could result in permanent stains on the instruments. Instruments must be completely submerged with hinged instruments in an open position so the solution can reach all parts of the instrument.

8. Procedural Step. Rinse each instrument thoroughly with warm, not hot, water (110° F [44° C]) for at least 20 to 30 seconds to remove all traces of the detergent. Open and close hinged instruments while

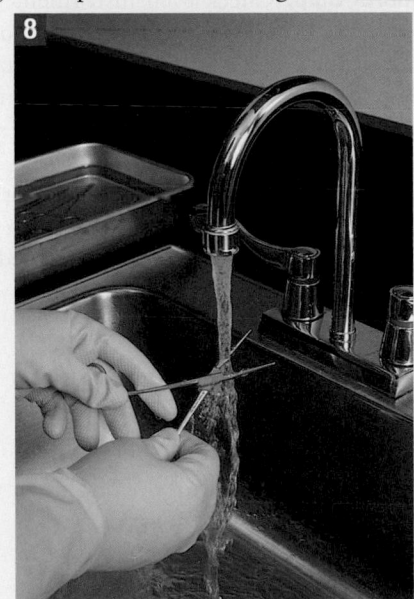

Rinse thoroughly with warm water.

Continued

PROCEDURE 18-1

PROCEDURE 18-1 Sanitization of Instruments—cont'd

rinsing to ensure the solution is completely rinsed out of every part of the instrument.

Principle. Detergent residue left on the instrument could cause stains, which could build up and interfere with proper functioning of the instrument. Using warm water helps to remove the cleaning solution and facilitates the drying process.

9. Procedural Step. Dry each instrument with a paper towel, and place the instrument on a cloth towel for additional air drying.

Principle. If the instrument is not completely dry, stains may occur on the instrument.

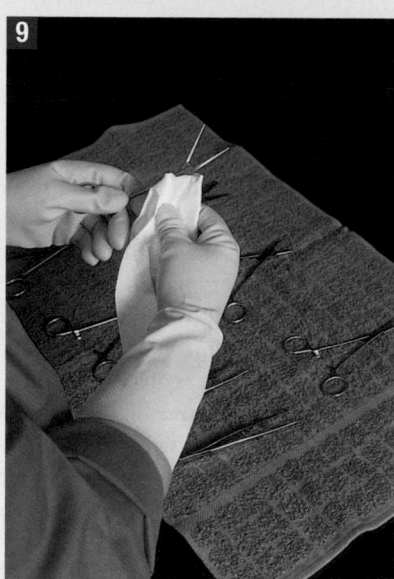

Dry the instrument with a paper towel.

10. Procedural Step. Check each instrument for defects and proper working condition. Scissors should cut all the way to the end of a thin piece of gauze without catching. If defects are noted, or the instrument is not working properly, it must be discarded or sent to the manufacturer for repair.

Principle. Instruments that have defects or are not in proper working condition are unsafe to use on a patient during a medical or surgical procedure.

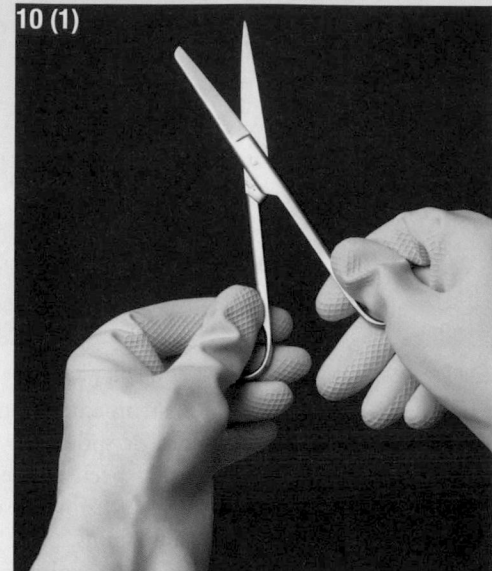

Check the instrument for defects and proper working order.

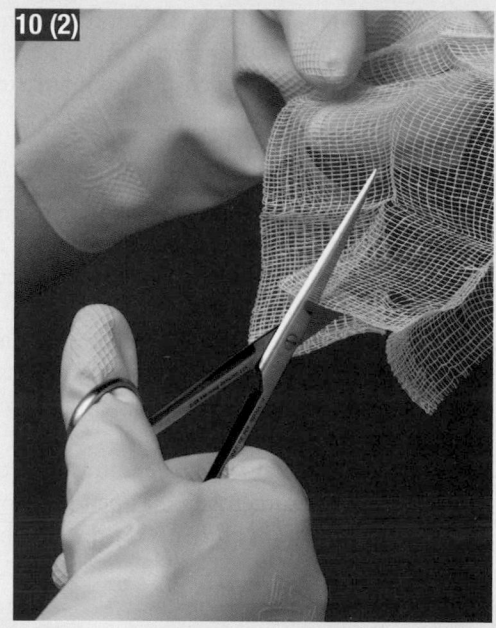

Scissors should cut through gauze without catching.

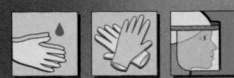

PROCEDURE 18-1 Sanitization of Instruments—cont'd

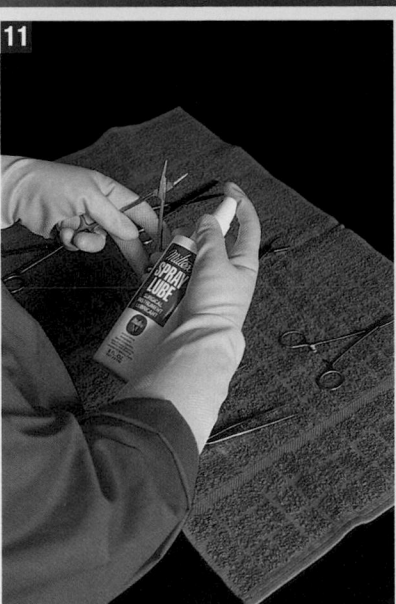

Lubricate hinged instruments.

11. Procedural Step. Lubricate hinged instruments using a steam-penetrable lubricant as follows:

a. Apply the lubricant to a hinged instrument in its open position.

b. Open and close the instrument after applying the lubricant so it reaches all parts of the hinged area.

c. Place the instrument back on the towel and allow it to drain. Rinsing or wiping is unnecessary.

Principle. Lubricating an instrument makes it function better and last longer.

12. Procedural Step. Dispose of the cleaning solution according to the manufacturer's instructions. Remove both sets of gloves, and sanitize your hands.

13. Procedural Step. Wrap the instruments and sterilize them in the autoclave according to the medical office policy.

Table 18-1 Disinfectants Used in the Medical Office

Disinfectant	Common Names	Use in the Medical Office
Glutaraldehyde	Cidex MetriCide ProCide Omnicide Wavicide	Disinfection of flexible fiberoptic sigmoidoscopes.
Alcohol	Isopropyl alcohol	Disinfection of stethoscopes, blood pressure cuffs, tuning forks, and percussion hammers; isopropyl alcohol wipes are used to disinfect rubber stoppers of multiple-dose medication vials.
Chlorine and chlorine compounds	Sodium hypochlorite (household bleach)	Recommended by OSHA for decontamination of blood spills.
Phenolics	Carbolic acid Hydroxybenzene Phenic acid Phenyl hydroxide Phenylic acid	Disinfection of walls, furniture, floors, and laboratory work surfaces.
Quaternary ammonium compounds	Benzalkonium chloride	Disinfection of walls, furniture, floors, and laboratory work surfaces.

From Bonewit-West K: *Clinical procedures for medical assistants*, ed 8, St Louis, 2011, Saunders.

DISINFECTION

Disinfection is the process of destroying pathogenic microorganisms, but it does not kill bacterial spores. Disinfection is accomplished in the medical office through the use of liquid chemical agents that are applied to inanimate objects. Chemical disinfection has been discussed with respect to its role in the sanitization process to decontaminate surgical instruments and make them safe to handle. This section discusses the use of chemical disinfection to disinfect semicritical and noncritical items so they can be used for patient care.

Table 18-1 lists disinfectants most frequently used in the medical office, along with common names and uses for each.

Levels of Disinfection

Based on killing action, disinfection can be classified according to three levels.

High-Level Disinfection

High-level disinfection is a process that destroys all microorganisms with the exception of bacterial spores. High-level disinfection is used to disinfect semicritical items. A **semicritical**

PROCEDURE 18-1

item is an item that comes in contact with nonintact skin or intact mucous membranes, such as a flexible fiberoptic sigmoidoscope. A frequently used high-level disinfectant is 2% glutaraldehyde (e.g., Cidex, MetriCide). A newer high-level disinfectant that is growing in popularity is Cidex OPA (*ortho*phthalaldehyde). Cidex OPA does not contain glutaraldehyde, which means it is less toxic and is safer to handle.

Intermediate-Level Disinfection

Intermediate-level disinfection is a process that inactivates tubercle bacilli (the causative agents of tuberculosis), all vegetative bacteria, most viruses, and most fungi, but it does not kill bacterial spores. Intermediate-level disinfection is used to disinfect noncritical items. **Noncritical items** are items that come in contact with intact skin but not with mucous membranes, including stethoscopes, blood pressure cuffs, tuning forks, percussion hammers, and crutches. A common intermediate-level disinfectant is isopropyl alcohol, which is frequently used in the form of alcohol wipes.

Low-Level Disinfection

Low-level disinfection is a process that kills most bacteria, some viruses, and some fungi, but it cannot be relied on to kill resistant microorganisms, such as tubercle bacilli, and it cannot kill bacterial spores. Low-level disinfectants typically are used to disinfect surfaces such as examining tables, laboratory countertops, and walls. Low-level disinfectants used in the medical office include sodium hypochlorite (household bleach) and phenolics.

STERILIZATION

Sterilization is the process of destroying all forms of microbial life, including bacterial spores. An item that is sterile is free of all living microorganisms and spores. Sterilization must be used to process all critical items. A **critical item** is an item that comes in contact with sterile tissue or the vascular system.

As previously described, a semicritical item (one that comes in contact with nonintact skin or with intact mucous membranes) can be chemically disinfected using a high-level disinfectant. Most offices prefer instead to sterilize

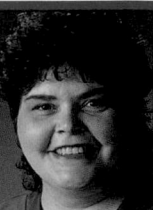

Memories *from* Externship

Kara VanDyke: During my externship experience, I was placed in a pediatrician's office. I wanted to go to a pediatric site because I love being around children. One day I was in the examining room with my patient, a 4-year-old boy who was there with his mother. It was standard procedure at this office to take every patient's temperature. I started getting out our electronic thermometer to take his temperature when I noticed he looked a little frightened. He was looking at the thermometer funny, and he said, "Can you do it in my ear?" I said I was sorry but we didn't have that kind of thermometer. I told him I could do it under his arm or under his tongue. His mom looked at him, and he said, "But I want it in my ear." He finally agreed to let me do it under his arm. When I was finished taking his temperature, he smiled and said, "You're the nicest doctor!" ■

semicritical items in the autoclave (e.g., vaginal specula, nasal specula). The autoclave provides a convenient, efficient, safe, and inexpensive method for destroying microorganisms. Chemical disinfectants not only are more expensive to use, but also are more hazardous and create problems regarding their proper disposal. The exception is any semicritical item that is heat sensitive. Flexible fiberoptic sigmoidoscopes would be damaged by the heat of an autoclave and must be chemically disinfected.

Sterilization Methods

Sterilization involves the use of physical or chemical methods. Each method of sterilization has advantages and disadvantages. The method used to achieve sterility depends primarily on the nature of the item to be sterilized. The most common physical and chemical sterilization methods include the following:

Physical Methods	Chemical Methods
Steam under pressure (autoclave)	Ethylene oxide gas
Hot air (dry heat oven)	Cold sterilization (chemical agents)
Radiation	

The most common method for sterilizing articles in the medical office is steam under pressure using an autoclave. The autoclave is discussed in detail in this chapter; the other methods of sterilization are briefly described.

Autoclave

The autoclave is dependable, efficient, and economical and can be used to sterilize items that are not harmed by moisture or high temperature. Refer to the box *Items Sterilized in the Autoclave* for a list of heat-resistant items that can be sterilized in the autoclave.

Items Sterilized in the Autoclave

Surgical instruments	Brushes
Medical instruments	Dressings
Minor office surgery trays	Glassware
Liquids	Reusable syringes

An **autoclave** consists of an outer jacket surrounding an inner sterilizing chamber. Under pressure, distilled water is converted to steam, which fills the inner sterilizing chamber. The pressure plays no direct part in killing microorganisms; rather, it functions to attain a higher temperature than could be reached by the steam from boiling water (212° F [100° C]). The cooler, drier air already in the chamber is forced out through the air exhaust valve.

It is important that all the air in the chamber be replaced by steam. When air is present, the temperature in the autoclave is reduced, and a temperature that is adequate for sterilization is not reached. When all the air has been removed, the air exhaust valve seals off the inner chamber, and the temperature in the autoclave begins to increase.

During the sterilization process, the steam penetrates the materials in the sterilizing chamber. The materials are cooler, so the steam condenses into moisture on them, giving up its heat. This heat serves to kill all microorganisms and their spores.

The autoclave is usually operated at approximately 15 pounds of pressure per square inch (psi) at a temperature of 250° F (121° C). Vegetative forms of most microorganisms are killed in a few minutes at temperatures ranging from 130° F to 150° F (54° C to 65° C), but certain bacterial spores can withstand a temperature of 240° F (115° C) for longer than 3 hours. No organism, however, can survive direct exposure to saturated steam at 250° F (121° C) for 15 minutes or longer.

The sterilization process using the autoclave is discussed in this section (with the exception of sanitization, which was already presented). The sterilization process consists of the following components:
- Monitoring program
- Sanitizing articles
- Wrapping articles
- Operating the autoclave (autoclave cycle)
- Handling and storing packs
- Maintaining the autoclave

Monitoring Program

To ensure that instruments and supplies are sterile when used, the Centers for Disease Control and Prevention (CDC) recommends that the medical office establish and maintain a monitoring program of the sterilization process. The monitoring program should consist of the following:

1. Written policies and procedures for each step of the sterilization process.
2. Sterilization indicators to ensure that minimum sterilizing conditions have been achieved.
3. Records for each cycle maintained in an autoclave log (Figure 18-6).

The information that should be recorded for each autoclave cycle includes the following:
- Date and time of the cycle
- Description of the load
- Exposure time
- Exposure temperature
- Results of the sterilization indicator
- Initials of the operator

Some autoclaves have recorders that automatically print out a portion of this information at the end of the cycle (Figure 18-7).

Sterilization Indicators

Materials that are being sterilized must be exposed to steam at a sufficient temperature and for a proper length of time. Sterilization indicators are available to determine the effectiveness of the procedure and to check against improper wrapping of articles, improper loading of the autoclave, and faulty operation of the autoclave.

An article is not considered sterile unless the steam has penetrated to its center; most sterilization indicators are placed in the center of the pack. The medical assistant should carefully read the instructions that come with the sterilization indicators. The most reliable indicators check for the attainment of the proper temperature and indicate the duration of the temperature.

If an indicator does not change properly, a problem may be present in the sterilization technique or in the working condition of the autoclave. The manufacturer's guidelines for proper sterilization techniques should be reviewed, and the articles should be resterilized while following these guidelines. If the indicator still does not change properly, the autoclave is in need of repair and should not be used until it has been serviced.

Sterilization indicators should be stored in a cool, dry area. Excessive heat or moisture can damage the indicator. The most common sterilization indicators are chemical indicators and biologic indicators, which are described next.

What Would You Do? What Would You *Not* Do?

Case Study 3

Cassie Augusta is in the examining room and is being prepared for the removal of a sebaceous cyst. Cassie is concerned about the instruments that the physician will be using to perform the procedure. She wants to know if they are "safe." Cassie says that her friend Mackenzie got a tattoo several years ago and developed hepatitis 3 weeks later. Mackenzie thinks she got hepatitis from the instruments that were used for her tattoo procedure. Cassie wants to know if it is possible for an instrument to give someone hepatitis. She says she heard that hepatitis can cause liver cancer and wants to know if this is true. Cassie also wants to know if there is a vaccine to prevent hepatitis. ■

AUTOCLAVE LOG						
Date/Time	Description of the Load	Cycle Time (min)	Temperature (° F)	Indicator* (+/−)	Initials	Comments
7/25/XX 4:00 PM	Surgical instruments	20	250	—	KV	
7/26/XX 3:00 PM	MOS tray setups	30	250	—	KV	

*Indicator Interpretation:
Positive (+): Spores not killed, indicating sterilization conditions have not been met.
Negative (−): Spores killed, indicating sterilization conditions have been met.

MAINTENANCE: (Indicate date, vendor name, service, etc.)

Figure 18-6 Example of an autoclave log.

Chemical Indicators

Chemical indicators are impregnated with a **thermolabile** dye that changes color when exposed to the sterilization process. If the chemical reaction of the indicator does not show the expected results, the item may not be sterile and must be resterilized. Chemical indicators include autoclave tape and sterilization strips.

Autoclave Tape. Autoclave tape contains a chemical that changes color if it has been exposed to steam. The tape is available in a variety of colors, can be written on, and is useful for closing and identifying the wrapped article (Figure 18-8). Autoclave tape has some limitations as an indicator. Because it is placed on the outside of the pack, it cannot ensure that steam has penetrated to the center of the pack. It also does not ensure that the item has been sterilized; it merely indicates that an article has been in the autoclave and that a high temperature has been attained.

Sterilization Strips. Sterilization strips are commercially prepared paper or plastic strips that contain a thermolabile dye and that change color when exposed to steam under

pressure for a certain length of time (Figure 18-9). Most sterilization strips are designed to change color after being exposed to a temperature of 250° F (121° C) for 15 minutes. The indicator strip should be placed in the center of the wrapped pack, with the end containing the dye placed in an area of the pack considered to be the hardest for steam to penetrate.

Biologic Indicators

Biologic indicators are the best means available for determining the effectiveness of the sterilization procedure. The CDC recommends that medical office personnel use a biologic indicator to monitor all autoclaves at least once a week.

A biologic indicator is a preparation of living bacterial spores. Biologic indicators are commercially available in the form of dry spore strips in small glassine envelopes. Biologic monitoring of an autoclave requires the use of a preparation of spores of *Geobacillus stearothermophilus,* a microorganism whose spores are particularly resistant to moist heat and are not harmful to humans.

```
READY

BEGIN

SET TEMP:      270 F        ← Temperature
SET TIME:      015          ← Time
RUN #          011          ← Cycle number

DATE   7/25/12

HEAT UP
DEG       PSI        MIN
066       00.0       000
066       00.0       002
074       00.0       004      ┐ Heat-up
164       00.0       006      │ phase
219       04.1       008
234       09.4       010
261       22.6       012

STERILIZE
DEG       PSI        MIN
272       30.2       000
272       30.7       001
273       31.3       002
274       31.0       003
273       30.7       004
273       30.4       005
273       30.1       006
272       30.0       007   ┐ Sterilization
272       30.1       008   │ phase
272       30.4       009
272       30.4       010
272       30.7       011
273       31.0       012
273       30.8       013
274       31.0       014
273       30.7       015

VENT
COMPLETE
```

Figure 18-7 Example of a printout of an autoclave cycle.

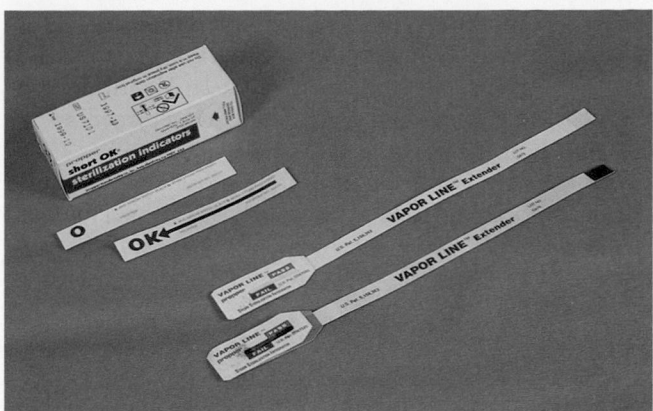

Figure 18-9 Sterilization strips. Sterilization strips contain a thermolabile dye and change color when exposed to steam under pressure for a certain length of time.

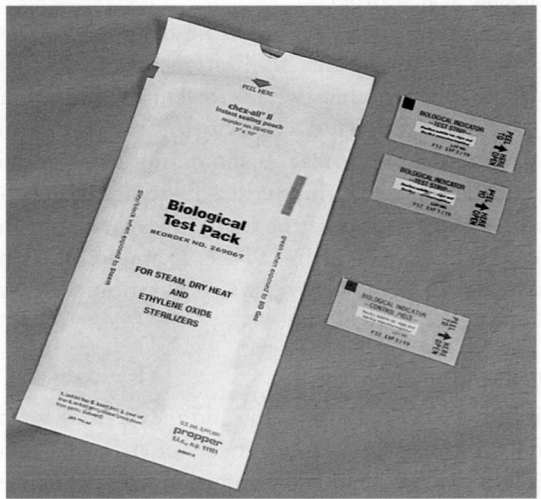

Figure 18-10 Biologic indicator. A biologic indicator includes two spore tests that are sterilized *(top right)* and one spore control that is not sterilized *(bottom right)*.

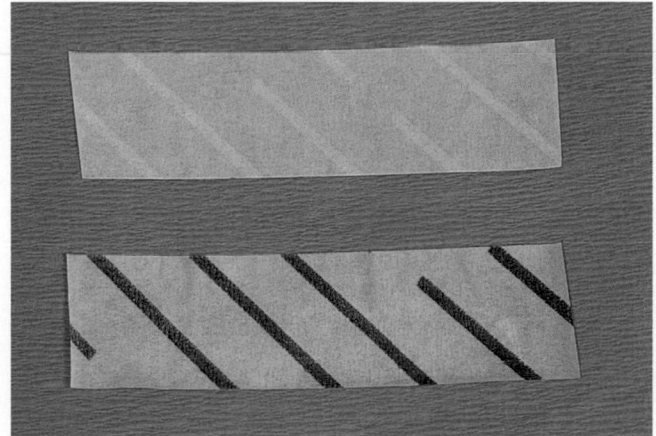

Figure 18-8 Autoclave tape. *Top,* Autoclave tape as it appears before the sterilization process. *Bottom,* Diagonal lines appear on the tape during autoclaving and indicate that the wrapped article has been autoclaved.

Each biologic testing unit includes two spore tests that are sterilized and one spore control that is not sterilized (Figure 18-10). The biologic indicator is placed in the center of two wrapped articles. The articles are placed in areas of the autoclave that are the least accessible to steam

penetration, such as on the bottom tray of the autoclave, near the front of the autoclave, and in the back of the autoclave.

After the indicators have been exposed to sterilization conditions, they must be processed before the results can be obtained. The two methods for processing results are the in-house method and the mail-in method.

In-house method. The in-house method involves processing and interpreting the results at the medical office. After sterilization, the processed spores are incubated for 24 to 48 hours. If sterilization conditions have been met, the color or condition of the processed spores is different from those of the control, and the spore test is interpreted as negative. If sterilization conditions have not been met, the processed spores and the unprocessed control display the same color or condition, and the spore test is interpreted as positive.

Mail-in method. With this method, the processed bacterial spores and the (unprocessed) control are mailed to a processing laboratory. The test is performed by the laboratory, and the results are returned to the medical office.

If spores are not killed in routine spore tests, the autoclave should be checked immediately for proper use and function, and the spore test should be repeated. If the spore test remains positive, the autoclave should not be used until it is serviced.

Wrapping Articles

Articles to be sterilized in the autoclave first must be thoroughly sanitized (see Procedure 18-1). Next, the articles are prepared for autoclaving by wrapping them. The purpose of wrapping articles is to protect them from recontamination during handling and storage. Articles that are wrapped and handled correctly remain sterile after autoclaving until the package seal is broken.

The wrapping material should be made of a substance that is not affected by the sterilization process and should allow steam to penetrate while preventing contaminants, such as dust, insects, and microorganisms, from entering during handling and storage. It should not tear or puncture easily and should allow the sterilized package to be opened without contamination of the contents. A wrapper should not be used if it is torn or has a hole. Examples of wrapping materials used for autoclaving are sterilization paper, sterilization pouches, and muslin.

Sterilization Paper

Sterilization paper is a disposable and inexpensive wrapping material. It consists of square sheets of paper of different sizes (Figure 18-11). The most common sizes (in inches) are 12×12, 15×15, 18×18, 24×24, 30×30, and 36×36. Articles must be wrapped in such a way that they do not become contaminated when the pack is opened. The proper method for wrapping instruments using sterilization paper is outlined in Procedure 18-2. This method of wrapping can be used for all types of instruments and supplies.

The disadvantage of sterilization paper is that it is difficult to spread open for removal of the contents. It has a "memory" and tends to flip back easily, so it may not open flat to provide a sterile field. (*Memory* is the ability of a material to retain a specific shape or configuration.) Because sterilization paper is opaque, it is impossible to view the contents of a pack before opening it.

Sterilization Pouches

Sterilization pouches typically consist of a combination of paper and plastic; paper makes up one side of the pouch, and a plastic film makes up the other side (Figure 18-12). Sterilization pouches are available in different sizes; the most common sizes (in inches) are 3×9, 5×10, and 7×12.

Most pouches have a peel-apart seal on one end that is used later to open the pouch for removal of the sterile item. The other end of the pouch is open and is used to insert the item into the pouch. When the article has been inserted, this end is sealed with heat or adhesive tape. The proper method for wrapping an instrument by using a pouch is outlined in Procedure 18-3.

Sterilization pouches provide good visibility of the contents on the plastic side. Most manufacturers include a sterilization indicator on the outside of the pouch. After removing a pouch from the autoclave, the medical assistant should check the indicator for proper color change. If the indicator does not change to the appropriate color (as specified by the manufacturer), the contents of the pouch must be resterilized.

Muslin

Muslin is a reusable woven fabric that is available in different sizes. Muslin is flexible and easy to handle and is considered the most economical sterilization wrap because it can be reused. Because of its durability, muslin is frequently used to wrap large packs, such as tray setups for minor office surgery. Muslin is "memory free," so it lies flat when opened. A pack wrapped in muslin may be opened on a table so that the wrapper becomes a sterile field. The procedure for wrapping an article with muslin is the same as that for sterilization paper (see Procedure 18-2).

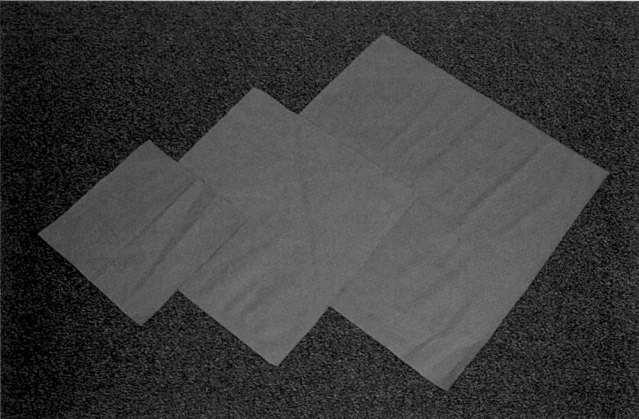

Figure 18-11 Sterilization paper wraps. Sterilization paper consists of square sheets of paper that are available in different sizes.

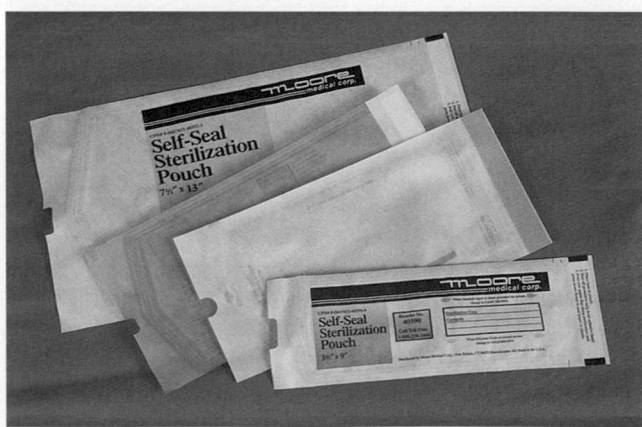

Figure 18-12 Sterilization pouches. Sterilization pouches consist of a combination of paper and plastic and are available in different sizes.

PROCEDURE 18-2   Wrapping Instruments Using Paper or Muslin

Outcome Wrap an instrument for autoclaving.

Equipment/Supplies

- Sanitized instrument
- Appropriate-sized wrapping material (sterilization paper or muslin)
- Sterilization indicator strip
- Autoclave tape
- Permanent marker

1. **Procedural Step.** Sanitize your hands.
2. **Procedural Step.** Assemble the equipment. Select the appropriate-sized wrapping material for the instrument being wrapped. Check the expiration date on the sterilization indicator box. If the sterilization strips are outdated, do not use them.
   Principle. Instruments are wrapped so they are protected from recontamination after they have been sterilized. Outdated strip indicators may not provide accurate test results.
3. **Procedural Step.** Place the wrapping material on a clean, flat surface. Turn the wrap in a diagonal position to your body so that it resembles a diamond shape.

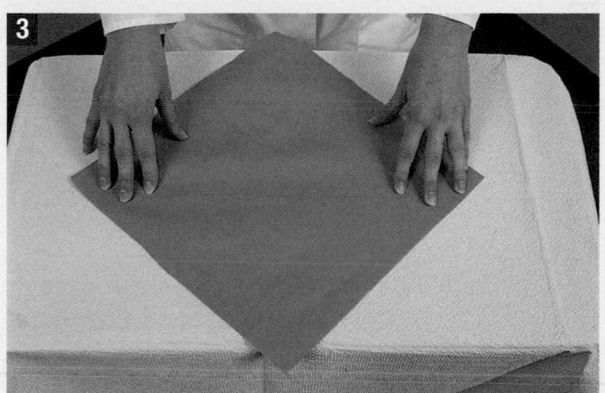

Turn the wrap in a diagonal position.

4. **Procedural Step.** Place the instrument in the center of the wrapping material with the longest part of the instrument pointing toward the two side corners. If the instrument has a movable joint, place it on the wrap in a slightly open position. If necessary, a gauze square can be used to hold the instrument in an open position.
   Principle. Instruments with movable joints must be in an open position to allow steam to reach all parts of the instrument. If the instrument is in a closed position, heat exposure could cause the instrument to crack at its weakest part, such as the lock area.

5. **Procedural Step.** Place a sterilization indicator in the center of the pack next to the instrument.
   Principle. Sterilization indicators assess the effectiveness of the sterilization process.

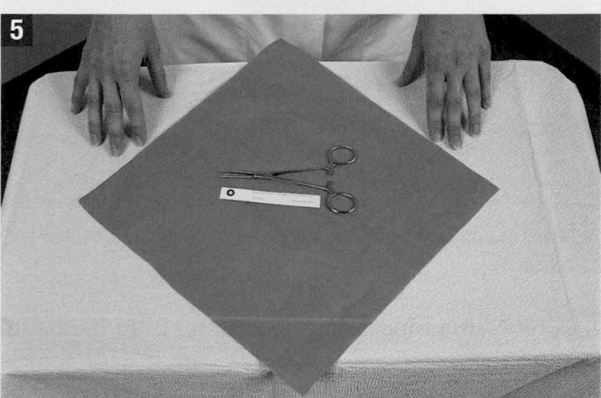

Place a sterilization indicator in the center of the pack next to the instrument.

6. **Procedural Step.** Fold the wrapping material up from the bottom, and double-back a small corner, creating a flap. This flap will later be used to open the sterile pack without contaminating the instrument.

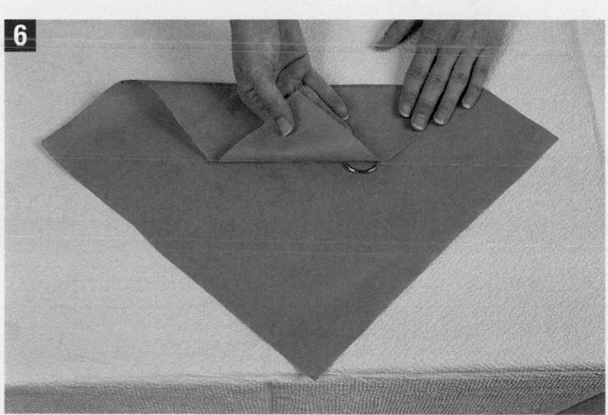

Fold the wrapping material up from the bottom, and double-back a small corner.

Continued

PROCEDURE 18-2

PROCEDURE 18-2   Wrapping Instruments Using Paper or Muslin—cont'd

7. **Procedural Step.** Fold over one edge of the wrapping material, and double-back the corner.
8. **Procedural Step.** Fold over the other edge of the wrapping material, and double-back the corner.

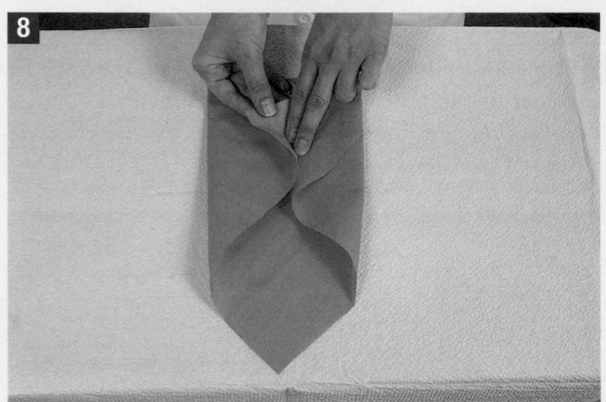

Fold over the other edge of the wrapping material, and double-back the corner.

9. **Procedural Step.** Fold the pack up from the bottom, pull the top flap down, and secure it with autoclave tape. Ensure that the pack is firm enough for handling but loose enough to permit proper circulation of steam.
Principle. Instruments must be wrapped properly to permit full penetration of steam and to prevent contaminating them when the wrap is opened. Using autoclave tape indicates that the pack has been through the autoclave cycle and prevents mix-ups with packs that have not been processed.

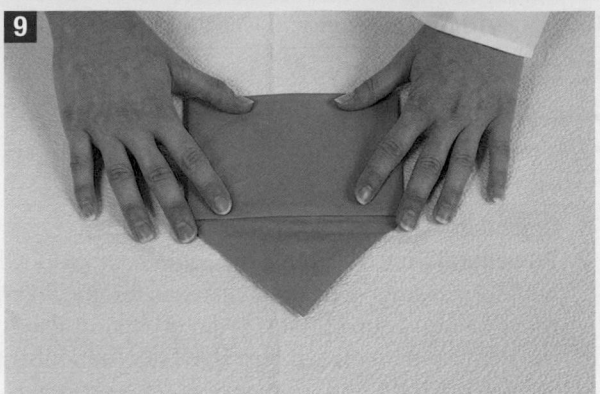

Fold the pack up from the bottom.

10. **Procedural Step.** Label the pack according to its contents. Mark the pack with the date of sterilization and your initials.
Principle. Dating the pack ensures that the most recently sterilized packs are stored in back of previously sterilized packs.

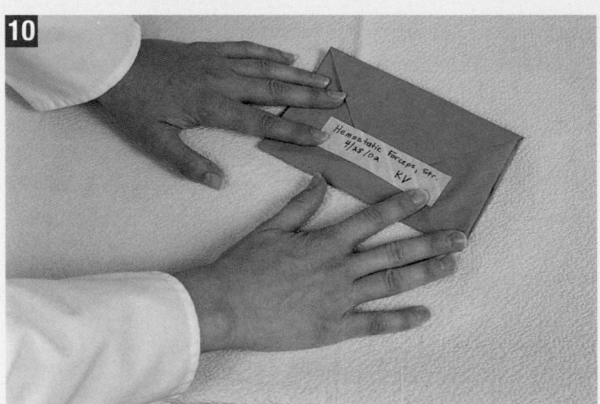

Label and date the pack. Include your initials.

PROCEDURE 18-3   Wrapping Instruments Using a Pouch

Outcome Wrap an instrument for autoclaving.

Equipment/Supplies

- Sanitized instrument
- Appropriate-sized sterilization pouch

- Permanent marker

1. **Procedural Step.** Sanitize your hands.
2. **Procedural Step.** Assemble the equipment. Select the appropriate-sized sterilization pouch for the instrument being wrapped. For hinged instruments, use a bag wide enough so the instrument can be placed in a slightly open position inside the bag.
Principle. Instruments are wrapped so they are protected from recontamination after they have been sterilized.

3. **Procedural Step.** Place the sterilization pouch on a clean, flat surface.
4. **Procedural Step.** Label the pack according to its contents. Mark the pack with the date of sterilization and your initials.
Principle. Dating the pack ensures that the most recently sterilized packs are stored in back of previously sterilized packs.

PROCEDURE **18-3** Wrapping Instruments Using a Pouch—cont'd

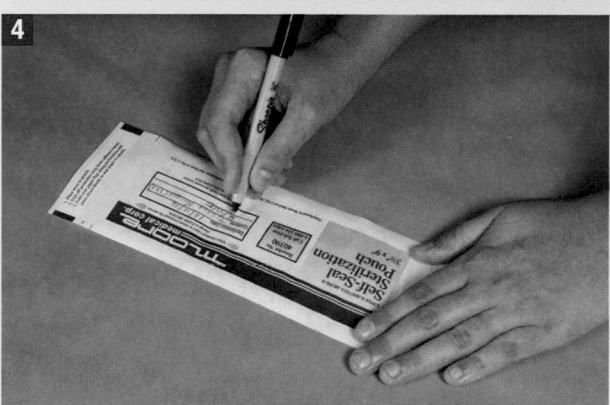

Label and date the pack. Include your initials.

5. Procedural Step. Insert the instrument to be sterilized into the unsealed, open end of the pouch. If the instrument has a movable joint, place it in the pouch in a slightly open position.

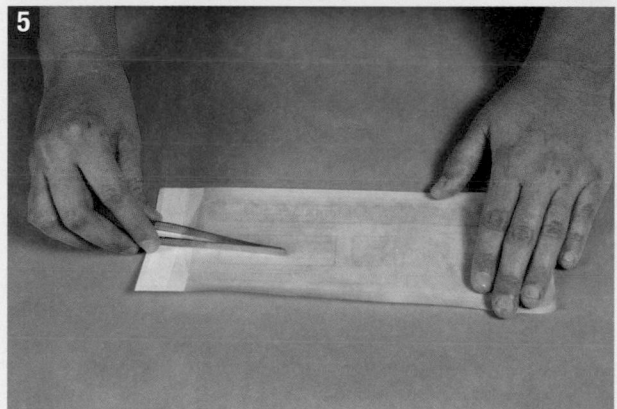

Insert the instrument into the pouch.

6. Procedural Step. Seal the open end of the pouch as follows:

Adhesive Closure. Peel off the paper strip located above the perforation to expose the adhesive. Fold along the perforation and press firmly to seal the paper to the plastic. Ensure that the seal is secure by running your fingers back and forth on both sides of the pouch over the entire sealing area.

Heat Closure. Seal the pouch using a heat-sealing device.

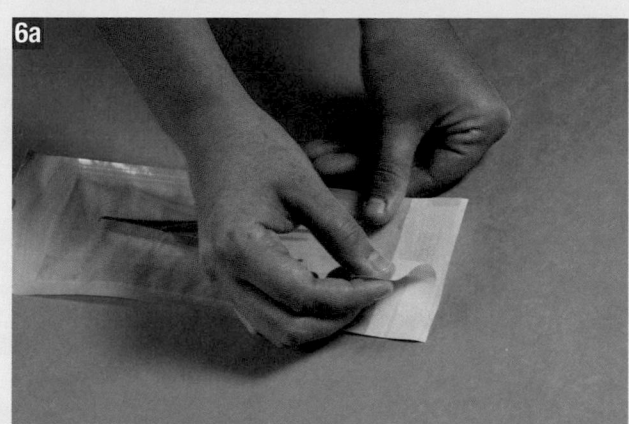

Peel off the paper strip.

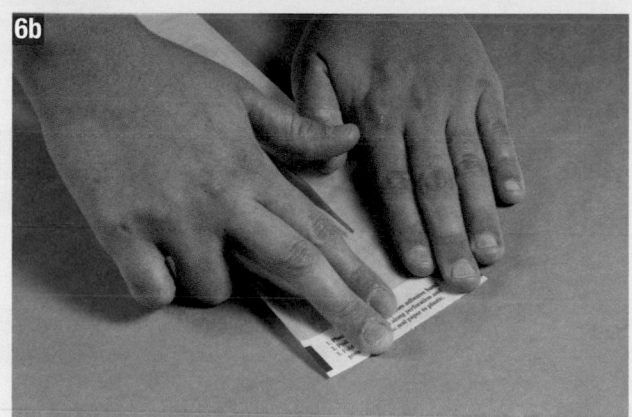

Press firmly to seal the pack.

7. Procedural Step. Sterilize the pack in the autoclave.

PROCEDURE 18-3

Operating the Autoclave

The autoclave must be operated according to the manufacturer's instructions. The medical assistant should read the operating manual carefully before running the autoclave for the first time. Thereafter, the manual should be kept in an accessible location so that it is available if needed as a reference. Procedure 18-4 outlines a general procedure for sterilizing articles in the autoclave.

The steps involved in achieving sterilization using an autoclave are known as the *autoclave cycle.* Accomplishment of each step varies based on whether the autoclave is operated manually or automatically. Figure 18-13 illustrates the autoclave cycle for manual and automatic autoclave operation.

Guidelines for Autoclave Operation

Location of the Autoclave

The autoclave must be placed on a level surface to ensure that the chamber fills correctly. The front of the autoclave should be near the front of the support surface so that water can be easily drained from the drain tube into a container when the autoclave is being flushed.

Filling the Water Reservoir

Distilled water is used to fill the water reservoir of the autoclave. Normal tap water contains minerals, such as chlorine, which have corrosive effects on the stainless-steel chamber of the autoclave. In addition, using tap water may cause a mineral buildup that can block the air exhaust valve.

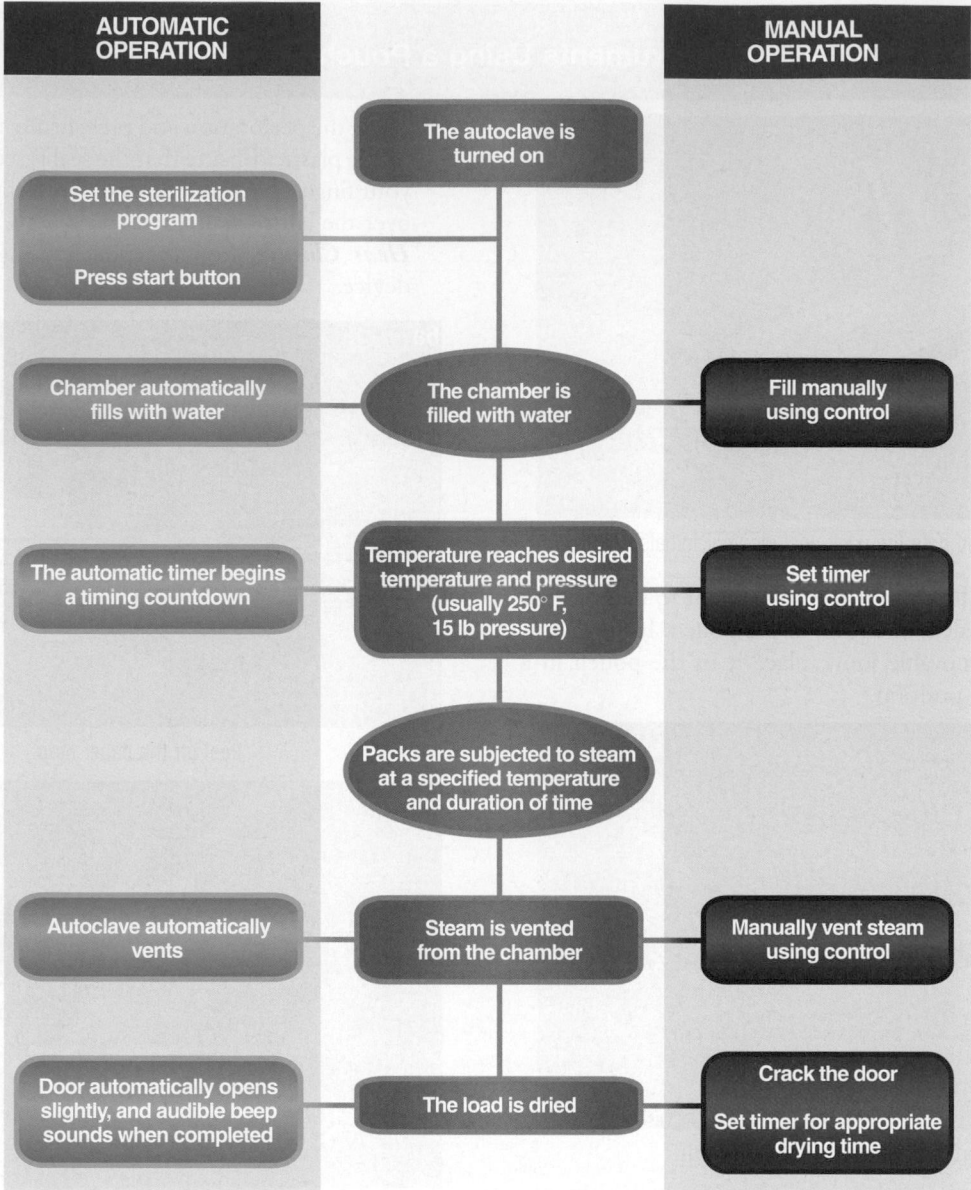

Figure 18-13 The autoclave cycle for manual and automatic operation.

This causes air pockets, which prevent the temperature from increasing in the autoclave. The water reservoir is filled to the proper level as indicated in the operating manual. An autoclave malfunction may occur if the reservoir is overfilled or if there is not enough water in the reservoir.

Loading the Autoclave

For an item to attain sterility, steam must penetrate every fiber and reach every surface of the item at a required temperature and for a specified time. To accomplish this, all packs must be positioned in the chamber to allow free circulation and penetration of steam. The following guidelines should be followed when loading the autoclave:

1. Small packs are best because steam penetrates them more easily; it takes longer for steam to reach the center of a large pack to ensure sterilization. A pack should be no larger than $12 \times 12 \times 20$ inches.

2. To allow for proper steam penetration, the packs should be packed as loosely as possible inside the autoclave, with approximately 1 to 3 inches between small packs and 2 to 4 inches between large packs. Packs should not be allowed to touch surrounding walls, and at least 1 inch should separate the autoclave trays. Placing the articles too close together retards the flow of steam (Figure 18-14).

3. Jars and glassware should be placed on their sides in the autoclave with their lids removed. If they are placed upright, air may be trapped in them, and they would not be sterilized. Trapped air must flow out and be replaced by steam during the sterilization process (Figure 18-15).

4. Packs that contain layers of fabric, such as dressings, should be placed in a vertical position. Because steam

Wrong method   Right method

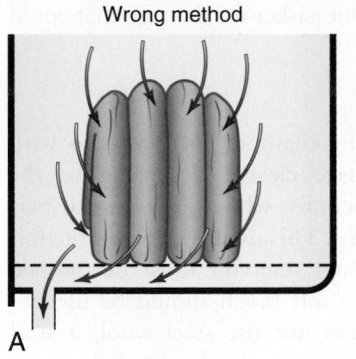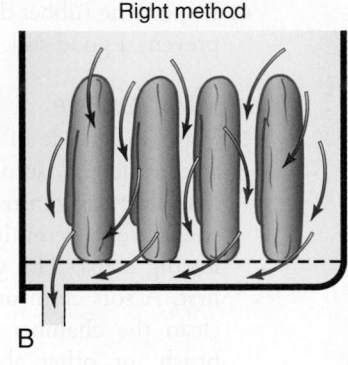

A   B

Figure 18-14 Arrangement of packs in the autoclave. **A,** Improper arrangement of packs in the autoclave. This arrangement prevents adequate penetration of steam, resulting in failure to sterilize the portions in the center of the mass. **B,** Proper arrangement of packs in the autoclave. The packs are separated from each other, and steam can now permeate each pack quickly and in the much shorter period of exposure needed.

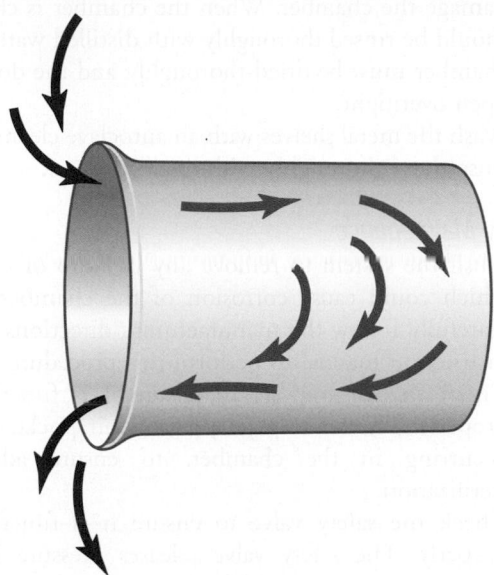

Figure 18-15 Jars and glassware should be placed on their sides in the autoclave with their lids removed.

Table 18-2 Minimum Sterilizing Times

Items (Manual Operation)*	Program (Automatic Operation)†	Time (Min at 250° F [121° C])
Unwrapped nonsurgical instruments	Unwrapped	15
Open glass or metal canisters		
Nonsurgical rubber tubing		
Wrapped instruments	Wrapped	20
Fabric or muslin		
Wrapped trays of loose instruments		
Rubber tubing		
Minor office surgery tray setup (wrapped)	Packs	30
Liquids or gels	Liquids	30

From Bonewit-West K: *Clinical procedures for medical assistants*, ed 8, St Louis, 2011, Saunders.
*Manual operation: The sterilizing time is selected on the basis of the items being sterilized, as indicated in this column. The sterilizing time is set by using the manual timing control when the autoclave has reached a temperature of 250° F (121° C).
†Automatic operation: The sterilization program selected from this column is based on the item being autoclaved. This program is selected by pressing the appropriate program button on the front of the autoclave (i.e., unwrapped, wrapped, packs, liquids). The autoclave automatically begins the proper timing countdown when it reaches 250° F (121° C).

flows from top to bottom, this method allows the steam to penetrate the layers of fabric.

5. Sterilization pouches should be positioned on their sides to maximize steam circulation and to facilitate the drying process. Pouches can also be placed on the autoclave tray with the paper side up and the plastic side down.

Timing the Load

The autoclave is operated at approximately 15 psi with a temperature of 250° F (121° C). The length of time required for sterilization varies according to the item that is being sterilized (Table 18-2). Steam can easily reach the surfaces of hard, nonporous items such as unwrapped instruments (e.g., vaginal specula) to kill microorganisms; these items require approximately 15 minutes of sterilization time. A large minor office surgery pack requires a longer sterilization time, about 30 minutes, because more time is needed for steam to penetrate to the center of the pack. Rubber goods may be damaged, however, by exposure to excessive heat. To prevent this, the medical assistant should sterilize rubber items for only the prescribed length of time.

The sterilizing time should not begin until the desired temperature in the autoclave has been reached. Timing the load is accomplished automatically or manually. Autoclaves with automatic operation begin timing the load automatically when the desired temperature has been reached. With the manual method of operation, the medical assistant must set the timer by hand using a timing control on the front of the autoclave. The medical assistant should not set the timer until the temperature gauge reaches the desired temperature. The articles in the load are not considered sterile unless they have been subjected to steam for the proper length of time at the proper temperature.

Drying the Load

The sterilized articles are moist and must be allowed to dry before they are removed from the autoclave. Microorganisms can move quickly through the moisture on a wet wrap and onto the sterile article inside, resulting in contamination.

When the load has been subjected to steam for the proper length of time and temperature, the chamber must be vented of steam. Venting the chamber permits the pressure in the autoclave to decrease to zero and the chamber to cool, making it safe for the door to be opened. Most autoclaves are designed to vent automatically, which eliminates having to vent them manually.

The door of the autoclave should be opened approximately $\frac{1}{2}$ inch but no more than 1 inch. Opening the door more than 1 inch causes cold air from the outside to rush into the autoclave, resulting in condensation of water on the packs. Cracking the door allows the moisture on the articles to change from a liquid to a vapor and to escape through the crack. The residual heat in the inner chamber also helps to dry the articles. The load should be allowed to dry for 15 to 60 minutes, depending on the type of autoclave and the load. Loads that contain large packs require a longer drying time than loads with smaller packs. The medical assistant should follow the manufacturer's recommendations for proper drying times of various loads.

Handling and Storing Packs

Sterilized wrapped articles should be handled carefully and as little as possible. If a wrapped article is crushed, compressed, or dropped, the sterility of the contents cannot be assumed, and the pack must be resterilized. This is known as *event-related sterility,* meaning that a sterile pack is considered sterile indefinitely, unless an event occurs that interferes with the sterility of the article.

Sterilized packs should be stored in clean, dry areas that are free from dust, insects, and other sources of contamination. Wrapped articles should be stored with the most recently sterilized articles placed in the back. The medical assistant should thoroughly check each sterilized pack at least twice: before storing it and before using it. If the pack is torn or opened, or if it is wet, it is no longer sterile and must be rewrapped and resterilized.

Maintaining the Autoclave

For the autoclave to work efficiently, it must be maintained properly. The operating manual that accompanies the autoclave provides specific information for the care and maintenance of that type of autoclave.

Safety precautions should be followed when performing maintenance procedures. Before proceeding with preventive maintenance, the autoclave must be cool, the pressure gauge at zero, and the power cord disconnected from the wall socket. Autoclave maintenance is performed on a daily, weekly, and monthly basis as follows.

Daily Maintenance

1. Wipe the outside of the autoclave with a damp cloth and a mild detergent.
2. Wipe the interior of the autoclave and the trays with a damp cloth.
3. Clean the rubber gasket on the door of the autoclave with a damp cloth.

4. Inspect the rubber door gasket for damage that could prevent a good seal.

Weekly Maintenance

1. Wash the inside of the chamber and the trays with a commercial autoclave cleaner according to the manufacturer's instructions, while observing all personal safety precautions. This usually involves the following steps: The water reservoir must be drained first. A soft cloth or a soft brush should be used to clean the chamber. Do not use steel wool, a steel brush, or other abrasive agents because they can damage the chamber. When the chamber is clean, it should be rinsed thoroughly with distilled water. The chamber must be dried thoroughly and the door left open overnight.
2. Wash the metal shelves with an autoclave cleaner, and rinse them thoroughly with distilled water.

Monthly Maintenance

1. Flush the system to remove any buildup of residue, which could cause corrosion of the chamber lines. Carefully follow the manufacturer's directions in the instruction manual to perform this procedure.
2. Check the air trap jet to ensure it is functioning properly. The air trap jet prevents air pockets from occurring in the chamber, to ensure adequate sterilization.
3. Check the safety valve to ensure it is functioning properly. The safety valve releases pressure in the chamber if it gets too high.

Other Sterilization Methods

In addition to the autoclave, other methods can be used to sterilize articles. These methods are not generally used in the medical office and are discussed only briefly in this chapter.

Dry Heat Oven

Dry heat ovens are used to sterilize articles that cannot be penetrated by steam or may be damaged by it. Dry heat is less corrosive than moist heat for instruments with sharp edges; it does not dull their sharp edges. Oil, petroleum jelly, and powder cannot be penetrated by steam and must be sterilized in a dry heat oven. Moist heat sterilization tends to erode the ground-glass surfaces of reusable syringes, whereas dry heat does not.

Dry heat ovens operate similarly to ordinary cooking ovens. A longer exposure period is needed with dry heat because microorganisms and spores are more resistant to dry heat than to moist heat and because dry heat penetrates more slowly and unevenly than moist heat. The most commonly used temperature for dry heat sterilization is 320° F (160° C) for 1 to 2 hours, depending on the article being sterilized. The recommended wrapping material for dry heat sterilization is aluminum foil because it is a good conductor of heat, and it protects against recontamination during handling and storage. Dry heat sterilization indicators are available to determine the effectiveness of the sterilization process.

Ethylene Oxide Gas Sterilization

Ethylene oxide is a colorless gas that is toxic and flammable. It is used to sterilize heat-sensitive items that cannot be sterilized in an autoclave. After items are sterilized with this gas, they must be aerated to remove the toxic residue of the ethylene oxide.

Ethylene oxide sterilization is a more complex and expensive process than steam sterilization. It frequently is used in the medical manufacturing industry for producing prepackaged, presterilized disposable items, such as syringes, sutures, catheters, and surgical packs.

Cold Sterilization

Cold sterilization involves the use of a chemical agent for an extended length of time. Only chemicals that are designated *sterilants* by the U.S. Environmental Protection Agency (EPA) can be used for sterilizing articles. If a chemical agent holds this status, the word *sterilant* is printed on the front of the container.

The item to be sterilized must be completely submerged in the chemical for a long time (6 to 24 hours depending on the manufacturer's instructions). Prolonged immersion of instruments can damage them. In addition, each time an instrument is added to the instrument container, the clock must be restarted for the entire amount of time. For these reasons, and because this method involves the use of a hazardous chemical, cold sterilization should be used only when an autoclave, gas, or a dry heat oven is not indicated or is unavailable.

Radiation

Radiation uses high-energy ionizing radiation to sterilize articles. Medical manufacturers use radiation to sterilize prepackaged surgical equipment and instruments that cannot be sterilized by heat or chemicals.

PROCEDURE 18-4

PROCEDURE 18-4 Sterilizing Articles in the Autoclave

Outcome Sterilize a load of contaminated articles in the autoclave.

Equipment/Supplies

- Autoclave and instruction manual
- Distilled water
- Wrapped articles
- Heat-resistant gloves

1. **Procedural Step.** Assemble the equipment.
2. **Procedural Step.** Check the level of water in the autoclave and add distilled water, if needed.

   Principle. Water contained in the water reservoir of the autoclave is converted to steam during the sterilization process. Distilled water is used to prevent corrosion of the stainless-steel chamber of the autoclave.

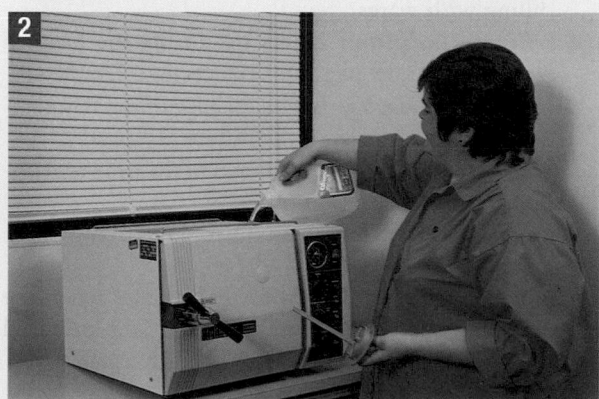

If needed, add distilled water to the autoclave.

3. **Procedural Step.** Properly load the autoclave while following these guidelines:
   a. Do not overload the chamber. Small packs should be placed 1 to 3 inches apart, and large packs should be placed 2 to 4 inches apart. The packs should not touch the chamber walls.

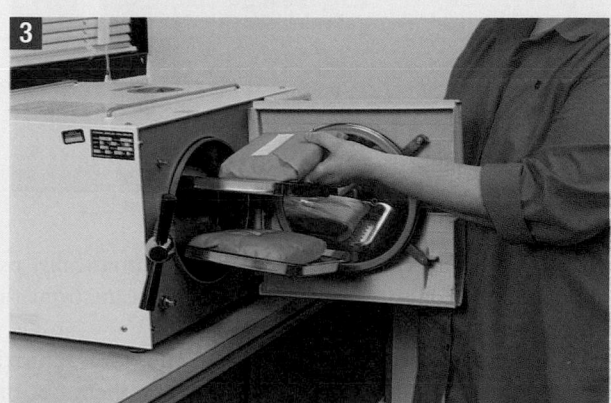

Properly load the autoclave.

Continued

b. Ensure that at least 1 inch separates the autoclave trays.

c. Place jars and glassware on their sides.

d. Place dressings in a vertical position.

e. When sterilizing dressings and hard goods together, place dressings on the top shelf and hard goods on the lower shelf.

f. When using sterilization pouches, set the pouches on their sides to maximize steam circulation and to facilitate drying.

Principle. The autoclave must be loaded properly to ensure adequate steam penetration of all articles.

4. Procedural Step. Operate the autoclave according to the procedure described in the instruction manual. A general procedure for the manual and the automatic methods of operation follows.

Manually Operated Autoclave

a. Determine the sterilizing time for the types of articles being autoclaved (see Table 18-2).

b. Turn on the autoclave.

c. Fill the chamber with water using the appropriate control.

d. Securely close and latch the door of the autoclave.

e. Set the timing control when the temperature gauge reaches the desired temperature (usually 250° F [121° C]). At the end of the steam exposure time, an indicator light usually comes on, or a beeper sounds.

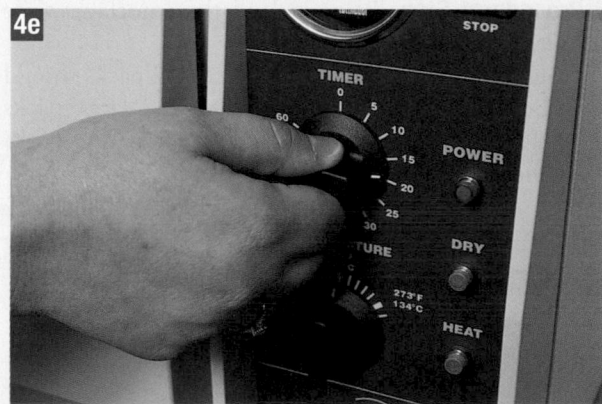

Set the timing control.

f. If the autoclave does not vent automatically, use the appropriate control to release steam from the chamber.

g. Dry the load by cracking open the door approximately ½ inch but no more than 1 inch. Set the drying time using the timing control. The drying

time varies between 15 and 60 minutes, depending on the autoclave and the type of load.

Principle. To ensure sterilization, the load should not be timed until the proper temperature has been reached. The sterility of wrapped packs cannot be ensured unless the wrapped articles are allowed to dry fully. Microorganisms can move through the moisture on a wet wrap and contaminate the sterile article inside.

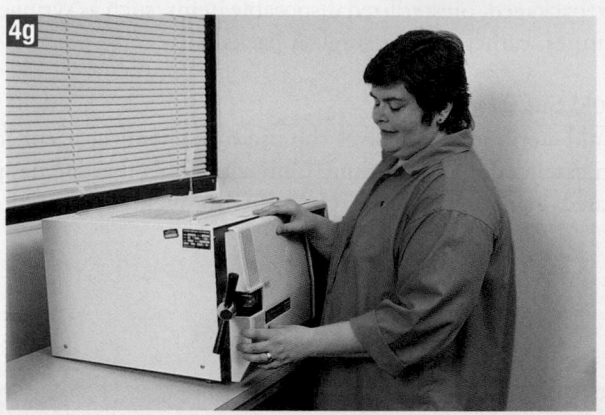

Crack the door to dry the load.

Automatically Operated Autoclave

a. Securely close and latch the door of the autoclave.

b. Turn on the autoclave.

c. Determine the sterilization program according to what is being autoclaved (see Table 18-2). Press the appropriate program button on the front of the autoclave to select the program. Press the start button.

d. Indicators on the front of the autoclave tell you what is happening (automatically) in the autoclave:

Filling Indicator. Lights up when the chamber is filling with water

Sterilizing Indicator. Lights up during the heat-up and sterilization phases of the cycle

Temperature Display. Digital display of the temperature in the autoclave

Time Display. Digital countdown of the time remaining in the sterilization program

Drying Indicator. Lights up during the drying phase of the cycle

Complete or Ready Indicator. Illuminates when the autoclave has completed the cycle and sterilized articles can be removed from the autoclave

PROCEDURE 18-4 Sterilizing Articles in the Autoclave—cont'd

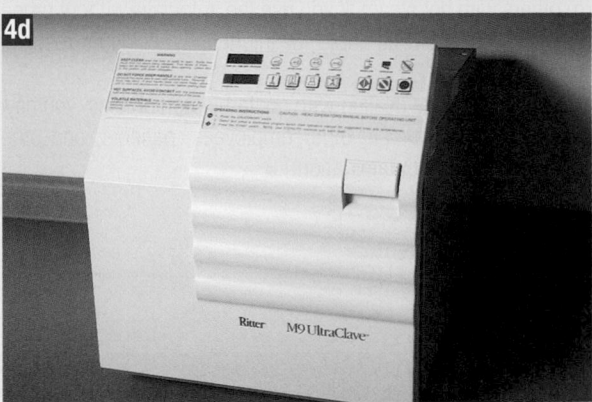

Automatic autoclave buttons and indicators.

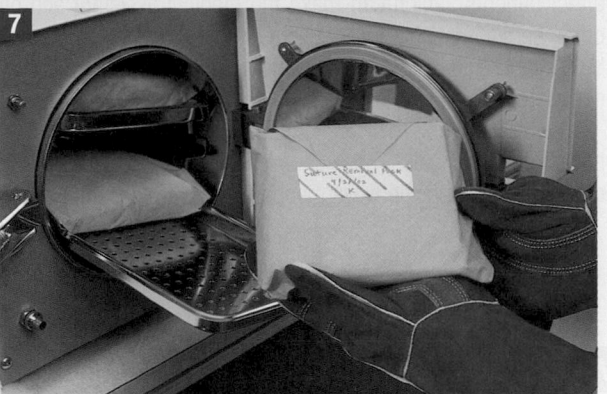

Check the sterilization indicator on the outside of the pack.

5. Procedural Step. Turn off the autoclave. Wearing heat-resistant gloves, remove the load. Do not touch the inner chamber of the autoclave with your bare hands.
Principle. Heat-resistant gloves protect the medical assistant's hands when the warm packs from the chamber of the autoclave are being removed. The inner chamber of the autoclave is hot and could burn bare skin

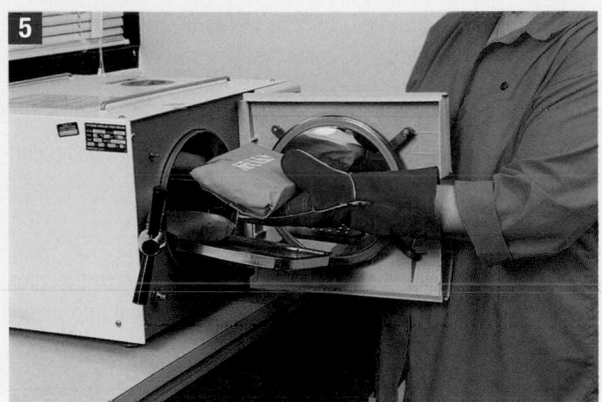

Remove the load with heat-resistant gloves.

6. Procedural Step. Inspect the packs as you take them out of the autoclave. If the packs show any damage, such as holes or tears, the articles should be rewrapped and resterilized.

7. Procedural Step. Check the sterilization indicators located on the outside of the pack to ensure the proper response has occurred.
Principle. Autoclave tape indicates only that the article has been through the autoclave cycle; it does not ensure that sterilization has taken place. Sterilization is confirmed when the pack is opened for use and the sterilization strip indicator in the center of the pack is checked for its proper response.

8. Procedural Step. Record monitoring information in the autoclave log. Include the date and time of the cycle, a description of the load, and the exposure time and temperature. If a biologic indicator has been included in the load, process it according to the medical office policy, and record results on the autoclave log.

9. Procedural Step. Store the packs in a clean, dustproof area with the most recently sterilized packs placed behind previously sterilized packs.

10. Procedural Step. Maintain appropriate daily care of the autoclave, while following the manufacturer's recommendations. Daily care of the autoclave includes the following:
a. Wipe the outside of the autoclave with a damp cloth and a mild detergent.
b. Wipe the interior of the autoclave and the trays with a damp cloth.
c. Clean the rubber gasket located on the door of the autoclave with a damp cloth.
d. Inspect the rubber door gasket for damage that could prevent a good seal.
Principle. For the autoclave to work efficiently, it must be properly maintained.

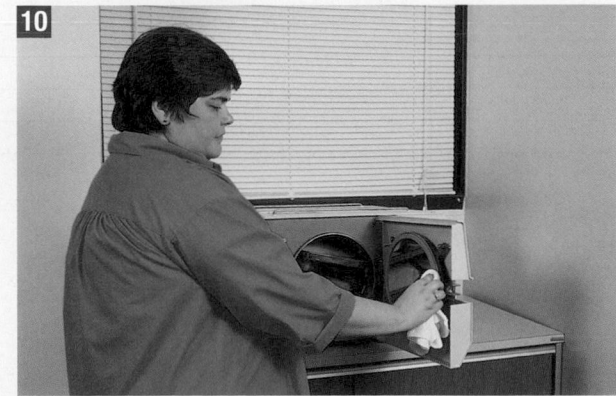

Clean the rubber gasket with a damp cloth.

MEDICAL PRACTICE *and the* LAW

If not performed properly, sterilization and disinfection can adversely affect patients, which can make the medical assistant and other office personnel liable for resultant injuries. Meticulous care must be taken to ensure that all procedures are performed correctly and completely.

Sterilization and disinfection procedures include the use of hazardous chemicals. These chemicals must be stored, used, and disposed of in specific ways mandated by law. The autoclave can be a dangerous machine if it is not used correctly, and it could harm others with hot steam. If you use the autoclave without proper instruction, you could be liable for injuries or accidents resulting from misuse.

Whenever you are dealing with contaminated articles, you have a duty to protect yourself, other employees, patients, and other articles from cross-contamination. ■

What Would You Do? What Would You *Not* Do? RESPONSES

Case Study 1
Page 270

What Did Kara Do?

❑ Complimented Mrs. Cordera for her concern and efforts to baby-proof her home.
❑ Gave Mrs. Cordera a patient information brochure on baby-proofing the home.
❑ Told Mrs. Cordera that she should assume that all cleaning products are poisonous. Got out a disinfectant container and showed Mrs. Cordera the information on the label that tells what to do in case of an accidental poisoning.
❑ Gave the National Poison Control hotline number (1-800-222-1222) to Mrs. Cordera and told her that was the fastest way to obtain information on what to do in case of an accidental poisoning. Told her to keep this number by her phone.

What Did Kara Not Do?

❑ Did not take Mrs. Cordera's question lightly.

What Would You Do/What Would You Not Do?
Review Kara's response and place a checkmark next to the information you included in your response. List additional information you included in your response.

_____
_____
_____
_____
_____
_____

Case Study 2
Page 280

What Did Kara Do?

❑ Explained to Mrs. Scout that toys are in the waiting room for children to play with to make their visit more comfortable and less stressful.
❑ Reassured Mrs. Scout that the medical office personnel do everything they can to prevent the spread of germs in the office and that the toys are sanitized every day.
❑ Relayed to Mrs. Scout that only toys that can be sanitized are kept in the medical office.
❑ Told Mrs. Scout that her concern would be brought up at the weekly office meeting.

What Did Kara Not Do?

❑ Did not get defensive because Mrs. Scout was just being concerned about her child's health.

What Would You Do/What Would You Not Do?
Review Kara's response and place a checkmark next to the information you included in your response. List additional information you included in your response.

_____
_____
_____
_____
_____

What Would You Do? What Would You *Not* Do? RESPONSES—cont'd

Case Study 3
Page 281

What Did Kara Do?
❑ Told Cassie through verbal and nonverbal behavior that her concern was valid.
❑ Told Cassie that hepatitis can be transmitted through dirty instruments.
❑ Reassured Cassie that all instruments are sterilized in the autoclave, which has special indicators to ensure all germs have been killed.
❑ Gave Cassie a patient information brochure on hepatitis. Told her that individuals with chronic hepatitis can develop liver cancer and that the best way to avoid hepatitis is through measures and behaviors recommended for prevention.
❑ Told Cassie that a vaccine is available to prevent hepatitis B, but not hepatitis C.

What Did Kara Not Do?
❑ Did not dismiss her concern about dirty instruments as unimportant.
❑ Did not overly alarm her about the consequences of chronic hepatitis.

What Would You Do/What Would You Not Do?
Review Kara's response and place a checkmark next to the information you included in your response. List additional information you included in your response.

_____
_____
_____
_____
_____
_____
_____

TERMINOLOGY REVIEW

Antiseptic A substance that kills disease-producing microorganisms but not their spores. An antiseptic is usually applied to living tissue.

Autoclave An apparatus for the sterilization of materials, using steam under pressure.

Contaminate To soil, stain, or pollute; to make impure.

Critical item An item that comes in contact with sterile tissue or the vascular system.

Decontamination The use of physical or chemical means to remove or destroy pathogens on an item so that it is no longer capable of transmitting disease; this makes the item safe to handle.

Detergent An agent that cleanses by emulsifying dirt and oil.

Disinfectant An agent used to destroy pathogenic microorganisms but not their spores. Disinfectants are usually applied to inanimate objects.

Hazardous chemical Any chemical that presents a threat to the health and safety of an individual coming into contact with it.

Incubate To provide proper conditions for growth and development.

Load The articles that are being sterilized.

Material safety data sheet (MSDS) A sheet that provides information regarding a chemical, its hazards, and measures to take to prevent injury and illness when handling the chemical.

Noncritical item An item that comes into contact with intact skin, but not with mucous membranes.

Sanitization A process to remove organic matter from an article and to reduce the number of microorganisms to a safe level as determined by public health requirements.

Semicritical item An item that comes into contact with nonintact skin or intact mucous membranes.

Spore A hard, thick-walled capsule formed by some bacteria that contains only the essential parts of the protoplasm of the bacterial cell.

Sterilization The process of destroying all forms of microbial life, including bacterial spores.

Thermolabile Easily affected or changed by heat.

ON THE WEB

For information on infection control in the health care setting:

Centers for Disease Control and Prevention: www.cdc.gov

Environmental Protection Agency: www.epa.gov

National Institute of Environmental Health Sciences: www.niehs.nih.gov

National Institute for Occupational Safety and Health: www.cdc.gov/niosh

Infection Control Today: www.infectioncontroltoday.com

Association for Professionals in Infection Control and Epidemiology: www.apic.com

To locate a material safety data sheet:

MSDS-Search: www.msdssearch.com

HazCom: www.hazard.com/msds

 Check out the Evolve site at http://evolve.elsevier.com/Bonewit/today/ to actively Prepare for your Certification, and to access additional interactive activities and exercises to help you study and prepare for success.

19

Vital Signs

LEARNING OBJECTIVES	PROCEDURES

Temperature

1. Define a *vital sign*.
2. Explain the reasons for taking vital signs.
3. Explain how body temperature is maintained.
4. List examples of how heat is produced in the body.
5. List examples of how heat is lost from the body.
6. State the normal body temperature range and the average body temperature.
7. List and explain factors that can cause variation in the body temperature.
8. List and describe the three stages of a fever.
9. List the sites for taking body temperature, and explain why these sites are used.

Measure oral body temperature.
Measure axillary body temperature.
Measure rectal body temperature.
Measure aural body temperature.
Measure temporal artery body temperature.

Pulse

10. Explain the mechanism of pulse.
11. List and explain the factors that affect the pulse rate.
12. Identify a specific use for each of the eight pulse sites.
13. State the normal range of pulse rate for each age group.
14. Explain the difference between pulse rhythm and pulse volume.

Measure radial pulse.
Measure apical pulse.

Respiration

15. Explain the purpose of respiration.
16. State what occurs during inhalation and exhalation.
17. State the normal respiratory rate for each age group.
18. List and explain the factors that affect the respiratory rate.
19. Explain the difference between rhythm and depth of respiration.
20. Describe the character of each of the following abnormal breath sounds: crackles, rhonchi, wheezes, and pleural friction rub.

Measure respiration.

Pulse Oximetry

21. Explain the purpose of pulse oximetry.
22. State the normal oxygen saturation level of a healthy individual.
23. List and describe the functions of the controls, indicators, and displays on a pulse oximeter.
24. Describe the difference between a reusable and a disposable oximeter probe.
25. List and describe factors that may interfere with an accurate pulse oximetry reading.

Perform pulse oximetry.

Blood Pressure

26. Define blood pressure.
27. State the normal range of blood pressure for an adult.
28. List and describe factors that affect the blood pressure.
29. Identify the different parts of a stethoscope and a sphygmomanometer.
30. Identify the Korotkoff sounds.
31. State the advantages and disadvantages of an automated oscillometric blood pressure device.
32. Explain how to prevent errors in blood pressure measurement.

Measure blood pressure.
Determine systolic pressure by palpation.

CHAPTER OUTLINE

KEY TERMS

adventitious (ad-ven-TISH-us) sounds
afebrile (uh-FEB-ril)
alveolus (al-VEE-oh-lus)
antecubital (AN-tih-CYOO-bi-tul) space
antipyretic (AN-tih-pye-REH-tik)
aorta (ay-OR-tuh)
apical-radial pulse
apnea (AP-nee-uh)
axilla (aks-ILL-uh)
bounding pulse
bradycardia (BRAY-dee-CAR-dee-uh)
bradypnea (BRAY-dip-NEE-uh)
Celsius (SELL-see-us) scale
conduction (kon-DUK-shun)
convection (kon-VEK-shun)
crisis
cyanosis (sye-an-OH-sus)
diastole (dye-AS-toh-lee)
diastolic (DYE-uh-STOL-ik) pressure
dyspnea (DISP-nee-uh)
dysrhythmia (dis-RITH-mee-uh)

eupnea (YOOP-nee-uh)
exhalation (EKS-hal-AY-shun)
Fahrenheit (FAIR-en-hite) scale
febrile (FEH-bril)
fever
frenulum linguae (FREN-yoo-lum
   LIN-gway)
hyperpnea (HYE-perp-NEE-uh)
hyperpyrexia (HYE-per-pye-REK-see-uh)
hypertension (HYE-per-TEN-shun)
hyperventilation (HYE-per-ven-til-AY-shun)
hypopnea (hye-POP-nee-uh)
hypotension (HYE-poe-TEN-shun)
hypothermia (HYE-poe-THER-mee-uh)
hypoxemia (hye-pok-SEE-mee-uh)
hypoxia (hye-POKS-ee-uh)
inhalation (IN-hal-AY-shun)
intercostal (IN-ter-KOS-tul)
Korotkoff (kuh-ROT-kof) sounds
malaise (mal-AYZE)
manometer (man-OM-uh-ter)

meniscus (men-IS-kus)
orthopnea (orth-OP-nee-uh)
pulse deficit
pulse oximeter
pulse oximetry
pulse pressure
pulse rhythm
pulse volume
radiation (RAY-dee-AY-shun)
SaO2
sphygmomanometer
   (SFIG-moe-man-OM-uh-ter)
SpO2
stethoscope (STETH-uh-skope)
systole (SIS-toh-lee)
systolic (sis-TOL-ik) pressure
tachycardia (TAK-ih-KAR-dee-uh)
tachypnea (TAK-ip-NEE-uh)
threadypulse

INTRODUCTION TO VITAL SIGNS

Vital signs are objective guideposts that provide data to determine a person's state of health. Vital signs include temperature, pulse, respiration (collectively called TPR), and blood pressure (BP). Another indicator of a patient's health status is pulse oximetry. Although some physicians order this measurement routinely on all patients as part of the patient workup, most physicians order this vital sign only when the patient complains of respiratory problems (e.g., shortness of breath).

The normal ranges of the vital signs are finely adjusted, and any deviation from normal may indicate disease. During the course of an illness, variations in the vital signs may occur. The medical assistant should be alert to any significant changes and report them to the physician because they indicate a change in the patient's condition. When patients visit the medical office, vital signs are routinely checked to establish each patient's usual state of health and to establish baseline measurements against which future measurements can be compared. The medical assistant should have a thorough knowledge of the vital signs and should attain proficiency in taking them to ensure accurate findings.

General guidelines that the medical assistant should follow when measuring the vital signs are as follows:

1. Be familiar with the normal ranges for all vital signs. Keep in mind that normal ranges vary based on the different age groups (infant, child, adult, elder).
2. Make sure that all equipment for measuring vital signs is in proper working condition to ensure accurate findings.
3. Eliminate or minimize factors that affect the vital signs, such as exercise, food and beverage consumption, smoking, and emotional state.
4. Use an organized approach when measuring the vital signs. If all of the vital signs are ordered, they are usually measured starting with temperature, followed by pulse, respiration, blood pressure, and pulse oximetry.

TEMPERATURE

Regulation of Body Temperature

Body temperature is maintained within a fairly constant range by the hypothalamus, which is located in the brain. The hypothalamus functions as the body's thermostat. It normally allows the body temperature to vary by only about 1° to 2° Fahrenheit (F) throughout the day.

Body temperature is maintained through a balance of the heat produced in the body and the heat lost from the body (Figure 19-1). A constant temperature range must be maintained for the body to function properly. When minor changes in the temperature of the body occur, the hypothalamus senses this and makes adjustments as necessary to ensure that the body temperature stays within a normal and safe range. If an individual is playing tennis on a hot day, the body's heat-cooling mechanism is activated to remove excess heat from the body through perspiration.

Heat Production

Most of the heat produced in the body is through voluntary and involuntary muscle contractions. Voluntary muscle contractions involve the muscles over which a person has control, for example, the moving of legs or arms. Involuntary muscle contractions involve the muscles over which a person has no control; examples are physiologic processes such as digestion, the beating of the heart, and shivering.

Body heat also is produced by cell metabolism. Heat is produced when nutrients are broken down in the cells. Fever and strong emotional states also can increase heat production in the body.

Heat Loss

Heat is lost from the body through the urine and feces and in water vapor from the lungs. Perspiration also contributes to heat loss. Perspiration is the excretion of moisture through the pores of the skin. When the moisture evaporates, heat is released and the body is cooled.

Radiation, conduction, and convection all cause loss of heat from the body. **Radiation** is the transfer of heat in the form of waves; body heat is continually radiating into cooler surroundings. **Conduction** is the transfer of heat from one object to another by direct contact; heat can be transferred by conduction from the body to a cooler object it touches. **Convection** is the transfer of heat through air currents; cool air currents can cause the body to lose heat. These processes are illustrated in Figure 19-2.

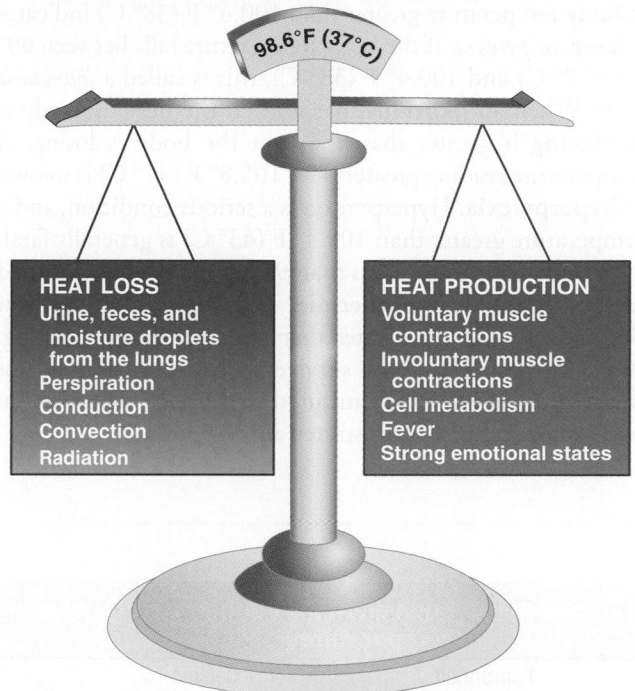

Figure 19-1 Body temperature represents a balance between the heat produced in the body and the heat lost from the body.

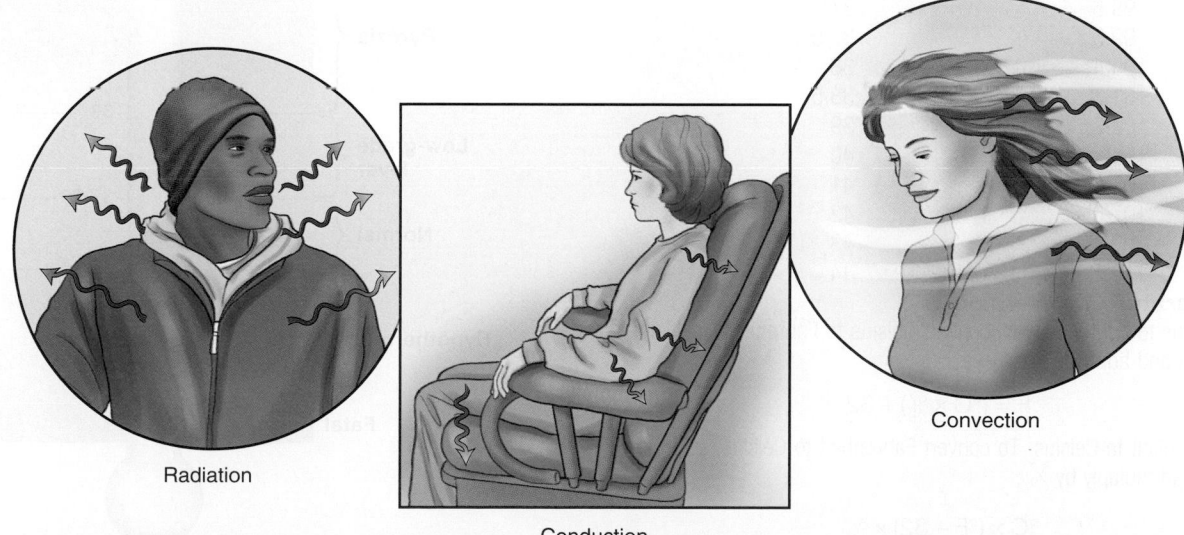

Figure 19-2 Heat loss from the body. With **radiation,** the body gives off heat in the form of waves to the cooler outside air. With **conduction,** the chair becomes warm as heat is transferred from the individual to the chair. With **convection,** air currents move heat away from the body.

Body Temperature Range

The purposes of measuring body temperature are to establish the patient's baseline temperature and to monitor an abnormally high or low body temperature. The normal body temperature range is 97° F to 99° F (36.1° C to 37.2° C), the average temperature being 98.6° F (37° C). Body temperature is usually recorded using the Fahrenheit system of measurement. Table 19-1 lists comparable **Fahrenheit** and **Celsius** temperatures and explains how to convert temperatures from one scale to the other.

Alterations in Body Temperature

A body temperature greater than 100.4° F (38° C) indicates a **fever,** or *pyrexia*. If the body temperature falls between 99° F (37.2° C) and 100.4° F (38° C), this is called a *low-grade fever*. When an individual has a fever, the heat the body is producing is greater than the heat the body is losing. A temperature reading greater than 105.8° F (41° C) is known as **hyperpyrexia.** Hyperpyrexia is a serious condition, and a temperature greater than 109.4° F (43° C) is generally fatal.

A body temperature less than 97° F (36.1° C) is classified as subnormal, or **hypothermia.** This means that the heat the body is losing is greater than the heat it is producing. A person usually cannot survive with a temperature less than 93.2° F (34° C). Terms used to describe alterations in body temperature are illustrated in Figure 19-3.

Variations in Body Temperature

During the day-to-day activities of an individual, normal fluctuations occur in the body temperature. The body temperature rarely stays the same throughout the course of a day. The medical assistant should take the following points into consideration when evaluating a patient's temperature.

1. **Age.** Infants and young children normally have a higher body temperature than adults because their thermoregulatory system is not yet fully established. Elderly individuals usually have a lower body temperature owing to factors such as loss of subcutaneous fat, lack of exercise, and loss of thermoregulatory control. Table 19-2 shows the normal ranges of body temperature according to age group.
2. **Diurnal variations.** During sleep, body metabolism slows down, as do muscle contractions. The body's temperature is lowest in the morning before metabolism and muscle contractions begin increasing.
3. **Emotional states.** Strong emotions, such as crying and extreme anger, can increase the body temperature. This is important to consider when working with young children, who frequently cry during examination procedures or when they are ill.
4. **Environment.** Cold weather tends to decrease the body temperature, whereas hot weather increases it.

Table 19-1 Equivalent Fahrenheit and Celsius Temperatures	
Fahrenheit	**Celsius**
93.2	34
95	35
96.8	36
97.7	36.5
98.6	37
99.5	37.5
100.4	38
101.3	38.5
102.2	39
104	40
105.8	41
107.6	42
109.4	43
111.2	44

Temperature Conversion

1. Celsius to Fahrenheit: To convert Celsius to Fahrenheit, multiply by $\frac{9}{5}$ and add 32:

$$°F = (°C \times \tfrac{9}{5}) + 32$$

2. Fahrenheit to Celsius: To convert Fahrenheit to Celsius, subtract 32 and multiply by $\frac{5}{9}$:

$$°C \times (°F - 32) \times \tfrac{5}{9}$$

From Bonewit-West K: *Clinical procedures for medical assistants*, ed 8, St Louis, 2011, Saunders.

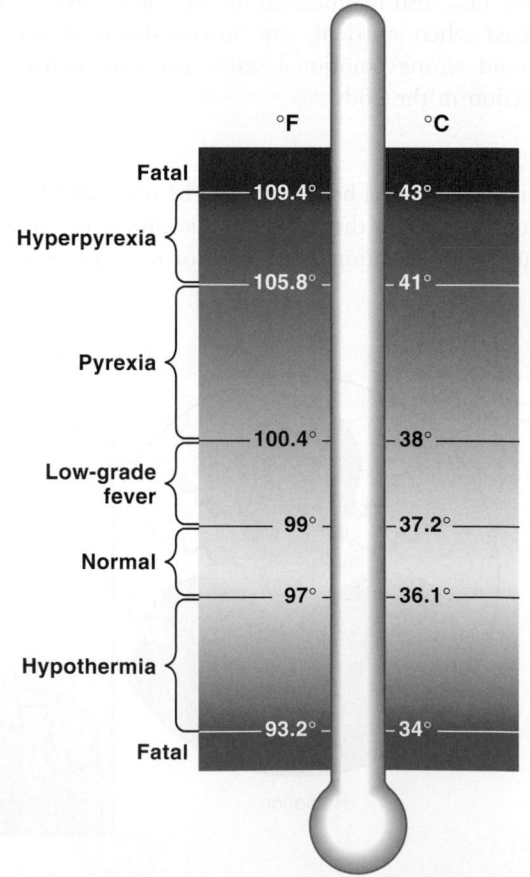

Figure 19-3 Terms that describe alterations in body temperature (adult oral temperature).

5. **Exercise.** Vigorous physical exercise causes an increase in voluntary muscle contractions, which elevates the body temperature.
6. **Patient's normal body temperature.** Some patients normally run a low or high temperature. The medical assistant should review the patient's past vital sign recordings.
7. **Pregnancy.** Cell metabolism increases during pregnancy, and this elevates body temperature.

Fever

Fever, or pyrexia, denotes that a patient's temperature has increased to greater than 100.4° F (38° C). An individual who has a fever is said to be **febrile;** one who does not have a fever is **afebrile.**

Fever is a common symptom of illness, particularly inflammation and infection. When there is an infection in the body, the invading pathogen functions as a *pyrogen,* which is any substance that produces fever. Pyrogens reset the hypothalamus, causing the body temperature to increase

to above normal. Fever is not an illness itself, but rather a sign that the body may have an infection. Most fevers are self-limited, that is, the body temperature returns to normal after the disease process is complete.

Stages of a Fever

A fever can be divided into the following three stages:
1. The *onset* is when the temperature first begins to increase. This increase may be slow or sudden, the patient often experiences coldness and chills, and the pulse and respiratory rate increase.
2. During the *course of a fever,* the temperature rises and falls in one of the following three fever patterns: continuous, intermittent, or remittent. Fever patterns are described and illustrated in Table 19-3. During this stage the patient has an increased pulse and respiratory rate and feels warm to the touch. The patient also may experience one or more of the following: flushed appearance, increased thirst, loss of appetite, headache, and malaise. **Malaise** refers to a vague sense of body discomfort, weakness, and fatigue.
3. During the *subsiding stage,* the temperature returns to normal. It can return to normal gradually or suddenly (known as a **crisis**). As the body temperature is returning to normal, the patient usually perspires and may become dehydrated.

Assessment of Body Temperature

Assessment Sites

There are five sites for measuring body temperature: mouth, **axilla,** rectum, ear, and forehead. The locations in which temperatures are taken should have an abundant blood supply so that the temperature of the entire body is obtained, not the temperature of only a part of the body. In addition, the site must be as closed as possible to prevent air currents

Table 19-2 Variations in Body Temperature by Age			
Age	**Site**	**Average Temperature**	
Newborn	Axillary	97° F-100° F	36.1° C-37.8° C
1 yr	Oral	99.7° F	37.6° C
5 yr	Oral	98.6° F	37° C
Adult	Oral	98.6° F	37° C
	Rectal	99.6° F	37.5° C
	Axillary	97.6° F	36.4° C
	Aural	98.6° F	37° C
Elderly (over 70 yr)	Oral	96.8° F	36° C

From Bonewit-West K: *Clinical procedures for medical assistants*, ed 8, St Louis, 2011, Saunders.

Table 19-3 Fever Patterns		
Pattern	**Description**	**Illustration**

Continuous fever	Body temperature fluctuates minimally but always remains elevated.
	Occurs with:
	    Scarlet fever
	    Pneumococcal pneumonia
		98.6°F (37°C)

Intermittent fever	Body temperature alternately rises and falls and at times returns to normal or becomes subnormal.
	Occurs with:
	    Bacterial infections
	    Viral infections
		98.6°F (37°C)

Remittent fever	Wide range of temperature fluctuations occur, all of which are above normal.
	Occurs with:
	    Influenza
	    Pneumonia
	    Endocarditis
		98.6°F (37°C)

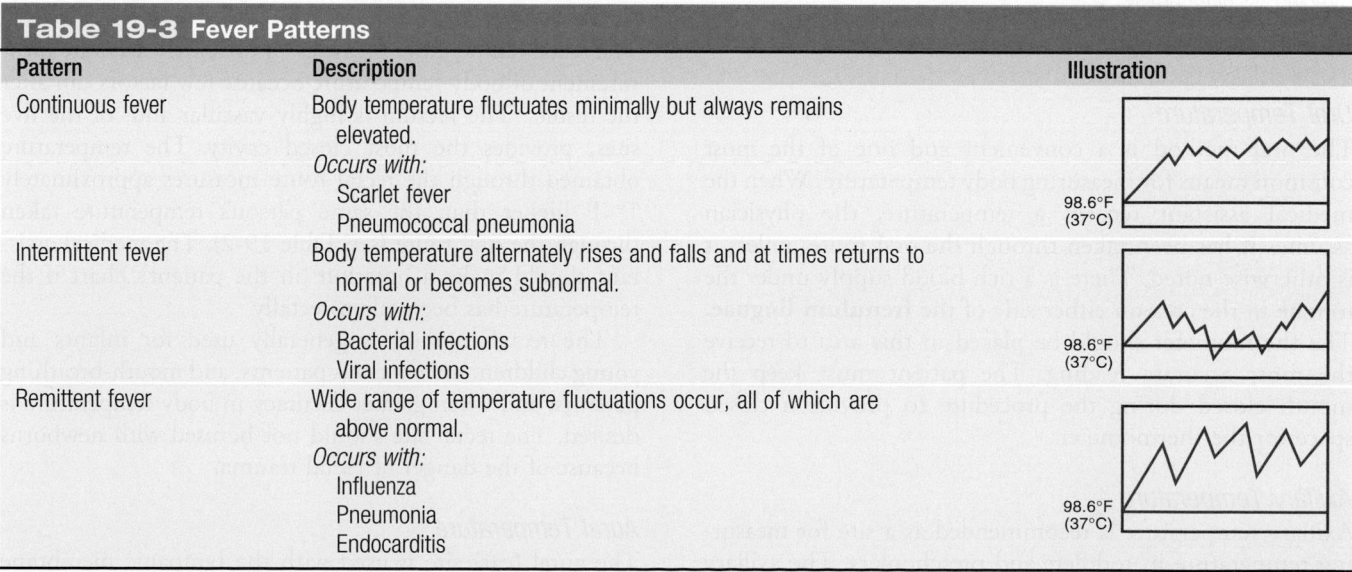

From Bonewit-West K: *Clinical procedures for medical assistants*, ed 8, St Louis, 2011, Saunders.

from interfering with the temperature reading. The site chosen for measuring a patient's temperature depends on the patient's age, condition, and state of consciousness; the type of thermometer available; and the medical office policy.

Highlight on Fever

Although most fevers indicate an infection, not all do. Noninfectious causes of fever include heatstroke, drug hypersensitivity, neoplasms, and central nervous system damage.

A fever usually is not harmful if it remains less than 102° F (38.9° C). Research suggests that fever may serve as a defense mechanism to destroy pathogens that are unable to survive above the normal body temperature range.

The level of the fever is not related to the seriousness of the infection. A patient with a temperature of 104° F (40° C) may not be any sicker than a patient with a temperature of 102° F (38.9° C).

In children, fever often is one of the first signs of illness and has a tendency to become highly elevated. In contrast, in elderly patients, fever may be elevated to only 1° F to 2° F above normal, even with a severe infection.

During a fever, the body's basal metabolism increases by 7% for each degree of temperature elevation. Heart and respiratory rates also increase to meet this metabolic demand.

Chills during a fever result when the hypothalamus has been reset at a higher temperature. In an attempt to reach this temperature, involuntary muscle contractions (chills) occur, which produce heat, causing the temperature of the body to increase. After the higher temperature has been reached, the chills subside, and the individual then feels warm.

Increased perspiration during a fever occurs when the hypothalamus has been reset at a lower temperature, for example, after taking an **antipyretic** or after the cause of the fever has been removed. To cool the body and reach this lower temperature, the body perspires, often profusely; profuse perspiration is known as *diaphoresis*. ∎

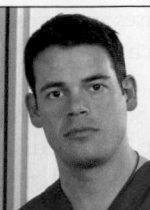

Putting It All Into Practice

My name is Sergio Martinez, and I am a registered medical assistant. I work in a large clinic that is associated with a medical school. At present, I work in the family medicine department, but I also have worked in dermatology and internal medicine. Family medicine is the area I enjoy most because of the wide variety of tasks that are performed. There is rarely a dull moment.

I focus primarily on clinical medical assisting. Taking vital signs is a big part of my job responsibilities. It is routine at my clinic to take height, weight, temperature, pulse, respiration, and blood pressure on every patient seen at the clinic, no matter what the reason for his or her visit. I assist the physician with various procedures, examinations, and minor office surgery, and I administer injections, run electrocardiograms, and perform various laboratory tests.

Taking vital signs and length and weight on small children can be very challenging at times. Some children start to cry as soon as they are put on the scale. Taking a temperature on an uncooperative toddler can be very difficult. I try to calm the child as much as possible, and for good behavior, I give a lot of praise. Stickers also are a great reward for cooperative behavior. Usually when small children learn that they can trust you, they are not as frightened by the experience. It is rewarding when a child learns not to be afraid of being evaluated for routine vital signs. ∎

Oral Temperature

The oral method is a convenient and one of the most common means for measuring body temperature. When the medical assistant records a temperature, the physician assumes it has been taken through the oral route, unless it is otherwise noted. There is a rich blood supply under the tongue in the area on either side of the **frenulum linguae.** The thermometer should be placed in this area to receive the most accurate reading. The patient must keep the mouth closed during the procedure to provide a closed space for the thermometer.

Axillary Temperature

Axillary temperature is recommended as a site for measuring temperature in toddlers and preschoolers. The axillary site also should be used for mouth-breathing patients and

for patients with oral inflammation or who have had oral surgery.

The temperature obtained through the axillary method measures approximately 1° F lower than the same person's temperature taken through the oral route (see Table 19-2). The medical assistant should make a notation to tell the physician that the temperature was taken through the axillary route.

Rectal Temperature

The rectal temperature provides an extremely accurate measurement of body temperature because few factors can alter the results. The rectum is highly vascular and, of the five sites, provides the most closed cavity. The temperature obtained through the rectal route measures approximately 1° F higher than the same person's temperature taken through the oral route (see Table 19-2). The medical assistant should make a notation on the patient's chart if the temperature has been taken rectally.

The rectal method is generally used for infants and young children, unconscious patients, and mouth-breathing patients, and when greater accuracy in body temperature is desired. The rectal site should not be used with newborns because of the danger of rectal trauma.

Aural Temperature

The aural (ear) site is used with the tympanic membrane thermometer. The ear provides a closed cavity that is easily accessible. Tympanic membrane thermometers provide instantaneous results, are easy to use, and are comfortable for the patient. They make it easier to measure the temperature of children younger than 6 years, uncooperative patients, and patients who are unable to have their temperatures taken orally.

Forehead Temperature

The temporal artery is a major artery of the head that runs laterally across the forehead and down the side of the neck. In the area of the forehead, it is located approximately 2 mm below the surface of the skin. Because the temporal artery is located so close to the skin surface and is easily accessible, the forehead provides an ideal site for obtaining a body temperature measurement. In addition, the temporal artery has a constant steady flow of blood, which assists in providing an accurate measurement of the patient's body temperature.

The forehead site can be used to measure body temperature using a temporal artery thermometer in individuals of all ages (newborns, infants, children, adults, elderly). The results compare in accuracy with other methods used to measure body temperature. The temperature obtained through the forehead site is about the same as a rectal temperature measurement. The temporal artery reading measures approximately 1° higher than oral body temperature and 2° higher than axillary temperature on the Fahrenheit scale.

Types of Thermometers

The four types of thermometers available for measuring body temperature are electronic thermometers, tympanic membrane thermometers, temporal artery thermometers, and chemical thermometers. Mercury glass thermometers are no longer used in the medical office because they break easily and release mercury. Mercury is a chemical that is dangerous to the human body because it can cause damage to the nervous system. If mercury is released into the environment, it can be harmful to wildlife. Many cities have banned the sale or use of mercury because of its potential hazards.

Electronic Thermometer

An electronic thermometer is often used in the medical office to measure body temperature. Electronic thermometers are portable and measure oral, axillary, and rectal temperatures ranging from 84° F to 108° F (28.9° C to 42.2° C).

An electronic thermometer measures body temperature in a brief time, which varies between 4 and 20 seconds, depending on the brand of thermometer used. The temperature results are digitally displayed on an LCD screen. An electronic thermometer consists of interchangeable oral and rectal probes attached to a battery-operated portable unit (Figure 19-4). The probes are color-coded for ease in identifying them. The oral probe is color-coded with blue on its collar and is used to take oral and axillary temperatures; the rectal probe is color-coded with red on its collar and is used to take rectal temperatures only.

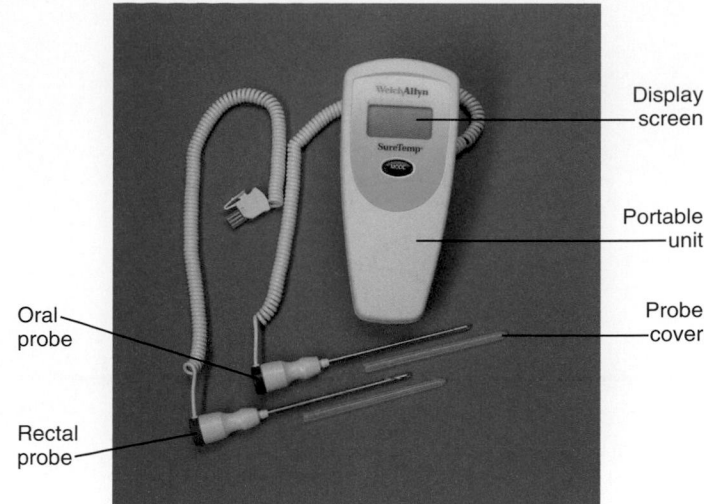

Figure 19-4 Electronic thermometer.

A disposable plastic cover is placed over the probe to prevent the transmission of microorganisms among patients. Depending on the method of taking the temperature, the probe may be inserted into the mouth, axilla, or rectum and is left in place until an audible tone is emitted from the thermometer. When the tone sounds, the patient's temperature in degrees Fahrenheit is displayed on the screen. The medical assistant ejects the plastic probe cover into a regular waste container.

The casing, probes, and attached cords of the electronic thermometer should be periodically cleaned with a soft cloth slightly dampened with a solution of warm water and a disinfectant cleaner.

Procedures 19-1, 19-2, and 19-3 outline the methods for measuring oral, axillary, and rectal temperatures using an electronic thermometer.

Tympanic Membrane Thermometer

The tympanic membrane thermometer is used at the aural site. The tympanic membrane thermometer functions by detecting thermal energy that is naturally radiated from the body. As with the rest of the body, the tympanic membrane gives off heat waves known as *infrared waves*. The tympanic thermometer functions like a camera by taking a "picture" of these infrared waves, which are considered a documented indicator of body temperature (Figure 19-5). The thermometer calculates the body temperature from the energy generated by the waves and converts it to an oral or rectal equivalent.

The tympanic membrane thermometer is battery operated and consists of a small handheld device with a sensor probe (Figure 19-6). To operate the thermometer, the probe is covered with a disposable soft plastic cover and is placed in the outer third of the external ear canal. An activation button is depressed momentarily, and the results are displayed in 1 to 2 seconds on a digital screen. The probe cover is ejected into a regular waste container. The procedure for taking aural body temperature using a tympanic membrane thermometer is presented in Procedure 19-4.

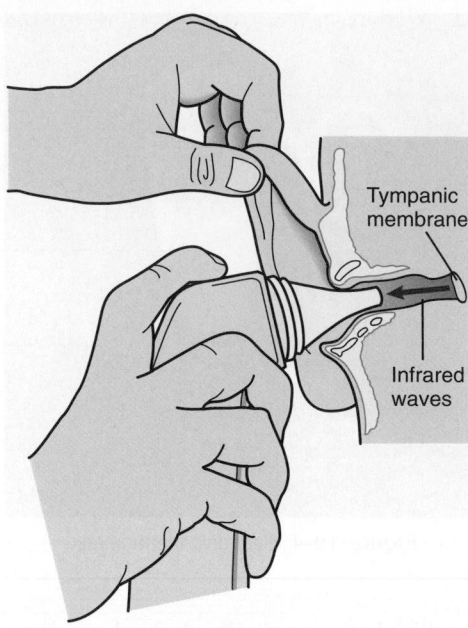

Figure 19-5 The tympanic membrane thermometer functions by detecting thermal energy that is naturally radiated from the tympanic membrane.

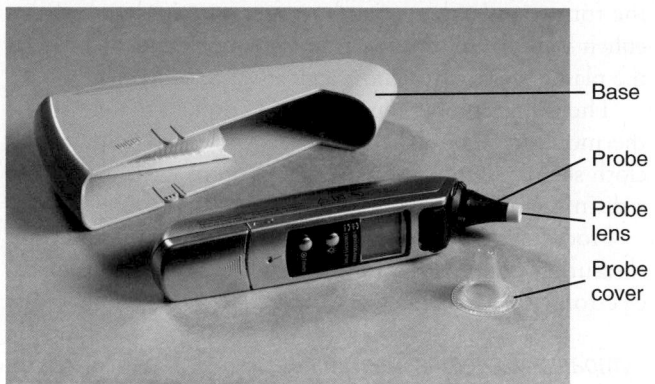

Figure 19-6 Tympanic membrane thermometer.

Temporal Artery Thermometer

Measuring temperature using a temporal artery thermometer is the newest method for assessing body temperature. A temporal artery thermometer is an electronic device consisting of a probe attached to a portable unit (Figure 19-7).

To perform the procedure, a scan button is continually depressed while the probe is gently and slowly moved across the patient's forehead. During this process, the probe sensor scans the forehead for the infrared heat given off by the temporal artery. The probe sensor captures the highest temperature or *peak temperature* in the area being scanned. The peak temperature represents the temperature given off by the temporal artery, or body temperature.

Along with measuring the peak temperature, the probe sensor automatically measures the *ambient temperature,* which is the surrounding air temperature. This is done because there is a small heat loss from the forehead that occurs as a result of cooling by ambient temperature.

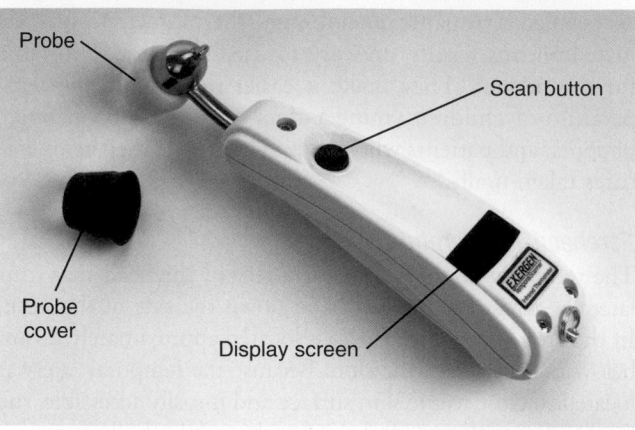

Figure 19-7 Temporal artery thermometer.

The thermometer's computer determines and automatically corrects for any effect from ambient temperature. An accurate body temperature reading is digitally displayed on the screen on the thermometer. The procedure for measuring temperature using a temporal artery thermometer is presented in Procedure 19-5.

Earlobe Temperature Measurement

Sweating of the forehead can cause an inaccurate temporal artery temperature reading. This is because perspiration causes the skin of the forehead to cool, resulting in a falsely low temperature reading. Sweating of the forehead occurs when a patient's fever breaks. It also occurs when a patient's skin is clammy; in this instance, forehead sweating may be present but not readily visible. To avoid this problem, the temperature of the neck area located just behind the earlobe also must be measured.

The area behind the earlobe is less affected by sweating than the forehead. During sweating, the blood vessels behind the earlobe dilate, resulting in a constant, steady flow of blood, which provides an accurate measurement of body temperature. After scanning the forehead, the medical assistant must place the probe of the thermometer in the soft depression of the neck just below the mastoid process of the ear. If the patient's forehead has cooled from sweating, the earlobe temperature automatically registers as the peak temperature, thereby overriding the forehead temperature.

The area behind the earlobe does not normally provide an accurate body temperature measurement and supersedes the forehead measurement only when the patient is in a diaphoretic state. Additional guidelines for temporal artery temperature measurement are presented in Box 19-1.

Care and Maintenance

The temporal artery thermometer should be stored in a clean, dry area. The thermometer must be protected from extremes in temperature, direct sunlight, and dust. The casing of the thermometer should be cleaned periodically with a soft cloth moistened with a solution of warm water and a disinfectant cleaner; never splash water on or immerse the unit in water because this could damage the internal components of the thermometer.

To obtain an accurate measurement, the probe lens must be clean and shiny. Dust and other minute particles of environmental debris can build up on the probe lens during normal use, preventing the probe sensor from getting an accurate "view" of the heat emitted by the temporal artery and resulting in a falsely low reading. The lens should be cleaned if it becomes dirty and as a part of routine maintenance. The lens is cleaned by gently wiping its surface with an antiseptic wipe and immediately wiping it dry with a cotton-tipped applicator stick.

Chemical Thermometers

Chemical thermometers contain chemicals that are heat sensitive and include disposable chemical single-use thermometers and temperature-sensitive strips. They are used most often by patients at home to measure body temperature. Although chemical thermometers are less accurate than other types of thermometers, they assist in providing a general assessment of body temperature. Because of their chemical makeup, they should be stored in a cool area, preferably colder than 86° F (30° C), and should not be exposed to direct sunlight because heat may cause the thermometer to register a higher temperature. Each type of chemical thermometer is described here.

Disposable Chemical Single-Use Thermometers

The disposable chemical single-use thermometer has small chemical dots at one end that respond to body heat by changing color (Figure 19-8, *A* and *B*). Each thermometer comes in its own wrapper. The protective wrapper must be peeled back to expose the handle of the thermometer. The thermometer is removed from the wrapper by pulling on the handle, taking care not to touch the dotted area. The thermometer is inserted under the tongue and is left in place for the duration of time recommended by the manufacturer (generally 60 seconds). After removal of the thermometer, the dots are observed for a change in color. The thermometer is read by noting the highest reading among the dots that have changed color (Figure 19-8, *C*). The thermometer is discarded after use.

Temperature-Sensitive Strips

A temperature-sensitive strip consists of a reusable plastic strip that contains heat-sensitive liquid crystals designed to measure body temperature. The plastic strip is pressed onto the forehead and is held in place until the colors stop changing, generally for 15 seconds. The results are read by observing the color change and noting the corresponding temperature indicated on the strip (Figure 19-9).

Text continued on p. 315

PROCEDURE 19-1 Measuring Oral Body Temperature—Electronic Thermometer

Outcome Measure oral body temperature.

Equipment/Supplies

- Electronic thermometer
- Oral probe (blue collar)
- Plastic probe cover
- Waste container

1. **Procedural Step.** Sanitize your hands, and assemble the equipment.
2. **Procedural Step.** Remove the thermometer unit from its storage base, and attach the oral (blue collar) probe to it. This is accomplished by inserting the latching plug (at the end of the coiled cord of the oral probe) to the plug receptacle on the thermometer unit until it clicks into place. Insert the probe into the face of the thermometer.

   Principle. The oral probe is color-coded with a blue collar for ease in identifying it.

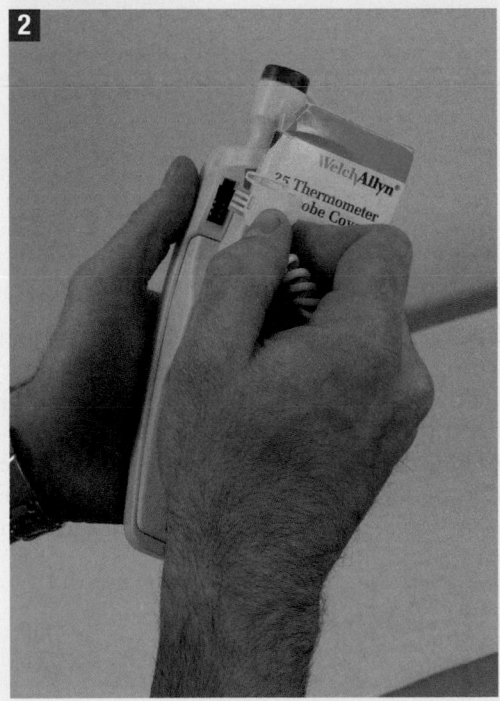

Attach the oral probe to the thermometer.

Continued

**PROCEDURE 19-1   Measuring Oral Body Temperature—
                              Electronic Thermometer—cont'd**

3. **Procedural Step.** Greet the patient and introduce yourself. Identify the patient and explain the procedure. If the patient has recently ingested hot or cold food or beverages or has been smoking, you must wait 15 to 30 minutes before taking the temperature.
Principle. Ingestion of hot or cold food or beverages and smoking change the temperature of the mouth, which could result in an inaccurate reading.

4. **Procedural Step.** Grasp the probe by the collar, and remove it from the face of the thermometer. Slide the probe into a disposable plastic probe cover until it locks into place.
Principle. Removing the probe from the thermometer automatically turns on the thermometer. The probe cover prevents the transfer of microorganisms from one patient to another.

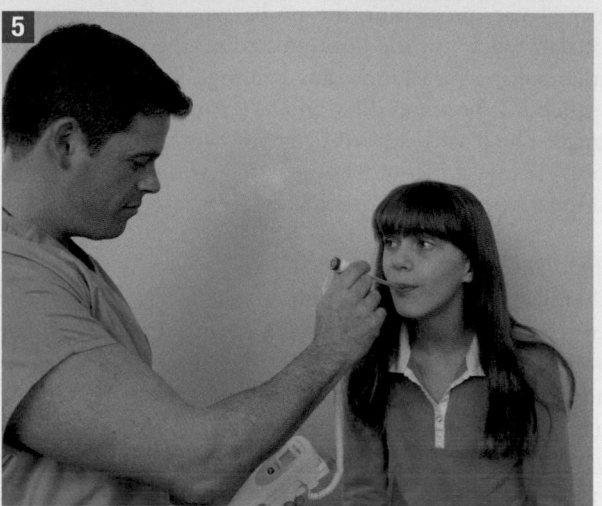

Insert the probe under the patient's tongue.

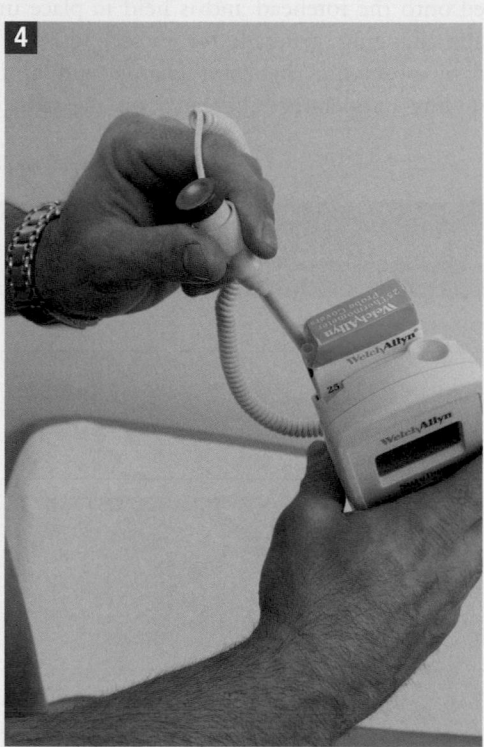

Slide the probe into a probe cover.

5. **Procedural Step.** Take the patient's temperature by inserting the probe under the patient's tongue in the pocket located on either side of the frenulum linguae. Instruct the patient to keep the mouth closed.
Principle. There is a good blood supply in the tissue under the tongue. The mouth must be kept closed to prevent cooler air from entering and affecting the temperature reading.

6. **Procedural Step.** Hold the probe in place until you hear the tone. At that time, the patient's temperature appears as a digital display on the screen. Make a mental note of the temperature reading. (The temperature indicated on this thermometer is 98.2° F [36.8° C]).

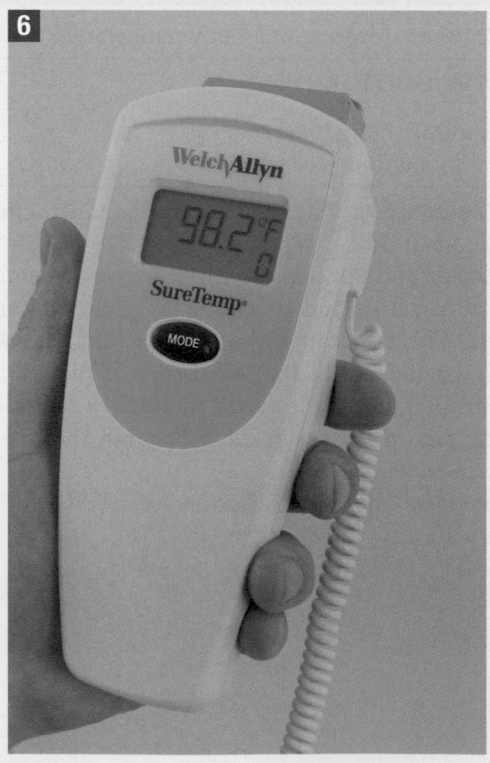

The patient's temperature appears as a digital display on the screen.

7. Procedural Step. Remove the probe from the patient's mouth. Discard the probe cover by firmly pressing the ejection button while holding the probe over a regular

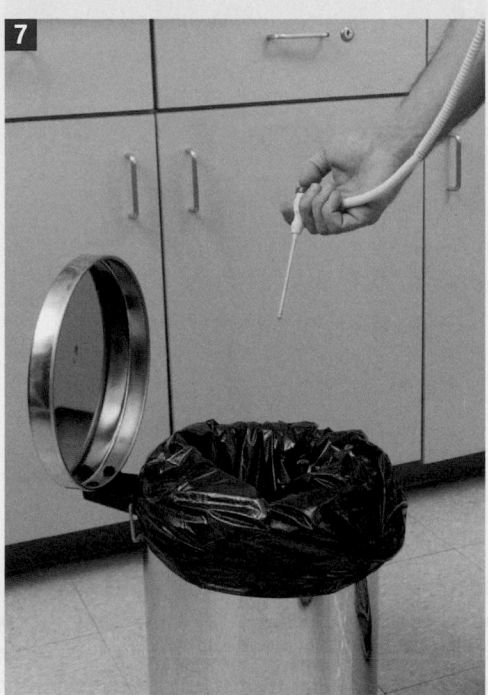

Discard the probe cover by pressing the ejection button.

waste container. Do not allow your fingers to come in contact with the probe cover.

Principle. The probe cover should not be touched so as to prevent the transfer of microorganisms from the patient to the medical assistant. Saliva is not considered regulated medical waste; the probe can be discarded in a regular waste container.

8. Procedural Step. Return the probe to its stored position in the thermometer unit. Return the thermometer unit to its storage base.

Principle. Returning the probe to the unit automatically turns off and resets the thermometer.

9. Procedural Step. Sanitize your hands, and chart the results. Include the date, the time, and the temperature reading.

Principle. Patient data must be recorded properly to aid the physician in the diagnosis and to provide future reference.

CHARTING EXAMPLE

Date	
10/15/XX	2:15 p.m. T: 98.2° F.——— S. Martinez, RMA

---

see DVD

Outcome Measure axillary body temperature. *NOTE:* Many of the principles for taking a temperature already have been stated and are not included in this procedure.

Equipment/Supplies

- Electronic thermometer
- Oral probe (blue collar)
- Plastic probe cover
- Waste container

1. **Procedural Step.** Sanitize your hands, and assemble the equipment.
2. **Procedural Step.** Remove the thermometer unit from its storage base, and attach the oral (blue collar) probe to it. This is accomplished by inserting the latching plug (on the end of the coiled cord of the oral probe) to the plug receptacle on the thermometer unit until it locks into place. Insert the probe into the face of the thermometer.
3. **Procedural Step.** Greet the patient and introduce yourself. Identify the patient and explain the procedure.
4. **Procedural Step.** Remove clothing from the patient's shoulder and arm. Ensure that the axilla is dry. If it is wet, pat it dry with a paper towel or a gauze pad.
   Principle. Clothing removal provides optimal exposure of the axilla for proper placement of the

thermometer. Rubbing the axilla causes an increase in the temperature in that area owing to friction, resulting in an inaccurate temperature reading.

5. **Procedural Step.** Grasp the probe by the collar, and remove it from the face of the thermometer. Slide the probe into a disposable probe cover until it locks into place.
6. **Procedural Step.** Take the patient's temperature by placing the probe in the center of the patient's axilla. Instruct the patient to hold the arm close to the body. Hold the arm in place for small children and other patients who cannot maintain the position themselves.
   Principle. Interference from outside air currents is reduced when the arm is held in the proper position.

Continued

PROCEDURE **19-2**   Measuring Axillary Body Temperature— Electronic Thermometer—cont'd

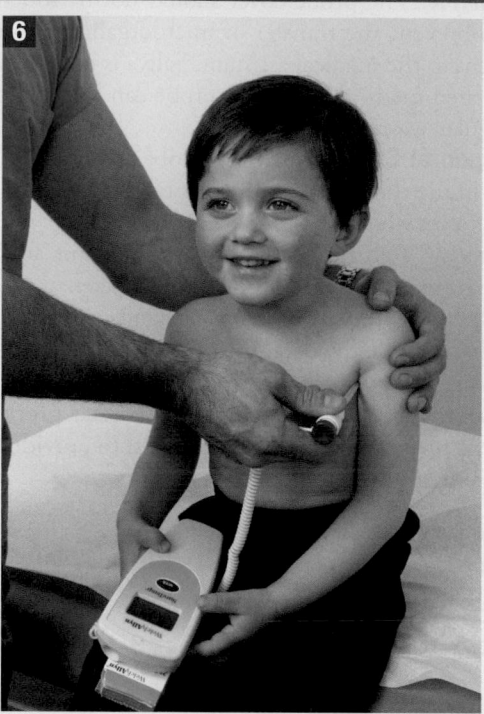

Place the probe in the center of the patient's axilla.

7. **Procedural Step.** Hold the probe in place until you hear the tone. At that time, the patient's temperature appears as a digital display on the screen. Make a mental note of the temperature reading.
8. **Procedural Step.** Remove the probe from the patient's axilla. Discard the probe cover by firmly pressing the ejection button while holding the probe over a regular waste container. Do not allow your fingers to come in contact with the probe cover.
9. **Procedural Step.** Return the probe to its stored position in the thermometer unit. Return the thermometer unit to its storage base.

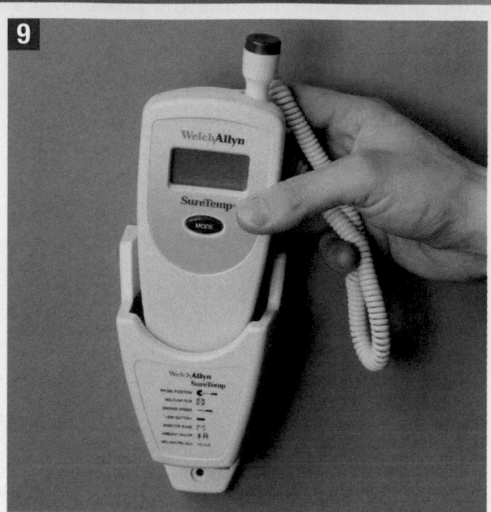

Return the thermometer to its base.

10. **Procedural Step.** Sanitize your hands, and chart the results. Include the date, the time, and the axillary temperature reading. The symbol (A) must be charted next to the temperature reading to tell the physician that an axillary reading was taken.

CHARTING EXAMPLE

Date	
10/15/XX	9:30 a.m. T: 97.4° F(A) –S. Martinez, RMA

PROCEDURE **19-3**   Measuring Rectal Body Temperature— Electronic Thermometer

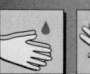

Outcome   Measure rectal body temperature.

Equipment/Supplies

- Electronic thermometer
- Rectal probe (red collar)
- Plastic probe cover
- Lubricant

- Disposable gloves
- Tissues
- Waste container

1. **Procedural Step.** Sanitize your hands, and assemble the equipment.
2. **Procedural Step.** Remove the thermometer unit from its storage base. Attach the rectal (red collar) probe to it. This is accomplished by inserting the latching plug (on the end of the coiled cord of the rectal probe) to

the plug receptacle on the thermometer unit. Insert the probe into the face of the thermometer.
   Principle. The rectal probe is color-coded with a red collar for ease in identifying it.
3. **Procedural Step.** Greet the patient and introduce yourself. Identify the patient and explain the

PROCEDURE 19-3   Measuring Rectal Body Temperature—Electronic Thermometer—cont'd

procedure. If a patient is a child or an adult, provide him or her with a patient gown. Instruct the patient to remove enough clothing to provide access to the anal area and to put on the gown with the opening in the back. If the patient is an infant, ask the parent to remove his or her diaper.

Principle. It is important to explain what you will be doing, because body temperature may be higher in a fearful or apprehensive patient. The patient gown provides the patient with modesty and comfort.

4. **Procedural Step.** Apply gloves. Position the patient. *Adults and children:* Position the patient in the Sims position, and drape the patient to expose only the anal area. *Infants:* Position the infant on his or her abdomen.

Principle. Gloves protect the medical assistant from microorganisms in the anal area and feces. Correct positioning allows clear viewing of the anal opening and provides for proper insertion of the thermometer. Draping reduces patient embarrassment and provides warmth.

5. **Procedural Step.** Grasp the probe by the collar, and remove it from the face of the thermometer. Slide the probe into a disposable plastic probe cover until it locks into place. Apply a lubricant to the tip of the probe cover up to a level of 1 inch.

Principle. A lubricated thermometer can be inserted more easily and does not irritate the delicate rectal mucosa.

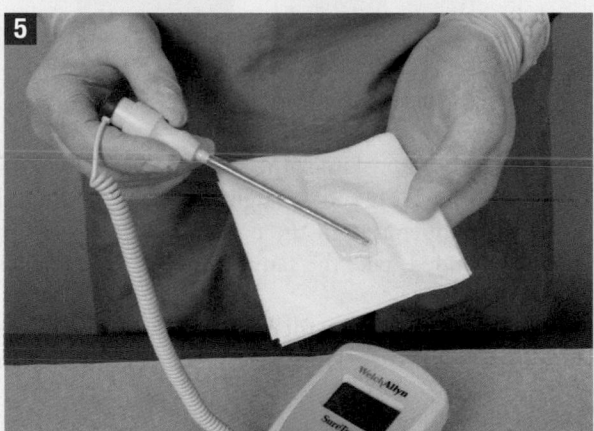

Apply a lubricant to the tip of the probe cover.

6. **Procedural Step.** Instruct the patient to lie still. Separate the buttocks to expose the anal opening, and gently insert the thermometer probe approximately 1 inch into the rectum of an adult, ⅝ inch in children, and ½ inch in infants. Do not force insertion of the probe. Hold the probe in place until the temperature registers.

Principle. The probe must be inserted correctly to prevent injury to the tissue of the anal opening. The

probe should be held in place to prevent damage to the rectal mucosa.

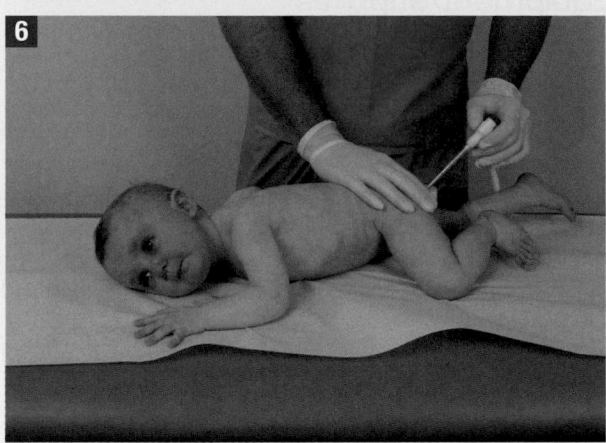

Gently insert the probe ½ inch into the rectum.

7. **Procedural Step.** Hold the probe in place until you hear the tone. At that time, the patient's temperature appears as a digital display on the screen. Make a mental note of the temperature reading.

8. **Procedural Step.** Gently remove the probe from the rectum in the same direction as it was inserted. Avoid touching the probe cover. Discard the probe cover by firmly pressing the ejection button while holding the probe over a regular waste container. Return the probe to its stored position in the thermometer unit. Return the thermometer unit to its storage base.

Principle. Fecal material is not considered regulated medical waste; the probe can be discarded in a regular waste container.

9. **Procedural Step.** Wipe the patient's anal area with tissues to remove excess lubricant. Dispose of the tissues in a regular waste container.

Principle. Wiping the anal area makes the patient more comfortable.

10. **Procedural Step.** Remove gloves, and sanitize your hands. Chart the results. Include the date, the time, and the rectal temperature reading. The symbol Ⓡ must be charted next to the temperature reading to tell the physician that a rectal reading was taken.

CHARTING EXAMPLE	
Date	
10/15/XX	11:15 a.m. T: 99.8° F Ⓡ — S. Martinez, RMA

PROCEDURE 19-3

PROCEDURE 19-4   **Measuring Aural Body Temperature—Tympanic Membrane Thermometer**

Outcome Measure aural body temperature.

Equipment/Supplies

- Tympanic membrane thermometer
- Probe cover
- Waste container

1. Procedural Step. Sanitize your hands, and assemble the equipment.
Principle. Your hands should be clean and free from contamination.

2. Procedural Step. Greet the patient and introduce yourself. Identify the patient and explain the procedure.
Principle. It is important to explain what you will be doing, because body temperature may be higher in a fearful or apprehensive patient.

3. Procedural Step. Remove the thermometer from its storage base. Ensure that the probe lens is clean and intact. To clean the lens, gently wipe its surface with an antiseptic wipe and immediately wipe it dry with a cotton swab. After cleaning, allow at least 5 minutes before taking a temperature.
Principle. A dirty or damaged probe lens could result in a falsely low temperature reading.

4. Procedural Step. Attach a cover on the probe by pressing the probe tip straight down into the cover box. You will be able to see and feel the cover snap securely into place on the probe. This procedure automatically turns on the thermometer.
Principle. The probe cover protects the lens and provides infection control. The cover must be seated securely on the probe to activate the thermometer.

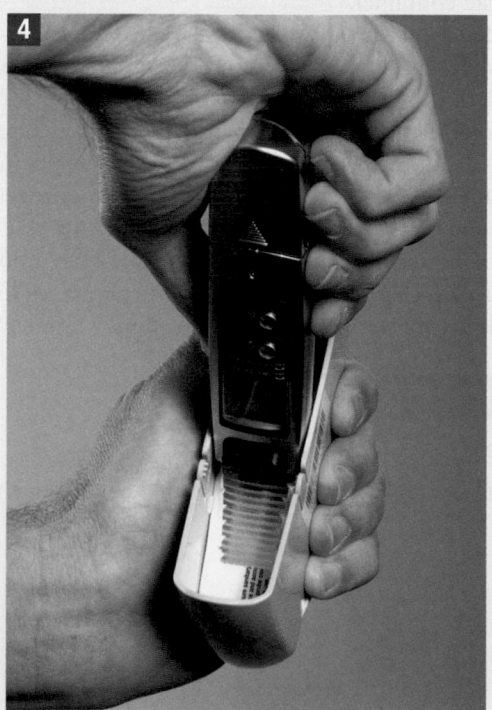

Place a cover on the probe.

5. Procedural Step. Pull the probe straight up from the cover box. Look at the digital display to see if the thermometer is ready to use.

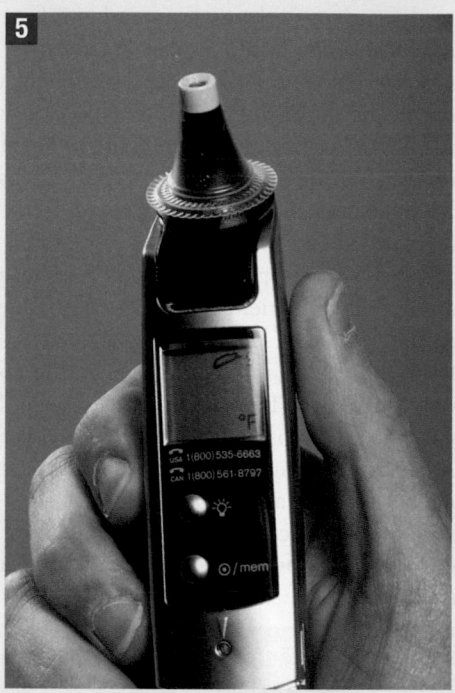

When the thermometer is ready, it displays the word READY.

6. Procedural Step. Hold the thermometer in your dominant hand. If you are right-handed, you should take the temperature in the patient's right ear. If you are left-handed, take the temperature in the patient's left ear.
Principle. Taking the temperature with the dominant hand assists in the proper placement of the probe in the patient's ear.

7. Procedural Step. Straighten the patient's external ear canal with your nondominant hand, as follows:
Adults and Children Older Than 3 Years Old. Gently pull the ear auricle upward and backward.
Children Younger Than 3 Years Old. Gently pull the ear pinna downward and backward.
Principle. Straightening the ear canal allows the probe sensor to obtain a clear picture of the tympanic membrane, resulting in an accurate temperature measurement.

PROCEDURE **19-4** Measuring Aural Body Temperature—Tympanic Membrane Thermometer—cont'd

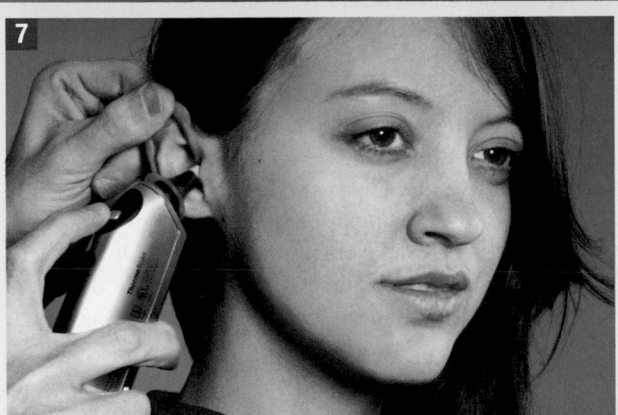

Straighten the canal of adults and children older than 3 years by pulling the ear auricle upward and backward.

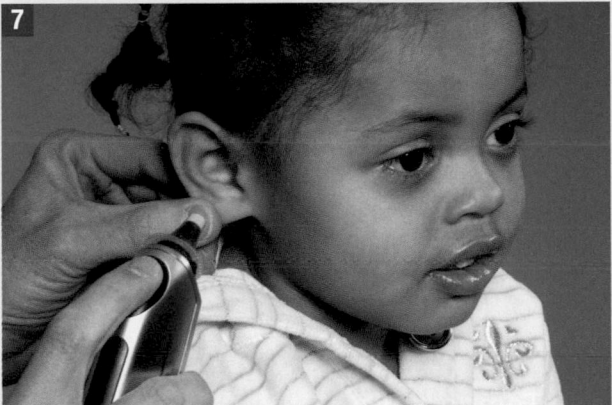

Straighten the canal of children younger than 3 years by pulling the ear auricle downward and backward.

8. Procedural Step. Insert the probe into the patient's ear canal tightly enough to seal the opening, but without causing patient discomfort. Point the tip of the probe toward the opposite temple (approximately midway between the opposite ear and eyebrow).
Principle. Sealing the ear canal prevents cooler external air from entering the ear, which could result in a falsely low reading. Correct positioning of the probe optimizes the sensor's view of the tympanic membrane, leading to an accurate temperature reading.

9. Procedural Step. Ask the patient to remain still. Hold the thermometer steady, and depress the activation button. Depending on the brand of the thermometer, perform one of the following:

a. Hold the button down for one full second, and then release it, or
b. Hold down the button down until an audible tone is heard.
Principle. The thermometer cannot take a temperature unless the activation button is depressed for 1 full second. When the button is depressed, the infrared sensor in the probe scans the thermal energy radiated by the tympanic membrane.

10. Procedural Step. Remove the thermometer from the ear canal. Turn the digital display of the thermometer toward you, and read the temperature. Make a mental note of the temperature reading. If the temperature seems to be too low, repeat the procedure to ensure that you have used the proper technique. The temperature indicated on this thermometer is 99.8° F (37.7° C). The temperature remains on the display screen for 30 to 60 seconds or until another cover is inserted on the probe (whichever occurs first).
Principle. The temperature remains on the display screen until another cover is inserted on the probe. Improper technique can result in a falsely low temperature reading.

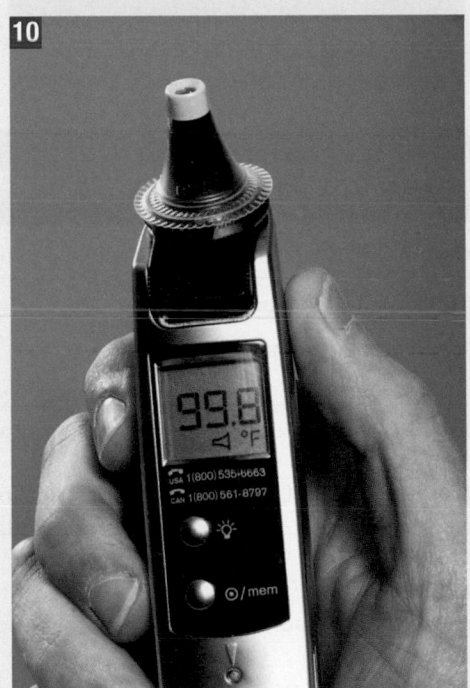

Read the temperature on the digital display.

Continued

PROCEDURE 19-4

PROCEDURE **19-4** Measuring Aural Body Temperature—Tympanic Membrane Thermometer—cont'd

11. **Procedural Step.** Dispose of the probe cover by ejecting it into a regular waste container.

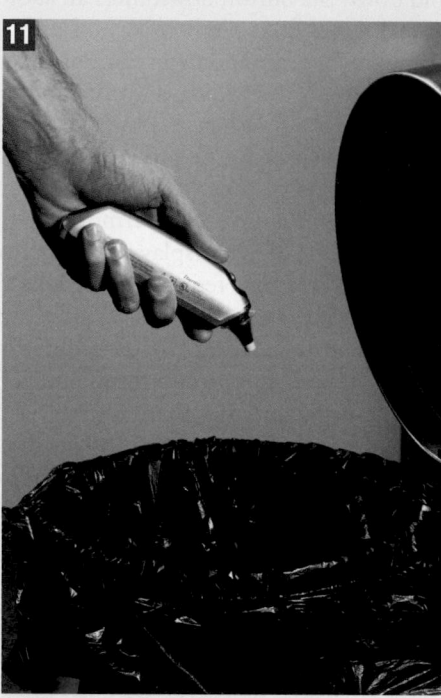

Dispose of the probe cover.

12. **Procedural Step.** Replace the thermometer in its storage base.
Principle. The thermometer should be stored in its base to protect the probe lens from damage and dirt.

13. **Procedural Step.** Sanitize your hands.

14. **Procedural Step.** Chart the results. Include the date, the time, the aural temperature reading, and which ear was used to take the temperature (AD: right ear; AS: left ear). When these abbreviations are used, the physician knows that the temperature was taken through the aural route.

CHARTING EXAMPLE	
Date	
10/15/XX	3:00 p.m. T: 99.8° F, AD — S. Martinez, RMA

PROCEDURE **19-5** Measuring Temporal Artery Body Temperature

Outcome Measure temporal artery body temperature.

Equipment/Supplies

- Temporal artery thermometer
- Probe cover
- Antiseptic wipe
- Waste container

1. **Procedural Step.** Sanitize your hands, and assemble the equipment.

2. **Procedural Step.** Greet the patient and introduce yourself. Identify the patient and explain the procedure.

3. **Procedural Step.** Examine the probe lens of the temporal artery thermometer to ensure that the lens is clean and intact.
Principle. A dirty or damaged probe lens could result in a falsely low temperature reading.

4. **Procedural Step.** Place a disposable cover over the probe. If the thermometer does not use disposable covers, clean the probe with an antiseptic wipe, and allow it to dry.
Principle. Applying a probe cover or cleaning the probe with an antiseptic wipe provides infection control.

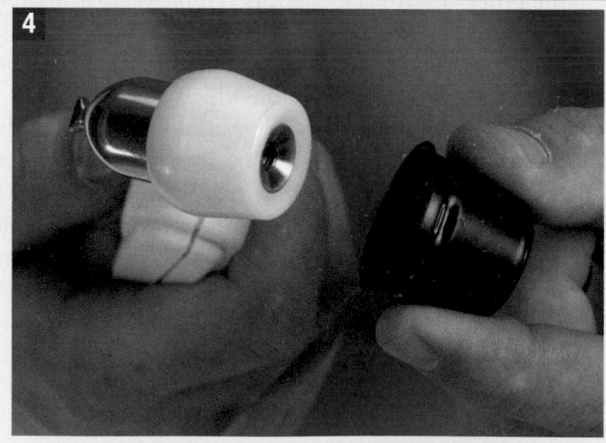

Place a disposable probe cover on the thermometer.

PROCEDURE 19-5   Measuring Temporal Artery Body Temperature—cont'd

5. **Procedural Step.** Select an appropriate site; the right or left side of the forehead can be used. The site selected should be fully exposed to the environment.
   Principle. The temporal artery is located in the center of each side of the forehead, approximately 2 mm below the surface of the skin.

6. **Procedural Step.** Prepare the patient by brushing away any hair that is covering the side of the forehead to be scanned and the area behind the earlobe on the same side.
   Principle. Hair covering the area to be measured traps body heat, resulting in a falsely high temperature reading.

7. **Procedural Step.** Hold the thermometer in your dominant hand with your thumb on the scan button.

8. **Procedural Step.** Gently position the probe of the thermometer on the center of the patient's forehead, midway between the eyebrow and the hairline.

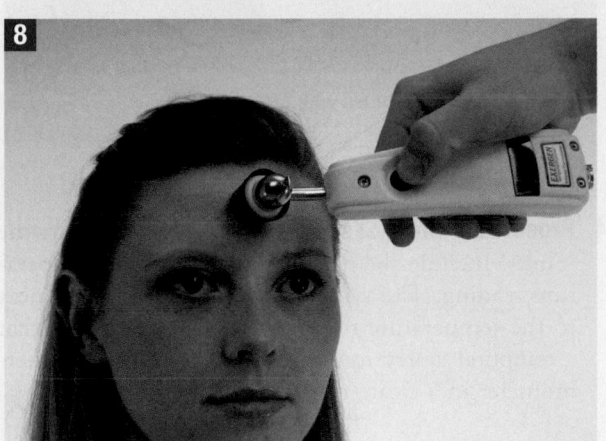

Position the probe on the center of the patient's forehead.

9. **Procedural Step.** Depress the scan button, and keep it depressed for the entire measurement.
   Principle. Not keeping the scan button depressed can result in a falsely low temperature reading.

10. **Procedural Step.** Slowly and gently slide the probe straight across the forehead, midway between the eyebrow and the upper hairline. Continue until the hairline is reached. Keep the scan button depressed and the probe flush (flat) against the forehead. During this time, a beeping sound occurs and a red light blinks to indicate that a measurement is taking place. Rapid beeping and blinking indicate a rise to a higher temperature. Slow beeping indicates that the ther-

mometer is still scanning but is not finding a higher temperature.
   Principle. The thermometer continually scans for the peak temperature as long as the scan button is depressed. The probe must be held flat against the forehead to ensure accurate scanning of the temporal artery.

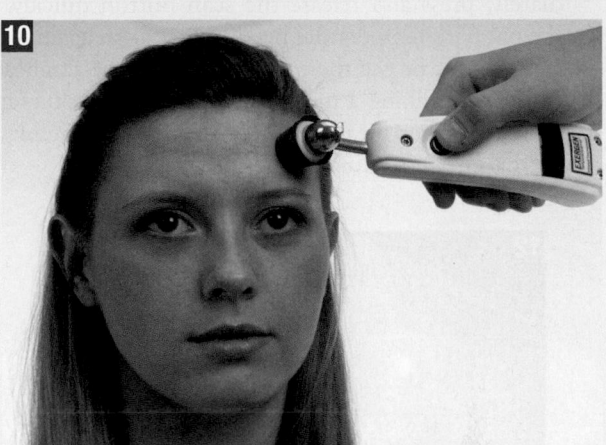

Slowly slide the probe straight across the patient's forehead.

11. **Procedural Step.** Keeping the button depressed, lift the probe from the forehead, and gently place the probe behind the earlobe in the soft depression of the neck just below the mastoid process. Hold the probe in place for 1 to 2 seconds.
    Principle. Taking the patient's temperature behind the earlobe prevents an error in temperature measurement in the event that the patient is sweating.

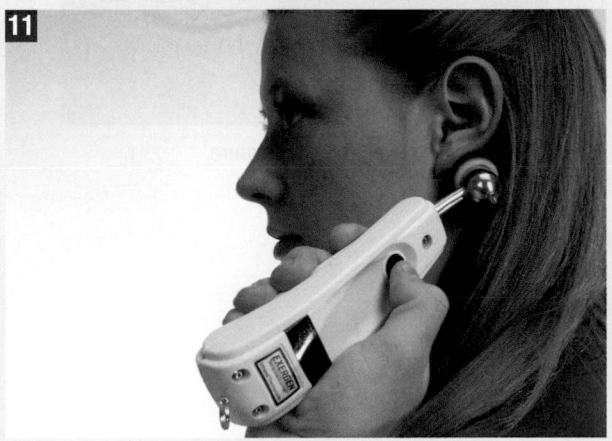

Place the probe behind the ear lobe.

Continued

PROCEDURE 19-5   Measuring Temporal Artery Body Temperature—cont'd

12. Procedural Step. Release the scan button on the digital display, and read the temperature. Make a mental note of the temperature reading (The temperature indicated on this thermometer is 99.1° F [37.3° C]). The reading remains on the display for approximately 15 to 30 seconds after the button is released. The thermometer shuts off automatically after 30 seconds. To turn the thermometer off immediately, press and release the scan button quickly. If the patient's temperature needs to be taken again, wait 60 seconds, or use the opposite side of the forehead. *Principle.* Taking a measurement cools the skin, and taking another measurement too soon may result in an inaccurate reading.

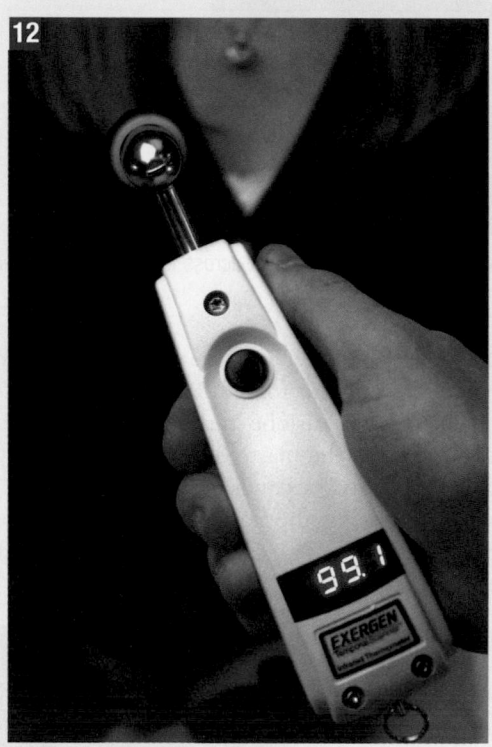

Read the temperature.

13. Procedural Step. Dispose of the probe cover by pushing it off the probe with your thumb and ejecting it into a regular waste container. Wipe the probe with an antiseptic wipe, and allow it to dry.

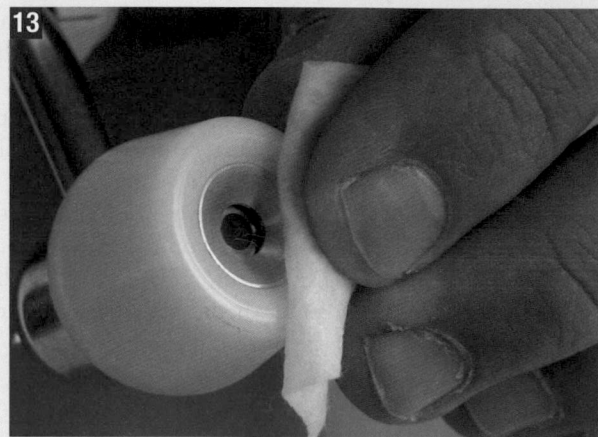

Wipe the probe with an antiseptic wipe.

14. Procedural Step. Sanitize your hands, and chart the results. Include the date, the time, and the temperature reading. The symbol (TA) must be charted next to the temperature reading to tell the physician that a temporal artery reading was taken. Store the thermometer in a clean, dry area.

CHARTING EXAMPLE

Date	
10/15/XX	9:15 a.m. T: 99.1° F (TA)— S. Martinez, RMA

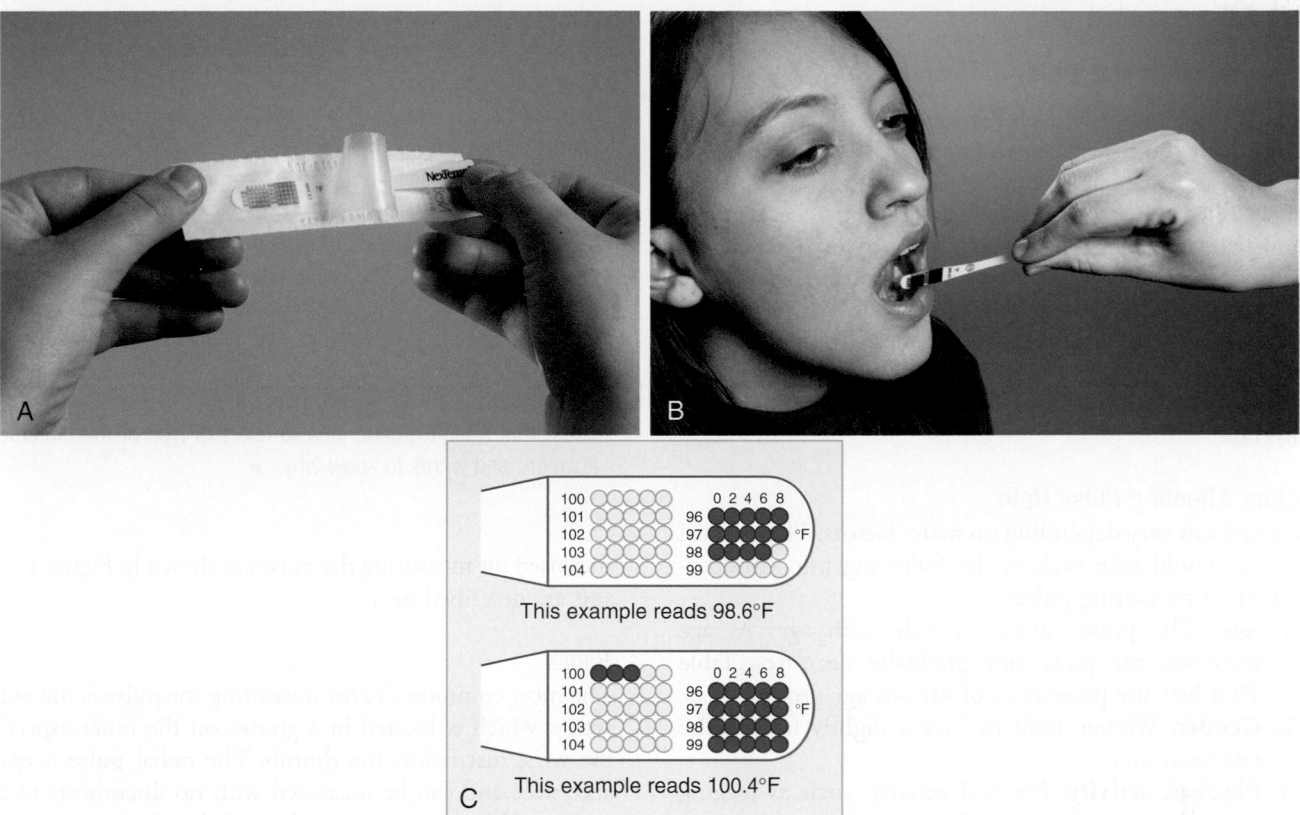

Figure 19-8 Disposable chemical single-use thermometers. **A,** The thermometer is removed from the wrapper by pulling on the handle. **B,** The thermometer is inserted under the tongue and is left in place for 60 seconds. **C,** The thermometer is read by noting the highest reading among the dots that have changed color.

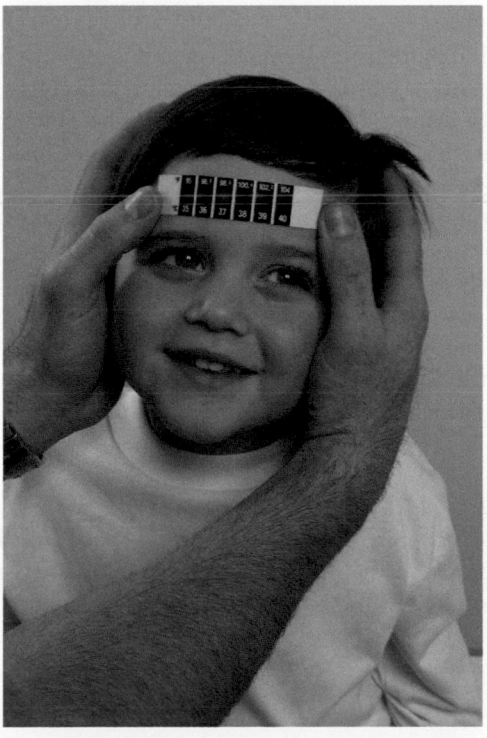

Figure 19-9 Temperature-sensitive strip. The plastic strip is pressed onto the forehead and is held in place until the color stops changing (generally for 15 seconds). The results are read by observing the color and noting the corresponding temperature indicated on the strip.

BOX 19-1 Temporal Artery Thermometer Guidelines

1. The operating environmental temperature for a temporal artery thermometer is 60° F to 104° F (15.5° C to 40° C).
2. Do not take temperature over scar tissue, open sores, or abrasions.
3. Ensure that the side of the head to be measured is exposed to the environment. Anything covering the area to be measured (e.g., hair, hat, wig, bandages) traps body heat, resulting in a falsely high reading.
4. A falsely low temporal artery reading can result from the following:
   • A dirty probe lens
   • Sweating of the forehead (in this instance, the earlobe measurement becomes the overriding temperature reading)
   • Scanning the forehead too quickly
   • Not keeping the button depressed while scanning the forehead and the area behind the earlobe

From Bonewit-West K: *Clinical procedures for medical assistants,* ed 8, St Louis, 2011, Saunders.

PULSE

Mechanism of the Pulse

When the left ventricle of the heart contracts, blood is forced from the heart into the **aorta,** which is the major trunk of the arterial system of the body. The aorta is already filled with blood and must expand to accept the blood being pushed out of the left ventricle. This creates a pulsating wave that travels from the aorta through the walls of the arterial system. This wave, known as the *pulse,* can be felt as a light tap by an examiner. The pulse rate is measured by counting the number of "taps," or beats per minute. The heart rate can be determined by taking the pulse rate.

Factors Affecting Pulse Rate

Pulse rate can vary depending on many factors. The medical assistant should take each of the following into consideration when measuring pulse:

1. **Age.** The pulse varies inversely with age. As age increases, the pulse rate gradually decreases. Table 19-4 lists the pulse rates of various age groups.
2. **Gender.** Women tend to have a slightly faster pulse rate than men.
3. **Physical activity.** Physical activity, such as jogging and swimming, increases the pulse rate temporarily.
4. **Emotional states.** Strong emotional states, such as anxiety, fear, excitement, and anger, temporarily increase the pulse rate.
5. **Metabolism.** Increased body metabolism, such as occurs during pregnancy, increases the pulse rate.
6. **Fever.** Fever increases the pulse rate.
7. **Medications.** Medications may alter the pulse rate. For example, digitalis decreases the pulse rate, and epinephrine increases it.

Pulse Sites

The pulse is felt most strongly when a superficial artery is held against a firm tissue, such as bone. The locations of

Table 19-4 Pulse Rates of Various Age Groups		
Age Group	Pulse Range (beats/min)	Average Pulse (beats/min)
Infant (birth to 1 yr)	120-160	140
Toddler (1-3 yr)	90-140	115
Preschool child (3-6 yr)	80-110	95
School-age child (6-12 yr)	75-105	90
Adolescent (12-18 yr)	60-100	80
Adult (after 18th yr)	60-100	80
Adult (after 60th yr)	67-80	74
Well-trained athletes	40-60	50

From Bonewit-West K: *Clinical procedures for medical assistants,* ed 8, St Louis, 2011, Saunders.

What Would You Do? What Would You *Not* Do?

Case Study 1

Marcela Mason comes in with Olivia, her 5-year-old daughter. Olivia has had a fever and sore throat for the past 2 days. Olivia's aural temperature is taken in her left ear, and it measures 103.3° F. Mrs. Mason says that she has an ear thermometer at home, but when she took Olivia's temperature with it, the readings were always below 97° F. She knew that could not be right because Olivia felt so warm. Mrs. Mason would like to be able to use her ear thermometer, but she thinks that it might be broken because of the low readings. Mrs. Mason says that she is thinking of switching back to a mercury glass thermometer, but she has heard that it isn't a good idea to use this type of thermometer anymore and wants to know why. ■

sites used for measuring the pulse are shown in Figure 19-10 and are described next.

Radial

The most common site for measuring the pulse is the radial artery, which is located in a groove on the inner aspect of the wrist just below the thumb. The radial pulse is easily accessible and can be measured with no discomfort to the patient. This site is also used by individuals at home monitoring their own heart rates, such as athletes, patients taking heart medication, and individuals starting an exercise program. The procedure for measuring radial pulse is outlined in Procedure 19-6.

Apical

The apical pulse has a stronger beat and is easier to measure than the other pulse sites. If the medical assistant is having difficulty feeling the radial pulse, or if the radial pulse is irregular or abnormally slow or rapid, the apical pulse should be taken (Procedure 19-7). This pulse site is often used to measure pulse in infants and in children up to 3 years old because the other sites are difficult to palpate accurately in these age groups. The apical pulse is measured using a stethoscope. The chest piece of the stethoscope is placed lightly over the apex of the heart, which is located in the fifth **intercostal** (between the ribs) space at the junction of the left midclavicular line (Figure 19-11).

Brachial

The brachial pulse is in the **antecubital space,** which is the space located at the front of the elbow. This site is used to take blood pressure, to measure pulse in infants during cardiac arrest, and to assess the status of the circulation to the lower arm.

Ulnar

The ulnar pulse is located on the ulnar (little finger) side of the wrist. It is used to assess the status of circulation to the hand.

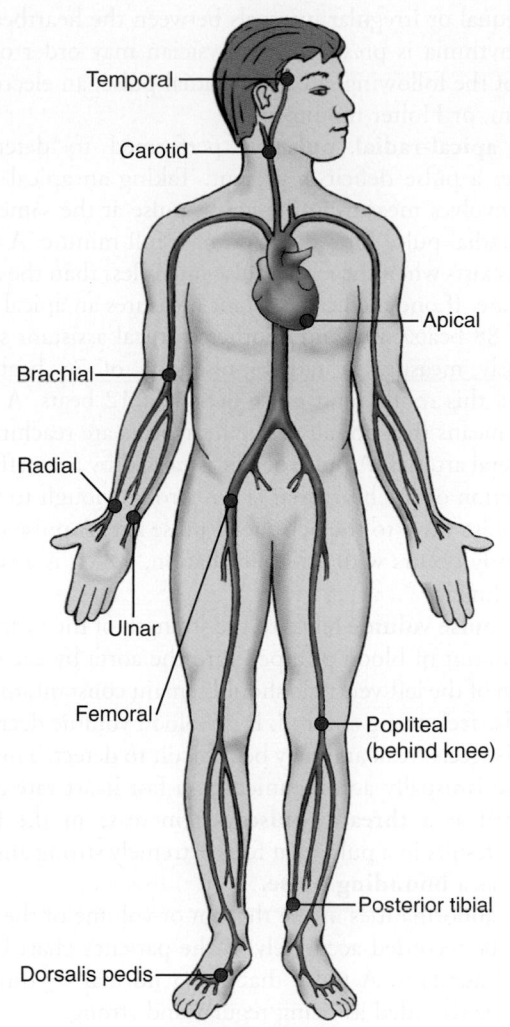

Figure 19-10 Pulse sites.

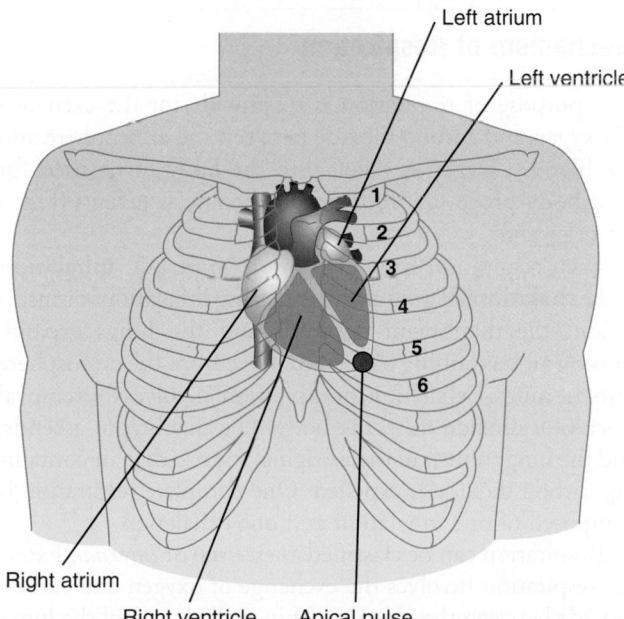

Figure 19-11 The apical pulse is found over the apex of the heart, which is located in the fifth intercostal space at the junction of the left midclavicular line.

Temporal

The temporal pulse is located in front of the ear and just above eye level. This site is used to measure pulse when the radial pulse is inaccessible. It is also an easy access site to assess pulse in children.

Carotid

The carotid pulse is located on the anterior side of the neck, slightly to one side of the midline, and is the best site to find a pulse quickly. This site is used to measure pulse in children and adults during cardiac arrest. The carotid site also is commonly used by individuals to monitor pulse during exercise.

Femoral

The femoral pulse is in the middle of the groin. This site is used to measure pulse in infants and children and in adults during cardiac arrest and to assess the status of circulation to the lower leg.

Popliteal

The popliteal pulse is at the back of the knee and is detected most easily when the knee is slightly flexed. This site is used to measure blood pressure when the brachial pulse is inaccessible and to assess the status of circulation to the lower leg.

Posterior Tibial

The posterior tibial pulse is located on the inner aspect of the ankle just posterior to the ankle bone. This site is used to assess the status of circulation to the foot.

Dorsalis Pedis

The dorsalis pedis pulse is located on the upper surface of the foot, between the first and second metatarsal bones. This site is used to assess the status of circulation to the foot.

Assessment of Pulse

The purpose of measuring pulse is to establish the patient's baseline pulse rate and to assess the pulse rate after special procedures, medications, or disease processes that affect heart functioning. Pulse is measured using palpation at all of the pulse sites except the apical site.

Pulse is palpated by applying moderate pressure with the sensitive pads located on the tips of the three middle fingers. The pulse should not be taken with the thumb because the thumb has a pulse of its own. This could result in measurement of the medical assistant's pulse rather than the patient's pulse. Excessive pressure should not be applied when measuring pulse because this could obliterate, or close off, the

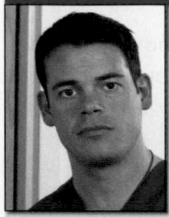
pulse. It may not be possible to detect the pulse if too little pressure is applied, however. An accurate assessment of pulse includes determinations of the pulse rate, the pulse rhythm, and the pulse volume.

Pulse Rate

The pulse rate is the number of heart pulsations or heartbeats that occur in 1 minute; therefore pulse rate is measured in beats per minute. Normal pulse rates vary widely in the various age groups, as shown in Table 19-4. For a healthy adult, the normal resting pulse rate ranges from 60 to 100 beats per minute, with the average falling between 70 and 80 beats per minute.

An abnormally fast heart rate of more than 100 beats per minute is known as **tachycardia.** Tachycardia may indicate disease states such as hemorrhaging or heart disease. Tachycardia usually occurs when an individual is involved in vigorous physical exercise or is experiencing strong emotional states.

Bradycardia is an abnormally slow heart rate—less than 60 beats per minute. A pulse rate of less than 60 beats per minute may occur normally during sleep. Trained athletes often have low pulse rates. If a patient exhibits tachycardia or bradycardia during radial pulse measurement, the apical pulse should also be measured.

Pulse Rhythm and Volume

In addition to measuring the pulse rate, the medical assistant should determine the rhythm and volume of the pulse. The **pulse rhythm** denotes the time interval between heartbeats; a normal rhythm has the same time interval between beats. Any irregularity in the heart's rhythm is known as a **dysrhythmia** (also termed *arrhythmia*) and is characterized

by unequal or irregular intervals between the heartbeats. If a dysrhythmia is present, the physician may order one or more of the following: an apical-radial pulse, an electrocardiogram, or Holter monitoring.

An **apical-radial pulse** is performed to determine whether a pulse deficit is present. Taking an apical-radial pulse involves measuring the apical pulse at the same time as the radial pulse for a duration of 1 full minute. A **pulse deficit** exists when the radial pulse rate is less than the apical pulse rate. If one medical assistant measures an apical pulse rate of 88 beats/min, and another medical assistant simultaneously measures a radial pulse rate of 76 beats per minute, this results in a pulse deficit of 12 beats. A pulse deficit means that not all of the heartbeats are reaching the peripheral arteries. A pulse deficit is caused by an inefficient contraction of the heart that is not strong enough to transmit a pulse wave to the peripheral pulse site. A pulse deficit frequently occurs with atrial fibrillation, which is a type of dysrhythmia.

The **pulse volume** refers to the strength of the heartbeat. The amount of blood pumped into the aorta by each contraction of the left ventricle should remain constant, making the pulse feel strong and full. If the blood volume decreases, the pulse feels weak and may be difficult to detect. This type of pulse is usually accompanied by a fast heart rate and is described as a **thready pulse.** An increase in the blood volume results in a pulse that feels extremely strong and full, known as a **bounding pulse.**

Any abnormalities in the rhythm or volume of the pulse should be recorded accurately in the patient's chart by the medical assistant. A pulse that has a normal rhythm and volume is recorded as being regular and strong.

RESPIRATION

Mechanism of Respiration

The purpose of respiration is to provide for the exchange of oxygen and carbon dioxide between the atmosphere and the blood. Oxygen is taken into the body to be used for vital body processes, and carbon dioxide is given off as a waste product.

Each respiration is divided into two phases: **inhalation** and **exhalation** (Figure 19-12). During inhalation, or inspiration, the diaphragm descends and the lungs expand, causing air containing oxygen to move from the atmosphere into the lungs. Exhalation, or expiration, involves the removal of carbon dioxide from the body. The diaphragm ascends, and the lungs return to their original state so that air containing carbon dioxide is expelled. One complete respiration is composed of one inhalation and one exhalation.

Respiration can be classified as *external* or *internal*. External respiration involves the exchange of oxygen and carbon dioxide between the **alveolus** (thin-walled sacs) of the lungs and the blood (Figure 19-13). The blood, located in small capillaries, comes in contact with the alveoli, picks up oxygen, and carries it to the cells of the body. At this point,

PATIENT TEACHING | Aerobic Exercise

Answer questions patients have about aerobic exercise.

What is aerobic exercise?
Aerobic exercise increases, sustains, and decreases your pulse over time. Aerobic exercise is accomplished through steady, nonstop activity, such as walking, jogging, cycling, or swimming. Each workout should include warm-up and cool-down periods of at least 5 minutes each. This is needed to prevent muscle or joint injuries.

What are the benefits of an aerobic exercise program?
The benefits of an aerobic exercise program include strengthening of the heart, a slower resting pulse rate, reduction of stress, increased energy, lowering of body fat, decreased "bad" (low-density lipoprotein) cholesterol, and increased "good" (high-density lipoprotein) cholesterol. The key to a safe and effective aerobic exercise program is the target heart rate (THR).

What is target heart rate?
Your THR is a safe and effective exercise pulse range that indicates that you are exercising at the right level for your age and for what you are trying to accomplish with exercise. Exercising at a level below your THR does little to promote fitness; exercising at a level above your THR may not be safe.

How do I determine my target heart rate?
The following formula is used to determine your THR:
1. Subtract your age from 220 to determine your maximum heart rate (MHR), which is the fastest your heart can beat safely for your age. The MHR of a 40-year-old person is calculated as follows:
   220 − 40 years old = 180 (MHR)
2. Determine the lower end of your THR range by multiplying your MHR by 0.6. For our example:
   180 × 0.60 = 108 (low end of THR)
3. Determine the upper end of your THR range by multiplying your MHR by 0.8. For our example:
   180 × 0.80 = 144 (upper end of THR)

Always exercise within your THR range. The 40-year-old person in our example should exercise with a THR between 108 and 144.

How often should aerobic exercise be performed?
To promote and maintain health, the American Heart Association recommends that healthy adults aged 18 to 65 spend at least 30 minutes a day, 5 days a week, in moderately intense aerobic exercise (e.g., brisk walking), or 20 minutes, 3 days each week, in vigorous-intensity exercise (e.g., jogging), or a combination of moderate and vigorous exercise. These moderate- and vigorous-intensity recommendations should be added to the light-intensity activities of daily living such as washing dishes and taking out the trash. In addition, the AHA recommends that adults perform activities that maintain or increase muscular strength and endurance a minimum of 2 days each week. The American Heart Association further recommends that children and adolescents engage in at least 60 minutes per day of moderate to vigorous physical activity. ∎

---

the oxygen is given off to the cells, and carbon dioxide is picked up by the blood to be transported as a waste product to the lungs. The exchange of oxygen and carbon dioxide between the body cells and the blood is known as *internal respiration.*

Control of Respiration
The medulla oblongata, located in the brain, is the control center for involuntary respiration. A buildup of carbon dioxide in the blood sends a message to the medulla, which triggers respiration to occur automatically.

To a certain extent, respiration is also under voluntary control. An individual can control respiration during activities such as singing, laughing, talking, eating, and crying. Voluntary respiration is ultimately under the control of the medulla oblongata. The breath can be held for only a certain length of time, after which carbon dioxide begins to build up in the body, resulting in a stimulus to the medulla that causes respiration to occur involuntarily. Small children may voluntarily hold their breath during a temper tantrum. A parent who does not understand the principles of respiration may be concerned that the child would cease to breathe. The medical assistant should be able to explain that involuntary respiration would eventually occur and the child would resume breathing.

Assessment of Respiration
Because an individual can control his or her respiration, the medical assistant should measure respirations without the patient's knowledge. Patients may change their respiratory rate unintentionally if they are aware that they are being measured. An ideal time to measure respiration is after the pulse is taken. Procedure 19-6 outlines the procedures for taking pulse and respiration in one continuous procedure.

Respiratory Rate
The respiratory rate of a normal healthy adult ranges from 12 to 20 respirations per minute. With most adults, there is a ratio of one respiration for every four pulse beats. If the respiratory rate is 18, the pulse rate would be approximately 72 beats per minute. An abnormal increase in the respiratory rate of more than 20 respirations per minute is

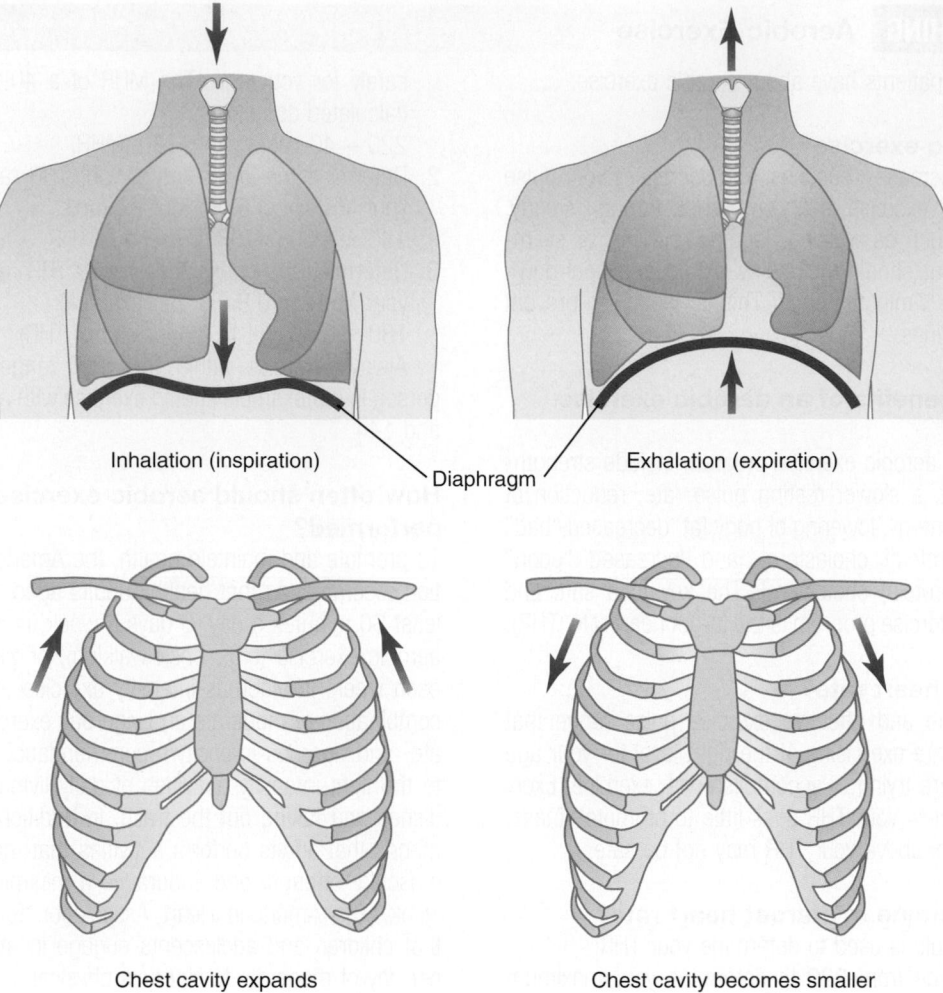

Inhalation (inspiration)   Exhalation (expiration)
                    Diaphragm

Chest cavity expands   Chest cavity becomes smaller

Figure 19-12 Inhalation and exhalation.

What Would You Do? What Would You *Not* Do?

Case Study 2

Alex Jacoby is 18 years old and a senior in high school. He comes to the office complaining of severe pain in his left shoulder. Alex is an outstanding competitive swimmer and is currently ranked first in the state in the 100-yard butterfly. Alex has a big meet coming up and must do well because he has a chance of getting an athletic scholarship to the University of Florida. He says he thinks he can take 2 seconds off his best time at this meet and he doesn't want anything to interfere with that. Alex wants the physician to do whatever he can to make his shoulder better and thinks that a steroid injection and OxyContin might be the answer. His vital signs are as follows: temperature 98.5° F, pulse 48 beats/min, respirations 12 breaths/min, and blood pressure 108/68 mm Hg. Alex asks why his pulse is so slow and wants to know if there is any medication that he can take to make it faster. ■

referred to as **tachypnea.** An abnormal decrease in the respiratory rate of less than 12 respirations per minute is known as **bradypnea.** When measuring the respiratory rate, the medical assistant should take into consideration the following factors:

1. **Age.** As age increases, the respiratory rate decreases. The respiratory rate of a child would be expected to be faster than that of an adult. Table 19-5 provides a chart of the respiratory rates for various age groups.
2. **Physical activity.** Physical activity increases the respiratory rate temporarily.
3. **Emotional states.** Strong emotional states temporarily increase the respiratory rate.
4. **Fever.** A patient with a fever has an increased respiratory rate. One way that heat is lost from the body is through the lungs; a fever causes an increased respiratory rate as the body tries to rid itself of excess heat.
5. **Medications.** Certain medications increase the respiratory rate, and others decrease it. If the medical assistant is unsure of what effect a particular drug may have on the respiratory rate, he or she should consult a drug reference, such as the *Physician's Desk Reference* (PDR).

External Respiration

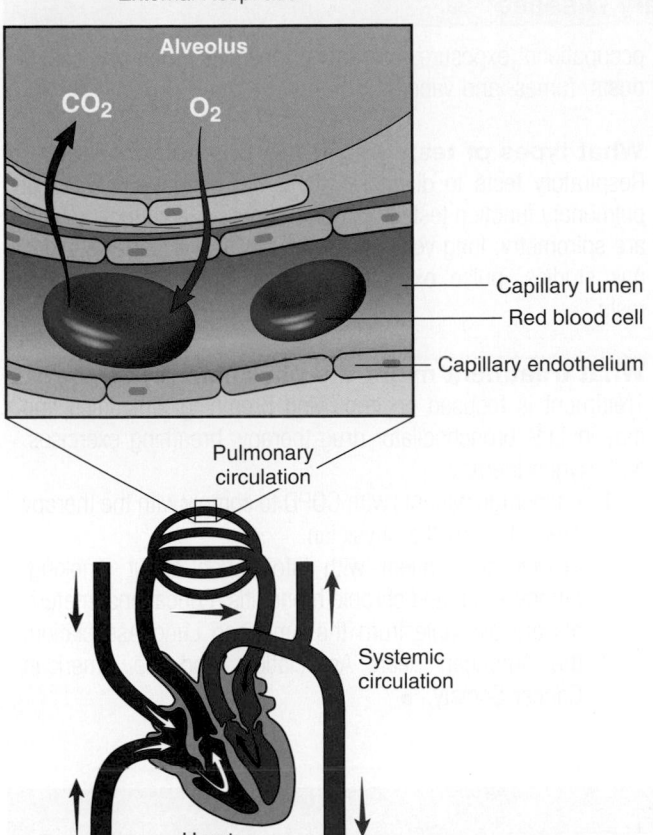

Figure 19-13 Exchange of oxygen and carbon dioxide between the alveoli of the lungs and the blood.

Table 19-5 Respiratory Rates of Various Age Groups

	Average Respiratory Range, breaths/min	Respiratory Average, breaths/min
Infant (birth to 1 yr)	30-40	35
Toddler (1-3 yr)	23-35	30
Preschool child (3-6 yr)	20-30	25
School-age child (6-12 yr)	18-26	22
Adolescent (12-18 yr)	12-20	16
Adult (after 18th yr)	12-20	16

From Bonewit-West K: *Clinical procedures for medical assistants*, ed 8, St Louis, 2011, Saunders.

Rhythm and Depth of Respiration

The *rhythm* and *depth* should be noted when measuring respiration. Normally, the rhythm should be even and regular, and the pauses between inhalation and exhalation should be equal. The depth of respiration indicates the amount of air that is inhaled or exhaled during the process of breathing. Respiratory depth is generally described as normal, deep, or shallow and is determined by observing the amount of movement of the chest. For normal respirations, the depth of each respiration in a resting state is approximately the same. Deep respirations are those in which a large volume of air is inhaled and exhaled, whereas shallow respirations involve the exchange of a small volume of air. Normal respiration is referred to as **eupnea.** The rate is approximately 12 to 20 breaths/min, the rhythm is even and regular, and the depth is normal.

Hyperpnea is an abnormal increase in the rate and depth of respirations. A patient with hyperpnea exhibits a very deep, rapid, and labored respiration. Hyperpnea occurs normally with exercise and abnormally with pain and fever. It also can occur with any condition in which the supply of oxygen is inadequate, such as heart disease and lung disease.

Hyperventilation is an abnormally fast and deep type of breathing that is usually associated with acute anxiety conditions, such as panic attacks. An individual who is hyperventilating is "overbreathing," which usually causes dizziness and weakness.

Hypopnea is a condition in which a patient's respiration exhibits an abnormal decrease in rate and depth. The depth is approximately half that of normal respiration. Hypopnea often occurs in individuals with sleep disorders.

Color of the Patient

The patient's color should be observed while the respiration is being measured. A reduction in the oxygen supply to the tissues (**hypoxia**) results in a condition known as **cyanosis**, which causes a bluish discoloration of the skin and mucous membranes. Cyanosis is first observed in the nail beds and lips because in these areas the blood vessels lie close to the surface of the skin. Cyanosis typically occurs in patients with advanced emphysema and in patients during cardiac arrest.

Apnea is a temporary absence of respirations. Some individuals experience apnea during sleep; this condition is known as *sleep apnea.* Apnea can be a serious condition if the individual's breathing ceases for more than 4 to 6 minutes because brain damage or death could occur.

Respiratory Abnormalities

A patient who is having difficulty breathing or shortness of breath has a condition known as **dyspnea.** Dyspnea may occur normally during vigorous physical exertion and abnormally in patients with asthma and emphysema. A patient with dyspnea may find it easier to breathe while in a sitting or standing position. This state is called **orthopnea** and occurs with disorders of the heart and lungs, such as asthma, emphysema, pneumonia, and congestive heart failure.

Breath Sounds

Breath sounds are caused by air moving through the respiratory tract. Normal breath sounds are quiet and barely audible. Abnormal breath sounds are referred to as **adventitious sounds** and generally signify the presence of a respiratory disorder. The causes and characters of abnormal breath sounds are presented in Table 19-6.

PATIENT TEACHING **Chronic Obstructive Pulmonary Disease**

Answer questions that patients have about chronic obstructive pulmonary disease (COPD).

What is COPD?
COPD is a chronic airway obstruction that results from emphysema or chronic bronchitis or a combination of these conditions. COPD is a chronic, debilitating, irreversible, and sometimes fatal disease.

How many people have COPD?
More than 12 million Americans have been diagnosed with COPD; however, it is estimated that an additional 12 million Americans have the disease but remain undiagnosed. COPD is the fourth leading cause of death in the United States behind heart disease, cancer, and stroke. Although COPD is much more common in men than in women, the greatest increase in death rates is occurring in women.

What causes COPD?
Cigarette smoking over a period of many years is the leading cause of COPD. Other causes include air pollution and occupational exposure to irritating inhalants, such as noxious dusts, fumes, and vapors.

What types of tests might the physician order?
Respiratory tests to diagnose COPD include various types of pulmonary function tests. Examples of pulmonary function tests are spirometry, lung volumes, diffusion capacity, arterial blood gas studies, pulse oximetry, and cardiopulmonary exercise tests.

What treatment might the physician prescribe?
Treatment is focused on improving breathing difficulties and may include bronchodilator drug therapy, breathing exercises, and oxygen therapy.
1. Encourage patients with COPD to comply with the therapy prescribed by the physician.
2. Provide the patient with information about smoking, emphysema, and chronic bronchitis. Educational materials are available from the American Lung Association, the American Heart Association, and the American Cancer Society. ■

Table 19-6 Abnormal Breath Sounds

Type	Cause	Character
Crackles* (rales)	Air moving through airways that contain fluid	Dry or wet intermittent sounds that vary in pitch (this sound can be duplicated by rubbing hair together next to ear)
Rhonchi*	Thick secretions, tumors, or spasms that partially obstruct air flow through large upper airways	Deep, low-pitched, rumbling sound more audible during expiration
Wheezes	Severely narrowed airways caused by partial obstruction in smaller bronchi and bronchioles; common symptom of asthma	Continuous, high-pitched, whistling musical sounds heard during inspiration and expiration
Pleural friction rub*	Inflamed pleurae rubbing together	High, grating sound similar to rubbing leather pieces together, heard on inspiration and expiration

From Bonewit-West K: *Clinical procedures for medical assistants*, ed 8, St Louis, 2011, Saunders.
*Audible only through a stethoscope.

PULSE OXIMETRY

Pulse oximetry is a painless and noninvasive procedure used to measure the oxygen saturation of hemoglobin in arterial blood. Hemoglobin is a complex compound found in red blood cells that functions in transporting oxygen in the body. Pulse oximetry provides the physician with information on a patient's cardiorespiratory status, in particular, the amount of oxygen being delivered to the tissues of the body. The procedure for performing pulse oximetry is presented in Procedure 19-8.

A **pulse oximeter** is the device used to measure and display the oxygen saturation of the blood. It is a computerized device that consists of a two-sided, cliplike probe connected by a cable to a monitor (Figure 19-14). A pulse oximeter also measures the patient's pulse rate in beats per minute. A constant-pitched audible beep is emitted with each pulse beat.

Assessment of Oxygen Saturation

Mechanism of Action

The probe of the pulse oximeter must be attached to a peripheral pulsating capillary bed, such as the tip of a finger. One side of the probe contains a **light-emitting diode (LED)** that transmits infrared light and red light through the patient's tissues to a light detector located on the other side of the probe, known as the *photodetector* (Figure 19-15).

Hemoglobin that is bright red in color has a high oxygen content (*oxygen-rich*) and absorbs more of the infrared light

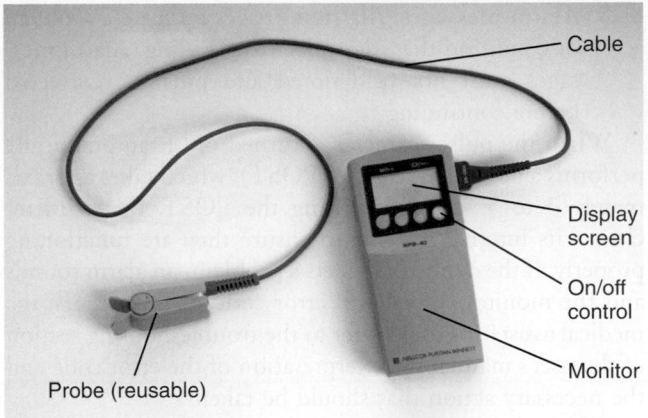

Figure 19-14 Pulse oximeter.

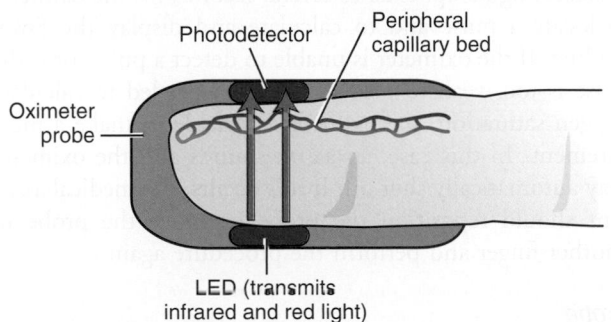

Figure 19-15 The probe of the pulse oximeter is attached to a peripheral capillary bed in the fingertip. The LED transmits light through the capillary bed to a light detector (photodetector) located on the other side of the probe to measure the oxygen saturation of hemoglobin.

emitted by the LED. Hemoglobin that is dark red in color is low in oxygen *(oxygen-poor)* and absorbs more of the red light. The computer of the oximeter compares and calculates the light transmitted from the oxygen-rich hemoglobin and the oxygen-poor hemoglobin and, from this ratio, is able to determine the oxygen saturation of the patient's hemoglobin. This measurement is converted to a percentage and is displayed as a digital readout on the screen of the monitor. Because the pulse oximeter measures the oxygen saturation of peripheral capillaries, the abbreviation SpO_2 *(saturation of peripheral oxygen)* is used to record the reading.

A more complete but invasive measurement of oxygen saturation is arterial blood gas analysis, which requires drawing a blood specimen from an artery. The abbreviation for this type of arterial oxygen saturation measurement is SaO_2 *(saturation of arterial oxygen).*

Interpretation of Results

The pulse oximetry reading represents the percentage of hemoglobin that is saturated (filled) with oxygen. Each molecule of hemoglobin can carry four oxygen molecules. If 100 molecules of hemoglobin were fully saturated with oxygen, they would be carrying 400 molecules of oxygen, and the oxygen saturation reading would be 100%. If these same 100 molecules of hemoglobin were carrying only 360

molecules of oxygen, however, the oxygen saturation reading would be 90%. The more hemoglobin that is saturated with oxygen, the higher the oxygen saturation of the blood.

The oxygen saturation level of most healthy individuals is 95% to 99%. Because the air we breathe is only 21% saturated with oxygen, it is unusual for an individual's hemoglobin to be fully or 100% saturated with oxygen. Patients on supplemental oxygen sometimes have a reading of 100%, however.

An oxygen saturation level of less than 95% typically results in an inadequate amount of oxygen reaching the tissues of the body, although patients with chronic pulmonary disease are sometimes able to tolerate lower saturation levels. Respiratory failure, resulting in tissue damage, usually occurs when the oxygen saturation decreases to a level between 85% and 90%. Cyanosis typically appears when an individual's oxygen saturation reaches a level of 75%, and an oxygen saturation of less than 70% is life-threatening.

A decrease in the oxygen saturation of the blood (less than 95%) is known as **hypoxemia.** Hypoxemia can lead to a more serious condition known as hypoxia. **Hypoxia** is defined as a reduction in the oxygen supply to the tissues of the body, and if not treated, it can lead to tissue damage and death. The first symptoms of hypoxia include headache, mental confusion, nausea, dizziness, shortness of breath, and tachycardia. The tissues most sensitive to hypoxia are the brain, heart, pulmonary vessels, and liver.

Purpose of Pulse Oximetry

In the medical office, pulse oximetry is often performed on patients complaining of respiratory problems (e.g., dyspnea). A decreased pulse oximetry reading (along with further testing and the patient's clinical signs and symptoms) assists the physician in proper diagnosis and treatment, which may include drug therapy and oxygen therapy.

Conditions that can cause a decreased SpO_2 value (hypoxemia) include the following:
- Acute pulmonary disease (e.g., pneumonia)
- Chronic pulmonary disease (e.g., emphysema, asthma, bronchitis)
- Cardiac problems (e.g., congestive heart failure, coronary artery disease)

In addition to assisting the physician in diagnosing a patient's condition, pulse oximetry is used to assess the following:
- Effectiveness of oxygen therapy
- Patient's tolerance to activity
- Effectiveness of treatment (e.g., bronchodilators)
- Patient's tolerance to analgesia and sedation

In the medical office, pulse oximetry is most often used as a "spot-check" measurement, in other words, as a single measurement of oxygen saturation. Occasionally, pulse oximetry may be used for the short-term *continuous monitoring* of a patient in the office for the following: to monitor a patient experiencing an asthmatic attack or to monitor a sedated patient during minor office surgery.

Components of the Pulse Oximeter

Most medical offices use a handheld pulse oximeter (see Figure 19-14), which is portable, lightweight, and battery operated. This is in contrast to a stand-alone oximeter, which is more apt to be used in a hospital setting for the continuous bedside monitoring of a patient's oxygen saturation level. A pulse oximeter not only measures oxygen saturation, it also measures the pulse rate in beats per minute. The two main parts of the pulse oximeter—the monitor and the probe—are described in detail next.

Monitor

The monitor contains controls, indicators, and displays (Figure 19-16). These may vary slightly depending on the brand of oximeter. Those that are found on most handheld pulse oximeters include the following:

1. **On/off control.** Turns the oximeter on and off.
2. **SpO₂% display.** A digital display of the patient's oxygen saturation expressed as a percent. This number is updated with each pulse beat.
3. **Pulse rate display.** This display indicates the patient's pulse rate in beats per minute. This number is updated with each pulse beat. Most oximeters emit a constant-pitched audible beep with each pulse beat.
4. **Pulse strength bar-graph indicator.** This indicator provides a visual display of the patient's pulse strength at the probe placement site. The pulse strength indicator consists of a segmented display of bars. The pulse strength indicator "sweeps" with each pulse beat, and the stronger the pulse, the more segments that light up on the bar graph.
5. **Pulse search indicator.** This indicator lights up when the oximeter is searching for the patient's pulse.
6. **Adjustable volume control.** This control is used to adjust the beep that sounds with each pulse beat. In most oximeters, the settings are high, low, and off.
7. **Low battery indicator.** This indicator is used to warn that the battery is getting low. The indicator lights up and the monitor sounds an alarm when approximately 30 minutes of battery use remains.

8. **Alarm messages.** Alarm messages indicate a problem or condition that may affect the reading. Alarm messages must not be ignored and must be corrected before continuing.

When the pulse oximeter is turned on, it automatically performs a power-on self-test (POST), which takes approximately 3 to 5 seconds. During the POST, the oximeter checks its internal systems to ensure they are functioning properly. If the oximeter detects a problem, an alarm sounds and the monitor displays an error code. If this occurs, the medical assistant should refer to the troubleshooting section of the user's manual for interpretation of the error code and the necessary action that should be taken.

When the POST is completed, the oximeter begins searching for a pulse. During this time, the pulse search indicator lights up. It takes several seconds for the oximeter to locate a pulse and to calculate and display the SpO₂ reading. If the oximeter is unable to detect a pulse, or if the pulse is too weak to provide the data needed to calculate oxygen saturation, the oximeter is unable to make a measurement. In this case, an alarm sounds and the oximeter may automatically shut off. If this occurs, the medical assistant should reposition the probe or move the probe to another finger and perform the procedure again.

Probe

The probe of the pulse oximeter may be reusable or disposable (Figure 19-17). Most offices use reusable clip-on probes. Reusable probes are convenient to use and easy to apply, but they are more susceptible to inaccurate readings

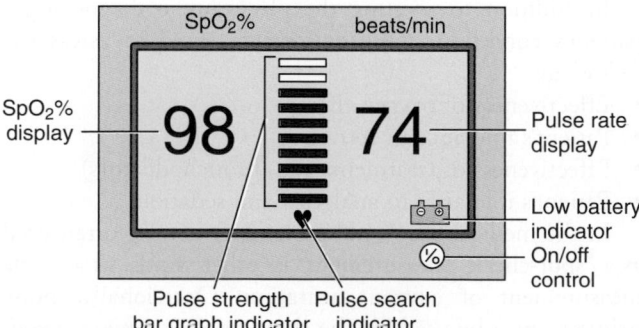

Figure 19-16 Pulse oximeter monitor: controls, indicators, and displays.

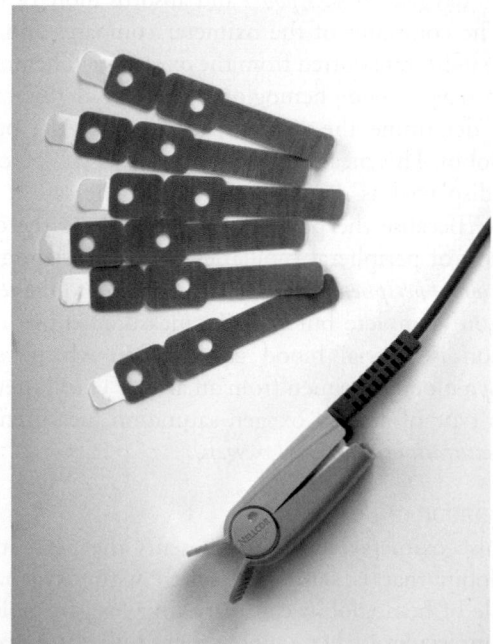

Figure 19-17 Disposable *(top)* and reusable *(bottom)* probes for the pulse oximeter.

owing to patient movement. Reusable probes must be cleaned and disinfected after each use. Disposable probes are expensive to use and are generally employed for the long-term monitoring of a patient's oxygen saturation level in a hospital setting. Disposable probes are made of an adhesive bandage–like material and are discarded after use.

It is important to handle reusable probes carefully. Hitting a probe against a hard object or dropping it may damage it. It is important to use the probe designed for the pulse oximeter that is being used. Mixing probes from different manufacturers can result in an inaccurate reading.

The probe must be attached to the patient at a peripheral site that is highly vascular and where the skin is thin. The most common site to apply a probe is the tip of a finger (Figure 19-18); other acceptable sites include the toe and earlobe. A specially designed probe is available for application to the earlobe; it is smaller than a finger probe and has a curved ear attachment to hold it in place.

A cable connects the probe to the monitor. The probe may be permanently attached to the cable, or it may be a separate device that requires connection to the cable. The pulse oximeter monitor should never be lifted or carried by the cable because this could damage the cable connections or could cause the cable to disconnect from the monitor and possibly drop on the floor or fall on the patient.

Factors Affecting Pulse Oximetry

Although pulse oximetry is an easy procedure to perform, the medical assistant must be aware of certain factors that may interfere with an accurate reading. These factors are listed, along with guidelines for correcting or preventing them.

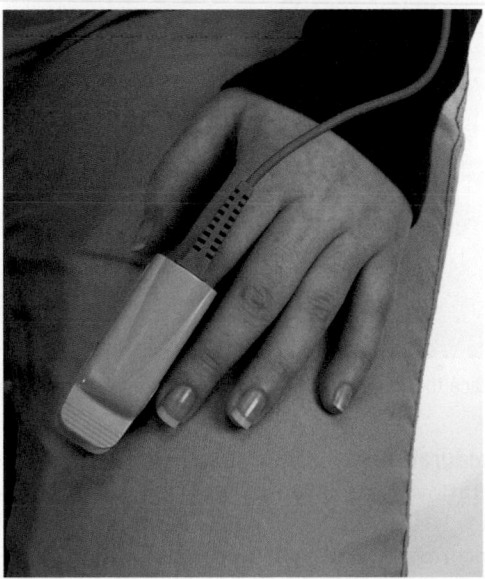

Figure 19-18 Applying a probe to the tip of a finger.

1. **Incorrect positioning of the probe.** As previously discussed, the oximeter probe consists of two parts: an LED and a photodetector. Because light is transmitted from the LED through the tissues to the photodetector, it is important that these two components be aligned directly opposite to each other during the measurement. In most cases, this automatically occurs when the clip-on probe is applied. Proper alignment of the probe may be impossible, however, with patients who have very small fingers (e.g., a thin individual, a child) or with patients who have very large fingers (e.g., an obese individual). To obtain an accurate reading, another site must be used, such as the earlobe. In addition, pediatric probes are available for use with thin patients or children.

2. **Fingernail polish or artificial nails.** A dark, opaque coating on the fingernail may result in a falsely low reading. This is because the coating interferes with proper light transmission through the finger. The darker the coating, the more likely that the SpO₂ reading will be affected. Blue, black, and green fingernail polishes tend to cause the most problems. If the patient is wearing fingernail polish, it should be removed with acetone or fingernail polish remover. If the patient has artificial fingernails, another site should be used to take the measurement, such as the earlobe or the toe. Oil, dirt, and grime on the fingertip can also interfere with proper light transmission. If the patient's fingertip is dirty, cleanse the site with soap and water and allow it to dry. Areas with bruises, burns, stains, or tattoos should be avoided as a probe placement site. Darkly pigmented skin and jaundice do not usually affect the ability of the oximeter to obtain an accurate reading.

3. **Poor peripheral blood flow.** A pulse oximeter works best when there is a good strong pulse in the finger to which the probe is applied. Poor peripheral blood flow may cause the pulse to be so weak that the oximeter cannot obtain a reading. Conditions resulting in poor blood flow include peripheral vascular disease, vasoconstrictor medications, severe hypotension, and hypothermia. In these situations, the medical assistant should try using the earlobe because it is less affected by decreased blood flow. Sometimes patients with cold fingers (but who are not hypothermic) may have enough constriction of the peripheral capillaries that it interferes with obtaining a reading. To solve this problem, the medical assistant should ask the patient to warm his or her fingers by rubbing the hands together. The probe should never be attached to the finger of an arm to which an automatic blood pressure cuff is applied because blood flow to the finger would be cut off when the cuff inflates, resulting in loss of the pulse signal.

4. **Ambient (surrounding) light.** Ambient light shining directly on the probe, such as bright fluorescent light, direct sunlight, or an overhead examination light,

may result in an inaccurate reading. This is because some of the ambient light may be picked up by the probe's photodetector and alter the reading. This problem can be corrected by one of the following: turning off the light, moving the patient's hand away from the light source, or covering the probe with an opaque material such as a washcloth.

5. **Patient movement.** Patient movement is a common cause of an inaccurate reading. Motion affects the ability of the light to travel from the LED to the photodetector and prevents the probe from picking up the pulse signal. To avoid this problem, it is important that the medical assistant instruct the patient to remain still during the procedure. Occasionally, patient movement cannot be eliminated, such as when the patient has tremors of the hands. In these instances, the oxygen saturation level should be measured at a site that is less affected by motion, such as the toe or the earlobe.

Pulse Oximeter Care and Maintenance

The pulse oximeter monitor and cable should be cleaned periodically using a cloth slightly dampened with a solution of warm water and a disinfectant cleaner. The medical assistant should make sure that the cloth is not too wet to prevent the solution from running into the monitor, which could damage the internal components. The probe should be cleaned periodically with a soft cloth moistened with warm water and a disinfectant cleaner. Cleaning the probe removes dirt and grime that could interfere with proper light transmission, leading to an inaccurate reading. The probe also should be disinfected after each use by wiping it thoroughly with an antiseptic wipe and allowing it to dry. The probe should never be soaked or immersed in a liquid solution because this would damage it. The probe is heat sensitive and cannot be autoclaved. The pulse oximeter should be stored at room temperature in a dry environment.

Text continued on p. 331

PROCEDURE 19-6   Measuring Pulse and Respiration

Outcome Measure pulse and respiration.

Equipment/Supplies

- Watch with a second hand

1. **Procedural Step.** Sanitize your hands. Greet the patient and introduce yourself. Identify the patient and explain the procedure. Observe the patient for any signs that might affect the pulse or respiratory rate.
   Principle. Pulse rate can vary according to the factors listed on Page 316.

2. **Procedural Step.** Have the patient sit down. Position the patient's arm in a comfortable position. The forearm should be slightly flexed to relax the muscles and tendons over the pulse site.
   Principle. Relaxed muscles and tendons over the pulse site make it easier to palpate the pulse.

3. **Procedural Step.** Place your three middle fingertips over the radial pulse site. Never use your thumb to take a pulse. The radial pulse is located in a groove on the inner aspect of the wrist just below the thumb.
   Principle. The thumb has a pulse of its own; using the thumb results in measurement of the medical assistant's pulse and not the patient's pulse.

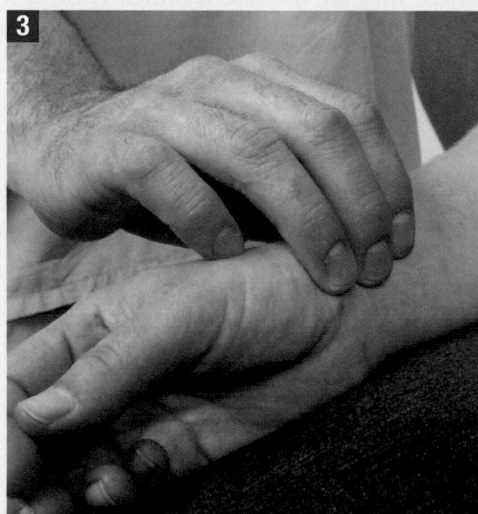

Place the three middle fingers over the radial pulse site.

4. **Procedural Step.** Apply moderate, gentle pressure directly over the site until you feel the pulse. If you cannot feel the pulse, this may be caused by:
   a. Incorrect location of the radial pulse: Move your fingers to a slightly different location in the groove of the wrist until you feel the pulse.

PROCEDURE 19-6   Measuring Pulse and Respiration—cont'd

   b. Applying too much pressure or not enough pressure: Vary the depth of your hold until you can feel the pulse.
      Principle. A normal pulse can be felt with moderate pressure. The pulse cannot be felt if not enough pressure is applied, whereas too much pressure applied to the radial artery closes it off, and no pulse is felt.

5. **Procedural Step.** Count the pulse for 30 seconds and make a mental note of this number. Note the rhythm and volume of the pulse. If abnormalities occur in the rhythm or volume, count the pulse for 1 full minute.
Principle. A longer time ensures an accurate assessment of abnormalities.

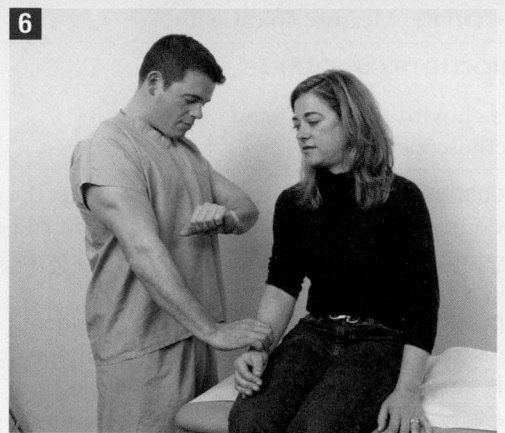

Count the number of respirations for 30 seconds.

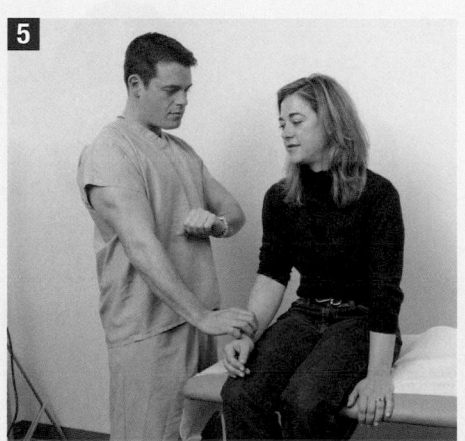

Count the pulse for 30 seconds.

6. **Procedural Step.** After taking the pulse, continue to hold three fingers on the patient's wrist with the same amount of pressure, and measure the respirations. This helps to ensure that the patient is unaware that respirations are being monitored.
Principle. If the patient is aware that respiration is being measured, the breathing may change.

7. **Procedural Step.** Observe the rise and fall of the patient's chest as the patient inhales and exhales.
Principle. One complete respiration includes one inhalation and one exhalation.

8. **Procedural Step.** Count the number of respirations for 30 seconds and make a mental note of this number; note the rhythm and depth of the respirations. Also observe the patient's color. If abnormalities occur in rhythm or depth, count the respiratory rate for 1 full minute.

9. **Procedural Step.** Sanitize your hands, and chart the results. If you counted the pulse and respirations for 30 seconds, multiply each of the numbers counted by 2. This will give you the pulse rate and respiratory rate for 1 full minute. Include the date; the time; the pulse rate, rhythm, and volume; and the respiratory rate, rhythm, and depth.

CHARTING EXAMPLE

Date	
10/15/XX	2:30 p.m. P: 74. Reg and strong. R: 18. Even and reg. ——————— S. Martinez, RMA

PROCEDURE 19-7 **Measuring Apical Pulse**

Outcome Measure apical pulse.

Equipment/Supplies

- Watch with a second hand
- Stethoscope
- Antiseptic wipe

1. **Procedural Step.** Sanitize your hands. Greet the patient and introduce yourself. Identify the patient and explain the procedure. Observe the patient for any signs that might increase or decrease the pulse rate.

2. **Procedural Step.** Assemble the equipment. If the stethoscope's chest piece consists of a diaphragm and a bell, rotate the chest piece to the bell position. Clean the earpieces and chest piece of the stethoscope with an antiseptic wipe.
   Principle. The bell position allows better auscultation of heart sounds. Cleaning the earpieces helps prevent the transmission of microorganisms.

3. **Procedural Step.** Ask the patient to unbutton or remove his or her shirt. Have the patient sit or lie down (supine).
   Principle. A sitting or supine position allows access to the apex of the heart.

4. **Procedural Step.** Warm the chest piece of the stethoscope with your hands. Insert the earpieces of the stethoscope into your ears, with the earpieces directed slightly forward, and place the chest piece over the apex of the patient's heart. The apex of the heart is located in the fifth intercostal space at the junction of the left midclavicular line.
   Principle. Warming the chest piece reduces the discomfort of having a cold object placed on the chest. In addition, a cold chest piece could startle the patient, resulting in an increase in pulse rate. The earpieces should be directed forward to follow the direction of the ear canal, which facilitates hearing.

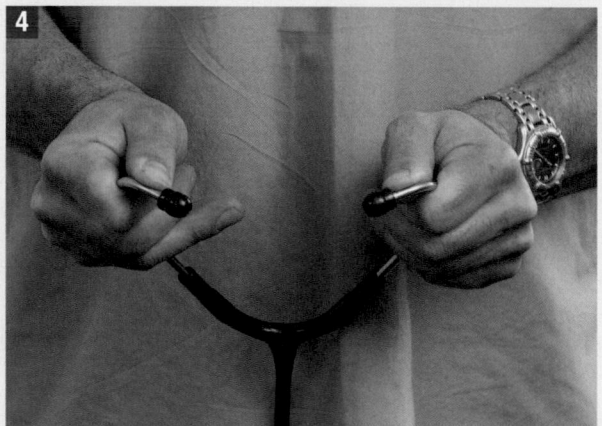

Insert the earpieces into your ears with the earpieces directed slightly forward.

5. **Procedural Step.** Listen for the heartbeat, and count the number of beats for 30 seconds (and multiply by 2) if the rhythm and volume are normal or if the apical pulse is being taken on an infant or child. If abnormalities occur in the rhythm or volume, count the pulse for 1 full minute. You will hear a "lubb-dupp" sound through the stethoscope. This sound is the closing of the heart's valves. Each "lubb-dupp" is counted as one beat.

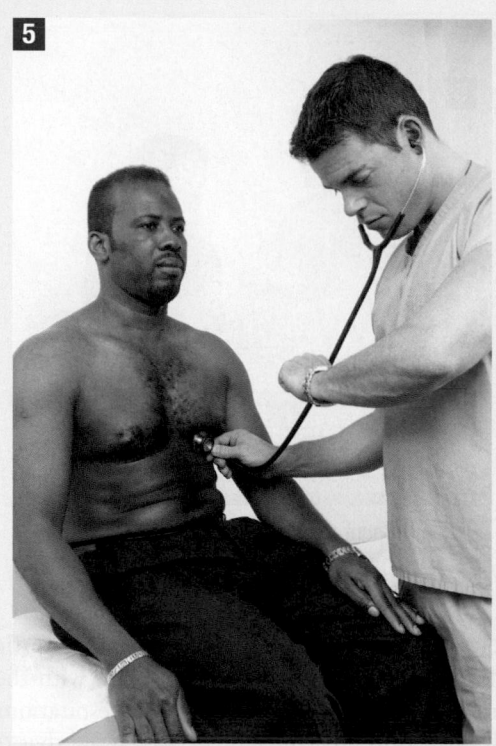

Count the number of beats for 30 seconds, and multiply by 2.

6. **Procedural Step.** Sanitize your hands, and chart the results. Include the date, the time, and the apical pulse rate, rhythm, and volume.

7. **Procedural Step.** Clean the earpieces and the chest piece of the stethoscope with an antiseptic wipe.

CHARTING EXAMPLE

Date	
10/15/XX	10:15 a.m. AP: 68. Reg and strong.————
	———————— S. Martinez, CMA (AAMA)

PROCEDURE 19-8   **Performing Pulse Oximetry**

Outcome Perform pulse oximetry.

Equipment/Supplies

- Handheld pulse oximeter
- Reusable finger probe
- Antiseptic wipe

1. Procedural Step. Sanitize your hands.

2. Procedural Step. Assemble the equipment. Handle the probe carefully, and perform the following:

a. Carefully inspect the probe to ensure it opens and closes smoothly. Inspect the probe windows (LED and photodetector) to ensure they are clean and free of lint.

b. Disinfect the probe windows and surrounding platforms with an antiseptic wipe, and allow them to dry.

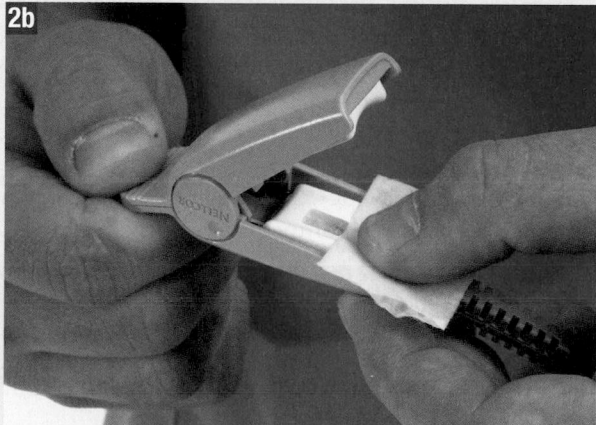

Disinfect the probe with an antiseptic wipe.

c. If necessary, connect the probe to the cable.

d. Connect the cable to the monitor by plugging it into the port on the monitor. Do not lift or carry the monitor by the cable.

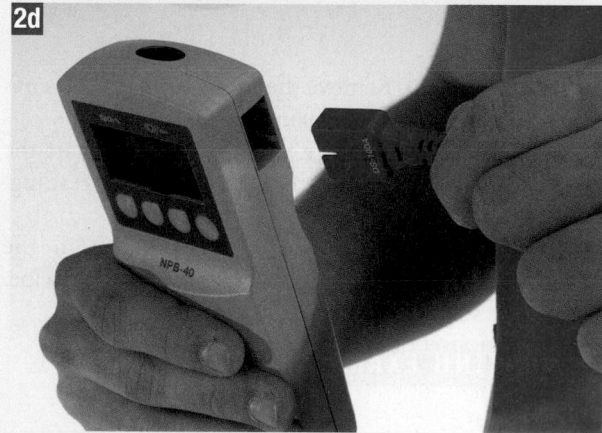

Connect the cable to the monitor by plugging it into the port on the monitor.

Principle. Misuse or improper handling of the probe could damage it. Dirt or lint on the probe windows could interfere with proper light transmission, leading to an inaccurate reading. Cross-contamination between patients is prevented by disinfecting the probe. Lifting the monitor by the cable could damage the cable connections.

3. Procedural Step. Greet the patient and introduce yourself. Identify the patient and explain the procedure. Explain to the patient that the clip-on probe does not hurt and feels similar to a clothespin attached to the finger. If the patient seems fearful, place the probe on your own finger first to reassure the patient that it is not painful.

4. Procedural Step. Seat the patient comfortably in a chair with the lower arm firmly supported and the palm facing down.

Principle. Supporting the lower arm helps prevent patient movement during the procedure.

5. Procedural Step. Select an appropriate finger to apply the probe. Use the tip of the patient's index, middle, or ring finger. If the patient's fingers are very small or very large, and the probe cannot seem to be aligned properly, use the earlobe to take the measurement. If the patient exhibits tremors of the hands, use the earlobe to obtain the reading.

Principle. The probe must be applied to a peripheral site with thin skin that is highly vascular. Very small or very large fingers may not allow for proper positioning of the probe on the finger.

6. Procedural Step. Observe the patient's fingernail. If the patient is wearing dark fingernail polish, ask him or her to remove it with acetone or nail polish remover. If the patient is wearing artificial nails, choose another probe site, such as the toe or earlobe.

Principle. An opaque coating on the fingernail may interfere with proper light transmission through the finger, leading to an inaccurate reading.

7. Procedural Step. Check to ensure that the patient's fingertip is clean. If it is dirty, cleanse the site with soap and water, and allow it to dry. Ensure that the patient's finger is not cold. If it is cold, ask the patient to rub his or her hands together.

Principle. Oils, dirt, or grime on the finger can interfere with proper light transmission through the finger, leading to an inaccurate reading. Sometimes patients with cold fingers may have enough constriction of the capillaries that it interferes with obtaining a reading.

8. Procedural Step. Ensure that ambient light does not interfere with the measurement. Position the probe securely on the fingertip as follows:

PROCEDURE 19-8

Continued

PROCEDURE 19-8   Performing Pulse Oximetry—cont'd

a. Ensure that the probe window is fully covered by placing the finger over the LED window, with the fleshy tip of the finger covering the window. The tip of the finger should touch the end of the probe stop.

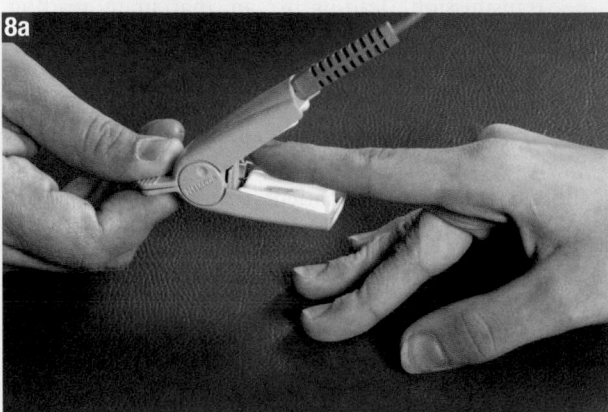

Position the probe securely on the fingertip.

b. Ensure that the light-emitting diode and the photodetector are aligned opposite to each other.

c. Allow the cable to lay across the back of the hand and parallel to the arm of the patient.
Principle. Ambient light can be picked up by the probe and alter the reading. Proper alignment of the LED and photodetector is necessary for an accurate reading.

9. Procedural Step. Instruct the patient to remain still and to breathe normally. Turn on the oximeter by pressing the on/off control. Wait while the oximeter goes through its power-on self-test (POST). If the monitor fails the POST, refer to the troubleshooting section of the user manual for interpretation of the error code and the necessary action that should be taken.
Principle. Patient movement may lead to an inaccurate reading. The monitor automatically conducts a POST to ensure that it is functioning properly.

10. Procedural Step. Allow several seconds for the pulse oximeter to detect the pulse and calculate the oxygen saturation of the blood. Ensure that the pulse strength indicator fluctuates with each pulsation and that the pulse signal is strong. If the oximeter sounds an alarm indicating that it was unable to locate a pulse, reposition the probe on the patient's finger or move the probe to another finger, and perform the procedure again.
Principle. The reading takes several seconds to display. The pulse strength indicator provides a quick assessment of pulse quality. If the oximeter is unable to locate a pulse, it will be unable to obtain a reading.

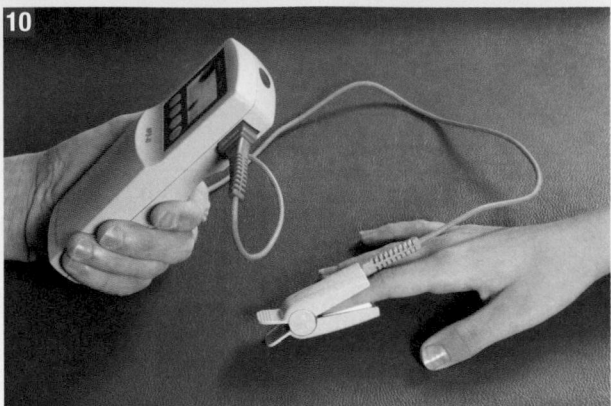

Allow several seconds for the pulse oximeter to detect the pulse.

11 Procedural Step. Leave the probe in place until the oximeter displays a reading. Read the oxygen saturation value and pulse rate, and make a mental note of these readings. On this pulse oximeter, the oxygen saturation reading is 100% and the pulse rate is 75. If the SpO$_2$ reading is less than 95%, reposition the probe on the finger, and perform the procedure again. *Principle.* A low SpO$_2$ reading may be caused by improper positioning of the probe on the finger.

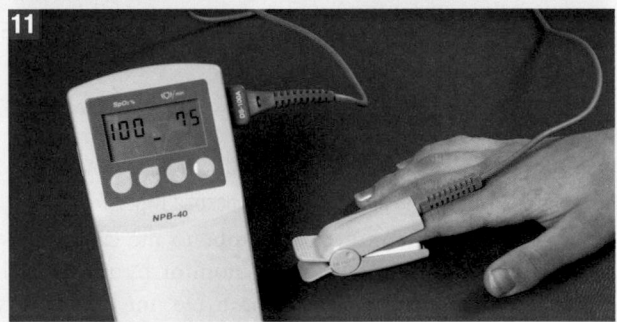

Read the oxygen saturation value and pulse rate.

12. Procedural Step. Remove the probe from the patient's finger, and turn off the oximeter.

13. Procedural Step. Sanitize your hands, and chart the results. Include the date, the time, the SpO$_2$ reading, and the pulse rate.

14. Procedural Step. Disconnect the cable from the monitor. Disinfect the probe with an antiseptic wipe. Properly store the monitor in a clean, dry area.

CHARTING EXAMPLE

Date	
10/15/XX	2:30 p.m. SpO$_2$: 100%. P: 75. —————————————————— S. Martinez, RMA

BLOOD PRESSURE

Mechanism of Blood Pressure

Blood pressure (BP) is a measurement of the pressure or force exerted by the blood on the walls of the arteries in which it is contained. Each time the ventricles contract, blood is pushed out of the heart and into the aorta and pulmonary aorta, exerting pressure on the walls of the arteries. This phase in the cardiac cycle is known as **systole,** and it represents the highest point of blood pressure in the body, or the **systolic pressure.** The phase of the cardiac cycle in which the heart relaxes between contractions is referred to as **diastole.** The **diastolic pressure** (recorded during diastole) is lower because the heart is relaxed. Contraction and relaxation of the heart result in two different pressures—systolic and diastolic.

Interpretation of Blood Pressure

Blood pressure measurement is expressed as a fraction. The numerator is the systolic pressure, and the denominator is the diastolic pressure. The standard unit for measuring blood pressure is millimeters of mercury (mm Hg). A blood pressure reading of 110/70 mm Hg means that there was enough force to raise a column of mercury 110 mm during systole and 70 mm during diastole.

Based on guidelines from the National Heart, Lung, and Blood Institute (NHLBI), a blood pressure reading of less than 120/80 mm Hg is classified as normal, whereas a blood pressure reading of 120/80 is classified as *prehypertension.* These guidelines were issued as a result of scientific studies showing that the risk of heart disease begins at a blood pressure reading lower than previously thought. The NHLBI guidelines are outlined in Table 19-7.

Blood pressure should be taken during every office visit to allow the physician to compare the patient's readings over time. This is a good preventive measure in guarding against serious illness. A single blood pressure reading taken on one occasion does not characterize an individual's blood pressure accurately. Several readings, taken on different occasions, provide a good index of an individual's baseline blood pressure.

Blood pressure readings always should be interpreted using a patient's baseline blood pressure. An increase or decrease of 20 to 30 mm Hg in a patient's baseline blood pressure is significant, even if it is still within the normal accepted blood pressure range.

The most common condition that causes an abnormal blood pressure reading is **hypertension.** Hypertension, or high blood pressure, results from excessive pressure on the walls of the arteries. Hypertension is determined by a sustained systolic blood pressure reading of 140 mm Hg or greater, or a sustained diastolic reading of 90 mm Hg or greater. See Table 19-7 for the NHLBI classifications for hypertension. **Hypotension,** or low blood pressure, results from reduced pressure on the arterial walls. Hypotension is determined by a blood pressure reading of less than 95/60 mm Hg.

Pulse Pressure

The difference between systolic and diastolic pressures is the **pulse pressure.** It is determined by subtracting the smaller number from the larger. If the blood pressure is 110/70 mm Hg, the pulse pressure would be 40 mm Hg. A pulse pressure between 30 and 50 mm Hg is considered to be within normal range.

Factors Affecting Blood Pressure

Blood pressure does not remain at a constant value. Numerous factors may affect it throughout the course of the day. An understanding of these factors helps to ensure an accurate interpretation of blood pressure readings.

1. **Age.** Age is an important consideration when determining whether a patient's blood pressure is normal. As age increases, the blood pressure gradually increases: A 6-year-old child may have a normal reading of 90/60 mm Hg, whereas a young, healthy adult may have a blood pressure reading of 116/76 mm Hg, and it would not be unusual for a 60-year-old man to have a reading of 130/90 mm Hg. As an individual gets older, there is a loss of elasticity in the walls of the blood vessels, causing this increase in pressure to occur. Table 19-8 is a chart of the average optimal blood pressure readings for various age groups.
2. **Gender.** After puberty, women usually have a lower blood pressure than men of the same age. After menopause, women usually have a higher blood pressure than men of the same age.

Table 19-7 Classification of Blood Pressure for Adults Age 18 and Older

Blood Pressure Classifications	Systolic Blood Pressure, mm Hg		Diastolic Blood Pressure, mm Hg
Normal	Less than 120	*and*	Less than 80
Prehypertension*	120-139	*or*	80-89
Hypertension*			
Stage 1	140-159	*or*	90-99
Stage 2	160 or higher	*or*	100 or higher

From National Heart, Lung, and Blood Institute: Seventh report of the Joint National Committee on Detection, Evaluation, and Treatment of High Blood Pressure. Bethesda, Md: NIH Publication No. 03-5231, May, 2003, U.S. Department of Health and Human Services.
*Based on the average of two or more properly measured, seated blood pressure readings taken at each of two or more visits.

3. **Diurnal variations.** Fluctuations in an individual's blood pressure are normal during the course of a day. When one awakens, the blood pressure is lower as a result of decreased metabolism and physical activity during sleep. As metabolism and activity increase during the day, the blood pressure rises.

4. **Emotional states.** Strong emotional states, such as anger, fear, and excitement, increase the blood pressure. If the medical assistant observes such a reaction, an attempt should be made to calm the patient before taking his or her blood pressure.

5. **Exercise.** Physical activity temporarily increases the blood pressure. To ensure an accurate reading, a patient who has been involved in physical activity should be given an opportunity to rest for 20 to 30 minutes before blood pressure is measured.

6. **Body position.** The blood pressure of a patient who is in a lying or standing position is usually different from that measured when the patient is sitting. For example, the diastolic pressure of an individual in a sitting position is higher than his or her diastolic pressure in a lying position. A notation should be made on the patient's chart if the reading was obtained in any position other than sitting, by using the following abbreviations: *L* (lying) and *St* (standing).

7. **Medications.** Many medications may increase or decrease the blood pressure. Because of this factor, it is important to record in the patient chart all prescription and over-the-counter medications that the patient is taking.

8. **Other factors.** Other factors that may increase the blood pressure include pain, a recent meal, caffeine, smoking, and bladder distention.

Assessment of Manual Blood Pressure

The equipment needed to measure manual blood pressure includes a stethoscope and a sphygmomanometer. The **stethoscope** amplifies sounds produced by the body and allows the medical assistant to hear them.

Table 19-8 Average Optimal Blood Pressure for Age	
Age	**Blood Pressure, mm Hg**
Newborn (6.6 lb)	40 (mean)
1 mo	85/54
1 yr	95/65
6 yr*	105/65
10-13 yr*	110/65
14-17 yr*	120/75
Adult	Less than 120/80

From National High Blood Pressure Education Program (NHBPEP); National Heart, Lung, and Blood Institute; National Institutes of Health: The seventh report of the Joint National Committees on Detection, Evaluation, and Treatment of High Blood Pressure, *JAMA* 239:2560, 2003.
*In children and adolescents, hypertension is defined as blood pressure that is, on repeated measurement, at the 95th percentile or greater adjusted for age, height, and gender (NHBPEP, 1997).

Stethoscope

The most common type of stethoscope used in the medical office is the acoustic stethoscope. It consists of four parts: earpieces, sidepieces known as *binaurals,* plastic or rubber tubing, and a chest piece (Figure 19-19, *A*).

What Would You Do? What Would You *Not* Do?

Case Study 3

Tyrone Jackson, 45 years old, is at the medical office to have his blood pressure checked. Three months ago, Tyrone started taking a diuretic and an antihypertensive prescribed by the physician to reduce his blood pressure. The last recording in his chart indicates that Tyrone's blood pressure decreased from 180/112 mm Hg to 126/84 mm Hg; however, his blood pressure at this visit is 158/98 mm Hg. Tyrone says that he has not been very good at taking his medication lately. He says it is really hard to remember to take all those pills every day. He also says that he felt just fine before being put on blood pressure pills, but when he started taking them, he felt awful. He had to urinate more often; when he got up fast, he felt dizzy; and he had some problems with headaches. Tyrone says that he decided to cut back on his pills to see if these problems got better, and sure enough, they went away altogether. Tyrone wants to know if there's anything he can do to lower his blood pressure other than taking pills. ■

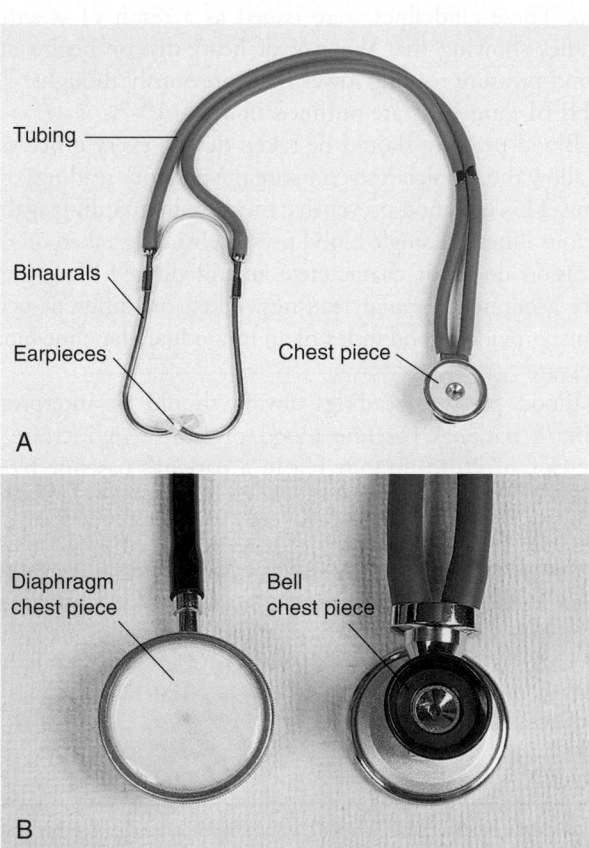

Figure 19-19 **A,** The parts of a stethoscope. **B,** Types of chest pieces.

Stethoscope Chest Piece

There are two types of chest pieces: a *diaphragm,* which is a large, flat disc, and a bell, which has a bowl-shaped appearance (Figure 19-19, *B*). The chest piece of a stethoscope consists of a diaphragm and a bell, or just a diaphragm. If a chest piece consists of a diaphragm and a bell, the medical assistant must ensure that the desired piece is rotated into position before use. Failure to do so would not allow the medical assistant to hear sound through the earpieces.

The diaphragm chest piece is more useful for hearing high-pitched sounds, such as lung and bowel sounds, whereas the bell chest piece is more useful for hearing low-pitched sounds, such as those produced by the heart and vascular system. Before using a stethoscope, the medical assistant should ensure that it is in proper working condition.

Sphygmomanometer

The **sphygmomanometer** is an instrument that measures the pressure of blood within an artery. It consists of a **manometer,** an inner inflatable bladder surrounded by a covering known as the *cuff,* and a pressure bulb with a control valve to inflate and deflate the inner bladder. The manometer contains a scale for registering the pressure of the air in the bladder.

Two types of sphygmomanometers are used—aneroid and mercury. The *aneroid sphygmomanometer* is lightweight and portable, but the *mercury sphygmomanometer* is more accurate.

Aneroid Sphygmomanometer

The aneroid sphygmomanometer (Figure 19-20) has a manometer gauge with a round scale. The scale is calibrated in millimeters, with a needle that points to the calibrations (Figure 19-21). To ensure an accurate reading, the needle must be positioned initially at zero. The manometer must be placed in the correct position for proper viewing. The medical assistant should be no farther than 3 feet from the scale on the gauge of the manometer, and the manometer

---

PATIENT TEACHING Hypertension

Answer questions patients have about hypertension.

What is high blood pressure?
Blood pressure is the force of blood against the walls of the arteries. High blood pressure, also called *hypertension,* means the pressure in the arteries is consistently above normal (140/90 mm Hg), resulting in excessive pressure on the walls of the arteries. Hypertension is the most common life-threatening disease among Americans. It is estimated that approximately 74 million adult Americans, age 20 and older, have high blood pressure, and another 25 million have blood pressure in the prehypertension range. Prehypertension is a reading higher than 120/80 but below 140/90. The incidence of hypertension in the United States has increased dramatically as a result of an aging population and an increased incidence of obesity.

What are the symptoms of high blood pressure?
Approximately 20% of individuals who have high blood pressure are unaware of it because there are few or no symptoms and, as a result, an individual with hypertension may go undiagnosed for many years. If symptoms do occur, they may include one or more of the following: headaches, dizziness, flushed face, fatigue, epistaxis (nosebleed), excessive perspiration, heart palpitations, frequent urination, and leg claudication (cramping in the legs with walking). The only way to know for sure whether you have high blood pressure is to have it checked regularly.

What causes high blood pressure?
In 90% to 95% of cases, the precise cause of high blood pressure is unknown. This type of hypertension is known as *essential* or *primary hypertension.* Certain factors seem to increase the risk of developing essential hypertension, however; these include the following:

Uncontrollable Risk Factors
- **Heredity.** A family history of high blood pressure increases an individual's risk of developing high blood pressure.
- **Ethnicity.** Research has shown that more black than white Americans develop high blood pressure.
- **Age.** Blood pressure normally increases as one grows older. High blood pressure occurs most often in individuals over the age of 35. Men tend to develop high blood pressure most often between the ages of 35 and 55, whereas women are more likely to develop it after menopause.

Controllable Risk Factors
- **Obesity.** Individuals with a BMI (body mass index) of 30 or higher are more likely to develop high blood pressure.
- **Sodium intake.** Sodium, found in salt and processed, canned, and most snack foods, does not cause high blood pressure; however, it can aggravate high blood pressure. Most Americans consume more sodium than they need. The current recommendation is to consume less than 2.4 g (2400 mg) of sodium per day. This is equivalent to 6 g (about 1 teaspoon) of salt.
- **Lack of physical exercise.** A sedentary lifestyle makes it easier to gain weight and increases the chance of developing high blood pressure.
- **Chronic stress.** Research indicates that people who are under continuous stress tend to develop more heart and circulatory problems than people who are not under stress.
- **Smoking.** Smoking tobacco constricts blood vessels, causing an increase in blood pressure.
- **Alcohol consumption.** Heavy and regular alcohol consumption can increase blood pressure.

The remaining 5% to 10% of individuals with hypertension have *secondary hypertension.* This means that high blood

Continued

pressure can be linked to a known cause, which includes chronic kidney disease, adrenal and thyroid diseases, narrowing of the aorta, steroid therapy, oral contraceptives, and pre-eclampsia associated with pregnancy.

What can happen if high blood pressure is not treated?

If high blood pressure is not brought under control, it can cause severe damage to vital organs, such as the heart, brain, kidneys, and eyes. This damage can result in a heart attack or heart failure, stroke, kidney damage, or damaged vision. Early detection and treatment of high blood pressure can prevent these complications. High blood pressure is often discovered during a routine medical examination or (less commonly) when an individual experiences one of the complications of hypertension caused by damage to a vital organ.

Can high blood pressure be cured?

Essential hypertension cannot be cured, but many treatments are used to bring it under control. These include lifestyle modifications, such as weight reduction, a healthy diet rich in fruits and vegetables and low in saturated fat, limitation of salt intake, regular aerobic exercise, cessation of smoking, limitation or elimination of alcohol consumption, and stress management. If lifestyle modifications alone are not enough, medications are available for reducing blood pressure, allowing the patient to lead a normal, healthy, active life.

How long will I undergo treatment?

Treatment for essential hypertension is usually lifelong. Even if you feel fine, you'll probably have to continue treatment for the rest of your life to maintain your blood pressure in a healthy range. If you discontinue your diet and lifestyle changes or stop taking your medication, your blood pressure will increase again.

- Encourage patients with hypertension to adhere to the treatment prescribed by the physician. Help patients remember to take their medication by telling them to associate their medication schedule with a daily routine, such as brushing their teeth or with meals.
- Provide the patient with educational materials about high blood pressure, available from sources such as the American Heart Association. ∎

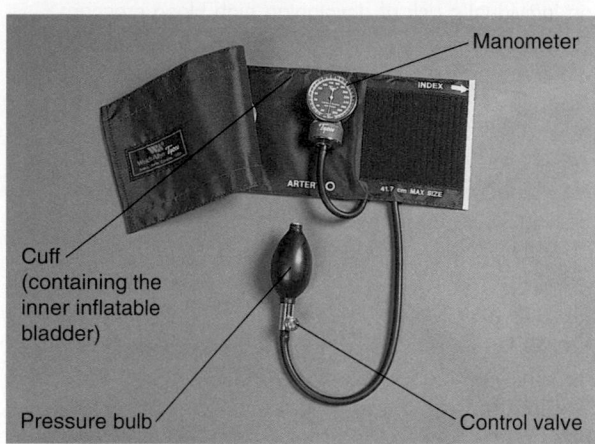

Figure 19-20   The parts of an aneroid sphygmomanometer.

should be placed so that it can be viewed directly. At least once a year, an aneroid sphygmomanometer should be recalibrated to ensure its accuracy.

Mercury Sphygmomanometer

The mercury sphygmomanometer (Figure 19-22) has a vertical tube calibrated in millimeters that is filled with mercury. Although more accurate than the aneroid sphygmomanometer, use of the mercury sphygmomanometer is being discouraged because mercury is a hazardous chemical that can be dangerous to humans and the environment.

If a mercury manometer is used to measure blood pressure, it must be placed in the correct position for proper viewing. The medical assistant should be no farther than 3 feet from the scale of the manometer. A portable mercury

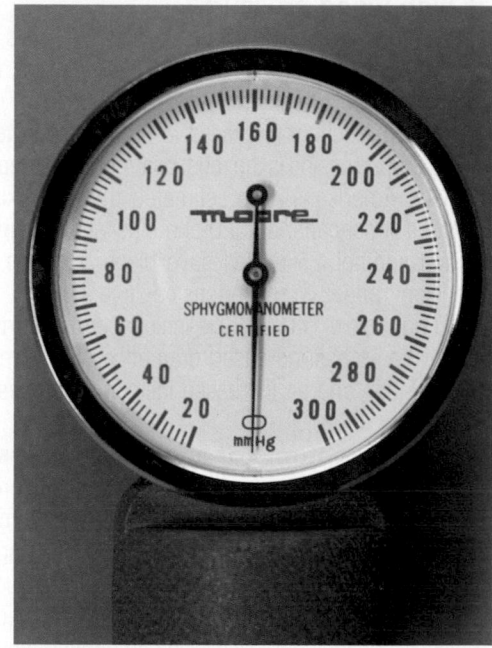

Figure 19-21 The scale of the gauge of an aneroid sphygmomanometer.

manometer should be placed on a flat surface so the mercury column is in a vertical position. The wall model mercury manometer is mounted securely on a wall, placing the mercury column in a vertical position.

The following guidelines must be followed when measuring blood pressure with a mercury sphygmomanometer. Before the blood pressure reading is obtained, the mercury must be even with the zero level at the base of the calibrated

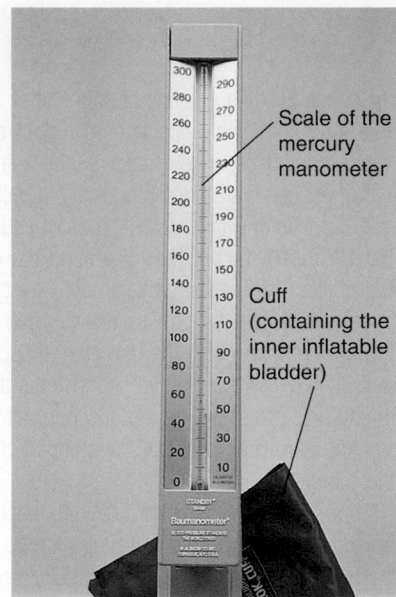

Figure 19-22 The parts of a mercury sphygmomanometer.

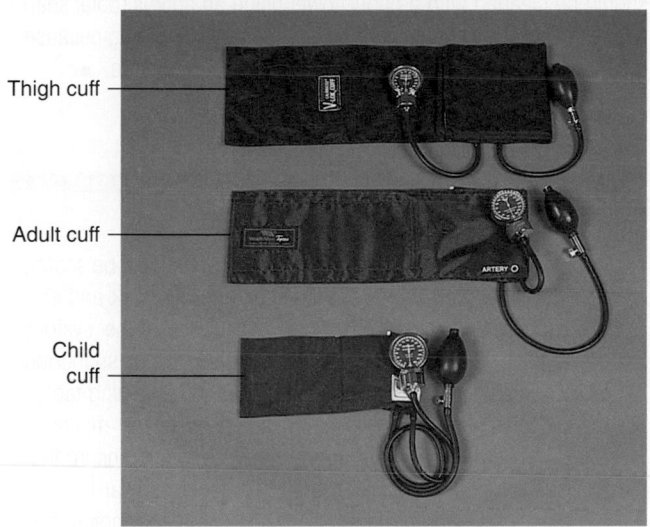

Figure 19-23 Blood pressure cuffs: child, adult, and thigh.

Table 19-9 Types of Blood Pressure Cuffs

Cuff	Bladder Length, cm	Bladder Width, cm	Acceptable Circumference, cm
Child arm	21	8	16-21
Small adult arm	24	10	22-26
Adult arm	30	13	27-34
Large adult arm	38	16	35-44
Adult thigh	42	20	45-52

From Bonewit-West K: *Clinical procedures for medical assistants*, ed 8, St Louis, 2011, Saunders.

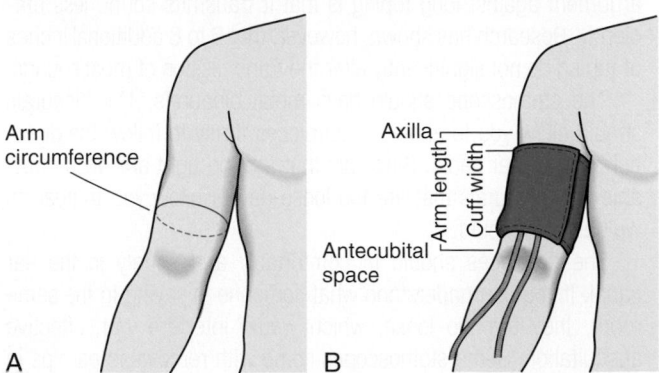

Figure 19-24 Determination of proper cuff size. **A,** The bladder of the cuff should be long enough to encircle 80% of the arm. **B,** The cuff should be wide enough to cover two thirds of the distance from the axilla to the antecubital space.

tube. Pressure created by inflation of the inner bladder causes the mercury to rise in the tube. The top portion of the mercury column, the **meniscus,** curves slightly upward. The blood pressure should be read at the top of the meniscus, with the eye at the same level as the meniscus of the mercury column.

Cuff Sizes

Blood pressure cuffs come in a variety of sizes and are measured in centimeters (cm) (Figure 19-23). The size of a cuff refers to its inner inflatable bladder, rather than its cloth cover. Table 19-9 lists the types of cuffs available and the size of the inner bladder of each cuff.

For accurate blood pressure measurement, the inner bladder of the cuff should encircle at least 80% (but not more than 100%) of the arm circumference and should be wide enough to cover two thirds of the distance from the axilla to the antecubital space (Figure 19-24). Child cuffs often must be used for adults with thin arms. The adult cuff is used for the average-sized adult arm, and the thigh cuff is used for taking blood pressure from the thigh or for adults with large arms. If the cuff is too small, the reading may be falsely high, as it would be, for example, when an adult cuff is used on a patient with a large arm. If the cuff is too large, the reading may be falsely low, as it would be when an adult cuff is used on a patient with a thin arm. The cuff should fit snugly and should be applied so that the center of the inflatable bag is directly over the brachial artery to allow for complete compression of the artery. The cuff has an interlocking, self-sticking substance (Velcro) that facilitates closing and fastening the cuff in place temporarily.

In obese patients with an arm circumference greater than 50 cm (20 inches), it may not be possible to fit even an adult thigh cuff around the patient's arm. In this situation, the American Heart Association (AHA) states that the patient's blood pressure can be measured using the forearm and radial artery; however, the AHA further states that this method may result in a falsely high systolic reading. When using this method, an appropriate sized cuff should be positioned midway between the elbow and the wrist, with the center of the bladder positioned over the radial

Highlight on Stethoscopes

The stethoscope was first introduced in the 1800s by a French physician named René Laennec. This early stethoscope consisted of a simple wooden tube with a bell-shaped opening at one end.

The selection of a stethoscope is an individual decision. One hears sounds differently when using different stethoscopes. The primary consideration in choosing a stethoscope should be that it is well made and fits well in your ears. Stethoscopes are available from uniform shops and medical supply companies.

The usual length of tubing on a stethoscope is 12 to 16 inches (30 to 40 cm), but you may prefer the longer 22-inch tubing. An argument against long tubing is that it transmits sound less efficiently. Research has shown, however, that 6 to 8 additional inches of tubing do not significantly alter the transmission of most sounds.

The stethoscope should have metal binaurals. The binaurals should allow you to angle the earpieces firmly to follow the direction of your ear canal. Binaurals that are too tight are uncomfortable and binaurals that are too loose do not allow you to hear as well as you should.

The earpieces should fit comfortably and snugly in the ear canal. If you can understand what someone is saying in the same room, they are too loose, which would interfere with effective auscultation. Some stethoscopes come with removable ear tips in different sizes. This offers the advantage of selecting an ear tip that fits your ear canal. Flexible ear tips of soft rubber are usually more comfortable than nonflexible tips of hard rubber or plastic.

The chest piece should be a key factor in the selection of a stethoscope. A stethoscope with a diaphragm and a bell offers the greatest versatility for listening to different types of sounds. Many stethoscopes have a rubber or plastic rim around the diaphragm and bell to avoid chilling the patient with a cold chest piece and to decrease air leaks between the chest piece and the patient.

The most common problem with the use of stethoscopes is air leaking. Air leaks interfere with effective sound transmission and allow environmental noise to enter the stethoscope. Air leaks may result from a cracked earpiece, a cracked or chipped chest piece, or a break in the tubing.

Stethoscopes must be cared for properly to ensure proper functioning and to prevent the transmission of disease in the medical office. The earpieces should be removed and cleaned regularly with a cotton-tipped applicator moistened with alcohol to remove cerumen. The chest piece should be cleaned with an antiseptic wipe to remove dirt, dust, lint, and oils. The tubing should be cleaned with a paper towel using an antimicrobial soap and water. Alcohol should not be used to clean the tubing because it can dry out the tubing and cause it to crack over time. ∎

Prevention of Errors in Blood Pressure Measurement

The following guidelines should be followed to prevent errors in blood pressure measurement:

1. *Instruct the patient* not to consume caffeine, use tobacco, or exercise for 30 minutes before blood pressure measurement.

2. *The patient should be comfortably seated* in a quiet room for at least 5 minutes before blood pressure is taken. Patient anxiety and apprehension can cause a spasm of the brachial artery, which can increase the blood pressure reading by as much as 30 to 50 mm Hg. This is known as the "white coat effect," which refers to the white lab coat worn by the physician. It tends to occur more frequently in older adults and young children.

3. *Always use the proper cuff size.* If the cuff is too small, it may come loose as the cuff is inflated, or the reading may be falsely high. If the cuff is too large, the reading may be falsely low. The inner inflatable bladder of the cuff should encircle at least 80% (but no more than 100%) of the patient's arm and should cover two thirds of the distance from the axilla to the antecubital space.

4. *Never take blood pressure over clothing.* Clothing interferes with the ability to hear Korotkoff sounds; this could result in an inaccurate blood pressure reading. Roll up the patient's sleeve approximately 5 inches above the elbow. If the sleeve is too tight after being rolled up, remove the arm from the sleeve. A tight sleeve causes partial compression of the brachial artery, resulting in an inaccurate reading.

5. *Position the patient properly.* The patient should be seated in a chair with the legs uncrossed and the back and arm supported. Crossing the legs can increase the systolic reading by 2 to 8 mm Hg. If the back is not supported (such as when a patient is seated on an examining table), the diastolic reading can be increased by as much as 6 mm Hg. Position the arm at heart level, and ensure that it is well supported with the palm facing upward. If the arm is above heart level, the blood pressure reading may be falsely low. If the arm is not supported or is placed below heart level, the blood pressure reading may be falsely high.

6. *Avoid extraneous sounds from the cuff.* Position the cuff approximately 1 to 2 inches above the bend in the elbow. The cuff should be up far enough to prevent the stethoscope from touching it; otherwise, extraneous sounds, which could interfere with an accurate measurement, may be picked up.

7. *Compress the brachial artery completely.* Center the inner bladder of the cuff directly over the artery to be compressed. Most cuffs are labeled with arrows indicating the center of the bladder for the right and left arms. Centering the inner bladder allows for complete compression of the brachial artery.

8. *Apply equal pressure over the brachial artery.* The cuff should be applied so that it fits smoothly and snugly around the patient's arm. This prevents bulging or slipping and permits application of an equal pressure over the

Prevention of Errors in Blood Pressure Measurement—cont'd

brachial artery. A loose-fitting cuff can cause a falsely high reading.

9. *Instruct the patient to relax as much as possible and to not talk during the procedure.* Patient anxiety and apprehension can increase the blood pressure reading. Talking interferes with the medical assistant's ability to hear the Korotkoff sounds.

10. *Position the earpieces so that you can hear the sounds clearly.* Place the earpieces of the stethoscope in your ears with the earpieces directed slightly forward. This allows the earpieces to follow the direction of the ear canal, which facilitates hearing.

11. *Avoid extraneous sounds from the tubing.* Make sure the tubing of the stethoscope hangs freely and is not permitted to rub against any object. If the stethoscope tubing rubs against an object, extraneous sounds may be picked up, and this could interfere with an accurate measurement.

12. *Position the chest piece properly.* Palpate the brachial pulse to provide good positioning of the chest piece over the brachial artery. Place the chest piece firmly, but gently, over the brachial artery to assist in transmitting clear and

audible sounds. Do not allow the chest piece to touch the cuff, to prevent extraneous sounds from being picked up, which could interfere with an accurate measurement.

13. *Release the pressure at a moderate steady rate.* Release the pressure in the cuff at a rate of 2 to 3 mm Hg/sec to ensure an accurate blood pressure measurement. Releasing the pressure too slowly is uncomfortable for the patient and could cause a falsely high diastolic reading. Releasing the pressure too quickly could cause a falsely low systolic reading.

14. *Avoid venous congestion.* If you need to take the blood pressure in the same arm again, wait 1 to 2 minutes to allow blood trapped in the veins (venous congestion) to be released. Venous congestion can result in a falsely high systolic reading and a falsely low diastolic reading.

15. *Measure and record the blood pressure in both arms during the initial blood pressure assessment of a new patient.* There may normally be a difference of 5 to 10 mm Hg between the two arms. During return visits, the blood pressure should be measured in the arm with the higher initial reading.

pulse. The medical assistant should then place the diaphragm of the stethoscope over the radial pulse and should measure the patient's blood pressure using the same technique presented in Procedure 19-9.

Korotkoff Sounds

Korotkoff sounds are used to determine systolic and diastolic blood pressure readings. When the bladder of the cuff is inflated, the brachial artery is compressed so that no audible sounds are heard through the stethoscope. As the cuff is deflated, at a rate of 2 to 3 mm Hg per second, the sounds become audible until the blood flows freely, at which point the sounds can no longer be heard (Table 19-10). The medical assistant should practice listening to these sounds and should be able to identify the various phases.

Procedure 19-9 outlines the procedure for taking blood pressure using an aneroid sphygmomanometer. Procedure 19-10 outlines the procedure for determining systolic pressure by palpation.

Automated Oscillometric Blood Pressure Device

Automated oscillometric devices (Figure 19-25) are being used in some medical offices to measure blood pressure. They are becoming especially popular for use in home monitoring of blood pressure by patients with high blood pressure. It is important to use an automated device that has undergone a formal clinical validation process to assess its accuracy. A current list of clinically validated automated blood pressure devices can be found at the following websites: British Hypertension Society (www.bhsoc.org) and

the Association for the Advancement of Medical Instrumentation (www.aami.org).

An automated oscillometric device uses an electronic sensor to measures oscillations from the wall of the brachial artery as the cuff gradually deflates. An oscillation is a back-and-forth movement that occurs in the brachial artery as the pulse wave travels through it. The point of maximum oscillation corresponds to the mean arterial pressure, which is an overall index of an individual's blood pressure. A computer in the device then uses this information to calculate the systolic blood pressure and the diastolic blood pressure. Results are then displayed on a screen. The automated blood pressure procedure takes approximately 30 seconds to complete from start to finish.

The medical assistant must make sure to follow the manufacturer's instructions for the particular brand and model of automated device used; these instructions are outlined in the user manual that accompanies the device. Many of the principles for the accurate measurement of blood pressure using an automated device are the same as those for manual measurement of blood pressure (refer to *Prevention of Errors in Blood Pressure Measurement*). The device should be calibrated periodically according to the manufacturer's recommendations. Automated oscillometric devices offer certain advantages and disadvantages, described as follows.

Advantages
1. The device can automatically determine how much the cuff should be inflated to reach a pressure that is approximately 30 mm Hg above the systolic pressure.

Table 19-10 Korotkoff Sounds

Phase	Description	Illustration
	Inflation of cuff compresses and closes off brachial artery so that no blood flows through the artery.	Cuff pressure inflated above systolic pressure (no pulse sounds heard) Brachial artery occluded by cuff, no blood flow No sound
Phase I	First faint but clear tapping sound is heard, and it gradually increases in intensity. First tapping sound is the systolic pressure.	SYSTOLIC PRESSURE Pressure in cuff is released to below systolic but higher than diastolic Blood spurts into constricted artery Sounds first heard 120 mm Hg Korotkoff sounds
Phase II	As cuff continues to deflate, sounds have murmuring or swishing quality.	DIASTOLIC PRESSURE Pressure in cuff below diastolic Blood flows freely 80 mm Hg Sounds disappear
Phase III	With further deflation, sounds become crisper and increase in intensity.	
Phase IV	Sounds become muffled and have soft, blowing quality.	
Phase V	Sounds disappear. This is recorded as the diastolic pressure.	

From Bonewit-West K: *Clinical procedures for medical assistants*, ed 8, St Louis, 2011, Saunders.

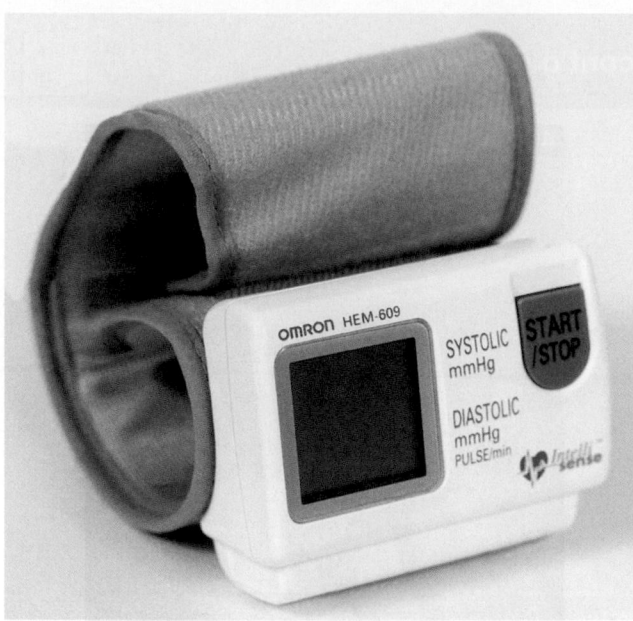

Figure 19-25 Automated oscillometric blood pressure device.

2. The cuff does not have to be manually inflated and deflated because this function is performed automatically by the device.

3. The patient's brachial artery does not need to be located, and the bladder of the cuff does not need to be centered over the brachial artery.

4. A stethoscope and user listening skills are not required to obtain the reading because the electronic sensor in the automated device measures oscillations from the wall of the brachial artery to obtain the reading.

5. Automated devices are less susceptible to external environmental noise than are manual devices.

6. The blood pressure measurement is easy to read because the systolic and diastolic readings are shown on a digital display screen.

7. The device allows multiple blood pressure measurements to be taken.

8. Most automated devices come equipped with an internal memory for storing multiple blood pressure measurements.

Disadvantages

1. There are certain factors that can cause an automated device to fail to obtain a reading. These include patient movement, muscle tremors, preeclampsia, dysrhythmias (such as atrial fibrillation), and a very weak pulse. If any of these conditions are present, an alternative method of blood pressure measurement should be used.

2. Because the device relies on brachial artery oscillations to obtain a reading, stiff arteries (especially in older patients) can interfere with obtaining an accurate reading.

3. Automated oscillometric devices are expensive.

PROCEDURE 19-9 Measuring Blood Pressure

Outcome Measure blood pressure.

Equipment/Supplies

- Stethoscope
- Sphygmomanometer
- Antiseptic wipe

1. **Procedural Step.** Sanitize your hands, and assemble the equipment. If the chest piece consists of a diaphragm and a bell, rotate it to the diaphragm position. Clean the earpieces and chest piece of the stethoscope with the antiseptic wipe.
   Principle. The chest piece must be rotated to the proper position for sound to be heard through the earpieces.

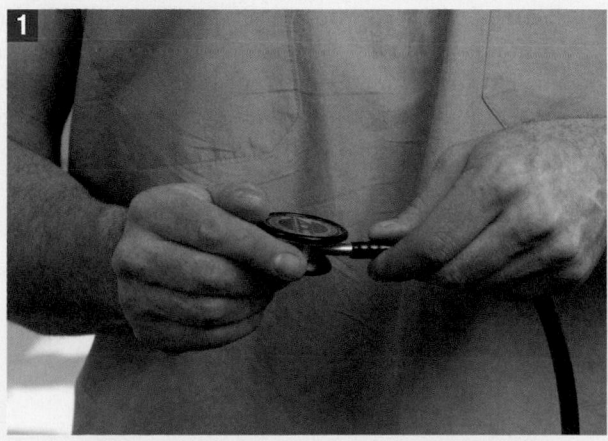

Rotate the chest piece to the diaphragm position.

Continued

2. **Procedural Step.** Greet the patient and introduce yourself. Identify the patient and explain the procedure. Explain to the patient that measuring blood pressure may normally cause a little numbing and tingling in the arm when the cuff is inflated. While explaining the procedure, observe the patient for signs that might influence the reading, such as anger, fear, pain, and recent physical activity. If it is not possible to reduce or eliminate these influences, list them in the patient's chart. Determine how high to pump the cuff by checking the patient's chart for previously measured systolic readings, or determine the patient's systolic pressure by palpation (see Procedure 19-10).

3. **Procedural Step.** Have the patient sit quietly in a comfortable position in a chair with the legs uncrossed and the back supported. The patient should relax in a sitting position for at least 5 minutes before measuring his or her blood pressure. Roll up the patient's sleeve approximately 5 inches above the elbow. If the sleeve does not roll up or is too tight after being rolled up, remove the arm from the sleeve. The arm should be positioned at heart level and well supported, with the palm facing up.
Principle. Patient anxiety can cause a significant increase in blood pressure. Clothing interferes with the ability to hear Korotkoff sounds, which could result in an inaccurate blood pressure reading. A tight sleeve causes partial compression of the brachial artery, resulting in an inaccurate reading. The position of the arm allows easy access to the brachial artery. Placing the arm above heart level may cause the reading to be falsely low. Not supporting the arm or placing it below heart level may cause the reading to be falsely high.

4. **Procedural Step.** Select the proper cuff size. The inner inflatable bladder of the cuff should be long enough to encircle at least 80% (but no more than 100%) of the patient's arm and wide enough to cover two thirds of the distance from the axilla to the antecubital space.
Principle. The appropriate-size cuff must be used to ensure an accurate measurement. If the cuff is too small, it may come loose as the cuff is inflated, or the reading may be falsely high. If the cuff is too large, the reading may be falsely low.

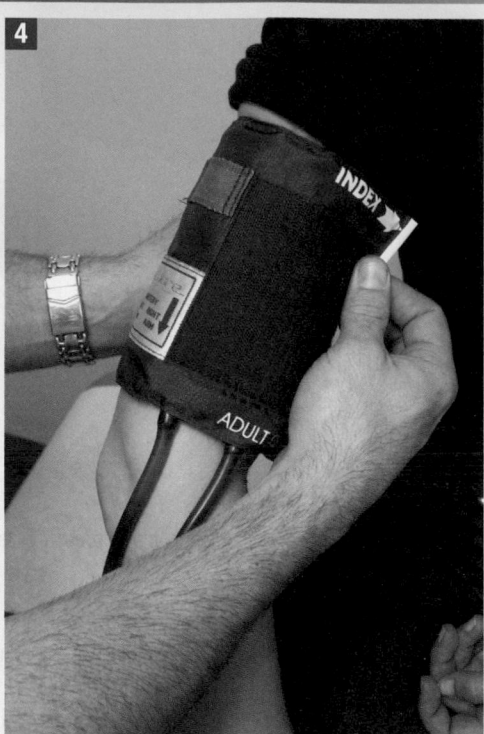

The inner bladder should encircle at least 80% of the patient's arm.

5. **Procedural Step.** Locate the brachial pulse with the fingertips. The brachial pulse is located near the center of the antecubital space but slightly toward the little finger–side of the arm. Center the inner bladder over the brachial pulse site. (*NOTE:* Place the cuff on the patient's arm so that the lower edge of the cuff is approximately 1 to 2 inches above the bend in the elbow. Most cuffs are labeled with right and left arrows indicating the center of the bladder. The right arrow should be placed over the brachial pulse site when you are using the right arm, and the left arrow should be placed over the brachial pulse site when you are using the left arm.)
Principle. The cuff should be placed high enough to prevent the stethoscope from touching it; otherwise, extraneous sounds, which could interfere with an accurate measurement, may be picked up. Centering the inner bladder over the pulse site allows complete compression of the brachial artery.

PROCEDURE 19-9 Measuring Blood Pressure—cont'd

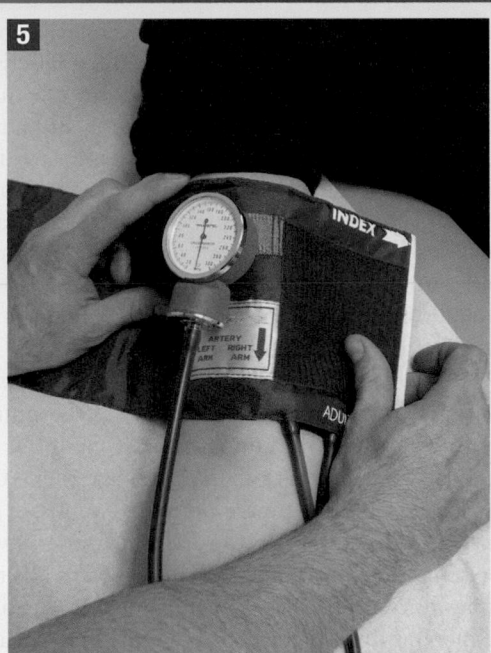

Center the inner bladder over the brachial pulse site.

6. **Procedural Step.** Wrap the cuff smoothly and snugly around the patient's arm, and secure the end of it.
   Principle. Applying the cuff properly prevents it from bulging or slipping. This technique permits application of an equal pressure over the brachial artery.

7. **Procedural Step.** Position the manometer for direct viewing and at a distance of no more than 3 feet.
   Principle. The medical assistant may have trouble seeing the scale on the manometer if it is placed more than 3 feet away.

8. **Procedural Step.** Instruct the patient not to talk or move. Place the earpieces of the stethoscope in your ears, with the earpieces directed slightly forward. During the blood pressure measurement, the tubing of the stethoscope should hang freely and should not be permitted to rub against any object.
   Principle. The earpieces should be directed forward, permitting them to follow the direction of the ear canal, which facilitates hearing. If the stethoscope tubing rubs against an object, extraneous sounds may be picked up; this would interfere with an accurate measurement.

9. **Procedural Step.** Making sure the arm is well extended, locate the brachial pulse again, and place the diaphragm of the stethoscope over the brachial pulse site. The diaphragm should be positioned to make a tight seal against the patient's skin. Enough pressure should be exerted to leave a temporary ring on the patient's skin when the disc is removed. Do not allow the chest piece to touch the cuff.

Principle. A well extended arm allows easier palpation of the brachial pulse. Locating the brachial pulse again is necessary for proper positioning of the chest piece over the brachial artery. Proper positioning of the diaphragm and good contact of the diaphragm with the skin help transmit clear and audible Korotkoff sounds through the earpieces of the stethoscope. If the diaphragm touches the cuff, extraneous sounds may be picked up; this would interfere with an accurate measurement.

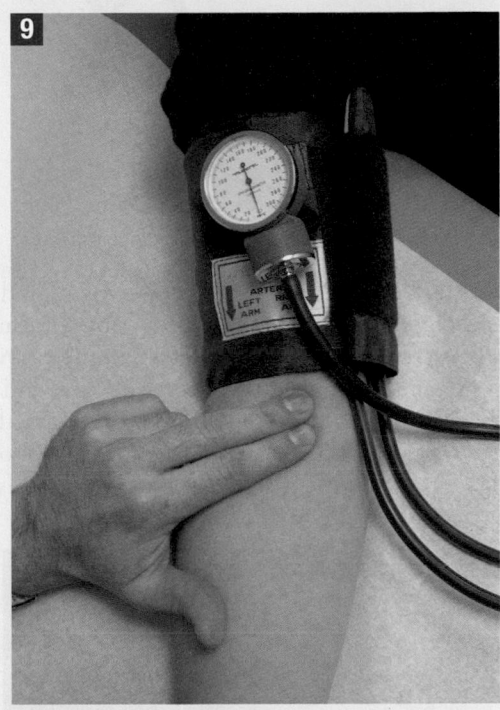

Locate the brachial pulse again before placing the diaphragm over the site.

10. **Procedural Step.** Close the valve on the bulb by turning the thumbscrew clockwise (to the right) with the thumb and forefinger of your dominant hand until it feels tight but can still be loosened with the thumb and forefinger of one hand when you need to deflate the cuff. Pump air into the cuff as rapidly as possible to at least 30 mm Hg above the previously measured or palpated systolic pressure.
    Principle. Inflation of the cuff compresses and closes off the brachial artery so that no blood flows through the artery. If the patient has had the blood pressure measured previously at the medical office, the recorded systolic pressure can be used to determine how high to inflate the cuff. Preliminary determination of the systolic pressure by palpation allows the medical assistant to estimate how high to inflate the cuff.

Continued

PROCEDURE 19-9

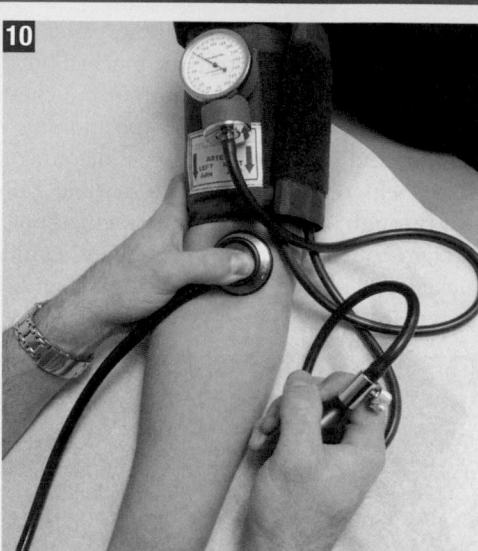

Pump air into the cuff as rapidly as possible.

11. **Procedural Step.** Release the pressure at a moderately steady rate of 2 to 3 mm Hg/sec by slowly turning the thumbscrew counterclockwise (to the left) with the thumb and forefinger. This opens the valve and allows the air in the cuff to escape slowly. Listen for the first clear tapping sound (phase I of the Korotkoff sounds). This represents the systolic pressure. Note this point on the scale of the manometer.

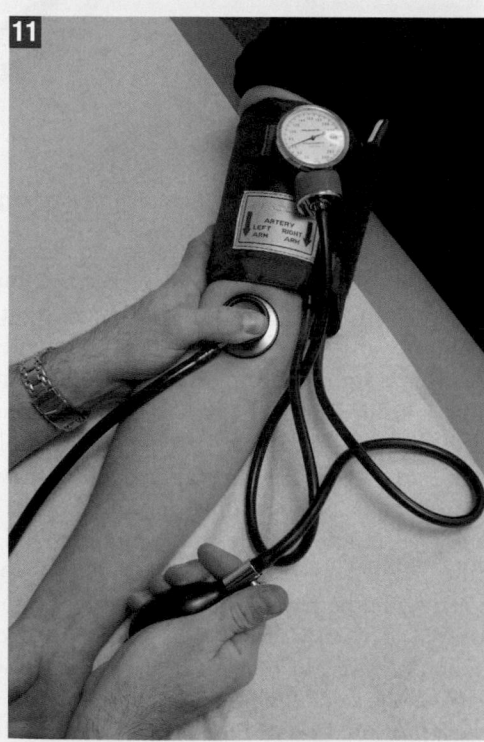

Release the pressure at a moderately steady rate.

Principle. Releasing the pressure too slowly is uncomfortable for the patient and could cause a falsely high diastolic reading. Releasing the pressure too quickly could cause a falsely low systolic reading and a falsely high diastolic reading. The systolic pressure is the point at which the blood first begins to spurt through the artery as the cuff pressure begins to decrease; it represents the pressure that occurs on the walls of the arteries during systole.

12. **Procedural Step.** Continue to deflate the cuff while listening to the Korotkoff sounds. Listen for the onset of the muffled sound that occurs during phase IV. Continue to deflate the cuff, and note the point on the scale at which the sound ceases (phase V). Continue to steadily deflate the cuff for another 10 mm Hg to ensure that there are no more sounds.

Principle. Phase V marks the diastolic pressure (which represents the pressure that occurs on the walls of the arteries during diastole); the cuff pressure is reduced, and blood is flowing freely through the brachial artery.

13. **Procedural Step.** Quickly and completely deflate the cuff to zero. If you could not obtain an accurate blood pressure reading, wait 1 to 2 minutes before taking another measurement on the same arm. Remove the earpieces of the stethoscope from your ears, and carefully remove the cuff from the patient's arm.

Principle. Venous congestion results when blood pressure is taken, which alters a second reading if it is taken too soon on the same arm.

14. **Procedural Step.** Sanitize your hands, and chart the results. Include the date, the time, and the blood pressure reading. Blood pressure is recorded using even numbers. Make a notation in the patient's chart if the lying or standing position was used to take blood pressure. Abbreviations that can be used are *L* (lying) and *St* (standing).

15. **Procedural Step.** Clean the earpieces and the chest piece of the stethoscope with an antiseptic wipe, and replace the equipment properly.

CHARTING EXAMPLE

Date	
10/20/XX	2:30 p.m. BP: 106/74.— S. Martinez, RMA

PROCEDURE **19-10** Determining Systolic Pressure by Palpation

Outcome Determine systolic pressure by palpation.

Equipment/Supplies

- Sphygmomanometer

1. **Procedural Step.** Sanitize your hands, and assemble the equipment.
2. **Procedural Step.** Locate the brachial pulse with the fingertips. Place the cuff on the patient's arm so that the inner bladder is centered over the brachial pulse site.
3. **Procedural Step.** Wrap the cuff smoothly and snugly around the patient's arm, and secure the end of it.
4. **Procedural Step.** Position the manometer for direct viewing and at a distance of no more than 3 feet.
5. **Procedural Step.** Locate the radial pulse with your fingertips.
6. **Procedural Step.** Close the valve on the bulb, and pump air into the cuff until the pulsation ceases.
7. **Procedural Step.** Release the valve at a moderate rate of 2 to 3 mm Hg per heartbeat while palpating the artery with your fingertips.
8. **Procedural Step.** Record the point at which the pulsation reappears as the palpated systolic pressure.
9. **Procedural Step.** Deflate the cuff completely, and wait 15 to 30 seconds before checking the blood pressure.

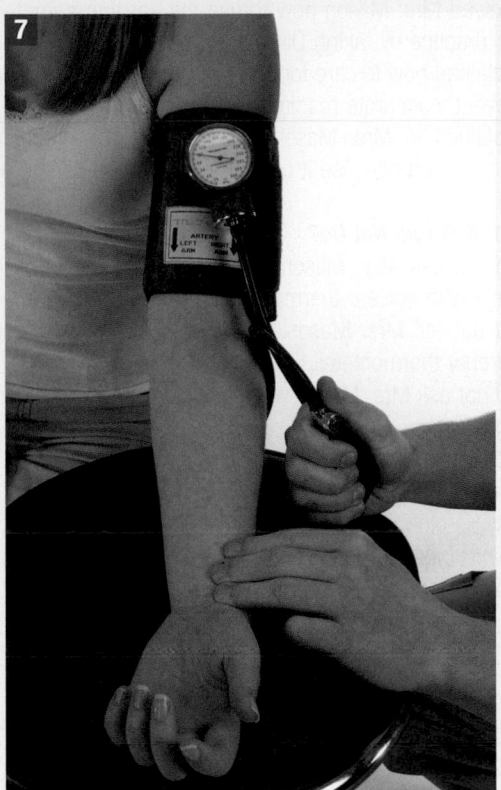

Release the valve while palpating the radial artery.

MEDICAL PRACTICE *and the* LAW

Measurement of vital signs is standard procedure for almost every patient in the physician's office. Because vital sign measurements are performed so frequently, the medical assistant may tend to minimize their importance. Changes in vital signs may be the first indicator of disease or illness, so meticulous attention must be paid to the performance and documentation of vital signs and to comparison of current measurements with past measurements for each patient.

Most patients want to know their vital signs, especially their blood pressure or temperature if febrile. Although the patient owns the information that you collect, be aware that you may not give this information to family members without the patient's consent. Some offices have a policy that indicates specific information that the medical assistant can give the patient; some physicians prefer to disclose this information themselves and discuss it with their patients.

Often, measurement of vital signs is the first contact patients have with the medical assistant. The most important factor in determining whether a patient will sue is not the skill of the practitioner, but the level of rapport with the patient. In everything you do, convey your caring and concern to every patient. ■

What Would You Do? What Would You *Not* Do? RESPONSES

Case Study 1
Page 316

What Did Sergio Do?
❑ Told Mrs. Mason that sometimes ear thermometers can be a little tricky to use.
❑ Showed Mrs. Mason how to use the ear thermometer and let her practice by taking Olivia's temperature.
❑ Explained how to care for and maintain the ear thermometer to prevent inaccurate readings.
❑ Explained to Mrs. Mason that the use of mercury is being discouraged because it can be toxic to humans and animals.

What Did Sergio Not Do?
❑ Did not ask Mrs. Mason if she had read the directions that came with her ear thermometer.
❑ Did not tell Mrs. Mason that she should switch back to the mercury thermometer.
❑ Did not ask Mrs. Mason why she waited so long to bring Olivia to the office.

What Would You Do/What Would You Not Do?
Review Sergio's response and place a checkmark next to the information you included in your response. List the additional information you included in your response.

_____
_____
_____
_____
_____
_____
_____

Case Study 2
Page 320

What Did Sergio Do?
❑ Recognized and congratulated Alex on his swimming achievements.
❑ Told Alex that it is normal for his pulse to be that slow because of his athletic training and it shows that he is in good shape.
❑ Assured Alex that the physician will do everything he can to help Alex.
❑ Stressed to Alex how important it is to follow the physician's advice so that his shoulder heals as soon as possible.

What Did Sergio Not Do?
❑ Did not comment on Alex's request for a steroid injection or OxyContin. Made sure to chart the information so that the physician could handle the situation.
❑ Did not criticize Alex for putting a swim meet before his health.

What Would You Do/What Would You Not Do?
Review Sergio's response and place a checkmark next to the information you included in your response. List the additional information you included in your response.

_____
_____
_____
_____
_____
_____
_____

Case Study 3
Page 332

What Did Sergio Do?
❑ Empathized with Tyrone about having to take so many pills. Suggested that he get a daily pill container to help him remember.
❑ Stressed to Tyrone the importance of taking his blood pressure medication. Explained to him that high blood pressure is a "silent disease." He may feel fine, but damage to his body organs can still be taking place if he does not take his pills.
❑ Gave Tyrone a brochure about high blood pressure and went over the long-term effects of hypertension and lifestyle changes that could help lower blood pressure.
❑ Encouraged Tyrone to call the office when he experiences side effects from medications because the physician may be able to do something to help.

What Did Sergio Not Do?
❑ Did not tell him it was all right to discontinue his medication.

What Would You Do/What Would You Not Do?
Review Sergio's response and place a checkmark next to the information you included in your response. List the additional information you included in your response.

_____
_____
_____
_____
_____
_____
_____

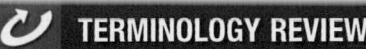

Medical Term	Word Parts	Definition
Adventitious sounds		Abnormal breath sounds.
Afebrile	*a-:* without	Without fever; the body temperature is normal.
Alveolus	*alveol/o:* air sac	A thin-walled air sac of the lungs in which the exchange of oxygen and carbon dioxide takes place.
Antecubital space	*ante-:* before *cubitum:* elbow	The space located at the front of the elbow.
Antipyretic	*anti-:* against *pyr/o:* fever *-ic:* pertaining to	An agent that reduces fever.
Aorta		The major trunk of the arterial system of the body. The aorta arises from the upper surface of the left ventricle.
Apnea	*a-:* without or absence of *-pnea:* breathing	The temporary cessation of breathing.
Axilla		The armpit.
Bounding pulse		A pulse with an increased volume that feels very strong and full.
Bradycardia	*brady-:* slow *cardi/o:* heart *-ia:* condition of diseased or abnormal state	An abnormally slow heart rate (less than 60 beats per minute).
Bradypnea	*brady-:* slow *-pnea:* breathing	An abnormal decrease in the respiratory rate of less than 10 respirations per minute.
Celsius scale		A temperature scale on which the freezing point of water is 0° and the boiling point of water is 100°; also called the *centigrade scale.*
Conduction		The transfer of energy, such as heat, from one object to another by direct contact.
Convection		The transfer of energy, such as heat, through air currents.
Crisis		A sudden falling of an elevated body temperature to normal.
Cyanosis	*cyan/o:* blue *-osis:* abnormal condition	A bluish discoloration of the skin and mucous membranes.
Diastole		The phase in the cardiac cycle in which the heart relaxes between contractions.
Diastolic pressure		The point of lesser pressure on the arterial wall, which is recorded during diastole.
Dyspnea	*dys-:* difficult, painful, abnormal *-pnea:* breathing	Shortness of breath or difficulty in breathing.
Dysrhythmia	*dys-:* difficult, painful, abnormal *rhythm:* rhythm *-ia:* condition of diseased or abnormal state	An irregular rhythm; also termed *arrhythmia.*
Eupnea	*eu-:* normal, good *-pnea:* breathing	Normal respiration. The rate is 16 to 20 respirations per minute, the rhythm is even and regular, and the depth is normal.
Exhalation	*-ex:* outside, outward	The act of breathing out.
Fahrenheit scale		A temperature scale on which the freezing point of water is 32° and the boiling point of water is 212°.
Febrile		Pertaining to fever.
Fever		A body temperature that is above normal; synonym for pyrexia.
Frenulum linguae		The midline fold that connects the undersurface of the tongue with the floor of the mouth.
Hyperpnea	*hyper-:* above, excessive *-pnea:* breathing	An abnormal increase in the rate and depth of respiration.
Hyperpyrexia	*hyper-:* above, excessive *pyr/o:* fever *-ia:* condition of diseased or abnormal state	An extremely high fever.
Hypertension	*hyper-:* above, excessive *tension:* pressure	High blood pressure.
Hyperventilation	*hyper-:* above, excessive	An abnormally fast and deep type of breathing, usually associated with acute anxiety conditions.

Continued

Medical Term	Word Parts	Definition
Hypopnea	*hypo-:* below, deficient *-pnea:* breathing	An abnormal decrease in the rate and depth of respiration.
Hypotension	*hypo-:* below, deficient *tension:* pressure	Low blood pressure.
Hypothermia	*hypo-:* below, deficient *therm/o:* heat *-ia:* condition of diseased or abnormal state	A body temperature that is below normal.
Hypoxemia	*hypo-:* below, deficient *ox/i:* oxygen *-emia:* blood condition	A decrease in the oxygen saturation of the blood. Hypoxemia may lead to hypoxia.
Hypoxia	*hypo-:* below, deficient *ox/i:* oxygen *-ia:* condition of diseased or abnormal state	A reduction in the oxygen supply to the tissues of the body.
Inhalation	*in-:* in, into	The act of breathing in.
Intercostal	*inter-:* between *cost/o:* rib *-al:* pertaining to	Between the ribs.
Korotkoff sounds		Sounds heard during the measurement of blood pressure that are used to determine the systolic and diastolic blood pressure readings.
Malaise	*-mal:* bad	A vague sense of body discomfort, weakness, and fatigue that often marks the onset of a disease and continues through the course of the illness.
Manometer	*-meter:* instrument used to measure	An instrument for measuring pressure.
Meniscus		The curved surface on a column of liquid in a tube.
Orthopnea	*orth/o:* straight *-pnea:* breathing	The condition in which breathing is easier when an individual is in a sitting or standing position.
Pulse oximeter	*ox/i:* oxygen *-meter:* instrument used to measure	A computerized device consisting of a probe and a monitor used to measure the oxygen saturation of arterial blood.
Pulse oximetry	*ox/i:* oxygen *-metry:* measurement	The use of a pulse oximeter to measure the oxygen saturation of arterial blood.
Pulse pressure		The difference between the systolic and diastolic pressures.
Pulse rhythm		The time interval between heartbeats.
Pulse volume		The strength of the heartbeat.
Radiation		The transfer of energy, such as heat, in the form of waves.
SaO$_2$ (saturation of arterial oxygen)		Abbreviation for the percentage of hemoglobin that is saturated with oxygen in arterial blood.
Sphygmomanometer	*sphygm/o:* pulse *-meter:* instrument used to measure	An instrument for measuring arterial blood pressure.
SpO$_2$ (saturation of peripheral oxygen)		Abbreviation for the percentage of hemoglobin that is saturated with oxygen in arterial blood as measured by a pulse oximeter.
Stethoscope	*steth/o:* chest *-scope:* to view, to examine	An instrument used for amplifying and hearing sounds produced by the body.
Systole		The phase in the cardiac cycle in which the ventricles contract, sending blood out of the heart and into the aorta and pulmonary aorta.
Systolic pressure		The point of maximum pressure on the arterial walls, which is recorded during systole.
Tachycardia	*tachy-:* fast, rapid *cardi/o:* heart *-ia:* condition of diseased or abnormal state	An abnormally fast heart rate (more than 100 beats/min).
Tachypnea	*tachy-:* fast *-pnea:* breathing	An abnormal increase in the respiratory rate of more than 20 breaths/min.
Thready pulse		A pulse with a decreased volume that feels weak and thin.

ON THE WEB

For information on hypertension:

American Heart Association: www.americanheart.org

National Heart, Lung, and Blood Institute: www.nhlbi.nih.gov

Cardiology Channel: www.cardiologychannel.com

Hypertension Education Foundation: www.hypertensionfoundation.org

American Society of Hypertension: www.ash-us.org

WebMD on Hypertension: www.webmd.com/hypertension-high-blood-pressure/default.htm

MedicineNet Hypertension: www.medicinenet.com/high_blood_pressure/article.htm

Mayo Clinic Hypertension: www.mayoclinic.com/health/high-blood-pressure/ds00100

For information on lung disease:

American Lung Association: www.lungusa.org

Pulmonology Channel: www.pulmonologychannel.com

Lung Cancer Online: www.lungcanceronline.org

Women's Health—Lung Disease: www.womenshealth.gov/FAQ/lung-disease.cfm

Check out the Evolve site at http://evolve.elsevier.com/Bonewit/today/ to actively Prepare for your Certification, and to access additional interactive activities and exercises to help you study and prepare for success.

20

The Physical Examination

LEARNING OBJECTIVES	PROCEDURES
Preparation for the Physical Examination	
1. Identify the three components of a complete patient examination.	Prepare the examining room.
2. List the guidelines that should be followed in preparing the examining room.	Operate and care for equipment and instruments used during the physical examination, according to the manufacturers' instructions.
3. Identify equipment and instruments used during the physical examination.	Prepare a patient for a physical examination.
Measuring Weight and Height	
4. Explain the purpose of measuring weight and height.	Measure weight and height.
5. List the guidelines that should be followed when measuring weight and height.	
Body Mechanics	
6. Explain the importance of using proper body mechanics.	Demonstrate proper body mechanics when standing, sitting, and lifting an object.
7. State the basic principles related to proper body mechanics that should be followed.	
Positioning and Draping	
8. Explain the purposes of positioning and draping.	
9. List one use of each patient position.	Position and drape a patient in each of the following positions:
	Sitting
	Supine
	Prone
	Dorsal recumbent
	Lithotomy
	Sims
	Knee-chest
	Fowler's
Wheelchair Transfer	
10. Explain the purpose of a wheelchair.	Transfer a patient from a wheelchair to the examining table and back again.
11. Describe the purpose of a transfer belt.	
Assessment of the Patient	
12. List and define the four techniques of examining the patient.	
13. State an example of the use of each examination technique during the physical examination of a patient.	
Assisting the Physician	
14. Describe the responsibilities of the medical assistant during the physical examination.	Assist the physician during the physical examination of a patient.

KEY TERMS

audiometer (aw-dee-OM-eh-ter)
auscultation (os-kul-TAY-shun)
bariatrics (BAR-ee-AT-riks)
body mechanics
clinical diagnosis
diagnosis

differential (diff-er-EN-shul) diagnosis
inspection
mensuration (men-soo-RAY-shun)
ophthalmoscope (off-THAL-meh-skope)
otoscope (AH-toh-skope)
palpation (pal-PAY-shun)

percussion (per-KUSH-un)
percussion hammer
prognosis
speculum (SPEK-yoo-lum)
symptom

INTRODUCTION TO THE PHYSICAL EXAMINATION

A complete patient examination consists of three parts: the *health history,* the *physical examination* of each body system, and *laboratory and diagnostic tests.* The physician uses the results to determine the patient's general state of health, to arrive at a diagnosis and prescribe treatment, and to observe any change in a patient's illness after treatment has been instituted.

An important and frequent responsibility of the medical assistant is to assist with a physical examination. Because health-promotion and disease-prevention activities have become an important focus of health care, individuals are becoming more aware of the need for a yearly physical examination to detect early signs of illness and to prevent serious health problems. Also, a physical examination may be a prerequisite for employment, participation in sports, attendance at summer camp, and admission to school. The physical examination is explained in detail in this chapter. Taking the health history, collecting specimens, and performing laboratory and diagnostic tests are discussed in other chapters.

DEFINITIONS OF TERMS

The medical assistant should know and understand the following terms related to the patient examination:

Final diagnosis. Often simply called the *diagnosis,* this term refers to the scientific method of determining and identifying a patient's condition through evaluation of the health history, the physical examination, laboratory tests, and diagnostic procedures. A final diagnosis is crucial because it provides a logical basis for treatment and prognosis.

Clinical diagnosis. The clinical diagnosis is an intermediate step in the determination of a final diagnosis. The clinical diagnosis of a patient's condition is obtained through evaluation of the health history and the physical examination without the benefit of laboratory or diagnostic tests. Laboratory and diagnostic imaging facilities provide a space to specify the clinical diagnosis on their request forms; this information assists the facility in correlating data from their test results with the physician's needs. When the physician has analyzed the test results, a final diagnosis can often be established.

Differential diagnosis. Two or more diseases may have similar symptoms. The differential diagnosis involves determining which of these diseases is producing the patient's symptoms so that a final diagnosis can be established. For example, streptococcal sore throat and pharyngitis have similar symptoms. A differential diagnosis is made by obtaining a throat specimen and performing a strep test.

Prognosis. The prognosis consists of the probable course and outcome of a patient's condition and the patient's prospects for recovery.

Risk factor. A risk factor is a physical or behavioral condition that increases the probability that an individual will develop a particular condition; examples are genetic factors, habits, environmental conditions, and physiologic conditions. The presence of a risk factor for a certain disease does not mean that the disease will develop; it means only that a person's chances of developing that disease are greater than those of a person without the risk factor. For example, cigarette smoking is a risk factor for developing lung cancer and heart disease. A person who smokes has a higher risk of developing lung cancer than a person who does not or who has stopped smoking.

Highlight on Health Screening

The chance of developing certain diseases is greater at different ages. Periodic health screening is recommended for the detection and early treatment of disease.

Test or Procedure	Gender	Recommended Frequency (for Individuals of Average Risk)
Beginning at Age 20 Years		
Blood pressure	M and F	Every year
Cholesterol levels	M and F	Every 5 years
Blood glucose level	M and F	Every 3-5 years
Breast self-examination	F	Every month
Beginning at the Age Specified		
Clinical breast examination (by a physician)	F	Every 3 years between the ages of 20 and 39 and then every year beginning at age 40
Pap test and pelvic examination	F	Begin within 3 years of the onset of vaginal intercourse or at age 21, whichever comes first, then every 1 to 2 years
Testicular self-examination	M	Every month beginning at age 15
Fecal occult blood test	M and F	Every year starting at age 50
Colonoscopy	M and F	Every 10 years beginning at age 50
Prostate cancer screening	M	Should be offered by a health provider every year beginning at age 50 to men with a life expectancy of at least 10 years
Mammography	F	Every year beginning at age 40
Electrocardiogram	M and F	One baseline recording starting at age 40 ■

Acute illness. An acute illness is characterized by symptoms that have a rapid onset, are usually severe and intense, and subside after a relatively short time. In some cases, the acute episode progresses into a chronic illness. Examples of acute illness include colds, influenza, strep throat, and pneumonia.

Chronic illness. A chronic illness is characterized by symptoms that persist for longer than 3 months and show little change over a long time. Examples of chronic illness include diabetes mellitus, hypertension, and emphysema.

Therapeutic procedure. A therapeutic procedure is performed to treat a patient's condition with the goal of eliminating it or promoting as much recovery as possible. Examples of therapeutic procedures include administration of medication, ear and eye irrigations, and application of heat and cold.

Laboratory testing. Laboratory testing involves the analysis and study of specimens obtained from patients to assist in diagnosing and treating disease. Examples of laboratory testing include the hemoglobin test, glucose test, urinalysis, and strep testing.

Diagnostic procedure. A diagnostic procedure is a procedure performed to assist in the diagnosis of a patient's condition; examples include electrocardiography, colonoscopy, and mammography.

PREPARATION OF THE EXAMINING ROOM

Proper preparation of the examining room provides a comfortable and healthy environment for the patient and facilitates the physical examination. The following guidelines should be followed in preparing the examining room:

1. Ensure that the examining room is free of clutter and well lit.
2. Check the examining rooms daily to ensure there are ample supplies. Restock supplies that are getting low.
3. Empty waste receptacles frequently.
4. Replace biohazard containers as necessary. When removing biohazard containers from the examining room (see Chapter 17), follow the OSHA Bloodborne Pathogens Standard.
5. Make sure the room is well ventilated, and install an air freshener to eliminate odors.
6. Maintain room temperatures that are comfortable not only for a fully clothed individual, but also for an individual who has disrobed.
7. Clean and disinfect examining tables, countertops, and faucets daily.
8. Remove dust and dirt from furniture and towel dispensers.
9. Change the examining table paper after each patient by unrolling a fresh length. Check to ensure there is an ample supply of gowns and drapes ready for use.
10. Ensure that the examining room door is closed during the examination because patient privacy is paramount.
11. Properly clean and prepare equipment, instruments, and supplies that are used for patient examinations so that they are ready for use by the physician. Table 20-1 lists the equipment and supplies, along with their uses, that may be employed during a physical examination.

Table 20-1 Equipment and Supplies for the Physical Examination

Item	Description and Purpose
Patient examination gown	Gown made of disposable paper or cloth that provides patient modesty, comfort, and warmth.
Drape	A length of disposable paper or cloth to cover a patient or parts of a patient to provide comfort and warmth and reduce exposure.
Sphygmomanometer	Instrument used to measure blood pressure.
Stethoscope	Instrument used to auscultate body sounds, such as blood pressure and lung and bowel sounds.
Thermometer	Instrument used to measure body temperature.
Upright balance scale	Device used to measure weight and height.
Otoscope	Lighted instrument with lens, used to examine external ear canal and tympanic membrane.
Tuning fork	Small metal instrument consisting of stem and two prongs, used to test hearing acuity.
Ophthalmoscope	Lighted instrument with lens, used for examining interior of eye.
Tongue depressor	Flat wooden blade used to depress patient's tongue during examination of mouth and pharynx.
Antiseptic wipe	Disposable pad saturated with antiseptic, such as alcohol, that is used to cleanse skin.
Tape measure	Flexible device calibrated in inches on one side and centimeters on the other side, used to measure patient (e.g., diameter of limb, head circumference).
Percussion hammer	Instrument with rubber head, used for testing neurologic reflexes.
Speculum	Instrument for opening body orifice or cavity for viewing (e.g., ear speculum, nasal speculum, vaginal speculum).
Disposable gloves	Gloves, usually latex, that are worn only once to provide protection from bloodborne pathogens and other potentially infectious materials.
Lubricant	Agent that is applied to physician's gloved hand or to speculum that reduces friction between parts to make insertion easier.
Specimen container	Container in which body specimen is placed for transport to laboratory (after it has been labeled).
Tissues	Used for wiping body secretions.
Cotton-tipped applicator	Small piece of cotton wrapped around the end of a slender wooden stick, used for collection of specimen from the body.
Overhead examination light	Light mounted on flexible movable stand to focus light on area for good visibility.
Basin	Container in which used instruments are deposited.
Biohazard container	Specially made container used for receiving items that contain infectious waste.
Waste receptacle	Container for used disposable articles that do not contain infectious waste.

From Bonewit-West K: *Clinical procedures for medical assistants*, ed 8, St Louis, 2011, Saunders.

12. Check equipment and instruments regularly to verify that they are in proper working condition. This protects the patient from harm caused by faulty equipment.
13. Have equipment and supplies ready for the examination and arranged for easy access by the physician. Equipment and supplies needed for the physical examination vary according to the type of examination and the physician's preference (Figure 20-1).
14. Know how to operate and care for each piece of equipment and each instrument. The manufacturer provides an operating manual, which should be read carefully and thoroughly and kept available for reference.

PREPARATION OF THE PATIENT

It is the medical assistant's responsibility to prepare the patient for the physical examination. After greeting and escorting the patient to the examining room, the medical assistant should identify the patient by asking the patient to state his or her full name and date of birth. This information should be compared with the demographic data indicated in the patient's chart. The patient should *not* be asked whether he or she is a certain patient. For example, the patient should not be asked: "Are you Mary Williams?" The

patient may not hear the medical assistant correctly or may not be paying attention and may answer in the affirmative even if he or she is not that patient. Proper identification is essential to avoid mistaking one patient for another. If the medical assistant performs a procedure on the wrong patient by mistake, he or she could be held liable. The medical assistant then takes vital signs and measures the weight and height of the patient. The results of these procedures are charted in the patient's medical record.

The medical assistant can reduce a patient's apprehension and embarrassment by addressing the patient by his or her name of choice, by adopting a friendly and supportive attitude, and by speaking clearly, distinctly, and slowly. The medical assistant should explain the purpose of the examination and offer to answer any questions. This also facilitates the physical examination of the patient.

The patient should be asked whether he or she needs to void before the examination. An empty bladder makes the examination easier and is more comfortable for the patient. If a urine specimen is needed, the patient is asked to void.

Instructions on disrobing for the examination should be specific so that the patient understands what items of clothing to remove and where to place the clothing. The disrobing area should be comfortable and should provide privacy. It is helpful to have a place for the patient to sit to make it

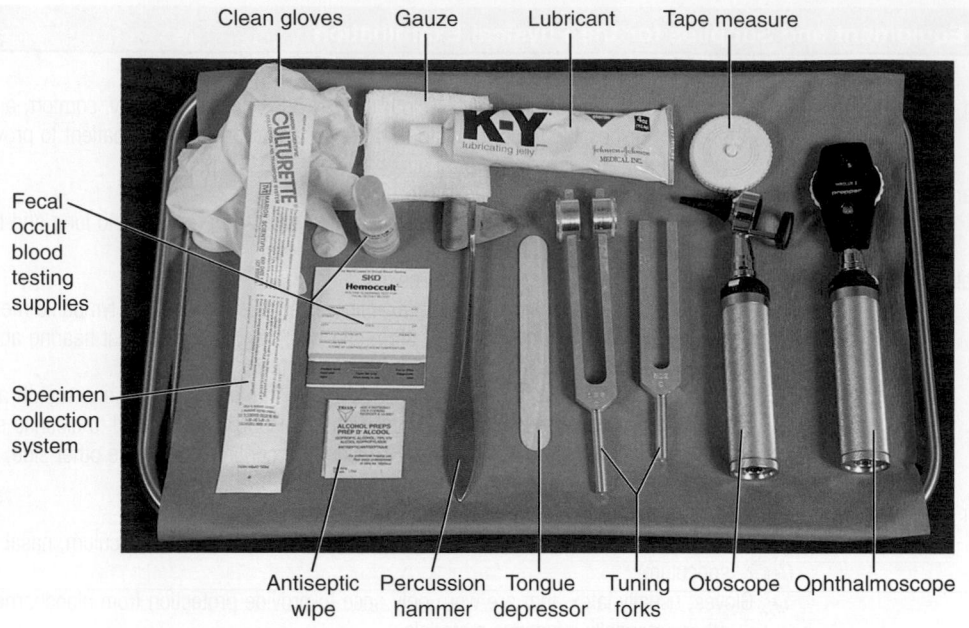

Figure 20-1 Common instruments and supplies used during the physical examination.

Highlight on Patient Teaching

The purpose of patient teaching is to help the patient develop habits, attitudes, and skills that enable the individual to maintain and improve his or her own health.

Fact: Patients who are active, informed participants in their health care are more apt to follow the physician's instructions than patients who are passive recipients of medical services.

Action: Provide patients with information on health care. Every patient interaction is an opportunity for teaching.

Fact: Adult learners are goal oriented and performance centered. They need and want information that would assist them in managing and improving their health.

Action: Review the information that you provide to patients, and determine whether it is nice to know or necessary to know. Select subject matter that is practical and useful and relates directly to the patient's needs.

Fact: The more information that is presented, the more the patient is likely to forget. Approximately one half of information presented to the patient is forgotten in the first 5 minutes after giving it.

Action: When teaching, use the following pointers to help patients learn and retain information:

- Keep it short and be specific.
- Speak in terms the patient can understand.
- Focus on "how," rather than "why."
- Repeat and reinforce important information.
- Give practical examples, and provide ample time for patient practice.

- Ask for feedback from the patient to determine whether he or she understands the information.
- Provide the patient with written information.

Fact: Each individual has a distinct style of learning and learns best when using his or her preferred learning style. The three main learning styles are reading, listening, and doing. People often use more than one style for learning.

Action: Use a variety of teaching strategies to engage the various learning styles of patients. Examples of teaching strategies include explanations, printed handouts, audiovisual aids, demonstrations, and discussions.

Fact: Only two thirds of patients comply with health care instructions prescribed by the physician. Factors that influence compliance include the patient's adaptation to illness, motivation to change, physical capability, and support systems.

Action: The following help increase patient compliance with prescribed treatment:

- Address the patient by his or her name of choice. (Keep in mind that many patients object to being called by their first name by strangers.)
- Encourage the patient to take an active role in personal health care.
- Help the patient set goals and objectives for change.
- Encourage care and support from family members.
- Make the patient aware of outside resources.
- Give positive reinforcement when the patient makes healthy changes. ■

easier to remove clothing and shoes. The area also should be equipped with hooks for hanging clothing. Instructions for putting on the examination gown and for locating the gown opening reduce patient confusion. If the medical assistant senses that the patient will have trouble undressing, assistance should be offered. Elderly and disabled patients sometimes have difficulty removing clothing.

The medical assistant is responsible for making the patient's medical record available for review by the physician. The medical office has a designated location where the record is placed, such as a small shelf mounted on the wall next to the outside of the examining room door or in a chart holder mounted on the outside of the examining room door. The medical assistant should ensure that the medical record is placed so that patient-identifiable information is not visible. This is required by the Health Insurance Portability and Accountability Act (HIPAA) Privacy Rule to protect a patient's health information.

The physical examination is performed with the patient positioned on an examining table, which is specially constructed to facilitate the examination. For safety, it is advisable to help the patient onto and off of the examining table.

What Would You Do? What Would You *Not* Do?

Case Study 1
Abbey Auden, 35 years old, is at the medical office. Her husband got a backyard trampoline for their two school-age children, and she decided to try it out. Abbey landed wrong on the trampoline and hurt her back and neck. For the past 5 days, she has been having headaches and back pain. Abbey refuses to have her weight taken because she has gained weight over the past several years and does not want to know how much she's gained. She does not understand why weight has to be taken at an office visit in the first place. Abbey says that many times when she should go to the doctor, she doesn't, just to avoid being weighed. She says she would not even be here now except that her husband insisted that she come. ■

MEASURING WEIGHT AND HEIGHT

The medical assistant routinely measures the weight and height of many types of patients. The process of measuring the patient is **mensuration**. A change in weight may be significant in the diagnosis of a patient's condition and in prescribing the course of treatment. Underweight and overweight patients who follow a diet therapy program should be weighed at regular intervals to determine their progress. Prenatal patients are weighed during each prenatal visit to assist in the assessment of fetal development and of the mother's health. Procedure 20-1 describes how to measure height and weight.

An adult's weight usually is measured during each office visit; an adult's height is typically measured only during the first visit or when a complete physical examination of the patient is requested. Children are weighed and their height

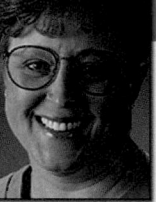

Putting It All into Practice

My Name is Hope Fauber, and I am a certified medical assistant. I work in a medical clinic with a family medicine department of 10 physicians and 10 residents and interns. My duties cover a broad spectrum, from pediatrics to geriatrics, and include prenatal care, allergy injections, minor office surgery, electrocardiograms, colposcopies, immunizations, and wound care.

At our clinic, many of the patients are elderly. I occasionally come across geriatric patients who are not very cooperative and are "set in their ways." One 90-year-old woman, in particular, had a reputation in the office for being cantankerous and difficult to work with. One day, when the physician ordered laboratory work on her, I prepared to draw blood from her tiny, frail body, praying that everything would go smoothly. As I helped her up after a successful "stick," she, of all people, reached to give me a hug and said to me, "I like you. That didn't even hurt!" She continued to hold my hand and talk to me as I walked her out of the office. This turned out to be the last time I would see her because she moved out of town, but not out of my heart, leaving a lasting impression on my life. ■

What Would You Do? What Would You *Not* Do?

Case Study 2
Karen Steiner drops her 17-year-old daughter, Mikayla, off at the medical office for her sports physical examination. Mikayla is captain of the varsity cheerleading squad and is getting ready to start her senior year in high school. Mikayla's vital signs are normal, and she measures 5 feet 6 inches tall and weighs 105 pounds. With some reluctance, Mikayla admits that she's been having problems with heartburn, and she's pretty sure she knows what's causing it. She says that she has to keep her weight down for cheerleading, and after eating dinner with her family, she makes herself vomit to get rid of the food in her stomach. Mikayla is not too concerned about doing this because a lot of the popular girls at school are doing the same thing. She says it's the easy way to stay slim, and she would like to lose another 10 pounds before football season starts. Mikayla wants some prescription drug samples to help with the heartburn because the over-the-counter pills that she's been taking are not working anymore. She does not want her parents to know about any of this because she's afraid that they would not understand and might make her drop out of cheerleading. ■

(or length) is measured during each office visit to observe their pattern of growth and to calculate medication dosage.

The patient's height is used to interpret body weight (see the box *Highlight on Interpreting Body Weight*). Weight and height are compared against a standardized chart that serves as a general guide to determine whether the patient's weight falls within normal limits (Figure 20-2).

Highlight on Cultural Diversity

Culture consists of the values, beliefs, and practices of a particular group of people. Culture is deeply rooted and is passed on from one generation to the next through communication. It includes areas such as religion, dietary practices, family lines of authority, family life patterns, beliefs, and health practices.

As the demographics of the United States continue to change, the medical assistant is faced with the challenge of providing care to an increasing number of cultural groups. It is important for the medical assistant to learn as much as possible about the cultural values of patients coming to the medical office. This is known as *cultural awareness* and can be accomplished by carefully observing and listening to patients to acquire knowledge of their cultural values.

Cultural sensitivity is respect and appreciation for cultural diversity, whereas *cultural competence* is understanding and using the cultural background of a patient to assist with the resolution of a problem. Because health practices are part of a patient's culture, changing them may have a negative impact on the patient. Whenever possible, the medical assistant should incorporate factors from a patient's cultural background into his or her health care.

Guidelines for Achieving Cultural Competence

The following guidelines help the medical assistant in developing cultural awareness and sensitivity and in achieving cultural competence:

1. **Respect the patient's values, beliefs, and practices.** Even if you do not agree with them, it is important to respect the patient's right to hold these values and to not dismiss them as strange or odd. Cultural values play an important role in a patient's lifestyle. Patients from some cultures believe that losing blood depletes the body's strength and provides a route for the soul to leave the body. If a blood specimen is needed, these patients may become highly distressed or refuse to have their blood drawn. Members of some cultural groups believe that illness results when the body's natural balance or harmony is disturbed. To restore the balance, alternative forms of medicine, such as herbal remedies and aromatherapy, are used.

2. **Refrain from cultural stereotypes.** Not all people of a cultural group have the same beliefs, practices, and values. Assuming that all members of a cultural group are alike is known as *stereotyping* and should be avoided. Just as one would never assume that all people in the United States like hamburgers and baseball, every individual must be approached according to his or her specific beliefs and practices.

3. **Always address patients by their last names (and Mr., Mrs., Miss, Ms.) unless they give you permission to use other names.** In many cultures, using a first name to address anyone other than family or friends is considered disrespectful. Most older people in the United States dislike being called by their first name and feel it shows a lack of respect.

4. **Speak slowly and clearly.** Communicating with a patient may be difficult if the patient has a limited knowledge of English. With these patients, you should speak slowly and clearly in a normal tone and volume of voice. Speaking loudly does not help the patient understand any better and may be offensive to the patient.

5. **Show respect for cultural lines of authority.** In many cultures, respect is given based on age and gender. In certain cultures, elders are considered the holders of the culture's wisdom and are highly respected. In other cultures, youth is valued over age. In certain cultures, the male dominates, and women have very little status. Because of this, a female patient from this type of culture may not be permitted to give her own health history or to answer questions. In addition, a male patient from this culture may not accept instructions from a female medical assistant.

6. **Use appropriate eye contact.** In most cultures, direct eye contact is important and generally shows that the other is attentive and listening. It conveys self-confidence, openness, interest, and honesty, whereas the lack of eye contact may be interpreted as secretiveness, shyness, guilt, or lack of interest. Other cultures consider eye contact impolite or an invasion of privacy; these patients show respect by avoiding direct eye contact.

7. **Be aware of cultural responses to illness.** The conditions under which an individual assumes the role of a (sick) patient and the way he or she performs in that role vary with culture. Individuals of some cultures resist the sick role and blame sickness on external forces as a means of punishment. These individuals may deny their illness and fail to provide much information when the medical assistant takes their symptoms. In other cultures, individuals take an optimistic view of the outcome of health care and, because of this, are more likely to elicit information and to follow the physician's instructions.

8. **Learn to appreciate the richness of diversity as an asset, rather than a hindrance, to communication and effective interaction with patients.** ■

Health Promotion and Disease Prevention

Teach patients the essentials of health promotion and disease prevention. Help patients become aware of the following patterns of behavior that promote and support health: ■
- Keeping up to date with immunizations
- Eating nutritiously from the food pyramid
- Exercising regularly
- Maintaining normal weight
- Managing stress
- Maintaining high self-esteem
- Avoiding tobacco and drugs
- Using alcohol wisely

- Understanding how the environment affects health and taking appropriate action to improve it
- Knowing the facts about cardiovascular disease, cancer, infections, sexually transmitted diseases, and accidents, and using this knowledge to protect against them
- Understanding the changes that occur through the natural processes of aging
- Developing a sense of responsibility for health by taking an active role in establishing and maintaining a healthy lifestyle ■

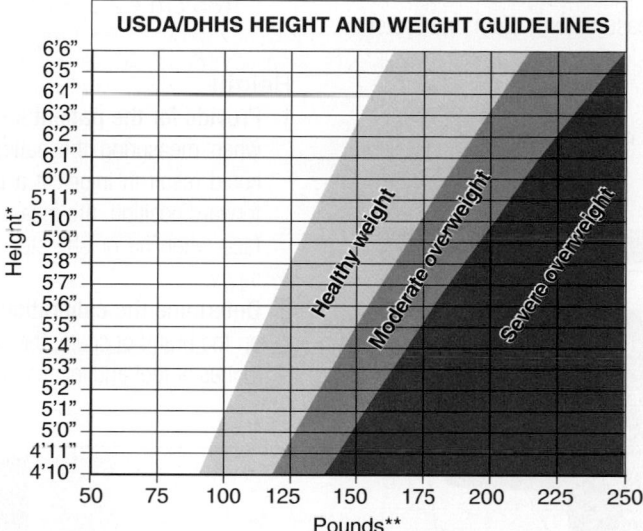

* Without shoes.
**Without clothes. The higher weights apply to people with more muscle and bone, such as many men.

Figure 20-2 U.S. Department of Agriculture (USDA)/Department of Health and Human Services (DHHS) height and weight guidelines.

Guidelines for Measuring Weight and Height

When using an upright balance scale to measure weight and height, use the following guidelines.

Weight
1. **Locate the scale to provide privacy for the patient.** Place the scale on a hard, level surface in a private location. Many patients are self-conscious about having their weight measured and prefer that it be done in privacy. Do not make weight-sensitive comments during the procedure. This is especially important for patients with weight control problems such as obesity and eating disorders.

2. **Balance the scale before measuring weight.** If the scale is not balanced, the weight measurement will be inaccurate. The scale is balanced when the upper and lower weights are on zero and the indicator point comes to a rest at the center of the balance area.
3. **Assist the patient.** Assist the patient onto and off of the scale platform. The scale platform moves slightly and may cause the patient to become unsteady.
4. **Obtain an accurate weight.** Always ask the patient to remove his or her shoes. Measure weight with the patient in normal

Continued

Guidelines for Measuring Weight and Height—cont'd

clothing. Ask the patient to remove heavy outer clothing, such as a sweater or a jacket.

5. **Interpret the calibration markings accurately.** The lower calibration bar is divided into 50-lb increments (Figure 20-3, *A*). The upper calibration bar is divided into pounds and quarter pounds. The longer calibration lines indicate pound increments, and the shorter calibration lines indicate quarter-pound and half-pound increments (Figure 20-3, *B*).

6. **Determine the patient's weight correctly.** Add the measurement on the lower scale to the measurement on the upper scale. The result should be rounded to the nearest quarter pound. Occasionally, the patient's weight may need to be converted to kilograms, which is the metric unit of measurement for weight. This may be required when determining medication dosage. The following formulas are used to convert weight and height measurements from one system to another.

Weight Conversion

Pounds to kilograms. Divide the number of pounds by 2.2:

$$136\ lb \div 2.2 = 61.8\ kg$$

Kilograms to pounds. Multiply the number of kilograms by 2.2:

$$75\ kg \times 2.2 = 165\ lb$$

Height Conversion

Inches to centimeters. Multiply the number of inches by 2.5:

$$64\ inches \times 2.5 = 160\ cm$$

Centimeters to inches. Divide the number of centimeters by 2.5:

$$185\ cm \div 2.5 = 74\ inches\ (or\ 6\ feet\ 2\ inches)$$

Height

1. **Provide for the patient's safety.** Follow the proper procedure when measuring the patient's height. An error in technique could result in injury. If a patient is placed on the scale in a forward position, the measuring bar could fall into the patient's face when he or she steps off of the scale, causing a facial injury.

2. **Determine the calibration markings accurately.** Depending on the brand of scale, the calibration markings are divided into inches or feet and inches. (Figure 20-4 is an example of a scale

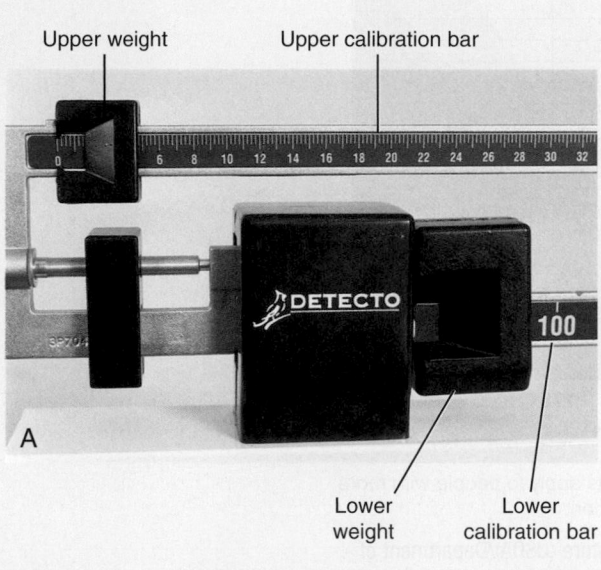

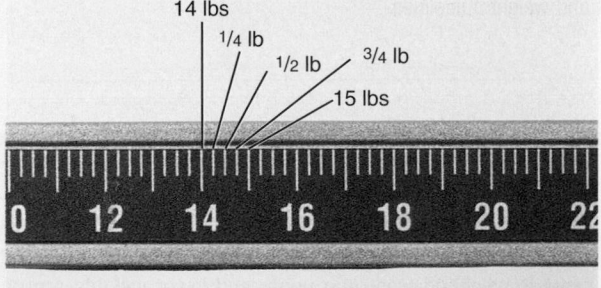

Figure 20-3 Calibration markings for measuring weight on an upright balance scale. **A,** The upper calibration bar is divided into pounds and quarter pounds. **B,** The longer calibration lines indicate pound increments, and the shorter calibration lines indicate quarter-pound and half-pound increments.

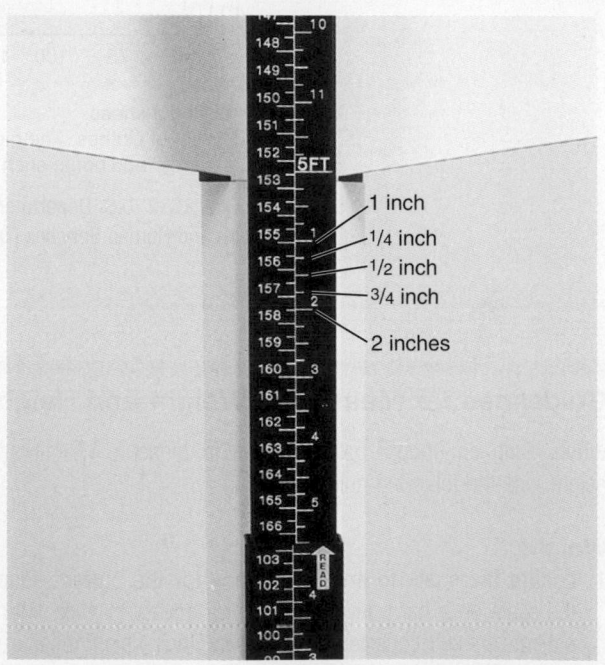

Figure 20-4 Calibration markings for measuring height on an upright balance scale.

Guidelines for Measuring Weight and Height—cont'd

divided into feet and inches.) The calibration rod also is calibrated into centimeters, which is the metric unit of measurement for height. This unit of measurement is not typically used to measure height in the United States.

3. **Read the measurement correctly.** The height measurement is read from the top of the bar down and should be read to the nearest quarter inch. For most patients, you can read the height measurement at the junction of the stationary calibration rod and the movable calibration rod (Figure 20-5, *A*). If the patient's height is less than the top value of the stationary calibration rod, however, you must read the measurement from the bottom of the bar up directly on the stationary rod. For example, on most scales the highest calibration on the stationary rod is 50 inches; patients with a height of 50 inches or less would have their height read directly from the stationary rod (Figure 20-5, *B*).

4. **Record the height measurement correctly.** Record the height measurement in feet and inches. If the scale is calibrated in inches, convert the reading to feet and inches by dividing the number of inches by 12. A height measurement of 60 inches is recorded as 5 feet (60 inches ÷ 12 = 5). If the patient's height measurement is 64 inches, the results would be recorded as 5 feet, 4 inches.

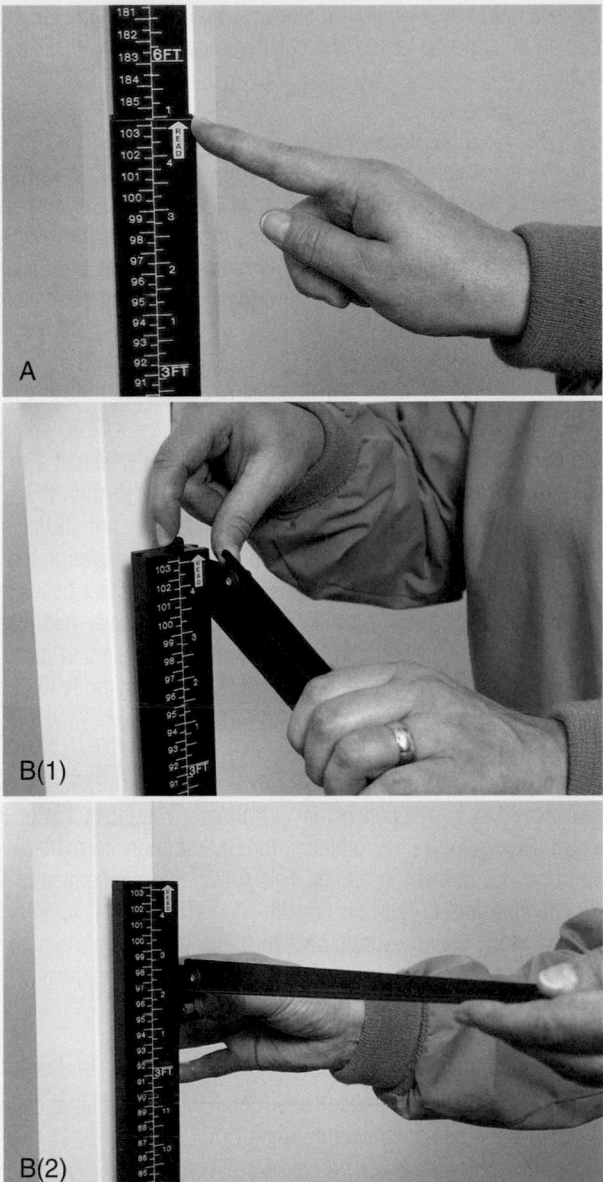

Figure 20-5 A, Reading a height measurement at the junction of the stationary calibration rod and the movable calibration rod. The height measurement in this illustration is 6 feet, 1 inch. **B(1),** Reading a height measurement on the stationary calibration rod. *NOTE:* The measuring bar must first be released and moved down to the stationary bar to measure the patient's height. **B(2),** Reading the height at the junction of the bar and the rod. The height measurement in this illustration is 3 feet, 2 inches.

Highlight on Interpreting Body Weight

The two common methods to interpret body weight are weight in relation to standard tables and calculation of the body mass index (BMI).

Height and Weight Tables

One way to interpret body weight is through the use of standardized height and weight tables. In 1959, the Metropolitan Life Insurance Company (MET) issued a set of tables indicating desirable height and weight ranges for men and women. In 1983, MET issued revised tables for men and women that showed height and weight ranges higher than those in the 1959 table. Many health experts believe that the desirable weight ranges of the revised tables are too high and do not represent healthy body weight.

In 1995, the U.S. Department of Agriculture (USDA) and the Department of Health and Human Services (DHHS) issued a set of weight guidelines (see Figure 20-2) that are lower than those of the MET tables. The USDA/DHHS guidelines do not distinguish between weights of men and women and must be interpreted by each individual as follows. Women usually have smaller bones and less muscle than men, so they should use the lower end of the range. Men and large-boned, muscular women should use the higher end of the weight range to find their healthy body weights.

Body Mass Index

Another method for interpreting body weight is the BMI. The BMI expresses the correlation of an individual's weight to his or her height. Except for trained athletes, the BMI strongly correlates with total body fat content in adults. This provides an indication of the risk of developing chronic health conditions associated with obesity. Many health experts believe that the BMI is a more accurate standard for interpreting body weight than are height and weight tables.

Method for Calculating BMI

a. Use the following website to have your BMI calculated automatically: www.cdc.gov/nccdphp/dnpa/bmi
b. Use the following steps to calculate your BMI:
  1. Multiply your weight in pounds (without clothes or shoes) by 703. For an individual who weighs 135 lb:
   $135 \times 703 = 94,905$
  2. Divide this number by your height in inches. If this individual is 66 inches tall: $94,905 \div 66 = 1438$
  3. Divide this amount again by your height in inches, and round off to the nearest whole number: $1438 \div 66 = 21.79$, or 22

The BMI of this individual is 22.

Interpretation of the BMI

In June 1998, the National Heart, Lung, and Blood Institute (NHLBI), a federal health agency, issued a set of guidelines for the classification of body weight in adults. One of these guidelines relates to interpretation of the BMI, as outlined here.

BMI	Interpretation
Below 18.5	Underweight
18.5-24.9	Healthy weight
25-29.9	Overweight
30-34.9	Obesity (I)
35.0-39.9	Obesity (II)
40 or more	Extreme obesity (III)

The NHLBI recommends that the BMI be determined in all adults. People of normal weight should have their BMI reassessed every 2 years.

Adult Obesity

The incidence of obesity in the United States has increased markedly, and obesity is now one of the most common problems encountered by primary care physicians. Approximately 66% of adults in the United States are either overweight or obese. That means that nearly two out of every three Americans are overweight or obese. Obesity is associated with premature death and, after smoking, is the second leading cause of preventable death in the United States today. Approximately 300,000 deaths in the United States each year are associated with obesity.

It has been determined that as the BMI increases to greater than 25, there is an increased risk of developing certain diseases associated with overweight and obesity, including the following:
- Hypertension
- Cardiovascular disease
- Dyslipidemia (high blood cholesterol levels, high blood triglyceride levels, or both)
- Type 2 diabetes
- Colon cancer
- Gallbladder disease
- Breast and endometrial cancers
- Sleep apnea and respiratory problems
- Osteoarthritis

Obesity is considered a chronic condition that requires a multiple treatment approach, including a behavioral therapy program, a low-calorie diet, and a suitable aerobic exercise program. Primary care physicians often manage individuals with mild and moderate obesity, but morbidly obese patients are usually referred to a bariatric specialist. **Bariatrics** is the branch of medicine that deals with the treatment and control of obesity and diseases associated with obesity. ■

PROCEDURE 20-1 Measuring Weight and Height

Outcome Measure weight and height.

Equipment/Supplies

- Upright balance scale
- Paper towel

Weight

1. Procedural Step. Sanitize your hands.

2. Procedural Step. Check the scale to ensure it is balanced as follows:

  a. Make sure the upper and lower weights are on zero. When the weights are on zero, they are all the way to the left of the calibration bars.

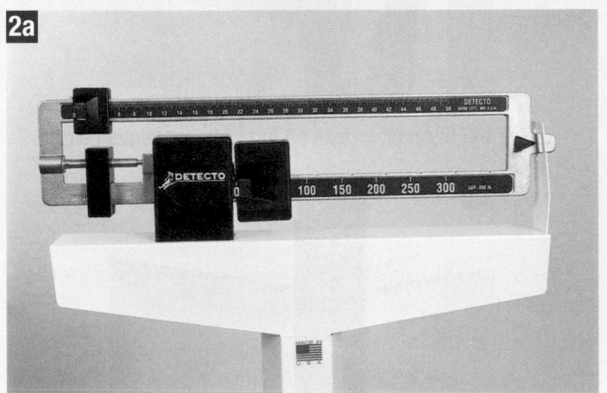

Ensure that the upper and lower weights are on zero.

  b. Look at the indicator point. If the scale is balanced, the indicator point is resting in the center of the balance area.

  c. If the indicator point rests below the center, adjust the screw on the balance knob by turning it clockwise (to the right) until the indicator point rests in the center of the balance area.

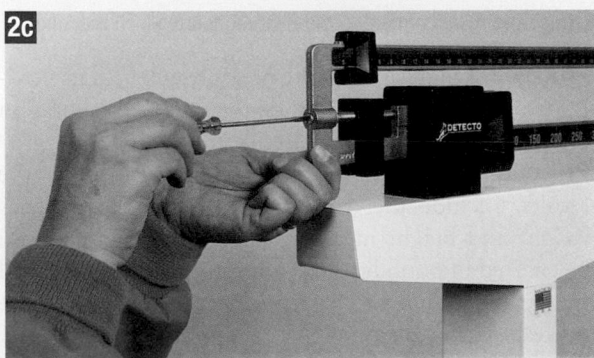

Correct the balance by adjusting the screw on the balance knob.

  d. If the indicator point rests above the center, adjust the screw on the balance knob by turning it counterclockwise (to the left) until the indicator point rests in the center of the balance area.

Principle. If the scale is not balanced, the weight measurement will be inaccurate.

3. Procedural Step. Greet the patient and introduce yourself.

4. Procedural Step. Identify the patient and explain to the patient that you will be measuring his or her height and weight.

5. Procedural Step. Instruct the patient to remove shoes and outer clothing such as a jacket or sweater. A good medical aseptic practice is to place a paper towel on the platform of the scale to protect the patient's feet.

Principle. Removing heavy clothing and shoes allows a more accurate measurement of the patient's weight.

6. Procedural Step. Assist the patient onto the scale, and instruct the patient not to move.

Principle. It is not possible to balance the scale if the patient is moving.

7. Procedural Step. Balance the scale as follows:

  a. Move the lower weight to the notched groove that does not cause the indicator point to drop to the bottom of the calibration area. Ensure that the lower weight is seated firmly in its groove.

  b. Slide the upper weight slowly along its calibration bar by tapping it gently until the indicator point comes to rest at the center of the balance area.

Principle. Not seating the lower weight firmly in its groove results in an inaccurate reading.

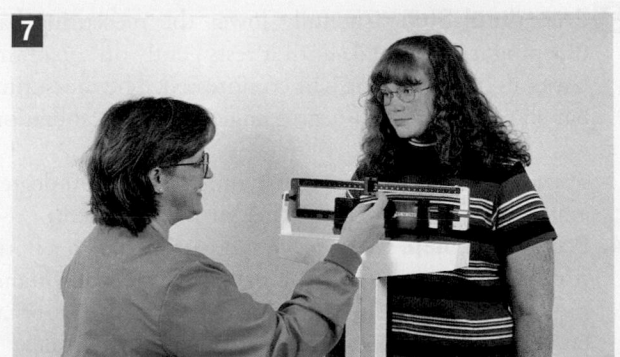

Slide the upper weight by tapping it gently.

8. Procedural Step. Read the results to the nearest quarter pound by adding the measurement on the lower scale to the measurement on the upper scale. Jot down this value or make a mental note of it.

9. Procedural Step. Ask the patient to step off of the scale platform. Provide assistance if needed.

Continued

PROCEDURE 20-1   **Measuring Weight and Height—cont'd**

Height

1. Procedural Step. Slide the movable calibration rod upward until the measuring bar is well above the patient's apparent height. Open the measuring bar to its horizontal position.

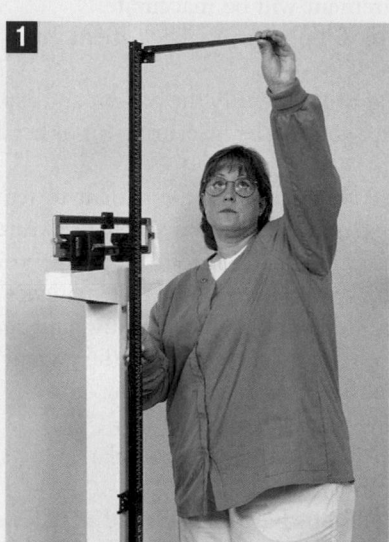

Slide the bar upward until it is well above the patient's height.

2. Procedural Step. Instruct the patient to step onto the scale platform with his or her back to the scale. Provide assistance if needed. Instruct the patient to stand erect and to look straight ahead.
Principle. Looking straight ahead helps the patient to stand erect and balanced, which ensures an accurate measurement.

3. Procedural Step. Carefully lower the measuring bar (keeping it horizontal) until it rests gently on top of the patient's head with the hair compressed. The measuring bar should form a 90-degree angle with the calibration rod.
Principle. The measuring bar must be at a 90-degree angle to ensure an accurate height measurement.

4. Procedural Step. Keeping the measuring bar in a horizontal position, instruct the patient to step down and put on his or her shoes. Hold the bar in a horizontal position until the patient has stepped off the scale.

5. Procedural Step. Read the height measurement from the top down to the nearest quarter-inch marking at the junction of the stationary calibration rod and the movable calibration rod. (*NOTE:* If the patient's height is less than the top value of the stationary rod, read the measurement from the bottom up directly on the stationary calibration rod.) Jot down this value or make a mental note of it.

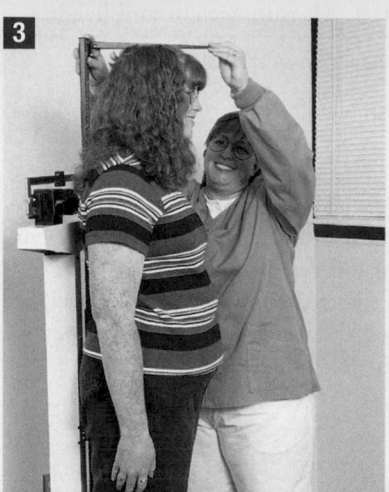

Lower the bar until it rests on top of the patient's head.

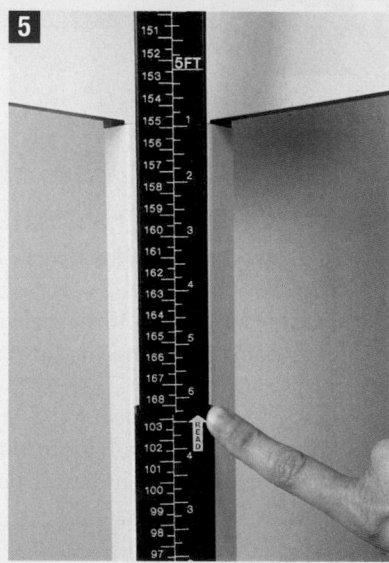

Read the measurement to the nearest quarter-inch marking.

6. Procedural Step. Return the measuring bar to its vertical (resting) position, and slide the movable calibration rod to its lowest position. Return the weights to zero.

7. Procedural Step. Sanitize your hands, and chart the results. Include the date and time and the patient's weight and height measurements. The weight should be charted in pounds to the nearest quarter pound, and the height should be charted in feet and inches to the nearest quarter inch.

CHARTING EXAMPLE

Date	
11/5/XX	10:15 a.m. Wt: 155. Ht: 5' 6¼" _____
	_____ Hope Fauber, CMA (AAMA)

BODY MECHANICS

Daily activities in a medical office sometimes carry the risk of acute or chronic musculoskeletal injury. Because of this, the medical assistant should have a thorough knowledge of the principles of proper body mechanics and know when to use them. **Body mechanics** is the utilization of the correct muscles to maintain proper balance, posture, and body alignment to accomplish a task safely and efficiently without undue strain on muscles or joints. Proper body mechanics should be used when the medical assistant performs the following: standing, walking, sitting, lifting, positioning a patient on the examining table, and transferring a patient. The medical assistant should also use proper body mechanics at home in his or her activities of daily living. Using proper body mechanics prevents musculoskeletal strains to the back and other body structures such as the knees, neck, shoulders, and wrists.

The primary benefits of proper body mechanics include the following:
1. Allows an individual to conserve energy, which makes it easier to perform a task
2. Protects the body from injury by reducing stress and strain on muscles, nerves, joints, tendons, ligaments, and soft tissues
3. Helps to maintain proper body control and balance
4. Promotes effective, efficient, and safe movement

Studies show that health care workers sustain a significantly higher incidence of back injuries as compared with other professions. To help prevent an injury to the back, a primary focus of proper body mechanics is to keep the natural curves of the spine or vertebral column in proper alignment. The vertebral column has four curvatures. These curvatures increase the strength and resilience of the vertebral column and include the cervical curvature, thoracic curvature, lumbar curvature, and sacral curvature (Figure 20-6). The vertebral column extends from the skull to the pelvis and consists of a series of bones known as *vertebrae*. The vertebrae are separated by shock-absorbing *intervertebral discs* (see Figure 20-6). These discs allow an individual to bend and twist. Over time, with improper and repeated bending and twisting (especially while carrying an object), the discs can deteriorate, which causes them to narrow, to harden, and even to crack and tear. This condition is known as *degenerative disc disease*. With degenerative disc disease, the discs lose their shock-absorbing ability and cause the patient to experience localized pain and stiffness in the area of disc deterioration. In addition, once a disc is weakened, it can bulge out or rupture; this is known as a *herniated disc*.

Principles

There are some basic principles related to proper body mechanics that should be followed:
1. Movements should be smooth and coordinated rather than jerky.

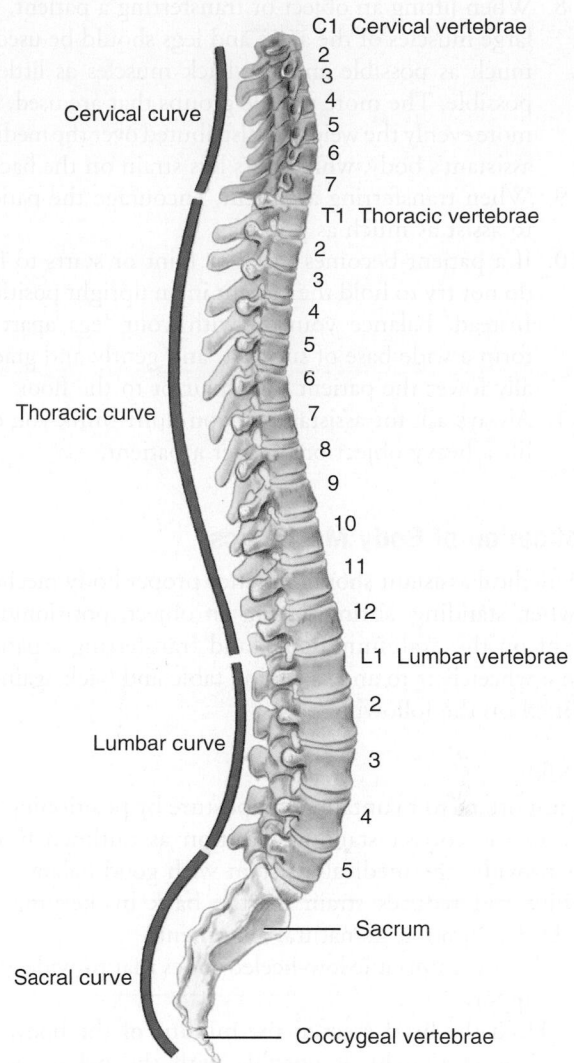

Figure 20-6 Vertebral column.

C1 Cervical vertebrae
2
3
4
5
6
7
Cervical curve

T1 Thoracic vertebrae
2
3
4
5
6
7
8
9
10
11
12
Thoracic curve

L1 Lumbar vertebrae
2
3
4
5
Lumbar curve

Sacrum
Sacral curve

Coccygeal vertebrae

2. Keeping the body in good physical condition through exercising, stretching, and weight training helps to prevent musculoskeletal injury.
3. To avoid straining the back, do not reach for something that is farther than 14 to 18 inches away.
4. Work at a comfortable height that avoids having to bend the neck or back forward to perform the task. People are usually most comfortable working at a height that falls between the waist and elbow levels.
5. If possible, push, pull, or slide an object rather than lift it. This conserves energy and places less strain on the back.
6. Lighter items should be stored on higher shelves or cabinets, and heavier items should be stored at or below waist level.
7. When an object from an overhead shelf or cabinet needs to be retrieved, use a step stool or chair to come up to the level of the object. Reaching for a stored overhead item can produce strain on the back.

8. When lifting an object or transferring a patient, the large muscles of the arms and legs should be used as much as possible and the back muscles as little as possible. The more muscle groups that are used, the more evenly the weight is distributed over the medical assistant's body, which puts less strain on the back.

9. When transferring a patient, encourage the patient to assist as much as possible.

10. If a patient becomes dizzy or faint or starts to fall, do not try to hold the patient in an upright position. Instead, balance yourself with your legs apart to form a wide base of support, and gently and gradually lower the patient to a chair or to the floor.

11. Always ask for assistance if you don't think you can lift a heavy object or transfer a patient.

Application of Body Mechanics

The medical assistant should practice proper body mechanics when standing, sitting, lifting an object, positioning a patient on the examining table, and transferring a patient from a wheelchair to an examining table and back again, as outlined on the following pages.

Standing

It is important to maintain good posture by positioning the body in the correct standing position as outlined below. This provides the medical assistant with good balance and stability and reduces strain on the back by keeping the vertebral column at its natural alignment.

1. Wear comfortable low-heeled shoes that provide good support.

2. Hold the head erect at the midline of the body, the back as straight as possible with the pelvis tucked inward, the chest forward with the shoulders back, and the abdomen drawn in and kept flat. This helps to maintain appropriate alignment of the vertebral column (Figure 20-7).

3. The knees should be slightly flexed with the feet pointing forward and parallel to each other about 3 inches apart. This provides a broad base of support and improves balance.

4. The arms should be positioned comfortably at the side, and the weight of the body should be evenly distributed over both feet.

Sitting

The medical assistant should use proper body mechanics when in a sitting position (Figure 20-8), as outlined below.

1. Sit in a chair with a firm back.

2. Sit firmly with the back and buttocks supported against the back of the chair; avoid slumping. The body weight should be evenly distributed over the buttocks and thighs.

3. Use a small pillow or a rolled towel to support the lower back.

4. The feet should be flat on the floor, and the knees should be level with the hips.

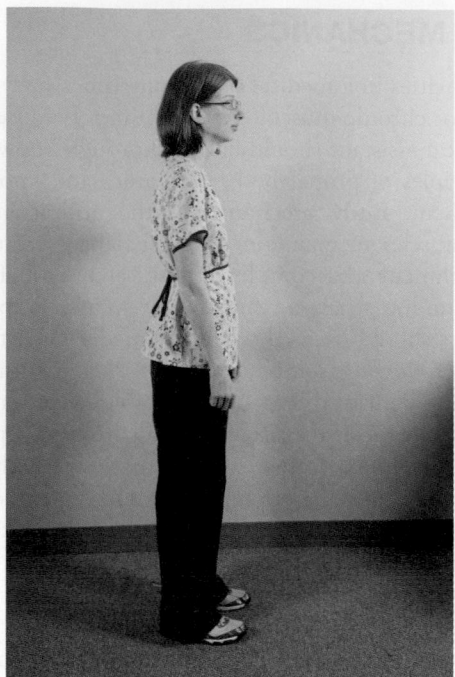

Figure 20-7 Proper standing position.

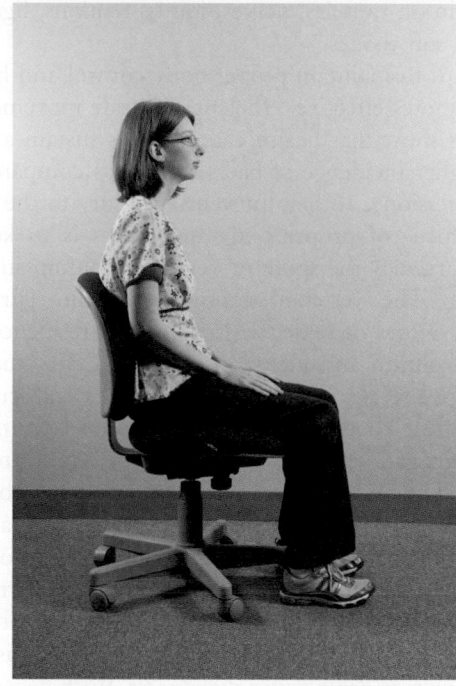

Figure 20-8 Proper sitting position.

5. If you need to sit for a prolonged period of time, use a footstool to raise one knee to reduce strain on the back.

6. Take frequent stretch breaks.

Lifting

The following steps outline the procedure for lifting an object while using proper body mechanics:

1. First determine the weight of the object to determine if you can safely lift it. Pushing the object with one foot can help you determine if you can lift it without assistance. Never lift anything heavier than you can easily manage.

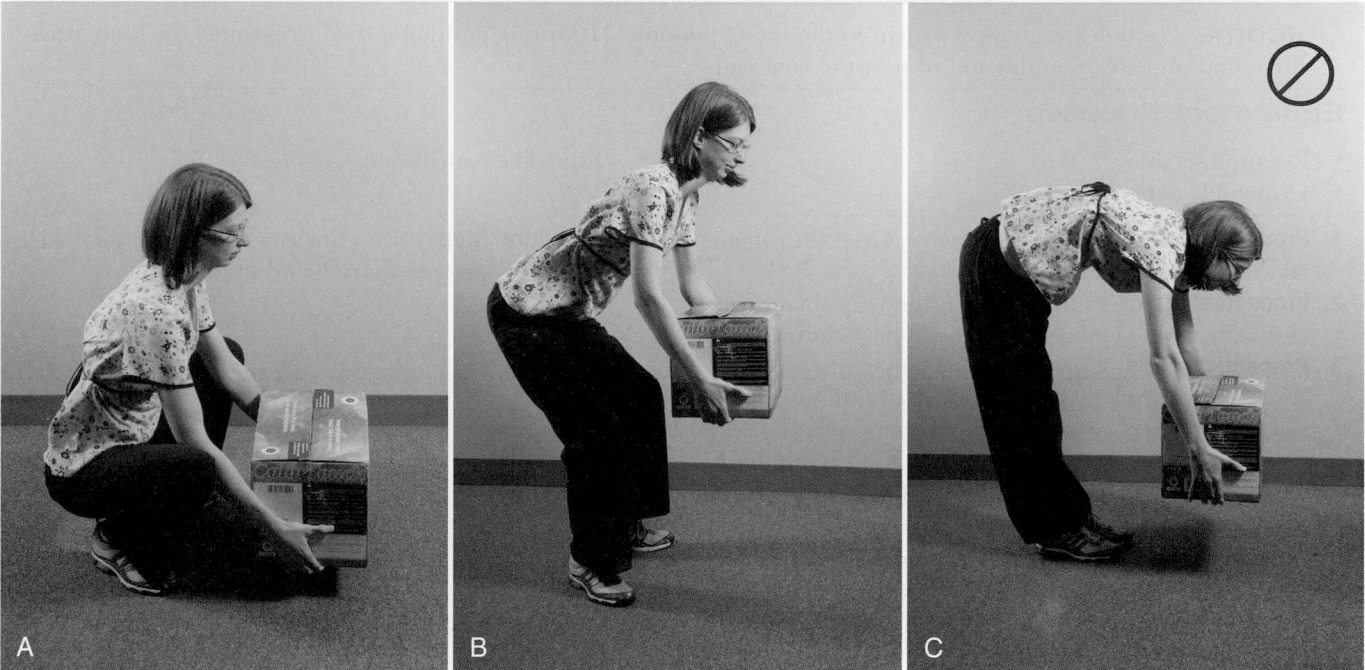

Figure 20-9 **A,** To lift the object, always bend the body at the knees and hips. **B,** Lift with the leg muscles, while keeping the back straight. **C,** Never bend from the waist.

2. Stand in front of the object and balance yourself with the feet about 6 to 8 inches apart, toes pointed outward, and one foot slightly forward to provide a wide base of support. Tighten the stomach and gluteal muscles in preparation for lifting the object.

3. To lift the object, always bend the body at the knees and hips (Figure 20-9, *A*). This helps to maintain your center of gravity and allows the strong muscles of the legs to do the lifting. Never bend from the waist (Figure 20-9, *C*).

4. Grasp the object firmly with both hands.

5. Keeping the back straight, lift the object smoothly with the leg muscles, not the back muscles (Figure 20-9, *B*). The muscles of the back are not as strong and are more easily injured than the leg muscles.

6. Hold the object as close to the body as possible and at waist level. This allows the weight of the object to be lifted by the arm and leg muscles rather than the back muscles. To prevent strain on the back, never lift anything higher than the level of the chest.

7. If you need to turn after lifting the object, don't twist. Turn by pivoting your whole body. Twisting the spine can cause a serious back injury.

8. If you need to carry the object to another location, make sure the area of transport is dry and free of clutter.

9. Lower the object slowly, making sure to bend from the knees to allow the leg muscles to do the work.

POSITIONING AND DRAPING

Correct positioning of the patient facilitates the examination by permitting better access to the part being examined or treated. The basic positions used in the medical office are sitting, supine, prone, dorsal recumbent, lithotomy, Sims, knee-chest, and Fowler's.

The position used depends on the type of examination or procedure to be performed. More than one position may be used to examine the same body part during the physical examination. The sitting and supine positions are both used to examine the chest. It is important to know the correct position for each examination or treatment. When positioning a patient, the medical assistant should explain the position to the patient and assist the patient in attaining it. The medical assistant should make sure to use proper body mechanics when positioning a patient to avoid musculoskeletal injuries.

It is important to take the patient's endurance and degree of wellness into consideration when positioning a patient. Patients who are weak or ill may be unable to assume a position or may require special assistance in attaining it. Some positions, such as the lithotomy and knee-chest positions, are embarrassing and uncomfortable. A patient should not be kept in these positions any longer than necessary. Some patients (especially the elderly) become dizzy after a time in certain positions, such as the knee-chest position. These patients should be allowed to rest before they get off the examining table. The medical assistant also should assist patients off the examining table to prevent falls.

The patient is draped during positioning to provide for modesty, comfort, and warmth. Only the part to be examined should be exposed. Patient gowns and drapes used in the medical office are usually made of paper but also may be made of cloth. Procedures 20-2 through 20-9 present proper positioning and draping of the patient.

Outcome Position and drape a patient in the sitting position. The sitting position is used to examine the head, neck, chest, and upper extremities and to measure vital signs.

Equipment/Supplies

- Examining table
- Disposable patient gown
- Disposable patient drape

1. **Procedural Step.** Sanitize your hands. Greet the patient and introduce yourself.
2. **Procedural Step.** Identify the patient and explain the type of examination or procedure that will be performed.
3. **Procedural Step.** Provide the patient with a patient gown. Instruct the patient to remove clothing as appropriate for the type of examination being performed and to put on the patient gown with the opening in front. The disrobing facility should provide privacy, a place to sit, and a place to hang clothing.
4. **Procedural Step.** Pull out the footrest of the examining table, and assist the patient into a sitting position. The patient's buttocks and thighs should be firmly supported on the edge of the table.

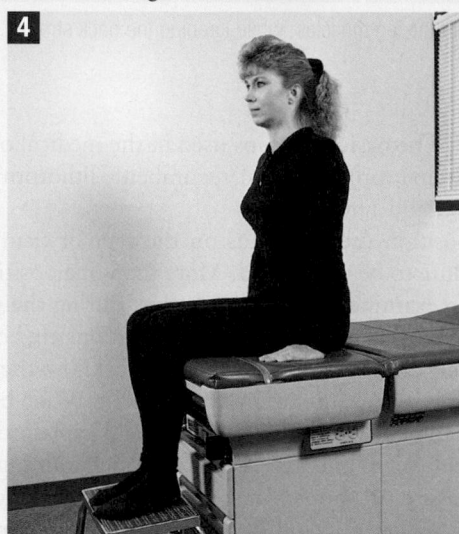
Sitting position.

5. **Procedural Step.** Place a drape over the patient's thighs and legs to provide warmth and modesty.

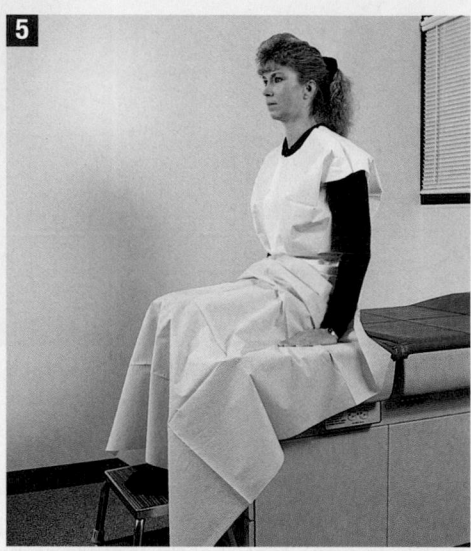
Place the drape over the patient's thighs and legs.

6. **Procedural Step.** After completion of the examination, assist the patient down from the table. Return the footrest to its normal position. Instruct the patient to get dressed. Discard the gown and drape in a waste container.

Outcome Position and drape a patient in the supine position. The supine position is used to examine the head, chest, abdomen, and extremities.

Equipment/Supplies

- Examining table
- Disposable patient gown
- Disposable patient drape

1. **Procedural Step.** Sanitize your hands. Greet the patient and introduce yourself.
2. **Procedural Step.** Identify the patient and explain the type of examination or procedure that will be performed.
3. **Procedural Step.** Provide the patient with a patient gown. Instruct the patient to remove clothing as appropriate for the type of examination being performed and

to put on the patient gown with the opening in front. The disrobing facility should provide privacy, a place to sit, and a place to hang clothing.

4. **Procedural Step.** Pull out the footrest of the examining table, and assist the patient into a sitting position. Place a drape over the patient's thighs and legs.
5. **Procedural Step.** Ask the patient to move back on the table. As the patient is doing this, pull out the

table extension while supporting the patient's lower legs.

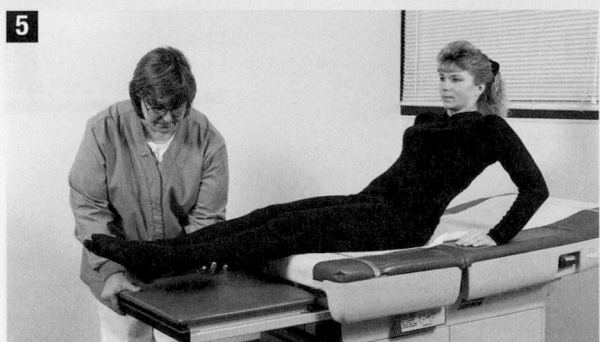

Pull out the table extension while supporting the patient's legs.

6. Procedural Step. Ask the patient to lie on his or her back with the legs together. Provide assistance if needed.

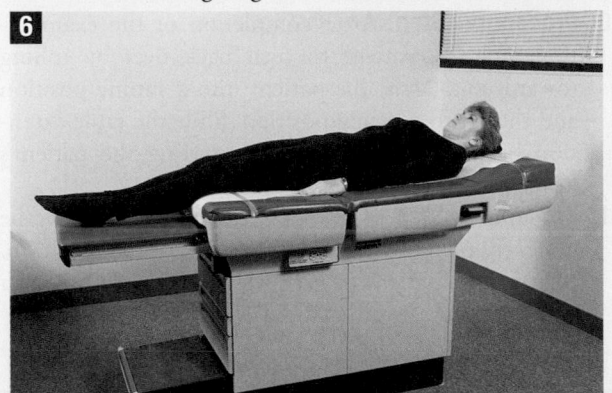

Position the patient on the back with the legs together.

The patient's arms may be placed above the head or alongside the body.

7. Procedural Step. Position the drape lengthwise over the patient to provide warmth and modesty. As the physician examines the patient, move the drape according to the body parts being examined.

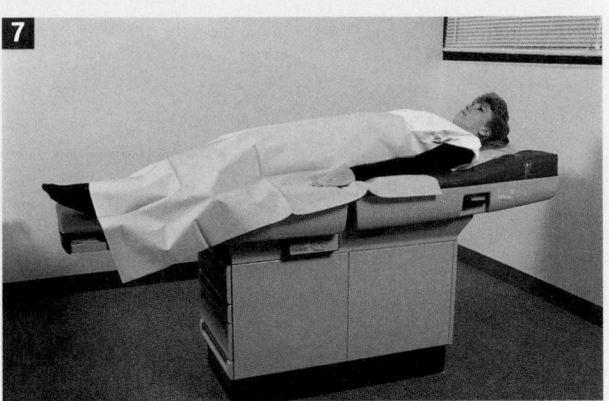

Place a drape lengthwise over the patient.

8. Procedural Step. After completion of the examination, assist the patient into a sitting position. Slide the table extension back into place while supporting the patient's lower legs.

9. Procedural Step. Assist the patient down from the table. Instruct the patient to get dressed. Return the footrest to its normal position. Discard the gown and drape in a waste container.

Outcome Position and drape a patient in the prone position. The prone position is used to examine the back and to assess extension of the hip joint.

Equipment/Supplies

- Examining table
- Disposable patient gown

- Disposable patient drape

1. Procedural Step. Sanitize your hands. Greet the patient and introduce yourself.

2. Procedural Step. Identify the patient and explain the type of examination or procedure that will be performed.

3. Procedural Step. Provide the patient with a patient gown. Instruct the patient to remove clothing as appropriate for the type of examination being performed and to put on the patient gown with the opening in back. The disrobing facility should provide privacy, a place to sit, and a place to hang clothing.

4. Procedural Step. Pull out the footrest of the examining table, and assist the patient into a sitting position. Place a drape over the patient's thighs and legs.

5. Procedural Step. Ask the patient to move back on the table. As the patient is doing this, pull out the table extension while supporting the patient's lower legs.

6. Procedural Step. Ask the patient to lie on his or her back. Provide assistance if needed. Position the drape lengthwise over the patient.

7. Procedural Step. Ask the patient to turn onto his or her stomach by rolling toward you. Provide assistance for this step by helping him or her turn and adjusting the drape to provide modesty.

Principle. This step prevents the patient from accidentally rolling off the table.

8. Procedural Step. Position the patient with the legs together and the head turned to one side. The arms can be placed above the head or alongside the body.

Continued

PROCEDURE 20-4   Prone Position—cont'd

8

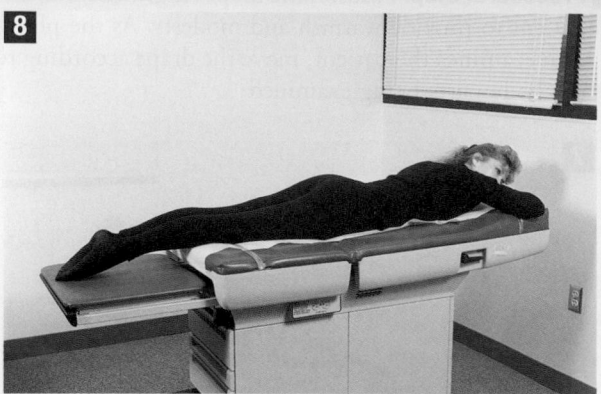

Position the patient's legs together with the head turned to one side.

9. Procedural Step. Adjust the drape as needed so that it is positioned lengthwise over the patient to provide warmth and modesty. As the physician examines the patient, move the drape according to the body parts being examined.

9

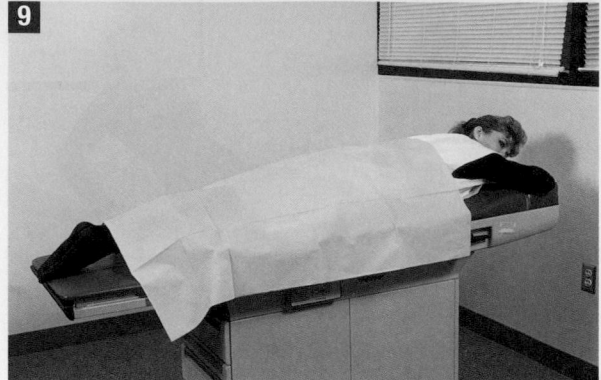

Place a drape lengthwise over the patient.

10. Procedural Step. After completion of the examination, ask the patient to turn back over by rolling toward you. Assist the patient into a supine position and then into a sitting position. Slide the table extension back into place while supporting the patient's lower legs.

11. Procedural Step. Assist the patient down from the table. Return the footrest to its normal position. Instruct the patient to get dressed. Discard the gown and drape in a waste container.

PROCEDURE 20-5   Dorsal Recumbent Position

Outcome Position and drape a patient in the dorsal recumbent position. The dorsal recumbent position is used to perform vaginal and rectal examinations; to insert a urinary catheter; and to examine the head, neck, chest, and extremities of patients who have difficulty maintaining the supine position. The supine position is an uncomfortable position for patients with respiratory problems, back injury, or lower back pain. Bending the legs (rather than lying flat) is more comfortable for these patients and is easier to maintain.

Equipment/Supplies

- Examining table
- Disposable patient gown

- Disposable patient drape

1. **Procedural Step.** Sanitize your hands. Greet the patient and introduce yourself.
2. **Procedural Step.** Identify the patient and explain the type of examination or procedure that will be performed.
3. **Procedural Step.** Provide the patient with a patient gown. Instruct the patient to remove clothing as appropriate for the type of examination being performed and to put on the patient gown with the opening in front. The disrobing facility should provide privacy, a place to sit, and a place to hang clothing.
4. **Procedural Step.** Pull out the footrest of the examining table, and assist the patient into a sitting position. Place a drape over the patient's thighs and legs.

5. **Procedural Step.** Ask the patient to move back on the table. As the patient is doing this, pull out the table extension while supporting the patient's lower legs.
6. **Procedural Step.** Ask the patient to lie on his or her back. Provide assistance if needed. The arms can be placed above the head or alongside the body. Position the drape diagonally over the patient.
7. **Procedural Step.** Ask the patient to bend the knees and place each foot at the edge of the examining table with the soles of the feet flat on the table. Provide assistance during this step. Push in the table extension and the footrest.

PROCEDURE 20-5 Dorsal Recumbent Position—cont'd

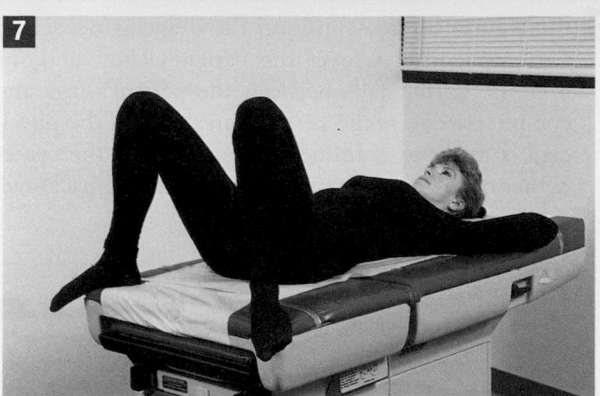

Ask the patient to bend the knees and place each foot at the edge of the examining table.

8. Procedural Step. Adjust the drape as needed to provide the patient with warmth and modesty. The drape should be positioned diagonally, with one corner over the patient's chest; the opposite corner falls between the patient's legs and completely covers the pubic area.

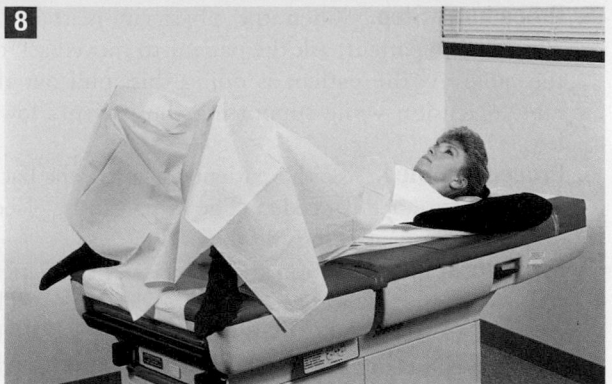

Place a drape diagonally over the patient.

9. Procedural Step. When the physician is ready to examine the genital area, the center corner of the drape is folded back over the abdomen.

10. Procedural Step. After completion of the examination, pull out the footrest and the table extension. Assist the patient into a supine position and then into a sitting position. Slide the table extension back into place while supporting the patient's lower legs.

11. Procedural Step. Assist the patient down from the table. Return the footrest to its normal position. Instruct the patient to get dressed. Discard the gown and drape in a waste container.

PROCEDURE 20-6 Lithotomy Position

Outcome Position and drape a patient in the lithotomy position. The lithotomy position is used for vaginal, pelvic, and rectal examinations. The lithotomy position is the same as the dorsal recumbent position except that the patient's feet are placed in stirrups. The lithotomy position provides maximal exposure to the genital area and facilitates insertion of a vaginal speculum. Because this is an uncomfortable position for the patient to maintain, the patient should not be put into this position until just before the examination.

Equipment/Supplies

- Examining table
- Disposable patient gown

- Disposable patient drape

1. Procedural Step. Sanitize your hands. Greet the patient and introduce yourself.

2. Procedural Step. Identify the patient and explain the type of examination or procedure that will be performed.

3. Procedural Step. Provide the patient with a patient gown. Instruct the patient to remove clothing as appropriate for the type of examination being performed and to put on the patient gown with the opening in front. If the patient is wearing socks, tell her that she may keep them on during the procedure.

The disrobing facility should provide privacy, a place to sit, and a place to hang clothing.

Principle. Socks help to keep the patient's feet warm after they are placed in the metal stirrups.

4. Procedural Step. Some medical offices use disposable stirrup covers. If this is the case, apply a cover to each stirrup. Pull out the footrest of the examining table, and assist the patient into a sitting position. Place a drape over the patient's thighs and legs.

Principle. Stirrup covers provide a soft, warm, non-slip surface for the patient's feet.

Continued

PROCEDURE **20-6** **Lithotomy Position—cont'd**

PROCEDURE 20-6

5. **Procedural Step.** When the physician is ready to examine the patient, ask the patient to move back on the table. As the patient is doing this, pull out the table extension while supporting the patient's lower legs.

6. **Procedural Step.** Ask the patient to lie on the back. Provide assistance if needed. The arms can be placed above the head or alongside the body.

7. **Procedural Step.** Position the drape over the patient to provide warmth and modesty. The drape should be positioned diagonally with one corner over the patient's chest and the opposite corner between the patient's feet.

8. **Procedural Step.** Pull out the stirrups and position them at an angle. Position the stirrups so that they are level with the examining table and pulled out approximately 1 foot from the edge of the table. Check to make sure the stirrups are not too far apart or too close together. Lock the stirrups into place.
   Principle. If the stirrups are too far apart, it is uncomfortable for the patient. If the stirrups are too close together, the patient will be unable to move her buttocks to the edge of the table as needed for the examination.

9. **Procedural Step.** Ask the patient to bend the knees and place each foot, one at a time, into a stirrup. Provide assistance during this step. Push in the table extension and the footrest.

10. **Procedural Step.** Instruct the patient to slide the buttocks all the way down to the edge of the examining table and to let her legs fall apart as far as is comfortable.

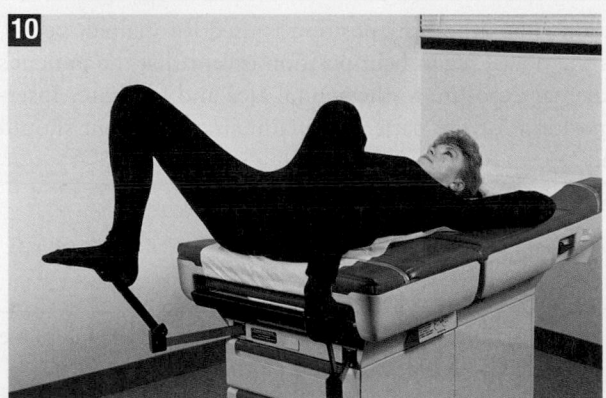

Ask the patient to slide the buttocks to the edge of the table and to rotate the thighs outward.

11. **Procedural Step.** Reposition the drape as needed so that one corner is over the patient's chest and the opposite corner falls between the patient's legs and completely covers the perineal area. When the physician is ready to examine the genital area, the center corner of the drape is pulled up and folded back over the knees.

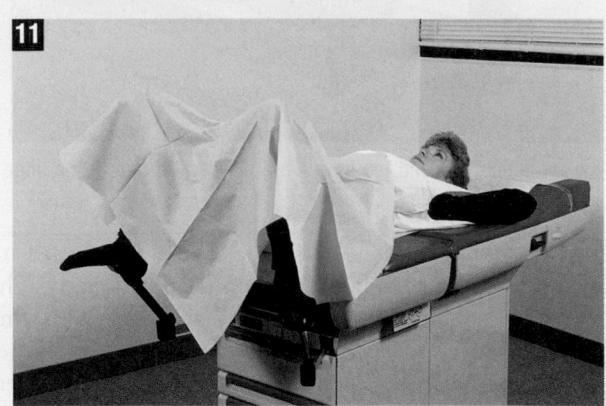

Position the drape diagonally.

12. **Procedural Step.** After completion of the examination, pull out the footrest and table extension. Ask the patient to slide the buttocks back from the end of the table. Lift the patient's legs out of the stirrups at the same time, and place them on the table extension (supine position). Remove the stirrup covers and discard them in a waste container. Return the stirrups to their normal position. Assist the patient into a sitting position. Slide the table extension back into place while supporting the patient's lower legs.
   Principle. Lifting both the patient's legs out of the stirrups at the same time avoids strain on the back and abdominal muscles.

13. **Procedural Step.** Assist the patient down from the table. Return the footrest to its normal position. Instruct the patient to get dressed. Discard the gown and drape in a waste container.

PROCEDURE 20-7 **Sims Position**

Outcome Position and drape a patient in the Sims position. Sims position, also known as the *left lateral position*, is used to examine the vagina and rectum, to measure rectal temperature, to perform a flexible sigmoidoscopy, and to administer an enema.

Equipment/Supplies

- Examining table
- Disposable patient gown
- Disposable patient drape

1. **Procedural Step.** Sanitize your hands. Greet the patient and introduce yourself.
2. **Procedural Step.** Identify the patient and explain the type of examination or procedure that will be performed.
3. **Procedural Step.** Provide the patient with a patient gown. Instruct the patient to remove clothing from the waist down and to put on the patient gown with the opening in back. The disrobing facility should provide privacy, a place to sit, and a place to hang clothing.
4. **Procedural Step.** Pull out the footrest of the examining table, and assist the patient into a sitting position. Place a drape over the patient's thighs and legs.
5. **Procedural Step.** Ask the patient to move back on the table. As the patient is doing this, pull out the table extension while supporting the patient's lower legs.
6. **Procedural Step.** Ask the patient to lie on his or her back. Provide assistance if needed.
7. **Procedural Step.** Position the drape lengthwise over the patient to provide warmth and modesty.
8. **Procedural Step.** Ask the patient to turn onto the left side. Provide assistance during this step to prevent the patient from accidentally rolling off the table and to adjust the drape to provide modesty. The patient's left arm should be positioned behind the body and the right arm forward with the elbow bent. Assist the patient in flexing the legs. The right leg is flexed sharply, and the left leg is flexed slightly.

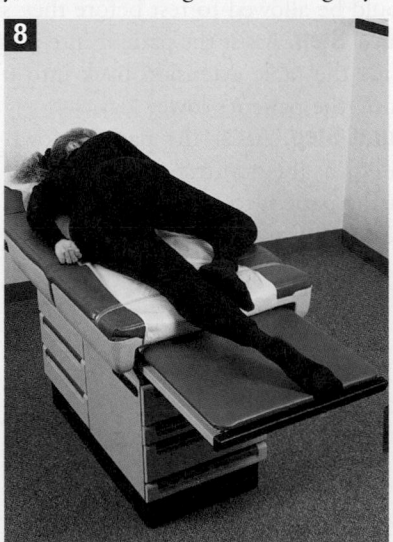

The right leg is flexed sharply, and the left leg is flexed slightly.

9. **Procedural Step.** Adjust the drape as needed. When the physician is ready to examine the patient, a small portion of the drape is folded back to expose the anal area.

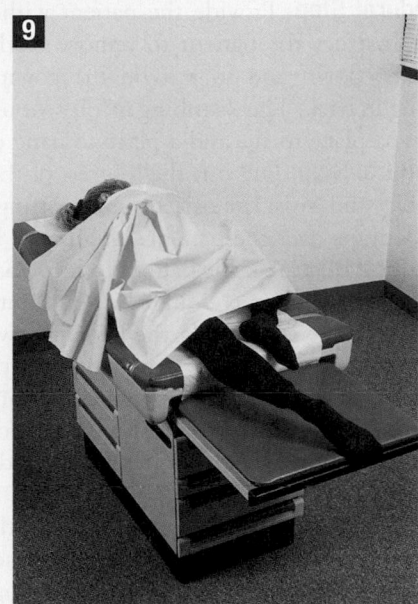

Adjust the drape as needed.

10. **Procedural Step.** After completion of the examination, assist the patient into a supine position and into a sitting position. Slide the table extension back into place while supporting the patient's lower legs.
11. **Procedural Step.** Assist the patient down from the table. Return the footrest to its normal position. Instruct the patient to get dressed. Discard the gown and drape in a waste container.

PROCEDURE 20-7

PROCEDURE 20-8 Knee-Chest Position

Outcome Position and drape a patient in the knee-chest position. The knee-chest position is used to examine the rectum and to perform a proctoscopic examination because it provides maximal exposure to the rectal area. This is a difficult position to maintain; the patient should not be put into this position until just before the examination.

Equipment/Supplies

- Examining table
- Disposable patient gown

- Disposable patient drape
- Pillow

1. **Procedural Step.** Sanitize your hands. Greet the patient and introduce yourself.
2. **Procedural Step.** Identify the patient and explain the type of examination or procedure that will be performed.
3. **Procedural Step.** Provide the patient with a patient gown. Instruct the patient to remove clothing from the waist down and to put on the gown with the opening in back. The disrobing facility should provide privacy, a place to sit, and a place to hang clothing.
4. **Procedural Step.** Pull out the footrest of the examining table, and assist the patient into a sitting position. Place a drape over the patient's thighs and legs.
5. **Procedural Step.** Ask the patient to move back on the table. As the patient is doing this, pull out the table extension while supporting the patient's lower legs.
6. **Procedural Step.** Assist the patient into the supine position and then into the prone position, making sure to have the patient roll toward you. Position the drape diagonally over the patient to provide warmth and modesty.
7. **Procedural Step.** Ask the patient to bend the arms at the elbows and rest them alongside the head. Ask the patient to elevate the buttocks while keeping the back straight. The patient's head should be turned to one side, and the weight of the body should be supported by the chest. A pillow under the chest can give additional support and aid in relaxation. The knees and lower legs are separated approximately 12 inches.

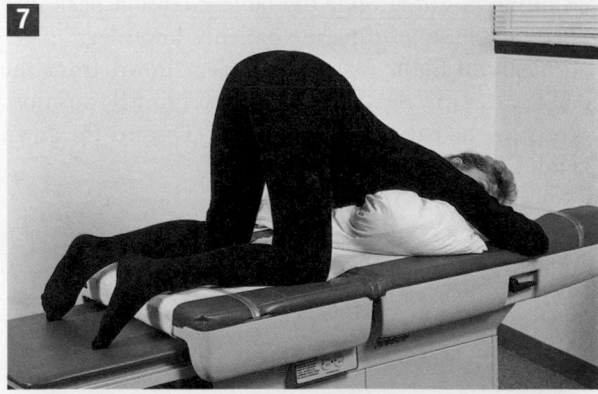

The buttocks are elevated, and the head is turned to one side.

8. **Procedural Step.** Adjust the drape diagonally as needed with one corner over the patient's back and the opposite corner over the buttocks and falling between the patient's legs. When the physician is ready to examine the patient, a small portion of the drape is folded back to expose the anal area.

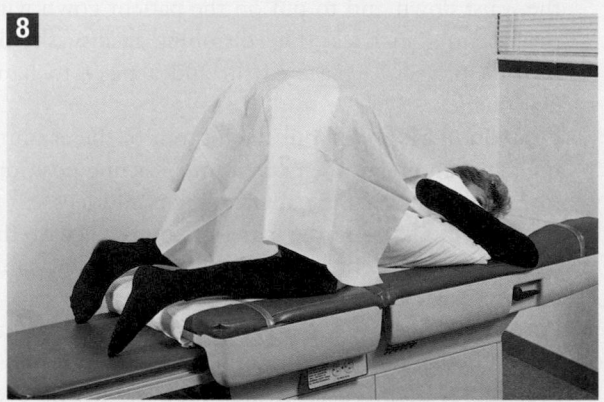

Position the drape diagonally.

9. **Procedural Step.** After completion of the examination, assist the patient into a prone position and then into a supine position. Allow the patient to rest in the supine position before he or she sits up.

    Principle. Patients (especially elderly ones) frequently become dizzy after being in the knee-chest position and should be allowed to rest before they sit up.

10. **Procedural Step.** Assist the patient into a sitting position. Slide the table extension back into place while supporting the patient's lower legs.

11. **Procedural Step.** Assist the patient down from the table. Return the footrest to its normal position. Instruct the patient to get dressed. Discard the gown and drape in a waste container.

PROCEDURE 20-9   Fowler's Position

Outcome Position and drape a patient in Fowler's position. Fowler's position is used to examine the upper body of patients with cardiovascular and respiratory problems, such as congestive heart failure, emphysema, and asthma. These patients find it easier to breathe in this position than in a sitting or supine position. This position also is used to draw blood from patients who are likely to faint.

Equipment/Supplies

- Examining table
- Disposable patient gown
- Disposable patient drape

1. **Procedural Step.** Sanitize your hands. Greet the patient and introduce yourself.
2. **Procedural Step.** Identify the patient and explain the type of examination or procedure that will be performed.
3. **Procedural Step.** Provide the patient with a patient gown. Instruct the patient to remove clothing as appropriate for the type of examination being performed and to put on the patient gown with the opening in front. The disrobing facility should provide privacy, a place to sit, and a place to hang clothing.
4. **Procedural Step.** Position the head of the table as follows:
   a. For the semi-Fowler's position, the table should be positioned at a 45-degree angle.
   b. For the full Fowler's position, the table should be positioned at a 90-degree angle.
5. **Procedural Step.** Pull out the footrest of the examining table, and assist the patient into a sitting position. Place a drape over the patient's thighs and legs.
6. **Procedural Step.** Pull out the table extension while supporting the patient's lower legs. Ask the patient to lean back against the table head. Provide assistance during this step.

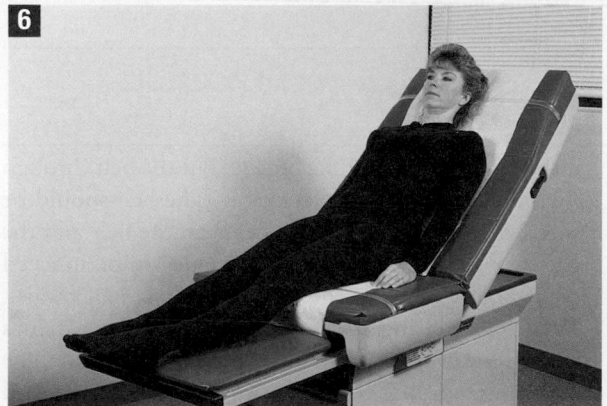

Ask the patient to lean back against the table head.

7. **Procedural Step.** Position the drape lengthwise over the patient to provide warmth and modesty. As the physician examines the patient, move the drape according to the body parts being examined.

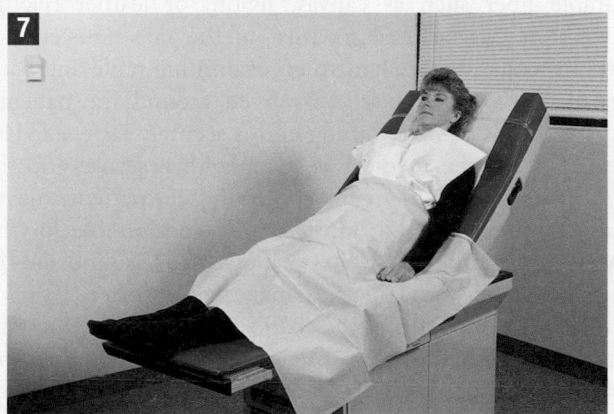

Position the table at a 45-degree angle for the semi-Fowler's position.

8. **Procedural Step.** After completion of the examination, assist the patient into a sitting position. Slide the table extension back into place while supporting the patient's lower legs.
9. **Procedural Step.** Assist the patient down from the table. Instruct the patient to get dressed. Return the head of the table and the footrest to their normal positions. Discard the gown and drape in a waste container.

PROCEDURE 20-9

PROCEDURE 20-10

WHEELCHAIR TRANSFER

A wheelchair is a chair mounted on wheels designed to make mobility easier for individuals who cannot walk or who are having difficulty walking because of illness or disability. Although some patients who come to the medical office in a wheelchair are able to transfer themselves from a wheelchair to an examining table, others may need assistance. The medical assistant plays an important role in the safe and efficient transfer of a patient from a wheelchair to an examining table and back again.

The Occupational Safety and Health Administration (OSHA) recommends that assistive devices be used whenever possible to transfer patients. A transfer belt (also known as a *gait belt*) is a safety device that is approximately $1\frac{1}{2}$ to 2 inches wide and 48 or 60 inches long and is made of a durable fiber such as canvas, nylon, or leather (Figure 20-10). It can be used to assist in the safe transfer of a patient from a wheelchair to an examining table and back again. The transfer belt is wrapped around the patient's waist over his or her clothing and is securely fastened. The belt provides the medical assistant with a secure grip for holding onto the patient and controlling the patient's movement. This makes the transfer more comfortable for the patient by not having to grasp the patient around the rib cage or under the axillae to make the transfer. Using a transfer belt also reduces the chance of the medical assistant hurting his or her musculoskeletal system while transferring a patient. Procedure 20-10 outlines the procedure for transferring a patient from a wheelchair to an examining table and back again using a transfer belt.

It is important for the medical assistant to realize that it may not always be possible to transfer a patient from a wheelchair to the examining table, even with the use of a transfer belt. Before transferring a patient, the medical assistant should carefully assess his or her ability to make the transfer. There are certain factors that may place undue strain on the medical assistant's musculoskeletal system. These factors include patients who are overweight or patients who have conditions that limit their mobility (e.g., leg paralysis), making it impossible for the patient to assist

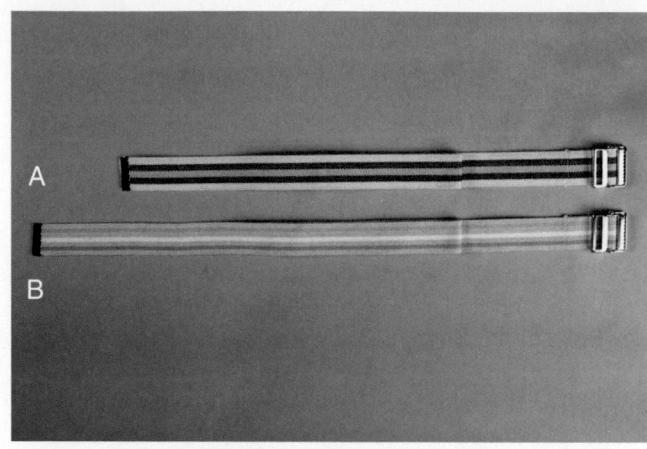

Figure 20-10 Transfer belts. **A,** Transfer belt that is 48 inches in length. **B,** Transfer belt that is 60 inches in length.

 PROCEDURE 20-10 Wheelchair Transfer

Outcome Transfer a patient from a wheelchair to the examining table and from an examining table to a wheelchair.

Equipment/Supplies

- Examining table
- Transfer belt

Transferring the Patient to the Examining Table

1. **Procedural Step.** Sanitize your hands.
2. **Procedural Step.** Greet the patient and introduce yourself. Identify the patient and explain the procedure.
3. **Procedural Step.** Evaluate the patient to determine his or her mental and physical capabilities to perform the transfer. Determine how heavy the patient is and if he or she is able to assist in the transfer. Assess whether or not you are able to perform the transfer safely. Do not perform the transfer if you think you may incur a musculoskeletal injury.
4. **Procedural Step.** Wrap the transfer belt snugly around the patient's waist over the patient's clothing with the buckle in front. Securely fasten the belt by threading

it through the teeth of the buckle. Put the belt through the other two openings to lock it. The belt should be snug with just enough space between the belt and the patient's clothing to allow your fingers to be inserted comfortably between the belt and the patient's waist. *Principle.* Placing the transfer belt over the patient's clothing prevents abrasions to the patient's skin. The belt must be snug to prevent it from sliding upward on the patient's body.

5. **Procedural Step.** With the patient's stronger side next to the examining table, position the wheelchair at a 45-degree angle to the end of the examining table.

PROCEDURE 20-10   Wheelchair Transfer—cont'd

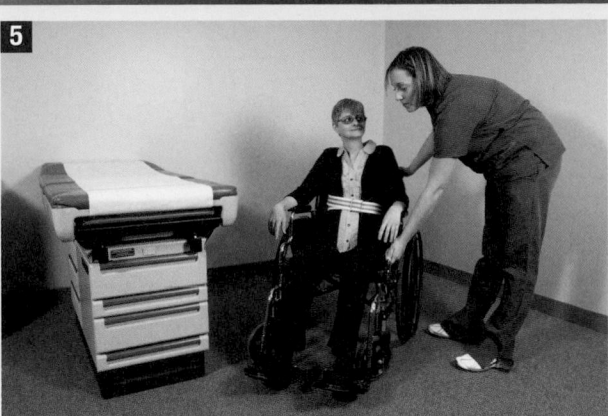

Position the wheelchair at a 45-degree angle.

6. Procedural Step. If the examining table is height-adjustable, lower it to the same height as the wheelchair or slightly lower. If it is not height-adjustable, pull out the footrest of the examining table.

7. Procedural Step. Lock the brakes of the wheelchair and fold back the wheelchair footrests.
Principle. The wheels must be locked to prevent the chair from moving during the transfer. The wheelchair footrests must be out of the way to provide an unobstructed path for making the transfer.

8. Procedural Step. Inform the patient of what he or she will be required to do during the transfer. During the transfer, clearly state in a step-by-step manner what the patient should do. Encourage the patient to help as much as possible during the transfer by using the muscles of his or her arms and legs.

9. Procedural Step. Make sure the patient's feet are positioned flat on the floor.
Principle. Making sure the patient's feet are flat on the floor provides the patient with balance and stability when he or she stands.

10. Procedural Step. Stand in front of the patient with the feet apart about 6 to 8 inches, the toes pointed outward, one foot slightly forward, and the knees bent.
Principle. This position conserves energy and provides a wide base of support for the transfer.

11. Procedural Step. Ask the patient to place his or her hands on the armrests of the wheelchair and to lean forward.

12. Procedural Step. Grasp the transfer belt on either side of the patient's waist using an underhand grasp.
Principle. The transfer belt provides a secure handle for holding onto the patient and controlling the patient's movement.

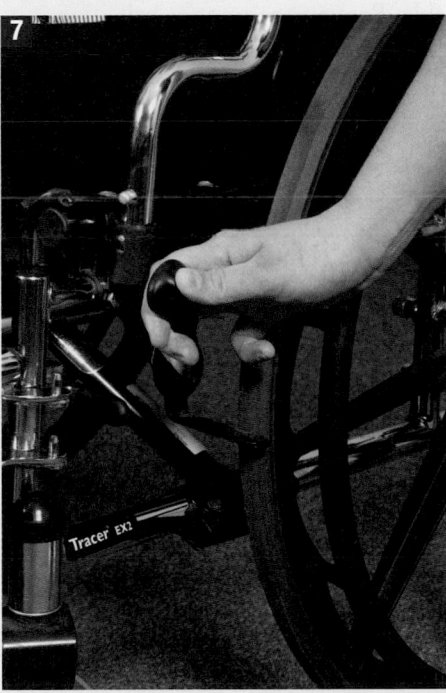

Lock the brakes.

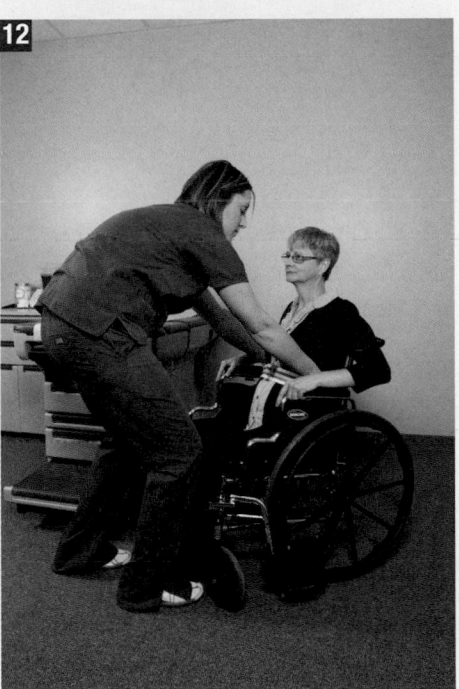

Grasp the transfer belt on either side of the patient's waist.

Continued

PROCEDURE 20-10   Wheelchair Transfer—cont'd

13. Procedural Step. Tighten your abdominal gluteal muscles in preparation for the transfer. Ask the patient to push off the armrests and into a standing position on the count of 3. At the same time, straighten your knees and assist the patient to a standing position by pulling upward on the transfer belt, making sure to keep your back straight.

Principle. The patient pushing upward with his or her arm and leg muscles provides an additional lifting force and reduces the chance of straining your back muscles. Lifting the patient using your knees and the transfer belt allows the strong muscles of the legs and arms to do the lifting rather than the back muscles.

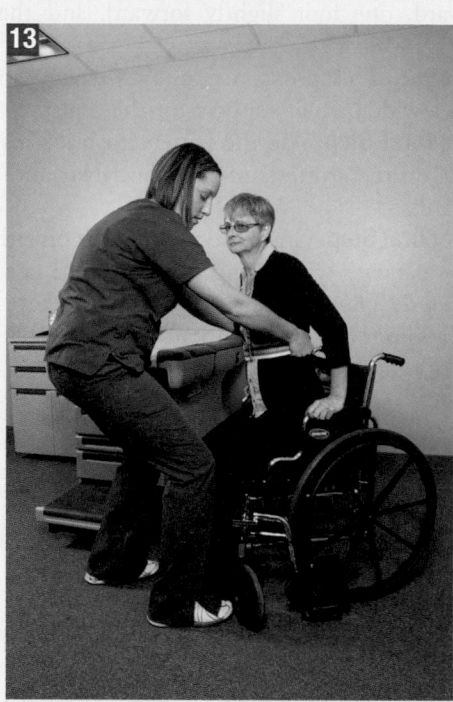

Assist the patient to a standing position.

14. Procedural Step. Pivot the patient toward the examining table. Position the patient's buttocks and backs of the knees toward the examining table. Instruct the patient to step onto the footrest (backward) one foot at a time.

Principle. Pivoting prevents twisting of the spine, which can result in a serious back injury.

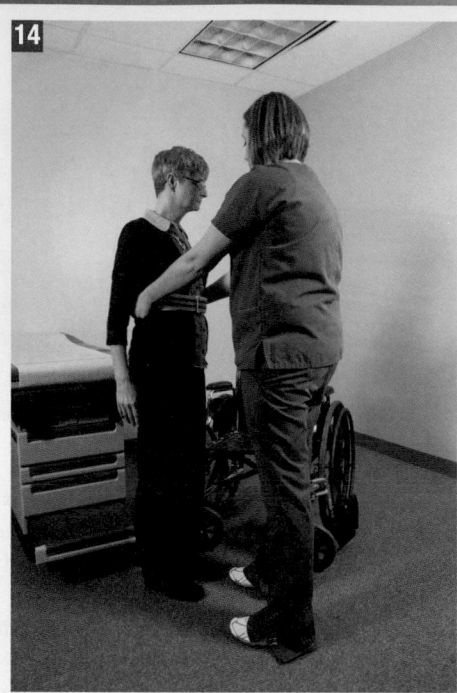

Position the patient toward the table.

15. Procedural Step. Gradually lower the patient into a sitting position on the examining table. Make sure the patient's buttocks and thighs are firmly supported on the table. Remove the transfer belt.

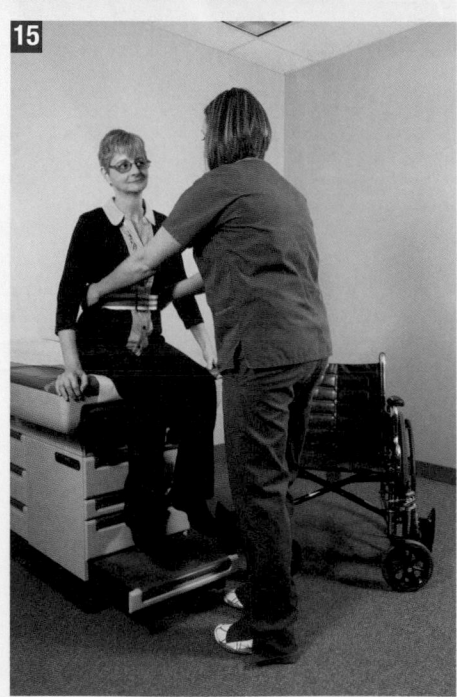

Gradually lower the patient onto the table.

PROCEDURE 20-10 Wheelchair Transfer—cont'd

16. **Procedural Step.** Unlock the wheelchair and move it out of the way of the examining table. Push in the footrest of the examining table.
17. **Procedural Step.** Stay with the patient to prevent falls.

Transferring the Patient to the Wheelchair

1. **Procedural Step.** Wrap the transfer belt snugly around the patient's waist and securely fasten it.
2. **Procedural Step.** Position the wheelchair at a 45-degree angle to the end of the examining table.
3. **Procedural Step.** If the examining table is height-adjustable, lower it to the same height as the wheelchair or slightly lower. If it is not height-adjustable, pull out the footrest of the examining table.
4. **Procedural Step.** Lock the wheelchair into place and fold back the footrests.
5. **Procedural Step.** Inform the patient of what he or she will be required to do during the transfer.
6. **Procedural Step.** Stand in front of the patient with the feet apart about 6 to 8 inches, the toes pointed outward, one foot slightly forward, and the knees bent.
7. **Procedural Step.** Ask the patient to place his or her arms on your shoulders. To prevent a neck injury, do not allow the patient to place his or her arms around your neck.

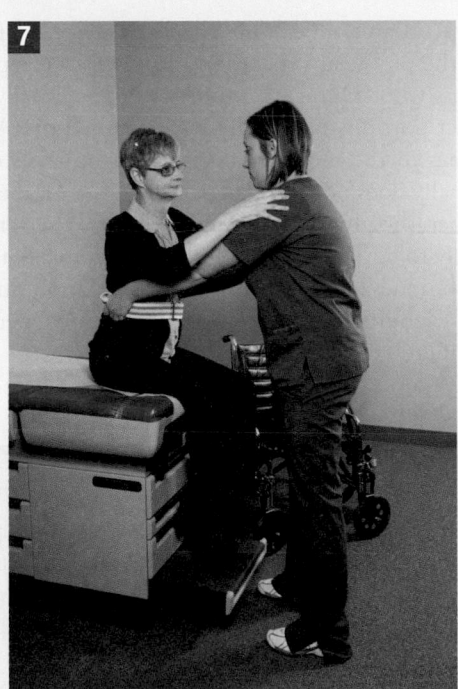

Ask the patient to put his or her arms on your shoulders.

8. **Procedural Step.** Grasp the transfer belt on either side of the patient's waist using an underhand grasp.

9. **Procedural Step.** Ask the patient to push to a standing position using his or her thigh and leg muscles on the count of 3. At the same time, straighten your knees and assist the patient to a standing position by pulling upward on the transfer belt.

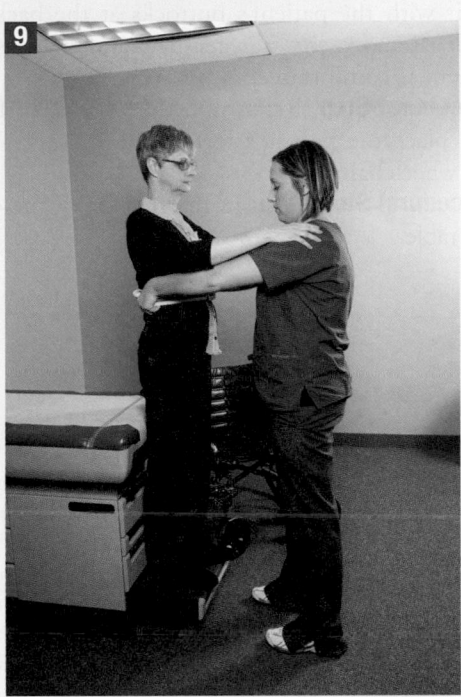

Assist the patient to a standing position.

10. **Procedural Step.** Instruct the patient to step down from the footrest, one foot at a time.

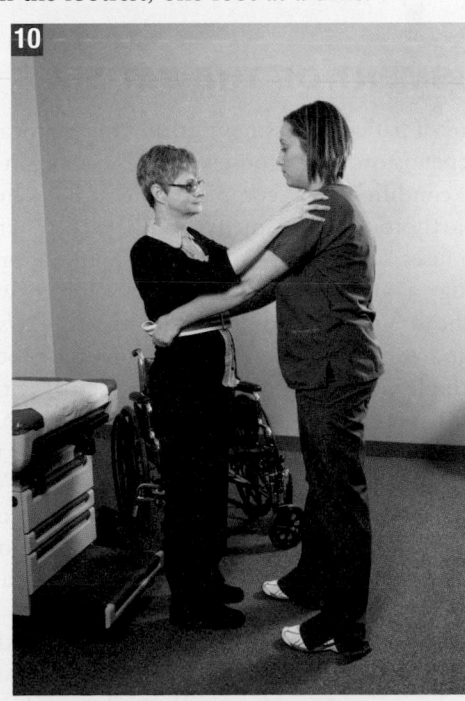

Instruct the patient to step down from the footrest.

PROCEDURE 20-10   Wheelchair Transfer—cont'd

11. **Procedural Step.** Pivot the patient toward the wheelchair. Position the backs of the patient's legs against the seat of the wheelchair.

12. **Procedural Step.** Bend at your knees and gradually lower the patient into a sitting position in the wheelchair with the patient's buttocks at the back of the chair. Remove the transfer belt and make sure the patient is comfortable.

13. **Procedural Step.** Reposition the wheelchair footrests and place the patient's feet in the footrests. Unlock the wheelchair.

14. **Procedural Step.** Push in the footrest of the examining table.

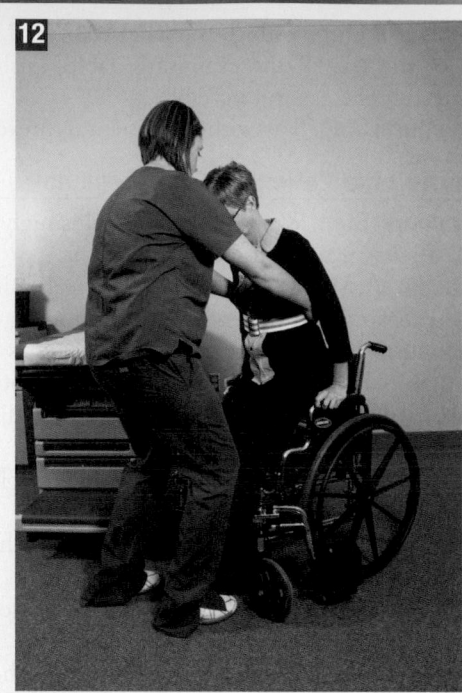

Gradually lower the patient into the wheelchair.

with the transfer. If factors exist that might cause strain to the medical assistant's musculoskeletal system, the medical assistant should ask for assistance or notify the physician that it is not possible to transfer the patient to the examining table.

ASSESSMENT OF THE PATIENT

The extent of patient assessment during the physical examination depends on the purpose of the examination and the patient's condition. A complete physical examination involves a thorough assessment of all body systems. The physician uses an organized and systematic approach in performing a physical examination, starting with the patient's head and proceeding toward the feet. Using this type of approach facilitates the examination process and requires the fewest position changes by the patient.

With a paper-based patient record (PPR), the physician notes the results of the physical examination in the patient's medical record, typically on a preprinted form. With an electronic medical record (EMR), the physician uses free-text entry, drop-down lists, and check-boxes to record findings on the screen of a computer monitor. The EMR program uses this information to generate the physical examination report. This means that by the end of the examination, the physical examination report is complete, and the physician does not need to dictate his or her

findings at a later time. This alleviates the need for transcribing the physician's dictation into a written report.

Patients who exhibit symptoms of illness usually require only select portions of the physical examination. A patient who comes to the medical office with symptoms of bronchitis usually does not require a complete physical examination; rather, the physician examines the body system that is most likely to be associated with the symptoms. Four assessment techniques are used to obtain information during the physical examination: inspection, palpation, percussion, and auscultation.

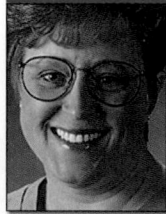

Memories *from* **Externship**

Hope Fauber: During my externship at a student health center at a 4-year college, I was responsible for working up patients for gynecologic examinations. The two-piece drapes had the top opening in the front and the bottom opening in the back. After explaining this to an Asian student who spoke very little English, I noticed that she had the openings opposite of what I had explained. I explained again, with words and gestures, that she needed to reverse the openings. To my surprise, she stood up, turned around in a circle, and sat down! ■

Inspection

Inspection involves observation of the patient for any signs of disease, and of the four assessment techniques, it is the one most frequently used. Good lighting, either natural or artificial, is important for effective observation. The patient's color, speech, deformities, skin condition (e.g., rashes, scars, warts), body contour and symmetry, orientation to the surroundings, body movements, and anxiety level are assessed through inspection. The medical assistant should develop a high level of detailed observational skills to assist the physician in assessing physical characteristics.

Palpation

Palpation is the examination of the body using the sense of touch (Figure 20-11). The physician uses palpation to determine the placement and size of organs; the presence of lumps; and the existence of pain, swelling, or tenderness. Examining the breasts and taking the pulse are performed by palpation. Palpation often helps verify data obtained by inspection. The patient's verbal and facial expressions also are observed during palpation to assist in the detection of abnormalities.

The two types of palpation—light and deep—are categorized by the amount of pressure applied. *Light palpation* of structures is performed to determine areas of tenderness. The fingertips are placed on the part to be examined and are gently depressed approximately one half inch. *Deep palpation* is used to examine the condition of organs such as those in the abdomen. Two hands are used for deep palpation. One hand is used to support the body from below, and the other hand is used to press over the area to be palpated. Deep palpation is used by the physician to perform a bimanual pelvic examination.

Percussion

Percussion involves tapping the patient with the fingers and listening to the sounds produced to determine the size, density, and locations of organs. This technique is often used to examine the lungs and abdomen.

The fingertips are used to produce a sound vibration similar to that of tapping a drumstick on a drum. The nondominant hand is placed directly on the area to be assessed, with the fingers slightly separated. The dominant hand is used to strike the joint of the middle finger placed on the patient to produce the sound vibration (Figure 20-12). Structures that are dense, such as the liver, spleen, and heart, produce a dull sound. Empty or air-filled

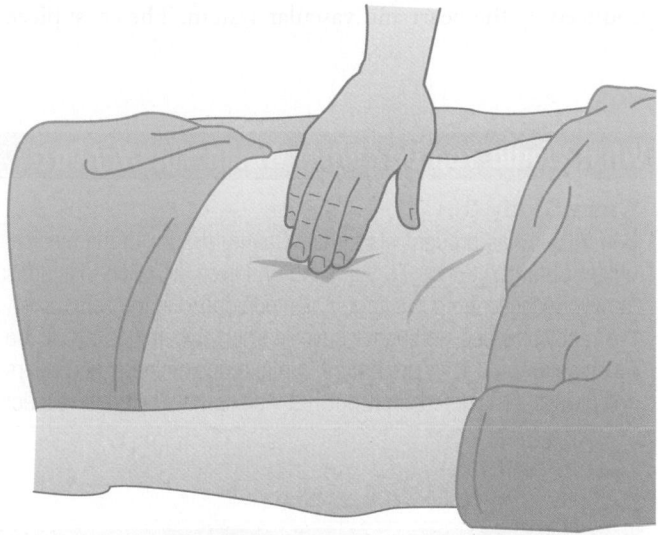

Figure 20-11 Palpation is examination of the body using the sense of touch.

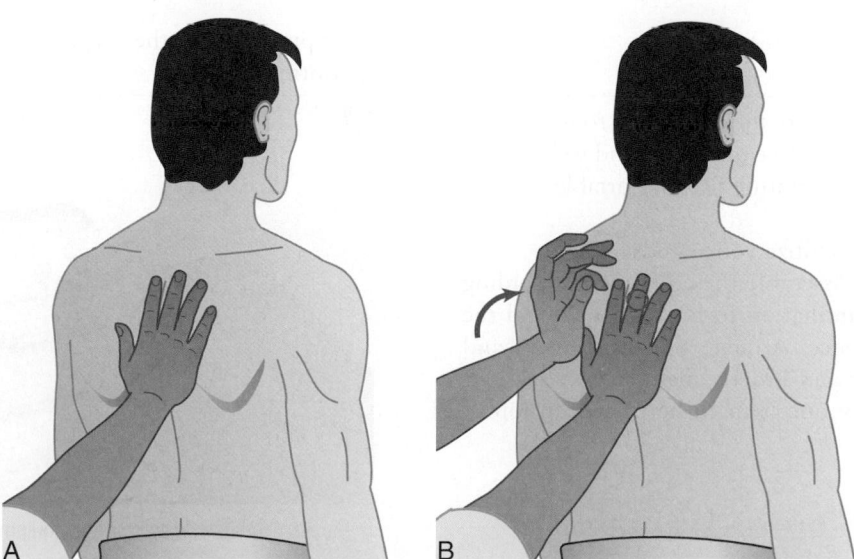

Figure 20-12 Percussion involves tapping the patient with the fingers. **A,** The nondominant hand is placed directly on the area to be assessed, with the fingers slightly separated. **B,** The fingers of the dominant hand are used to strike the joint of the middle finger to produce a sound vibration.

structures, such as the lungs, produce a hollow sound. Any condition that changes the density of an organ or tissue, such as fluid in the lungs, would change the quality of the sound.

Auscultation

Auscultation is an examination technique that involves listening with a stethoscope to the sounds produced within the body. This technique is used to listen to the heart and lungs or to measure blood pressure. Environmental noise interferes with effective auscultation of body sounds and should be minimized. The diaphragm of the stethoscope chest piece is used to assess high-pitched sounds, such as lung and bowel sounds; the bell of the stethoscope chest piece is used to assess low-pitched sounds, such as those produced by the heart and vascular system. The chest piece

should be cleaned with an antiseptic wipe and warmed with the hands before being placed on the patient.

ASSISTING THE PHYSICIAN

During the patient assessment, the medical assistant should assist the physician as required. This includes helping the patient change positions for the physician's examination of different parts of the body, handing the physician instruments and supplies, and reassuring the patient to reduce apprehension. When the examination is completed, the medical assistant should assist the patient off the examining table and provide additional information if needed, such as scheduling a return visit or patient education to promote wellness. Procedure 20-11 describes the procedure for assisting with the physical examination.

What Would You Do? What Would You *Not* Do?

Case Study 3

Ben-Yi Sun has brought his father, Chang-Yi Sun, to the medical office. Chang-Yi Sun is 76 years old and lives with Ben-Yi and his family. Because there is a large Asian population in the community, the medical office personnel have learned two things about the Asian culture: (1) They are brought up to respect elders, and elders are always considered first, and (2) Asians have a great respect

for harmony. If they do not understand something, they may not admit it to avoid disrupting harmony. Ben-Yi Sun speaks very good English, but his father understands only a few words of English. Chang-Yi Sun has been diagnosed with hypertension, and he needs education about going on a low-sodium diet. He also needs instructions on taking his blood pressure at home and recording the results. ∎

PROCEDURE 20-11   Assisting with the Physical Examination

Outcome Prepare the patient and assist with a physical examination.

Equipment/Supplies

- Examining table

- Equipment for the type of examination to be performed

1. **Procedural Step.** Prepare the examining room. Ensure that the room is clean, free of clutter, and well lit, and that the room temperature is comfortable for the patient.
2. **Procedural Step.** Sanitize your hands.
3. **Procedural Step.** Assemble the equipment according to the type of examination to be performed and the physician's preference. Arrange the instruments and supplies in a neat and orderly manner on a table or tray. Do not allow one item to be placed on top of another.

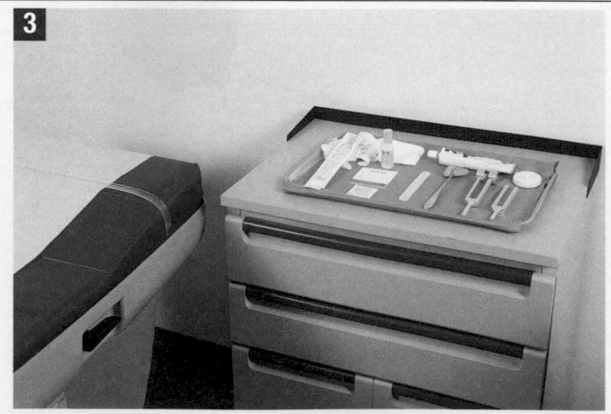

Assemble the equipment.

PROCEDURE 20-11   Assisting with the Physical Examination—cont'd

4. Procedural Step. Obtain the patient's medical record. Go to the waiting room and ask the patient to come back to the examining room.

5. Procedural Step. Escort the patient to the examining room.

6. Procedural Step. Ask the patient to be seated. Greet the patient and introduce yourself using a calm and friendly manner. Identify the patient by his or her full name and date of birth.
Principle. Identifying the patient correctly avoids mistaking one patient for another. Using a calm and friendly manner helps to put the patient at ease.

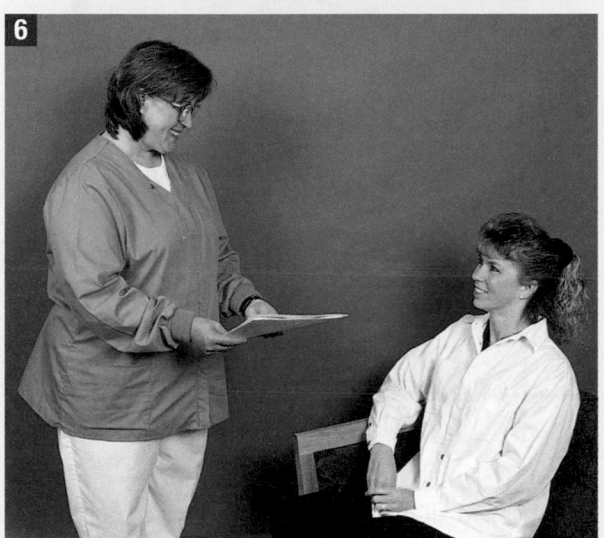

Greet and identify the patient by name and date of birth.

7. Procedural Step. Seat yourself so that you face the patient at a distance of 3 to 4 feet.

8. Procedural Step. Obtain and record the patient's symptoms while following the procedure outlined in Procedure 36-4 in Chapter 36.

9. Procedural Step. Measure the patient's vital signs, and chart the results.

10. Procedural Step. Measure the weight and height of the patient, and chart the results.

11. Procedural Step. Instruct and prepare the patient for the examination as follows:
a. Ask the patient whether he or she needs to empty the bladder before the examination. If a urine specimen is needed, the patient will be required to void into a urine container.
b. Provide the patient with a patient gown. Instruct the patient to remove all clothing and to put on the patient gown. Offer assistance if you sense the patient may have trouble undressing.
c. Tell the patient to have a seat on the examining table after putting on the patient gown. Inform the patient that the physician will be with him or her

soon, and leave the room to provide the patient with privacy.
Principle. An empty bladder makes the examination easier and is more comfortable for the patient.

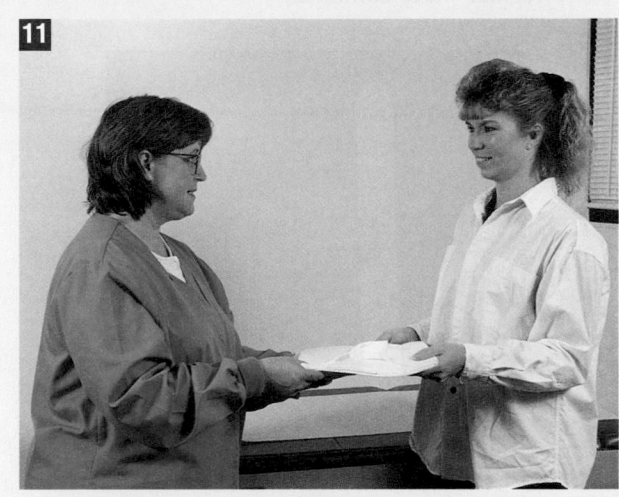

Instruct and prepare the patient for the examination.

12. Procedural Step. Make the medical record available to the physician. The medical office has a designated location where the record is placed, such as on a small shelf mounted on the wall next to the outside of the examining room door or in a chart holder on the outside of the examining room door. Position the medical record so that patient-identifiable information is not visible. Check to make sure that the patient is ready to be seen by the physician. Before entering a patient's room, knock lightly on the door to let the patient know that you are getting ready to enter the room. If a patient is ready to be seen, inform the physician. This may be done using a color-coded flagging system mounted on the wall next to the examining room.
Principle. HIPAA requires protection of a patient's health information.

13. Procedural Step. Assist the physician with examination of the body systems as follows:
a. Ensure that the patient is positioned correctly in a sitting position on the examining table. This allows the physician to examine the patient's head, eyes, ears, nose, mouth and pharynx, neck, chest, lungs, and heart.
b. Hand the physician the ophthalmoscope, otoscope, and tongue depressor.
c. Dim the light when the physician is ready to use the ophthalmoscope. The dim light helps dilate the patient's pupils, providing the physician better visualization of the interior of the eye.

Continued

PROCEDURE 20-11

PROCEDURE 20-11   Assisting with the Physical Examination—cont'd

d. After use, the tongue depressor should be transferred by holding it at the center to prevent contact with the patient's secretions, which may contain pathogens. Dispose of the tongue depressor in a regular waste container.

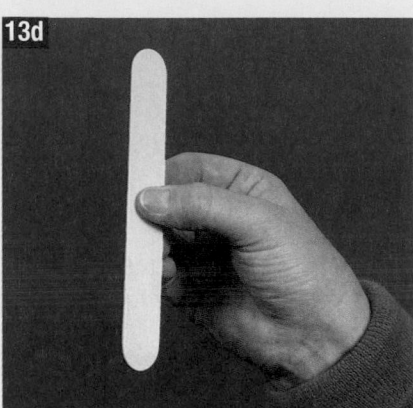

Transfer the tongue depressor by holding it at the center.

e. Offer reassurance to the patient to reduce apprehension.

14. Procedural Step. Position the patient as required for examination of the remaining body systems. Place and drape the patient in the proper position for examination of a particular part of the body using proper body mechanics.

15. Procedural Step. Assist and instruct the patient as follows:

a. Allow the patient to rest in a sitting position on the examining table before he or she gets off of it. Some patients become dizzy after being positioned on the examining table.

b. Assist the patient off the examining table to prevent falls.

c. Instruct the patient to get dressed. Provide assistance if needed.

d. Provide the patient with any necessary instructions, such as patient education and scheduling a return visit. Give instructions involving medical care in terms the patient can understand; do not use medical terms.

e. Sanitize the hands, and chart in his or her medical record any instructions given to the patient.

f. Escort the patient to the reception area.

16. Procedural Step. Clean the examining room in preparation for the next patient as follows:

a Discard the paper on the examining table. If body secretions have gotten on the examining table, apply gloves, and clean and disinfect the table. Unroll a fresh length of paper on the table.

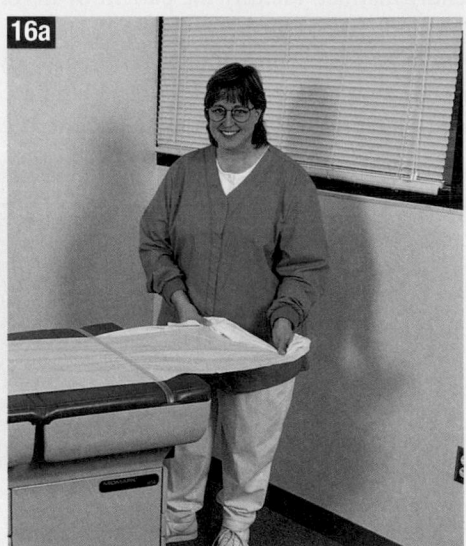

Unroll a fresh length of paper.

b. Discard all disposable supplies into an appropriate waste container.

c. Ensure that there are ample numbers of clean gowns and drapes and other supplies.

d. Remove reusable equipment to a work area for sanitization, sterilization, or disinfection as required by the medical office policy.

CHARTING EXAMPLE	
Date	
11/20/XX	11:30 a.m. CC. Shortness of breath x 2 days.
	T: 98.8° F AD, P: 78 reg and strong, R: 20
	even and reg, BP: 110/68, Wt: 126, Ht: 5' 6"
	—————————— H. Fauber, CMA (AAMA)

Activities involved in the physical examination can be sensitive for the patient. Information obtained while taking the patient history is confidential; revealing this information to anyone is unethical and illegal. A good rapport is essential for obtaining complete information, especially when asking sensitive questions. Complete information is necessary for accurate diagnosis and treatment.

Preparing the patient for a physical examination can be embarrassing for the patient. Keep in mind your duty to "do good" and "do no harm" to the patient. This involves proper knowledge and techniques and a professional, caring, and helpful attitude. Draping the patient correctly allows only minimal exposure. Incorrect draping or positioning that is unnecessarily uncomfortable could become a legal issue. Patients who are young, very old, or weak should never be left alone on an examining table. A fall from a table often results in harm and potential for a lawsuit.

Finally, while assisting the physician, be supportive of the patient as much as you are able. While the physician concentrates on the examination, you should continually assess the patient and provide for any needs, including assistance, encouragement, and physical comfort. Be patient, polite, and professional in all directions given to the patient. You may have done this many times, but this could be the first time for a frightened, ill patient. ∎

What Would You Do? What Would You *Not* Do? RESPONSES

Case Study 1
Page 353

What Did Hope Do?
- ❑ Empathized with Abbey and told her that a lot of patients feel just like she does about having their weight taken. Explained that the information in her medical record is strictly confidential.
- ❑ Told Abbey that weight is important so that the physician can properly diagnose and treat her condition, and that medication dosage is often based on a person's weight.
- ❑ Told Abbey that she could stand on the scale backward while her weight is being measured so that she would not see the reading on the scale.
- ❑ Returned the weights to zero before Abbey got off the scale.
- ❑ Recorded Abbey's weight in her chart without telling her the results.
- ❑ Encouraged Abbey to see the physician when she needs to so that she stays as healthy as possible.

What Did Hope Not Do?
- ❑ Did not make any comments about Abbey's body or weight after weighing her.
- ❑ Did not criticize Abbey for letting her weight stand in the way of coming in when she needed health care.

What Would You Do/What Would You Not Do?
Review Hope's response and place a checkmark next to the information you included in your response. List the additional information you included in your response.

_____
_____
_____
_____
_____
_____

Case Study 2
Page 353

What Did Hope Do?
- ❑ Listened carefully to Mikayla and showed concern verbally and nonverbally.
- ❑ Carefully charted the information relayed by Mikayla so that the physician would be aware of all aspects of Mikayla's problem.
- ❑ Told Mikayla that she needs to talk to the physician about wanting some medicine for heartburn.
- ❑ Encouraged Mikayla to talk to her parents about what's been going on with her.

What Did Hope Not Do?
- ❑ Did not agree with Mikayla that she needs to lose more weight.
- ❑ Did not make comments about Mikayla being too thin.

What Would You Do/What Would You Not Do?
Review Hope's response and place a checkmark next to the information you included in your response. List the additional information you included in your response.

_____
_____
_____
_____
_____
_____
_____

Case Study 3
Page 378

What Did Hope Do?
- ❑ Greeted Chang-Yi first before greeting his son.
- ❑ Spoke clearly and slowly to Ben-Yi in a normal tone of voice.
- ❑ Gave them a brochure on low-sodium diets and went over the foods that are low in sodium.

Continued

What Would You Do? What Would You *Not* Do?   RESPONSES—cont'd

❑ Asked Chang-Yi (via Ben-Yi's translating) to indicate the foods he likes that he thinks would be low in sodium. Determined whether these foods are low in sodium.

❑ Showed Ben-Yi how to take his father's blood pressure. Had Ben-Yi practice taking his father's blood pressure.

❑ Made sure that Chang-Yi and Ben-Yi understood all of the information before they left the office.

What Did Hope Not Do?

❑ Was careful not to ignore Chang-Yi.

What Would You Do/What Would You Not Do?
Review Hope's response and place a checkmark next to the information you included in your response. List the additional information you included in your response.

_____
_____
_____
_____
_____
_____

↻ TERMINOLOGY REVIEW

Medical Term	Word Parts	Definition
Audiometer	*audi/o:* hearing *-meter:* instrument used to measure	An instrument used to measure hearing.
Auscultation		The process of listening to the sounds produced within the body to detect signs of disease.
Bariatrics	*bar/o:* weight *-iatrics:* a branch of medicine	The branch of medicine that deals with the treatment and control of obesity and diseases associated with obesity.
Body mechanics		Utilization of the correct muscles to maintain proper balance, posture, and body alignment to accomplish a task safely and efficiently without undue strain on any muscle or joint.
Clinical diagnosis		A tentative diagnosis of a patient's condition obtained through evaluation of the health history and the physical examination, without the benefit of laboratory or diagnostic tests.
Diagnosis	*dia-:* through, complete *-gnosis:* knowledge	The scientific method of determining and identifying a patient's condition.
Differential diagnosis		A determination of which of two or more diseases with similar symptoms is producing a patient's symptoms.
Inspection		The process of observing a patient to detect signs of disease.
Mensuration		The process of measuring a patient.
Ophthalmoscope	*ophthalm/o:* eye *-scope:* to view, to examine	An instrument for examining the interior of the eye.
Otoscope	*ot/o:* ear *-scope:* to view, to examine	An instrument for examining the external ear canal and tympanic membrane.
Palpation		The process of feeling with the hands to detect signs of disease.
Percussion		The process of tapping the body to detect signs of disease.
Percussion hammer		An instrument with a rubber head, used for testing reflexes.
Prognosis	*pro-:* before *-gnosis:* knowledge	The probable course and outcome of a patient's condition and the patient's prospects for recovery.
Speculum		An instrument for opening a body orifice or cavity for viewing.
Symptom		Any change in the body or its functioning that indicates a disease might be present.

ON THE WEB

For information on nutrition:

American Dietetic Association: www.eatright.org

Ask the Dietitian: www.dietitian.com

For information on weight control and fitness:

American Obesity Association: www.obesity.org

Obesity Action Coalition: www.obesityaction.org

Weight Watchers: www.weightwatchers.com

E-Diets: www.ediets.com

Calorie Control Council: www.caloriecontrol.org

For information on accessing health information:

InteliHealth: www.intelihealth.com

Mayo Clinic: www.mayoclinic.com

U.S. Department of Health and Human Services: www.os.dhhs.gov

American Academy of Family Physicians: Family Doctor: www.familydoctor.org

Healthfinder: www.health.gov

WebMD: www.webmd.com

Medline Plus: www.nlm.nih.gov/medlineplus

For information on cultural diversity:

National Geographic Society: www.nationalgeographic.com

U.S. Department of the Interior: Workforce Diversity: www.doi.gov/diversity/workforce

Generations United: www.gu.org

 Check out the Evolve site at http://evolve.elsevier.com/Bonewit/today/ to actively Prepare for your Certification, and to access additional interactive activities and exercises to help you study and prepare for success.

21

Eye and Ear Assessment and Procedures

KEY TERMS

astigmatism (uh-STIG-muh-tizm)
audiometer (aw-dee-OM-eh-ter)
canthus (KAN-thus)
cerumen
hyperopia (HYE-per-OH-pee-uh)

impacted
instillation (IN-still-AY-shun)
irrigation (EAR-ih-GAY-shun)
myopia (mye-OH-pee-uh)
otoscope (AH-toh-skope)

presbyopia (PRESS-bee-OH-pee-uh)
refraction (ree-FRAK-shun)
tympanic membrane (tim-PAN-ik MEM-brane)

INTRODUCTION TO THE EYE

The medical assistant is responsible for performing a variety of assessments and procedures that involve the eye. An understanding of the structure and function of the eye is essential to mastering skills in these areas. Refer to Chapter 10 to review the structure and function of the eye.

A visual acuity test is usually part of the routine physical examination. This test is a screening test to detect deficiencies in vision.

The medical assistant may also be responsible for assessing color vision with the use of specially prepared colored plates. As a result of this testing, color blindness can be detected. Color blindness is an inability to distinguish certain colors; the most common problem is with the colors red and green. Color blindness is particularly significant if the patient is involved in an activity that relies on the ability to distinguish colors, such as electronics and interior decorating.

The medical assistant is responsible for performing or teaching the patient to perform eye irrigations and instillations. **Irrigation** is washing a body canal with a flowing solution. **Instillation** is dropping a liquid into a body cavity. Eye irrigations and instillations should be performed using the important principles of medical asepsis outlined in Chapter 17.

VISUAL ACUITY

Visual acuity refers to acuteness or sharpness of vision. A person with normal visual acuity can see clearly and is able to distinguish fine details close up and at some distance.

Errors of refraction are the most common causes of defects in visual acuity (Figure 21-1). **Refraction** refers to the ability of the eye to bend the parallel light rays coming into it so that they can be focused on the retina. An *error of refraction* means that the light rays are not being refracted or bent properly and are not adequately focused on the retina. A defect in the shape of the eyeball can cause a refractive error. Errors of refraction can be improved with corrective lenses.

A person who is nearsighted has a condition termed **myopia.** The eyeball is too long from front to back, causing the light rays to be brought to a focus in front of the retina. A myopic person has difficulty seeing objects at a distance and may squint and have headaches as a result of eyestrain. A corrective lens (e.g., eyeglasses, contact lenses) or laser eye surgery can correct this condition, which then allows the light rays to come to a focus on the retina.

A person who is farsighted has a condition known as **hyperopia.** The eyeball is too short from front to back, resulting in a different type of refractive error, in which the light rays are brought to a focus behind the retina. The individual has difficulty viewing objects at a reading or working distance. An individual with hyperopia may experience blurring, headaches, and eyestrain while performing up-close tasks. A corrective lens can correct this condition by causing the light rays to come to a focus on the retina.

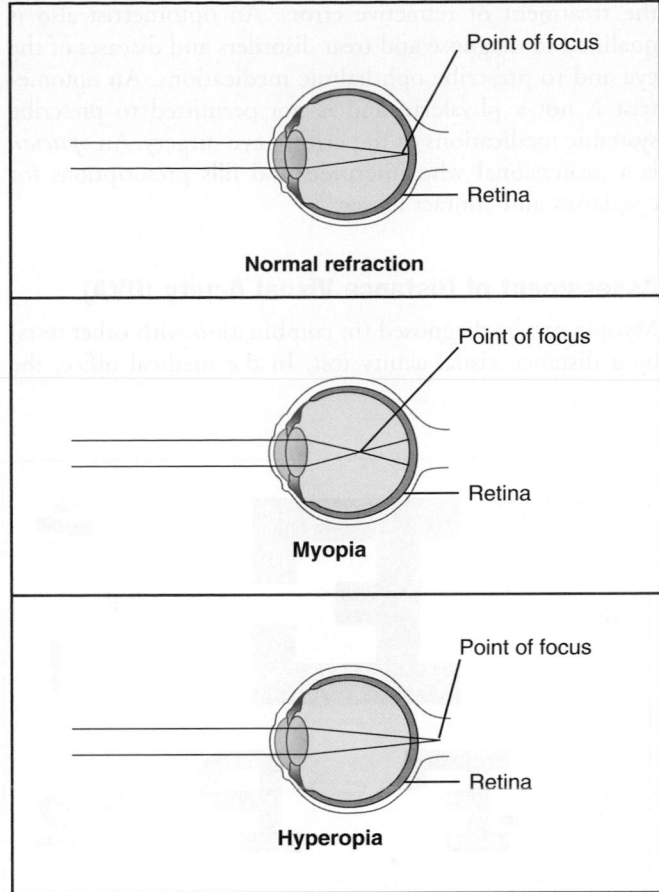

Errors of Refraction

Figure 21-1 Diagram of normal refraction compared with myopia (nearsightedness) and hyperopia (farsightedness), which are errors of refraction that cause visual defects.

Astigmatism is a refractive error that causes distorted and blurred vision for both near and far objects. A normal cornea has a round or spherical shape and is smooth. With astigmatism, the cornea is curved into an oval shape. This causes the light rays to focus on two different points on the retina, instead of just one, resulting in distorted and blurred vision. Astigmatism often occurs in combination with myopia or hyperopia and can be corrected with corrective lenses.

In most people, a decrease in the elasticity of the lens of the eye begins to occur after age 40 years. This condition, **presbyopia,** results in a decreased ability to focus clearly on close objects.

If a defect in visual acuity is detected, the patient is referred to an eye specialist for further evaluation. Several types of specialists are involved in the care of the eyes. An *ophthalmologist* is a physician who specializes in diagnosing and treating diseases and disorders of the eye. An ophthalmologist is qualified to prescribe ophthalmic and systemic medications and to perform eye surgery. An *optometrist* is a licensed primary health care provider who has expertise in measuring visual acuity and prescribing corrective lenses for the treatment of refractive errors. An optometrist also is qualified to diagnose and treat disorders and diseases of the eye and to prescribe ophthalmic medications. An optometrist is not a physician and is not permitted to prescribe systemic medications or to perform eye surgery. An *optician* is a professional who interprets and fills prescriptions for eyeglasses and contact lenses.

Assessment of Distance Visual Acuity (DVA)

Myopia can be diagnosed (in combination with other tests) by a distance visual acuity test. In the medical office, the

Snellen eye chart is most often used. Two types of charts are commonly used. One type is used for school-age children and adults and consists of a chart of letters in decreasing sizes (Figure 21-2). The other type is used for preschool children, non–English-speaking people, and nonreaders; it is composed of the capital letter *E* in decreasing sizes and arranged in different directions (Figure 21-3). Visual acuity charts with pictures of familiar objects also are available for use with preschool children. Testing with these charts tends to be less accurate than with the Snellen charts. Some children are unable to identify the objects because of lack of recognition, not because of a defect in visual acuity. It is

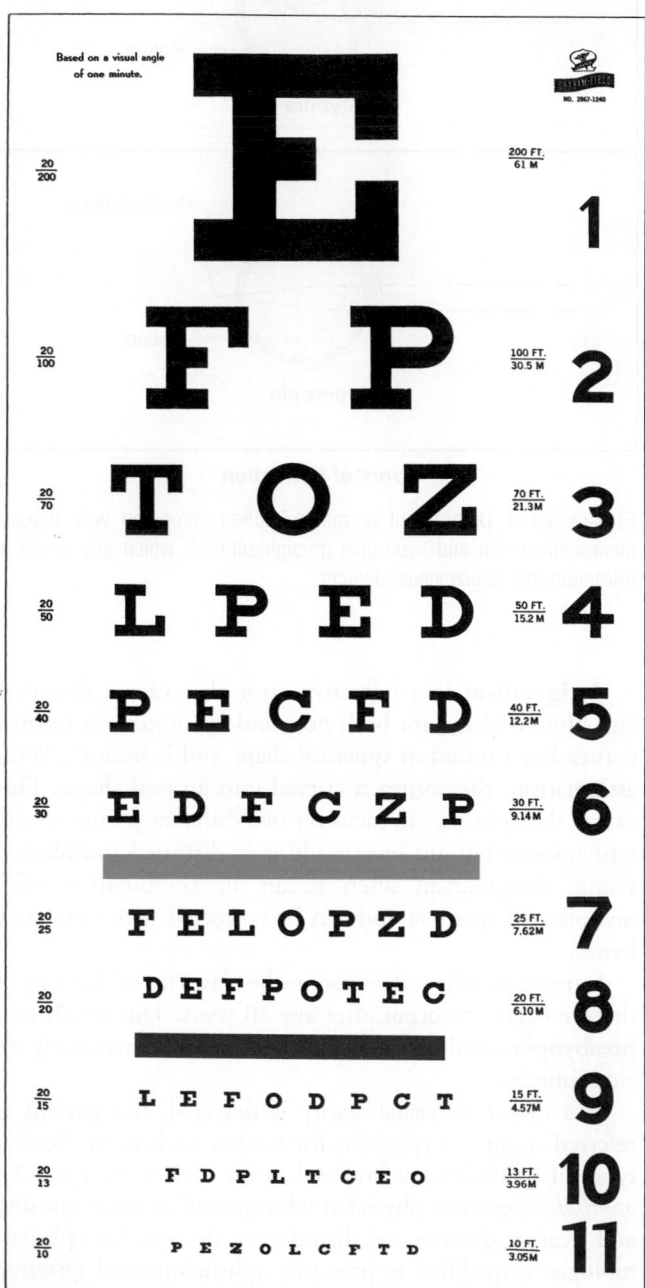

Figure 21-2 Snellen eye chart consisting of letters in decreasing sizes; this chart is used to measure distance visual acuity.

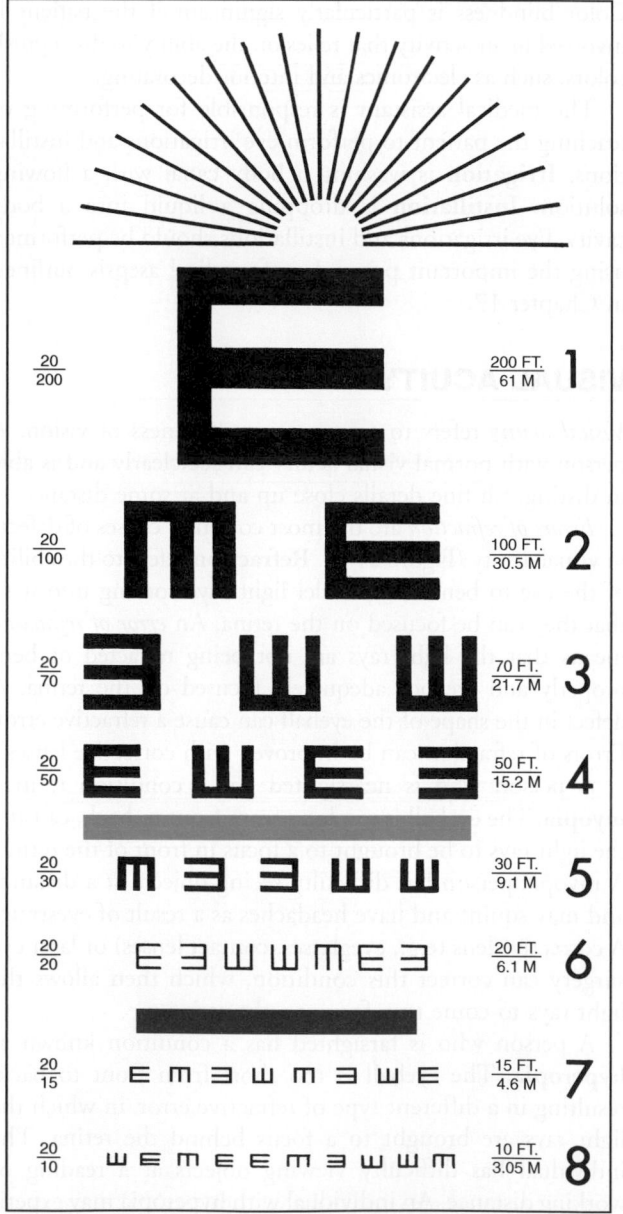

Figure 21-3 Snellen Big E eye chart consisting of the capital letter *E* in decreasing sizes and arranged in different directions; this chart is used to measure distance visual acuity.

suggested that the Snellen Big E chart be used with preschool children.

Conducting a Snellen Test

The visual acuity test should be performed in a well-lit room that is free of distractions. The test is usually performed at a distance of 20 feet; this can be conveniently marked off in the medical office with paint or a piece of tape so that it does not have to be remeasured every time the test is performed.

Two numbers, separated by a line, appear at the side of each row of letters on the chart. The number above the line represents the distance (in feet) at which the test is conducted. It is usually 20 feet because most eye tests are conducted at this distance. The number below the line represents the distance from which a person with normal visual acuity can read the row of letters. The line marked 20/20 indicates normal distance visual acuity, or 20/20 vision. This means a person could read what he or she was supposed to read at a distance of 20 feet.

A visual acuity reading of 20/30 means this was the smallest line that the individual could read at a distance of 20 feet. People with normal acuity would be able to read this line at a distance of 30 feet.

A visual acuity reading of 20/15 means this was the smallest line that the individual could read at a distance of 20 feet. It indicates above-average acuity for distance vision. People with normal acuity would be able to read this line at 15 feet.

The acuity of each eye should be measured separately, traditionally beginning with the right eye. Most physicians prefer that the patient wear his or her contact lenses or glasses, except reading glasses, during the test; the medical assistant should record in the patient's chart that corrective lenses were worn by the patient during the test. An eye occluder should be held over the eye not being tested. The patient's hand should not be used to cover the eye because this may encourage peeking through the fingers, especially in the case of children. The patient should be instructed to leave open the eye not being tested because closing it causes squinting of the eye that is being tested. The procedure for measuring distance visual acuity is outlined in Procedure 21-1.

Assessing Distance Visual Acuity in Preschool Children

With minor variations, Procedure 21-1 can be used to test distance visual acuity in preschool children. The Snellen Big E chart is used for this purpose.

A child needs a complete and thorough explanation of what is expected of him or her before beginning the test. Tell the child you will be playing a pointing game. Do not force the child to play the game because the results then tend to be inaccurate. Draw the capital letter E on an index card, and teach the child to point in the direction of the open part of the E by turning the card in different directions (up, down, to the right, and to the left). Using such phrases as "fingers" or the "legs of the table" to describe the open part of the E helps the child understand what is expected (Figure 21-4). Allow the child to practice the pointing game with the index card until you are sure this level of skill has been mastered. Be sure to praise the child when the correct response is given.

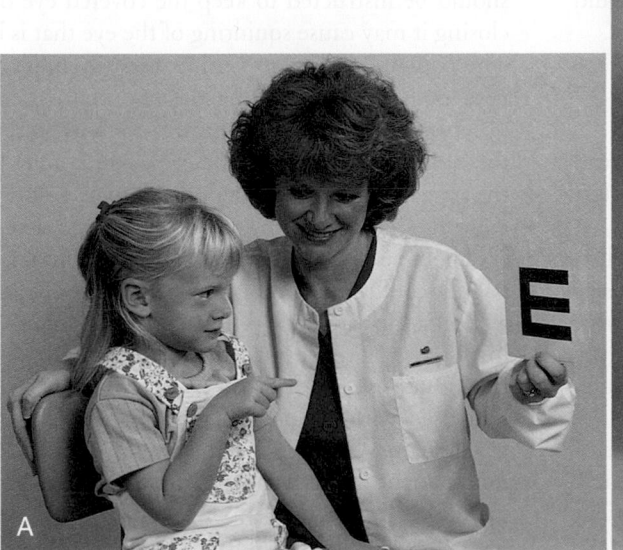
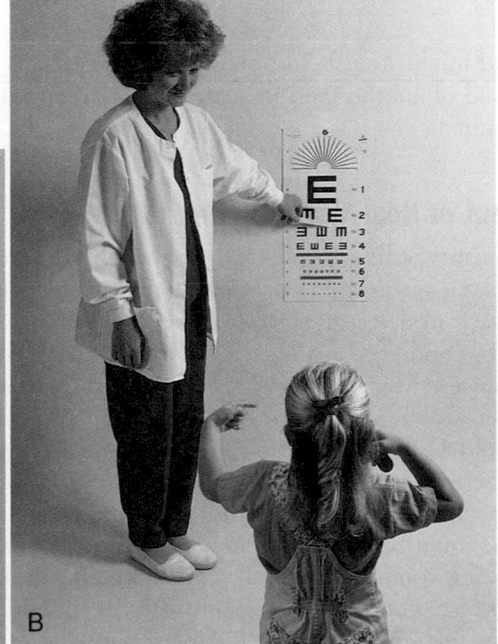

Figure 21-4 **A,** Cammie teaches a preschool child to point in the direction of the open part of the capital letter E. **B,** Cammie performs the Snellen Big E visual acuity test.

No. 1.
.37M

In the second century of the Christian era, the empire of Rome comprehended the fairest part of the earth, and the most civilized portion of mankind. The frontiers of that extensive monarchy were guarded by ancient renown and disciplined valor. The gentle but powerful influence of laws and manners had gradually cemented the union of the provinces. Their peaceful inhabitants enjoyed and abused the advantages of wealth.

No. 2.
.50M

fourscore years, the public administration was conducted by the virtue and abilities of Nerva, Trajan, Hadrian, and the two Antonines. It is the design of this, and of the two succeeding chapters, to describe the prosperous condition of their empire; and afterwards, from the death of Marcus Antoninus, to deduce the most important circumstances of its decline and fall; a revolution which will ever be remembered, and is still felt by

No. 3.
.62M

the nations of the earth. The principal conquests of the Romans were achieved under the republic; and the emperors, for the most part, were satisfied with preserving those dominions which had been acquired by the policy of the senate, the active emulations of the consuls, and the martial enthusiasm of the people. The seven first centuries were filled with a rapid succession of triumphs; but it was

No. 4.
.75M

reserved for Augustus to relinquish the ambitious design of subduing the whole earth, and to introduce a spirit of moderation into the public councils. Inclined to peace by his temper and situation, it was very easy for him to discover that Rome, in her present exalted situation, had much less to hope than to fear from the chance of arms; and that, in the prosecution of

No. 5.
1.00M

the undertaking became every day more difficult, the event more doubtful, and the possession more precarious, and less beneficial. The experience of Augustus added weight to these salutary reflections, and effectually convinced him that, by the prudent vigor of

No. 6.
1.25M

his counsels, it would be easy to secure every concession which the safety or the dignity of Rome might require from the most formidable barbarians. Instead of exposing his person or his legions to the arrows of the Parthinians, he obtained, by an honor-

No. 7.
1.50M

able treaty, the restitution of the standards and prisoners which had been taken in the defeat of Crassus. His generals, in the early part of his reign, attempted the reduction of Ethiopia and Arabia Felix. They marched near a thou-

No. 8.
1.75M

sand miles to the south of the tropic; but the heat of the climate soon repelled the invaders, and protected the unwarlike natives of those sequestered regions

No. 9.
2.00M

The northern countries of Europe scarcely deserved the expense and labor of conquest. The forests and morasses of Germany were

No. 10.
2.25M

filled with a hardy race of barbarians who despised life when it was separated from freedom; and though, on the first

No. 11.
2.50M

attack, they seemed to yield to the weight of the Roman power, they soon, by a signal

Figure 21-5 Example of a near visual acuity card.

The child might need help holding the eye occluder in place. The aid of another person such as the parent would then be required.

Assessment of Near Visual Acuity (NVA)

Near visual acuity testing assesses the patient's ability to read close objects (i.e., at a reading or working distance); the test results are used to detect hyperopia and presbyopia.

The test is conducted with a card similar to the Snellen eye chart; however, the size of the type ranges from the size of newspaper headlines down to considerably smaller print such as would be found in a telephone directory (Figure 21-5). The test card is available in a variety of forms, such as printed paragraphs, printed words, and pictures.

The test should be performed in a well-lit room free of distractions. It is conducted with the patient holding the test card at a distance between 14 and 16 inches. If the patient wears reading glasses, they should be worn during the test. The acuity should be measured in each eye separately, traditionally beginning with the right eye. An eye occluder

should be held over the eye not being tested. The patient should be instructed to keep the covered eye open because closing it may cause squinting of the eye that is being tested. The patient is asked to read or identify orally each line or paragraph of type. During the test, the patient should be observed for unusual symptoms, such as squinting, tilting the head, or watering of the eyes, which may indicate that the patient is having difficulty reading the card. The patient continues until reaching the smallest type that can be read.

The results are recorded as the smallest type that the patient could comfortably read with each eye at the distance at which the card is held (i.e., 14 to 16 inches). The recording is based on the type of test card used to conduct the test. One type of card uses a recording method similar to that used with the Snellen eye test. For this type of near visual acuity card, the results would be recorded as 14/14 for a patient with normal near visual acuity. This means the patient read what was supposed to be read at a distance of 14 inches. Also included in the recording should be the date and time, corrective lenses worn, and any unusual symptoms exhibited by the patient.

ASSESSMENT OF COLOR VISION

Defects in color vision may be classified as congenital or acquired. *Congenital defects* are more common and refer to a color vision deficiency that is inherited and is present at birth. Congenital color vision deficiencies most often affect males. *Acquired defects* refer to a color vision deficiency that is acquired after birth, resulting from such factors as an eye or brain injury, disease, and certain drugs. Color vision tests, such as the Ishihara test (Figure 21-6), detect congenital color vision disturbances and are commonly performed in the medical office. A basic screening for color vision can be performed by asking the patient to identify the red and green lines on the Snellen eye chart.

What Would You Do? What Would You *Not* Do?

Case Study 1

Nicole Neason brings her daughter, Haley, to the office for a camp physical. Haley has just completed the fourth grade and is going to summer camp for 2 weeks with Tess, her best friend. Tess wears glasses and Haley thinks they are really cool. She often asks to try on Tess's glasses and wishes she could wear glasses just like her best friend. When Haley is measured for visual acuity, she misses a few letters on the 20/70 line, the 20/50 line, the 20/40 line, and the 20/20 line. She is unable to read any of the letters on the 20/15 line. After the examination, Haley wants to know if she's missed enough letters to be able to get glasses. ■

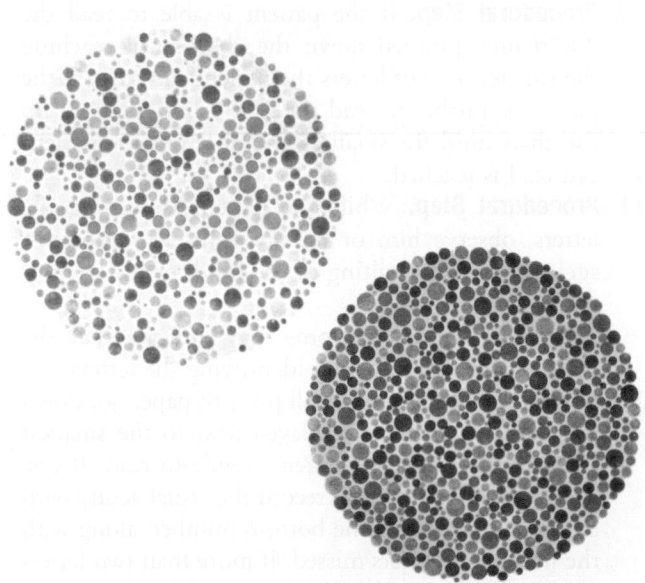

Figure 21-6 Ishihara color plates. Polychromatic plates. In the upper figure, a person with normal color vision reads 74, but a person with red-green color blindness reads 21. In the lower figure, a red-blind person (protanope) reads 2, but a green-blind person (deuteranope) reads 4. A normal-vision person reads 42. Reproduced plates are not good for testing for color deficiency.

Ishihara Test

The Ishihara test for color blindness is a convenient and accurate method to detect total congenital color blindness and red-green color blindness by assessing an individual's ability to perceive primary colors and shades of color. The Ishihara book contains a series of polychromatic plates of primary colored dots arranged to form a numeral against a background of similar dots of contrasting colors (see Figure 21-6). Patients with normal color vision are able to read the appropriate numeral; however, patients with color vision defects read the dots either as not forming a number at all or as forming a number different from the one identified by the individual with normal color vision. The first plate in the Ishihara book is designed to be read correctly by all individuals (with normal vision and exhibiting color vision deficiencies) and should be used to explain the procedure to the patient.

The book includes plates with winding colored lines for patients who are unable to identify the numbers by name, such as preschool children and non–English-speaking people. The patient should be asked to trace the line formed by the colored dots using a cotton swab or the eraser end of a pencil. The patient's finger should not be used to do the tracing because over time soiled fingers can degrade the polychromatic plates.

The Ishihara test should be conducted in a quiet room illuminated by natural daylight. If this is not feasible, a room lit with electric light may be used; however, the light should be adjusted to resemble the effect of natural daylight as much as possible. Using light other than just described, such as bright sunlight, may change the appearance of shades of color on the plates, leading to inaccurate test results.

The medical assistant is responsible for performing the color vision test and for recording results in the patient's chart. The physician assesses the results to determine whether the patient has a deficiency in color vision.

The Ishihara test consists of 14 color plates. Plates 1 through 11 are used to conduct the basic test, and plates 12, 13, and 14 are used to further assess patients who exhibit a red-green color deficiency. It is unnecessary to include these plates (12, 13, and 14) in the test of patients who exhibit normal color vision. In interpreting the results, if 10 or more plates are read correctly, the patient's color vision is considered normal. If 7 or fewer of the 11 Ishihara plates are read correctly, the patient is identified as having a color vision deficiency. It would be unusual for the medical assistant to obtain results in which the patient has read eight or nine plates correctly. The test is structured so that a patient with a color vision defect generally does not read eight or nine plates correctly and the rest incorrectly.

If a defect in color vision is detected, the patient is referred for additional assessment of color vision to an ophthalmologist or optometrist, who would use more precise color vision tests. The procedure for assessing color vision using the Ishihara color plates is outlined in Procedure 21-2.

PROCEDURE 21-1   Assessing Distance Visual Acuity—Snellen Chart

Outcome Assess distance visual acuity.

Equipment/Supplies

- Snellen eye chart
- Eye occluder

- Antiseptic wipe

1. Procedural Step. Sanitize your hands.

2. Procedural Step. Assemble the equipment. Perform the test in a well-lit room that is free of distractions. Wipe the eye occluder with an antiseptic wipe, and allow it to dry completely.

Principle. The eye occluder should be disinfected before use.

3. Procedural Step. Greet the patient and introduce yourself. Identify the patient and explain the procedure. Tell the patient that he or she will be asked to read several lines of letters. The patient should not have an opportunity to study or memorize the letters before beginning the test.

4. Procedural Step. Determine whether the patient wears contact lenses or glasses (other than reading glasses). If the patient wears such aids, he or she should be told to keep them on during the test.

5. Procedural Step. Ask the patient to stand on the marked line located 20 feet from the chart.

6. Procedural Step. Position the center of the Snellen chart at the patient's eye level. Stand next to the chart during the test to indicate to the patient the line to be identified.

Principle. Ensure that the chart is at the patient's eye level rather than at your eye level, to provide the most accurate results.

7. Procedural Step. Test the acuity of each eye separately. Measure the visual acuity of the right eye first.

Principle. The medical assistant should establish a pattern of beginning with the same eye (traditionally the right eye) every time the test is performed. This helps to reduce errors during the recording of results.

8. Procedural Step. Ask the patient to cover the left eye with the eye occluder. If the patient wears eyeglasses, tell him or her to place the occluder in front of the glasses gently to prevent the glasses from being moved out of their normal position. Instruct the patient to keep the left eye open. During the test, the medical assistant should check to make sure the patient is keeping the left eye open.

Principle. Eyeglasses moved out of normal position may lead to inaccurate test results. Keeping the left eye open prevents squinting of the right eye, which temporarily improves vision, leading to inaccurate test results.

9. Procedural Step. Instruct the patient not to squint during the test because squinting temporarily improves vision. Ask the patient to identify orally one line at a time on the Snellen chart, starting with the 20/70 line (or a line that is several lines above the 20/20 line).

Principle. It is best to start at a line above the 20/20 line to give the patient a chance to gain confidence and to become familiar with the test procedure.

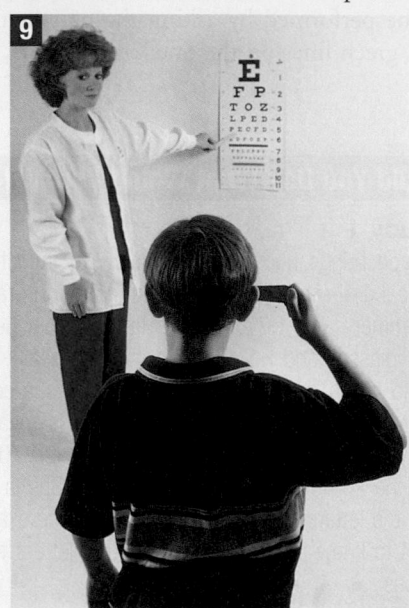

Ask the patient to identify one line at a time.

10. Procedural Step. If the patient is able to read the 20/70 line, proceed down the chart until reaching the smallest line of letters the patient can read. If the patient is unable to read the 20/70 line, proceed up the chart until the smallest line of letters the patient can read is reached.

11. Procedural Step. While the patient is reading the letters, observe him or her for unusual symptoms, such as squinting, tilting of the head, or watering of the eyes.

Principle. These symptoms may indicate that the patient is having difficulty identifying the letters.

12. Procedural Step. On a small piece of paper, jot down the numbers that are displayed next to the smallest line of letters that the patient is able to read. If one or two letters are missed, record the visual acuity with a minus sign next to the bottom number, along with the number of letters missed. If more than two letters are missed, the previous line is recorded.

13. Procedural Step. Ask the patient to cover the right eye with the eye occluder and to keep the right eye open. Measure the visual acuity in the left eye as described in steps 9 through 12. During the test, check to make sure the patient is keeping the right eye open.

PROCEDURE 21-1 Assessing Distance Visual Acuity—Snellen Chart—cont'd

Principle. Keeping the right eye open prevents squinting of the left eye.

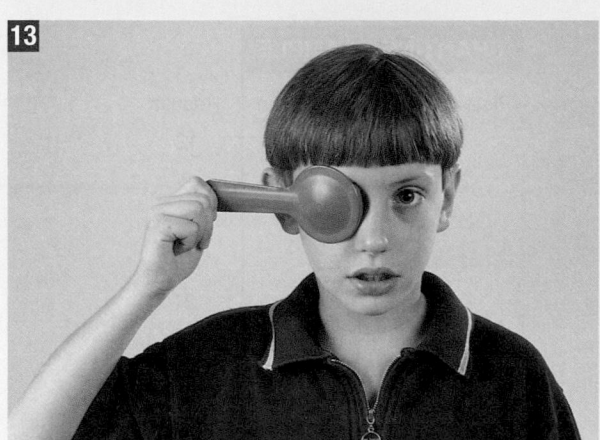

Ask the patient to cover the right eye and to keep the left eye open.

14. Procedural Step. Chart the procedure. Include the date and time, the name of the test (Snellen test), the visual acuity results, and any unusual symptoms the patient exhibited during the test. Also chart whether the patient was wearing corrective lenses during the test. Use the following abbreviations: $\overline{sc}$ without correction or $\overline{cc}$ with correction. Latin abbreviations are used to record visual acuity. The abbreviation for the right eye is *OD (oculus dexter),* the abbreviation for the left eye is *OS (oculus sinister),* and the abbreviation for both eyes is *OU (oculus uterque).*

15. Procedural Step. Disinfect the eye occluder with an antiseptic wipe, and sanitize your hands.

CHARTING EXAMPLE	
Date	
11/5/XX	3:30 p.m. Snellen test, $\overline{sc}$: OD 20/20-1.
	OS 20/25. Exhibited squinting, OD. ———————
	——————————— C. Lindner, CMA (AAMA)

PROCEDURE 21-2 Assessing Color Vision—Ishihara Test

Outcome Assess color vision.

Equipment/Supplies

- Ishihara book
- Cotton swab

1. Procedural Step. Sanitize your hands. Assemble the equipment.

2. Procedural Step. Conduct the test in a quiet room illuminated by natural daylight.

Principle. Using unnatural light may change the appearance of the shades of color on the plates, leading to inaccurate test results.

3. Procedural Step. Greet the patient and introduce yourself. Identify the patient and explain the procedure. Using the first (practice) plate as an example, instruct the patient to orally identify numbers formed by colored dots. Tell the patient that 3 seconds will be given to identify each plate.

Principle. The first plate is designed to be read correctly by all individuals and is used to explain the procedure to the patient.

4. Procedural Step. Hold the first color plate 30 inches (75 cm) from the patient, at a right angle to the patient's line of vision. The patient should keep both eyes open during the test.

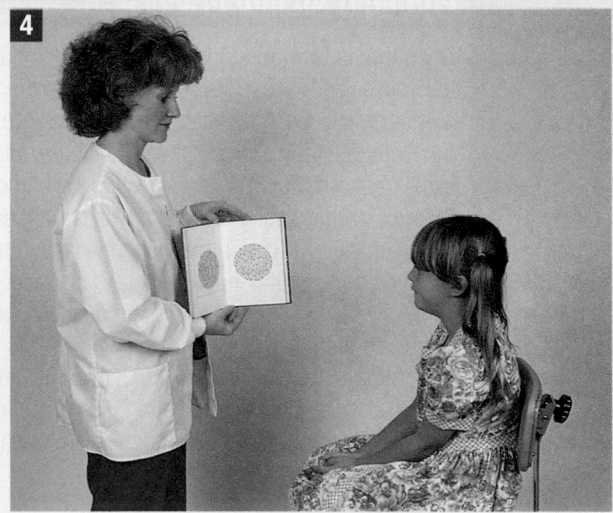

Hold the color plate 30 inches from the patient.

5. Procedural Step. Ask the patient to identify the number on the plate. If the plate consists of a traceable winding colored line, ask the patient to trace the line using a

Continued

PROCEDURE 21-2   Assessing Color Vision—Ishihara Test—cont'd

cotton swab or the eraser end of a pencil. The patient's finger should not be used to make the tracing.

Principle. The patient's finger should not be used to trace the line because soiled fingers can degrade the plate over time.

6. **Procedural Step.** Record results after each plate. Continue until the patient has viewed all the plates. To record color vision results, use the plate identification number and the number given by the patient. If the patient is unable to identify a number, the mark **X** should be recorded to indicate that the patient could not read the plate. Examples:

Plate 5: 21. This means the patient read the number 21 on plate 5 (instead of 74).

Plate 6: X. This means the patient could not identify a number on plate 6.

Plate 11: Traceable. This means that the patient correctly traced a winding line on plate 11.

As you can see from the results of this patient's color vision test, the patient correctly identified all 11 plates, which indicates normal color vision. Because the patient has normal color vision, the medical assistant did not need to include plates 12, 13, and 14 in the color vision test.

Principle. Reading 10 or more plates correctly indicates normal color vision. If 7 or fewer of the plates are read correctly, the patient is identified as having a color vision deficiency.

7. **Procedural Step.** Complete the charting entry. Include the date and time, the name of the test (Ishihara test), and any unusual symptoms the patient exhibited during the test, such as squinting or rubbing the eyes.

CHARTING EXAMPLE

Plate No.	Normal Person	Results
1	12	12
2	8	8
3	5	5
4	29	29
5	74	21
6	7	X
7	45	45
8	2	2
9	X	X
10	16	16
11	Traceable	Traceable
11/6/XX	10:00 a.m.	
	C. Lindner, CMA (AAMA)	

8. **Procedural Step.** Return the Ishihara book to its proper place. The book of color plates must be stored in a closed position to protect it from light.

Principle. Exposing the plates to excessive and unnecessary light results in fading of the color.

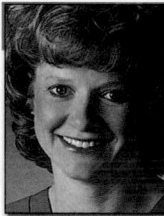

Putting It All into Practice

My name is Cammie Lindner, and I work for an ear, nose, and throat (ENT) surgeon. There are administrative responsibilities in my job; however, the focus is on the clinical aspects, including vital signs measurements, allergy testing, immunotherapy, and assisting with minor office surgeries, such as excision of skin lesions and tympanostomy tube insertions. Over past years in an ENT practice, there have been many challenging and rewarding situations. A recent incident was one that certainly falls into the rewards category.

A young girl came into the office from the emergency department for repair of a facial laceration. It had been quite a day for her, so it was understandable that she was a bit nervous and upset.

As the suturing was being performed, she grasped her mother's hand as I tried to discuss interests and school with her. She did fine and was very relieved when the last suture was done.

On her return visit for suture removal, her mother could not accompany her. As I was showing her to the examination room, she quietly asked if I would be in the room. I said, "If you would like, I certainly will." She anxiously nodded yes. As the sutures were removed, she squeezed my hand tighter and tighter. After all of them were out, she first checked her appearance in the mirror, then turned before going out the door and gave me a big hug and a "thank you." Days like this one are truly great rewards and make you feel you really can make a difference in someone's care. ∎

EYE IRRIGATION

An eye irrigation involves washing the eye with a flowing solution. Eye irrigations are performed for the following purposes: to cleanse the eye by washing away foreign particles, ocular discharges, or harmful chemicals; to relieve inflammation through the application of heat; and to apply an antiseptic solution. Procedure 21-3 shows how to perform an eye irrigation.

EYE INSTILLATION

An eye instillation involves the dropping of a liquid into the lower conjunctival sac of the eye. Eye instillations are performed to treat eye infections (with medication), to soothe an irritated eye, to dilate the pupil, and to anesthetize the eye during an eye examination or treatment. Medication to be instilled in the eye may come in the form of a liquid, as ophthalmic drops, or as an ophthalmic ointment. Eye drops are usually dispensed in a flexible plastic container with an attached dropper. Eye ointment is dispensed in a small metal tube with a small tip for applying the medication. Procedure 21-4 shows how to perform an eye instillation.

What Would You Do? What Would You *Not* Do?

Case Study 2

Peter Mitchell comes in with his 5-year-old son, Clive. Clive is diagnosed with conjunctivitis ("pink eye"), and the physician prescribes Polytrim ophthalmic suspension. Mr. Mitchell says that Clive does not cooperate very well when having drops put in his eyes and asks for any ideas that might make it less of an ordeal. Mr. Mitchell has 7-year-old twin girls at home and wants to know what can be done so they don't get pink eye. He asks if it would be all right to instill the drops in the twins' eyes as a preventive measure. ■

PATIENT TEACHING   Conjunctivitis

Answer questions that patients have about conjunctivitis.

What is conjunctivitis?

Conjunctivitis, often referred to as *pink eye,* is an inflammation of the conjunctiva (see illustration). The conjunctiva is a thin transparent membrane that covers the white of the eye. Conjunctivitis occurs when the conjunctiva becomes infected with a bacterium or virus. Other causes of conjunctivitis include allergies, prolonged wearing of contact lenses, and irritation from wind, dust, and smoke. Conjunctivitis is almost always harmless and clears up by itself within 2 weeks. If it is caused by a bacterium, the physician may prescribe antibiotic eye drops or ointment.

What are the symptoms of conjunctivitis?

Most types of conjunctivitis are relatively painless. The eye is red or pink because of irritation, and there is a feeling of sandiness or grittiness in the eye. A discharge is usually present, which dries at night when the eyes are closed. This may cause the eyelids to be stuck together in the morning. Other symptoms include tearing, itching, and sensitivity to light.

Is conjunctivitis contagious?

Conjunctivitis caused by a virus or bacterium is highly contagious. It can be spread easily from one eye to another and throughout a family or classroom in a matter of days.

How can we avoid spreading conjunctivitis?

The following measures help prevent the spread of conjunctivitis:

- Avoid touching or rubbing the infected eye, which can spread the infection to the other eye or to other people.
- Sanitize your hands frequently with soap, particularly after touching the eyes or face.
- Do not share washcloths, towels, or pillows with anyone.
- Do not wear contact lenses or eye makeup until the conjunctivitis is completely gone.
- Discard eye makeup that was used while you were infected to prevent reinfection.
- Encourage the patient to practice techniques that prevent the spread of conjunctivitis.
- If the physician has prescribed eye medication, teach the patient (or parent) the proper procedure for performing an eye instillation.
- Give the patient educational materials on conjunctivitis. ■

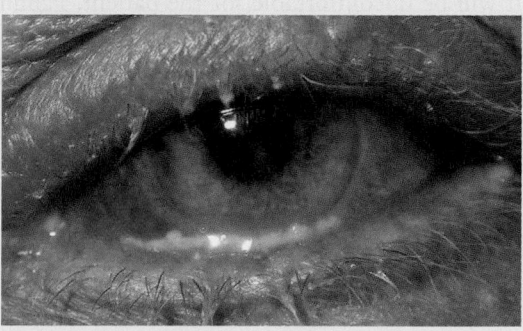
Bacterial conjunctivitis.

PROCEDURE 21-3 **Performing an Eye Irrigation**

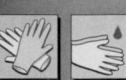

Outcome Perform an eye irrigation.

Equipment/Supplies

- Disposable gloves (nonpowdered)
- Irrigating solution
- Solution basin
- Bath thermometer

- Disposable rubber bulb syringe
- Basin
- Moisture-resistant towel
- Gauze pads

1. **Procedural Step.** Sanitize your hands.
2. **Procedural Step.** Assemble the equipment. If both eyes are to be irrigated, two sets of equipment must be used to prevent cross-infection from one eye to the other. Normal saline is generally used to irrigate the eye. Perform the following:
   a. Carefully check the label of the irrigating solution three times to make sure you have the correct solution. The first time is after you remove the solution container from the shelf. Compare the label of the solution container with the physician's instructions.
   b. Check the expiration date of the solution.
   c. Warm the irrigating solution to body temperature (98.6° F [37° C]) by placing the solution container in a basin of warm water. Use a bath thermometer to make sure the temperature of the water used to warm the solution does not exceed body temperature.
   d. Check the solution label a second time before pouring the solution.
   e. Pour the solution as follows:
   Palm the label of the container and remove the cap. Place the cap on a flat surface with the open end up. Pour the solution into the basin and replace the cap without contaminating it. Cover the basin to keep the solution warm.
   f. Check the solution label a third time before returning the container to its storage area.
   Principle. The solution label should be carefully checked three times to prevent an error. Outdated solutions may produce undesirable effects and should be discarded. If the solution is too cold or too warm, it will be uncomfortable for the patient. Palming the label prevents solution from dripping on the label and obscuring it or loosening the label. Placing the cap open end up prevents contamination.
3. **Procedural Step.** Greet the patient and introduce yourself. Identify the patient and explain the procedure and the irrigation. If the patient wears glasses or contact lenses, ask him or her to remove them.

4. **Procedural Step.** Position the patient. The patient may be placed in a sitting or lying position. Place a moisture-resistant towel on the patient's shoulder to protect the patient's clothing. Position a basin tightly against the patient's cheek under the affected eye to catch the irrigating solution, and ask the patient to hold it in place. Ask the patient to tilt the head in the direction of the affected eye.
   Principle. The patient is positioned so that the solution flows away from the unaffected eye to prevent cross-infection.
5. **Procedural Step.** Apply nonpowdered gloves. Cleanse the eyelids from inner to outer canthus with a moistened gauze pad to remove any discharge or debris on the lids. The inner canthus is the inner junction of the eyelids next to the nose. The outer canthus is the junction of the eyelids farthest from the nose. Normal saline or the solution ordered for the irrigation may be used. Discard the gauze pad after each wipe.
   Principle. Nonpowdered gloves avoid irritation of the patient's eye with powder that may have gotten on the outside of the glove. The eyelids should be clean to prevent foreign particles from entering the eye during the irrigation. Cleansing from inner to outer canthus prevents cross-infection.

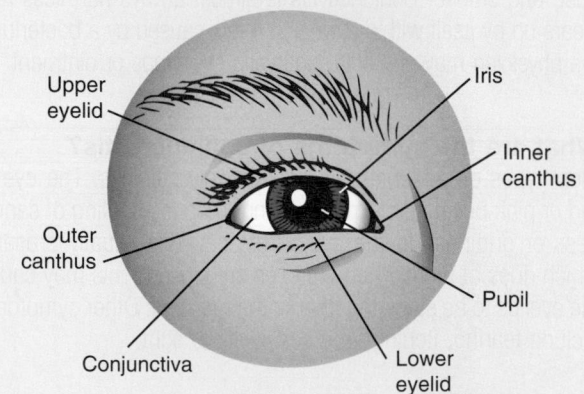

PROCEDURE 21-3   Performing an Eye Irrigation—cont'd

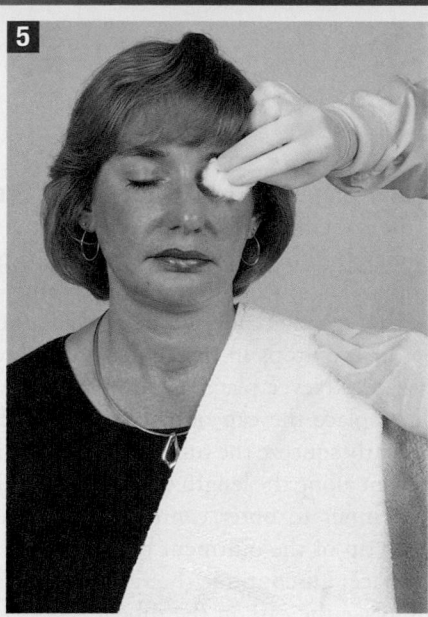

Cleanse the eyelids from inner to outer canthus.

6. **Procedural Step.** Fill the irrigating syringe with the solution by squeezing the bulb and slowly releasing it until the desired amount of solution enters the bulb. Instruct the patient to keep both eyes open and to find a focal point in the room and focus on it.
   Principle. Looking at a focal point helps the patient keep the irrigated eye open during the procedure.

7. **Procedural Step.** Separate the eyelids with the index finger and thumb to expose the lower conjunctiva and to hold the upper eyelid open.
   Principle. The medical assistant must hold the eye open during the procedure because the patient has a tendency to close it.

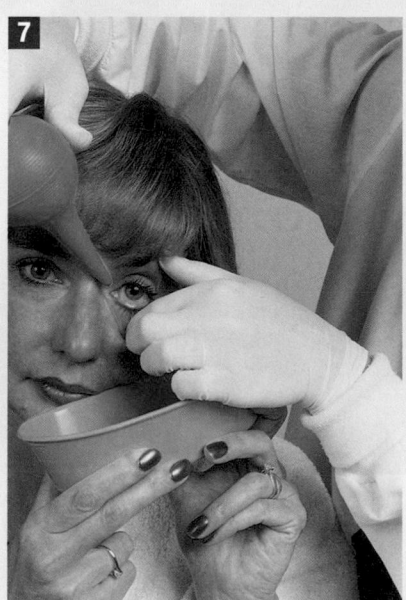

Separate the eyelids, and hold the tip of the syringe 1 inch above the eye.

8. **Procedural Step.** Hold the tip of the syringe approximately 1 inch above the eye. Gently release the solution onto the eye at the inner canthus. This allows the solution to flow over the eye at a moderate rate from the inner to the outer canthus. Direct the solution to the lower conjunctiva. To prevent injury, do not allow the tip of the syringe to touch the eye.
   Principle. The solution flows away from the unaffected eye to prevent cross-infection. The cornea is sensitive and can be harmed easily. The irrigating solution must be directed to the lower conjunctiva to prevent injury to the cornea.

9. **Procedural Step.** Refill the syringe, and continue irrigating until the desired results have been obtained or all the solution is used, depending on the purpose of the irrigation.

10. **Procedural Step.** Dry the eyelids from inner to outer canthus with a gauze pad.

11. **Procedural Step.** Remove the gloves, and sanitize your hands.

12. **Procedural Step.** Chart the procedure. Include the following: the date and time; which eye was irrigated; the type, strength, and amount of solution used; and any significant observations and patient reactions. Use one of these abbreviations to indicate which eye was irrigated:
    OU—Both eyes
    OD—Right eye
    OS—Left eye

CHARTING EXAMPLE

Date	
11/5/XX	10:30 a.m. Irrigated OS c̄ sterile saline @ 98.6° F. No complaints of discomfort.
	—————————— C. Lindner, CMA (AAMA)

13. **Procedural Step.** Remove reusable equipment to a work area for sanitization, sterilization, or disinfection as required by the medical office policy.

PROCEDURE 21-3

PROCEDURE 21-4   **Performing an Eye Instillation**

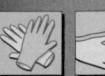 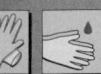

Outcome Perform an eye instillation.

- Disposable gloves (nonpowdered)
- Ophthalmic drops or ophthalmic ointment as ordered by the physician

- Tissues
- Gauze pads

1. **Procedural Step.** Sanitize your hands.
2. **Procedural Step.** Assemble the equipment, and perform the following:
   a. Check the drug label three times to make sure you have the correct medication. The first time should be when you remove the medication from the shelf. The medication label must bear the word *ophthalmic.*
   b. Check the medication label a second time against the physician's instructions. Also check the dosage ordered by the physician.
   c. Check the expiration date.
   d. Check the medication label a third time before the cap is removed to instill the medication.
   Principle. The drug label should be carefully checked three times to prevent a medication error. Medication not bearing the word *ophthalmic* must never be placed in the eye because it could injure the eye. An outdated medication may produce undesirable effects and should be discarded.
3. **Procedural Step.** Greet the patient and introduce yourself. Identify the patient and explain the procedure and the purpose of the instillation. If the patient wears glasses or contact lenses, ask him or her to remove them.
4. **Procedural Step.** Help the patient into a sitting or supine position.
5. **Procedural Step.** Apply nonpowdered gloves. Prepare the medication. **Eye drops:** If the medication requires mixing, shake the container well. Check the medication label for the third time, and remove the cap from the container. **Eye ointment:** Check the medication label for the third time, and remove the cap from the tip of the tube.
   Principle. Nonpowdered gloves avoid irritation of the patient's eyes with powder that may have gotten on the outside of the gloves.
6. **Procedural Step.** Ask the patient to look up at the ceiling, and expose the lower conjunctival sac by using the fingers of the nondominant hand placed over a tissue. The fingers should be placed on the patient's cheekbone just below the eye, and the skin of the cheek should be drawn gently downward.
   Principle. Looking up helps keep the patient from blinking when the drops are instilled.

7. **Procedural Step.** Insert the medication. **Eye drops:** Invert the container and hold the tip of the dropper approximately ½ inch above the eye sac. Do not allow the dropper to touch the eye or any other surface. Gently squeeze the container and place the correct number of eye drops in the center of the lower conjunctival sac. Never place the drops directly on the eyeball. Replace the cap on the container. **Eye ointment:** Gently squeeze the tube and place a thin ribbon of ointment along the length of the lower conjunctival sac from inner to outer canthus. Be careful not to touch the tip of the ointment tube to the eye or any other surface. Discontinue the ribbon by twisting the tube. Replace the cap on the tube.
   Principle. Touching the dropper or tip of the tube to the eye (or other surfaces) could injure the eye and contaminate the medication. Placing the medication in the conjunctival sac, rather than directly on the eyeball, is more comfortable for the patient.

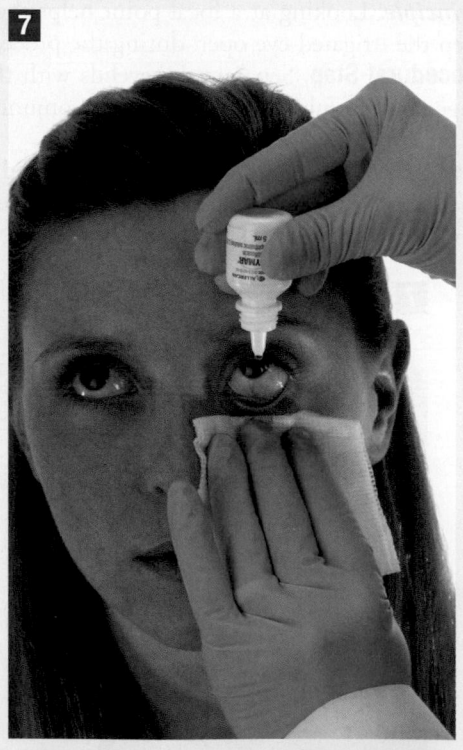

Ask the patient to look up, and insert the medication.

PROCEDURE 21-4   Performing an Eye Instillation—cont'd

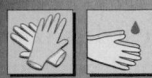

8. **Procedural Step.** Ask the patient to close his or her eyes gently and move the eyeballs. Instruct the patient not to shut the eyes tight or to blink and to keep the eyes closed for 1 to 2 minutes. Tell the patient that the instillation may blur the vision temporarily.
Principle. Moving the eyeballs helps distribute the medication over the entire eye. Keeping the eyes closed allows the medication to be absorbed. If the eyes are shut tightly or if the patient blinks, the drops or ointment may be pushed out of the eye.

9. **Procedural Step.** Dry the eyelid from inner to outer canthus with a gauze pad to remove excess medication.

10. **Procedural Step.** Remove the gloves, and sanitize your hands.

11. **Procedural Step.** Chart the procedure. The medication dosage for eye drops is recorded in the number of drops instilled. The abbreviation for drop is *gtt*; for

drops, *gtts*. The number of drops must be recorded in Roman numerals (e.g., i, ii) following the *gtt* abbreviation. The recording should include the date and time, the name and strength of the medication, the number of drops or amount of ointment, which eye received the instillation, your observations, and the patient's reaction.

CHARTING EXAMPLE

Date	
11/5/XX	2:30 p.m. Atropine sulfate, 1% gtts ii OU.
	Pt states a temporary blurring of vision. ——
	—————————— C. Lindner, CMA (AAMA)

12. **Procedural Step.** Return the medication to its proper storage area.

INTRODUCTION TO THE EAR

The medical assistant is responsible for performing a variety of procedures that involve the ear. An understanding of the structure and function of the ear is essential to mastering skill in these areas. Refer to Chapter 10 to review the structure and function of the ear.

Hearing tests also may be part of the routine physical examination. During contact with the patient, the medical assistant should be alert to signs that indicate the patient might be having difficulty hearing what is being said. A whispered voice next to the patient's ear can be a screening test for hearing acuity. The use of tuning forks or an audiometer provides a more accurate determination of hearing acuity. An **audiometer** is an instrument that emits sound waves at various frequencies. The patient is instructed to indicate when a sound at a given frequency can be heard.

The medical assistant is responsible for performing or teaching the patient to perform ear irrigations and instillations. Ear irrigations and instillations should be performed using the important principles of medical asepsis outlined in Chapter 17.

ASSESSMENT OF HEARING ACUITY

The assessment of hearing acuity is an integral part of a complete physical examination. It is possible for an individual to have hearing loss and not be aware of it. Early detection and treatment of hearing problems help prevent permanent hearing loss.

What Would You Do? What Would You *Not* Do?

Case Study 3
Willow Basil brings in her 6-year-old daughter, Jade. For the past 3 days, Jade has been running a fever and has had persistent pain and hearing loss in her left ear. Mrs. Basil practices alternative medicine and uses prescription medications as little as possible. She says that she has been trying herbal therapy and aromatherapy to make Jade better, but it does not seem to be helping. Jade is diagnosed with acute otitis media, and the physician prescribes amoxicillin for 10 days. Mrs. Basil wants to know if she has to give Jade the amoxicillin for the entire 10 days. She asks if she can stop using it when Jade starts feeling better. Mrs. Basil also wants to know if the ear infection will cause a permanent problem with Jade's hearing. ■

An individual with normal hearing should be able to hear the frequencies of normal speech, which range from 300 to 4000 Hz (hertz, or cycles per second) at a normal sound intensity. Patients who exhibit hearing loss are referred to an otolaryngologist or an audiologist for further evaluation.

Types of Hearing Loss

There are three types of hearing loss: conductive, sensorineural, and mixed. *Conductive hearing loss* results when there is a physical interference with the normal conduction of sound waves through the external and middle ear. Because of the interference, the amount of sound reaching the inner ear is less than normal, resulting in hearing impairment. Conductive loss in the external ear may be caused by an obstruction in the external ear canal, such as impacted cerumen, swelling from external otitis (swimmer's ear), foreign bodies, and benign growths such as polyps. Conductive loss in the middle ear may be caused by serous otitis media (fluid in the middle ear) or acute otitis media (infection in the middle ear), a perforated tympanic membrane, or otosclerosis. The cause of conductive hearing loss often can be detected by examining the external ear canal with an otoscope. Hearing is frequently restored by removing the obstruction (e.g., impacted cerumen) or treating the disorder (e.g., serous otitis media).

Sensorineural hearing loss results from damage to the inner ear or auditory nerve. With this type of hearing loss, sound is conducted normally through the outer and middle ear structures, but because of a problem with the perception of sound waves, a hearing deficit occurs. Specific causes of sensorineural loss include hereditary factors, degenerative changes from the normal aging process known as *presbycusis,* intense noise exposure over time, tumors, ototoxicity caused by certain medications, and infectious diseases, such as measles, mumps, and meningitis. The most common cause of sensorineural hearing loss in an adult is presbycusis. As an individual ages, nerves and sensory receptor cells in the inner ear deteriorate, leading to a gradual loss of hearing. *Mixed hearing loss* is a combination of conductive and sensorineural loss.

Hearing Acuity Tests

Numerous tests can be used to assess hearing acuity. Tests range from the simple gross screening test to qualitative tests using a tuning fork to highly specific quantitative tests using an audiometer. It is important to test only one ear at a time because a hearing deficit can exist in one ear only. The ear not being tested should be blocked by an earplug or masked. *Masking* involves the presentation of sound (usually noise) to the ear not being tested so that the patient's response is based only on hearing in the ear being tested.

Gross Screening Test

The gross hearing test is a simple and quick screening test used to identify a large hearing impairment. The physician performs the screening test during the physical examination. Hearing is assessed by asking the patient to repeat a simple word or series of numbers whispered from a distance of 1 to 2 feet from the ear. When a hearing loss is discovered, a tuning fork or audiometer is used for a more precise assessment of hearing.

Tuning Fork Tests

Tuning fork tests provide a general assessment of hearing acuity and may be part of the physical examination. A tuning fork with a frequency of 512 Hz or 1024 Hz is generally used because these frequencies fall within the range of normal speech. The Weber and Rinne tests are the tuning fork tests most commonly performed by the physician; they are used to identify conductive and sensorineural hearing loss.

The *Weber test* is a useful assessment of hearing loss when one ear hears better than the other. The tuning fork is set in vibration, and the base of the fork is placed on the center of the patient's head. The patient is asked to indicate where the sound is heard best. A patient with normal hearing would hear the sound equally in both ears or in the center of the head. Figure 21-7 illustrates the Weber test and describes the interpretation of results.

The *Rinne test* compares the duration of sound perception by air conduction with that of bone conduction. The tuning fork is set in vibration, and the base of the fork is placed against the bone of the mastoid process. The patient is instructed to indicate when the sound is no longer heard. The prongs of the fork (still vibrating) are placed in the air about 1 inch from the opening of the patient's ear canal, and the patient indicates when the sound is no longer heard. An individual with normal hearing is able to hear the sound at least twice as long through air conduction as through bone conduction. Figure 21-8 illustrates the Rinne test and describes the interpretation of results.

Audiometry

Audiometry is the measurement of hearing acuity using a special instrument called an **audiometer.** An audiometer quantitatively measures hearing for the various frequencies of sound waves. Audiometry is a more specific hearing acuity test because it provides information on how extensive a hearing loss is and which frequencies are involved. It is important that the test be conducted in a quiet room because outside noise may affect the results, especially in the lower frequencies. The patient wears headphones placed snugly over the ears (Figure 21-9). The audiometer delivers

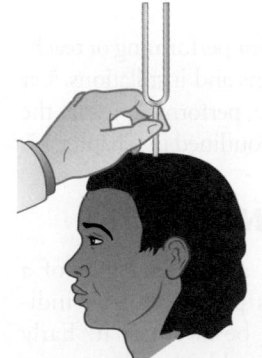

Normal Hearing
The patient hears the sound equally in both ears or in the center of the head.

Conductive Hearing Loss
The patient hears the sound better in the problem ear.

Sensorineural Hearing Loss
The patient does not hear the sound as well in the problem ear.

Figure 21-7 Weber test.

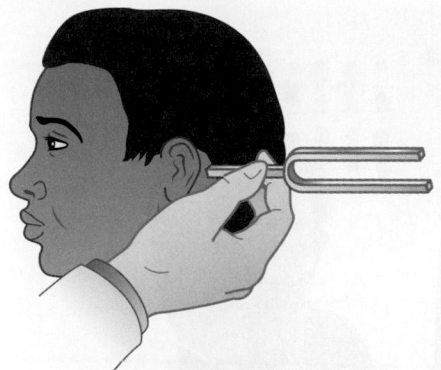

Bone conduction

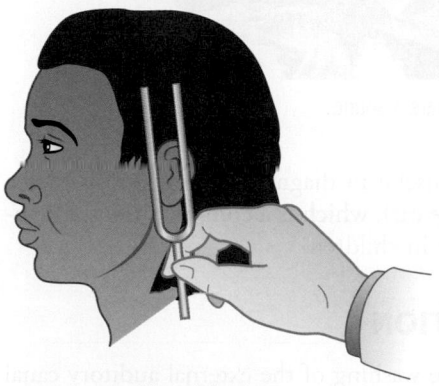

Air conduction

Normal Hearing
The patient hears the sound at least twice as long through air conduction as through bone conduction.

Conductive Hearing Loss
The patient hears the sound longer by bone conduction than by air conduction.

Sensorineural Hearing Loss
The sound is reduced. The patient will also hear the sound longer through air conduction than through bone conduction but not twice as long.

Figure 21-8 Rinne test.

Memories *from* Externship

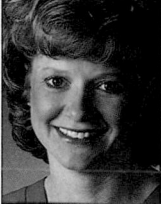

Cammie Lindner: There is one characteristic that is shared by all patients. I first noticed this during my externships, and it does not seem to matter what type of practice it is. Patients like to feel special and to be treated that way. They like consistency in their physician and in the office staff, and seeing familiar faces. This is especially hard during externship. The time spent is too short to truly get to know the patients, but it is a great learning experience.

It is important to observe the staff and patient communication and interaction skills. By doing this, you can decide which ones you admire and those that you do not wish to copy. The following are just a few of the guidelines that have helped me: (1) Call patients by name, and be sure that they know your name. (2) Follow through with what you have told patients you will do, and keep them updated if circumstances change. (3) Smile, and do not let one patient's negative attitude interfere with your care of others. (4) Take time to listen.

When you do begin your career, it does not take long to get into a routine and to start knowing your patients. When patients see a familiar face, they are more willing to share information that can contribute to improved communication and good health care. ■

a single frequency at a time at specific intensities, starting with low-frequency tones of 250 to 500 Hz and going to very high frequencies of 6000 to 8000 Hz. The patient is asked to signal when he or she hears a sound so that the patient's hearing threshold for each frequency can be determined. The hearing acuity in each ear is assessed separately, and the results are plotted on a graph known as an *audiogram*. The medical assistant may be responsible for performing audiometry in the medical office. Before operating an audiometer, however, the medical assistant must receive extensive on-site training by an audiologist to ensure that proper technique is used to conduct the test.

Tympanometry

Tympanometry is not a hearing test, but it does help determine the cause of hearing loss, so it is presented in this section. The tympanometer consists of an earpiece attached to an electronic device (Figure 21-10). The earpiece is placed snugly in the patient's ear, and low-frequency sound waves are directed against the eardrum while pressure is applied in the ear canal. With a normal ear, the eardrum exhibits mobility in response to the pressure, as indicated on a graphic readout known as a *tympanogram*. If there is fluid in the middle ear, the eardrum does not move but remains stiff, as indicated on the tympanogram.

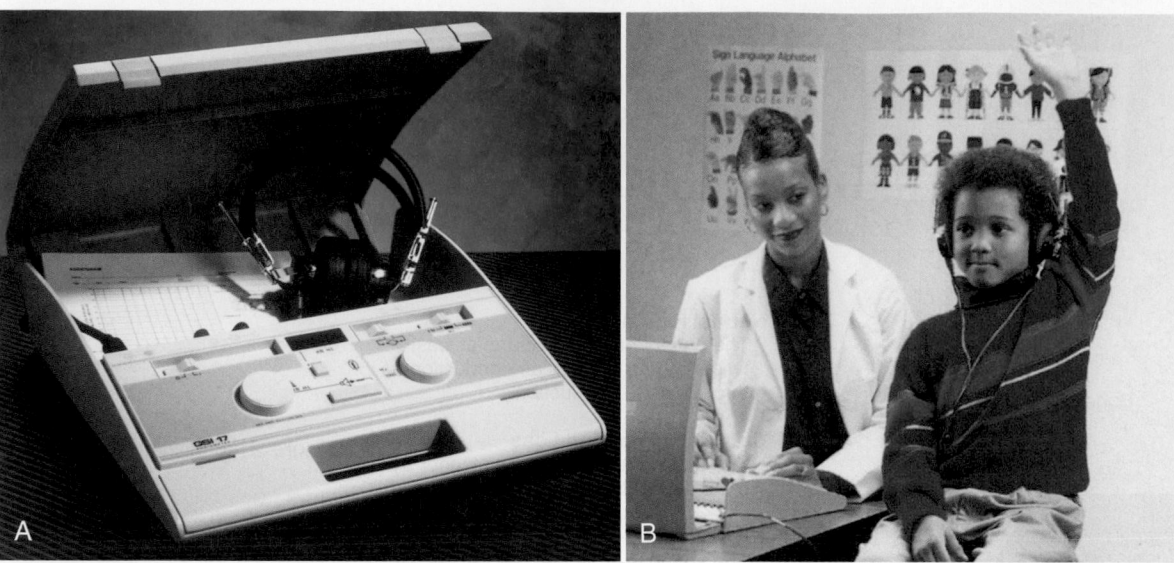

Figure 21-9 **A,** Audiometer. **B,** The patient signals when he hears a sound.

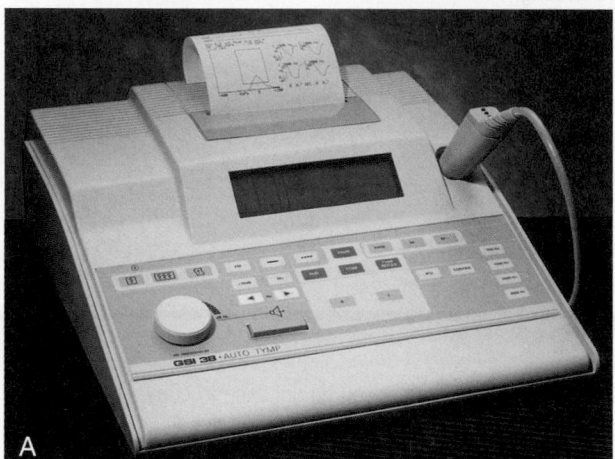

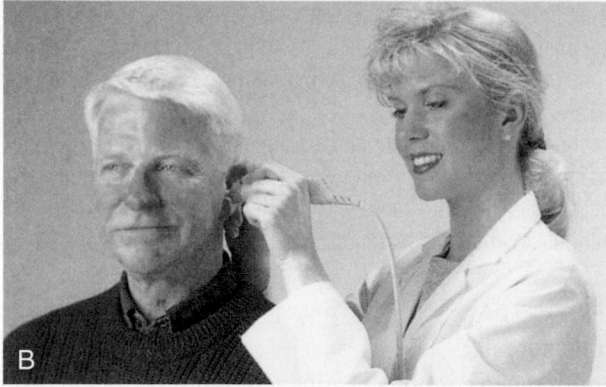

Figure 21-10 **A,** Tympanometer. **B,** The earpiece is placed snugly in the patient's ear.

Tympanometry is useful in diagnosing serous otitis media (fluid in the middle ear), which is a common cause of temporary hearing loss in children.

EAR IRRIGATION

Ear irrigation is the washing of the external auditory canal with a flowing solution. Ear irrigations are performed for the following purposes: to cleanse the external auditory canal to remove cerumen, discharge, or a foreign body; to relieve inflammation by applying an antiseptic solution; and to apply heat to the ear. Before irrigating, impacted cerumen must be softened by instilling warm mineral oil or hydrogen peroxide for 10 to 15 minutes. Procedure 21-5 shows how to perform an ear irrigation. An ear irrigation should not be performed if the tympanic membrane is perforated because this could result in severe irritation or infection of the middle ear.

EAR INSTILLATION

An ear instillation involves dropping a liquid into the external auditory canal. Ear instillations are performed to soften impacted cerumen, to combat infection with the use of antibiotic ear drops, and to relieve pain. The ear drops are usually dispensed in a flexible plastic container with an attached dropper. Procedure 21-6 shows how to perform an ear instillation.

PATIENT TEACHING Acute Otitis Media

Answer questions patients have about otitis media.

What is a middle ear infection?

An infection of the middle ear is medically referred to as *acute otitis media*. It is an inflammation of the middle ear caused by an infection and can occur in one or both ears. It is common in young children 3 months to 3 years old, but is unusual in adults. A middle ear infection is not serious if treated promptly and effectively. If not treated, however, middle ear infections can lead to serious complications, such as acute mastoiditis, meningitis, and permanent hearing loss.

What causes a middle ear infection?

A middle ear infection is often due to an upper respiratory infection or allergy that causes the eustachian tube to swell and become blocked. The blockage causes fluid to build up in the middle ear. This fluid is an ideal place for bacteria to grow. If this occurs, the result is acute otitis media.

What are the symptoms of a middle ear infection?

The most common symptoms are intense pain, fever, and temporary hearing loss. Other symptoms may include dizziness, nausea and vomiting, and (if the eardrum ruptures) drainage from the ear.

How does the physician know whether a middle ear infection is present?

The physician examines the ears with an otoscope. If a middle ear infection is present, the eardrum is red and swollen (see illustration) as a result of irritation from the infection, and pus and mucus can be seen behind the eardrum.

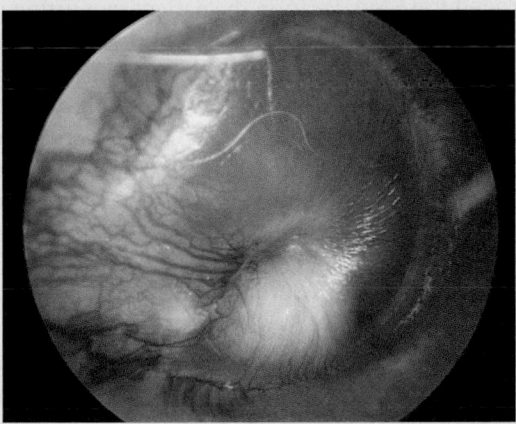

Chronic otitis media.

How is the infection treated?

A middle ear infection is usually treated with an oral antibiotic for 10 to 14 days. It is important to take all of the antibiotic prescribed; otherwise, the ear infection may recur. The physician also may recommend a decongestant to help open the blocked eustachian tube. After the acute infection is over, fluid may remain trapped in the middle ear. This condition is known as *serous otitis media* (see illustration) and, if not treated, may last for days, weeks, months, or even a year. Although fluid in the middle ear is painless, it may result in a feeling of fullness or pressure in the ears and temporary hearing loss.

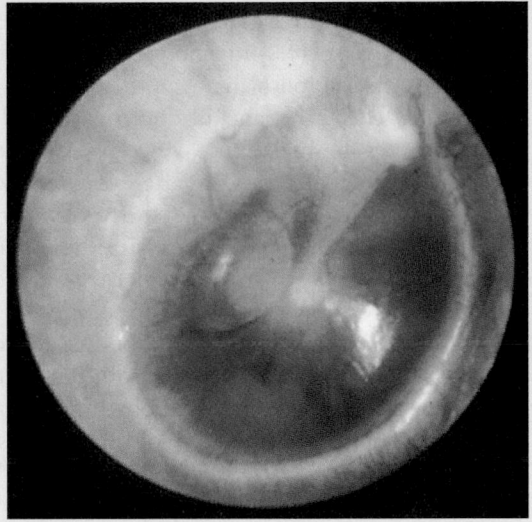

Serous otitis media.

Why are middle ear infections so common in children?

In children, the eustachian tube is positioned horizontally and is shorter and narrower than in adults. When a child has an upper respiratory infection, bacteria can travel easily to the middle ear. In addition, swelling from the respiratory infection can block this narrow tube, which causes fluid to build up in the middle ear.

- Encourage the patient to complete the entire prescribed course of antibiotics.
- If the physician has prescribed ear drops, teach the patient (or parent) the proper procedure for performing an ear instillation.
- Encourage early treatment of upper respiratory infections.
- Give the patient educational materials on otitis media. ∎

PROCEDURE 21-5   Performing an Ear Irrigation

Outcome Perform an ear irrigation.

Equipment/Supplies

- Disposable gloves
- Irrigating solution
- Solution basin
- Bath thermometer
- Irrigating syringe

- Ear basin
- Moisture-resistant towel
- Gauze pads
- Ear wick

1. **Procedural Step.** Sanitize your hands.
2. **Procedural Step.** Assemble the equipment. If both ears are to be irrigated, two sets of equipment must be used to prevent cross-infection from one ear to the other. Perform the following:
   a. Carefully check the label of the irrigating solution three times to make sure you have the correct solution. The first time is after you remove the solution container from the shelf. Compare the label of the solution container with the physician's instructions.
   b. Check the expiration date of the solution.
   c. Warm the irrigating solution to body temperature (98.6° F [37° C]) by placing the solution container in a basin of warm water. Use a bath thermometer to make sure the temperature of the water used to warm the solution does not exceed body temperature.
   d. Check the solution label a second time before pouring the solution.
   e. Pour the solution as follows:
   Palm the label of the container and remove the cap. Place the cap on a flat surface with the open end up. Pour the solution into the basin and replace the cap without contaminating it. Cover the basin to keep the solution warm.
   f. Check the solution label a third time before returning the container to its storage area.
   Principle. The solution label should be carefully checked three times to prevent an error. An outdated solution may produce undesirable effects. If the solution is too cold or too warm, it might stimulate the inner ear and the patient may become dizzy. Palming the label prevents the solution from dripping on the label and obscuring it or loosening the label. Placing the cap open end up prevents contamination.

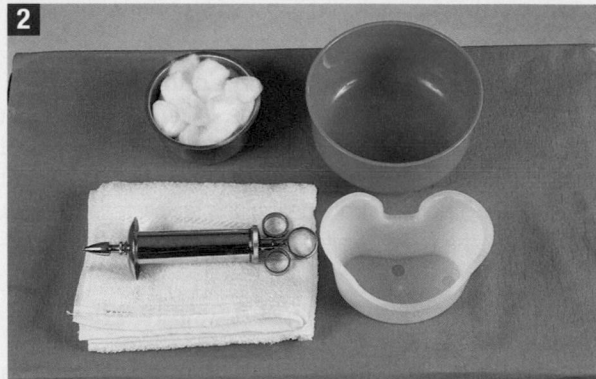

3. **Procedural Step.** Greet the patient and introduce yourself. Identify the patient and explain the procedure. Explain the purpose of performing the irrigation—for example, to remove cerumen. Tell the patient the procedure is not painful; however, he or she may feel a minimal amount of discomfort and occasional dizziness, fullness, and warmth as the ear solution comes in contact with the tympanic membrane.
4. **Procedural Step.** Position the patient in a sitting position. Place a moisture-resistant towel on the patient's shoulder under the ear to be irrigated to protect clothing and to prevent water from running down the neck. Position a basin tightly against the patient's neck under the affected ear to catch the irrigating solution, and ask the patient to hold it in place. Ask the patient to tilt the head in the direction of the affected ear.
   Principle. The patient is positioned so that gravity aids the flow of the solution out of the ear and into the basin.
5. **Procedural Step.** Apply gloves. Cleanse the outer ear with a moistened gauze pad to remove any discharge or debris present. Normal saline or the solution ordered for the irrigation may be used.
   Principle. The outer ear should be clean to prevent foreign particles from entering the ear canal during the irrigation.

PROCEDURE **21-5** Performing an Ear Irrigation—cont'd

6. **Procedural Step.** Fill the syringe with the irrigating solution (approximately 50 mL). Expel air from the syringe.
   Principle. Air forced into the ear is uncomfortable for the patient.

7. **Procedural Step.** Straighten the external ear canal. The canal is straightened by gently pulling the ear upward and backward for adults and children older than 3 years old and downward and backward for children 3 years old and younger.
   Principle. Straightening the canal permits the irrigating solution to reach all areas of the canal.

8. **Procedural Step.** Insert the syringe tip into the ear, but not too deeply. Make sure that the tip of the syringe does not obstruct the canal opening so that the solution can flow freely out of the canal.
   Principle. Inserting the tip of the syringe too deeply causes discomfort for the patient.
   Obstruction of the canal causes pressure to build up in the canal, resulting in patient discomfort and possible injury to the tympanic membrane.

9. **Procedural Step.** Inject the irrigating solution toward the roof of the ear canal. It is important that the solution be injected toward the roof of the canal to prevent it from being injected directly onto the tympanic membrane.
   Principle. The tip of the syringe should be directed at the roof of the canal to prevent injury to the tympanic membrane and to aid in the removal of foreign particles by allowing the solution to flow down the length of the canal and out the bottom. In addition, severe patient discomfort and dizziness may occur if the solution is injected directly onto the tympanic membrane.

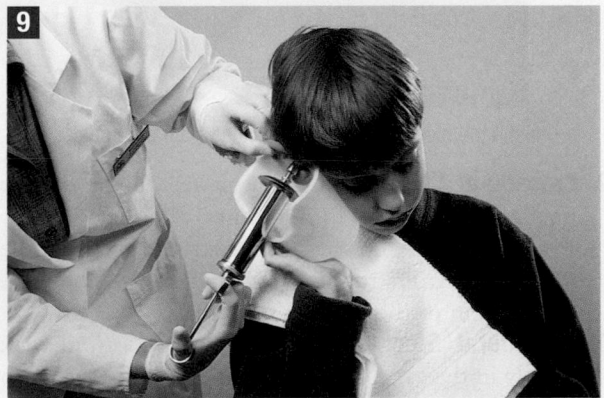

Inject the irrigating solution toward the roof of the ear canal.

10. **Procedural Step.** Refill the syringe, and continue irrigating until the desired results have been obtained or all the solution is used, depending on the purpose of the irrigation. Observe the returning solution to note the material present (e.g., cerumen, discharge, a foreign object) and the amount (small, moderate, or large).

11. **Procedural Step.** Dry the outside of the ear with a gauze pad. Have the patient lie on the affected side on the treatment table. Tell the patient that the ear will feel sensitive for a short time. Place a cotton wick loosely in the ear canal for 15 minutes if instructed to do so by the physician.
    Principle. Any solution remaining in the ear canal should be allowed to drain out. A cotton wick makes the patient's ear feel less sensitive after the irrigation.

12. **Procedural Step.** Remove the gloves, and sanitize your hands.

13. **Procedural Step.** Chart the procedure. Include the following: the date and time; which ear was irrigated; the type, strength, and amount of solution used; the amount and type of material returned in the irrigating solution; any significant observations; and patient reactions. Use one of these abbreviations to indicate which ear was irrigated:
    AU—Both ears
    AD—Right ear
    AS—Left ear

CHARTING EXAMPLE

Date	
11/15/XX	2:15 p.m. Irrigated AD c̄ saline, 200 ml @ 98.6° F. Mod amt of cerumen present in returned solution. Cotton wick placed in ear canal × 15 min. No complaints of discomfort. —————— C. Lindner, CMA (AAMA)

14. **Procedural Step.** Remove reusable equipment to a work area for sanitization, sterilization, or disinfection as required by the medical office policy.

PROCEDURE 21-5

PROCEDURE 21-6 *Performing an Ear Instillation*

Outcome Perform an ear instillation.

Equipment/Supplies

- Disposable gloves
- Otic drops

- Gauze pad

1. **Procedural Step.** Sanitize your hands.
2. **Procedural Step.** Assemble the equipment, and perform the following:
   a. Check the drug label three times to make sure you have the correct medication. The first time should be when you remove the medication from the shelf. The medication label must bear the word *otic.*
   b. Check the medication label a second time against the physician's instructions. Also check the dosage ordered by the physician.
   c. Check the expiration date.
   d. Check the medication label a third time before the cap is removed to instill the medication.
   Principle. The drug label should be carefully checked three times to prevent a medication error. Medication not bearing the word *otic* must never be placed in the ear because it could injure the ear. An outdated medication may produce undesirable effects and should be discarded.
3. **Procedural Step.** Greet the patient and introduce yourself. Identify the patient and explain the procedure and the purpose of the instillation.
4. **Procedural Step.** Position the patient in a sitting position.
5. **Procedural Step.** Warm the drops to body temperature by holding the medication container in the palms of your hands for a few minutes. Do not warm the drops by placing them in hot water.
   Principle. If the drops are too cold or too warm, they might stimulate the inner ear, causing the patient to become dizzy.
6. **Procedural Step.** Apply gloves. If the medication requires mixing, shake the container well. Check the medication label for the third time, and remove the cap from the container.
   Principle. Gravity aids in the flow of medication into the ear canal.
7. **Procedural Step.** Ask the patient to tilt his or her head in the direction of the unaffected ear. Straighten the external auditory canal. The canal is straightened by pulling the ear upward and backward for adults and

children older than 3 years old and downward and backward for children 3 years old and younger.
   Principle. Straightening the canal permits the medication to reach all areas of the canal.

8. **Procedural Step.** Invert the container and place the tip of the dropper at the opening of the ear canal. Gently squeeze the container and instill the correct number of drops along the side of the canal. Replace the cap on the container.

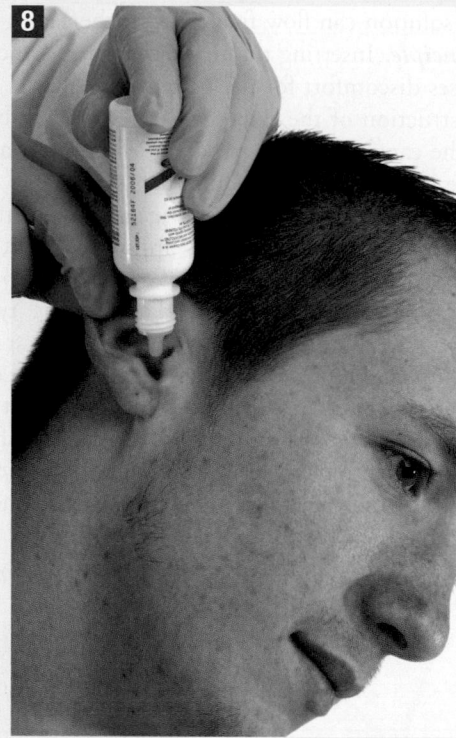

Instill the medication along the side of the ear canal.

9. **Procedural Step.** Instruct the patient to lie on the unaffected side for 2 to 3 minutes.
   Principle. Lying on the unaffected side prevents the medication from running out and allows complete distribution of the medication.
10. **Procedural Step.** Place a moistened cotton wick loosely in the ear canal for 15 minutes if instructed to do so by the physician.

PROCEDURE 21-6 Performing an Ear Instillation—cont'd

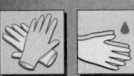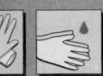

Principle. The cotton wick prevents the medication from running out when the patient is upright. Moistening the wick prevents the medication from being absorbed by the cotton.

11. **Procedural Step.** Remove the gloves, and sanitize your hands.

12. **Procedural Step.** Chart the procedure. Include the date and time, the name and strength of the medication, the number of drops, which ear received the instillation, any significant observations, and the patient's reaction.

CHARTING EXAMPLE

Date	
11/20/XX	9:30 a.m. Auralgan gtts ii , AD. No discharge present. Pt states a relief of pain. ———————————— C. Lindner, CMA (AAMA)

13. **Procedural Step.** Return the medication to its storage area.

Highlight on Hearing Impairment

The number of individuals with a hearing impairment has gradually increased over the past 20 years. Factors that contribute to this increase include an aging population and a noisier environment.

It is estimated that approximately 28 million people in the United States have a hearing loss severe enough to interfere with their daily activities, whereas another 2 million individuals are profoundly deaf.

Precise screening of preschool children for hearing loss is difficult. This is because tuning fork tests and audiometry require the ability to signal in response to sound, and children up to age 4 or 5 years have trouble mastering this skill.

Most state, county, and local school systems require hearing screening as a prerequisite for entrance to school and again at periodic intervals, usually during the first, third, fifth, and seventh grades.

Risk factors for hearing impairment in children include family history of deafness, premature birth, low birth weight, measles, mumps, high fevers, meningitis, recurrent or chronic ear infections, and the maternal rubella infection during pregnancy.

Signs of hearing impairment in children are poor attentiveness, delayed speech development, and persistent problems with articulation. Signs of hearing impairment in adults include frequent requests for words or statements to be repeated, leaning toward the speaker, turning the head, cupping the ears, and speaking in a loud or unvaried tone of voice.

The most common cause of conductive hearing loss in children is fluid in the middle ear, which prevents the tympanic membrane from vibrating freely. In adults, the most common cause of conductive loss is otosclerosis, a condition in which the stapes becomes fixed because of calcium deposits and less able to pass on vibrations when sound enters the ear.

The loudness of sound is measured in units called *decibels* (dB). Sounds of less than 75 dB, even after long exposure, are unlikely to cause hearing loss. Normal conversation is approximately 60 dB, and a whisper in a quiet library is 30 to 40 dB.

Permanent sensorineural hearing loss can result when the ear is repeatedly bombarded with loud sounds over time. Standards set by the Occupational Safety and Health Administration (OSHA) indicate that continued exposure to noise louder than 85 dB eventually harms an individual's hearing by damaging the tiny hair cells in the organ of Corti. The organ of Corti is a structure in the cochlea (inner ear) that converts sound waves into nerve impulses for transmission to the brain. This type of sensorineural hearing loss is known as *noise-induced hearing loss.* It is most often seen in individuals who frequently listen to loud music, fire guns without wearing ear protection, or are exposed to loud noise as part of their jobs. The following are examples of common noises and the decibel level of each:

Noise	Decibels
Normal breathing	10
Humming of a refrigerator	40
Television	70
Vacuum cleaner	60 to 85
Motorcycle	95 to 100
Personal stereo system with earphones (on high)	115
Rock concert	120
Chain saw	120
Auto stereo on high	125
Jet taking off	140
Firecracker	150
Firearms	140 to 170

Many hearing impairments can be helped with the use of a hearing aid. Individuals who benefit most from a hearing aid have mild to moderate conductive hearing loss. Individuals with sensorineural or mixed hearing loss have more trouble finding a suitable hearing aid and often get less satisfactory results. ∎

PROCEDURE 21-6

MEDICAL PRACTICE and the LAW

Legal issues concerning eye and ear assessment are similar to the legal issues that concern any assessment. Accurate assessments done properly are necessary for accurate diagnoses and treatment and to prevent injuries to these structures.

Patient Rights

Patients entering the office have six major rights, which are enforceable by law, as follows:

1. The right to have the physician and medical assistant *do good for them.*

2. The right to *be treated fairly.*
3. The right to *be free.*
4. The right *not to be harmed.*
5. The right of fidelity, or *being true.*
6. The right to *life.*

If any of these rights is violated, the patient has the right to sue. ■

What Would You Do? What Would You *Not* Do? RESPONSES

Case Study 1
Page 389

What Did Cammie Do?

❑ Talked with Haley (on her level) about why someone needs to wear glasses.

❑ Retested Haley with the Snellen chart to see if she missed the same letters.

❑ Tested Haley with the Big E chart to give the physician an additional measurement to make an interpretation of Haley's visual acuity.

What Did Cammie Not Do?

❑ Did not tell Haley that she needs glasses.

❑ Did not scold Haley for trying to miss letters on the test.

What Would You Do/What Would You *Not* Do?

Review Cammie's response and place a checkmark next to the information you included in your response. List the additional information you included in your response.

_____

_____

_____

_____

_____

_____

Case Study 2
Page 393

What Did Cammie Do?

❑ Gave Mr. Mitchell some suggestions on how to put drops in Clive's eyes so it is less scary. One idea is to have Clive lie down flat and close his eyes. Place the drops in the inner corner of his eye next to the bridge of his nose, letting them make a little lake there. When Clive relaxes and opens his eye, the drops will gently flow into his eye.

❑ Talked with Clive (on his level) about why he needs eye drops.

❑ Told Mr. Mitchell that the eye drops were prescribed for Clive, and they should be used only for Clive. Told him that if the twins developed conjunctivitis, he should call the office.

❑ Gave Mr. Mitchell suggestions for preventing the twins from getting conjunctivitis (not touching the infected eye, frequent handwashing, not sharing toys or towels).

What Did Cammie Not Do?

❑ Did not tell Mr. Mitchell to hold Clive down or force drops in his eyes.

❑ Did not tell Mr. Mitchell that he should know better than to think about giving the twins a medication not prescribed for them

What Would You Do/What Would You *Not* Do?

Review Cammie's response and place a checkmark next to the information you included in your response. List the additional information you included in your response.

_____

_____

_____

_____

_____

_____

Case Study 3
Page 397

What Did Cammie Do?

❑ Explained to Mrs. Basil that Jade may begin to feel better after several days of antibiotics, but not all of the germs causing her ear infection will have been killed by then. If she does not give Jade the full course of antibiotics, the infection could come back.

❑ Documented all the medications that Mrs. Basil has administered to Jade.

❑ Gave Mrs. Basil a patient information brochure on acute otitis media.

What Would You Do? What Would You *Not* Do? RESPONSES—cont'd

❑ Told Mrs. Basil that she needs to talk to the physician about her concern regarding hearing loss because he is most qualified to answer that question.

❑ Encouraged Mrs. Basil to bring Jade in sooner when she develops fever and ear pain.

What Did Cammie Not Do?

❑ Did not criticize Mrs. Basil for waiting so long to bring Jade in.

❑ Did not offer a personal opinion about alternative medicine.

What Would You Do/What Would You *Not* Do?

Review Cammie's response and place a checkmark next to the information you included in your response. List the additional information you included in your response.

_____

_____

_____

_____

_____

TERMINOLOGY REVIEW

Medical Term	Word Parts	Definition
Astigmatism	*a-:* without *stigma/a:* point *-ism:* state of	A refractive error that causes distorted and blurred vision for both near and far objects due to a cornea that is oval shaped.
Audiometer	*audi/o:* hearing *-meter:* instrument used to measure	An instrument used to measure hearing acuity quantitatively for the various frequencies of sound waves.
Canthus		The junction of the eyelids at either corner of the eye.
Cerumen		Earwax.
Hyperopia	*hyper-:* above, excessive *-opia:* vision	Farsightedness.
Impacted		Wedged firmly together so as to be immovable.
Instillation		The dropping of a liquid into a body cavity.
Irrigation		The washing of a body canal with a flowing solution.
Myopia	*-opia:* vision	Nearsightedness.
Otoscope	*ot/o:* vision *-scope:* to view	An instrument used to examine the external ear canal and tympanic membrane.
Presbyopia	*-opia:* vision	A decrease in the elasticity of the lens that occurs with aging, resulting in a decreased ability to focus on close objects.
Refraction		The deflection or bending of light rays by a lens.
Tympanic membrane	*tympan/o:* eardrum *-ic:* pertaining to	A thin, semitransparent membrane between the external ear canal and the middle ear that receives and transmits sound waves. Also known as the *eardrum*.

ON THE WEB

For information on the eye:

American Optometric Association: www.aoa.org

American Academy of Ophthalmology: www.aao.org

National Eye Institute: www.nei.nih.gov

All About Vision: www.allaboutvision.com

Sight and Hearing Association: www.sightandhearing.org

American Academy of Optometry: www.aaopt.org

American Association for Pediatric Ophthalmology and Strabismus: www.aapos.org

The Eyes Have It: www.aboutcataractsurgery.com

About Cataract Surgery: www.kellogg.umich.edu/theeyeshaveit/index.html

For information on the ear:

American Academy of Audiology: www.audiology.org

National Institute on Deafness and Other Communication Disorders: www.nidcd.nih.gov

Healthy Hearing: www.healthyhearing.com

Hear It: www.hear-it.org

League for the Hard of Hearing: www.lhh.org

 Check out the Evolve site at http://evolve.elsevier.com/Bonewit/today/ to actively Prepare for your Certification, and to access additional interactive activities and exercises to help you study and prepare for success.

22

Physical Agents to Promote Tissue Healing

KEY TERMS

ambulation (AM-byoo-LAY-shun)
ambulatory
compress (KOM-press)
edema (uh-DEE-muh)

erythema (err-uh-THEE-muh)
exudate (EKS-oo-date)
soak
sprain

strain
suppuration (SUP-er-AY-shun)

INTRODUCTION TO TISSUE HEALING

Physical agents are often employed in the medical office to promote tissue healing for individuals who experience a disability as a result of injury, disease, or loss of a body part. Physical agents are used therapeutically to improve circulation, provide support, and promote the return of motion so that the individual can perform the activities of daily living. Physical agents frequently used in the medical office include heat and cold applied locally and ambulatory aids, such as crutches, canes, and walkers.

LOCAL APPLICATION OF HEAT AND COLD

The application of heat and cold is used therapeutically to treat conditions such as infection and trauma. The medical assistant may be responsible for applying various forms of heat and cold at the medical office or for instructing patients in the proper procedure for applying heat or cold at home. The medical assistant should have a basic understanding of the physiologic effects of heat and cold on the body and of possible adverse reactions if they are not administered correctly.

Heat and cold can be applied in moist or dry forms. Common applications of dry and moist heat and cold are as follows:

1. *Dry heat:* heating pad, chemical hot pack
2. *Moist heat:* hot soak, hot compress
3. *Dry cold:* ice bag, chemical cold pack
4. *Moist cold:* cold compress

Heat and cold are applied for short periods (generally 15 to 30 minutes) to produce the desired therapeutic results. The application may be repeated at time intervals specified by the physician. Prolonged application of heat or cold is not recommended because it can result in adverse secondary effects. The type of heat or cold application used for a particular condition depends on the purpose of the application, the location and condition of the affected area, and the age and general health of the patient. The physician instructs the medical assistant to apply a heat or cold treatment based on these factors.

Heat and cold receptors in the skin readily adapt to changes in temperature, eventually resulting in diminished heat or cold sensations. The temperature actually remains the same and is providing the intended therapeutic effects. The patient, not perceiving the same degree of temperature, may want to increase the intensity of the application, however, without realizing the inherent dangers. Excessive heat or cold could result in tissue damage. A common example of this situation is a patient who turns up the setting of a heating pad from medium to high when the heating pad no longer feels warm. The medical assistant should fully explain to the patient the necessity

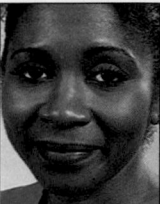

of maintaining a safe temperature range during the application.

Factors Affecting the Application of Heat and Cold

Before applying heat or cold, certain factors must be taken into consideration to prevent unfavorable reactions, such as tissue necrosis. The temperature may need to be adjusted based on the following conditions:

1. **The age of the patient.** Young children and elderly patients tend to be more sensitive to the application of heat or cold.
2. **Location of the application.** Certain areas of the body are more sensitive to the application of heat or cold, especially thin areas of the skin and areas that are usually covered by clothing, such as the chest, back, and abdomen. The skin on the hands and face is not as sensitive and is better able to tolerate temperature change. Broken skin, such as is found with an open wound, is more sensitive to heat and cold and is more prone to tissue damage.
3. **Impaired circulation.** Patients with impaired circulation tend to be more sensitive to heat and cold. This impairment may be at the site of the application or may be a systemic problem involving the entire body that is a result of certain conditions, such as peripheral vascular disease, diabetes mellitus, or congestive heart failure.
4. **Impaired sensation.** Patients with impaired sensation, such as diabetic patients, must be watched carefully

because tissue damage may occur from the application of heat or cold without the patient's awareness.

5. **Individual tolerance to change in temperature.** Some individuals cannot tolerate temperature change as easily as others.

The medical assistant should observe the area to which the heat or cold has been applied before, during, and after treatment for signs indicating that a modification of temperature is needed. Prolonged erythema or paleness, pain, swelling, and blisters should be reported to the physician. The medical assistant also should ask the patient whether the application feels comfortable or is too hot or too cold.

Heat

Local Effects of Heat

The application of moderate heat to a localized area of the body for a short time (approximately 15 to 30 minutes) produces *dilation,* or an increase in diameter, of the blood vessels in the area as the body tries to rid itself of excess heat (Figure 22-1). This results in an increased blood supply to the area, and tissue metabolism increases. Nutrients and oxygen are provided to the cells at a faster rate, and wastes and toxins are carried away faster. The skin in the area becomes warm and exhibits erythema. **Erythema** is reddening of the skin caused by dilation of superficial blood vessels in the skin.

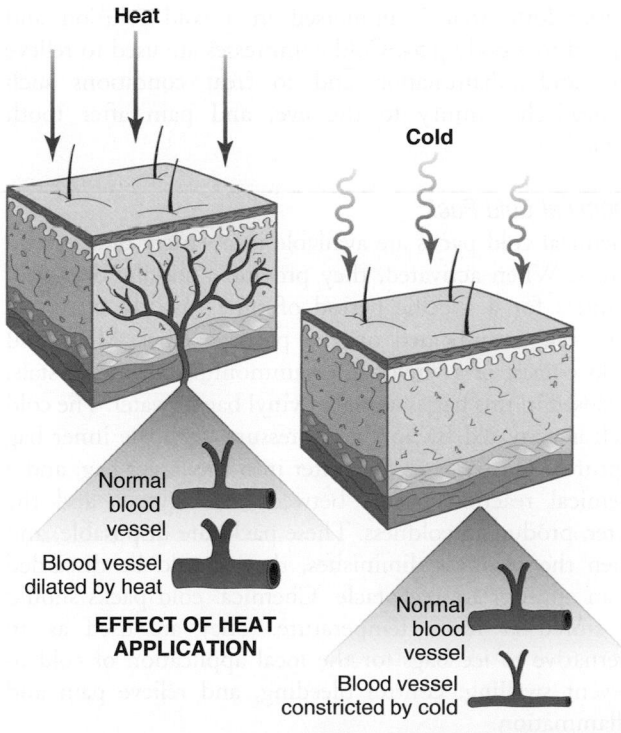

Figure 22-1 Effects of the local application of heat and cold.

These physiologic effects of moderate heat applied to a localized area promote healing. Prolonged application of heat (longer than 1 hour) produces secondary effects, however, that reverse this healing process. Blood vessels constrict, and blood supply to the area decreases. The medical assistant must be careful to apply heat for the length of time specified by the physician.

Purpose of Applying Heat

Heat functions in relieving pain, congestion, muscle spasms, and inflammation. Conditions for which the local application of heat is often prescribed are low back pain, arthritis, menstrual cramping, and localized abscesses.

Heat promotes muscle relaxation and is often used for the relief of pain caused by excessive contraction of muscle fibers. **Edema,** or swelling, in the tissues can be reduced through the application of heat because the increased blood supply functions to increase the absorption of fluid from the tissues through the lymphatic system.

Heat, usually in the form of a hot **compress,** can be used to soften exudates. An **exudate** is a discharge produced by the body's tissues. Exudates may sometimes form a hard crust over an area and require removal. Heat also increases **suppuration,** or the process of pus formation, to help in the relief of inflammation by breaking down infected tissues. Heat is not recommended, however, for the initial treatment of acute inflammation or trauma.

Types of Heat Applications

The most common types of heat applications are described next, along with the conditions they are often used to treat.

Heating Pad

The electric heating pad consists of a network of wires that function to convert electric energy into heat to provide a constant and even heat application. The wires must not be bent or crushed. This could damage the pad, resulting in overheating of parts of the pad and leading to burns or fire. Pins must not be inserted into the pad as a means of securing it; if a pin comes in contact with a wire, an electric shock could result. To prevent electric hazards, heating pads should not be used over areas that contain moisture, such as wet dressings. Heating pads are often used to relieve pain and muscle spasms.

Hot Soak

A **soak** is the direct immersion of a body part in water or a medicated solution. A soak can be applied to an extremity or a part of the torso. Hot soaks are used to cleanse open wounds, increase suppuration, increase the blood supply to an area to hasten the healing process, and apply a medicated solution to an area.

Hot Compress

A hot compress is a soft, moist, absorbent cloth, such as a washcloth, that is immersed in a warm solution and applied to a body part. Hot compresses are used to increase suppuration, to improve circulation to a body part to aid in healing, to promote drainage from infection, and to soften exudates. Applying a hot compress to an open wound requires the use of sterile technique.

Chemical Hot Pack

Chemical hot packs are available in a variety of sizes and shapes. When activated, they provide a specific degree of heat for a specific period of time (usually 30 to 60 minutes), as indicated on the package label. A chemical hot pack consists of a vinyl bag containing calcium chloride crystals and a smaller bag (encased in the vinyl bag) containing water. Pressure is applied with the hands to break the inner bag. The water in the inner bag combines with the calcium chloride crystals to produce heat. After using the pack, it should be discarded in an appropriate receptacle. Chemical hot packs should be stored at room temperature and are used as an alternative to a heating pad to relieve pain and muscle spasms.

Procedures 22-1, 22-2, 22-3, and 22-6 (see later) present the proper application of heat with a heating pad, a hot soak, a hot compress, and a chemical hot pack.

What Would You Do? What Would You *Not* Do?

Case Study 1

Aaron Collins is at the office. Aaron recently helped a friend move, and the next day he developed intense pain in his lower back. To alleviate the pain, he slept on a heating pad, but when he woke up, his back was red and blistered. Aaron says he turned the setting on the heating pad to high because his back was hurting so much and he thought that it would help his back feel better sooner. Aaron wants to know the best way to apply heat using a heating pad. He also wants to know what he can do to prevent low back pain in the future. ■

Cold

Local Effects of Cold

The application of moderate cold to a localized area produces *constriction,* or a decrease in diameter, of blood vessels in the area as the body attempts to prevent heat loss (see Figure 22-1). This constriction leads to decreased blood supply to the area. Tissue metabolism decreases, less oxygen is used, and fewer wastes accumulate. The skin becomes cool and pale. Prolonged application of cold (longer than 1 hour) has a reverse secondary effect. Blood vessels dilate, and tissue metabolism is increased. To prevent secondary effects, the medical assistant must apply cold for the recommended length of time only.

Purpose of Applying Cold

The application of moderate cold for a short time is used to prevent edema. Cold may be applied immediately after an individual has suffered direct trauma, such as a bruise, minor burn, **sprain, strain,** joint injury, or fracture. The cold limits the accumulation of fluid in the body tissues by constricting blood vessels and reducing the leakage of fluid into the tissues. Through constriction of peripheral blood vessels, cold can be used to control bleeding. Cold temporarily relieves pain through its anesthetic, or numbing, effect, which reduces stimulation of the pain receptors. Cold also slows the movement of blood and tissue fluids in the affected area, resulting in less pressure against pain receptors and therefore less pain. In the early stages of an infection, the local application of cold inhibits the activity of microorganisms. In this way, suppuration is decreased and inflammation is reduced. Cold applications should always be placed in a protective covering because applying cold directly to the skin could result in a skin burn.

Types of Cold Applications

Ice Bag

An ice bag consists of a waterproof bag with a screw-on cap. Before use, it must be filled with small pieces of ice and placed in a protective covering. Ice bags are used to prevent swelling, control bleeding, and relieve pain and inflammation.

Cold Compress

A cold compress is a soft, moist, absorbent cloth, such as a washcloth, that is immersed in a cold solution and applied to a body part. Cold compresses are used to relieve pain and inflammation and to treat conditions such as headache, injury to the eye, and pain after tooth extraction.

Chemical Cold Pack

Chemical cold packs are available in a variety of sizes and shapes. When activated, they provide a specific degree of coldness for a specific period of time (usually 30 to 60 minutes), as indicated on the package label. Most cold packs consist of a vinyl bag of ammonium nitrate crystals. Enclosed in this bag is a smaller vinyl bag of water. The cold pack is activated by applying pressure until the inner bag ruptures. This releases the water into the larger bag, and a chemical reaction occurs between the crystals and the water, producing coldness. These packs are disposable, and when the coldness diminishes, they should be discarded in an appropriate receptacle. Chemical cold packs should be stored at room temperature. They are used as an alternative to ice bags for the local application of cold to prevent swelling, control bleeding, and relieve pain and inflammation.

Procedures 22-4, 22-5, and 22-6 present proper application of cold with an ice bag, a cold compress, and a chemical cold pack.

Text continued on p. 418

PROCEDURE 22-1 Applying a Heating Pad

Outcome Apply a heating pad.

Equipment/Supplies

- Heating pad with a protective covering

1. **Procedural Step.** Sanitize your hands.
2. **Procedural Step.** Assemble the equipment.
3. **Procedural Step.** Greet the patient and introduce yourself. Identify the patient and explain the procedure. Explain the purpose of the application (e.g., to relieve pain).
4. **Procedural Step.** Place the heating pad in the protective covering.

   Principle. The protective covering provides more comfort for the patient and absorbs perspiration.

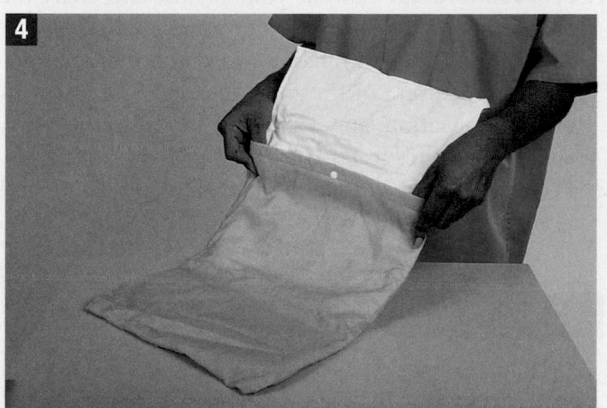

Place the heating pad in a protective covering.

5. **Procedural Step.** Connect the plug to an electric outlet. Set the selector switch at the proper setting, as designated by the physician (usually low or medium).
6. **Procedural Step.** Place the heating pad on the patient's affected body area. Ask the patient how the temperature feels. The heating pad should feel warm but not uncomfortable.
7. **Procedural Step.** Instruct the patient not to lie on the pad or turn the control higher to prevent burns.

Principle. Lying on the pad causes heat to accumulate and burn the patient. The patient's heat receptors eventually become adjusted to the temperature change, resulting in a decreased heat sensation, and the patient may be tempted to increase the temperature. Turning the control higher results in excessive heat on the patient's skin, which could burn the patient.

8. **Procedural Step.** Check the patient periodically for signs of an increase or decrease in redness or swelling, and ask the patient whether the site is painful. Administer the treatment for the proper length of time as designated by the physician.
9. **Procedural Step.** Sanitize your hands, and chart the procedure. Include the date and time, method of heat application (heating pad), temperature setting of the pad, location and duration of the application, appearance of the application site, and the patient's reaction. Also, chart any instructions provided to the patient on applying a heating pad at home.
10. **Procedural Step.** Properly care for equipment, and return it to its storage location.

CHARTING EXAMPLE

Date	
12/10/XX	10:15 a.m. Heating pad on medium setting applied to lower back x 20 min. Area appears pink following application. Pt states a relief of pain and better mobility. Provided instructions on the application of a heating pad at home. ———— M. Cooper, CMA (AAMA)

PROCEDURE 22-2 Applying a Hot Soak

Outcome Apply a hot soak.

Equipment/Supplies

- Soaking solution ordered by the physician
- Bath thermometer
- Basin
- Bath towels

1. **Procedural Step.** Sanitize your hands.
2. **Procedural Step.** Assemble the equipment. Check the label on the solution container to make sure you have the correct solution as ordered by the physician. Place the solution containers in a basin of warm water. Warm the soaking solution to a temperature between 105° F and 110° F (41° C and 44° C).
3. **Procedural Step.** Greet the patient and introduce yourself. Identify the patient and explain the procedure. Explain the purpose of the application (e.g., to apply a medicated solution).
4. **Procedural Step.** Fill the basin one-third to two-thirds full with the warmed soaking solution.
5. **Procedural Step.** Check the temperature of the solution with a bath thermometer. The temperature for

Continued

PROCEDURE 22-2 Applying a Hot Soak—cont'd

an adult should be 105° F to 110° F (41° C to 44° C).

6. **Procedural Step.** Assist the patient into a comfortable position to avoid fatigue and muscle strain. Pad the side of the basin with a towel for the patient's comfort.

7. **Procedural Step.** Slowly and gradually immerse the patient's affected body part in the solution. Ask the patient how the temperature feels.
Principle. The affected body part should gradually become accustomed to the change in temperature.

8. **Procedural Step.** Test the temperature of the solution frequently. To keep the solution at a constant temperature, remove cooler fluid every 5 minutes, and replace it with hot solution. Pour the hot solution in near the edge of the basin by placing your hand between the patient and the solution. Stir the solution as you pour.

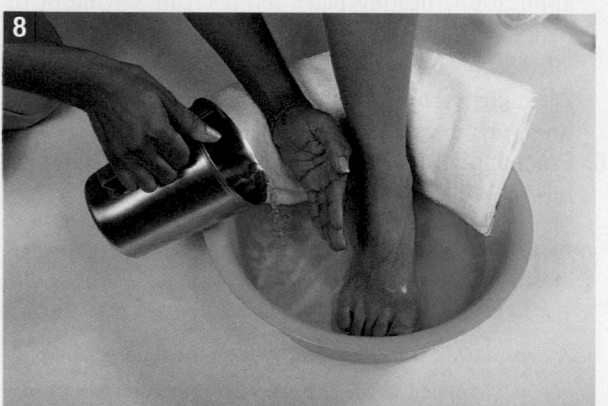

Replace cooler solution with hot solution.

Principle. The solution should be added away from the patient's body part to prevent splashing hot fluid on the patient. Stirring in the solution helps distribute the heat and keep the temperature constant.

9. **Procedural Step.** Check the patient's skin periodically for signs of an increase or decrease in redness or swelling, and ask the patient whether the site is painful. Apply the hot soak for the proper length of time as designated by the physician (usually 15 to 20 minutes).

10. **Procedural Step.** Dry the affected part completely and gently.

11. **Procedural Step.** Sanitize your hands, and chart the procedure. Include the date and time, method of heat application (hot soak), name and strength of the solution, temperature of the soak, location and duration of the application, appearance of the application site, and the patient's reaction.

12. **Procedural Step.** Properly care for equipment, and return it to its storage location.

CHARTING EXAMPLE

Date	
12/12/XX	1:15 p.m. Normal saline hot soak @ 105° F applied to ⓇR ankle x 20 min. Area appears pink following application. Pt states less stiffness in ankle. — M. Cooper, CMA (AAMA)

PROCEDURE 22-3 Applying a Hot Compress

Outcome Apply a hot compress.

Equipment/Supplies

- Solution ordered by the physician
- Bath thermometer
- Basin
- Washcloths
- Waterproof covering
- Towel

1. **Procedural Step.** Sanitize your hands.
2. **Procedural Step.** Assemble the equipment. Check the label on the solution container to make sure you have the correct solution as ordered by the physician. Place the solution containers in a basin of warm water. Warm the soaking solution to a temperature between 105° F and 110° F (41° C and 44° C).
3. **Procedural Step.** Greet the patient and introduce yourself. Identify the patient and explain the procedure. Explain the purpose of the application (e.g., to soften an exudate).
4. **Procedural Step.** Fill the basin half full with warmed solution. Check the temperature of the solution with

the bath thermometer. The temperature for an adult should be 105° F to 110° F (41° C to 44° C).

5. **Procedural Step.** Completely immerse the compress in the solution. Wring the compress to remove excess moisture. The compress should be wet but not dripping. Apply it lightly at first to the affected site to allow the patient to become used to the heat gradually. You may want to cover the compress with a waterproof cover to help hold in the heat. Ask the patient how the temperature feels. The compress should be as hot as the patient can comfortably tolerate.
Principle. The waterproof cover prevents cool air currents from coming into contact with the compress and

PROCEDURE 22-3 Applying a Hot Compress—cont'd

reduces the number of times the compress needs to be changed.

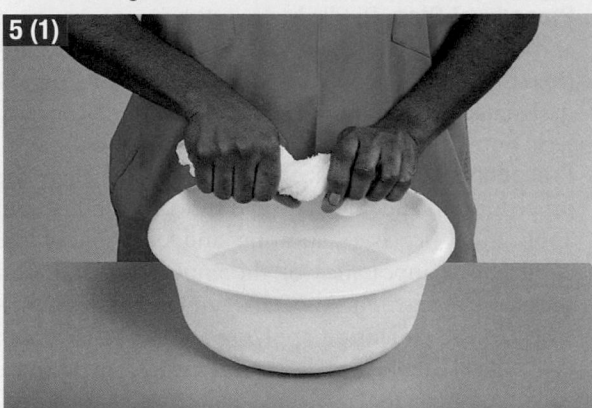

Wring out the compress.

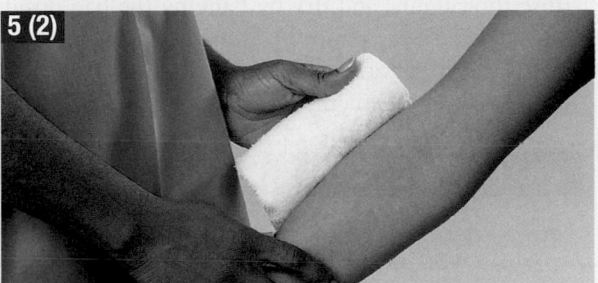

Apply the compress to the affected site.

6. **Procedural Step.** Place additional compresses in the solution so that they are ready for use.

7. **Procedural Step.** Repeat the application of the compress every 2 to 3 minutes for the duration of time specified by the physician (usually 15 to 20 minutes). Check the patient's skin periodically for signs of an increase or decrease in redness or swelling, and ask the patient whether the site is painful.

8. **Procedural Step.** Check the temperature of the solution periodically. Remove cooler fluid and replace it with hot solution if needed. Administer the treatment for the proper length of time as designated by the physician.

9. **Procedural Step.** Dry the affected part thoroughly and gently.

10. **Procedural Step.** Sanitize your hands, and chart the procedure. Include the date and time, method of heat application (hot compress), name and strength of the solution, temperature of the solution, location and duration of the application, appearance of the application site, and the patient's reaction.

11. **Procedural Step.** Properly care for equipment, and return it to its storage location.

CHARTING EXAMPLE

Date	
12/20/XX	10:30 a.m. Normal saline hot compress @ 110° F applied to Ⓡ forearm x 20 min. No complaints of discomfort. ——————— ———————— M. Cooper, CMA (AAMA)

PROCEDURE 22-4 Applying an Ice Bag

Outcome Apply an ice bag.

Equipment/Supplies

- Ice bag with a protective covering
- Small pieces of ice (ice chips or crushed ice)

1. **Procedural Step.** Sanitize your hands.
2. **Procedural Step.** Assemble the equipment.
3. **Procedural Step.** Greet the patient and introduce yourself. Identify the patient and explain the procedure. Explain the purpose of applying the ice bag (e.g., to prevent swelling).
4. **Procedural Step.** Check the ice bag for leakage.
   Principle. A leaking bag would get the patient wet and cause chilling.

5. **Procedural Step.** Fill the bag one-half to two-thirds full with small pieces of ice.
   Principle. Small pieces of ice work better than large pieces because they reduce the air spaces in the bag, resulting in better conduction of cold. In addition, small pieces of ice allow the bag to mold better to the body area.
6. **Procedural Step.** Expel air from the bag by squeezing the empty top half of the bag together and screwing on the stopper.

Continued

PROCEDURE 22-4 Applying an Ice Bag—cont'd

Principle. Air is a poor conductor of cold and makes it difficult to mold the ice bag to the body area.

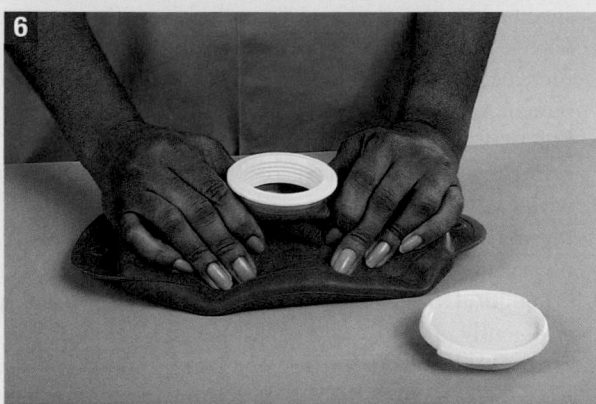

Expel air from the bag.

7. Procedural Step. Place the bag in the protective covering.
Principle. The protective covering provides for patient comfort and absorbs the moisture that condenses on the outside of the bag.

8. Procedural Step. Place the bag on the patient's affected body area. Ask the patient how the temperature feels. The application of ice is usually uncomfortable, but most patients tolerate it when they know how much benefit may be derived from it.
Principle. Individuals vary in their ability to tolerate cold.

9. Procedural Step. Check the patient's skin periodically for signs of an increase or decrease in redness or swelling, and ask the patient whether the site is painful. If extreme paleness and numbness or a mottled blue appearance occur at the application site, remove the bag, and notify the physician.

10. Procedural Step. Refill the bag with ice as necessary, and change the protective covering if needed. Administer the treatment for the proper length of time, as designated by the physician (usually until the area feels numb, approximately 15 to 30 minutes).

11. Procedural Step. Sanitize your hands, and chart the procedure. Include the date and time, method of cold application (ice bag), location and duration of the application, appearance of the application site, and the patient's reaction. Also, chart any instructions provided to the patient on applying an ice bag at home.

12. Procedural Step. Properly care for the ice bag. Dispose of or launder the protective covering as required. Cleanse the ice bag with a warm detergent solution, rinse thoroughly, and dry by hanging the bag upside down with the top removed. Store the bag by screwing on the stopper, leaving air inside to prevent the sides from sticking together.

CHARTING EXAMPLE

Date	
12/22/XX	11:30 a.m. Ice bag applied to Ⓡ knee x 20 min. Pt complained of slight discomfort during the application. Area appears less swollen following application. Provided instructions on the application of an ice bag at home. _____ M. Cooper, CMA (AAMA)

PROCEDURE 22-5 Applying a Cold Compress

Outcome Apply a cold compress.

Equipment/Supplies

- Ice cubes
- Basin
- Washcloths
- Towel
- Ice bag

1. Procedural Step. Sanitize your hands.

2. Procedural Step. Assemble the equipment. Check the label on the solution container to make sure you have the correct solution as ordered by the physician.

3. Procedural Step. Greet the patient and introduce yourself. Identify the patient and explain the procedure. Explain the purpose of the application (e.g., to treat an eye injury).

4. Procedural Step. Place large ice cubes in the basin. Add the solution until the basin is half full.
Principle. Using larger pieces of ice prevents them from sticking to the compress and slows the rate at which they melt in the solution.

PROCEDURE 22-5   Applying a Cold Compress—cont'd

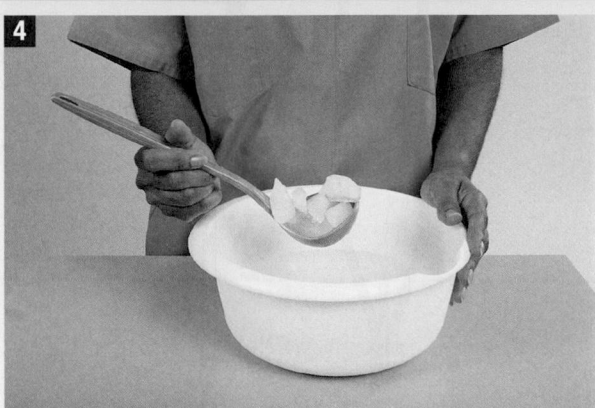

Place large ice cubes in the basin.

5. Procedural Step. Completely immerse the compress in the solution. Wring the compress to rid it of excess moisture. The compress should be wet but not dripping. Apply it lightly at first to the affected site to allow the patient to become used to the cold gradually. The compress can be covered with an ice bag to help keep it cold and to reduce the number of times it needs to be changed. Ask the patient how the temperature feels.

6. Procedural Step. Place additional compresses in the solution to be ready for use.

7. Procedural Step. Repeat the application of the compress every 2 to 3 minutes for the duration of time specified by the physician (usually 15 to 20 minutes). Check the patient's skin periodically for signs of an increase or decrease in redness or swelling, and ask the patient whether the site is painful.

8. Procedural Step. Add ice if needed to keep the solution cold. Administer the treatment for the proper length of time designated by the physician.

9. Procedural Step. Thoroughly dry the affected part.

10. Procedural Step. Sanitize your hands, and chart the procedure. Include the date and time, method of cold application (cold compress), location and duration of the application, appearance of the application site, and the patient's reaction.

11. Procedural Step. Properly care for equipment, and return it to its storage location.

CHARTING EXAMPLE

Date	
12/27/XX	9:15 a.m. Normal saline cold compress applied to bridge of nose x 15 min. Nose appears less swollen following application. Tolerated application well.—————————
	————————— M. Cooper, CMA (AAMA)

PROCEDURE 22-6   Applying a Chemical Pack

Outcome Apply a chemical cold pack and a chemical hot pack.

The procedure for applying a chemical cold or hot pack is as follows:

1. Procedural Step. Shake the crystals to the bottom of the bag.

2. Procedural Step. Squeeze the bag firmly with your hands to break the inner water bag.

3. Procedural Step. Shake the bag vigorously to mix the contents.

4. Procedural Step. Cover the bag with a protective covering.

5. Procedural Step. Apply the bag to the affected area. Check the patient's skin periodically.

6. Procedural Step. Administer the treatment for the proper length of time.

7. Procedural Step. Discard the bag in an appropriate receptacle.

8. Procedural Step. Sanitize your hands, and chart the procedure. Include the date and time, method of application (chemical cold or hot pack), location and duration of the application, appearance of the application site, and the patient's reaction.

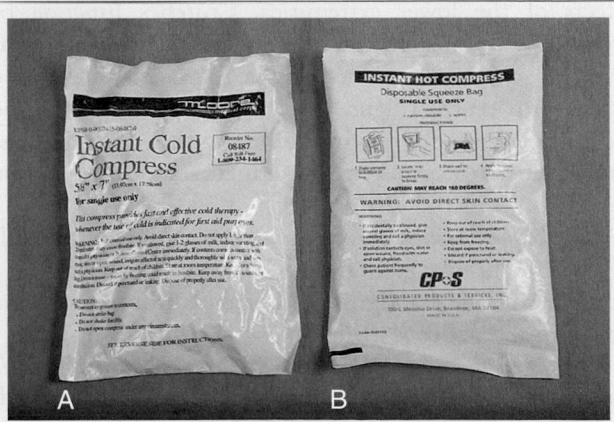

Chemical packs. **A,** Chemical cold pack; **B,** Chemical hot pack.

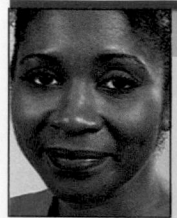

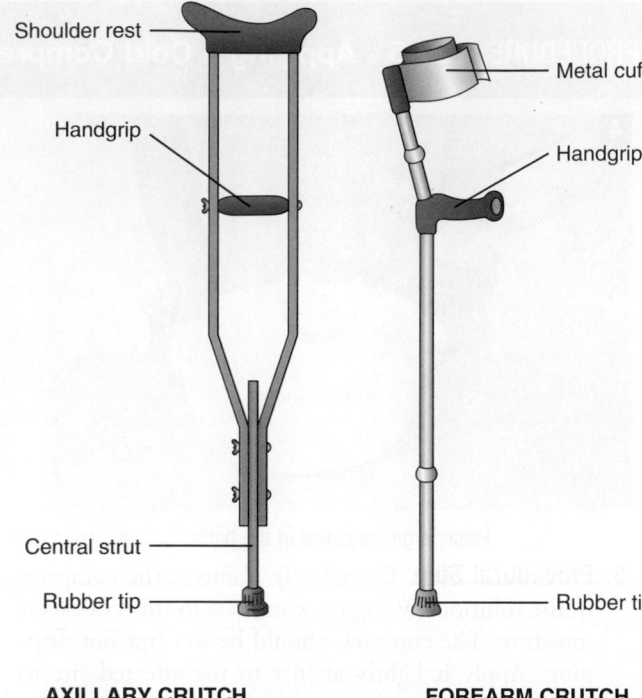

Figure 22-2 Types of crutches.

AMBULATORY AIDS

Mechanical assistive devices are used by individuals who require aid in ambulation. The word **ambulation** means walking; patients who are **ambulatory** are able to walk as opposed to being confined to a wheelchair or a bed. Ambulatory aids include crutches, canes, and walkers. The device used depends on factors such as the type and severity of the disability, the amount of support required, and the patient's age and degree of muscular coordination. The ambulatory aid may be prescribed for a temporary condition, such as a fracture, a sprain to a lower extremity, and disability after orthopedic surgery. It also may be prescribed for a long-term condition, such as paralysis, deformity, and permanent weakness of the lower extremities.

Crutches

Crutches are artificial supports that consist of wood or tubular aluminum. They are used for patients who require assistance in walking as a result of disease, injury, or birth defects of the lower extremities. Crutches function by removing weight from the legs and transferring it to the arms. The two main crutch types are the axillary crutch and the forearm crutch (Figure 22-2). The axillary crutch and the forearm crutch require rubber tips, which increase surface tension, to prevent the crutches from slipping on the floor.

The *axillary crutch* is used most frequently and is made of wood or tubular aluminum. This type of crutch has a shoulder rest and handgrips and extends from the ground almost to the patient's axilla.

The *forearm crutch,* also known as a *Lofstrand crutch,* consists of a single adjustable tube of aluminum that extends to the forearm. A metal cuff attached to the crutch fits securely around the patient's forearm, and a handgrip covered with rubber extends from the crutch for weight bearing. The metal cuff and the handgrip stabilize the patient's wrists to make walking safer and easier. One advantage of the forearm crutch is that the individual can release

the handgrip, enabling use of the hand, while the metal cuff holds the crutch in place. Individuals who are paraplegic or have cerebral palsy use the forearm crutch most often.

Axillary Crutch Measurement

The patient must be measured for axillary crutches to ensure the correct crutch length and proper placement of the handgrip. Incorrectly fitted crutches increase the patient's risk of developing back pain, nerve damage, and injuries to the axillae and palms of the hands. Procedure 22-7 presents the correct way to measure a patient for axillary crutches.

If the crutches are too long, the shoulder rests exert pressure on the patient's axillae. This can injure the radial nerve in the brachial plexus, which eventually may lead to *crutch palsy,* a condition of muscular weakness in the forearm, wrist, and hand. In addition, crutches that are too long force the patient's shoulders forward, preventing the patient from pushing his or her body off the ground. Crutches that are too short force the patient to be bent over and uncomfortable, also making them awkward to use. If the handgrips are too low, pressure is put on the patient's axillae, whereas handgrips that are too high are awkward.

Wooden crutches are made with bolts and wing nuts, which allow proper adjustment of the length and handgrip level. Aluminum crutches consist of aluminum tubes. Spring-loaded pushbuttons on an inner tube "pop out" into holes on an outer tube to allow proper adjustment of the crutch length.

Crutch Guidelines

It is important that the patient receive specific guidelines to ensure safety while using crutches, to prevent injuries and

Highlight on Ambulatory Aids

Many people who could benefit from ambulatory aids are not using them. The primary reason is that they do not know how to use them correctly, become discouraged, and quit using them.

Other types of aids available to assist individuals with physical disabilities include raised toilet seats, handle bars, carrying devices, tub seats, over-bed tables, and swivel cushions for assistance in getting into and out of cars.

If an individual needs help in learning to drive with a physical disability, the local bureau of vocational rehabilitation or the state motor vehicle department can provide information on qualified instruction available in the community.

Walking with an ambulatory aid is a physiologic stressor to the body because it requires more energy than normal walking. Because of this, individuals need to rest frequently when using an ambulatory aid.

Many people need to have their crutches lengthened after they have had them for a while. This is because their posture improves as they gain confidence in walking with them. Children and teenagers who use crutches for a long time also need frequent adjustments as they grow.

A cane can provide security to the individual using it; however, it can be more trouble than it is worth if it is the incorrect size. It is estimated that two thirds of people who buy canes select one that is too long.

Some walkers are designed to fit over chairs and toilets, allowing the user additional support when rising or sitting. Folding walkers are available, and they are easy to store and transport. ■

PATIENT TEACHING Crutches

- Teach patients the guidelines for the proper use of crutches.
  - Provide the patient with an exercise sheet that illustrates exercises to strengthen arm muscles before beginning crutch walking.
  - Teach the patient the crutch gaits prescribed by the physician, and have the patient demonstrate the gaits before leaving the office.
  - Provide the patient with a list of local vendors who provide crutch services, such as repairs and supplies (e.g., rubber tips, crutch pads).
  - Provide the patient with printed educational materials on the use of crutches and crutch gaits.

falls. The medical assistant is responsible for instructing the patient in the following guidelines:

1. Wear well-fitting flat shoes with firm, nonskid soles to provide good traction and stability.
2. Use correct posture to prevent strain on muscles and joints and to maintain proper body balance.
3. Support your weight with your hands on the handgrips and the axillary pads pressing against the sides of the rib cage. The body weight should not be supported by the axillae because pressure on the axillae may cause crutch palsy.
4. Look ahead when walking, rather than down at your feet.
5. Be aware of the surface on which you are walking. It should be clean, flat, dry, and well lighted. Throw rugs and objects serving as obstacles should temporarily be removed from your environment to prevent falls.
6. Keep the crutches about 4 to 6 inches out from the sides of your feet when walking to prevent obstruction of the pathway for the feet.

7. Take steps by moving the crutches forward a safe and comfortable distance, preferably 6 inches. When first learning to use the crutches, take small steps rather than large ones. Do not move forward more than 12 to 15 inches with each step. A greater distance might cause the crutches to slide forward and you to lose your balance.
8. Report tingling or numbness in the upper body to the physician. You might be using the crutches incorrectly, or they might be the wrong size for you.
9. Extra padding can be added to the shoulder rests of your crutches to make them more comfortable. If you do this, ensure that the extra padding does not press against your axillae, but rather against your lateral rib cage. The handgrips also can be padded for increased comfort.
10. To prevent slipping, keep the crutch tips dry to maintain their surface friction. If they become wet, dry them completely before use.
11. Inspect the crutch tips regularly. They should be securely attached. If the crutch tips are worn down, they should be replaced with tips of the proper size.
12. For wooden crutches, periodically check the wing nuts holding the central strut and handgrips in place to ensure that they are tight.

Crutch Gaits

The type of crutch gait used depends on the amount of weight the patient is able to support with one or both legs and the patient's physical condition and muscular coordination. The patient should learn a fast and a slow gait. The faster gait is used for making speed in open areas, and the slower one is used in crowded places. In addition, learning more than one gait reduces patient fatigue because a different combination of muscles is used for each gait. Procedure 22-8 provides guidelines and charts for use in instructing the patient on how to walk with crutches.

Canes

A cane is a lightweight, easily movable device made of wood or aluminum with a rubber tip and is used to help provide balance and support. Canes are generally used by patients who have weakness on one side of the body, such as patients with hemiparesis, joint disabilities, or defects of the neuro-muscular system. The three main types of canes are the *standard cane,* the *tripod cane,* and the *quad cane* (Figure 22-3). The standard cane provides the least amount of support and is used by patients who require only slight assistance in walking. The tripod and quad canes have three and four legs, respectively, a bent shaft, and a T-shaped handle with grips. They are easier to hold and provide greater stability than a standard cane because of the wider base of support. In addition, multilegged canes are able to stand alone, which frees the arms when the patient is getting up from a chair. The disadvantage of a multilegged cane is that it is bulkier and more difficult to move.

A cane is held on the side of the body that is opposite to the side that needs support. The cane length must be properly adjusted to ensure optimal stability. The cane handle should be approximately level with the greater trochanter, and the elbow should be flexed at a 25- to 30-degree angle. The patient should be instructed to stand erect and not lean on the cane to ensure good balance. Procedure 22-9 presents guidelines on instructing the patient on how to walk with a cane.

Walkers

A walker is an ambulatory aid consisting of an aluminum frame with handgrips and four widely placed legs with rubber suction tips and one open side (Figure 22-4). A walker is light and easily movable. Walkers are available with wheels that facilitate movement of the walker. They are also available with a fold-up feature that allows them to be easily transported in a vehicle. For proper ambulation, the walker should extend from the ground to approximately the level of the patient's hip joint. Procedure 22-10 presents guidelines on instructing the patient on how to walk with a walker.

Walkers are used most often by geriatric patients with weakness or balance problems. Walkers also are used during the healing process for patients who have had knee or hip joint replacement surgery. These patients need more help with balance and walking than can be provided by crutches or a cane. Because of its wide base, a walker provides the patient with a great amount of stability and security. Disadvantages of a walker include a slow pace and difficulty in maneuvering the walker in a small room.

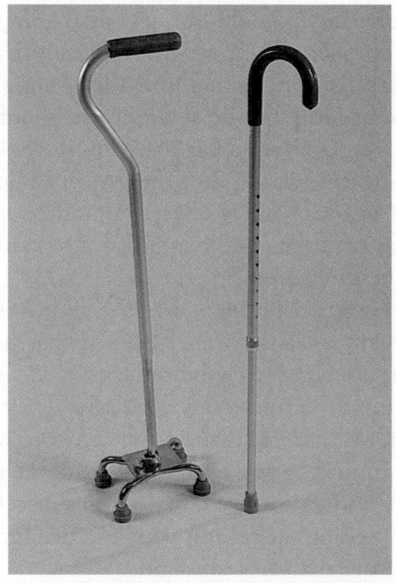

Figure 22-3 Examples of a quad cane *(left)* and a standard cane *(right).*

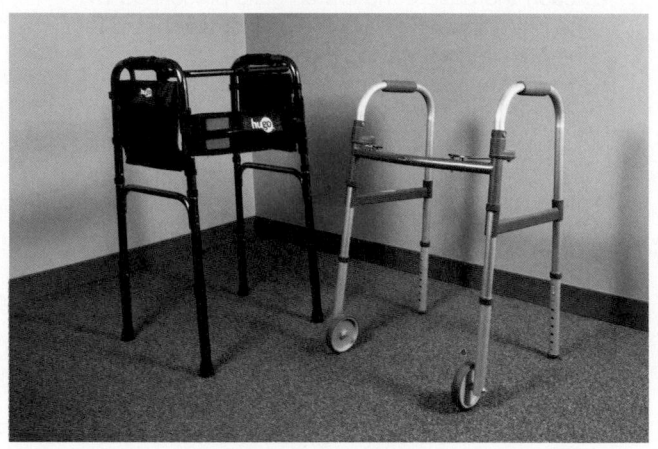

Figure 22-4 Walkers.

What Would You Do? What Would You *Not* Do?

Case Study 2

Thaddeus Bernard calls the office. Thaddeus fractured the femur of his left leg 2 weeks ago in a skiing accident. The physician applied a long leg fiberglass cast, and Thaddeus was properly fitted with aluminum crutches. Thaddeus says that he is having some problems with his crutches. He is complaining of weakness in his forearms and hands and some tingling and numbness in his fingers. He also says that he has bruises under his arms. Thaddeus says that after he got home, his crutches didn't seem to fit right, so he readjusted them. Thaddeus is getting ready to return to college and wants to know the best way to carry his books while using crutches. ■

PROCEDURE 22-7 **Measuring for Axillary Crutches**

Outcome Measure an individual for axillary crutches.

Determining Crutch Length

For you to determine crutch length correctly, the patient must wear shoes while being measured. The measurement can be taken while the patient is standing.

1. **Procedural Step.** Ask the patient to stand erect.
2. **Procedural Step.** Position the crutches with the crutch tips at a distance of 2 inches (5 cm) in front of and 4 to 6 inches (15 cm) to the side of each foot. (The large dots in the figure represent crutch tips.)
3. **Procedural Step.** Adjust the crutch length so that the shoulder rests are approximately 1½ to 2 inches (about 2 finger widths) below the axillae.
   Wooden crutches. The length of the crutch is adjusted by removing the bolt and wing nut and sliding the central strut (support piece) at the bottom upward or downward as necessary to attain the proper length. The strut is secured by replacing the bolt and securely fastening the wing nut.
   Tubular aluminum crutches. The length of the crutch is adjusted by pressing the spring-loaded push button with your thumb and sliding the outer tube upward or downward as necessary to attain the proper length. The spring-loaded button on the inner tube should be allowed to "pop out" into the appropriate hole on the outer tube.

Handgrip Positioning

When the crutch length has been adjusted, correct placement of the handgrips must be determined.

1. **Procedural Step.** Ask the patient to stand erect with a crutch under each arm and to support his or her weight by the handgrips.
2. **Procedural Step.** Adjust the handgrips on the crutches so that the patient's elbow is flexed to an angle of approximately 30 degrees. The handgrip level is adjusted by removing the bolt and wing nut and sliding the handgrip upward or downward, as required. The handgrip is secured by replacing the bolt and tightly fastening the wing nut. The angle of elbow flexion can be verified by using a measuring device known as a *goniometer.* A goniometer is an instrument that measures the angle of a joint.
3. **Procedural Step.** Check the fit of the crutches. If the crutches are measured correctly, the medical assistant should be able to insert two fingers between the top of the crutches and the axillae when the patient is standing erect with the crutches under the arms.

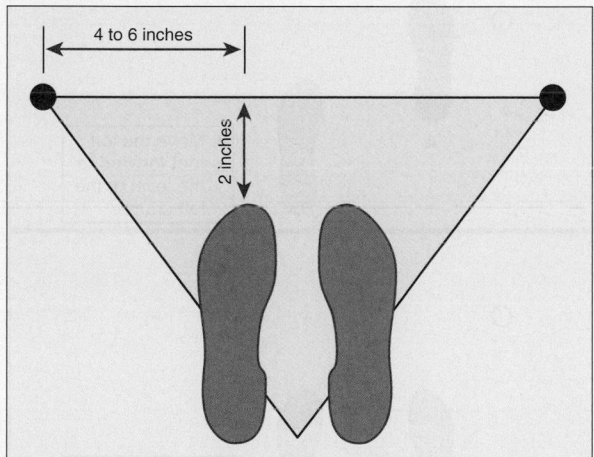

Position for measuring for crutches.

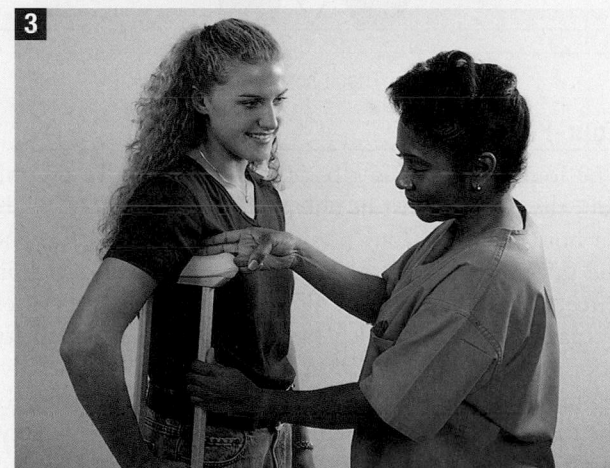

Insert two fingers between the top of the crutch and the axilla.

PROCEDURE 22-7

PROCEDURE 22-8 Instructing a Patient in Crutch Gaits

Outcome Instruct a patient in the following crutch gaits: four-point, two-point, three-point, swing-to, and swing-through.

Tripod Position

The tripod position is the basic crutch stance used before crutch walking. It provides a wide base of support and enhances stability and balance.

Instruct the patient in the tripod position as follows:

1. **Procedural Step.** Stand erect, and face straight ahead.
2. **Procedural Step.** Place the tips of the crutches 4 to 6 inches (15 cm) in front of the feet and 4 to 6 inches (10 to 15 cm) to the side of each foot. (The large dots in the figure represent crutch tips.)

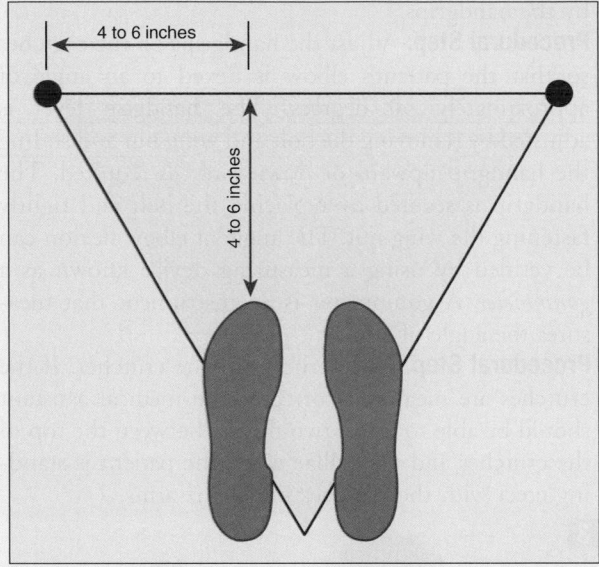

Tripod position.

Four-Point Gait

The four-point gait is a basic and slow gait. To use this gait, the patient must be able to bear considerable weight on both legs. The four-point gait is the most stable and the safest of the crutch gaits because it provides at least three points of support at all times. It is used most often by patients who have leg muscle weakness or spasticity, poor muscular coordination or balance, or degenerative leg joint disease. Instruct the patient in the procedure for the four-point gait, following the steps in the accompanying figure.

CHARTING EXAMPLE

Date	
12/15/XX	1:30 p.m. Instructed pt in four-point gait. Pt
	was able to demonstrate four-point gait. ————
	———————— M. Cooper, CMA (AAMA)

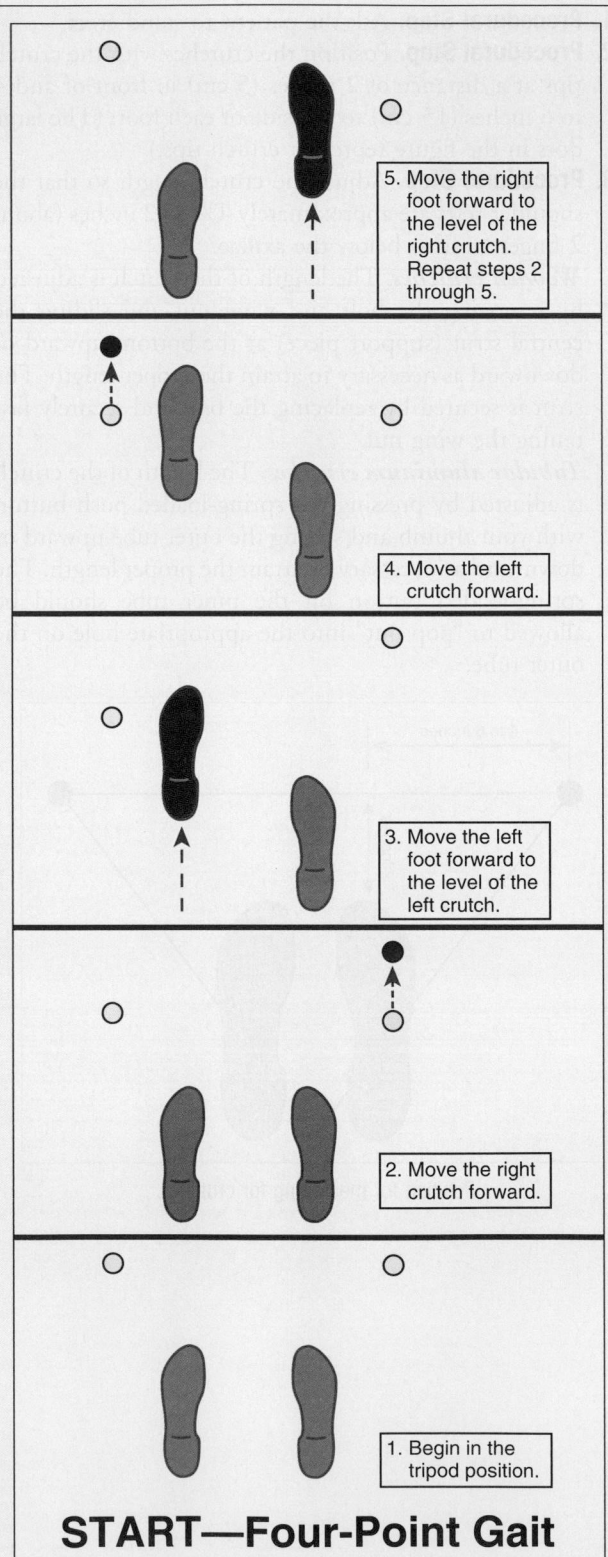

5. Move the right foot forward to the level of the right crutch. Repeat steps 2 through 5.

4. Move the left crutch forward.

3. Move the left foot forward to the level of the left crutch.

2. Move the right crutch forward.

1. Begin in the tripod position.

START—Four-Point Gait

PROCEDURE 22-8 **Instructing a Patient in Crutch Gaits—cont'd**

Two-Point Gait

The two-point gait is similar to, but faster than, the four-point gait. This gait requires better balance because only two points support the body at one time. The two-point gait is used when the patient is capable of partial weight bearing on each foot and has good muscular coordination. Instruct the patient in the procedure for the two-point gait, following the steps in the accompanying figure.

Three-Point Gait

The three-point gait is used by patients who cannot bear weight on one leg. The patient must be able to support his or her full weight on the unaffected leg. With this gait, the crutches and the unaffected leg alternately bear the patient's weight. This gait is used most often by amputees without a prosthesis, patients with musculoskeletal or soft tissue trauma to a lower extremity (e.g., fracture, sprain), patients with acute leg inflammation, and patients who have had recent leg surgery. To use this gait, the patient must have good muscular coordination and arm strength. Instruct the patient in the procedure for the three-point gait, following the steps in the accompanying figure.

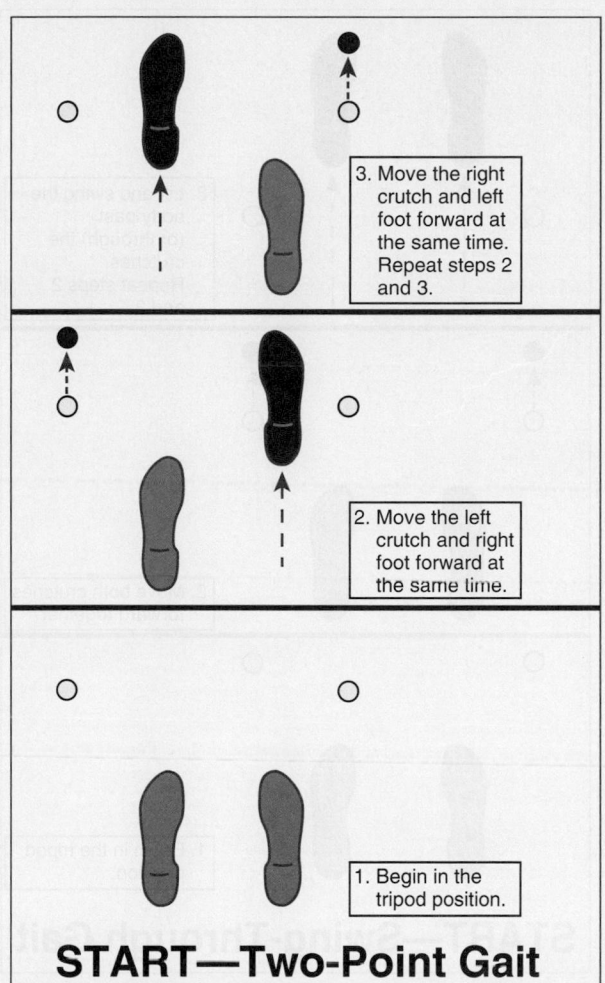

3. Move the right crutch and left foot forward at the same time. Repeat steps 2 and 3.

2. Move the left crutch and right foot forward at the same time.

1. Begin in the tripod position.

START—Two-Point Gait

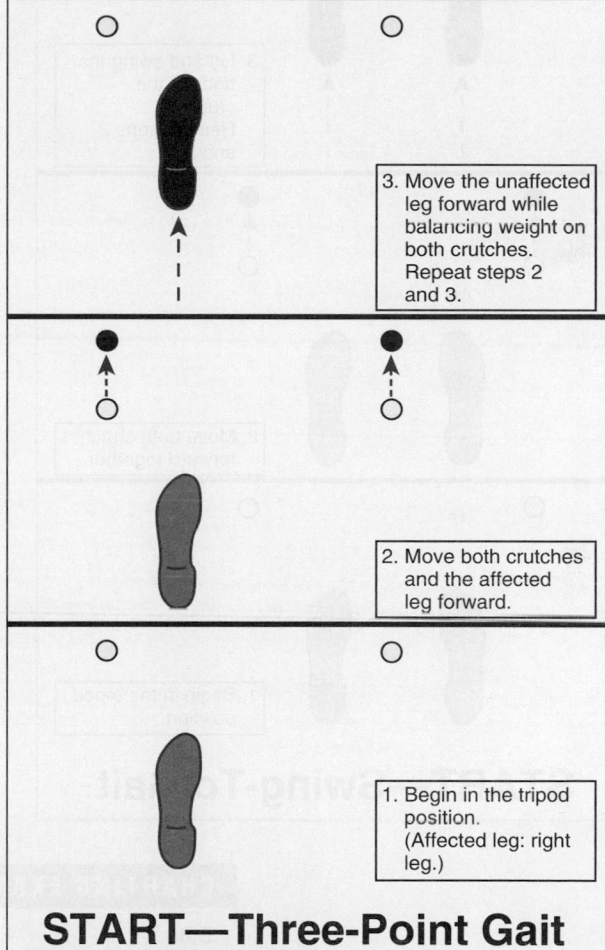

3. Move the unaffected leg forward while balancing weight on both crutches. Repeat steps 2 and 3.

2. Move both crutches and the affected leg forward.

1. Begin in the tripod position. (Affected leg: right leg.)

START—Three-Point Gait

CHARTING EXAMPLE

Date	
12/16/XX	2:30 p.m. Instructed pt in two-point gait. Pt was able to demonstrate two-point gait. —————————— M. Cooper, CMA (AAMA)

CHARTING EXAMPLE

Date	
12/17/XX	2:30 p.m. Instructed pt in three-point gait. Pt was able to demonstrate three-point gait. —————————— M. Cooper, CMA (AAMA)

PROCEDURE 22-8

Continued

PROCEDURE 22-8   Instructing a Patient in Crutch Gaits—cont'd

Swing Gaits

The swing gaits include the swing-to gait and the swing-through gait and are used by patients with severe lower extremity disabilities, such as paralysis, and by patients who wear supporting braces on their legs.

Instruct the patient in the procedures for the swing-to and the swing-through crutch gaits, following the steps in the accompanying figures.

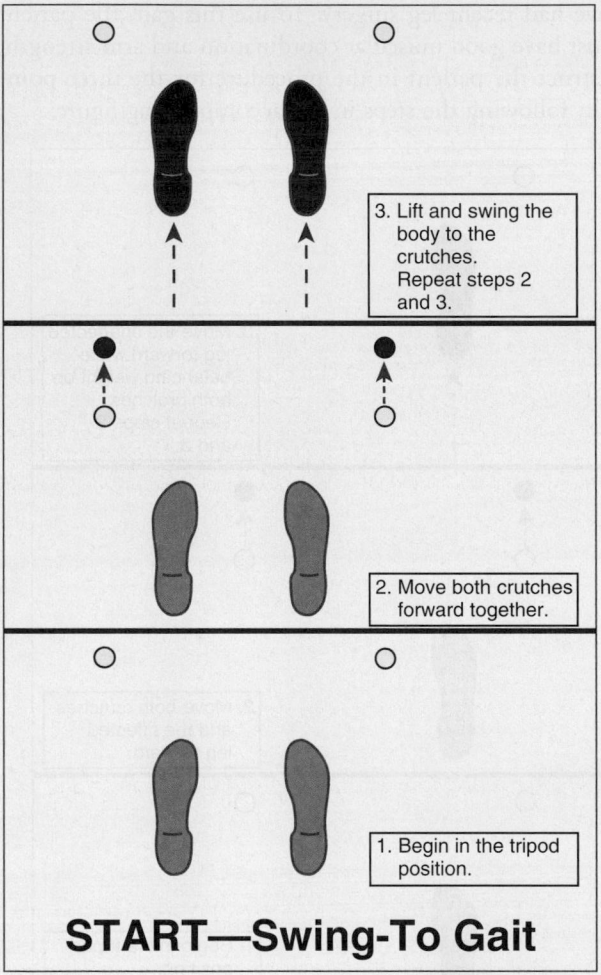

3. Lift and swing the body to the crutches. Repeat steps 2 and 3.

2. Move both crutches forward together.

1. Begin in the tripod position.

START—Swing-To Gait

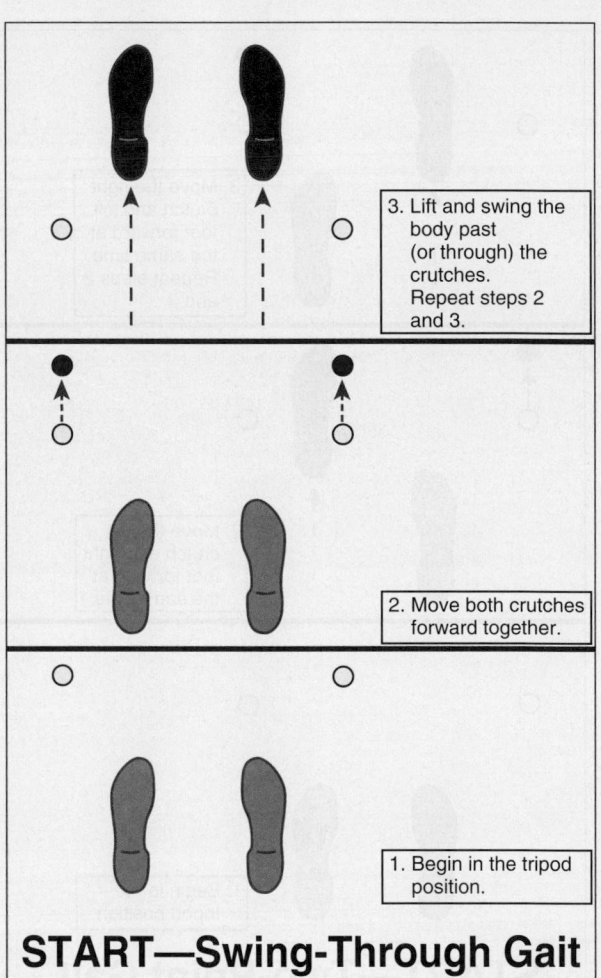

3. Lift and swing the body past (or through) the crutches. Repeat steps 2 and 3.

2. Move both crutches forward together.

1. Begin in the tripod position.

START—Swing-Through Gait

CHARTING EXAMPLE	
Date	
12/18/XX	3:30 p.m. Instructed pt in swing-to and swing-through gaits. Pt was able to demonstrate swing gaits.— M. Cooper, CMA (AAMA)

PROCEDURE 22-9   Instructing a Patient in Use of a Cane

Outcome Instruct the patient in the use of a cane.

1. **Procedural Step.** Hold the cane on the strong side of the body (i.e., in the hand opposite the affected extremity).
2. **Procedural Step.** Place the tip of the cane 4 to 6 inches to the side of the foot.
3. **Procedural Step.** Move the cane forward approximately 12 inches (1 foot).

4. **Procedural Step.** Move the affected leg forward to the level of the cane.
5. **Procedural Step.** Move the strong leg forward and ahead of the cane and weak leg.
6. **Procedural Step.** Repeat steps 3 through 5.
   NOTE: The cane and the affected leg can be moved forward simultaneously (steps 3 and 4); however, the patient has less support with this method.

PROCEDURE 22-10   Instructing a Patient in Use of a Walker

Outcome Instruct the patient in the use of a walker.

1. **Procedural Step.** Pick up the walker, and move it forward approximately 6 inches.

2. **Procedural Step.** Move the right foot and then the left foot up to the walker.
3. **Procedural Step.** Repeat steps 1 and 2.

MEDICAL PRACTICE *and the* LAW

The procedures described in this chapter deal with the goal of returning full function to an injured area. Sometimes, despite correct treatment, full function does not return. This problem can become a legal issue if the patient believes that he or she should have healed fully or cannot return to work. To protect yourself, follow each procedure to the letter, and record the patient's progress (or lack of progress) carefully in the medical record. Sometimes the patient is involved in insurance fraud and falsely complains of pain or impaired function to continue receiving disability benefits. If you suspect this is the case, objectively document the functions you have seen the patient perform.

The application of heat and cold must be performed precisely to maximize effectiveness of the treatment without injury to the patient. Failure to follow procedures correctly or to obtain the correct temperature could leave you legally liable.

Ambulatory aids used correctly can help the patient regain mobility. If crutches are used improperly, the patient could fall or develop nerve or other injuries. When instructing about ambulation aid use, allow enough time for the patient to give a return demonstration, and send home written instructions in case the patient forgets what was taught. ■

What Would You Do? What Would You *Not* Do? RESPONSES

Case Study 1
Page 412

What Did Marlyne Do?
❑ Empathized with Aaron for being in so much pain.
❑ Explained to Aaron that he should never sleep on a heating pad because the heat builds up and causes the type of burn he experienced.
❑ Explained to Aaron that it is best to apply heat for 15 to 30 minutes at a time with the pad set no higher than the medium setting. Told him the pad may not feel warm after his body gets used to it, but that it is still helping him. Told Aaron that the high setting could burn his skin.
❑ Told Aaron how to prevent low back pain by using good body mechanics, especially during lifting.

What Did Marlyne Not Do?
❑ Did not criticize Aaron for sleeping on the heating pad or turning the pad to the high setting.

What Would You Do?/What Would You Not Do?
Review Marlyne's response and place a checkmark next to the information you included in your response. List the additional information you included in your response.

_____
_____
_____
_____
_____
_____
_____

Case Study 2
Page 420

What Did Marlyne Do?
❑ Listened carefully and empathetically to Thaddeus's problems with and concerns about his crutches.

Continued

PROCEDURES 22-9 and 22-10

What Would You Do? What Would You *Not* Do? RESPONSES—cont'd

❑ Explained to Thaddeus that the crutches were adjusted to fit him properly at the office and that he may have caused some problems by readjusting them.

❑ Scheduled an appointment for Thaddeus to come in that day so the physician could examine him and his crutches could be checked for proper length.

❑ Went over crutch guidelines and crutch gaits with Thaddeus again when he came to the office for his appointment.

❑ Told Thaddeus that he should use a backpack to carry his books to keep his hands free to move on his crutches. Stressed that he should keep his backpack as light as possible and keep the weight evenly distributed on his back (i.e., use both straps).

What Did Marlyne Not Do?

❑ Did not tell Thaddeus to readjust the crutches himself.

❑ Did not tell Thaddeus that he should have paid more attention when he was being instructed in crutch guidelines.

What Would You Do?/What Would You *Not* Do?

Review Marlyne's response and place a checkmark next to the information you included in your response. List the additional information you included in your response.

_____
_____
_____
_____
_____
_____
_____

TERMINOLOGY REVIEW

Medical Term	Word Parts	Definition
Ambulation		Walking or moving from one place to another.
Ambulatory		Able to walk as opposed to being confined to bed or a wheelchair.
Compress		A soft, moist, absorbent cloth that is folded in several layers and applied to a part of the body in the local application of heat or cold.
Edema		The retention of fluid in the tissues, resulting in swelling.
Erythema	hem/o: blood	Reddening of the skin caused by dilation of superficial blood vessels in the skin.
Exudate		A discharge produced by the body's tissues.
Soak		The direct immersion of a body part in water or a medicated solution.
Sprain		Trauma to a joint that causes injury to the ligaments.
Strain		An overstretching of a muscle caused by trauma.
Suppuration		The process of pus formation.

ON THE WEB

For information on rehabilitation and disability:

National Rehabilitation Information Center (NARIC): www.naric.com

American Academy of Orthopaedic Surgeons: www.aaos.org

About.com: Orthopedics: orthopedics.about.com

American Physical Therapy Association: www.apta.org

American Chiropractic Association: www.amerchiro.org

American Occupational Therapy Association: www.aota.org

National Stroke Association (NSA): www.stroke.org

Arthritis Foundation: www.arthritis.org

National Institute of Arthritis and Musculoskeletal and Skin Diseases: www.niams.nih.gov

American Academy of Physical Medicine and Rehabilitation: www.aapmr.org

Check out the Evolve site at http://evolve.elsevier.com/Bonewit/today/ to actively Prepare for your Certification, and to access additional interactive activities and exercises to help you study and prepare for success.

23

The Gynecologic Examination and Prenatal Care

Obstetric Terminology
Prenatal Visits
First Prenatal Visit
Prenatal Record

Special Tests and Procedures
Medical Assistant Responsibilities

Breast Examination
Pelvic Examination
Inspection of External Genitalia, Vagina, and Cervix
Pap Test

Rectal-Vaginal Examination
Vaginal Infections
Trichomoniasis

LEARNING OBJECTIVES

Gynecologic Examination
1. State the purpose of the gynecologic examination.
2. Identify the components of the gynecologic examination.

Breast Examination
3. Explain the purpose of a breast examination.

Pelvic Examination
4. Explain the purpose of a pelvic examination.
5. List and describe the four parts of the pelvic examination.
6. State the purpose of a Pap test.
7. List the advantages and disadvantages of the liquid-based Pap test.
8. List and describe each category on a cytology request for a Pap test.

Vaginal Infections
9. Identify the symptoms of each of the following:
   Trichomoniasis
   Candidiasis
   Chlamydia
   Gonorrhea
10. Explain how each of the above-listed infections is diagnosed.

Prenatal Visits
11. Explain the purpose of each part of the prenatal record.
12. List and explain the purpose of each procedure included in the initial prenatal examination.
13. List and explain the purpose of each prenatal laboratory test.
14. Explain the purpose of return prenatal visits.
15. Explain the purpose of each of the following:
   Triple screen test
   Ultrasound scan
   Amniocentesis
   Fetal heart rate monitoring

PROCEDURES

Instruct patient in the procedure for a breast self-examination.

Prepare patient for a gynecologic examination.
Assist the physician with a gynecologic examination.
Complete a cytology requisition form.

Assist in the collection of a vaginal microbiologic specimen.

Calculate the expected date of delivery (EDD).

Complete a prenatal health history.
Assist with an initial prenatal examination.
Assist with a return prenatal examination.

CHAPTER OUTLINE

INTRODUCTION TO THE GYNECOLOGIC EXAMINATION AND PRENATAL CARE
GYNECOLOGIC EXAMINATION
Gynecology
Terms Related to Gynecology
Breast Examination
Pelvic Examination
Inspection of External Genitalia, Vagina, and Cervix
Pap Test
Bimanual Pelvic Examination
Rectal-Vaginal Examination
Vaginal Infections
Trichomoniasis
Candidiasis

Chlamydia
Gonorrhea
PRENATAL CARE
Obstetrics
Obstetric Terminology
Prenatal Visits
First Prenatal Visit
Prenatal Record
Initial Prenatal Examination
Return Prenatal Visits
Special Tests and Procedures
Medical Assisting Responsibilities

KEY TERMS

Gynecology
adnexal (ad-NEKS-al)
amenorrhea (AY-men-ah-REE-ah)
atypical (ay-TIP-ih-kul)
cervix (SER-viks)
colposcopy (kol-POS-koe-pee)
cytology (sy-TOL-oh-jee)
dysmenorrhea (DIS-men-ah-REE-ah)
dyspareunia (DIS-pah-ROO-nee-ah)
dysplasia (dis-PLAY-shah)
ectocervix (EK-toe-SER-viks)
endocervix (EN-doe-SER-viks)
external os (eks-TER-nal AHS)
gynecology (gie-nuh-KOL-oh-jee)
menopause (MEN-oh-paws)
menorrhagia (men-uh-RAY-jee-ah)
metrorrhagia (met-ro-RAY-jee-ah)
perimenopause (PEAR-ee-MEN-oh-paws)

perineum (pear-ih-NEE-um)
risk factor
vulva (VUL-va)
Obstetrics
abortion (ah-BOR-shun)
Braxton Hicks contractions (BRAK-stun
   HIKS con-TRAK-shuns)
dilation (die-LAY-shun) (of the cervix)
effacement (eh-FAYS-ment)
embryo (EM-bree-oh)
engagement
expected date of delivery (EDD)
fetal heart rate
fetal heart tones
fetus (FEE-tus)
fundus (FUN-dus)
gestation (jess-TAY-shun)
gestational (jess-TAY-shun-al) age

infant
multigravida (MUL-tee-GRAV-ih-duh)
multipara (mul-TIH-pear-uh)
nullipara (nul-IH-pear-uh)
obstetrics (ob-STEH-triks)
position
postpartum (poest-PAR-tum)
preeclampsia (PREE-ih-KLAMP-see-ah)
prenatal (pree-NAY-tul)
presentation
primigravida (PRIH-mih-GRAV-ih-duh)
primipara (prih-MIH-pear-uh)
puerperium (PYOO-ur-PEER-ee-um)
quickening
toxemia (tok-SEE-mee-uh)
trimester (try-MES-ter)

INTRODUCTION TO THE GYNECOLOGIC EXAMINATION AND PRENATAL CARE

The medical assistant should have knowledge of gynecology and obstetrics to assist in examinations and treatments in these specialties. Gynecologic examinations are frequently and routinely performed in the medical office. Prenatal care consists of a series of scheduled medical office visits for the promotion of the health of the mother and fetus during the pregnancy. Obtaining the patient's cooperation makes the gynecologic or prenatal examination proceed more smoothly and, as a result, makes the patient feel more comfortable. The medical assistant can help by explaining the purpose of the procedure to the patient. If the patient understands the beneficial results to be derived from the examination, she is more likely to participate as required. This chapter discusses the gynecologic examination and prenatal care and the procedures involved in both.

GYNECOLOGIC EXAMINATION

GYNECOLOGY

Gynecology is the branch of medicine that deals with diseases of the reproductive organs of women. The gynecologic examination is frequently and routinely performed in the medical office and generally includes a *breast examination* and a *pelvic examination*.

The purpose of the gynecologic examination is to assess the health of the female reproductive organs to detect early signs of disease, leading to early diagnosis and treatment. This examination may be part of a general physical examination, or it may be performed by itself. Although assisting with the gynecologic examination is a routine procedure for the medical assistant, the patient may not consider it a routine examination. To reduce apprehension or embarrassment, the medical assistant should fully explain the procedure to the patient and offer to answer any questions.

Terms Related to Gynecology

The medical assistant should have a thorough knowledge of the female reproductive system (refer to Chapter 16) and the following terms associated with the female reproductive system:

Amenorrhea Absence or cessation of the menstrual period. Amenorrhea occurs normally before puberty, during pregnancy, and after menopause.

Cervix The lower narrow end of the uterus that opens into the vagina.

Colposcopy Examination of the cervix using a colposcope (a lighted instrument with a magnifying lens).

Dysmenorrhea Pain associated with the menstrual period.

Dyspareunia Pain in the vagina or pelvis experienced by a woman during sexual intercourse.

Dysplasia The growth of abnormal cells. Dysplasia is a precancerous condition that may or may not develop into cancer.

Menopause The permanent cessation of menstruation, which usually occurs between the ages of 45 and 55 with an average age of 51.

Menorrhagia Excessive bleeding during a menstrual period, in the number of days, the amount of blood, or both. Also called *dysfunctional uterine bleeding* (DUB).

Metrorrhagia Bleeding between menstrual periods.

Perimenopause Before the onset of menopause, the phase during which a woman with regular periods changes to irregular cycles and increased periods of amenorrhea.

Perineum The external region between the vaginal orifice and the anus in a female and between the scrotum and the anus in a male.

Risk factor Anything that increases an individual's chance of developing a disease. Some risk factors (e.g., smoking) can be avoided, but others cannot (e.g., age and family history).

BREAST EXAMINATION

The physician usually begins the gynecologic examination with the breast examination. The medical assistant is responsible for assisting the patient into the supine position. The physician inspects the breasts and nipples for swelling, dimpling, puckering, and change in skin texture. The nipples are checked for abnormalities such as bleeding and discharge. The breasts and axillary lymph nodes are palpated for lumps, hard knots, and thickening.

The patient should know how to examine her breasts at home for the presence of lumps and other changes with a breast self-examination (BSE). Most breast cancers are first discovered by women themselves. The American College of Obstetricians and Gynecologists recommends that women 20 years of age and older examine their breasts once every month. The medical assistant may be responsible for instructing the patient in this procedure at the medical office (Procedure 23-1). If a lump or other change is discovered, the woman should schedule an appointment with her physician as soon as possible. Most breast lumps are not cancerous, but the physician must make that diagnosis.

PELVIC EXAMINATION

The purpose of the pelvic examination is to assess the size, shape, and location of the reproductive organs and to detect the presence of disease. The pelvic examination consists of the following components:

- Inspection of the external genitalia, vagina, and cervix
- Collection of a specimen for a Pap test
- Bimanual pelvic examination
- Rectal-vaginal examination

For the pelvic examination, the patient is positioned in the lithotomy position. The patient lies on the table on her back, with her feet in the stirrups and her buttocks at the bottom edge of the table. The stirrups should be level with the examining table and pulled out approximately 1 foot from the edge of the table. The patient's knees should be bent and relaxed, and her thighs should be rotated outward as far as is comfortable. This position helps relax the vulva and perineum and facilitates insertion of the vaginal speculum. The patient should be properly draped to reduce exposure and to provide warmth. The lithotomy position is difficult to maintain, and the patient should not be placed in this position until the physician is ready to begin the examination.

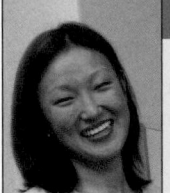

Putting It All into Practice

My name is Yin-Ling Wu, and I am a Registered Medical Assistant. I work with 10 physicians in a large clinic. My primary job responsibilities include documenting patient histories and complaints, taking vital signs, and assisting physicians with patient examinations and procedures.

One experience that has probably affected me more than any other occurred while I was working in obstetrics and gynecology. A full-term prenatal patient came in for a routine weekly appointment late one afternoon. By this stage of the pregnancy, you have seen the patients often enough to develop a more personal relationship. I was obtaining her vital signs and asking the routine questions when she said, "I haven't felt the baby move for 2 days." This immediately sent up a red flag, but I was careful to hide my concern until I was out of her room. The physician was unable to pick up any fetal heart tones, so she immediately did an ultrasound. It showed that the fetus had died. The patient was alone and extremely upset. I stayed with her until her family came.

Although little medical treatment was given during this time, I do believe that my medical assisting training and experience made a difference in my knowing what to do and say to help comfort the patient through this crisis. ■

PATIENT TEACHING Breast Self-Examination

Answer questions that patients have about breast self-examination.

When should I examine my breasts?

Beginning at age 20, the American College of Obstetricians and Gynecologists recommends that you examine your breasts once a month according to your reproductive status as follows:

- **Regular periods:** Approximately 2 to 3 days after your menstrual period has ended. At this time, your breasts are least likely to be tender or swollen, and it will be easier to perform the examination.
- **No periods (because of menopause or hysterectomy):** Any day of the month is fine; however, it helps to choose a particular day, such as the first day of the month or an easy-to-remember date such as your birthday.
- **Hormone therapy:** If you are taking hormones, talk to your physician about when to examine your breasts.

Why is it important to examine my breasts every month?

The purpose of a breast self-examination is not just to find lumps, but also to notice when there are changes in your breasts. The best way to do this is to become as familiar as possible with your breasts. By examining your breasts once every month, you will learn what is normal for you, and it will be easier to notice changes.

What is considered normal?

Breast tissue normally feels a little lumpy and uneven. The left and right breasts may not be the same size; most women's breasts are slightly different in size. Many women have a normal thickening or ridge of firm tissue under the lower curve of the breast where it attaches to the chest wall. Throughout your life, changes also can occur in the size, shape, and feel of your breasts because of aging, weight changes, the menstrual cycle, pregnancy, breastfeeding, and use of birth control pills or other hormones.

What should be reported to the physician?

Early breast cancer does not usually cause pain. When breast cancer first develops, there may be no symptoms at all. As the cancer grows, it can cause changes that should be reported to the physician. Contact your physician immediately if any of the following changes occurs:

- Any new lump, hard knot, or thickening in the breast or underarm area
- A change in the size or shape of the breast
- A puckering or dimpling of the skin of the breast or nipple
- A change in skin texture of the breast or nipple
- A nipple that becomes retracted (pulled in)
- A discharge or bleeding from the nipple ∎

What Would You Do? What Would You *Not* Do?

Case Study 1

Carol Wooster, 42 years old, has come to the office for a gynecologic examination. She has not had a gynecologic examination in 10 years. Mrs. Wooster picked up a BSE brochure at a local health fair and performed a breast self-examination at home. She is now concerned because she found some unusual things. Her right breast is slightly larger than her left breast, her left nipple is pulled in, and she found some freckles on her right breast. Mrs. Wooster explains that she has not had a gynecologic examination in such a long time because her periods have been normal and regular. She also says that the physician will probably want her to have a mammogram, and she has heard that it hurts to have one. Mrs. Wooster is afraid that the physician will be annoyed with her for not having had a gynecologic examination sooner. ∎

The medical assistant can help the patient relax during the examination by telling her to breathe deeply, slowly, and evenly through the mouth. If the patient is relaxed, it is easier for the physician to insert the vaginal speculum and to perform the bimanual pelvic examination; it also is more comfortable for the patient. It is recommended that the medical assistant remain in the room during the pelvic examination to provide legal protection for the physician,

to reassure the patient, and to assist the physician. Procedure 23-2 outlines the medical assistant's role in assisting the physician with a gynecologic examination.

Inspection of External Genitalia, Vagina, and Cervix

The physician begins the pelvic examination with inspection of the external genitalia. The **vulva** is inspected for swelling, ulceration, and redness.

Next, the physician inserts a vaginal speculum into the vagina. Specula are available in two forms—metal and plastic. Metal specula are reusable and must be sanitized and sterilized after each use. Plastic specula are disposable and are designed to be used only once. Vaginal specula come in three sizes—small, medium, and large. The physician determines the size required based on the physical and sexual maturity of the patient. The function of the speculum is to hold the walls of the vagina apart to allow visual inspection of the vagina and cervix (Figure 23-1).

A metal vaginal speculum is cold and should be warmed before use by placing it on a heating pad or by storing it in a warming drawer. A warmed speculum is more comfortable for the patient. It is important not to overheat the speculum, however; one that is too hot is just as uncomfortable as one that is too cold. A disposable plastic speculum does not hold the cold and does not need to be warmed.

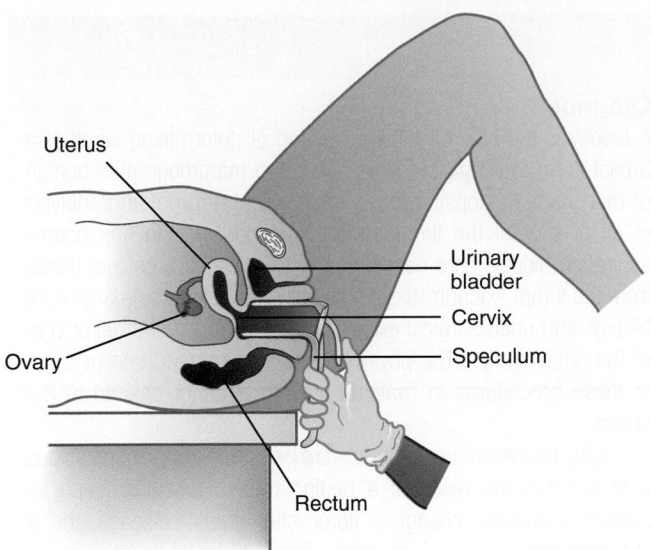

Figure 23-1 Insertion of the vaginal speculum for visualization of the vagina and cervix.

The physician inspects the vagina and cervix for color, lacerations, ulcerations, redness, nodules, and discharge. If an abnormal discharge is present, the physician obtains a specimen for microbiologic examination. Examples of pathologic conditions that produce a discharge include vaginal infections such as *trichomoniasis, candidiasis, chlamydia,* and *gonorrhea,* which are discussed in detail later.

Pap Test

A Pap test is usually part of the pelvic examination. It is a simple and painless **cytology** evaluation named after its developer, Dr. George Papanicolaou (1883-1962). It is used for the early detection of cervical cancer. Almost all cancers of the cervix can be cured if detected early enough. The Pap test also is used to detect abnormal (**atypical**) cells of the cervix that might develop into cancer if not treated. In some cases, the Pap test can detect cancer of the endometrium; however, it is less reliable in doing so.

Highlight on Breast Cancer

Breast cancer is one of the most common types of cancer among American women. The American Cancer Society estimates that one of every eight women in the United States develops breast cancer at some point in her lifetime. Every year, more than 200,000 women learn they have breast cancer, and about 40,000 of them die from the disease. Most women (82%) diagnosed with breast cancer are older than 50 years old, but breast cancer does occur in younger women.

Survival rate

The 5-year survival rate for breast cancer that has spread to a distant site in the body (metastasized) is only 21%. The 5-year survival rate for small, localized tumors is 94%. If the cancer has spread to lymph nodes in the region of the breast, the 5-year survival rate is 73%. These encouraging statistics are the result of advances in the early detection of breast cancer and better treatment, including improved surgical procedures, radiation therapy, chemotherapy, hormonal therapy, and biologic therapy.

Recommendations for early detection

A three-point program is recommended for the early detection of breast cancer: (1) monthly breast self-examination, (2) periodic clinical breast examination by a physician, and (3) screening mammography.

Risk factors

Breast cancer results from the abnormal growth of cells in breast tissue. It occurs more often in the left breast than in the right, and more often in the upper outer quadrant of the breast. The cause of abnormal growths in the breasts is unknown; therefore, every woman should consider herself at risk for breast cancer. Certain factors seem to place a woman at higher than normal risk for breast cancer, however, including the following:

- **Gender.** Women are much more likely than men to develop breast cancer.

- **Age.** The risk of breast cancer increases as women get older. Most women diagnosed with breast cancer are older than age 50.
- **Personal history.** Women with cancer in one breast have a greater chance of developing a new cancer in the other breast or in another part of the same breast.
- **Family history.** A woman's risk of developing breast cancer increases if her mother, sister, or daughter had breast cancer, especially at a young age.
- **Dense breast tissue.** Women with dense breast tissue (meaning they have more glandular tissue than fat tissue as seen on a mammogram) have a higher risk of developing breast cancer.
- **Breast biopsy.** Women who have had a breast biopsy that indicated certain types of benign breast disease (characterized by atypical hyperplasia) have an increased risk of developing breast cancer.
- **Breast cancer genes.** A woman who has inherited mutations in breast cancer genes (mutations of the *BRCA1* and *BRCA2* genes) from either parent is more likely to develop breast cancer.
- **Reproductive history.** Women who began menstruating at an early age (before age 12) or who went through menopause at a late age (after age 55) have a slightly increased risk of breast cancer.
- **Childbearing.** Women who have never had a child or women who had their first child late (after age 30) have a slightly increased risk of developing breast cancer.
- **Hormone replacement therapy (HRT).** Studies indicate that the long-term use of estrogen and progesterone combination hormone replacement therapy for relief of menopausal symptoms increases the risk of breast cancer.

Continued

Highlight on Breast Cancer—cont'd

- **Radiation treatment.** Women who have had radiation of the chest before age 30 as treatment for another type of cancer (e.g., Hodgkin disease) have a significantly increased risk of developing breast cancer.
- **Race.** Caucasian women are diagnosed more frequently than Hispanic, Asian, or African American women.
- **Lifestyle factors.** Studies suggest that the use of alcohol (more than two drinks per day) increases the risk of breast cancer. Obesity, especially for women after menopause, also may increase the risk of breast cancer.

Warning signs

The warning signs of possible breast cancer include a lump, hard knot, or thickening in the breast or armpit; a change in breast color or texture; dimpling or puckering; nipple discharge; changes in the size or shape of the breast; and an enlargement of the lymph nodes.

Diagnosis

A biopsy is the only conclusive method of determining whether a breast lump or suspicious area seen on a mammogram is benign or malignant. A biopsy involves the surgical removal and analysis of all or part of the lump. Biopsy methods include fine needle aspiration biopsy, core needle biopsy (removal of a core of tissue from the lump), vacuum-assisted biopsy (Mammotome), large core biopsy, and open surgical excisional biopsy (removal of all or part of the entire lump). The physician may recommend one or more of these procedures to evaluate a lump or other change in the breast.

Eighty percent of breast lumps are benign. A lump or suspicious area is often the result of a benign breast condition, such as normal hormonal changes, fibrocystic breast disease, or a fibroadenoma. ∎

The American Cancer Society (ACS) recommends a woman have her first Pap test beginning within 3 years of having vaginal intercourse or at 21 years of age, whichever is earlier. Screening should be performed every year with the direct smear Pap test or every 2 years with the liquid-based Pap test. The ACS guidelines further state that beginning at age 30, women who have tested negative for three or more consecutive Pap tests may be screened every 2 to 3 years. Women who are at high risk for cervical cancer or who have had abnormal Pap test results should continue to be screened annually. Factors that place a woman at a higher risk for cervical cancer include diethylstilbestrol (DES) exposure before birth, human immunodeficiency virus (HIV) infection, and a weakened immune system due to organ transplantation, chemotherapy, or long-term steroid use.

Patient Instructions

A Pap specimen must not be collected from a woman during her menstrual period because the red blood cells obscure the specimen and interfere with an accurate evaluation. The patient should be instructed to schedule her Pap test 10 to 20 days after the first day of her last menstrual period. The patient should be told not to douche or insert tampons, medications, or contraceptive spermicides into the vagina for 2 days before having a Pap test. Douching and tampon insertion reduce the number of cells available for analysis, and vaginal medications and spermicides change the pH of the vagina, making the specimen nonrepresentative or invalid. The patient also should be told to abstain from sexual intercourse for 2 days before the Pap test. Recent sexual intercourse can produce inflammatory changes that can interfere with visualization of abnormal cells that may be present.

Specimen Collection

The outermost layer of the cervix consists of a thin, flat layer of cells, approximately 10 layers thick, known as *squamous*

epithelial cells. With the speculum in place, the physician collects a sampling of these cells for evaluation by the laboratory. A scraping of epithelial cells is taken from the ectocervix and the endocervix. A scraping of cells also can be collected from the vagina; however, this is not usually done unless the physician has observed a lesion on the vaginal wall, or the maturation index is to be determined. The technique used by the physician to collect the epithelial cells is described next.

Vaginal Specimen

If a vaginal specimen is needed, it is collected first, before the cervical and endocervical specimens are obtained. The rounded end of the plastic spatula is used to collect the specimen. If a routine vaginal specimen is being obtained, it is collected from the vaginal pool in the posterior fornix of the vagina, which is located just below the cervix (Figure 23-2, *A*). If the physician is collecting a specimen from a lesion on the vaginal wall, a scraping of cells is taken from the area of the lesion. To obtain a specimen for determination of the maturation index (discussed later), the physician obtains the vaginal specimen from the upper one third of the lateral vaginal wall.

Cervical Specimen

The physician obtains the cervical specimen by placing the S-shaped end of the plastic spatula just inside the cervical canal at the **external os** and rotating the blade 360 degrees over the surface of the ectocervix at the squamocolumnar junction, where cervical cancer is most often found (Figure 23-2, *B*). The ectocervix is the part of the cervix that projects into the vagina and is lined with stratified squamous epithelium.

Endocervical Specimen

The physician collects this specimen from the endocervix. The endocervix consists of the mucous membrane lining the endocervical canal. This is accomplished by inserting an

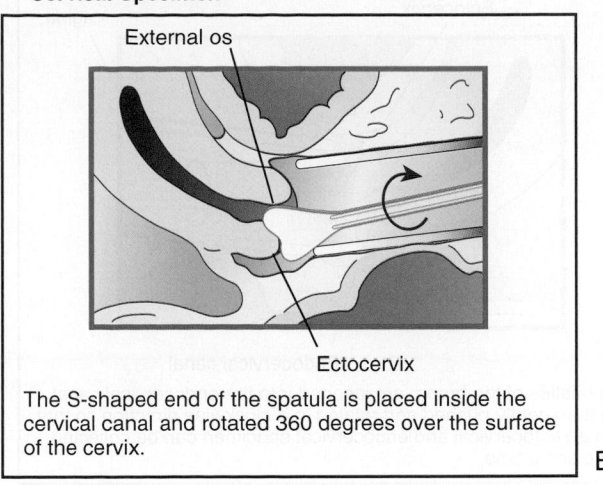

Vaginal Specimen

Vaginal speculum

Posterior fornix

The rounded end of the spatula is used to obtain the vaginal specimen from the posterior fornix of the vagina.

A

Cervical Specimen

External os

Ectocervix

The S-shaped end of the spatula is placed inside the cervical canal and rotated 360 degrees over the surface of the cervix.

B

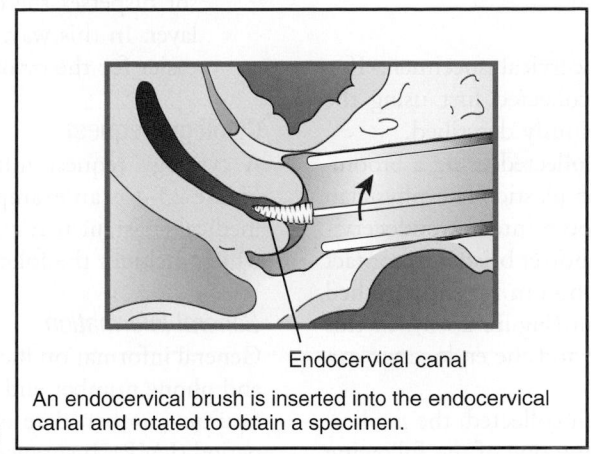

Endocervical Specimen

Endocervical canal

An endocervical brush is inserted into the endocervical canal and rotated to obtain a specimen.

C

Figure 23-2 Obtaining the Pap specimen.

endocervical brush into the endocervical canal and rotating the brush (Figure 23-2, *C*). The endocervical brush is made up of soft bristles designed to be inserted into the canal without causing damage to it.

Preparation Methods

Two methods are used to prepare a specimen for a Pap test. The traditional method is the *direct smear* (Pap smear), and the newer method is the *liquid-based preparation.*

Direct Smear

With the direct smear method, a thin smear of each specimen is spread on a glass slide that has a frosted edge. The medical assistant must label each slide on its frosted edge with a lead pencil according to the source of the specimen as follows: *V* (vaginal), *C* (cervical), or *E* (endocervical). Slides on which all three specimens can be placed also are available. These slides are divided into thirds and are prelabeled with *V, C,* and *E.*

The smears must be fixed immediately by flooding the slides with 95% ethyl alcohol or by lightly spraying the slides with a commercial cytology spray fixative. The slides

must be fixed before they dry to avoid inaccurate results. The purposes of the fixative are to maintain the normal appearance of the cells; to protect the slides from contaminants in the air, such as dust and bacteria; and to attach the smear firmly to the slide. The cytology fixative must be allowed to dry thoroughly; the slides are then ready for transport to a laboratory for evaluation. To protect the slides during transport, they must be placed in a slide container designed especially for this purpose.

Liquid-Based Preparation

A newer method to prepare the specimen for evaluation is the liquid-based preparation. Brand names include Thin-Prep, AutoCyte, and SurePath. Using the liquid-based method improves the quality of the specimen, resulting in fewer slides that are unsatisfactory for evaluation. A better quality specimen also reduces the occurrence of false-negative test results.

The specimen for a liquid-based preparation can be obtained by using the specimen collection technique described earlier. A plastic spatula (S-shaped end) is used to collect the ectocervical specimen, and an endocervical

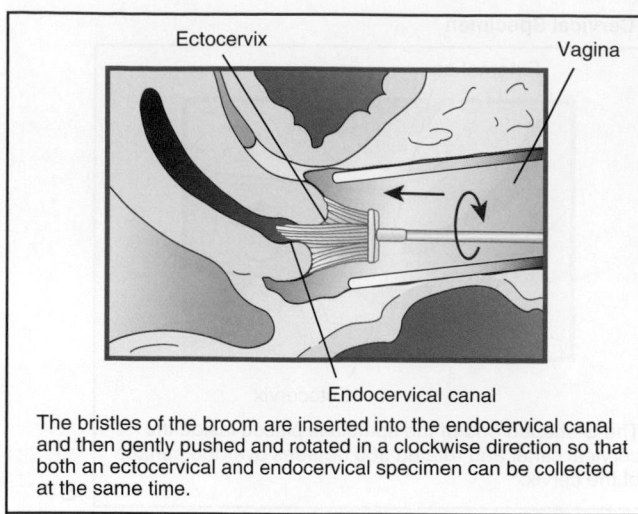

The bristles of the broom are inserted into the endocervical canal and then gently pushed and rotated in a clockwise direction so that both an ectocervical and endocervical specimen can be collected at the same time.

Figure 23-3 Collecting a Pap specimen using a broom.

brush is used to collect the endocervical specimen. If a vaginal specimen is needed, it is collected first using the rounded end of the spatula as previously described.

The Pap specimen also can be collected using a broom, a collection device made of flexible plastic. The physician inserts the central bristles of the broom into the endocervical canal deep enough to allow the shorter bristles to contact the outside of the cervix fully. The broom is gently pushed and rotated in a clockwise direction (Figure 23-3). In this way, specimens from the ectocervix and the endocervix can be collected at the same time.

When the Pap specimen has been collected, the medical assistant is responsible for performing one of the following steps depending on the brand of liquid-based preparation being used:

1. Rinse the collection device in the vial of liquid preservative, and discard the collection device (performed with ThinPrep).
2. Remove the tip of the collection device, and deposit it in the vial of preservative. Discard the handle (performed with SurePath).

The preservative maintains the specimen and prevents it from drying out during transport to the laboratory. After it is received by the laboratory, the vial is placed in an automated slide preparation processor. The automated processor performs several important functions. First, it separates the cells from debris present in the specimen, and then it disperses a representative cell sample onto a slide in a thin, uniform layer. The slide is next immersed in a fixative to maintain the normal appearance of the cells.

The ways in which the liquid-based method provides a better-quality specimen than the direct smear method are as follows:

• With the direct smear method, only a small portion of the specimen is smeared on the slide; most of it is thrown away with the collection device. With the liquid-based method, the collection device is rinsed or the tip is deposited in a vial of liquid that preserves all or

most of the specimen. Having more of the specimen available allows the laboratory to evaluate it better.

• When a Pap specimen is collected, it includes unnecessary debris, such as blood, mucus, and inflammatory cells. With the direct smear method, the debris is smeared on the slide along with the cells. This debris may obscure the cells in the specimen, making it difficult to evaluate them. With the liquid-based method, the automated processor removes a large portion of the debris from the specimen and transfers the cells to a glass slide. This provides the cytotechnologist with a clear, unobstructed view of the epithelial cells.

• With the direct smear method, the cells have a tendency to clump together when they are smeared on the slide, making them more difficult to evaluate. With the liquid-based method, the automated processor disperses the cells onto the slide in a thin, even layer. In this way, the cells are spread out, making it easier for the cytotechnologist to evaluate them.

Cytology Request

A cytology request must accompany all Pap specimens. Figure 23-4 is an example of a cytology request form. The medical assistant is responsible for completing the request, which includes the following categories.

General Information

General information includes the physician's name, address, and phone number and the patient's name, address, identification number, date of birth, and date of last menstrual period (LMP). Insurance information also is required in this section for third-party billing.

Date and Time of Collection

The date and time of collection indicate to the laboratory the number of days that have passed since the collection, providing the laboratory with information regarding the freshness of the specimen.

Collection Method

Under the collection method category, the medical assistant must indicate whether the specimen is a direct smear (Pap smear) or a liquid-based preparation.

Source of the Specimen

The purpose of this category is to identify the origin of the specimen because it is impossible for the laboratory to obtain this information by looking at the specimen. The medical assistant checks one or more of the following boxes on the form: cervical, endocervical, or vaginal.

Collection Technique

The collection device or devices used to obtain the specimen must be indicated. The medical assistant checks one or more of the following boxes on the form: spatula, brush, or broom.

GYN CYTOLOGY REQUISITION

THOMAS WOODSIDE, MD
501 MAIN ST
ST. LOUIS, MO 63146
(314) 555–0093

PATIENT INFO

Patient's Name (Last)	(First)	(MI)	Date of Birth MO DAY YR	Collection Time AM : PM	Collection Date MO DAY YR	Patient's ID #

Patient's Address   Phone

City   State   ZIP

RESP. PARTY

Name of Responsible Party (if different from patient)

Address of Responsible Party   APT #

City   State   ZIP

INSURANCE

Patient's Relationship to Responsible Party   ☐ 1. Self   ☐ 2. Spouse   ☐ 3. Child   ☐ 4. Other

Insurance Comany Name	Plan	Carrier Code
Subscriber/Member #	Location	Group #
Insurance Address		Physician's Provider #
City	State	ZIP
Employer's Name or Number	Insured SSN	

Diagnosis/Signs/Symptoms in ICD-9 Format (Highest Specificity)

R E Q U I R E D

ICD-9 codes are the internationally accepted method of describing the clinical picture of the patient. All diagnoses should be provided by the ordering physician or his or her authorized designee. The following is a partial list of of common diagnoses in ICD-9 format. Most third party payers require an ICD-9 code to indicate the medical necessity of the test(s) and or profile(s) ordered. For a complete list of all ICD-9 codes, please refer to a current ICD-9 manual.

V76.2	Routine Cervical Pap Smear	616.0	Cervicitis	626.8	Abnormal Bleeding
V15.89	High Risk Cervical Screening	616.10	Vaginitis	627.1	Postmenopausal Bleeding
V22.2	Pregnancy	617.0	Endometriosis, Uterus	627.3	Atrophic Vaginitis
079.4	Human Papillomavirus	622.1	Dysplasia, Cervix	795.0	Abnormal Cervical Pap Smear
180.0	Malignant Neoplasm, Cervix	623.0	Dysplasia, Vagina		

COLLECTION METHOD	SOURCE OF SPECIMEN	COLLECTION TECHNIQUE

Liquid-Based Prep

192055 ☐ ThinPrep Pap Test

192039 ☐ ThinPrep Pap Test w/reflex to HPV Hybrid Capture when ASC-US or SIL

192047 ☐ ThinPrep Pap Test w/reflex to high-risk only HPV Hybrid Capture when ASC-US

Pap Smear
009100 ☐ 1 Slide   009191 ☐ 2 Slides

Pap Smear and Maturation Index
009209 ☐ 1 Slide   190074 ☐ 2 Slides

☐ Cervical
☐ Endocervical
☐ Vaginal

Date LMP
___ / ___ / ___
Mo   Day   Year

☐ Spatula
☐ Brush
☐ Broom
☐ Other _____

PATIENT HISTORY	PREVIOUS TREATMENT	Date/Results

☐ Pregnant
☐ Lactating
☐ Oral Contraceptives
☐ Postmenopausal
☐ Hormone Replacement Therapy

☐ PMP Bleeding
☐ Postpartum
☐ IUD
☐ Postcoital Bleeding
☐ DES Exposure
☐ Previous Abnormal Pap Test

☐ Other _____

☐ None
☐ Colposcopy and Bx _____
☐ Cryosurgery _____
☐ LEEP _____
☐ Laser Vaporization _____
☐ Conization _____
☐ Hysterectomy _____
☐ Radiation _____
☐ Chemotherapy _____

Figure 23-4 Cytology request form.

Patient History

Information on the present and past health status of the patient is specified under the patient history category. The medical assistant must check the following boxes that apply to the patient: pregnant, lactating, oral contraceptives, post-menopausal, hormone replacement therapy, postmeno-pausal bleeding, postpartum, intrauterine device (IUD), postcoital bleeding, DES (diethylstilbestrol) exposure, and previous abnormal smear. This information assists the laboratory in evaluating the specimen.

Previous Treatment

Any previous treatment for a precancerous or cancerous condition of the cervix is indicated under this category. The medical assistant checks the appropriate box on the form if any of the following procedures have been performed on the patient: colposcopy and biopsy, cryosurgery, loop electrocautery excision procedure (LEEP), laser vaporization, conization, hysterectomy, radiation, and chemotherapy.

Evaluation of the Pap Specimen

Before a Pap slide can be evaluated, it must be stained by a laboratory technician. Staining is performed on slides prepared by the direct smear method and the liquid-based method. The purpose of staining is to allow better viewing of the morphology of the epithelial cells. The slide is studied under a microscope for evidence of abnormalities by a specially trained technician, known as a *cytotechnologist*. When an abnormality is detected, it is reviewed by a *cytopathologist* (a physician specializing in pathology), who makes a final evaluation. The findings are recorded on a cytology report and returned to the medical office.

A more recent development in the evaluation of Pap slides is the use of automated cytology computer-imaging devices. An abnormal slide may contain only a few abnormal cells among thousands of normal cells. Because of this, these abnormal cells may be missed during the evaluation by the cytotechnologist. A cytology computer-imaging device is able to examine every cell on the slide and select and display cells that appear "most abnormal." The cytotechnologist can evaluate these cells further under a microscope. In this way, the cytotechnologist is able to focus his or her expertise and decision making on preselected areas of the slide.

Maturation Index

The maturation index must be performed on a sampling of cells taken from the upper third of the lateral vaginal wall. The *maturation index* refers to the percentage of parabasal, intermediate, and superficial cells present in the specimen. The maturation index provides the physician with an endocrine evaluation of the patient, which can assist in evaluating the cause of infertility, menopausal or postmenopausal bleeding, or amenorrhea and can help assess the results of treatment with hormones. If the physician orders a maturation index along with the Pap test, the medical assistant must indicate this on the cytology request by checking the box labeled *Maturation Index* (see Figure 23-4). Numerous factors affect the results of the maturation index; it is important to indicate on the cytology request the presence of abnormal bleeding; hormone treatment; or treatment with digitalis, corticosteroids, or thyroid medication.

Cytology Report

The Bethesda System (TBS) is the standard for reporting the results of a Pap test on the cytology report (Figure 23-5). The National Cancer Institute in Bethesda, Maryland, developed this system. It provides a detailed cytologic description (Table 23-1), rather than a numerical result (as with the previous class I through V system). For this reason, TBS is a more effective means of communicating the results of the Pap test to the physician.

Bimanual Pelvic Examination

After obtaining the smear for the Pap test, the physician withdraws the speculum and performs a bimanual pelvic examination. The physician inserts the index and middle fingers of a lubricated gloved hand into the vagina. The fingers of the other hand are placed on the woman's lower abdomen. Between the two hands, the physician can palpate

Table 23-1 Pap Test Results	
Test Result	**Interpretation**
Negative for intraepithelial lesion or malignancy	Epithelial cells were normal, and there were no precancerous or cancerous findings.
Atypical squamous cells of undetermined significance (ASC-US)	Cells are only slightly abnormal. Nature and cause of abnormality cannot be determined. These slightly altered cells usually return to normal on their own, resulting in negative results on subsequent Pap tests.
Atypical squamous cells of higher risk (ASC-H)	Minor abnormal changes in cells with unknown causes, but at risk of progressing to high-grade lesion (HSIL). Further testing is required to determine whether this is a minor condition or one that may progress to HSIL.
Low-grade squamous intraepithelial lesion (LSIL)	Abnormal cells that show definite minor changes but are unlikely to progress to cancer (general term for this is *mild dysplasia*). LSIL may be caused by HPV infection, but of a type that is not likely to lead to cervical cancer.
High-grade squamous intraepithelial lesion (HSIL)	Abnormal cell changes that have a higher likelihood of progressing to cancer. Although not cancerous yet, abnormal cells may become cancerous if treatment is not obtained (general term for this is *moderate-to-severe dysplasia*). HSIL is often caused by HPV infection of a type associated with cervical cancer.
Carcinoma	Usually means patient has cervical cancer. Most women with cervical cancer also test positive for HPV infection.

From Bonewit-West K: *Clinical procedures for medical assistants*, ed 8, St Louis, 2011, Saunders.
HPV, Human papillomavirus.

GYN CYTOLOGY REPORT

RIVERVIEW MEDICAL LABORATORY **DEPARTMENT OF PATHOLOGY** **2501 GRANT AVENUE** **ST. LOUIS, MO 63146** **(314) 555–3443**	**PATIENT:** Heather Jones **PATIENT NO:** 45876 **DOB:** 10/20/65 **SUBMITTING:** T. Woodside, MD

	SPECIMEN TYPE
Date of Specimen: 7/01/10	
Date Received: 7/02/10	☒ ThinPrep ☐ Conventional Pap Smear
Date Reported: 7/06/10	

Performed By: Richard McVay, Cytotechnologist   **Checked By:** Melissa Wagner, Pathologist

SPECIMEN ADEQUACY	GENERAL CATEGORIZATION
☒ **Satisfactory for Evaluation** ☐ **Unsatisfactory for Evaluation**	☐ **Negative for Intraepithelial Lesion** **or Malignancy (*see Interpretation/Result*)** ☒ **Epithelial Cell Abnormality (*see Interpretation/Result*)** ☐ **Other (*see Interpretation/Result*)**

INTERPRETATION/RESULT

A. BENIGN CELLULAR CHANGES

☐ Infection:
- ☐ Trichomonas vaginalis
- ☐ Fungal organisms morphologically compatible w/ Candida species
- ☐ Cellular changes associated with herpes simplex virus
- ☐ Bacterial infection morphologically compatible with gardnerella
- ☐ Cytoplasmic inclusions suggestive of chlamydia

☐ Reactive changes
- ☐ Without inflammation
- ☐ With inflammation
- ☐ Atrophy with inflammation (atrophic vaginitis)
- ☐ Radiation effect
- ☐ Repair
- ☐ Hyperkeratosis
- ☐ Parakeratosis

B. EPITHELIAL CELL ABNORMALITIES

☒ Squamous Cell
- ☒ Atypical Squamous Cells of Undetermined Significance (ASC-US)
- ☐ Atypical Squamous Cells of Higher Risk (ASC-H)
- ☐ Low-Grade Squamous Intraepithelial Lesion (LSIL)
- ☐ High-Grade Squamous Intraepithelial Lesion (HSIL)
- ☐ Squamous Cell Carcinoma

☐ Glandular Cell
- ☐ Atypical Glandular Cells of Undetermined Significance (AGUS)
- ☐ Adenocarcinoma

Figure 23-5 Cytology report form (The Bethesda System).

the size, shape, and position of the uterus and ovaries and can detect tenderness or lumps (Figure 23-6).

Rectal-Vaginal Examination

The last part of the pelvic examination is a rectal-vaginal examination. The physician inserts one gloved finger into the vagina and another gloved finger into the rectum to obtain information about the tone and alignment of the pelvic organs and the **adnexal** region (ovaries, fallopian tubes, and ligaments of the uterus). The presence of hemorrhoids, fistulas, and fissures also can be noted. During this examination, the physician may want to obtain some fecal material from the rectum to test for occult blood in the stool, which requires a guaiac slide test (e.g., Hemoccult). This is typically performed on women beginning at 40 years of age. The medical assistant is responsible for assisting with the collection and testing the specimen for occult blood. This procedure (fecal occult blood testing) is presented in detail in Chapter 28.

Text continued on p. 444

PROCEDURE 23-1 Breast Self-Examination Instructions

Outcome Instruct a patient in the procedure for performing a breast self-examination.

Equipment/Supplies

- Small pillow

1. Procedural Step. Greet the patient and introduce yourself. Identify the patient and inform the patient that you will be showing her how to perform a breast self-examination. Discuss with her the purpose of a breast self-examination and when to examine the breasts (see the box *Patient Teaching: Breast Self-Examination*).

2. Procedural Step. Explain to the patient that a complete breast self-examination should be performed in three ways—before a mirror, lying down, and in the shower.

Principle. Using three methods results in a thorough examination, making it more likely that breast changes will be detected.

Instruct the patient in the procedure for performing a breast self-examination as follows:

Before a Mirror

3. Procedural Step. Remove clothing from the waist up. Stand in front of a large mirror with your arms relaxed at your sides. Observe each breast for the following:
  a. Change in size or shape
  b. Swelling, puckering, or dimpling of the skin
  c. Change in skin texture
  d. Retraction of the nipple
  e. Changes in size or position of one nipple compared with the other
  Principle. Puckering and dimpling of the skin or retraction of the nipple may mean that a tumor is pulling the skin inward.

4. Procedural Step. Slowly raise your arms over your head, and repeat the same inspection listed in Procedural Step 3.

Principle. When the arms are moved at the same time into the same positions, both breasts and nipples should react to the movement in the same way. A change in one breast (e.g., dimpling or puckering of the skin) and not the other should be reported to your physician.

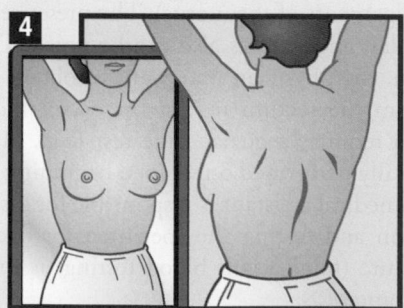

Raise your arms over your head.

5. Procedural Step. Rest your palms on your hips and press down firmly to flex your chest muscles. Repeat the inspection in Procedural Step 3.

Principle. Flexing the chest muscles allows abnor-

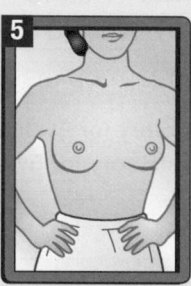

Press down firmly to flex the chest muscles.

malities to become more apparent.

6. Procedural Step. Gently squeeze the nipple of each breast with your fingertips and look for a discharge.

Lying Down

7. Procedural Step. To examine the right breast, lie on your back and place a small pillow (or folded towel) under your right shoulder. Place your right hand behind your head.

Principle. The purpose of this step is to flatten the breast and distribute the breast tissue more evenly on the chest, making it easier to palpate the breast tissue.

8. Procedural Step. Extend your left hand with the fingers held flat. The pads of the middle three fingers of the left hand are used to perform the examination. The finger pads include the top third of each finger. Do not use the tips of the fingers. Use small rotating motions (about the size of a dime) and continuous firm pressure with the finger pads.

Principle. The finger pads are more sensitive than the fingertips, making it easier to detect an abnormality.

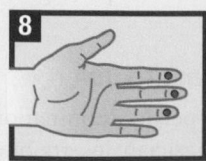

Use the pads of the middle three fingers.

PROCEDURE 23-1 Breast Self-Examination Instructions—cont'd

9. **Procedural Step.** Use one of the following patterns to move around the breast: circular, vertical strip, or wedge. Choose the pattern that is easiest for you. When you have chosen a pattern, use the same pattern each time you examine your breasts.

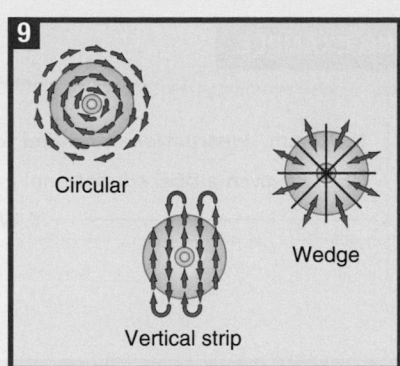

Use one of three patterns to examine the breasts.

Circular

a. Visualize the breast as a clock face.
b. Start at the outside top edge of the breast.
c. Proceed clockwise around the entire outer rim of the breast until your fingers return to the starting point.
d. Move in about 1 inch toward the nipple, and make the same circling motion again.
e. Move around the breast in smaller and smaller circles until you reach the nipple.

Vertical Strip

a. Mentally divide the breast into strips.
b. Start in the underarm area and slowly move your fingers downward until they are below the breast.
c. Move your fingers about 1 inch toward the middle, and slowly move back up.
d. Repeat until the entire breast has been examined.

Wedge

a. Mentally divide your breast into wedges, similar to the pieces of a pie.
b. Starting at the outer edge of the breast, move your fingers toward the nipple and back to the edge of the breast.
c. Check your entire breast, covering one small wedge-shaped section at a time.
   Principle. Using a specific pattern ensures that the entire breast is examined.

10. **Procedural Step.** Holding the middle three fingers of your hand together with the thumb extended, use your finger pads and the pattern you selected to examine the right breast thoroughly. Press firmly enough to feel the different breast tissues. The breast should be palpated for lumps, hard knots, and thickening. Breast tissue normally feels a little lumpy and uneven.

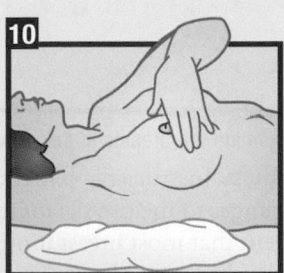

Examine the right breast.

11. **Procedural Step.** Examine the entire chest area from your collarbone to the base of a properly fitted bra and from the breastbone to the underarm. Pay special attention to the area between the breast and the underarm, including the underarm itself. A ridge of firm tissue in the lower curve of the breast is normal. Continue the examination until every part of the breast has been examined, including the nipple.
Principle. An enlarged node in the armpit also can be a sign of breast cancer even if nothing can be felt in the breast.

12. **Procedural Step.** Repeat this procedure on the left breast. Place a small pillow (or folded towel) under the left shoulder, and place your left hand behind your head. Use the finger pads of the right hand to examine the left breast.

In the Shower

13. **Procedural Step.** Gently lather each breast.
Principle. Fingers glide easily over wet, soapy skin, making it easier to detect changes in the breast.

14. **Procedural Step.** Place your right hand behind your head. Extend your left hand with the fingers held flat. With the finger pads of the middle three fingers, use small rotating motions (about the size of a dime) and continuous firm pressure with the finger pads to examine the right breast. Use your preferred pattern (circular, vertical strip, or wedge) to palpate for lumps, hard knots, and thickening. Examine the area between the breast and the underarm, including the underarm itself.
Principle. The upright position makes it easier to examine the upper and outer portions of the breast.

15. **Procedural Step.** Repeat the procedure on the left breast. Place the left arm behind the head, and use the right fingers to examine the left breast.

Continued

PROCEDURE 23-1 Breast Self-Examination Instructions—cont'd

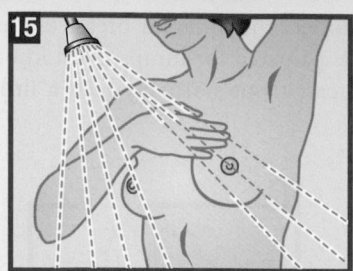

Examine the breasts in the shower.

16. **Procedural Step.** Instruct the patient to report lumps and other changes to the physician immediately. Reassure the patient that most breast lumps are not cancerous, but the only way to know for sure is to see the physician as soon as possible.

17. **Procedural Step.** Chart the procedure. Include the date and time and the type of instructions given to the patient. If you gave a printed instruction sheet or educational brochure to the patient, document this as well.

CHARTING EXAMPLE

Date	
9/7/XX	11:00 a.m. Instructions provided for a
	BSE. Pt given a BSE educational brochure.
	———————————— Y. Wu, RMA

PROCEDURE 23-2 Assisting with a Gynecologic Examination

Outcome Assist with a gynecologic examination. The following procedure describes the medical assistant's role in assisting with a gynecologic examination consisting of breast and pelvic examinations, including a Pap test and a fecal occult blood test.

Equipment/Supplies

- Disposable gloves
- Examining gown and drape
- Disposable vaginal speculum
- Water-based lubricant
- Gauze pads

- Hemoccult slide and developing solution
- Tissues
- Cytology request form
- Biohazard specimen transport bag

Direct Smear Method

- Glass slides with frosted edge
- Cytology fixative
- Plastic spatula

- Endocervical brush
- Slide container

Liquid-Prep Method

- Vial with preservative (ThinPrep, SurePath)

- Plastic spatula and endocervical brush or cytology broom

1. **Procedural Step.** Sanitize your hands.
2. **Procedural Step.** Assemble the equipment. Complete as much of the cytology request form as possible. Some information on the form, such as the last menstrual period (LMP), requires input from the patient and must be completed later. Prepare the collection materials as follows:
Pap Smear Method. Using a lead pencil, identify the slides on the frosted edge with the patient's name and date of birth, the date, and the source of the specimen using the following abbreviations: *V* (vaginal), *C* (cervical), and *E* (endocervical).
Liquid-Prep Method. Check the expiration date on the vial. Label the vial with the date and the patient's name, date of birth, and identification number. The

identification number is located on the cytology request form.

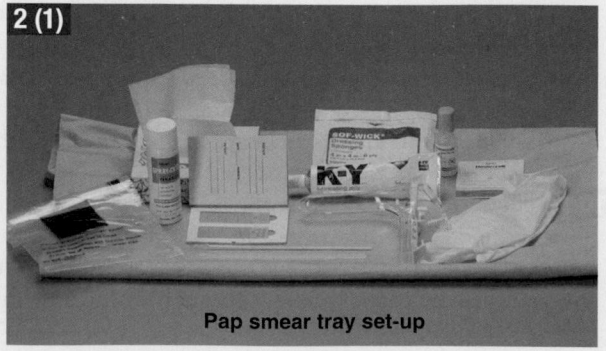
Pap smear tray set-up

Assemble equipment.

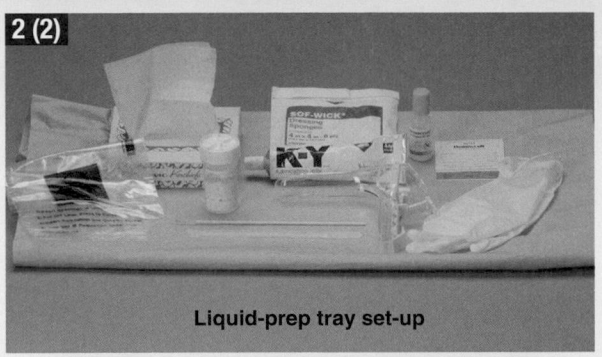

Liquid-prep tray set-up

Assemble equipment.

Principle. If the vial is outdated, it should be discarded because it may lead to inaccurate test results.

3. **Procedural Step.** Greet the patient and introduce yourself.

4. **Procedural Step.** Escort the patient to the examining room and ask her to be seated. Identify the patient. Seat yourself so that you are facing the patient. Ask the patient whether she has any problems or concerns, and record the information in the patient's chart. Ask the patient the necessary questions to complete the rest of the cytology request form.

5. **Procedural Step.** Measure the patient's vital signs, height, and weight, and chart the results.

6. **Procedural Step.** Instruct and prepare the patient for the examination as follows:

   a. Ask the patient whether she needs to empty the bladder before the examination. If a urine specimen is needed, instruct the patient in the proper collection of the specimen.

   b. Provide the patient with a patient gown. Instruct the patient to remove all clothing and to put on the patient gown with the opening in front. If the patient is wearing socks, tell her she can keep them on. Offer assistance if you sense the patient may have trouble undressing.

   c. Tell the patient to have a seat on the examining table after she has put on the examining gown.

   d. Inform the patient that the physician will be with her soon, and leave the room to give her privacy.

   Principle. An empty bladder makes the examination easier and is more comfortable for the patient. Wearing socks helps keep the patient's feet warm during the examination.

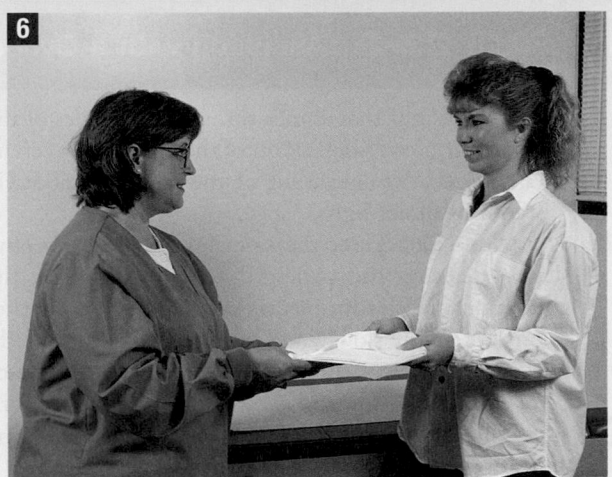

Instruct and prepare the patient for the examination.

7. **Procedural Step.** Make the medical record available for review by the physician. The medical office has a designated location where the record is placed, such as a small shelf mounted on the wall next to the outside of the examining room door or a chart holder on the outside of the examining room door. Position the medical record so that patient-identifiable information is not visible.

   Principle: Before going into the room, the physician will want to review the patient's measurements and urine test results documented by the medical assistant. The Health Insurance Portability and Accountability Act (HIPAA) requires protection of a patient's health information.

8. **Procedural Step.** Check to make sure the patient is ready to be seen by the physician. Before entering a patient's room, always knock lightly on the door to let the patient know you are getting ready to enter the room. Inform the physician that the patient is ready. This may be done using a color-coded flagging system mounted on the wall next to the examining room.

9. **Procedural Step.** Assist the patient into a supine position, and properly drape her for the breast examination.

10. **Procedural Step.** Assist the patient into the lithotomy position for the pelvic examination.

11. **Procedural Step.** Prepare the vaginal speculum by removing it from the warming drawer and performing one of the following:

    Pap Smear Method: Moisten the blades of the speculum with warm water.

    Liquid Prep Method: Thinly lubricate the blades of the speculum with a water-based lubricant. Never apply lubricant to the tip of the speculum.

    Principle. Preparing the vaginal speculum facilitates its insertion into the vagina.

12. **Procedural Step.** Prepare the light for the physician as follows:

    a. *Overhead examination lamp:* Adjust and focus the light for the physician.

    b. *Speculum-illumination system:* Snap the light source device into the light holder on the vaginal speculum and turn it on. The lighting system produces a

Continued

beam of light that shines through the blades of the speculum for visualization of the vagina and cervix. *Principle.* Visualization of the vagina and cervix requires direct light.

13. **Procedural Step.** Hand the vaginal speculum to the physician. Reassure the patient, and help her relax the abdominal muscles during the examination by telling her to breathe deeply, slowly, and evenly through the mouth. *Principle.* If the patient is relaxed, the examination proceeds more smoothly and is more comfortable for her.

14. **Procedural Step.** Apply gloves, and assist with the collection of the Pap specimen as follows:

a. *Direct Smear Method*

(1) Hold each slide so that the physician can smear the specimen on it.

(2) Fix each slide immediately after collection by flooding it with 95% ethyl alcohol or by spraying it with a cytology fixative. The slide should be sprayed lightly with a continuous motion from a distance of 5 to 6 inches.

(3) Allow the slides to air dry for 5 to 10 minutes, and place them in a protective slide container.

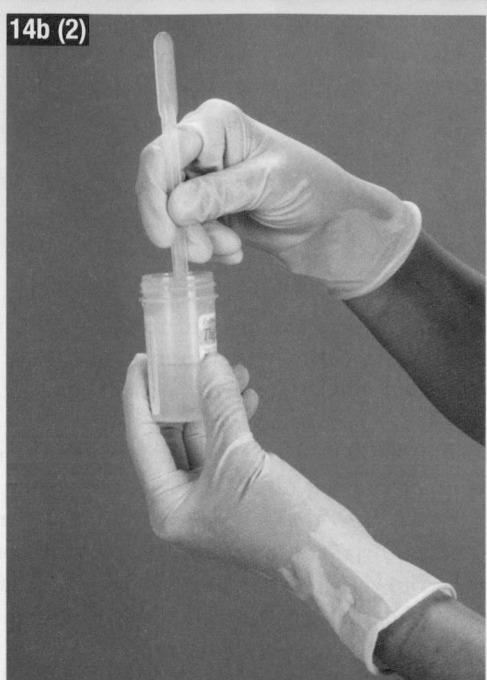

Vigorously swirl the spatula in the preservative.

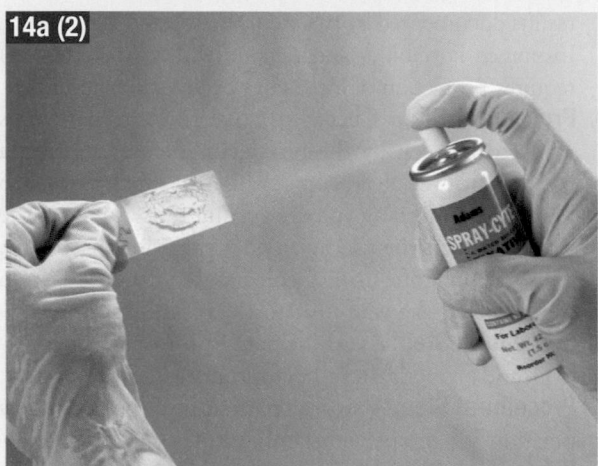

Spray lightly from a distance of 5 to 6 inches.

b. *Liquid-Prep Method (ThinPrep)*

Spatula and Brush Method

(1) Remove the cap from the ThinPrep vial, and hold it so that the physician can insert the spatula into the vial.

(2) Rinse the plastic spatula in the liquid preservative by vigorously swirling it around in the solution 10 times.

(3) Discard the spatula in a biohazard waste container.

(4) Hold the vial so that the physician can insert the endocervical brush into the vial.

(5) Rinse the brush in the liquid preservative by vigorously rotating it in the solution 10 times

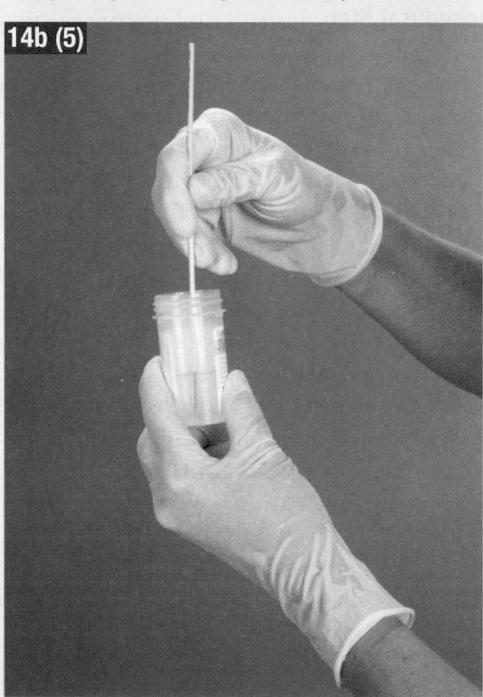

Rotate the brush in the preservative.

while pushing the brush against the vial wall. Swirl the brush in the solution to further release cellular material.

(6) Discard the brush in a biohazard waste container. Securely tighten the cap so that the torque line on the cap passes the torque line on the vial.

PROCEDURE 23-2 Assisting with a Gynecologic Examination—cont'd

Broom Method

(1) Remove the cap from the ThinPrep vial, and hold it so that the physician can insert the broom into the vial.

(2) Rinse the broom in the liquid preservative by pushing the broom vigorously into the bottom of the vial 10 times. This motion forces the broom bristles apart, releasing cervical cells into the solution. Swirl the broom vigorously in the liquid preservative to further release cellular material.

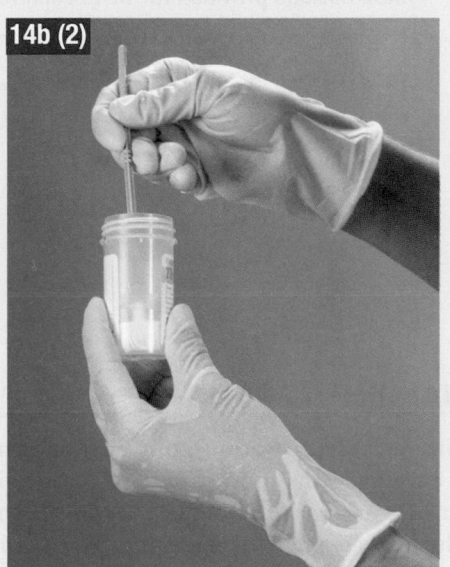

Push the broom vigorously into the bottom of the vial.

(3) Discard the broom in a biohazard waste container. Tighten the cap so that the torque line on the cap passes the torque line on the vial.

c. *Liquid-Prep Method (SurePath)*

(1) Remove the cap from the SurePath vial, and hold it so that the physician can insert the collection device into the vial.

(2) Break off or disconnect the tip of the collection device from the handle.

(3) Discard the handle of the collection device in a waste container.

(4) Repeat the above steps until the physician has collected all of the specimens needed for the Pap test.

(5) Securely tighten the cap on the vial.

15. Procedural Step. Turn off the examining lamp or disconnect the light source from the vaginal speculum. Discard the disposable vaginal speculum in a biohazard waste container. Apply lubricant to a gauze square. Hold it out so that the physician can apply lubricant to his or her gloves to perform the bimanual and rectal-vaginal examinations. Assist with the collection of the fecal specimen for the fecal occult blood test.

Principle. Applying lubricant to a gauze square (rather than directly to the physician's gloved fingers) prevents the opening of the tube of lubricant from touching the physician's gloves and contaminating the contents of the tube.

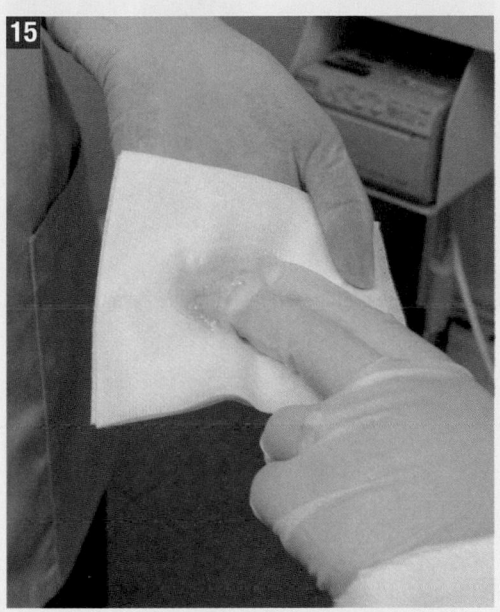

Hold the gauze with the lubricant for the physician.

16. Procedural Step. After the examination, assist the patient into a sitting position, and allow her the opportunity to rest for a moment. Offer the patient tissues to remove excess lubricant from the perineum. Assist the patient off the examining table.

Principle. Some patients (especially geriatric) become dizzy after lying on the examining table and should be allowed to rest after sitting up.

17. Procedural Step. Instruct the patient to get dressed. Tell the patient how and when she will be notified of Pap test results.

18. Procedural Step. Test the fecal occult blood specimen, and chart the results.

19. Procedural Step. Prepare the Pap specimen for transport to the laboratory. Place the specimen (slide container or vial) in a biohazard specimen transport bag, and seal the bag. Insert the cytology requisition into the outside pocket of the bag, and tuck the top of the

PROCEDURE 23-2   **Assisting with a Gynecologic Examination—cont'd**

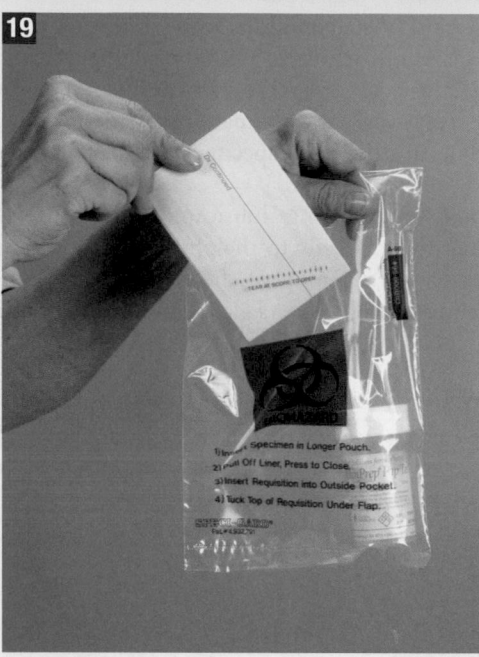

Insert the laboratory request into the outside pocket.

requisition under the flap. Place the bag in the appropriate location for pickup by the laboratory.

20. **Procedural Step.** Chart the transport of the Pap specimen to an outside laboratory.

21. **Procedural Step.** Clean the examining room.

CHARTING EXAMPLE

Date	
9/7/XX	10:00 a.m. Hemoccult: negative.
	Instructions provided for BSE. ThinPrep
	Pap specimen to Medical Center Laboratory
	for cytology. ——————— Y. Wu, RMA

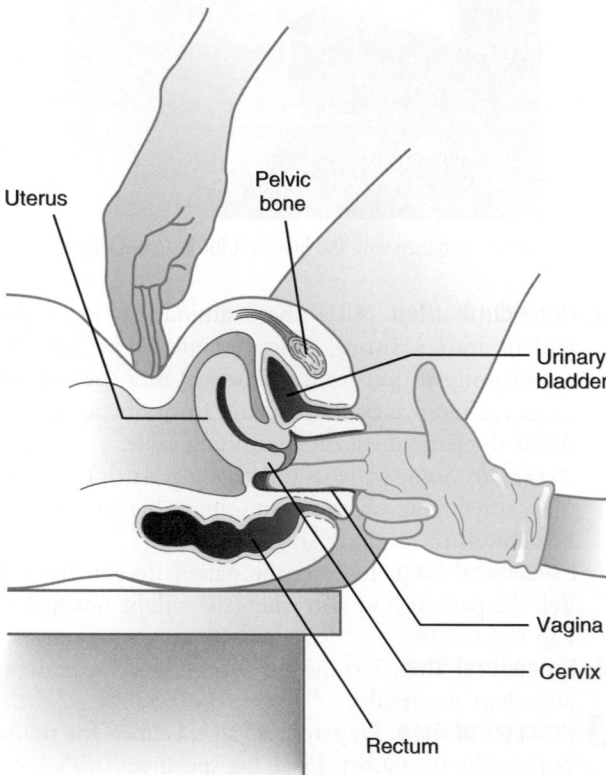

Figure 23-6 The bimanual pelvic examination.

Uterus

Pelvic bone

Urinary bladder

Vagina

Cervix

Rectum

VAGINAL INFECTIONS

The vagina provides a warm, moist environment, which tends to encourage the growth of various organisms that can result in a vaginal infection, or *vaginitis*. If an unusual vaginal discharge is present, suggesting a vaginal infection, a specimen is obtained to identify the invading organism. A specimen of the discharge is collected at the medical office and is evaluated there or placed in a transport medium that is picked up by a laboratory courier and transported to an outside medical laboratory for evaluation.

The medical assistant is responsible for assembling the appropriate supplies for the collection and evaluation of the suspected invading organism. The medical assistant must label all specimens with the patient's name and date of birth, the date, and the source of the specimen. If the specimen is to be transported to an outside medical laboratory for evaluation, a laboratory request form must be completed. The request form indicates the source of the specimen, the physician's clinical diagnosis, the microbiologic examination requested, and other pertinent information, such as medications the patient is taking. The physician's clinical assessment of the patient's signs and symptoms, along with the results of the laboratory evaluation of the specimen, are used to diagnose the presence of a vaginal infection.

Medical assistants should protect themselves from infection with a pathogen while assisting with the collection and evaluation of the specimen by practicing good techniques of medical asepsis. Methods used to identify the invading organism and supplies required for the collection and evaluation of organisms that cause common vaginal infections are presented next.

Trichomoniasis

Trichomonas vaginalis, the causative agent of trichomoniasis (trich), is a pear-shaped protozoan with four flagella, which allow for the motility of the organism (Figure 23-7). Trichomoniasis is usually, but not always, spread through sexual intercourse. Symptoms of this infection include a profuse, frothy vaginal discharge that is usually yellowish green and has an unpleasant odor; itching and irritation of the vulva and vagina; dyspareunia; and dysuria. The cervix may exhibit small red spots, a condition known as "strawberry cervix."

Trichomonas may be identified at the medical office by a wet preparation, which involves placing a small amount of the discharge on a microscope slide using a sterile swab, adding a drop of isotonic saline to it, and placing a coverslip over the mixture to protect it (Figure 23-8). The slide is examined under the microscope and observed for the presence of the lashing movements of the flagella and the motility of the organism.

If the physician prefers to have an outside laboratory evaluate the specimen, it must be placed in a tube containing a transport medium. The specimen must be transported as soon as possible (within 24 hours) to prevent it from dying, which would impede visualization of the motility of the organism.

Candidiasis

Candida albicans is a yeastlike fungus normally found in the intestinal tract and is a frequent contaminant of the vagina; however, it usually does not produce symptoms indicating a vaginal infection. Conditions such as pregnancy, diabetes mellitus, and prolonged antibiotic therapy produce changes in the vagina that may precipitate a candidal infection of the vagina, commonly referred to as a "yeast infection." Symptoms of candidiasis include white patches on the mucous membrane of the vagina; a thick, odorless, cottage cheese–like discharge; vulval irritation; and dysuria. The discharge is extremely irritating and usually results in burning and intense itching.

Candida may be identified microscopically in the medical office by placing a specimen of the vaginal discharge on a slide using a sterile swab and adding a drop of a 10% solution of potassium hydroxide (KOH). The KOH dissolves cellular debris present in the smear and allows better visualization of yeast buds, spores, or hyphae (fungus filaments) indicating the presence of *C. albicans* (Figure 23-9). If the specimen is to be transported to a medical laboratory for

Wet Preparation

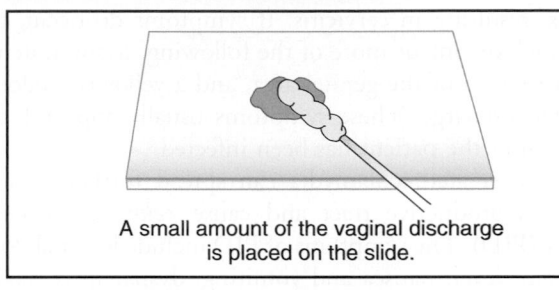

A small amount of the vaginal discharge is placed on the slide.

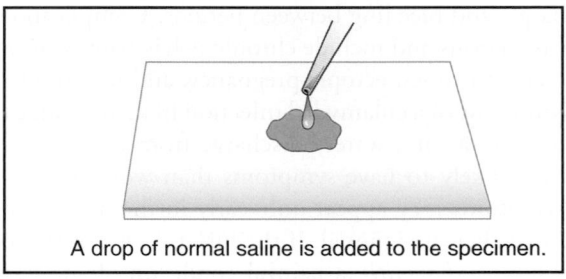

A drop of normal saline is added to the specimen.

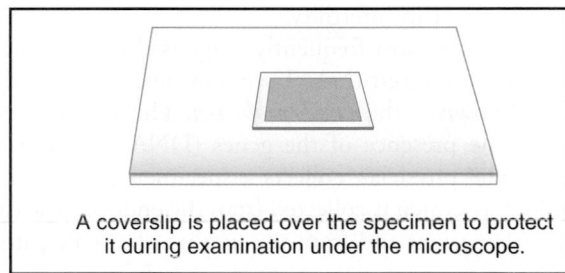

A coverslip is placed over the specimen to protect it during examination under the microscope.

Figure 23-8 Preparing a wet preparation for the identification of *Trichomonas vaginalis.*

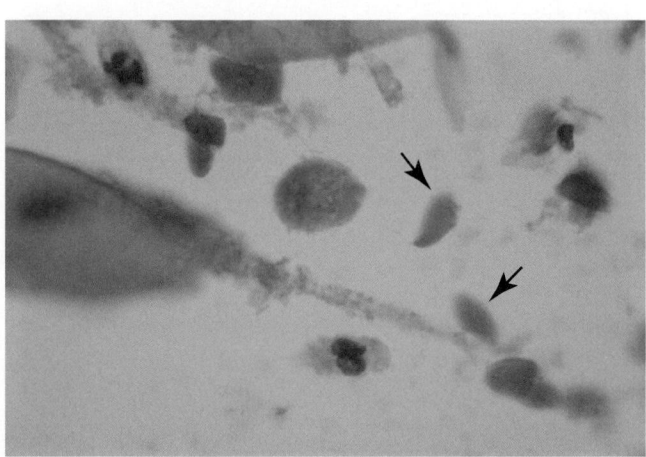

Figure 23-7 *Trichomonas vaginalis* under a microscope.

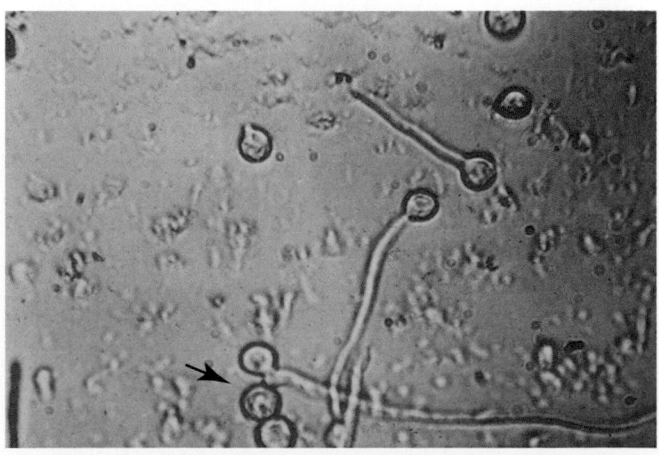

Figure 23-9 *Candida albicans* under a microscope.

identification, it must be placed in a transport medium to prevent drying and death of the organism.

Chlamydia

Chlamydia is caused by the bacterium *Chlamydia trachomatis.* Chlamydia is the most frequently reported and fastest spreading sexually transmitted disease in the United States, particularly among adolescent girls and young women.

Most women with chlamydia have no symptoms and are not aware of having the condition. Because of this, many women do not seek medical care until serious complications have occurred. After infection, chlamydia first attacks the cervix, resulting in cervicitis. If symptoms do occur, they may include one or more of the following: dysuria, itching and irritation of the genital area, and a yellowish, odorless vaginal discharge. These symptoms usually appear 1 to 3 weeks after the patient has been infected.

If not treated, chlamydia can spread further into the female reproductive tract and cause *pelvic inflammatory disease* (PID). The symptoms of PID include lower abdominal pain, fever, nausea and vomiting, dyspareunia, vaginal discharge, and bleeding between periods. Complications of PID are serious and include chronic pelvic pain, scarring of the fallopian tubes, ectopic pregnancy, and infertility.

Symptoms of a chlamydial infection in men include mild dysuria and a thin, watery discharge from the penis. Men are more likely to have symptoms than women; however, the symptoms may appear only early in the day and be so mild that they are ignored. If the infection is not treated, it can cause *epididymitis,* a painful condition of the testicles that could result in infertility.

Chlamydia is most frequently diagnosed using a nucleic acid amplification test (NAAT) or a nucleic acid hybridization test known as the *DNA-probe test.* These tests are able to detect the presence of the genes (DNA) of chlamydia bacteria. The physician collects a specimen using a sterile swab. The specimen is collected from the endocervical canal of a female patient and from the urethra of a male patient.

Male patients should be instructed not to void for 1 hour before the collection of the specimen to prevent chlamydia organisms from being washed out of the urethra. After collection, the specimen is placed in a tube containing a transport medium to preserve the specimen until it reaches the laboratory. See the box *Chlamydia and Gonorrhea Specimen Collection* for detailed instructions on how to assist with the collection of a chlamydia specimen.

Gonorrhea

Gonorrhea is caused by the bacterium *Neisseria gonorrhoeae,* which is a gram-negative diplococcus. Gonorrhea is an infection of the genitourinary tract that is transmitted through sexual intercourse. Chlamydia often occurs in association with gonorrhea; approximately 25% to 40% of patients infected with gonorrhea also have chlamydia.

Women who have contracted gonorrhea may have no symptoms or may exhibit dysuria and a yellow vaginal discharge. The symptoms of gonorrhea (if they occur) appear 2 to 10 days after infection and may be so mild that they are ignored. As the disease progresses, it can spread farther into the reproductive tract, resulting in PID. As mentioned previously, PID can lead to serious complications such as infertility.

Men who have contracted gonorrhea exhibit more symptoms than women, including dysuria and a whitish discharge from the penis, which may progress to a thick and creamy discharge. The burning and pain experienced during urination are often severe, which usually prompts an infected man to seek early treatment. If not treated, gonorrhea may cause epididymitis, which could lead to infertility.

The medical office most frequently uses a DNA-probe test or a nucleic acid amplification test (NAAT) to diagnose gonorrhea. These tests detect the presence of the genes of the gonorrhea bacterium. The procedure for obtaining a specimen for the DNA-probe test is outlined in the box *Chlamydia and Gonorrhea Specimen Collection.*

Chlamydia and Gonorrhea Specimen Collection

DNA-Based Detection Test

The procedure for collecting a specimen for the DNA test is outlined below. Chlamydia and gonorrhea tests can be performed on the same specimen.

1. The medical assistant assembles supplies needed to collect the specimen, including a vaginal speculum, clean disposable gloves, and the DNA-probe collection kit. The collection kit includes cotton-tipped swabs and a tube of transport medium.

2. The transport tube must be labeled with the following information: patient's name, date of birth, and identification number, date and time of collection, and physician's name and telephone number.

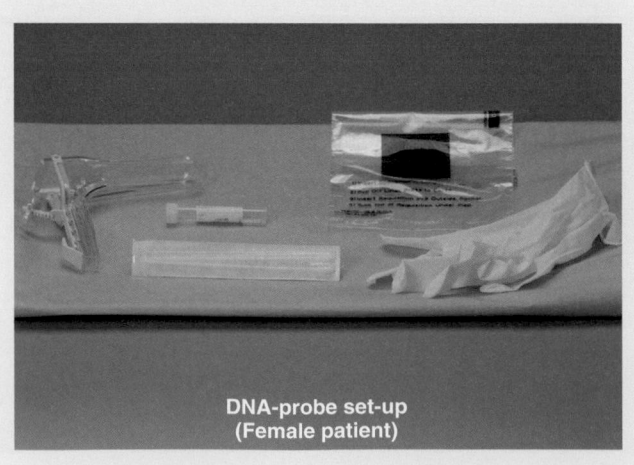

DNA-probe set-up
(Female patient)

Chlamydia and Gonorrhea Specimen Collection—cont'd

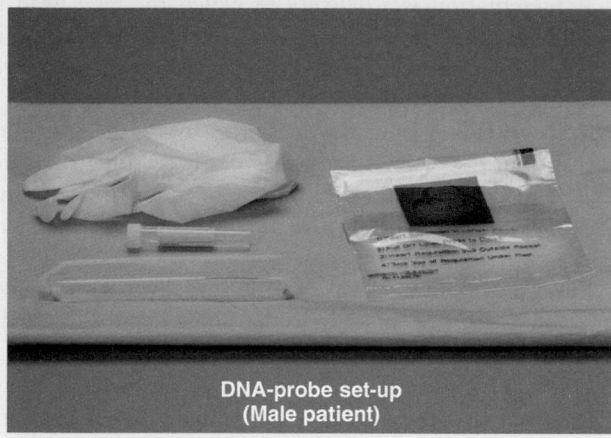

DNA-probe set-up
(Male patient)

3. The physician collects the specimen as follows:
   - **Female Patient:** The physician inserts a vaginal speculum into the vagina. Using a cotton-tipped swab, the physician first removes excess mucus or discharge from the cervix. Next, the physician collects the specimen by inserting another cotton-tipped swab into the endocervical canal and rotating it for 5 to 10 seconds. This ensures a good sampling of the specimen.
   - **Male Patient:** The patient must not urinate for 1 hour before the collection to prevent any urethral discharge from being washed away. The physician inserts a small-tipped cotton swab 2 to 4 cm into the penis. The swab is gently rotated for 3 to 5 seconds to dislodge cells and to ensure contact with all urethral surfaces.

4. The physician withdraws the swab.
5. The medical assistant should ensure that the transport medium is at the bottom of the tube. The medical assistant unscrews the cap and holds the tube for the physician.
6. The physician inserts the swab into the transport tube and breaks off the shaft of the swab at the score line.

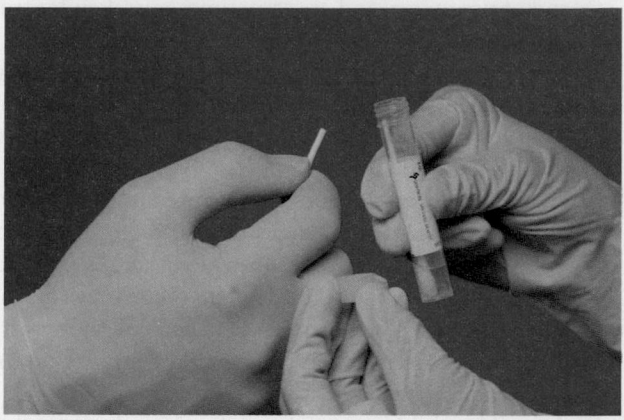

The physician inserts the swab into the tube and breaks off the shaft.

7. The medical assistant places the cap on the tube and twists it until it clicks into place. The tube is placed in a biohazard specimen transport bag along with the laboratory requisition for pickup by the laboratory.

What Would You Do? What Would You *Not* Do?

Case Study 2

Dagny Fairchild comes to the office. She is 16 years old, and her father is a lawyer and her mother is a chemical engineer. Her boyfriend was diagnosed 2 weeks ago with chlamydia. Dagny was hesitant to come in because she does not have any symptoms and her boyfriend always uses a condom. She is worried about her parents finding out that she is sexually active and what they will think if she has one of "those diseases." Dagny also is afraid and extremely embarrassed about what will be "done to her" to determine whether she has chlamydia. She tells Yin-Ling that she is thinking of leaving the office and not seeing the physician at all. (*NOTE:* Dagny lives in a state that allows minors to receive health care services without parental consent.) ■

Memories *from* Externship

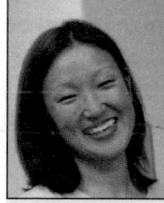

Yin-Ling Wu: During my externship, I was assigned to an OB/GYN clinic. They had an ultrasound technician working there who ran all the scans on prenatal patients. She would always bring the pictures out so we could all look at them. They always looked like a big blob to me—I could never see anything.

One day, a patient that one of the medical assistants knew really well came into the office. The patient agreed to let us all come in for her ultrasound. It was her first time getting an ultrasound. When the technician put the ultrasound probe on her abdomen, we could see the outline of the whole baby. You could even see a tiny arm and fingers, and it looked like the baby was waving. The look of joy and amazement on the mom's face was unforgettable. After that, I knew I was in the right profession. ■

PRENATAL CARE

OBSTETRICS

Obstetrics is the branch of medicine that deals with the supervision of women's health during pregnancy, childbirth, and the puerperium. **Prenatal** refers to the care of a pregnant woman before delivery of the infant. Prenatal care consists of a series of scheduled medical office visits for promotion of the health of the mother and fetus through prevention of disease and early detection, diagnosis, and treatment of problems common to pregnancy (e.g., anemia, urinary tract infection, and preeclampsia). Early detection of medical problems helps prevent serious complications in the mother and the fetus.

Obstetric Terminology

The medical assistant should know the common terms related to obstetrics, as follows:

Braxton Hicks contractions Intermittent and irregular painless uterine contractions that occur throughout pregnancy. They occur more frequently toward the end of pregnancy and are sometimes mistaken for true labor pains.

Dilation Stretching of the external os (of the cervix) from an opening of a few millimeters to an opening large enough to allow the passage of an infant (approximately 10 cm).

Effacement Thinning and shortening of the cervical canal from its normal length of 1 to 2 cm to a structure with paper-thin edges in which there is no canal at all. Effacement occurs late in pregnancy, during labor, or both. The purpose of effacement, along with dilation, is to permit the passage of the infant into the birth canal.

Embryo The child in utero from the time of conception to the beginning of the first trimester (i.e., the first 2 months of development).

Engagement The entrance of the fetal head or the presenting part into the pelvic inlet.

Fetus The child in utero, from the third month after conception to birth; during the first 2 months of development, it is called an *embryo.*

Fundus The dome-shaped upper portion of the uterus between the fallopian tubes.

Gestation The period of intrauterine development from conception to birth; the period of pregnancy. The average pregnancy lasts about 280 days, or 40 weeks, from the date of conception to childbirth.

Gestational age The age of the fetus between conception and birth.

Infant A child from birth to 12 months old.

Multigravida A woman who has been pregnant more than once.

Multipara A woman who has completed two or more pregnancies to the age of viability regardless of whether they ended in live infants or stillbirths.

Nullipara A woman who has not carried a pregnancy to the point of fetal viability (20 weeks of gestation).

Position The relation of the presenting part of the fetus to the maternal pelvis.

Postpartum Occurring after childbirth.

Preeclampsia A major complication of pregnancy, the cause of which is unknown, characterized by increasing hypertension, albuminuria, and edema. If the condition is neglected or is not treated properly, preeclampsia may develop into eclampsia, which could cause maternal convulsions and coma. Preeclampsia generally occurs between the 20th week of pregnancy and the end of the first week postpartum.

Presentation Indication of the part of the fetus that is closest to the cervix and is delivered first. A cephalic presentation is a delivery in which the fetal head is presenting against the cervix. A breech presentation is a delivery in which the buttocks or feet are presented instead of the head.

Primigravida A woman who is pregnant for the first time.

Primipara A woman who has carried a pregnancy to fetal viability (20 weeks of gestation) for the first time regardless of whether the infant was stillborn or alive at birth.

Puerperium The period of time (usually 4 to 6 weeks) after delivery in which the uterus and the body systems are returning to normal.

Quickening The first movements of the fetus in utero as felt by the mother, which usually occurs between 16 and 20 weeks of gestation and is felt consistently thereafter.

Toxemia A condition that can occur in pregnant women that includes preeclampsia and eclampsia. If preeclampsia goes undiagnosed or is not satisfactorily controlled, it could develop into eclampsia, which is characterized by convulsions and coma.

Trimester Three months, or one third, of the gestational period. The 9 months of pregnancy are divided into three trimesters, each consisting of 3 months. From conception to 3 months is the first trimester, from 4 to 6 months is the second trimester, and from 7 to 9 months is the third trimester.

PRENATAL VISITS

Medical office visits for prenatal and postpartum care of the pregnant woman can be grouped into three major categories as follows:

1. First prenatal visit
2. Return prenatal visits
3. 6 weeks postpartum visit

First Prenatal Visit

The first prenatal visit generally occurs after the woman has missed her second menstrual period; if problems exist, the woman is seen after missing her first menstrual period. Regardless of whether or not the patient is happy and excited about the pregnancy, the first visit is often a stressful experience for the patient. The medical assistant plays an important role in relaxing the patient and relieving her anxiety.

The first prenatal visit requires more time than subsequent prenatal visits; sufficient time should be scheduled to allow a complete and accurate initial assessment of the pregnant woman. The components of the first prenatal visit vary depending on the medical office, but they generally include the following:

• Completion of a prenatal record form.
• Initial prenatal examination, consisting of a complete physical examination. Of particular importance are the breast, abdominal, and pelvic examinations. Pelvic

measurements may be taken at this time or during a return prenatal visit.

- Prenatal patient education.
- Laboratory tests.

Prenatal Record

The prenatal record provides information regarding the past and present health of the patient and serves as a database and flow sheet for subsequent prenatal visits. The prenatal record is essential in helping identify high-risk patients. The medical assistant is usually responsible for collecting a portion of the information required for the prenatal record. Many types of printed prenatal record forms are available (Figure 23-10). The specific form used in the medical office is based on the physician's preference and the method used for conducting the prenatal examination.

Obtaining and recording information in the prenatal record from one visit to the next provides an opportunity for the medical assistant to develop a rapport with the patient. It is also an excellent time to relay information to her regarding various aspects of the prenatal and postnatal periods, such as an explanation of the changes occurring in her body,

PRENATAL HEALTH HISTORY

PATIENT INFORMATION

Date: _____ EDD: _____   Referred By: _____

Name: _____   Phone (home): _____
        LAST   FIRST   MIDDLE   Phone (work): _____

Address: _____   Emergency Contact: _____
        _____   Phone: _____
        CITY   STATE   ZIP

Date of Birth: ____/____/____ Age: ____ Marital Status: _____
Occupation: _____
Education: ☐ High School   ☐ College   ☐ Post-graduate

PAST MEDICAL HISTORY

	O Neg + Pos	DETAIL POSITIVE REMARKS INCLUDE DATE AND TREATMENT		O Neg + Pos	DETAIL POSITIVE REMARKS INCLUDE DATE AND TREATMENT
1. DIABETES			16. D (Rh) SENSITIZED		
2. HYPERTENSION			17. PULMONARY (TB, ASTHMA)		
3. HEART DISEASE			18. RHEUMATIC FEVER		
4. AUTOIMMUNE DISORDER			19. BLEEDING TENDENCY		
5. KIDNEY DISEASE/UTI			20. GYN SURGERY		
6. NEUROLOGIC/EPILEPSY					
7. PSYCHIATRIC			21. OPERATIONS/HOSPITALIZATIONS (YEAR AND REASON)		
8. HEPATITIS/LIVER DISEASE					
9. VARICOSITIES/PHLEBITIS					
10. THYROID DYSFUNCTION			22. ANESTHETIC COMPLICATIONS		
11. TRAUMA/DOMESTIC VIOLENCE			23. HISTORY OF ABNORMAL PAP		
12. BLOOD TRANSFUSION			24. UTERINE ANOMALY/DES		

	AMT/DAY PREPREG.	AMT/DAY PREG.	# YEARS USE		
				25. INFERTILITY	
				26. SEXUALLY TRANSMITTED DISEASE	
13. TOBACCO					
14. ALCOHOL					
15. STREET DRUGS				27. OTHER	

IMMUNIZATIONS: ALLERGIES:

Mark an X next to those you have had.   List all allergies (foods, drugs, environment). ☐ None

☐ Influenza   ☐ Chickenpox   _____
☐ Hepatitis B   ☐ Pneumococcal   _____
☐ Hib   ☐ Tuberculin Test   _____
☐ Polio   ☐ Tetanus Booster   _____
☐ MMR   _____

MENSTRUAL HISTORY

Menarche: Age of Onset _____   GYN Disorders (List): _____
Frequency: Q _____ Days   _____
Duration: _____ Days   _____
Amount of Flow: ☐ Small ☐ Moderate ☐ Large   On contraceptive at conception? ☐ Yes ☐ No

Figure 23-10 Example of a prenatal record form.

Continued

OBSTETRIC HISTORY

G _____ (Total Pregnancies)   T _____ (Term)   P _____ (Preterm)   A _____ (Abortions)   L _____ (Living Children)

PREVIOUS PREGNANCIES:

DATE MONTH/ YEAR	WEEKS GEST.	LENGTH OF LABOR	BIRTH WEIGHT	SEX M/F	TYPE DELIVERY	ANES.	MATERNAL COMPLICATIONS	INFANT COMPLICATIONS

PRESENT PREGNANCY HISTORY

NAUSEA			ABDOMINAL PAIN		
VOMITING			URINARY COMPLAINTS		
FATIGUE			VAGINAL BLEEDING		
BREAST CHANGES			VAGINAL DISCHARGE		
INDIGESTION			PRURITIS		
CONSTIPATION			ACCIDENTS		
PERSISTENT HEADACHES			SURGERY		
DIZZINESS			X-RAYS		
VISUAL DISTURBANCE			RUBELLA EXPOSURE		
EDEMA (SPECIFY AREA)			OTHER VIRAL INFECTIONS		

LMP ____/____/____ Mo Day Year   Amount of Flow: ☐Small ☐Moderate ☐Large

CURRENT MEDICATIONS: (Include prescription, OTC, herbal, and vitamins). ☐None

Medication _____ Frequency _____

INITIAL PHYSICAL EXAMINATION

DATE ____/____/____

1. HEENT	☐NORMAL	☐ABNORMAL	12. VULVA	☐NORMAL	☐CONDYLOMA	☐LESIONS
2. FUNDI	☐NORMAL	☐ABNORMAL	13. VAGINA	☐NORMAL	☐INFLAMMATION	☐DISCHARGE
3. TEETH	☐NORMAL	☐ABNORMAL	14. CERVIX	☐NORMAL	☐INFLAMMATION	☐LESIONS
4. THYROID	☐NORMAL	☐ABNORMAL	15. UTERUS SIZE	____ WEEKS		☐FIBROIDS
5. BREASTS	☐NORMAL	☐ABNORMAL	16. ADNEXA	☐NORMAL	☐MASS	
6. LUNGS	☐NORMAL	☐ABNORMAL	17. RECTUM	☐NORMAL	☐ABNORMAL	
7. HEART	☐NORMAL	☐ABNORMAL	18. DIAGONAL CONJUGATE	☐REACHED	☐NO	____CM
8. ABDOMEN	☐NORMAL	☐ABNORMAL	19. SPINES	☐AVERAGE	☐PROMINENT	☐BLUNT
9. EXTREMITIES	☐NORMAL	☐ABNORMAL	20. SACRUM	☐CONCAVE	☐STRAIGHT	☐ANTERIOR
10. SKIN	☐NORMAL	☐ABNORMAL	21. SUBPUBIC ARCH	☐NORMAL	☐WIDE	☐NARROW
11. LYMPH NODES	☐NORMAL	☐ABNORMAL	22. GYNECOID PELVIC TYPE	☐YES	☐NO	

COMMENTS (Number and explain abnormals): _____

_____

_____ EXAM BY _____

Figure 23-10, cont'd

PATIENT'S NAME _____

INTERVAL PRENATAL HISTORY

Date 20___	Weeks Gestation	Height of Fundus (cm)	Weight	B/P	Urine Glucose	Urine Protein	FHT	Vaginal Examination	Presentation	Edema	Discharge	Bleeding	Contractions	Fetal Activity	NST	Next Appt.	Initials

PLANS/EDUCATION   (COUNSELED ☑)

☐ ANESTHESIA PLANS _____
☐ TOXOPLASMOSIS PRECAUTIONS (CATS/RAW MEAT) _____
☐ CHILDBIRTH CLASSES _____
☐ PHYSICAL/SEXUAL ACTIVITY _____
☐ LABOR SIGNS _____
☐ NUTRITION COUNSELING _____
☐ BREAST OR BOTTLE FEEDING _____
☐ NEWBORN CAR SEAT _____
☐ POSTPARTUM BIRTH CONTROL _____
☐ ENVIRONMENTAL/WORK HAZARDS _____

☐ TUBAL STERILIZATION _____
☐ VBAC COUNSELING _____
☐ CIRCUMCISION _____
☐ TRAVEL _____
☐ LIFESTYLE, TOBACCO, ALCOHOL _____
REQUESTS _____
_____

TUBAL STERILIZATION   DATE   INITIALS
CONSENT SIGNED   ___/___/___   _____

Figure 23-10, cont'd

Continued

LABORATORY		PATIENT'S NAME _____			
INITIAL LABS	**DATE**	**RESULTS**		**REVIEWED**	**COMMENTS**
BLOOD TYPE	/ /	A B AB O			
Rh FACTOR	/ /	☐ Pos ☐ Neg			
Rh ANTIBODY SCREEN	/ /	☐ Pos ☐ Neg			
HCT/HGB	/ /	_____% _____ g/dL			
RUBELLA ANTIBODY TITER	/ /	Immune Nonimmune			
VDRL	/ /	☐ NR ☐ R			
HBsAg (HEPATITIS B)	/ /	☐ Pos ☐ Neg			
HIV	/ /	☐ Pos ☐ Neg ☐ Declined			
URINE CULTURE/SCREEN	/ /				
PAP TEST	/ /	☐ Normal ☐ Abnormal			
CHLAMYDIA (DNA PROBE)	/ /	☐ Pos ☐ Neg			
GONORRHEA (DNA PROBE)	/ /	☐ Pos ☐ Neg			
7–20 WEEK LABS (WHEN INDICATED/ELECTED)	**DATE**	**RESULTS**		**REVIEWED**	**COMMENTS**
ULTRASOUND #1 (7–12 WEEKS)	/ /	EDD:			
ULTRASOUND #2 (18–20 WEEKS)	/ /	EFW:			
TRIPLE SCREEN (15–20 WEEKS)	/ /				
CVS	/ /				
AMNIOCENTESIS	/ /				
24–28 WEEK LABS (WHEN INDICATED)	**DATE**	**RESULTS**		**REVIEWED**	**COMMENTS**
HCT/HGB	/ /	_____ % _____ g/dL			
GCT (24–28 WKS)	/ /	1 Hour _____			
GTT (IF SCREEN ABNORMAL)	/ /	_____ FBS _____ 1 Hour _____ 2 Hour _____ 3 Hour			
D (Rh) ANTIBODY SCREEN	/ /				
D IMMUNE GLOBULIN (RhIG) GIVEN (28 WKS)	/ /	SIGNATURE			
32–36 WEEK LABS	**DATE**	**RESULTS**		**REVIEWED**	**COMMENTS**
HCT/HGB (32 WKS)	/ /	_____ % _____ g/dL			
ULTRASOUND #3 (34 WKS)	/ /	EFW:			
GROUP B STREP (35–37 WKS)	/ /	☐ Pos ☐ Neg			
ADDITIONAL LAB TESTS	**DATE**	**RESULTS**		**REVIEWED**	**COMMENTS**
	/ /				
	/ /				
	/ /				
	/ /				
	/ /				

Figure 23-10, cont'd

the signs and symptoms of labor, nutrition of the infant (breastfeeding and bottle feeding), and care of the newborn infant. The prenatal record form should be completed in a quiet setting that is free from distractions. This gives the patient the confidence to discuss areas of concern openly, which helps ensure a complete and accurate prenatal history.

Past Medical History

The past medical history focuses on conditions that could affect the health of the mother and fetus, such as diabetes, hypertension, heart disease, autoimmune disorders, kidney disease, liver disease, varicosities or phlebitis, alcohol and tobacco intake, drug addiction, Rh sensitization, pulmonary disease (e.g., tuberculosis, asthma), bleeding tendencies, surgeries, anesthetic complications, previous abnormal Pap tests, infertility problems, sexually transmitted diseases, and drug allergies. In addition, the medical assistant solicits information

from the patient regarding immunizations and childhood diseases to provide the physician with the information needed to assess her antibody protection against such diseases.

Menstrual History

A menstrual history is obtained from the patient. It includes the date of onset of menstruation, the menstrual interval cycle, the duration, the amount of flow (recorded as small, moderate, or large), and any gynecologic disorders. The form also includes a space for the patient to indicate whether or not she was using a method of contraception when she became pregnant.

Obstetric History

A thorough obstetric history is a component of the prenatal record and provides the opportunity to obtain information from the patient related to previous pregnancies.

If a woman is a multigravida, information about each pregnancy is obtained, including the date of delivery, gestation in weeks, length of labor in hours, birth weight and sex of the newborn, type of delivery (vaginal or cesarean section), type of anesthesia, and any maternal or infant complications. The obstetric history assists in identifying areas that may need to be investigated further or monitored during the prenatal period. Women with previous complications, such as premature labor, gestational diabetes, or postpartum hemorrhaging, are at risk for having these problems again.

Present Pregnancy History

The present pregnancy history establishes a baseline for the present health status of the prenatal patient. In addition, the patient is queried regarding any warning signs that may be present and that may place the mother or fetus in jeopardy, such as persistent headaches, visual disturbances, abdominal pain, vaginal bleeding, or discharge. The patient also is asked whether she has experienced any of the early signs of pregnancy, such as nausea, vomiting, fatigue, and breast changes.

All prescribed or over-the-counter medications (including vitamin supplements and herbal products) the patient is taking must be recorded. Certain medications cross the placental barrier and could be harmful to the developing fetus. The patient should be instructed not to take any medications without first checking with the physician.

In the space provided under the present pregnancy history, the medical assistant needs to record the date of the first day of the patient's last menstrual period (LMP). The LMP is used to calculate due date, or **expected date of delivery (EDD)**, by using the Nägele rule: Add 7 days to the date of the LMP, subtract 3 months, and add 1 year (EDD = LMP + 7 days − 3 months + 1 year). For example, if the date of the patient's LMP was June 10, 2011, the EDD is March 17, 2012. The problem is set up as follows:

6	10	2011	(LMP)
−3	+7	+1	(Applying Nägele rule)
3	17	2012	(Delivery date)

Using the Nägele rule, approximately 4% of patients deliver spontaneously on the EDD; most patients deliver during the period extending from 7 days before to 7 days after the EDD.

Gestation calculators are commercially available that can be used to determine the delivery date by lining up an arrow and the date of the LMP, using a movable inner cardboard wheel (Figure 23-11). These calculators require less time to determine the EDD than using the Nägele rule, and they provide information on the probable size (length and weight) of the fetus on any given date. The accuracy of gestation calculators is comparable with that of the Nägele rule. If the patient is unsure of the date of her LMP, the

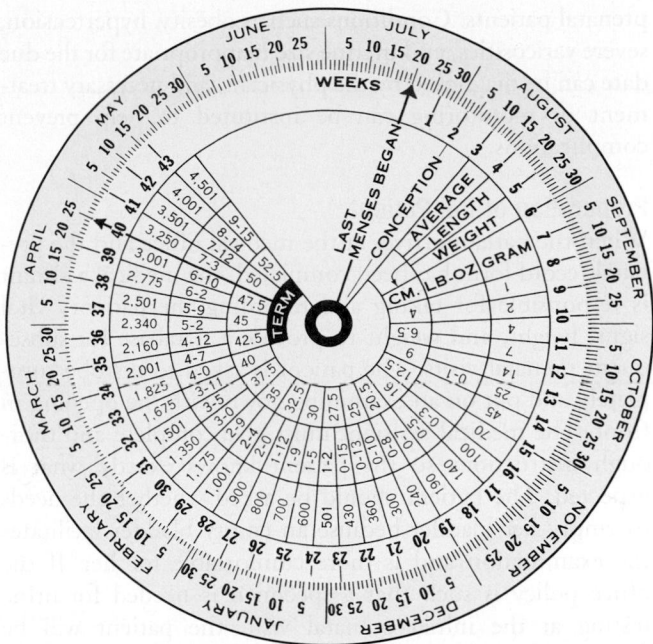

Figure 23-11 Gestation calculator. The last menstrual period is July 20, and the expected date of delivery is April 25.

physician estimates the length of gestation by other methods, such as fundal height measurement and sonography.

Interval Prenatal History

The interval prenatal history also is included in the prenatal record form; its purpose is to update the record. During every return visit, essential data, including weight, blood pressure, urine testing results, fundal height measurement, and fetal heart rate, are collected and recorded in this section. A general inquiry is made regarding the occurrence of additional signs of pregnancy, such as fetal movement or Braxton Hicks contractions, and how the patient is feeling and any concerns or symptoms since the last prenatal visit.

This information is recorded and assists the medical staff in planning, implementing, and evaluating individual needs. Particular attention is focused on risk factors, such as hypertension, thrombophlebitis, and uterine bleeding, which could influence the course of the pregnancy.

Initial Prenatal Examination

Purpose

The initial prenatal examination is of particular importance because it results in confirmation of the pregnancy and establishes a baseline for the woman's state of health. It includes a thorough gynecologic examination (breast and pelvic examinations) and a general physical examination of the other body systems, although the latter may be performed during a subsequent prenatal visit, depending on the medical office routine.

Women often have little or no medical supervision during their childbearing years; the physical examination is of particular importance in establishing a baseline for the woman's general state of health and in identifying high-risk prenatal patients. Conditions such as obesity, hypertension, severe varicosities, and uterine size inappropriate for the due date can be diagnosed by the physician, and necessary treatment or monitoring can be instituted to help prevent complications.

Preparation of the Patient

When the patient arrives at the medical office and the prenatal record form has been completed, the medical assistant is responsible for taking and recording the patient's vital signs, height, and weight to provide a database for subsequent prenatal visits. The patient is asked to disrobe completely and put on an examining gown with the opening in front. The medical assistant must give complete and thorough instructions so the patient knows exactly what is expected. The patient should be asked whether she needs to empty her bladder because an empty bladder facilitates the examination and is more comfortable for her. If the office policy is such that a specimen is needed for urine testing at the initial prenatal visit, the patient will be required to void.

Special precautions should be taken in assisting the prenatal patient. The medical assistant should support the patient as she gets onto and off the scale and examining table to ensure her safety and comfort. This is especially important as the pregnancy progresses and the patient becomes more awkward and off balance.

The medical assistant is responsible for setting up the tray required for the examination. The setup includes the equipment and supplies required for the procedures to be performed. During the prenatal examination, the medical assistant is responsible for positioning the patient as required for each aspect of the examination and assisting the physician as necessary.

Patient Education

At the conclusion of the initial prenatal examination and after the patient is dressed, the physician talks with her regarding instructions on diet, weight gain, rest, sleep, employment, exercise, travel, sexual intercourse, dental care, smoking, alcohol, and drugs. Many offices have a prenatal guidebook designed especially for this purpose that is given to each patient to use as a reference. Some offices also use a series of teaching films that the patient views during the return prenatal visit while waiting to see the physician. The physician also prescribes a daily vitamin supplement to be taken during the prenatal period to ensure that the mother and fetus obtain an adequate supply of vitamins and minerals.

When the physician is finished talking with the patient, the medical assistant is responsible for scheduling the next prenatal visit and for ensuring that the patient understands the instructions for maintaining health and preventing disease during the pregnancy. The medical assistant should tell the patient to report the occurrence of any warning signs during the pregnancy (see the *Warning Signs during Pregnancy* box) and not to take any medications without first checking with the physician. The patient also should be encouraged to contact the medical office should any questions or problems arise.

Warning Signs during Pregnancy

Signs of Infection
- Fever
- Vaginal discharge
- Dysuria
- Increased frequency of urination
- Marked decrease in urinary output

Signs of Spontaneous Abortion
- Vaginal bleeding
- Persistent low back pain
- Abdominal pain and cramping

Signs of Preeclampsia
- Severe, persistent headache
- Dizziness
- Blurred vision
- Sudden swelling of hands, feet, or face
- Sudden rapid weight gain
- Abdominal pain

Signs of Placental or Fetal Problems
- Vaginal spotting or bleeding
- Abdominal pain and cramping
- Back pain
- Noticeable decrease in fetal activity
- No fetal movement

Signs of Preterm Labor
- Regular or frequent contractions (more than four to six per hour)
- Recurring low, dull backache
- Menstrual-like cramping
- Unusual pressure in the pelvis, low back, abdomen, or thighs

---

Laboratory Tests

The physician orders many laboratory tests to assist in the assessment of the patient's state of health and to detect problems that may put the pregnancy at risk. Several tests, such as the Pap test and the chlamydia and gonorrhea tests, require the physician to collect the specimens at the medical office and have them transported by laboratory courier to an outside laboratory for evaluation. The specimen required for the prenatal blood tests (known as a *prenatal profile*) must be obtained through a venipuncture to provide a sufficient quantity of blood for the number of tests ordered. The blood specimen is collected at the medical office or at an outside laboratory.

It is important to have these initial tests completed as soon as possible to provide the physician with the test results by the time of the next scheduled prenatal visit. Based on the results of the prenatal examination and the laboratory tests, the physician may order additional tests to assess the patient's condition. Certain tests and procedures, such as the glucose challenge test (GCT) and the group B streptococcus (GBS) test, are scheduled later in the pregnancy. The prenatal laboratory tests that are usually performed on a pregnant woman are described next.

Urine Tests

Urinalysis

A complete urinalysis, including physical, chemical, and microscopic analyses of the urine, is performed; a clean-catch midstream urine specimen is generally required for the test. If bacteria are found in the urine specimen, the physician usually requests a urine culture and sensitivity test to determine the possible presence of a urinary tract infection. A pregnancy test also may be performed on the urine specimen, if ordered by the physician.

Swab Tests

Pap Test

A Pap test is done for the detection of abnormalities of cell growth to diagnose precancerous or cancerous conditions of the cervix. This test also can be used for hormonal assessment (maturation index) and to assist in the detection of vaginal infections.

Chlamydia and Gonorrhea

Specimens are taken from the endocervical canal and sent to the laboratory to rule out chlamydia and gonorrhea. Chlamydia can be passed from an infected woman to her infant during childbirth, resulting in conjunctivitis and pneumonia in the newborn. If a gonorrheal infection is present at the time of delivery, the *N. gonorrhoeae* organism could infect the infant's eyes during passage through the birth canal. This may result in *ophthalmia neonatorum,* which, if not treated, could lead to blindness. For this reason, most states require that pregnant women be tested for gonorrhea, and that the eyes of newborns be treated with antibiotic drops immediately after birth to kill any gonococcal bacteria that may be present. A patient who is diagnosed with chlamydia or gonorrhea requires immediate treatment with an appropriate antibiotic to prevent problems for herself and her child.

Trichomoniasis and Candidiasis

If an excessive irritating vaginal discharge is present, the physician obtains a specimen to rule out trichomoniasis and candidiasis. It is important to control candidiasis before delivery to prevent the development of thrush, a yeastlike infection of the infant's mucous membranes of the mouth or throat.

Group B Streptococcus

Group B streptococcus (GBS) is a common bacterium often found in the vagina and rectum of healthy women. Normally, one in four pregnant women carries GBS. GBS is not harmful to a pregnant woman, but it can cause life-threatening infections in the newborn. While passing through the birth canal, a newborn can become infected with the bacteria carried by the mother. When infected, the infant may develop an infection of the blood (septicemia), pneumonia, or meningitis.

To prevent GBS infection of the newborn, a pregnant woman is tested for the bacteria between 35 and 37 weeks of gestation. Using two swabs, the physician collects specimens from the vagina and the rectum. The specimen swabs are placed in a transport tube and sent to the laboratory to be cultured for GBS. If GBS is found, intravenous antibiotics are administered to the woman every 4 hours during labor until delivery. In most cases, this antibiotic administration prevents the newborn from becoming infected with GBS. In situations in which the newborn does become infected with GBS, antibiotics are administered immediately, and the infant is closely monitored.

Blood Tests

Complete Blood Count

The complete blood count (CBC) is a basic screening test used to assist in assessing the patient's state of health. It includes a hemoglobin, hematocrit, white blood cell count, red blood cell count, differential white blood cell count, platelet count, and red blood cell indices. Of particular importance with respect to the prenatal patient are the hemoglobin and hematocrit evaluations, which are described here.

Hemoglobin and Hematocrit

Low hemoglobin or hematocrit values are seen in cases of anemia. Prenatal patients have a tendency to develop anemia because there is an increased demand for and correlating increased production of red blood cells during pregnancy; the physician carefully reviews the results of these tests. If the hemoglobin or hematocrit value is low, further hematologic evaluation is usually required. If necessary, therapy is instituted, which usually consists of an iron supplement and nutritional counseling. The hemoglobin and hematocrit values are checked again at approximately 32 weeks of gestation as a precaution against anemia before delivery.

What Would You Do? What Would You *Not* Do?

Case Study 3

Johanna Kruger is 24 years old and pregnant with her first child. She is at the office for her first prenatal visit. She is quite upset. Her best friend just had her first baby, and the baby died 24 hours later from a group B strep infection. Johanna is afraid that the same thing will happen to her baby. She wants to be tested for GBS as soon as possible. She has some antibiotics at home and is thinking of taking them. Johanna is worried because she has been experiencing some problems with her pregnancy. She is sick all day, her breasts hurt, and yesterday she had some spotting. Johanna is hesitant to tell all of this to the physician because he might think she worries too much. ■

Rh Factor and ABO Blood Type

Tests are performed to anticipate ABO blood type and Rh factor incompatibilities. If the patient is Rh-negative, the father's blood type also must be evaluated. If the father's blood type is Rh-positive, the possibility of an Rh incompatibility exists. This situation warrants the performance of an Rh antibody titer test and repeat antibody titers throughout the pregnancy to determine whether the mother's antibody level is increasing. An increased Rh antibody level could be dangerous to the developing fetus. It can result in severe anemia, jaundice, brain damage, heart failure, and sometimes death of the fetus.

Glucose Challenge Test

A glucose challenge test is performed between 24 and 28 weeks of gestation to screen for gestational diabetes mellitus (GDM). This test works by assessing the body's response to a measured glucose solution. The patient does not need to fast for this test, and no preparation is required other than arriving at the laboratory at the scheduled time. To perform the glucose challenge test, the patient is asked to drink 50 g of a glucose solution, and her glucose level is measured 1 hour later. A woman with a glucose level of less than 140 mg/dL does not have GDM and requires no further testing. If the glucose level is greater than 140 mg/dL, the test is abnormal. Not all women with elevated results have diabetes, however, and further testing using the 3-hour oral glucose tolerance test (OGTT) must be performed before a final diagnosis can be made. (*NOTE:* Refer to Chapter 33 for information on the OGTT.)

Syphilis Test

The microorganism that causes syphilis, *Treponema pallidum,* is able to cross the placental barrier and infect the fetus; this could result in intrauterine death or could cause the fetus to be born with congenital syphilis. Infants with congenital syphilis are often born with deformities and may become blind, deaf, paralyzed, or insane. The tests most commonly employed to screen for the presence of syphilis are the Venereal Disease Research Laboratory (VDRL) test and the rapid plasma reagin (RPR) test. The test results are reported as nonreactive, weakly reactive, or reactive. Because these tests are screening tests, a weakly reactive or reactive test result warrants more specific testing to arrive at a diagnosis for syphilis. Examples of these tests are the fluorescent treponemal antibody absorption (FTA-ABS) test and the *T. pallidum* particle agglutination assay (TPPA) test.

A prenatal test for syphilis is mandated by most states and should be performed early in the pregnancy, before fetal damage occurs. A patient who has contracted syphilis requires treatment with an appropriate antibiotic.

Rubella Antibody Titer

The rubella antibody titer assesses the level of antibody against rubella (German measles) in the patient's blood and is used to determine whether the woman is immune to rubella. If the mother contracts rubella during pregnancy, serious congenital abnormalities can occur in the fetus. Patients who lack immunity should be immunized against rubella within 6 weeks of delivery.

Rh Antibody Titer (on Rh-Negative Blood Specimens)

An Rh antibody titer detects the quantity of circulating Rh antibodies against red blood cells. These antibodies can occur in a pregnant woman who is Rh-negative and is carrying an Rh-positive fetus; an Rh antibody titer is performed on all Rh-negative blood specimens. Repeat antibody titer levels also are performed during the pregnancy to determine whether the woman's antibody level is increasing. As was previously indicated, an increased Rh antibody level could be dangerous to the developing fetus. As a preventive measure, Rh-negative women with the potential of having an Rh-positive infant and who test negative for Rh antibodies are given two injections of Rh immune globulin (RhoGAM). The Rh immune globulin prevents the formation of Rh antibodies in the mother, which avoids Rh incompatibility complications during the next pregnancy. The first injection is given at 28 weeks of gestation, and the second injection is administered within 72 hours of delivery.

Hepatitis B and Human Immunodeficiency Virus

The Centers for Disease Control and Prevention (CDC) recommends that pregnant women have the hepatitis B surface antigen (HBsAg) test to screen for hepatitis B virus. Women who have positive HBsAg test results have an increased risk of spontaneous abortion or preterm labor. In addition, the mother may transmit hepatitis B to the infant, particularly during delivery or in the first few days of life. This risk can be greatly reduced by administering hepatitis B immune globulin (HBIG) and the hepatitis B vaccine within 12 hours of birth to the newborns of women who have tested positive for hepatitis B.

Infants born to women who are human immunodeficiency virus (HIV) positive are at risk of developing the disease. If antiretroviral drugs are taken during pregnancy and the infant is delivered by cesarean section, the chance of transmitting HIV to the infant is reduced significantly. Because of this, the CDC recommends that testing for HIV be included in the routine panel of prenatal screening tests for all pregnant women, and that separate written consent is not required. The CDC further recommends that the patient should be notified that HIV testing will be performed unless the patient declines the test. The CDC recommends that repeat HIV screening be performed in the third trimester in geographic areas that have elevated rates of HIV infection among pregnant women.

Return Prenatal Visits

Return prenatal visits provide the opportunity for a continuous assessment of the health of the mother and the fetus. During each visit, essential data are collected and recorded in the prenatal record, resulting in an updated record at each visit, as is discussed in this section. If signs or symptoms of a pathologic condition are present, the physician performs select aspects of the physical examination as necessary to diagnose and treat the condition. In addition, diagnostic and laboratory tests may be ordered to assist in diagnosis and treatment. The usual schedule of visits for prenatal care is listed below. A patient who exhibits complications is seen more frequently for closer monitoring.

- 0 to 28 weeks of gestation: Every 4 weeks
- 29 to 35 weeks: Every 2 weeks
- 36 weeks until delivery: Every week

The return prenatal visit also provides the opportunity for the physician and the medical assistant to lend support to the mother, to provide her with ongoing prenatal education to reduce apprehension and anxiety, and to ensure that the mother is well informed and prepared during her pregnancy, childbirth, and the postpartum period. The medical assistant plays an important role in prenatal education and should take the necessary time with each patient to provide appropriate information and to allow the patient to ask questions. Procedure 23-3 outlines the medical assistant's role in the return prenatal visit.

The patient is asked to provide a urine specimen during each return prenatal visit. The medical assistant is responsible for testing the specimen for glucose and protein using a reagent strip and for recording results in the prenatal record. A positive reaction to glucose may indicate the development of gestational diabetes mellitus or a prediabetic condition, and a positive reaction to protein may indicate a urinary tract infection or preeclampsia. Further testing usually is needed to arrive at a final diagnosis and to institute treatment. Hypertension is the most common medical disorder of pregnancy and occurs in 10% to 12% of all pregnancies. Because of this, the medical assistant must make sure to obtain an accurate blood pressure measurement.

During the return visit, the physician performs one or more of the following procedures, depending on the stage of the pregnancy: (1) palpation of the woman's abdomen to measure fundal height, (2) measurement of the fetal heart rate, and (3) a vaginal examination. These procedures are discussed in detail next.

Fundal Height Measurement

The pregnant uterus rises gradually into the abdominal cavity, and the fundus is palpable between 8 and 13 weeks of gestation. The first fundal height measurement, which is usually performed during the first prenatal visit, is used as a guideline for all subsequent measurements. The physician measures the fundal height by placing one end of a flexible, nonstretchable centimeter tape measure on the superior aspect of the symphysis pubis and measuring to the crest or top of the uterine fundus (Figure 23-12). The measurement is recorded on a flow chart in the patient's prenatal record. By 20 weeks, the fundus reaches the lower border of the umbilicus, and between 36 and 37 weeks, it reaches the tip of the sternum. During the first and second trimesters, measuring the fundal height provides a rough estimate of the duration of the pregnancy (Figure 23-13).

Because fetal weights vary considerably during the third trimester, it is difficult to use fundal height measurements as an estimate of the duration of the pregnancy in the last trimester.

In addition to assessing the duration of the pregnancy, the fundal height measurements permit variations from normal to become apparent and are used to assess whether fetal growth is progressing normally. Growth that is too

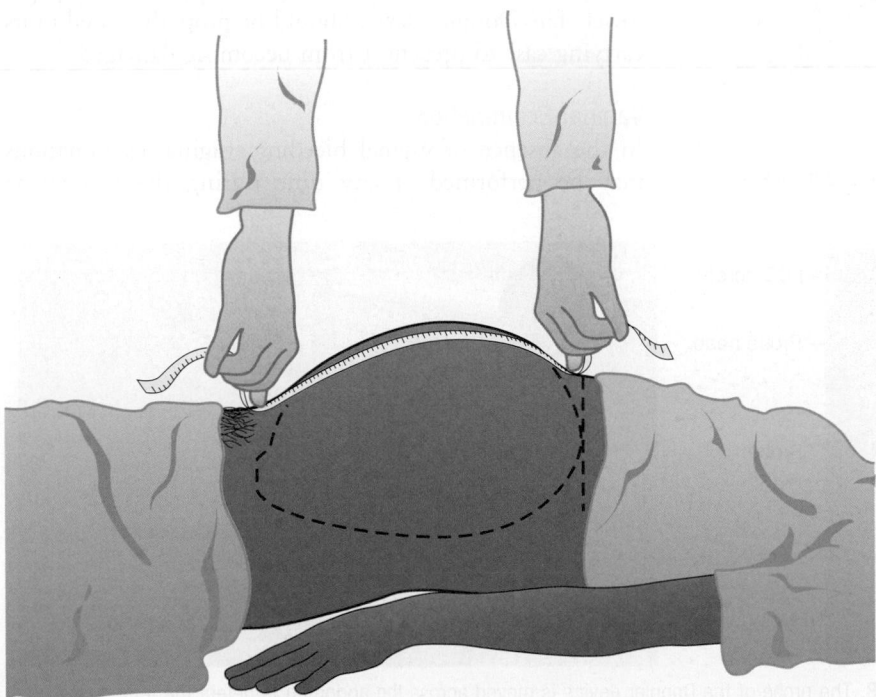

Figure 23-12 Measurement of fundal height. The physician places one end of a centimeter tape measure on the superior aspect of the symphysis pubis and measures to the top of the uterine fundus.

rapid or too slow must be evaluated further by the physician as a possible indication of high-risk conditions, such as multiple pregnancies, polyhydramnios, ovarian tumor, and intrauterine growth retardation, intrauterine death, or an error in estimating the fetal progress.

Fetal Heart Tones

The normal **fetal heart rate** is between 120 and 160 beats per minute with a regular rhythm. A very slow or rapid fetal heart rate usually indicates fetal distress. The term **fetal heart tones** refers to the heartbeat of the fetus as heard through the mother's abdominal wall. The fetal heart tones can be heard with a Doppler fetal pulse detector between 10 and 12 weeks of gestation. The Doppler fetal pulse detector converts ultrasonic waves into audible sounds of the fetal pulse.

The Doppler device consists of a main control unit and a probe (Figure 23-14, *A*). The probe head contains a transducer and electronic components, which generate the sound waves. The probe head is delicate and must be handled carefully, making sure not to drop or knock the head to prevent damaging it.

Because air is a poor conductor of sound, an ultrasound coupling gel must first be spread on the mother's abdomen in the area to be examined. The gel is usually applied by the medical assistant, and its purpose is to increase conductivity of the sound waves between the abdomen and the transducer.

The physician places the head of the probe into the gel on the mother's abdomen and slowly moves it until the fetal heart tones are located. The Doppler device amplifies the fetal heart tones, and they are broadcast through a built-in loudspeaker in the main unit. A volume control provides adjustment of the sound level as required. (Fetal heart tones sound like the hoofbeats of a galloping horse, and when the probe is over the placenta, a windlike sound is heard.) The Doppler device also may have an LCD screen, which provides a digital display of the fetal pulse rate. Stereo headphones come with the Doppler device to allow private listening. The loudspeaker is muted when the headphones are connected (Figure 23-14, *B*).

After the procedure, the medical assistant should remove excess gel from the mother's abdomen with a paper towel. The probe head is cleaned using a damp cloth or a paper towel. The Doppler device should be properly stored in its carrying case to prevent it from becoming damaged.

Vaginal Examination

In the absence of vaginal bleeding, vaginal examinations may be performed at any time during the pregnancy;

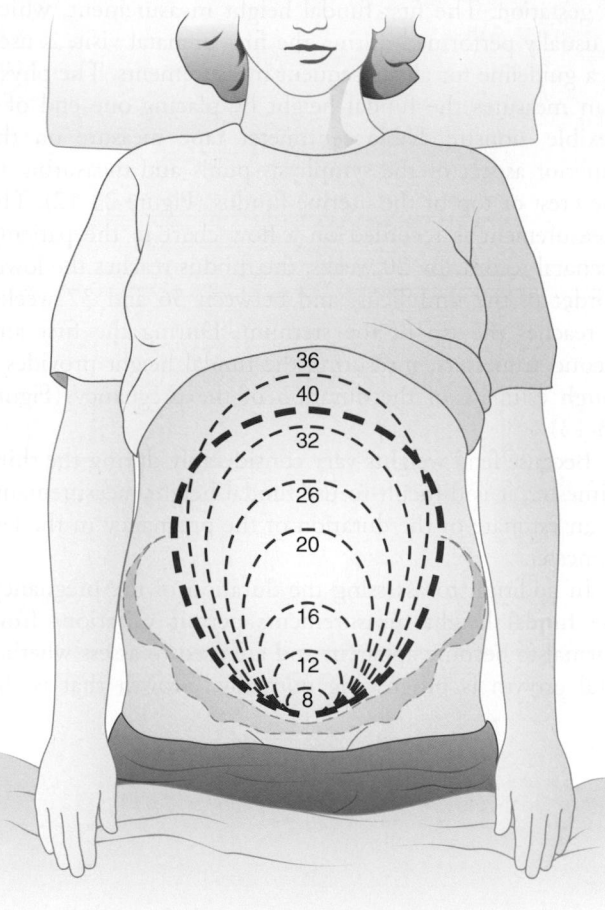

Figure 23-13 Fundal height showing gestational age in weeks.

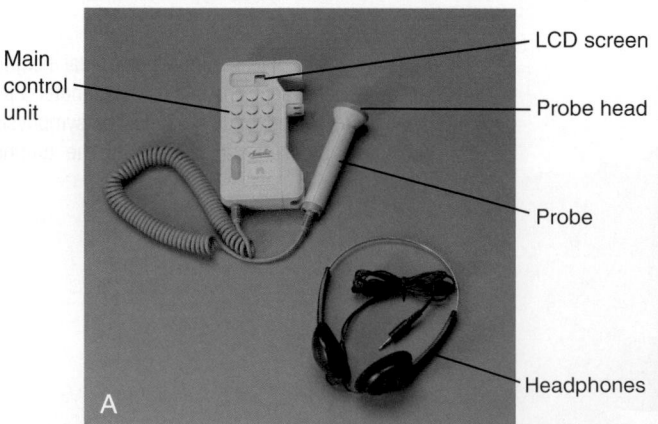

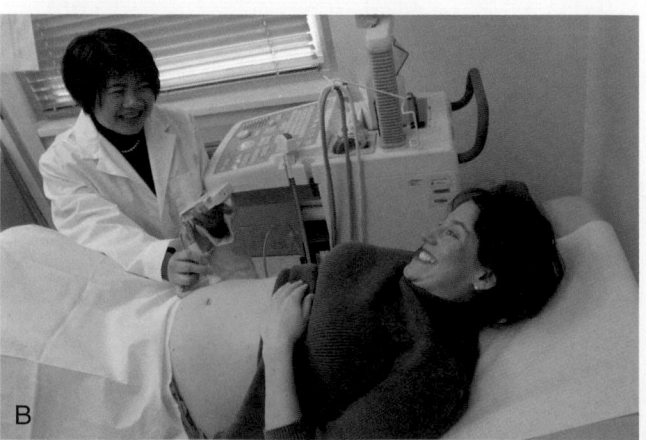

Figure 23-14 **A,** Parts of a Doppler device. **B,** The probe of the Doppler device is moved across the abdomen to detect the fetal pulse.

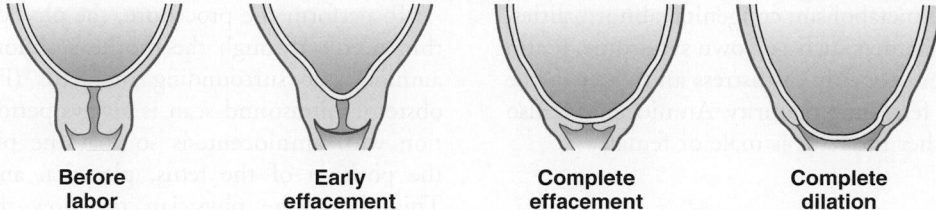

Before labor   **Early effacement**   **Complete effacement**   **Complete dilation**

Figure 23-15 Effacement and dilation occur to permit the passage of the infant into the birth canal. The cervical canal shortens from its normal length of 1 to 2 cm to a structure with paper thin edges in which there is no canal at all. The cervix dilates from an opening a few millimeters wide to an opening large enough to allow the passage of the infant (approximately 10 cm).

however, in a normal pregnancy, there is usually no need to perform a vaginal examination until the patient nears term. The vaginal examination is usually begun approximately 2 to 3 weeks from the EDD and is performed to confirm the presenting part and to determine the degree, if any, of cervical dilation and effacement. The purpose of dilation and effacement is to permit the passage of the infant from the uterus into the birth canal (Figure 23-15).

What Would You Do? What Would You *Not* Do?

Case Study 4

Wynita Lopez is at the office with her husband. She is 32 years old and 18 weeks pregnant. It took Wynita a long time—almost 6 years—to get pregnant. She is excited and happy about being pregnant but, at the same time, sad and confused. Her test results on her triple screen test came back indicating the possibility that her baby has Down syndrome. A repeat test was done with the same results. Wynita just got finished having an ultrasound that showed a normal baby, but Wynita and her husband understand that the only way to know for sure is to have an amniocentesis. Wynita does not know what to do. She is afraid of having an amniocentesis because of the chance of miscarriage. She also knows her triple screen test could be a false-positive. Wynita is unsure what her decision would be if the baby did have Down syndrome. Her husband is visibly distressed and wants Wynita to make all the decisions, saying he will be supportive of whatever she decides. Right now she wants as much information as she can get about all of this before she makes a decision. She feels "safer" being at the medical office and does not want to go home just yet. ■

Special Tests and Procedures

The pregnancy can be evaluated with one or more of the following special tests and procedures: triple screen test, obstetric ultrasound scan, amniocentesis, and fetal heart rate monitoring. These are not considered routine procedures; however, they involve little or no risk to the mother or the fetus. Because some of these tests may be performed in the obstetric medical office, the medical assistant should have a general knowledge of these procedures.

Triple Screen Test

The triple screen test (also known as the *multiple marker test*) is a laboratory test available to pregnant women

between 15 and 20 weeks of gestation. Its purpose is to screen for the presence of certain fetal abnormalities, which include neural tube defects, Down syndrome, trisomy 18, and ventral wall defect. Because the triple screen test has a high incidence of false-positive test results, it is not a mandatory prenatal test; however, the American College of Obstetricians and Gynecologists believes that this test should be offered to all pregnant women regardless of maternal age.

The triple screen test is a screening test. Abnormal test results always require further testing, such as an ultrasound or amniocentesis, to determine whether a fetal abnormality actually exists.

Obstetric Ultrasound Scan

An obstetric ultrasound scan is a diagnostic imaging technique, similar to sonar, used to view the fetus in utero. It allows continuous viewing of the fetus and shows fetal movement. The physician or an ultrasound technologist performs the procedure. The primary purpose of an ultrasound scan is to evaluate the health of the fetus and to determine gestational age. This is accomplished by viewing the image of the fetus and by taking various measurements of the image, such as crown-rump length; biparietal diameter, which is a side-to-side measurement of the fetal head; femur length; and abdominal circumference.

Obstetric ultrasound scanning uses high-frequency sound waves that are directed into the uterus through a transducer. When the sound waves reach the uterus, they "bounce" back to the transducer, similar to an echo. These reflected sound waves are converted into an image, or *sonogram* (Figure 23-16), which is displayed on a monitor screen. The monitor is usually positioned so the mother can observe the image on the screen if she wishes. Although an obstetric ultrasound scan can be performed at any time during the pregnancy, it is often performed at between 7 and 12 weeks of gestation and again at between 18 and 20 weeks. A third scan is sometimes done around 34 weeks of gestation. Box 23-1 outlines this schedule and what can be assessed at these times.

Amniocentesis

Amniocentesis is a diagnostic procedure that can be performed between 15 and 18 weeks of gestation. Amniocentesis aids in prenatal diagnosis of certain genetically transmitted errors of metabolism, congenital abnormalities, and chromosomal disorders such as Down syndrome. It also is used to detect fetal jeopardy or distress and, later in the pregnancy, to assess fetal lung maturity. Amniocentesis also can determine whether the fetus is male or female.

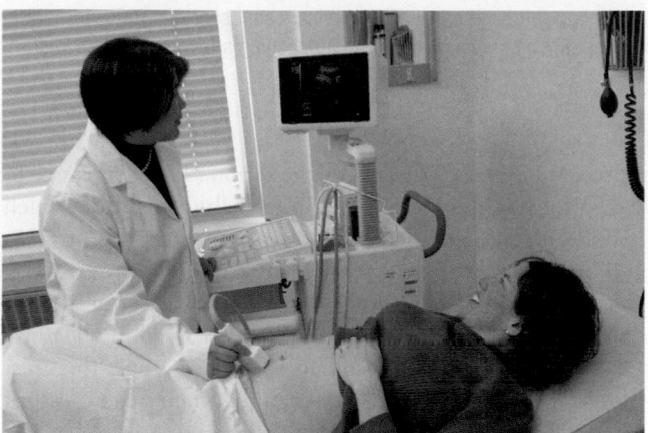

Figure 23-16 Obstetric ultrasound scan.

To perform the procedure, the physician inserts a long, thin needle through the mother's abdomen and into the amniotic sac surrounding the fetus (Figure 23-17). An obstetric ultrasound scan is always performed in conjunction with amniocentesis so that the physician can view the position of the fetus, placenta, and amniotic fluid. This allows the physician to know the exact place to insert the needle. The physician withdraws a sample (about 1 tablespoon) of fluid, which contains fetal cells. The fluid is sent to a laboratory for study. It usually takes 1 to 3 weeks to evaluate the amniotic fluid and report the results.

Although the complication rate for an amniocentesis is extremely low, the procedure is not risk free. There is a slight risk of bleeding, leakage of fluid, and infection of the amniotic fluid. There also is a slight possibility of miscarriage. Because of these risks, amniocentesis is offered only to women whose pregnancies are at risk for fetal abnormalities. This includes women who are 35 years old or older, women who have a child with a genetic or neural tube defect, women who have abnormal triple screen test results, women who have or whose partner has a chromosomal abnormality,

---

BOX 23-1 Purpose of Obstetric Ultrasound Scanning

Between 7 and 12 Weeks
- To confirm pregnancy by detecting fetal heart motion
- To determine gestational age by taking measurements of the embryo and embryonic sac
- To detect an ectopic pregnancy

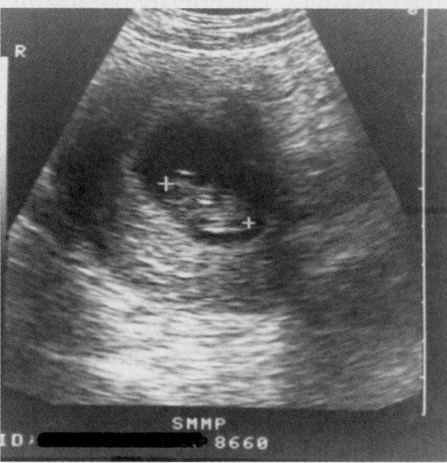

Embryo at approximately 9 weeks of gestation.

Between 18 and 20 Weeks
- To determine fetal growth, size, and weight by taking measurements of the fetus
- To detect the presence of multiple fetuses
- To examine the brain, spinal cord, heart, lungs, gastrointestinal tract, reproductive organs, kidneys, bladder, bowel, and extremities of the fetus
- To detect congenital abnormalities
- To determine the location of the placenta

- To determine the cause of bleeding or spotting

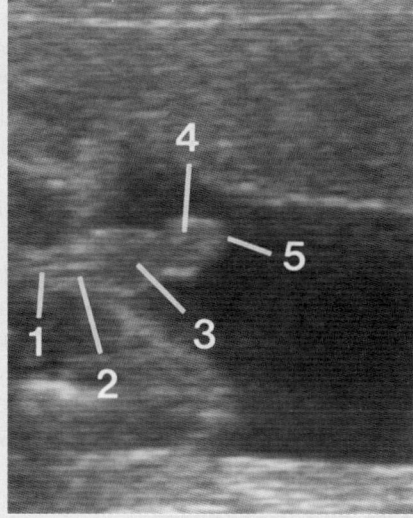

Erect fetal penis. *1,* Urethra; *2,* corpus cavernosum; *3,* shaft; *4,* glans; *5,* foreskin.

At 34 Weeks
- To evaluate fetal growth, size, and weight by taking measurements of the fetus
- To verify the location of the placenta
- To confirm fetal presentation in uncertain cases

Other Purposes
- To diagnose uterine and pelvic abnormalities during pregnancy

BOX 23-1 Purpose of Obstetric Ultrasound Scanning—cont'd

- To view the fetus, placenta, and amniotic fluid during tests such as amniocentesis and chorionic villus sampling
- To confirm intrauterine death

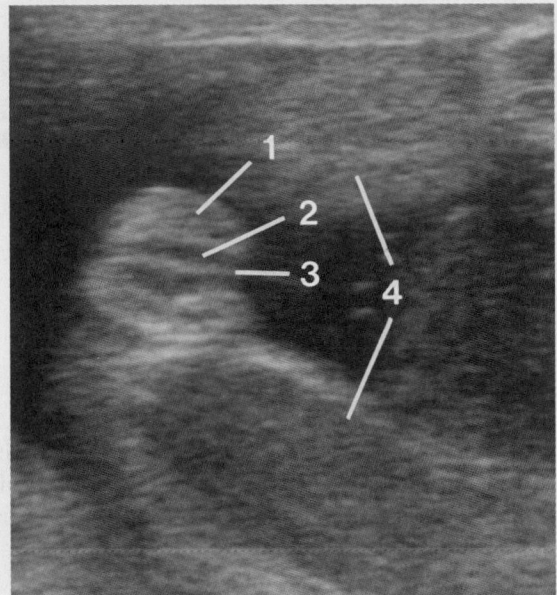

External female genitalia. *1,* Major labium; *2,* minor labium; *3,* vaginal cleft; *4,* thighs.

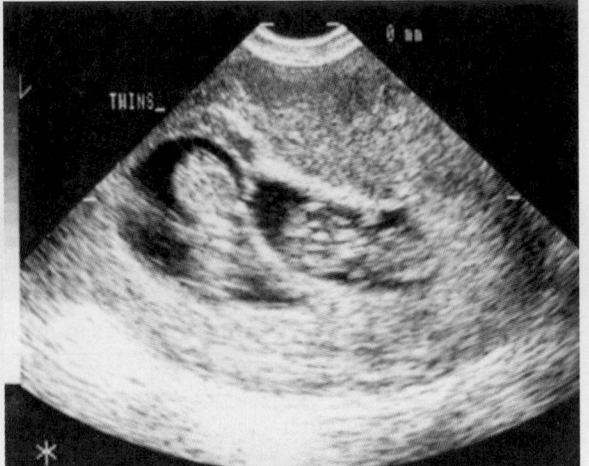

Twins.

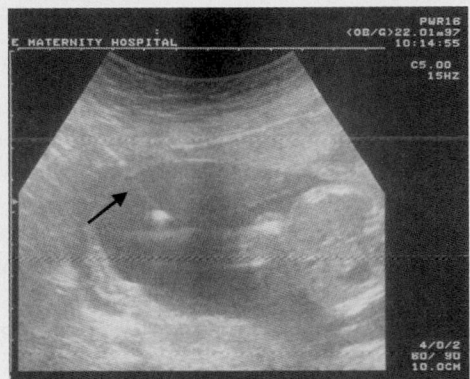

Amniocentesis being performed under ultrasound guidance.

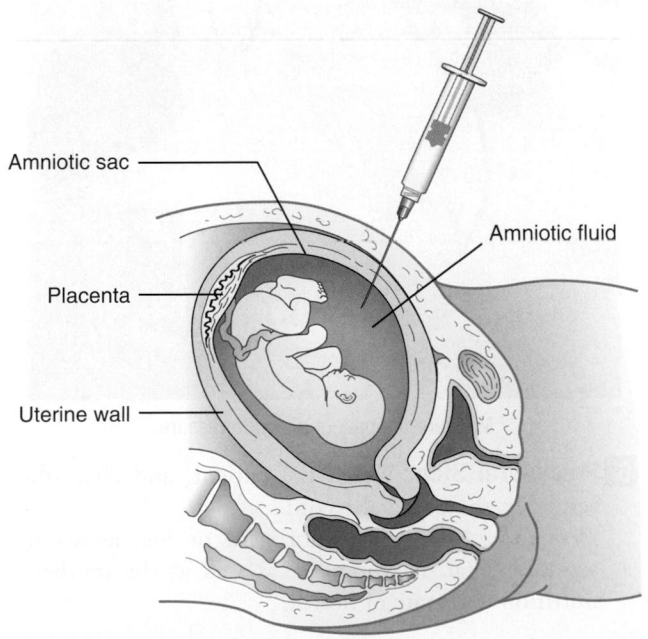

Figure 23-17 Amniocentesis.

and women who are or whose partner is a carrier for a metabolic disease.

Fetal Heart Rate Monitoring

Fetal heart rate (FHR) monitoring is performed later in the pregnancy to obtain information on the physical condition of the fetus. Specific conditions that may warrant this procedure are fetal growth that is not progressing well, decreased amniotic fluid, decreased fetal activity, elevation of the mother's blood pressure, gestational diabetes, and an overdue infant.

To perform the procedure, an electronic microphone is strapped to the mother's abdomen to amplify the fetal heartbeat. A gel is usually applied under the microphone to make the sounds clearer. The fetal heartbeat is heard and displayed on a screen and printed on special paper.

Medical Assisting Responsibilities

The medical assistant has many important responsibilities in the return prenatal examination, which are outlined in Procedure 23-3. The medical assistant is responsible for assembling the equipment and supplies required for the examination, for obtaining information to update the prenatal record, for preparing the patient for the examination, and for assisting the physician during the examination.

The physician depends on the medical assistant to have the urine test results and certain measurements, such as blood pressure and weight, completed and recorded in advance to allow him or her the opportunity to review these measurements before examining the patient.

PROCEDURE 23-3   Assisting with a Return Prenatal Examination

Outcome Assist with a return prenatal examination.

Equipment/Supplies

- Urine specimen container
- Centimeter tape measure
- Doppler fetal pulse detector
- Ultrasound coupling gel
- Paper towel

- Disposable vaginal speculum
- Disposable gloves
- Water-based lubricant
- Gauze pads
- Examining gown and drape

1. Procedural Step. Sanitize your hands.

2. Procedural Step. Set up the tray for the prenatal examination. The equipment and supplies depend on the procedures to be included in the examination, which may include one or more of the following:
a. Fundal height measurement
b. Measurement of fetal heart tones
c. Examination of the legs, feet, and face for edema and development of varicosities
d. Taking a specimen for the diagnosis of a vaginal infection
e. Vaginal examination

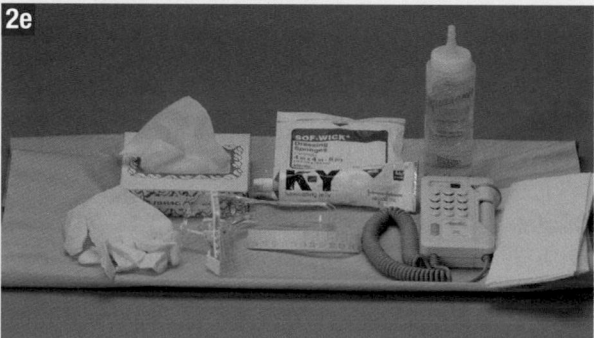

Set up the prenatal tray.

3. Procedural Step. Greet the patient and introduce yourself. Identify the patient and explain the procedure. Provide the patient with a urine specimen container, and ask her to obtain a urine specimen.
Principle. A urine specimen is needed to test for glucose and protein at each prenatal visit. In addition, an empty bladder makes the examination easier and is more comfortable for the patient.

4. Procedural Step. Escort the patient to the examining room, and ask her to be seated. Seat yourself so that

you are facing the patient. Ask the patient whether she has experienced any problems since the last prenatal visit, and record information in the appropriate section in her prenatal record.
Principle. The physician investigates any unusual or abnormal signs or symptoms relayed by the patient.

5. Procedural Step. Measure the patient's blood pressure, and chart the results in the prenatal record. If the blood pressure is elevated, allow the patient to relax, and then measure the blood pressure again.
Principle. Taking the blood pressure again gives the opportunity to determine whether the elevation was due to emotional excitement.

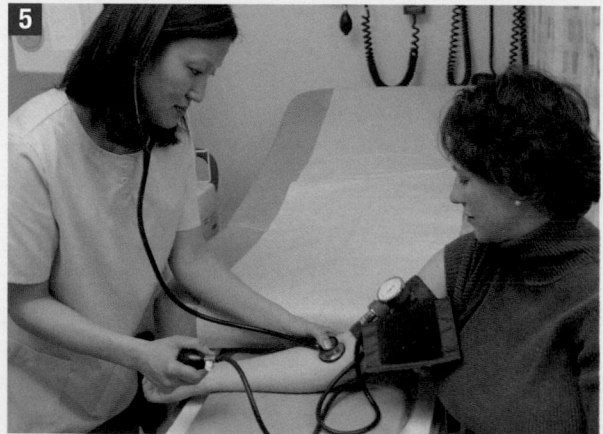

Measure the patient's blood pressure.

6. Procedural Step. Weigh the patient, and chart the results in the prenatal record.
Principle. Maternal weight gain or loss assists in assessing fetal development, as well as the mother's nutrition and state of health.

PROCEDURE 23-3   Assisting with a Return Prenatal Examination—cont'd

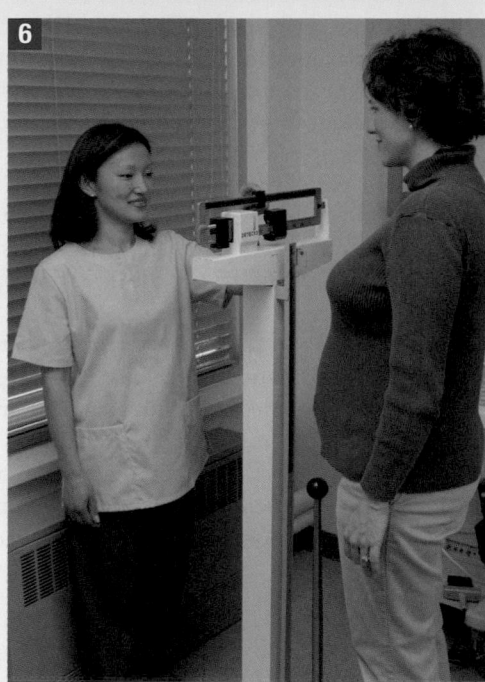

Weigh the patient.

7. Procedural Step. Instruct and prepare the patient for the examination. Have her remove or pull up her outer clothing to expose the abdominal area. If the physician will be performing a vaginal examination, the patient also must remove her panties; otherwise, she may leave them on. Tell the patient to have a seat on the examining table when she is finished getting ready for the examination. Inform the patient that the physician will be with her soon, and leave the room to give her privacy.

8. Procedural Step. Using a reagent strip, test the urine specimen for glucose and protein, and chart the results. *Note:* The urine specimen may be tested at any time before the physician examines the patient; however, a convenient time to test the specimen is while the patient is disrobing.
Principle. The prenatal patient's urine must be tested at every visit to assist in early detection and prevention of disease.

9. Procedural Step. Make the medical record available for review by the physician. The medical office has a designated location where the record is placed, such as a small shelf mounted on the wall next to the outside of the examining room door or in a chart holder on the outside of the examining room door. Position the medical record so that patient-identifiable information is not visible.
Principle. Before going into the room, the physician will want to review the patient's chart and information documented by the medical assistant. HIPAA requires protection of a patient's health information.

10. Procedural Step. Check to make sure the patient is ready to be seen by the physician. Before entering a patient's room, always knock lightly on the door to let the patient know you are getting ready to enter the room. Inform the physician. This may be done using a color-coded flagging system mounted on the wall next to the examining room.

11. Procedural Step. Assist the patient into a supine position, and properly drape her. Provide support and reassurance to the patient to help her relax during the examination.
Principle. The patient should be properly draped so that she is warm and comfortable.

12. Procedural Step. Assist the physician as required for the prenatal examination, as follows:
   a. *Fundal Height Measurement:* Hand the physician the tape measure for determination of the fundal measurement.
   b. *Fetal Heart Tones:* Apply a liberal amount of coupling gel to the patient's abdomen. Turn on the Doppler fetal pulse detector and hand it to the physician. When the physician is finished, remove excess gel from the patient with a paper towel. Clean the probe head of the Doppler device with a damp cloth or a paper towel. Place the probe head back in its holder.

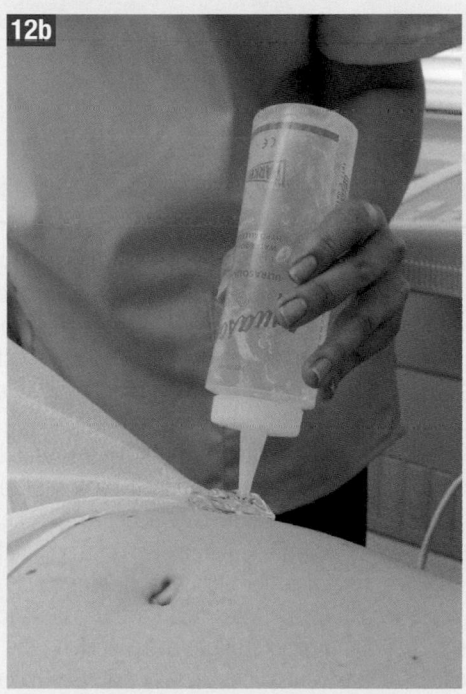

Apply a liberal amount of coupling gel.

   c. *Vaginal Specimen:* Assist the patient into the lithotomy position if a specimen is to be taken for the detection of a vaginal infection. Assist with collection of the specimen as required.

Continued

PROCEDURE **23-3**   Assisting with a Return Prenatal Examination—cont'd

d. *Vaginal Examination:* Assist the patient into the lithotomy position if a vaginal examination is to be performed.

13. **Procedural Step.** After the examination, assist the patient into a sitting position, and allow her the opportunity to rest for a moment. If a vaginal

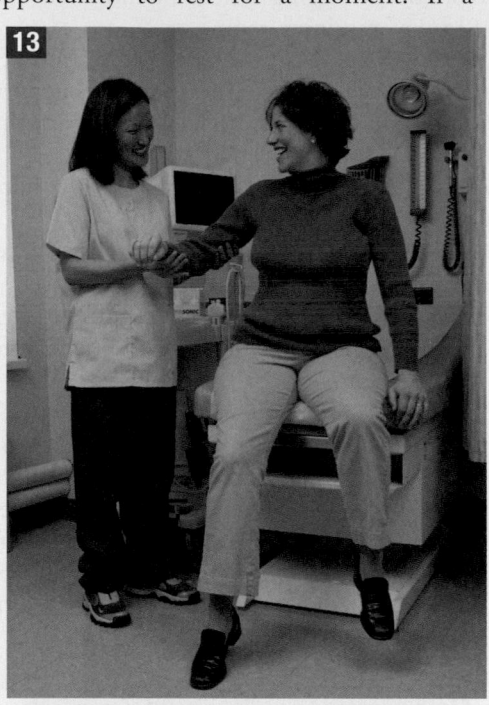

Assist the patient off the examining table.

examination was performed, offer the patient tissues to remove excess lubricating jelly from the perineum. Assist her off the examining table to prevent falls. Instruct the patient to get dressed. Leave the room to provide the patient with privacy.

Principle. The patient may become dizzy after being on the examining table and should be allowed to rest before getting off the table. The medical assistant must provide for the safety of the prenatal patient while she is getting off the examining table.

14. **Procedural Step.** Provide the prenatal patient teaching and further explanation of the physician's instructions as required to meet individual patient needs. Escort the patient to the reception area.

15. **Procedural Step.** Clean the examining room in preparation for the next patient, and, if necessary, prepare specimens for transport to an outside medical laboratory.

MEDICAL PRACTICE *and the* LAW

Mature minor

A difficult and complex issue facing policymakers today involves whether a minor should be able to obtain health care services without a parent's consent. A minor is an individual who has not reached the age of majority; in most states, minors reach majority at 18 years old (at that time, individuals are legally able to make their own decisions regarding health care).

Over the past 3 decades, many states have passed legislation permitting minors to receive some health care services without parental consent. These include contraceptive services, testing and treatment for sexually transmitted diseases, prenatal care and delivery services, treatment for alcohol and drug abuse, and outpatient mental health care. States that have passed such legislation reason that some minors might avoid seeking the care that they need for certain conditions if they have to have parental consent. The one major exception to this is abortion. Most states have laws that require the involvement of at least one parent in a minor's decision to have an abortion.

In recent years, some states have given minors even greater authority to make health care decisions for themselves by adopting what is known as the *mature minor rule*. This allows an individual in the middle to late teens who exhibits the intelligence and maturity to understand the nature and consequences of a medical treatment to consent to such treatment without parental consent.

It is important for the medical assistant to become familiar with the laws in his or her state regarding a minor's right to consent to health care to help the medical assistant in making appropriate decisions with respect to minors. For example, if a state does not allow a minor to obtain prenatal care without parental consent, the medical assistant would not be permitted to make an appointment for a minor who is pregnant; rather, the appointment would have to be scheduled by the minor's parent. Consent by minors to health care services will continue to be a complex issue; the medical assistant must keep up-to-date with changes in his or her state. ■

What Would You Do? What Would You *Not* Do? RESPONSES

Case Study 1
Page 430

What Did Yin-Ling Do?
- ❒ Reassured Mrs. Wooster that the physician is there to help her and stressed that he will be pleased that she has come to the office for an examination.
- ❒ Commended Mrs. Wooster on performing a breast self-examination at home and encouraged her to continue performing a BSE each month. Asked her whether she had any questions on how to perform a BSE.
- ❒ Told Mrs. Wooster that some breast changes are normal and others are not normal, and the only way to know for sure is to be examined by the physician.
- ❒ Told Mrs. Wooster that it is important to have a periodic gynecologic examination even if her periods are normal. Explained to her that some conditions can be present without symptoms. Took plenty of time with her so that she would feel comfortable coming back again in the future for a gynecologic examination. Gave Mrs. Wooster a patient information brochure on gynecologic examinations.
- ❒ Gave Mrs. Wooster a patient information brochure on mammograms, and explained the mammogram procedure to reduce her apprehension. Explained that the procedure is not painful, but there may be some minor discomfort. Provided her with some tips on reducing discomfort that may occur, such as avoiding caffeine several days before the procedure and having the office schedule the mammogram a week after her menstrual period.

What Did Yin-Ling Not Do?
- ❒ Did not criticize Mrs. Wooster for waiting so long to schedule a gynecologic examination.
- ❒ Did not tell Mrs. Wooster that there is no discomfort involved with a mammogram.

What Would You Do?/What Would You Not Do?
Review Yin-Ling's response and place a checkmark next to the information you included in your response. List additional information you included in your response.

_____

_____

_____

_____

_____

Case Study 2
Page 447

What Did Yin-Ling Do?
- ❒ Stressed to Dagny how important it is that she be seen by the physician. Explained that she could be infected with chlamydia and not know it because chlamydia often has no symptoms, especially in women.
- ❒ Explained to Dagny that state law allows her to be treated for a sexually transmitted disease without permission from her parents. Told her the law was created to encourage minors to seek treatment for sexually transmitted diseases.
- ❒ Commended Dagny on practicing safe sex. Relayed to her that if a condom is not used correctly, or if it tears, she might not be protected from getting a sexually transmitted disease. That is another reason she should be tested.
- ❒ Explained to Dagny what will occur during the examination and what the physician will be doing. Relayed techniques that Dagny could use to relax during the procedure.

What Did Yin-Ling Not Do?
- ❒ Did not tell Dagny everything would be all right and that she probably does not have chlamydia.
- ❒ Did not ask Dagny whether she knew how her boyfriend got chlamydia.
- ❒ If Dagny still insisted on leaving, did not try to prevent her from doing so.

What Would You Do?/What Would You Not Do?
Review Yin-Ling's response and place a checkmark next to the information you included in your response. List additional information you included in your response.

_____

_____

_____

_____

_____

Case Study 3
Page 455

What Did Yin-Ling Do?
- ❒ Tried to calm Johanna by telling her that it is normal for her to be worried and concerned. Explained that the purpose of her prenatal visits is so that the physician can keep a close watch on her and detect any problems that might occur.
- ❒ Reassured Johanna that she does not need to be afraid to tell the physician any of her concerns because he is there to help her and her baby.
- ❒ Told Johanna that it is important not to take any medications during her pregnancy without first checking with the physician because some medications could be harmful to her baby.
- ❒ Told Johanna that her problems and concerns would be relayed to the physician and that he would want to talk to her about them. Explained that the physician also would talk with her about being tested for group B streptococcus.

What Did Yin-Ling Not Do?
- ❒ Did not tell Johanna that it was all right to take the antibiotics.

Continued

What Would You Do? What Would You *Not* Do? RESPONSES—cont'd

What Would You Do?/What Would You Not *Do?*
Review Yin-Ling's response and place a checkmark next to the information you included in your response. List additional information you included in your response.

_____
_____
_____
_____
_____
_____

Case Study 4
Page 459

What Did Yin-Ling Do?
❐ Escorted Mr. and Mrs. Lopez to a private room in the office. Tried to relax them and told them that whatever they choose to do will be the right decision for them. Reassured them that they could stay at the office for as long as they wanted.
❐ Gave Mrs. Lopez the information she requested that was available at the office and provided her with a list of resources

approved by the physician that she could contact for further information.
❐ Asked Mr. and Mrs. Lopez whether they had any more questions they wanted to ask the physician.

What Did Yin-Ling Not Do?
❐ Did not give Mr. and Mrs. Lopez advice on what they should do.

What Would You Do?/What Would You Not *Do?*
Review Yin-Ling's response and place a checkmark next to the information you included in your response. List additional information you included in your response.

_____
_____
_____
_____
_____
_____

TERMINOLOGY REVIEW

Medical Term	Word Parts	Definition
Abortion		The termination of the pregnancy before the fetus reaches the age of viability (20 weeks).
Adnexal		Adjacent.
Amenorrhea	*a-:* without *men/o:* menstruation *-orrhea:* flow, excessive discharge	The absence or cessation of the menstrual period. Amenorrhea occurs normally before puberty, during pregnancy, and after menopause.
Atypical	*a-:* without	Deviation from the normal.
Braxton Hicks contractions		Intermittent and irregular painless uterine contractions that occur throughout pregnancy. They occur more frequently toward the end of pregnancy and are sometimes mistaken for true labor pains.
Cervix		The lower narrow end of the uterus that opens into the vagina.
Colposcopy	*colp/o:* vagina *-scopy:* visual examination	Examination of the cervix using a colposcope (a lighted instrument with a magnifying lens).
Cytology	*cyt/o:* cell *-ology:* study of	The science that deals with the study of cells, including their origin, structure, function, and pathology.
Dilation (of the cervix)		The stretching of the external os from an opening a few millimeters wide to an opening large enough to allow the passage of an infant (approximately 10 cm).
Dysmenorrhea	*dys-:* difficult, painful, abnormal *men/o:* menstruation *-orrhea:* flow, excessive discharge	Pain associated with the menstrual period.
Dyspareunia	*dys-:* difficult, painful, abnormal	Pain in the vagina or pelvis experienced by a woman during sexual intercourse.
Dysplasia	*dys-:* difficult, painful, abnormal *plasia:* a growth	The growth of abnormal cells. Dysplasia is a precancerous condition that may or may not develop into cancer.
Ectocervix	*ecto-:* outside, outer	The part of the cervix that projects into the vagina and is lined with stratified squamous epithelium.

TERMINOLOGY REVIEW—cont'd

Medical Term	Word Parts	Definition
Effacement		The thinning and shortening of the cervical canal from its normal length of 1 to 2 cm to a structure with paper-thin edges in which there is no canal at all. Effacement occurs late in pregnancy, during labor, or both. The purpose of effacement along with dilation is to permit the passage of the infant into the birth canal.
Embryo		The child in utero from the time of conception to the beginning of the first trimester.
Endocervix	*endo-:* within	The mucous membrane lining the cervical canal.
Engagement		The entrance of the fetal head or the presenting part into the pelvic inlet.
Expected date of delivery (EDD)		Projected birth date of the infant.
External os		The opening of the cervical canal of the uterus into the vagina.
Fetal heart rate		The number of times per minute the fetal heart beats.
Fetal heart tones		The sounds of the heartbeat of the fetus heard through the mother's abdominal wall.
Fetus		The child in utero from the third month after conception to birth; during the first 2 months of development, it is called an *embryo.*
Fundus		The dome-shaped upper portion of the uterus between the fallopian tubes.
Gestation		The period of intrauterine development from conception to birth; the period of pregnancy. The average pregnancy lasts about 280 days, or 40 weeks, from the date of conception to childbirth.
Gestational age		The age of the fetus between conception and birth.
Gynecology	*gynec/o:* woman *-ology:* study of	The branch of medicine that deals with the diseases of reproductive organs of women.
Infant		A child from birth to 12 months of age.
Menopause	*men/o:* menstruation	The permanent cessation of menstruation, which usually occurs between the ages of 45 and 55.
Menorrhagia	*men/o:* menstruation *-orrhagia:* rapid flow of blood	Excessive bleeding during a menstrual period, in the number of days or the amount of blood or both. Also called *dysfunctional uterine bleeding (DUB).*
Metrorrhagia	*metr/o:* uterus *-orrhagia:* rapid flow of blood	Bleeding between menstrual periods.
Multigravida	*multi-:* many *gravid/o:* pregnancy	A woman who has been pregnant more than once.
Multipara	*multi-:* many *par/o:* bear, give birth to	A woman who has completed two or more pregnancies to the age of fetal viability regardless of whether they ended in live infants or stillbirths.
Nullipara	*nulli-:* none *par/o:* bear, give birth to	A woman who has not carried a pregnancy to the point of fetal viability (20 weeks of gestation).
Obstetrics		The branch of medicine concerned with the care of the woman during pregnancy, childbirth, and the postpartal period.
Perimenopause	*peri-:* surrounding *men/o:* menstruation	Before the onset of menopause, the phase during which the woman with regular periods changes to irregular cycles and increased periods of amenorrhea.
Perineum		The external region between the vaginal orifice and the anus in a female and between the scrotum and the anus in a male.
Position		The relation of the presenting part of the fetus to the maternal pelvis.
Postpartum	*post-:* after *par/o:* bear, give birth to	Occurring after childbirth.
Preeclampsia		A major complication of pregnancy, the cause of which is unknown, characterized by increasing hypertension, albuminuria, and edema. If this condition is neglected or is not treated properly, it may develop into eclampsia, which could cause maternal convulsions and coma. Preeclampsia generally occurs between the 20th week of pregnancy and the end of the first week postpartum.
Prenatal	*pre-:* in front of, before *nat/o:* birth *-al:* pertaining to	Before birth.

Continued

⟳ TERMINOLOGY REVIEW—cont'd

Medical Term	Word Parts	Definition
Presentation		Indication of the part of the fetus that is closest to the cervix and is delivered first. A cephalic presentation is a delivery in which the fetal head is presenting against the cervix. A breech presentation is a delivery in which the buttocks or feet are presented instead of the head.
Primigravida	*prim/i:* first *gravid/o:* pregnancy	A woman who is pregnant for the first time.
Primipara	*prim/i:* first *par/o:* bear, give birth to	A woman who has carried a pregnancy to fetal viability (20 weeks of gestation) for the first time regardless of whether the infant was stillborn or alive at birth.
Puerperium		The period of time, usually 4 to 6 weeks after delivery, in which the uterus and the body systems are returning to normal.
Quickening		The first movements of the fetus in utero as felt by the mother, which usually occur between 16 and 20 weeks of gestation and are felt consistently thereafter.
Risk factor		Anything that increases an individual's chance of developing a disease. Some risk factors (e.g., smoking) can be avoided, but others cannot (e.g., age and family history).
Toxemia		A condition that can occur in pregnant women that includes preeclampsia and eclampsia. If preeclampsia goes undiagnosed or is not satisfactorily controlled, it could develop into eclampsia, characterized by convulsions and coma.
Trimester	*tri-:* three	Three months, or one third, of the gestational period of pregnancy.
Vulva		The region of the external female genital organs.

🔖 ON THE WEB

For information on sexually transmitted diseases:

National Institute of Allergy and Infectious Diseases: Sexually Transmitted Infections: www3.niaid.nih.gov/topics/sti

Centers for Disease Control and Prevention: Sexually Transmitted Diseases: www.cdc.gov/std

Planned Parenthood: www.plannedparenthood.org

Medline Plus Sexually Transmitted Diseases: www.nlm.nih.gov/medlineplus/sexuallytransmitteddiseases.html

WebMD Sexual Conditions: www.webmd.com/sexual-conditions

Your STD Help: yourstdhelp.com

STD Support Website: herpes-coldsores.com/support/std.htm

American Social Health Association: www.ashastd.org

Herpes Information: www.gotherpes.com

HPV Information: www.gothpv.com

For information on women's health:

The National Women's Health Information Center: www.4women.gov

The Universe of Women's Health: www.obgyn.net

Women's Health: www.womenshealth.gov

For information on contraceptives:

Planned Parenthood: www.plannedparenthood.org

Mayo Clinic Birth Control Options: www.mayoclinic.com/health/birth-control/BI99999

Ultimate Birth Control Links: www.ultimatebirthcontrol.com

Reproductive Health Online: www.reproline.jhu.edu/index.htm

ON THE WEB—cont'd

For information on menopause:

North American Menopause Society: www.menopause.org

Everything Menopause: www.menopauseinfo.org

Power Surge: www.power-surge.com

Project Aware: www.project-aware.org

Mayo Clinic Menopause Information: www.mayoclinic.com/health/menopause/DS00119

WebMD Menopause Health Center: www.webmd.com/mcnopause

Medline Plus Menopause: www.nlm.nih.gov/medlineplus/menopause.html

For information on pregnancy and childbirth:

Pregnancy and Childbirth: www.childbirth.org

Pregnancy and Childbirth: pregnancy.about.com

Childbirth Connection: www.childbirthconnection.org

Pregnancy: www.pregnancy.org

My Pregnancy Guide: www.mypregnancyguide.com

WebMD Health and Pregnancy: www.webmd.com/baby

StorkNet's Pregnancy Guide: www.pregnancyguideonline.com

What to Expect: www.whattoexpect.com

The American College of Obstetricians and Gynecologists: www.acog.com

American Baby: www.americanbaby.com

Baby Zone: www.babyzone.com

Baby Center: www.babycenter.com

Lamaze International: www.lamaze.org

LaLeche League International: http://www.llli.org

 Check out the Evolve site at http://evolve.elsevier.com/Bonewit/today/ to actively Prepare for your Certification, and to access additional interactive activities and exercises to help you study and prepare for success.

24

The Pediatric Examination

Pediatric Office Visits

1. List the components of the well-child visit.
2. State the usual schedule for well-child visits.
3. Explain the purpose of the sick-child visit.
4. List the procedures performed by the medical assistant during pediatric office visits.
5. Explain why it is important to develop a rapport with the pediatric patient.

Growth Measurements

6. State the importance of measuring the child's weight, height (or length), and head circumference during each office visit.
7. State the functions served by a growth chart.

Pediatric Blood Pressure Measurement

8. State the importance of measuring a child's blood pressure.
9. List the three factors that determine whether a child has hypertension.

Collection of a Urine Specimen

10. List the reasons for collecting a urine specimen from a child.

Pediatric Injections

11. State the range for the gauge and length of needles used for intramuscular and subcutaneous pediatric injections.
12. Explain the use of each of the following pediatric injection sites: vastus lateralis and deltoid.

Immunizations

13. Describe the schedule for immunization of infants and children recommended by the American Academy of Pediatrics.
14. State the information that must be provided to parents as required by the National Childhood Vaccine Injury Act.
15. List the information that must be recorded in the medical record after administering an immunization.

Newborn Screening Test

16. Explain the purpose of a newborn screening test.
17. List the symptoms of phenylketonuria.
18. State what occurs if phenylketonuria is left untreated.

Carry an infant using the following positions:
 Cradle
 Upright

Plot pediatric growth values on a growth chart.
Measure the weight and length of an infant.
Measure the head and chest circumference of an infant.

Measure the blood pressure of a child.

Collect a urine specimen using a pediatric urine collector.

Locate the following pediatric intramuscular injection sites:
 Vastus lateralis
 Deltoid
Administer an intramuscular injection to an infant.
Administer a subcutaneous injection to an infant.

Read and interpret a vaccine information statement.
Record information on an immunization administration record.

CHAPTER OUTLINE

KEY TERMS

adolescent
immunity (ih-MYOO-nih-tee)
immunization (IM-yoo-nih-ZAY-shun)
infant
length

pediatrician (PEE-dee-uh-TRIH-shun)
pediatrics (pee-dee-AT-riks)
preschool (PREE-skool) child
school-age child
toddler (TOD-ler)

toxoid (TOKS-oid)
vaccine (vak-SEEN)
vertex (VER-teks)

INTRODUCTION TO THE PEDIATRIC EXAMINATION

Pediatrics is the branch of medicine that deals with the care and development of children and the diagnosis and treatment of diseases in children. A **pediatrician** is a physician who specializes in pediatrics. Many physicians in general practice accept pediatric patients. It is essential that the medical assistant develop the skills needed to assist the physician in the care and treatment of children.

PEDIATRIC OFFICE VISITS

There are two broad categories of pediatric patient office visits. The first is the *well-child visit* (also termed *health maintenance visit*), in which the physician progressively evaluates the growth and development of the child. A physical examination is performed during each well-child visit and is directed toward discovering any abnormal conditions commonly associated with the stage of development reached by the child. Table 24-1 provides an outline of normal development during infancy. The child also receives necessary immunizations during these visits.

Another important component of the well-child visit is *anticipatory guidance*. Anticipatory guidance is the process of providing parents with information to prepare them for anticipated developmental events and to assist them in promoting their children's well-being. Topics that are commonly included are safety, nutrition, sleep, play, exercise, development, and discipline.

The interval between well-child visits depends on the medical office, but it frequently follows this schedule after

Table 24-1 Milestones of Gross and Fine Motor Development in Infancy

Average Age (mo)	Gross Motor	Fine Motor
1	Turns head from side to side	Grasping reflex present
2	Holds head at 45-degree angle when prone	Holds rattle briefly
3	Begins rolling over	Grasps rattle or dangling objects
4	Slight head lag when pulled to sitting position	Brings objects to mouth
5	No head wobble when held in sitting position	Transfers objects from hand to hand
6	Sits without support	Manipulates and examines large objects with hands
7	Stands while holding on	Reaches for, grabs, and retains object
8	Pulls self to stand	Grasps objects with thumb and finger
9	Crawls backward	Begins to show hand preference
10	Creeps on hands and knees	Hits cup with spoon
11	Walks using furniture for support	Picks up small objects with thumb and forefinger (pincer grasp)
12	Stands alone easily	Puts three or more objects into container
12-16	Walks alone easily	Turns two or three pages in large cardboard book

From Leahy JM, Kizilay PE: *Foundations of nursing practice*, Philadelphia, 1998, Saunders.

birth: 1 month, 2 months, 4 months, 6 months, 9 months, 12 months, 15 months, 18 months, 24 months, and yearly thereafter.

The second category of pediatric patient office visits is the *sick-child visit*. The child is exhibiting the signs and symptoms of disease, and the physician evaluates the patient's condition to arrive at a diagnosis and to prescribe treatment.

During well-child and sick-child visits, the medical assistant performs many of the same procedures that have been presented in previous chapters (e.g., measurement of temperature, pulse, respiration, and blood pressure; measurement of weight and height; measurement of visual acuity; assisting with the physical examination). This chapter discusses procedures specifically related to the pediatric patient and variations in procedures previously presented.

DEVELOPING A RAPPORT

The medical assistant must establish a rapport with the pediatric patient. If the medical assistant gains the child's trust and confidence, the child is likely to cooperate during an examination or procedure. Interacting with children requires special techniques. The techniques employed depend on the age of the child. Toddlers and preschool children often respond well to making a game of the procedure. Explaining the purpose of an instrument (e.g., the stethoscope) to a school-age child and allowing him or her to hold the instrument or even to help during the procedure may overcome fears in that age group (Figure 24-1).

The medical assistant should always explain the procedure to children who are able to understand. Each child must be approached at his or her level of understanding. To do this, the medical assistant should know what to expect from a child at a particular age, in terms of motor and social development. Each child has his or her own individual rate of development; the descriptions of normal development based on age are meant to serve as a guide only and may have to be modified to meet individual needs. In addition, it is normal for an ill child to regress to an earlier level of behavior. Table 24-2 outlines techniques that can be used with various age groups to gain their cooperation during an examination or procedure.

What Would You Do? What Would You *Not* Do?

Case Study 1

My-Lai Chang comes into the office with Christopher Chang, her 2-month-old son. Christopher is here for his 2-month well-child visit. Mrs. Chang is very distraught. She says that Christopher has episodes of nonstop crying every day that last 2 to 3 hours at a time. She is breastfeeding Christopher and says that the crying is worse after he nurses. Although Mrs. Chang realizes that Christopher has colic, she feels guilty because it seems "her milk" is making it worse. She also is having problems with sore nipples and engorgement. She really wanted to breastfeed Christopher, but she is thinking of stopping because it just seems too hard to do. Christopher measures in the 50th percentile for weight and length. Mrs. Chang is worried that he is not growing enough and thinks it is because she is not producing enough milk. ■

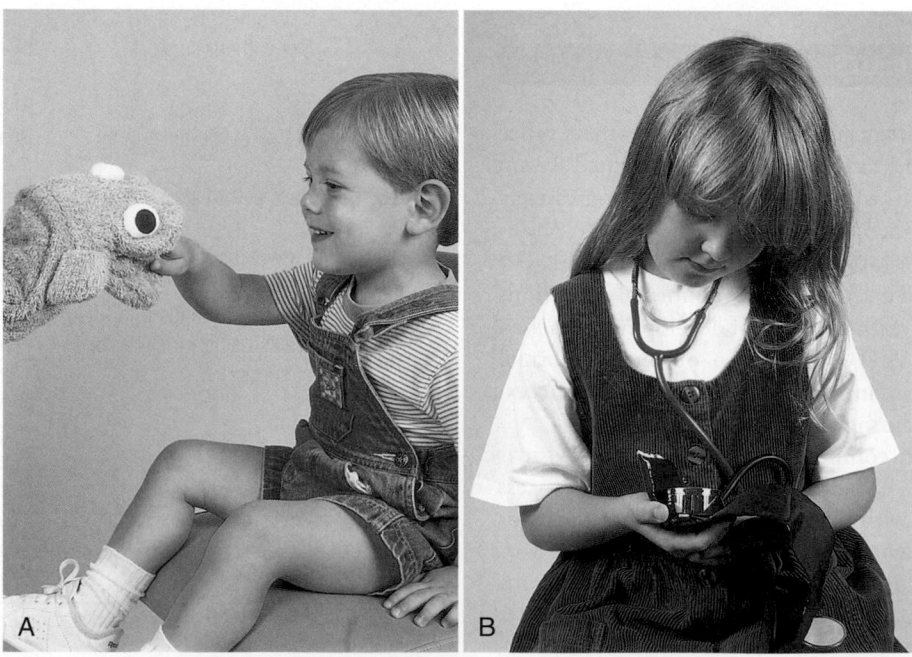

Figure 24-1 The medical assistant should develop a rapport with children to gain their trust and cooperation. Making a game of the procedure **(A)** and explaining the purpose of the stethoscope and allowing the child to hold it **(B)** help the child overcome fears.

Table 24-2 Techniques for Interaction with Children

Technique	Infant (Birth-1 yr)	Toddler (1-3 yr)	Preschool (3-6 yr)	School Age (6-12 yr)	Adolescent (12-18 yr)
Avoid sudden motion and loud or abrupt noises.	♥		♥		
Limit number of strangers in room.	♥				
Use distractions, bright objects, rattles, and talking to gain cooperation.	♥				
Physically restrain child if necessary to ensure safety.	♥	♥	♥		
Allow physical contact with parent during procedure.	♥	♥	♥		
Encourage parent to comfort child after procedure.	♥	♥	♥		
Use play to explain procedure (e.g., dolls, puppets).		♥	♥		
Perform procedures quickly, if possible.		♥	♥		
Use concrete terms, rather than abstract terms.		♥	♥		
Avoid words that have more than one meaning (e.g., shot).		♥	♥		
Give child permission to cry, yell, or otherwise express pain verbally.		♥	♥		
Praise child for cooperative behavior.		♥	♥	♥	
Allow child to handle equipment, if possible.			♥	♥	
Make sure child understands body part to be involved.			♥	♥	
Try to describe how procedure will feel.			♥	♥	
Tell child about any discomfort that may be felt, but don't dwell on it.			♥	♥	
Stress benefits of anything child may find pleasurable afterward (e.g., stickers, feeling better).			♥	♥	
Give child choices when possible (e.g., arm to use).			♥	♥	
Suggest ways to maintain control (e.g., counting, deep breathing, relaxation).			♥	♥	
Use drawing and diagrams to illustrate parts of body that will be involved.			♥	♥	
Encourage participation such as holding instrument during procedure.			♥	♥	
Include child in decision-making process.				♥	♥
Discuss risks of procedure.					♥
Provide information about appearance changes that might result.					♥
Give child educational brochures or have him or her view videos about procedure.					♥
Ask parent to step out if child does not want parent in examining room.					♥

From Bonewit-West K: *Clinical procedures for medical assistants,* ed 8, St Louis, 2011, Saunders.

CARRYING THE INFANT

The medical assistant needs to lift and carry the infant to perform various procedures, such as measurement of length and weight. The infant should be lifted and carried in a manner that is safe and comfortable. Proper positions include the cradle and upright positions.

Cradle Position

The medical assistant slides the left hand and arm under the infant's back and grasps the infant's arm from behind. The thumb and fingers should encircle the infant's forearm. The infant's head, shoulders, and back are supported by the medical assistant's arm. Next, the medical assistant slips the right arm up and under the infant's buttocks. The infant is cradled in the arm with his or her body resting against the medical assistant's chest (Figure 24-2).

Upright Position

The medical assistant slips the right hand under the infant's head and shoulders. The fingers should be spread apart to support the infant's head and neck. The left forearm is slipped under the infant's buttocks to help support the infant's weight. The infant should be allowed to rest against the medical assistant's chest with the cheek resting on the medical assistant's shoulder (Figure 24-3).

GROWTH MEASUREMENTS

One of the best methods to evaluate the progress of a child is to measure his or her growth. The weight, height (or length), and head circumference (up to age 3 years) of a child should be measured during each office visit and plotted on a growth chart.

Weight

A child's weight is often used to determine nutritional needs and the proper dosage of a medication to administer to the child. The medical assistant should exercise care in measuring weight. Infants are weighed in a recumbent position, as outlined in Procedure 24-1. Older children are weighed in a standing position, as presented in Chapter 20.

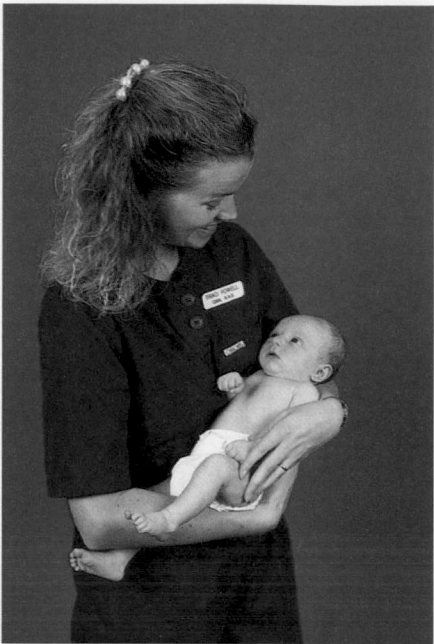

Figure 24-2 Traci holds the infant in the cradle position.

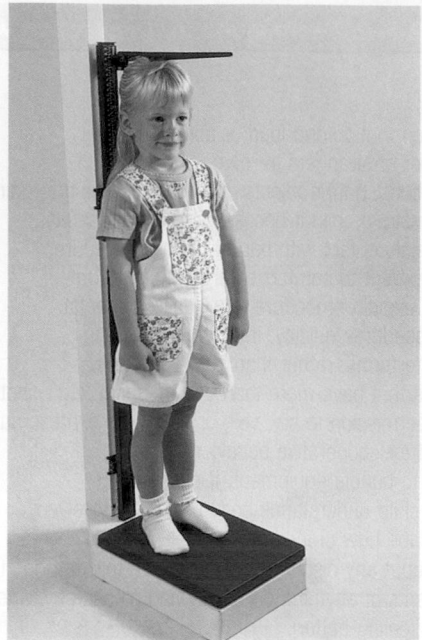

Figure 24-4 Measuring the height of a child.

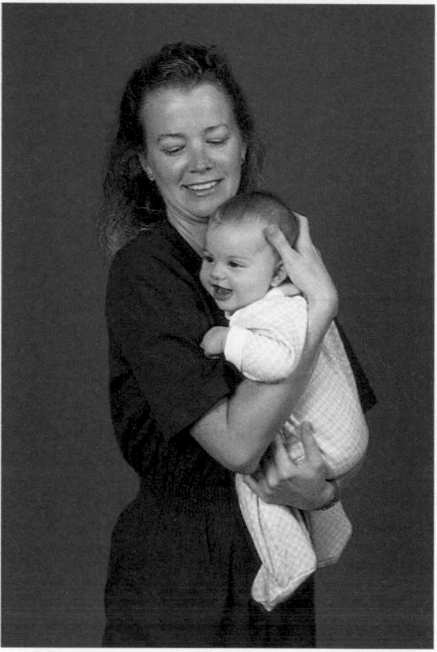

Figure 24-3 Traci holds the infant in the upright position.

Length and Height

Another measure of a child's growth is **length,** or height (stature). Length is measured in children younger than 24 months. The recumbent length is a measurement from the **vertex** of the head to the heel of the infant in a supine position, as outlined in Procedure 24-1. Two people are often needed to determine the length of an infant accurately. The parent's help can be requested; the medical assistant must provide the parent with thorough instructions on what is to be done. Older children have their height measured in a standing position (Figure 24-4), as presented in Chapter 20.

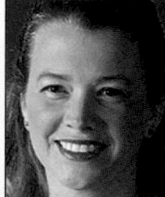

Putting It All into Practice

My name is Traci Powell, and I am a Certified Medical Assistant. I work in the pediatrics department of a large multispecialty clinic. My job responsibilities are mostly clinical; however, I do assist in the front office when needed. I love working with the children and have enjoyed watching them grow over the years.

A co-worker and I recently organized a local AAMA (American Association of Medical Assistants) chapter. Our chapter provides AAMA continuing education units (CEUs). Our members attend state and national conventions every year, and they hold state and national leadership positions. It is my goal to see the medical assisting profession continue to grow and advance in the health care field.

It is interesting how your education, training, and experience all come together, especially in a crisis. Early one morning when I arrived at work, a mother was waiting with a small child who was approximately 2 years old. The child was dusky in color, panicky, and having trouble breathing. Apparently the child had gotten into some dry beans the previous night and had inhaled one into her lung. None of the physicians was in the building yet, and this child was in respiratory distress. We immediately called a Code Blue, put her on oxygen, and made arrangements for a squad car to take her to Children's Hospital, where a surgeon was waiting. All went well, and she is a healthy little girl today.

Looking back, I am grateful for a good, solid medical assisting education; a PALS (Pediatric Advance Life Support) certification; and experience in working with children so that I was able to help that child through a life-threatening experience. I firmly believe that no matter how long a person has been in the medical field or what his or her profession is, continuing education is essential to stay current in the ever-changing health care field. ■

Head and Chest Circumference

Infancy is a period of rapid brain growth. Because of this, the head circumference is an important measurement. The head circumference for a newborn ranges from 32 to 38 cm, or 12½ to 15 inches. A 10-cm (4-inch) increase in head circumference occurs within the first year of life.

The head circumference of children younger than 3 years old should be routinely measured and plotted on a head circumference growth chart. Measurement of head circumference is an important screening measure for microencephaly and macroencephaly.

At birth a newborn's head circumference is about 2 cm larger than his or her chest circumference. The chest grows at a faster rate than the cranium, and between 6 months and 2 years of age, the measurements are about the same. After age 2 years, the chest circumference is greater than the head circumference. The measurement of the chest circumference is valuable in a comparison with the head circumference, but not by itself. The chest circumference is not typically measured on a routine basis; this measurement is done only when a heart or lung abnormality is suspected. Procedure 24-2 outlines the procedure for measuring the head and chest circumference of an infant.

Growth Charts

Growth charts should be part of every child's permanent record. The National Center for Health Statistics developed growth charts to assist physicians in determining whether the growth of a child is normal. The charts can be used to identify children with growth or nutritional abnormalities. The medical assistant is usually responsible for plotting the child's measurements on the growth chart (Procedure 24-3).

Growth charts provide a means of comparing a child's weight and length (or height) with those of other children of the same age. For example, the medical assistant calculates the growth percentile of an 18-month-old boy and finds that he is in the 25th percentile for weight and the 80th percentile for length. This means that 75% of 18-month-old boys weigh more than he does, and 25% weigh less than he does. It also means that 20% of 18-month-old boys are taller, and 80% are shorter. Although comparing a child with other children of the same age is one use of growth charts (particularly by parents), it is not the most important use.

The primary use of growth charts is to look at the child's growth pattern. If a child has always hovered around a certain percentile in height and weight, there is no need for

Text continued on p. 481

Highlight on Childhood Obesity

Statistics

An epidemic of childhood obesity is occurring in the United States; the incidence of obesity in children has doubled over the past 20 years. Approximately 25% of Americans younger than age 19 are overweight or obese, which equates to one of every four children. A child is considered overweight if his or her weight falls in the 85th to 95th percentile for age, gender, and height on the National Center for Health Statistics growth charts. When a child's weight exceeds the 95th percentile for age, gender, and height, he or she is considered obese.

Causes

The primary causes of childhood obesity are overeating and inadequate exercise. Other causes include hormonal and genetic problems, but these are much less likely, occurring in only 5% of obese children. The risk of obesity tends to be greater among children who have obese parents. After age 3, the likelihood that obesity will persist into adulthood increases as an obese child gets older. When an obese child reaches age 6, the probability is more than 50% that obesity will persist into adulthood. Of obese adolescents, 70% to 80% remain obese as adults.

Related Problems

Problems associated with childhood obesity include high blood pressure, type 2 diabetes, orthopedic problems caused by increased stress on weight-bearing joints, skin disorders such as dermatitis, sleep apnea, low self-esteem, social isolation, and feelings of rejection and depression. Some authorities believe that the social and psychological problems are the most significant consequences of childhood obesity.

Prevention

It is much easier to prevent childhood obesity than to treat it after it has occurred. Authorities believe that the primary focus should be on educating parents about the problems associated with childhood obesity and helping them employ preventive measures. Guidelines for preventing childhood obesity include the following:

- Provide a healthy diet, with 30% or fewer calories coming from fat.
- Encourage active play.
- Do not use food for reward, comfort, or bribes.
- Limit television, video, and computer time.
- Limit the amount of "junk" food kept in the home.
- Do not make the child eat when he or she is not hungry.
- Do not offer dessert as a reward for finishing a meal.
- Encourage the child to drink water instead of sweet beverages.
- Do not frequently eat at fast-food restaurants.

Treatment

The treatment of childhood obesity is difficult, and the success rate is not particularly high. Children seem to be most successful at losing weight and keeping it off when the entire family is involved. Parents should eat healthy meals and snacks with their children. The most successful diets are those that use ordinary foods in controlled portions, rather than diets that require the avoidance of specific foods. Parents also should spend time being active with their children. Activities should stress self-improvement rather than competition. ∎

PROCEDURE 24-1   Measuring the Weight and Length of an Infant

Outcome Measure the weight and length of an infant.

Equipment/Supplies

- Pediatric balance scale (table model)

1. **Procedural Step.** Sanitize your hands.
2. **Procedural Step.** Greet the infant's parent and introduce yourself. Identify the infant and explain the procedure to the parent. The weight of the infant is usually measured first. Depending on the medical office policy, ask the parent to perform one of the following:
   a. Remove the infant's clothing and put a dry diaper on the infant.
   b. Remove the infant's clothing, including the diaper.
   Principle. The infant should not be weighed with a wet diaper because it could increase the infant's weight considerably. Also, growth charts for infants and young children base their percentiles on the weight of the child without clothing.
3. **Procedural Step.** Unlock the pediatric scale, and place a clean paper protector on it. Check the balance scale for accuracy, making sure to compensate for the weight of the paper.
   Principle. The paper protector prevents cross-contamination and reduces the spread of disease from one patient to another.
4. **Procedural Step.** Gently place the infant on his or her back on the table of the scale. Place one hand slightly above the infant as a safety precaution.
5. **Procedural Step.** Balance the scale as follows:
   a. Move the lower weight to the notched groove that does not cause the indicator point to drop to the bottom of the calibration area. Ensure that the lower weight is seated firmly in its groove.
   b. Slowly slide the upper weight along its calibration bar by tapping it gently until the indicator point comes to rest at the center of the balance area.
   Principle. Not seating the lower weight firmly in its groove results in an inaccurate reading.

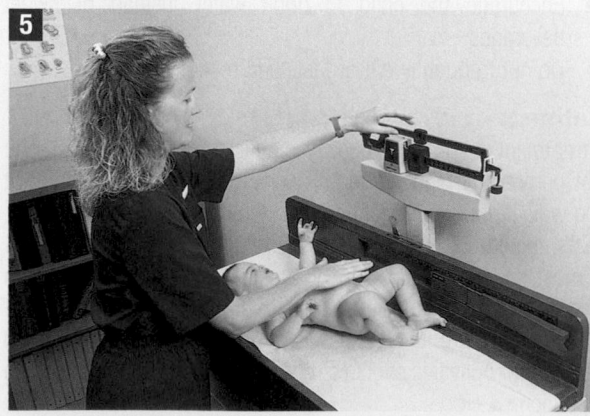

Balance the scale.

6. **Procedural Step.** Read the results in pounds and ounces while the infant is lying still. Jot down this value or make a mental note of it. (***NOTE:*** The result on the pictured scale is 15 lb and 2 oz.)

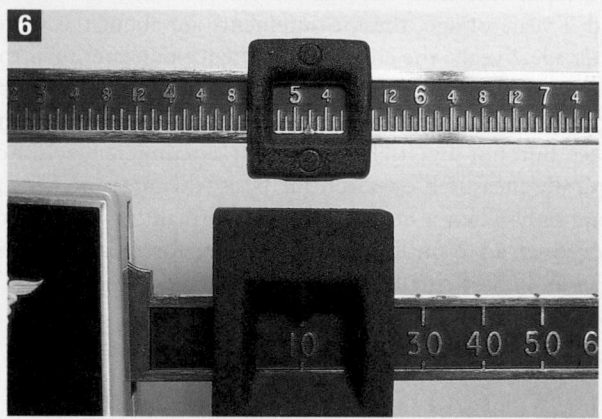

Read the results in pounds and ounces.

7. **Procedural Step.** Return the balance to its resting position, and lock the scale.
8. **Procedural Step.** Place the vertex (top) of the infant's head against the headboard at the zero mark. Ask the parent to hold the infant's head in this position.

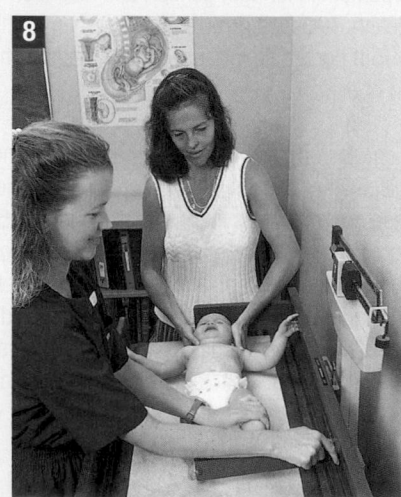

Properly position the infant.

9. **Procedural Step.** Straighten the infant's knees, and place the soles of his or her feet firmly against the upright footboard (to create a right angle).
10. **Procedural Step.** Read the infant's length in inches (to the nearest ⅛ inch) from the measure. Jot down

PROCEDURE 24-1   Measuring the Weight and Length of an Infant—cont'd

this value or make a mental note of it. (*NOTE:* The result on this scale is 25½ inches.)

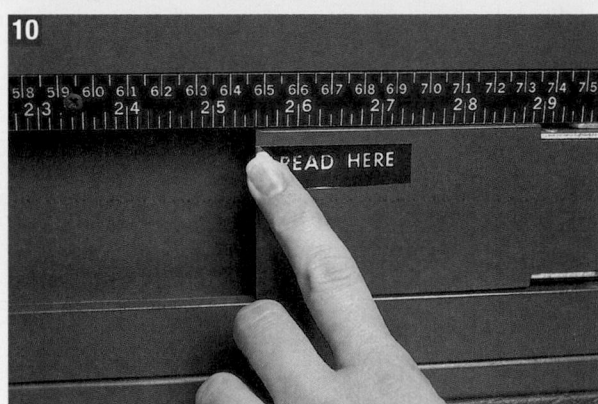

Read the length in inches.

11. **Procedural Step.** Gently remove the infant from the table, and hand him or her to the parent. Return the headboard and footboard to their resting positions.
12. **Procedural Step.** Sanitize your hands, and chart the results.

CHARTING EXAMPLE

Date	
8/10/XX	9:30 a.m. Wt. 15 lb 2 oz. Length 25 ½ in. —————— T. Powell, CMA (AAMA)

PROCEDURE 24-2   Measuring Head and Chest Circumference of an Infant

Outcome Measure the head and chest circumference of an infant.

Equipment/Supplies

• Flexible nonstretch tape measure

Measurement of Head Circumference

1. **Procedural Step.** Sanitize your hands, and assemble the equipment.
2. **Procedural Step.** Position the infant. The infant should be placed on his or her back on the examining table. An alternative position is to have the parent hold the infant.
3. **Procedural Step.** Position the tape measure around the infant's head at the greatest circumference. This is usually accomplished by placing the tape slightly above the eyebrows and pinna of the ears and around the occipital prominence at the back of the skull.

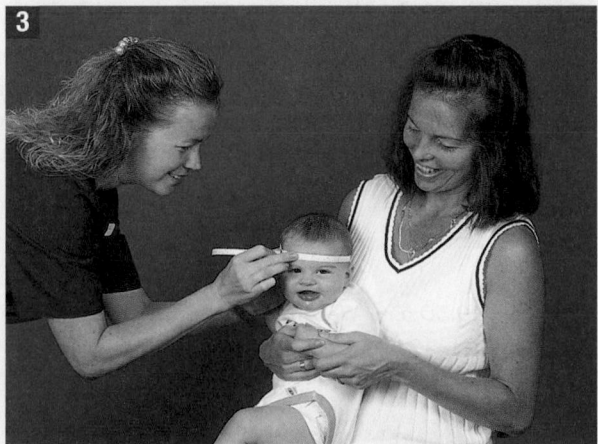

Position the tape measure around the infant's head.

4. **Procedural Step.** Read the results in centimeters (or inches) to the nearest 0.5 cm (or ¼ inch). Jot down this value or make a mental note of it. Sanitize your hands, and chart the results.

CHARTING EXAMPLE

Date	
8/10/XX	10:00 a.m. Head circumference: 42 ½ cm. —————— T. Powell, CMA (AAMA)

Measurement of Chest Circumference

1. **Procedural Step.** Position the infant on his or her back on the examining table.
2. **Procedural Step.** Encircle the tape around the infant's chest at the nipple line. It should be snug, but not so tight that it leaves a mark.

Continued

PROCEDURE 24-2 Measuring Head and Chest Circumference of an Infant—cont'd

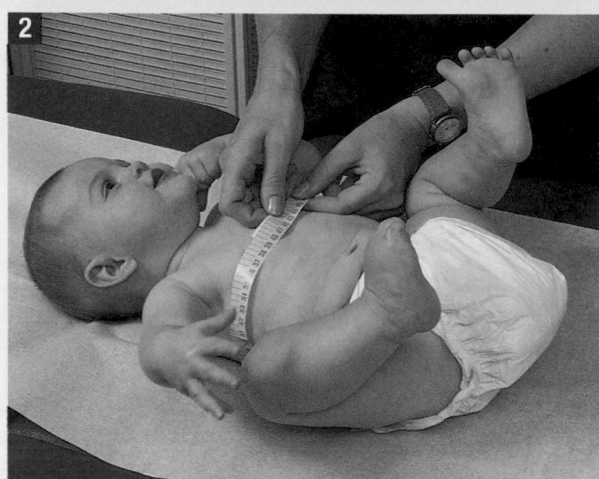

Encircle the tape around the infant's chest.

3. **Procedural Step.** Read the results in centimeters (or inches) to the nearest 0.5 cm (or ¼ inch). Jot down this value or make a mental note of it. Sanitize your hands, and chart the results.

CHARTING EXAMPLE	
Date	
8/15/XX	10:00 a.m. Chest circumference: 42 cm. ___
	_____ T. Powell, CMA (AAMA)

PROCEDURE 24-3 Calculating Growth Percentiles

Outcome Plot a pediatric growth value on a growth chart.

Equipment/Supplies

• Pediatric growth chart

1. **Procedural Step.** Select the proper growth chart.
2. **Procedural Step.** Locate the child's age in the horizontal column at the bottom of the chart.
3. **Procedural Step.** Locate the growth value in the vertical column under the appropriate category (weight, length or stature, and head circumference).
4. **Procedural Step.** Draw an imaginary vertical line from the child's age mark and an imaginary horizontal line from the child's growth mark. Find the site at

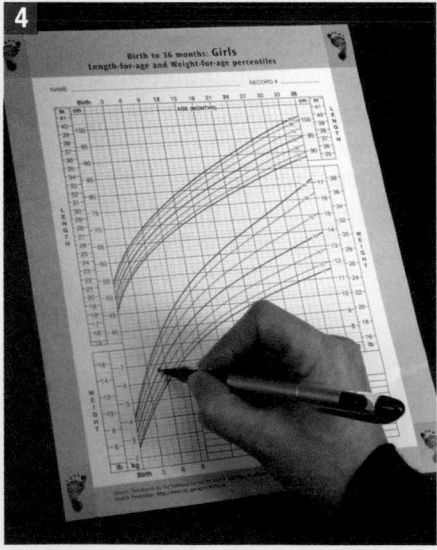

which the two lines intersect on the graph, and place a dot on this site.

5. **Procedural Step.** To determine the percentile in which the child falls, follow the curved percentile line upward to read the value located on the right side of the chart. Interpolation is needed if the value does not fall exactly on a percentile line. (*Interpolation* means that you must estimate a percentile that falls between a larger and a smaller known percentile.)

6. **Procedural Step.** Chart the results. Include the date and time and each growth percentile.
   NOTE: The weight (15 lb, 2 oz), length (25½ inches), and head circumference (42.5 cm) of the child in Procedures 24-1 and 24-2 have been plotted on a growth chart. This child is 5 months old. Locate these values on the appropriate growth chart to ensure you obtain the same percentiles.

CHARTING EXAMPLE	
Date	
10/22/XX	10:30 a.m. Weight: 55%. Length: 70%. _____
	Head Circum: 67% ___ T. Powell, CMA (AAMA)

PROCEDURE 24-3 Calculating Growth Percentiles—cont'd

Birth to 36 months: Girls NAME ______________

Length-for-age and Weight-for-age percentiles RECORD # ______________

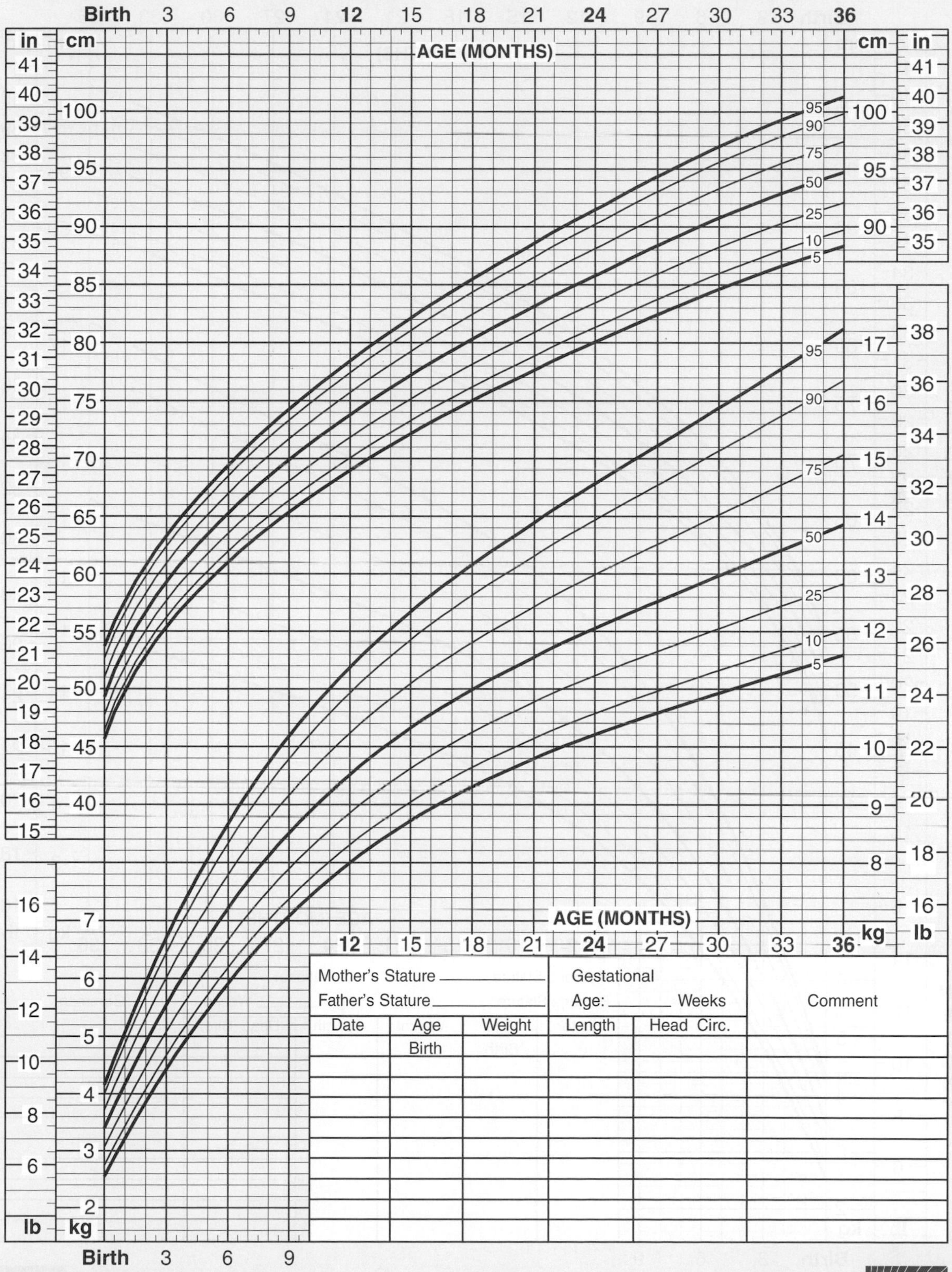

Mother's Stature ______			Gestational		Comment
Father's Stature ______			Age: ______ Weeks		
Date	Age	Weight	Length	Head Circ.	
	Birth				

Published May 30, 2000 (modified 4/20/01).

SOURCE: Developed by the National Center for Health Statistics in collaboration with the National Center for Chronic Disease Prevention and Health Promotion (2000).
http://www.cdc.gov/growthcharts

CDC

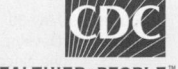

SAFER • HEALTHIER • PEOPLE™

PROCEDURE **24-3**   Calculating Growth Percentiles—cont'd

Birth to 36 months: Boys
Length-for-age and Weight-for-age percentiles

NAME _____

RECORD# _____

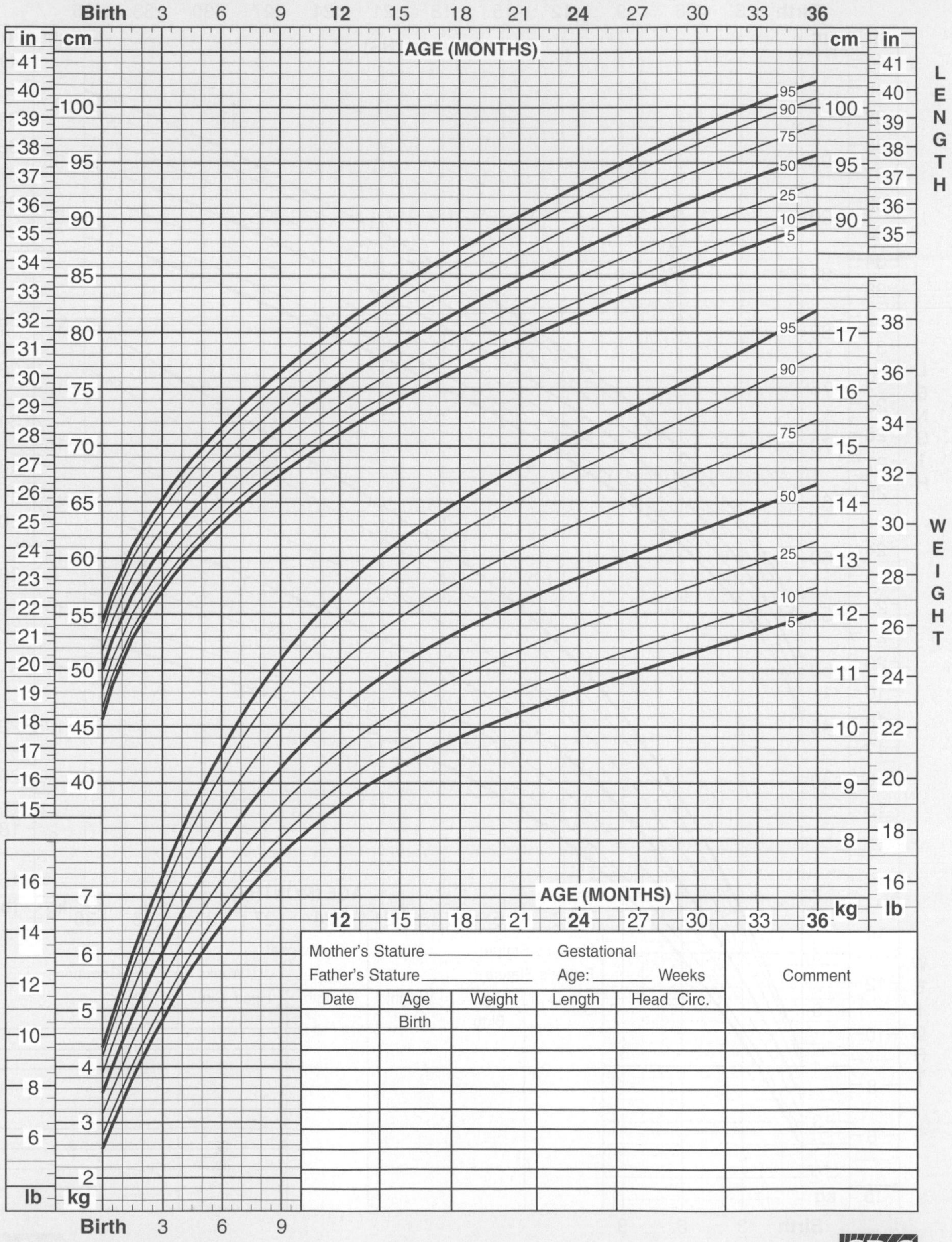

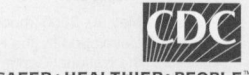

Published May 30, 2000 (modified 4/20/01).
SOURCE: Developed by the National Center for Health Statistics in collaboration with
the National Center for Chronic Disease Prevention and Health Promotion (2000).
http://www.cdc.gov/growthcharts

SAFER · HEALTHIER · PEOPLE™

concern. If a child is in the 20th percentile for weight but has always been in this percentile, he is likely growing normally. It would be more of a concern if the child had been in the 75th percentile and dropped to the 20th percentile. The physician investigates any significant change or rapid increase or decrease in a child's growth pattern.

PEDIATRIC BLOOD PRESSURE MEASUREMENT

The American Academy of Pediatrics recommends that all children 3 years old and older have their blood pressure measured annually. Measuring pediatric blood pressure helps to identify children at risk for developing hypertension as adults. High blood pressure in children can be caused by kidney disease and, to a lesser degree, by heart disease. When the condition is treated, the blood pressure usually returns to normal. Overweight children usually have higher blood pressure than children of normal weight. Losing weight through a prescribed diet and regular physical activity often reduces blood pressure in these children.

Special Guidelines for Children

The procedure for measuring blood pressure in children is the same as that for adults and is presented in Chapter 19. Some special pediatric guidelines must be taken into consideration.

Correct Cuff Size

The most important criterion in obtaining an accurate pediatric blood pressure measurement is selecting the correct cuff size. If the cuff is too small, the reading may be falsely high. If the cuff is too large, the reading may be falsely low. Blood pressure cuffs come in a variety of sizes and are measured in centimeters (cm). The size of a cuff refers to its inner inflatable bladder, rather than its cloth cover. Table 24-3 lists the range of cuff sizes commercially available. The name of the cuff (e.g., child, adult) does not imply that it is appropriate for that age. An 8-year-old overweight child may need an adult-sized cuff.

For an accurate blood pressure measurement, the bladder of the cuff should encircle 80% to 100% of the arm. The child's arm circumference should be assessed midpoint between the acromion process (shoulder) and the olecranon process (elbow). Figure 24-5 shows how to determine the correct pediatric cuff size.

Cooperation of the Child

Another important factor to consider when taking pediatric blood pressure is preparing the child for the procedure. It is important to gain the child's cooperation and to ensure that the child is relaxed. Apprehension can cause the blood pressure to be falsely high. To reduce a child's anxiety level, carefully explain the procedure to the child, and, if appropriate, allow him or her to handle the equipment before measuring blood pressure. The blood pressure should be measured after the child has been sitting quietly for 3 to 5 minutes (Figure 24-6).

Table 24-3 Acceptable Bladder Dimensions for Arms of Different Sizes		
Cuff	Bladder Length (cm)	Arm Circumference Range at Midpoint (cm)
Newborn	6	Less than 6
Infant	15	6-15
Child	21	16-21
Small adult	24	22-26
Adult	30	27-34
Large adult	38	35-44
Adult thigh	42	45-52

From Bonewit-West K: *Clinical procedures for medical assistants,* ed 8, St Louis, 2011, Saunders.

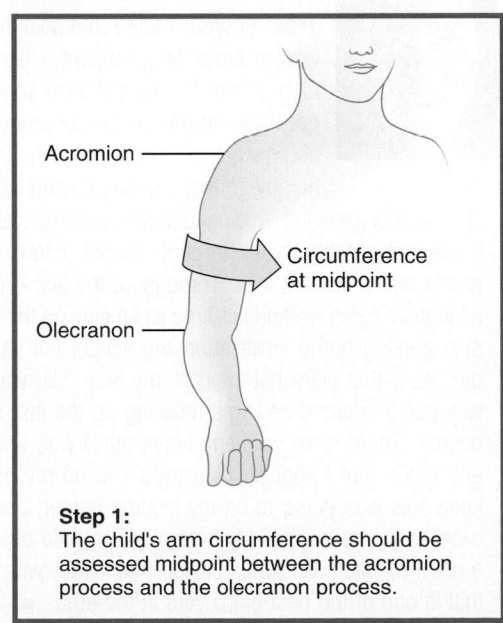

Step 1:
The child's arm circumference should be assessed midpoint between the acromion process and the olecranon process.

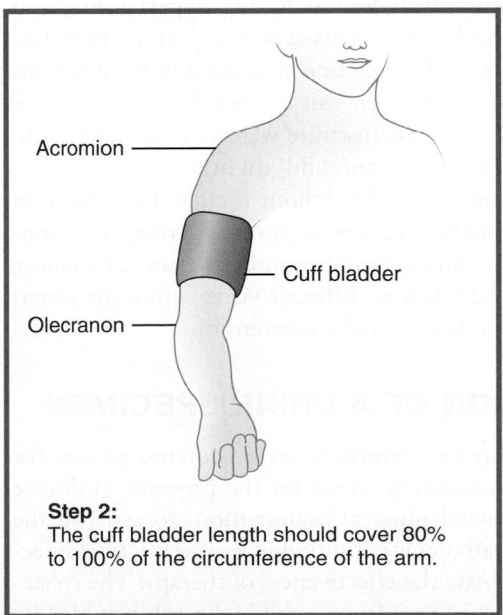

Step 2:
The cuff bladder length should cover 80% to 100% of the circumference of the arm.

Figure 24-5 Determination of proper blood pressure cuff size.

What Would You Do? What Would You *Not* Do?

Case Study 2

Wanda Tilley comes to the office with her 10-year-old daughter, Courtney. Courtney has a skin condition on her legs that needs to be evaluated by the physician. Courtney has been obese since she was 4 years old. Mrs. Tilley also is obese and is not too concerned about Courtney's weight. She says that Courtney must have inherited her "fat gene," and there's not much that can be done about it. Courtney's favorite activities are playing video games and reading. She would like to join the community swim team, but she's too embarrassed for anyone to see her in a bathing suit. Courtney says the other kids are always making fun of her at school. She says that they call her "two-ton Tilley" and "double-roll," and they don't want to sit with her at lunch. Courtney wants her mom to home-school her because she's getting to the point where she can't take it anymore. She doesn't want the doctor to examine her because he'll see how fat she is and say bad things about it. ■

Blood Pressure Classifications

Blood pressure varies depending on the age of the child and his or her height and gender. The National High Blood Pressure Education Program (NHBPEP) prepared a set of tables that physicians use to determine whether a child's blood pressure is higher than the average among children of the same age and height. If a child has a blood pressure that is higher than 90% to 95% of most other children of the same age, height, and gender, the child may have high blood pressure.

The NHBPEP tables (one for boys and one for girls) allow precise classification of blood pressure according to body size, which avoids misclassifying children at the extreme ends of normal growth. A very tall child would not be mistakenly diagnosed as having hypertension, and hypertension would not be missed in a very short child. The NHBPEP tables used by physicians to assist in the diagnosis of hypertension in children can be found at the National Heart, Lung, and Blood Institute website (www.nhlbi.nih.gov/guidelines/hypertension/child_tbl.htm).

Blood pressure varies throughout the day in children as a result of normal fluctuations in physical activity and emotional stress. If a child's blood pressure is elevated, two more readings must be taken at different visits before the physician can make a diagnosis of hypertension.

COLLECTION OF A URINE SPECIMEN

A urinalysis may be performed on a pediatric patient for the following reasons: to screen for the presence of disease as part of a general physical examination, to assist in the diagnosis of a pathologic condition (e.g., urinary tract infection), or to evaluate the effectiveness of therapy. The collection of a urine specimen from a child who exhibits bladder

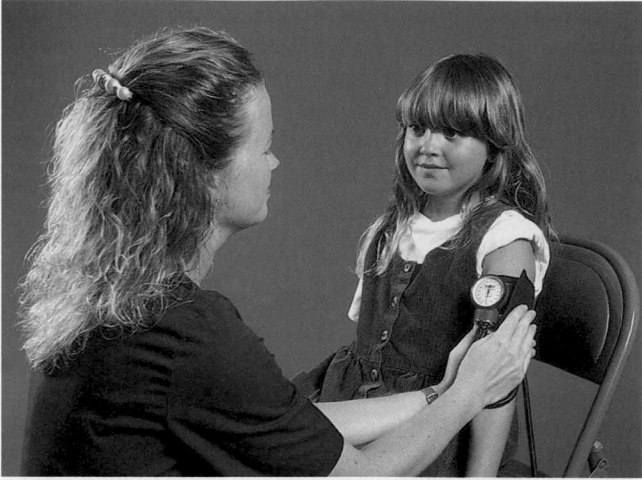

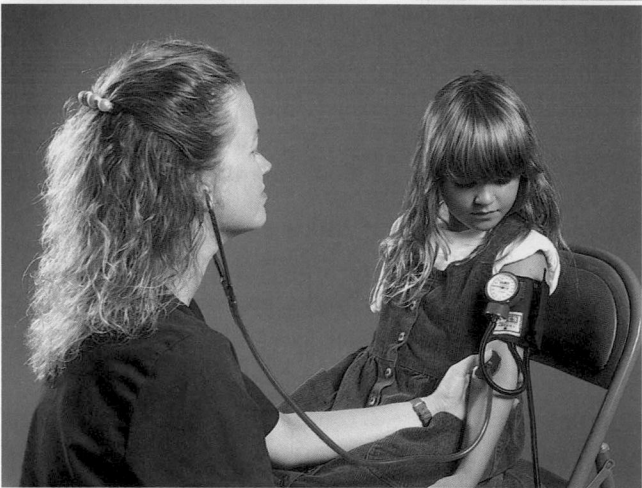

Figure 24-6 Traci measures the blood pressure of a pediatric patient.

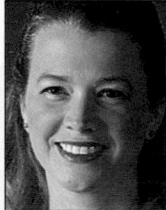

Memories *from* Externship

Traci Powell: I still remember how difficult it was at times as a student. I had been out of high school for more than a year, so I had to get back into the routine of studying. I worried about whether I would do well, whether I would be able to find a good job, and whether I would like medical assisting. Adding to these concerns was the financial burden of putting myself through school. I took advantage of grants and a student loan. Throughout the last 6 months of my education, I also worked full-time as an aide on the midnight shift at a nursing home while attending school full-time during the day. As if that were not enough, my first child was well on her way into this world as I was finishing up the last quarter of my degree. There were so many times that I was tired, frustrated, and broke, but I kept pushing myself to do my best because I knew this was going to be my lifetime career, and I wanted to excel in my profession. My determination paid off. Today I have a great medical assisting position that I love, with an institution that is one of the best employers in the area. ■

control is performed using the technique outlined in Chapter 30. Collecting a urine specimen from an infant or young child who cannot urinate voluntarily involves the use of a pediatric urine collector. Pediatric urine collectors are designed to be used with both sexes. The urine collector consists of a clear plastic disposable bag containing a hypoallergenic pressure-sensitive adhesive around the opening of the bag. The adhesive firmly attaches the urine collector to the genitalia. Procedure 24-4 outlines the procedure for applying a pediatric urine collector.

PROCEDURE 24-4   Applying a Pediatric Urine Collector

Outcome Apply a pediatric urine collector.

Equipment/Supplies
- Disposable gloves
- Personal antiseptic wipes
- Pediatric urine collector bag
- Urine specimen container and label
- Regular waste container

1. **Procedural Step.** Sanitize your hands.
2. **Procedural Step.** Assemble the equipment.
3. **Procedural Step.** Greet the infant's parent and introduce yourself. Identify the infant and explain the procedure to the parent.
4. **Procedural Step.** Apply gloves. Position the child. The child should be placed on his or her back with the legs spread apart. The medical assistant may need another individual to hold the child's legs apart.
   Principle. This position facilitates cleansing of the genitalia and permits proper application of the urine collector bag.
5. **Procedural Step.** Cleanse the child's genitalia.
   Female: Using a front-to-back motion (pubis to anus), cleanse each side of the meatus with a separate wipe. With a third wipe, cleanse directly down the middle (directly over the urinary meatus). Discard each wipe after cleansing. Allow the area to dry completely.
   Male: If the child is not circumcised, retract the foreskin of the penis. Cleanse the area around the meatus and the urethral opening (meatal orifice) in a manner similar to that used to cleanse the female patient. Use a separate wipe for each swipe. Cleanse the scrotum last, using a fresh wipe. Discard each wipe after cleansing. Allow the area to dry completely.
   Principle. The urinary meatus and surrounding area must be cleansed to prevent contaminants, such as baby powder, fecal material, and microorganisms, from entering the urine specimen, which could affect the test results. A front-to-back motion must be used to prevent drawing microorganisms from the anal area into the area being cleansed. The area must be completely dry to ensure an airtight adhesion of the collection bag to prevent leakage of urine.
6. **Procedural Step.** Remove the paper backing from the urine collector bag. This exposes the hypoallergenic adhesive surface around the opening of the bag. Firmly attach the bag in the following manner:
   Female: Stretch the perineum taut, and firmly place the bottom of the adhesive surface on the infant's perineum. Starting at the perineum and working upward, firmly press the adhesive surface to the skin surrounding the external genitalia, ensuring there is no puckering. The opening of the bag should be directly over the urinary meatus. The excess of the bag should be positioned toward the child's feet.
   Male: Position the bag so that the child's penis and scrotum are projected through the opening of the bag. Starting at the perineum and working upward, firmly press the adhesive surface to the skin surrounding the penis and scrotum, ensuring there is no puckering. The excess of the bag should be positioned toward the child's feet.
   Principle. The adhesive surface of the bag must be attached securely with no puckering to prevent leakage.

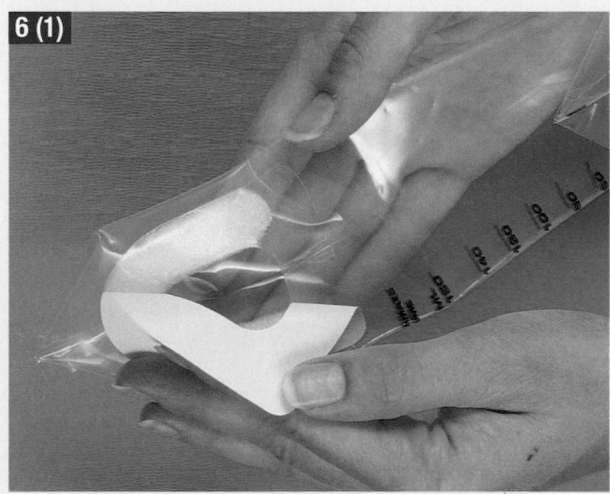
6 (1)
Remove paper backing from the urine collector bag.

Continued

PROCEDURE 24-4 **Applying a Pediatric Urine Collector—cont'd**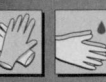

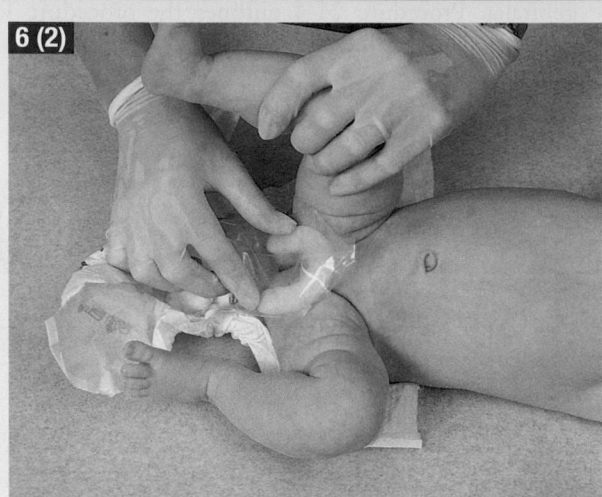

6 (2)

Firmly press the adhesive surface to the skin surrounding the external genitalia.

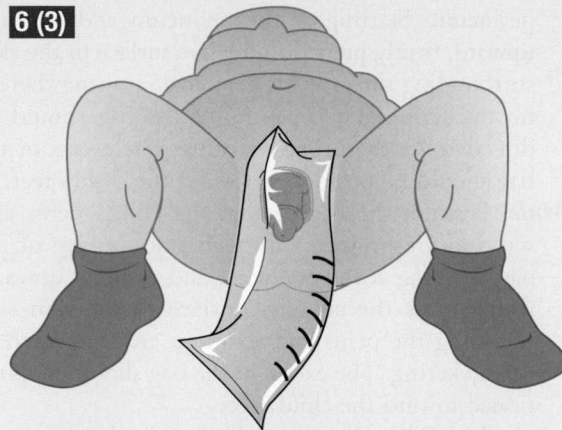

6 (3)

Male: The penis and scrotum are projected through the opening of the bag.

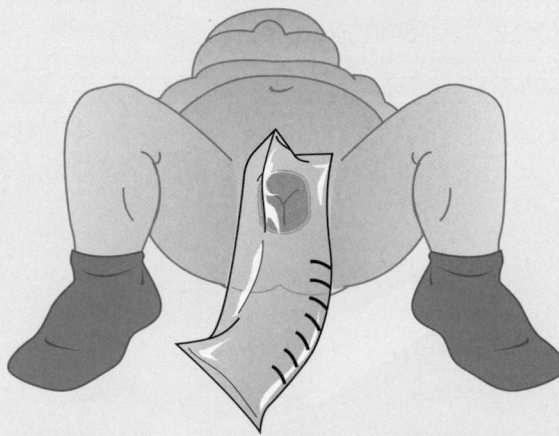

Female: The opening of the bag should be directly over the urinary meatus.

7. **Procedural Step.** Loosely diaper the child. Check the urine collector bag every 15 minutes until a urine specimen is obtained.
   Principle. The diaper helps hold the urine collector bag in place. The bag must be checked frequently. Once the infant has urinated, moisture from the urine may cause the adhesive surface to become loose and leak, especially with an active infant.

8. **Procedural Step.** When the child has voided, gently remove the urine collector bag by holding the bottom of the adhesive surface against the infant's skin and carefully peeling the bag off from the top to the bottom.
   Principle. The bag must be removed gently because pulling the adhesive away too quickly may cause discomfort and irritation of the child's skin.

9. **Procedural Step.** Cleanse the genital area with a personal antiseptic wipe. Rediaper the child.

10. **Procedural Step.** Transfer the urine specimen into a urine specimen container, and tightly apply the lid. Label the container with the child's name and date of birth, the date, the time of collection, and the type of specimen (i.e., urine). Dispose of the collector bag in a regular waste container. (*NOTE:* The urine collector bag can be used as a urine container to transport the specimen to the laboratory. This is accomplished by folding the adhesive sponge ring in half along its vertical axis and pressing the adhesive surfaces firmly together to ensure a tight seal.)

11. **Procedural Step.** Based on the medical office routine, test the urine specimen, or prepare it for transfer to an outside laboratory; be sure to include a completed laboratory request form. If the specimen cannot be tested or transferred immediately, preserve it by placing it in the refrigerator.
    Principle. Changes occur in a urine specimen that is left sitting out at room temperature, which can lead to inaccurate test results.

12. **Procedural Step.** Remove the gloves, and sanitize your hands.

13. **Procedural Step.** Chart the procedure. Include the date, the time of collection, and the type of specimen (i.e., urine). If the specimen is to be transported to an outside laboratory, indicate this information, including the laboratory tests ordered.

CHARTING EXAMPLE	
Date	
8/12/XX	10:15 a.m. Urine specimen collected for culture. Picked up by Medical Center Lab on 8/12/10. ——————— T. Powell, CMA (AAMA)

PEDIATRIC INJECTIONS

Administering an injection to a child is an important responsibility. The experience a child has with early injections influences the child's attitude toward later ones. If the child is old enough to understand, the procedure should be explained. The medical assistant should be honest and should attempt to gain the child's trust and cooperation. The child should be told the truth about the injection—that it will hurt, but only for a short time. It also is advisable to explain that the medicine will help him or her get better. Another person should be present to assist. The assistant can help position the child and can divert or restrain him or her if necessary. If the child struggles and fights excessively, the medical assistant should delay the injection and consult the physician.

The administration of injections is presented in Chapter 26. Before undertaking the study of pediatric injections, the medical assistant should review this chapter thoroughly, concentrating on the locations of injection sites and the procedures for preparing and administering injections. The same basic technique is used to administer an injection to an adult and a child. Variations in procedure are explained in the following section.

Types of Needles

The gauge and length of the needle used for intramuscular injections vary, depending on the consistency of the medication to be administered and the size of the child. Thick or oily preparations require a larger needle lumen, and the needle must be long enough to reach muscle tissue. A needle length ranging from ⅝ inch to 1 inch is generally used to administer an intramuscular injection to a child, and the gauge of the needle generally ranges between 22 and 25, depending on the viscosity of the medication. The length of the needle used to administer a pediatric subcutaneous injection ranges from ⅜ inch to ½ inch, and the gauge of the needle ranges from 23 to 25.

Intramuscular Injection Sites

Pediatric injection sites vary based on the age of the child. The specific site to be injected is stated in the package insert accompanying the medication. Until the child is walking, the gluteus muscle is small and not well developed, and is covered with a thick layer of fat. An injection in the dorsogluteal site (Figure 24-7) may come dangerously close to the sciatic nerve. The danger is increased if the child is squirming or fighting. Because serious trauma can result from incorrect administration of an injection in this area, the dorsogluteal site should not be used as an injection site for an infant or young child.

The vastus lateralis muscle site is recommended for injections of infants and young children. It is located on the anterior surface of the midlateral thigh, away from major nerves and blood vessels, and it is large enough to accommodate the injected medication (Figure 24-8, *A*). To locate

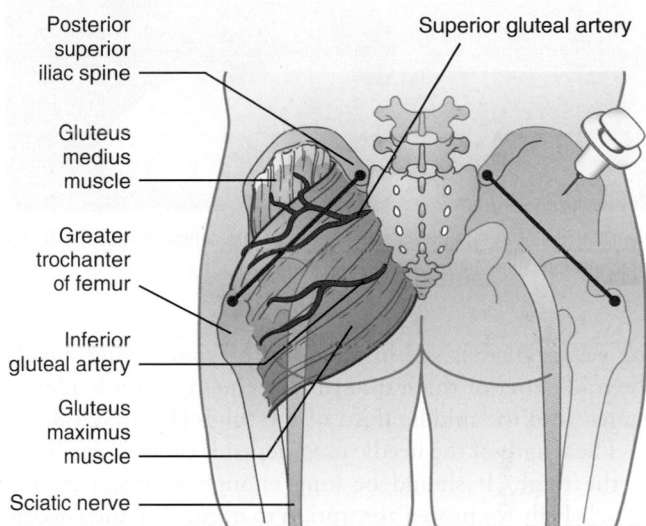

Figure 24-7 Dorsogluteal intramuscular injection site.

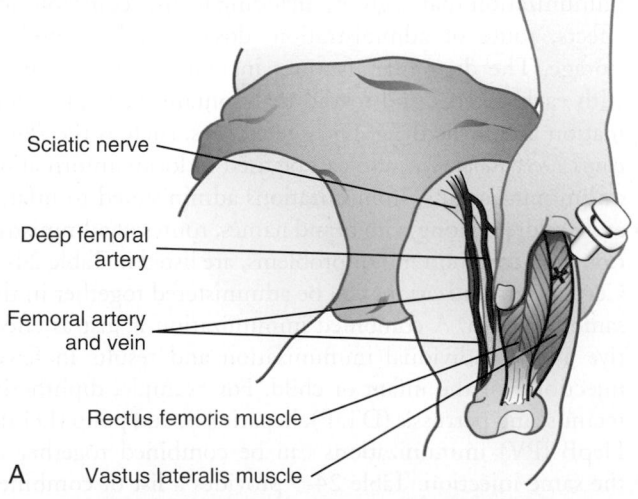

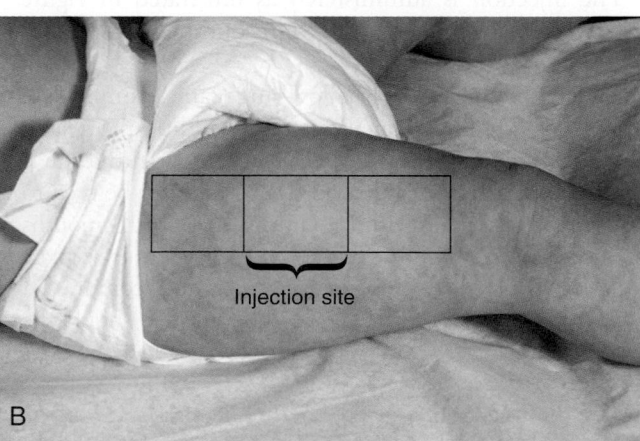

Figure 24-8 A, Vastus lateralis intramuscular injection site. **B,** Location of the vastus lateralis injection site in an infant. Divide the mid-anterior thigh into thirds. The injection is administered into the middle third of the thigh.

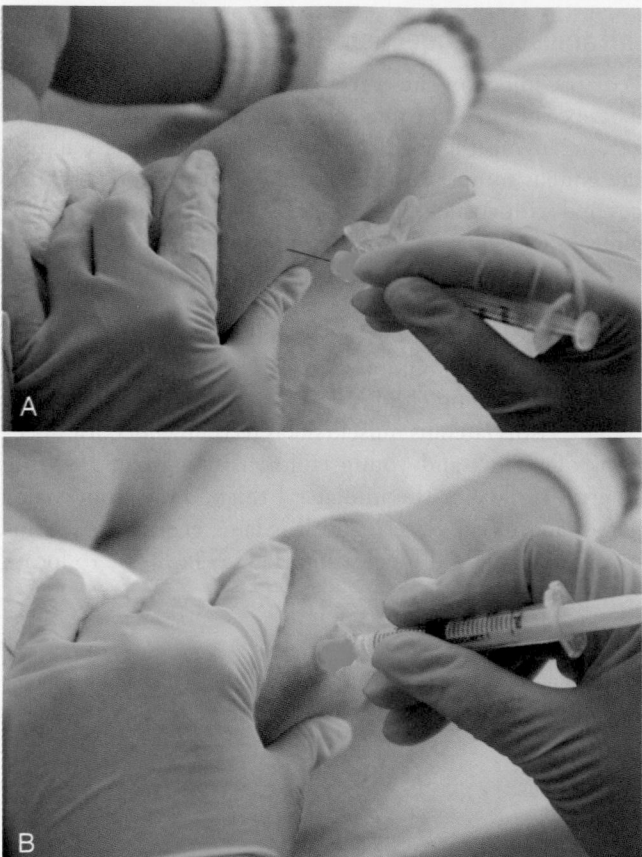

Figure 24-9 **A,** Compression of the vastus lateralis muscle. **B,** IM injection into the vastus lateralis injection site.

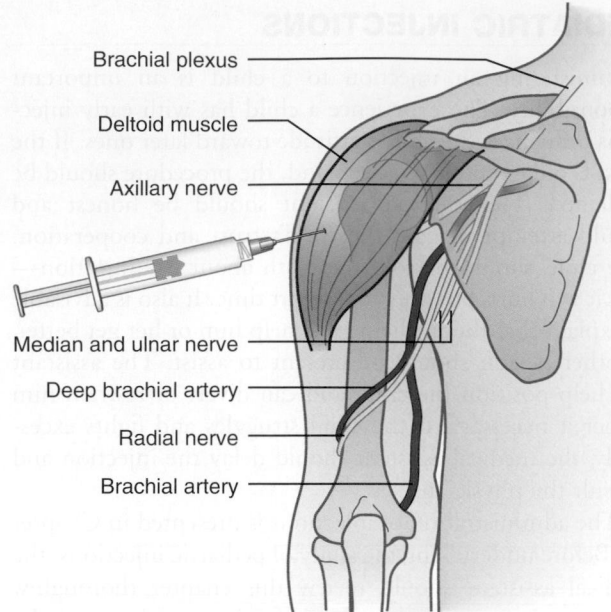

Figure 24-10 Deltoid intramuscular injection site.

the vastus lateralis site in an infant or young child, divide the mid–anterior thigh into thirds. The injection is administered into the middle third of the thigh (Figure 24-8, *B*).

The length of the needle used depends on the overall size of the thigh. It should be long enough to penetrate the muscle belly for proper absorption to occur. A 1-inch needle is often used. To administer the injection, the infant is placed on his or her back. The thigh is grasped to compress the muscle tissue and to stabilize the extremity (Figure 24-9, *A*). The injection is administered as illustrated in Figure 24-9, *B*, by following the procedure outlined in Chapter 26.

The deltoid muscle is shallow and can accommodate only a small amount of medication. In addition, repeated injections at this site are painful. Because the deltoid site is so small in an infant, the deltoid site should not be used to administer an injection until a child is at least 18 months old. To administer the injection, the deltoid muscle mass should be grasped at the injection site and compressed between the thumb and fingers. The needle should be inserted pointing slightly upward toward the shoulder (Figure 24-10).

After the injection is given, the medical assistant or the child's parent should hold the infant and provide comfort and show approval so that the child associates something other than pain with this procedure.

IMMUNIZATIONS

Immunity is the resistance of the body to the effects of harmful agents, such as pathogenic microorganisms and their toxins. The process of becoming immune or rendering an individual immune through the use of a **vaccine** or **toxoid** is known as active, artificial **immunization.** Immunizations build the body's defenses and protect an individual from attack by certain infectious diseases.

Immunizations should be administered to infants and young children during well-child visits according to an immunization schedule. The American Academy of Pediatrics recommends that the schedule outlined in Figure 24-11 should be followed. This schedule is intended as a guide to be used with any modifications needed to meet the requirements of an individual or group.

The medical assistant should be familiar with every immunization that is given, including its use, common side effects, route of administration, dosage, and method of storage. The drug manufacturer includes a package insert with each vaccine and toxoid that contains valuable information about the drug. Drug references, such as the *Physician's Desk Reference,* also can be used to locate information on immunizations. Immunizations administered to infants and children, along with brand names, routes of administration, and common minor problems, are listed in Table 24-4. Certain immunizations can be administered together in the same injection. A combined immunization is just as effective as the individual immunization and results in fewer injections for the infant or child. For example, diphtheria, tetanus, and pertussis (DTaP), hepatitis B, and polio (DTaP-HepB-IPV) immunizations can be combined together in the same injection. Table 24-5 provides a list of combined immunizations administered to infants and children, along with brand names and the routes of administration.

Recommended Immunization Schedule for Persons Aged 0–6 Years—UNITED STATES • 2012

For those who fall behind or start late, see the catch-up schedule

Vaccine ▼ / Age ►	Birth	1 month	2 months	4 months	6 months	9 months	12 months	15 months	18 months	19–23 months	2–3 years	4–6 years
Hepatitis B[1]	Hep B	HepB			HepB							
Rotavirus[2]			RV	RV	RV[2]							
Diphtheria, tetanus, pertussis[3]			DTaP	DTaP	DTaP		see footnote[3]	DTaP	DTaP			DTaP
Haemophilus influenzae type b[4]			Hib	Hib	Hib[4]		Hib	Hib				
Pneumococcal[5]			PCV	PCV	PCV		PCV	PCV			PPSV	PPSV
Inactivated poliovirus[6]			IPV	IPV	IPV							IPV
Influenza[7]					Influenza (Yearly)							
Measles, mumps, rubella[8]							MMR	MMR		see footnote[8]		MMR
Varicella[9]							Varicella	Varicella		see footnote[9]		Varicella
Hepatitis A[10]							Dose 1[10]				HepA Series	HepA Series
Meningococcal[11]							MCV4 — see footnote[11]					

Legend:
- Range of recommended ages for all children
- Range of recommended ages for certain high-risk groups
- Range of recommended ages for all children and certain high-risk groups

This schedule includes recommendations in effect as of December 23, 2011. Any dose not administered at the recommended age should be administered at a subsequent visit, when indicated and feasible. The use of a combination vaccine generally is preferred over separate injections of its equivalent component vaccines. Vaccination providers should consult the relevant Advisory Committee on Immunization Practices (ACIP) statement for detailed recommendations, available online at http://www.cdc.gov/vaccines/pubs/acip-list.htm. Clinically significant adverse events that follow vaccination should be reported to the Vaccine Adverse Event Reporting System (VAERS) online (http://www.vaers.hhs.gov) or by telephone (800-822-7967).

Figure 24-11 Immunization schedule.

Table 24-4 Infant and Childhood Immunizations

Immunization (and Abbreviation)	Brand Names	Route of Administration	Common Minor Problems after Administration
Hep B (hepatitis B vaccine)	Engerix-B, Recombivax HB	IM	Mild fever; Soreness at injection site
DTaP (diphtheria and tetanus toxoids and acellular pertussis vaccine)	Acel-Imune, Certiva, Daptacel, Infanrix, Tripedia	IM	Fever, irritability, tiredness, poor appetite, and vomiting; Redness or swelling at injection site; Soreness or tenderness at injection site (occurs 1-3 days after the injection and occurs more often after the 4th or 5th dose in the series than after earlier doses)
Hib (Haemophilus influenzae type b vaccine)	ActHIB, HibTITER, PedvaxHIB	IM	Redness, swelling, and warmth at injection site; fever greater than 101° F (38.3° C) (occurs within 1 day after injection; may last 2-3 days)
IPV (inactivated polio vaccine)	IPOL	IM or SC	Soreness at the injection site
PCV (pneumococcal conjugate vaccine)	Prevnar	IM	Redness, swelling, and tenderness at the injection site; fever; Irritability and drowsiness; Loss of appetite
RV (rotavirus vaccine)	Rotarix, RotaShield, RotaTeq	Oral	Irritability, temporary diarrhea, and vomiting
MMR (measles, mumps, and rubella vaccines)	M-M-R II	SC	Fever, mild rash, swelling of glands in the cheeks or neck (occur 7-12 days after administration)
Var (varicella) (chickenpox vaccine)	Varivax	SC	Fever, mild rash; Soreness or swelling at injection site
Hep A (hepatitis A vaccine)	Havrix, Vaqta	IM	Soreness at the injection site; Headache, loss of appetite, and tiredness (usually last 1-2 days)
MCV4 (meningococcal vaccine)	Menactra	IM	Pain and redness at injection site; Fever (usually lasts 1-2 days)
HPV (human papillomavirus vaccine)	Gardasil	IM	Pain, redness, swelling, or itching at injection site; Fever
Influenza vaccine (injection)	Afluria, Fluarix, FluLaval, FluShield, Fluvirin, Fluzone	IM	Soreness, redness, or swelling at the injection site, fever and malaise; Hoarseness; sore, red, or itchy eyes; Cough, fever, aches (occur soon after injection and usually last 1-2 days)
Influenza vaccine (nasal spray)	FluMist	IN	Runny nose, nasal congestion or cough; Headache, muscle aches, abdominal pain, or occasional vomiting or diarrhea; Fever; wheezing

From Bonewit-West K: *Clinical procedures for medical assistants*, ed 8, St Louis, 2011, Saunders.
IM, Intramuscular; *IN,* intranasal; *SC,* subcutaneous.

Table 24-5 Infant and Childhood Combination Immunizations

Combined Immunization	Brand Name	Route of Administration
DTaP-HepB-IPV	Pediarix	IM
DTaP-Hib-IPV	Pentacel	IM
DTaP-IPV	Kinrix	IM
DTaP-Hib	TriHIBit	IM
Hib-HepB	Comvax	IM
MMRV	ProQuad	SC

From Bonewit-West K: *Clinical procedures for medical assistants,* ed 8, St Louis, 2011, Saunders.

DTaP, Diphtheria, tetanus, and pertussis; *HepB,* hepatitis B; *Hib, Haemophilus influenzae* type b; *IM,* intramuscular; *IPV,* inactivated polio vaccine; *MMRV,* measles, mumps, rubella, varicella; *SC,* subcutaneous.

NOTE: See Table 24-4 for the common minor problems that may occur following administration of each individual immunization.

Parents should be provided with an immunization record card (Figure 24-12) at their infant's first well-child visit. They should be instructed to bring this card to every visit so that their child's immunizations can be recorded. Parents should be informed of the possible normal side effects of each immunization and given instructions on how to respond if they occur.

National Childhood Vaccine Injury Act

The National Childhood Vaccine Injury Act (NCVIA), which became effective in 1988, requires that parents be provided with information about the benefits and risks of childhood immunizations. To help medical offices comply with these regulations, the Centers for Disease Control and Prevention developed a set of vaccine information statements. A vaccine information statement (VIS) explains, in lay terminology, the benefits and risks of a vaccine. It also contains information about reporting an adverse reaction, the National Vaccine Injury Compensation Program, and how to get more information about childhood diseases and vaccines. See Figure 24-13 for a DTaP vaccine information statement.

The NCVIA requires that the appropriate VIS be given to the child's parent or guardian each and every time before the child receives a dose of any immunization listed in Table 24-4. The medical assistant must give the parent or guardian enough time to read the VIS and an opportunity to ask questions before the immunization is administered. In addition, the medical assistant must chart the following information in the patient's medical record: the name and publication date of each VIS provided to the parent, and the date the VIS was given to the parent. The publication date of the VIS is located at the bottom left or right corner of the VIS. Vaccine information statements also are available for pneumococcal polysaccharide, shingles (herpes zoster), rabies, yellow fever, typhoid, Japanese encephalitis, anthrax, and smallpox. Their use is strongly encouraged by the NCVIA, but is not required, because these vaccines are not administered to children on a routine basis.

The NCVIA also requires that the following information be recorded in each patient's medical record or on a permanent office log after administration of the vaccine: the date of administration of the vaccine, the manufacturer and lot number of the vaccine, the signature and title of the health care provider who administered the vaccine, and the name and address of the medical office where the vaccine was administered. Figure 24-14 shows an example of an immunization administrative record that is included in a patient's medical record.

What Would You Do? What Would You *Not* Do?

Case Study 3

Stacy Jones, a legal secretary, brings her 5-year-old son, Matthew, in for a kindergarten physical. Stacy has read the vaccine information statements for the DTaP, IPV, and MMR immunizations that Matthew will be getting at this visit and has some questions. She wants to know why polio is not given orally anymore. She also wants to know why children are immunized against chickenpox because it is such a harmless disease. She is annoyed because she thinks that children are receiving too many unnecessary injections these days. Matthew is extremely afraid of "shots" and says that no one with a needle is getting anywhere near him. Stacy is protective of Matthew and knows that he will be hard to handle. She wants to know whether this set of immunizations could just be skipped. She says that most of these diseases do not even exist anymore and that she noticed, from reading the vaccine sheets, that there are a lot of possible side effects. ■

NEWBORN SCREENING TEST

A newborn screening test is performed on an infant to screen for the presence of certain metabolic and endocrine diseases. The diseases that are screened vary by state but typically include phenylketonuria (PKU), biotinidase deficiency, congenital adrenal hyperplasia, maple sugar urine disease, congenital hypothyroidism, galactosemia, homocystinuria, and sickle cell anemia. The most important of these is PKU, which is discussed in greater detail in the following paragraphs.

PKU is a congenital hereditary disease caused by a lack of the enzyme *phenylalanine hydroxylase.* This enzyme is needed to convert phenylalanine, an amino acid, into tyrosine, which is an amino acid needed for normal metabolic functioning. Without this enzyme, phenylalanine accumulates in the blood and, if the accumulation is left untreated, causes mental retardation and other abnormalities, such as tremors and poor muscle coordination. In most cases, on early detection, a special low-phenylalanine diet and close periodic monitoring can prevent adverse effects. Normal development usually occurs if treatment is started before the child reaches 3 to 4 weeks of age. To promote the best

PEDIATRIC VACCINE ADMINISTRATION RECORD

Name _____
    (first)   (MI)   (last)

DOB _____

Physician _____

Address _____

_____

SITE ABBREVIATIONS:

RVL: Right vastus lateralis

LVL: Left vastus lateralis

RD: Right deltoid

LD: Left deltoid

Vaccine	Type of Vaccine[1] (generic abbreviation)	Date Given (mo/day/yr)	Dose	Site	Vaccine		Vaccine Information Statement		Signature of Vaccinator
					Lot #	Mfr.	Date on VIS	Date Given	
Hepatitis B[2] (e.g., HepB, Hib-HepB, DTaP-HepB-IPV) Give IM.									
Diphtheria, Tetanus, Pertussis[2] (e.g., DTaP, DTaP-Hib, DTaP-HepB-IPV, DT, Tdap, Td) Give IM.									
Haemophilus influenzae type b[2] (e.g., Hib, Hib-HepB, DTaP-Hib) Give IM.									
Polio[2] (e.g., IPV, DTaP-HepB-IPV) Give IPV SC or IM. Give DTaP-HepB-IPV IM.									
Pneumococcal (e.g., PCV, conjugate; PPV, polysaccharide) Give PCV IM. Give PPV SC or IM.									
Measles, Mumps, Rubella[5] (e.g., MMR, MMRV) Give SC.									
Varicella[5] (e.g., Var, MMRV) Give SC.									
Meningococcal (e.g., MCV4, conjugate; MPSV4, polysaccharide) Give MCV4 IM and MPSV4 SC.									
Influenza[5] (e.g., TIV, inactivated; LAIV, live attenuated) Give TIV IM. Give LAIV IN.									
Other									

1. Record the generic abbreviation for the type of vaccine given (e.g., DTaP-Hib, PCV), *not* the trade name.
2. For combination vaccines, fill in a row for each separate antigen in the combination.

Figure 24-12 Immunization record card.

DIPHTHERIA TETANUS & PERTUSSIS VACCINES

WHAT YOU NEED TO KNOW

1 | Why get vaccinated?

Diphtheria, tetanus, and pertussis are serious diseases caused by bacteria. Diphtheria and pertussis are spread from person to person. Tetanus enters the body through cuts or wounds.

DIPHTHERIA causes a thick covering in the back of the throat.
• It can lead to breathing problems, paralysis, heart failure, and even death.

TETANUS (Lockjaw) causes painful tightening of the muscles, usually all over the body.
• It can lead to "locking" of the jaw so the victim cannot open his mouth or swallow. Tetanus leads to death in up to 2 out of 10 cases.

PERTUSSIS (Whooping Cough) causes coughing spells so bad that it is hard for infants to eat, drink, or breathe. These spells can last for weeks.
• It can lead to pneumonia, seizures (jerking and staring spells), brain damage, and death.

Diphtheria, tetanus, and pertussis vaccine (DTaP) can help prevent these diseases. Most children who are vaccinated with DTaP will be protected throughout childhood. Many more children would get these diseases if we stopped vaccinating.

DTaP is a safer version of an older vaccine called DTP. DTP is no longer used in the United States.

2 | Who should get DTaP vaccine and when?

Children should get <u>5 doses</u> of DTaP vaccine, one dose at each of the following ages:

2 months	15-18 months
4 months	4-6 years
6 months	

DTaP may be given at the same time as other vaccines.

3 | Some children should not get DTaP vaccine or should wait

• Children with minor illnesses, such as a cold, may be vaccinated. But children who are moderately or severely ill should usually wait until they recover before getting DTaP vaccine.

• Any child who had a life-threatening allergic reaction after a dose of DTaP should not get another dose.

• Any child who suffered a brain or nervous system disease within 7 days after a dose of DTaP should not get another dose.

• Talk with your doctor if your child:
  - had a seizure or collapsed after a dose of DTaP,
  - cried non-stop for 3 hours or more after a dose of DTaP,
  - had a fever over 105°F after a dose of DTaP.

Ask your health care provider for more information. Some of these children should not get another dose of pertussis vaccine, but may get a vaccine without pertussis, called **DT**.

4 | Older children and adults

DTaP is not licensed for adolescents, adults, or children 7 years of age and older.

But older people still need protection. A vaccine called **Tdap** is similar to DTaP. A single dose of Tdap is recommended for people 11 through 64 years of age. Another vaccine, called **Td**, protects against tetanus and diphtheria, but not pertussis. It is recommended every 10 years. There are separate Vaccine Information Statements for these vaccines.

Diphtheria/Tetanus/Pertussis	5/17/2007

Figure 24-13 Vaccine information statement for diphtheria, tetanus, and pertussis (DTaP).

5 | What are the risks from DTaP vaccine?

Getting diphtheria, tetanus, or pertussis disease is much riskier than getting DTaP vaccine.

However, a vaccine, like any medicine, is capable of causing serious problems, such as severe allergic reactions. The risk of DTaP vaccine causing serious harm, or death, is extremely small.

Mild Problems (Common)

- Fever (up to about 1 child in 4)
- Redness or swelling where the shot was given (up to about 1 child in 4)
- Soreness or tenderness where the shot was given (up to about 1 child in 4)

These problems occur more often after the 4th and 5th doses of the DTaP series than after earlier doses. Sometimes the 4th or 5th dose of DTaP vaccine is followed by swelling of the entire arm or leg in which the shot was given, lasting 1-7 days (up to about 1 child in 30).

Other mild problems include:

- Fussiness (up to about 1 child in 3)
- Tiredness or poor appetite (up to about 1 child in 10)
- Vomiting (up to about 1 child in 50)

These problems generally occur 1-3 days after the shot.

Moderate Problems (Uncommon)

- Seizure (jerking or staring) (about 1 child out of 14,000)
- Non-stop crying, for 3 hours or more (up to about 1 child out of 1,000)
- High fever, over 105°F (about 1 child out of 16,000)

Severe Problems (Very Rare)

- Serious allergic reaction (less than 1 out of a million doses)
- Several other severe problems have been reported after DTaP vaccine. These include:
  - Long-term seizures, coma, or lowered consciousness
  - Permanent brain damage.
  These are so rare it is hard to tell if they are caused by the vaccine.

Controlling fever is especially important for children who have had seizures, for any reason. It is also important if another family member has had seizures. You can reduce fever and pain by giving your child an *aspirin-free* pain reliever when the shot is given, and for the next 24 hours, following the package instructions.

6 | What if there is a moderate or severe reaction?

What should I look for?

Any unusual conditions, such as a serious allergic reaction, high fever or unusual behavior. Serious allergic reactions are extremely rare with any vaccine. If one were to occur, it would most likely be within a few minutes to a few hours after the shot. Signs can include difficulty breathing, hoarseness or wheezing, hives, paleness, weakness, a fast heart beat or dizziness. If a high fever or seizure were to occur, it would usually be within a week after the shot.

What should I do?

- **Call** a doctor, or get the person to a doctor right away.
- **Tell** your doctor what happened, the date and time it happened, and when the vaccination was given.
- **Ask** your doctor, nurse, or health department to report the reaction by filing a Vaccine Adverse Event Reporting System (VAERS) form.

Or you can file this report through the VAERS web site at **www.vaers.hhs.gov**, or by calling **1-800-822-7967**. *VAERS does not provide medical advice*

7 | The National Vaccine Injury Compensation Program

In the rare event that you or your child has a serious reaction to a vaccine, a federal program has been created to help pay for the care of those who have been harmed.

For details about the National Vaccine Injury Compensation Program, call **1-800-338-2382** or visit the program's website at **www.hrsa.gov/vaccinecompensation.**

8 | How can I learn more?

- Ask your health care provider. They can give you the vaccine package insert or suggest other sources of information.

- Call your local or state health department's immunization program.

- Contact the Centers for Disease Control and Prevention (CDC):
  - Call **1-800-232-4636 (1-800-CDC-INFO)**
  - Visit the National Immunization Program's website at **www.cdc.gov/nip**

 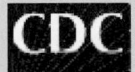

U.S. DEPARTMENT OF HEALTH & HUMAN SERVICES
Centers for Disease Control and Prevention

Vaccine Information Statement	
DTaP (5/17/07)	42 U.S.C. § 300aa-26

Figure 24-13, cont'd

---

development of cognitive abilities, most authorities recommend lifelong dietary restriction of phenylalanine. Although PKU is not a common condition (affecting 1 in every 12,000 births), early diagnosis and treatment lead to a better prognosis.

Phenylalanine can be detected in the blood of an affected infant only after the infant has been receiving breast or formula milk. Infants taking formula can be tested earlier than breastfed infants because formula contains phenylalanine, whereas the "first breast milk," or colostrum, does not.

IMMUNIZATION ADMINISTRATION RECORD

Name _____
    (first)   (MI)   (last)

DOB _____

Physician _____

Address _____

_____

SITE ABBREVIATIONS:

RVL: Right vastus lateralis

LVL: Left vastus lateralis

RD: Right deltoid

LD: Left deltoid

PO: By mouth

IN: Intranasal

Vaccine	Type of Vaccine[1] (generic abbreviation)	Date Given (mo/day/yr)	Dose	Site	Vaccine		Vaccine Information Statement		Signature and Title of Vaccinator
					Lot #	Mfr.	Date on VIS	Date Given	
Hepatitis B[2] (e.g., HepB, Hib-HepB, DTaP-HepB-IPV) Give IM.									
Diphtheria, Tetanus, Pertussis[2] (e.g., DTaP, DTaP-Hib, DTaP-HepB-IPV, DT, DTaP-Hib-IPV, Tdap, DTaP-IPV, Td) Give IM.									
Haemophilus influenzae **type b**[2] (e.g., Hib, Hib-HepB, DTaP-Hib-IPV, DTaP-Hib) Give IM.									
Polio[2] (e.g., IPV, DTaP-HepB-IPV, DTaP-Hib-IPV, DTaP-IPV) Give IPV SC or IM. Give all others IM.									
Pneumococcal (e.g., PCV, conjugate; PPV, polysaccharide) Give PCV IM. Give PPV SC or IM.									
Rotovirus Give oral.									
Measles, Mumps, Rubella[5] (e.g., MMR, MMRV) Give SC.									
Varicella[5] (e.g., Var, MMRV) Give SC.									
Hepatitis A Give IM									
Meningococcal (e.g., MCV4, MPSV4) Give MCV4 IM and MPSV4 SC.									
Human papillomavirus (e.g., HPV) Give IM									
Influenza[5] (e.g., TIV, inactivated; LAIV, live attenuated) Give TIV IM. Give LAIV IN.									
Other									

1. Record the generic abbreviation for the type of vaccine given (e.g., DTaP-Hib, PCV), *not* the trade name.
2. For combination vaccines, fill in a row for each separate antigen in the combination.

Figure 24-14 Immunization administration record included in a patient's medical record.

The test results of breastfed infants are usually invalid until the mother begins producing milk.

All states require by law that infants undergo newborn screening. The best time to perform the test is between 1 and 7 days after birth. In most states, the newborn screening test is performed before the infant leaves the hospital. If test results come back indicating abnormal or invalid results, the infant needs to be retested. Most repeat tests are required because of invalid test results due to the collection of an inadequate amount of the blood specimen. Newborn screening retesting is usually performed at a hospital laboratory but may sometimes be performed in the medical office.

The newborn screening test card (Figure 24-15) includes an information section that must be completed before the test is performed. The newborn screening test is performed on capillary blood obtained from the fleshy part of the lateral or medial posterior curve of the plantar surface of the infant's heel (Figure 24-16, *A* and *B*). The blood specimen is placed on a special filter paper attached to the newborn screening test card (Figure 24-17) and is mailed to an outside laboratory for analysis. The results are ready in a few days. If one of the newborn screening test results is positive, further testing is performed.

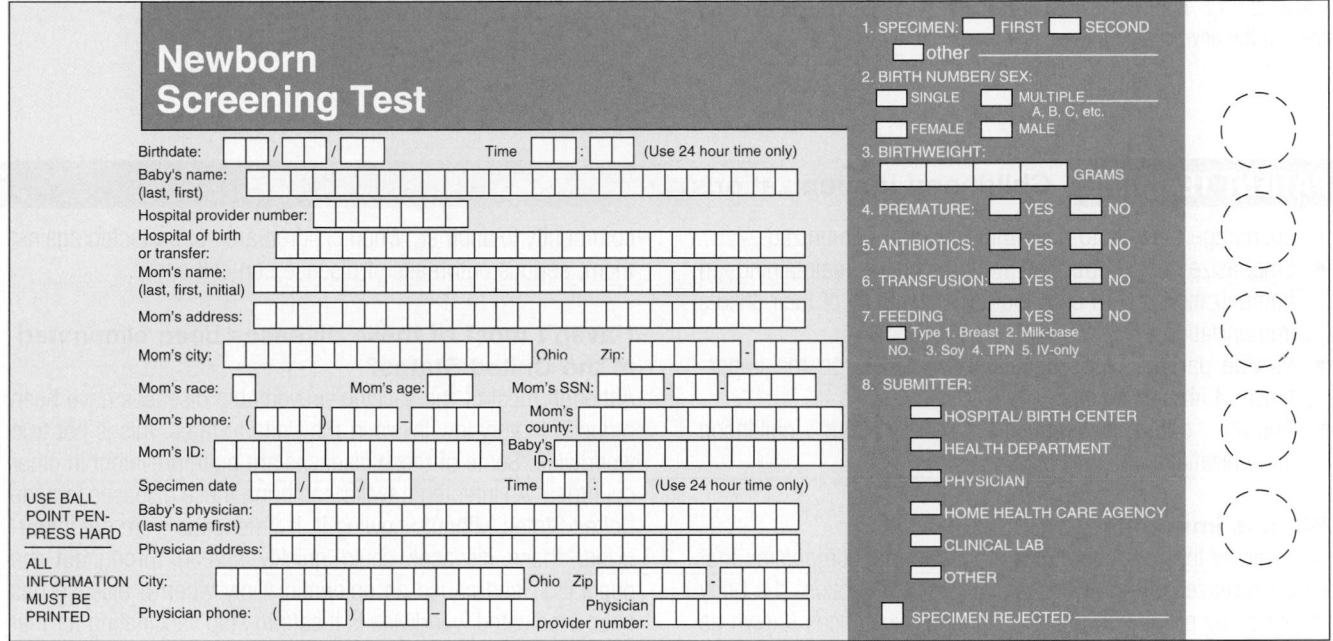

Figure 24-15 Newborn screening test card.

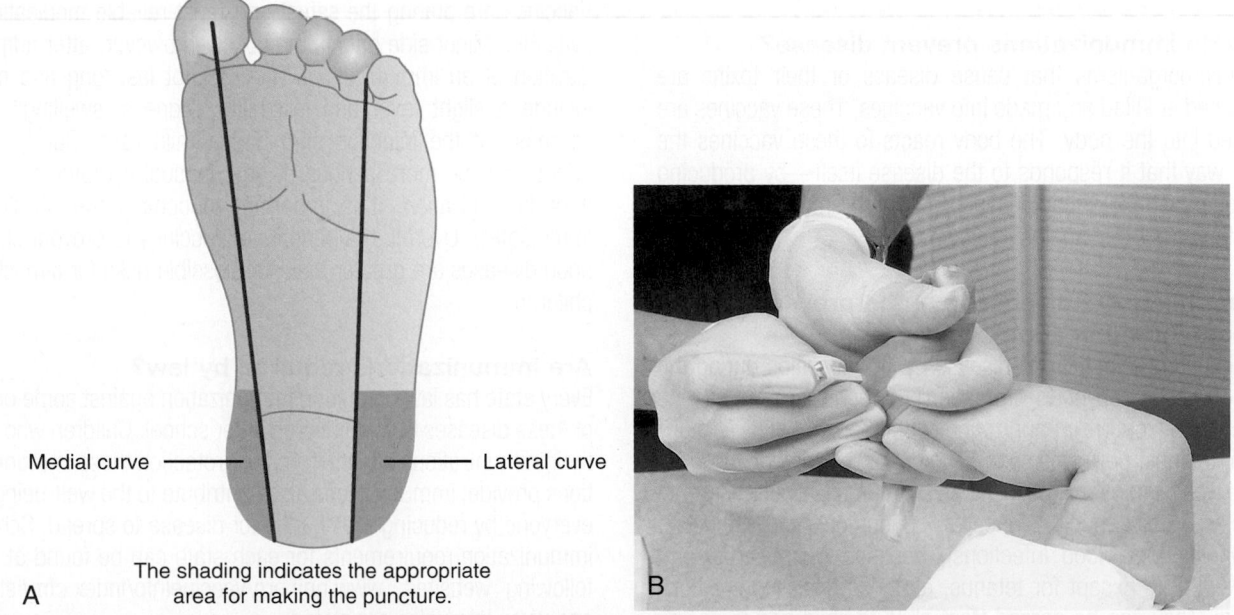

Figure 24-16 **A,** Heel puncture sites for a pediatric patient. **B,** Puncture of the medial posterior curve of the plantar surface of an infant's heel.

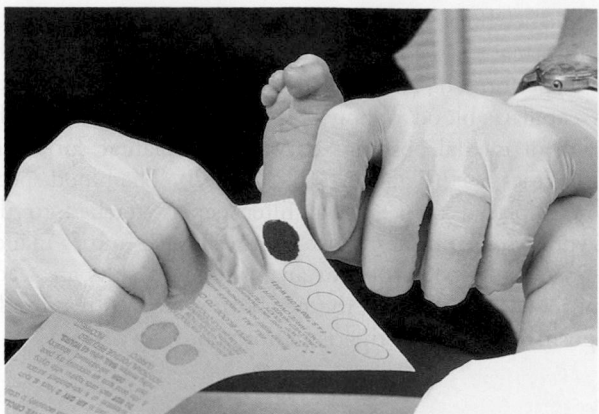

Figure 24-17 Applying a drop of blood to the first circle on the filter paper on the newborn screening test card.

PATIENT TEACHING   Childhood Immunizations

- Encourage parents to have their children immunized.
- Emphasize to parents the importance of maintaining an immunization record card that documents all of their child's immunizations.
- Provide parents with educational materials on the importance of immunizations.
- Answer questions patients have about childhood immunizations.

What is immunity?
Immunity is the resistance of the body to microorganisms that cause disease. When an individual has an infection, the body responds by producing disease-fighting substances known as *antibodies.* Antibodies usually remain in the body even after the individual has recovered from the disease. This protects the individual from getting that disease again.

How do immunizations prevent disease?
The microorganisms that cause disease or their toxins are weakened or killed and made into vaccines. These vaccines are injected into the body. The body reacts to these vaccines the same way that it responds to the disease itself—by producing antibodies. These antibodies last for a long time, often for life, to defend the body against disease.

What childhood diseases can be prevented through immunization?
The reduction of childhood disease by immunization during the past 40 years has been dramatic. Fourteen diseases can be prevented by routine immunization of children: hepatitis B, diphtheria, tetanus, pertussis (whooping cough), *Haemophilus influenzae* type b infections, polio, measles, mumps, rubella (German measles), chickenpox (varicella), pneumococcal infections (meningitis and blood infections), hepatitis A, rotavirus, and influenza (flu). Except for tetanus, all these diseases are contagious. They can be spread from child to child and from one community to another. When children are not protected against them, serious outbreaks of disease can still occur.

Haven't most of these diseases been eliminated in the United States?
Although most of the vaccine-preventable diseases have been reduced to very low levels in the United States, this is not true worldwide. Some of these diseases are quite prevalent in other countries. An infected traveler can bring these diseases into the United States without knowing it. If Americans were not immunized, these diseases could quickly spread throughout the population and cause an epidemic. Only when a disease has been eradicated worldwide is it safe to stop vaccinating for that particular disease.

Do immunizations have side effects?
Vaccines are among the safest and most reliable medications available. Minor side effects may occur, however, after administration of an immunization. They do not last long and may include a slight fever and irritability; redness, swelling, and soreness at the injection site; and a mild rash. Rarely, the effects can be more serious; if any unusual symptoms occur after immunization, it is important to contact the physician immediately. Overall, the benefits of vaccines to prevent childhood diseases are greater than the possible risks for almost all children.

Are immunizations required by law?
Every state has laws requiring immunization against some or all of these diseases before children enter school. Children who get their immunizations benefit from the protection these immunizations provide; immunizations also contribute to the well-being of everyone by reducing the chance for disease to spread. School immunization requirements for each state can be found at the following websites: www.nnii.org/vaccineInfo/index.cfm#state and www.immunize.org/states. ■

Case Study 1
Page 472

What Did Traci Do?

❏ Listened patiently to Mrs. Chang and allowed her to vent her frustrations.

❏ Reassured Mrs. Chang that her milk is very nutritious for Christopher. Gave her a brochure on breastfeeding that included information on what to do for sore nipples and engorgement.

❏ Gave Mrs. Chang the names and phone numbers of community resources for nursing mothers.

❏ Told Mrs. Chang that Christopher's weight and length do not fall in the underweight category on his growth chart. Showed her Christopher's growth chart so that she could see that Christopher is progressing normally.

What Did Traci Not Do?

❏ Did not tell Mrs. Chang to cheer up because the colic would eventually go away on its own.

❏ Did not give a personal opinion on whether Mrs. Chang should breastfeed or bottle feed her infant.

What Would You Do?/What Would You Not Do?

Review Traci's response and place a checkmark next to the information you included in your response. List additional information included in your response.

_____

_____

_____

_____

_____

_____

Case Study 2
Page 482

What Did Traci Do?

❏ Explained to Mrs. Tilley that childhood obesity has doubled in the past 20 years and has become a serious health concern.

❏ Told Mrs. Tilley that she could have a big impact on Courtney's life by preparing healthy meals and eating them with her and by becoming involved in activities with Courtney, such as taking walks.

❏ Spent some time talking with Courtney about her interests and complimented Courtney on her achievements.

❏ Encouraged Courtney to join the swim team. Told her that lots of people do not like to be seen in a bathing suit and encouraged her not to let that stand in her way of doing something she wants to do.

❏ Reassured Courtney that the doctor wants to help her and that he would never say anything bad about her weight.

What Did Traci Not Do?

❏ Did not agree with Mrs. Tilley that there is nothing that can be done about Courtney's weight problem.

❏ Did not tell Courtney that she needs to lose weight or she might develop serious health problems such as diabetes.

What Would You Do?/What Would You Not Do?

Review Traci's response and place a checkmark next to the information you included in your response. List additional information included in your response.

_____

_____

_____

_____

_____

_____

Case Study 3
Page 488

What Did Traci Do?

❏ Explained to Stacy that it is rare, but sometimes a child develops polio from getting the oral polio vaccine. Told her that this does not occur with the injectable polio vaccine.

❏ Explained to Stacy that chickenpox is usually a mild disease, but it can be serious, especially in young infants and adults.

❏ Explained to Stacy that most side effects from vaccines are mild, and that complications from the diseases far outweigh the possible side effects.

❏ Told Stacy that these diseases have been reduced to very low levels in the United States, but they still occur in other countries. Explained that infected travelers can bring these diseases to the United States and infect individuals who are not immunized.

❏ Reminded Stacy that these immunizations are required for Matthew to start kindergarten.

❏ Talked with Matthew on his level about why he needs to be immunized.

❏ Told Matthew that they would play a game so that it wouldn't hurt as much. Taught him to hold up his finger and pretend that it was a birthday candle; when the injection was given, told him to keep blowing out the candle until he was told to stop.

❏ Told Matthew that he could choose a prize from the treasure chest after he had his immunizations.

What Did Traci Not Do?

❏ Did not ignore or minimize Stacy's concerns.

❏ Did not tell Stacy that the answers to all her questions are in the vaccine information sheets that she was just given.

❏ Did not tell Stacy it would be all right to skip Matthew's immunizations.

❏ Did not refer to the immunizations as "shots" when talking with Matthew.

❏ Did not tell Matthew that it would not hurt when he gets his immunizations.

What Would You Do?/What Would You Not Do?

Review Traci's response and place a checkmark next to the information you included in your response. List additional information included in your response.

_____

_____

_____

_____

TERMINOLOGY REVIEW

Medical Term	Word Parts	Definition
Adolescent		An individual 12 to 18 years old.
Immunity		The resistance of the body to the effects of a harmful agent, such as a pathogenic microorganism and its toxins.
Immunization (active, artificial)		The process of becoming immune or of rendering an individual immune through the use of a vaccine or toxoid.
Infant		A child from birth to 12 months old.
Length (recumbent)		The measurement from the vertex of the head to the heel of the foot in a supine position.
Pediatrician	*pedi/a:* child	A physician who specializes in the care and development of children and the diagnosis and treatment of children's diseases.
Pediatrics	*pedi/a:* child	The branch of medicine that deals with the care and development of children and the diagnosis and treatment of children's diseases.
Preschool child	*pre-:* in front of; before	A child 3 to 6 years old.
School-age child		A child 6 to 12 years old.
Toddler		A child 1 to 3 years old.
Toxoid		A toxin (a poisonous substance produced by a bacterium) that has been treated by heat or chemicals to destroy its harmful properties. It is administered to an individual to prevent an infectious disease by stimulating the production of antibodies in that individual.
Vaccine		A suspension of attenuated (weakened) or killed microorganisms administered to an individual to prevent an infectious disease by stimulating the production of antibodies in that individual.
Vertex		The top of the head.

ON THE WEB

For information on child health:

KidsHealth: www.kidshealth.org

Baby Center: www.babycenter.com

Pediatric on Call: www.pediatriconcall.com

Kids Source Online: www.kidsource.com

American Academy of Pediatrics: www.aap.org

Child and Youth Health: www.cyh.com

Girl's Health: www.girlshealth.gov

For information on childhood conditions:

Attention-Deficit/Hyperactivity Disorder: www.add-adhd.org

Attention Deficit Disorder Association: www.add.org

Cerebral Palsy: www.about-cerebral-palsy.org

American Academy for Cerebral Palsy and Developmental Medicine: www.aacpdm.org

Child Abuse: www.preventchildabuse.org

American Professional Society on the Abuse of Children: www.apsac.org

Cystic Fibrosis: www.cysticfibrosis.com

ON THE WEB—cont'd

Cystic Fibrosis Foundation: www.cff.org

Dental Health: Colgate World of Care: www.colgate.com

American Dental Association: www.ada.org

The Tooth Fairy Online: www.asis.com/toothfairy

Diabetes: American Diabetes Association: www.diabetes.org

Children with Diabetes: www.childrenwithdiabetes.com

Down Syndrome: downsyndrome.com

National Down Syndrome Society: www.ndss.org

Spina Bifida Association of America: www.sbaa.org

National Sudden and Unexpected Infant/Child Death and Pregnancy Loss Resource Center: www.sidscenter.org

Influenza Information: www.cdc.gov/flu

SIDS Alliance: www.sidsalliance.org

For information on immunizations:

Immunization Action Coalition: www.immunize.org

Centers for Disease Control and Prevention: Vaccines and Immunizations: www.cdc.gov/vaccines

American Academy of Pediatrics Childhood Immunization Support Program: www.cispimmunize.org

American Academy of Family Physicians: Recommendations for Immunizations: www.aafp.org

Vaccine Information: www.vaccineinformation.org

The Children's Hospital of Philadelphia Vaccine Education Center: www.chop.edu

Every Child by Two: www.ecbt.org

National Network for Immunization Information: www.immunizationinfo.org

Drug Information Online: www.drugs.com

 Check out the Evolve site at http://evolve.elsevier.com/Bonewit/today/ to actively Prepare for your Certification, and to access additional interactive activities and exercises to help you study and prepare for success.

25

Minor Office Surgery

LEARNING OBJECTIVES

PROCEDURES

Surgical Asepsis

1. State the characteristics of a minor surgical procedure.
2. Identify procedures that require the use of surgical asepsis.
3. Describe the medical assistant's responsibilities during a minor surgical procedure.
4. List the guidelines to follow to maintain surgical asepsis during a sterile procedure.
5. Identify and explain the use and care of instruments commonly used for minor office surgery.

Apply and remove sterile gloves.
Open a sterile package.
Add an article to a sterile field.
Pour a sterile solution.

Wound Healing

6. Explain the differences between a closed and an open wound, and give examples.
7. List and explain the three phases of the healing process.
8. List and describe the different types of wound drainage.
9. List the functions of a dressing.

Change a sterile dressing.

Sutures

10. Explain the method used to measure the diameter of suturing material.
11. Describe the two types of sutures (absorbable and nonabsorbable), and give examples of their uses.
12. Categorize suturing needles according to type of point and shape.

Remove sutures.
Remove surgical staples.
Apply and remove adhesive skin closures.
Set up a tray for each of the following minor surgical procedures:
    Suture insertion
    Sebaceous cyst removal
    Incision and drainage of a localized infection
    Mole removal
    Needle biopsy
    Ingrown toenail removal
    Colposcopy
    Cervical punch biopsy
    Cryosurgery

Medical Office Surgical Procedures

13. Explain the purpose of and procedure for each of the following minor surgical operations: sebaceous cyst removal, incision and drainage of a localized infection, mole removal, needle biopsy, ingrown toenail removal, colposcopy, cervical punch biopsy, and cryosurgery.
14. Explain the principles underlying each step in the minor office surgery procedures.

Assist the physician with minor office surgery.

LEARNING OBJECTIVES

Bandaging

15. State the functions of a bandage, and list the guidelines for applying a bandage.
16. Identify the common types of bandages used in the medical office.

PROCEDURES

Apply each of the following bandage turns:
  Circular
  Spiral
  Spiral-reverse
  Figure-eight
  Recurrent

CHAPTER OUTLINE

KEY TERMS

abrasion (ah-BRAY-shun)
abscess (AB-sess)
absorbable suture (ab-SOR-ba-bul SOO-chur)
approximation (ah-PROKS-ih-MAY-shun)
bandage
biopsy (BYE-op-see)
capillary action (KAP-ill-air-ee AK-shun)
colposcope (KOL-poh-skope)
colposcopy (kol-POS-koh-pee)
contaminate (kon-TAM-in-ate)
contusion (kon-TOO-shun)
cryosurgery (KRY-oh-SURJ-er-ee)
exudate (EKS-oo-date)
fibroblast (FYE-broh-blast)

forceps (FORE-seps)
furuncle (FYOOR-un-kul)
hemostasis (hee-moe-STAY-sis)
incision (in-SIH-shun)
infection (in-FEK-shun)
infiltration (in-fill-TRAY-shun)
inflammation (in-flah-MAY-shun)
laceration (lass-ur-AY-shun)
ligate (LIH-gate)
local anesthetic (LOE-kul an-es-STET-ik)
Mayo (MAY-oe) tray
needle biopsy (NEE-dul BYE-op-see)
nonabsorbable suture (non-ab-SOR-ba-bul SOO-chur)
postoperative (post-OP-er-uh-tiv)

preoperative (pree-OP-er-uh-tiv)
puncture (PUNK-shur)
scalpel (SKAL-pul)
scissors
sebaceous cyst (suh-BAY-shus SIST)
serum (SEER-um)
sterile (STARE-ul)
surgery
surgical asepsis (SUR-jih-kul ay-SEP-sis)
sutures (SOO-churz)
swaged (SWAYJD) needle
wound

INTRODUCTION TO MINOR OFFICE SURGERY

The term *surgery* is defined as the branch of medicine that deals with operative and manual procedures for correction of deformities and defects, repair of injuries, and diagnosis and treatment of certain diseases. *Minor office surgery* (also known as *minor surgery*) refers to a surgical procedure that is restricted to the management of minor conditions and injuries that does not require the use of general anesthesia. Minor surgical procedures have the following characteristics:

- Are performed in an ambulatory health care facility, such as a physician's office or clinic

- Can be performed in a short period of time, usually in less than 1 hour
- Require a local anesthetic, a topical anesthetic, or no anesthetic
- Can be performed safely with a minimum of discomfort to the patient
- Do not, under normal circumstances, pose a major risk to life, or function of an organ or body parts

Various types of minor surgical operations are performed in the medical office, such as insertion of sutures, sebaceous cyst removal, incision and drainage of infections, mole removal, needle biopsies, cervical biopsies, and ingrown toenail removal. The physician explains the nature of the surgical procedure and any risks to the patient and offers to answer questions. The medical assistant is responsible for explaining the patient preparation required for the procedure and for obtaining the patient's signature on a written consent to treatment form, which grants the physician permission to perform the surgery (Figure 25-1).

Additional responsibilities of the medical assistant include preparing the treatment room, preparing the patient, preparing the minor surgery tray, assisting the physician during the procedure, administering postoperative care to the patient, and cleaning the treatment room after the procedure.

The treatment room must be spotlessly clean, and the medical assistant should ensure that the physician has adequate lighting for the procedure. The patient is positioned and draped according to the procedure to be performed. The skin is prepared as specified by the physician. Hair around the operative site is a contaminant and may need to be removed by shaving. The skin is cleansed, and an appropriate antiseptic is applied to the area to reduce the number of microorganisms present.

The medical assistant prepares the minor surgery tray using **sterile** technique. The specific instruments and supplies included in each setup vary, depending on the type of surgery to be performed and the physician's preference. The medical assistant must become familiar with the instruments and supplies required for each surgical procedure performed in the medical office.

During the minor surgery, the medical assistant is present to assist the physician as needed and to lend support to the patient. The medical assistant should become completely familiar with the assisting techniques (e.g., swabbing blood from the operative site) required for each surgical procedure performed in the medical office and should learn to anticipate the physician's needs to help the procedure go quickly and smoothly.

After the minor surgery, the medical assistant should remain with the patient as a safety precaution to prevent

---

(attach label or complete blanks)

First name: _____   Last name: _____

Date of Birth: _____ Month _____ Day _____ Year

Account Number: _____

Procedure Consent Form

I, _____ , hereby consent to have

Dr. _____ perform _____ .

I have been fully informed of the following by my physician:

1. The nature of my condition.
2. The nature and purpose of the procedure.
3. An explanation of risks involved with the procedure.
4. Alternative treatments or procedures available.
5. The likely results of the procedure.
6. The risks involved with declining or delaying the procedure.

My physician has offered to answer all questions concerning the proposed procedure.

I am aware that the practice of medicine and surgery is not an exact science, and I acknowledge that no guarantees have been made to me about the results of the procedure.

Patient _____   Date _____
(or guardian and relationship)

Witnessed _____   Date _____

Figure 25-1 Consent to treatment form.

accidental falls and other injuries and to make sure the patient understands the postoperative instructions. The medical assistant removes and properly cares for all used instruments and supplies and cleans the treatment room in preparation for the next patient.

SURGICAL ASEPSIS

Surgical asepsis, also known as *sterile technique,* refers to practices that keep objects and areas sterile, or free from all living microorganisms and spores. Surgical asepsis protects the patient from pathogenic microorganisms that may enter the body and cause disease. It is always employed under the following circumstances: when caring for broken skin, such as open wounds and suture punctures; when a skin surface is being penetrated, as by a surgical incision for a mole removal or the administration of an injection (the needle must remain sterile); and when a body cavity is entered that is normally sterile, such as during the insertion of a urinary catheter. Sterility of instruments and supplies is achieved through the use of disposable sterile items or by sterilizing reusable articles.

A sterile object that touches any unsterile object is automatically considered contaminated and must not be used. If the medical assistant is in doubt or has a question concerning the sterility of an article, he or she should consider it contaminated and replace it with a sterile article.

Sterility of the hands cannot be attained. Sanitizing the hands renders them medically aseptic and must be performed before and after every surgical procedure using proper technique (see Chapter 17). To prevent contamination of sterile articles, sterile gloves must be worn while picking up or transferring articles during a sterile procedure. Procedure 25-1 describes the procedure for applying and removing sterile gloves.

Specific guidelines must be observed during a sterile procedure to maintain surgical asepsis. See the accompanying box, Guidelines for Surgical Asepsis.

INSTRUMENTS USED IN MINOR OFFICE SURGERY

A variety of surgical instruments are used for minor office surgery. Most instruments are made of stainless steel and have either a bright, highly polished finish or a dull finish. The medical assistant should become familiar with the name, use, and proper care of all instruments used in the medical office. Surgical instruments are named by one or more of the following: (1) function (e.g., splinter forceps); (2) design (e.g., mosquito hemostatic forceps); and (3) the individual who developed the instrument (e.g., Kelly hemostatic forceps). The parts of an instrument are illustrated in Figure 25-2; some common instruments are described here and are illustrated in Figure 25-3.

Scalpels

A **scalpel** is a small straight surgical knife consisting of a handle and a thin, sharp steel blade. A scalpel is used to make surgical incisions and can divide tissue with the least

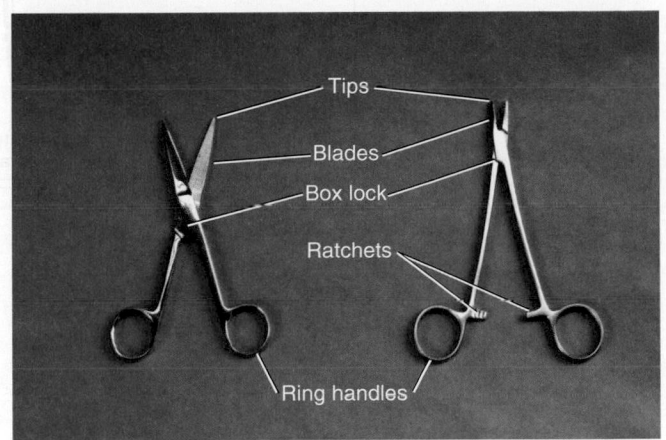

Figure 25-2 Parts of an instrument.

Guidelines for Surgical Asepsis

1. Take precautions to prevent sterile packages from becoming wet. Wet packages draw microorganisms into the package owing to the capillary action of the liquid, resulting in contamination of the sterile package. If a sterile package that has been prepared at the medical office becomes wet, it must be rewrapped and resterilized; if a disposable sterile package becomes wet, it must be discarded.
2. A 1-inch border around the sterile field is considered contaminated or unsterile because this area may have become contaminated while the sterile field was being set up.
3. Always face the sterile field. If you must turn your back to it or leave the room, a sterile towel must be placed over the sterile field.
4. Hold all sterile articles above waist level. Anything out of sight might become contaminated. The sterile articles also should be held in front of you and should not touch your uniform.

5. To avoid contamination, place all sterile items in the center, not around the edges, of the sterile field.
6. Be careful not to spill water or solutions on the sterile field. The area beneath the field is contaminated, and microorganisms are drawn up onto the field by the capillary action of the liquid, resulting in contamination of the field.
7. Do not talk, cough, or sneeze over a sterile field. Water vapor from the nose, mouth, and lungs is carried outward by the air and contaminates the sterile field.
8. Do not reach over a sterile field. Dust or lint from your clothing may fall onto it, or your unsterile clothing may accidentally touch it.
9. Do not pass soiled dressings over the sterile field.
10. Always acknowledge if you have contaminated the sterile field so that proper steps can be taken to regain sterility.

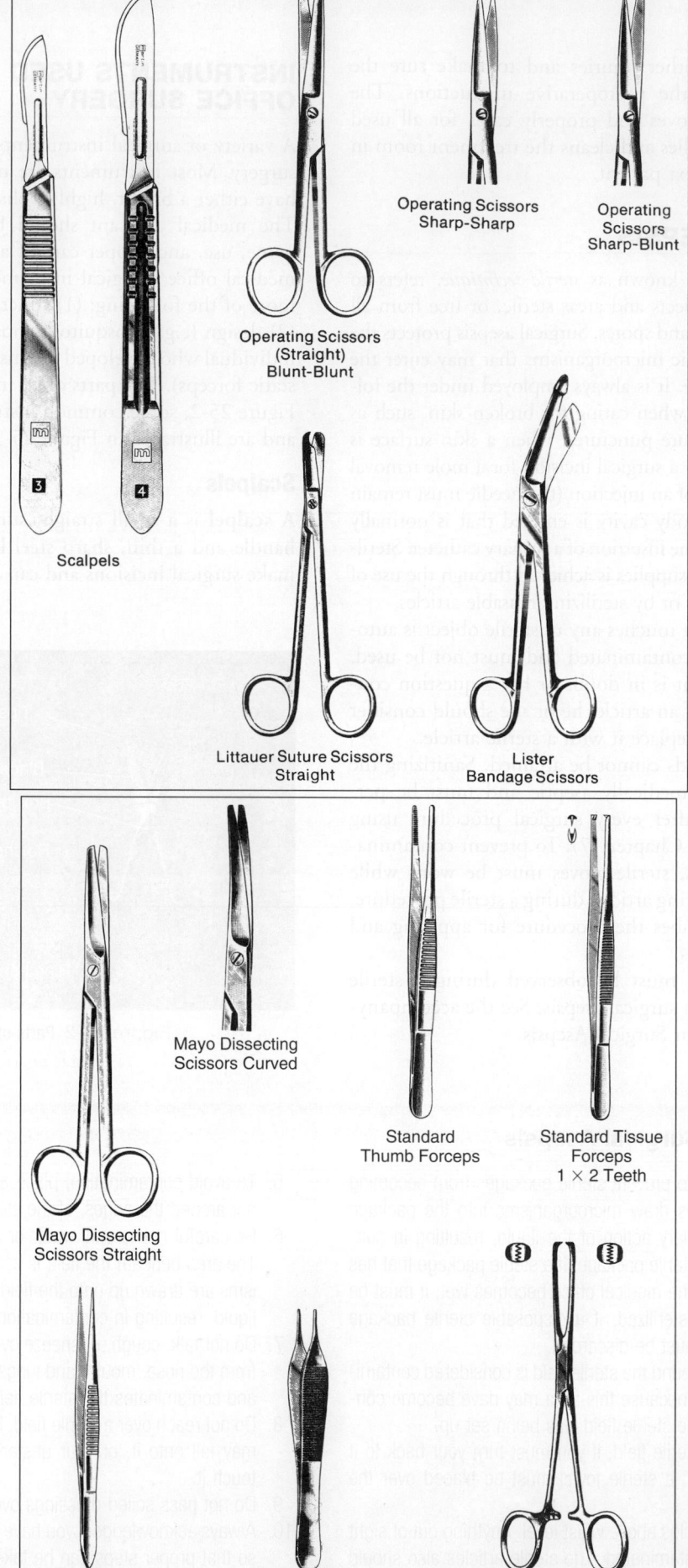

Operating Scissors
Sharp-Sharp

Operating
Scissors
Sharp-Blunt

Operating Scissors
(Straight)
Blunt-Blunt

Scalpels

Littauer Suture Scissors
Straight

Lister
Bandage Scissors

Mayo Dissecting
Scissors Curved

Standard
Thumb Forceps

Standard Tissue
Forceps
1 × 2 Teeth

Mayo Dissecting
Scissors Straight

Plain Splinter
Forceps

Adson Dressing
Forceps

Allis Tissue Forceps

Figure 25-3 Instruments used in minor office surgery.

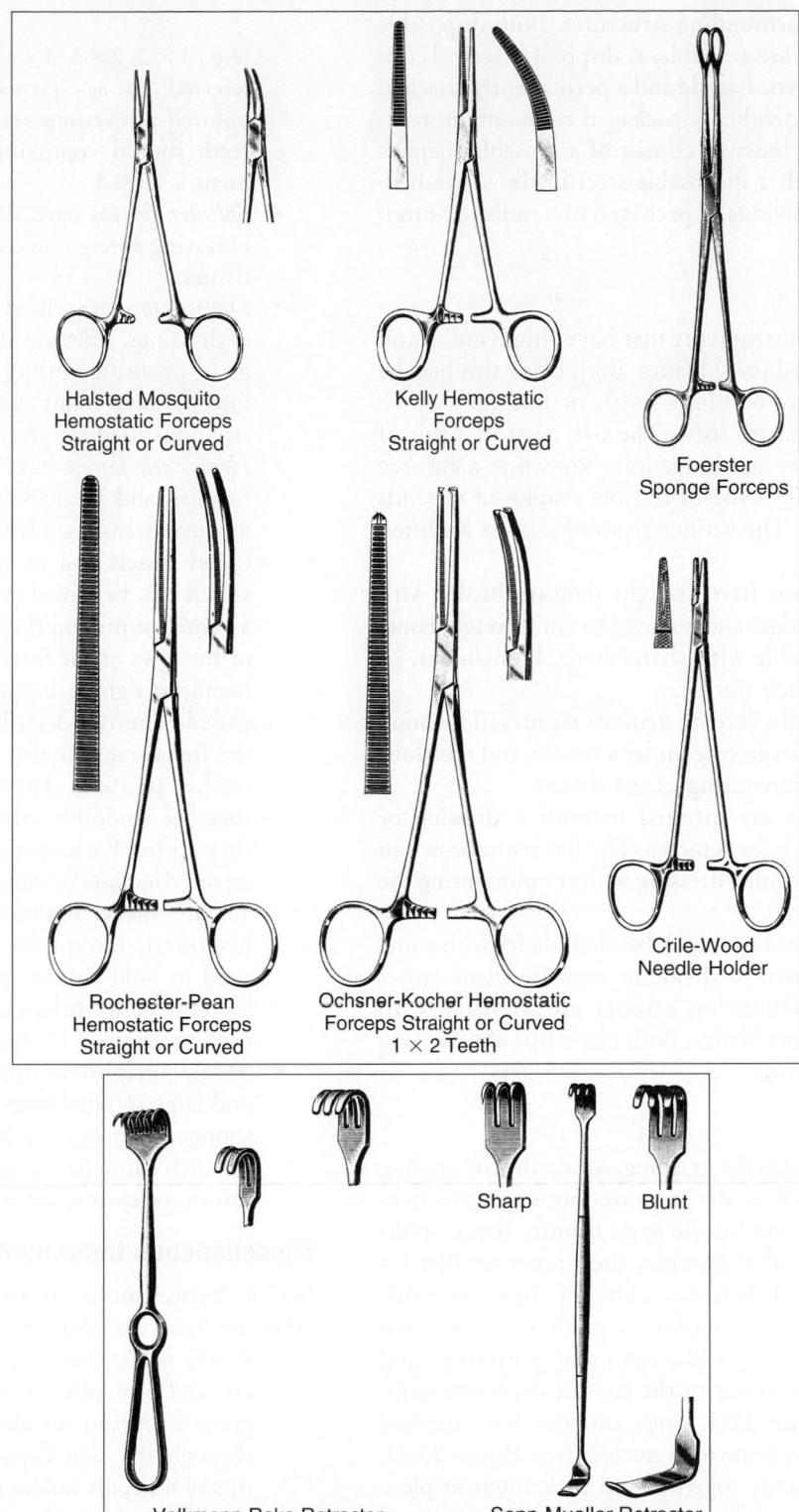

Halsted Mosquito
Hemostatic Forceps
Straight or Curved

Kelly Hemostatic
Forceps
Straight or Curved

Foerster
Sponge Forceps

Rochester-Pean
Hemostatic Forceps
Straight or Curved

Ochsner-Kocher Hemostatic
Forceps Straight or Curved
1 × 2 Teeth

Crile-Wood
Needle Holder

Sharp   Blunt

Volkmann Rake Retractor

Senn-Mueller Retractor

Figure 25-3, cont'd

possible trauma to surrounding structures. Both disposable and reusable scalpels are available. A disposable scalpel consists of a non-slip plastic handle and a permanently attached steel blade that is individually packaged to maintain sterility. Scalpels that are reusable consist of a reusable stainless steel handle to which a disposable steel blade is attached. The blade comes individually packaged in a moisture-proof sterile package.

Scissors

Scissors are cutting instruments that have ring handles and straight (str) or curved (cvd) blades. Both blade tips may be sharp (s/s), both may be blunt (b/b), or one tip may be blunt and the other sharp (b/s). The two parts of a pair of scissors come together at a hinge joint known as a *box lock* (see Figure 25-2). The type of scissors employed depends on the intended use. The various types of scissors are listed and described next.

- *Operating scissors* have straight delicate blades with sharp cutting edges and are used to cut through tissue. They are available with sharp/sharp, blunt/blunt, or blunt/sharp blade tips.
- *Suture scissors* are used to remove sutures. The hook on the tip aids in getting under a suture, and the blunt end prevents puncturing of the tissues.
- *Bandage scissors* are inserted beneath a dressing or bandage to cut it for removal. The flat blunt prow can be inserted beneath a dressing without puncturing the skin.
- *Dissecting scissors* have thick beveled blades with a fine cutting edge used to divide or separate tissue rather than cut it. Dissecting scissors are available with straight or curved blades. Both blade tips of dissecting scissors are blunt.

Forceps

Forceps are instruments for grasping, squeezing, or holding tissue or an item such as sterile gauze. Some forceps have two prongs and a spring handle (e.g., thumb, tissue, splinter, dressing forceps) that provides the proper tension for grasping an object such as tissue, a foreign object, or sterile gauze. Some forceps have serrations (e.g., thumb and hemostatic forceps), which are sawlike teeth that grasp tissue and prevent it from slipping out of the jaws of the instrument. As is shown in Figure 25-3, some varieties have toothed clasps on the handle, known as *ratchets* (see Figure 25-2), to hold the tips securely together and lock them in place (e.g., Allis tissue forceps, hemostatic forceps). The ratchets are designed to allow locked closure of the instrument at two or more positions. The various types of forceps are listed and described next.

- *Thumb forceps* have serrated tips and are used to pick up tissue or to hold tissue between adjacent surfaces.
- *Tissue forceps* have teeth, which are used to grasp tissue and prevent it from slipping. Tissue forceps are identified by the number of apposing teeth on each jaw

(e.g., 1×2, 2×3, 3×4). Tissue forceps are sometimes referred to as "rat-toothed" forceps because the pointed projections resemble the teeth of a rat. The teeth should approximate tightly when the instrument is closed.
- *Splinter forceps* have sharp points that are useful in removing foreign objects, such as splinters, from the tissues.
- *Dressing forceps* are used in the application and removal of dressings. They are also used to hold or grasp sterile gauze or sutures during a surgical procedure. Dressing forceps have blunt ends that contain coarse cross-striations used for grasping.
- *Hemostatic forceps* have serrated blades, ratchets, ring handles, and box locks and are available with straight or curved blades. Hemostats are used to clamp off blood vessels and to establish **hemostasis** until the vessels can be closed with sutures. The serrations on a hemostat prevent the blood vessel from slipping out of the jaws of the instrument. The ratchets keep the hemostat tightly shut and locked in place when it is closed. The ring handles allow for a secure grasp of the hemostat and also are used to select the desired ratchet position. The serrated blades should mesh together smoothly when the hemostat is closed; if they spring back open, the instrument is in need of repair. *Mosquito hemostatic forceps* have small, fine tips and are smaller and more delicate than standard Kelly hemostatic forceps. Mosquito hemostatic forceps are used to hold delicate tissue or to clamp off smaller blood vessels, whereas standard hemostatic forceps are used to grasp and compress larger blood vessels.
- *Sponge forceps* have ring handles, ratchets, box locks, and large serrated rings on the blade tips for holding sponges. A *sponge* is a porous, absorbent pad, such as a 4-inch gauze pad, used to absorb fluids, apply medication, or cleanse an area.

Miscellaneous Instruments

Various miscellaneous instruments used in the medical office are listed and described next.

- *Needle holders* have serrated tips, ring handles, ratchets, and box locks. A needle holder is used to firmly grasp a curved needle for insertion of the needle through the skin flaps of an incision. The serrated tips of a needle holder are designed to hold a curved needle securely without damaging it. A needle holder is sometimes referred to as a "driver" because it functions to "drive" the curved needle through the skin.
- *Retractors* are used to hold tissues aside to improve the exposure of the operative area.

Care of Surgical Instruments

Surgical instruments are expensive, are delicate yet durable, and last for many years if handled and maintained properly.

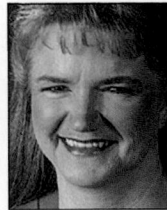
The care an instrument receives depends to a large degree on the parts making up the instrument (e.g., box lock, ratchet, cutting edge, serrations). The medical assistant works with instruments while setting up a sterile tray, performing certain procedures such as suture removal and sterile dressing change, and cleaning up after minor office surgery and during the sanitization and sterilization process. During each of these procedures, guidelines must be followed to prolong the life span of each instrument and to ensure its proper functioning:

1. Always handle instruments carefully. Dropping an instrument on the floor or throwing an instrument into a basin could damage it.
2. Do not pile instruments in a heap because they become entangled and might be damaged when separated.
3. Keep sharp instruments separate from the rest of the instruments to prevent damaging or dulling the cutting edge. Also, keep delicate instruments, such as lensed instruments, separate to protect them from damage.
4. To prolong the proper functioning of the ratchet, keep instruments with a ratchet in an open position when not in use.
5. Rinse blood and body secretions off an instrument as soon as possible to prevent them from drying and hardening on the instrument.
6. When performing procedures that require surgical instruments, always use the instrument for the purpose for which it was designed. Substituting one type of instrument for another could damage it.
7. Sanitize and sterilize instruments using proper technique.

COMMERCIALLY PREPARED STERILE PACKAGES

Commercially prepared disposable packages are used frequently and may contain one particular article (e.g., sterile dressing) or a complete sterile setup (e.g., one for the removal of sutures). The directions for opening the package are stated on the outside of the package; they should be followed carefully to prevent contamination of the sterile contents. Procedure 25-2 describes opening a sterile package.

One type of commercially prepared package is the peel-apart package (commonly referred to as a *peel-pack*). This type of sterile package has an edge with two flaps that can be pulled apart in the following manner: Grasp each unsterile flap between your bent index finger and extended thumb, and, rolling your hands outward, pull the package apart (Figure 25-4, *A*). The inside of the wrapper and the contents are sterile, and to prevent contamination, they must not be touched with the bare hands. The medical assistant can place the contents of the peel-pack directly on the sterile field by stepping back slightly from the field and gently ejecting or "flipping" the contents onto the center of the sterile field (Figure 25-4, *B*). Stepping back prevents the unsterile outer wrapper and the medical assistant's hands from crossing over the sterile field, which would result in contamination.

The contents of the package also can be removed with a sterile gloved hand. This technique is useful during minor office surgery, when the physician needs additional supplies, such as gauze pads and sutures. The medical assistant opens the sterile package, and the physician removes the sterile contents from the package using a gloved hand (Figure 25-4, *C*). The inside of the package can be used as a sterile field by opening the peel-apart package completely and laying it flat on a clean dry surface (Figure 25-4, *D*).

Once a sterile package has been opened and set up, the medical assistant may need to pour a sterile solution, such as an antiseptic, into a container located on the field. To do so, the steps of surgical asepsis outlined in Procedure 25-3 should be followed.

Text continued on p. 510

PROCEDURE 25-1   Applying and Removing Sterile Gloves

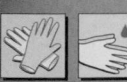

Outcome Apply and remove sterile gloves.

The medical assistant must wear sterile gloves to perform a sterile procedure, such as a dressing change, or to assist the physician during minor office surgery. The medical assistant must learn to put on the gloves using the principles of surgical asepsis so as not to contaminate them.

Gloves must be removed in a manner that protects the medical assistant from contaminating the clean hands with pathogens that might be on the outside of the gloves. This is accomplished by not allowing the bare hands to come in contact with the outside of the gloves.

Equipment/Supplies

- Sterile gloves

Applying Sterile Gloves

1. **Procedural Step.** Remove all rings and put them in a safe place. Wash your hands with an antimicrobial soap.
Principle. Rings may cause the gloves to tear. The warm, moist environment inside gloves provides ideal growing conditions for the multiplication of transient microorganisms on the hands. Washing the hands with an antimicrobial removes these microorganisms and also deposits an antibacterial film on your hands to discourage the growth of bacteria. This prevents the transmission of pathogens.

2. **Procedural Step.** Choose appropriate-sized gloves; they should not be too small or too large. The gloves should fit snugly but not be too tight.
Principle. If your gloves are too small, they may rip as you apply them or become uncomfortable to wear. If they are too large, you may find it difficult to perform your tasks.

3. **Procedural Step.** Place the glove package on a clean flat surface. Open the glove package without touching the inside of the wrapper. The tops of the gloves are turned down to form a cuff.
Principle. The hands are not sterile, and the inside of the wrapper is sterile.

4. **Procedural Step.** Pick up the first glove on the inside of the cuff with the fingers of the opposite hand, being sure not to touch the outside of the glove with your ungloved hand.
Principle. After applying the gloves, the inside of the cuff lies next to your skin and does not remain sterile; therefore it is permissible to pick up the glove by the cuff. The outside of the glove is sterile, and touching it would contaminate it. If a glove becomes contaminated, you must obtain a new pair of gloves and repeat the procedure.

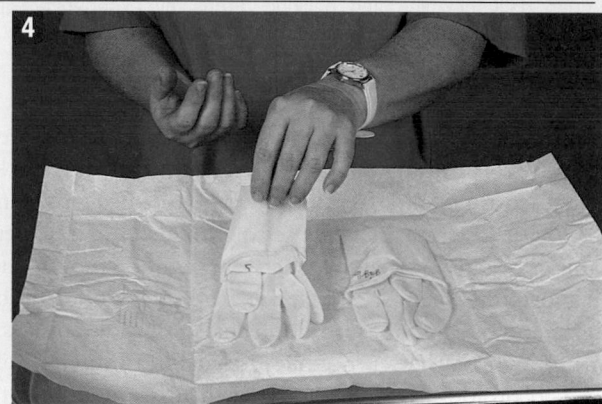

Pick up the first glove on the inside of the cuff.

5. **Procedural Step.** Step back and pull the glove on. Allow the cuff to remain turned back on itself.
Principle. Stepping back prevents your unsterile hand from passing over the glove still in the glove package, which would contaminate it.

6. **Procedural Step.** Pick up the second glove by slipping your sterile gloved fingers under its cuff and grasping the opposite side of the cuff with your thumb.
Principle. The cuff is sterile and may be touched by the sterile gloved hand.

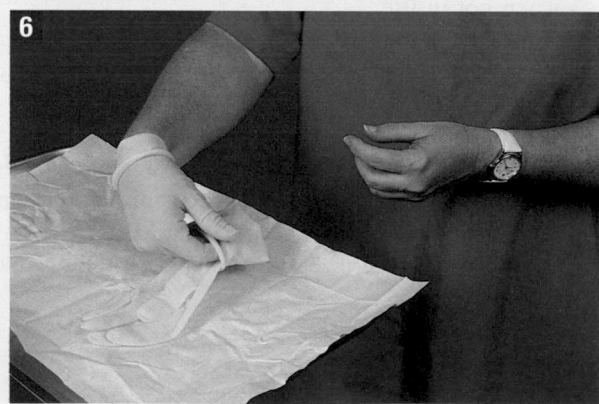

Pick up the second glove.

7. **Procedural Step.** Remove your thumb from the cuff and pull the glove on. Turn back the cuff.

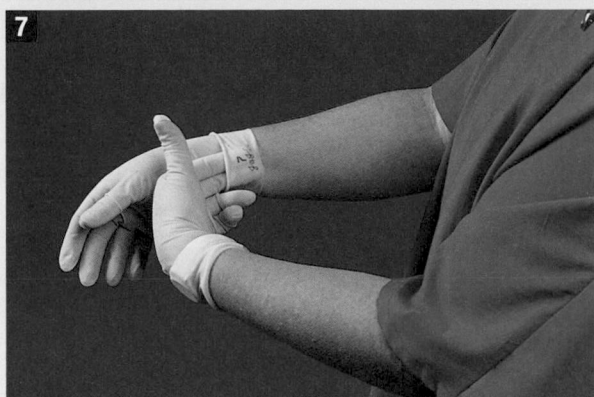

Turn back the cuff.

8. **Procedural Step.** Turn back the cuff of the first glove by reaching under the cuff with the other gloved hand. Do not allow your sterile gloved hand to come in contact with the inside of the cuff. Adjust the gloves to a comfortable position. Inspect the gloves for tears. *Principle.* The area under the folded cuff is sterile and may be touched by the sterile gloved hand. The inside of the cuff has previously been touched by your clean hands and is not sterile. If a tear is present, a new pair of gloves must be applied.

Removing Sterile Gloves

1. **Procedural Step.** With your gloved left hand, grasp the outside of the right glove 1 to 2 inches from the top. (*NOTE:* It does not matter which glove is removed first—you may start with the left glove if you prefer.)

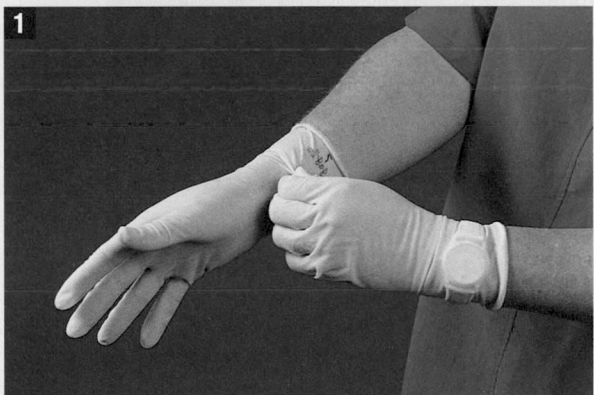

Grasp the outside of the glove.

2. **Procedural Step.** Slowly pull the right glove off the hand. It turns inside out as it is removed from your hand.

3. **Procedural Step.** Pull the right glove free, and scrunch it into a ball with your gloved left hand.

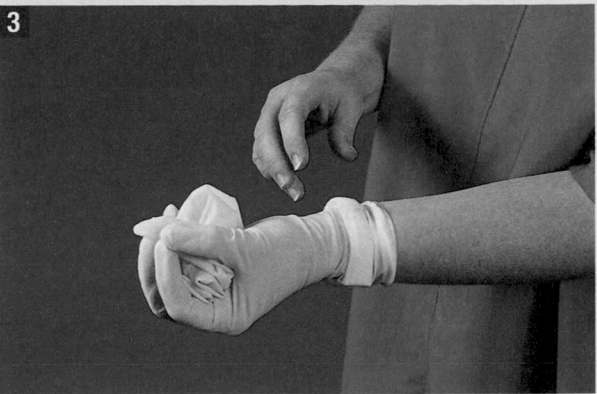

Scrunch the glove into a ball.

4. **Procedural Step.** Place the index and middle fingers of the right hand on the inside of the left glove. Do not allow your clean hand to touch the outside of the glove.

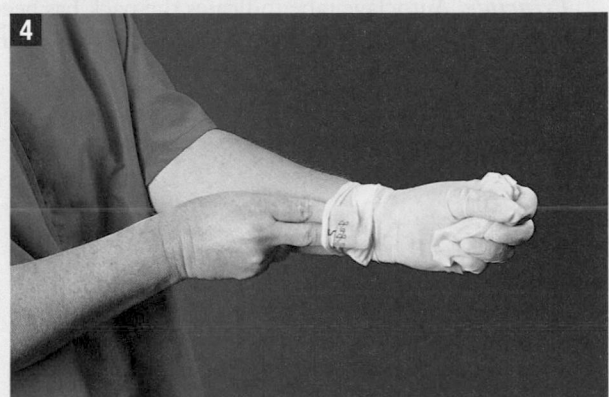

Place the fingers on the inside of the glove.

5. **Procedural Step.** Pull the second glove off the left hand. It turns inside out as it is removed from your hand, enclosing the balled-up right glove. Discard both gloves in an appropriate waste container. If your gloves are visibly contaminated with blood or other potentially infectious materials, discard them in a biohazard waste container; otherwise, they can be discarded in a regular waste container.

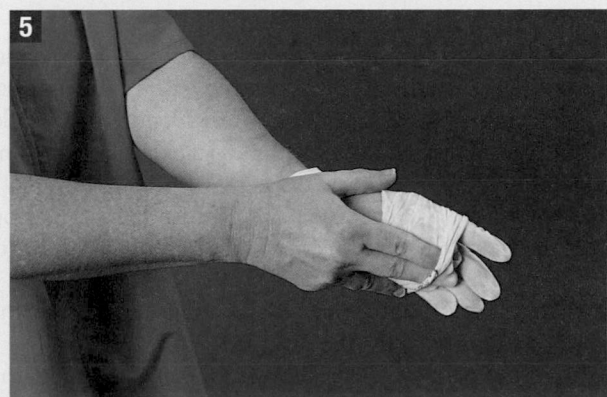

Pull the glove off the hand.

6. **Procedural Step.** Sanitize your hands thoroughly to remove any microorganisms that may have come in contact with your hands.

PROCEDURE **25-2**   Opening a Sterile Package

Outcome Open a sterile package. A sterile package that has been wrapped after the procedure for wrapping presented in Chapter 18 is opened using the procedure outlined here. The sterile package may be in the form of a commercially prepared disposable package (e.g., sterile dressing change) or a pack that has been assembled and sterilized at the medical office (e.g., sebaceous cyst removal pack); in both cases, the inside of the sterile wrapper serves as the sterile field.

Equipment/Supplies

- Sterile package

1. **Procedural Step.** Sanitize your hands.
2. **Procedural Step.** Assemble the equipment.
3. **Procedural Step.** Check the pack to make sure it is not wet, torn, or opened. These factors cause contamination of the sterile contents and the pack must not be used. If autoclave tape has been used to close the pack, check to make sure the tape has changed color. *Principle.* Autoclave tape indicates the pack has been through the sterilization process, but it does not verify that the contents of the pack are sterile.

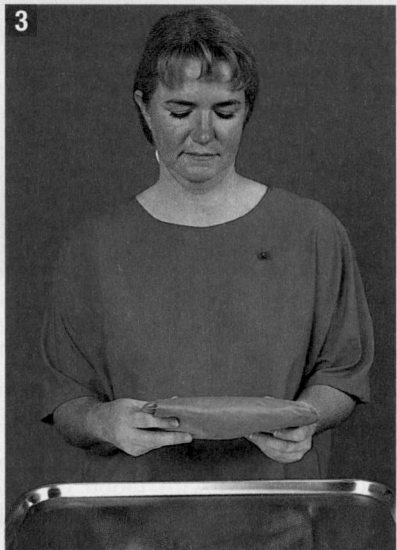

Check the sterilization indicator.

4. **Procedural Step.** Place the wrapped package on the table so that the top flap of the wrapper opens away from you. Always face the sterile field, and do not talk, laugh, cough, or sneeze over the field. These actions contaminate the sterile field.
5. **Procedural Step.** Loosen and remove the fastener on the wrapped package, and discard it in a waste container.
6. **Procedural Step.** Open the first flap away from the body. Handle only the outside of the wrapper. *Principle.* The medical assistant should open the sterile package so as not to reach over the sterile contents. Otherwise, dust or lint from unsterile clothing may fall on the contents of the package and cause contamination.

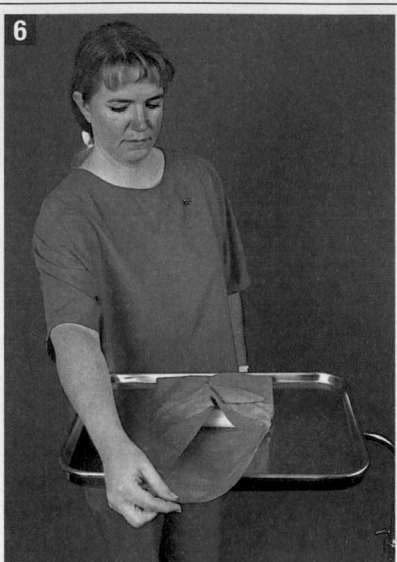

Open the first flap away from the body.

7. **Procedural Step.** Without crossing over the sterile field, open the left and right flaps.

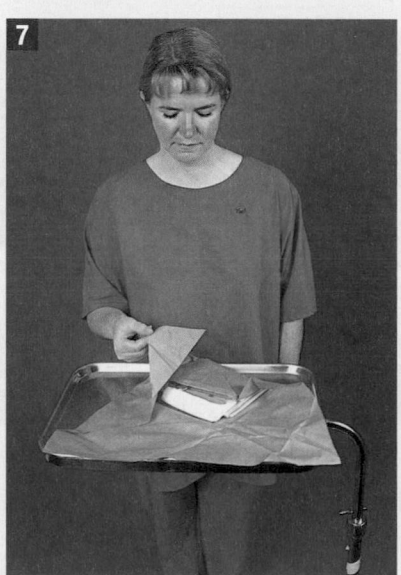

Open the left and right flaps.

8. **Procedural Step.** Open the flap closest to the body by lifting it toward you. Touch only the outside of the wrapper.

PROCEDURE 25-2   **Opening a Sterile Package—cont'd**

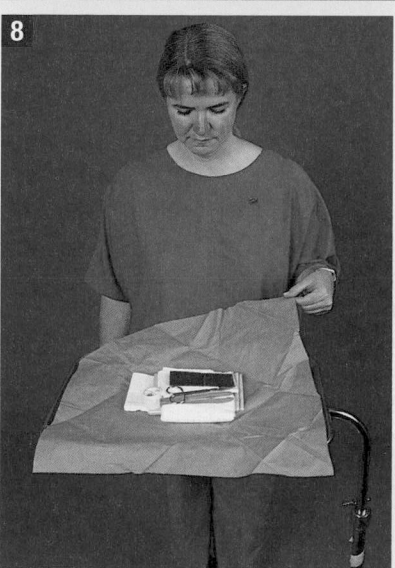

Open the flap closest to the body.

9. **Procedural Step.** Adjust the sterile wrapper by the corners as needed to make sure it lies in proper position on the tray or table.

10. **Procedural Step.** Check the sterilization indicator on the inside of the pack to make sure it has changed appropriately. This indicates that the contents of the pack are sterile.

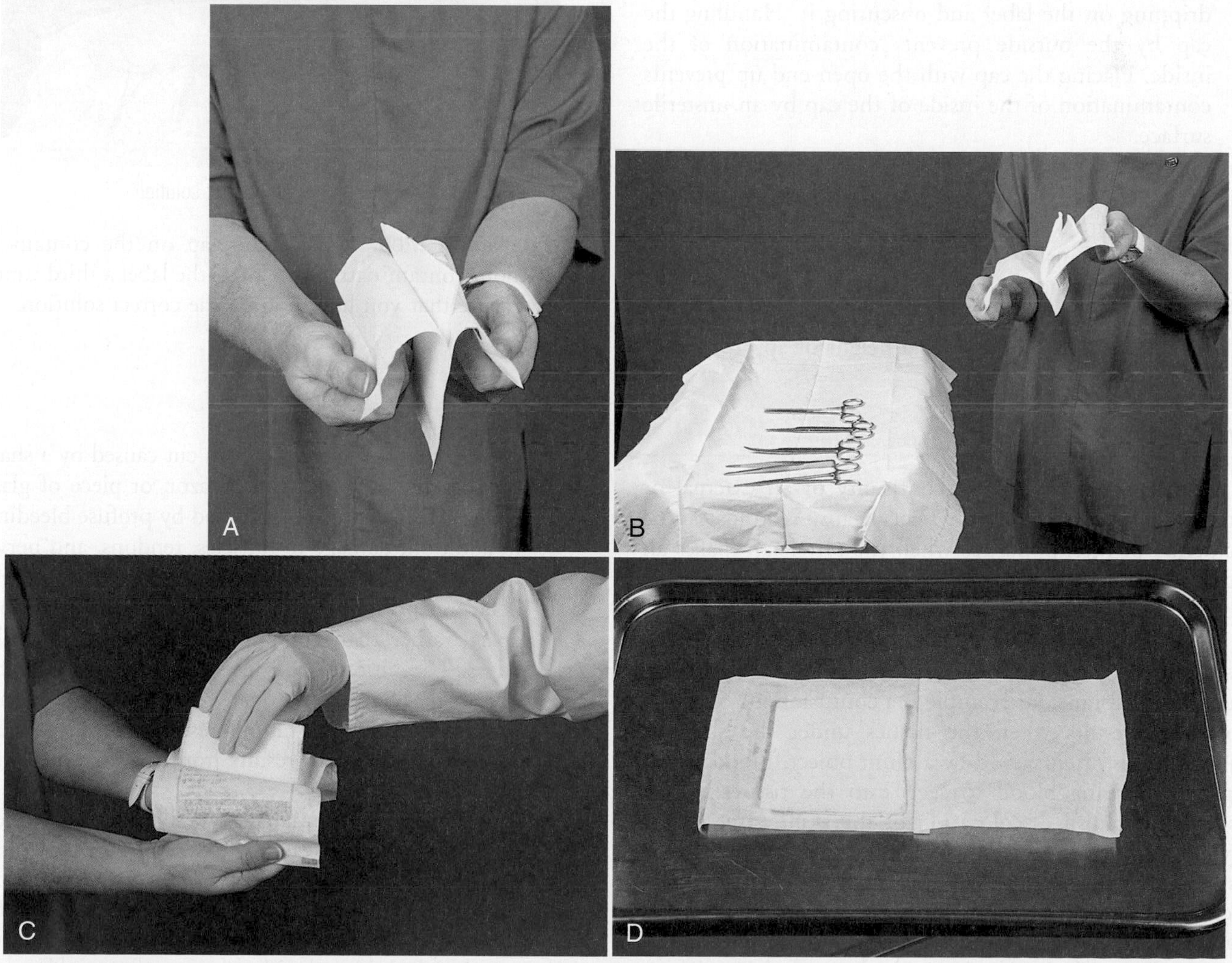

Figure 25-4 Methods for removing the sterile contents of a peel-apart package so that sterility is maintained. **A,** Grasp each flap between a bent index finger and an extended thumb, and roll hands outward to pull apart. **B,** Step back and eject the contents onto the field. **C,** The medical assistant opens the pack, and the physician removes the sterile contents with a gloved hand. **D,** The inside of the peel-apart package can be used as a sterile field.

PROCEDURE 25-3   Pouring a Sterile Solution

Outcome Pour a sterile solution.

Equipment/Supplies

* Sterile solution
* Sterile container
* Sterile towel

1. **Procedural Step.** Read the label of the solution to ensure that you have the correct solution.
2. **Procedural Step.** Check the expiration date on the solution. Do not use an outdated solution.
   Principle. Outdated solutions may produce undesirable effects and should be discarded.
3. **Procedural Step.** Check the solution label a second time to make sure you have the correct solution.
4. **Procedural Step.** Place the palm of your hand over the label. Remove the cap by touching only the outside, and place the cap on a flat surface with the open end up. Do not place the cap on the sterile field, as the outside of the cap is contaminated.
   Principle. Palming the label prevents the solution from dripping on the label and obscuring it. Handling the cap by the outside prevents contamination of the inside. Placing the cap with the open end up prevents contamination of the inside of the cap by an unsterile surface.
5. **Procedural Step.** Rinse the lip of the bottle (if it has been previously used) by pouring a small amount of solution into a separate container.
   Principle. Rinsing the lip washes away any microorganisms that may be on it.
6. **Procedural Step.** Pour the proper amount of solution into the sterile container at a height of approximately

6 inches. Do not allow the neck of the bottle to come in contact with the sterile container, and be careful not to splash solution onto the sterile field.
Principle. Pouring from a height of approximately 6 inches reduces splashing and prevents contamination of the sterile container with the outside of the (unsterile) bottle.

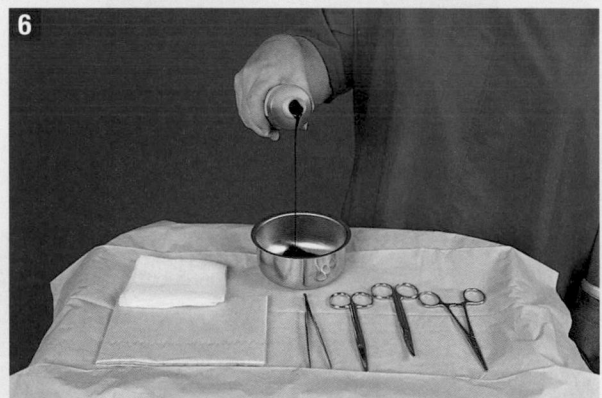

Pour the proper amount of solution.

7. **Procedural Step.** Replace the cap on the container without contaminating it. Check the label a third time to ensure that you have poured the correct solution.

WOUNDS

A **wound** is a break in the continuity of an external or internal surface caused by physical means. Wounds can be accidental or intentional (as when the physician makes an incision during a surgical operation). There are two basic types of wounds: closed and open.

A *closed wound* involves an injury to the underlying tissues of the body without a break in the skin surface or mucous membrane; an example is a contusion, or bruise. A **contusion** results when the tissues under the skin are injured and is often caused by a blunt object. Blood vessels rupture, allowing blood to seep into the tissues, which results in a bluish discoloration of the skin. After several days, the color of the contusion turns greenish yellow as a result of oxidation of blood pigments. Bruising commonly occurs with injuries such as fractures, sprains, strains, and black eyes. *Open wounds* involve a break in the skin surface or mucous membrane that exposes the underlying tissues; examples include incisions, lacerations, punctures, and abrasions. Figure 25-5 illustrates specific wounds.

* An **incision** is a clean, smooth cut caused by a sharp instrument, such as a knife, razor, or piece of glass. Deep incisions are accompanied by profuse bleeding; in addition, damage to muscles, tendons, and nerves may occur.
* A **laceration** is a wound in which the tissues are torn apart, rather than cut, leaving ragged and irregular edges. Lacerations are caused by dull knives, large objects that have been driven into the skin, and heavy machinery. Deep lacerations result in profuse bleeding, and a scar often results from the jagged tearing of the tissues.
* A **puncture** is a wound made by a sharp-pointed object piercing the skin layers, for example, a nail, splinter, needle, wire, knife, bullet, or animal bite. A puncture wound has a very small external skin opening, and for this reason bleeding is usually minor. A tetanus booster may be administered with this type of wound because the tetanus bacteria grow best in a warm anaerobic environment, such as the one in a puncture.

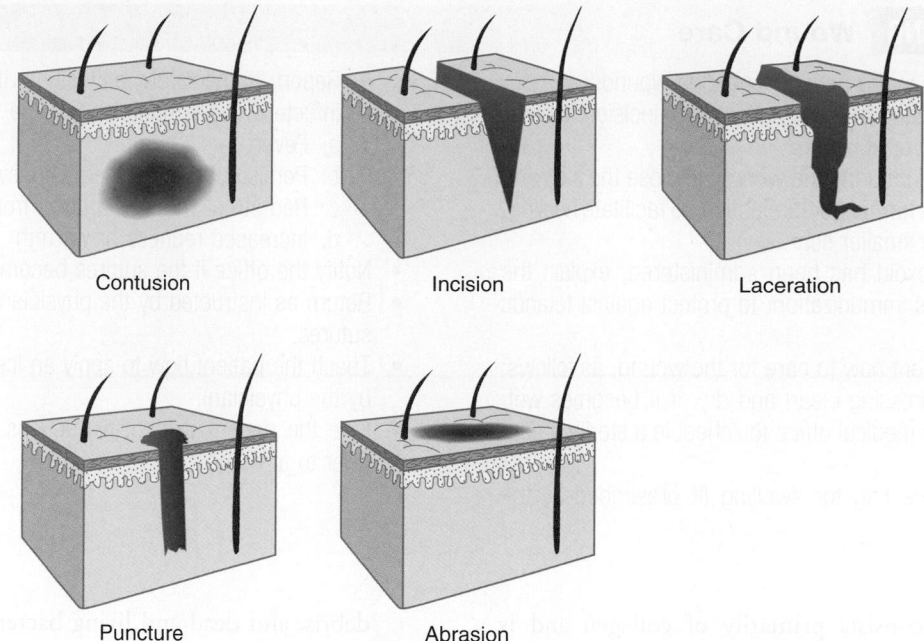

Figure 25-5 Types of wounds.

- An **abrasion** or scrape is a wound in which the outer layers of the skin are scraped or rubbed off, resulting in oozing of blood from ruptured capillaries. Abrasions are often caused by falling on gravel and floors (floor burn). These falls can result in skinned knees and elbows.

Wound Healing

The skin is a protective barrier for the body and is considered its first line of defense. When the surface of the skin has been broken, it is easy for microorganisms to enter and cause **infection.** The body has a natural healing process that works to destroy invading microorganisms and to restore the structure and function of damaged tissues, as is described next.

Phases of Wound Healing

Wound healing occurs in three phases, which are described here and illustrated in Figure 25-6.

Phase 1

Phase 1, also called the *inflammatory phase,* begins as soon as the body is injured. This phase lasts approximately 3 to 4 days. During this phase, a fibrin network forms, resulting in a blood clot that "plugs" up the opening of the wound and stops the flow of blood. The blood clot eventually becomes the scab. The inflammatory process also occurs during this phase. **Inflammation** is the protective response of the body to trauma, such as cuts and abrasions, and to the entrance of foreign matter, such as microorganisms. During inflammation, the blood supply to the wound increases, which brings white blood cells and nutrients to the site to assist in the healing process. The four local signs of inflammation are redness, swelling, pain, and warmth. The purpose of inflammation is to destroy invading microorganisms and to remove damaged tissue debris from the area so that proper healing can occur.

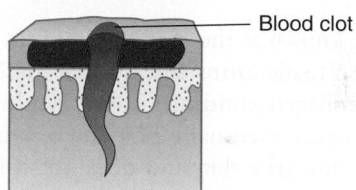

Phase 1: Inflammatory Phase

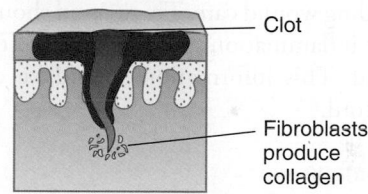

Phase 2: Granulation Phase

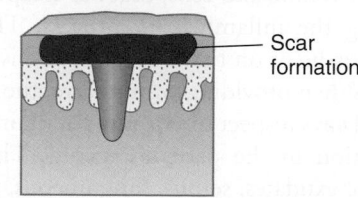

Phase 3: Maturation Phase

Figure 25-6 Phases of wound healing.

Phase 2

Phase 2 is also called the *granulation phase* and typically lasts 4 to 20 days. During this phase, **fibroblasts** migrate to the wound and begin to synthesize collagen. Collagen is a white protein that provides strength to the wound. As the amount of collagen increases, the wound becomes stronger, and the chance that the wound will open decreases. There also is a growth of new capillaries during this phase to provide the damaged tissue with an abundant supply of blood. As the capillary network develops, the tissue becomes a translucent red color. This tissue is known as *granulation tissue.*

Explain the following to the patient regarding wounds:
- The type of wound that the patient has: incision, laceration, puncture, or abrasion.
- The purpose of suturing the wound: to close the skin and protect against further contamination, to facilitate healing, and to leave a smaller scar.
- If a tetanus toxoid has been administered, explain the purpose of this immunization: to protect against tetanus (lockjaw).
- Teach the patient how to care for the wound, as follows:
  - Keep the dressing clean and dry. If it becomes wet, contact the medical office to schedule a sterile dressing change.
  - Apply an ice bag for swelling (if prescribed by the physician).

- Report immediately any signs that the wound is infected. These signs include the following:
  a. Fever
  b. Persistent or increased pain, swelling, or drainage
  c. Red streaks radiating away from the wound
  d. Increased redness or warmth
- Notify the office if the sutures become loose or break.
- Return as instructed by the physician for the removal of sutures.
- Teach the patient how to apply an ice bag (if prescribed by the physician).
- Give the patient written instructions on wound care to refer to at home. ■

Granulation tissue consists primarily of collagen and is fragile and shiny and bleeds easily.

Phase 3

Phase 3, also known as the *maturation phase,* begins as soon as granulation tissue forms and can last for 2 years. During this phase, collagen continues to be synthesized, and the granulation tissue eventually hardens to white scar tissue. Scar tissue is not true skin and does not contain nerves or have a blood supply.

The medical assistant should always inspect the wound when providing wound care. The wound should be observed for signs of inflammation and the amount of healing that has occurred. This information should be charted in the patient's record.

Wound Drainage

The medical term for drainage is **exudate**. An exudate is material, such as fluid and cells, that has escaped from blood vessels during the inflammatory process. The exudate is deposited in tissue or on tissue surfaces and is often present in a wound. When providing wound care, the medical assistant should always inspect the wound for drainage and chart this information in the patient's record. There are three major types of exudates: serous, sanguineous, and purulent.
- Serous exudate. A serous exudate consists chiefly of **serum,** which is the clear portion of the blood. Serous drainage is clear and watery. An example of a serous exudate is the fluid in a blister from a burn.
- Sanguineous exudate. A sanguineous exudate is red and consists of red blood cells. This type of drainage results when capillaries are damaged, allowing the escape of red blood cells, and is frequently seen in open wounds. A bright-red sanguineous exudate indicates fresh bleeding, and a dark exudate indicates older bleeding.
- Purulent exudate. A purulent exudate contains pus, which consists of leukocytes, dead liquefied tissue

debris, and dead and living bacteria. Purulent drainage is usually thick and has an unpleasant odor. It is white in color, but may acquire tinges of pink, green, or yellow depending on the type of infecting organism. The process of pus formation is *suppuration.*

In addition to the exudates just described, mixed types of exudates are often observed in a wound. A *serosanguineous exudate* consists of clear and blood-tinged drainage and is commonly seen in surgical incisions. A *purosanguineous exudate* consists of pus and blood and is often seen in a new wound that is infected.

STERILE DRESSING CHANGE

Surgical asepsis must be maintained when one is caring for and applying a dry sterile dressing (abbreviated as *DSD*) to an open wound. The medical assistant must take care to prevent infection in clean wounds and to decrease infection in wounds already infected. The function of a sterile dressing is to protect the wound from contamination and trauma, to absorb drainage, and to restrict motion, which may interfere with proper wound healing. The size, type, and amount of dressing material used during a sterile dressing change depend on the size and location of the wound and the amount of drainage.

Sterile folded *gauze pads* are used in the medical office for a sterile dressing change. This type of dressing absorbs drainage, but the gauze has a tendency to stick to the wound when the drainage dries. Gauze pads come in a variety of sizes, including 4×4, 3×3, and 2×2; the 4×4 size is used most frequently.

Nonadherent pads also are used as a sterile dressing; they have one surface impregnated with agents that prevent the dressing from sticking to the wound. One brand of this type of material is Telfa pads. The nonadherent side, which is shiny, is placed next to the wound. Telfa dressings are often used to cover burned skin. Procedure 25-4 presents the procedure for changing a sterile dressing.

PROCEDURE 25-4 Changing a Sterile Dressing

Outcome Change a sterile dressing.

Equipment/Supplies

- Mayo stand
- Biohazard waste container

Side Table

- Clean disposable gloves
- Antiseptic swabs
- Sterile gloves
- Plastic waste bag
- Surgical tape
- Scissors

Sterile Field

- Sterile dressing
- Sterile thumb forceps

1. **Procedural Step.** Wash your hands with an antimicrobial soap.
2. **Procedural Step.** Assemble the equipment. Set up the nonsterile items on a side table or counter. Position the waterproof waste bag in a location convenient for disposal of contaminated items.

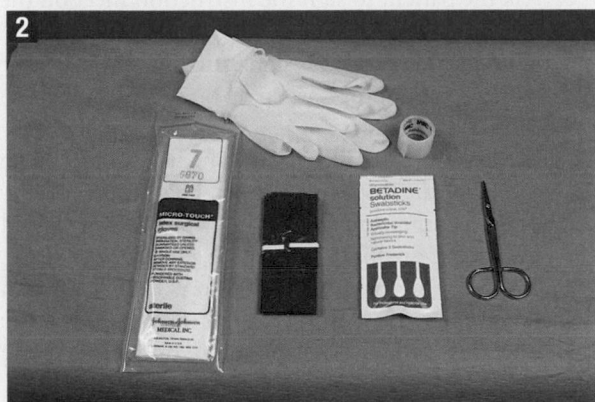

Prepare the side table.

3. **Procedural Step.** Greet the patient and introduce yourself. Identify the patient by full name and date of birth and explain the procedure. Instruct the patient not to move during the procedure. Adjust the light so that it is focused on the dressing.
4. **Procedural Step.** Apply clean gloves. Loosen the tape on the dressing, and pull it toward the wound. Carefully and gently remove the soiled dressing by pulling it upward. Do not touch the inside of the dressing that was next to the open wound. If the dressing is stuck to the wound, it can be loosened by moistening it with a normal saline solution. Place the soiled dressing in the waste bag without allowing the dressing to touch the outside of the bag.

Principle. Gentle dressing removal avoids unnecessary stress on the wound. Touching the inside of the dressing can transfer an infected discharge to your gloves.

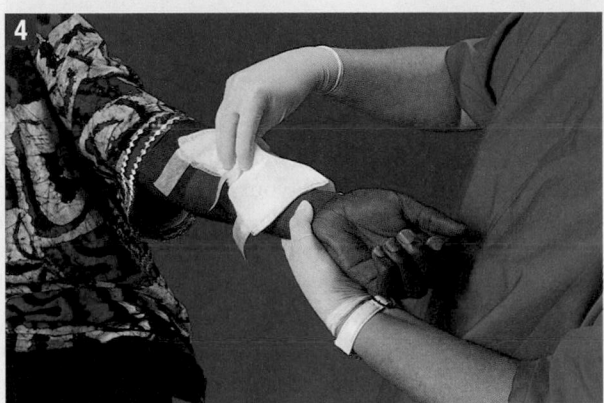

Remove the soiled dressing.

5. **Procedural Step.** Inspect the wound, and observe for the following: amount of healing; presence of inflammation; and presence of drainage, including the amount (scant, moderate, or profuse) and type of drainage.
Principle. Drainage is classified as serous (containing serum), sanguineous (red and composed of blood), serosanguineous (containing serum and blood), or purulent (containing pus and appearing white with tinges of yellow, pink, or green, depending on the type of infecting microorganism). Purulent drainage is usually thick and has an unpleasant odor.
6. **Procedural Step.** Open the pouch containing the sterile antiseptic swabs, and place it in a convenient location or hold it in your nondominant hand.
7. **Procedural Step.** Using the antiseptic swabs, apply the antiseptic to the wound. Apply the antiseptic from

Continued

the top to the bottom of the wound, working from the center to the outside of the wound. Use a new swab for each motion. Discard each contaminated swab in the waste bag after use.

Principle. The purpose of the antiseptic is to decrease the number of microorganisms in the wound.

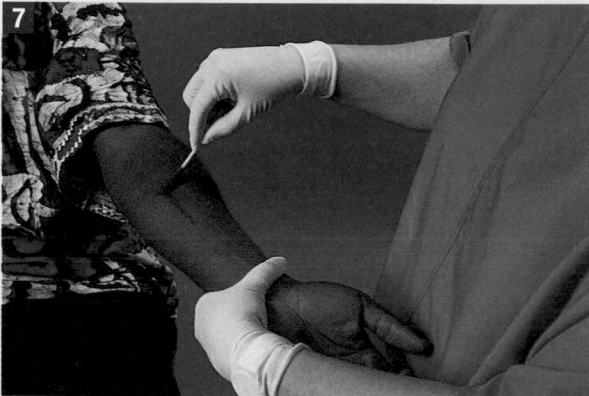

Apply an antiseptic to the wound.

8. Procedural Step. Remove the clean disposable gloves, and discard them in the waste bag without contaminating yourself. Sanitize your hands and prepare the sterile field using surgical asepsis. Items are either placed onto a sterile field or are contained in a prepackaged setup. Instruct the patient not to talk, laugh, sneeze, or cough over the sterile field.

Principle. Microorganisms are carried in water vapor from the mouth, nose, and lungs, and can be transferred onto the sterile field.

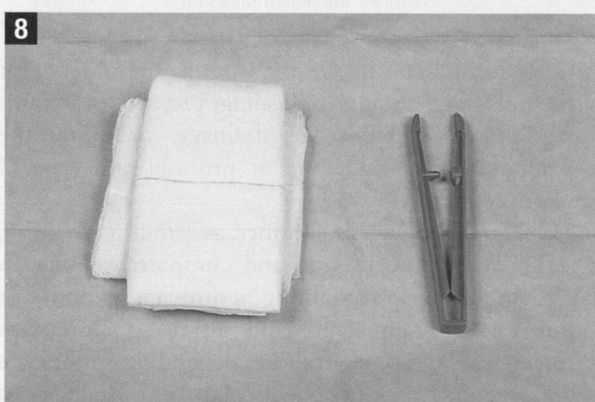

Prepare the sterile field.

9. Procedural Step. Open a package of sterile gloves, and apply them.

10. Procedural Step. Pick up the sterile dressing with your gloved hand or sterile forceps. Place the sterile dressing over the wound by lightly dropping it in place. Do not move the dressing once you have dropped it into place. Discard the gloves or forceps in the waste bag.

Principle. Dropping the dressing over the wound and not moving it prevent the transfer of microorganisms from the skin to the center of the wound.

11. Procedural Step. Apply hypoallergenic adhesive tape to hold the dressing in place. The tape must be long enough to adhere to the skin, but not so long that it loosens when the patient moves. The strips of tape should be evenly spaced, with strips at each end of the dressing.

12. Procedural Step. Instruct the patient in wound care as follows:

a. Provide the patient with written wound care instructions (see the patient teaching box on wound care in this chapter).

b. Explain the wound care instructions, and ask the patient whether he or she has any questions. Tell the patient to keep the wound clean and dry and to contact the office if signs of infection occur such as excessive swelling, pain, or discharge.

c. Ask the patient to sign the instruction sheet on the appropriate line.

d. Witness the patient's signature by signing your name in the appropriate space on the form. Include today's date.

e. Before the patient leaves the medical office, make a copy of the instruction sheet. Give a signed copy of the wound care instructions to the patient, and file the original in the patient's medical record.

Principle. The filed copy protects the physician legally in the event that the patient fails to follow the instructions and causes further harm or damage to the wound.

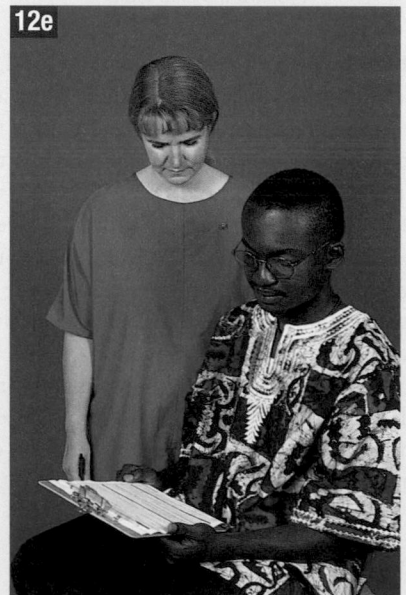

Instruct the patient in wound care.

PROCEDURE 25-4   Changing a Sterile Dressing—cont'd

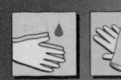

13. Procedural Step. Return the equipment. Tightly secure the bag containing the soiled dressing and contaminated articles, and dispose of it in a biohazard waste container.
Principle. Contaminated items must be disposed of properly to prevent the spread of infection.

14. Procedural Step. Sanitize your hands.

15. Procedural Step. Chart the procedure. Include the date and time, location of the dressing, condition of the wound, type and amount of drainage, care of the wound, and any problems the patient experienced with the wound. Also chart the instructions given to the patient on wound care.

CHARTING EXAMPLE

Date	
9/20/XX	10:30 a.m. Dressing changed (L) ant forearm.
	Scant amt of serous drainage noted. Sl
	redness around incision line. Sutures intact
	and suture line in good approximation. Incision
	cleaned c̄ Betadine and DSD applied. No
	complaints of pain or discomfort. Explained
	wound care. Written instructions provided.
	Signed copy filed in chart. To return in 2 days
	for suture removal. ———————
	——————— T. Browning, CMA (AAMA)

SUTURES

Insertion and removal of **sutures** are commonly performed in the medical office. Sutures may be required to close a surgical incision or to repair an accidental wound. They **approximate**, or bring together, the edges of the wound with surgical stitches and hold them in place until enough healing has taken place so that the wound can withstand ordinary stress and no longer needs support from the sutures. Sutures also protect the wound from further contamination and minimize the amount of scar formation. A **local anesthetic** is necessary to numb the area before the sutures are inserted.

Types of Sutures

Sutures are available in two types: absorbable and nonabsorbable. **Absorbable sutures** are made of a material that is gradually digested and absorbed by the body in a relatively short period of time. The amount of time can range from 7 days to several months, depending on the type of tissue being sutured and the size and type of absorbable suture being used.

Absorbable sutures consist of surgical gut (Surgigut) or synthetic materials, such as polyglycolic acid (Dexon), polyglactin 910 (Vicryl), polydioxanone (PDS II), polyglyconate (Maxon), and poliglecaprone (Monocryl), lactomer (Polysorb), and Caprosyn (Figure 25-7, *A*). Surgical gut is made from sheep or cow intestine. This type of suturing material is gradually digested by tissue enzymes and is absorbed by the body's tissues 7 to 21 days after insertion, depending on the kind of surgical gut employed. *Plain surgical gut* has a rapid absorption time, whereas *chromic surgical gut* is treated to slow down its rate of absorption in the tissues. Absorbable sutures frequently are used to suture subcutaneous tissue, fascia, intestines, bladder, and peritoneum, and to **ligate,** or tie off, vessels. Because suturing of this type of

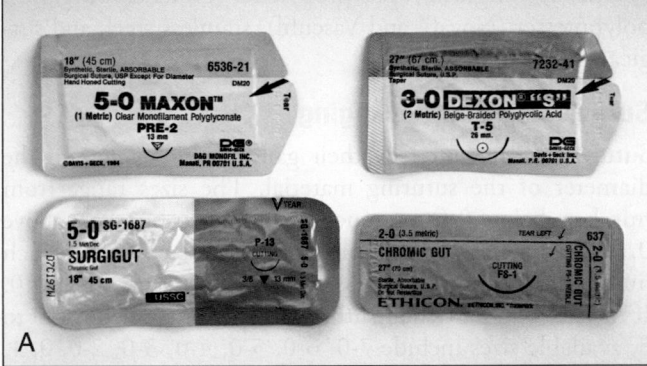
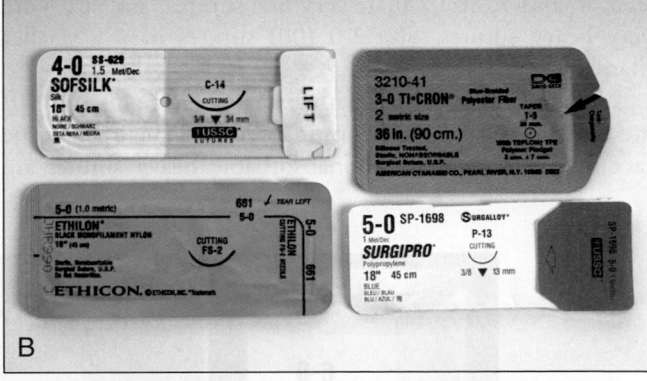

Figure 25-7 Swaged suture packets. **A,** Absorbable sutures. **B,** Nonabsorbable sutures.

tissue is generally done during surgery performed by the physician in the hospital with the patient under a general anesthetic, the medical office may not stock absorbable suture material.

Nonabsorbable sutures (Figure 25-7, *B*) are not absorbed by the body and may remain permanently in the body tissues and become encapsulated by fibrous tissue or may be removed (e.g., skin sutures). Nonabsorbable sutures are used to suture skin; this type of suture is used frequently

PROCEDURE 25-4

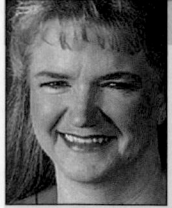

in the medical office. Nonabsorbable sutures are made from materials that are not affected by tissue enzymes. These materials include silk (Sofsilk), nylon (Ethilon), polyester (Ti-Cron, Surgidac), polypropylene (Prolene, Surgipro), polybutester (Novafil and Vascufil), stainless steel, and surgical skin staples.

Suture Size and Packaging

Sutures are measured by their gauge, which refers to the diameter of the suturing material. The sizes range from numbers below 0 (pronounced "aught") to numbers above 0. The diameter of the suture material increases with each number above 0 and decreases with each number below 0. If the size of a particular suture material ranges from 7-0 to 5, available sizes include 7-0, 6-0, 5-0, 4-0, 3-0, 2-0, 0, 1, 2, 3, 4, and 5. Size 7-0 are very fine sutures, and size 5 are very heavy sutures. Size 2-0 (00) sutures have a smaller diameter than size 0 sutures.

Nonabsorbable sutures with a smaller gauge (5-0 to 6-0) are used for suturing incisions in delicate tissue, such as the face and neck, whereas nonabsorbable heavy sutures are used for firmer tissue, such as the chest and abdomen. Finer sutures leave less scar formation and are used when cosmetic results are desired.

Sutures come in a box of individually packaged sutures (Figure 25-8, *A*). The box of sutures is stamped with an expiration date that must be checked each time a suture package is removed from the box. Each individual suture package consists of an outer peel-apart envelope and a sterile inner packet (Figure 25-8, *B*). Packages are labeled according to the type of suture material (e.g., surgical silk), the size (e.g., 4-0), the length of the suturing material (e.g., 18 inches), the date of manufacture, and the expiration date of the suture. The type and size of material used are based on the nature and location of the tissue being sutured and the physician's preference. To repair a laceration of the arm, the physician might use a 4-0 surgical silk suture. The physician informs the medical assistant of the type and size of sutures needed.

Suture Needles

Needles used for suturing are made from stainless steel alloys and are categorized according to their type of point

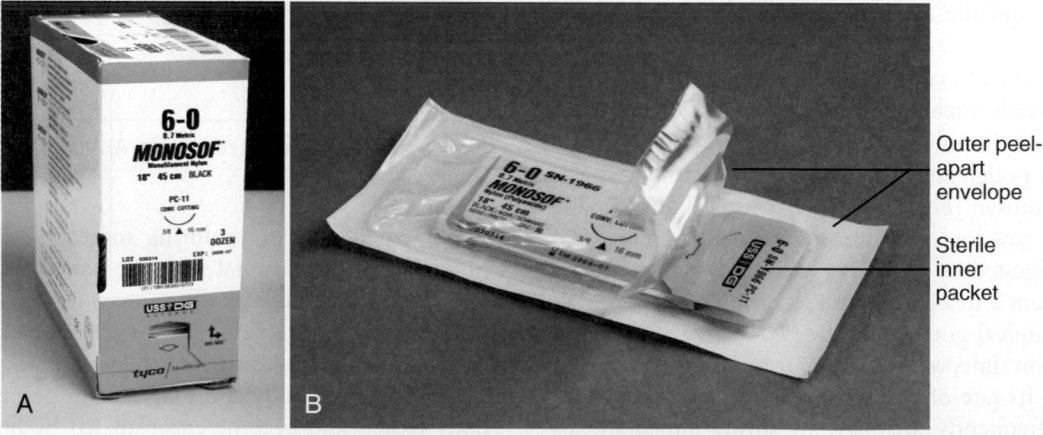

Figure 25-8 A, Sutures come in a box of individually packaged sutures. **B,** Each individual suture package consists of an outer peel-apart envelope and a sterile inner packet.

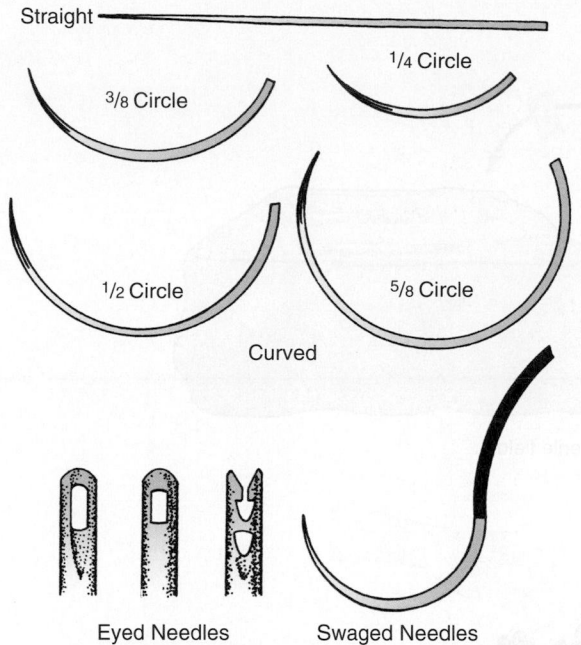

Figure 25-9 Common suture needles. **A,** Needles with a cutting point. **B,** Eyed needles and a swaged needle.

and their shape. A needle with a sharp point is a *cutting needle,* and one with a round point is a *noncutting needle.* Cutting needles (Figure 25-9, *A*) are used for firm tissues such as skin; the sharp point helps push the needle through the tissue. Noncutting or blunt needles are used to penetrate tissues that offer a small amount of resistance, such as the fascia, intestine, liver, spleen, kidneys, subcutaneous tissue, and muscle.

A suture needle may be curved or straight (see Figure 25-9, *A*). *Curved needles* permit the physician to dip in and out of the tissue. A needle holder must be used with a curved needle. A *straight needle* is used when the tissue can be displaced sufficiently to permit the needle to be pushed and pulled through the tissue. Straight needles do not require the use of a needle holder.

Some needles have an eye through which the suture material is inserted; however, most needles are **swaged** (Figure 25-9, *B*). *Swaged* means that the suture and needle are one continuous unit; the needle is permanently attached to the end of the suture. Swaged needles are used frequently because they offer several advantages over eyed needles. One advantage is that the suture material does not slip off the needle, as might occur with suture material threaded through the eye of a needle. Another advantage is that tissue trauma is reduced because a swaged needle has only a single strand of suture that must be pulled through the tissue compared with a double strand in an eyed needle. The swaged needle can be pulled through the tissue with less resulting trauma. Swaged suture packets are labeled to specify the gauge, type, and length of suture material, the

type of needle point (cutting or noncutting), and the needle shape (curved or straight) (see Figure 25-7).

Insertion of Sutures

The medical assistant may be responsible for preparing the suture tray and for assisting the physician during the insertion of the sutures. The physician designates the size and type of suture material and needle required. Because sutures, needles, and suture-needle combinations (swaged needles) are contained in peel-apart packages, they can be added to the sterile field by flipping them onto the sterile field or by placing them there with a sterile gloved hand (Figure 25-10).

Suture Insertion Setup

The items required for a suture insertion setup are listed next.

Items Placed to the Side of the Sterile Field
- Clean disposable gloves
- Antiseptic solution
- Surgical scrub brush
- Antiseptic swabs
- Sterile gloves
- Local anesthetic
- Antiseptic wipe to cleanse the vial
- Tetanus toxoid with needle and syringe

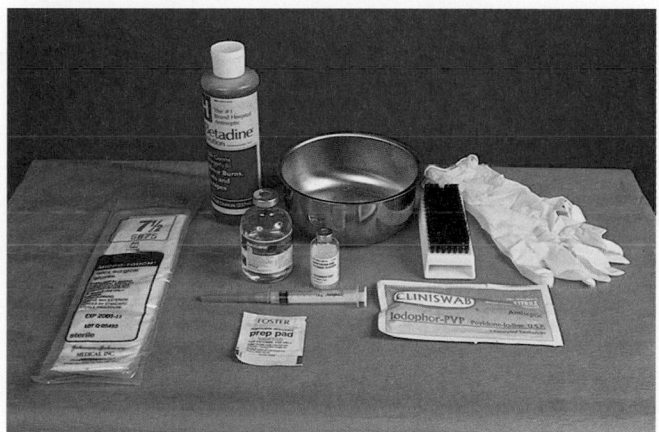

Suture insertion side table.

Items Included on the Sterile Field
- Fenestrated drape
- Syringe and needle for drawing up the local anesthetic
- Hemostatic forceps
- Thumb forceps
- Tissue forceps
- Dissecting scissors
- Operating scissors
- Needle holder
- Suture
- Sterile 4 × 4 gauze

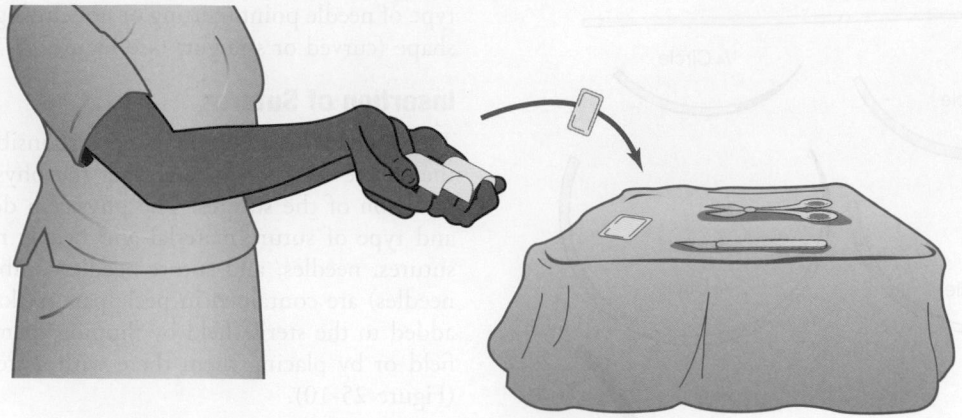

Flipping sutures onto the sterile field.

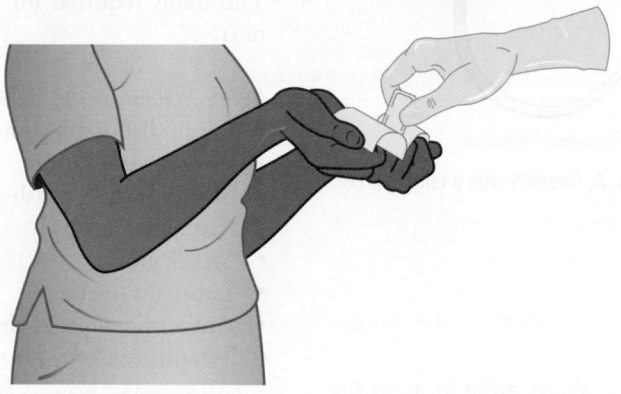

The physician removing the sutures with a sterile gloved hand.

Figure 25-10 Adding sutures to a sterile field.

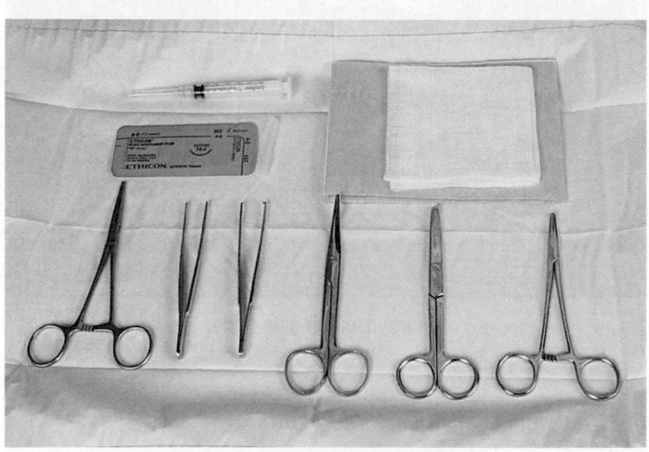

Suture insertion sterile field.

Procedure: Suture Insertion

Sutures are inserted as follows:

1. A local anesthetic is used to numb the area.
2. The physician inserts sutures to close a surgical incision or to repair an accidental wound.
3. A sterile dressing may be applied to the operative site.

Postoperative Instructions: Suture Insertion

Postoperative instructions include the following:

1. Keep the dressing clean and dry.
2. Contact the medical office if any signs of infection occur at the incision site, including excessive redness, swelling, discharge, or an increase in pain.
3. Notify the medical office if the sutures become loose or break.

Provide the patient with written instructions on wound care to refer to at home, and instruct the patient when to return for removal of the sutures.

Suture Removal

When the wound has healed such that it no longer needs the support of nonabsorbable suture material, the sutures must be removed. The length of time the sutures remain in place depends on their location and the amount of healing that must occur. Some areas of the body, such as the head and neck, have a good blood supply; the sutures do not need to remain there as long as they do in other areas because this area heals more rapidly.

Sutures must always be left in place long enough for proper healing to occur. The physician determines the length of time, but in general, skin sutures inserted in the face and neck are removed in 3 to 5 days, and sutures inserted in other areas, such as the skin of the chest, arms, legs, hands, and feet, are removed in 7 to 14 days.

What Would You Do? What Would You *Not* Do?

Case Study 1

Kerry Ventura brings her 6-year-old son Cory to the medical office. Cory got a new bike for his birthday and just learned how to ride it without training wheels. While going around a corner, he lost his balance and fell and cut his left knee. The incision is about 1½ inches long. Cory is going to need sutures to approximate the wound. Mrs. Ventura is very upset and blames herself. She says that she should have been watching him more closely. Mrs. Ventura wants to know why Steri-Strips can't be used to close the incision. She says that it would be a lot less painful for Cory than having stitches. When asked to sign the consent to treatment form for Cory, Mrs. Ventura says she does not want to sign the form until her husband has a chance to read it. She says that right now he is in Japan for 2 weeks on a business trip. ■

Surgical Skin Staples

Surgical skin staples are often used to close wounds. Stapling is the fastest method of closure of long skin incisions. In addition, trauma to the tissue is reduced because the tissue does not have to be handled much when the staples are inserted. Surgical staples are stainless steel and are inserted into the skin using a special skin stapler. Skin staplers are available as reusable or disposable devices. The skin stapler holds a cartridge that contains a prescribed number and size of staples (Figure 25-11).

The physician inserts the staples by gently approximating the tissues with tissue forceps. The skin stapler is held over the site, and the staple is inserted into the skin. Skin stapling produces excellent cosmetic results, and the staples are easy to remove with a specially designed staple remover.

The medical assistant is frequently responsible for removing sutures and staples. This procedure should be done only after the physician has given a written or verbal order to the medical assistant. Procedure 25-5 presents the method used to remove sutures and skin staples.

Adhesive Skin Closures

Adhesive skin closures may be used for wound repair to approximate the edges of a laceration or incision. Skin closures consist of sterile, hypoallergenic tape that is commercially available in a variety of widths and lengths and is strong enough to approximate a wound until healing occurs. Brand names for adhesive skin closures are Steri-Strip (3M Corporation, St Paul, Minn) and Proxi-Strip (Ethicon, Inc., Bridgewater, NJ) (Figure 25-12).

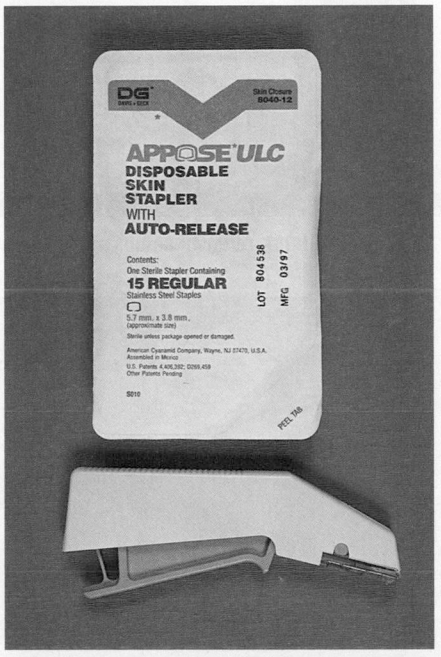

Figure 25-11 Disposable skin stapler.

PROCEDURE 25-5 Removing Sutures and Staples

 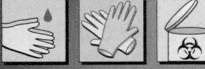

Outcome Remove sutures and staples.

Equipment/Supplies

- Antiseptic swabs
- Clean disposable gloves
- Sterile 4 × 4 gauze
- Surgical tape
- Mayo stand
- Biohazard waste container

For Suture Removal

- Suture removal kit, which includes the following:
- Suture scissors
- Thumb forceps
- Sterile 4 × 4 gauze

For Staple Removal

- Staple removal kit, which includes:
- Staple remover
- Sterile 4 × 4 gauze

Continued

PROCEDURE 25-5   Removing Sutures and Staples—cont'd

1. Procedural Step. Wash your hands with an antimicrobial soap. Assemble the equipment.
Principle. Washing the hands with an antimicrobial soap removes microorganisms from the hands and also deposits an antimicrobial film on your hands to discourage the growth of bacteria.

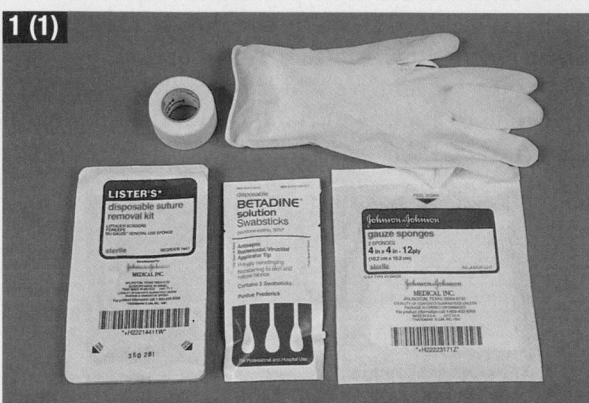

Suture removal setup.

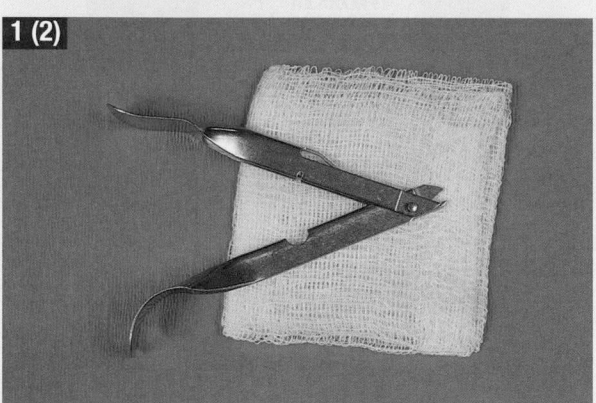

Staple removal setup.

2. Procedural Step. Greet the patient and introduce yourself. Identify the patient by full name and date of birth and explain the procedure.

3. Procedural Step. Position the patient as required to provide good access to the site. Adjust the light so that it is focused on the wound. Verify that the sutures (or staples) are intact and that the incision line is approximated and not gaping. Check that the incision line is not infected. If the incision line is not approximated, or if redness, swelling, or a discharge is present, do not remove the sutures; notify the physician.
Principle. The sutures (or staples) should not be removed unless the incision line is approximated and free from infection.

4. Procedural Step. Open the suture or staple removal kit, keeping the contents of the kit sterile. Most kits are opened by peeling back a top cover, which exposes a plastic tray that holds the necessary instruments and supplies.

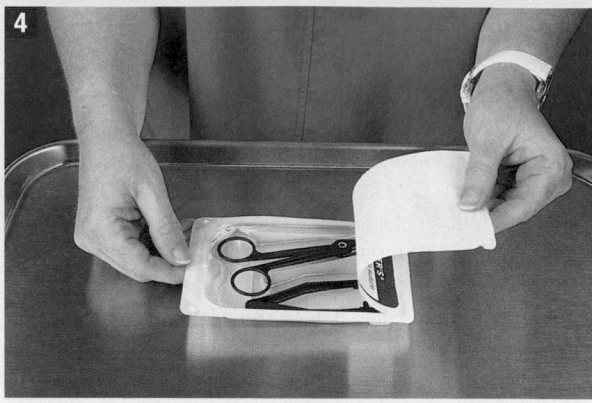

Open the suture removal kit.

5. Procedural Step. Apply clean gloves. Cleanse the incision line with an antiseptic swab to destroy microorganisms and to remove any dried exudate encrusted around the sutures or staples. Clean the wound from the top to the bottom, working from the center to the outside of the wound. Use a new swab for each cleansing motion. Allow the skin to dry.
Principle. Dried exudate must be removed to allow unimpeded removal of the sutures or staples.

6. Procedural Step. Remove the sutures or staples. Tell the patient that he or she will feel a pulling or tugging sensation as each suture (or staple) is removed, but that it will not be painful. Count the number of sutures or staples removed. Check the patient's chart to make sure the same number is removed as was inserted by the physician.
To remove sutures:

a. Using the sterile thumb forceps provided in the kit, pick up the knot of the first suture.

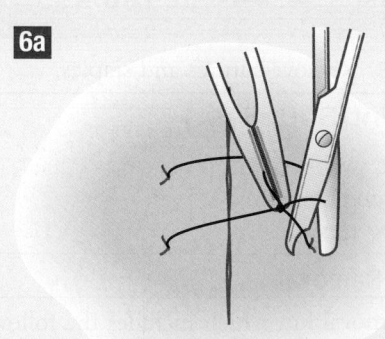

Cut the suture below the knot on the side closest to the skin.

b. Place the curved tip of the suture scissors under the suture. Using the sterile suture scissors, cut the

PROCEDURE 25-5   Removing Sutures and Staples—cont'd

suture below the knot on the side of the suture closest to the skin. Cut the suture as close to the skin as possible.

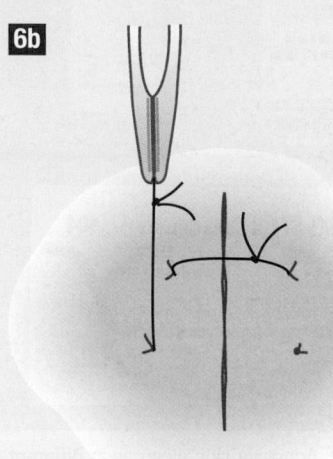

6b

Gently pull the suture out.

c. Using a smooth, continuous motion, gently pull the suture out of the skin. Remove the suture without allowing any portion that was previously outside to be pulled back through the tissue lying beneath the incision line. Place the suture on the 4 × 4 gauze included in the suture kit.

d. Continue in this manner until all the sutures have been removed.

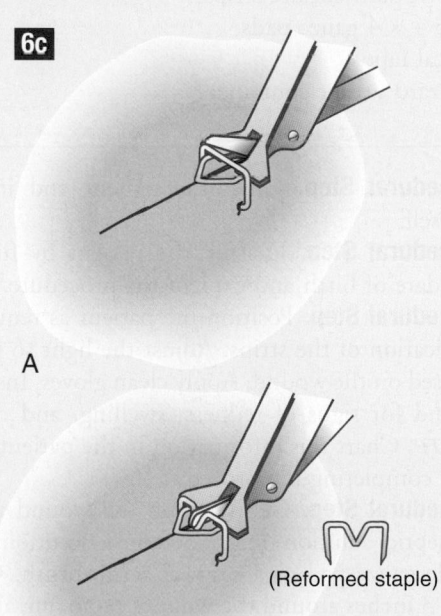

6c

A

(Reformed staple)

B

A, Place the bottom jaws of the staple remover under the staple.
B, Firmly squeeze the staple handles until they are fully closed.

Principle. To prevent infection, the suture must be removed without pulling any portion that has been outside the skin back through the tissue lying beneath the incision line.

To remove staples:

a. Gently place the bottom jaws of the staple remover under the staple to be removed.

b. Firmly squeeze the staple handles until they are fully closed.

c. Carefully lift the staple remover upward to remove the staple from the incision line. Place the staple on the 4 × 4 gauze included in the staple kit.

d. Continue in this manner until all the staples have been removed.

7. **Procedural Step.** Cleanse the site with an antiseptic swab. Some physicians want the medical assistant to apply adhesive skin closures after removing the sutures or staples to provide additional support to the wound as it continues to heal.

8. **Procedural Step.** Apply a dry sterile dressing if indicated by the physician.

9. **Procedural Step.** Dispose of the sutures (or staples) and the gauze in a biohazard waste container.

10. **Procedural Step.** Remove the gloves, and sanitize your hands.

11. **Procedural Step.** Chart the procedure. Include the date and time, the status of the sutures (or staples) and incision line, the number of sutures (or staples) removed, the location of the site, care of the wound (i.e., application of an antiseptic or dressing), and the patient's reaction. Chart any instructions given to the patient.

CHARTING EXAMPLE

Date	
9/20/XX	10:30 a.m. Sutures intact and incision line in good approximation. No signs of infection. Sutures x6 removed from Ⓡ ant forearm. Incision line cleaned c̄ Betadine and DSD applied. Instructions provided on dressing care. ———————— T. Browning, CMA (AAMA)

Adhesive skin closures may be used when not much tension exists on the skin edges. The strips of tape are applied transversely across the line of incision to approximate the skin edges. The advantages of adhesive skin closures are that they eliminate the need for sutures and a local anesthetic, they are easy to apply and remove, they have a lower incidence of wound infection compared with sutures, and they result in less scarring than sutures. The disadvantage of this method is that there is less precision in bringing the wound edges together compared with suturing the wound. In addition, adhesive skin closures cannot be used on certain areas of the body where the adhesive has difficulty adhering to the skin. This includes areas that harbor moisture (e.g., palms of the hands, soles of the feet, axillae) and hairy areas of the body (e.g., scalp, a man's chest).

The medical assistant frequently is responsible for applying adhesive skin closures. Procedure 25-6 outlines this procedure. Approximately 5 to 10 days after application, the skin closures usually loosen and fall off on their own. If they require removal by the medical assistant, the method presented at the end of Procedure 25-6 should be followed.

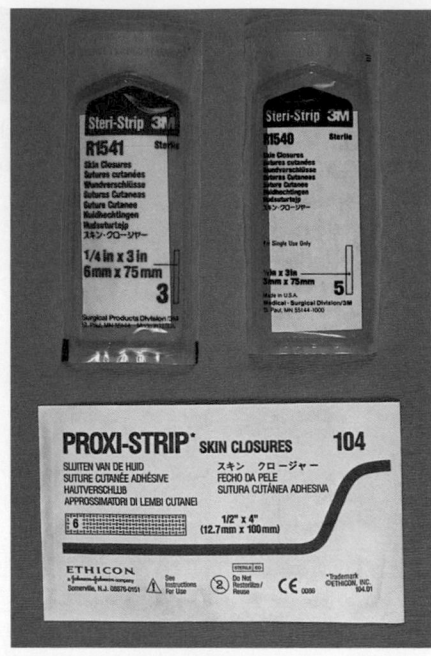

Figure 25-12 Adhesive skin closures in different sizes.

PROCEDURE 25-6 Applying and Removing Adhesive Skin Closures

Outcome Apply and remove adhesive skin closures.

Equipment/Supplies

- Clean disposable gloves
- Sterile gloves
- Antiseptic solution
- Surgical scrub brush
- Antiseptic swabs
- Tincture of benzoin

- Sterile cotton-tipped applicator
- Adhesive skin closure strips
- Sterile 4 × 4 gauze pads
- Surgical tape
- Biohazard waster container

Application of Adhesive Skin Closures

1. Procedural Step. Wash your hands with an antimicrobial soap and assemble the equipment. Check the expiration date on the adhesive skin closures.

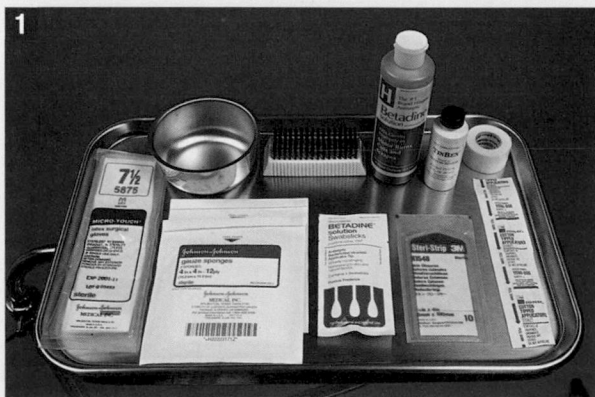

Assemble the equipment.

2. Procedural Step. Greet the patient and introduce yourself.

3. Procedural Step. Identify the patient by full name and date of birth and explain the procedure.

4. Procedural Step. Position the patient as required for application of the strips. Adjust the light so that it is focused on the wound. Apply clean gloves. Inspect the wound for signs of redness, swelling, and drainage. (*NOTE*: Chart this information in the patient's record after completing the procedure.)

5. Procedural Step. Gently scrub the wound using an antiseptic solution (e.g., Betadine solution) and a sterile gauze pad or a surgical scrub brush. Clean at least 3 inches around the wound, removing all debris, skin oil, and exudates. Allow the skin to dry or pat dry with gauze pads. (*NOTE*: Change gloves as needed to maintain cleanliness.)

PROCEDURE 25-6 Applying and Removing Adhesive Skin Closures—cont'd

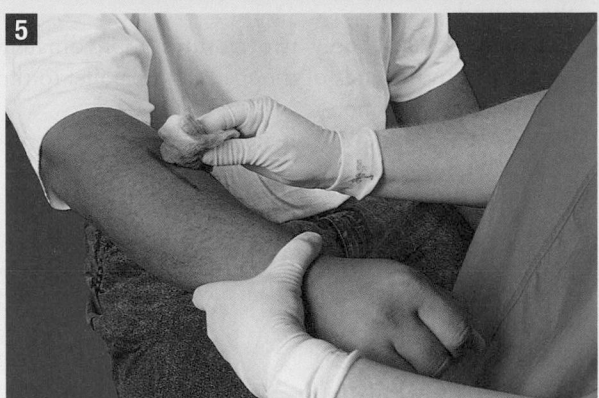

Clean the wound.

6. Procedural Step. Apply an antiseptic to the site using antiseptic swabs such as Betadine swabs. Apply the antiseptic from the top to the bottom of the wound, working from the center to the outside of the wound. Use a new swab for each motion. Allow the skin to dry completely.

Principle. The antiseptic decreases the number of microorganisms in the wound. The skin must be completely dry to ensure adhesion of the skin closures to the skin.

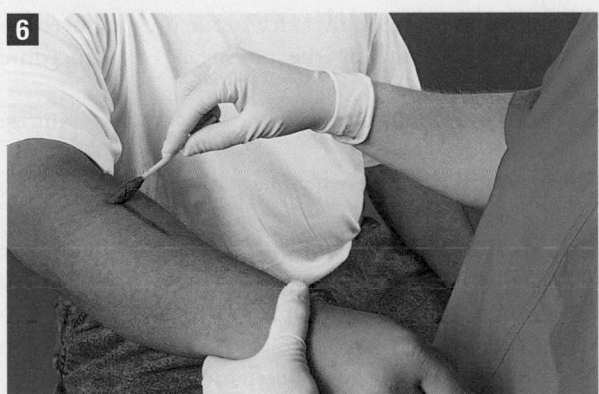

Apply an antiseptic to the wound.

7. Procedural Step. If dictated by the medical office policy, apply a thin coat of tincture of benzoin to the skin parallel to each side of the wound with a sterile cotton-tipped applicator. Do not allow the tincture of benzoin to touch the wound. Allow the skin to dry. Remove the gloves, and wash your hands with an antimicrobial soap.

Principle. Tincture of benzoin facilitates adhesion of the strips to the skin.

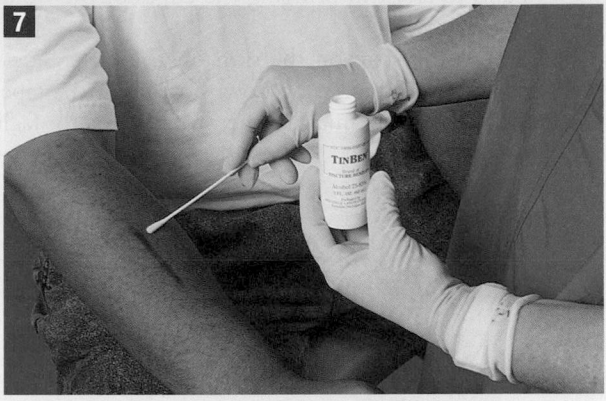

Apply tincture of benzoin.

8. Procedural Step. Open the plastic peel-apart package of strips using sterile technique as follows:
a. Grasp each flap of the package between the thumbs and bent index fingers. Pull the package apart.
b. Peel back the package until it is completely open.
c. Lay the opened package flat on a clean dry surface. The inside of the package serves as the sterile field.

9. Procedural Step. Apply sterile gloves. Fold the card of strips along its perforated tab, and tear off the tab, which exposes the ends of the strips, making them easier to grasp. Peel a strip of tape off the card at a 45-degree angle to the card.

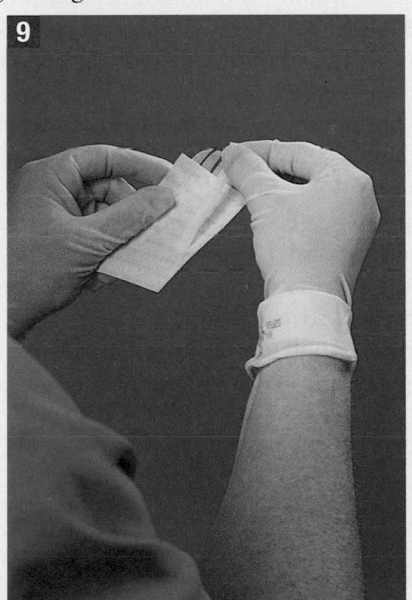

Peel a strip of tape off the card.

10. Procedural Step. Check that the skin surface is dry. Position the first strip over the center of the wound as follows:
a. Secure one end of the strip of tape to the skin on one side of the wound by pressing down firmly on the tape.
b. Stretch the strip transversely across the line of the incision until the edges of the wound are

Continued

approximated exactly. If necessary, use your gloved hand to assist in bringing the edges of the wound together.

c. Secure the strip on the skin on the other side of the wound by pressing down firmly on the tape.

Principle. Approximating the wound exactly facili-

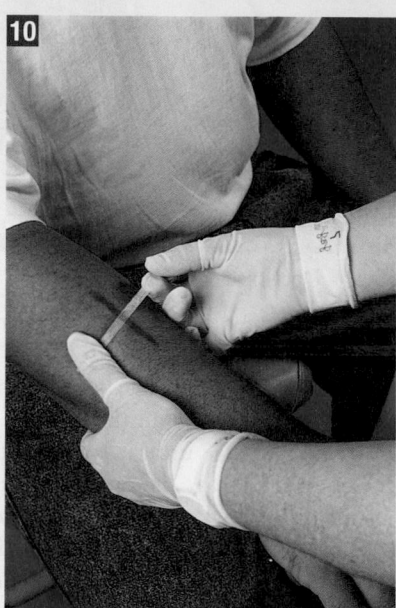

Position the first strip over the center of the wound.

tates good healing and minimizes scar formation.

11. Procedural Step. Apply the second strip perpendicular to the wound on one side of the center strip. The space between the strips should be approximately ⅛ inch. Apply a third strip on the other side of the center strip at a ⅛-inch interval. Continue applying the strips at ⅛-inch intervals until the edges of the wound are approximated. If at any time the skin surfaces become moist with perspiration, blood, or serum, wipe the area dry with a sterile gauze pad before applying the next strip.

Principle. Applying the strips in this manner facilitates good approximation of the wound. Spacing the

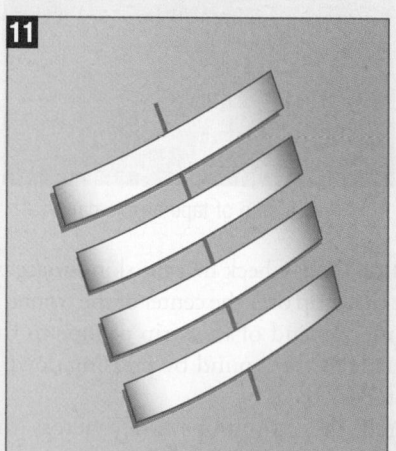

Apply the strips until the edges of the wound are approximated.

strips at ⅛-inch intervals allows proper drainage of the wound.

12. Procedural Step. Apply two closures approximately ½ inch from the ends of the strips and parallel to the wound (ladder fashion).

Principle. Applying a strip along each edge redistrib-

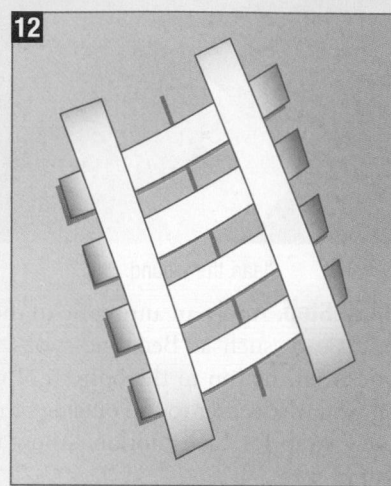

Apply a strip along each edge.

utes the tension and assists in holding the strips firmly in place.

13. Procedural Step. Apply a dry sterile dressing over the strips if indicated by the physician (see Procedure 25-4).

14. Procedural Step. Remove the gloves, and sanitize your hands.

15. Procedural Step. Instruct the patient in wound care as follows:

a. Provide the patient with written wound care instructions (see the patient teaching box on wound care in this chapter).

b. Explain the wound care instructions, and ask the patient whether he or she has any questions.

c. Ask the patient to sign the instruction sheet on the appropriate line.

d. Witness the patient's signature by signing your name in the appropriate space on the form. Include today's date.

e. Before the patient leaves the medical office, make a copy of the instruction sheet. Give a signed copy of the wound care instructions to the patient, and file the original in the patient's medical record.

Principle. An instruction sheet signed by the patient provides legal documentation that wound care instructions were provided to the patient in the event that the patient fails to follow the instructions and causes further harm or damage to the wound.

PROCEDURE 25-6   Applying and Removing Adhesive Skin Closures—cont'd

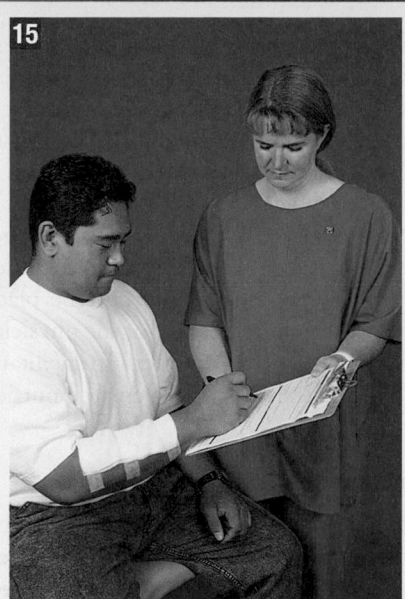

Ask the patient to sign the instruction sheet.

16. **Procedural Step.** Chart the procedure. Include the date and time, the appearance of the wound, wound preparation, the number of strips applied, the location of the wound, the care of the wound, and the patient's reaction. Chart verbal and written instructions given to the patient concerning wound care.

CHARTING EXAMPLE

Date	
9/20/XX	10:30 a.m. Incision approx 5 cm long located on ℞ post forearm. Redness noted on edge of wound. Sl amt of serous drainage noted. Wound scrubbed c̄ Betadine sol and Betadine antiseptic applied. Applied Steri-Strips x4. Incision in good approximation. Applied DSD. Explained wound care. Written instructions provided. Signed copy filed in chart. To return in 5 days for removal of strips. _____
	_____ T. Browning, CMA (AAMA)

Removal of Adhesive Skin Closures

Adhesive skin closures usually loosen and fall off on their own approximately 5 to 10 days following application. If they require removal, the procedure outlined below should be followed by the medical assistant.

1. **Procedural Step.** Sanitize your hands. Greet the patient and introduce yourself. Identify the patient by full name and date of birth and explain the procedure.
2. **Procedural Step.** Position the patient as required. Adjust the light so that it is focused on the wound.

Check that the skin closures are intact and that the incision line is approximated and not gaping. Check that the incision line is not infected. If the incision line is not approximated, or if redness, swelling, or a discharge is present, do not remove the skin closures; notify the physician.

3. **Procedural Step.** Position a 4 × 4 gauze pad in a convenient location. Apply clean gloves.
4. **Procedural Step.** Remove the skin closures as follows:
   a. Gently grasp one end of a strip of tape with the dominant hand.
   b. Stabilize the skin with one finger of the nondominant hand.
   c. Slowly loosen and peel off one half of the strip of tape from the outside to the wound margin, keeping the peeled-off section of the strip close to the skin surface and pulled back over itself. As you remove the strip from the skin, continue moving the finger as necessary to support the newly exposed skin. Always pull the strip toward the wound. Never pull the strip away from the wound because tension on the wound site could disrupt the healing process.
   d. Remove the other half of the strip of tape from the outside to the wound margin in the manner just described.
   e. When both halves of the strip are completely loosened, gently lift the strip up and away from the wound surface. Place the strip on a 4 × 4 gauze pad.
   f. Continue in this manner until all the skin closures have been removed.
5. **Procedural Step.** Cleanse the site with an antiseptic swab. Apply a dry sterile dressing if indicated by the physician (see Procedure 25-4).
6. **Procedural Step.** Dispose of the strips and gauze in a biohazard waste container. Remove the gloves, and sanitize your hands.
7. **Procedural Step.** Chart the procedure. Include the date and time, the status of the skin closures, the number of skin closures removed, the location of the site, the care of the wound, and the patient's reaction. Chart any instructions given to the patient.

CHARTING EXAMPLE

Date	
9/25/XX	10:30 a.m. Skin closures intact and in good approximation. No signs of infection. Strips x 4 removed from ℞ post forearm. Incision line cleaned c̄ Betadine and DSD applied. Instructions provided on dressing care.
	_____ T. Browning, CMA (AAMA)

ASSISTING WITH MINOR OFFICE SURGERY

Tray Setup

Assisting with minor office surgery requires a thorough knowledge of the instruments and supplies for each tray setup and the type of assistance required by the physician during the surgery. The medical assistant must be able to work quickly and efficiently and to anticipate the physician's needs.

The instruments and supplies for the surgery must be set on a sterile field. Many offices maintain index cards indicating the appropriate instruments and supplies for each minor office surgery tray setup. The card also may include information regarding the type of skin preparation, the position of the patient, the physician's glove size, the type of suture material, preoperative instructions, and postoperative instructions. The index cards are generally kept in a file box and are filed alphabetically by the type of surgery. The medical assistant should pull the card before setting up for the minor office surgery and use it as a guide to ensure that all required articles are placed on the sterile field. The medical assistant may set up the sterile tray before or after preparing the patient's skin. The sterile tray setup must not become contaminated. If the medical assistant must turn away from the sterile tray or leave the room after setting up, a sterile towel must be placed over the tray to maintain sterility.

Methods Used to Set up a Sterile Tray

A common method used to set up a sterile tray is to use prepackaged sterile setups wrapped in disposable sterilization paper or muslin that are prepared by the medical office through autoclave sterilization (see Procedure 25-2). These setups are labeled according to use (e.g., suture pack, cyst removal pack) and contain most of the instruments and supplies required for the minor office surgery indicated on the label. The medical assistant opens the wrapped package on a flat surface, such as a **Mayo tray.** A Mayo tray is a broad, flat metal tray placed on a stand that can be used to hold sterile instruments and supplies; the inside of the wrapped package is sterile and serves as the sterile field. Several additional articles not contained in the prepackaged setup (e.g., an antiseptic, sterile 4 × 4 gauze pads, disposable syringes and needles, sutures) may need to be added to the sterile field when the package is opened. If an antiseptic solution is poured into a basin on the sterile field, this is performed according to Procedure 25-3. Items in peel-apart packages are added by flipping them onto the sterile field or by placing them on the field using a sterile gloved hand.

Another method used to set up a sterile tray is to place all necessary articles on the sterile field by flipping them onto the sterile field from peel-apart packages. With this method, the sterile field is prepared by placing a sterile towel over a tray such as a Mayo tray or another flat surface. The sterile towel must be handled by the corners only so as not to contaminate it. It must not be fanned through the air,

but instead must be laid down gently and slowly to prevent airborne contamination.

Side Table

Some articles required for minor office surgery are not placed on the sterile field but are set on an adjacent table or counter. These articles, such as a surgical scrub brush, are not sterile and must not be placed on the sterile field. The local anesthetic, which is a sterile solution, is in a vial that is not sterile and must *not* be placed on the sterile field. The physician needs to apply gloves to perform the surgery. Although the gloves are sterile, the outside wrapper is not; the package of gloves must not be placed on the sterile field. In addition, it is easier for the physician to apply gloves from a side table or counter. To facilitate applying the gloves, the medical assistant opens the outside wrapper for the physician.

Skin Preparation

The patient's skin must be prepared before the minor office surgery because the skin contains an abundance of microorganisms. If these microorganisms were to enter the body through the operative site, a wound infection could develop. It is impossible to sterilize skin because chemical agents required to kill all living microorganisms are too strong to be placed on the skin surfaces. The operative site and an area surrounding it must be cleaned and prepared in such a way as to remove as many microorganisms as possible to reduce the risk of surgical wound contamination.

Shaving the Site

Hair supports the growth of microorganisms, and the physician may want the medical assistant to shave the skin at and around the operative site. Shave preparation trays are commercially available and include several gauze sponges, a measured amount of antiseptic soap, a container for soapy water, and a disposable safety razor. The skin should be pulled taut as it is shaved, and the medical assistant must be careful to prevent nicks. When all the hair has been removed, the shaved area should be rinsed and dried thoroughly.

Cleansing the Site

The operative site must be cleaned with an antiseptic solution such as povidone-iodine (Betadine Surgical Scrub) or chlorhexidine gluconate (Hibiclens) (Figure 25-13). The medical assistant should scrub the operative area with a surgical scrub brush using a firm circular motion, moving from the inside outward. The area is rinsed using gauze pads saturated with water and is blotted dry with sterile gauze.

Antiseptic Application

When the patient's skin has been shaved (if required) and cleansed, an antiseptic is applied to the operative area, followed by the application of a sterile drape. The antiseptic decreases the number of microorganisms on the patient's skin; a common antiseptic is Betadine. A disposable sterile *fenestrated drape* (Figure 25-14) is the type of drape most

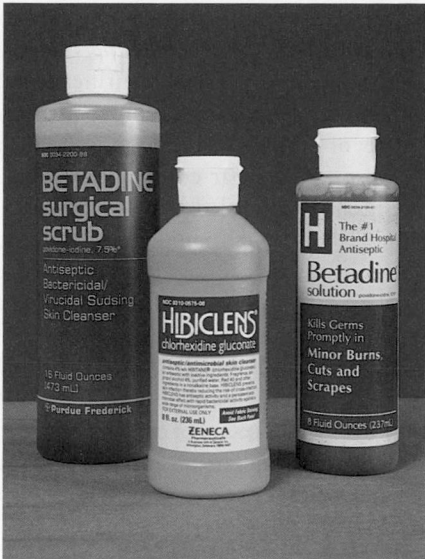

Figure 25-13 Cleansing solutions.

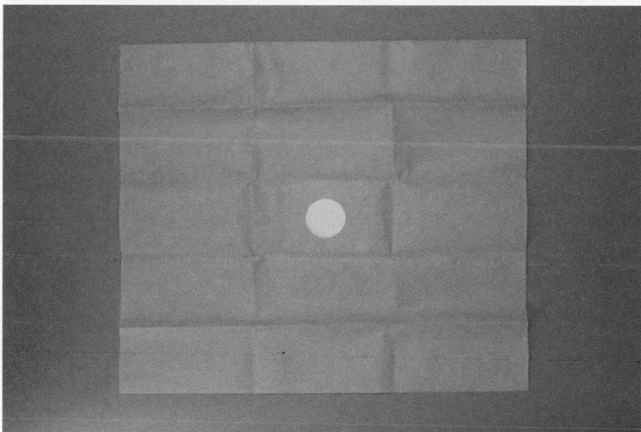

Figure 25-14 Fenestrated drape.

commonly used. It has an opening that is placed directly over the operative site. A fenestrated drape covers a wide area of skin around the operative area, leaving only the operative site exposed. This provides a sterile area around the operative site and decreases contamination of the patient's surgical wound.

Local Anesthetic

Minor office surgeries often require the use of a local anesthetic; the local anesthetic most frequently used in the medical office is lidocaine hydrochloride (Xylocaine). The physician injects the local anesthetic into the tissue surrounding the operative site, a process termed **infiltration,** to produce a loss of sensation in that area and prevent the patient from feeling pain during the surgery. When first injected into the tissues, lidocaine causes the patient to experience a brief burning or stinging sensation at the injection site. The local anesthetic begins working in 5 to 15 minutes and has a duration of action of 1 to 3 hours, depending on the type of anesthetic.

Some physicians prefer to use a local anesthetic containing *epinephrine.* Epinephrine is a vasoconstrictor that prolongs

the local effect of the anesthetic and decreases the rate of systemic absorption of the local anesthetic. It accomplishes this by constricting blood vessels at the operative site. The physician informs the medical assistant of the type, strength, and amount of local anesthetic needed for the minor office surgery. Xylocaine is available in 0.5%, 1%, 1.5%, and 2% solutions. The physician may order 1 mL of Xylocaine 2% with epinephrine to suture a laceration of the forearm.

Preparing the Anesthetic

The local anesthetic is drawn up into the syringe according to the procedure presented in Chapter 26. The vial must first be cleansed using an antiseptic wipe. The correct amount of anesthetic solution is withdrawn into the syringe. This may be performed by the medical assistant or the physician. The medical assistant withdraws the anesthetic into the syringe and hands it to the physician, who has not yet applied sterile gloves. The physician injects the anesthetic into the patient's tissues and then applies sterile gloves to begin the surgery.

The physician may prefer to draw the anesthetic solution into the syringe after he or she has applied sterile gloves. The medical assistant should first show the label of the vial to the physician and should then hold the vial securely while the physician withdraws the medication (Figure 25-15). The medical assistant must hold the vial because the outside of the vial is medically aseptic and cannot be touched by the physician's sterile gloved hand.

If the medical assistant prepares the anesthetic injection, the needle and syringe are not placed on the sterile field, but are assembled off to the side. If the physician withdraws the anesthetic, the needle and syringe are placed on the sterile field.

Assisting the Physician

The type of assistance required by the physician during minor office surgery is based on the type of surgery and the physician's preference. Some physicians want the medical assistant to apply sterile gloves and assist directly by handing instruments and supplies from the sterile field. An instrument should be handed to the physician in a firm, confident manner so that the instrument does not slip out of the physician's hand and drop on the floor. The instrument should be placed in the physician's hand in its functional position, that is, the position in which it is to be used (Figure 25-16). If the instrument is handed correctly, the physician should not have to reposition the instrument to use it.

The medical assistant is responsible for adding any instruments or supplies to the sterile field that the physician requires after the surgery has begun, such as another hemostat, additional 4 × 4 gauze pads, and sutures. This is generally accomplished using peel-apart packages and by either flipping the contents onto the sterile field or by holding the package open and allowing the physician to remove the contents with a gloved hand. In assisting with minor office surgery, it is essential to know all steps in the procedure, so that the physician's needs are anticipated, and the surgery proceeds smoothly and efficiently.

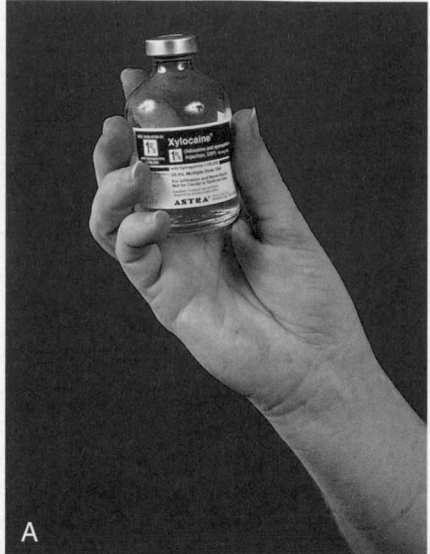

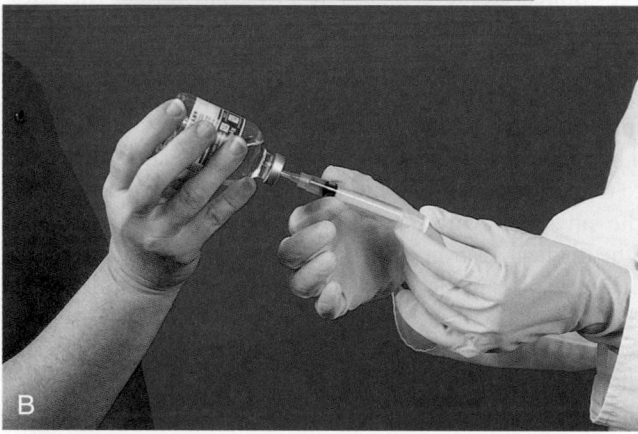

Figure 25-15 Drawing up the local anesthetic. **A,** Trudy holds up the vial so that the physician can verify the name and strength of the local anesthetic. **B,** Trudy holds the vial securely while the physician withdraws the medication.

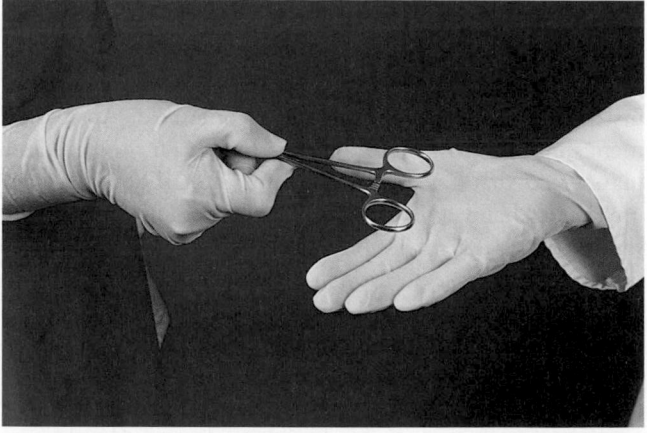

Figure 25-16 Trudy hands a hemostat to the physician in its functional position.

The physician may obtain a tissue specimen that is sent to the laboratory for histologic examination. The specimen must be placed in an appropriate-sized container with a preservative. The medical assistant is responsible for labeling the specimen container. An unlabeled specimen is a cause for rejection of the specimen by an outside laboratory. Two *unique identifiers* should be used to label the specimen. A unique identifier is information that clearly identifies a specific patient, such as the patient's name and date of birth. A specimen can be labeled by attaching a computerized bar code label to the specimen. A specimen can also be labeled by hand-writing the information on the label, which should include the patient's name and date of birth, the date and time of collection, the medical assistant's initials, and any other information required by the laboratory, such as the source of the specimen. The information should be printed legibly, and the medical assistant should be certain that the information is accurate to avoid a mix-up of specimens. The medical assistant also must complete a laboratory requisition to accompany the specimen; this is known as a *biopsy requisition* (Figure 25-17).

What Would You Do? What Would You *Not* Do?

Case Study 2

Abbey Mendy is having a sebaceous cyst removed from her neck. She wants to know why the antiseptic applied to her neck is orange, and whether it is going to stain her skin permanently. During the procedure, Abbey reaches her hand up to adjust her hair and accidentally touches the physician's gloved hand. After the procedure, a sterile dressing is applied to her neck, and she is given an appointment to return to have her sutures removed. Abbey becomes alarmed when she is told that the cyst will be sent to the laboratory for a biopsy. She wants to know whether the physician is not telling her everything about her condition, and is concerned that maybe he thinks she has cancer. Abbey asks if her neighbor can take out her sutures. She says that he has worked as a veterinary assistant for the past 8 years and has lots of experience in removing stitches. ∎

When the minor office surgery is completed, the physician may want the medical assistant to place a dry sterile dressing over the surgical wound to protect it from contamination or injury or to absorb drainage. The medical assistant also is responsible for assisting the patient and cleaning the examining room.

Procedure 25-7 describes the medical assistant's responsibilities while assisting with minor office surgery. Specific instruments and supplies required for the minor office surgery depend on the type of surgery being performed and the physician's preference. Knowing the name and function of the surgical instruments shown in Figure 25-3 enables the medical assistant to set up for each type of minor surgery performed in the medical office. If the medical office uses prepackaged sterile setups, the medical assistant should have already assembled the instruments and supplies in the package during the sanitization and sterilization process; however, the instruments and supplies should be checked after the pack is opened to ensure that all the sterile articles are included.

Text continued on p. 534

Highlight on the History of Surgery

Primitive Surgery

Surgery evolved from very primitive beginnings. The first record of a surgical operation dates back to 350,000 BC. Primitive humans believed that headaches were caused by demons that had gained entrance to the head and were unable to get out. To release the demons, a hole was chiseled through the patient's skull with a sharp flint. Early operating instruments consisted of sharpened flints and crude hammers. Sharpened animal teeth were used for bloodletting and drainage of abscesses. Ancient records show that suturing materials consisted of dried gut, dried tendon, strips of hide, horsehair, and fibers from tree bark. To help form a clot, bleeding wounds were covered with materials such as rabbit fur, shredded tree bark, egg yolk, and cobwebs.

Early 1800s

In the early 1800s, surgical instruments were still almost nonexistent. Kitchen knives and penknives doubled as scalpels, and table forks were used as retractors. Physicians would use household pincushions to hold their suturing needles. The same sponges were used for every patient to wipe away blood and other secretions. Because of these conditions, the most trivial operations were likely to be followed by infection, and death occurred in half of all surgical operations. Joseph Lister, an English surgeon, was one of the first individuals to advocate the use of antiseptics during surgery. Lister insisted on the use of antiseptics on the hands of his surgical team, instruments, wounds, and dressings. Many surgeons ridiculed Lister's ideas, but in 1879 his antiseptic principles were, at long last, formally adopted by the medical profession. Today, Lister is known as the father of modern surgery.

Mid-1800s

Anesthetic agents, such as ether and chloroform, were discovered in the mid-1800s. Before this time, various methods were used to subdue and restrain patients during surgery, such as having the patient consume alcohol before the operation and strapping the patient to the operating table. With the advent of anesthetics, new surgical procedures never before considered possible came into existence. This resulted in new demands for surgical instruments and the necessity for smaller and more delicate instruments.

Late 1800s and Early 1900s

The late 1800s and early 1900s saw dramatic advances in surgical operations and techniques. The most notable include the invention of the steam sterilizer, which permitted sterilization of surgical instruments and supplies; the use of surgical gowns, caps, masks, and gloves during surgery; the monitoring of a patient's condition while under anesthesia; the development of stainless steel, which provided a superior material for manufacturing surgical instruments; and the establishment of standards for manufacturing and packaging sutures. Other discoveries important to surgery during this time included the discovery of x-rays by Wilhelm Röntgen; the discovery of penicillin by Alexander Fleming; the discovery by William Halsted that cocaine could be used as a local anesthetic; and the development of endoscopic instruments, such as the laryngoscope, bronchoscope, and sigmoidoscope, for viewing internal structures of the body.

Breakthroughs in surgical technology established through the ages laid the foundation for present-day complex surgical procedures, such as laser surgery, open-heart surgery, and microsurgery. It is incredible to think that it all started with a sharpened flint! ■

DIAGNOSTIC PATHOLOGY ASSOCIATES, INC

HISTOPATHOLOGY/CYTOPATHOLOGY REQUISITION

BILL TO: ❑ ACCOUNT ❑ MEDICARE ❑ BLUE SHIELD ❑ PATIENT ❑ MEDICAID ❑ OTHER | PATIENT NAME (LAST, FIRST, MIDDLE INITIAL) | PATIENT ID | ROOM NO.

SEX | BIRTHDATE / / | DATE COLLECTED | TIME COLLECTED A.M. P.M. | REQUESTING PHYSICIAN | SPECIAL INSTRUCTIONS

RESPONSIBLE PARTY NAME | RESPONSIBLE PARTY ADDRESS | CITY, STATE, ZIP

PHONE | MEDICAID ID NUMBER | MEDICARE HIC NUMBER | INSURANCE COMPANY NAME

INSURANCE COMPANY ADDRESS | GROUP NUMBER | CONTRACT NUMBER | COVERAGE CODE | PATIENT/INSURED RELATIONSHIP ❑ SELF ❑ SPOUSE ❑ DEPEND.

PATIENT AUTHORIZATION: I AUTHORIZE THE RELEASE OF ANY MEDICAL INFORMATION NECESSARY TO PROCESS A CLAIM, I PERMIT A COPY OF THIS AUTHORIZATION TO BE USED IN PLACE OF THE ORIGINAL AND REQUEST PAYMENT OF ANY MEDICAL INSURANCE BENEFITS EITHER TO ME OR TO THE PARTY WHO ACCEPTS ASSIGNMENT. | SIGNED X______________ | DATE ______

TISSUE EXAM:
❑ GROSS & MICROSCOPIC
❑ GROSS ONLY
SPECIMEN TYPE:
❑ BIOPSY
❑ SCRAPING
❑ BRUSHING
❑ WASHING
❑ FLUIDS
❑ FINE NEEDLE
❑ OTHER ____________

SOURCE OF SPECIMEN:

❑ PHONE REPORT
(NEXT WORKING DAY)
COPIES TO:__________

CLINICAL DIAGNOSIS:

PATIENT HISTORY:

Figure 25-17 Biopsy requisition.

PROCEDURE 25-7   Assisting with Minor Office Surgery

Outcome Set up a surgical tray, and assist with minor office surgery.

Equipment/Supplies

- Mayo stand
- Instruments and supplies for the type of surgery to be performed
- Biohazard waste container

Preparing the Tray

1. **Procedural Step.** Determine the type of minor office surgery to be performed. The physician instructs the medical assistant as to the type of surgery and provides any additional information needed to set up for the surgery, such as the type of local anesthetic and sutures to be used. If the medical office maintains a minor office surgery filing system, pull the file card that indicates the instruments and supplies required for the type of surgery to be performed.

2. **Procedural Step.** Prepare the examining room. Make sure the room is clean and well lighted.

3. **Procedural Step.** Sanitize your hands.

4. **Procedural Step.** Set up nonsterile articles on a side table or counter. If a specimen container is included in the setup, perform one of the following (based on the medical office policy):

   a. Attach a computer-generated bar code label to the specimen container **or**

   b. Clearly label the tubes and containers with the patient's name and date of birth, the date, your initials, and any other information required by the laboratory, such as the source of the specimen.

   Principle. Articles that are not sterile cannot be placed on the sterile field because they would contaminate it. Two unique identifiers should be used when labeling the specimen (e.g., patient's name and date of birth).

5. **Procedural Step.** Wash your hands with an antimicrobial soap and set up the minor office surgery tray on a clean, dry, flat surface, using the principles of surgical asepsis. The sterile tray can be set up as follows:

   Prepackaged setup:

   a. Select the appropriate package from the supply shelf, and place it on a Mayo tray or other flat surface

   b. Open the prepackaged setup using the inside of the wrapper as the sterile field. Check the sterilization indicator to make sure the contents of the pack are sterile.

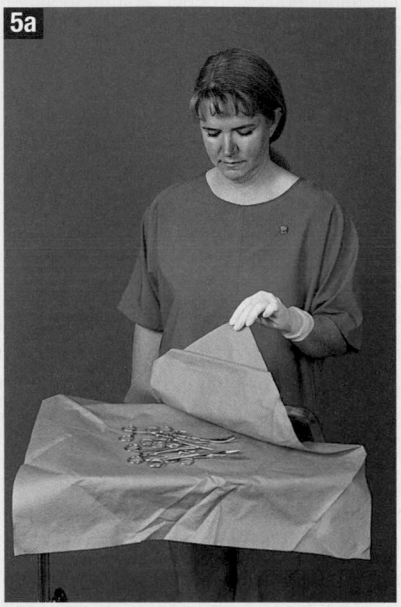

Open the sterile pack using the inside of the wrapper as the sterile field.

   c. Add other articles to the sterile field that are needed for the surgery but not contained in the sterile package, such as 4 × 4 gauze, sutures, and a fenestrated drape. If sutures are required for the setup, make sure to check the expiration date of the sutures.

   Transferring articles to a sterile field:

   a. Pick up the folded sterile towel by two corner ends and allow it to unfold; make sure it does not touch an unsterile surface.

   b. Lay the sterile towel down gently and slowly over the Mayo tray, making sure it does not brush against an unsterile surface such as your uniform. Do not allow your arms to pass over the towel as you lay it down because this would result in contamination of the sterile field.

   c. Transfer instruments and supplies to the sterile field from wrapped or peel-apart packages.

   Principle. The principles of surgical asepsis must be followed to prevent contamination of the sterile field.

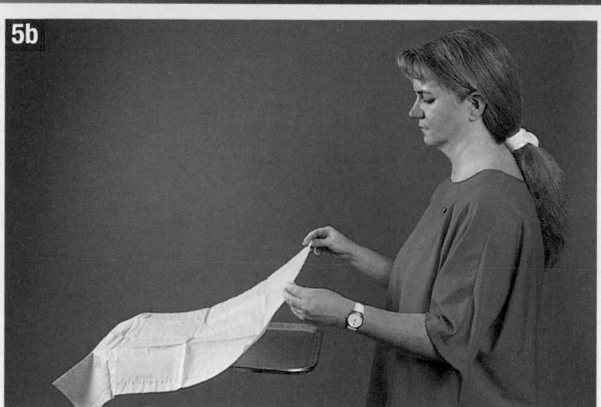

Lay the sterile towel down gently and slowly.

6. Procedural Step. Apply a sterile glove, and arrange the articles neatly on the sterile field. Do not allow one article to lie on top of another. Check that all the instruments and supplies required for the surgery are available on the sterile field.

Principle. Instruments and supplies can be located quickly and efficiently on a neat and orderly sterile field. Sterile gloves must be used to prevent contamination of the sterile articles.

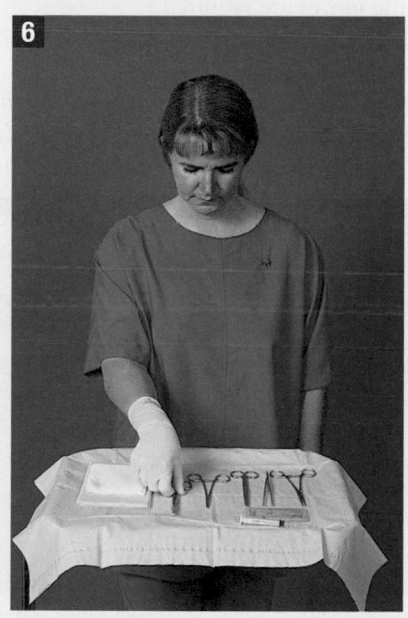

Arrange the articles neatly on the sterile field.

7. Procedural Step. Cover the tray setup with a sterile towel by picking up the towel by two corner ends and placing it gently and slowly over the setup. Do not allow your arms to pass over the sterile field as you lay it down.

Principle. The towel prevents the sterile tray from becoming contaminated. The towel must be picked up by the corner ends to prevent contaminating it and

should be moved slowly and not fanned through the air to prevent airborne contamination. Passing the arms over the sterile field results in contamination of the field.

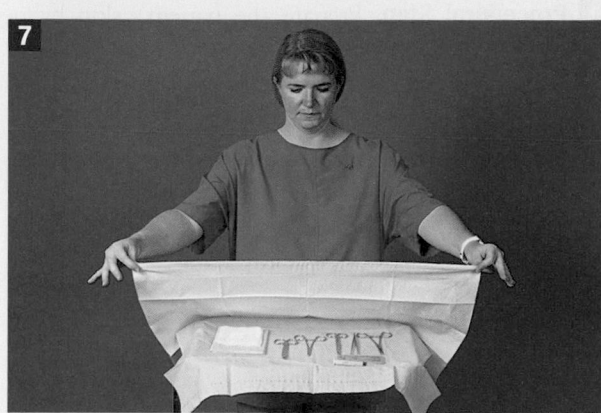

Cover the tray setup with a sterile towel.

Preparing the Patient

8. Procedural Step. Greet the patient and introduce yourself. Identify the patient by full name and date of birth. Explain the procedure, and prepare the patient for the minor office surgery as outlined below:

a. Try to allay the patient's fear or anxiety.

b. Ask the patient whether he or she needs to void before the surgery.

c. Provide instructions to the patient about any clothing that must be removed and putting on an examination gown, if required. Enough clothing must be removed to expose the operative area completely and to avoid getting the antiseptic or blood on the patient's clothing.

d. Instruct the patient not to move during the procedure and not to talk, laugh, sneeze, or cough over the sterile field.

Principle. Minor office surgery is often a frightening experience for the patient, and reassurance should be offered to reduce apprehension. The amount of clothing that must be removed depends on the type of minor office surgery being performed. By moving, the patient may accidentally contaminate the sterile field or touch the operative site. Microorganisms are carried in water vapor from the mouth, nose, and lungs and can be transferred onto the sterile field.

9. Procedural Step. Position the patient. The position is determined by the type of minor office surgery to be performed. The patient is positioned in such a way as to provide the best possible exposure and accessibility to the operative site. *NOTE:* If a difficult position must be maintained, such as the knee-chest position, the

Continued

PROCEDURE 25-7

patient should not be positioned until the physician is ready to begin the minor office surgery.

10. Procedural Step. Adjust the light so that it is focused on the operative site.

11. Procedural Step. Prepare the patient's skin by performing the following:

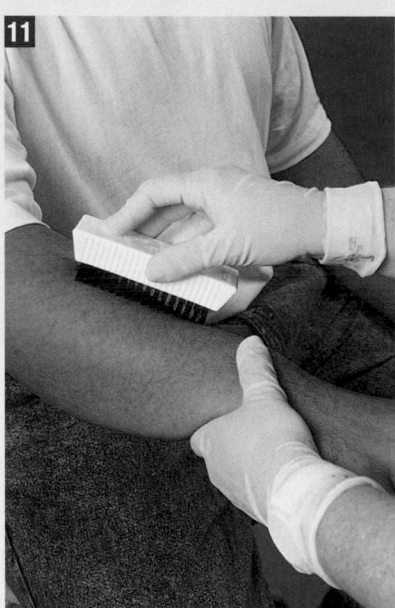

Cleanse the patient's skin with an antiseptic solution.

a. Apply clean disposable gloves.

b. If hair is present, the skin at and around the operative site may need to be shaved. The skin should be pulled taut as it is shaved. The area is rinsed and dried thoroughly.

c. Cleanse the patient's skin with an antiseptic solution and a surgical scrub brush using a firm, circular motion and moving from the inside outward. Do not return to an area just cleansed. The area is rinsed using gauze pads saturated with water and blotted dry with a sterile gauze pad.

d. Apply an antiseptic to the site using antiseptic swabs such as Betadine. Allow the skin to dry. Alternatively, the physician may place a fenestrated drape over the operative site and then apply the antiseptic.

e. Remove the gloves, and sanitize your hands.

12. Procedural Step. Verify that everything is prepared for the minor office surgery, and inform the physician that the patient is ready.

Assisting the Physician

13. Procedural Step. Assist the physician as required during the minor office surgery, following the principles of surgical asepsis. The physician drapes the

patient, injects the local anesthetic, and performs the surgery. The responsibilities of the medical assistant may include the following:

a. Uncover the sterile tray setup by picking up the sterile towel covering it. The towel should be picked up by two corner ends and removed slowly and gently without allowing the arms to pass over the sterile field.

b. Open the outer glove wrapper for the physician to facilitate the application of sterile gloves.

c. Withdraw the local anesthetic into a syringe and hand it to the physician, or hold the vial while the physician withdraws the local anesthetic. If lidocaine (Xylocaine) is used, the physician or medical assistant should inform the patient to expect a brief burning or stinging sensation as it is injected into the tissues.

d. Adjust the light as needed by the physician for good visualization of the operative site.

e. Restrain patients such as children.

f. Relax and reassure the patient during the minor office surgery.

g. Hand instruments and supplies to the physician. (Sterile gloves are required.)

h. Keep the sterile field neat and orderly. (Sterile gloves are required.)

i. Hold a basin in which the physician can deposit soiled instruments and supplies, such as hemostats and gauze sponges. (Clean gloves are required.)

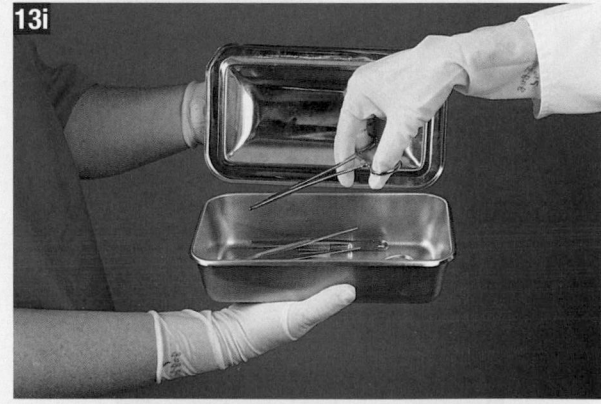

Hold a basin for the physician to deposit soiled instruments.

j. Retract tissue from an area to allow the physician the best access to and visibility of the operative site. (Sterile gloves are required.)

k. Sponge blood from the operative site. (Sterile gloves are required.)

l. Add instruments and supplies to the sterile field as required by the physician.

PROCEDURE 25-7 Assisting with Minor Office Surgery—cont'd

m. Hold the specimen container to accept a tissue specimen received from the physician. (Clean gloves are required.) Do not touch the inside of the container because it is sterile. After the physician inserts the specimen, replace the container lid and close it tightly.

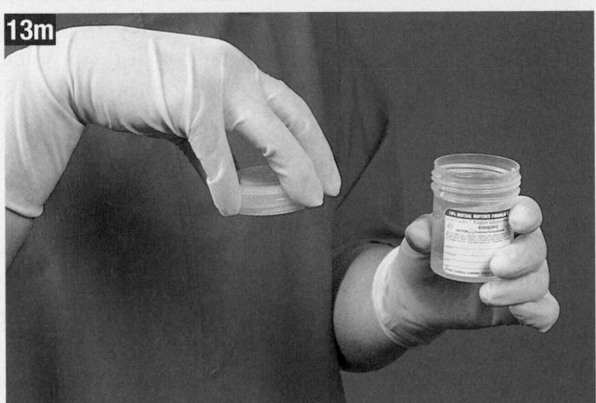

13m

Hold the container to accept a tissue specimen.

n. After the physician has inserted a suture, cut the ends of the suture material approximately ⅛ inch above the knot of the suture. (Sterile gloves are required.)

14. Procedural Step. Apply a sterile dressing to the surgical wound, if ordered by the physician (see Procedure 25-4).

Principle. The sterile dressing protects the wound from contamination and injury and absorbs drainage.

15. Procedural Step. After the surgery, perform the following:

a. Stay with the patient as a safety precaution and to assist and instruct the patient.

b. Ensure that postoperative instructions regarding any type of medical care to be administered at home are understood. If the patient has a wound or if sutures have been inserted, he or she should be told to keep the area clean and dry and to report any signs of infection, such as excessive redness, swelling, discharge, or increased pain. Provide the patient with written wound care instructions (see the patient teaching box on wound care in this chapter). Ask the patient if he or she has any questions. Have the patient sign the instruction sheet. Witness the patient's signature. Before the patient leaves the office, make a copy of the instruction sheet. Give a copy to the patient and file the original in the patient's chart.

c. Relay information regarding the return visit for postoperative care, such as the removal of sutures or a dressing change.

d. Help the patient off the table to prevent falls.

e. Instruct the patient to get dressed, offering assistance if needed.

f. Any instructions or information given must be charted in the patient's medical record.

Principle. The patient (especially an elderly one) may become dizzy after the minor office surgery and may fall when getting off the examining table. The filed copy protects the physician legally, in the event that the patient fails to follow instructions and causes harm or damage to the operative site.

16. Procedural Step. If a specimen was collected, it must be transferred to the laboratory in a tightly closed, properly labeled specimen container. Prepare the specimen for transport. Complete a biopsy request form to accompany the specimen. Place the specimen container in a biohazard specimen bag and seal it. Insert the biopsy request in the outer pocket of the bag and tuck the requisition under the flap. Place the bag in the appropriate location for pickup by the laboratory. Record information in the patient's chart, including the date the specimen was picked up or sent to the laboratory and the name of the laboratory.

Principle. Recording information regarding transport of the specimen documents that the specimen was sent to the laboratory.

17. Procedural Step. Clean the examining room. Handle the instruments carefully so as not to damage them. Be especially careful with sharp instruments to prevent cutting yourself. Blood and body secretions should be rinsed off the instruments immediately to prevent them from drying and hardening. The instruments must be sanitized and sterilized when it is convenient to do so; follow the procedures presented in Chapter 18. Discard disposable articles contaminated with blood or other potentially infectious materials in a biohazard waste container.

Principle. Surgical instruments are expensive and must be handled carefully to prolong their life span. Hardened blood and secretions on an instrument are difficult to remove. Disposable articles must be discarded in an appropriate manner to prevent the spread of infection.

CHARTING EXAMPLE

Date	
9/25/XX	2:00 p.m. Applied DSD to Ⓡ post forearm.
	Instructed patient on suture care. Written
	instructions provided. Signed copy filed in
	chart. To return in 5 days for removal of
	sutures. Sebaceous cyst specimen sent to
	Medical Center Laboratory for biopsy on
	9/25/XX. ——— T. Browning, CMA (AAMA)

PROCEDURE 25-7

MEDICAL OFFICE SURGICAL PROCEDURES

The most common surgical procedures performed in the medical office are presented on the following pages. A discussion of the procedure and the items required for each tray setup are included. The medical assistant should take into account, however, that the instruments and supplies may vary slightly from those listed here, based on the physician's preference.

Sebaceous Cyst Removal

A **sebaceous cyst** (also known as an epidermal cyst) is a thin, closed sac or capsule located just under the surface of the skin. A sebaceous cyst forms when the outlet of a sebaceous (oil) gland becomes obstructed. The cyst contains *sebum,* which is made up of secretions from the sebaceous gland. The built-up secretion of sebum causes swelling, and the lining of the cyst consists of the stretched sebaceous gland. A sebaceous cyst is usually white or yellow in appearance and varies in size from less than ¼ inch (0.6 cm) in diameter to nearly 2 inches (5 cm) in diameter. It is usually a movable, dome-shaped mass with a smooth surface that is filled with a thick, fatty-white, cheesy material that has a foul odor. This type of cyst can occur anywhere on the body except on the palms of the hands and the soles of the feet—these areas do not contain sebaceous glands. Sebaceous cysts tend to occur most frequently on the scalp, face (Figure 25-18), ears, neck, back, and genital area.

A sebaceous cyst is usually slow-growing, painless, and nontender and may disappear on its own. A sebaceous cyst usually does not require surgical removal unless it becomes infected. An infected cyst is painful, tender, red, and swollen and may have a grayish-white, foul-smelling discharge. Because it is difficult to remove an infected sebaceous cyst, the physician usually drains the cyst and allows it to heal and

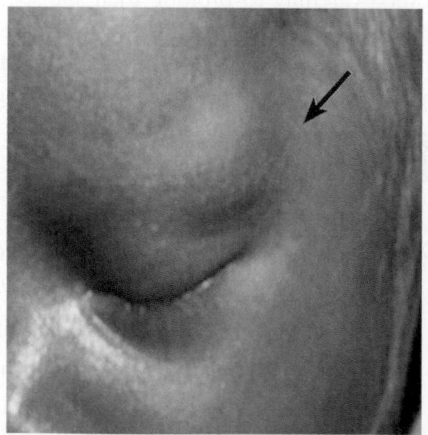

Figure 25-18 Sebaceous cyst.

then performs the cyst excision at a later time. Other reasons for removing a sebaceous cyst include cosmetic concerns and the need to reduce discomfort from a cyst that is located in a body area that is easily irritated, such as the armpit.

Surgical excision of a sebaceous cyst is a simple procedure that involves complete removal of the sac wall and its contents. Most sebaceous cysts are benign and are not usually biopsied unless they have an unusual appearance that may indicate a more serious problem. The side tray setup presented below includes the items needed for a tissue biopsy (specimen container and laboratory request form); however, these items would not be placed on the tray if the physician determines that a biopsy of the sebaceous cyst is not warranted.

Procedure: Sebaceous Cyst Removal

A sebaceous cyst is removed as follows:
1. A local anesthetic is used to numb the area.
2. The physician makes an incision using either a single cut down the center or an oval cut on both sides of the cyst. The physician then removes the cyst and sutures the surgical incision (Figure 25-19).
3. If the cyst is to be biopsied, it is placed in a specimen container with a preservative and sent to the laboratory for examination by a pathologist.
4. A sterile dressing is applied to the operative site.

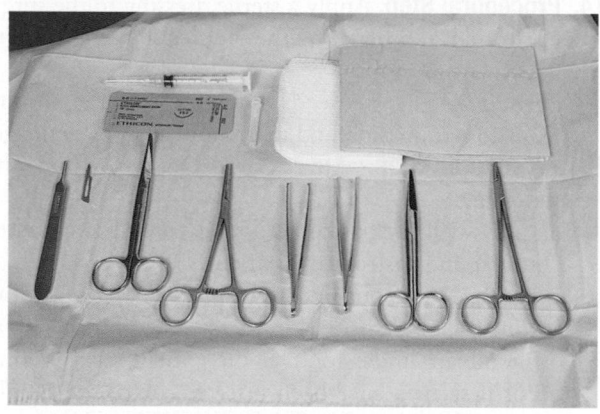

Sebaceous cyst removal sterile field.

Postoperative Instructions: Sebaceous Cyst Removal

Postoperative instructions include the following:
1. Keep the dressing clean and dry.
2. Report any signs that the wound is infected, which include fever, increased pain, swelling, redness, warmth, and discharge.
3. Notify the medical office if the sutures become loose or break.

Provide the patient with written instructions on wound care to refer to at home, and instruct the patient when to return for removal of the sutures.

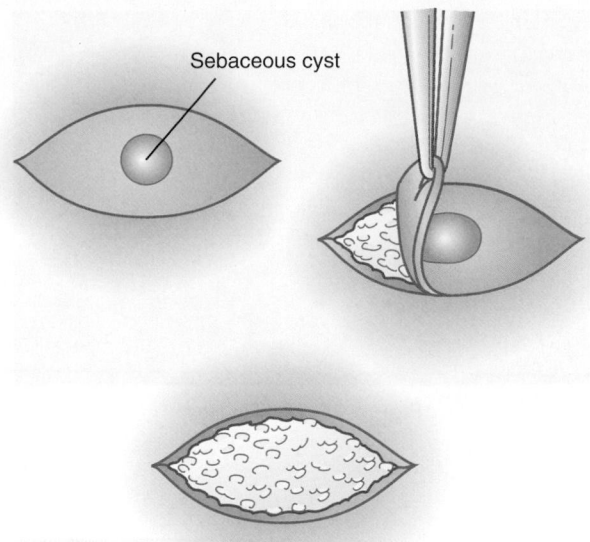

Figure 25-19 Sebaceous cyst removal. The physician makes an incision, removes the cyst, and sutures the surgical incision.

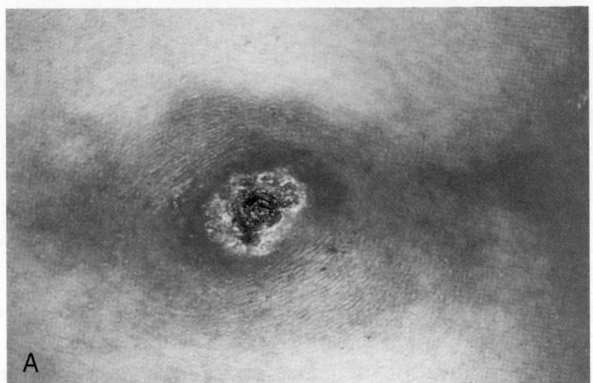

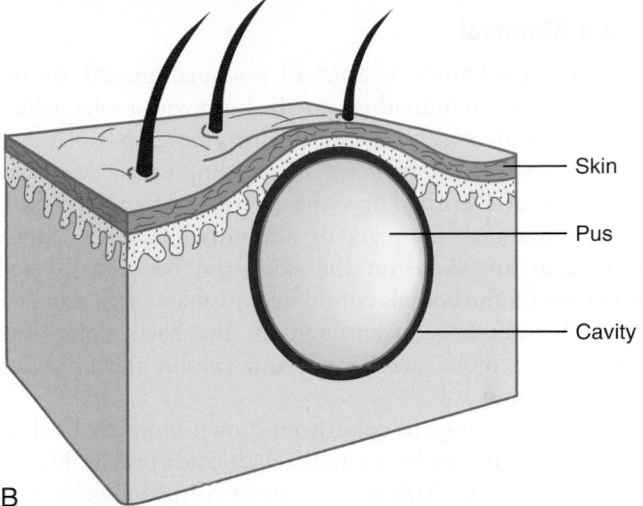

Figure 25-20 **A,** *Staphylococcus* skin abscess. **B,** An abscess is a collection of pus in a cavity surrounded by inflamed tissue.

Surgical Incision and Drainage of Localized Infections

An **abscess** is a collection of pus in a cavity surrounded by inflamed tissue (Figure 25-20, *A*). It is caused by a pathogen that invades the tissues, usually via a break in the skin. An abscess serves as a defense mechanism of the body to keep an infection localized by walling off the microorganisms, preventing them from spreading through the body (Figure 25-20, *B*). A **furuncle,** also known as a *boil,* is a localized staphylococcal infection that originates deep within a hair follicle (Figure 25-21). Furuncles produce pain and itching. The skin initially becomes red and then turns white and necrotic over the top of the furuncle. Erythema and induration usually surround it.

Procedure: Incision and Drainage

Localized infections, such as abscesses, furuncles, and infected sebaceous cysts, that do not rupture and drain naturally may need to be incised and drained by the physician as follows:

1. A local anesthetic is generally used for the procedure.
2. A scalpel is used to make the incision. The physician then allows the pus to drain out using gauze to absorb pus and blood. Either gauze packing or a rubber Penrose drain is inserted into the wound to keep the edges of the tissues apart; this facilitates drainage of the exudate. The exudate contains pathogenic microorganisms; the medical assistant should be careful to avoid contact with the exudate while assisting with the minor surgery.

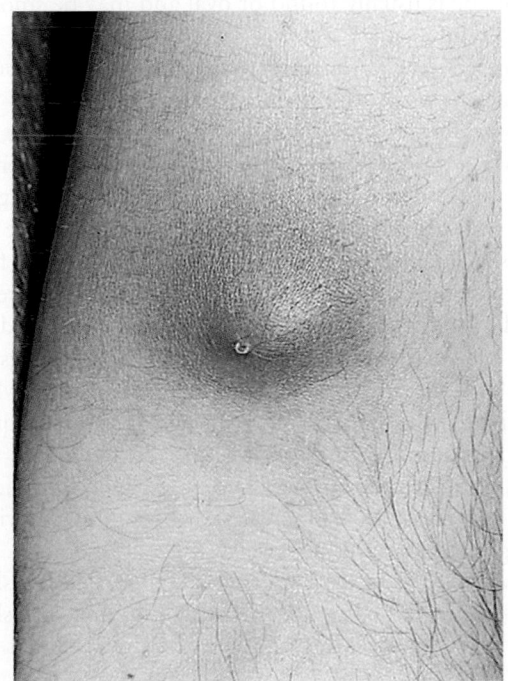

Figure 25-21 Furuncle resulting from a *Staphylococcus aureus* infection.

3. A sterile dressing of several thicknesses is applied over the operative site to absorb the drainage.

Postoperative Instructions: Incision and Drainage

Postoperative instructions include the following:

1. Keep the dressing clean and dry.
2. Report any signs that the wound is infected, which include fever, increased pain, swelling, redness, warmth, and discharge.

Provide the patient with written instructions on wound care to refer to at home, and instruct the patient when to return for removal of the gauze packing or Penrose drain.

Mole Removal

A mole (also known as a *nevus*) is a small growth on the human skin. An individual may be born with moles, which are known as *congenital nevi*, but may develop moles over time, known as *acquired nevi*. According to the American Academy of Dermatology, the majority of moles appear during the first 20 years of an individual's life. Moles can occur anywhere on the skin, and between 10 and 40 moles on the body is considered normal. Large numbers of moles can be concentrated on the back, chest, and arms. Most moles are benign and exhibit the following characteristics:

- Usually range in color from brown to nearly black in color but can be a pinkish flesh color to dark blue or even black. Dark-colored moles consist of a cluster of melanocytes. Melanocytes produce the pigment *melanin,* which is responsible for the dark color of moles.
- Shape is usually round or oval and may be smooth or rough.
- Size is usually smaller than a pencil eraser but can range from barely visible to quite a large area.
- May form a raised area on the skin or may be flat
- May sometimes have hairs growing out of them

The most common types of moles are skin tags, flat moles, and raised moles. *Skin tags* or *acrochordon* are small, painless, benign growths that project from the skin from a small narrow stalk known as a *peduncle.* They are flesh colored or slightly darker, often appear in groups, and range from 1 mm to 5 mm in size (Figure 25-22). Skin tags occur most often during and after middle age in adults who are overweight or have diabetes. Skin tags are most frequently found in body areas where the skin creases, such as the eyelids, neck, armpits, upper chest, and groin. Occasionally, a skin tag becomes irritated as the result of shaving or rubbing from clothing or jewelry.

A *flat mole* is any dark spot or irregularity in the skin. A *raised mole,* as the name implies, extends above the skin. It can be a variety of colors and runs deeper than flat moles (Figure 25-23).

Although most moles are benign, some moles may be precancerous and are known as *dysplastic nevi* (Figure 25-24). Dysplastic nevi are usually larger than normal moles and

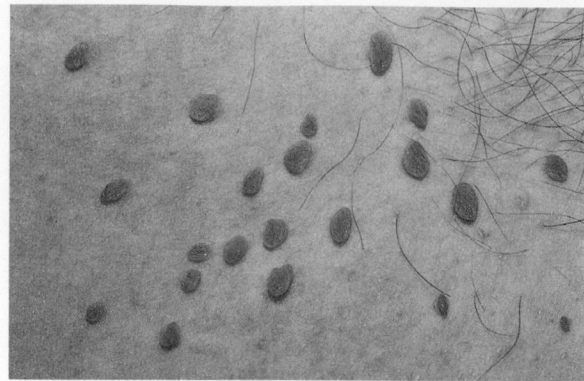

Figure 25-22 Skin tags.

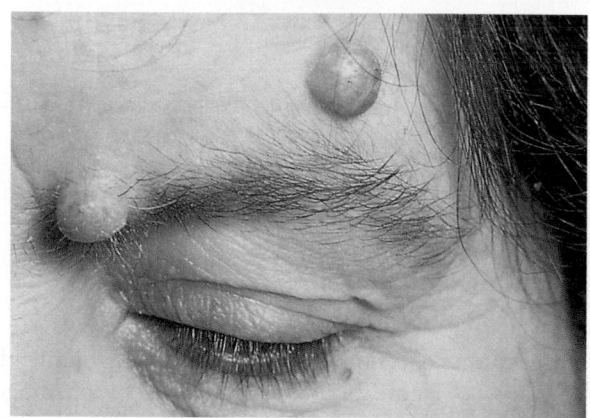

Figure 25-23 Raised moles.

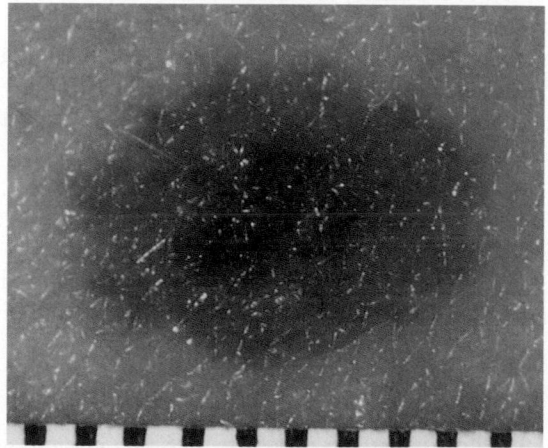

Figure 25-24 Dysplastic nevi.

have an irregular coloration and shape. The center of dysplastic nevi may be raised and darkened. According to the National Cancer Institute, dysplastic nevi are more likely than ordinary moles to develop into malignant melanoma. Because of this, dysplastic nevi are often biopsied or removed and biopsied to determine whether they are malignant.

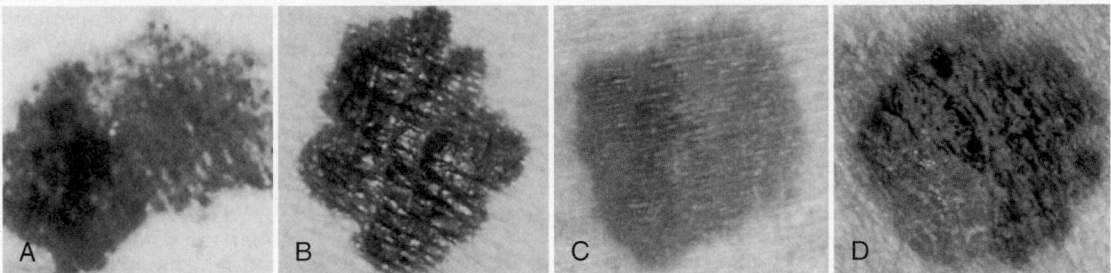

Figure 25-25 The ABCDs of melanoma. A: Asymmetry (one half unlike the other half). B: Border (edges of mole are notched, uneven, or blurred). C: Color varied from one area to another; shades of tan, brown, and black, and sometimes white, red, or blue. D: Diameter larger than ¼ inch or 6 mm (diameter of a pencil eraser).

Melanoma is a very serious type of skin cancer that can sometimes develop within a mole. Melanoma is most apt to be found on the upper backs of men and on the lower legs of women. Studies show that excessive sun exposure, especially severe blistering sunburns early in life, increase the risk of developing certain melanomas. If discovered early, it may be possible to completely remove the melanoma and reduce the spread of skin cancer. Left untreated, melanoma can be fatal.

Any moles exhibiting the following characteristics common to melanoma (Figure 25-25) should be evaluated by a physician:

- Asymmetric: one half of the mole is different from the other half.
- Irregular border: the edges of the mole are notched, uneven, or blurred rather than round or distinct.
- Color varies from one area of the mole to another: various shades of tan, brown, and black (and sometimes white, red, or blue) are present.
- Diameter is larger than ¼ inch (6 mm), which is about the diameter of a pencil eraser.
- Other signs: the mole is painful or tender, itches, bleeds, oozes, or has a scaly appearance.

Moles are removed for a variety of reasons, which include the following: cosmetic (to improve an individual's appearance), and to reduce irritation and discomfort from a mole that is rubbing against clothing or that is in the way when shaving. A more serious reason for removing a mole is that the mole is suspected of being precancerous (dysplastic nevus) or cancerous (melanoma). Several methods may be used for mole removal. The most common methods include shave excision, surgical excision, and laser surgery. The method used depends on the type of mole being removed, including its size, shape and color, and location. In some cases, a biopsy of the mole is taken before the mole is removed to determine whether the mole is benign or malignant.

Procedure: Mole Shave Excision

A shave excision is most commonly used to remove protruding moles. It can also be used to remove skin tags. This procedure is not used to remove dysplastic nevi because it might leave mole cells beneath the surface of the skin, which could cause the mole to grow back again. Sutures are not generally required for a shave excision. After the numbing effect of the anesthetic wears off, the area will be tender and sore. As healing occurs, a scab forms, which usually falls off within 1 to 2 weeks, leaving a red mark. As healing progresses, a flat, white mark usually remains in the place of the mole, which is approximately the same size as the mole. Over time, it fades to a barely visible scar. A mole is removed using the shave excision procedure as follows:

1. The physician numbs the area with a local anesthetic.
2. The physician uses a scalpel to shave off the protruding part of the mole until the area is flush with the level of the surrounding skin.
3. The physician may use an electrocautery instrument to destroy the tissue below the surface of the mole and to control bleeding.
4. A topical antibiotic is applied to the area.
5. A sterile dressing is applied to the operative site.
6. The mole shavings may be placed in a specimen container with a preservative and sent to the laboratory for examination by a pathologist.

Procedure: Surgical Mole Excision

The surgical excision procedure is often used when the physician suspects that a mole is precancerous or cancerous. A scalpel is used to remove the entire mole, as well as a border of surrounding skin and tissue underlying the mole, to remove all the mole cells. A scar commonly forms after this procedure; however, it usually fades over time. A mole is removed using the surgical excision procedure as follows:

1. The physician numbs the area with a local anesthetic.
2. The physician uses a scalpel to cut an oval border surrounding the mole and removes the mole with tissue forceps.
3. The physician may use an electrocautery instrument to control bleeding.
4. The physician inserts sutures to close the surgical incision.
5. A sterile dressing is applied to the operative site.

6. The mole is placed in a specimen container with a preservative and is sent to the laboratory for examination by a pathologist.

Postoperative Instructions: Shave Excision and Surgical Excision

Postoperative instructions for both a shave excision and a surgical excision of a mole include the following:
1. Keep the dressing clean and dry.
2. Report any signs that the wound is infected, which include fever, increased pain, swelling, redness, warmth, and discharge.
3. If sutures have been inserted, notify the medical office if they become loose or break.
4. To reduce scarring, protect the area from the ultraviolet (UV) rays of the sun by staying out of the sun or using a good sunscreen with a sun protection factor (SPF) of 15 or higher.
5. Provide the patient with written instructions on wound care to refer to at home. If sutures have been inserted, instruct the patient when to return for removal of the sutures.

Laser Mole Surgery

Laser surgery is used to remove small or flat moles that are brown or black in color. This procedure involves the use of a laser beam of light, which evaporates the mole tissue. The laser beam also seals off blood vessels, which avoids the need for sutures. Because the laser light cannot penetrate deeply enough, this method generally is not used on raised moles, deep moles, large moles, or dysplastic nevi.

Removing a mole with a laser reduces the amount of tissue destruction in the surrounding tissue, which minimizes scarring. This procedure does not require a local anesthetic. No pain is involved during the procedure; the patient feels only a mild tingling when the laser pulses. A scab forms, which usually falls off within 1 to 2 weeks. Once the scab falls off, the area is usually reddish, and it may take several weeks before normal skin color returns. Repeated treatments (one to three) may be required before the mole is completely removed.

The medical assistant should instruct the patient to keep the area clean and dry. The area should also be protected from the UV rays of the sun by staying out of the sun or by using a good sunscreen with an SPF of 15 or higher.

Needle Biopsy

A **biopsy** is the removal and examination of tissue from the living body. The tissue usually is examined under a microscope. Biopsies are most often performed to determine whether a tumor is malignant or benign; however, a biopsy also may be used as a diagnostic aid for other conditions, such as infections. A **needle biopsy** is a type of biopsy in which tissue from deep within the body is obtained by the insertion of a biopsy needle through the skin. The

advantage of a needle biopsy is that a sample of tissue can be obtained that might otherwise require a major surgical operation.

Procedure: Needle Biopsy
1. The procedure is performed with the patient under a local anesthetic, and because an incision is not required, the patient does not have to undergo the discomfort and inconvenience of an operative recovery.
2. The tissue specimen is placed in a container with a preservative and is sent to the laboratory for examination by a pathologist.
3. A small dressing, placed over the needle puncture site, is usually sufficient to protect the operative site and promote healing.
4. After the procedure, the patient should be observed for any evidence of complications related to the procedure.

Postoperative Instructions: Needle Biopsy
1. A bruise typically occurs at the biopsy site and will gradually disappear within several weeks.
2. Keep the dressing clean and dry.
3. Rest and avoid strenuous activity and heavy lifting for 2 days following the procedure.
4. Report any signs that the wound is infected, which include fever, increased pain, swelling, redness, warmth, and discharge.

Ingrown Toenail Removal

An ingrown toenail occurs when the edge of the toenail grows deeply into the nail groove and penetrates the surrounding skin, resulting in pain and discomfort to the patient (Figure 25-26, *A*). An ingrown nail can occur in both the nails of the hands and feet; however, it is most apt to occur in the toenails. External pressure, such as from tight shoes, or from trauma, improper nail trimming, or infection, can cause an ingrown toenail. The protruding nail acts as a foreign body, usually resulting in secondary infection and inflammation. In mild cases, this condition is treated by inserting a small piece of cotton packing under the toenail to raise the nail edge away from the tissue of the nail groove (Figure 25-26, *B*). In severe and recurring cases, part of the nail must be surgically removed (Figure 25-26, *C* and *D*). Severe cases cause pain, swelling, redness, and drainage (Figure 25-27). The toenail removal procedure relieves pain by decreasing nail pressure on the soft tissues.

Procedure: Ingrown Toenail
An ingrown toenail is removed as follows:
1. Before the surgical procedure is performed, the affected foot must be soaked in tepid water containing an antibacterial skin solution for 10 to 15 minutes to soften the nail plate and decrease the possibility of bacterial infection.

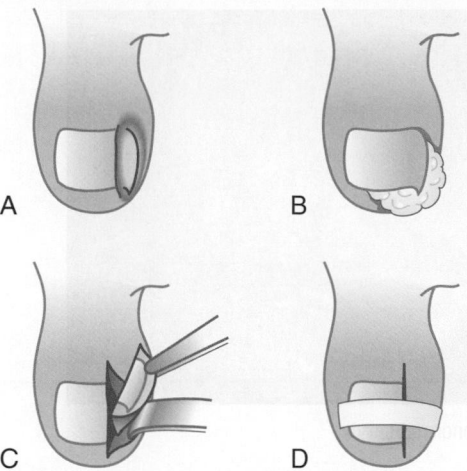

Figure 25-26 Ingrown toenail. **A,** The edge of the toenail grows deeply into the nail groove. **B,** In mild cases, treatment consists of inserting a small piece of cotton packing under the toenail. **C,** In severe and recurring cases, a wedge of the nail is surgically removed. **D,** A strip of surgical tape is applied over the area.

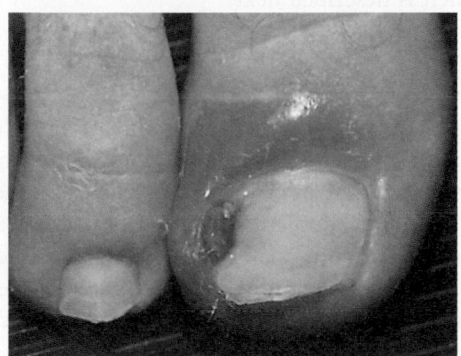

Figure 25-27 Ingrown toenail.

2. The patient is placed in a reclining position with the foot adequately supported, and the toe is shaved to remove hair, which would act as a contaminant.
3. An antiseptic is applied to the affected toe, which is then numbed using a local anesthetic.
4. Using surgical toenail scissors, the physician surgically removes a wedge of the nail (see Figure 25-26, *C*).
5. An antibiotic ointment is applied to the area.
6. A sterile gauze dressing or a strip of surgical tape is applied over the area to protect the operative site and to promote healing (see Figure 25-26, *D*).

Postoperative Instructions: Ingrown Toenail
Postoperative instructions include the following:
1. Elevate the foot for 25 hours following the procedure.
2. Keep the area clean and dry.
3. Cleanse the toe daily with warm water and gently dry the area.
4. Apply an antibiotic ointment daily until the wound has completely healed.

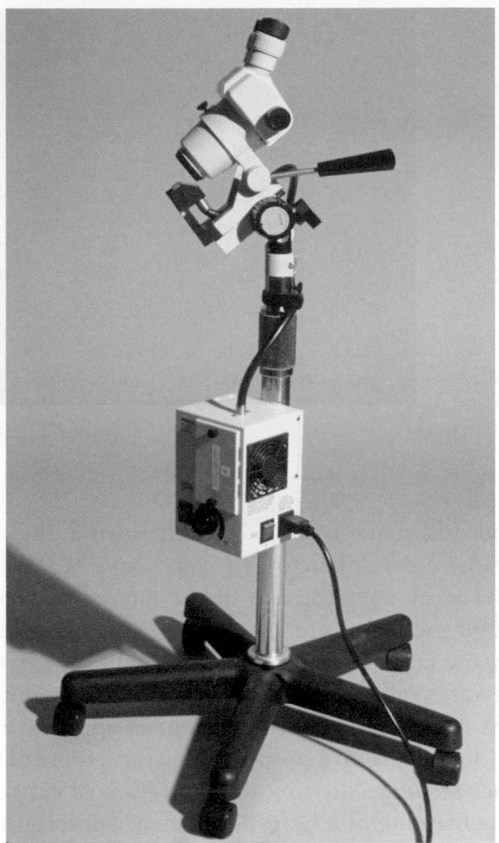

Figure 25-28 A colposcope.

5. Wear loose-fitting shoes for 2 weeks following the procedure.
6. Avoid strenuous exercise for 2 weeks following the procedure.
7. Contact the medical office if any signs of infection occur, which include increasing pain, redness, swelling, and drainage from the toe.

Provide the patient with written instructions on wound care to refer to at home, and instruct the patient on the importance of wearing properly fitting shoes and on the proper procedure for nail trimming. The nail should be cut straight across with the corners of the nail protruding from the end of the toe.

Colposcopy
Colposcopy is the visual examination of the vagina and cervix by means of a lighted instrument with a binocular magnifying lens, known as a **colposcope** (Figure 25-28). The purpose of colposcopy is to examine the vagina and cervix to detect areas of abnormal tissue growth that may not be visible with the naked eye (Figure 25-29). Colposcopy is performed following abnormal Pap test results and to evaluate a vaginal or cervical lesion observed during a pelvic examination. The primary goal of colposcopy is to prevent cervical cancer by detecting precancerous lesions early and treating them.

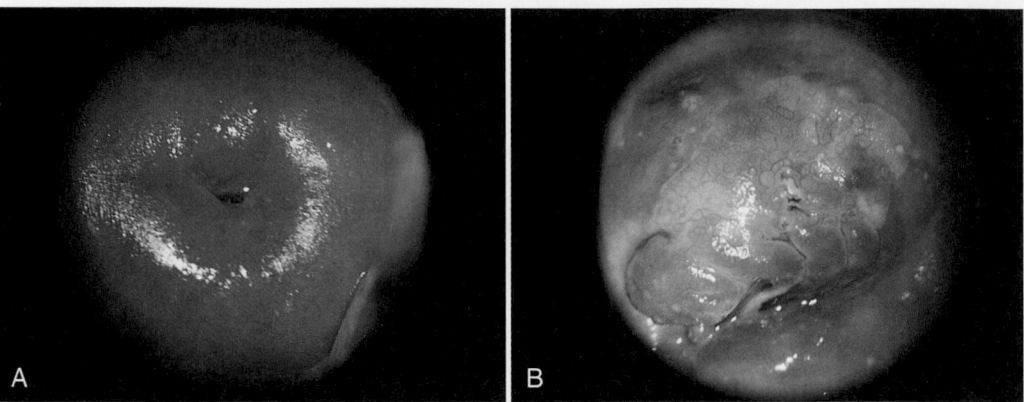

Figure 25-29 **A,** Normal cervix. **B,** Abnormal cervix.

Blood cells make it more difficult for the physician to observe the cervix; therefore, a colposcopy is usually performed 1 week after the end of the menstrual period. To prepare for the procedure, the patient should be told not to douche; use tampons, vaginal medications, or spermicides; or have intercourse for 25 hours before the examination. The lens of the colposcope is positioned approximately 12 inches (30 cm) from the opening of the vagina. The lens magnifies tissue, facilitating the inspection of cervical cells and the obtaining of a biopsy specimen. For a routine colposcopic examination, a magnification ranging from 6× to 15× is generally used. The colposcope may be placed on an adjustable stand or attached to the side of the examining table and swung out before use.

Procedure: Colposcopy
Colposcopy is performed as follows:
1. The patient is assisted into a lithotomy position and is prepared as for a pelvic examination.
2. The physician inserts a vaginal speculum into the vagina.
3. A long, cotton-tipped applicator moistened with saline is used to wipe the cervix to remove the mucous film that normally covers it. The saline also provides better visualization of the cervical epithelium because dry cervical epithelium is not transparent and does not allow satisfactory viewing of the vascular pattern of the cervix.
4. The colposcope is focused on the cervix, and the physician inspects the saline-moistened cervix.
5. The cervix is swabbed with acetic acid, using a long, cotton-tipped applicator. The acetic acid dissolves cervical mucus and other secretions. It also causes abnormal tissue to turn white, which allows easier visualization of abnormal areas of the cervix.
6. The cervical epithelium also may be stained with Lugol iodine solution using a long, cotton-tipped applicator. This provides another means to identify unhealthy epithelium. The healthy epithelium of the cervix contains glycogen, which is able to absorb the iodine, causing the epithelium to stain a dark brown

color. Conversely, abnormal epithelium, such as would constitute a malignancy, does not contain glycogen and is unable to absorb the iodine.
7. If an abnormal area is observed, the physician obtains a cervical biopsy specimen using punch biopsy forceps, which is described next.

Cervical Punch Biopsy
A cervical biopsy is performed in combination with colposcopy to remove a cervical tissue specimen for examination by a pathologist. The purpose of the biopsy is to detect the presence of cervical dysplasia or cancer of the cervix. *Cervical dysplasia* is an abnormal growth of cells on the surface of the cervix that are precancerous. *Precancerous* means that abnormal cells have the potential to develop into cancer in the future. Cervical dysplasia can range from mild, to moderate, to severe. A cervical punch biopsy can also be used to diagnose polyps on the cervix and genital warts. Genital warts may indicate infection with human papillomavirus (HPV), which is a risk factor for developing cervical cancer. Performing a cervical punch biopsy helps the physician determine the type of abnormal tissue present on the cervix, so that the physician can determine the best form of treatment for the patient's condition.

Cervical biopsies are most frequently performed following abnormal Pap test results. Although an abnormal Pap test result is a cause for concern, the majority of abnormal Pap tests are not caused by cervical cancer, but rather by a vaginal infection. To prevent inaccurate test results, the cervical biopsy is usually performed 1 week after the end of the menstrual period, when the cervix is the least vascular. To prepare for the procedure, the patient should be told not to douche; use tampons, vaginal medications, or spermicides; or have intercourse for 25 hours before the procedure to prevent inaccurate test results.

Procedure: Cervical Punch Biopsy
A cervical punch biopsy is performed as follows:
1. The patient is positioned and draped in a lithotomy position. An anesthetic is not needed because the

cervix has few pain receptors. The patient may experience no discomfort during the procedure or a certain amount of discomfort ranging from mild to moderate in intensity. Some patients experience mild cramping and pinching when the specimen is being removed from the cervix.

2. The physician inserts a vaginal speculum into the vagina for proper visualization of the cervix.

3. The cervix is wiped with saline and then swabbed with ascetic acid.
4. To assist in obtaining the specimen, the physician may stain the cervix with Lugol iodine solution.
5. The colposcope is focused on the cervix, and the physician inspects the cervix.
6. Using cervical biopsy punch forceps, the physician obtains several tissue specimens (Figure 25-30, *A*) from the abnormal cervical epithelium (Figure 25-30, *B*). The patient may feel a pinching sensation and mild cramps each time a specimen is removed from the cervix.
7. The specimen is placed in a container with a preservative and is sent to the laboratory for examination by a pathologist.
8. If bleeding occurs, the physician controls it with gauze packing, a hemostatic solution (e.g., Monsel solution), or electrocautery.
9. The patient is given a sanitary pad at the office after the procedure to absorb any discharge.

Postoperative Instructions: Cervical Punch Biopsy
Postoperative instructions include the following:
A minimum amount of cramping and bleeding may follow the procedure and last up to 1 week. Contact the medical office if the bleeding lasts longer than 2 weeks.

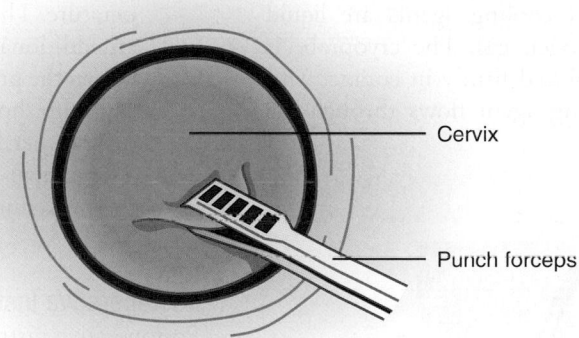

A

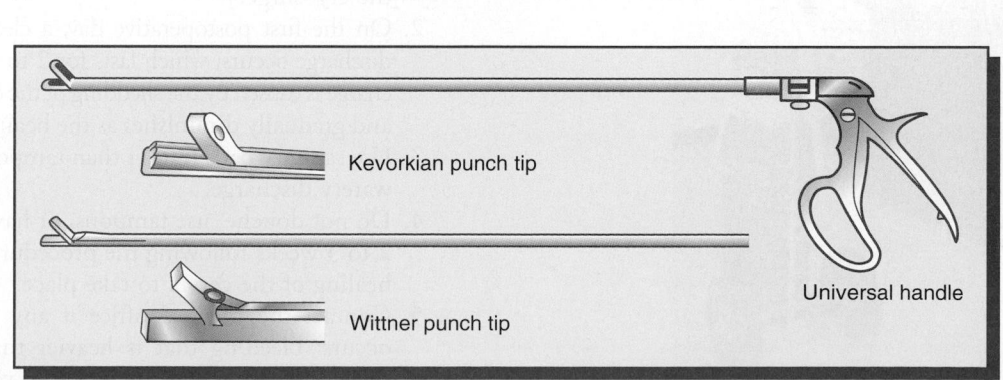

B

Figure 25-30 Cervical punch biopsy. **A,** Obtaining a tissue specimen from the cervix using cervical biopsy punch forceps. **B,** Cervical biopsy punch forceps.

If Monsel solution is used to control bleeding, a thick, dark-colored vaginal discharge may occur following the procedure and may last for several days.

Do not douche, use tampons, or have intercourse for 1 week following the procedure to allow proper healing of the cervix to take place.

Contact the medical office if any of the following occurs: bleeding that is heavier than normal menstrual bleeding, a foul-smelling vaginal discharge, fever, or lower abdominal pain.

Provide the patient with written instructions to refer to at home. An appointment is scheduled approximately 1 week following the procedure to make sure that healing is taking place and to discuss the biopsy results.

Cryosurgery

Cervical Cryosurgery

Cervical **cryosurgery,** also known as *cryotherapy,* uses freezing temperatures to treat certain gynecologic conditions. Cryosurgery is most often performed as a treatment for cervical dysplasia to destroy abnormal cervical cells that show changes that may lead to cancer. Cryosurgery is done only after a colposcopy confirms the presence of cervical dysplasia. Cryosurgery is also used for the treatment of chronic cervicitis, which is inflammation of the cervix.

Cervical cryosurgery can be performed without an anesthetic, although occasionally a mild analgesic is necessary immediately afterward. The cryosurgery unit consists of a long metal cryoprobe attached to a cooling-agent tank (Figure 25-31). The principal cooling agents are liquid nitrogen and compressed nitrogen gas. The cryoprobe is inserted into the vagina and placed firmly in contact with the abnormal area. The cooling agent flows through the

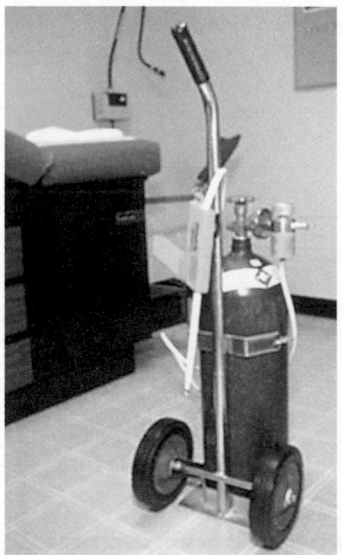

Figure 25-31 Cryosurgery unit.

cryoprobe, freezing the cervical tissue to −20° C. This causes the abnormal cells to die and slough off so that the cervical covering can eventually be replaced with new, healthy epithelial tissue. Regeneration of cervical tissue occurs within approximately 4 to 6 weeks after the procedure. Following cryosurgery, the patient will be required to have a Pap test every 3 to 6 months for a period of time determined by the physician.

Procedure: Cervical Cryosurgery

Cryosurgery is performed as follows:
1. The patient is draped and assisted into the lithotomy position.
2. The physician inserts a vaginal speculum for proper visualization of the cervix.
3. The cervix is swabbed with an acid-saline solution to remove mucus and other contaminants.
4. The metal cryoprobe is inserted into the vagina and placed firmly in contact with the affected area, and the cryosurgery unit is turned on.
5. The cooling agent flows through the cryoprobe and causes the metal probe to freeze and destroy superficial abnormal cervical tissue. The physician allows the cryoprobe to come in contact with the cervical area for approximately 3 minutes. During the procedure, the patient may experience some pain resembling menstrual cramping.
6. The cryoprobe is removed for 3 to 5 minutes to permit the cervical tissue to return to its normal temperature. The freezing procedure is then repeated for an additional 3 minutes.
7. When the procedure has been completed, the medical assistant should assist the patient as necessary and observe her for signs of discomfort or vertigo.
8. The patient is given a sanitary pad at the office after the procedure to absorb any discharge.

Postoperative Instructions: Cervical Cryosurgery

Postoperative instructions include the following:
1. Normal activities can be resumed the day following the cryosurgery.
2. On the first postoperative day, a clear, watery vaginal discharge occurs, which lasts for 2 to 4 weeks. The discharge is caused by the shedding of the dead cervical tissue and gradually diminishes as the healing progresses.
3. Use sanitary pads (rather than tampons) to absorb the watery discharge.
4. Do not douche, use tampons, or have intercourse for 2 to 3 weeks following the procedure to allow proper healing of the cervix to take place.
5. Contact the medical office if any of the following occurs: bleeding that is heavier than normal menstrual bleeding, a foul-smelling vaginal discharge, fever, or lower abdominal pain.

Provide the patient with written instructions to refer to at home. The patient must schedule a return visit 6 weeks after the procedure to ensure that proper healing has occurred.

Skin Lesions

In the medical office, cryosurgery also may be used to remove benign skin lesions, such as common warts and skin tags. Only a small amount of cooling agent is required for skin lesions, so the cryosurgery unit is considerably smaller than the one described for cervical cryosurgery. Most physicians use liquid nitrogen contained in a small, pressurized, stainless steel canister with an attached probe. The physician applies the liquid nitrogen to the skin lesion until it turns white, which indicates that freezing of the tissue has occurred. During the procedure, the patient feels a slight burning or stinging sensation as the cooling agent is applied. After cryosurgery, a blister develops and dries to a scab in 1 week to 10 days and eventually sloughs off. The patient should be told to keep the area clean and dry until the scab has sloughed off. In some cases, the treatment may not result in complete destruction of the lesion; two or more treatments may be required to remove the lesion.

BANDAGING

A **bandage** is a strip of woven material used to wrap or cover a part of the body. The function of the bandage may be to apply pressure to control bleeding, to protect a wound from contamination, to hold a dressing in place, or to protect, support, or immobilize an injured part of the body.

Guidelines for Application

The bandage should be applied so that it feels comfortable to the patient, and it must be fastened securely with metal clips or adhesive tape. Guidelines for applying a bandage are as follows:

1. Observe the principles of medical asepsis during the application of a bandage.
2. Ensure that the area to which a bandage is applied is clean and dry.
3. Do not apply a bandage directly over an open wound. To prevent contamination of the wound, apply first a sterile dressing and then the bandage. The bandage should extend at least 2 inches (5 cm) beyond the edge of the dressing.
4. To prevent irritation, do not allow the skin surfaces of two body parts (e.g., two fingers) to touch. In addition, the patient's perspiration provides a moist environment that encourages the growth of microorganisms. A piece of gauze should be inserted between the two body parts.
5. Ensure that joints and prominent parts of bones are padded to prevent the bandage from rubbing the skin and causing irritation.
6. Bandage the body part in its normal position with joints slightly flexed to avoid muscle strain.
7. Apply the bandage from the distal to the proximal part of the body to aid the venous return of blood to the heart.
8. As you apply the bandage, ask the patient whether it feels comfortable. The bandage should fit snugly enough that it does not fall off, but not so tightly that it impedes circulation.
9. If possible, leave the fingers and toes exposed when bandaging an extremity. This provides the opportunity to check them for signs of impairment in circulation. Signs indicating that the bandage is too tight include coldness, pallor, numbness, cyanosis of the nail beds, swelling, pain, and tingling sensations. If any of these signs occurs, loosen the bandage immediately.
10. If a bandage roll is dropped during the procedure, obtain a new bandage and begin again.

Types of Bandages

Three basic types of bandages are used in the medical office. A *roller bandage* is a long strip of soft material wound on itself to form a roll. It ranges from ½ to 6 inches (1.3 to 15.2 cm) wide and from 2 to 5 yards (1.83 to 4.57 m) long. The width used depends on the part being bandaged. Roller bandages usually are made of sterilized gauze. Gauze is porous and lightweight, molds easily to a body part, and is relatively inexpensive and easily disposed of. Because it is made of loosely woven cotton, however, it may slip and fray easily. *Kling gauze* is a special type of gauze that stretches; this allows it to cling, and, as a result, it molds and conforms better to the body part than does regular gauze.

Elastic bandages are made of woven cotton that contains elastic fibers. One brand name of elastic bandages is the Ace bandage. Although elastic bandages are expensive, they can be washed and used again. The medical assistant must be extremely careful when applying an elastic bandage because it is easy to apply it too tightly and impede circulation. Elastic adhesive bandages also may be used; these have an adhesive backing to provide a secure fit.

Bandage Turns

Five basic bandage turns are used, alone or in combination. The type of turn used depends on which body part is to be bandaged, and whether the bandage is used for support or immobilization or for holding a dressing in place.

The *circular turn* is applied to a part of uniform width, such as toes, fingers, or the head. Each turn completely overlaps the previous turn. Two circular turns are used to anchor a bandage at the beginning and end of a spiral, spiral-reverse, figure-eight, or recurrent turn (Figure 25-32).

The *spiral turn* is applied to a part of uniform circumference, such as the fingers, arms, legs, chest, or abdomen.

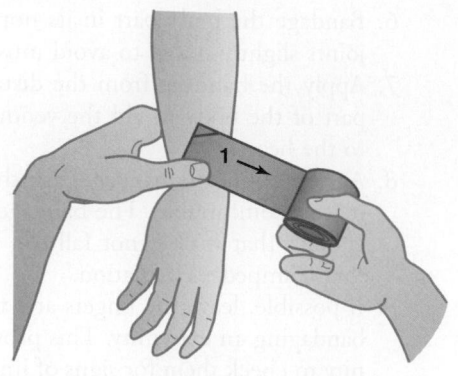

1. Place the end of the roller bandage on a slant.

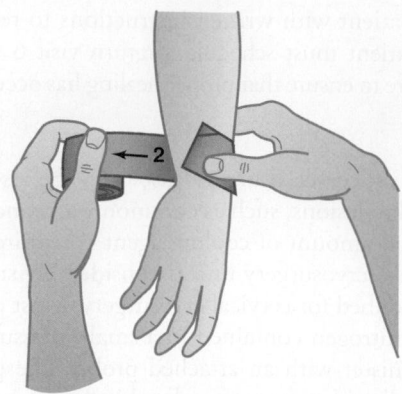

2. Encircle the part while allowing the corner of the bandage to extend.

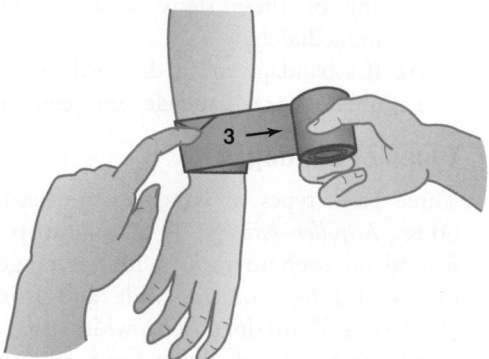

3. Turn down the corner of the bandage.

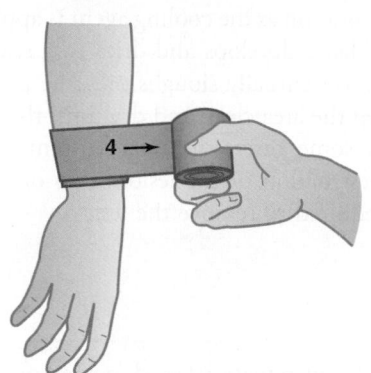

4. Make another circular turn around the part.

Figure 25-32 Procedure for anchoring a bandage.

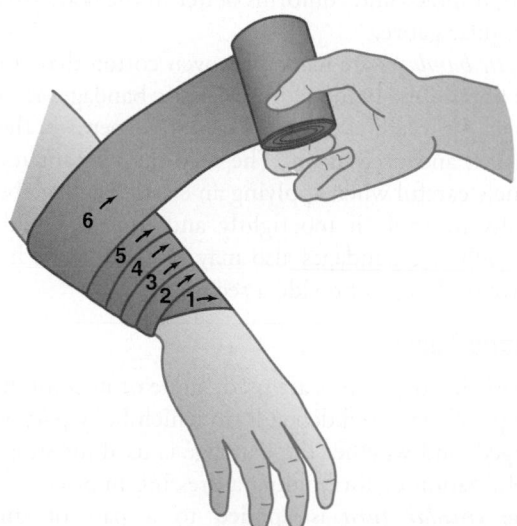

Figure 25-33 Procedure for making the spiral turn.

Each spiral turn is carried upward at a slight angle and should overlap the previous turn by one-half to two-thirds the width of the bandage (Figure 25-33).

The *spiral-reverse turn* is useful for bandaging a part that varies in width, such as the forearm or lower leg. Reversing each spiral turn allows for a smoother fit and prevents gaping caused by variation in the contour of the limb. The thumb is used to make the reverse halfway through each spiral turn. The bandage is directed downward and folded on itself while it is kept parallel to the lower edge of the previous turn. Each turn should overlap the previous one by two-thirds the width of the bandage. The reverse turn is used as often as necessary to provide a uniform fit (Figure 25-34).

The *figure-eight turn* generally is used to hold a dressing in place or to support and immobilize an injured joint, such as the ankle, knee, elbow, or wrist. The figure-eight turn consists of slanting turns that alternately ascend and descend around the part and cross over one another in the middle, resembling the figure eight. Each turn overlaps the previous one by two-thirds the width of the bandage (Figure 25-35).

The *recurrent turn* is a series of back-and-forth turns used to bandage the tips of fingers or toes, the stump of an amputated extremity, or the head. The bandage is anchored by using two circular turns and is passed back and forth over the tip of the part to be bandaged, first on one side and then on the other side of the first center turn. Each turn should overlap the previous turn by two-thirds the width of the bandage (Figure 25-36).

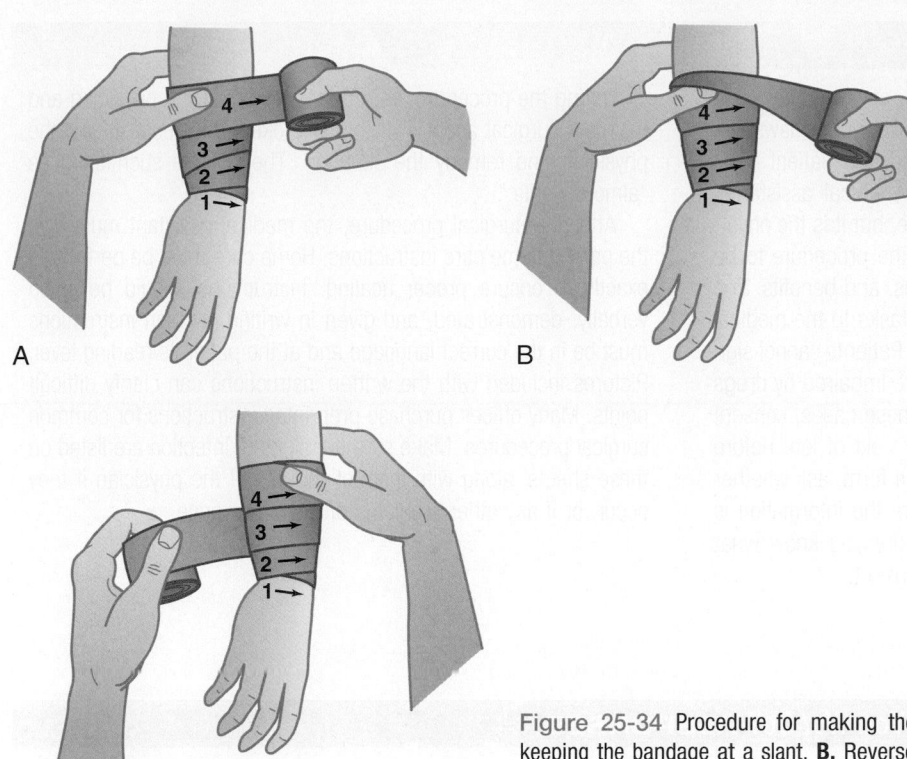

Figure 25-34 Procedure for making the spiral-reverse turn. **A,** Encircle the part while keeping the bandage at a slant. **B,** Reverse the spiral turn using the thumb or index finger, and direct the bandage downward to fold it on itself. **C,** Keep the bandage parallel to the lower edge of the previous turn.

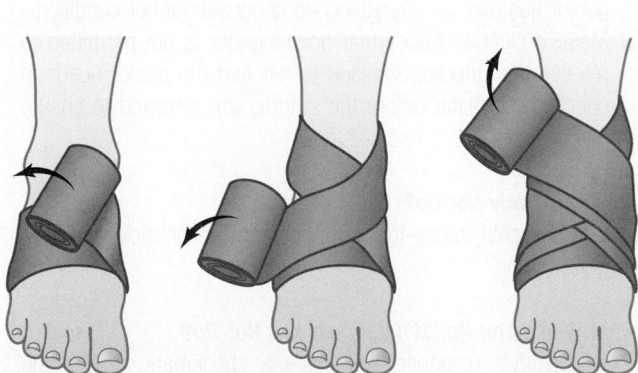

Figure 25-35 Procedure for applying an elastic bandage around the ankle using a figure-eight turn.

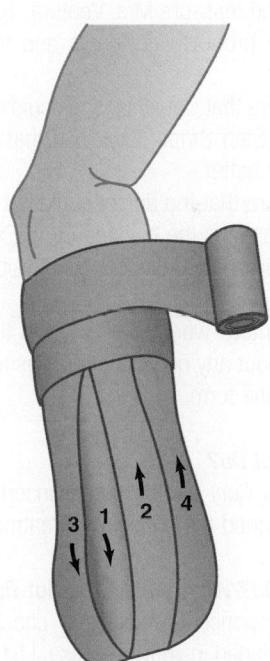

Figure 25-36 Procedure for using the recurrent turn to bandage the end of a stump.

MEDICAL PRACTICE *and the* LAW

Surgical procedures are invasive and painful, and they have the potential for harmful complications and subsequent lawsuits. Before having a surgical procedure performed, the patient must sign a consent to treatment form. It is the medical assistant's responsibility to witness the patient's signature, but it is the physician's responsibility to inform the patient of the procedure to be performed and its risks, alternative procedures, and benefits. The physician may delegate some or all of these tasks to the medical assistant, but *do not* accept this responsibility. Patients cannot sign for themselves if they are minors or if they are impaired by drugs or disease, such as Alzheimer's disease. In these cases, consent must be obtained from the legal guardian or next of kin. Before asking a patient to sign a consent to treatment form, ask whether he or she has any questions. If so, make sure the information is given before the consent is signed. Make sure you know what procedures in your office require informed consent.

During the procedure, your duty is to assist the physician and maintain surgical asepsis. If this is broken, you must inform the physician and remedy the situation. There is no such thing as "almost sterile."

After the surgical procedure, the medical assistant must give the patient home care instructions. Home care must be performed exactly to ensure proper healing. Instructions should be given verbally, demonstrated, and given in writing. Written instructions must be in the correct language and at the patient's reading level. Pictures included with the written instructions can clarify difficult points. Many offices purchase preprinted instructions for common surgical procedures. Make sure the signs of infection are listed on these sheets, along with instructions to call the physician if they occur, or if any other problems or questions arise. ■

What Would You Do? What Would You *Not* Do? RESPONSES

Case Study 1
Page 519

What Did Trudy Do?
❑ Tried to calm and reassure Mrs. Ventura. Told her that children at this age are prone to accidents and that she should not blame herself.
❑ Told Mrs. Ventura that Cory's wound could not be held together effectively with Steri-Strips. Explained that sutures would help the wound heal better.
❑ Told Mrs. Ventura that the doctor could not perform the procedure unless she signs the consent form. Explained that Cory's wound should be sutured as soon as possible to prevent infection and to minimize scarring.
❑ Asked Mrs. Ventura whether she would like to talk with the doctor again about any questions she has about the procedure before signing the form.

What Did Trudy Not Do?
❑ Did not prepare Cory for the suture insertion procedure until Mrs. Ventura signed the consent to treatment form.

What Would You Do?/What Would You Not Do?
Review Trudy's response and place a checkmark next to the information you included in your response. List additional information you included in your response.

_____
_____
_____
_____
_____
_____

Case Study 2
Page 528

What Did Trudy Do?
❑ Explained to Abbey that the antiseptic contains iodine, which appears orange when it is applied to the skin. Assured her that the iodine would not stain her skin permanently and that it would wear off in a few days.
❑ Calmly and discreetly opened a new pair of sterile gloves so that the physician could reapply sterile gloves. Reminded Abbey not to move during the procedure.
❑ Told Abbey that all tissues removed from patients are routinely sent to the laboratory for a biopsy. Reassured her that the doctor has told her everything he knows about her condition.
❑ Made it clear to Abbey that her neighbor is not permitted to remove her sutures. Stressed to her that the doctor needs to check her incision before the sutures are removed to ensure that proper healing has occurred.

What Did Trudy Not Do?
❑ Did not scold Abbey for contaminating the physician's sterile gloved hand.

What Would You Do?/What Would You Not Do?
Review Trudy's response and place a checkmark next to the information you included in your response. List additional information you included in your response.

_____
_____
_____
_____
_____

What Would You Do? What Would You *Not* Do? RESPONSES—cont'd

Case Study 3
Page 541

What Did Trudy Do?

❑ Listened empathetically to Sadira, and tried to calm and reassure her.

❑ Spent some time going over the colposcopy procedure and what to expect.

❑ Answered as many of Sadira's questions as possible. Reassured her that a lot of people do not know what a cervix is, and that she was asking some very good questions.

❑ Asked the physician to spend some time talking with Sadira before the procedure to answer the questions that Trudy was not qualified to answer.

❑ Ensured that Sadira understood all of the information about the procedure before asking her to sign a consent to treatment form.

What Did Trudy Not Do?

❑ Did not tell Sadira that her family physician and staff should have spent some time explaining the procedure to her so that she did not have to worry so much.

❑ Did not tell Sadira that she does not have cancer.

What Would You Do?/What Would You Not Do?

Review Trudy's response and place a checkmark next to the information you included in your response. List additional information you included in your response.

_____

_____

_____

_____

_____

_____

_____

↻ TERMINOLOGY REVIEW

Medical Term	Word Parts	Definition
Abrasion		A wound in which the outer layers of the skin are damaged; a scrape.
Abscess		A collection of pus in a cavity surrounded by inflamed tissue.
Absorbable suture		Suture material that is gradually digested and absorbed by the body.
Approximation		The process of bringing two parts, such as tissue, together through the use of sutures or other means.
Bandage		A strip of woven material used to wrap or cover a part of the body.
Biopsy	*bi/o:* life *-opsy:* to view	The surgical removal and examination of tissue from the living body. Biopsies are generally performed to determine whether a tumor is benign or malignant.
Capillary action		The action that causes liquid to rise along a wick, a tube, or a gauze dressing.
Colposcope	*colp/o:* vagina *-scope:* instrument used for visual examination	A lighted instrument with a binocular magnifying lens used to examine the vagina and cervix.
Colposcopy	*colp/o:* vagina *-scopy:* visual examination	The visual examination of the vagina and cervix using a colposcope.
Contaminate		As it relates to sterile technique, to cause a sterile object or surface to become unsterile.
Contusion		An injury to the tissues under the skin that causes blood vessels to rupture, allowing blood to seep into the tissues; a bruise.
Cryosurgery	*cry/o:* cold	The therapeutic use of freezing temperatures to destroy abnormal tissue.
Exudate		A discharge produced by the body's tissues.
Fibroblast	*fibr/o:* fibrous tissue *blast:* developing cell	An immature cell from which connective tissue can develop.
Forceps		A two-pronged instrument for grasping and squeezing.
Furuncle		A localized staphylococcal infection that originates deep within a hair follicle. Also known as a *boil.*
Hemostasis	*hem/o:* blood *stasis:* control, stop	The arrest of bleeding by natural or artificial means.
Incision		A clean cut caused by a cutting instrument.
Infection		The condition in which the body, or part of it, is invaded by a pathogen.
Infiltration		The process by which a substance passes into and is deposited within the substance of a cell, tissue, or organ.

Continued

TERMINOLOGY REVIEW—cont'd

Medical Term	Word Parts	Definition
Inflammation		A protective response of the body to trauma and the entrance of foreign matter. The purpose of inflammation is to destroy invading microorganisms and to remove damaged tissue debris from the area so that proper healing can occur.
Laceration		A wound in which the tissues are torn apart, leaving ragged and irregular edges.
Ligate		To tie off and close a structure such as a severed blood vessel.
Local anesthetic		A drug that produces a loss of feeling and an inability to perceive pain in only a specific part of the body.
Mayo tray		A broad, flat metal tray placed on a stand and used to hold sterile instruments and supplies when it has been covered with a sterile towel.
Needle biopsy	*bi/o:* life	A type of biopsy in which tissue from deep within the body is obtained by the insertion of a
	-opsy: to view	biopsy needle through the skin.
Nonabsorbable suture		Suture material that is not absorbed by the body and either remains permanently in the body tissue and becomes encapsulated by fibrous tissue or is removed.
Postoperative	*post-:* after	After a surgical operation.
Preoperative	*pre-:* before	Preceding a surgical operation.
Puncture		A wound made by a sharp-pointed object piercing the skin.
Scalpel		A surgical knife used to divide tissues.
Scissors		A cutting instrument.
Sebaceous cyst		A thin, closed sac or capsule that contains fatty secretions from a sebaceous gland.
Serum		The clear, straw-colored part of the blood that remains after the solid elements have been separated out of it.
Sterile		Free of all living microorganisms and bacterial spores.
Surgery		The branch of medicine that deals with operative and manual procedures for correction of deformities and defects, repair of injuries, and diagnosis and treatment of certain diseases.
Surgical asepsis	*a:* without or absence of	Practices that keep objects and areas sterile or free from microorganisms.
	-sepsis: infection	
Sutures		Material used to approximate tissues with surgical stitches.
Swaged needle		A needle with suturing material permanently attached to its end.
Wound		A break in the continuity of an external or internal surface caused by physical means.

ON THE WEB

For information on surgery and emergency medicine:

American College of Surgeons: www.facs.org

American Red Cross: www.redcross.org

Ethicon Incorporated: www.ethicon.com

Federal Emergency Management Agency: www.fema.gov

 Check out the Evolve site at http://evolve.elsevier.com/Bonewit/today/ to actively Prepare for your Certification, and to access additional interactive activities and exercises

26

Administration of Medication and Intravenous Therapy

LEARNING OBJECTIVES

Introduction to the Administration of Medication

1. Explain the difference among administering, prescribing, and dispensing medication.
2. State the common routes for administering medication.
3. List and describe the six sections of the PDR.
4. List and describe the categories of information in a drug package insert.
5. Describe the Food and Drug Administration's responsibilities with respect to drugs.
6. List and define the four names of drugs.
7. Classify drugs according to preparation.
8. Classify drugs according to the action they have on the body.
9. List the guidelines for writing metric and apothecary notations.
10. List and describe the five schedules for controlled drugs.
11. List and explain the parts of a prescription.
12. Describe the functions performed by an electronic medical record (EMR) prescription program.
13. Explain the purpose of a medication record.
14. Describe the factors that affect the action of drugs in the body.
15. List and describe the possible adverse effects of medication.
16. List the guidelines for preparing and administering medication.

Oral Administration

17. Explain why the oral route is most frequently used to administer medication.
18. State where the absorption of most oral medications occurs.

Parenteral Administration

19. State the advantages and disadvantages of the parenteral route of administration.
20. Identify the parts of a needle and syringe and explain their functions.
21. State the ranges of gauge and length of needles for each of the following injections: intradermal, subcutaneous, and intramuscular.
22. State the purpose of safety-engineered syringes.
23. Describe the dispensing units available for injectable medications.
24. State which tissue layers of the body are used for intradermal, subcutaneous, and intramuscular injections.
25. List the medications commonly administered through each of the following routes: intradermal, subcutaneous, and intramuscular.
26. Explain the reason for administering medication with the Z-track method.

PROCEDURES

Research a drug using the *Physician's Desk Reference* (PDR).
Interpret a drug package insert.
Calculate drug dosage.
Complete a prescription form.
Complete a medication record form.

Prepare and administer oral medications.

Reconstitute a powdered drug for parenteral administration.
Withdraw medication from a vial.
Withdraw medication from an ampule.
Locate appropriate subcutaneous injection sites.
Administer a subcutaneous injection.
Locate each of the following intramuscular injection sites: dorsogluteal, deltoid, vastus lateralis, and ventrogluteal.
Administer an intramuscular injection.
Administer an injection using the Z-track method.
Administer an intradermal injection.

LEARNING OBJECTIVES

PROCEDURES

Tuberculin Testing

27. Explain the difference between active and latent tuberculosis.
28. Explain the purpose of tuberculin skin testing.
29. Identify the categories of individuals who should have a tuberculin test.
30. Explain the significance of a positive reaction to a tuberculin test.
31. List the diagnostic procedures that might be performed following a positive tuberculin test.
32. State the guidelines that should be followed when administering and reading a Mantoux test.
33. State the advantages of the tuberculosis blood test.

Administer a Mantoux test, and read the test results.
Complete a tuberculosis test record card.

Allergy Testing

34. Define an allergy, and name common allergens.
35. Explain what occurs during an allergic reaction.
36. List the guidelines for direct skin allergy testing.
37. State the purpose of each of the following types of allergy tests: patch testing, skin-prick testing, intradermal skin testing, and in vitro blood testing.

Perform allergy skin testing.

Intravenous Therapy

38. Explain the advantages of outpatient intravenous (IV) therapy.
39. Identify the role of the entry-level medical assistant in IV therapy.
40. State the indications for outpatient IV therapy.

CHAPTER OUTLINE

INTRODUCTION TO THE ADMINISTRATION OF MEDICATION
Administering, Prescribing, and Dispensing Medication
Legal Aspects
Routes of Administration
Drug References
Food and Drug Administration
Drug Nomenclature
Classification of Drugs Based on Preparation
Liquid Preparations
Solid Preparations
Classification of Drugs Based on Action
Systems of Measurement for Medication
Metric System
Apothecary System
Household System
Converting Units of Measurement
Controlled Drugs
Prescription
Parts of a Prescription
Generic Prescribing
Completing a Prescription Form
EMR Prescription Program
Medication Record
Factors Affecting Drug Action
Therapeutic Effect
Undesirable Effects of Drugs
Guidelines for Preparation and Administration of Medication

Oral Administration
Parenteral Administration
Parts of a Needle and Syringe
Safety-Engineered Syringes
Preparation of Parenteral Medication
Storage
Reconstitution of Powdered Drugs
Subcutaneous Injections
Intramuscular Injections
Intradermal Injections
Tuberculin Skin Testing
Tuberculosis
Purpose of Tuberculin Testing
Tuberculin Skin Test Reactions
Tuberculin Skin Testing Methods
Mantoux Test
Two-Step Tuberculin Skin Test
Tuberculosis Blood Test
Allergy Testing
Allergy
Allergic Reaction
Diagnosis and Treatment
Types of Allergy Tests
Intravenous Therapy
Advantages of Outpatient Intravenous Therapy
Medical Office–Based Intravenous Therapy
Indications for Outpatient Intravenous Therapy

adverse reaction (AD-vers ree-AK-shun)
allergen (AL-er-jen)
allergy (AL-er-jee)
ampule (AM-pyool)
anaphylactic reaction (an-uh-ful-AK-tik ree-AK-shun)
autoimmune disease
chemotherapy
controlled drug
conversion (kon-VER-shun)
cubic centimeter (KYOO-bik SEN-tih-mee-ter)
DEA number
dose

drug
enteral nutrition
gauge (GAYJ)
hemophilia
immune globulin
induration (in-dur-AY-shun)
infusion
inhalation (in-hal-AY-shun)
inscription (in-SKRIP-shun)
intradermal injection (in-tra-DER-mal in-JEK-shun)
intramuscular (in-tra-MUS-kyoo-lar) injection
intravenous (in-tra-VEE-nus) (IV) therapy

oral (OR-ul) administration
parenteral (par-EN-ter-al)
pharmacology (far-ma-KOL-oh-jee)
prescription
signatura (sig-na-CHUR-ah)
subcutaneous (sub-kyoo-TAY-nee-us) injection
sublingual (sub-LIN-gwal) administration
subscription (sub-SKRIP-shun)
superscription (soo-per-SKRIP-shun)
topical (TOP-ih-kul) administration
transfusion
vial (VIE-ul)
wheal (WEE-ul)

INTRODUCTION TO THE ADMINISTRATION OF MEDICATION

Pharmacology is the study of drugs and includes the preparation, use, and action of drugs in the body. A **drug** is a chemical that is used for the treatment, prevention, or diagnosis of disease. Most drugs are produced synthetically, but they also can be obtained from other sources, such as animals, plants, and minerals.

ADMINISTERING, PRESCRIBING, AND DISPENSING MEDICATION

Medication may be administered, prescribed, or dispensed in the medical office. Medication that is *administered* is actually given to a patient at the office. Medication is *prescribed* when a physician provides a patient with a handwritten or computer-generated prescription for a drug to be filled at a pharmacy. Prescriptions also can be telephoned or faxed to the pharmacy by the physician, depending on the preference of the patient. *Dispensed* medication is given to a patient at the office to be taken at home; for example, the physician gives a patient drug samples to take home.

LEGAL ASPECTS

An important responsibility of the medical assistant is the administration of medication. (One should check the laws of the state to ensure that it is legally permissible for the medical assistant to administer medication.) The medical assistant should administer medication only under the direction of the physician. In all states, it is unlawful to administer medication in the medical office without the consent of the physician.

ROUTES OF ADMINISTRATION

Common routes of administration of medication are oral, sublingual, inhalation, rectal, vaginal, topical, intradermal, subcutaneous (SC), intramuscular (IM), and intravenous (IV). The route of administration depends on the type of drug being given, the dosage form, the intended action, and the rapidity of response desired. The route by which medication is most commonly administered in the medical office is the parenteral route. **Parenteral** refers to sites outside the gastrointestinal tract; this term is most commonly used to refer to the administration of medication by injection.

DRUG REFERENCES

The medical assistant is obligated to become familiar with the drugs that are most frequently used in his or her office. It is essential to know their indications, adverse reactions, routes of administration, dosage, and storage. With each drug (including drug samples and injectable medications), the manufacturer includes a *package insert* (PI), which contains valuable information regarding the drug. In addition, many drug references are available. The *Physician's Desk Reference* (PDR) is frequently used in the medical office. The PDR contains information on most major prescription pharmaceutical products available in the United States. The drug information in the PDR consists of the actual drug package insert. Figure 26-1 provides guidelines for using the PDR. These guidelines not only assist in learning how to use the PDR, but they also provide the necessary information for understanding how to interpret drug package inserts. Drug information is also available on the Internet on certain recognized websites; many of these sites are listed at the end of the chapter under the section entitled *On the Web: For Information on Pharmacology.*

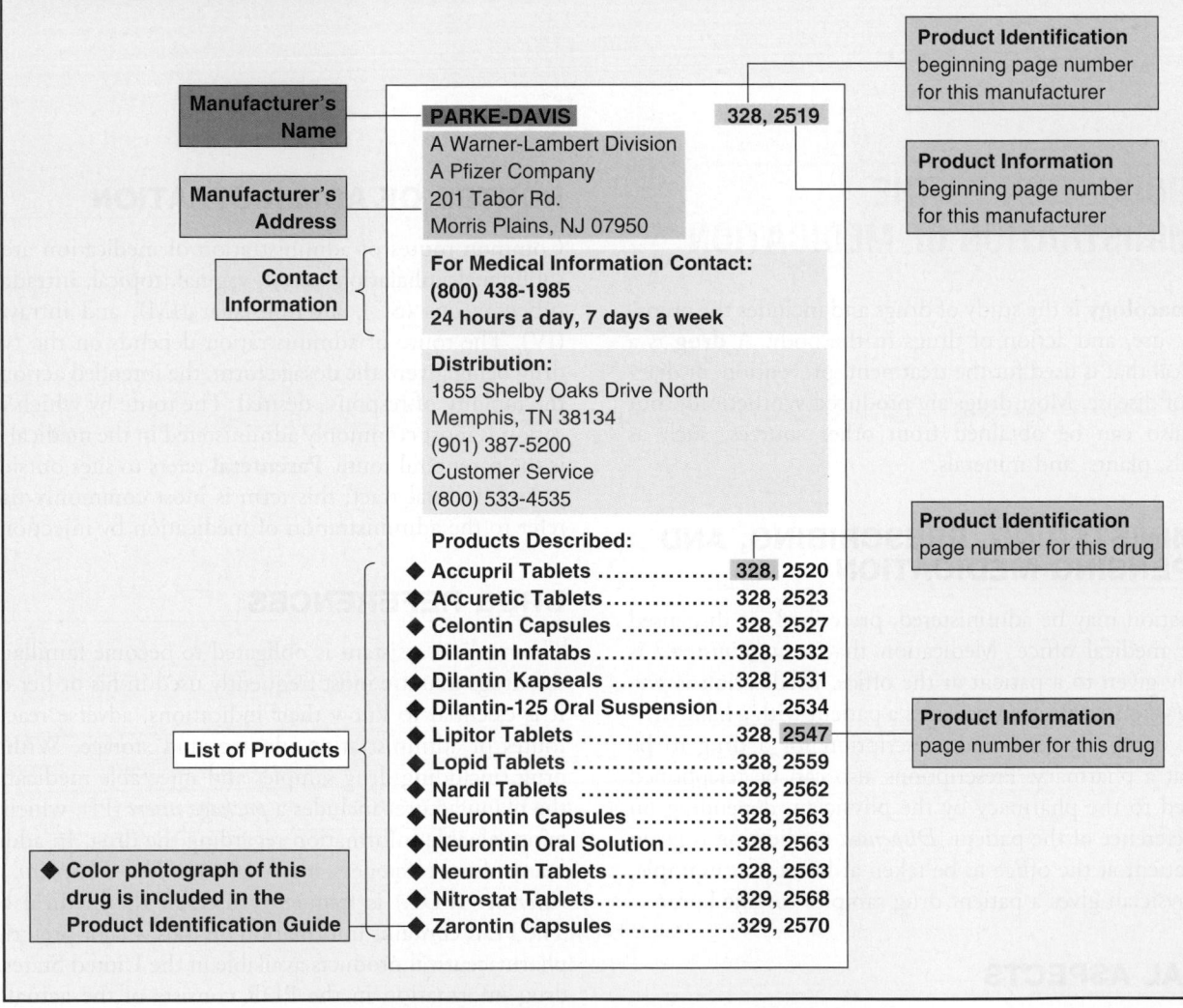

GUIDELINES FOR USING THE PHYSICIAN'S DESK REFERENCE

The *Physician's Desk Reference* (PDR) is published anually by the Medical Economics Company with the cooperation of the pharmaceutical manufacturers whose products are included in it. This reference includes essential information on most major prescription pharmaceutical products available in the United States. The PDR is divided into sections, which are described below.

SECTION 1: MANUFACTURER'S INDEX

The Manufacturer's Index lists pharmaceutical manufacturers in alphabetical order along with a list of drugs that are manufactured by each company. This index provides all of the necessary information, should the manufacturer need to be contacted regarding a particular drug.

Product Identification
beginning page number
for this manufacturer

Manufacturer's Name

PARKE-DAVIS   328, 2519
A Warner-Lambert Division
A Pfizer Company
201 Tabor Rd.
Morris Plains, NJ 07950

Product Information
beginning page number
for this manufacturer

Manufacturer's Address

Contact Information
For Medical Information Contact:
(800) 438-1985
24 hours a day, 7 days a week

Distribution:
1855 Shelby Oaks Drive North
Memphis, TN 38134
(901) 387-5200
Customer Service
(800) 533-4535

Products Described:
◆ Accupril Tablets 328, 2520
◆ Accuretic Tablets 328, 2523
◆ Celontin Capsules 328, 2527
◆ Dilantin Infatabs 328, 2532
◆ Dilantin Kapseals 328, 2531
◆ Dilantin-125 Oral Suspension 2534
◆ Lipitor Tablets 328, 2547
◆ Lopid Tablets 328, 2559
◆ Nardil Tablets 328, 2562
◆ Neurontin Capsules 328, 2563
◆ Neurontin Oral Solution 328, 2563
◆ Neurontin Tablets 328, 2563
◆ Nitrostat Tablets................. 329, 2568
◆ Zarontin Capsules 329, 2570

Product Identification
page number for this drug

Product Information
page number for this drug

List of Products

◆ Color photograph of this drug is included in the Product Identification Guide

Figure 26-1 Guidelines for using the *Physician's Desk Reference.*

SECTION 2: BRAND AND GENERIC NAME INDEX

This section consists of an alphabetical listing of the drugs included in the PDR by both generic and brand names. This section allows for the quick and easy location of drug information.

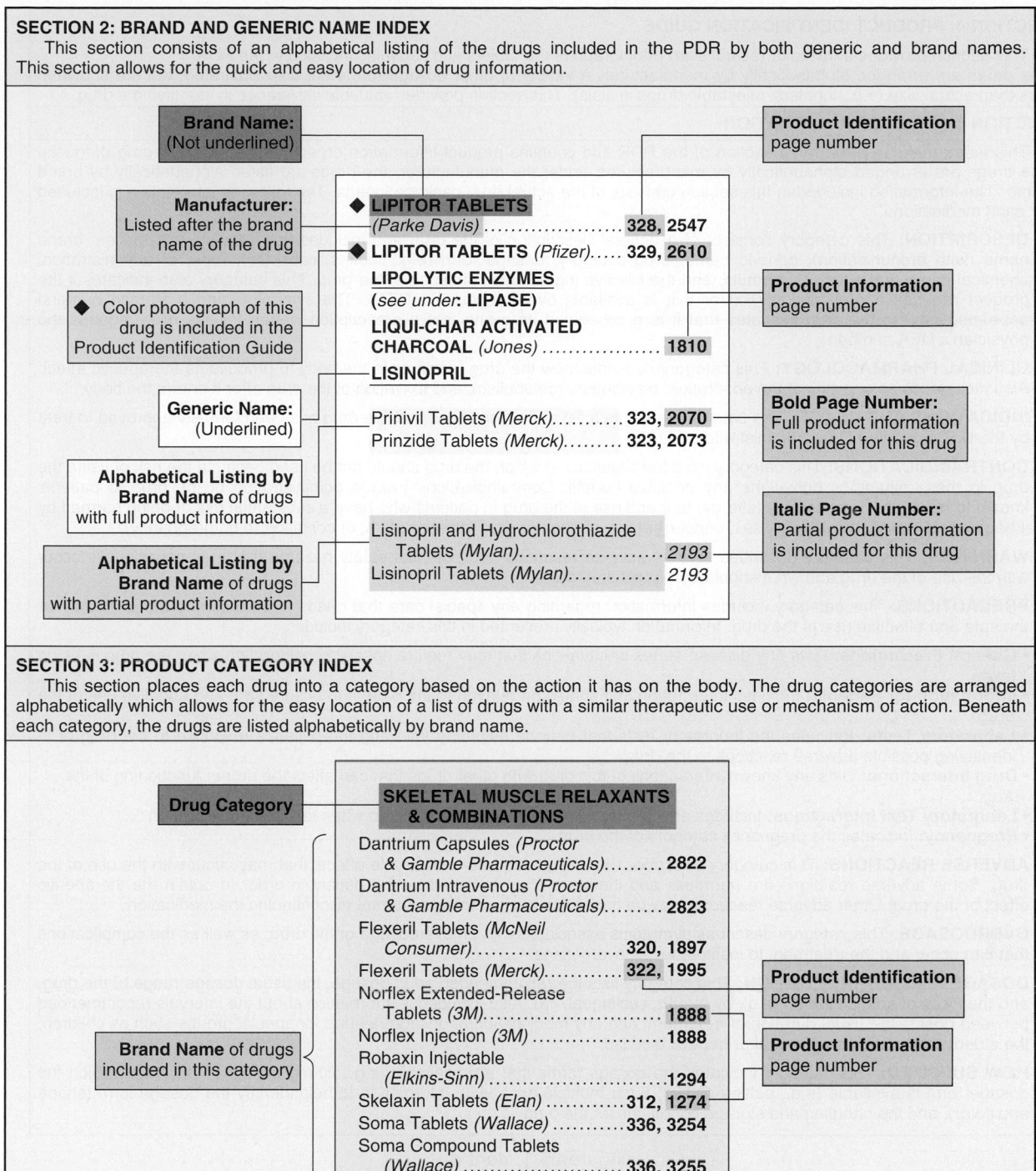

SECTION 3: PRODUCT CATEGORY INDEX

This section places each drug into a category based on the action it has on the body. The drug categories are arranged alphabetically which allows for the easy location of a list of drugs with a similar therapeutic use or mechanism of action. Beneath each category, the drugs are listed alphabetically by brand name.

Figure 26-1, cont'd

Continued

SECTION 4: PRODUCT IDENTIFICATION GUIDE

This section provides a full-color (actual size) photograph of the tablets and capsules included in the PDR. The drugs are arranged alphabetically by manufacturer. A variety of other dosage forms are also illustrated, but are shown in less than actual size (e.g., inhalers, injectable drugs in vials). This section provides valuable assistance in identifying a drug.

SECTION 5: PRODUCT INFORMATION

This index makes up the main section of the PDR and contains product information on approximately 3000 drug products. The drugs are arranged alphabetically by manufacturer; under the manufacturer, the drugs are listed alphabetically by brand name. The information included in this section consists of the actual drug package inserts. The following information is included for each medication:

DESCRIPTION: This category consists of a general description of the drug and includes the following information: brand name (with pronunciation), generic name, drug category, dosage form (e.g., tablets, capsules), route of administration, chemical name and structural formula, and the inactive ingredients contained in the drug. This category also indicates if the product requires a prescription (Rx) or if it is available over-the-counter (OTC). The symbol C and a Roman numeral appearing next to the drug indicates that it is a scheduled drug and that a prescription written for this drug requires the physician's DEA number.

CLINICAL PHARMACOLOGY: This category describes how the drug functions in the body to produce its therapeutic effect. Also included is an analysis of the absorption, distribution, metabolism, and excretion of the drug after it enters the body.

INDICATIONS AND USAGE: This category presents a list of the conditions that the drug has been formally approved to treat by the U.S. Food and Drug Administration (FDA).

CONTRAINDICATIONS: This category includes situations in which the drug should not be used because the risk of using the drug in these situations outweighs any possible benefit. Contraindications include administration of the drug to patients known to have a hypersensitivity (allergy) to it and use of the drug in patients who have a substantial risk of being harmed by it because of their particular age, sex, concurrent use of another drug, disease state, or condition (e.g., pregnancy).

WARNINGS: This category describes serious adverse reactions and potential safety hazards that may occasionally occur with the use of the drug and what should be done if they occur.

PRECAUTIONS: This category includes information regarding any special care that needs to be taken by the physician for the safe and effective use of the drug. Information typically presented in this category includes:

- **General Precautions:** Lists any disease states or situations that may require special consideration when the drug is being taken.
- **Information for Patients:** Includes information that should be relayed to the patient to ensure safe and effective use of the drug.
- **Laboratory Tests:** Indicates the laboratory tests that may be helpful in following the patient's response to the drug or in identifying possible adverse reactions to the drug.
- **Drug Interactions:** Lists any known interactions of this drug with other drugs that can affect the proper functioning of the drug.
- **Laboratory Test Interactions:** Includes any laboratory tests that may be affected when taking the medication.
- **Pregnancy:** Indicates the pregnancy category of the drug.

ADVERSE REACTIONS: This category describes the unintended and undesirable effects that may occur with the use of the drug. Some adverse reactions are harmless and therefore often tolerated by the patient in order to obtain the therapeutic effect of the drug. Other adverse reactions may be harmful to the patient and warrant discontinuing the medication.

OVERDOSAGE: This category describes symptoms associated with an overdosage of the drug, as well as the complications that can occur and the treatment to institute for an overdosage.

DOSAGE AND ADMINISTRATION: This category lists the recommended adult dosage, the usual dosage range of the drug, and the route of administration (e.g., by mouth, sublingual, IM). Also included is information about the intervals recommended between doses, the usual duration of treatment, and any modification of dosage needed for special groups such as children, the elderly, and patients with renal or hepatic disease.

HOW SUPPLIED: This category indicates the dosage forms that are available (e.g., 20-mg tablets), the units in which the dosage form is available (e.g., bottles of 100; 5-mL multiple-dose vial), information to help identify the dosage form (shape and color), and the handling and storage conditions for the drug.

Figure 26-1, cont'd

FOOD AND DRUG ADMINISTRATION

The U.S. Food and Drug Administration (FDA) is a federal agency in the Department of Health and Human Services. The FDA is responsible for determining whether new food products, drugs, vaccines, medical devices, cosmetics, and other products are safe before they are released for human use.

The FDA determines the safety and effectiveness of prescription and nonprescription (over-the-counter [OTC]) drugs. Pharmaceutical manufacturers are required to submit new drug applications to the FDA for review and approval before products can be released for human use.

The FDA also is responsible for determining whether a medication will be available with or without a prescription. Medications that require a prescription have been determined by the FDA to be safe and effective when used under the guidance of a physician. Prescription medication labels must bear the following statement: *Caution: Federal law prohibits dispensing without a prescription.*

Nonprescription medications are drugs that the FDA determines to be safe and effective for use without physician supervision. Nonprescription medications have a low incidence of adverse reactions when the consumer follows the directions and warnings on the label. Examples of nonprescription medications include mild pain relievers, topical antibiotics, topical corticosteroids, cold medications, and laxatives.

DRUG NOMENCLATURE

Each drug has four names: chemical, generic, official, and brand (also known as *trade*) names.

1. **Chemical name.** The chemical name provides a precise description of the drug's chemical composition; pharmaceutical manufacturers and pharmacists are most concerned with the chemical makeup of a drug.
2. **Generic name.** The generic name is assigned by the pharmaceutical manufacturer who develops the drug, before it receives official approval by the FDA. The generic name is often a shortened derivative of the chemical name.
3. **Official name.** The official name is the name under which the drug is listed in official publications, such as the *United States Pharmacopeia* (USP) and the *National Formulary* (NF). Official publications set specific standards to regulate the strength, purity, packaging, safety, labeling, and dosage form of each drug. The generic name is frequently used for the official name.
4. **Brand name.** The brand name is the name under which a pharmaceutical manufacturer markets a drug. Because a drug may be manufactured by more than one pharmaceutical company, it may have several brand names. The generic name of a common analgesic is acetaminophen; brand names for this drug include Tylenol, Tempra, Datril, Exdol, Panadol, and Liquiprin.

The medical assistant should be familiar with the generic and brand names of medications commonly prescribed and administered in the medical office.

What Would You Do? What Would You *Not* Do?

Case Study 1

Carol Okasinski, 56 years old, is a new patient. She was a patient of another physician in the community; however, his receptionist was often rude to her, and she decided not to go there anymore. Mrs. Okasinski is obese and has hypertension, type 2 diabetes, osteoarthritis in her hands and knees, and problems with depression. While filling in the health history form, she says she cannot fill in the names of the medications she is taking. She is on a lot of medications prescribed by her previous physician. She says she could not get the childproof pill containers open because of the arthritis in her hands, so she had her husband throw away the childproof containers and transfer each medication into an easy-to-open plastic container. She knows when to take her medications, but she does not know the names of them or why she is taking them. She has brought in a bag with all her medications in their plastic containers. ∎

CLASSIFICATION OF DRUGS BASED ON PREPARATION

Drugs are available in two basic forms: liquid and solid. A medication may be available in both these forms (liquid and solid), which permits it to be administered to different types of patients. A liquid preparation of an antibiotic is administered to young children, and the solid preparation (e.g., tablets) of the same medication is administered to older children and adults. The following list includes the common categories of drugs based on preparation.

Liquid Preparations

Elixir A drug that is dissolved in a solution of alcohol and water. Elixirs are sweetened and flavored and are taken orally. *Example:* Dimetapp elixir.

Emulsion A mixture of fats or oils in water. *Example:* Durezol ophthalmic emulsion.

Liniment A drug combined with oil, soap, alcohol, or water. Liniments are applied externally, using friction, to produce a feeling of heat or warmth. *Example:* Heet liniment.

Lotion An aqueous preparation that contains suspended ingredients. Lotions are used to treat external skin conditions. They work to soothe, protect, and moisten the skin and to destroy harmful bacteria. *Example:* Caladryl lotion.

Solution A liquid preparation that contains one or more completely dissolved substances. The dissolved substance is known as the *solute,* and the liquid in which it is dissolved is known as the *solvent.* Most drugs administered parenterally (by injection) consist of solutions. *Example:* Depo-Provera injectable solution.

Spirit A drug combined with an alcoholic solution that is volatile (a substance that is volatile evaporates readily). *Example:* Aromatic spirit of ammonia.

Spray A fine stream of medicated vapor, usually used to treat nose and throat conditions. *Example:* Dristan nasal spray.

Suspension A drug that contains solid insoluble drug particles in a liquid; the preparation must be shaken before administration. *Example:* Amoxicillin oral suspension.

Suspension aerosol A pressurized form in which solid aerosol or liquid drug particles are suspended in a gas to be dispensed in a cloud or mist. *Example:* Proventil inhalation aerosol.

Syrup A drug dissolved in a solution of sugar, water, and sometimes a flavoring to disguise an unpleasant taste. *Example:* Robitussin cough syrup.

Tincture A drug dissolved in a solution of alcohol or alcohol and water. *Example:* Tincture of iodine.

Solid Preparations

Tablet A powdered drug that has been pressed into a disc. Some tablets are scored, that is, they are marked with an indentation so that they can be broken into halves or quarters for proper dosage. *Example:* Tylenol tablets.

Chewable tablet A powdered drug that has been flavored and pressed into a disc. Chewable tablets are often used for antacids, antiflatulents, and children's medications. *Example:* Pepto-Bismol chewable tablets.

Sublingual tablet A powdered drug that has been pressed into a disc and is designed to dissolve under the tongue, which permits its rapid absorption into the bloodstream. *Example:* Nitroglycerin sublingual tablets (Nitrostat).

Enteric-coated tablet A tablet coated with a substance that prevents it from dissolving until it reaches the intestines. The coating protects the drug from being destroyed by gastric juices and prevents it from irritating the stomach lining. To prevent the active ingredients from being released prematurely in the stomach, enteric-coated tablets must not be crushed or chewed. *Example:* Ecotrin enteric-coated aspirin.

Capsule A drug contained in a gelatin capsule that is water-soluble and functions to prevent the patient from tasting the drug. *Example:* Benadryl capsules.

Sustained-release capsule A capsule that contains granules that dissolve at different rates to provide a gradual and continuous release of medication. This reduces the number of doses that must be administered. (Sustained-release medication also comes in other preparations, such as tablets and caplets.) *Example:* Sudafed 12-hour sustained-release capsules.

Caplet A drug contained in an oblong tablet with a smooth coating to make swallowing easier. *Example:* Advil caplets.

Lozenge A drug contained in a candy-like base. Lozenges are circular and are designed to dissolve on the tongue. *Example:* Chloraseptic throat lozenges.

Cream A drug combined in a base that is generally nongreasy, resulting in a semisolid preparation. Creams are applied externally to the skin. *Example:* Hydrocortisone topical cream.

Ointment A drug with an oil base, resulting in a semisolid preparation. Ointments are applied externally to the skin and are usually greasy. *Example:* Cortisporin topical ointment.

Suppository A drug mixed with a firm base, such as cocoa butter, that is designed to melt at body temperature. A suppository is shaped into a cylinder or a cone for easy insertion into a body cavity, such as the rectum or vagina. *Example:* Preparation H suppositories.

Transdermal patch A patch with an adhesive backing, which contains a drug, that is applied to the skin. The drug enters the circulation after being absorbed through the skin. *Example:* Nitroglycerin patches (Nitro-Dur).

CLASSIFICATION OF DRUGS BASED ON ACTION

Drugs also can be classified according to the action they have on the body. The medical assistant should know in which category a particular drug belongs and its primary uses and major therapeutic effects. Table 26-1 contains classifications based on action and examples of drugs that are commonly administered and prescribed in the medical office.

Text continued on p. 566

Table 26-1 Classification of Drugs Based on Action

Drug Category	Primary Use and Major Therapeutic Effects	COMMONLY PRESCRIBED DRUGS	
		Generic	Brand
Analgesics (Opioid)	**Used** to manage moderate to severe pain **Work** by altering perception of and response to painful stimuli	codeine/APAP	▸ Tylenol w/ Codeine (III)
		fentanyl	Actiq
		hydrocodone/APAP	▸ Vicodin (III)
		hydrocodone/ASA	Lortab/ASA (III)
		hydrocodone/ibuprofen	▸ Vicoprofen (III)
		meperidine	Demerol (II)
		oxycodone	▸ OxyContin (II)
		oxycodone/APAP	▸ Percocet (II)
		oxycodone/ASA	Percodan (II)
		propoxyphene	Darvon (IV)
		propoxyphene N/APAP	▸ Darvocet-N (IV)
		tramadol	▸ Ultram
Analgesics (Barbiturate)	**Used** to manage moderate to severe pain of tension headaches **Work** by relieving pain and relaxing muscle contractions	butalbital/APAP/caffeine butalbital/ASA/caffeine	▸ Fioricet (III) Fiorinal (III)
Analgesics/ Antipyretics	**Used** to manage mild to moderate pain and to reduce fever **Work** by relieving pain and reducing fever	acetaminophen aspirin	Tylenol* Bayer* Ecotrin*

Table 26-1 Classification of Drugs Based on Action—cont'd

Drug Category	Primary Use and Major Therapeutic Effects	COMMONLY PRESCRIBED DRUGS	
		Generic	Brand
Analgesics/ Antipyretics		**NSAIDs** diclofenac ibuprofen	Voltaren Advil* ► Motrin* Aleve*
		naproxen	► Anaprox ► Naprosyn
Anesthetics (Local)	*Used* to produce local anesthesia through loss of feeling to a body part *Work* by preventing initiation and conduction of normal nerve impulses in body part	lidocaine dibucaine	Xylocaine Nupercainal ointment*
Antacids	*Used* to treat heartburn, hyperacidity, indigestion, and gastroesophageal reflux disease, and to promote healing of ulcers *Work* by neutralizing gastric acid to relieve gastric pain and irritation	aluminum hydroxide/magnesium hydroxide calcium carbonate sodium bicarbonate/ASA	Maalox* Mylanta* Tums* Alka-Seltzer*
Anti-Alzheimer Agents	*Used* to treat mild to moderate dementia associated with Alzheimer disease *Work* by elevating acetylcholine concentration in the cerebral cortex	donepezil memantine rivastigmine	► Aricept ► Namenda Exelon
Antianemics	**Iron Supplements** *Used* to prevent or cure iron-deficiency anemia *Work* by increasing amount of iron in body	ferrous sulfate iron dextran	Feosol* DexFerrum InFed
	Vitamin B$_{12}$ Injections *Used* to treat pernicious anemia *Work* by increasing amount of vitamin B$_{12}$ in body	cyanocobalamin	Cobex Cyanoject
	Folic Acid Supplements *Used* to promote normal fetal development *Work* by stimulating production of red blood cells, white blood cells, and platelets	folic acid	► Folvite
Antianginals	*Used* to relieve or prevent angina attacks *Work* by increasing blood supply to myocardial tissue	**Nitrates** isosorbide dinitrate isosorbide mononitrate nitroglycerin	Sorbitrate ► Imdur Nitro-Bid Nitro-Dur Nitrostat
		Beta-Blockers atenolol propranolol metoprolol	Tenormin Inderal ► Toprol-XL
		Calcium Channel Blockers amlodipine bepridil diltiazem nifedipine verapamil	► Norvasc Vascor Cardizem Dilacor XR Adalat Procardia XL ► Calan Isoptin Verelan

Continued

Table 26-1   Classification of Drugs Based on Action—cont'd

Drug Category	Primary Use and Major Therapeutic Effects	Generic	Brand
		COMMONLY PRESCRIBED DRUGS	
Antianxiety Agents	**Used** to treat anxiety **Work** at many levels in central nervous system to produce anxiolytic (anxiety-relieving) effect	alprazolam buspirone chlordiazepoxide diazepam lorazepam	▸ Xanax (IV) BuSpar Librium (IV) ▸ Valium (IV) ▸ Ativan (IV)
Anticholinergics	**Used** to decrease preoperatively oral and respiratory secretions **Work** by blocking effects of acetylcholine in autonomic nervous system	atropine	Atro-Pen
Anticoagulants	**Used** to prevent and treat venous thrombosis, pulmonary embolism, and myocardial infarction by preventing clot extension and formation **Work** by delaying or preventing blood coagulation	heparin enoxaparin warfarin	 ▸ Lovenox ▸ Coumadin
Anticonvulsants	**Used** to prevent or relieve seizures **Work** by decreasing incidence and severity of seizures	carbamazepine clonazepam divalproex gabapentin lamotrigine phenytoin pregabalin topiramate	Tegretol ▸ Klonopin (IV) ▸ Depakote ▸ Neurontin ▸ Lamictal ▸ Dilantin ▸ Lyrica ▸ Topamax
Antidepressants	**Used** to prevent, cure, or alleviate depression, and to treat anxiety disorders (panic attacks) and obsessive-convulsive disorder **Work** by inhibiting reuptake of neurotransmitters in the central nervous system	**Selective Serotonin Reuptake Inhibitors (SSRIs)** citalopram escitalopram fluoxetine fluvoxamine paroxetine sertraline **Serotonin-Norepinephrine Reuptake Inhibitors (SNRIs)** desvenlafaxine duloxetine venlafaxine **Miscellaneous** amitriptyline bupropion mirtazapine nefazodone trazodone	 ▸ Celexa ▸ Lexapro ▸ Prozac Luvox ▸ Paxil ▸ Zoloft Pristiq ▸ Cymbalta ▸ Effexor XR ▸ Elavil ▸ Wellbutrin SR ▸ Remeron Serzone ▸ Desyrel
Antidiabetics	**Oral Hypoglycemics** **Used** to manage non–insulin-dependent type 2 diabetes mellitus **Work** by stimulating release of insulin from pancreas and increasing sensitivity to insulin	glimepiride glipizide glyburide metformin pioglitazone rosiglitazone	▸ Amaryl ▸ Glucotrol XL ▸ Micronase ▸ Glucophage ▸ Actos ▸ Avandia
Antidiabetics	**Insulins** **Used** to manage diabetes mellitus **Work** by reducing blood glucose levels	regular insulin NPH insulin NPH/regular insulin insulin glargine insulin lispro	Humulin R* Novolin R* Humulin N* Novolin N* Humulin 70/30* Novolin 70/30* ▸ Lantus Humalog

Table 26-1 Classification of Drugs Based on Action—cont'd

Drug Category	Primary Use and Major Therapeutic Effects	COMMONLY PRESCRIBED DRUGS	
		Generic	**Brand**
Antidiarrheals	**Used** to control and relieve diarrhea **Work** by inhibiting peristalsis, reducing fecal volume, and preventing loss of fluids and electrolytes	bismuth subsalicylate diphenoxylate/atropine kaolin/pectin loperamide	Pepto-Bismol* Lomotil (V) Kaopectate* Imodium*
Antidysrhythmics	**Used** to control or prevent cardiac dysrhythmias **Work** by decreasing myocardial excitability and slowing conduction velocity	metoprolol procainamide propranolol	▸ Lopressor ▸ Toprol-XL Pronestyl Inderal
Antiemetics	**Used** to prevent or relieve nausea and vomiting **Work** by depressing chemoreceptor trigger zone in central nervous system to inhibit nausea and vomiting	dronabinol ondansetron prochlorperazine promethazine meclizine	Marinol (III) Zofran Compazine ▸ Phenergan Bonine*
Antiflatulents	**Used** to relieve discomfort of excess gas and bloating in gastrointestinal tract **Work** by causing coalescence of gas bubbles in intestinal tract	simethicone	Gas-X* Mylanta Gas*
Antifungals	**Used** to treat fungal infections **Work** by killing or inhibiting growth of susceptible fungi	amphotericin B clotrimazole fluconazole itraconazole ketoconazole miconazole nystatin terbinafine	Fungizone Gyne-Lotrimin* ▸ Diflucan Sporanox Nizoral Monistat* Mycostatin* ▸ Lamisil
Antigout Agents	**Used** to prevent attacks of gout **Work** by inhibiting production of uric acid	allopurinol colchicine	▸ Zyloprim Colchicine tablets
Anthelmintics	**Used** to treat worm infections (pinworms, roundworms, hookworms) **Work** by destroying worms	mebendazole	Vermox
Antihistamines	**Used** to relieve symptoms associated with allergies (increased sneezing; rhinorrhea; itchy eyes, nose, and throat) **Work** by blocking effects of histamine at histamine receptor sites	brompheniramine cetirizine chlorpheniramine desloratadine diphenhydramine fexofenadine/pseudoephedrine levocetirizine loratadine promethazine	Dimetane* ▸ Zyrtec* Chlor-Trimetron* Teldrin* ▸ Clarinex Benadryl* ▸ Allegra Xyzal ▸ Claritin* ▸ Phenergan
Antihypertensives	**Used** to manage hypertension **Work** by causing systemic vasodilation to reduce blood pressure	**Angiotensin-Converting Enzyme (ACE) Inhibitors** benazepril captopril enalapril lisinopril quinapril ramipril **Peripherally Acting Adrenergic Blockers** clonidine doxazosin prazosin	 Lotensin Capoten ▸ Vasotec ▸ Prinivil ▸ Accupril ▸ Altace ▸ Catapres Cardura Minipress

Continued

Table 26-1 Classification of Drugs Based on Action—cont'd

Drug Category	Primary Use and Major Therapeutic Effects	COMMONLY PRESCRIBED DRUGS Generic	Brand
Antihypertensives, cont'd		**Angiotensin II Receptor Antagonists**	
		candesartan	Atacand
		irbesartan	▸ Avapro
		losartan	▸ Cozaar
		olmesartan	▸ Benicar
		telmisartan	Micardis
		valsartan	▸ Diovan
		Beta-Blockers	
		atenolol	▸ Tenormin
		carvedilol	▸ Coreg
		metoprolol	▸ Lopressor
			▸ Toprol-XL
		propranolol	Inderal
		sotalol	Betaspace
		Calcium Channel Blockers	
		amlodipine	▸ Norvasc
		diltiazem	▸ Cardizem
		felodipine	Plendil
		Vasodilators	
		hydralazine	Apresoline
		Miscellaneous	
		amlodipine/atorvastatin	Caduet
		amlodipine/benazepril	▸ Lotrel
		bisoprolol/hydrochlorothiazide	Ziac
		irbesartan/hydrochlorothiazide	▸ Avalide
		losartan/hydrochlorothiazide	▸ Hyzaar
		olmesartan/hydrochlorothiazide	▸ Benicar HCT
		triamterene/hydrochlorothiazide	▸ Maxzide
		valsartan/hydrochlorothiazide	Diovan HCT
Antiimpotence Agents	*Used* to treat erectile dysfunction *Work* by promoting increased blood flow to penis	sildenafil	▸ Viagra
		tadalafil	▸ Cialis
		vardenafil	Levitra
Antiinfectives	*Used* to treat infections *Work* by killing or inhibiting growth of bacteria	**Penicillins**	
		amoxicillin	▸ Amoxil
			▸ Trimox
		amoxicillin/clavulanate	▸ Augmentin
		ampicillin	Omnipen
		benzathine penicillin	Bicillin
		penicillin V	▸ Veetids
		procaine penicillin	Wycillin
		Macrolides	
		azithromycin	▸ Zithromax
		clarithromycin	Biaxin
		erythromycin	Ery-Tab
		Cephalosporins	
		cefaclor	Ceclor
		cefdinir	▸ Omnicef
		cefprozil	▸ Cefzil
		ceftriaxone	Rocephin
		cefuroxime	Ceftin
		cephalexin	▸ Keflex

Table 26-1 Classification of Drugs Based on Action—cont'd

Drug Category	Primary Use and Major Therapeutic Effects	COMMONLY PRESCRIBED DRUGS Generic	Brand
Antiinfectives, cont'd		**Fluoroquinolones** ciprofloxacin levofloxacin moxifloxacin ofloxacin	‣ Cipro ‣ Levaquin Avelox Floxin
		Tetracyclines doxycycline minocycline tetracycline	Doryx ‣ Vibramycin Arestin Achromycin Sumycin
		Aminoglycosides gentamicin kanamycin neomycin tobramycin	Garamycin Kantrex Neobiotic Nebcin
		Sulfonamides sulfamethoxazole trimethoprim/sulfamethoxazole	Gantanol ‣ Bactrim
		Miscellaneous clindamycin chloramphenicol nitrofurantoin vancomycin	Cleocin Chloromycetin ‣ Macrobid Macrodantin Vancocin
Antiinflammatory Agents	**Used** to relieve signs and symptoms of osteoarthritis and rheumatoid arthritis in adults **Work** by decreasing pain and inflammation	aspirin celecoxib etodolac ibuprofen indomethacin meloxicam nabumetone naproxen piroxicam valdecoxib	Bayer* Ecotrin* ‣ Celebrex Lodine Advil* Motrin* Indocin ‣ Mobic ‣ Relafen Aleve* Anaprox Naprosyn Feldene Bextra
Antimanics	**Used** to treat bipolar affective disorders **Work** by altering cation transport in nerves and muscles	lithium	Eskalith Eskalith CR
Antimigraines	**Used** in acute treatment of migraine attacks **Work** by causing vasoconstriction in large intracranial arteries	sumatriptan	‣ Imitrex

Continued

Table 26-1   Classification of Drugs Based on Action—cont'd

Drug Category	Primary Use and Major Therapeutic Effects	COMMONLY PRESCRIBED DRUGS	
		Generic	Brand
Antineoplastics	**Used** to treat tumors **Work** by preventing development, growth, or proliferation of malignant cells	cyclophosphamide methotrexate	Cytoxan Mexate Folex
Anti-Parkinson Agents	**Used** to treat symptoms of Parkinson disease **Work** by restoring balance between acetylcholine and dopamine in central nervous system	carbidopa/levodopa ropinirole	Sinemet Requip
Antiprotozoals	**Used** to treat protozoal infections **Work** by destroying protozoa	metronidazole	Flagyl
Antipsychotics	**Used** to treat psychotic disorders **Work** by blocking dopamine and serotonin receptors in central nervous system	haloperidol aripiprazole olanzapine risperidone quetiapine	Haldol ‣ Abilify ‣ Zyprexa ‣ Risperdal ‣ Seroquel
Antiretrovirals	**Used** to manage human immunodeficiency virus (HIV) infections and to reduce maternal-fetal transmission of HIV **Work** by inhibiting replication of retroviruses	efavirenz emtricitabine lamivudine ritonavir tenofovir zidovudine	Sustiva Emtriva Epivir Norvir Viread Retrovir
Antispasmodics	**Used** to control hypermotility in irritable bowel syndrome, spastic colitis, spastic bladder, and pylorospasm **Work** by preventing or relieving spasms of gastrointestinal or genitourinary tract	dicyclomine hyoscyamine	Bentyl Levsin
Antituberculars	**Used** to treat tuberculosis **Work** by killing or inhibiting growth of mycobacteria	isoniazid rifampin	INH Rifadin
Antitussives	**Used** in prevention or relief of coughs caused by minor viral upper respiratory infections or inhaled irritants **Work** by suppressing cough reflex by direct effect on cough center in central nervous system	benzonatate chlorpheniramine/hydrocodone dextromethorphan guaifenesin/codeine	Tessalon Tussionex (III) Robitussin DM* Robitussin A-C (V)
Antiulcers	**Used** to manage ulcers, gastroesophageal reflux disease, heartburn, indigestion, and gastric hyperacidity **Work** by preventing accumulation of acid in stomach	**Proton Pump Inhibitors** esomeprazole lansoprazole omeprazole pantoprazole rabeprazole **H$_2$-Receptor Antagonists** cimetidine famotidine ranitidine	 ‣ Nexium ‣ Prevacid ‣ Prilosec* ‣ Protonix ‣ AcipHex Tagamet* ‣ Pepcid AC* ‣ Zantac*
Antivirals	**Used** to manage herpes infections **Work** by inhibiting viral replication	acyclovir famciclovir valacyclovir	‣ Zovirax Famvir ‣ Valtrex
Bone Resorption Inhibitors	**Used** to treat and prevent osteoporosis **Work** by inhibiting resorption of bone	alendronate ibandronate raloxifene risedronate	‣ Fosamax Boniva ‣ Evista ‣ Actonel

Table 26-1 Classification of Drugs Based on Action—cont'd

Drug Category	Primary Use and Major Therapeutic Effects	COMMONLY PRESCRIBED DRUGS	
		Generic	**Brand**
Bronchodilators	***Used*** to manage reversible airway obstruction caused by asthma or chronic obstructive pulmonary disease ***Work*** by relaxing smooth muscle of respiratory tract resulting in bronchodilation	albuterol fluticasone/salmeterol formoterol ipratropium/albuterol levalbuterol montelukast salmeterol theophylline tiotropium	‣ Proventil ‣ Advair Diskus Foradil ‣ Combivent Xopenex ‣ Singulair Serevent Bronkodyl ‣ Spiriva
Cardiac Glycosides	***Used*** to treat congestive heart failure and cardiac arrhythmias ***Work*** by increasing strength and force of myocardial contractions and slowing heart rate	digitoxin digoxin	Crystodigin ‣ Digitek Lanoxicaps ‣ Lanoxin
Central Nervous System Stimulants	***Used*** to treat narcolepsy and manage attention-deficit/hyperactivity disorder ***Work*** by increasing level of catecholamines in central nervous system	atomoxetine dextroamphetamine dextroamphetamine saccharate and sulfate lisdexamfetamine methylphenidate	‣ Strattera Dexedrine (II) ‣ Adderall (II) Vyvanse (II) ‣ Ritalin (II) ‣ Concerta (II)
Contraceptives (Hormonal)	***Used*** to prevent pregnancy and to regulate menstrual cycle ***Work*** by inhibiting ovulation	**Oral Contraceptives** ethinyl estradiol/drospirenone ethinyl estradiol/levonorgestrel ethinyl estradiol/norethindrone ethinyl estradiol/norgestimate **Injectable Contraceptives** medroxyprogesterone **Transdermal Contraceptives** ethinyl estradiol/norelgestromin **Vaginal Ring Contraceptives** ethinyl estradiol/etonogestrel	 ‣ Yasmin Yaz Alesse Levien Kariva ‣ Ortho-Novum ‣ Loestrin Fe ‣ Ortho Tri-Cyclen Tri-Sprintec ‣ Depo-Provera ‣ Ortho Evra NuvaRing
Corticosteroids	Systemic Corticosteroids ***Used*** to treat inflammation, allergies, asthma, and autoimmune disorders and as replacement therapy in adrenal insufficiency ***Work*** by suppressing inflammation and modifying normal immune response Nasal Corticosteroids ***Used*** to treat chronic nasal inflammatory conditions (e.g., allergic rhinitis) ***Work*** by suppressing inflammation and reducing hypersecretions of respiratory tract	cortisone fluticasone hydrocortisone methylprednisolone triamcinolone fluticasone mometasone prednisone triamcinolone	Cortone ‣ Flovent Cortef Mcdrol Depo-Medrol Aristocort ‣ Flonase ‣ Nasonex ‣ Deltasone ‣ Nasacort

Continued

Table 26-1 **Classification of Drugs Based on Action—cont'd**

Drug Category	Primary Use and Major Therapeutic Effects	COMMONLY PRESCRIBED DRUGS Generic	Brand
Decongestants	**Used** to decrease nasal congestion **Work** by producing vasoconstriction in respiratory tract mucosa	oxymetazoline phenylephrine pseudoephedrine	Afrin* Dristan* Neo-Synephrine* Sudafed*
Diuretics	**Used** to manage hypertension, edema in congestive heart failure, and renal disease **Work** by removing excess fluid from the body by increasing urine output	**Loop Diuretics** bumetanide furosemide **Thiazide Diuretics** chlorthalidone hydrochlorothiazide **Potassium-Sparing Diuretics** spironolactone triamterene	 Bumex ▸ Lasix Hygroton ▸ Microzide Aldactone Dyrenium
Electrolyte Replacements	**Used** to treat or prevent electrolyte depletion **Work** by replacing electrolytes in body	**Potassium Supplements** potassium chloride	 ▸ K-Dur ▸ Klor-Con
Emetics	**Used** to treat poisoning **Work** by inducing vomiting	syrup of ipecac	
Expectorants	**Used** to manage coughs by expelling mucus **Work** by decreasing viscosity of bronchial secretions to promote clearance of mucus from respiratory tract	guaifenesin	Robitussin* Mucinex* Naldecon*
Hormone Replacements	**Used** to treat moderate to severe vasomotor symptoms of menopause **Work** by restoring hormonal balance	conjugated estrogens conjugated estrogen/ progesterone estradiol/norethindrone	▸ Premarin ▸ Prempro Activella
Immunizations	**Used** to prevent (vaccine-preventable) diseases **Work** by stimulating body to produce antibodies	diphtheria, tetanus toxoids, and acellular pertussis vaccine *Haemophilus* b conjugate vaccine hepatitis A vaccine hepatitis B vaccine human papillomavirus vaccine inactivated polio vaccine influenza virus vaccine types A and B measles, mumps, and rubella vaccine meningococcal conjugate vaccine pneumococcal conjugate vaccine rotavirus rubella vaccine varicella vaccine	Acel-Imune Certiva Daptacel Infanrix Tripedia ActHIB HibTITER Havrix Vaqta Engerix-B Recombivax HB Gardasil IPOL Afluria FluShield Fluzone FluMist M-M-R II Menactra Prevnar Pneumovax II Rotarix RotaShield Meruvax II Varivax

Table 26-1 Classification of Drugs Based on Action—cont'd

Drug Category	Primary Use and Major Therapeutic Effects	COMMONLY PRESCRIBED DRUGS	
		Generic	Brand
Immunosuppressants	**Used** to treat severe rheumatoid arthritis and to prevent and treat rejection of transplanted organs **Work** by inhibiting body's normal immune response	cyclosporine methotrexate	Sandimmune Neoral Rheumatrex
Laxatives	**Used** to relieve constipation **Work** by promoting defecation of normal, soft stool	bisacodyl docusate phenolphthalein psyllium	Dulcolax* Colace* Phenolax* Metamucil*
Lipid-Lowering Agents	**Used** to lower cholesterol to reduce risk of myocardial infarction and stroke **Work** by inhibiting enzyme needed to synthesize cholesterol in body	atorvastatin ezetimibe ezetimibe/simvastatin fenofibrate fluvastatin gemfibrozil lovastatin pravastatin rosuvastatin simvastatin	▸ Lipitor ▸ Zetia ▸ Vytorin ▸ Tricor Lescol Lopid ▸ Mevacor ▸ Pravachol ▸ Crestor ▸ Zocor
Muscle Relaxants (Skeletal)	**Used** to treat acute painful musculoskeletal conditions **Work** by relaxing skeletal muscles	baclofen carisoprodol cyclobenzaprine metaxalone methocarbamol tizanidine	▸ Lioresal ▸ Soma ▸ Flexeril Skelaxin Robaxin ▸ Zanaflex
Ophthalmic Antiinfectives	**Used** to treat eye infections **Work** by destroying bacteria	dexamethasone/tobramycin moxifloxacin polymyxin/bacitracin polymyxin/neomycin polymyxin/trimethoprim tobramycin	TobraDex Vigamox Polysporin Neosporin Polytrim Tobrex
Otic Preparations	**Used** to treat ear conditions Analgesics **Work** by relieving ear pain Antiinfectives **Work** by treating otitis externa Cerumenolytics **Work** by softening cerumen	benzocaine neomycin/polymyxin/ hydrocortisone ofloxacin carbamide peroxide	Auralgan Cortisporin Otic Floxin Otic Debrox*
Platelet Inhibitors	**Used** to reduce incidence of myocardial infarction and stroke **Work** by interfering with ability of platelets to adhere to each other	clopidogrel salicylates	▸ Plavix Aspirin*
Sedatives and Hypnotics	**Used** for short-term treatment of insomnia **Work** by promoting sleep by central nervous system depression	eszopiclone flurazepam hydroxyzine phenobarbital temazepam zolpidem	▸ Lunesta (IV) Dalmane (IV) Atarax Vistaril Luminal (IV) ▸ Restoril (IV) ▸ Ambien (IV)

Continued

Table 26-1   Classification of Drugs Based on Action—cont'd

| Drug Category | Primary Use and Major Therapeutic Effects | COMMONLY PRESCRIBED DRUGS | |
		Generic	Brand
Smoking Deterrents	**Used** to manage nicotine withdrawal to cease cigarette smoking **Work** by providing nicotine during controlled withdrawal from cigarette smoking	bupropion nicotine	Zyban Nicorette Gum* Nicotrol Inhaler Nicoderm Patch* Commit Lozenges*
		varenicline	Chantix
Thrombolytic Agents	**Used** for acute management of coronary thrombosis (myocardial infarction) **Work** by dissolving existing clots	alteplase anistreplase reteplase streptokinase	Activase Eminase Retavase Streptase
Thyroid Preparations	**Thyroid Hormones** **Used** as replacement or substitute therapy for diminished or absent thyroid functioning of many causes **Work** by increasing basal metabolic rate	levothyroxine	▶ Levoxyl ▶ Synthroid
	Antithyroid Agents **Used** to treat hyperthyroidism **Work** by inhibiting thyroid hormone synthesis, reducing basal metabolic rate	methimazole	Tapazole
Urinary Tract–Antispasmodics	**Used** to treat overactive bladder function **Work** by inhibiting bladder contractions	oxybutynin tolterodine	Ditropan ▶ Detrol
Vasopressors	**Used** to treat severe allergic reactions and cardiac arrest **Work** by increasing blood pressure and cardiac output and by dilating bronchi	epinephrine	Adrenalin EpiPen
Weight Control Agents	**Used** to manage obesity **Appetite Suppressants** **Work** by suppressing appetite center in central nervous system	diethylpropion phentermine sibutramine orlistat	Tenuate (IV) Fastin (IV) Meridia (IV) Xenical Alli*
	Lipase Inhibitors **Work** by inhibiting action of lipase to decrease absorption of dietary fats		

Modified from Bonewit-West K: *Clinical procedures for medical assistants*, ed 8, St Louis, 2011, Saunders.
*Available OTC (over-the-counter).
▶ Top-200 most prescribed drugs.
(II), Schedule II drug; *(III)*, Schedule III drug; *(IV)*, Schedule IV drug.

SYSTEMS OF MEASUREMENT FOR MEDICATION

Three systems of measurement are used in the United States for prescribing, administering, and dispensing medication: the metric system, the apothecary system, and the household system. The metric system is the most common system used to measure medication because it provides a more exact measurement and is easier to use. Some physicians occasionally use the apothecary system; the medical assistant should be familiar with this system. The third system of measurement, the household system, is the least accurate and generally is used only when a patient takes liquid medication at home.

Systems of measurement have units of weight, volume, and length. *Weight* refers to the heaviness of an item, and *volume* refers to the amount of space occupied by a substance. *Length* is a unit of linear measurement of the distance from one point to another. Although length is not used to administer medication, it is used in other aspects of the medical office. The head circumference of infants is measured in centimeters (cm), a metric unit of linear measurement.

To prepare and administer medication properly and to avoid medication errors, the medical assistant must have a thorough knowledge of the specific units of measurement for these three systems and must be able to convert within each and from one system to another. A basic discussion of the metric, apothecary, and household systems is presented next. A more thorough study of these systems, including conversion of units and dose calculation, is included in Chapter 26 of the Study Guide.

Metric System

The metric system was developed in France in the latter part of the 18th century in an effort to simplify measurement. Most European countries are required by law to use this system for the measurement of weight, volume, and length. Overall, the metric system is used for most scientific and medical measurements. Pharmaceutical companies use the metric system to measure and label medications.

The metric system employs a uniform decimal scale based on units of 10, making it very flexible and logical. The basic metric units of measurement are the gram, liter, and meter. The *gram* is a unit of weight used to measure solids, the *liter* is a unit of volume used to measure liquids, and the *meter* is a linear unit used to measure length or distance. The metric units used most often in the administration of medication in the medical office are the milligram, gram, milliliter, and cubic centimeter. Because a **cubic centimeter (cc)** is the amount of space occupied by 1 milliliter (mL), these two units can be used interchangeably (i.e., 1 mL = 1 cc).

Prefixes added to the words *gram, liter,* and *meter* designate smaller or larger units of measurement in the metric system. The same prefixes are used with all three units. For example, *milli-* is used as follows: *milli*gram, *milli*liter, and *milli*meter. A prefix changes the value of the basic unit of measurement by the same amount. The prefix *milli-* describes a unit that is $\frac{1}{1000}$ of the basic unit: 1 gram is equal to 1000 milligrams, 1 liter is equal to 1000 milliliters, and 1 meter is equal to 1000 millimeters. The box *Metric Notation Guidelines* lists the metric units of measurement and equivalent values in different units. Specific guidelines are used in the medical notation of metric units and doses, which also are presented in the box. To read prescriptions and medication orders, to record medication administration, and, most important, to avoid medication errors, the medical assistant must be familiar with and be able to follow these guidelines.

Metric Notation Guidelines

Follow these guidelines when using the metric notation of measurement and dosage.

1. The units of metric measurement are written using the following abbreviations.

Weight
>   microgram: mcg or µg
>   milligram: mg
>   gram: g
>   kilogram: kg

Volume
>   milliliter: mL (or ml)
>   liter: L

2. Do not use a period with the abbreviations for metric units because it might be mistaken for another letter or symbol.
   Correct: mg
>   mL
   Incorrect: mg.
>   mL.

3. Use Arabic numerals (e.g., 1, 2, 3, 4) to express the quantity of the dose.
   Correct: 4 mg
   Incorrect: iv mg

4. Place the numeral that expresses the quantity of the dose in front of the abbreviation. To make it easier to read, leave a (single) space between the quantity and the abbreviation.
   Correct: 5 mL
   Incorrect: mL 5
>   5mL

5. Write a fraction of a dose as a decimal.
   Correct: 0.5 g
   Incorrect: ½ g

6. If the dose is a fraction of a unit, place a zero before the decimal point as a means of focusing on the fractional dose. This reduces the possibility of misreading the dose as a whole number.
   Correct: 0.5 g (this reduces the possibility of not seeing the decimal point and reading the dose as 5 grams)
   Incorrect: .5 g

7. Do not place a decimal point and a zero after a whole number. The decimal point may be overlooked, resulting in a 10-fold overdose error.
   Correct: 1 mL (this reduces the possibility of not seeing the decimal point and reading the dose as 10 mL)
   Incorrect: 1.0 mL

Metric System: Conversion of Equivalent Values
Weight
1000 micrograms = 1 milligram
1000 milligrams = 1 gram
1000 grams = 1 kilogram
Volume
1000 milliliters = 1 liter
1000 liters = 1 kiloliter
1 milliliter = 1 cubic centimeter

Apothecary System

The apothecary system is older and less accurate than the metric system. It was brought to the United States from England during the 18th century. Pharmacists used this system during the colonial period to compound and measure medications. This system is gradually being phased out for measurement of medication in favor of the metric system. Until that process is completed, however, the medical assistant must be familiar with this system and be able to use it to administer medication.

The basic unit of weight in the apothecary system is the *grain*, derived from the weight of a large grain of wheat, which was used to balance the material being weighed. The next largest unit of measurement is the *scruple;* however, this unit is not used to administer medication. The remaining units, in order of increasing weight, are *dram, ounce,* and *pound.* The pound is not generally used in the administration of medication. The medical assistant should note,

however, that in the apothecary system the pound is equal to 12 ounces, in contrast to the more familiar *avoirdupois* pound used to measure body weight, which is equal to 16 ounces.

Measures of liquid volume in the apothecary system correlate closely with measures of dry weight in the same system. The smallest unit of measurement is the *minim,* meaning "the least." A minim is approximately equivalent to a volume of water that weighs 1 grain. A minim glass or a syringe calibrated in minims must be used to measure with this unit. The remaining units of liquid volume in the apothecary system, in order of increasing volume, are *fluid dram, fluid ounce, pint, quart,* and *gallon.* The basic unit of linear measurement is the *inch,* followed by *foot, yard,* and *mile.* Most Americans are familiar with apothecary units of measurement because of their use in everyday life. For example, milk is available in pints, quarts, and gallons, and height is measured in feet and inches.

Apothecary Notation Guidelines

Follow these guidelines when using the medical notation of apothecary units and dosage.

1. The units of apothecary measurement are usually written with abbreviations and symbols as follows.

Weight

    grain: gr

    dram: dr or ʒ

    ounce: oz or ℥

Volume

    minim: ♍

    fluid dram: fʒ; fluid ounce: f℥

    pint: pt

    quart: qt

    gallon: gal

2. When writing symbols and abbreviations to express apothecary units, use lowercase roman numerals to express the dose quantity.

    Correct: ℥ v̄i (6 ounces)

    Incorrect: 6 ℥

            ℥6

3. Place the roman numeral expressing dose quantity after the symbol or abbreviation.

    Correct: ʒ ïi (2 drams)

            gr v (5 grains)

    Incorrect: ïi ʒ

            v gr

4. A line may be placed over the roman numerals. Dots are placed above the line for emphasis as a safeguard against error.

    Correct: f ʒ ïïi (3 fluid drams)

    Incorrect: f ʒ lll

5. Write ss to designate one half of a dose, and place it after the apothecary symbol or abbreviation.

    Correct: gr ss

    Incorrect: gr ½

6. Write fractions (other than ½) in Arabic numerals, and place them after the apothecary symbol or abbreviation.

    Correct: gr ¼

    Incorrect: gr 0.25; ¼ gr

    Note: If abbreviations and symbols are not used to express apothecary units of measurement, Arabic numerals must be used to express dose quantity and are placed before the unit of measurement. *Example:* ¼ grain.

Apothecary System: Conversion of Equivalent Values

Weight

60 grains = 1 dram

8 drams = 1 ounce

12 ounces = 1 pound

Volume

60 minims = 1 fluid dram

8 fluid drams = 1 fluid ounce

16 fluid ounces = 1 pint

2 pints = 1 quart

4 quarts = 1 gallon

The box *Apothecary Notation Guidelines* lists the units of measurement in the apothecary system and equivalent values in different units. It also includes guidelines for the medical notation of apothecary units.

Household System

The household system is more complicated and less accurate for administering liquid medication than either the metric or the apothecary system. Nevertheless, most individuals are familiar with this system because of its frequent use in the United States. This system of measurement may be the only one the patient can understand and safely use to take liquid medication at home. Most patients are more comfortable measuring medication in drops and teaspoons than in minims and milliliters. In addition, the patient is more likely to have household measuring devices on hand than to have metric measuring devices. If a precise measurement is needed, however, the metric system must be used, and the medical assistant should instruct the patient in the use of the metric measuring device.

Volume is the only household unit of measurement used to administer medication. The basic unit of liquid volume in the household system is the *drop (gtt),* which is approximately equal to 0.6 mL in the metric system and 1 minim in the apothecary system. These units cannot be considered exact equivalents because the size of the drop varies based on temperature, the viscosity of the liquid, and the size of the dropper. The remaining units, in order of increasing volume, are *teaspoon, tablespoon, ounce (fluid ounce), cup,* and *glass.* Table 26-2 lists the units of liquid volume measurement in the household system and equivalent values in different units.

Table 26-2 Household System: Conversion of Common Values

Abbreviations	
drop	gtt
teaspoon	tsp
tablespoon	T
ounce	oz
cup	c
Volume	
60 gtt =	1 tsp
3 tsp =	1 T
6 tsp =	1 oz
2 T =	1 oz
6 oz =	1 teacup
8 oz =	1 glass

From Bonewit-West K: *Clinical procedures for medical assistants,* ed 8, St Louis, 2011, Saunders.

CONVERTING UNITS OF MEASUREMENT

Changing from one unit of measurement to another is known as **conversion.** Conversion is required when medication is ordered in a unit of measurement that differs from the medication's label. The dose quantity must be mathematically translated or converted to the unit of measurement of the medication on hand. If the physician orders 5 grams of an oral solid medication, and the medication label expresses the drug strength in milligrams, the medical assistant would need to convert the grams into milligrams to know how much medication to administer. Converting units of measurement can be classified into the following categories: (1) conversion of units within a measurement system, and (2) conversion of units from one measurement system to another.

Converting units within a measurement system allows a quantity to be expressed in two different but equal units of measurement within *one* system. An example of converting units of weight within the metric system is as follows: 1 gram is equal to 1000 milligrams. Converting from one measurement system to another allows a quantity written in one measurement system to be expressed in an equivalent unit of measurement in *another* system. An example of a conversion from the apothecary system to the metric system is as follows: 1 grain (apothecary system) is equivalent to 60 milligrams (metric system).

Conversion requires the use of a conversion table to indicate the equivalent values of various units of measurement. Conversion tables of equivalent values in these three measurement systems are included in this chapter:

Metric conversion—*Metric Notation Guidelines* box
Apothecary conversion—*Apothecary Notation Guidelines* box
Household conversion—Table 26-2

Tables used to convert from one system to another consist of approximate rather than exact equivalents, and a 10% error usually occurs in making these conversions. Conversion tables used to convert from one system to another are presented in Table 26-3.

The medical assistant must be careful when using conversion tables to avoid errors in interpolation. The numbers on conversion tables are small and close together; it is easy to misread the chart from one column to the other. To reduce this possibility, a straightedge, such as a ruler, should be used when reading a conversion table.

CONTROLLED DRUGS

By means of federal and state legislation, restrictions are placed on drugs that have potential for abuse. These drugs are known as **controlled drugs.** They are classified into five categories, called *schedules,* which are based on their abuse potential. Table 26-4 lists, describes, and provides examples of the schedules for controlled drugs.

Table 26-3 Conversion Charts for Systems of Measurement

CONVERSION CHART FOR METRIC AND APOTHECARY SYSTEMS (COMMON APPROXIMATE EQUIVALENTS)

Metric System to Apothecary System			Apothecary System to Metric System		
Weight			**Weight**		
60 mg	=	1 gr	15 gr	=	1000 mg (1 g)
1 g	=	15 gr	10 gr	=	600 mg
29 g	=	1 dr	7½ gr	=	500 mg
30 g	=	1 oz	5 gr	=	300 mg
1 kg	=	2.2 lb	3 gr	=	200 mg
			1½ gr	=	100 mg
Volume			**Volume**		
0.06 mL	=	1 ♏	1 gr	=	60 mg
1 mL (cc)	=	15 ♏	¾ gr	=	50 mg
4 mL	=	1 fℨ	½ gr	=	30 mg
30 mL	=	1 fℨ	¼ gr	=	15 mg
500 mL	=	1 pt	⅙ gr	=	10 mg
1000 mL (1 L)	=	1 qt	⅛ gr	=	8 mg
			1/12 gr	=	5 mg
			1/15 gr	=	4 mg
			1/20 gr	=	3 mg
			1/30 gr	=	2 mg
			1/40 gr	=	1.5 mg
			1/50 gr	=	1.2 mg
			1/60 gr	=	1 mg
			1/100 gr	=	0.6 mg
			1/120 gr	=	0.5 mg
			1/150 gr	=	0.4 mg
			1/200 gr	=	0.3 mg
			1/300 gr	=	0.2 mg
			1/600 gr	=	0.1 mg

EQUIVALENCES IN HOUSEHOLD, APOTHECARY, AND METRIC UNITS (VOLUME)

Household	Apothecary	Metric
1 gtt	= 1 ♏	= 0.06 mL
15 gtts	= 15 ♏	= 1 mL (1 cc)
1 tsp	= ⅙ fℨ	= 5 (4) mL*
1 T	= ½ fℨ	= 15 mL
2 T	= 1 fℨ	= 30 mL
1 oz	= 1fℨ	= 30 mL
1 teacup	= 6fℨ	= 180 mL
1 glass	= 8fℨ	= 240 mL

From Bonewit-West K: *Clinical procedures for medical assistants,* ed 8, St Louis, 2011, Saunders.
*The American standard teaspoon is accepted as 5 mL; however, 4 mL can be used as the equivalent to provide a more accurate conversion.

To administer, prescribe, or dispense controlled drugs, the physician must register every year with the Drug Enforcement Administration (DEA). The physician is assigned a registration number known as the **DEA number.** Every time a prescription for a controlled drug is written, the physician must put his or her DEA number in the appropriate space on the prescription blank.

PRESCRIPTION

A **prescription** is a physician's order authorizing the dispensing of a drug by a pharmacist. Prescriptions can be authorized in different forms, including hand-written, computer-generated, and telephoned or faxed to a pharmacy.

Table 26-4 Classification of Controlled Drugs

Classification	Description and Prescription Regulations	EXAMPLES	
		Generic	Brand
Schedule I	High potential for abuse Currently no accepted medical use in treatment in the United States There is a lack of accepted safety for use of the drug under medical supervision Use may lead to severe physical or psychological dependence May be used for research with appropriate limitations Not available for prescribing	GHB heroin LSD marijuana MDMA (Ecstasy) mescaline methaqualone (Quaalude) psilocybin	
Schedule II	High potential for abuse Currently accepted medical use in treatment in the United States or a currently accepted medical use with severe restrictions Abuse may lead to severe psychological or physical dependence Prescription must be in writing in indelible ink or typed Emergency telephone order permitted only for immediate amount needed to treat patient; written prescription must be provided to pharmacist within 7 days No refills allowed Manufacturer's label marked C-II	**Analgesics** cocaine codeine fentanyl hydrocodone hydromorphone meperidine methadone morphine oxycodone oxycodone/APAP oxycodone/ASA **Central Nervous System Stimulants** dextroamphetamine lisdexamfetamine methylphenidate methamphetamine **Sedatives/Hypnotics** amobarbital glutethimide pentobarbital secobarbital	 Duragesic Dilaudid Demerol Dolophine Roxanol OxyContin Percocet Percodan Adderall Vyvanese Ritalin, Concerta Desoxyn Amytal Doriden Nembutal Seconal
Schedule III	Less potential for abuse than drugs in Schedules I and II Currently accepted medical use in treatment in the United States Abuse may lead to moderate or low physical dependence or high psychological dependence Telephone and fax orders permitted If authorized by physician, prescription can be refilled five times within 6 months from issue date Prescription expires 6 months from issue date Manufacturer's label marked C-III	**Anabolic Steroids** oxandrolone oxymetholone analgesics buprenorphine butalbital compound codeine combined with nonopioid analgesic hydrocodone combined with nonopioid analgesic **Central Nervous System Stimulant** benzphetamine **Male Hormone** testosterone **Sedative/Hypnotic** butabarbital	 Anavar Anapolon Buprenex Fioricet, Fiorinal Tylenol w/ codeine, Empirin w/ codeine Vicodin, Lortab, Lorcet, Tussionex, Vicoprofen Didrex Depotest, Delatestryl Butisol
Schedule IV	Lower potential for abuse than drugs in Schedule III Currently accepted medical use in treatment in the United States Abuse may lead to limited physical or psychological dependence Telephone and fax orders permitted	**Analgesics** butorphanol pentazocine propoxyphene **Antianxiety Agents** alprazolam chlordiazepoxide	 Stadol Talwin Darvon, Darvocet-N Xanax Librium

Continued

Table 26-4 Classification of Controlled Drugs—cont'd

Classification	Description and Prescription Regulations	EXAMPLES	
		Generic	Brand
	If authorized by physician, prescription can be refilled five times within 6 months of issue date Prescription expires 6 months from issue date Manufacturer's label marked C-IV	diazepam halazepam lorazepam meprobamate oxazepam	Valium Paxipam Ativan Equanil Serax
		Anticonvulsant clonazepam	Klonopin
		Central Nervous System Stimulants modafinil pemoline	Provigil Cylert
		Sedatives/Hypnotics chloral hydrate eszopiclone ethchlorvynol flurazepam midazolam phenobarbital temazepam triazolam zaleplon zolpidem	Noctec Lunesta Placidyl Dalmane Versed Luminal Restoril Halcion Sonata Ambien
		Weight Control Agents diethylpropion phentermine sibutramine	Tenuate Fastin Meridia
Schedule V	Low potential for abuse Accepted medical use in United States Abuse may lead to limited physical or psychological dependence Telephone and fax orders permitted Prescribing policies determined by state and local regulations. In most states: Number of refills determined by physician Prescription expires 1 year from issue date Some are available without prescription to patients older than 18 years of age (with proper identification) Manufacturer's label marked C-V	Cough suppressants with small amounts of codeine Antidiarrheals containing paregoric diphenoxylate/atropine	Robitussin A-C, Cheracol syrup Parepectolin, Kapectolin PG Lomotil

From Bonewit-West K: *Clinical procedures for medical assistants*, ed 8, St Louis, 2011, Saunders.

Abbreviations and symbols are usually used to write a prescription. They also are used to record medication information in the patient's chart. Common abbreviations used in the medical office for writing prescriptions are included in Table 26-5.

The medical assistant should ensure that all prescription pads are kept in a safe place and out of reach of individuals who may want to obtain drugs illegally. The stock supply of prescription pads should be locked in a drawer.

Parts of a Prescription

A prescription is a handwritten (Figure 26-2) or computer-generated document that includes directions to the pharmacist for filling the prescription and instructions to the patient for taking the medication. The specific information that the prescription must include follows:

- **Date.** A pharmacist cannot fill a prescription unless the date the prescription was issued is indicated on the prescription. The reason for this is that a prescription expires after a certain length of time. In most states, a prescription for a drug (with the exception of controlled drugs) expires 1 year from the date of issue. After this time, the prescription (or any refills left on the prescription) cannot be filled.

- **Physician's name, address, telephone number, and fax number.** This information is preprinted on prescription forms that are handwritten and automatically printed on

Table 26-5 Common Abbreviations and Symbols Used in Medication Documentation

Abbreviation or Symbol	Meaning	Abbreviation or Symbol	Meaning
$\overline{aa}$	of each	OS	left eye
ac	before meals	OTC	over-the-counter
AD	right ear	OU	in each eye
ad lib	as desired	ʒ or oz	ounce
aq	water	$\overline{p}$	after
admin	administer, administration	pc	after meals
am or a.m.	morning	Pt or pt	patient
APAP	acetaminophen	per	by
AS	left ear	pm or p.m.	evening
ASA	aspirin	po or PO	by mouth
AU	in each ear	prn	as needed
bid	twice a day	qam	every morning
$\overline{c}$	with	qd	every day
cap(s)	capsule(s)	qh	every hour
cc	cubic centimeter	q (2, 3, 4) h	every (2, 3, 4) hours
DAW	dispense as written	qid	four times a day
dil	dilute	qod	every other day
ʒ or dr	dram	qs	of sufficient quantity
elix	elixir	Rx	take
g̊	gram	$\overline{s}$	without
gr	grain	SC or SQ	subcutaneous
gtt(s)	drop(s)	SL	sublingual
h or hr	hour	sol	solution
hs	at bedtime	ss	one half
ID	intradermal	STAT	immediately
IM	intramuscular	T	tablespoon
IN	inhalation	tab(s)	tablet(s)
IV	intravenous	tid	three times a day
kg	kilogram	tsp	teaspoon
L	liter	#	number
liq	liquid	×	times
♏	minim	Ø	no, none
med(s)	medication(s)	ī	one
mg	milligram	ïi	two
min	minute	ïïi	three
mL (or ml)	milliliter	īV	four
NPO	nothing by mouth	V̄	five
OD	right eye		

From Bonewit-West K: *Clinical procedures for medical assistants,* ed 8, St Louis, 2011, Saunders.

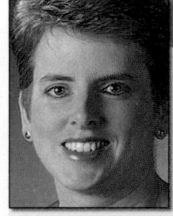

Putting It All into Practice

My name is Theresa Cline, and I work for four physicians in a family practice medical office. I have worked there ever since I graduated from college with an associate's degree in medical assisting. One experience that I will never forget taught our entire office staff a valuable lesson. It involved a woman who came to our office because she had lacerated her wrist while using a butcher knife. After the wound was sutured, I gave her a tetanus injection because she was past due for one. Shortly thereafter, she became very nauseated and dizzy, and I made her lie down on the examining table. She asked me to get her a cold drink of water, and I left the room to do so. Apparently, while I was gone, she must have tried to sit up or turn over

because she rolled off the table and struck the back of her head on the floor. She sustained a laceration to her scalp, which also had to be sutured. Owing to her persistent symptoms of severe nausea, vomiting, and headache, it was decided that she should be admitted to the hospital for neurologic observation and x-ray studies.

The vital lesson that this experience taught everyone in our office was that you must never leave a patient alone, not even for a minute to get something, if there is the slightest indication that he or she is not feeling perfectly fine. Another staff member should be called to obtain whatever is needed. From that point on, this has been our office policy and procedure. ■

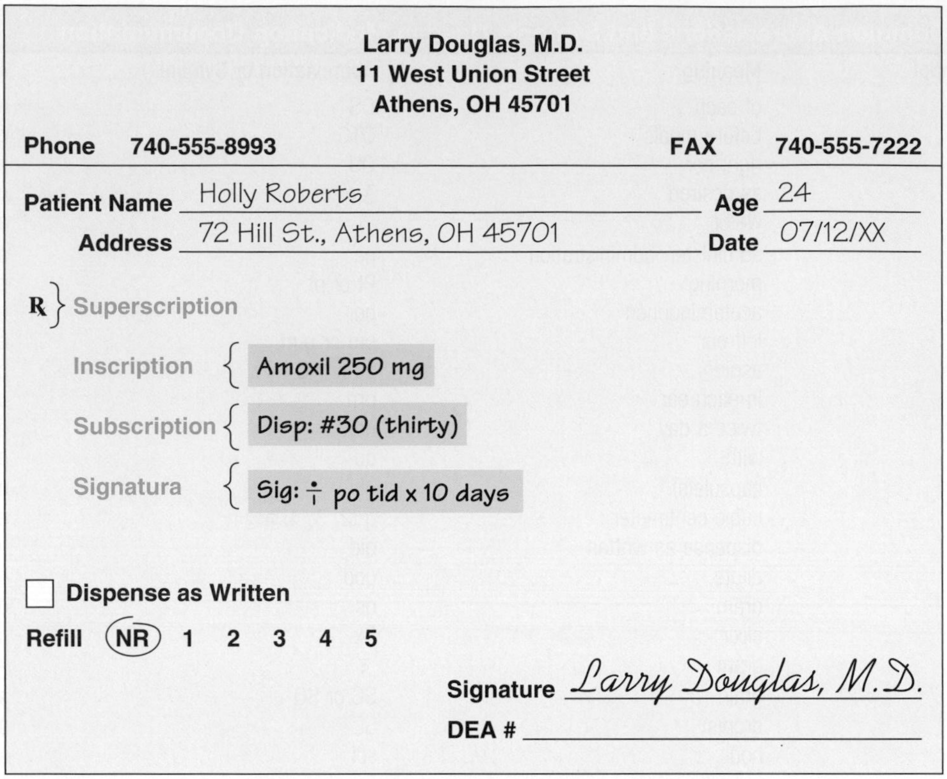

```
                    Larry Douglas, M.D.
                    11 West Union Street
                    Athens, OH 45701

Phone    740-555-8993                    FAX    740-555-7222
```

Patient Name ___Holly Roberts_____ Age __24____

     Address ___72 Hill St., Athens, OH 45701_____ Date __07/12/XX__

R } Superscription

Inscription { Amoxil 250 mg

Subscription { Disp: #30 (thirty)

Signatura { Sig: ÷ po tid x 10 days

☐ **Dispense as Written**

Refill (NR) 1 2 3 4 5

Signature _Larry Douglas, M.D._

DEA # _____

Figure 26-2 Example of a handwritten prescription.

forms that are computer generated. This information identifies the physician issuing the prescription and provides the necessary information should the pharmacist have a question and need to contact the medical office.

- **Patient's name and address.** This information is important for insurance billing and for properly dispensing the medication.
- **Patient's age.** The patient's age is important to the pharmacist when he or she double checks the physician's order to ensure that the proper dose is being dispensed. The most common errors in dosage occur among children and the elderly, who may not require the standard dose of a drug because these age groups metabolize drugs differently. The patient's age also allows the pharmacist to double check that the drug is age appropriate for the patient. For example, *ciprofloxacin* (e.g., Cipro) should not be taken by children and adolescents because this antibiotic can damage cartilage in individuals younger than 18 years old.
- **Superscription.** The superscription consists of the symbol *Rx.* This symbol comes from the Latin word *recipe* and means "take."
- **Inscription.** The inscription states the name of the drug and the dose (e.g., Amoxil 250 mg). Most drugs are available in various doses; it is important that the correct dose be prescribed. For example, Amoxil comes in the following doses: 125 mg, 250 mg, and 500 mg.

- **Subscription.** The subscription gives directions to the pharmacist. At present, it is generally used to designate the number of doses to be dispensed. To prevent a prescription from being altered illegally, it is recommended that numbers and letters be used to indicate the quantity to be dispensed (e.g., #30 [thirty]).
- **Signatura.** The signatura (abbreviated *Sig.*) comes from the Latin term *signa*, which means "write" or "label." The signatura indicates the information to be included on the medication label. It consists of directions to the patient for taking the medication. The name of the medication also is included on the label so that the patient can identify the medication.
- **Refill.** This part of the prescription indicates the number of times the prescription may be refilled.
- **Physician's signature.** A prescription cannot be filled unless it is signed by the physician.
- **DEA number.** The number assigned to the physician by the Drug Enforcement Administration must appear on the prescription for a controlled drug. See Table 26-4 for examples of controlled drugs.

Generic Prescribing

Generic prescribing means that the physician writes the prescription using the generic rather than the brand name of the drug. Because many pharmaceutical manufacturers may produce the same generic drug and sell it under different brand names, price competition often results. If the physician prescribes a drug using its generic name, the pharmacist is permitted to fill it with the drug that offers the best savings to the patient. In addition, most states allow the pharmacist the option of filling the prescription with a chemically equivalent generic drug, even if the drug has been prescribed by brand name. If the physician wants the prescription to be filled with a specific brand of drug, instructions must be indicated on the prescription form, such as "Dispense as Written (DAW)," or words of a similar meaning (see Figure 26-2).

Completing a Prescription Form

The physician is responsible for having accurate and pertinent information on the prescription form. If delegated by the physician, a prescription form can be completed by the medical assistant and signed by the physician. The physician must review the prescription thoroughly before signing it to ensure all of the information is correct. If the medical

assistant is delegated this responsibility, he or she must carefully follow the important guidelines presented in the box *Guidelines for Completing a Prescription Form.*

EMR Prescription Program

Electronic medical record (EMR) software includes a prescription program, which greatly reduces the amount of time needed to prescribe and refill medication. The prescription program generates and prints a prescription(s) on a regular sheet of $8\frac{1}{2} \times 11$-inch paper, which is then signed by the physician and given to the patient (Figure 26-3). The program can also transmit the prescription electronically (by e-fax or e-mail) to the patient's pharmacy. Both of these features eliminate the need for the pharmacist to decipher the physician's handwriting.

The EMR prescription program also has the capability to quickly refill a prescription and print a list of medications being taken by the patient. The patient can use this list to keep track of the medication he or she is taking (Figure 26-4).

Guidelines for Completing a Prescription Form

- Work in a quiet, well-lit area that is free of distractions.
- Use an indelible black ink pen to write on the form.
- Print all information on the form.
- Ensure that all information is spelled correctly.
- Review the metric notation guidelines presented in the box *Metric Notation Guidelines.* (Most prescriptions are written in metric units.)
- Always ask the physician if you have questions about the prescription.
- Complete all of the required information on the form; it includes the following:
  1. **Patient's name, address, and age**
     - Clearly print all of this information on the form. Never leave the address and age categories blank.
  2. **Date**
     - Indicate today's date on the prescription form.
  3. **Name of the medication**
     - The physician may prescribe the medication using either the generic or the brand name.
     - Make sure to spell the name of the drug correctly. If you are unsure, use a drug reference to find the correct spelling of a drug.
  4. **Medication dosage**
     - Never leave a decimal point "naked." If the dosage is a fraction of a unit, a zero must be placed before the decimal point as a means of focusing on the fractional dose. This reduces the possibility of misreading the dose as a whole number. *Example:* 0.5 mL (*not* .5 mL).

- Never place a decimal point and a zero after a whole number because the decimal point may be overlooked, resulting in a 10-fold overdose error. *Example:* 5 mg (*not* 5.0 mg).
  5. **Quantity to dispense**
     - Use numbers and letters to indicate the quantity to be dispensed. *Example:* Disp: #30 (thirty).
     - Ensure that the quantity is correct. The number of prescribed pills should match the duration of treatment. *Example:* If the patient has been prescribed 3 tablets a day for 7 days, the quantity should be written as follows: Disp: #21 (twenty-one).
  6. **Directions for taking the medication**
     - Clearly indicate the directions for taking the medication. Many authorities recommend writing the directions without abbreviations. *Example:* Sig: Take 1 capsule 3 times a day for 10 days.
     - If abbreviations are used, use only commonly accepted abbreviations, and print the information clearly. *Example:* Sig: cap po tid × 10 days.
  7. **Refills**
     - Never leave this category blank.
     - If there are no refills, indicate this clearly on the form. The method for doing this is based on the setup of the preprinted form.
     Example: Refill: (NR) 1 2 3 4 5
     (on this form, the information is circled)
     Example: Refill: 0
     (on this form, the information is written in)

Continued

Guidelines for Completing a Prescription Form—cont'd

8. **Dispense as written**
   - If the physician does not allow a substitution (e.g., generic equivalent) for this medication, check this category.
9. **DEA number**
   - If the prescription is for a controlled drug, clearly indicate the physician's DEA number on the form.
10. **Group practice**
    - If there is more than one physician in the practice, circle (or check) the name of the physician prescribing the medication. This avoids confusion if the pharmacist cannot read the physician's signature.

Example:

James Ortman, MD, (Mark Rothstein, MD), Richard Bontrager, MD

- Give the prescription to the physician to review and sign.
- Document the prescription order in the patient's medication record if directed by the physician. Some offices use multiple-copy prescription pads. In this case, file the copy of the prescription in the patient's medical record.
- Give the prescription to the patient. Provide the patient with guidelines for taking the medication (see patient teaching box on prescription medications).
- Ask the patient whether he or she has any questions about the medication.

PATIENT TEACHING **Prescription Medications**

To avoid adverse reactions, teach patients the proper guidelines for taking prescription medication. These guidelines are as follows:

Know the names of all your prescription and nonprescription medications. Know the generic and brand names of each of your medications. Nonprescription drugs are known as *over-the-counter* (OTC) drugs; they are drugs that can be purchased without a prescription. Vitamin supplements and herbal products are considered OTC drugs.

Know why you are taking each medication. It is important to know the desired therapeutic outcome, dosage, frequency and time of administration, and common side effects of each medication, and guidelines ("do's and don't's") to follow when taking the medication. Never take your medication in the dark or without your reading glasses (if needed for close vision).

Take your medication exactly as prescribed, at the right times and in the right amounts. The medication may not work properly if it is not taken as directed. If the dose is too small, the drug may not produce its intended therapeutic effect; exceeding the recommended dosage could result in a toxic effect. Make sure you know what to do if you are late in taking a dose or miss a dose of your medication. It is also important to know if any other medication or food interferes with your medication and should be avoided.

Inform the physician if new symptoms or adverse effects develop when you are taking the medication. The physician may need to change your dosage or prescribe a different medication. There are usually alternative medications that the physician can prescribe to treat your condition.

Take the medication for the prescribed duration of time, even after you begin to feel better. If you do not complete the entire course of drug therapy, your condition may recur. Not taking all of a prescribed antibiotic may cause an infection to return, and it may be worse than the first infection.

Tell the physician if you decide not to take your medication. Otherwise, the physician may think your medication is not working. Not taking a medication prescribed by the physician could be serious because this may allow your condition to worsen.

Do not take additional medications, including OTC medications, without checking with the physician. All drugs, including OTC medications, are designed to have an effect on the body. Some combinations of drugs cause serious reactions. In some cases, one drug cancels the effects of another and prevents it from working.

Never take a medication that was prescribed for someone else. Physicians prescribe medication based on an individual's age, weight, sex, and condition. Taking a medication prescribed for someone else can have serious results.

Keep all medications in their original containers to avoid taking the wrong medication by mistake. Store your medications in their original containers from the pharmacy. Basic information about your medication is on the original container. Medications that are not clearly marked may be taken inadvertently by the wrong person.

Store your medications in a safe place, away from the reach of children. If you have young children, make sure your medication is dispensed in containers with child-resistant safety closures. After taking your medication, make sure that the cap of the container is closed tightly. Accidental drug poisoning in children is a common and preventable problem. Also, do not take your medication in front of young children because they may want to mimic your behavior.

Store medications in a cool, dry place or as stated on the label. Do not store capsules or tablets in the bathroom or kitchen because heat or moisture may cause the medication to break down.

Discard unused portions of prescription medications and outdated OTC medications. Medications should be discarded by flushing them down the toilet. Medications that are past their expiration dates may produce adverse effects in the body. ∎

PRESCRIPTION: (Give to the pharmacist)	PRESCRIPTION: (Give to the pharmacist)
Huntington Clinic 701 Concord Ave Lexington, KY 48710 614-871-0033 Doctor: John Blauser, MD For: Danielle Travis Age: 28 DOB: 08/08/84 Date: 10/27/20XX Address: 101 Coventry Lane Lexington, KY 48710 Rx: Amoxil (Generic - amoxicillin) (Dose/unit - 250 mg) (Form - Caps) (Disp - #30) (Frequency - One three times daily for 10 days) (Route - By mouth) (Refills-0). Dr: _____ *John Blauser, MD* _____	Huntington Clinic 701 Concord Ave Lexington, KY 48710 614-871-0033 Doctor: John Blauser, MD For: Danielle Travis Age: 28 DOB: 08/08/84 Date: 10/27/20XX Address: 101 Coventry Lane Lexington, KY 48710 Rx: Tylenol-3 (Generic - Acetaminophen/Codeine) (Dose/unit - 1 to 2) (Form - Tabs) (Disp - #15)(fifteen) (Frequency - Every 4 hours as needed for moderate to severe pain) (Route - By mouth) (Refills-0). Dr: _____ *John Blauser, MD* _____

Figure 26-3 Example of a computer-generated prescription.

MEDICATION RECORD

A medication record form (Figure 26-5) includes detailed information about each medication, so that the physician can tell at a glance what medications and how much the patient is taking. Both prescription medication and over-the-counter (OTC) medication, including vitamin supplements and herbal products, must be recorded in the medication record.

The medication record is part of the patient's medical record. The medical assistant is often responsible for documenting medication information in the medication record. Care must be taken to ensure the information is correct and clearly stated.

In a paper-based patient record (PPR), the medical office may use a preprinted form to record the medication that a patient is taking. With an EMR, the medical assistant enters this information into a digital form on the screen of the monitor using free-text entry, drop-down lists, and check-boxes.

A medication record typically includes the following information:

- Patient's name and date of birth
- Any drug allergies
- Date the medication was prescribed (Rx) or date the patient started taking the medication (OTC)
- Name and dose of the medication
- Frequency of administration of the medication
- Route of administration
- Prescription or OTC medication category
- Refills (Rx medication only)
- Date the patient stopped taking the medication

What Would You Do? What Would You *Not* Do?

Case Study 2

Linda Cardwell calls the medical office. Her daughter Rachel, 9 years old, was seen in the office 10 days ago. Rachel was diagnosed with strep throat, and the physician ordered Amoxil 250 mg tid × 7 days. Mrs. Cardwell says that after 3 days of taking the medication, Rachel was much better, so she stopped giving her the Amoxil because it was causing her to have diarrhea. Mrs. Cardwell says that her 12-year-old son started feeling achy all over and she gave him the Amoxil for 2 days, and it seemed to help. She also says that her husband started complaining of sinus problems, so she also gave him the Amoxil for 2 days. Mrs. Cardwell says that now Rachel's throat is hurting again, and she has a fever. She wants to know whether Rachel has developed another case of strep throat. Mrs. Cardwell says she does not know what to do because she does not have any Amoxil left to give Rachel. ■

FACTORS AFFECTING DRUG ACTION

Therapeutic Effect

Each drug has an intended therapeutic effect—the reason the patient takes the medication. Certain factors affect the therapeutic action of drugs in the body, causing patients to respond differently to the same drug. Because of this, the drug therapy may need to be adjusted to meet these variations, which include the following.

Huntington Clinic
701 Concord Ave
Lexington, KY 48710
614-871-0033

Patient: Clare Andrews
      352 Pinewood Dr.
      Lexington, KY 48710

Age/DOB: 12/25/1970
EMRN: 7016780

Medication List

Medication	Refills	Start
Abilify 15 mg tablet	0	24Sep20XX
TAKE 1 TABLET DAILY		
Acetaminophen-Codeine #3 300-30 mg tablet	0	23Sep20XX
TAKE 1 TABLET EVERY 6 TO 8 HOURS AS NEEDED FOR PAIN		
Clonazepam 1 mg tablet	0	24Sep20XX
TAKE 1 TABLET EVERY 8 HOURS PRN		
Etodolac CR 500 mg tablet extended release 24 hour	0	21Sep20XX
1-2 TABLETS PO ONCE DAILY WITH FOOD		
Fish Oil 1000 mg capsule	11	7Apr20XX
TAKE 1 CAPSULE DAILY		
Flovent HFA 44 mcg/act aerosol	3	6Jan20XX
INHALE 2 PUFFS TWICE DAILY		
Fluticasone Propionate 50 mcg/act suspension	3	9Sep20XX
USE 2 SPRAYS IN EACH NOSTRIL ONCE DAILY		
Lamictal 200 mg tablet	0	24Sep20XX
TAKE 2 TABLETS DAILY		
Omeprazole 20 mg capsule delayed release	11	24Sep20XX
TAKE 1 TABLET DAILY		
Pamine 2.5 mg tablet	0	6Jan20XX
TAKE 1 TABLET 3 TIMES DAILY		
Proventil HFA 108 (90 base) mcg/act aerosol solution	3	21Jul20XX
INHALE 1-2 PUFFS EVERY 4-6 HOURS AS NEEDED AND AS DIRECTED		
Tramadol HCl 50 mg tablet	0	29Apr20XX
TAKE 1 TABLET EVERY 6 HOURS		
Voltaren 1% gel	6	24Sep20XX
APPLY 2 GRAMS TOPICALLY 4 TIMES DAILY		
WelChol 625 mg tablet	11	29Apr20XX
TAKE 3 TABLETS TWICE DAILY WITH MEALS		

Figure 26-4 Example of a computer-generated patient medication list.

Age

Children and the elderly tend to respond more strongly to drugs than young and middle-aged adults. The physician may calculate smaller doses for very young and geriatric patients.

Route of Administration

Medications administered by different routes are absorbed at different rates. Drugs administered orally are absorbed slowly because they must be digested first. Parenterally administered drugs are absorbed more quickly than orally administered drugs because they are injected directly into the body.

Size

A patient's body size has an effect on drug action. A thin individual may require a smaller quantity of a drug, and an obese individual may require more.

Time of Administration

A drug administered through the oral route is absorbed more rapidly when the stomach is empty than when it contains food. A drug may not produce the desired effect or may be absorbed too slowly if it is taken when food is present. Some drugs irritate the stomach's lining, however, and must be taken with food. The drug package insert or a drug reference should always be consulted to determine when a drug should be taken.

Tolerance

A patient taking a certain drug over a period of time may develop a tolerance to it. This means that the same dose of a drug no longer produces the desired effect after prolonged administration. The physician should be notified to determine whether a change of drug or dosage is needed.

Undesirable Effects of Drugs

A drug may cause undesirable effects, which may occur immediately or may be delayed hours or even days after administration of the medication.

MEDICATION RECORD

Patient _John Walsh_
Birthdate _6/10/49_

ALLERGY
Ø

DATE	MEDICATION AND DOSAGE	FREQUENCY	RX	OTC	REFILLS			STOP
2/18/XX	Cipro 250 mg	÷ q 12 h po x 10 days	X					2/28/XX
6/10/XX	Prevacid 15 mg	÷ qd po	X					7/10/XX
6/10/XX	Lipitor 10 mg	÷ qd po	X		1/6/XX			
6/10/XX	Prozac 20 mg	÷ qd po	X		1/6/XX			
12/3/XX	Tobrex Ophthalmic Solution	÷ gtt q 3 h OD	X					12/10/XX
2/5/XX	Echinacea	÷ qd po		X				
3/15/XX	Nitrostat 0.4 mg	÷ prn pain SL Rep q 5 min prn pain, not to exceed 3 tabs	X					
3/15/XX	Inderal 40 mg	÷ bld po	X					
3/15/XX	St Joseph ASA Enteric Coated 81 mg	÷ qd po		X				

Figure 26-5 Example of a medication record.

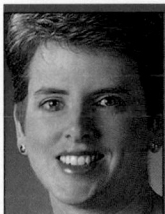

Memories *from* Externship

Theresa Cline: I can clearly remember the first time I gave an injection at my externship site. I was worried that I would forget how to give an injection and look bad in front of my externship supervisor and the patient. What made things worse is that the patient was a woman with very thin arms. I was giving her a flu shot, and I was so scared that the needle would hit her bone even though I was only using a 1-inch needle. When I walked into the room, my supervisor told the woman that I was a student and asked her if it was all right if I gave her the flu injection. The woman laughed and said, "Well, I guess so." That made me feel even more nervous. The patient then asked if it was my first shot. I told her "yes" and she said, "Just don't hurt me." When it came time to give the injection, everything that I had ever learned about injections came back to me. I gave the injection, and the woman told me I did a good job and that she didn't even feel it. That made me feel so good! My supervisor said, "If you can give a shot to her, you can give a shot to anyone." Every injection after that was a "piece of cake." I've learned just to take a deep breath before each difficult situation encountered in the office, and everything will work out. ∎

Adverse Reactions

Most drugs produce unintended and undesirable effects known as **adverse reactions.** Adverse reactions are secondary effects that occur along with the therapeutic effect of the drug. Some adverse reactions, referred to as *side effects,* are harmless and are often tolerated by the patient to obtain the therapeutic effect of the drug. Most patients are willing to tolerate the dry mouth and drowsiness that may accompany an antihistamine to obtain its therapeutic effect. Other adverse reactions, such as a decrease in blood pressure or an allergic reaction, can be harmful to the patient and warrant discontinuing the medication.

Drug Interactions

When certain medications are used at the same time, drug interactions may produce undesirable effects. The medical assistant should inquire about other medications the patient is taking and record this information in the patient's chart for review by the physician.

Allergic Drug Reaction

The patient may exhibit an allergic reaction to a drug. The reaction is usually mild and takes the form of a rash, rhinitis, or pruritus. Occasionally, a patient has a severe allergic reaction that occurs suddenly and immediately. This is known as an **anaphylactic reaction.**

An anaphylactic reaction is the least common but the most serious type of allergic reaction. Symptoms begin with sneezing, urticaria (hives), itching, erythema, angioedema, and disorientation. Erythema is reddening of the skin caused by dilation of superficial blood vessels in the skin. Angioedema is a localized urticaria of the deeper tissues of the body. If not treated, the symptoms of anaphylaxis quickly increase in severity and progress to dyspnea, cyanosis, and shock. Blood pressure decreases, and the pulse becomes weak and thready. Convulsions, loss of consciousness, and death may occur if treatment is not initiated promptly.

To prevent an anaphylactic reaction to a drug or to reduce its danger, the medical assistant should stay with the patient after administration of the medication. The medical assistant should be especially alert for signs of an anaphylactic reaction after administering allergy skin tests or a penicillin or allergy injection. If a reaction occurs, the physician should be notified immediately so that he or she can begin treatment immediately. Treatment generally consists of one or more injections of epinephrine, depending on the severity of the reaction. Epinephrine goes to work immediately to reverse the life-threatening symptoms of anaphylaxis. When the patient is stabilized, he or she is usually given an injection of an antihistamine. The antihistamine takes longer to begin working but helps alleviate urticaria, itching, angioedema, and erythema. The medical assistant must ensure that an ample supply of epinephrine is on hand at all times. Many offices maintain emergency crash carts for this purpose.

Idiosyncratic Reaction

An idiosyncratic reaction is an abnormal or peculiar response to a drug that is unexplained and unpredictable. Elderly patients are most prone to idiosyncratic reactions to drugs and should be monitored closely when they are taking a new medication.

GUIDELINES FOR PREPARATION AND ADMINISTRATION OF MEDICATION

To prevent medication errors, the medical assistant should follow these guidelines when preparing and administering any drug:

1. Work in a quiet, well lit atmosphere that is free of distractions.
2. Always ask if you have a question about the medication order.
3. Know the drug to be given.
4. Select the proper drug. Check the label of the medication three times—as it is taken from its storage location, before preparing the medication, and after preparing the medication. Do not use a drug if the label is missing or is difficult to read.
5. Do not use a drug if the color has changed, if a precipitate has formed, or if it has an unusual odor.

6. Check the expiration date before preparing the drug for administration.
7. Prepare the proper dose of the drug. The term **dose** refers to the quantity of a drug to be administered at one time. Each medication has a dose range, or range of quantities of the drug that can produce therapeutic effects. It is important to administer the exact dose of the drug. A dose that is too small would not produce a therapeutic effect, and a dose that is too large could be harmful or even fatal to the patient.
8. Correctly identify the patient so that the drug is administered to the intended patient. When medication is administered, the patient should be identified by his or her full name and date of birth.
9. Before administering the medication, check the patient's records or question the patient to ensure that he or she is not allergic to the medication.
10. If you are giving an injection, determine the appropriate route and site at which to administer the injection; the route and site are dictated by the type of injection being given. An allergy injection is given through the SC route, and an antibiotic injection is given through the IM route. The site must be free from abrasions, lesions, bruises, and edema.
11. Use the proper technique to administer the medication.
12. Stay with the patient after administering the medication.
13. Document information properly in the patient's medical record immediately after administering the drug. Include the date and time, the name of the medication, the lot number (if required), the dose given, the route of administration, the site of administration, and any unusual observations or patient reactions. Sign the recording with your name and credentials. If you administer a medication that contains a fraction of a unit, place a 0 before the decimal point (e.g., 0.5 mg, not .5 mg) so that the dosage is not misread as 5 mg. A decimal point and a zero should never be placed after a whole number. The decimal point may be overlooked and misread, resulting in a 10-fold overdose error (e.g., 20 mg, not 20.0 mg).
14. Always follow the seven "rights" of preparing and administering medication in the medical office:
    Right drug
    Right dose
    Right time
    Right patient
    Right route
    Right technique
    Right documentation

ORAL ADMINISTRATION

The oral route is the most convenient and most used method of administering medication. **Oral administration** means that the drug is given by mouth in either a solid form (e.g., tablet, capsule) or a liquid form (e.g., suspension, syrup). Absorption of most oral medications occurs in the small intestine, although some may be absorbed in the mouth and stomach.

Many patients find it easier to swallow a tablet or a capsule with a glass of water. Water should not be offered after the patient has received a cough syrup, however, because the water would dilute the medication's beneficial effects. Unless the patient has a malabsorption problem or is unable to swallow, the oral route is considered the safest and most desirable route for administering medication. Procedure 26-1 outlines the procedure for the administration of oral medications.

PROCEDURE 26-1 Administering Oral Medication

Outcome Administer oral solid and liquid medications.

Equipment/Supplies

- Medication ordered by the physician
- Medicine cup
- Medication tray

1. **Procedural Step.** Sanitize your hands.
2. **Procedural Step.** Assemble the equipment.
3. **Procedural Step.** Work in a quiet, well-lit atmosphere.
   Principle. Good lighting aids the medical assistant in reading the medication label.
4. **Procedural Step.** Select the correct medication from the shelf. Compare the medication with the physician's instructions. Check the drug label three times—while removing the medication from storage, while preparing the medication, and after preparing the medication. Check the expiration date.
   Principle. If the medication is outdated, consult the physician because it may produce undesirable effects for which the medical assistant could be held responsible. To prevent a drug error, the medication should be carefully compared with the physician's instructions.

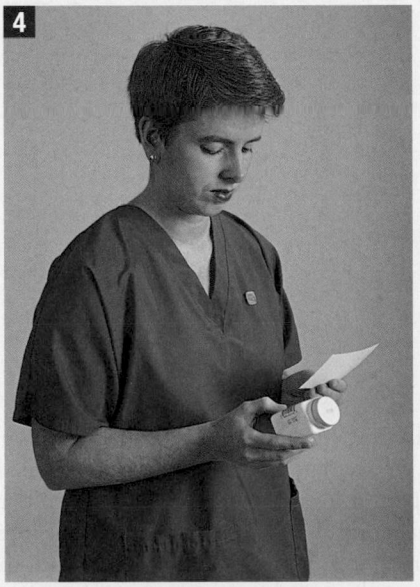

Compare the medication with the physician's instructions.

5. **Procedural Step.** Calculate the correct dose to be given, if necessary.
6. **Procedural Step.** Remove the bottle cap, touching the outside of the lid only.
   Principle. Touching the inside of the lid contaminates it.
7. **Procedural Step.** Check the drug label again, and pour the medication.
   Solid Medications. Pour the correct number of capsules or tablets into the bottle cap. Transfer the medication to a medicine cup, being careful not to touch the inside of the cup.
   Principle. Pouring the medication into the lid prevents contamination of the medication and lid.
   Liquid Medications. Place the lid of the bottle on a flat surface with the open end facing up. Palm the surface of the label.
   With the opposite hand, place the thumbnail at the proper calibration on the medicine cup, and hold the cup at eye level. Pour the medication, and read the dose at the lowest level of the meniscus. (The meniscus is the curved surface of the liquid in a container. When a liquid is poured into a medicine cup, capillary action causes the liquid in contact with the cup to be drawn upward, resulting in a curved surface in the middle.)
   Principle. Placing the bottle cap with the open end up prevents contamination of the inside of the cap. Palming the medication label prevents the medication from dripping on the label and obscuring it.

Continued

PROCEDURE 26-1   Administering Oral Medication—cont'd

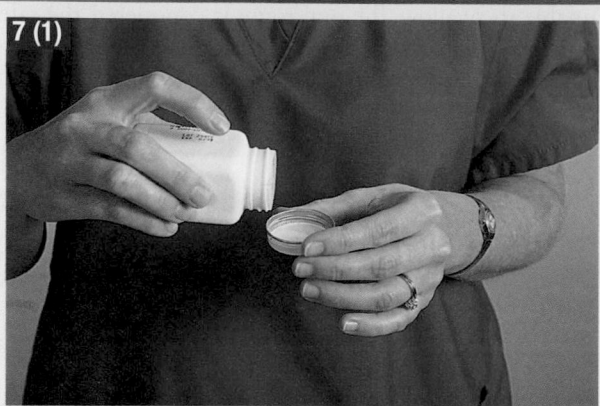

Pour the correct number of capsules or tablets into the bottle cap.

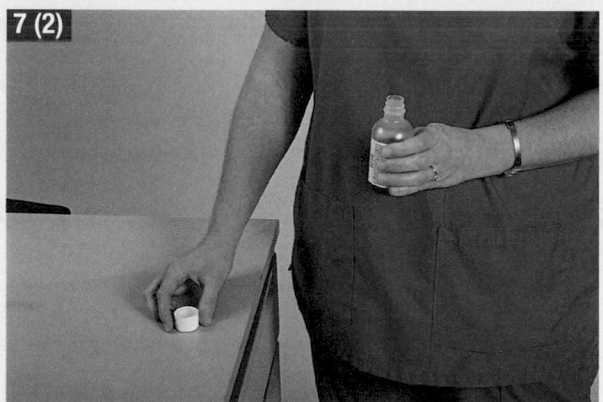

Place the lid of the bottle on a flat surface with the open end facing up.

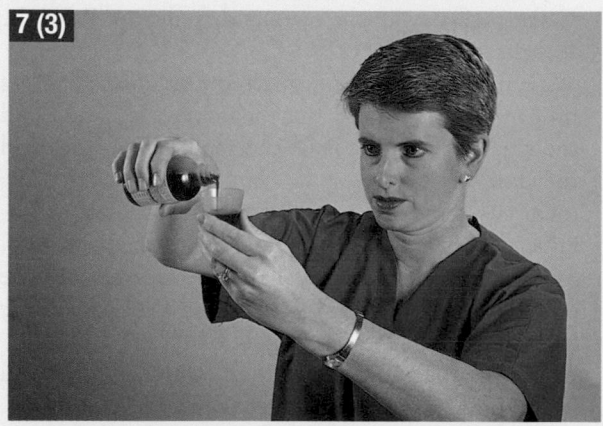

Hold the cup at eye level, and pour the medication.

8. **Procedural Step.** Replace the bottle cap, and check the drug label a third time to ensure it is the correct medication. Return the medication to its storage location.

9. **Procedural Step.** Greet the patient and introduce yourself. Identify the patient by full name and date of birth and explain the procedure. Explain the purpose of administering the medication.
   Principle. It is crucial that no error be made in patient identity.

10. **Procedural Step.** Hand the medicine cup containing the medication to the patient, along with a glass of water. (If the medication is a cough syrup, do not offer water.)
    Principle. Water helps the patient swallow the medication.

11. **Procedural Step.** Remain with the patient until the medication is swallowed. If the patient experiences any unusual reaction, notify the physician.

12. **Procedural Step.** Sanitize your hands.

13. **Procedural Step.** Chart the procedure. Include the date and time, the name of the medication, the dosage given, the route of administration, and any significant observations or patient reactions. The Latin abbreviation *po,* which means "by mouth," can be used to indicate the route of administration.

CHARTING EXAMPLE	
Date	
2/12/XX	9:30 a.m. Acetaminophen, 650 mg, po.
	———————— T. Cline, CMA (AAMA)

PARENTERAL ADMINISTRATION

The parenteral route of drug administration has several advantages. Medications given subcutaneously, intramuscularly, and intravenously are absorbed more rapidly and completely than medications given orally. In some cases, the parenteral route is the only way a drug can be given (e.g., insulin, most immunizations). If the patient is unconscious or has a gastric disturbance, such as nausea or vomiting, the parenteral route may be used to administer medication. If state laws permit, the medical assistant is usually responsible for administering SC, IM, and intradermal injections. IV medications are sometimes administered in the medical office and are discussed in greater detail later in the section on IV therapy.

The parenteral route also has disadvantages, such as pain and the possibility of infection as a result of breaking the skin. The medical assistant can minimize pain by inserting and withdrawing the needle quickly and smoothly and by withdrawing the needle at the same angle as for insertion. If injections are given repeatedly (e.g., allergy injections), the sites should be rotated to prevent the overuse of one site, which may cause irritation and tissue damage. Rotating sites also allows for better absorption of the drug.

When recording the administration of a medication in the patient's chart, the medical assistant must include the site of injection (e.g., right upper arm, left dorsogluteal). This assists in proper site rotation for patients who receive repeated injections. In addition, the information provides a reference point should a problem arise with the injection site.

Medical asepsis must be used when parenteral medications are administered. In addition, the needle and the inside of the syringe must remain sterile. These practices reduce the danger of microorganisms entering the patient's body during the administration of medication. The medical assistant must follow the Occupational Safety and Health Administration (OSHA) standard when administering medication as a means of protecting himself or herself from bloodborne pathogens (see Chapter 17). Procedure 26-2 describes how to prepare an injection.

Parts of a Needle and Syringe

Needle

The needle consists of several parts (Figure 26-6). The *hub* of the needle fits onto the top of the syringe. The *shaft* is inserted into the body tissue. The opening in the shaft of the needle, known as the *lumen,* is continuous with the needle hub. Medication flows from the syringe and through the lumen of the needle. The *point* of the needle is located at the end of the needle shaft. The point is sharp so that it can penetrate body tissues easily. The top of the needle is slanted and is called the *bevel.* The bevel is designed to make a narrow, slitlike opening in the skin. This narrow opening closes quickly when the needle is removed to prevent leakage of medication, and it heals quickly.

The length of the needle ranges between $\frac{3}{8}$ and 3 inches; the length used is based on the type of injection being given and the size of the patient. Refer to Figure 26-7 for examples of various needle lengths. Administering an IM injection to an obese adult requires a longer needle to reach the muscle tissue than would be required for a normal-size adult. Administering an IM injection to a thin patient requires a shorter needle to avoid inserting a needle too deeply and possibly penetrating the bone. The needle used to give an IM injection must be longer than the one used for an SC injection so that it penetrates deeply enough to reach the muscle tissue.

Each needle has a certain **gauge;** needle gauges for administering medication range between 18 G and 27 G. The gauge of a needle is determined by the diameter of the lumen: As the size of the gauge increases, the diameter of

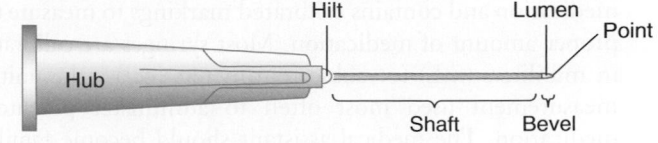

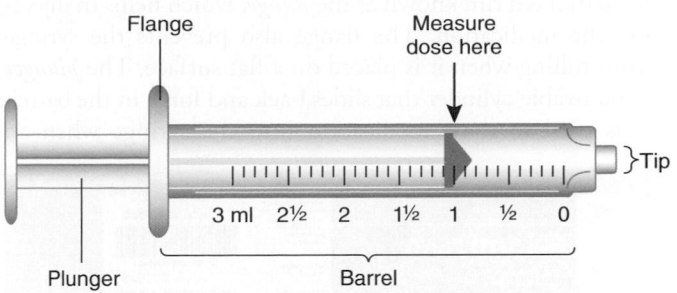

Figure 26-6 Diagram of a needle and a 3-mL syringe, with parts identified.

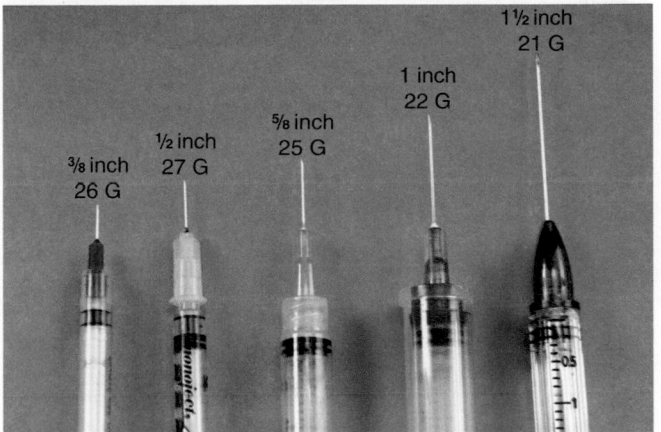

Figure 26-7 Needle lengths and gauges.

the lumen decreases (see Figure 26-7). A needle with a gauge of 23 has a smaller lumen diameter than a needle with a gauge of 21. Thick or oily preparations must be given with a large lumen because they are too thick to pass through a smaller one. A needle with a larger lumen makes a larger needle track in the tissues. To reduce pain and tissue damage, a needle with the smallest gauge appropriate for the solution and route of administration is always chosen.

Syringe

The syringe is used for inserting fluids into the body. It is made of plastic and must be disposed of after one use. The syringe with an attached needle is packaged in a cellophane wrapper or a rigid plastic container. Information regarding the syringe's capacity and the needle's length and gauge is printed on the wrapper of the syringe and needle (Figure 26-8). Syringes and needles also are available in separate packages. In this case, the medical assistant must attach a needle to the syringe before drawing medication into the syringe.

The parts of a syringe are the barrel, flange, and plunger (see Figure 26-6). The *barrel* of the syringe holds the medication and contains calibrated markings to measure the proper amount of medication. Most syringes are calibrated in milliliters (mL) (or cubic centimeters [cc])—the unit of measurement used most often to administer parenteral medication. The medical assistant should become familiar with reading the graduated scales on syringes. At the end of the barrel is a rim known as the *flange,* which helps in injecting the medication. The flange also prevents the syringe from rolling when it is placed on a flat surface. The *plunger* is a movable cylinder that slides back and forth in the barrel. It is used to draw medication into the syringe when an

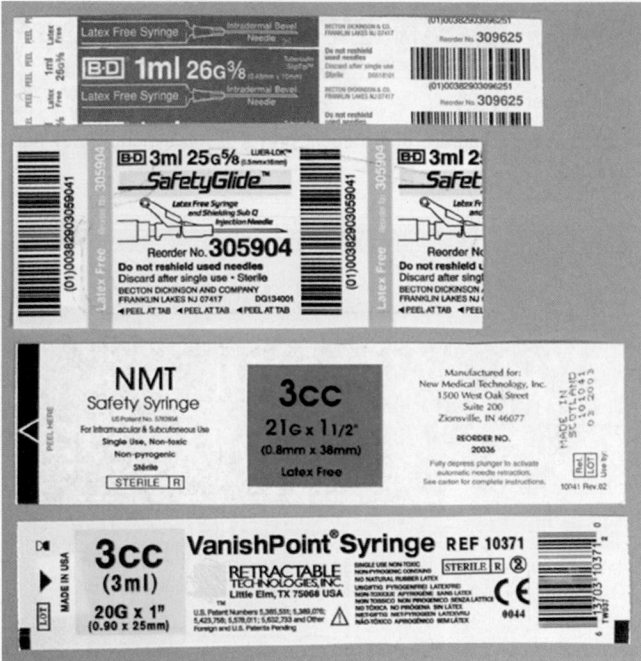

Figure 26-8 Examples of syringe and needle packages labeled according to contents.

injection is prepared and to push medication out of the syringe when an injection is administered.

Various types of syringes are available to administer injections. The choice is based on the type of injection being given (e.g., tuberculin skin test, allergy injection, antibiotic injection) and the amount of medication being administered. The types of syringes used most often in the medical office include hypodermic, insulin, and tuberculin (Figure 26-9).

Hypodermic syringes are available in 2-, 2.5-, 3-, and 5-mL sizes and are calibrated in milliliters (or cubic centimeters). They are commonly used to administer IM injections.

The *insulin syringe* is designed especially for the administration of an insulin injection, and the barrel is calibrated in units. The most common type is the U-100 syringe, which is calibrated into 100 units in increments of 2.

Tuberculin syringes are employed to administer a small dose of medication, such as when administering a tuberculin skin test. The tuberculin syringe has a capacity of 1 mL, and the calibrations are divided into tenths (0.10) and hundredths (0.01) of a milliliter.

Syringes also are available with capacities of 10, 20, 30, 50, and 60 mL; however, they are not used for administering medication, but rather for medical treatments, such as irrigating wounds and draining fluid from cysts.

Safety-Engineered Syringes

The Occupational Safety and Health Administration (OSHA) stipulates requirements to reduce needlestick and other sharps injuries among health care workers. As was discussed in Chapter 17, employers are required to evaluate and implement commercially available safer medical devices that reduce occupational exposure to the lowest extent feasible.

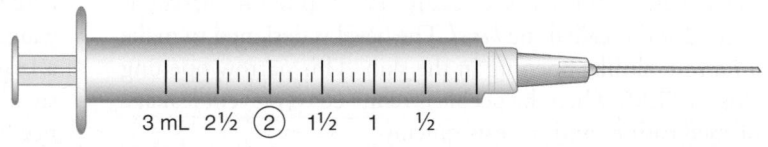

A Hypodermic syringe

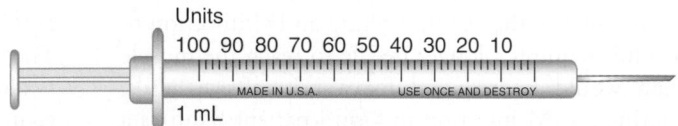

B Insulin syringe

Figure 26-9 Various syringes used to administer injections. **A,** Hypodermic. **B,** Insulin (U-100). **C,** Tuberculin.

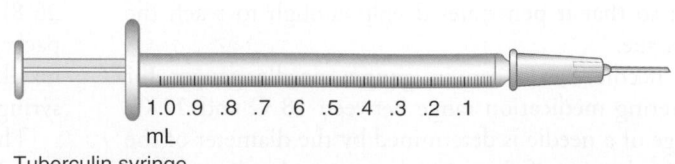

C Tuberculin syringe

Safer medical devices include safety-engineered syringes. *Safety-engineered syringes* incorporate a built-in safety feature to reduce the risk of a needlestick injury. Figure 26-10 illustrates types of safety-engineered syringes and the methods for using them.

Preparation of Parenteral Medication

Medication used for injections is available in various types of dispensing units—vials, ampules, and prefilled syringes and cartridges.

Vials

A **vial** is a closed glass container with a rubber stopper; a soft metal or plastic cap protects the rubber stopper and must be removed the first time the medication is used. An injectable medication may be available in a single-dose vial, a multiple-dose vial, or both (Figure 26-11). A vial is labeled with specific information as illustrated in Figure 26-12.

Before the medication can be withdrawn, some vials require mixing (e.g., reconstituting a powdered drug, mixing a vial that separates on standing). Vials that require

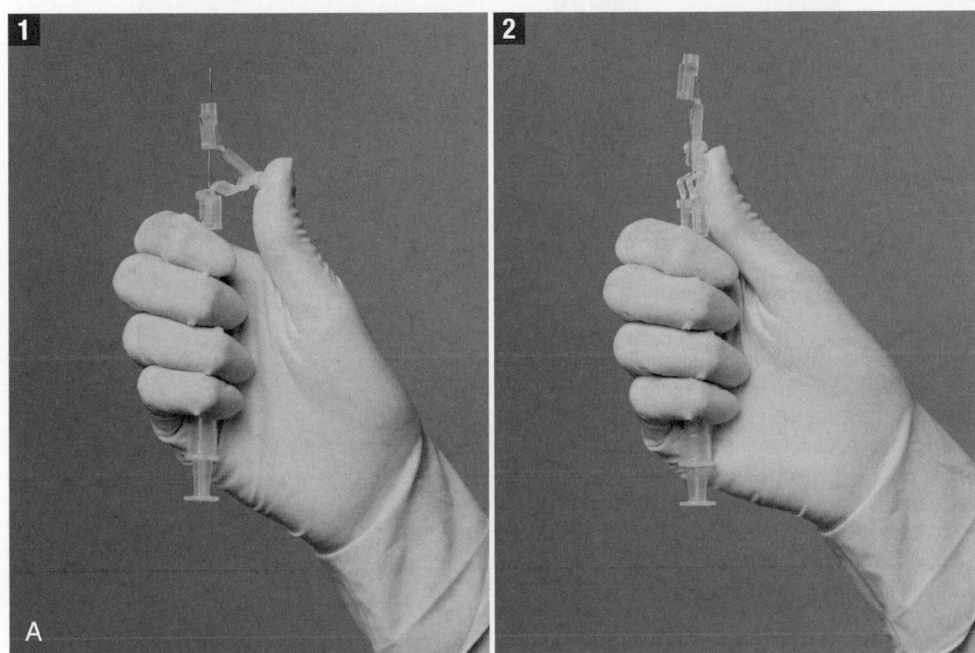

A, Hinged-shield syringe.
1. After administering the injection, push the lever of the hinged shield forward.
2. Continue pushing until the needle tip is fully covered by the shield, then discard the syringe in a biohazard sharps container.

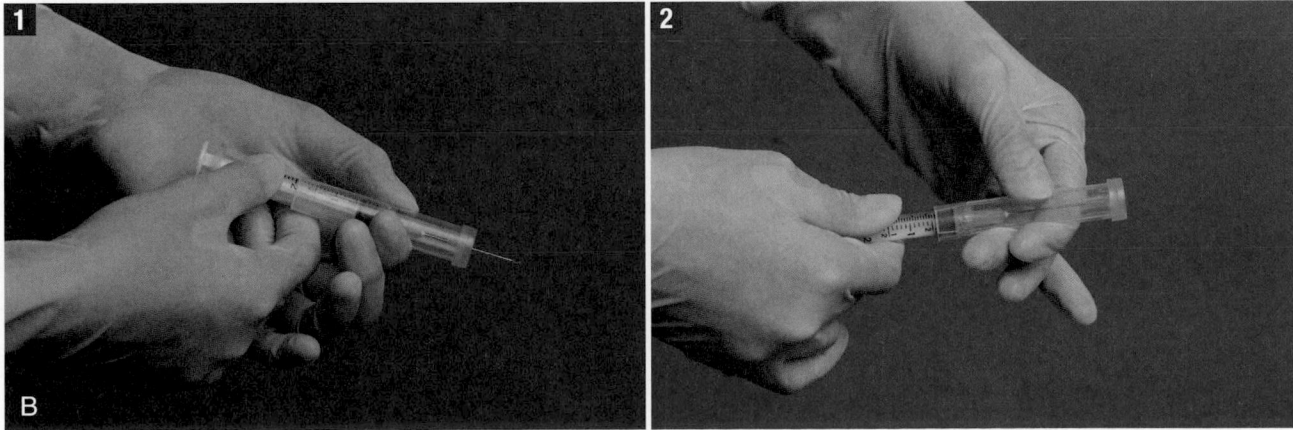

B, Sliding-shield syringe.
1. After administering the injection, extend the sliding shield forward fully until a click is heard.
2. Lock the shield by twisting it in either direction until a click is heard. Discard the syringe in a biohazard sharps container.

Figure 26-10 Safety-engineered syringes.

Continued

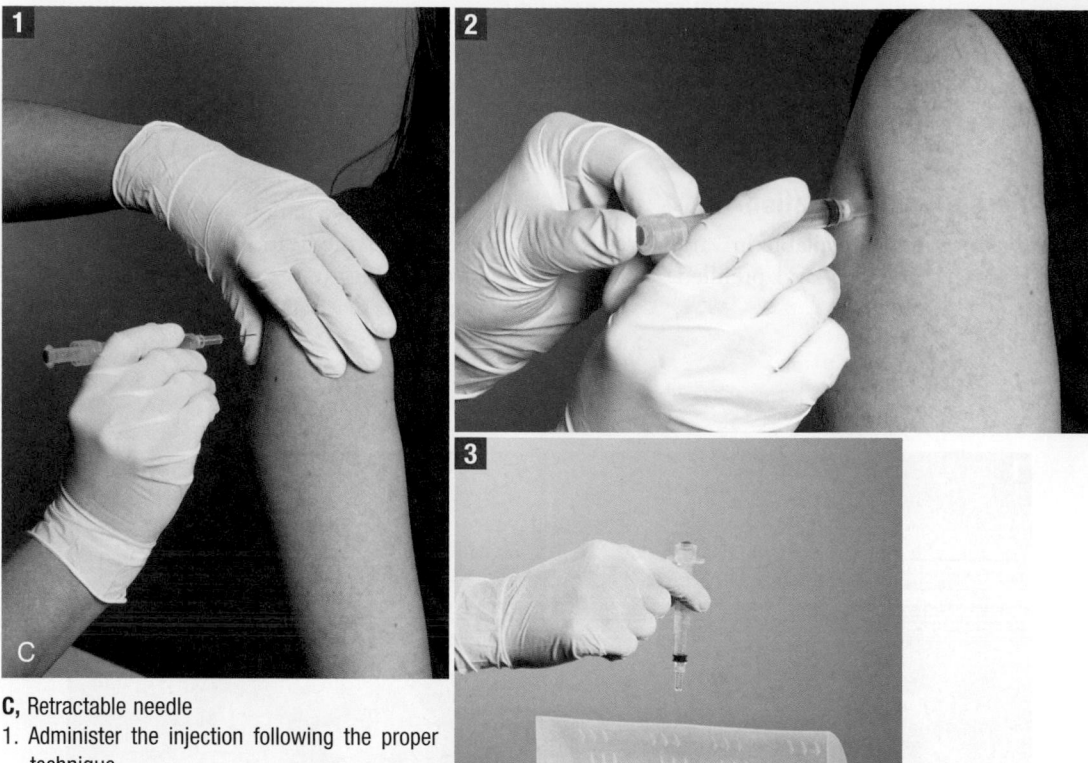

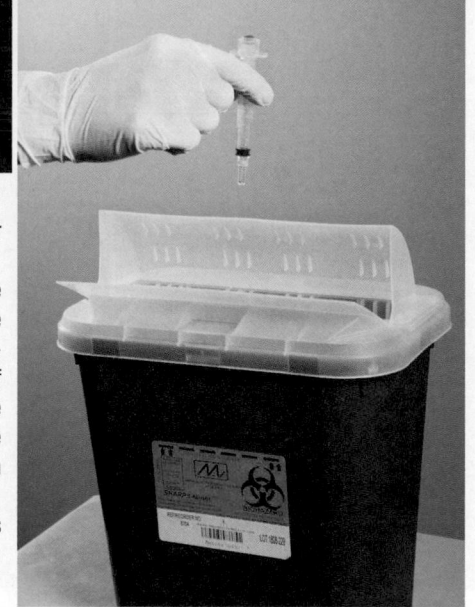

C, Retractable needle

1. Administer the injection following the proper technique.
2. After administering the medication, continue depressing the plunger with the thumb. Use firm pressure past the point of initial resistance. This action delivers the full dose of medication to the patient and activates the needle retraction device, causing the needle to retract automatically from the patient's skin and into the barrel of the syringe.
3. Discard the syringe in a biohazard sharps container.

Figure 26-10, cont'd

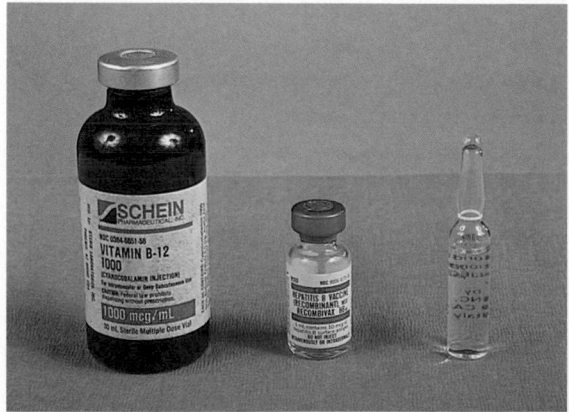

Figure 26-11 The multiple-dose vial *(left)* and the single-dose vial *(middle)* consist of a closed glass container with a rubber stopper. The ampule *(right)* consists of a small, sealed glass container that holds a single dose of medication.

mixing should be rolled between the hands rather than shaken because shaking would cause the medication to foam, creating air bubbles that may enter the syringe when the medication is withdrawn.

To remove medication from a vial, an amount of air exactly equal to the amount of liquid to be removed is injected into the vial. The air should be inserted above the fluid level to avoid creating bubbles in the medication. If air is not injected first, a partial vacuum is created, and it is difficult to remove the medication. During the withdrawal of medication, the needle opening should be inserted below the fluid level to prevent the entrance of air bubbles. Air bubbles can be removed by tapping the barrel of the syringe with the fingertips. If the bubbles are allowed to remain, they take up space that the medication should occupy, which would prevent the patient from receiving the full dose of medication.

Ampules

An **ampule** is a small, sealed glass container that holds a single dose of medication (see Figure 26-11). An ampule has a constriction in the stem, known as the *neck,* which

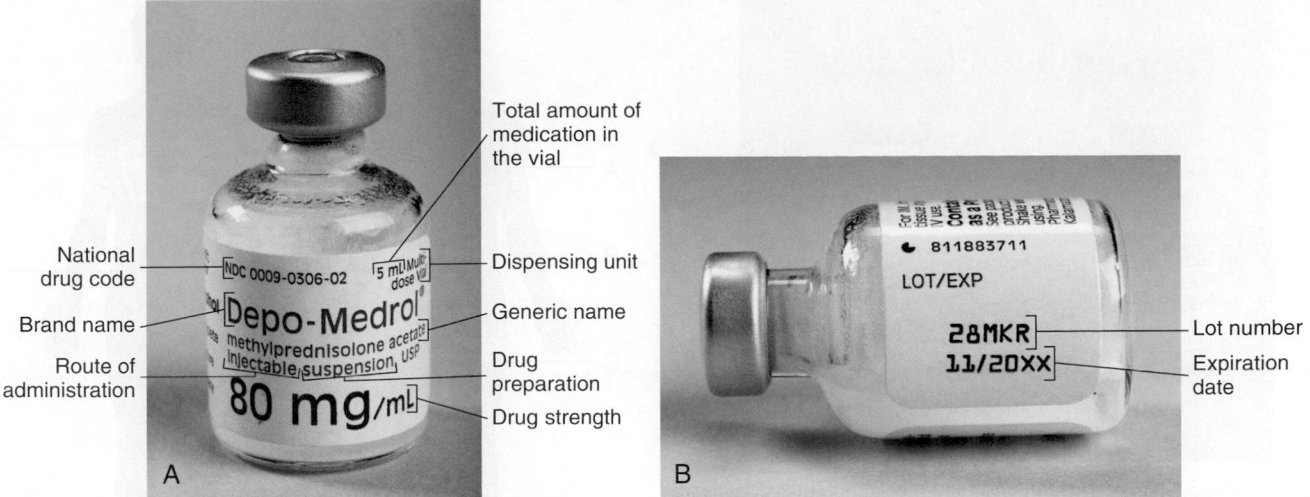

Figure 26-12 Information included on the label of a medication vial.

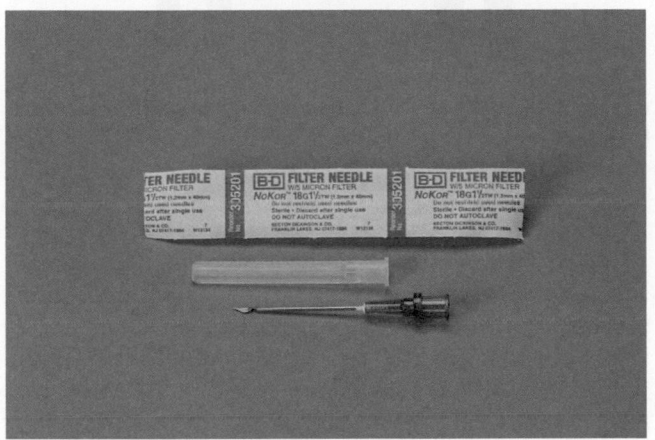

Figure 26-13 Filter needle used to withdraw medication from an ampule.

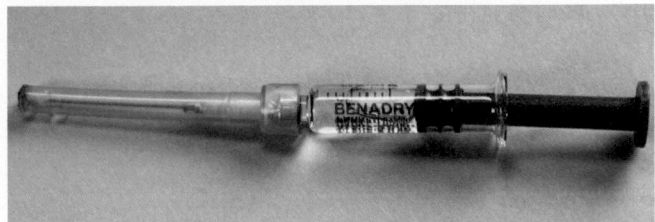

Figure 26-14 A prefilled disposable syringe of medication.

helps in opening it. Before opening, the medical assistant must ensure that there is no medication in the stem by tapping it lightly. A colored ring around the neck indicates where the ampule is prescored for easy opening. The ampule is opened by holding it firmly with gauze and breaking off the stem with a strong steady pressure.

A hazard with medication in ampules is the possibility of small glass particles getting into the ampule as the stem is broken off. When the medication is withdrawn into the syringe, the glass particles also might be withdrawn. To prevent this problem, a needle with a filter should be used that filters out small glass particles (Figure 26-13).

The needle opening is inserted into the base of the ampule below the fluid level to withdraw medication. To prevent contamination, the needle should not be permitted to touch the outside of the ampule. Air should never be injected into the ampule because it could force out some of the medication.

Prefilled Syringes

Some drugs come in *prefilled disposable syringes.* Using this type of dispensing unit does not require drawing up the

medication. The name of the drug, the dose, and the expiration date are printed on the syringe (Figure 26-14).

Storage

The medical assistant should always read the drug package insert to determine the proper method for storing each parenteral medication because improper storage may alter the effectiveness of the medication.

Reconstitution of Powdered Drugs

Some parenteral medications are stable for only a short time in liquid form; these medications are prepared and stored in powdered form and require the addition of a liquid before administration. The process of adding a liquid to a powdered drug is known as *reconstitution.* The liquid used to reconstitute a powdered drug is known as the *diluent* and usually consists of sterile water or normal saline. The powdered drug is contained in a single-dose or multiple-dose vial and is accompanied by specific instructions for reconstitution. An example of a parenteral medication that requires reconstitution is the measles, mumps, and rubella (MMR) immunization (Figure 26-15). The procedure for reconstituting powdered drugs is outlined in Procedure 26-3.

Subcutaneous Injections

A **subcutaneous injection** is made into the subcutaneous tissue, which consists of adipose (fat) tissue and is located just under the skin (Figure 26-16). Subcutaneous tissue is

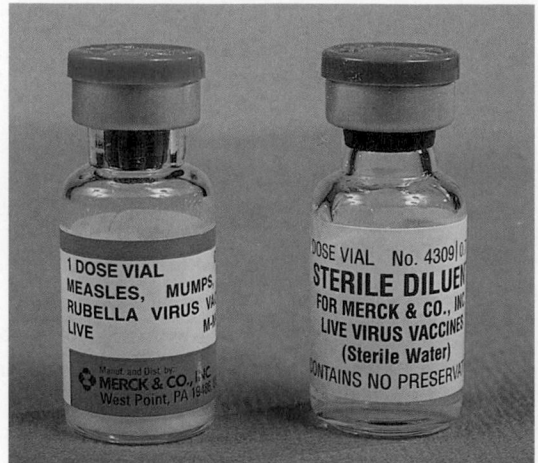

Figure 26-15 The measles, mumps, and rubella (MMR) vaccine is a parenteral medication that requires reconstitution before administration. The vial on the left contains the medication in powdered form, and the vial on the right contains the sterile diluent.

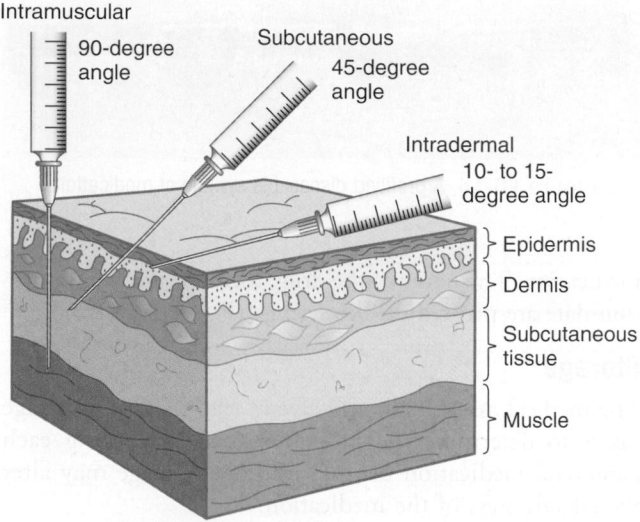

Figure 26-16 Angle of insertion for intradermal, subcutaneous, and intramuscular injections.

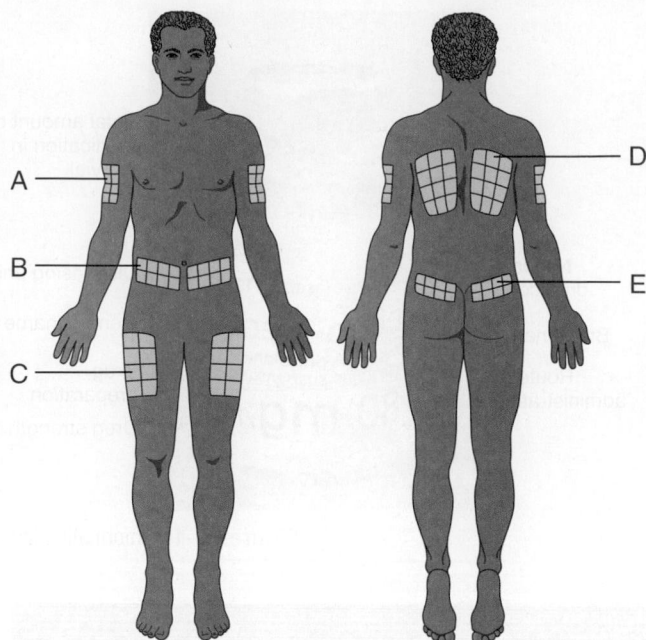

Figure 26-17 Common sites for subcutaneous injections. **A,** Upper outer arm. **B,** Lower abdomen. **C,** Upper outer thigh. **D,** Upper back. **E,** Flank region.

located all over the body; however, certain sites are more commonly used because they are located where bones and blood vessels are not near the surface of the skin. These sites include the upper lateral part of the arms, the anterior thigh, the upper back, and the abdomen (Figure 26-17). Absorption of medication from an SC injection occurs mainly through capillaries, resulting in a slower absorption rate than with IM injections. To ensure proper absorption, tissue that is grossly adipose, hardened, inflamed, or edematous should not be used as an injection site.

The needle length varies from ½ to ⅝ inch, and the gauge ranges from 23 G to 25 G. Elderly and dehydrated patients tend to have less SC tissue, and obese patients have more. The length of the needle should be adjusted accordingly to ensure the medication is administered into the subcutaneous tissue and not into muscle tissue.

Subcutaneous tissue is sensitive to irritating solutions and large volumes of medications; therefore, drugs given subcutaneously must be isotonic, nonirritating, nonviscous, and water-soluble. The amount of medication injected through the SC route should not exceed 1 mL. More than this amount results in pressure on sensory nerve endings, causing discomfort and pain.

Medications commonly administered through the SC route include epinephrine, insulin, and allergy injections. Patients who receive allergy injections must wait in the medical office for 15 to 20 minutes after the injection to be observed for an allergic reaction. Procedure 26-4 outlines the administration of a subcutaneous injection.

Intramuscular Injections

Intramuscular injections are made into the muscular layer of the body, which lies below the skin and subcutaneous layers (see Figure 26-16). The amount of medication that can be injected into muscle tissue is more than the amount that can be injected into subcutaneous tissue. An amount of up to 3 mL can be injected into the gluteal or vastus lateralis muscles, although older and very thin adults are able to tolerate only 2 mL or less in these sites.

Absorption is more rapid by this route than by the SC route because there are more blood vessels in muscle tissue. Medication that is irritating to subcutaneous tissue is often given intramuscularly because there are fewer nerve endings in deep muscle tissue. Most parenteral medications administered in the medical office are given through the IM route; examples include immunizations, antibiotics, injectable contraceptives, vitamin B_{12}, and corticosteroids.

The needle for an adult must be long enough to reach muscle tissue and varies in length from 1 to 3 inches. A 1½-inch needle is typically used for an average-sized adult, whereas a 1-inch needle is often used for a thin adult or a child, and a needle of 2 to 3 inches may be needed for an obese adult. The gauge of the needle used ranges from 18 G to 23 G, depending on the viscosity of the medication. Procedure 26-5 outlines the technique for the administration of an IM injection.

Intramuscular Injection Sites

The sites chosen for IM injections are away from large nerves and blood vessels. The medical assistant should practice locating these sites to become familiar with them. The area should always be fully exposed to permit clear visualization of the injection site.

Dorsogluteal Site

The dorsogluteal site is often used to administer IM injections in the medical office. In adults and children older than 3 years of age, the gluteal muscles are well developed and can absorb a large amount of medication. The patient should lie on the abdomen with the toes pointed inward,

which aids in relaxation of the gluteal muscles. The medication is injected into the upper outer quadrant of the gluteal area. This site is located by palpating the greater trochanter and the posterior superior iliac spine. An imaginary line is then drawn between these two points, and the injection is administered above and outside of this area (Figure 26-18, *A*). The dorsogluteal site can also be located by dividing the buttocks into quadrants. The site is located in the upper outer quadrant approximately 2 to 3 inches below the iliac crest. The medical assistant must be *extremely* careful to maintain the proper boundary lines to avoid injection into the sciatic nerve or the superior gluteal artery (see Figure 26-18, *A*).

Deltoid Site

The deltoid area is easily accessible and can be used when the patient is sitting or lying down. This site is small because major nerves and blood vessels surround it, and large amounts of medication (no more than 1 mL) and repeated injections should not be given in this area. The medication is injected into the deltoid muscle.

The medical assistant should ensure that the entire arm is exposed by having the patient's sleeve completely pulled

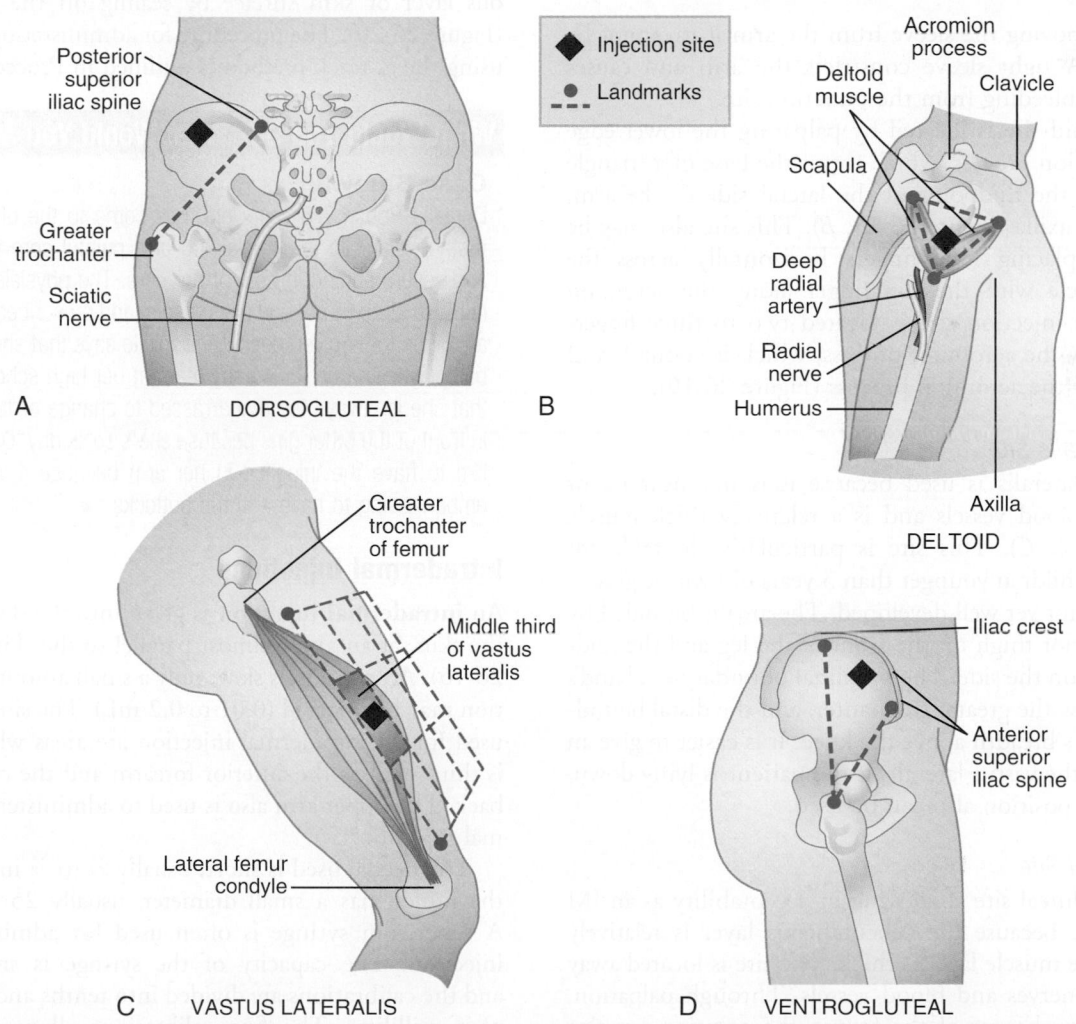

Figure 26-18 Sites of intramuscular injections. **A,** Dorsogluteal muscle. **B,** Deltoid muscle. **C,** Vastus lateralis. **D,** Ventrogluteal muscle.

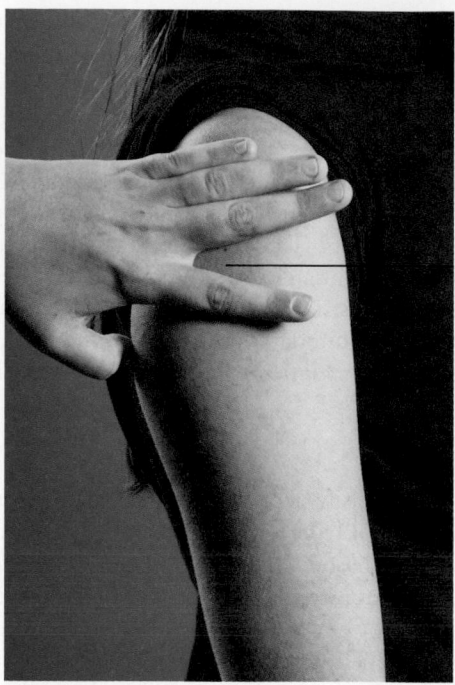

Figure 26-19 Location of the deltoid site.

up or by removing the sleeve from the arm if it cannot be pulled up. A tight sleeve constricts the arm and causes unnecessary bleeding from the puncture site.

The deltoid site is located by palpating the lower edge of the acromion process, which forms the base of a triangle in line with the midpoint of the lateral side of the arm, opposite the axilla (Figure 26-18, *B*). This site also may be located by placing four fingers horizontally across the deltoid muscle with the top finger along the acromion process. The injection site is located two to three finger-widths below the acromion process, which is about 1 to 2 inches below the acromion process (Figure 26-19).

Vastus Lateralis Site

The vastus lateralis is used because it is not near major nerves and blood vessels and is a relatively thick muscle (Figure 26-18, *C*). This site is particularly desirable for infants and children younger than 3 years old whose gluteal muscles are not yet well developed. The area is bounded by the midanterior thigh on the front of the leg and the midlateral thigh on the side. The proximal boundary is a hand's breadth below the greater trochanter, and the distal boundary is a hand's breadth above the knee. It is easier to give an injection in the vastus lateralis if the patient is lying down, but a sitting position also can be used.

Ventrogluteal Site

The ventrogluteal site is growing in acceptability as an IM injection site because the subcutaneous layer is relatively small and the muscle layer is thick. The site is located away from major nerves and blood vessels. Through palpation, the greater trochanter of the femur, the anterior superior iliac spine, and the iliac crest can be located. If the injection is being made into the patient's left side, the palm of the

right hand is placed on the greater trochanter, and the index finger is placed on the anterior superior iliac spine. The middle finger is spread posteriorly as far as possible away from the index finger, to touch the iliac crest. The hand position is reversed if the injection is being made into the patient's right side. The triangle formed by the fingers is the area into which the injection is given. An injection into the ventrogluteal site can be administered when the patient is lying prone or on one side (Figure 26-18, *D*).

Z-Track Method

Medications that are irritating to subcutaneous and skin tissue or that discolor the skin must be given intramuscularly using the Z-track method; one medication that is administered by this method is iron dextran (Imferon). The dorsogluteal, ventrogluteal, and vastus lateralis sites all can be used as areas to administer a Z-track injection.

The Z-track method is similar to the IM injection procedure except that the skin and subcutaneous tissue at the injection site are pulled to the side before the needle is inserted. This causes a zigzag path through the tissues when the needle is removed and the skin is released. The zigzag path prevents the medication from reaching the subcutaneous layer or skin surface by sealing off the needle track (Figure 26-20). The procedure for administering medication using the Z-track method is outlined in Procedure 26-6.

What Would You Do? What Would You *Not* Do?

Case Study 3

Danielle Roush, 16 years old, has come to the office with her mother. Danielle is complaining of a painful sore throat, fever, and severe aching in both of her ears. The physician diagnoses her with strep throat and otitis media, and prescribes a parenteral antibiotic to be given deep IM. Danielle says that she's a basketball player and on the varsity team at her high school. She says that she is always too embarrassed to change or take a shower in front of the other girls because she's so skinny. Danielle would like to have the injection in her arm because it would be too embarrassing to have it in the buttocks. ■

Intradermal Injections

An **intradermal injection** is given into the dermal layer of the skin, at an angle almost parallel to the skin (see Figure 26-16). Absorption is slow; only a small amount of medication may be injected (0.01 to 0.2 mL). The sites most often used for an intradermal injection are areas where the skin is thin, such as the anterior forearm and the middle of the back. The upper arm also is used to administer an intradermal injection.

The needle used is short, usually ⅜ to ⅝ inch long, and the lumen has a small diameter, usually 25 G to 27 G. A tuberculin syringe is often used for administering the injection. The capacity of the syringe is small (1 mL), and the calibrations are divided into tenths and hundredths of a milliliter. The fine calibrations allow a very small amount of medication to be administered, which is required with an intradermal injection. Procedure 26-7 outlines the

Text continued on p. 600

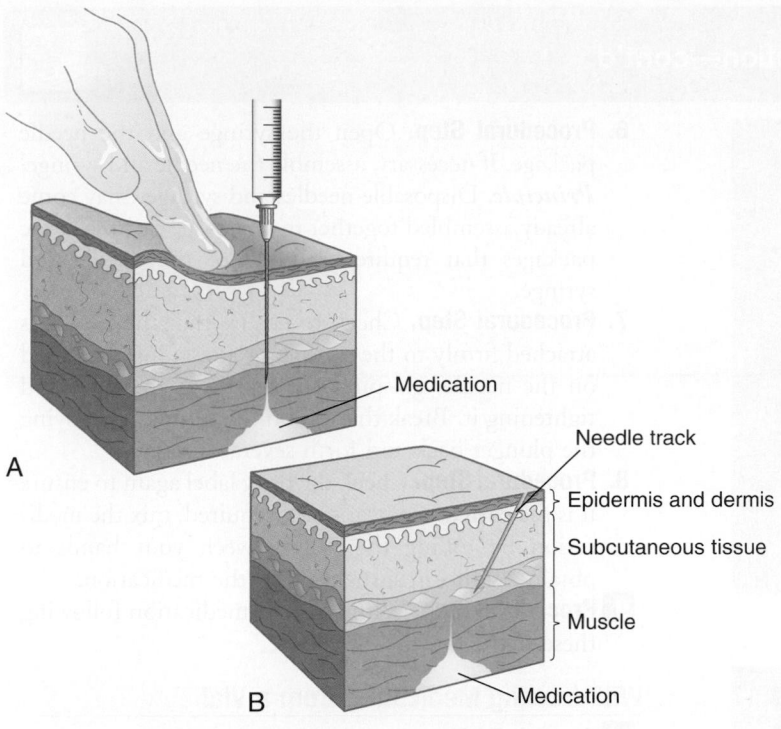

A

B

- Medication
- Needle track
- Epidermis and dermis
- Subcutaneous tissue
- Muscle
- Medication

Figure 26-20 Z-track intramuscular injection method. **A,** The skin and subcutaneous tissue are pulled to the side before the needle is inserted. **B,** This causes a zigzag path through the tissue when the skin is released, which seals off the needle track.

PROCEDURE 26-2

PROCEDURE 26-2 Preparing an Injection

Outcome Prepare an injection from an ampule and a vial.

Equipment/Supplies

- Medication ordered by the physician
- Appropriate needle and syringe
- Antiseptic wipe
- Medication tray

1. **Procedural Step.** Sanitize your hands.
2. **Procedural Step.** Assemble the equipment.
3. **Procedural Step.** Work in a quiet and well lit atmosphere.
   Principle. Good lighting aids the medical assistant in reading the medication label.
4. **Procedural Step.** Select the proper medication. Compare the medication with the physician's instructions. Check the drug label three times—while removing the medication from storage, before withdrawing the medication into the syringe, and after preparing the medication. Check the expiration date.
   Principle. The medication should be carefully identified to prevent administration of the wrong medication. Outdated medication should not be used because it could produce undesirable effects.

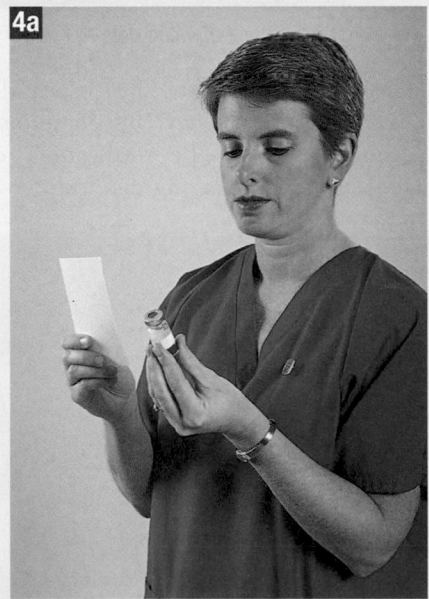

4a

Compare the medication with the physician's instructions.

Continued

PROCEDURE 26-2   Preparing an Injection—cont'd

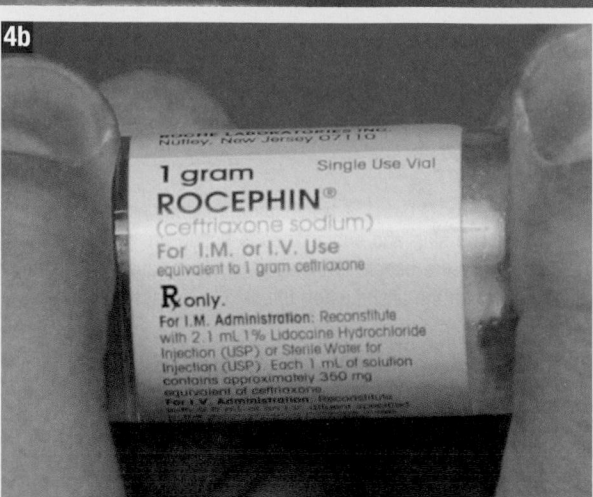

Check the drug label three times.

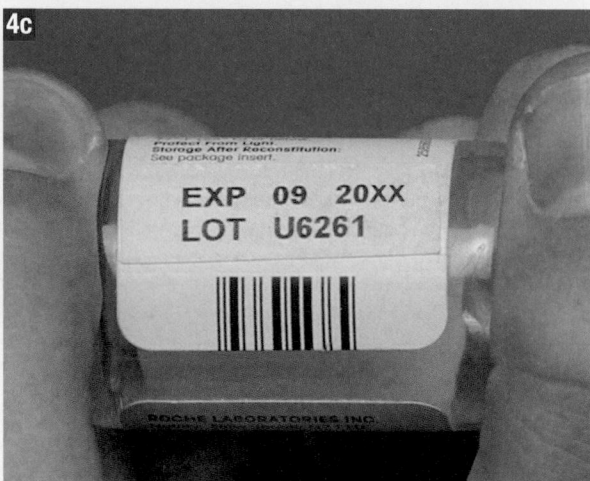

Check the expiration date.

5. Procedural Step. Calculate the correct dose to be given, if necessary. If you have any questions regarding the administration of the medication, check the package insert accompanying the drug.

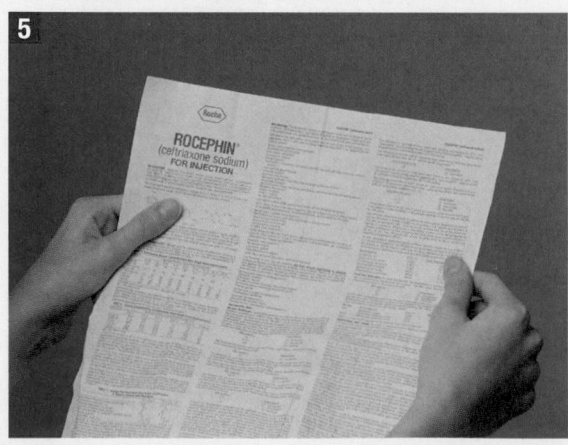

Check the package insert.

6. Procedural Step. Open the syringe and the needle package. If necessary, assemble the needle and syringe. *Principle.* Disposable needles and syringes may come already assembled together in a package or in separate packages that require assembly of the needle and syringe.

7. Procedural Step. Check to ensure that the needle is attached firmly to the syringe by loosening the guard on the needle, grasping the needle at the hub, and tightening it. Break the seal on the syringe by moving the plunger back and forth several times.

8. Procedural Step. Check the drug label again to ensure it is the correct medication. If required, mix the medication by rolling the vial between your hands to obtain a uniform suspension of the medication.

9. Procedural Step. Withdraw the medication following these steps.

Withdrawing Medication from a Vial

a. Procedural Step. Remove the soft metal or plastic cap protecting the rubber stopper of an unused vial to expose the rubber stopper. Open the antiseptic; wipe and cleanse the rubber stopper and allow it to dry. *Principle.* Cleansing the top of the vial removes dust and bacteria. The alcohol must be allowed to dry to prevent it from adhering to the needle and mixing with the medication.

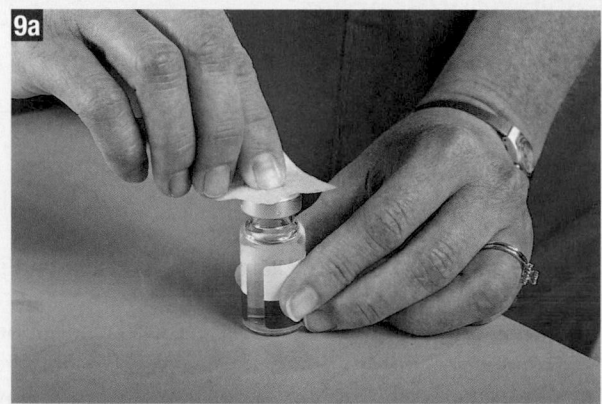

Cleanse the rubber stopper.

b. Procedural Step. Place the vial in an upright position on a flat surface. Remove the needle guard. Pull back on the plunger to draw an amount of air into the syringe equal to the amount of medication to be withdrawn from the vial. *Principle.* Air must be injected into the vial first to prevent the formation of a partial vacuum in the vial, which would make it difficult to remove medication.

PROCEDURE 26-2 Preparing an Injection—cont'd

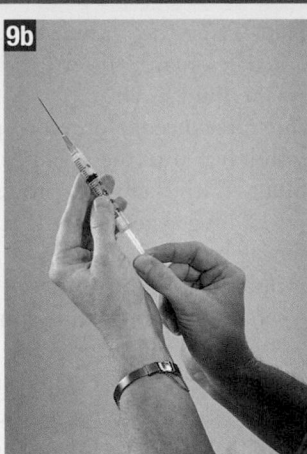

Draw air into the syringe.

c. Procedural Step. With the vial on a flat surface, use moderate pressure on the barrel of the syringe to insert the needle through the center of the rubber stopper at a 90-degree angle. Continue to apply pressure until the needle reaches the empty space between the stopper and fluid level. Be careful not to bend the needle. Push down on the plunger to inject the air into the vial, keeping the needle opening above the fluid level. (*NOTE:* If you are using a retractable safety syringe, do not push too hard on the plunger to avoid activating the retracting mechanism prematurely.)
Principle. The center of the rubber stopper is thinner and easier to penetrate. The air must be inserted above the fluid level to avoid creating air bubbles in the medication.

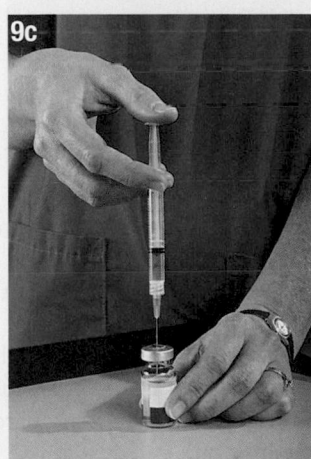

Inject air into the vial.

d. Procedural Step. Invert the vial while holding onto the syringe and plunger. Hold the syringe at eye level,

and withdraw the proper amount of medication. Keep the needle opening below the fluid level.
Principle. The needle opening must be below the fluid level to prevent the entrance of air bubbles into the syringe.

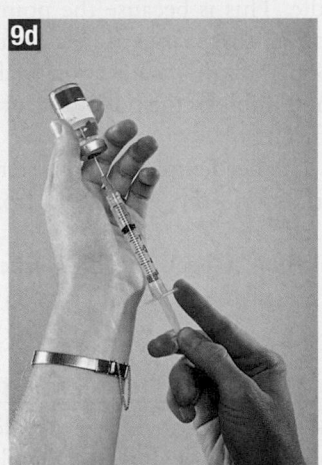

Withdraw the proper amount of medication.

e. Procedural Step. Remove any air bubbles in the syringe by holding the syringe in a vertical position and tapping the barrel carefully with the fingertips until they disappear.
Principle. Tapping the barrel too forcefully could cause the needle to bend. Air bubbles take up space the medication should occupy, preventing the patient from getting the proper dose of medication.

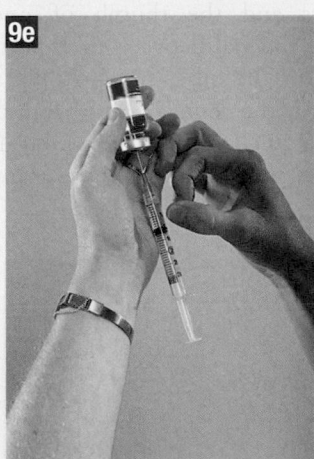

Tap the barrel with the fingertips to remove air bubbles.

f. Procedural Step. Remove any air remaining at the top of the syringe by slowly pushing the plunger forward and allowing the air to flow back into the vial.

Continued

PROCEDURE 26-2 Preparing an Injection—cont'd

g. **Procedural Step.** Carefully remove the needle from the rubber stopper, and replace the needle guard. (*NOTE:* After drawing up the medication, some facilities require that the needle used to draw up the medication be removed from the syringe and replaced with a new sterile needle. This is because the point of the needle may not be as sharp after it has been inserted into rubber stopper of the medication vial. The medical assistant should follow the policy set forth by his or her medical office.)
Principle. The needle must remain sterile. The needle guard prevents the needle from becoming contaminated.

h. **Procedural Step.** Check the drug label for the third time, and return the medication to its proper storage location.

Withdrawing Medication from an Ampule

a. **Procedural Step.** Remove the needle (and needle guard) from the syringe, and attach a filter needle (and needle guard).

b. **Procedural Step.** Open the antiseptic wipe, and cleanse the neck of the ampule.
Principle. Cleansing the neck of the ampule removes dust and bacteria.

c. **Procedural Step.** Tap the stem of the ampule lightly to remove any medication in the neck of the ampule.

d. **Procedural Step.** Check the medication label a second time and place a piece of gauze around the neck of the ampule. Hold the base of the ampule between the first two fingers and the thumb of one hand. Hold the neck of the vial between the first two fingers and the thumb of the other hand. Apply a strong steady pressure with the thumbs, and break off the stem by snapping it quickly and firmly away from the body. Discard the stem and gauze in a biohazard sharps container.

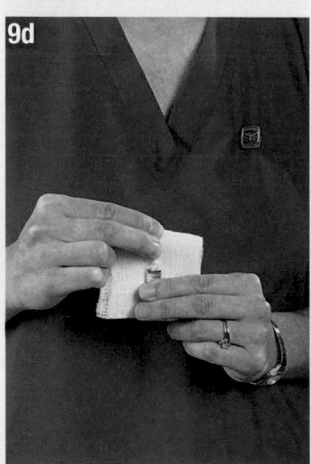

Snap off the stem away from the body.

e. **Procedural Step.** Place the ampule on a flat surface. Remove the needle guard. Insert the filter needle opening below the fluid level.
Principle. The filter needle prevents glass particles from being withdrawn into the syringe.

f. **Procedural Step.** Withdraw the proper amount of medication by pulling back on the plunger. Keep the needle opening below the fluid level to prevent the entrance of air bubbles into the syringe. Tilt the ampule as needed to keep the needle opening immersed in the fluid.

NOTE: There is another method that can be used to remove medication from an ampule. Choose the method that is easiest for you. To perform this method, invert the ampule, making sure to keep the needle opening below the fluid level. Withdraw the proper amount of medication by pulling back on the plunger. Move the needle downward as necessary to keep the needle opening immersed in the fluid.

Principle. Air bubbles take up space the medication should occupy, resulting in an inaccurate measurement of medication.

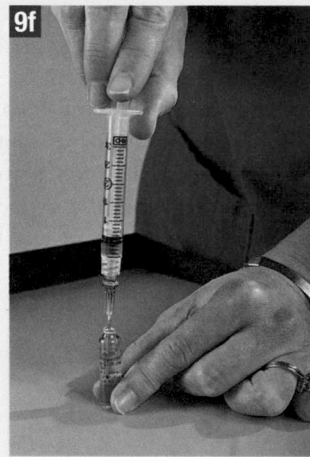

Withdraw the medication.

g. **Procedural Step.** Remove the needle from the ampule, and replace the needle guard. Check the drug label for the third time, and dispose of the glass ampule in a biohazard sharps container.

h. **Procedural Step.** Remove the filter needle (and guard) from the syringe, and discard it in a biohazard sharps container. Reapply the needle (and guard) for administering the medication.

i. **Procedural Step.** If air bubbles are in the syringe, remove the needle guard, hold the syringe in a vertical position, and tap the barrel with the fingertips until the bubbles disappear. Remove the air at the top of the syringe by slowly pushing the plunger forward. If the syringe contains excess fluid, hold the syringe vertically over a sink with the needle tip up and slanted toward the sink. Slowly eject the excess fluid into the sink. Replace the needle guard.

PROCEDURE 26-3 **Reconstituting Powdered Drugs**

Outcome Reconstitute a powdered drug for parenteral administration.

Equipment/Supplies

- Medication ordered by the physician
- Appropriate needle and syringe
- Antiseptic wipe
- Medication tray

1. **Procedural Step.** Follow steps 1 through 8 of Procedure 26-2.
2. **Procedural Step.** From the vial of the powdered drug, withdraw an amount of air equal to the amount of liquid to be injected into the vial.
   Principle. Removing air from the powdered drug vial allows room for injection of the diluent.
3. **Procedural Step.** Inject the air removed from the powdered drug vial into the vial of diluent.
   Principle. Air must be injected into the vial to prevent formation of a partial vacuum in the vial, which would make it difficult to remove the diluent.
4. **Procedural Step.** Invert the diluent vial, and withdraw the proper amount of liquid into the syringe. Remove air bubbles from the syringe, and carefully remove the needle from the vial.
5. **Procedural Step.** Insert the needle into the powdered drug vial, and inject the diluent into the vial. Remove the needle from the vial, and replace the needle guard.

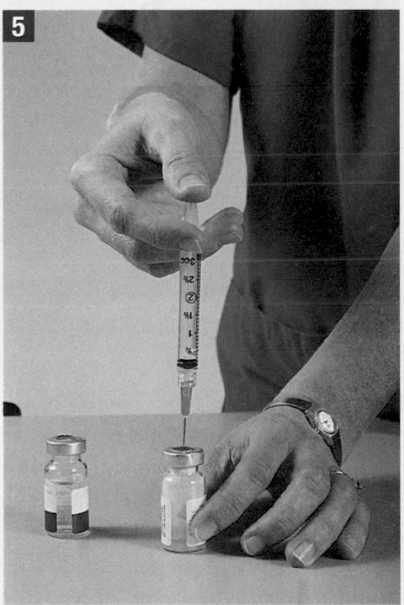

Inject the diluent into the vial.

6. **Procedural Step.** Roll the vial between the hands to mix the powdered drug and liquid (unless indicated otherwise by the drug package insert).
   Principle. Shaking the vial may cause air bubbles to form.

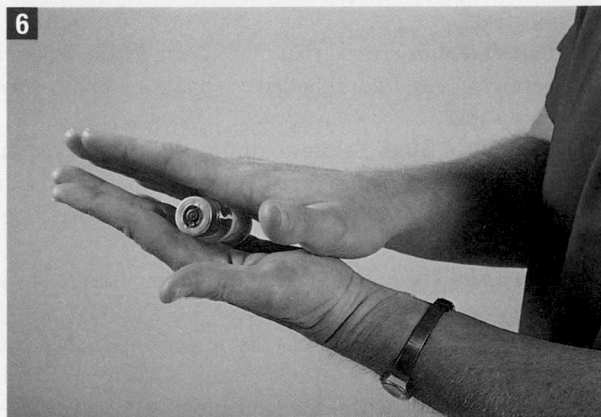

Roll the vial between the hands.

7. **Procedural Step.** Label multiple-dose vials with the date of preparation and your initials.
8. **Procedural Step.** Administer the injection.
9. **Procedural Step.** Store multiple-dose vials as indicated by the manufacturer's instructions. Because reconstituted drugs are stable for a short time, carefully check the date of preparation on the multiple-dose vial before administering it again.

PROCEDURE 26-3

PROCEDURE 26-4 **Administering a Subcutaneous Injection**

Outcome Administer a subcutaneous injection.

Equipment/Supplies

- Medication ordered by the physician
- Appropriate needle and syringe
- Antiseptic wipe
- Sterile 2 × 2 gauze pad
- Disposable gloves
- Biohazard sharps container

1. **Procedural Step.** Sanitize your hands, and prepare the injection (see Procedure 26-2).

2. **Procedural Step.** Greet the patient and introduce yourself. Identify the patient by full name and date of birth. Explain the procedure and the purpose of the injection.
   Principle. It is crucial that no error be made in patient identity. An apprehensive patient may need reassurance.

3. **Procedural Step.** Select an appropriate injection site. The upper arm, thigh, back, and abdomen are recommended sites for a subcutaneous injection. See Figure 26-17.
   Principle. The entire area should be exposed to ensure a safe and comfortable injection.

4. **Procedural Step.** Prepare the injection site. Cleanse the area with an antiseptic wipe. Using a circular motion, start with the injection site, and move outward. Do not touch the site after cleansing it.
   Principle. Using a circular motion carries contaminants away from the injection site. Touching the site after cleansing contaminates it, and the cleansing process needs to be repeated.

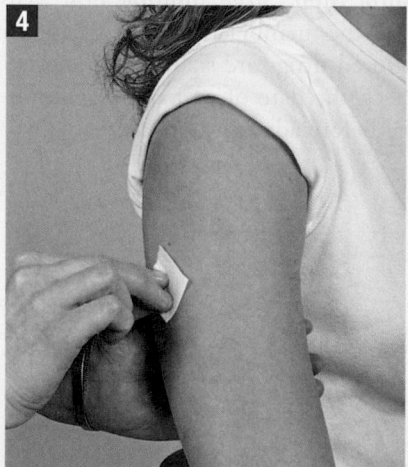

Cleanse the area with an antiseptic wipe.

5. **Procedural Step.** Allow the area to dry completely.
   Principle. If the area is not permitted to dry, the antiseptic may enter the tissues when the skin is pierced, resulting in irritation and patient discomfort.

6. **Procedural Step.** Apply gloves, and remove the needle guard. Position your nondominant hand on the area surrounding the injection site. The skin may be held taut, or the area surrounding the injection site may be grasped and held in a cushion fashion.
   Principle. Gloves provide a barrier against bloodborne pathogens. In normal adults, the needle enters the subcutaneous tissue when the skin is held taut. Grasping the area around the injection site is recommended for a thin or dehydrated patient. This ensures that the subcutaneous tissue, and not muscle tissue, is entered.

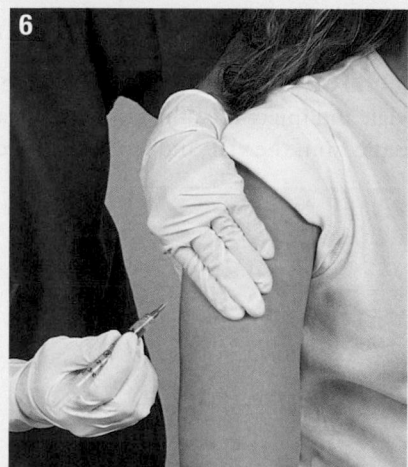

Grasp the area surrounding the injection site.

7. **Procedural Step.** Hold the barrel of the syringe between your thumb and index finger. Insert the needle quickly and smoothly at a 45-degree or 90-degree angle, depending on the length of the needle. With a ½-inch needle, a 90-degree angle should be used; with a ⅝-inch needle, a 45-degree angle should be used. Insert the needle to the hub.
   Principle. Inserting the needle quickly and smoothly minimizes tissue trauma and pain. Needle length determines the angle of insertion to ensure placement of the medication in subcutaneous tissue.

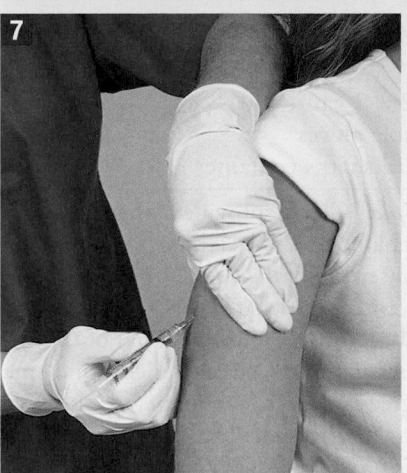

Insert the needle at a 45-degree angle.

8. **Procedural Step.** Remove your hand from the skin.
   Principle. Medication injected into compressed tissue causes pressure against nerve fibers and is uncomfortable for the patient.

9. **Procedural Step.** Hold the syringe steady and pull back gently on the plunger to determine whether the needle is in a blood vessel, in which case blood would appear in the syringe. If blood appears, withdraw the needle, prepare a new injection, and begin again.
   Principle. Moving the syringe after the needle has entered the tissue causes patient discomfort. Drugs intended for subcutaneous administration but injected into a blood vessel are absorbed too quickly, and undesirable results may occur.

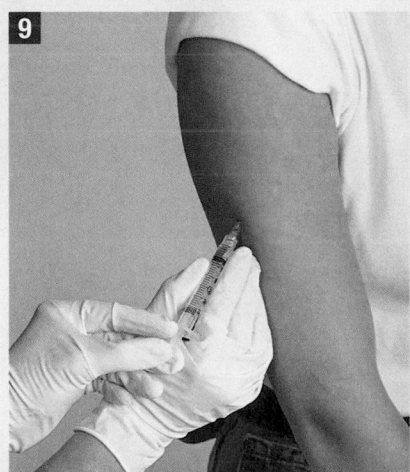

Pull back gently to determine whether the needle is in a blood vessel.

10. **Procedural Step.** Inject the medication slowly and steadily by depressing the plunger. If you are using a retractable safety syringe, activate it at this time following the steps outlined in Figure 26-10, *C*, and continue to step 12.
    Principle. Rapid injection creates pressure and destroys tissue, both of which are uncomfortable for the patient.

11. **Procedural Step.** Place the antiseptic wipe or a gauze pad gently over the injection site and quickly remove the needle, keeping it at the same angle as for insertion.
    Principle. Withdrawing the needle quickly and at the same angle as for insertion reduces patient discomfort. The antiseptic wipe or gauze pad placed over the injection site helps prevent tissue movement as the needle is withdrawn, reducing patient discomfort. Using a gauze pad prevents a stinging sensation from the alcohol.

12. **Procedural Step.** Apply gentle pressure to the injection site with the antiseptic wipe or gauze pad. If you are using a safety syringe with a shield, activate the safety feature at this time following the steps outlined in Figure 26-10.
    Principle. Gentle pressure helps distribute the medication so that it is completely absorbed. Avoid vigorous massaging because this could damage underlying tissue.

13. **Procedural Step.** Properly dispose of the needle and syringe in a biohazard sharps container.
    Principle. Proper disposal is required by the Occupational Safety and Health Administration (OSHA) standard to prevent accidental needlestick injuries.

14. **Procedural Step.** Remove gloves, and sanitize your hands.

15. **Procedural Step.** Chart the procedure. Include the date and time, the name of the medication, the lot number (if required), the dosage given, the route of administration, the injection site used, and any significant observations or patient reactions.
    Principle. The lot number indicates the batch in which the medication was made. Should a problem arise with that batch, the drug can be recalled, and the individuals who received it can be identified.

16. **Procedural Step.** Stay with the patient to ensure that he or she is not experiencing any unusual reactions. (*NOTE:* If an allergy injection has been given, the patient should remain at the medical office for 15 to 20 minutes to ensure that an allergic reaction does not occur.) Check the patient's arm after the waiting period, and observe for induration and redness. If the patient experiences such a reaction, notify the physician immediately.

CHARTING EXAMPLE

Date	
2/17/XX	3:30 p.m. Ragweed allergy inj, 0.20 mL, SC ⓡ upper arm. Arm checked 15 min. after admin. No reaction noted. —— T. Cline, CMA (AAMA)

PROCEDURE 26-4

Outcome Administer an intramuscular injection.

Equipment/Supplies

- Medication ordered by the physician
- Appropriate needle and syringe
- Antiseptic wipe
- Sterile 2 × 2 gauze pad
- Disposable gloves
- Biohazard sharps container

1. **Procedural Step.** Sanitize your hands, and prepare the injection (see Procedure 26-2).

2. **Procedural Step.** Greet the patient and introduce yourself. Identify the patient by his or her full name and date of birth. Explain the procedure and purpose of the injection.
   Principle. Make sure that you administer the medication to the right patient. Explain the purpose of the injection. Assistance may be needed for restraining infants and children.

3. **Procedural Step.** Select an appropriate intramuscular (IM) injection site. See Figure 26-18 for the recommended IM injection sites. Remove the patient's clothing as necessary to ensure the entire area is exposed.
   Principle. Major nerves and blood vessels may lie in close proximity to the intramuscular injection sites. The medical assistant should develop skill and accuracy in locating the proper sites.

4. **Procedural Step.** Prepare the injection site. Cleanse the area with an antiseptic wipe. Using a circular motion, start with the injection site and move outward. Do not touch the site after cleansing it.
   Principle. Using a circular motion carries contaminants away from the injection site. Touching the site after cleansing contaminates it, and the cleansing process needs to be repeated.

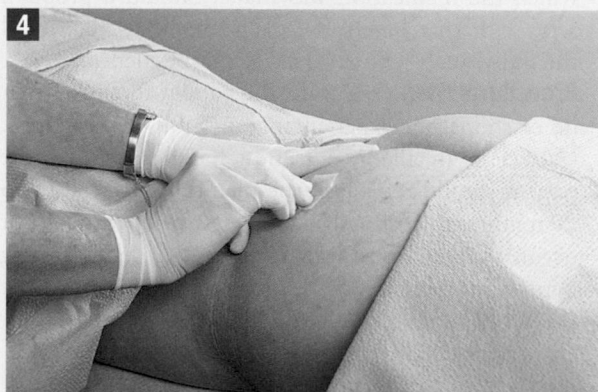

Cleanse the site with an antiseptic wipe.

5. **Procedural Step.** Allow the area to dry completely.
   Principle. If the area is not permitted to dry, the antiseptic may enter the tissues when the skin is pierced, resulting in irritation and patient discomfort.

6. **Procedural Step.** Apply gloves, and remove the needle guard. Using the thumb and first two fingers of the nondominant hand, stretch the skin taut over the injection site.

Principle. Gloves provide a barrier against blood-borne pathogens. Stretching the skin taut permits easier insertion of the needle and helps ensure that the needle enters muscle tissue.

7. **Procedural Step.** Hold the barrel of the syringe like a dart, and insert the needle quickly and smoothly at a 90-degree angle to the patient's skin with a firm motion. Insert the needle to the hub.
   Principle. The needle is inserted at a 90-degree angle and to the hub to ensure that it reaches muscle tissue. Inserting the needle quickly and smoothly minimizes tissue trauma and pain.

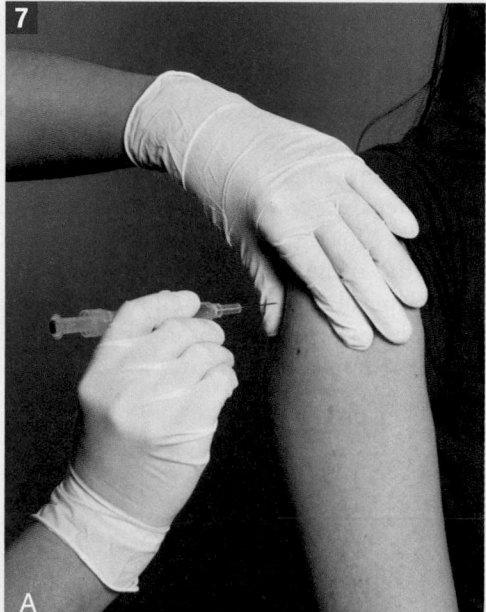

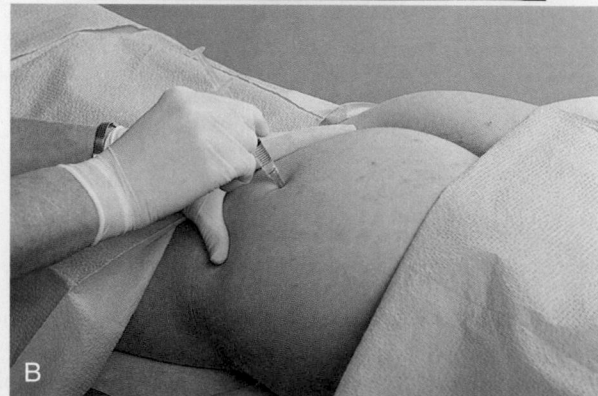

Insert the needle at a 90-degree angle.

8. **Procedural Step.** Hold the syringe steady, and pull back gently on the plunger to determine whether the needle is in a blood vessel. If blood appears, withdraw the needle, prepare a new injection, and begin again.

Principle. Moving the syringe after the needle has penetrated the tissue causes patient discomfort. If drugs intended for intramuscular administration are injected into a blood vessel, the result is faster absorption of the medication. This may produce undesirable results.

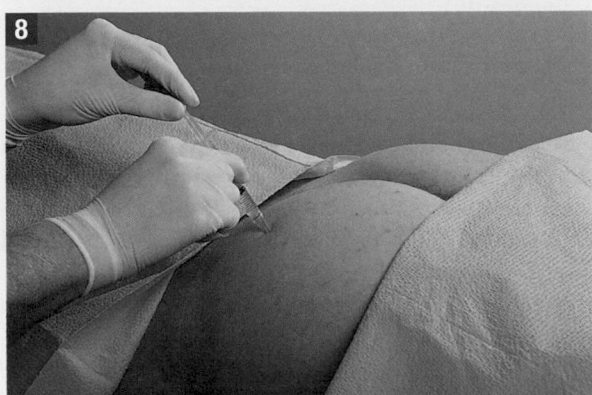

Aspirate to determine whether the needle is in a blood vessel.

9. **Procedural Step.** Inject the medication slowly and steadily by depressing the plunger. If you are using a retractable safety syringe, activate it at this time while following the steps outlined in Figure 26-10, *C,* and continue to step 11.
   Principle. Rapid injection creates pressure and destroys tissue, causing discomfort for the patient.

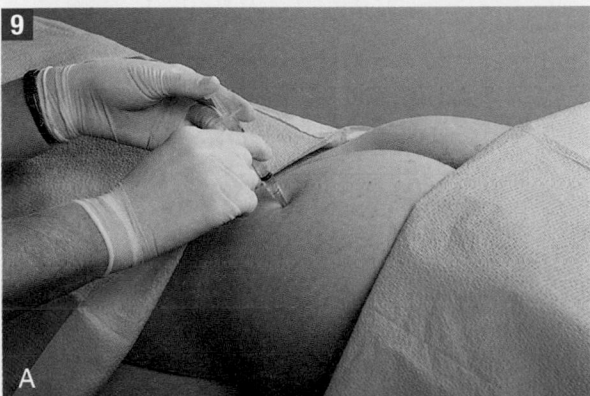

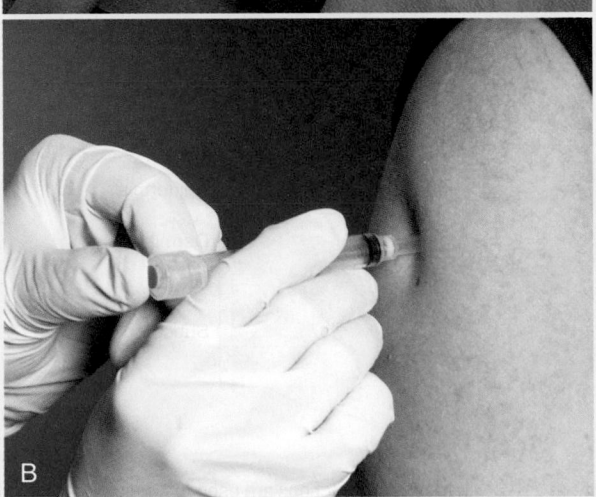

Inject the medication slowly and steadily.

10. **Procedural Step.** Place the antiseptic wipe or gauze pad gently over the injection site and remove the needle quickly, keeping it at the same angle as for insertion.
    Principle. Withdrawing the needle quickly and at the same angle as for insertion reduces patient discomfort. Placing the antiseptic wipe or gauze pad over the injection site helps prevent tissue movement as the needle is withdrawn, also reducing patient discomfort. Using a gauze pad prevents a stinging sensation from the alcohol.

11. **Procedural Step.** Apply gentle pressure to the injection site with an antiseptic wipe or gauze pad. If you are using a safety syringe with a shield, activate the safety feature at this time following the steps outlined in Figure 26-10.
    Principle. Gentle pressure helps distribute the medication so that it is absorbed by the muscle tissue. Avoid vigorous massaging because this could damage underlying tissues.

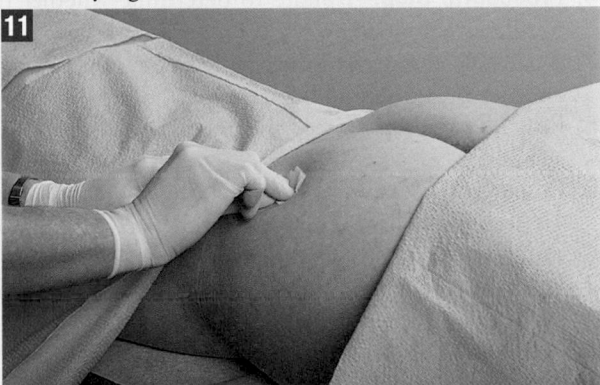

Apply gentle pressure to the injection site.

12. **Procedural Step.** Properly dispose of the needle and syringe in a biohazard sharps container.
    Principle. Proper disposal is required by the OSHA standard to prevent accidental needlestick injuries.

13. **Procedural Step.** Remove the gloves, and sanitize your hands.

14. **Procedural Step.** Chart the procedure. Include the date and time, the name of the medication, the lot number (if required), the dosage given, the route of administration, the injection site used, and any significant observations or patient reactions.
    Principle. The lot number indicates the batch in which the medication was made. Should a problem arise with that batch, the drug can be recalled, and individuals who received it can be identified.

15. **Procedural Step.** Stay with the patient to ensure he or she is not experiencing any unusual reactions. If the patient experiences an unusual reaction, notify the physician immediately.

CHARTING EXAMPLE	
Date	
2/20/XX	9:30 a.m. Rocephin (Lot #: U6261). Admin 1 gram, IM, Ⓛ dorsogluteal. Tolerated injection well.
	—————— T. Cline, CMA (AAMA)

PROCEDURE 26-6 Z-Track Intramuscular Injection Technique

Outcome Administer an intramuscular injection using the Z-track method.

Equipment/Supplies

- Medication ordered by the physician
- Appropriate needle and syringe
- Antiseptic wipe

- Disposable gloves
- Biohazard sharps container

1. **Procedural Step.** Follow steps 1 through 5 of Procedure 26-5.

2. **Procedural Step.** Apply gloves, and remove the needle guard. With the nondominant hand, pull the skin away laterally from the injection site approximately 1 to 1½ inches.

3. **Procedural Step.** Insert the needle quickly and smoothly at a 90-degree angle.

4. **Procedural Step.** Aspirate to determine whether the needle is in a blood vessel. If blood appears, withdraw the needle and discard the needle and syringe. Prepare another injection and begin again.

5. **Procedural Step.** Inject the medication slowly and steadily.

6. **Procedural Step.** After injecting the medication, wait 10 seconds before withdrawing the needle to allow initial absorption of the medication.

7. **Procedural Step.** Withdraw the needle quickly, keeping it at the same angle as for insertion.

8. **Procedural Step.** Release the traction on the skin to seal off the needle track; doing so prevents the medication from reaching the subcutaneous tissue and skin surface.

9. **Procedural Step.** Do not apply pressure to the site because this could cause the medication to seep out.

10. **Procedural Step.** If you are using a safety syringe with a shield, activate the safety feature at this time following the steps outlined in Figure 26-10.

11. **Procedural Step.** Properly dispose of the needle and syringe in a biohazard sharps container.

12. **Procedural Step.** Remove your gloves, and sanitize your hands.

13. **Procedural Step.** Chart the procedure. Include the date and time, the name of the medication, the lot number (if required), the dosage given, the route of administration, the injection site used, and any significant observations or patient reactions.

14. **Procedural Step.** Stay with the patient to ensure he or she is not experiencing any unusual reactions. If the patient experiences an unusual reaction, notify the physician immediately.

CHARTING EXAMPLE

Date	
2/20/XX	10:30 a.m. Iron dextran (Lot #: 1445). Admin 100 mg, IM, Z-track into Ⓡ dorsogluteal. No complaints of discomfort.
	———————— T. Cline, CMA (AAMA)

---

technique for the administration of an intradermal injection.

The most frequent use of intradermal injections is to administer a skin test, such as an allergy test or a tuberculin test. The medication for the appropriate test is placed into the skin layers, and a small, raised area known as a **wheal** is produced at the injection site, owing to distention of the skin (Figure 26-21). At a time dictated by the type of test being administered, the results are read and interpreted. Most allergy tests can be read and interpreted at the medical office a short time (usually 15 to 20 minutes) after administration of the test, whereas tuberculin testing requires 48 hours before the results can be read.

The skin testing medication interacts with the body tissues; if no reaction occurs, the wheal disappears within a short time, and the only visible sign left is the puncture site.

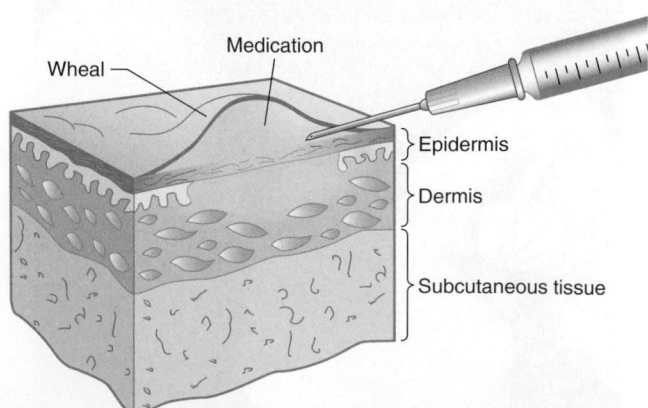

Figure 26-21 Intradermal injections are used to administer skin tests. Enough medication must be deposited in the skin layers to form a wheal.

If a reaction to the skin test occurs, induration results, indicating a positive reaction. Erythema also may be present at the test site; however, for most skin tests, the extent of induration is the only criterion used to assess a positive reaction.

TUBERCULIN SKIN TESTING

Tuberculosis

Tuberculosis (TB) is an infectious bacterial disease that can occur in almost any part of the body but usually attacks the lungs. Tuberculosis affecting the lungs is known as *pulmonary tuberculosis,* whereas tuberculosis occurring in other parts of the body is known as *extrapulmonary tuberculosis* and is most apt to occur in the brain, spine, kidneys, bones, and joints. The name of the bacterium that causes tuberculosis is *Mycobacterium tuberculosis,* which is a rod-shaped bacterium. Shortly (within weeks) after infection, a small percentage of individuals infected with the TB bacteria develop active pulmonary tuberculosis. In these individuals, the TB bacteria are able to overcome the body's defense system. This is most apt to occur in young children and individuals with a weakened immune system. The TB bacteria then begin to multiply and attack the body, resulting in the destruction of tissue.

Symptoms of active pulmonary tuberculosis include a chronic cough lasting 3 weeks or longer that produces a mucopurulent sputum, occasional hemoptysis (coughing up blood), and chest pain. Systemic symptoms include fatigue, loss of appetite, weakness, unexplained weight loss, chills, low-grade fever, and sweating at night. If active tuberculosis is left untreated, it can result in serious complications such as permanent lung damage and even death.

Most people (90%) infected with the TB bacterium do not develop the active disease because their body defenses protect them. Body defenses may be able to destroy the TB bacteria immediately after they enter the body and completely clear them from the body. If this is not possible, the TB bacteria are engulfed by white blood cells known as macrophages. The body then builds a fibrous wall of tissue around these macrophages (infected with TB bacteria) to encapsulate them. Some of the TB bacteria may remain alive inside the capsule in a dormant or inactive state. During this time, the individual experiences no symptoms and cannot spread the disease to others. Individuals are said to have a latent tuberculosis infection (LTBI), and the only sign indicating that they have been infected with tuberculosis is a positive reaction to a TB test.

Individuals with latent tuberculosis may go on to develop active tuberculosis. This occurs in approximately 10% of individuals with LTBI. About half of these individuals develop active tuberculosis within 2 years after the initial infection, and the other half develop tuberculosis many years, even decades, after becoming infected. The TB bacteria break out of the capsule and cause the symptoms of active tuberculosis (described previously). The development of LTBI into active tuberculosis is most apt to occur when the body's immune system is weakened, such as during a serious illness, or in patients who have an immune disorder such as human immunodeficiency virus (HIV) infection. The difference between active tuberculosis and latent tuberculosis is outlined in Table 26-6.

Purpose of Tuberculin Skin Testing

The purpose of tuberculin skin testing (TST) is to identify individuals who are infected with *M. tuberculosis.* TST is recommended for individuals who are at higher risk for TB exposure or infection, or at higher risk for progressing from latent tuberculosis to active tuberculosis. Examples include individuals who have close day-to-day contact with someone with active tuberculosis, individuals who have immigrated from a country with a high incidence of TB, and individuals who work or reside in facilities or institutions with people who are at high risk for TB (e.g., hospitals and other health care facilities, correctional facilities, and nursing homes). Tuberculin skin testing may also be required as a

Table 26-6 Differences between Active TB and Latent TB		
Characteristics	**Active TB**	**Latent TB**
Symptoms	Patient usually feels sick and has symptoms of TB such as cough, fever, and weight loss.	Patient feels fine and has no symptoms.
TB bacterial status	Active TB bacteria are present in the body.	TB bacteria are present in the body that are alive but inactive.
TB test results	Patient usually has a positive TST or QFT-G blood test result.	Patient usually has a positive TST or QFT-G blood test result.
Diagnostic tests	Patient may have an abnormal chest x-ray and a positive sputum test.	Patient has a normal chest x-ray and a negative sputum test.
Ability to infect others	Patient is infectious and may spread the disease to others.	Patient is not infectious and cannot spread the TB to others.
Treatment	Patient needs treatment for active TB.	Physician may consider treatment for latent TB to prevent active TB disease.

From Bonewit-West K: *Clinical procedures for medical assistants,* ed 8, St Louis, 2011, Saunders.
QFT, QuantiFERON-TB Gold; *TB,* tuberculosis; *TST,* tuberculin skin testing.

prerequisite for employment, college entrance, entrance into the military service, and so on. A positive reaction to a tuberculin skin test occurs 2 to 10 weeks after an individual is infected with tuberculosis. Because of this, a patient recently infected with TB bacteria may show a false-negative test result and should be retested 10 weeks later.

The medical assistant is responsible for administering the tuberculin test and for reading the test results. Although tuberculin skin testing is relatively easy to perform, the procedure must be followed exactly to ensure accurate results. A patient with a tuberculous infection may fail to react to the test if it is not performed correctly.

Tuberculin Skin Test Reactions

The substance used in the skin test is tuberculin, which consists of a purified protein derivative (PPD) extracted from a culture of *M. tuberculosis* (the causative agent of tuberculosis), to test for sensitivity to the TB organism. The tuberculin PPD solution contains no live tuberculosis organisms and is completely harmless, making it safe to administer to people of all ages.

When introduced into the skin of an individual with an active or latent case of tuberculosis, tuberculin causes localized thickening of the skin, resulting in induration. **Induration,** which indicates a positive reaction, is an abnormally raised hardened area with clearly defined margins caused by an accumulation of small, sensitized lymphocytes (a type of white blood cell) that occurs in the area in which the tuberculin was injected into the skin (Figure 26-22). Tuberculin skin test reactions are based on the amount of induration present and are interpreted according to the manufacturer's instructions that accompany the test.

A positive reaction to a tuberculin skin test indicates the presence of a tuberculous infection; however, it does not differentiate between active and latent forms of the infection. Therefore, a positive reaction warrants additional diagnostic procedures before the physician can make a final diagnosis. Other procedures used to detect an active tuberculous infection include chest x-ray and microbiologic examination and culture of the patient's sputum for TB bacteria.

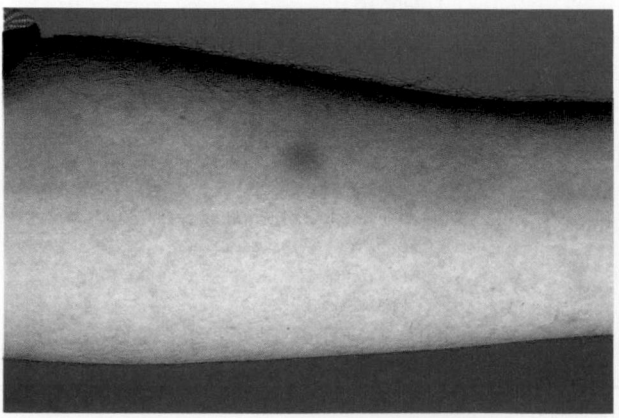

Figure 26-22 Positive tuberculin skin test.

Tuberculin Skin Testing Methods

Two methods are available for tuberculin skin testing: the Mantoux test and the Tine multiple puncture test. The Mantoux test is the most common method used for tuberculin skin testing. The Mantoux test is administered using an intradermal needle and syringe. The Mantoux test is considered a more specific and accurate test because a known amount of tuberculin is used to perform the test.

The Tine multiple puncture test uses a sterile plastic unit containing four stainless-steel tines for puncturing the skin. The tines are approximately 2 mm long and are impregnated with tuberculin. The patient is inoculated intradermally to a depth of 1 to 2 mm by pressing the disc onto the skin, causing the tuberculin on the tines to be deposited into the skin layers. The amount of tuberculin injected into the patient's skin cannot be precisely controlled with the Tine multiple puncture test; therefore, it is rarely used anymore. Because of this, this section will focus on the Mantoux test.

Mantoux Test

The Mantoux test is named after Charles Mantoux, the French physician who developed the test. The Mantoux test is administered through an intradermal injection using a tuberculin syringe with a capacity of 1.0 mL and a short (⅜ to ½ inch) needle with a gauge of 26 to 27. The standard injected dose is 0.1 mL of tuberculin PPD solution containing 5 TU (tuberculin units). Brand names for Mantoux tests include Tubersol and Aplisol. Once opened, a vial of tuberculin PPD solution expires after 30 days and must be discarded. This is because oxidation and degradation of tuberculin reduce its potency, which can lead to inaccurate test results. The medical assistant should write the expiration date on the vial upon opening. Before withdrawing tuberculin from the vial, the medical assistant should check both the manufacturer's expiration date and the 30-day expiration date marked by the medical assistant on the vial.

It is important to properly store the tuberculin PPD solution because it can be adversely affected by exposure to light and heat. The vial should be stored in the dark as much as possible; exposure to bright light should be avoided because this can diminish the potency of the PPD solution. A vial that has been exposed to light for an extended period of time should be discarded. The vial must be stored in the refrigerator at a temperature between 35° F to 46° F (2° C to 8° C). The vial should be returned to its refrigerated storage area as soon as possible after the proper dosage is drawn up into a syringe.

It is important that the medical assistant draw up the proper amount of tuberculin PPD solution. Injecting too much of the solution might elicit a reaction not caused by a tuberculous infection, and injecting too little of the solution results in insufficient solution being injected into the skin to elicit a reaction. This will invalidate the test because if no reaction occurs, it cannot be accepted as a negative reaction.

The medical assistant must make sure to inject the tuberculin solution into the superficial skin layers to form a tense, pale, raised area known as a **wheal.** If the injection is made into the subcutaneous layer, a wheal will not form and the test will yield a false-negative result, whereas a too-shallow injection may cause leakage of the tuberculin solution onto the skin. In either case, the medical assistant must repeat the test at a site at least 2 inches (5 cm) away.

The medical assistant should not apply pressure to the site after injecting the tuberculin PPD solution because the solution is not intended to be absorbed into the tissues. In addition, applying pressure may cause leakage of the solution through the needle puncture site. The wheal will disappear on its own within a few minutes and should not be covered with an adhesive bandage.

Guidelines for Administering a Mantoux Test

1. Use the anterior forearm, approximately 4 inches (10 cm) below the bend in the elbow, as the site of administration of the test. Avoid the following areas because they make the test harder to perform and interfere with good visualization and palpation of test reactions:
   - Hairy areas of the skin
   - Areas with visible veins
   - Scar tissue
   - Red or swollen areas
   - Bruised areas
   - Areas with lesions, dermatitis, or other skin irritations
   - Muscle ridges
2. Cleanse the skin thoroughly with an antiseptic wipe and allow it to dry completely before administering the test.
3. Be sure to inject the tuberculin slowly into the superficial layers of the skin. If the injection is performed correctly, a wheal should appear that is approximately 6 to 10 mm (⅜ inch) in diameter. If blood appears at the puncture site once the test has been administered, this is not significant and will not interfere with the test. The blood can be removed by gently blotting the area with a gauze pad, making sure not to apply pressure.
4. Once the test has been administered, the results must be read within 48 to 72 hours.

Guidelines for Reading Mantoux Test Results

1. The test results must be read in good lighting within 48 to 72 hours.
2. Use both inspection and palpation to read the test results. Induration may not always be visible and therefore must be assessed through palpation.
3. If induration is present, rub your fingertip lightly from the area of normal skin (without induration) to the indurated area to assess its size. The diameter of induration must be assessed and measured transversely to the long axis of the forearm (left to right, not up and down). Measure the widest diameter of induration in millimeters using a flexible millimeter ruler. (*NOTE:* If

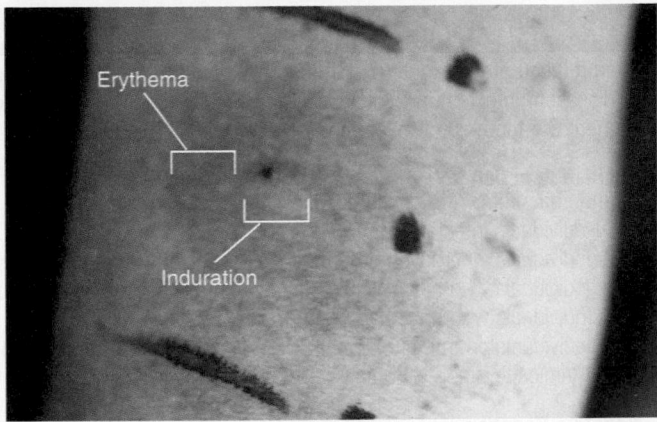

Figure 26-23 Positive tuberculin skin test showing induration and erythema. Induration is the only criterion used to determine a positive reaction.

you have difficulty locating the edges of the induration, the following technique will help. Take a ballpoint pen and place the tip of it on normal skin adjacent to the induration at a 45-degree angle. Then push the pen toward the indurated area. The pen will make an ink line on the normal skin and then will stop at the edge of the induration. Repeat this technique on the opposite side of the induration.
4. The extent of induration present is the only criterion used to determine a positive reaction (Figure 26-23). If erythema is present without induration, the results are interpreted as negative.
5. Record all reactions in millimeters to the nearest millimeter. If no induration is present, the results should be recorded as 0 mm. Results should never be recorded as positive or negative.
6. The interpretation of the test results depends on:
   a. Measurement (in mm) of the induration
   b. The individual's risk of being infected with tuberculosis (e.g., close contact with an individual with active TB increases the risk of being infected)
   c. The individual's risk of progression to disease if infected (e.g., HIV-infected individuals are more apt to progress from LTBI to active TB)
7. Mantoux tuberculin test results are interpreted according to the guidelines presented in Table 26-7. The procedure for administering and reading a Mantoux test is presented in Procedure 26-7.

Two-Step Tuberculin Skin Test

The two-step tuberculin test is recommended by the Centers for Disease Control and Prevention (CDC) for the initial baseline testing of adults who are required to undergo periodic tuberculin skin testing. For example, most health care workers are required to have an initial tuberculin skin test when hired and then a yearly test thereafter. On employment, the initial tuberculin skin test should consist of a baseline two-step test.

Table 26-7 Interpretation of the Tuberculin Mantoux Skin Test*

Interpretation of the Mantoux skin test results is based on the individual's risk of being infected with tuberculosis and the risk of progression to disease if infected. Individuals with impaired immunity are more likely to have a weaker response to a tuberculin skin test. Because of this, there are three cutoff points for identifying a positive reaction to a Mantoux test.

Positive Reaction
An induration of 5 mm or more is classified as positive in individuals with the following high-risk factors for developing TB:
1. Individuals infected with HIV
2. Individuals who have had recent close contact with individuals who have active TB
3. Individuals who have fibrotic changes on a chest radiograph consistent with previously healed TB
4. Individuals who have had organ transplants
5. Individuals on immunosuppressive drug therapy (e.g., prolonged high-dose corticosteroid therapy, TNF/alpha-antagonist drug therapy [Remicade, Enbrel, Humira])

Negative Reaction
An induration of 4 mm or less

Positive Reaction
An induration of 10 mm or more is classified as positive in individuals who do not meet the above criteria but who have other risk factors for TB, including the following:
1. Individuals who inject illegal drugs
2. Individuals with the following conditions that weaken the immune system: diabetes mellitus, chronic renal failure, being 10% or more below ideal body weight, silicosis, gastrectomy, jejunoileal bypass, certain hematologic disorders such as leukemias and lymphomas, carcinoma of the head, neck, or lungs
3. Residents and employees of the following high-risk congregate settings: hospitals and other health care facilities, correctional facilities, nursing homes, homeless shelters, drug rehabilitation centers, residential facilities for patients with AIDS
4. Recent immigrants from countries with a high incidence of TB (countries in Asia, Africa, the Caribbean, Latin America, and Eastern Europe and Russia)
5. Children younger than 4 years of age
6. Infants, children, and adolescents exposed to adults at high risk for developing TB
7. Mycobacteriology laboratory personnel

Negative Reaction
An induration of 9 mm or less

Positive Reaction
An induration of 15 mm or more is classified as positive in individuals at low risk for developing TB, including the following:
Individuals with no known risk factors for TB

Negative Reaction
An induration of 14 mm or less

From Bonewit-West K: *Clinical procedures for medical assistants*, ed 8, St Louis, 2011, Saunders.
AIDS, Acquired immunodeficiency syndrome; *HIV*, human immunodeficiency virus; *TB*, tuberculosis; *TNF*, tumor necrosis factor.
*The cutoff point may sometimes vary from state-to-state from those presented in this table.

To understand the purpose of a two-step tuberculin skin test, it is first necessary to understand what can sometimes occur in individuals who were infected with tuberculosis many years ago. Over a period of years, the ability of the immune system of an individual with a previous TB infection to react to the tuberculin solution may gradually diminish. When a tuberculin skin test is administered to such an individual, the body does not react at all or only weakly reacts, resulting in a false-negative test result. For example, a 42-year-old individual who was infected with tuberculosis during childhood may have a negative test result to an initial tuberculin skin test.

Administering a tuberculin skin test to an individual with a previous TB infection causes stimulation or "boost-

ing" of the patient's immune system that takes place over several days following administration of the test. Basically, the first test "jogs the memory" of the immune system to recognize and react to the tuberculin. If another test is administered following the first test, there is often a strong reaction to the tuberculin, resulting in a positive test result. This boosted reaction is caused by an old TB infection and should not be interpreted as a newly acquired infection. Misinterpretation could result in an unnecessary investigation to identify the source of the infection and unnecessary treatment of individuals. Although the booster effect can occur in an individual in any age group, it is most apt to occur in older individuals who were infected with tuberculosis at a younger age.

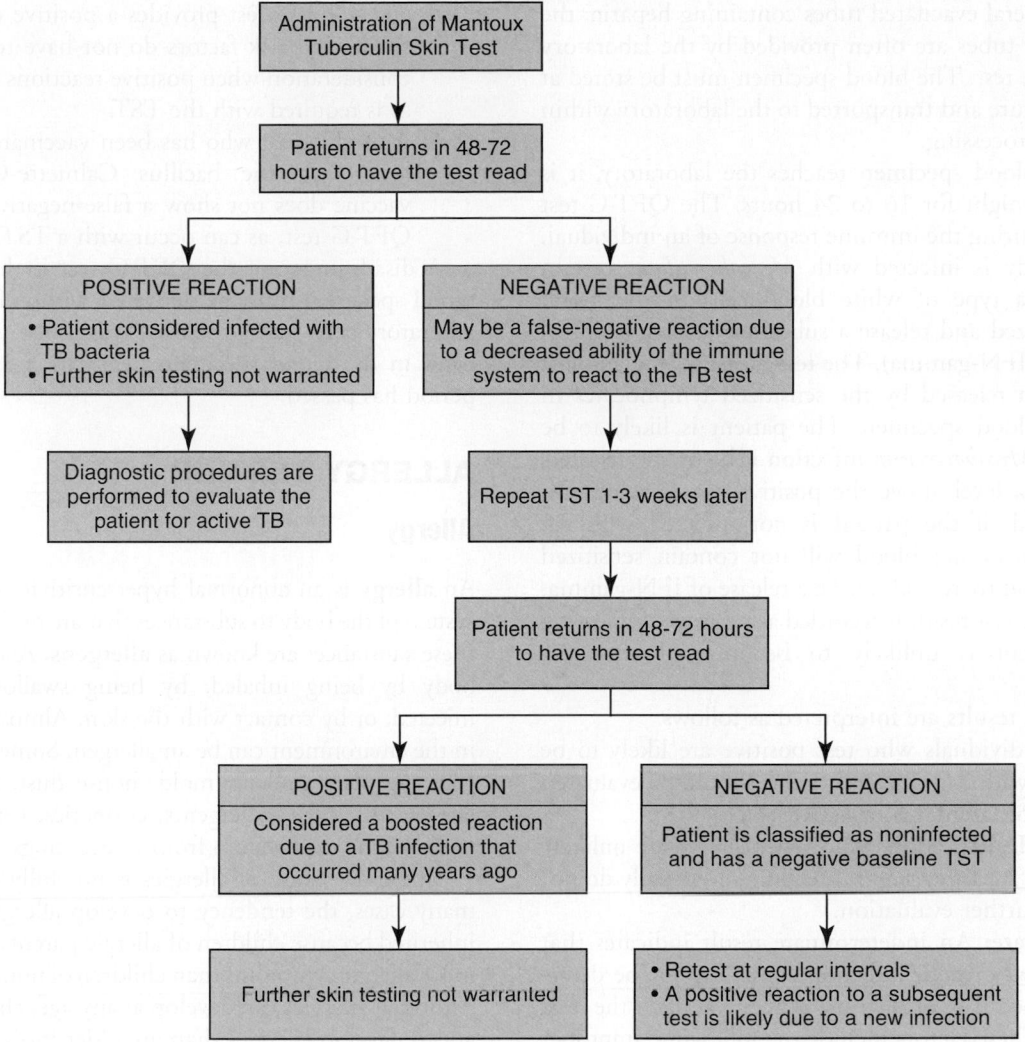

Figure 26-24 Interpretation of the two-step Mantoux tuberculin skin test.

To perform a two-step tuberculin test, the medical assistant administers the Mantoux test and instructs the patient to return to have the test read within 48 to 72 hours as outlined in Procedure 26-7. If the test result is positive, the individual is considered infected with TB bacteria, and further skin testing is not warranted. If the test result is negative, a second test is performed 1 to 3 weeks after the first test. If the second test result is negative, the patient is classified as noninfected, and a positive reaction later on to a subsequent test is likely to represent a new infection. If the second test result is positive, this is most likely caused by a boosted reaction indicating the patient was previously infected with *M. tuberculosis*. Refer to Figure 26-24 for a diagram to assist in interpreting two-step tuberculin skin testing.

When periodic TB testing is required, the two-step tuberculin skin test needs to be completed only *once*. The initial test (consisting of two tests) indicates the true baseline reading of the individual's tuberculosis status. Any subsequent tuberculin skin test performed on a periodic basis (after a two-step test) needs to consist of only one skin test.

Tuberculosis Blood Test

The QuantiFERON-TB Gold (QFT-G) test is a new blood test used to identify individuals who are infected with *M. tuberculosis* (the causative agent of tuberculosis). As with the tuberculin skin test, the QFT-G test cannot differentiate between active and latent forms of the infection. Therefore, a positive result warrants additional diagnostic procedures, such as a chest x-ray and microbiologic examination and culture of the patient's sputum, before the physician can make a diagnosis.

The QFT-G test was approved for use in the United States by the Food and Drug Administration (FDA) in 2005. The CDC recently came out with guidelines indicating that the QFT-G test can be used in all situations in which the Mantoux tuberculin skin test is currently being used. A number of laboratories across the United States perform QFT-G blood testing for tuberculosis.

If the blood specimen for the QFT-G test is drawn in the medical office, several guidelines must be followed to ensure accurate test results. The blood specimen must be drawn into several evacuated tubes containing heparin; the blood drawing tubes are often provided by the laboratory performing the test. The blood specimen must be stored at room temperature and transported to the laboratory within 12 hours for processing.

Once the blood specimen reaches the laboratory, it is incubated overnight for 16 to 24 hours. The QFT-G test works by measuring the immune response of an individual. When the body is infected with *M. tuberculosis,* certain lymphocytes (a type of white blood cell) in the blood become sensitized and release a substance known as interferon gamma (IFN-gamma). The test measures the amount of IFN-gamma released by the sensitized lymphocytes in the patient's blood specimen. The patient is likely to be infected with *Mycobacterium* infection if he or she registers an IFN-gamma level above the positive cutoff value. On the other hand, if the patient is not infected with *M. tuberculosis,* his or her blood will not contain sensitized lymphocytes and there will not be a release of IFN-gamma. In this case, the test result is recorded as negative, indicating that the patient is unlikely to be infected with *M. tuberculosis.*

QFT-G test results are interpreted as follows:

Positive: Individuals who test positive are likely to be infected with *M. tuberculosis* and should be evaluated further for latent TB or active TB.

Negative: Healthy adults who test negative are unlikely to have a *M. tuberculosis* infection and usually do not require further evaluation.

Indeterminate: An indeterminate result indicates that the *M. tuberculosis* infection status cannot be determined because of factors that invalidate the test results. These factors include the following: improper handling and storage of the blood specimen, a delay of longer than 12 hours in transporting the specimen to the laboratory, and the inability of the patient's blood to respond to the test because of a severely weakened immune system, such as in a patient undergoing chemotherapy. If a test result is indeterminate, the QFT-G test should be repeated using a fresh blood specimen.

The QFT-G test offers several advantages over the Mantoux tuberculin skin test (TST), which include the following:

1. The patient needs to visit the office only one time to have his or her blood drawn. This alleviates the problem that sometimes occurs with patients undergoing the TST, in which a patient does not return for the second visit to have the results read.
2. The results are available within 24 hours compared with the 48 to 72 hours required for a TST.
3. The QFT-G test is an objective evaluation, whereas the TST is a subjective evaluation. If the TST test is not measured correctly, inaccurate test results may occur.
4. The QFT-G test is not affected by the booster effect, which can occur with TST, thus eliminating the need for two-step tuberculin skin testing.

5. The QFT-G test provides a positive or negative test result, and risk factors do not have to be taken into consideration when positive reactions are interpreted, as is required with the TST.
6. An individual who has been vaccinated for tuberculosis with the bacillus Calmette-Guérin (BCG) vaccine does not show a false-negative result on the QFT-G test, as can occur with a TST.

A disadvantage of the QFT-G test is that the patient's blood specimen must be delivered within 12 hours to the laboratory performing the test. This is because the lymphocytes in the blood specimen begin to die after this time period has passed.

ALLERGY TESTING

Allergy

An **allergy** is an abnormal hypersensitivity of the immune system of the body to substances that are ordinarily harmless; these substances are known as **allergens.** Allergens enter the body by being inhaled, by being swallowed, by being injected, or by contact with the skin. Almost any substance in the environment can be an allergen. Some common allergens are plant pollens, mold, house dust, animal dander, latex, dyes, soaps, detergents, cosmetics, certain foods and medications, and venom from insect stings.

The exact cause of allergies is not fully understood. In many cases, the tendency to develop allergies seems to be inherited because children of allergic parents tend to exhibit more allergic symptoms than children of nonallergic parents. Although allergies can develop at any age, children are more apt to develop allergies than are older individuals.

Allergic Reaction

The immune system of an individual with allergies interprets certain allergens (e.g., pollen, mold, house dust) as invaders. The first time the allergen enters the body of an allergic individual, it stimulates the body to produce antibodies to that allergen. These antibodies are usually of a type known as *immunoglobulin (Ig)E antibodies.* After the initial sensitization, allergic antibodies combine with the allergen in the body, resulting in an allergen-antibody reaction. When such a reaction occurs, histamine is released in significant amounts, causing allergic symptoms (e.g., sneezing, watery eyes, runny nose). Allergen-antibody reactions may involve any system of the body; however, they most frequently affect the respiratory and integumentary systems. Allergic symptoms can range from mild to very severe, as is the case with the potentially fatal anaphylactic reaction.

Depending on the allergen and the body system affected, allergies appear in different forms in an individual and commonly include allergic rhinitis, asthma, urticaria, contact dermatitis, eczema, and food allergies. Symptoms exhibited by an allergic individual depend on an individual's form of allergy.

Diagnosis and Treatment

The best way to prevent allergic symptoms is to identify and avoid the offending allergen or allergens. The first and most important step in this process is the completion of a careful and detailed medical history by the physician. Of particular importance to the diagnosis of an allergy are the patient's home and work environments, diet, and living habits. The physician also performs a thorough physical examination to detect conditions resulting from allergies, such as nasal polyps, wheezing, skin rashes, and urticaria.

When the medical history and physical examination have been completed, the physician may order diagnostic tests. Allergy testing is performed to confirm information obtained through the medical history and physical examination. The allergy tests ordered most often are direct skin testing and in vitro blood testing, which are described in greater detail in the following section. The general treatment of allergies includes avoiding the allergen(s) (if possible); alleviating the symptoms through drug therapy such as antihistamines, decongestants, bronchodilators, and inhaled steroids; and decreasing the sensitivity of the body to the allergen by the administration of allergy injections, or desensitization injections (known as *immunotherapy*).

Types of Allergy Tests

The purpose of allergy testing is to determine the specific substances or allergens that are causing the patient's allergic symptoms. The two main categories of allergy tests are direct skin tests and the in vitro blood test. The medical assistant is often responsible for performing direct skin testing in the medical office. The in vitro blood test is performed on a blood specimen by an outside laboratory. The medical assistant may be responsible for performing a venipuncture to obtain the blood specimen.

Direct Skin Testing

Direct skin testing involves applying extracts of common allergens to the skin and observing the body's reaction to them. The extract is applied either topically to the skin (patch testing) or into the superficial skin layers (skin-prick testing and intradermal testing). The advantage of direct skin testing is that test results are obtained immediately. This in vivo administration of allergens has the potential, however, to cause adverse reactions, the least common but most serious being an anaphylactic reaction. The medical assistant should have a thorough knowledge of the symptoms of an anaphylactic reaction and should alert the physician immediately if the patient begins to exhibit them.

Regardless of the specific type of direct skin test used (patch, skin-prick, or intradermal), some general guidelines should be followed:

1. Instruct the patient to discontinue the use of antihistamines for 3 days before the skin testing. Antihistamines block the response of histamine, which may suppress skin testing reactions and lead to false-negative test results. Certain medications decrease the immune response of the body to skin testing, which could cause a false-negative test result. These medications include tricyclic antidepressants, corticosteroids, theophylline, beta-blockers, angiotensin-converting enzyme (ACE) inhibitors, and nifedipine. If the patient is taking any of these medications, the physician must determine if it is possible to take the patient off of the medication. If it is not feasible, the physician may order in vitro allergy blood testing, which is not affected by medication.

2. Verify that the area of application is free from hair, scar tissue, and dermatitis to permit good visualization and palpation of test reactions. Recommended sites include the anterior forearm, the upper arm, and the middle of the back. The back is usually used for patch and skin-prick testing, and the upper arm and forearm are typically used for intradermal skin testing.

3. Cleanse the area of application thoroughly with an antiseptic wipe, and allow it to dry completely.

4. Wear gloves when the allergy testing involves puncture of the skin, which includes skin-prick testing and intradermal skin testing. Gloves protect the medical assistant from exposure to bloodborne pathogens, as required by the OSHA standard.

5. Space the allergen extracts at least 1 inch apart to provide enough surface area for a sizable reaction. If not enough surface area is available, large adjacent reactions may run together, making it difficult to read test results.

6. Label the test sites so that the application site of each allergen extract can be identified later when reading results.

7. Closely observe the patient after the procedure for a systemic reaction to the skin testing. The patient should remain at the office for at least 30 minutes following the procedure for observation.

8. Make the patient aware that the skin testing may cause a mild allergic reaction, such as a runny nose, sneezing, and mild wheezing 8 to 24 hours after skin-prick and intradermal skin testing. Instruct the patient to contact the physician immediately if a more severe reaction than this occurs, such as difficulty in breathing, dizziness, or swelling of the face, lips, or mouth.

Quality Control

Positive and negative controls should be performed with each skin testing procedure to ensure reliable and valid test results. Controls are performed at the same time and in the same way that the allergy skin testing is performed.

Negative Control: To perform a negative skin test control, a substance that should not cause a reaction in a normal person is inserted into the patient's superficial skin layers. The negative control usually consists of normal saline. Some patients have a condition known as *dermographism,* which causes them to have a reaction just from the irritating effect of a needle pricking their skin. Running a negative control ensures that positive skin test reactions are truly positive and are not due to another factor, such as dermographism.

Positive Control: To perform a positive control, a substance that should cause a reaction in a nonallergenic patient is inserted into the patient's superficial skin layers. The substance used for the positive control is histamine. The positive control should produce a reaction that consists of at least 3 mm of induration surrounded by erythema. Patients who are taking an antihistamine or who have a depressed immune system due to a disease or immunosuppressive medication may have a false-negative reaction to a skin test. Running a positive control ensures that negative skin test reactions are truly negative and are not just due to another factor, as in a patient who has taken an antihistamine.

Types of Direct Skin Tests

Patch Testing

Patch testing is primarily used to identify allergens that cause contact dermatitis. Patch testing involves the topical application of each allergen to the skin, using a "patch." A patch consists of a small piece of gauze or filter paper impregnated with the allergen, which is applied to the skin and taped in place with hypoallergenic tape (Figure 26-25). Allergens commonly applied include plants, topical drugs,

---

Highlight on Allergens

House Dust

There are many components in house dust to which an individual may be allergic; the most significant of these is the house dust mite. Dust mites thrive in warm humid conditions and feed on scales shed from human skin; they are often found in mattresses, carpets, stuffed animals, and upholstered furniture. An individual who is allergic to house dust reacts to the waste products of these dust mites.

There is no shortage of food for the dust mite because one person sheds up to 1 g of scales per day, which is enough to feed thousands of mites for months. *Dermatophagoides pteronyssinus* and *Dermatophagoides farinae* are the most common house dust mites and are present in varying numbers in virtually every home. Mites occur in greatest numbers in bedding, particularly in mattresses; there may be 5000 mites in each gram of dust from a mattress. Sufferers often notice that symptoms become much worse when the bedding is disturbed and allergenic material becomes airborne. Practices that eliminate dust also reduce the number of dust mites in a household.

Insect Stings

It is estimated that 1 of every 125 Americans is allergic to the venom from insect stings. Approximately 40 people in the United States die each year from a severe allergic reaction to insect venom. The incidence of deaths is low because most people know they need to obtain medical attention immediately if an allergic reaction begins.

Almost all insects whose venom can cause allergic reactions belong to the group Hymenoptera, which includes honeybees and bumblebees, wasps, yellow jackets, and hornets. When a honeybee stings, its stinger remains embedded in the victim's skin, causing the bee to die as it tries to tear itself away. Wasps, yellow jackets, and hornets are more aggressive than bees and can sting repeatedly. Hornets are the most aggressive of the group and may sting even when not provoked. Yellow jackets are close behind in aggressiveness, but wasps usually sting only if someone interferes with them near their nest.

If an insect sting does not cause an allergic reaction within 30 minutes, chances are excellent that no problem will occur. A normal reaction to an insect sting includes localized pain, redness, swelling, and itching lasting 1 to 2 days. Any generalized reaction not arising directly from the area of the sting is almost certain to be an anaphylactic reaction, which begins with such symptoms as sneezing, urticaria, itching, angioedema, erythema, and disorientation and progresses to difficulty in breathing, dizziness, faintness, and loss of consciousness. Medical care should be sought immediately because most fatalities occur within 2 hours following the sting. Because time is a factor, individuals who are known to have a severe allergy to insect stings are provided with an anaphylactic emergency treatment kit that contains epinephrine in a prefilled syringe and oral antihistamines. They can carry the kit with them so that treatment for a severe allergic reaction can be started as soon as possible.

Penicillin

Penicillin is a common cause of allergic drug reactions. Approximately 2% to 5% of individuals are allergic to penicillin. The reaction may be mild and completely overlooked or confused with the symptoms of the disease being treated with penicillin, or it can be more serious and take the form of severe dermatitis or an anaphylactic reaction. Death as a result of a severe anaphylactic reaction is rare, occurring in only 0.01% of patients being treated with penicillin.

Penicillin was discovered in 1929 by Sir Alexander Fleming, but it was not used as a therapeutic drug until 1940. By 1944, it was evident that some of the side effects of penicillin were allergic reactions; the first recorded death as a result of an anaphylactic reaction to penicillin occurred in 1945.

Oral administration of penicillin is safer than a penicillin injection because it has a lower frequency of severe allergic reactions. There have been only six reported deaths from oral administration of penicillin.

Approximately 95% of serious reactions occur within 1 hour after a penicillin injection. The best preventive measure is to keep the patient under direct observation for at least 30 minutes after administration of the injection. ■

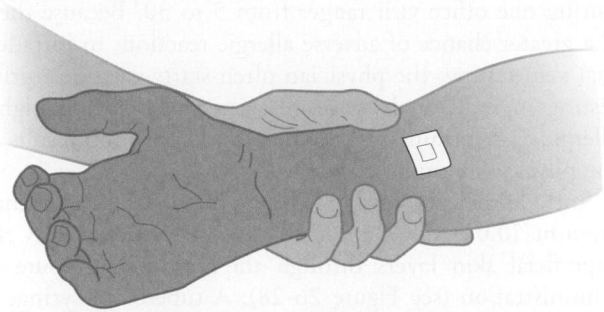

Figure 26-25 Patch testing. A patch consists of a small piece of gauze or filter paper impregnated with the allergen, which is applied to the skin and taped in place.

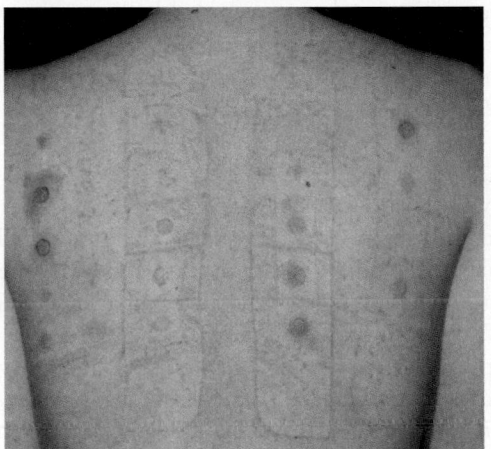

Figure 26-26 Patch test showing positive results.

Table 26-8 Guidelines for Recording Direct Skin Test Results

Patch Test

—	No reaction
+1	Presence of erythema and edema, possibly papules
+2	Presence of erythema, edema, and vesicles, possibly papules
+3	Erythema, vesicles, and severe edema

Skin-Prick Testing and Intradermal Testing

—	No reaction
±1	Induration 1 mm or less
+1	Induration greater than 1 mm and up to 5 mm in diameter
+2	Induration greater than 5 mm and up to 10 mm in diameter
+3	Induration greater than 10 mm and up to 15 mm in diameter
+4	Induration greater than 15 mm in diameter

From Bonewit-West K: *Clinical procedures for medical assistants*, ed 8, St Louis, 2011, Saunders.

latex, resins, metals, cosmetics, dyes, and chemicals. The patient should be instructed to leave the patches in place, keep them dry, and return to the medical office in 48 hours to have the results read. When the patient returns to the office, the patches are carefully removed, and the results are read 20 minutes later. The delayed reading time allows lessening of redness that may occur from the tape removal.

Test results are recorded as positive or negative. Positive reactions cause a small area of contact dermatitis characterized by itching, erythema, induration, and vesiculation (Figure 26-26). In strongly positive responses, the reaction may extend beyond the margins of the patch. Positive results are graded further on a quantitative 1+ to 3+ scoring system according to the type of reaction (Table 26-8).

Skin-Prick Testing

Skin-prick testing usually is performed to diagnose allergies to common allergens, particularly those that are inhaled, such as house dust, pollens, and molds. It is also used to test for food allergies; the most common foods that cause allergies are milk, soy, eggs, peanuts, tree nuts (e.g., walnuts), fish, shellfish, and wheat.

Skin-prick testing involves the application of numerous allergen extracts to the skin, followed by the pricking of each with a sterile needle or another sharp instrument

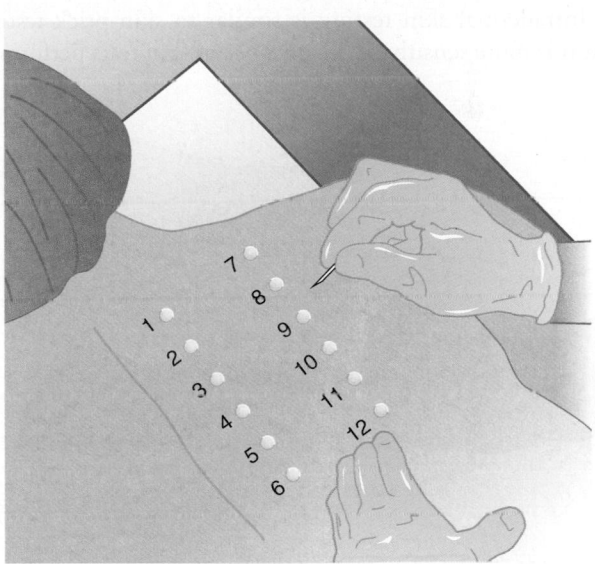

Figure 26-27 Skin-prick testing. Skin-prick testing involves the application of numerous allergen extracts to the skin, followed by the pricking of each with a sterile needle.

(Figure 26-27). The number of allergen extracts applied during one office visit usually ranges between 20 and 30. Pricking the skin deposits the allergens in the outer layers of the skin to allow each to react with the body tissues.

The following guidelines should be followed for skin-prick testing: The extracts should be placed on the skin in rows in a specific pattern. This, along with labeling the test sites with a felt-tipped pen, tracks the location of each extract. Only a single drop of extract should be placed on the skin; more than this amount may cause the extracts to diffuse and run together. A sterile needle should be passed through the drop, and the point should lightly lift the top layer of skin without causing bleeding. It is important to wipe the needle dry with a sterile swab between pricks to prevent one extract from mixing with the next, leading to inaccurate test results.

The maximum reaction is usually seen in 15 to 20 minutes. During this time, the test sites should be left uncovered, and the patient should be instructed not to touch them. These areas should not be wiped because this removes the allergen extract, resulting in false-negative results. The results are read (after 15 to 20 minutes) using a millimeter ruler.

An area of induration surrounded by redness and itching characterizes a positive reaction. Positive results are recorded by measuring the size of the induration in millimeters and converting it to a numeric scale based on the extent of the induration (see Table 26-8). Any redness should be ignored. See Figure 26-28 for an illustration of skin test results. If a negative or only a mild reaction occurs and the physician still suspects the presence of an allergy, the physician may order intradermal skin testing.

Intradermal Skin Testing

Intradermal skin testing is similar to skin-prick testing but it is more sensitive. The number of skin tests performed

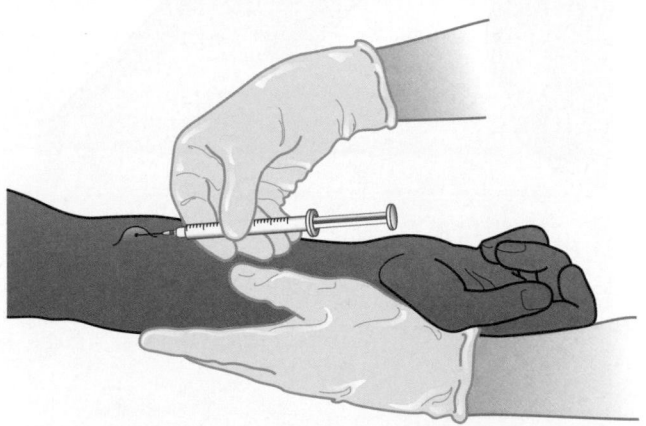

Figure 26-28 Intradermal skin testing. Intradermal testing involves the injection of a small amount of allergen extract into the superficial skin layers through the intradermal route of administration.

during one office visit ranges from 5 to 30. Because there is a greater chance of adverse allergic reactions to intradermal skin testing, the physician often starts with skin-prick testing in individuals who are suspected of being highly allergic as determined by the medical history and results of the physical examination.

Intradermal skin testing involves the injection of a small amount (0.02 to 0.05 mL) of allergen extract into the superficial skin layers through the intradermal route of administration (see Figure 26-28). A tuberculin syringe is used to administer the test, and the allergen extract is injected until a wheal forms (see Procedure 26-7). After 15 to 20 minutes, the test sites are observed for reactions. Positive reactions are characterized by an area of induration surrounded by redness and itching. As with skin-prick testing, positive results are recorded by measuring the size of the induration in millimeters and converting it to a numeric scale based on the amount of induration present (Figure 26-29; see Table 26-8).

In Vitro Allergy Blood Testing

An in vitro allergy blood test measures the amount of IgE antibodies in the blood that respond to common allergens. Examples of in vitro blood tests include enzyme-linked immunosorbent assay (ELISA), the radioallergosorbent test (RAST), and ImmunoCAP. To perform the test, a sample of the patient's blood is sent to an outside laboratory, where it is exposed to allergens suspected of causing an allergic reaction in that patient. A detection device is used to measure the level of IgE antibodies that respond to each allergen being tested, and the results are reported as a numeric value. An elevated level of IgE antibodies responding to an allergen indicates the patient is allergic to that allergen.

Advantages of the in vitro blood test over direct skin testing are as follows: The results are not affected by medication (e.g., antihistamines); there is no danger of adverse allergic reactions because the test is performed in vitro, meaning outside the body; and in vitro blood testing can be performed on patients who have skin eruptions and are unable to undergo direct skin testing because of the lack of an intact skin surface area. In vitro blood testing is expensive, however, and does not provide immediate test results, which

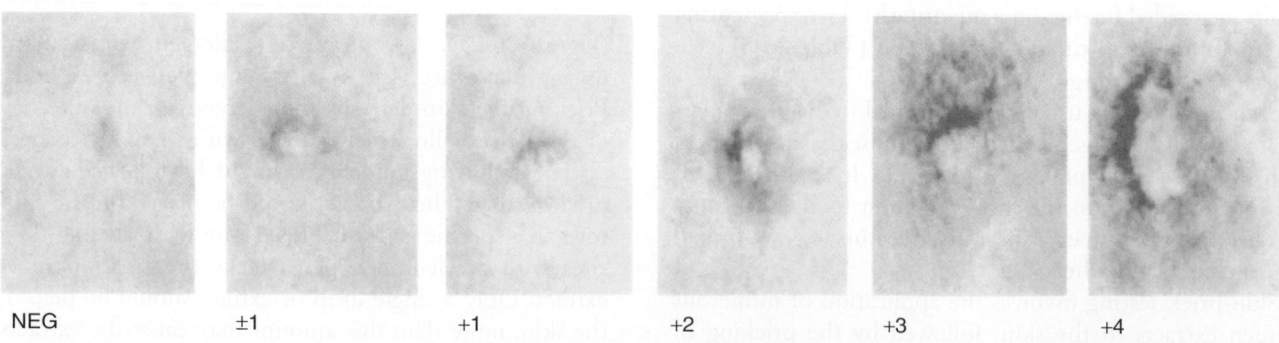

| NEG | ±1 | +1 | +2 | +3 | +4 |

Figure 26-29 Skin-prick and intradermal skin test results.

are available with direct skin testing. Blood testing is often used to test for allergies when it is not possible to perform skin testing. These situations include the following:

1. The physician does not want the patient to be taken off of a medication that interferes with skin test results.

2. The physician suspects that skin testing could result in an anaphylactic reaction in that patient.

3. The patient suffers from a severe skin condition such as widespread dermatitis.

4. The skin testing may be difficult to perform, as in a child younger than 4 years of age.

 PROCEDURE 26-7 **Administering an Intradermal Injection**

Outcome Administer an intradermal injection and read the test results.

Equipment/Supplies

- Skin test solution ordered by the physician
- Appropriate needle and syringe
- Antiseptic wipe
- Sterile 2 × 2 gauze pad

- Disposable gloves
- Millimeter ruler
- TB skin test record card
- Biohazard sharps container

1. **Procedural Step.** Sanitize your hands and prepare the injection (see Procedure 26-2).

2. **Procedural Step.** Greet the patient and introduce yourself. Identify the patient by full name and date of birth. Explain the procedure and purpose of the injection.
   Principle. It is crucial that no error be made in patient identity. Explain the purpose of the injection to reassure an apprehensive patient.

3. **Procedural Step.** Select an appropriate injection site. The anterior forearm and the middle of the back are recommended sites for an intradermal injection. If using the anterior forearm, position the arm on a firm surface with the palm facing upward.
   Principle. The entire area should be exposed to ensure a safe and comfortable injection.

4. **Procedural Step.** Prepare the injection site. Cleanse the area with an antiseptic wipe. Using a circular motion, start with the injection site and move outward. Do not touch the site after cleansing it.
   Principle. Using a circular motion will carry material away from the injection site. Touching the site after cleansing will contaminate it, and the cleansing process will need to be repeated.

5. **Procedural Step.** Allow the area to dry completely.
   Principle. If the area is not permitted to dry, the antiseptic may enter the tissue when the skin is pierced, resulting in irritation and patient discomfort. In addition, the antiseptic may cause a reaction that could be mistaken for a positive test response.

6. **Procedural Step.** Apply gloves, and remove the needle guard. With the nondominant hand, stretch the skin taut at the proposed site of administration. Insert the needle at a 10- to 15-degree angle (almost parallel to the skin), with the bevel upward. The needle should be inserted about ⅛ inch until the bevel of the needle just penetrates the skin. Slight resistance may be felt as the needle is inserted. No aspiration is needed.

Principle. Gloves provide a barrier against blood-borne pathogens. Stretching the patient's skin taut will permit easier insertion of the needle. The needle should be inserted at an angle almost parallel to the skin, to ensure penetration within the dermal layer of the skin. The needle must be inserted with the bevel facing up to allow proper wheal formation. If the needle is inserted with the bevel facing down, the skin test solution will be absorbed into the underlying subcutaneous tissue, and a wheal will not form.

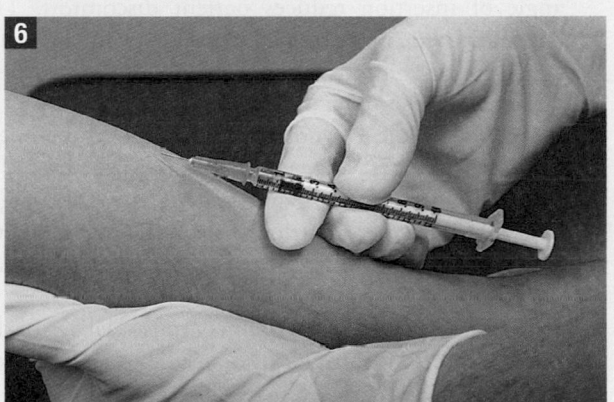

Insert the needle at a 10- to 15-degree angle with the bevel upward.

7. **Procedural Step.** Release the stretched skin. Hold the syringe steady, and inject the skin test solution slowly and steadily by depressing the plunger until a firm, tense, pale wheal forms (approximately 6 to 10 mm in diameter). Expect to feel a certain amount of resistance as you inject the solution; this helps in indicating that the needle is properly located in the superficial skin layers rather than in the deeper subcutaneous tissue. If a wheal does not form, the test must be repeated at another site that is at least 2 inches (5 cm) from the first site. If you are using a retractable safety syringe, activate it at this time following the steps outlined in Figure 26-10, *C,* and continue to Step 9.

Continued

PROCEDURE 26-7   Administering an Intradermal Injection—cont'd

Principle. Moving the syringe once the needle has entered the skin causes patient discomfort. Test results are considered reliable only if a wheal forms.

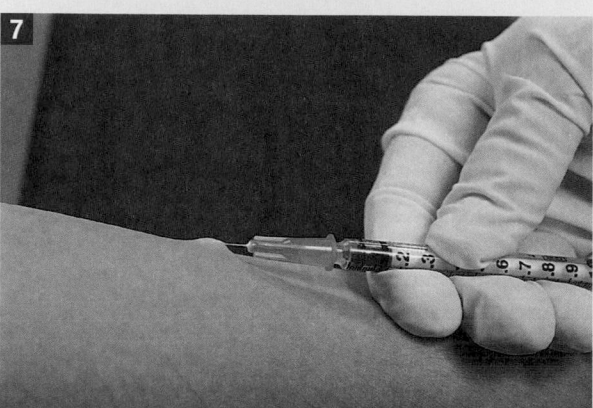

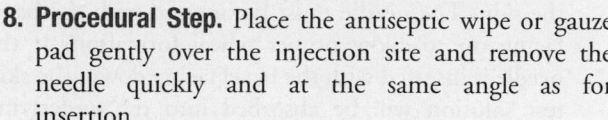
Inject the medication to form a wheal.

8. **Procedural Step.** Place the antiseptic wipe or gauze pad gently over the injection site and remove the needle quickly and at the same angle as for insertion.
   Principle. Withdrawing the needle quickly and at the angle of insertion reduces patient discomfort. The antiseptic wipe or gauze pad placed over the injection site helps prevent tissue movement as the needle is withdrawn, also reducing patient discomfort.

9. **Procedural Step.** Do not apply pressure to the injection site. If blood appears at the injection site, blot the site lightly with a gauze pad. If you are using a safety syringe with a shield, activate the safety feature at this time following the steps outlined in Figure 26-10.
   Principle. Applying pressure may cause leakage of the testing solution through the needle puncture site, resulting in inaccurate test results.

10. **Procedural Step.** Properly dispose of the needle and syringe in a biohazard sharps container.
    Principle. Proper disposal of the needle and syringe is required by the Occupational Safety and Health Administration (OSHA) Standard to prevent accidental needlestick injuries.

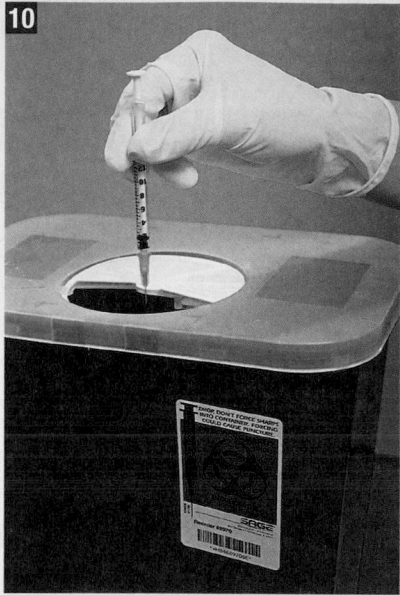
Properly dispose of the needle and syringe.

11. **Procedural Step.** Remove gloves and sanitize your hands.

12. **Procedural Step.** Stay with the patient to make sure that he or she is not experiencing any unusual reactions. The medical assistant should be especially careful and alert for any sign of a patient reaction when administering allergy skin tests. If the patient experiences an unusual reaction, notify the physician immediately.

13. **Procedural Step.** Perform one of the following, based on the type of skin test being administered.

Allergy Skin Tests

a. Read the test results within 20 to 30 minutes, using inspection and palpation at the site of the injection to assess the presence of and to determine the amount of induration. Interpret the skin test results according to the information outlined in Table 26-8.

b. Chart the procedure. Include the date and time, the injection site used, the names of the skin tests, the skin test results, and any significant observations or patient reactions.

CHARTING EXAMPLE	
Date	
2/15/XX	Allergy skin tests, ID, Ⓡ ant forearm.
	Results: House dust +2
	Cat dander +4
	Dog dander −
	Ragweed +4
	Mixed fungi +3
	———— T. Cline, CMA (AAMA)

PROCEDURE 26-7 **Administering an Intradermal Injection—cont'd**

Mantoux Tuberculin Skin Test

1. Inform the patient of the date and time to return to the medical office to have the results read. Results must be read within 48 to 72 hours after the test has been administered. Stress the importance of returning to the office to have the results read, even if the test site does not exhibit a reaction. Failure to return warrants having to repeat the test.

2. Chart the procedure. Include the date and time, the name of the tuberculin purified protein derivative (PPD) solution, the dosage given, the manufacturer and lot number, the route of administration, the injection site used, and any significant observations or patient reactions. The lot number indicates the batch in which the tuberculin solution was made. Should a problem arise with that batch, the tuberculin solution can be recalled and the individuals who received it can be identified.

CHARTING EXAMPLE	
Date	
2/15/XX	10:00 a.m. Tubersol Mantoux test 5 TU,
	0.10 mL, ID. Connaught Laboratories,
	Lot #: C0832AA. Admin Ⓡ ant forearm.
	Pt to return on 2/17/XX to have results
	read. ———————— T. Cline, CMA (AAMA)

3. Instruct the patient in the care of the test site as follows:
   - Continue your normal daily personal hygiene activities.
   - Do not cover the test site with an adhesive bandage.
   - Avoid the use of ointments, lotions, and sunscreens.
   - Mild itching, swelling, or irritation may normally occur at the test site.
   - Do not touch, scratch, press on, or rub the test site. This could alter the test results. If the test site itches, apply a cold compress to the area.
   - Pat the arm dry after washing it. Do not rub it dry.

Reading Mantoux Test Results

Equipment/Supplies

- Millimeter ruler
- Disposable gloves
- Tuberculin test record card

1. **Procedural Step.** Greet the patient and introduce yourself. Identify the patient by full name and date of birth and explain the procedure.
2. **Procedural Step.** Work in a quiet well-lit atmosphere. Check the patient's chart to determine which arm was used to administer the test.
3. **Procedural Step.** Sanitize your hands and apply gloves.

4. **Procedural Step.** Position the patient's arm on a firm surface with the arm flexed at the elbow.
5. **Procedural Step.** Locate the application site. The result should be read transversely to the long axis of the forearm, meaning "across" the forearm.
6. **Procedural Step.** Gently rub your fingertip over the test site and lightly palpate for the presence of induration. If induration is present, the area should be lightly rubbed from the area of normal skin (without induration) to the indurated area to assess the size of the area of induration. If the margins of induration are irregular, assess the widest diameter of induration across the forearm.
   Principle. Induration is the only criterion used in determining a positive reaction. If erythema is present without induration, the results are interpreted as negative.

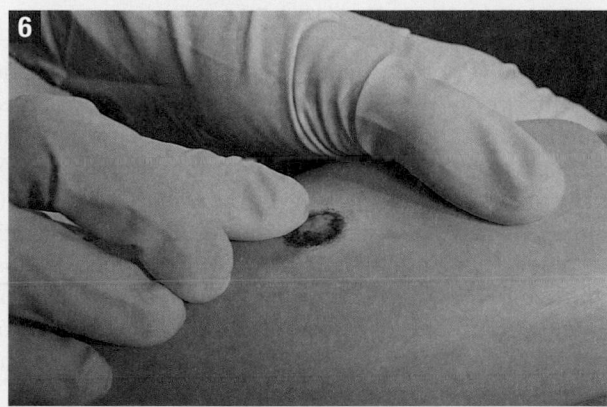
Lightly palpate for induration.

7. **Procedural Step.** Measure the diameter of the induration with a flexible millimeter ruler (supplied by the manufacturer).

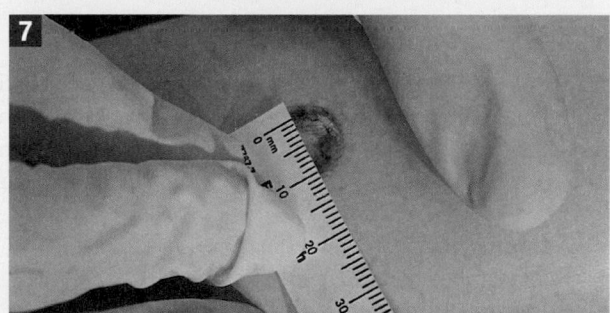
Measure the induration.

8. **Procedural Step.** Remove gloves and sanitize your hands.
9. **Procedural Step.** Chart the results. Include the date and time, the name of the test (Mantoux), and the test results (recorded in millimeters). If no induration is present, 0 mm should be recorded. The results of the Mantoux test are interpreted according to the guidelines outlined in Table 26-7.

Continued

PROCEDURE 26-7

PROCEDURE 26-7 Administering an Intradermal Injection—cont'd

CHARTING EXAMPLE	
Date	
2/17/XX	3:00 p.m. Tubersol Mantoux test: 9mm.
	Pt provided c̄ TB record card. Scheduled
	for TB retesting on 2/28/XX.
	———————— T. Cline, CMA (AAMA)

10. Procedural Step. Complete a tuberculin test record card and give it to the patient.
Principle. The record card provides the patient with a permanent record of the test results.

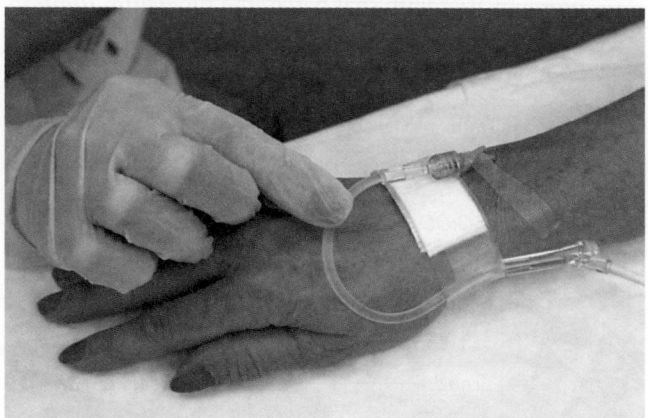

10
TUBERCULOSIS TEST RECORD

Name	Date Admin: 2/15/XX
Carrie Fee	Date Read: 2/17/XX
MANTOUX TEST	**RESULT**
Tubersol, 5 TU	9 mm

Logan Family Practice
401 St. George St.
St. Augustine, FL 32084
(904) 555-3933

Performed by ___*T. Cline*___, *CMA* (AAMA)

INTRAVENOUS THERAPY

Intravenous (IV) therapy is the administration of a liquid agent directly into a patient's vein, where it is distributed throughout the body by way of the circulatory system (Figure 26-30). The veins most commonly used for IV therapy are the peripheral veins of the arm and hand. The liquid agent may consist of basic fluids, medication, nutrients, blood, or blood products. When fluids, medications, or nutrients are administered through the IV route, the technique is called an **infusion.** When whole blood or blood products are administered through the IV route, the procedure is called a **transfusion.**

Most IV therapy occurs in a hospital setting on both an inpatient and an outpatient basis. IV therapy also is administered in outpatient ambulatory settings, such as medical offices and clinics, urgent care centers, ambulatory infusion clinics, and the patient's home (Figure 26-31).

Advantages of Outpatient Intravenous Therapy

Administration of IV therapy in an outpatient setting is growing in acceptance by patients and the medical community. IV therapy may be administered in an outpatient setting for a variety of reasons which include the following:

- Administration of IV medication
- Replacement of fluids and electrolytes
- Administration of nutritional supplements
- Administration of blood products
- Emergency administration of IV medication and fluids

Outpatient IV therapy is more convenient for the patient and reduces medical costs through earlier discharge from the hospital or avoidance of hospitalization altogether.

Earlier Hospital Discharge

When a hospitalized patient is receiving IV therapy and requires continued therapy, it is not always necessary or

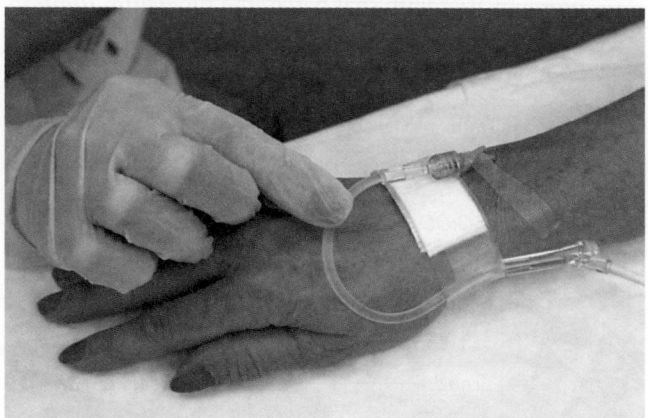

Figure 26-30 IV therapy.

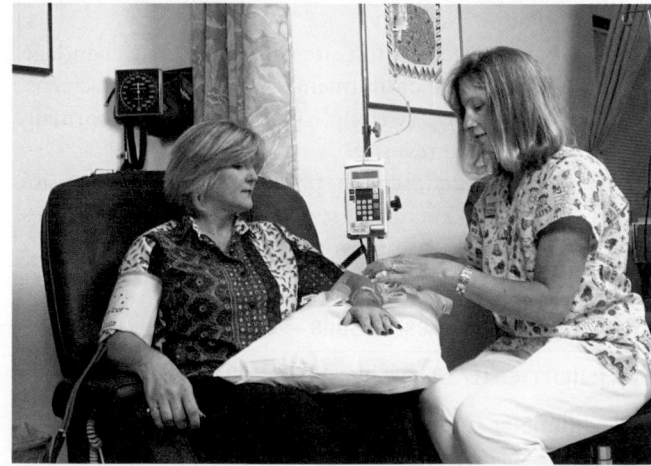

Figure 26-31 Patient receiving IV therapy in an outpatient setting.

cost-effective to keep the patient in the hospital. If the patient is medically stable, he or she may no longer need the careful observation and daily nursing care provided by a hospital. By receiving IV therapy in an outpatient setting, the patient can be discharged earlier. Most patients,

CHAPTER 26 Administration of Medication and Intravenous Therapy **615**

particularly children, are more comfortable in their home environment, which often contributes to faster healing. An example of this is a hospitalized patient with an infection who still needs IV antibiotic therapy but no longer needs to be hospitalized, and receives the therapy at an infusion clinic.

Avoidance of Hospitalization

Outpatient IV therapy provides an alternative to patients with an acute or chronic illness that requires IV therapy. Patients who do not require hospitalization for their condition are able to obtain their IV therapy in an outpatient setting. This allows patients the option of being able to continue their daily routine without major interruptions and provides them with greater independence and control over their condition. An example of this is a patient with rheumatoid arthritis who needs IV infliximab (Remicade) therapy and receives that therapy at the rheumatology medical office.

Medical Office–Based Intravenous Therapy

Some medical offices provide outpatient IV therapy. Outpatient IV therapy may be provided in an oncology office for the administration of IV chemotherapy. With the advent of newer rheumatology medications that must be given intravenously, some rheumatology offices have started to provide this service. There are distinct advantages to medical office–based IV therapy. It allows the physician to provide closer monitoring of a patient's response to the IV therapy and any adverse reactions exhibited by the patient. These benefits have prompted more physicians to consider office-based IV therapy.

Based on the potential future growth of IV therapy in the medical office and the current growth of other IV outpatient settings, such as infusion clinics and the patient's home, there is a need for medical assistants to acquire some basic knowledge in IV therapy. The medical assistant is often responsible for scheduling IV therapy and providing the patient with IV therapy instructions and information, such as the length of time required for the therapy. In addition, patients may have questions that the medical assistant may need to answer (or refer to the proper individual for answering) regarding their outpatient IV therapy. The entry-level medical assistant should be familiar with the basic theory of outpatient IV therapy, which is presented here.

Advanced IV theory and initiating, maintaining, and discontinuing IV therapy are not entry-level medical assisting competencies and are not addressed in this text. Certain requirements must be met before the medical assistant can perform IV therapy in the medical office. The medical assistant first should check the laws of his or her state to determine whether it is legally permissible for the medical assistant to perform this procedure. The medical assistant must

acquire the proper training (theory and skills) by completing a recognized IV therapy training program, including supervised clinical practice. Although the IV procedure can appear simple when performed by an expert, it is a difficult skill that requires considerable practice to perfect.

Indications for Outpatient Intravenous Therapy

Outpatient IV therapy has been shown to be a safe and effective alternative to inpatient IV therapy for the treatment of certain conditions. Before prescribing outpatient IV therapy, the physician assesses the need for the therapy by determining whether the following criteria are met: The patient's condition warrants the use of IV therapy, no alternative routes are feasible or appropriate to deliver the therapy, and the patient does not need to be hospitalized to receive the IV therapy. After determining the need for outpatient IV therapy, the physician prescribes the appropriate medication or fluid and treatment plan, orders laboratory tests to monitor the patient's progress, and assesses the patient after the IV therapy.

Scheduling the IV Therapy

If the patient receives the IV therapy at an outpatient site other than the medical office (e.g., an infusion clinic), the medical assistant may be responsible for scheduling the necessary services and providing the patient with IV therapy instructions, such as the length of time required for the therapy, any dietary restrictions, whether to wear loose-fitting comfortable clothing, and whether someone needs to transport the patient to and from the appointment.

Medical Office Guidelines

Medical offices that provide IV therapy on-site usually set up a special room to deliver the therapy, which often includes a lounge chair to provide for patient comfort during the therapy. With office-based IV therapy, the entry-level medical assistant is responsible for scheduling the IV therapy and providing the patient with the IV therapy instructions listed previously. The medical office employs an IV practitioner, such as a nurse or a specially trained medical assistant, to initiate, maintain, and discontinue the IV therapy. This practitioner must be completely familiar with all aspects of the IV therapy, including indications and uses, actions, dose and rate of infusion, incompatibilities, contraindications and precautions, antidote, and adverse effects. During the IV therapy, the practitioner must monitor carefully the patient's response to the therapy and be alert for adverse or allergic reactions. After the therapy is completed, the IV practitioner provides the patient with follow-up instructions, such as information on normal side effects that may occur when the patient returns home and any adverse reactions that need to be reported to the medical office.

MEDICAL PRACTICE and the LAW

Medications have the potential to do great good and great harm. Many lawsuits are medication related, so the medical assistant has a tremendous responsibility to follow all procedures to avoid doing harm.

Many patients are prescribed multiple medications from various physicians. When performing a medication evaluation, ask the patient to bring in all medications he or she is currently taking. Include over-the-counter medications such as aspirin, vitamins, and herbal products.

When administering medications, first check a current medication reference to determine potential adverse effects. See the *Physician's Desk Reference* or package insert for this information. This information also may be available on a computer program. Next check for patient allergies. Check the chart, then ask the patient about allergies before administering the medication. Be sure the

patient knows why the drug is being given, its name, and common side effects. Watch the patient take the drug if given orally. If given parenterally, use proper technique to prevent injury. Follow the seven "rights" of medication administration, and check the medication label three times before administering any medication. This all may seem cumbersome, but if any steps are omitted and the patient has a serious adverse reaction, you could be held liable.

Controlled drugs have specific laws that regulate their ordering, storing, and dispensing. Failure to adhere to these regulations could cause the physician to lose his or her license. Be aware of drug-seeking behaviors of patients and physical symptoms of addiction. You also have a duty to be aware of co-workers' behavior and to report to the physician any individual who appears chemically impaired or whom you suspect of diverting medications for personal use. ■

What Would You Do? What Would You *Not* Do?   RESPONSES

Case Study 1
Page 555

What Did Theresa Do?
❏ Asked Mrs. Okasinski what pharmacy she uses. Called the pharmacy and asked them to fax a copy of her medications to the medical office. Used the information from the pharmacy and the Product Identification section of the PDR to identify Mrs. Okasinski's medications.
❏ Wrote the names of her medications in her chart for the physician to review.
❏ Explained to Mrs. Okasinski that when she has her prescriptions filled, she should request nonchildproof containers so that she will be able to use the original containers, which have the name and prescription information on them. This will make it easier to tell her medications apart.
❏ After the physician was finished with Mrs. Okasinski, made a list of all the medications she would be taking based on the physician's order. Went over each medication with Mrs. Okasinski, and gave her a copy of the medication list to keep as a reference.

What Did Theresa Not Do?
❏ Did not criticize Mrs. Okasinski for taking her medications out of their original containers.

What Would You Do?/What Would You Not Do?
Review Theresa's response and place a checkmark next to the information you included in your response. List additional information you included in your response.

_____
_____
_____
_____

Case Study 2
Page 577

What Did Theresa Do?
❏ Explained to Mrs. Cardwell that for the infection to be completely eliminated from Rachel's body, she needed to be given all of the medication.
❏ Stressed to Mrs. Cardwell that medication prescribed to one person should never be given to someone else because it might cause him or her to have a bad reaction.
❏ Explained to Mrs. Cardwell that if side effects of medication ever occur, it is important to call the medical office for information on what to do.
❏ Told Mrs. Cardwell that Rachel needs to be seen by the doctor again and scheduled an appointment for her. Asked if any other family members needed an appointment with the doctor.

What Did Theresa Not Do?
❏ Did not tell Mrs. Cardwell that she should have known better than to give Rachel's antibiotic to the other family members.

What Would You Do?/What Would You Not Do?
Review Theresa's response and place a checkmark next to the information you included in your response. List additional information you included in your response.

_____
_____
_____
_____
_____

Case Study 3
Page 590

What Did Theresa Do?
❐ Explained to Danielle that if the injection were given in her arm, it would not be absorbed very well and she might not get better.
❐ Explained to Danielle that injections are given to patients every day at the office and that Danielle does not need to be embarrassed.
❐ Told Danielle that she would be draped extra well and that it would only take a minute to give the injection.

What Did Theresa Not Do?
❐ Did not disregard Danielle's concerns.
❐ Did not give the injection in the deltoid.

What Would You Do?/What Would You Not *Do?*
Review Theresa's response and place a checkmark next to the information you included in your response. List additional information you included in your response.

_____
_____
_____
_____
_____

TERMINOLOGY REVIEW

Medical Term	Word Parts	Definition
Adverse reaction		An unintended and undesirable effect produced by a drug.
Allergen		A substance that is capable of causing an allergic reaction.
Allergy		An abnormal hypersensitivity of the body to substances that are ordinarily harmless.
Ampule		A small sealed glass container that holds a single dose of medication.
Anaphylactic reaction		A serious allergic reaction that requires immediate treatment.
Autoimmune disease	*auto-:* self	A condition in which the body's immune system produces antibodies that attack the body's own cells. The cause is unknown.
Chemotherapy	*chem/o-:* chemical *-therapy:* treatment	The use of chemicals to treat disease. Chemotherapy is most often used to refer to the treatment of cancer using antineoplastic medications.
Controlled drug		A drug that has restrictions placed on it by the federal government because of its potential for abuse.
Conversion		Changing from one system of measurement to another.
Cubic centimeter		The amount of space occupied by 1 milliliter (1 mL = 1 cc).
DEA number		A registration number assigned to physicians by the Drug Enforcement Administration for prescribing or dispensing controlled drugs.
Dose		The quantity of a drug to be administered at one time.
Drug		A chemical used for the treatment, prevention, or diagnosis of disease.
Enteral nutrition	*enter/o-:* intestines *-al:* pertaining to	The delivery of nutrients through a tube inserted into the gastrointestinal tract.
Gauge		The diameter of the lumen of a needle used to administer medication.
Hemophilia	*hem/o-:* blood *-philia:* love	An inherited bleeding disorder caused by a deficiency of a clotting factor needed for proper coagulation of the blood.
Immune globulin		A blood product consisting of pooled human plasma containing antibodies.
Induration		An abnormally raised, hardened area of the skin with clearly defined margins.
Infusion		The administration of fluids, medications, or nutrients into a vein.
Inhalation administration		The administration of medication by way of air or other vapor being drawn into the lungs.
Inscription		The part of a prescription that indicates the name of the drug and the drug dosage.
Intradermal injection	*intra-:* within *derm/o:* skin *-al:* pertaining to	Introduction of medication into the dermal layer of the skin.
Intramuscular injection	*intra-:* within *muscul/o:* muscle *-ar:* pertaining to	Introduction of medication into the muscular layer of the body.
Intravenous (IV) therapy	*intra-:* within *ven/o:* vein *-ous:* pertaining to	The administration of a liquid agent directly into a patient's vein, where it is distributed throughout the body by way of the circulatory system.

Continued

TERMINOLOGY REVIEW—cont'd

Medical Term	Word Parts	Definition
Oral administration		Administration of medication by mouth.
Parenteral		Administration of medication by injection.
Pharmacology	*pharmac/o-:* drugs *-ology:* study of	The study of drugs.
Prescription		A physician's order authorizing the dispensing of a drug by a pharmacist.
Signatura		The part of a prescription that indicates the information to print on the medication label.
Subcutaneous injection	*sub-:* under, below *cutane/o:* skin *-ous:* pertaining to	Introduction of medication beneath the skin, into the subcutaneous or fatty layer of the body.
Sublingual administration	*sub-:* under, below *lingu/o:* tongue *-al:* pertaining to	Administration of medication by placing it under the tongue, where it dissolves and is absorbed through the mucous membrane.
Subscription	*sub-:* under, below	The part of the prescription that gives directions to the pharmacist and usually designates the number of doses to be dispensed.
Superscription	*super-:* over, above	The part of a prescription consisting of the symbol Rx (from the Latin word recipe, meaning "take").
Topical administration		Application of a drug to a particular spot, usually for a local action.
Transfusion	*trans-:* through, across	The administration of whole blood or blood products through the intravenous route.
Vial		A closed glass container with a rubber stopper that holds medication.
Wheal		A tense, pale, raised area of the skin.

ON THE WEB

For information on pharmacology:

Food and Drug Administration: www.fda.gov

Drug Enforcement Administration: www.usdoj.gov/dea

RxList: The Internet Drug Index: www.rxlist.com

Drug Topics: www.drugtopics.com

Medline Plus: www.medlineplus.gov

Health Square: www.healthsquare.com

For information on alcohol and drug abuse:

Alcoholics Anonymous (AA): www.aa.org

National Institute on Alcohol Abuse and Alcoholism (NIAAA): www.niaaa.nih.gov

National Council on Alcoholism and Drug Dependence (NCADD): www.ncadd.org

National Institute on Drug Abuse: www.nida.nih.gov

National Clearinghouse for Alcohol and Drug Information: http://ncadi.samhsa.gov

Substance Abuse and Mental Health Services Administration: www.samhsa.gov

Partnership for a Drug Free America: www.drugfree.org

Institute for a Drug-Free Workplace: www.drugfreeworkplace.org

Al-Anon/Alateen: www.al-anon.alateen.org

Mothers Against Drunk Driving (MADD): www.madd.org

For information on tuberculosis:

American Lung Association: www.lungusa.org

American Thoracic Society: www.thoracic.org

National Center for TB Prevention: www.cdc.gov/nchstp/tb

For information on allergies:

American Academy of Allergy, Asthma, and Immunology: www.aaaai.org

National Institute of Allergy and Infectious Diseases (NIAID): www3.niaid.nih.gov

Asthma and Allergy Foundation of America: www.aafa.org

 Check out the Evolve site at http://evolve.elsevier.com/Bonewit/today/ to actively Prepare for your Certification, and to access additional interactive activities and exercises to help you study and prepare for success.

27

Cardiopulmonary Procedures

LEARNING OBJECTIVES

Peak Flow Measurement
15. Identify the symptoms of an asthma attack.
16. List examples of asthma triggers.
17. Explain the difference between long-term control and quick-relief asthma medications.
18. Describe the purpose of a peak flow meter.

Home Oxygen Therapy
19. Explain why oxygen is needed by the body.
20. Describe what occurs when the body cannot maintain an adequate blood oxygen level.
21. Identify the conditions that may require home oxygen therapy.
22. List and describe the three common types of oxygen delivery systems.
23. List and describe the two types of devices used to administer home oxygen therapy.
24. Describe oxygen safety guidelines.

PROCEDURES

Measure a patient's peak flow rate.

CHAPTER OUTLINE

INTRODUCTION TO ELECTROCARDIOGRAPHY
Cardiac Cycle
Waves
Baseline, Segments, and Intervals
Electrocardiograph Paper
Standardization of the Electrocardiograph
Electrocardiograph Leads
Electrodes
Bipolar Leads
Augmented Leads
Chest Leads
Paper Speed
Patient Preparation
Maintenance of the Electrocardiograph
Electrocardiographic Capabilities
Three-Channel Recording Capability
Teletransmission
Interpretive Electrocardiograph
EMR Connectivity
Artifacts
Muscle Artifact

Wandering Baseline Artifact
60-Cycle Interference Artifact
Interrupted Baseline Artifact
Holter Monitor Electrocardiography
Purpose
Digital Holter Monitor
Evaluating Results
Cardiac Dysrhythmias
Pulmonary Function Tests
Spirometry
Post-Bronchodilator Spirometry
Peak Flow Measurement
Asthma
Peak Flow Meter
Peak Flow Rate
Home Oxygen Therapy
Oxygen Delivery Systems
Oxygen Administration Devices
Oxygen Safety Guidelines

KEY TERMS

amplitude (AM-pli-tood)
artifact (AR-tih-fakt)
atherosclerosis (ath-roe-skler-OH-sus)
baseline
cardiac cycle
dysrhythmia (dis-RITH-mee-ah)
ECG cycle
electrocardiogram (ee-LEK-troe-KAR-dee-oh-gram) (ECG)

electrocardiograph
   (ee-LEK-troe-KAR-dee-oh-graf)
electrode (ee-LEK-trode)
electrolyte (ee-LEK-troe-lite)
flow rate
hypoxemia
hypoxia
interval (IN-ter-val)
ischemia (is-KEEM-ee-ah)

normal sinus rhythm
oxygen therapy
peak flow rate
segment
spirometer (spih-ROM-ih-ter)
spirometry (spih-ROM-ih-tree)
wheezing

INTRODUCTION TO ELECTROCARDIOGRAPHY

The **electrocardiograph** is an instrument used to record the electrical activity of the heart. The **electrocardiogram (ECG)** is the graphic representation of this activity. The ECG exhibits the amount of electrical activity produced by the heart and the time required for the impulse to travel through the heart.

Cardiovascular disorders can cause abnormal changes to occur on the ECG. Because of this, electrocardiography is used for the following purposes:

- To evaluate the following symptoms: chest pain, shortness of breath, dizziness, or heart palpitations
- To detect an abnormality in the heart's rate or rhythm (**dysrhythmia**)
- To detect the presence of impaired blood flow to the heart muscle (**cardiac ischemia**)
- To help diagnose damage to the heart caused by a myocardial infarction
- To determine the presence of hypertrophy (enlargement) of the heart
- To detect inflammation of the heart muscle (**myocarditis**) or the lining of the heart (**pericarditis**)
- To assess the effect on the heart of digitalis and other cardiac drugs
- To determine the presence of electrolyte disturbances
- To assess the progress of rheumatic fever
- To detect congenital heart defects
- Performed before surgery to assess cardiac risk during surgery
- As part of a complete physical examination

A 12-lead resting ECG cannot detect all cardiovascular disorders nor can it always detect impending heart disease such as a myocardial infarction. An ECG is taken with the patient in a resting state and records only about 10 seconds of the heart's electrical activity. If a patient has a dysrhythmia that occurs intermittently, the abnormal heartbeat may not occur during this brief time period. A patient who experiences angina pectoris does not typically have symptoms while in a resting state, and an ECG run on such a patient may appear normal. Because of this, an ECG must be used in combination with the patient's symptoms, health history, physical examination, and other diagnostic and laboratory tests to obtain a complete assessment of cardiac functioning.

The medical assistant is frequently responsible for recording ECGs in the medical office. The medical assistant must acquire knowledge, and skill must be acquired in the following aspects of electrocardiography: preparation of the patient, operation of the electrocardiograph, identification and elimination of artifacts, and care and maintenance of the electrocardiograph.

Electrocardiographs are available in single-channel and three-channel recording formats. Because most medical offices use a three-channel ECG, the information in this

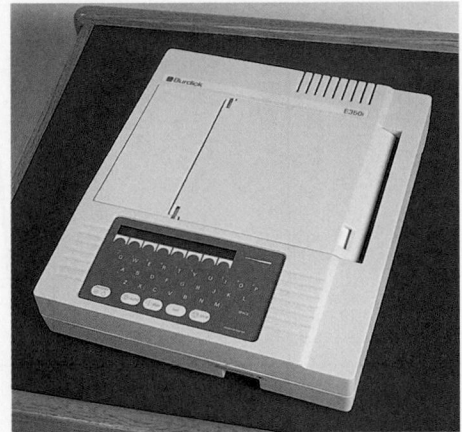

Figure 27-1 A three-channel electrocardiograph.

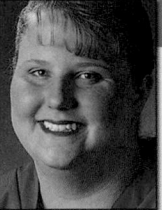

Putting It All into Practice

My name is Janet Canterbury, and I work in the medical laboratory of an internal medicine office. I also run electrocardiograms, apply and remove Holter monitors, perform pulmonary function tests, and assist with cardiac stress testing.

One of my most rewarding experiences was when a young woman came into the office with severe chest pain. I immediately helped her back to an examining room. I ran an electrocardiogram, as ordered by the physician. After the physician read the electrocardiogram, he indicated the results did not look good and that the patient would have to be transported to the hospital. I went into the patient's room to comfort her. She asked me if she was going to have to go to the hospital. I replied, "Possibly." She immediately said, "No!" Then I began to explain to her how important it was to have more tests to make sure she would be alright. She finally agreed to go. After being taken to the hospital by an ambulance, she was later transferred to another hospital for a heart catheterization. A few weeks passed, and she came into the office. She hugged me and thanked me for possibly saving her life. It felt so good that I could help make a difference in a patient's life. ■

chapter focuses on the three-channel electrocardiograph (Figure 27-1).

CARDIAC CYCLE

The **cardiac cycle** represents one complete heartbeat. It consists of the contraction of the atria, the contraction of the ventricles, and the relaxation of the entire heart (as described previously). The electrocardiograph records the electrical activity that causes these events in the cardiac cycle. The **ECG cycle** is the graphic representation of the cardiac cycle (Figure 27-2).

Waves

The normal ECG cycle consists of a P wave; the Q, R, and S waves (known as the *QRS complex*); and a T wave. The

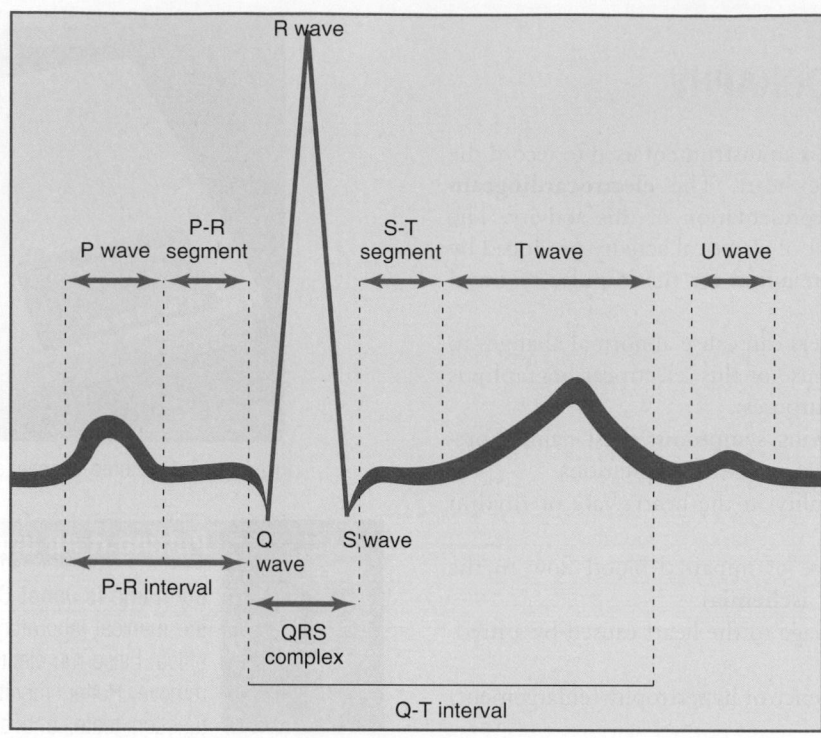

Figure 27-2 ECG cycle.

ECG cycle is recorded from left to right, beginning with the P wave.

P wave The P wave represents the electrical activity associated with the contraction of the atria, or *atrial depolarization.*

QRS complex The QRS complex represents the electrical activity associated with the contraction of the ventricles, or *ventricular depolarization,* and consists of the Q wave, the R wave, and the S wave. The ventricles are larger than the atria and therefore require a stronger electrical stimulus to depolarize the ventricles. That is why the R wave is taller than the P wave on the ECG graph cycle.

T wave The T wave represents the electrical recovery of the ventricles, or *ventricular repolarization.* The muscle cells are recovering in preparation for another impulse. (*NOTE:* Electrical recovery, known as *atrial repolarization,* occurs following the P wave. This repolarization occurs at the same time as ventricular depolarization [QRS complex]. Because of this, atrial repolarization is masked or hidden by the QRS complex and does not appear as a separate wave on the ECG cycle.)

U wave Occasionally, a U wave follows a T wave. It is a small wave that is associated in some as yet undefined way with repolarization of the Purkinje fibers or repolarization of the papillary muscles of the heart.

Baseline, Segments, and Intervals

The flat, horizontal line that separates the various waves is known as the **baseline.** Following the U wave, the heart is at rest or *polarized.* Because no electrical activity is occurring in the heart during this time, the electrocardiograph does not have anything to record, which is why the baseline is flat.

The waves deflect either upward (positive deflection) or downward (negative deflection) from the baseline. The ECG cycle between the P wave and the T wave is divided into segments and intervals for the purpose of interpretation and analysis of the ECG by the physician. A **segment** is the portion of the ECG between two waves, and an **interval** is the length of a wave or the length of a wave with a segment.

Segments

P-R segment The P-R segment represents the time interval from the end of the atrial depolarization to the beginning of the ventricular depolarization. It is the time needed for the impulse to be delayed at the AV node and then travel through the bundle of His and Purkinje fibers to the ventricles.

S-T segment The S-T segment represents the time interval from the end of the ventricular depolarization to the beginning of repolarization of the ventricles.

Intervals

P-R interval The P-R interval represents the time interval from the beginning of the atrial depolarization to the beginning of the ventricular depolarization.

Q-T interval The Q-T interval is the time interval from the beginning of the ventricular depolarization to the end of repolarization of the ventricles.

Baseline The baseline after the T wave (or U wave, if present) represents the period when the entire heart returns to its resting, or polarized, state.

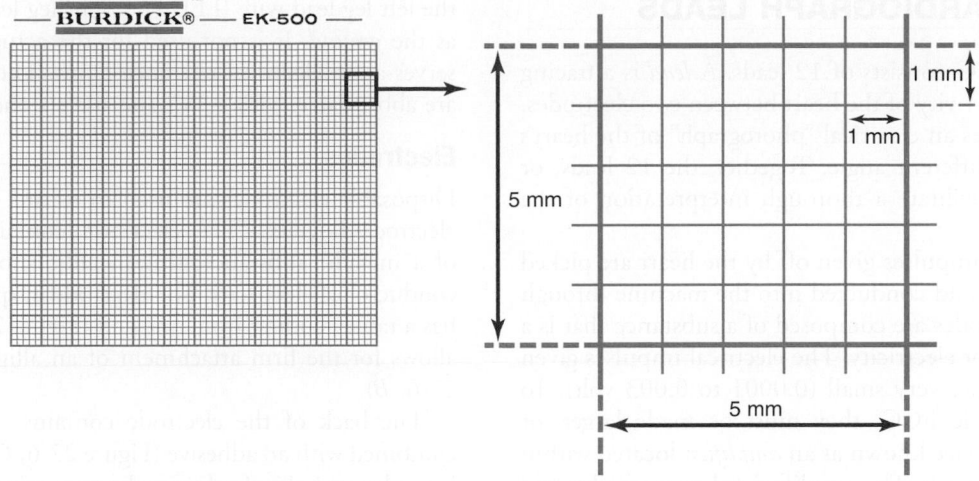

Figure 27-3 Diagram of ECG paper with a section enlarged to indicate the sizes of the large and small squares.

ELECTROCARDIOGRAPH PAPER

Electrocardiograph paper is divided into two sets of squares for the accurate and convenient manual measurement of the waves, intervals, and segments (Figure 27-3). Each small square is 1 mm high and 1 mm wide. Each large square (made up of 25 small squares) is 5 mm high and 5 mm wide. By manually measuring the various waves, intervals, and segments of the ECG graph cycle with ECG calipers or an ECG ruler, the physician is able to determine whether the electrical activity of the heart falls within normal limits. Heart disease can trigger abnormal changes in the ECG cycle, causing the results to fall outside of normal limits. For example, cardiac ischemia (often due to coronary artery disease) can cause a depressed S-T segment and an inverted T wave. A myocardial infarction can cause a larger than normal Q wave and an elevated S-T segment.

Electrocardiograph paper contains a thermosensitive coating. A black or red graph is printed on top of this coating. The electrocardiograph uses a thermal print head to produce the ECG tracing. The print head has the ability to generate heat in a prescribed pattern. When the thermosensitive paper comes in contact with the heated print head, the coating turns black in the areas where it is heated, producing the ECG tracing. In addition to being heat sensitive, ECG paper is pressure sensitive and should be handled carefully to avoid making impressions that would interfere with proper reading of the ECG.

STANDARDIZATION OF THE ELECTROCARDIOGRAPH

The electrocardiograph machine must be standardized, or calibrated, when an ECG is recorded. This is a quality control measure that ensures an accurate and reliable recording. It also means that an ECG run on one electrocardiograph compares in accuracy with a recording run on another machine. An ECG run on a properly calibrated

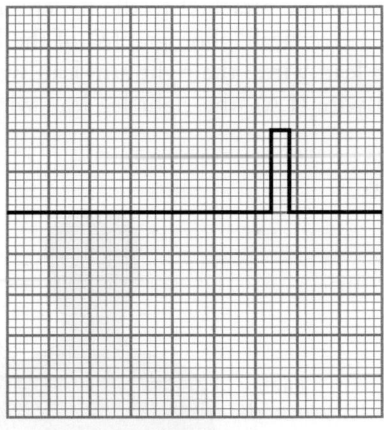

Normal Standard
Standardization mark is
10 mm high

Figure 27-4 Standardization mark.

electrocardiograph results in an accurate and reliable representation of the electrical activity of the patient's heart.

By international agreement, 1 millivolt (mV) of electricity should cause the stylus to move 10 mm high in **amplitude** (10 small squares). During the recording, the machine allows 1 mV to enter the electrocardiograph machine, which should result in an upward deflection of 10 mm. The marking that occurs on the ECG paper is known as a *standardization mark* (Figure 27-4). The width of the mark made by the machine is approximately 2 mm (two small squares). A three-channel electrocardiograph automatically records standardization marks on the ECG; a standardization mark is recorded at the beginning and end of each of the ECG strips included in the three-channel recording (see Figure 27-9). If the standardization mark is more or less than 10 mm in amplitude, it must be adjusted; otherwise, the ECG recording may not be accurate. The manufacturer's operating manual must be consulted for proper adjustment information. An electrocardiograph must never be adjusted without use of the operating manual.

ELECTROCARDIOGRAPH LEADS

The standard ECG consists of 12 leads. A *lead* is a tracing of the electrical activity of the heart between two electrodes. Each lead provides an electrical "photograph" of the heart's activity from a different angle. Together, the 12 leads, or "photographs," facilitate a thorough interpretation of the heart's activity.

The electrical impulses given off by the heart are picked up by **electrodes** and conducted into the machine through lead wires. Electrodes are composed of a substance that is a good conductor of electricity. The electrical impulses given off by the heart are very small (0.0001 to 0.003 volt). To produce a readable ECG, they must be made larger, or amplified, by a device known as an *amplifier,* located within the electrocardiograph. The amplified voltages are changed into mechanical motion by the *galvanometer* and recorded on the electrocardiograph paper by a thermal print head (Figure 27-5).

Ten lead wires are attached to the patient and are used to take the 12 electrical "photographs" of the heart. There are four limb lead wires: the right arm lead wire (RA), the left arm lead wire (LA), the right leg lead wire (RL), and the left leg lead wire (LL). The right leg lead wire is known as the *ground.* It is not used for the actual recording, but serves as an electrical reference point. The chest lead wires are abbreviated with a "V" and use six chest lead wires.

Electrodes

Disposable electrodes are used to record a resting 12-lead electrocardiogram. The electrode contains a thin layer of a metallic substance; this metallic substance is a good conductor of electricity. The electrode is square in shape and has a tab extending from one end (Figure 27-6, *A*). The tab allows for the firm attachment of an alligator clip (Figure 27-6, *B*).

The back of the electrode contains an electrolyte gel combined with an adhesive (Figure 27-6, *C*). An **electrolyte** is a substance that facilitates the transmission of the heart's electrical impulse. Skin is a poor conductor of electricity; therefore, an electrolyte must be used when recording an ECG. The adhesive allows for firm adherence of the electrode to the patient's skin. There is no adhesive on the tab of the electrode to allow for attachment of the alligator clip. The electrode is applied to the skin and held in place with its adhesive backing; it is thrown away after use.

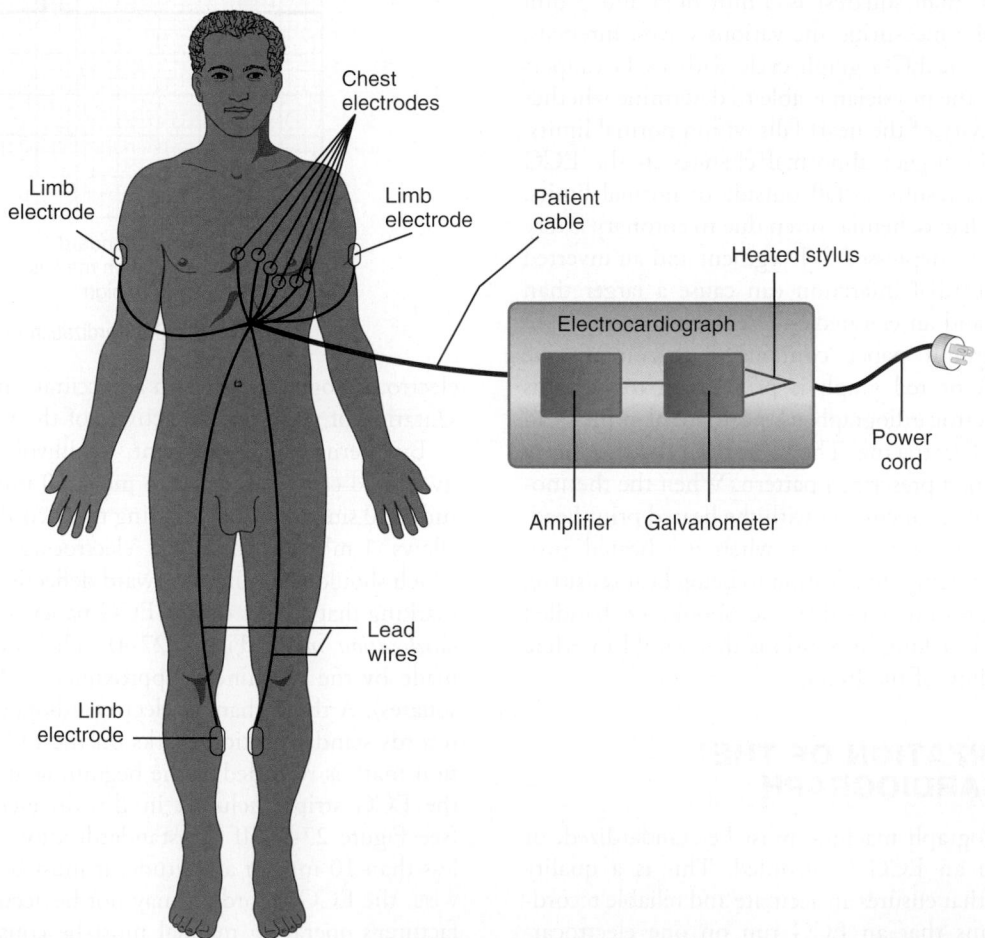

Figure 27-5 Diagram of the basic components of the electrocardiograph. The limb electrodes are attached to the fleshy parts of the limbs, and the lead wires are arranged to follow body contour. The patient cable is not dangling, and the power cord points away from the electrocardiograph.

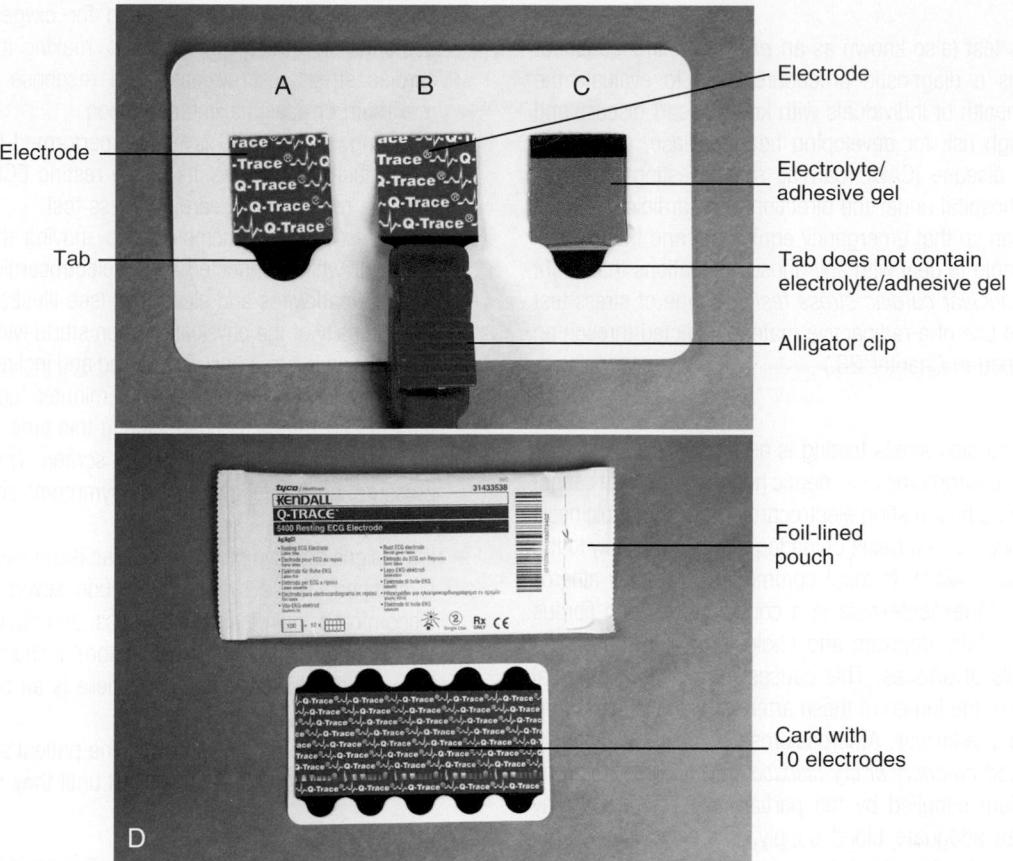

Figure 27-6 Resting 12-lead ECG electrodes. **A,** Disposable resting 12-lead electrode. **B,** The tab allows for attachment of the alligator clip. **C,** The back of the electrode contains an electrolyte gel combined with an adhesive. **D,** Disposable 12-lead electrodes are packaged in a foil-lined pouch and come on a card that contains 10 electrodes.

Disposable 12-lead electrodes come on a card containing 10 electrodes (Figure 27-6, *D*). A foil-lined pouch is used to hold 10 cards of electrodes (or 100 electrodes per pouch). The foil-lined pouch preserves moisture to prevent the electrolyte from drying out.

Each electrode pouch (and the box containing the pouches) is stamped with an expiration date. The medical assistant must always check the expiration date of the electrodes before applying them. The electrolyte gel on outdated electrodes may be dried out; a dried out electrolyte is unable to transmit a good ECG signal.

Electrodes are sensitive to environmental conditions and must be stored properly to prevent electrolyte drying. Electrodes should be stored in a cool area (less than 75° F or 24° C) away from sources of heat. When an electrode pouch is opened, the medical assistant should seal the pouch by folding over the end of it and then place the pouch (containing the remaining electrode cards) in a zipper-lock plastic bag to preserve moisture.

Bipolar Leads

The first three leads of the 12-lead ECG are the bipolar leads; they are leads I, II, and III. The bipolar leads use two of the limb electrodes to record the heart's electrical activity. Lead I records the electrical current traveling between the right arm and the left arm, lead II records the electrical current traveling between the right arm and the left leg, and lead III records the electrical current traveling between the left arm and the left leg (Figure 27-7).

Lead II shows the heart's rhythm more clearly than the other leads. Because of this, the physician often requests a *rhythm strip,* which is a longer recording (approximately 12 inches) of lead II (see Figure 27-9).

AUGMENTED LEADS

The next three leads are the augmented leads: aVR (augmented voltage—right arm), aVL (augmented voltage—left arm), and aVF (augmented voltage—left leg or foot). Lead aVR records the electrical current traveling between the right arm electrode and a central point between the left arm and left leg. Lead aVL records the electrical current traveling between the left arm electrode and a central point between the right arm and left leg. Lead aVF records the electrical current traveling between the left leg electrode and a central point between the right and left arms. Leads I, II, III, aVR, aVL, and aVF provide an electrical "photograph" of the heart's activity from side to side and from the top to the bottom of the heart (see Figure 27-7).

Highlight on Cardiac Stress Testing

Description

A cardiac stress test (also known as an *exercise tolerance test* or *exercise ECG*) is a diagnostic procedure used to evaluate the cardiovascular health of individuals with known heart disease and individuals at high risk for developing heart disease, particularly coronary artery disease (CAD). Cardiac stress testing is usually performed in a hospital under the direction of a cardiologist and a cardiac technician so that emergency equipment and trained personnel are available to deal with any unusual situations that might arise. (NOTE: A *nuclear cardiac stress test* is a type of stress test that employs the use of a radioactive material injected through an IV and is described in Chapter 28.)

Purpose

The purpose of cardiac stress testing is as follows:

1. To evaluate symptoms of ischemic heart disease that cannot be assessed by a resting electrocardiogram. Ischemic heart disease occurs as a result of inadequate blood supply to the myocardium, which is most commonly caused by atherosclerosis. **Atherosclerosis** is a condition in which fibrous plaques of fatty deposits and cholesterol build up on the inner walls of arteries. This causes narrowing and partial blockage of the lumen of these arteries, along with hardening of the arterial wall. Atherosclerosis in the coronary arteries is called *coronary artery disease (CAD)*. During rest, the myocardium supplied by the partially blocked artery may receive an adequate blood supply. If the individual exercises, however, the artery may not be able to supply enough blood to the myocardium, resulting in myocardial ischemia. Myocardial ischemia can cause chest discomfort and certain abnormal changes on the ECG.
2. To assist in evaluating symptoms indicating the presence of cardiac dysrhythmias.
3. To assess the effectiveness of cardiac drug therapy.
4. To follow the course of rehabilitation after a myocardial infarction or a cardiac surgical procedure, such as a coronary bypass operation or a coronary stent placement.
5. To determine an individual's fitness level for a strenuous exercise program, such as jogging.

Patient Preparation

Patient preparation for a cardiac stress test includes the following:

1. Refrain from smoking for 4 hours before the test.
2. Avoid strenuous physical activities for 8 to 12 hours before the test.
3. Do not consume alcohol or food and beverages containing caffeine for 12 hours before the test. These substances may interfere with obtaining accurate results.
4. Do not eat or drink anything except water for 4 hours before the test. This reduces the likelihood of nausea that may accompany strenuous activity after a meal.
5. Certain cardiac medications may need to be discontinued 1 to 2 days before the test; this determination is made by the physician.
6. Wear loose, comfortable clothing and sports shoes suitable for exercising.

How the Test Works

- Cardiac stress testing involves the continuous electrocardiographic monitoring of an individual during physical exercise.

During exercise, the body's need for oxygen places added demands or "stress" on the heart, making it work harder. A cardiac stress test evaluates the response of the heart to maximum or near-maximum exertion.

- A resting 12-lead ECG is usually performed before a cardiac stress test, and the results of the resting ECG are compared with the results of the cardiac stress test.
- The stress test is accomplished by having the patient use a treadmill while connected to an electrocardiograph machine through lead wires and electrodes (see illustration).
- The intensity of the physical exertion starts with a slow "warm-up" walk on the treadmill. The speed and incline of the treadmill are gradually increased every 3 minutes until the patient's target heart rate is reached. During this time, the ECG is continuously displayed on a computer screen. The patient's blood pressure, heart rate, and physical symptoms are also monitored during the test.
- If the signs and symptoms of cardiac ischemia appear, the test is stopped. These symptoms include severe dyspnea, chest discomfort or pain, pallor, weakness, and dizziness. The test is also stopped if the ECG shows abnormal changes, if a serious, irregular heartbeat occurs, or if there is an abnormal change in blood pressure.
- Once the exercising is complete, the patient's blood pressure, heart rate, and ECG are monitored until they return to normal.

Interpretation of Results

The patient's response to the cardiac stress test is used to determine normal or abnormal results. A normal response is a gradual increase in the patient's blood pressure as physical exertion increases, whereas an abnormal response is a sudden increase or decrease in the patient's blood pressure. The electrocardiogram of a normal individual undergoing exercise exhibits a shortened P-R interval and a compressed QRS complex. An abnormal tracing indicative of myocardial ischemia results in a depressed S-T segment and an inverted T wave. An abnormal cardiac stress test usually warrants further testing, such as coronary angiography, to assess the extent and severity of the heart disease. ∎

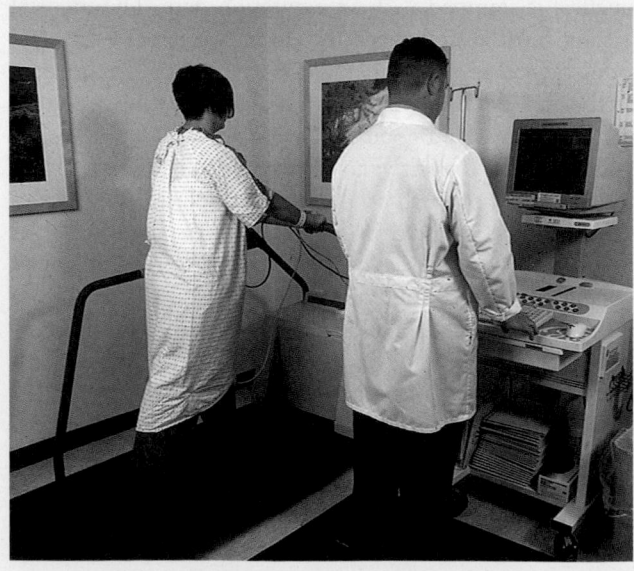

Cardiac treadmill stress test.

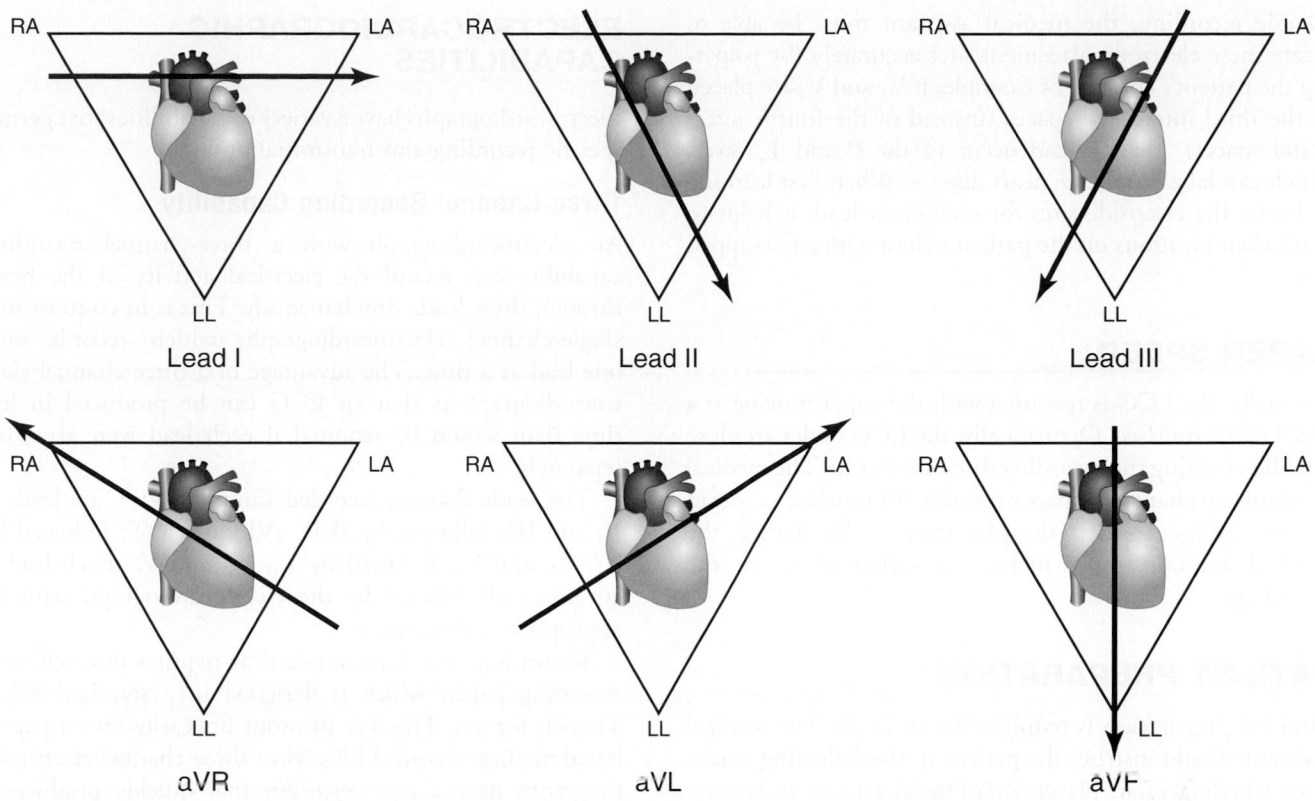

Figure 27-7 Diagram of the heart's voltage for leads I, II, III, aVR, aVL, and aVF.

Chest Leads

The last six leads are the chest, or precordial, leads: V_1, V_2, V_3, V_4, V_5, and V_6. These leads record the heart's voltage from front to back. The electrical current traveling through the heart is recorded from a central point "inside" the heart to a point on the chest wall where the electrode is placed. These points correspond to the chest electrode placement sites. Figure 27-8 shows the proper location of the electrodes for the six chest leads. To ensure an accurate and

What Would You Do? What Would You *Not* Do?

Case Study 1

Camilla Rossi is 22 years old and works at a Waffle House during the day and goes to business school at night. She comes to the office because she has been experiencing some heart problems. Over the past month, she has had three episodes of tachycardia, palpitations, trouble breathing, and profuse sweating. She is really scared that she has heart disease. Her grandfather just died from a heart attack, and she is afraid she will die next. The physician orders an ECG, but Camilla is reluctant to have the procedure. She is embarrassed about having to disrobe from the waist up, and she is worried that she will get shocked by all the wires coming out of the machine. She says that she does not have health insurance, and she does not know how she would pay for such a fancy test. She wants to know whether there is a less expensive way to find out what is wrong with her. ■

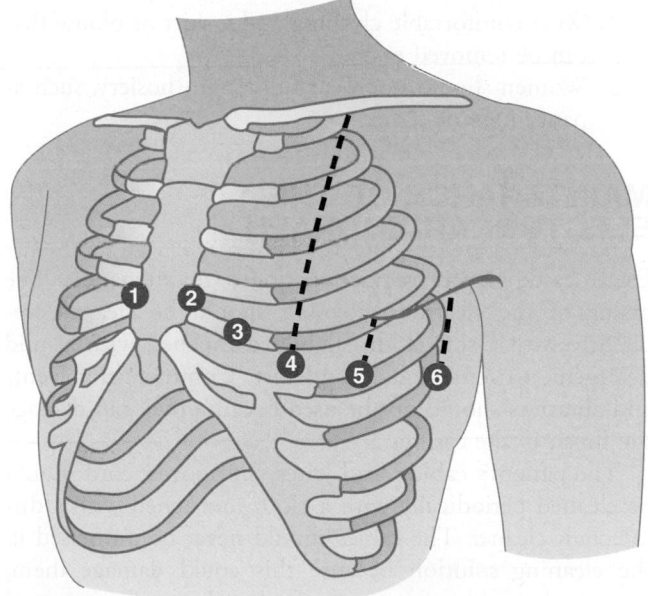

Figure 27-8 Recommended positions for ECG chest electrodes:
1. V_1, fourth intercostal space at right margin of sternum
2. V_2, fourth intercostal space at left margin of sternum
3. V_3, midway between positions 2 and 4
4. V_4, fifth intercostal space at junction of left midclavicular line
5. V_5, at horizontal level of position 4 at left anterior axillary line
6. V_6, at horizontal level of position 4 at left midaxillary line

reliable recording, the medical assistant must be able to locate these electrode placement sites accurately (by palpating the patient's chest). For example, if V_1 and V_2 are placed in the third intercostal spaces (instead of the fourth intercostal spaces), changes can occur to the P and T waves, which can falsely indicate heart disease. When first learning to locate the electrode sites for each chest lead, it helps to mark their locations on the patient's chest with a felt-tipped pen.

PAPER SPEED

Normally, the ECG is recorded with the paper moving at a speed of 25 mm/sec. Occasionally, the ECG cycles are close together, making the recording difficult to read. The medical assistant can change the paper speed to 50 mm/sec to spread out the cycles. To alert the physician to the change, the medical assistant must make a notation of it on the recording.

PATIENT PREPARATION

Minimal preparation is required for an ECG. The medical assistant should instruct the patient in the following guidelines, which facilitate placement of the electrodes and ensure good adhesion of the electrodes to the patient's skin.

1. Do not apply body lotion, oil, or powder on the day of the test. This may make it more difficult to apply the electrodes.
2. Wear comfortable clothing and a shirt or blouse that can be removed easily.
3. Women should not wear full-length hosiery, such as panty hose or tights.

MAINTENANCE OF THE ELECTROCARDIOGRAPH

Electrocardiographs require periodic maintenance. The casing of the electrocardiograph should be cleaned frequently with a soft cloth, slightly dampened with a mild detergent, to remove dust and dirt. Commercial solvents and abrasives should not be used because they can damage the finish of the casing.

The patient's cables, lead wires, and power cord should be cleaned periodically with a cloth moistened with a disinfectant cleaner. The cables should never be immersed in the cleaning solution because this could damage them. Inspect the cables frequently for cracks or fraying, and replace them if needed. Check the metal tip of each lead wire for adhesive/electrolyte gel residue, which can interfere with the transmission of a good ECG signal from the electrode. Remove any residue with an alcohol wipe using pressure and friction.

The reusable alligator clips should be cleaned thoroughly with an alcohol wipe after patient use. Check the alligator clips periodically to make sure they fit snugly on the metal tip of each lead wire.

ELECTROCARDIOGRAPHIC CAPABILITIES

Electrocardiographs have a variety of capabilities that permit specific recording and transmittal options.

Three-Channel Recording Capability

An electrocardiograph with a three-channel recording capability can record the electrical activity of the heart through three leads simultaneously. This is in contrast to a single-channel electrocardiograph, which records only one lead at a time. The advantage of a three-channel electrocardiograph is that an ECG can be produced in less time than would be required if each lead were recorded separately.

The leads that are recorded simultaneously are leads I, II, and III; followed by aVR, aVL, and aVF; followed by V_1, V_2, and V_3; followed by V_4, V_5, and V_6. Each lead is automatically labeled by the electrocardiograph with its appropriate abbreviation.

Recording three leads at one time requires three-channel recording paper, which is designed in a standard $8\frac{1}{2} \times$ 11-inch format. This size printout fits easily into a paper-based medical record (PPR). Most three-channel electrocardiographs have a *copy capability* that quickly produces a duplicate copy of an ECG that has just been recorded. Some three-channel electrocardiographs have a memory storage capability in which a specified number of ECGs can be stored in the machine for later retrieval. In this way, an ECG that has been misplaced can be retrieved from the electrocardiograph's memory and printed out again. Figure 27-9 is an example of a three-channel ECG recording that also includes a rhythm strip. Procedure 27-1 describes how to run a 12-lead three-channel ECG.

Teletransmission

An electrocardiograph with teletransmission capabilities can transmit a recording performed at the medical office electronically to an ECG data interpretation site. The recording is interpreted by a cardiologist (often along with a computer analysis) at the interpretation site, and the ECG recording, along with its interpretation, is electronically transmitted to the sending office the same day. Patient information (e.g., age, sex, height, weight, medications) must be relayed to the ECG site to assist in the interpretation. This information is entered into the electrocardiograph by the medical assistant (using a keyboard) and is transmitted automatically with the ECG recording.

Interpretive Electrocardiograph

An electrocardiograph with interpretive capabilities has a built-in computer program that analyzes the recording as it is being run. Interpretive electrocardiographs provide immediate information on the heart's activity, leading to earlier diagnosis and treatment. Patient data are used in the interpretation of the ECG and must be entered into the electrocardiograph using a keyboard before running the

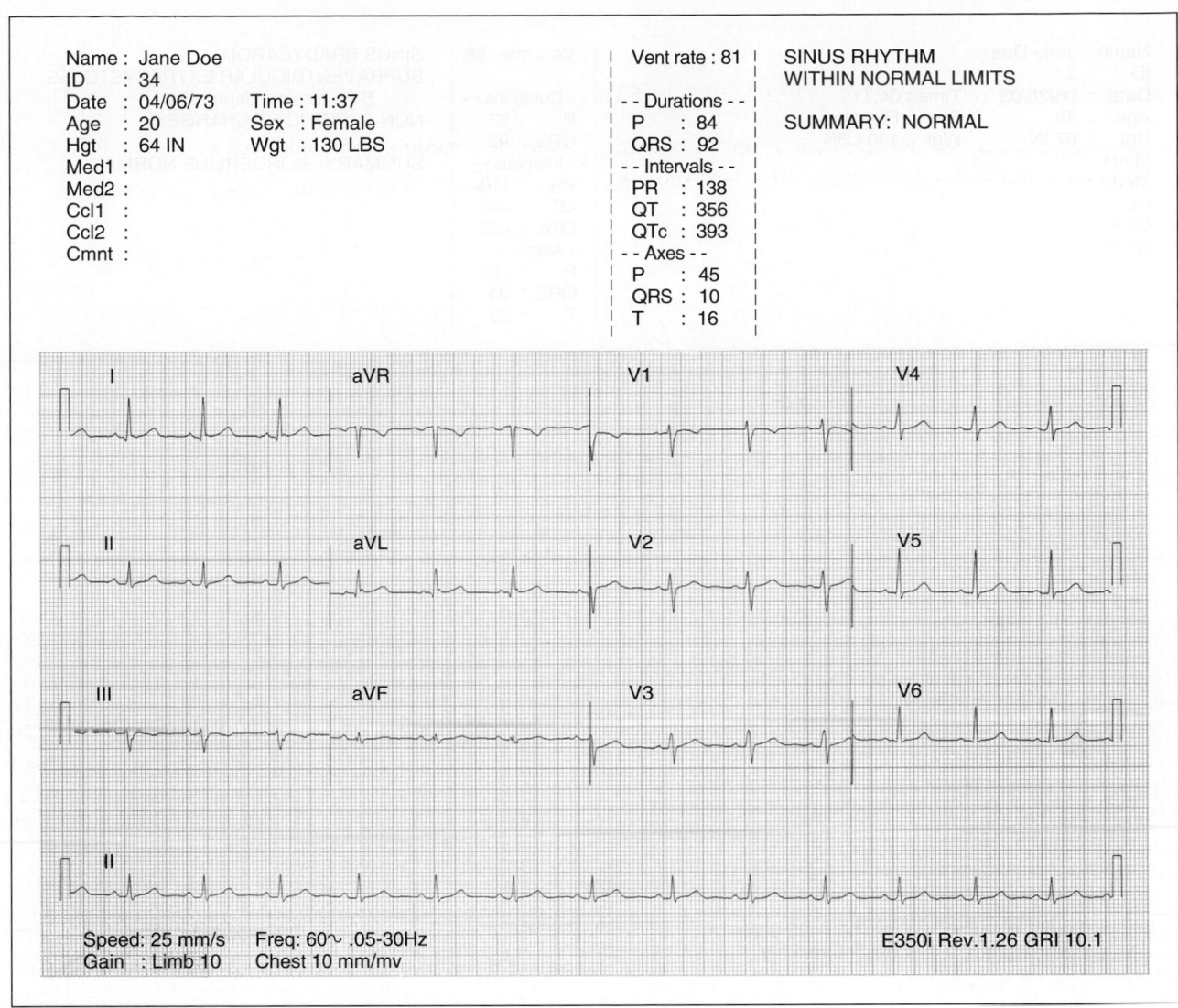

Name : Jane Doe
ID   : 34
Date : 04/06/73   Time : 11:37
Age   : 20   Sex : Female
Hgt   : 64 IN   Wgt : 130 LBS
Med1 :
Med2 :
Ccl1 :
Ccl2 :
Cmnt :

| Vent rate : 81 |
| - - Durations - - |
| P   : 84 |
| QRS : 92 |
| - - Intervals - - |
| PR   : 138 |
| QT   : 356 |
| QTc : 393 |
| - - Axes - - |
| P   : 45 |
| QRS : 10 |
| T   : 16 |

SINUS RHYTHM
WITHIN NORMAL LIMITS

SUMMARY: NORMAL

I   aVR   V1   V4

II   aVL   V2   V5

III   aVF   V3   V6

II

Speed: 25 mm/s   Freq: 60~ .05-30Hz   E350i Rev.1.26 GRI 10.1
Gain : Limb 10   Chest 10 mm/mv

Figure 27-9 A three-channel ECG with a rhythm strip.

recording. The data generally required are the patient's age, sex, height, weight, and medications, which are presented at the top of the recording. The computer analysis of the ECG is also printed at the top of the recording, along with the reason for each interpretation (Figure 27-10). The results are reviewed and interpreted further by the physician before a diagnosis is made and treatment is initiated.

EMR Connectivity

EMR (electronic medical record) connectivity allows the electrocardiograph machine to be linked with the office's computer system, either wirelessly or through a USB port. This enables a digital image of the recording to be sent from the electrocardiograph machine to the computer. EMR software can display the digital image of the ECG on the screen of the computer. The software also analyzes the ECG and displays this information along with the reason for each interpretation. If needed, a copy of the ECG report can be printed out on a regular sheet of paper using an ink-jet or laser printer. The ECG report is reviewed and interpreted further by the physician before a diagnosis is made and treatment is initiated. The ECG report is then stored electronically in the patient's EMR.

ARTIFACTS

The medical assistant is responsible for producing a clear and concise ECG recording that can be read and interpreted by both a computer and the physician. Structures sometimes appear in the recording that are not natural and interfere with the normal appearance of the ECG cycles. They are known as **artifacts** and represent additional electrical activity that is picked up by the electrocardiograph. The presence of artifacts affects the quality of the recording, making it difficult to manually measure the ECG cycles. Artifacts can also sometimes cause a false-positive result on an ECG that is analyzed by a computer. The medical assistant should be able to identify artifacts and correct them.

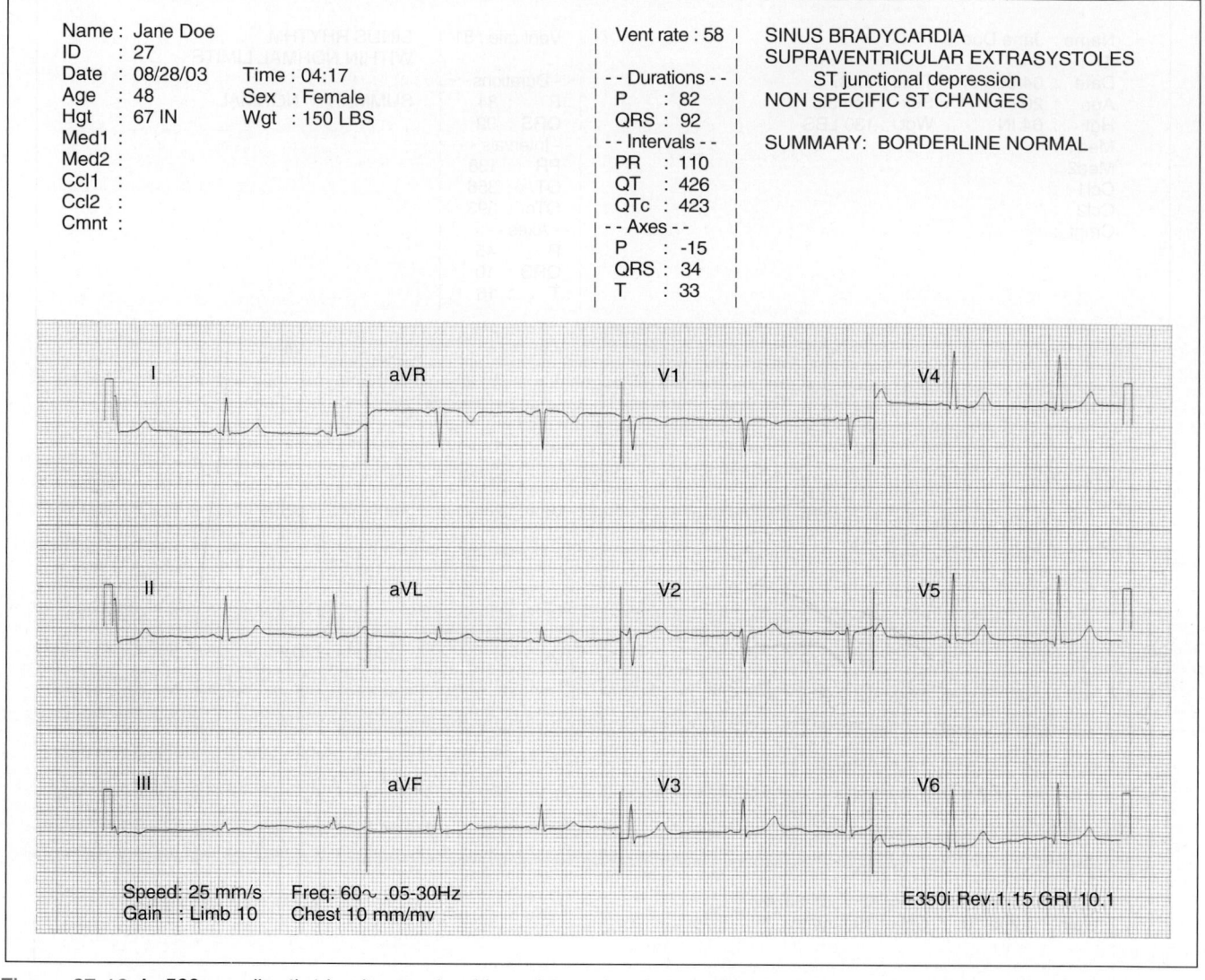

Figure 27-10 An ECG recording that has been analyzed by an interpretive electrocardiograph. The computer analysis is printed at the top of the recording, along with the reason for each interpretation.

There are several types of artifacts; the most common are muscle, wandering baseline, and 60-cycle interference (also known as *AC artifacts*).

In some circumstances, as when individuals have trouble holding still or in buildings with older electrical systems, normal methods to eliminate muscle and 60-cycle interference artifacts may be unsuccessful. Electrocardiographs have an artifact filter that can reduce artifacts when all else fails. Because the *artifact filter* also affects the diagnostic accuracy of the ECG, it should be used as little as possible.

If the medical assistant is unable to correct an artifact, the physician should be consulted. It is possible that the machine is broken. If an electrocardiograph service technician has to be contacted, the medical assistant should have the following information available to aid the service technician in locating the problem:

1. What already has been done to locate and correct the problem

2. Leads in which the artifact occurs
3. A sample of the artifact recorded by the machine

Muscle Artifact

A muscle artifact (Figure 27-11, *A*) can be identified by its fuzzy, irregular baseline. There are two types of muscle artifacts: those caused by involuntary muscle movement (somatic tremor) and those caused by voluntary muscle movement. Muscle artifacts may be caused by the following:

1. **An apprehensive patient.** To reduce the patient's apprehension and relax muscles, explain the procedure and reassure the patient that having an ECG recorded is a painless procedure.
2. **Patient discomfort.** Ensure that the table is wide enough to support the patient's arms and legs adequately. The patient can be made more comfortable by placing a pillow under his or her head. Check that the room temperature is comfortable for the patient. A

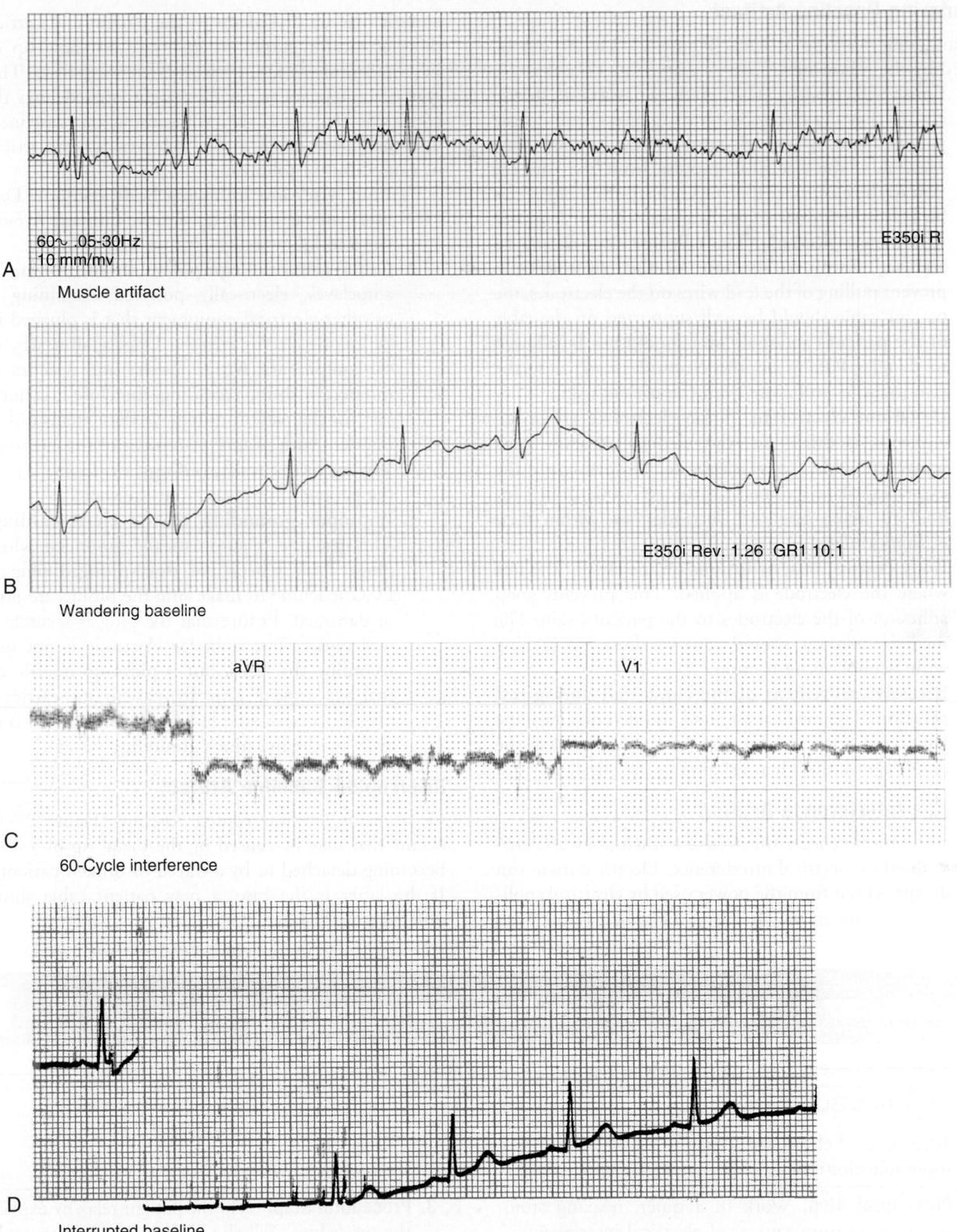

A Muscle artifact

B Wandering baseline

C 60-Cycle interference

D Interrupted baseline

Figure 27-11 Examples of ECG artifacts.

temperature that is warm enough for the medical assistant may be too cold for the patient who has removed clothing. This could result in shivering, which also would produce a muscle artifact on the ECG.

3. **Patient movement.** The patient must be instructed to lie still and not talk during the recording.

4. **A physical condition.** Several nervous system disorders, such as Parkinson disease, prevent relaxation, and the patient trembles continually. For these individuals, it is difficult to obtain an ECG that is free of artifacts. The artifacts can be reduced, however, by asking the patient to place his or her hands under the buttocks with the palms facing downward.

Wandering Baseline Artifact

A wandering baseline artifact (Figure 27-11, *B*) can be caused by the following:

1. **Loose electrodes.** The medical assistant should ensure that the electrodes are attached firmly to the patient's skin. A loose electrode results in poor transmission of the electrical impulse from the patient's skin to the electrode. If an electrode pulls loose, it can be reattached with hypoallergenic tape or replaced with a new electrode. The alligator clips should be attached firmly to the tabs of the electrodes. To prevent pulling of the lead wires on the electrodes, the patient cable should be well supported on the table or the patient's abdomen and should not be allowed to dangle. Pulling on the electrodes can cause the electrodes to pull away from the patient's skin.

2. **Dried-out electrolyte.** If the electrolyte gel on an electrode is dried out, the medical assistant must replace it with a new electrode. Always check the expiration date stamped on the electrode pouch (or box) to make sure the electrodes are within their expiration date.

3. **Body creams, oils, or lotions** on the skin in the area where the electrode is applied. This prevents good adhesion of the electrodes to the patient's skin. The medical assistant should remove these by rubbing with alcohol, using friction.

4. **Excessive movement of the chest wall during respiration.** The medical assistant should encourage the patient to relax and breathe more calmly, using the diaphragm rather than expanding the chest.

60-Cycle Interference Artifact

A 60-cycle interference artifact (also known as an *AC artifact*) is caused by electrical interference. Electric current can "leak" or spread out from the power used by electrical appliances in the room in which the ECG is being run. This current may be picked up by the patient and carried into the electrocardiograph, where it would show up on the ECG recording as a 60-cycle interference artifact. This type of artifact appears as small, straight, spiked lines that are consistent (Figure 27-11, *C*), causing the baseline to be thick and unreadable. A 60-cycle interference artifact can be caused by the following:

1. **Lead wires not following body contour.** Dangling lead wires can pick up electric current. Arrange the wires to follow body contour and to lie flat.

2. **Other electrical equipment in the room.** Lamps, autoclaves, electrically powered examining tables, or other electrical equipment that is plugged in may be leaking electric current. Unplug all nearby electrical equipment. (*NOTE:* Jewelry and watches do not interfere with the recording, therefore it is not necessary for the patient to remove these items unless they interfere with proper placement of the electrodes.)

3. **Wiring in the walls, ceilings, or floors.** Try moving the patient table away from the walls.

4. **Improper grounding of the electrocardiograph.** The machine is automatically grounded when it is plugged in. Check the three-pronged plug of the ECG machine to make sure the prongs are not loose or damaged. Ensure that the plug is securely in the wall outlet. The right leg electrode is not used for recording the leads, but it picks up electric current that has "leaked" onto the patient and carries it into the electrocardiograph. The electric current is carried away by the machine's grounding system.

Interrupted Baseline Artifact

Occasionally, an interrupted baseline (Figure 27-11, *D*) occurs that may be caused by the metal tip of a lead wire becoming detached or by a frayed or broken patient cable. If the latter is the case, a new patient cable should be ordered from the manufacturer.

PROCEDURE **27-1**   Running a 12-Lead, Three-Channel Electrocardiogram

Outcome Record a 12-lead electrocardiogram.

Equipment/Supplies

- Three-channel electrocardiograph
- Disposable electrodes

- ECG paper

1. **Procedural Step.** Work in a quiet, relaxing atmosphere away from sources of electrical interference.

2. **Procedural Step.** Sanitize your hands, and assemble the equipment. Check the expiration date of the electrodes. Greet the patient and introduce yourself. Identify the patient by full name and date of birth.
   Principle. The electrolyte gel on outdated electrodes may be dried out, which can cause artifacts on the ECG.

3. **Procedural Step.** Help the patient relax by explaining the procedure. Tell the patient that having an ECG recording is painless. Explain that he or she must lie still, breathe normally, and not talk while the ECG is being recorded so that an accurate ECG can be obtained.
   Principle. Explaining the procedure helps reassure apprehensive patients. The patient should be mentally and physically relaxed for an accurate ECG recording;

PROCEDURE 27-1   Running a 12-Lead, Three-Channel Electrocardiogram—cont'd

an apprehensive or moving patient produces muscle artifacts. Heavy breathing or sighing can cause a wandering baseline artifact.

4. **Procedural Step.** Prepare the patient. Ask him or her to remove clothing from the waist up. The lower legs also must be uncovered. Provide a female patient with a gown, and instruct her to put it on with the opening in front. Assist the patient into a supine position on the table. The table should support the arms and legs adequately so that they do not dangle. Properly drape the patient to prevent exposure and to provide warmth. A pillow can be used to support the patient's head.

   Principle. The chest, upper arms, and lower legs must be uncovered to allow proper placement of the electrodes. The patient should be kept warm, and the arms and legs should not be allowed to dangle; otherwise, muscle artifacts could result.

5. **Procedural Step.** Position the electrocardiograph so that the power cord points away from the patient and does not pass under the table. It is usually easier for the medical assistant to work on the left side of the patient.

   Principle. Proper positioning of the electrocardiograph reduces 60-cycle interference artifacts.

6. **Procedural Step.** Prepare the patient's skin for application of the disposable electrodes. If the patient has sweaty or oily skin or has used lotion, rub the area to which the electrode will be applied with alcohol, and allow it to dry. If the patient's chest is hairy, dry shave it at each electrode site before applying the electrode.

   Principle. The patient's skin must be dry and free of oil and body hair so that the adhesive backing of the electrodes sticks to the patient's skin and stays on during the procedure.

7. **Procedural Step.** Remove a card containing 10 electrodes from its foil-lined pouch and reseal the pouch. Apply the limb electrodes. Firmly apply the adhesive backing of the electrodes to the fleshy part of each of the four limbs (upper arms and lower legs). The electrode tabs should point toward the center of the body. The tabs of the arm electrodes should point downward, and the tabs of the leg electrodes should point upward. The adhesive backing of the electrode allows it to adhere firmly to the patient's skin.

   Principle. The pouch should be resealed to preserve moisture and prevent the electrolyte on the remaining

electrodes from drying out. The electrodes must be firmly attached to permit good transmission of the electrical impulse from the patient's skin to the electrode. Loose electrodes can cause artifacts to occur on the recording, making it difficult to analyze the recording. The tabs of the electrodes should be positioned toward the center of the body to provide a more stable connection when the lead wire is attached to the electrode and to prevent the lead wires from pulling onto the electrodes and causing artifacts.

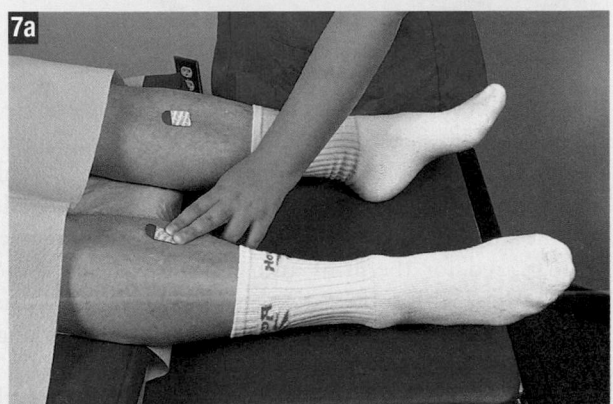

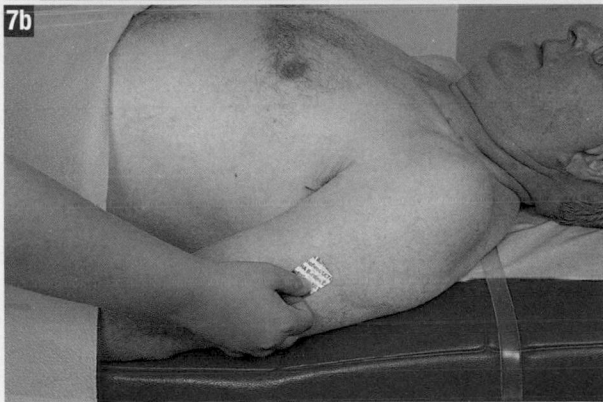

A, Apply the leg electrodes. **B,** Apply the arm electrodes.

8. **Procedural Step.** Apply the chest electrodes. Properly locate each electrode placement site using palpation, and apply the electrode with the tab pointing downward. Continue until all six of the chest electrodes have been applied.

   Principle. Positioning the tabs of the electrodes downward prevents the lead wires from pulling and causing artifacts.

Continued

634 CHAPTER 27 Cardiopulmonary Procedures

PROCEDURE 27-1 Running a 12-Lead, Three-Channel Electrocardiogram—cont'd

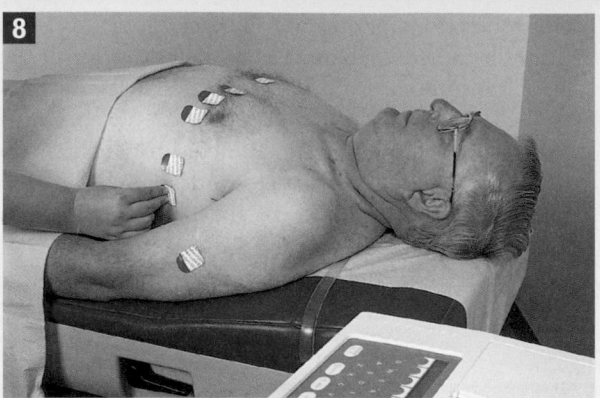

Apply the chest electrodes.

9. Procedural Step. Connect the lead wires to the electrodes. This is accomplished by inserting an alligator clip onto the metal tip of each lead wire. Next, firmly attach an alligator clip to the tab of each electrode. The ends of the lead wires are usually color-coded (e.g., red for the arms and green for the legs) and identified with abbreviations to help the medical assistant connect the proper lead to each electrode. Arrange the lead wires to follow body contour.

Principle. The lead wires must be attached correctly to ensure an accurate and reliable ECG. Arranging the lead wires to follow body contour reduces the possibility of 60-cycle interference artifacts.

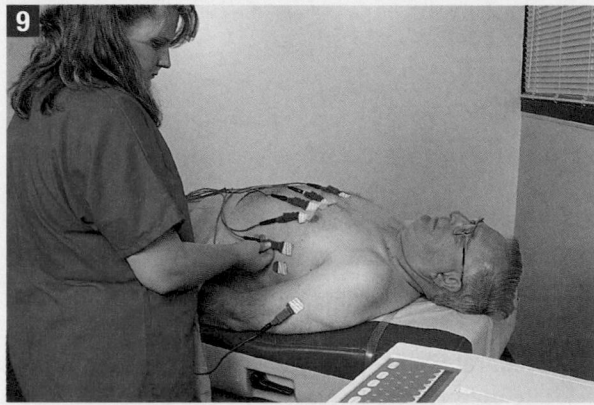

Connect the lead wires to the electrodes.

10. Procedural Step. Plug the patient cable into the machine. The cable should be supported on the table or on the patient's abdomen to prevent pulling of the lead wires on the electrodes.

Principle. Pulling of the lead wires on the electrodes can cause the electrodes to pull away from the skin, resulting in artifacts.

11. Procedural Step. Turn on the electrocardiograph. Enter patient data using the soft-touch keypad. Always

use your fingertips to enter the data. Pencils and other sharp objects can damage the keyboard. As the data are entered, they are displayed on the LCD screen. Patient data to be entered generally include the patient's name, a patient identification number, age, sex, height, weight, and medications.

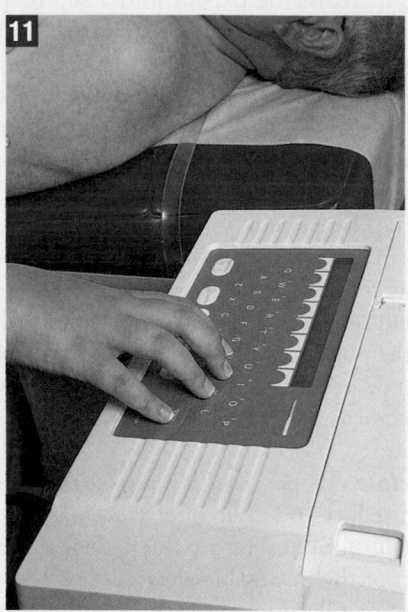

Enter patient data.

12. Procedural Step. Remind the patient to lie still, breathe normally, and not talk. Press the AUTO (automatic) button, and run the recording. The machine automatically inserts a standardization mark at the beginning of each ECG strip, followed by the recording of the 12-lead ECG in a three-channel format. Another standardization mark is inserted at the end of each ECG strip.

(*NOTE:* With most three-channel electrocardiographs, the machine checks for a clear ECG signal after the AUTO button is pressed. If the signal is "noisy," this may indicate that an electrode does not have a good connection with the patient's skin. The machine usually indicates which electrode is causing the problem [e.g., "V_6 noisy"]. Apply firm pressure to the electrode causing the problem. If this does not correct the problem, replace the electrode with a new one and/or place a piece of nonallergenic tape over the electrode.)

13. Procedural Step. After the ECG has been recorded:
a. Check the printout to ensure the standardization mark is 10 mm high. If it is more or less than 10 mm, adjust the standardization mark according

PROCEDURE 27-1 Running a 12-Lead, Three-Channel Electrocardiogram—cont'd

to the manufacturer's instructions, and run another ECG.

b. Check the direction of the R wave in lead I. If your patient's limb leads are attached correctly, the R wave on lead I should have a positive deflection. If it has a negative deflection, the limb leads are not attached correctly. Reattach the limb leads properly and run another recording.

c. Observe the recording for artifacts. If an artifact is present, determine the cause of the artifact, correct the problem, and run another ECG.

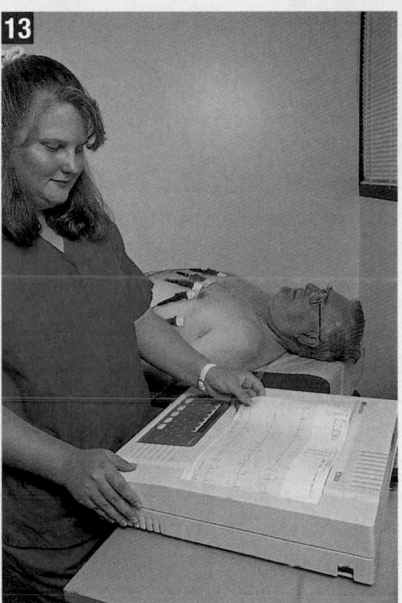

Check the standardization mark.

14. **Procedural Step.** Inform the patient that you are finished and he or she can now talk or move. Turn the machine off. Disconnect the lead wires. Remove and discard the electrodes.

15. **Procedural Step.** Assist the patient in stepping down from the table.

16. **Procedural Step.** Sanitize your hands. Chart the procedure. Include the date and time and the name of the procedure (12-lead ECG). Place the recording in the patient's medical record, and put the record in the appropriate place to be reviewed by the physician.

17. **Procedural Step.** Return all equipment to its proper storage place.

CHARTING EXAMPLE

Date	
6/12/XX	10:30 a.m. Completed a 12-lead ECG.
	Recording to physician for review. ———
	——— J. Canterbury, CMA (AAMA)

HOLTER MONITOR ELECTROCARDIOGRAPHY

A Holter monitor is a portable ambulatory monitoring system for the continuous recording of the electrical activity of the heart for 24 hours or longer (Figure 27-12). The monitor is named for Dr. Norman Holter, an American biophysicist who invented this cardiac monitoring device. The original Holter monitor consisted of a large pack of equipment worn on the patient's back.

A Holter monitor is also known as an *ambulatory electrocardiographic monitor* (AEM). The purpose of a Holter monitor is to detect cardiac abnormalities that occur while the patient is engaged in his or her normal daily routine. Because of this, the Holter system is designed so that the patient is able to maintain his or her usual daily activities with minimal inconvenience while being monitored.

A Holter monitor is similar to a resting 12-lead ECG in that the electrical impulses given off by the heart are picked up by electrodes and transmitted through lead wires to a

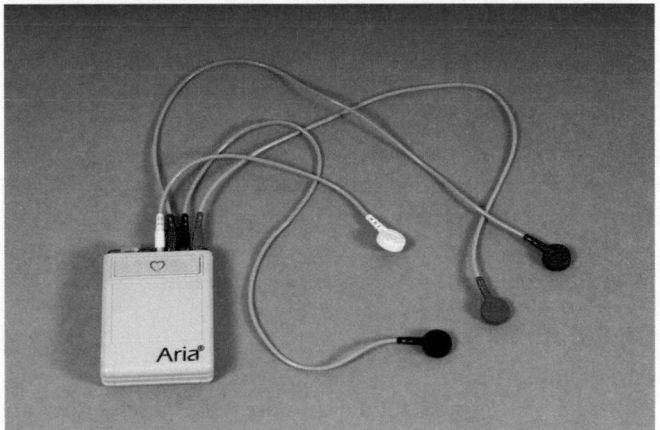

Figure 27-12 Digital Holter monitor.

recording device (Figure 27-13). It is different from a resting 12-lead ECG in that only about 10 seconds of the heart's activity are recorded with a 12-lead ECG, whereas a Holter monitor records the heartbeat continuously for an extended period of time. This allows the Holter monitor to pick up

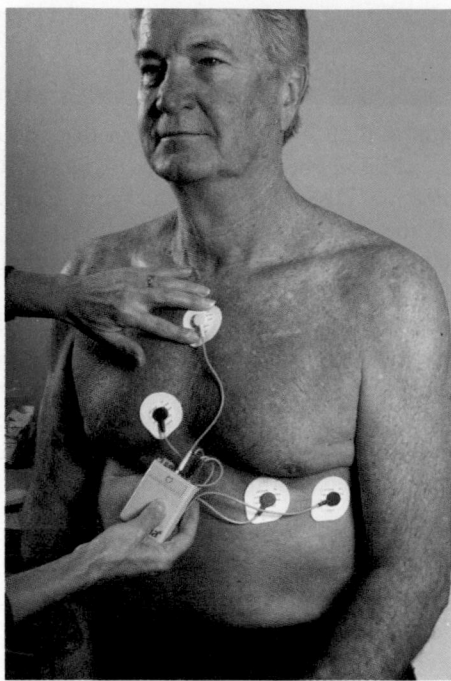

Figure 27-13 Digital Holter monitor. Electrical impulses given off by the heart are picked up by electrodes placed on the patient's chest.

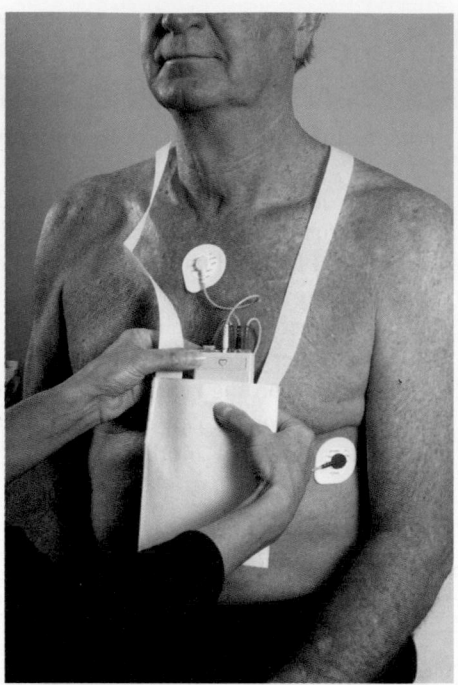

Figure 27-14 The digital Holter monitor is placed in a pouch hung around the patient's neck by a strap.

cardiac abnormalities that do not occur during the brief recording period of a resting 12-lead ECG.

Purpose

Holter monitor electrocardiography is an important noninvasive procedure used to diagnose cardiac rate, rhythm, and conduction abnormalities. Specifically, it is most frequently used for the following purposes:

- To assess the rate and rhythm of the heart during daily activities.
- To evaluate patients with unexplained chest pain, dizziness, or syncope (fainting).
- To discover intermittent cardiac dysrhythmias not picked up on a routine resting 12-lead ECG. A resting ECG records only between 40 and 50 heartbeats, whereas a Holter monitor records approximately 100,000 heartbeats in a 24-hour period.
- To detect myocardial ischemia.
- To assess the effectiveness of antidysrhythmic medications (e.g., digitalis, antianginal medications).
- To assess the effectiveness of a pacemaker.

Digital Holter Monitor

Holter monitors are available in two formats. The newer format consists of a digital monitor that uses either an external (removable) or an internal (nonremovable) memory card to document the heart's activity (see Figure 27-12). The older type of Holter monitor consists of a magnetic tape monitor that uses a cassette tape to record the activity of the heart. Most facilities have phased out the magnetic tape monitor in favor of the digital monitor.

A digital Holter monitor is lightweight and battery-powered. The monitor can be clipped onto a belt around the patient's waist. It can also be held in a protective pouch, which is hung around the patient's neck with a strap known as a *lanyard* (Figure 27-14). Digital monitors can continuously record the electrical activity of the heart for 24 hours, 48 hours, or 72 hours. Most physicians order a 24-hour recording, but they may occasionally order a 48- or 72-hour recording when the heart's activity needs to be recorded for a longer period of time. Throughout the monitoring period, the system continuously records the electrical activity of the heart and stores it on the memory card. The Holter monitor automatically stops recording after the monitoring period has been completed.

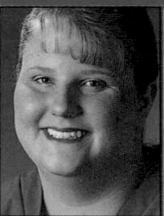

Memories *from* Externship

Janet Canterbury: During my externship, I was at an office where electrocardiograms were one of the many procedures that were performed. For my first electrocardiogram, the patient was a man who had a lot of hair on his chest, and I would need to shave the electrode placement sites on his chest. I was very nervous, but the procedure went well. When the electrocardiogram was run, he told me that I did a wonderful job and that it did not hurt at all to have his chest shaved. I realized then that it was not so bad after all. That patient made me feel so good about what I do and helped me feel confident in the procedures I had ahead of me. ■

Evaluating Results

At the end of the monitoring period, the Holter monitor system is removed from the patient. The information on the memory card is then uploaded to a computer. Specialized ECG software performs calculations on the data and prepares an ECG summary report of the monitoring period, which is then displayed on the screen of the computer.

The computer-generated ECG report summarizes information about the patient's heart rate and rhythm and any abnormalities that occurred during the monitoring period. The report also includes selected samples of the patient's cardiac activity, including patient event strips and any abnormal cardiac activity exhibited by the patient, such as dysrhythmias. The results of the ECG summary report are reviewed and interpreted further by the physician. The ECG report can be printed out on regular sheets of paper using an ink-jet or laser printer and stored in a PPR (patient-based paper record). It can also be stored electronically in the patient's EMR (electronic medical record).

CARDIAC DYSRHYTHMIAS

The normal ECG graph cycle consists of a P wave, a QRS complex, and a T wave, which repeat in a regular pattern (see Figure 27-2). The term **normal sinus rhythm** refers to an ECG that is within normal limits. This means that the waves, intervals, segments, and cardiac rate fall within the normal range. The normal heart rate ranges from 60 to 100 beats/min. A rate slower than 60 beats/min is *sinus bradycardia,* and a rate faster than 100 beats/min is *sinus tachycardia.*

Cardiac **dysrhythmia** is the term used to describe abnormal electrical activity in the heart causing an irregular heartbeat. Cardiac dysrhythmias can be classified into one of the following categories: (1) extra beats, (2) an abnormal rhythm, or (3) an abnormal heart rate. Cardiac dysrhythmias include atrial premature contraction, paroxysmal atrial tachycardia, atrial flutter, atrial fibrillation, premature ventricular contraction, ventricular tachycardia, and ventricular fibrillation.

PULMONARY FUNCTION TESTS

The purpose of a pulmonary function test (PFT) is to assess lung functioning, assisting in the detection and evaluation of pulmonary disease. Pulmonary function tests include spirometry, lung volumes, diffusion capacity, arterial blood gas studies, pulse oximetry, peak flow measurement, and cardiopulmonary exercise tests. The most frequently performed pulmonary function test is spirometry, which is described in the next section.

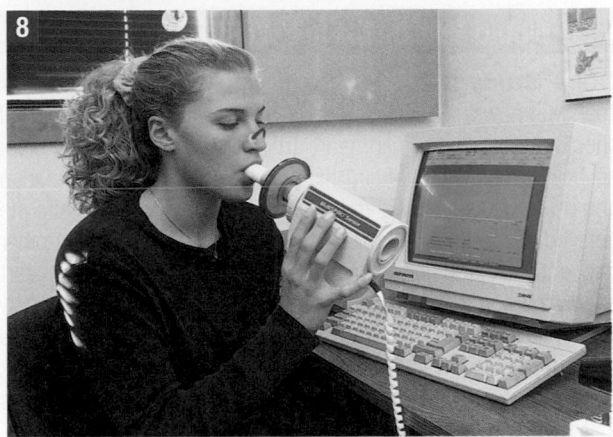
Figure 27-15 Spirometer.

Spirometry

Spirometry is a simple, noninvasive screening test that is often performed in the medical office. A computerized electronic instrument known as a **spirometer** is used to conduct the test (Figure 27-15). A spirometer measures how much air is pushed out of the lungs and how fast it is pushed out. The spirometry report is printed out as a table and graph. Spirometry is considered a screening test, and abnormal test results require that the patient undergo additional pulmonary function tests and possibly a computed tomography scan before a diagnosis can be made. Indications for performing spirometry include the following:

1. Patients who exhibit symptoms of lung dysfunction such as dyspnea
2. Individuals at high risk for lung disease because of smoking or exposure to environmental pollutants such as coal dust, asbestos, and exhaust fumes
3. Patients with lung disease, such as asthma, chronic bronchitis, and emphysema
4. Patients who are to undergo surgery (to assess probable lung performance during an operation)
5. Patients who need to be evaluated for lung disability or impairment for a compensation program (e.g., coal miners)

Patient Preparation

Patient preparation is essential to obtain accurate test results. To prepare for the test, the patient should be instructed to do the following:

1. Do not eat a heavy meal for 8 hours before the test. (The patient must exert the diaphragm muscles, and a full stomach may interfere with this action.)
2. Stop smoking at least 8 hours before the test.
3. Do not take bronchodilators for 4 hours before the test.
4. Do not engage in strenuous activity for 4 hours before the test.
5. Wear loose, nonrestrictive clothing to keep the chest area as free as possible, which makes it easier to perform the breathing maneuver.

What Would You Do? What Would You *Not* Do?

Case Study 2

Joel Matthews, 48 years old, is at the office for a biannual checkup. Joel had a mild heart attack 2 years ago. Since then, he has completely changed his life. He's become a vegetarian and practices yoga every morning before going to work. After he gets home, he jogs 10 miles. He also lifts weights every other day and takes herbal vitamin supplements. Since his heart attack, he has lost 40 lb and says that he has never felt better. The only thing he cannot seem to do is give up smoking. He started smoking when he was 17 years old and has cut back from 2 packs to 1 pack a day. He keeps trying to stop but says that he has been smoking so long that it might not be possible. Besides, with all the other healthy stuff he is doing, he thinks it probably cancels out the bad effect of the cigarettes. Joel is very concerned that if he does stop smoking, he will gain back all of the weight that it took him so long to lose. ∎

Post-Bronchodilator Spirometry

If the results of the spirometry test indicate a possible obstruction, the physician usually orders a post-bronchodilator spirometry test. This test is performed by having the patient inhale a bronchodilator and running a spirometry test approximately 10 to 15 minutes later. The purpose of this test is to inform the physician as to how treatment would work in patients whose airways are obstructed.

PEAK FLOW MEASUREMENT

Asthma

Asthma is a chronic lung disease that affects the smaller bronchi and the bronchioles of the lungs.

Asthma can occur at any age but is more common in children and young adults. Asthma affects boys more

Highlight on Smoking and Chronic Obstructive Pulmonary Disease

COPD Defined

Chronic obstructive pulmonary disease (COPD) is a chronic airway obstruction that results from emphysema or chronic bronchitis or a combination of these conditions. COPD is a chronic, debilitating, irreversible, and sometimes fatal disease.

More than 12 million Americans have been diagnosed with COPD; however, it is estimated that an additional 12 million Americans have the disease and remain undiagnosed. Smoking tobacco is the primary cause of COPD. In the United States, approximately 80% to 90% of deaths due to COPD are caused by smoking. According to the American Lung Association, COPD is the fourth leading cause of death in the United States, behind heart disease, cancer, and stroke. COPD claims the lives of more than 120,000 Americans each year.

Emphysema

Emphysema is most often seen in older individuals with a long history of smoking. Emphysema due to smoking is caused by irreversible damage to the alveoli in the lungs from toxins present in cigarette smoke (see illustration). As alveoli continue to be damaged, the lungs are able to transfer less and less oxygen to the bloodstream. In addition, air becomes trapped in the damaged alveoli, making it difficult to remove during exhalation. Because of this, the primary symptom of emphysema is shortness of breath. Other symptoms include chronic cough, tiredness, and limited exercise tolerance. More than 3 million people in the United States have been diagnosed with emphysema; of these, 52% are men and 48% are women. The reason is not yet understood, but fortunately only 10% to 15% of long-term smokers develop emphysema.

Chronic Bronchitis

Chronic bronchitis is an inflammation of the lining of the bronchiole tubes that causes swelling and excess production of mucus. Swelling and excess mucus narrow the bronchiole tubes and restrict

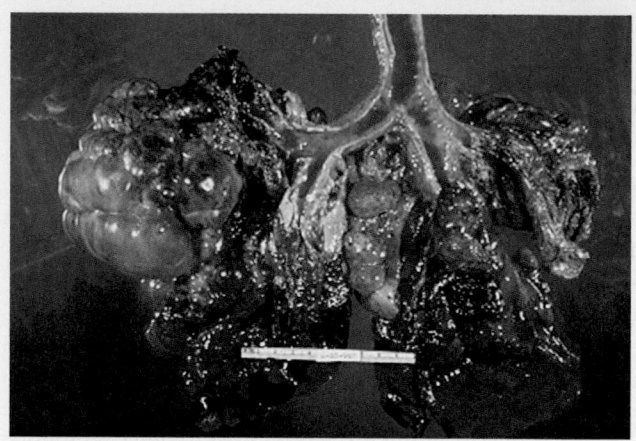

Emphysema caused by smoking.

airflow into and out of the lungs. Symptoms include chronic cough, shortness of breath, and coughing up of mucus. To be classified as chronic bronchitis, the symptoms must last 3 or more months out of the year for at least 2 years. As the disease progresses, the lips and skin may exhibit cyanosis resulting from lack of oxygen in the blood. Chronic bronchitis is most often caused by long-term irritation of the bronchial tubes due to cigarette smoking; other causes include air pollution and exposure to dust or toxic gases in the workplace (e.g., coal mines). Chronic bronchitis often precedes or accompanies emphysema. It is estimated that 12 million Americans have chronic bronchitis. This condition affects individuals of all ages but has a higher incidence in individuals over 45 years of age. Women are more than twice as likely to be diagnosed with chronic bronchitis as men.

Symptoms of COPD

Damage to the lungs caused by COPD occurs gradually over many years. In fact, more than 90% of patients who have COPD are over

Highlight on Smoking and Chronic Obstructive Pulmonary Disease—cont'd

the age of 45 at the time of their diagnosis. Because there are no early symptoms, many people do not know they have COPD. By the time an individual experiences symptoms, it is usually a sign that irreversible lung damage has already occurred. The first symptoms of COPD include mild shortness of breath on exertion and occasional coughing. The disease slowly becomes more pronounced with severe episodes of dyspnea and coughing even after modest activity. As the disease progresses, the heart also can be affected and shortness of breath is present all the time, even while sitting quietly. At this point, the individual's quality of life is greatly diminished. When the lungs and the heart are no longer able to deliver oxygen to the body's tissues, death occurs.

Treatment for COPD

The best treatment for COPD caused by smoking is for the patient to stop smoking. Continued smoking makes the COPD worse; quitting smoking slows the disease process. There are programs, support groups, and stop-smoking aids (e.g., nicotine patch, Zyban) to help individuals quit smoking. Other forms of treatment depend on the patient's condition and degree of lung impairment and may include the following:

1. Bronchodilators to relax and widen the bronchial tubes to increase airflow. They may be inhaled as aerosol sprays or taken orally.
2. Expectorants to thin the mucus so that it is easier to expel.
3. Antibiotics to treat infections that could interfere further with breathing and lung function.
4. Corticosteroids to reduce inflammation in the airways.
5. Breathing exercises to strengthen the muscles used to breathe.
6. Maintaining overall good health habits, which include proper nutrition, adequate sleep, and regular exercise.
7. Oxygen therapy for patients with low blood oxygen to help with shortness of breath, allowing them to be more active.
8. Special measures include avoiding extremes (heat and cold) of temperature, getting an annual influenza immunization, avoiding individuals with respiratory infection, and reducing exposure to air pollution.
9. Lung transplantation surgery is being performed on some patients who are in the later stages of COPD. ∎

frequently before puberty and girls more frequently after puberty. In the United States, there are approximately 20 million individuals with asthma; of these, 6 million are children. Each year, more than 4000 deaths result from asthma.

Asthma is characterized by chronic inflammation of the small airways of the lungs and recurrent attacks of coughing, chest tightness, shortness of breath, and wheezing. **Wheezing** is a continuous, high-pitched, whistling, musical sound heard particularly during exhalation and sometimes during inhalation. In most patients, an asthma attack is followed by a symptom-free period. Asthma can be controlled by recognizing the warning signs and symptoms of an attack and treating them when they first occur. Failure to treat asthma can lead to serious complications, such as permanent lung damage.

Asthma Attack

Asthma attacks are highly individualized. Depending on the patient, asthma attacks vary in frequency and severity and may come on suddenly or gradually. An asthma attack may last for only 10 to 15 minutes or it may last for hours or even days.

In a normal individual, the airways to the lungs are fully open, allowing air to move easily into and out of the lungs. In a patient with asthma, the airways are always inflamed and hypersensitive to certain stimuli that do not affect the airways of normal individuals. These stimuli are known as *asthma triggers* because they can "trigger" an asthma attack.

Asthma triggers vary from one patient to another and may also vary from one season to the next. Examples of common allergens that may trigger an asthma attack include house dust, pollens, molds, animal danders, and cockroaches. Asthma attacks can also be triggered by environmental irritants, activities, or events, including air pollutants, tobacco smoke, chemical fumes (e.g., perfume, paint, gasoline), vigorous physical exercise, upper respiratory viral infections, exposure to cold, and emotional stress. It is sometimes difficult to determine what specific triggers cause a patient's asthma attack.

When the inflamed airways of a patient with asthma are stimulated by a trigger, a series of reactions occur that affect the bronchial tubes. The bronchial tubes begin to constrict and swell, causing the patient to experience asthma symptoms. Sometimes the symptoms are mild and go away, either on their own or with minimal treatment with medication. At other times, the symptoms become worse, leading to a full-blown asthma attack. During a severe asthma attack, the bronchial tubes continue to constrict and swell and become clogged with mucus (Figure 27-16). This results in less air moving into and out of the lungs, which leads to a decrease in the amount of oxygen available to the body. The narrowed bronchial tubes and decreased oxygen supply cause the patient to experience coughing, chest tightness, shortness of breath, and wheezing. It is important to treat symptoms when they first begin to occur to prevent them from getting worse and causing a severe asthma attack, which may require emergency care.

Diagnosis and Treatment

The physician diagnoses asthma through a careful and detailed medical history. Of particular importance to the diagnosis of asthma are the patient's symptoms, family history of asthma, home and work environment, and living habits. The physician also performs a thorough physical examination to detect symptoms resulting from asthma,

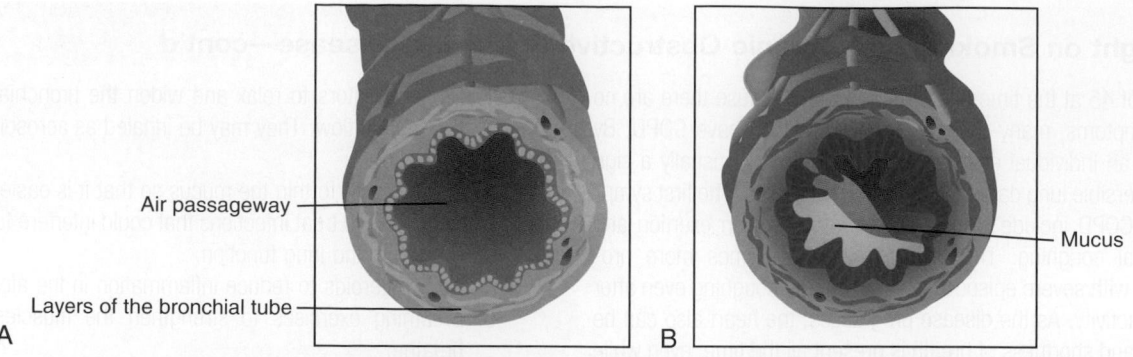

Figure 27-16 **A,** Normal bronchial tube. **B,** Bronchial tube during an asthma attack.

such as wheezing. When the medical history and physical examination have been completed, the physician usually orders laboratory and diagnostic tests, which may include pulmonary function tests (such as spirometry), allergy testing, and arterial blood gas studies.

Although asthma is a chronic disease with no cure, most patients with asthma are able to lead a normal life through proper management and treatment. The general treatment of asthma includes identifying and avoiding asthma triggers (if possible) and preventing and alleviating the symptoms through drug therapy. Two general categories of medication are prescribed for asthma: long-term control medication and quick-relief medication.

Long-term control medication helps relieve bronchial inflammation and prevents symptoms from occurring. Control medication helps the patient have fewer and milder asthma attacks and is typically taken every day. Corticosteroids are an example of a control medication; brand names include Flovent, Azmacort, Vanceril, and AeroBid. Other examples of long-term control medication include Singulair, Accolate, Serevent, Alupent, and Advair.

Quick-relief medication (also called *rescue medication*) opens the airways quickly by dilating the bronchial tubes. It is taken when the patient is experiencing symptoms to prevent or control an asthma attack. Fast-acting bronchodilators are an example of quick-relief medication; brand names include Proventil, Ventolin, and Xopenex.

Many asthma medications are delivered through an *inhaler* (Figure 27-17), which allows the medication to go directly to the lungs. Quick-relief medications can be used in a breathing machine known as a *nebulizer* to treat an asthma attack at home. Other asthma medications are administered orally; however, they take longer to work because they first have to travel through the digestive and circulatory systems before reaching the lungs.

Peak Flow Meter

A peak flow meter is a portable, handheld manual or digital device used to measure a breathing maneuver performed by the patient. *A manual peak flow meter* consists of a plastic tube with a sliding indicator that manually moves along a scale of numbers when the patient performs the breathing maneuver (Figure 27-18). A *digital peak flow*

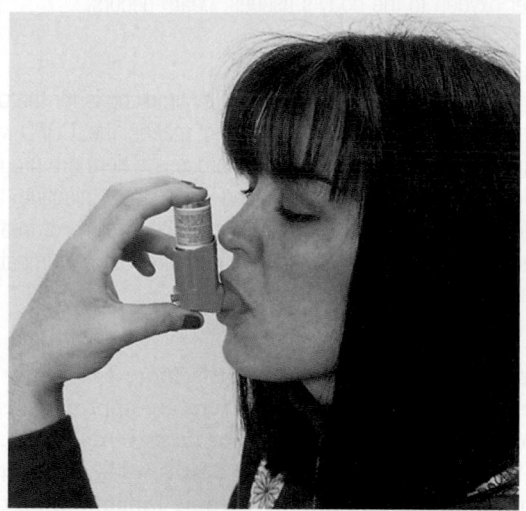

Figure 27-17 An inhaler is often used to deliver asthma medication to the bronchial tubes of the lungs.

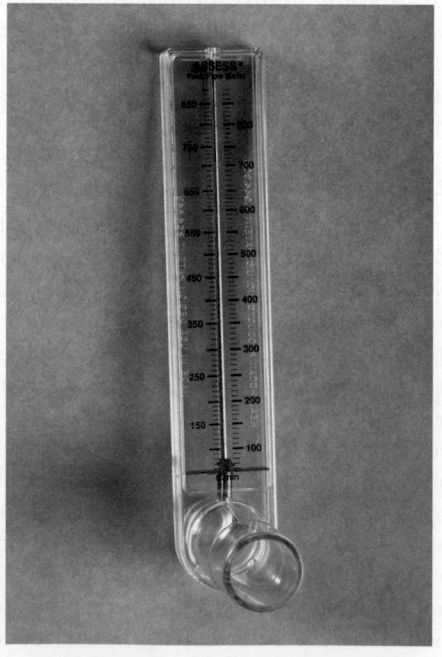

Figure 27-18 Manual peak flow meter.

meter automatically measures the breathing maneuver and displays the measurement digitally on a screen (Figure 27-19). Because the manual meter is currently used most often, the remainder of this unit will focus on the manual peak flow meter.

A peak flow meter is used to measure how quickly air flows out of the lungs when the patient exhales forcefully. Peak flow meters are frequently used by patients with asthma and are recommended for patients with moderate to severe asthma. The measurements obtained from a peak

flow meter are not as accurate as those obtained by spirometry; however, a peak flow meter can be used easily by a patient at home.

Peak flow measurements provide patients with important information such as when to take their medication and how severe an asthma attack is. Several different brands of peak flow meters are available, and peak flow measurements between brands may vary. Because of this, a patient who purchases more than one meter should always buy the same brand to provide consistency between measurements.

Peak flow meters can be purchased over-the-counter and are available in two ranges: a low range and a full range. The *low-range meter* has a range from zero to 300 and is used by young children and some older patients. The *full-range meter* has a range from zero to 800 and is used by older children, teenagers, and adults (Figure 27-20). An adult has much larger bronchial tubes than a child and needs the wider range.

Peak Flow Rate

The **peak flow rate** (PFR) is the maximum volume of air measured in liters per minute (L/min) that can be exhaled when the patient blows into a peak flow meter as forcefully and as rapidly as possible. The PFR is obtained by having the patient perform a breathing maneuver.

The patient is instructed to take a deep breath until the lungs are completely full. Following this, the patient is told to blow all the air out of the lungs and into the mouthpiece of the peak flow meter as hard and as fast as possible. When the patient blows into the peak flow meter, his or her breath causes the sliding indicator to move up the scale of the meter. The indicator stops and remains at the patient's peak

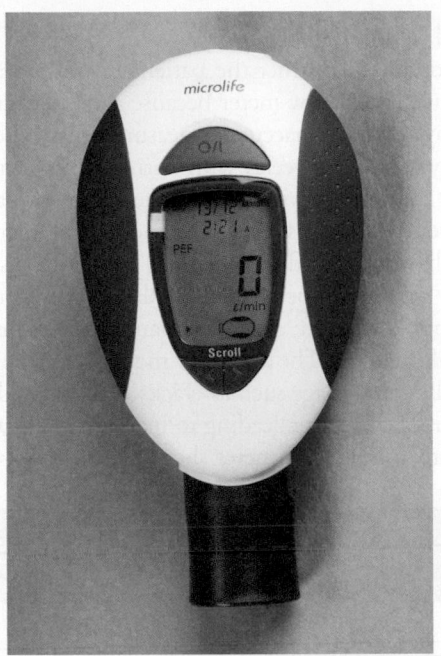

Figure 27-19 Digital peak flow meter.

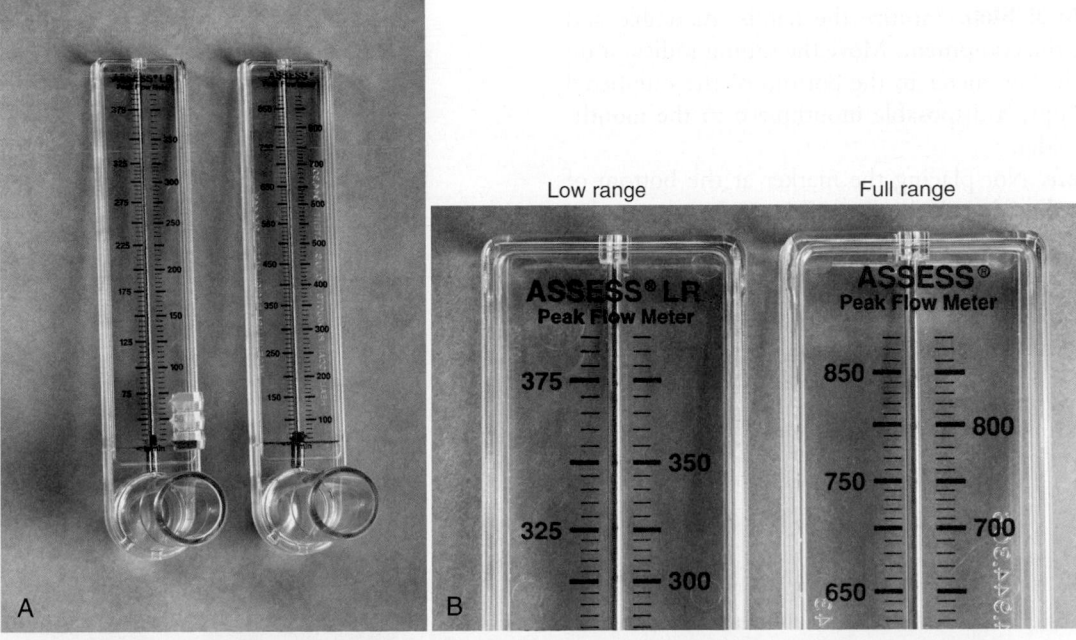

Figure 27-20 Comparison of a low-range (**A, B:** *left*) and full-range (**A, B:** *right*) peak flow meter.

flow rate. To obtain the most accurate PFR, the patient should perform three acceptable breathing maneuvers, and then record the highest of the three measurements. The three measurements should be about the same to show that an acceptable breathing maneuver was performed each time. This is especially important to note when parents are evaluating a child's peak flow measurement.

The medical assistant is often responsible for instructing a newly diagnosed asthma patient in the procedure for using a peak flow meter. In addition, the medical assistant may be responsible for obtaining the peak flow rate of a patient with asthma at the medical office. The procedure for measuring peak flow rate is outlined in Procedure 27-2.

Schedule of Use

A peak flow meter should be used on a regular schedule by patients with moderate to severe asthma to determine how well their asthma is being controlled. The physician determines each patient's schedule based on the severity and frequency of asthma symptoms. Most physicians recommend that the patient use a peak flow meter at least once a day, preferably in the morning before taking asthma medication. A peak flow measurement should also be obtained when the patient is having symptoms. If the patient has a more severe form of asthma, the physician may want the patient to use a peak flow meter twice a day—in the morning and in the evening.

Purpose of Peak Flow Measurements

Peak flow measurements allow physicians and patients to monitor changes in the patient's airflow to determine how well the patient's asthma is being controlled. A high number usually means that air is moving easily out of the patient's lungs. A low number usually means that the airways are narrowed and air cannot move easily through them, resulting in a decrease in oxygen available to the body.

Care and Maintenance

It is important to instruct the patient in the proper care of the (manual) peak flow meter because dirt collecting on the meter may result in inaccurate measurements. The meter is cleaned by washing it weekly with warm soapy water and then rinsing it thoroughly with warm water. Excess water should be removed by gently shaking the meter. The meter should then be allowed to air-dry completely before it is used. Many peak flow meters can be cleaned by placing them in the dishwasher on the top shelf; check the manufacturer's instructions for this information. The peak flow meter should be inspected periodically for damage such as cracks, which could cause air to leak out of the meter, leading to inaccurate readings. With proper care, a peak flow meter should last 2 to 3 years.

PROCEDURE **27-2**   **Measuring Peak Flow Rate**

Outcome Measure a patient's peak flow rate.

Equipment/Supplies

- Peak flow meter
- Disposable mouthpiece

- Waste container

1. Procedural Step. Sanitize the hands. Assemble and prepare the equipment. Move the sliding indicator on the peak flow meter to the bottom of the numbered scale. Apply a disposable mouthpiece to the mouthpiece holder.

Principle. Not placing the marker at the bottom of the numbered scale leads to inaccurate test results. The disposable mouthpiece prevents the spread of microorganisms from one patient to another.

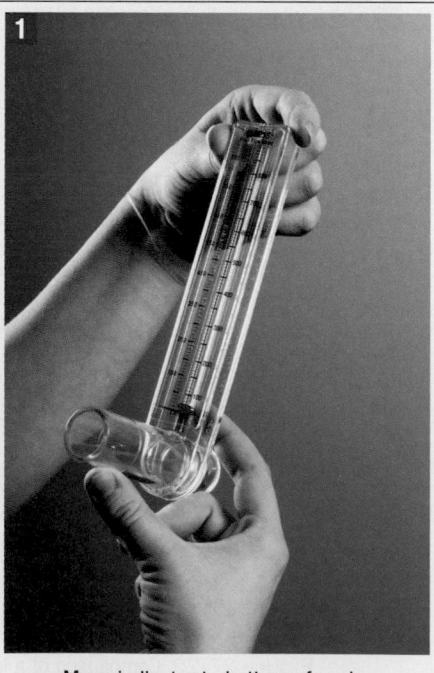

Move indicator to bottom of scale.

PROCEDURE 27-2 Measuring Peak Flow Rate—cont'd

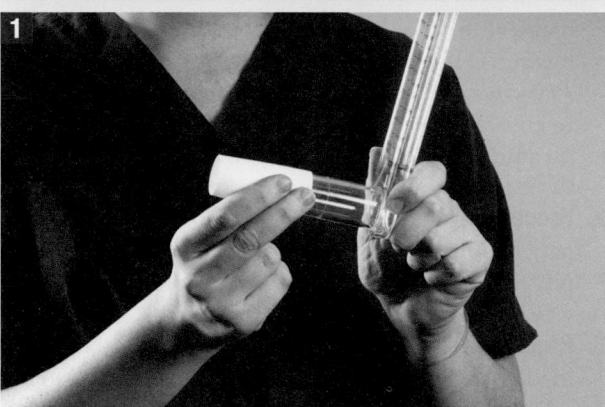

Apply a disposable mouthpiece.

2. Procedural Step. Greet the patient and introduce yourself. Identify the patient and explain the procedure. Tell the patient that he or she will be performing a breathing maneuver several times to see how well his or her lungs are functioning.

3. Procedural Step. Prepare the patient. Have the patient remove any heavy or constricting clothing, such as a jacket or a sweater. Also, ask the patient to loosen tight clothing, such as a necktie or a tight collar. If the patient is chewing gum, ask him or her to discard it in a waste container.
Principle. Heavy outer clothing, tight clothing, or gum may make it difficult for the patient to perform the breathing maneuver.

4. Procedural Step. Instruct the patient in the breathing maneuver. The following procedure should be described and demonstrated to the patient.
a. Relax and take the deepest breath possible until your lungs are completely filled with air.

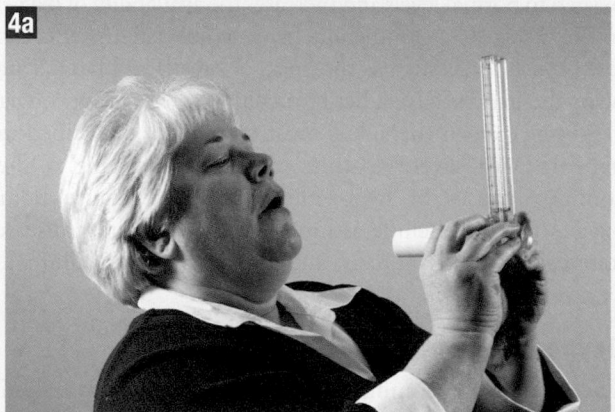

The patient takes a deep breath.

b. Place the mouthpiece in your mouth, and seal your lips tightly around it.

c. Blow out as hard and fast as you can until your lungs are completely empty. Try to move the marker as high as you can on the numbered scale. Do not block the opening of the mouthpiece with your tongue.

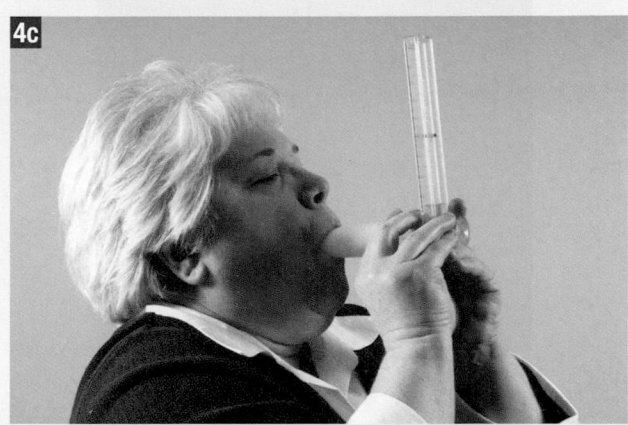

The patient blows out hard and fast.

d. Remove the mouthpiece from your mouth.
Principle. The lips must be tightly sealed around the mouthpiece so that all of the air leaving the mouth enters the mouthpiece. The force of the air coming out of the patient's lungs causes the marker to move upward on the scale. The reading depends on how hard the patient blows out the air in his or her lungs.

5. Procedural Step. Tell the patient you will repeat the instructions during the test. Encourage the patient to remain calm during the procedure.
Principle. Fear or anxiety can make the results less reliable.

6. Procedural Step. Place a new disposable mouthpiece on the peak flow meter, and slide the marker to the bottom of the numbered scale. Hand the peak flow meter to the patient.

7. Procedural Step. Instruct the patient to stand up straight and look straight ahead.

8. Procedural Step. Begin the test. Actively coach the patient …
a. "Now relax and take in a big breath—in—in—in—"
b. "Put the mouthpiece in your mouth and blow hard."
c. "Take out the mouthpiece and rest for a while. You did a great job."

9. Procedural Step. Note the number where the indicator stopped on the scale of the peak flow meter. Jot down the number on a piece of paper.

Continued

PROCEDURE 27-2

PROCEDURE 27-2   Measuring Peak Flow Rate—cont'd

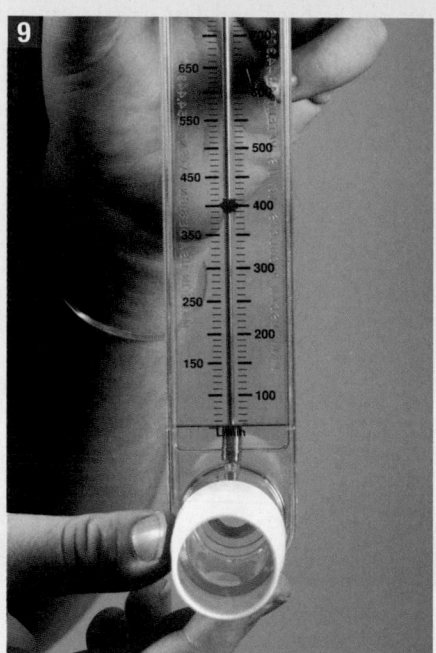

Note where the indicator stopped on the scale.

10. Procedural Step. If the patient coughs or does not perform the breathing maneuver correctly, do not write down the number. Inform the patient of what modifications are needed for the next effort.

11. Procedural Step. Continue until three acceptable efforts have been obtained. Make sure to slide the marker to the bottom of the scale before each measurement.

Principle. Three acceptable efforts must be obtained to ensure valid test results. If the patient performs the breathing maneuver correctly, the numbers from the three tests should be about the same.

12. Procedural Step. Take the peak flow meter from the patient, and remove the mouthpiece from the mouthpiece holder. Dispose of the mouthpiece in a regular waste container.

13. Procedural Step. Sanitize your hands. Note the highest of the three peak flow measurements. (Do not calculate an average.) Chart the procedure. Include the date, the time, the name of the procedure, and the highest peak flow expiratory reading.

14. Procedural Step. Clean the peak flow meter by washing it in warm soapy water, rinsing it thoroughly, and allowing it to dry completely.

CHARTING EXAMPLE

Date	
6/21/XX	10:30 a.m. PFR: 400 L/min. Pt stated she was tired following the test. ———————— ———————— D. Brown, CMA (AAMA)

HOME OXYGEN THERAPY

Oxygen is a colorless, odorless, and tasteless gas that is vital to the human body. Oxygen is transported by the blood to various tissues of the body. When it reaches the tissues, oxygen is taken into the cells, where it combines with glucose to produce energy. Energy is necessary to the body for carrying out all metabolic processes that sustain life such as breathing and beating of the heart.

When the lungs cannot deliver enough oxygen to the body, there is a reduction in the amount of oxygen in the blood, resulting in hypoxemia. **Hypoxemia** is defined as a decrease in the oxygen saturation of the blood. Hypoxemia, in turn, leads to **hypoxia,** which is a reduction in the oxygen supply to the tissues of the body. Failure to maintain an adequate blood oxygen level can result in progressive deterioration of the patient, beginning with the death of cells and, if prolonged, organ failure and eventually body system failure and death.

There are certain conditions, such as severe chronic obstructive pulmonary disease (COPD), that reduce the amount of oxygen in the body, resulting in hypoxemia. In these cases, the physician may write a prescription for home oxygen therapy. **Oxygen therapy** is the administration of supplemental oxygen at concentrations greater than room air to treat or prevent hypoxemia. Oxygen therapy increases the oxygen supply to the lungs, which, in turn, raises blood oxygen to normal levels and increases the availability of oxygen to the tissues. Oxygen therapy helps to alleviate the effects of low oxygen levels such as shortness of breath and fatigue and helps the patient have a better quality of life and live longer.

Home oxygen therapy is most commonly prescribed for patients with severe COPD caused by smoking. Other common causes of hypoxemia that may require home oxygen therapy include asthma, occupational lung disease, lung cancer, cystic fibrosis, and congestive heart failure.

Oxygen Delivery Systems

There are three common delivery systems for providing supplemental oxygen to a patient: compressed oxygen gas, liquid oxygen, and an oxygen concentrator.

The amount of supplemental oxygen prescribed for a patient is known as the **flow rate,** which is measured in liters per minute (L/min). For example, if a patient has been prescribed 2 L/min, each minute, 2 liters of oxygen will flow from the patient's oxygen delivery system into tubing, and then into the patient's upper airway.

The type of delivery system prescribed by the physician is based on the patient's condition, the patient's personal preference, the ease of equipment use, and cost. Each of these delivery systems can be used alone or in combination with another system to meet the oxygen needs of the patient. These systems are described in greater detail below.

Compressed Oxygen Gas

Compressed oxygen gas is oxygen gas compressed under high pressure and then stored in a container referred to as a *cylinder* or *tank*. Compressed oxygen cylinders vary in size from very large stationary cylinders to small portable cylinders that can be carried around (Figure 27-21, *A*). A large cylinder of compressed oxygen is used at home by the patient. A small cylinder is placed in a carrying device such as a shoulder bag and is used when the patient goes outside the home.

The cylinder is equipped with a regulator and a flow meter that control the flow rate of the oxygen (Figure 27-21, *B*). The flow of oxygen out of the cylinder is constant. To conserve oxygen and avoid waste, an oxygen-conserving device may be attached to the system. An oxygen-conserving device releases the oxygen gas only when the patient inhales and cuts off the release of oxygen when the patient exhales.

Liquid Oxygen

When oxygen gas is subjected to an extremely cold temperature, it changes from a gas to a very cold liquid. The liquid oxygen is stored in an insulated tank with a lining similar to a thermos. Oxygen in a liquid form takes up much less space than compressed oxygen gas, for example, 1 liter of liquid oxygen is equal to 860 liters of compressed oxygen gas. Because of this, a container of liquid oxygen lasts four times longer than compressed oxygen gas of the same weight.

A liquid oxygen system consists of a large stationary tank that serves as the primary reservoir of oxygen (Figure 27-22). A small portable tank weighing between 5 and 13 pounds is filled from the large primary tank for use outside the home (see Figure 27-22). The portable tank can be hung over the shoulder or pulled on a roller cart. When liquid oxygen is released from its tank, it changes into a gas and the patient breathes it in, similar to breathing in compressed oxygen gas.

Oxygen Concentrator

An oxygen concentrator is an electrically powered device that weighs about 35 pounds and is about the size of a large suitcase (Figure 27-23, *A*). It works by separating oxygen out of the air, concentrating it, and then storing it for use by the patient. The oxygen concentrator is equipped with a built-in flow meter, which allows the prescribed flow rate to be set.

Small, portable, battery-powered oxygen concentrator systems weighing about 10 pounds have recently been developed (Figure 27-23, *B*). They can provide a patient with oxygen for about 8 hours when used at a flow rate of 2 L/min. For many patients, portable oxygen concentrators have replaced the need to use liquid oxygen or compressed gas cylinders for mobility.

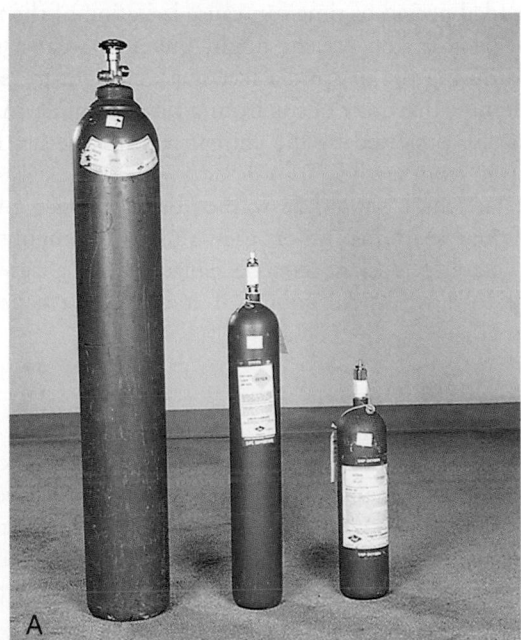

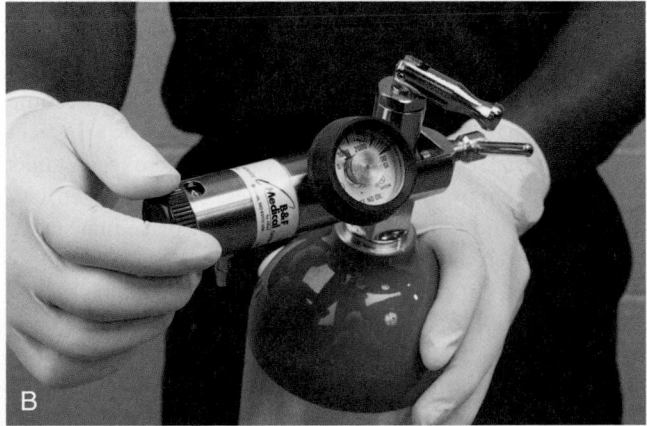

Figure 27-21 A, Compressed oxygen cylinders. **B,** Oxygen cylinder with regulator and flow meter attached.

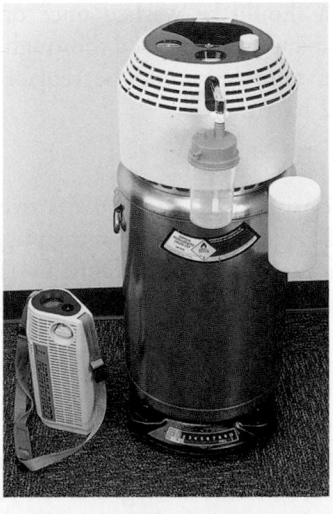

Figure 27-22 Liquid oxygen tank (stationary tank and portable tank).

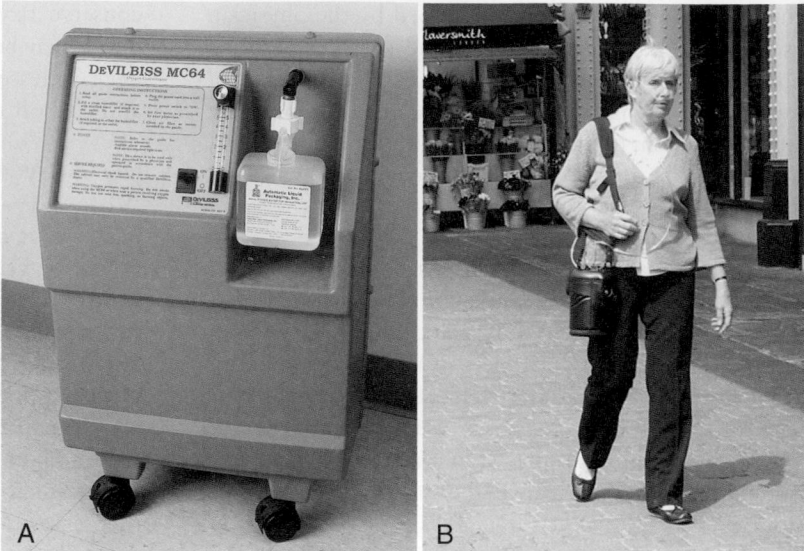

Figure 27-23 **A,** Stationary oxygen concentrator. **B,** Portable oxygen concentrator.

Oxygen Administration Devices

A device must be used to administer the oxygen to the upper airway of the patient from the delivery system. The device used depends on the expected duration of therapy and the personal preference and needs of the patient. The most commonly used devices to administer home oxygen therapy are a nasal cannula and a face mask, which are described in greater detail below.

Nasal Cannula

A nasal cannula is the most frequently used device for administering home oxygen therapy. A nasal cannula consists of soft plastic tubing with a two-pronged device that is inserted into the patient's nose (Figure 27-24, *A*). The tubing of the prongs loops over the patient's ears and is secured under the chin (Figure 27-24, *B*). The tubing connects to the delivery system (i.e., compressed oxygen cylinder, liquid oxygen, or oxygen concentrator). The primary advantage of a nasal cannula is that it does not interfere with the patient's ability to talk, eat, or drink.

The cannula should be washed once or twice a week using liquid soap and water, rinsed thoroughly, and allowed to air-dry. The cannula should be replaced with a new cannula every 2 to 4 weeks.

Face Mask

A face mask consists of plastic and fits over the patient's nose and mouth. A face mask strap is then tightened around the patient's head to ensure a secure fit (Figure 27-25). Oxygen tubing is used to connect the face mask to the oxygen delivery system. A face mask is not used as frequently as a nasal cannula to administer oxygen because it is bulky and must be removed for eating or drinking and to communicate effectively.

A face mask is often used for patients who need a high flow of oxygen. It can deliver oxygen to the patient at a flow

rate between 5 and 15 L/min. Wearing a nasal cannula for an extended period of time can cause irritation of the nose. Because of this, the patient might prefer to wear a nasal cannula during the day and a face mask at night to reduce the irritation that may occur from a nasal cannula. A face mask is also preferred by the patient if he or she has nasal congestion from a cold.

The face mask should be washed once or twice a week using liquid soap and water, then rinsed thoroughly and dried. The face mask should be replaced with a new one every 2 to 4 weeks, or sooner if it becomes cracked or discolored.

Oxygen Safety Guidelines

Oxygen is a safe gas as long as it is used properly. Oxygen itself is not flammable, nor will it explode; however, it greatly increases the combustion rate of a fire. If something catches fire, oxygen will make the flame hotter and cause it to burn faster and more vigorously. The result is that a fire involving oxygen can appear explosive-like.

1. Store oxygen in a clean, dry, well-ventilated room. If kept in a closed area such as a closet, the small amount of oxygen gas that is continually vented from these units can accumulate in a confined space and become a fire hazard.
2. Compressed oxygen cylinders and liquid oxygen tanks must remain upright at all times. Secure oxygen cylinders and tanks to a fixed object, or place in a stand.
3. Never smoke while using oxygen. Do not allow smoking in the room where the oxygen is kept. Post "No Smoking: Oxygen in Use" signs where oxygen is kept.
4. Keep the oxygen supply at least 6 to 8 feet away from open flames such as gas stoves, lighted fireplaces, and candles.

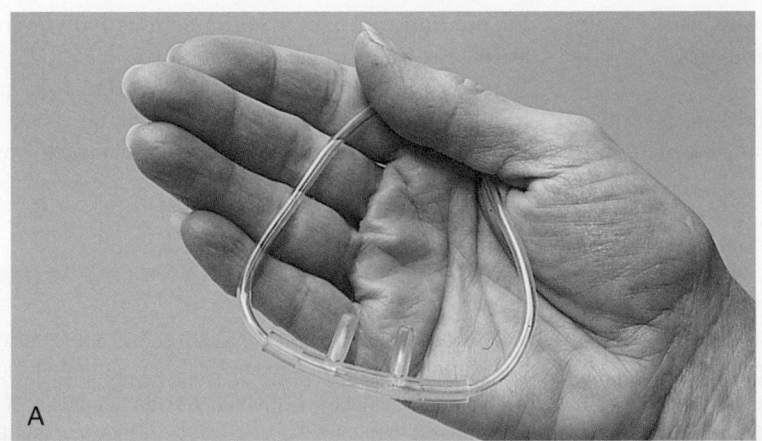

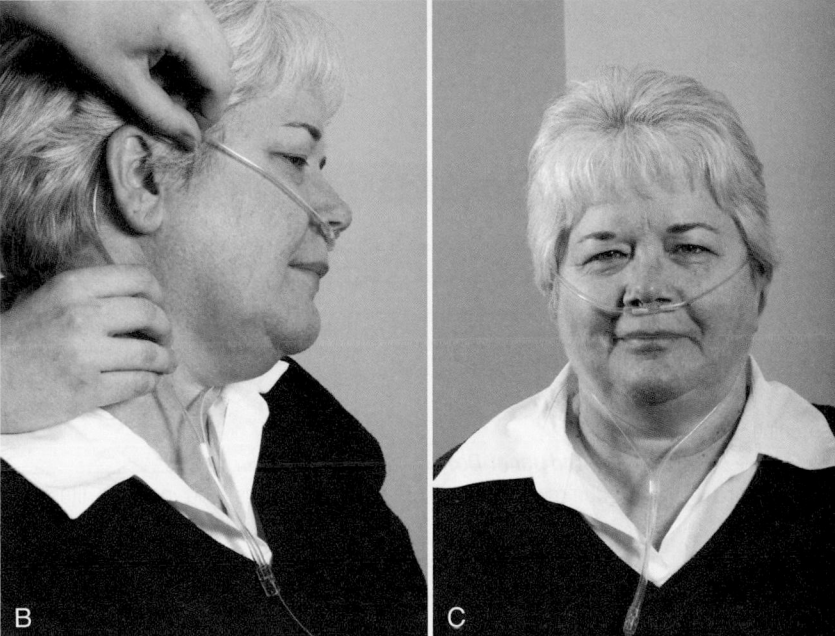

Figure 27-24 **A,** Nasal cannula showing prongs. **B and C,** The tubing of the prongs loops over the patient's ears and is secured under the chin.

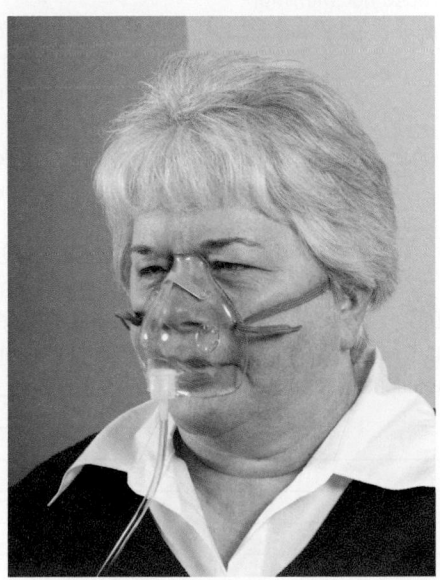

Figure 27-25 Face mask.

5. Keep the oxygen supply at least 6 to 8 feet away from intense heat such as radiators, furnaces, and space heaters.
6. Keep the oxygen supply away from flammable products such as cleaning fluid, paint thinner, and aerosol sprays.

7. Do not lubricate oxygen equipment with oil or grease, as these substances are flammable.
8. Be sure to have functioning smoke detectors in the home.
9. Buy a fire extinguisher, and be familiar with how to use it.

MEDICAL PRACTICE and the LAW

Cardiopulmonary procedures are frightening for many patients because of the potential for unfavorable results. These results must never be given to the patient by the medical assistant. Only a physician can interpret results of electrocardiographic and pulmonary function tests. If results indicate a life-threatening condition, your duty is to calmly notify the physician at once, without alarming the patient. All offices have emergency supplies; be sure you know where they are and how to use them. While you are attending to the machinery and technology, remember the human dignity of the patient, and attend to all of his or her needs for privacy, comfort, respect, and caring. ■

What Would You Do? What Would You *Not* Do? RESPONSES

Case Study 1
Page 627

What Did Janet Do?
❑ Tried to reduce Camilla's fears by talking with her calmly and quietly.
❑ Explained to Camilla that an ECG is the best screening test available to check for heart problems.
❑ Reassured Camilla that she would be draped during the procedure and that she would be exposed as little as possible.
❑ Told Camilla that the wires may look a little scary, but there is no chance of being shocked by them. Explained that she won't feel anything when the test is being run.
❑ Told Camilla that she could talk with the billing clerk about setting up a payment plan for the test. Provided her with information about community resources that might help her pay for the test.

What Did Janet Not Do?
❑ Did not tell Camilla that she was too young to have heart problems.
❑ Did not tell Camilla that she needed to act more mature about being tested.

What Would You Do?/What Would You Not Do?
Review Janet's response and place a checkmark next to the information you included in your response. List additional information you included in your response.

_____
_____
_____
_____

Case Study 2
Page 638

What Did Janet Do?
❑ Commended Joel on his weight loss and positive lifestyle changes.
❑ Shared a positive story with Joel about a patient who stopped smoking and did not gain weight.
❑ Asked Joel whether he would like any of the latest information on smoking cessation.

What Did Janet Not Do?
❑ Did not agree that Joel's positive lifestyle changes would counteract the bad effects of smoking.
❑ Did not lecture Joel on the dangers of smoking because if he has been smoking since age 17 and has been trying to quit, he already knows what they are.

What Would You Do?/What Would You Not Do?
Review Janet's response and place a checkmark next to the information you included in your response. List additional information you included in your response.

_____
_____
_____
_____
_____

↻ TERMINOLOGY REVIEW

Medical Term	Word Parts	Definition
Amplitude		Refers to amount, extent, size, abundance, or fullness.
Artifact		Additional electrical activity picked up by the electrocardiograph that interferes with the normal appearance of the ECG cycles.
Atherosclerosis	*ather/o-:* yellowish, fatty plaque *-sclerosis:* hardening of	Buildup of fibrous plaques of fatty deposits and cholesterol on the inner walls of an artery that causes narrowing, obstruction, and hardening of the artery.
Baseline		The flat horizontal line that separates the various waves of the ECG cycle.
Cardiac cycle	*cardi/o:* heart	One complete heartbeat.
Dysrhythmia	*dys-:* difficult, painful, abnormal *rhythm:* rhythm *-ia:* condition of diseased or abnormal state	An irregular heart rate or rhythm; also termed *arrhythmia.*
ECG cycle		The graphic representation of a heartbeat.
Electrocardiogram (ECG)	*electr/o-:* electrical, electrical activity *cardi/o:* heart *-gram:* record of	The graphic representation of the electrical activity of the heart.
Electrocardiograph	*electr/o-:* electrical, electrical activity *cardi/o:* heart *-graph:* instrument used to record	The instrument used to record the electrical activity of the heart.
Electrode	*electr/o-:* electrical, electrical activity	A conductor of electricity, which is used to promote contact between the body and the electrocardiograph.
Electrolyte	*electr/o-:* electrical, electrical activity	A chemical substance that promotes conduction of an electrical current.
Flow rate		The number of liters of oxygen per minute that come out of an oxygen delivery system.
Hypoxemia	*hypo-:* below, deficient *ox/i:* oxygen *-emia:* blood condition	A decrease in the oxygen saturation of the blood.
Hypoxia	*hypo-:* below, deficient *ox/i:* oxygen *-ia:* condition of diseased or abnormal state	A reduction in the oxygen supply to the tissues of the body.
Interval		The length of a wave or the length of a wave with a segment.
Ischemia	*isch/o-:* deficiency, blockage *-emia:* blood condition	Deficiency of blood in a body part.
Normal sinus rhythm		Refers to an ECG that is within normal limits.
Oxygen therapy		The administration of supplemental oxygen at concentrations greater than room air to treat or prevent hypoxemia.
Peak flow rate		The maximum volume of air that can be exhaled when the patient blows into a peak flow meter as forcefully and as rapidly as possible.
Segment		The portion of the ECG between two waves.
Spirometer	*spir/o-:* breathe, breathing *-meter:* instrument used to measure	An instrument for measuring air taken into and expelled from the lungs.
Spirometry	*spir/o-:* breathe, breathing *-metry:* measurement	Measurement of an individual's breathing capacity by means of a spirometer.
Wheezing		A continuous, high-pitched whistling musical sound heard particularly during exhalation and sometimes during inhalation.

ON THE WEB

For information on heart disease:

American Heart Association: www.americanheart.org

National Heart, Lung, and Blood Institute: www.nhlbi.nih.gov

American Association of Cardiovascular and Pulmonary Rehabilitation: www.aacvpr.org

My Heart Central: www.healthcentral.com/heart-disease

Cardiology Channel: www.cardiologychannel.com

American College of Cardiology: www.acc.org

The National Coalition for Women with Heart Disease: www.womenheart.org

For information on lung disease:

American Lung Association: www.lungusa.org

Pulmonary Channel: www.pulmonarychannel.com

Lung Cancer Online: www.lungcanceronline.org

American Association for Respiratory Care: www.aarc.org

Emphysema: emphysema.org

For information on smoking cessation:

Quit Net: www.quitnet.com

Smoking Cessation: www.smoking-cessation.org

National Center for Tobacco-free Kids: www.tobaccofreekids.org

Why Quit.com: www.whyquit.com

Quit Smoking Now: www.smokefree.gov

The Quit Smoking Company: www.quitsmoking.com

 Check out the Evolve site at http://evolve.elsevier.com/Bonewit/today/ to actively Prepare for your Certification, and to access additional interactive activities and exercises to help you study and prepare for success.

28

Specialty Examinations and Procedures: Colon Procedures, Male Reproductive Health, and Radiology and Diagnostic Imaging

LEARNING OBJECTIVES

Fecal Occult Blood Testing

1. Explain the purpose of a fecal occult blood test.

2. Describe the patient preparation for fecal occult blood testing (guaiac slide method).
3. Explain the purpose of each type of preparation for fecal occult blood testing (guaiac slide method).

Sigmoidoscopy

4. Explain the purpose of a digital rectal examination before a sigmoidoscopic examination.
5. Explain the purpose of a sigmoidoscopy.
6. Describe the patient preparation for a sigmoidoscopy.

Colonoscopy

7. Explain the purpose of a colonoscopy.

8. List the conditions that can be detected and assessed during a colonoscopy.
9. Describe the patient preparation for a colonoscopy.

Male Reproductive Health

10. List the symptoms of prostate cancer.

11. Explain the purpose of the digital rectal examination (DRE).
12. Explain the purpose of the prostate-specific antigen (PSA) test.
13. State the risk factors for testicular cancer.

14. Describe the TSE schedule.

PROCEDURES

Instruct a patient in the preparation and procedure for a fecal occult blood test (guaiac slide test).
Develop a fecal occult blood test.

Instruct a patient in the preparation required for a sigmoidoscopy.
Assist the physician with sigmoidoscopy.

Instruct a patient in the preparation required for a colonoscopy.

Assist the physician with a digital rectal examination.
Instruct a patient in the preparation for a PSA test.

Teach a patient how to perform a testicular self-examination (TSE).

LEARNING OBJECTIVES

Radiology

15. State the function of radiographs in medicine.
16. Explain the importance of proper patient preparation for a radiographic examination.
17. Explain the function of a contrast medium.
18. Describe the purpose of a fluoroscope.
19. Explain the purpose of each of the following types of radiographic examinations:
    Mammography
    Bone density scan
    Upper gastrointestinal radiography
    Lower gastrointestinal radiography
    Intravenous pyelography

Diagnostic Imaging

20. Explain the purpose of each of the following diagnostic imaging procedures:
    Ultrasonography
    Computed tomography
    Magnetic resonance imaging
    Nuclear medicine
21. Explain how nuclear medicine is used to produce an image of a body part or organ.
22. State the guidelines that may be required for nuclear medicine.

Digital Radiology

23. Explain the advantages of digital radiology.

PROCEDURES

Instruct a patient in the proper preparation necessary for each of the following types of radiographic examinations:
Mammography
Bone density scan
Upper gastrointestinal radiography
Lower gastrointestinal radiography
Intravenous pyelography

Instruct a patient on the purpose and advance preparation for each of the following diagnostic imaging procedures:
Ultrasonography
Computed tomography
Magnetic resonance imaging
Nuclear medicine

CHAPTER OUTLINE

biopsy (BIE-op-see)
colonoscope (KOL-un-oh-skope)
colonoscopy (KOL-un-OS-koe-pee)
contrast medium
echocardiogram
  (EK-oh-KAR-dee-oh-gram)
endoscope (EN-doe-skope)
enema (EN-em-ah)

fluoroscope (FLOOR-oh-skope)
fluoroscopy (floor-OS-koe-pee)
insufflate (IN-suf-flate)
melena (ma-LEE-na)
occult (ah-KULT) blood
peroxidase (per-OKS-ih-dase)
radiograph (RAY-dee-oh-graf)
radiography (ray-dee-OG-rah-fee)

radiologist (ray-dee-AH-lah-jist)
radiology (ray-dee-AH-lah-jee)
radiolucent (ray-dee-oh-LOO-sent)
radiopaque (ray-dee-oh-PAYK)
sigmoidoscope (sig-MOYD-oh-skope)
sigmoidoscopy (sig-moyd-OS-koe-pee)
sonogram (SON-oh-gram)
ultrasonography (ul-trah-son-AH-grah-fee)

Colon Procedures

INTRODUCTION TO COLON PROCEDURES

Colon procedures are performed in the medical office or clinic and include the fecal occult blood test (FOBT), sigmoidoscopy, and sometimes colonoscopy, which are presented in this chapter. The FOBT is a screening test used to detect blood in the stool for the early detection of colorectal cancer. Stool specimens must be collected by the patient at home. Some patients initially may be reluctant to comply with the FOBT patient preparation requirements and collection of the stool specimens. The medical assistant can help by explaining the purpose of the test to the patient. If the patient understands the benefits to be derived from the test, he or she is more likely to participate as required.

Medical assistants are often responsible for explaining to a patient the preparation required for a sigmoidoscopy and colonoscopy. The medical assistant should make sure the patient thoroughly understands the instructions. If the patient does not prepare properly, the procedure must be cancelled, which requires the patient to go through the preparation procedure again. The medical assistant assists the physician during a sigmoidoscopy, and he or she should have a thorough knowledge of the responsibilities accompanying this procedure.

BLOOD IN THE STOOL

Blood in the stool can indicate a number of gastrointestinal conditions, including hemorrhoids, diverticulitis, polyps, colitis, upper gastrointestinal ulcers, and colorectal cancer. Some of these conditions (e.g., hemorrhoids) produce visible red blood on the outside of the stool, making it easy to detect. Blood entering the stool in an amount of 50 mL or greater from conditions affecting the upper gastrointestinal tract (e.g., peptic ulcers) causes the stool to exhibit **melena,** meaning it is black and tarlike. The dark color is a result of oxidation of the iron in the blood (heme) by intestinal and bacterial enzymes. If a minute quantity of blood is present, however, it is not possible to detect it with the unaided eye. This hidden, or nonvisible, blood is termed **occult blood,** and its presence can be determined by testing the stool for blood.

Colorectal cancer is one of the most common forms of cancer in individuals older than the age of 50 years (see *Highlight on Colorectal Cancer*). During the early asymptomatic stages, almost all lesions (e.g., benign and malignant tumors) of the colon and rectum bleed a small amount on an intermittent basis, and this is usually in the form of occult blood. Discovery of occult blood in the stool does not mean that a patient has colorectal cancer. It does, however, warrant further diagnostic procedures, such as a colonoscopy, to determine if colorectal cancer is present. Early diagnosis and treatment of colorectal cancer increase the patient's survival rate. In most cases, when more pronounced symptoms of colorectal cancer start to appear (e.g., visible bleeding from the rectum, a change in bowel habits, abdominal pain), the cancer has reached an advanced stage.

FECAL OCCULT BLOOD TEST

Guaiac Slide Test

Routine screening of stool specimens for occult blood is frequently performed in the medical office. The guaiac slide test is a chemical test used to screen for fecal occult blood and is discussed in detail in this chapter. This test is commercially available with the brand names of Hemoccult, ColoScreen (Figure 28-1), and Seracult.

Fecal blood loss greater than 5 mL per day results in a positive reaction on a guaiac slide test. Individuals normally may lose up to 3 mL per day of blood in the feces, owing to minor insignificant abrasions of the nasopharynx and gastrointestinal tract, such as from brushing the teeth. To allow for normal blood loss, the guaiac slide test does not show a positive reaction until the blood in the stool reaches a level of 5 mL (or more) per day.

The guaiac slide test is a simple and inexpensive method to screen for the presence of fecal occult blood; however, care must be taken to reduce the occurrence of false-positive and false-negative test results. This test is designed to assess the presence of blood in stool specimens collected from three bowel movements on three different days. The purpose of using three specimens is to provide for the detection of blood from gastrointestinal lesions that exhibit intermittent bleeding, meaning they do not bleed every day. The patient must collect the three specimens at home and return the prepared slides to the medical office for developing. The medical assistant is responsible for providing the patient with instructions on patient preparation and collection and proper care and storage of the slides until they are returned to the medical office.

Purpose

The primary use of the guaiac slide test is to screen for the presence of occult blood caused by colorectal cancer. Other conditions that can cause blood in the stool include the following:

- Hemorrhoids
- Anal fissures
- Colorectal polyps
- Diverticulitis

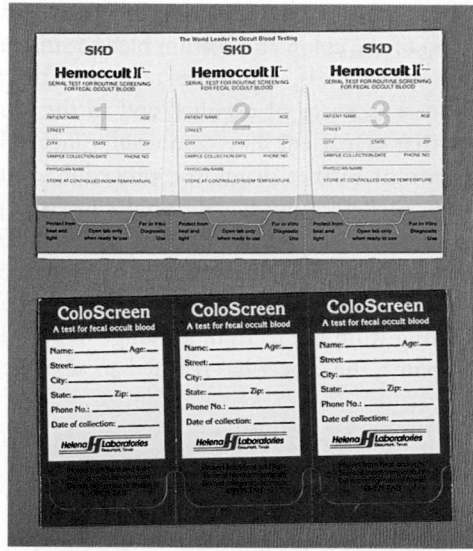

Figure 28-1 Examples of fecal occult blood testing kits. Hemoccult *(top)* and ColoScreen *(bottom)*.

- Peptic ulcers
- Ulcerative colitis
- Gastroesophageal reflux disease (GERD)
- Crohn disease

A positive test result on the guaiac slide test indicates only the presence of blood in the stool; the source and cause of the bleeding must still be determined. This means that additional diagnostic procedures must be performed before the physician can make a final diagnosis. These procedures may include colonoscopy, sigmoidoscopy, a double-contrast barium enema radiographic study, computed tomography (CT) colonography, and a newer procedure known as *capsule endoscopy*, which uses a tiny wireless camera (that the patient swallows as a pill) to take photographs of the digestive tract.

Patient Preparation

Patient preparation for a guaiac slide test plays an important role in ensuring accurate test results. The patient must follow a special diet, beginning 3 days before the test, and must continue the diet until all three slides have been prepared. The patient is placed on a high-fiber, meat-free diet. Meat contains animal blood, which could lead to a false-positive test result. A high-fiber diet is used because it encourages bleeding from lesions that may bleed only occasionally. In addition, fiber adds bulk, which promotes bowel elimination and ensures adequate specimen collection.

Certain medications irritate the gastrointestinal tract, which may result in a small amount of bleeding, and thus could result in a false-positive result on the guaiac slide test. Medications that should be avoided include ibuprofen (Motrin, Advil), naproxen (Aleve), and more than one adult aspirin per day. In addition, an iron supplement may cause a false-positive result, and a vitamin C supplement (greater than 250 mg per day) can cause a false-negative result. All

---

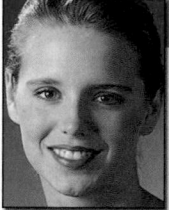

Putting It All into Practice

My name is Megan Baer, and I work in a large clinic that includes the specialties of family practice, gastroenterology, allergies, and dermatology. I am the clinical supervisor and oversee all of the clinical medical assistants and our "in-house" laboratory. I work closely with all physicians to meet the growing needs of the clinic.

Working with a gastroenterologist has been interesting and educational. When preparing a patient for a sigmoidoscopy, you must help the patient feel relaxed. This is an embarrassing situation for the patient, so you need to make him or her feel as comfortable as possible and maintain the patient's privacy and modesty. During the procedure, I talk to patients about the weather, their pets, and other interests to make them feel more relaxed and comfortable. This can help take their mind off the procedure.

One day I was assisting with a sigmoidoscopic examination, and a few minutes into the procedure the look on the physician's face told me something was wrong. When the examination was

finished, the physician and I left the room and went back to his office. He informed me that what he saw on his examination was colorectal cancer, and at this stage, not much could be done for the patient. The worst thing a physician has to do is give unpleasant news to a patient and see the look on the patient's face. Going into the room of a patient who has just received life-threatening information is something you don't forget. All you can do is be sympathetic and understanding and be a good listener. You have to be strong and not show your emotions even though your heart is breaking for the patient and the family. Always let patients know you are there for them.

Being with a patient who receives bad news about his or her health can make you think about your own life, and how it affects not only you, but also your family and friends. I often think of how I would feel about receiving such news. I try to put myself in the patient's place and to be sincere and understanding and willing to lend an ear. ■

Table 28-1 Patient Preparation for the Fecal Occult Guaiac Slide Test

Dietary and Medication Guidelines

Beginning 3 days before obtaining the first stool specimen, the patient should follow certain diet and medication modifications. These modifications should be followed until all three slides have been prepared.

Meats	Eat no red or rare meat (beef and lamb) or liver. Small amounts of well-cooked pork, poultry, and fish are permitted. Red meat contains animal blood that could cause a false-positive test result.
Vegetables	Eat moderate amounts of raw and cooked vegetables. Especially advised are lettuce, spinach, corn, and celery. Do not consume horseradish, turnips, broccoli, cauliflower, and radishes. These foods contain peroxidase, which sometimes can cause a false-positive test result.
Fruits	Eat moderate amounts of apples, bananas, oranges, peaches, pears, and plums. Avoid vitamin C in excess of 250 mg a day from citrus fruits and juices. Do not consume melons, because they contain peroxidase.
Miscellaneous high-fiber foods	Eat moderate amounts of whole-wheat bread, bran cereal, and popcorn. Foods high in fiber provide roughage to promote bowel elimination and encourage bleeding from "silent" lesions that bleed only occasionally.
Medications	Do not take medications or vitamin supplements that contain iron or vitamin C in excess of 250 mg for 3 days before and during the collection period. In addition, based on the patient's medication therapy, the physician may stipulate additional medication restrictions. Certain medications cause irritation of the gastrointestinal tract, which may result in a small amount of bleeding. Nonsteroidal antiinflammatory drugs (NSAIDs) and more than one adult aspirin a day should be avoided for at least 7 days before and continuing through the test period. Examples of NSAIDs include ibuprofen (Advil, Motrin) and naproxen (Aleve). Acetaminophen (Tylenol) can be taken as needed.
Special guidelines	Inform the physician, and do not consume any of the food items listed previously if you know, from past experience, that they cause you severe gastrointestinal discomfort or serious diarrhea. Ensure that the diet modifications have been followed for 3 days before collecting the first stool specimen.
	Do not initiate the test during a menstrual period or in the first 3 days after a menstrual period. The test should not be conducted when blood is visible in the stool or urine, such as from bleeding from hemorrhoids or a urinary tract infection. These conditions would result in false-positive test results. Store the slides with the flaps in a closed position at room temperature, and protect them from heat, sunlight, and fluorescent light. The slides must also be stored away from volatile chemicals such as ammonia, bleach, and other household cleaners. Improper storage can result in deterioration of the active reagents on the slides, leading to inaccurate test results.

of these substances should be discontinued before testing. Table 28-1 lists the specific patient preparation requirements for fecal occult blood testing using the guaiac slide test.

Quality Control

Quality control methods must be employed with the guaiac slide test to ensure reliable and valid results. It is important to properly store the box containing the guaiac slides and developing solution. Adverse storage conditions can result in deterioration of the developing solution and the active reagents impregnated on the filter paper of the slides, leading to inaccurate test results. The box must be stored at a room temperature between 59° F (15° C) and 86° F (30° C). The contents of the box must be protected from heat, sunlight, and strong fluorescent light. In addition, the box should not be stored in close proximity to volatile chemicals such as ammonia, bleach, bromine, iodine, and disinfectant cleaners. If stored properly, the slides and developer will remain effective until the expiration date that is stamped on the side of the box, each slide itself, and the container of developing solution.

A quality control procedure must be performed *after* the patient's test has been developed, read, and interpreted. This ensures that the test results are accurate and valid. The

Hemoccult slide test contains an on-slide performance monitor that consists of positive and negative monitor areas. This monitor is located on the developing side of the filter paper under the back flap of the cardboard slide. The positive monitor area contains a control chemical that has been impregnated into the filter paper during the manufacturing process.

The medical assistant should apply 1 drop of the developing solution between the positive and negative performance monitor areas on each of the three slides. The results must be read within 10 seconds after application of the developer. If the slides and developer are functioning properly, the positive area turns blue, whereas the negative area shows no color change. Failure of the expected control results to occur indicates an error, and the test results are not considered valid; possible causes include the use of outdated slides or developing solution; an error in technique; and subjection of the slides to heat, sunlight, strong fluorescent light, or volatile chemicals. Procedure 28-1 outlines the medical assistant's responsibilities related to fecal occult blood testing using the Hemoccult guaiac slide test. Procedure 28-2 describes the development of a Hemoccult slide test.

Text continued on p. 661

Case Study 1
Beatrice Bernard is 52 years old and has come to the office for a physical examination. The physician wants Mrs. Bernard to perform a Hemoccult test. After being told the purpose of the test and how to prepare for it, Mrs. Bernard expresses some concerns. She does not like the idea of what she has to do to perform the test because it does not seem sanitary to her. She also thinks it will be a lot of work to prepare for the test. She has red meat for dinner at least four times a week, and she does not understand why she has to eliminate it from her meals. She says she takes a baby aspirin every day for "heart health" and would prefer not to stop taking it. Mrs. Bernard says that she has always taken very good care of herself, and she has never had problems with her colon. She also says no history of colon cancer has been reported in her family. Mrs. Bernard is too embarrassed to talk about this topic with the physician. She says she may just throw the test away when she gets home. ■

Highlight on Colorectal Cancer

Incidence
Colorectal cancer is used to describe both cancer of the colon and cancer of the rectum. Based on what area is affected, these cancers are often referred to separately as *colon cancer* (see illustration below) and *rectal cancer*. Colorectal cancer is the third leading cause of cancer-related deaths in the United States for both men and women. According to the American Cancer Society, every year approximately 150,000 people are diagnosed with colorectal cancer, and approximately 50,000 people die every year from this disease. As the U.S. population of baby boomers ages, these numbers may increase.

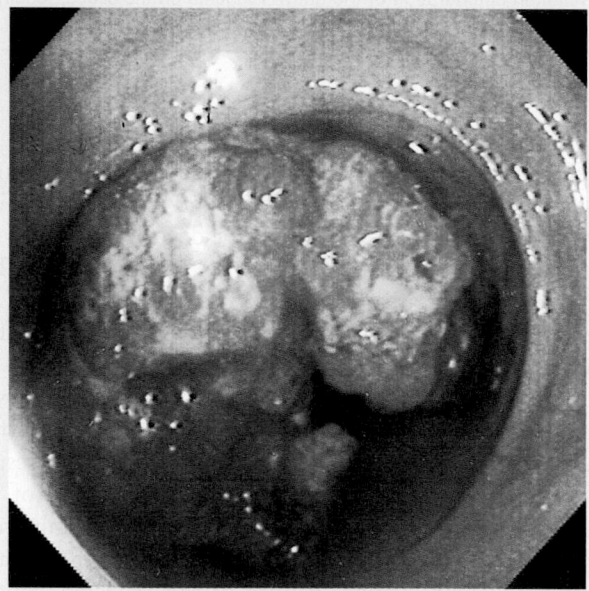
Colon cancer.

Risk factors
The following factors increase the risk of developing colorectal cancer:
- *Age.* The risk of colorectal cancer increases significantly after 50 years of age and reaches a peak from ages 60 to 75 years. More than 90% of individuals diagnosed with colorectal cancer are older than 50 years of age.
- *Colorectal polyps.* A colorectal *polyp* is a grapelike growth that protrudes from the inner lining (mucosa) of the colon or rectum (see Figure 28-7). Individuals with large polyps or numerous polyps are particularly at risk for colorectal cancer. Most cases of colorectal cancer arise from *adenomatous* polyps that gradually become malignant over many years. Colorectal polyps are fairly common in individuals older than 50 years of age. Approximately 1 in 20 colorectal polyps can become cancerous if not removed.
- *Personal history of colorectal cancer.* Individuals who have been diagnosed previously with colorectal cancer are at higher risk for developing it in other parts of the colon and rectum, even if it was completely removed.
- History of inflammatory bowel disease of long duration, such as ulcerative colitis and Crohn disease
- Strong family history of colorectal cancer
- Known family history of hereditary colorectal cancer syndromes such as familial adenomatous polyposis (FAP) or hereditary nonpolyposis colon cancer (HNPCC)
- Other factors that have been associated with a higher incidence of colorectal cancer include smoking; heavy alcohol consumption; obesity; a diet high in fat, red meat, and processed meats (e.g., hot dogs, luncheon meats); low intake of fresh fruits and vegetables; and physical inactivity.

Symptoms
No or very few symptoms occur during the early stages of colorectal cancer. If colorectal cancer is detected and treated while the patient is still asymptomatic, the patient has a 90% chance of 5-year survival. By comparison, the 5-year survival rate for patients in whom colorectal cancer is diagnosed after symptoms appear is only 40%, and the 5-year survival rate when the cancer has spread to distant organs (metastasized) such as the liver or lungs is only 11%.

Symptoms that occur when colorectal cancer is more developed include the following:
- Bleeding from the rectum
- Blood in the stool
- A change in the shape of the stool (e.g., stools that are narrower than usual)
- A change in bowel habits (e.g., diarrhea, constipation)
- General abdominal discomfort (e.g., aches, pains, cramps)
- Unexplained weight loss
- Constant fatigue

Highlight on Colorectal Cancer—cont'd

Recommendations for early detection

For the early prevention and detection of colorectal cancer, the American Cancer Society recommends that all adults 50 years old and older who are at average risk for colorectal cancer be screened using one of the screening tests listed below. Tests that detect both polyps and cancer are preferred over those tests that detect just cancer. Individuals with risk factors for colorectal cancer should be screened at an earlier age and with greater frequency. For example, an individual who has a family history of colorectal cancer should begin colorectal cancer screening at 40 years of age.

Tests that detect both polyps and cancer include the following:
- Sigmoidoscopy: every 5 years*
- Colonoscopy: every 10 years

- Double-contrast barium enema: every 5 years*
- CT colonography (virtual colonoscopy): every 5 years*

Tests that detect cancer only include these:
- Fecal occult blood test: every year*
- Fecal immunochemical test: every year*
- Fecal DNA test: interval uncertain*

Cause

The cause of colorectal cancer is unknown, but studies have shown a higher incidence of this disease in countries, such as the United States, whose populations have a diet that is high in meat and animal fat and low in fiber. This finding is supported by the fact that in countries such as Japan, in which the diet is high in fiber and low in fat, the incidence of colorectal cancer is much lower. ■

*Colonoscopy should be performed if test results are positive.

PROCEDURE 28-1   Fecal Occult Blood Testing: Guaiac Slide Test

Outcome   Instruct a patient in specimen collection for a Hemoccult guaiac slide test.

Equipment/Supplies

- Hemoccult slide testing kit

1. Procedural Step. Obtain a Hemoccult testing kit. Check the expiration date on the slides.
Principle. Outdated slides can lead to inaccurate test results.

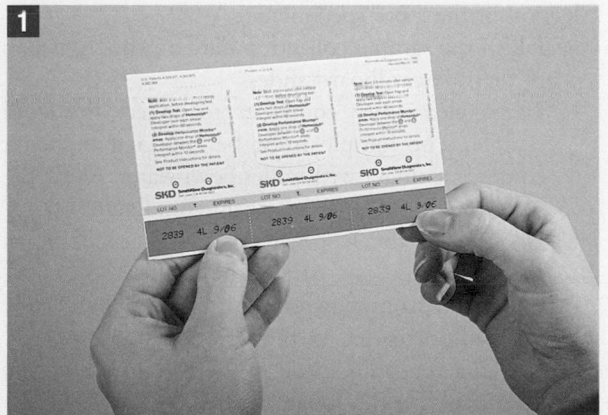

Check the expiration date.

2. Procedural Step. Greet the patient and introduce yourself. Identify the patient and explain the purpose of the test. Tell the patient that the test should not be conducted during a menstrual period or when hemorrhoids are bleeding or a urinary tract infection is present.
Principle. Bleeding from other (identifiable) sources causes a false-positive test result.

3. Procedural Step. Instruct the patient in proper preparation for the test. See the box *Highlight on Colorectal Cancer* for the specific guidelines the patient should follow. Tell the patient to begin the diet modifications 3 days before collecting the first stool specimen. Encourage the patient to adhere to the diet modifications.
Principle. The diet modifications may discourage patient compliance. The medical assistant should reinforce the importance of adhering to the diet requirements. Improper patient preparation can lead to inaccurate test results.

4. Procedural Step. Provide the patient with the Hemoccult testing kit. The kit consists of three identical cardboard slides attached to one another; each slide contains two squares, labeled "A" and "B." Three wooden applicator sticks and written instructions also are included in the testing kit.

Continued

PROCEDURE 28-1

PROCEDURE 28-1 Fecal Occult Blood Testing: Guaiac Slide Test—cont'd

Principle. Three slides are provided so that three stool specimens can be collected. The two squares in each slide (A and B) contain filter paper impregnated with guaiac, a chemical necessary for detection of blood in the stool.

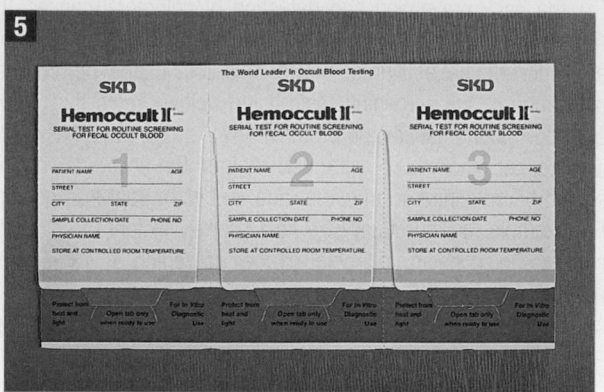

Instruct the patient on how to complete the information section on the slides.

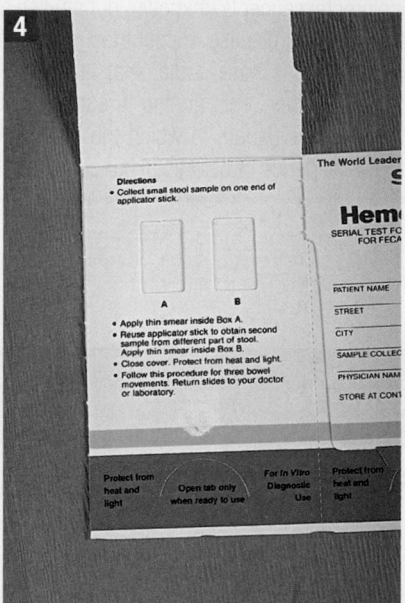

Each slide contains two squares labeled "A" and "B."

5. **Procedural Step.** Instruct the patient on completion of the information required on the front flap of each card. This includes the patient's name, address, phone number, and age and the date of the specimen collection. A ballpoint pen should be used to write this information.

6. **Procedural Step.** Provide instructions on proper care and storage of the slides. Make it clear that the slides must be stored (with the flaps in a closed position) at room temperature and protected from heat, sunlight, strong fluorescent light, and volatile chemicals.

Principle. Adverse storage conditions can result in deterioration of the active reagents impregnated on the filter paper, leading to inaccurate test results.

7. **Procedural Step.** Instruct the patient on initiation of the test by telling him or her to begin the diet modifications and then to collect a stool specimen from the first bowel movement after the 3-day preparatory period.

8. **Procedural Step.** Instruct the patient on proper collection of the stool specimen:

a. Fill in the sample collection date on the front flap of the first cardboard slide.

b. Use a clean, dry container to collect the stool sample. The sample must be collected before it comes in contact with toilet bowl water. Allow the stool to fall into the collection container.

c. Use one of the wooden applicators to obtain a specimen from one part of the stool sample.

d. Open the front flap of the first cardboard slide (located on the left in the series of three).

e. Spread a very thin smear of the specimen over the filter paper in the square labeled "A."

f. Using the same wooden applicator, obtain another specimen from a different area of the stool.

g. Spread a thin smear of the specimen over the filter paper in the square labeled "B."

h. Close the front flap of the cardboard slide.

PROCEDURE 28-1   Fecal Occult Blood Testing: Guaiac Slide Test—cont'd

i. Discard the wooden applicator in a waste container. Do not flush it down the toilet.

j. Place the slides in a regular paper envelope to air-dry overnight.

Principle. Two squares are included in each slide to allow specimen collection from different parts of the stool because occult blood is not always uniformly distributed throughout the stool. Thick specimens prevent adequate light penetration through the filter paper, making it difficult to interpret the test results.

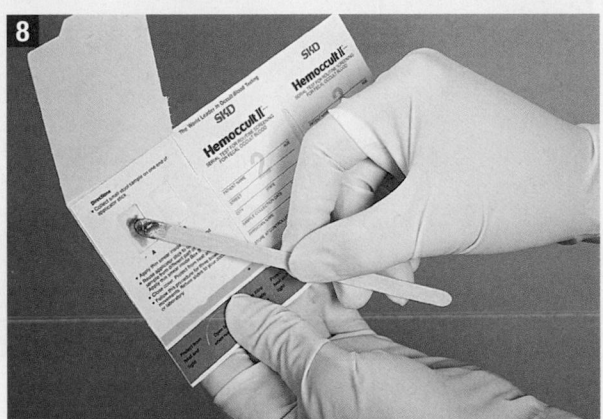

Spread a thin smear of the specimen over the filter paper.

9. **Procedural Step.** Instruct the patient to continue the testing period on 3 different days until all three specimens have been obtained as follows.

a. Repeat Procedural Step 8 after the second bowel movement the next day. If you do not have a bowel movement on the next day, then collect the specimen on the following day. The specimens should be collected on 3 different days. Use the cardboard slide located in the middle of the series of three.

b. Repeat Procedural Step 8 after the third bowel movement, using the cardboard slide located to the right in the series of three.

c. Allow the completed slides to air-dry overnight in the paper envelope.

10. **Procedural Step.** Instruct the patient to place the cardboard slides in the envelope lined with foil, seal carefully, and return them as soon as possible to the medical office. Emphasize to the patient that only the foil-lined envelope can be used to mail the slides; a standard envelope cannot be used. Inform the patient that the slides must be returned no later than 14 days after the first specimen is collected.

Principle. Standard paper envelopes are not approved by U.S. postal regulations for mailing fecal occult blood testing slides. Slides should not be developed after 14 days, as the test results may not be accurate.

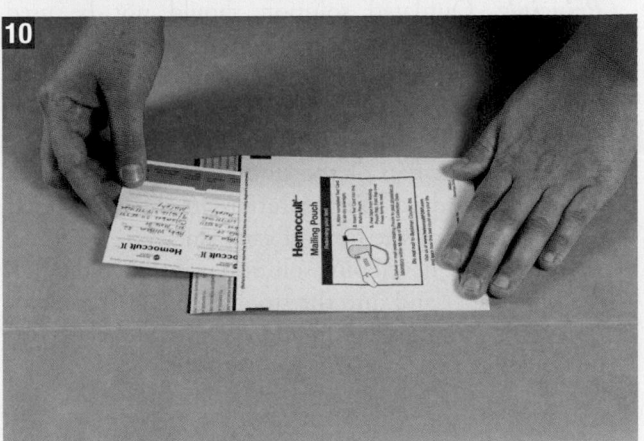

Place the cardboard slides in the envelope.

11. **Procedural Step.** Give the patient an opportunity to ask questions; ensure that the patient understands the instructions for patient preparation and collection of the stool specimen and for storage of the slides.

Principle. Improper patient preparation and poor collection technique can lead to inaccurate test results.

12. **Procedural Step.** Record in the patient's chart. Include the date and documentation that the Hemoccult test and instructions were given to the patient.

Note: The ColoScreen and Seracult guaiac slide tests use a procedure similar to that of the Hemoccult test.

OTHER TYPES OF STOOL TESTS

Two types of newer tests are now available to screen for colorectal cancer. They include the fecal immunochemical test and the fecal DNA test.

Fecal Immunochemical Test

The fecal immunochemical test (FIT) is a fecal occult blood test that uses antibodies to detect blood in the stool. Examples of brand names for this test are Hemoccult ICT and QuickVue iFOB (Figure 28-2). The stool specimen for an FIT is collected by the patient at home in a similar manner to the guaiac slide test. Although the FIT is more expensive than the guaiac slide test, it is more sensitive to the presence of lower gastrointestinal (GI) bleeding than is the guaiac test. This test is not affected by drugs or food and therefore does not require medication or dietary restrictions. In addition, FIT has fewer false-positive test results

PROCEDURE 28-2   Developing the Hemoccult Slide Test

Outcome Develop a Hemoccult slide test.

Equipment/Supplies

- Disposable gloves
- Prepared cardboard slides
- Hemoccult developing solution
- Waste container

1. Procedural Step. Assemble the equipment. Check the expiration date on the developing solution bottle. The developing solution contains hydrogen peroxide and must be stored away from heat and light. It must be tightly capped when not in use.

Principle. Outdated solution should not be used because it can lead to inaccurate test results. The solution should be stored properly because it is flammable and evaporates easily.

2. Procedural Step. Sanitize your hands and apply gloves. Open the back flap of the cardboard slides. Apply 2 drops of the developing solution to the guaiac test paper underlying the back of each smear.

Principle. The developing solution is absorbed through the filter paper and into the stool specimen. This solution could irritate the skin and eyes; if contact occurs, immediately rinse the area with water.

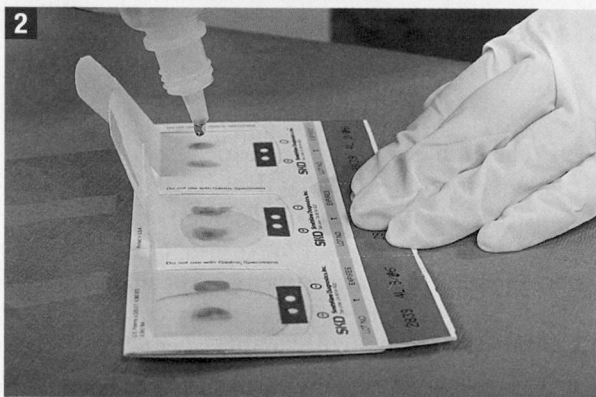

Apply 2 drops of developing solution.

3. Procedural Step. Read the results within 60 seconds. Fecal blood loss greater than 5 mL per day results in a positive reaction, which is indicated by any trace of blue on or at the edge of the fecal smear. If no detectable color change occurs, the result is considered negative.

Principle. In the presence of hydrogen peroxide, the heme compound in hemoglobin oxidizes guaiac, causing it to turn blue within 60 seconds after the developer is added. The reading time is important because the color reaction may fade after 2 to 4 minutes.

4. Procedural Step. Perform the quality control procedure as follows:

a. Apply 1 drop of developing solution between the positive and negative control performance indicators on each of the three slides.

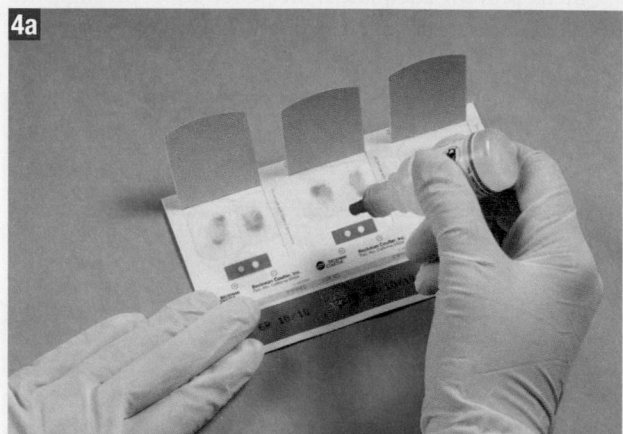

Apply 1 drop of developing solution to the control area.

b. Read the results within 10 seconds.

c. The positive area should turn blue and the negative area should show no color change. Failure of the expected control results to occur indicates an error and that the test results are invalid.

Principle. The quality control procedure must be performed after developing, reading, and interpreting the slides. Quality control procedures ensure the accuracy and reliability of the test results.

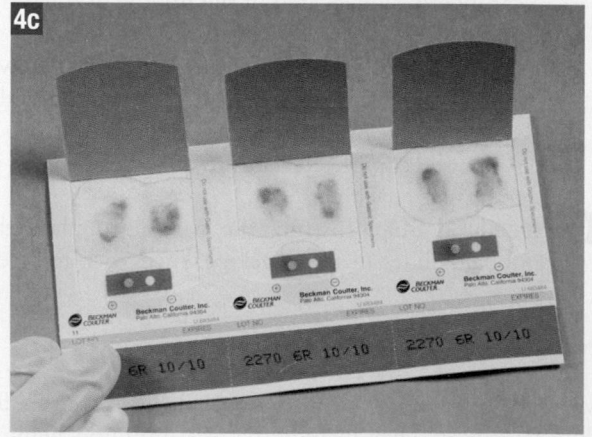

The positive control area should turn blue, and the negative control++ area should show no color change.

PROCEDURE 28-2 Developing the Hemoccult Slide Test—cont'd

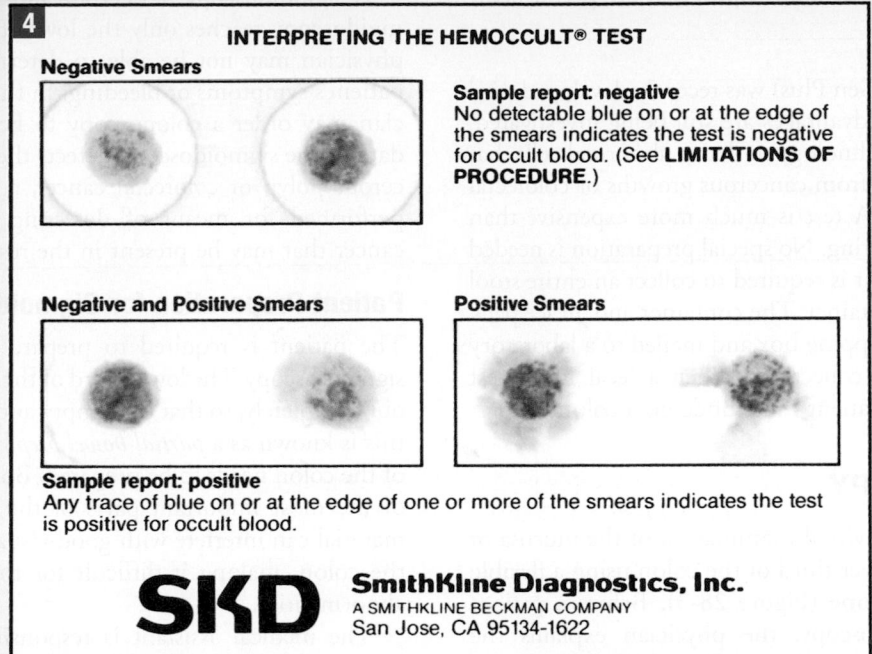

4

INTERPRETING THE HEMOCCULT® TEST

Negative Smears

Sample report: negative
No detectable blue on or at the edge of the smears indicates the test is negative for occult blood. (See **LIMITATIONS OF PROCEDURE**.)

Negative and Positive Smears

Positive Smears

Sample report: positive
Any trace of blue on or at the edge of one or more of the smears indicates the test is positive for occult blood.

SKD **SmithKline Diagnostics, Inc.**
A SMITHKLINE BECKMAN COMPANY
San Jose, CA 95134-1622

5. **Procedural Step.** Properly dispose of the Hemoccult slides in a regular waste container.
Principle. Fecal material is not considered regulated medical waste and can be discarded in a regular waste container.

6. **Procedural Step.** Remove gloves and sanitize your hands. Chart the results. Include the date and time, the brand name of the test (Hemoccult), and the test results for each slide (recorded as positive or negative).

CHARTING EXAMPLE

Date	
9/08/XX	9:00 a.m. Pt provided with a Hemoccult test and instructions for the procedure.
	———————— M. Baer, CMA (AAMA)
9/14/XX	10:30 a.m. Hemoccult test:
	Slide 1: Negative
	Slide 2: Negative
	Slide 3: Negative
	———————— M. Baer, CMA (AAMA)

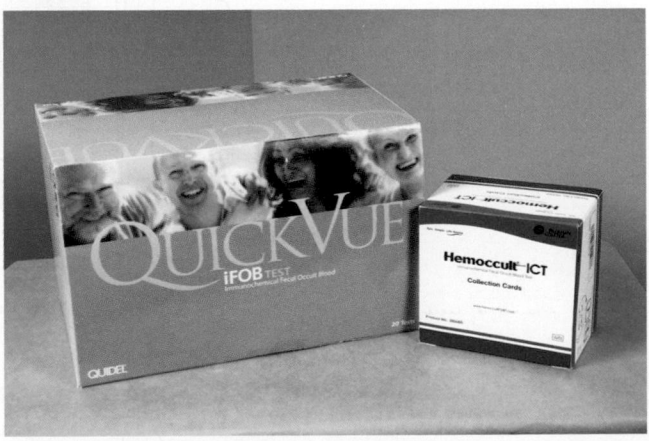

Figure 28-2 Fecal immunochemical tests: QuickVue iFOB *(left)* Hemoccult ICT *(right).*

than the guaiac slide test. When a fecal occult blood test is positive, the patient must undergo a colonoscopy. Reducing the number of false-positive test results, in turn, reduces the number of unnecessary colonoscopies that are performed.

Fecal DNA Test

A fecal DNA test (PreGen Plus) was recently developed, and its advantages and disadvantages are still being investigated. This test uses DNA technology to detect abnormal cells that are shed into the stool from cancerous growths or colorectal polyps. The fecal DNA test is much more expensive than other forms of stool testing. No special preparation is needed for this test. The patient is required to collect an entire stool sample in a special container. The container and an ice pack are then placed in a shipping box and mailed to a laboratory within 24 hours after collection. When a fecal DNA test result is positive, the patient must undergo a colonoscopy.

SIGMOIDOSCOPY

Sigmoidoscopy is the visual examination of the mucosa of the rectum and the lower third of the colon using a flexible fiberoptic **sigmoidoscope** (Figure 28-3). Before a patient undergoes a sigmoidoscopy, the physician explains the nature of the procedure and any risks to the patient and offers to answer questions. The medical assistant is responsible for obtaining the patient's signature on a written consent to treatment form, which grants the physician permission to perform the procedure.

Purpose

Sigmoidoscopy may be performed following a positive fecal occult blood test result to determine the source and cause of the bleeding. It is also performed to evaluate patient symptoms related to the colon such as lower abdominal pain, diarrhea, or constipation. Conditions that can be detected and assessed during a sigmoidoscopy include lesions (benign or malignant tumors), polyps, hemorrhoids,

fissures, infection, and inflammation. It is especially valuable as a diagnostic procedure for detecting inflammatory bowel disease such as ulcerative colitis and Crohn disease.

A sigmoidoscopy has certain limitations. Because a sigmoidoscopy reaches only the lower third of the colon, the physician may not be able to determine the cause of the patient's symptoms or bleeding. In this situation, the physician may order a colonoscopy to be performed at a later date. If the sigmoidoscopy detects the presence of a precancerous polyp or colorectal cancer, a colonoscopy must be performed for means of detecting additional polyps or cancer that may be present in the rest of the colon.

Patient Preparation for Sigmoidoscopy

The patient is required to prepare the colon before the sigmoidoscopy. The lower third of the colon must be flushed out completely, so that it is empty and free of fecal material; this is known as a *partial bowel prep* because only a portion of the colon needs to be prepared. Bowel preparation is one of the most important parts of the sigmoidoscopy. Fecal material can interfere with good visualization of the wall of the colon, making it difficult for the physician to detect abnormalities.

The medical assistant is responsible for providing the patient with instructions on preparing the colon. The medical assistant should encourage the patient to follow the instructions exactly. If the patient does not prepare properly, the sigmoidoscopy is usually cancelled and must be rescheduled, which requires the patient to go through the bowel preparation procedure again. The patient preparation instructions may vary slightly from one facility to another. General patient preparation recommendations for a sigmoidoscopy are outlined in Table 28-2.

Digital Rectal Examination

A digital examination of the anal canal and rectum is performed before a sigmoidoscopy. Using a well lubricated, gloved index finger, the physician palpates the rectum for

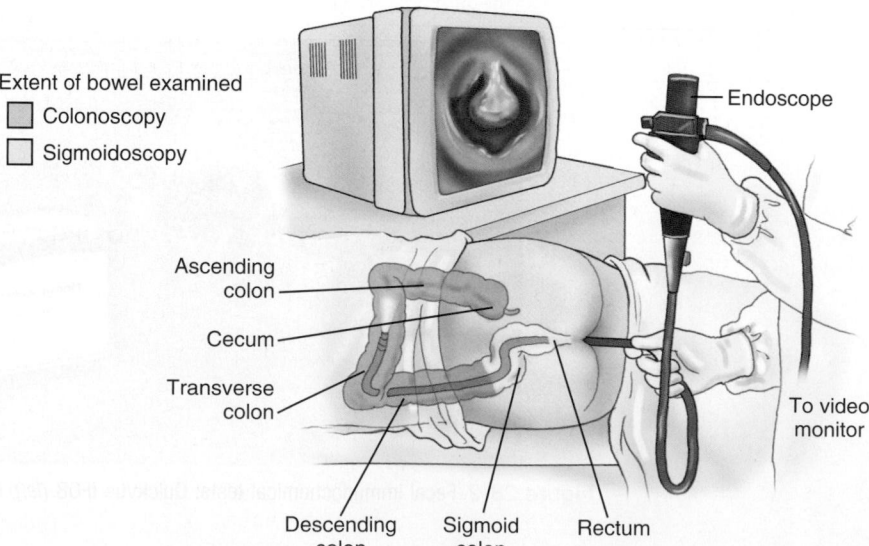

Figure 28-3 Sigmoidoscopy and colonoscopy.

Extent of bowel examined
☐ Colonoscopy
☐ Sigmoidoscopy

Endoscope

Ascending colon
Cecum
Transverse colon
To video monitor
Descending colon
Sigmoid colon
Rectum

Table 28-2 Patient Preparation for Sigmoidoscopy

It is important to follow the patient preparation requirements as carefully as possible to ensure accurate results. The following preparation is required for a sigmoidoscopy:

Beginning 5 days before the procedure	Discontinue taking iron, aspirin, and aspirin products. Iron can alter the color of the wall of the colon, and aspirin may cause bleeding if a polyp is removed from the colon.
Beginning 2 days before the procedure	Discontinue taking nonsteroidal antiinflammatory drugs such as ibuprofen and naproxen to minimize the risk of bleeding if a polyp is removed.
Medication restrictions	The physician will advise the patient of any other medication restrictions that need to be followed.
The day before the procedure and continuing until your examination is completed	a. Do not consume any solid food or milk products. b. Consume only gelatin (Jell-O) or popsicles (except purple or red, which could be mistaken for blood in the colon). c. Drink only clear liquids (water, apple juice, sport drinks [e.g., Gatorade], soft drinks, clear broth). Do not drink alcohol. d. Coffee or tea is permitted with no milk or cream.
The evening before the procedure	a. Drink the following laxative between 5 and 7 PM: one 10-ounce bottle of magnesium citrate. b. Continue drinking plenty of clear liquids throughout the evening.
The day of the procedure	a. You may continue drinking clear liquids until 4 hours before the procedure. b. Two hours before the examination: Insert one Fleet's enema rectally by following the package instructions. One hour before the procedure: Insert another Fleet's enema.

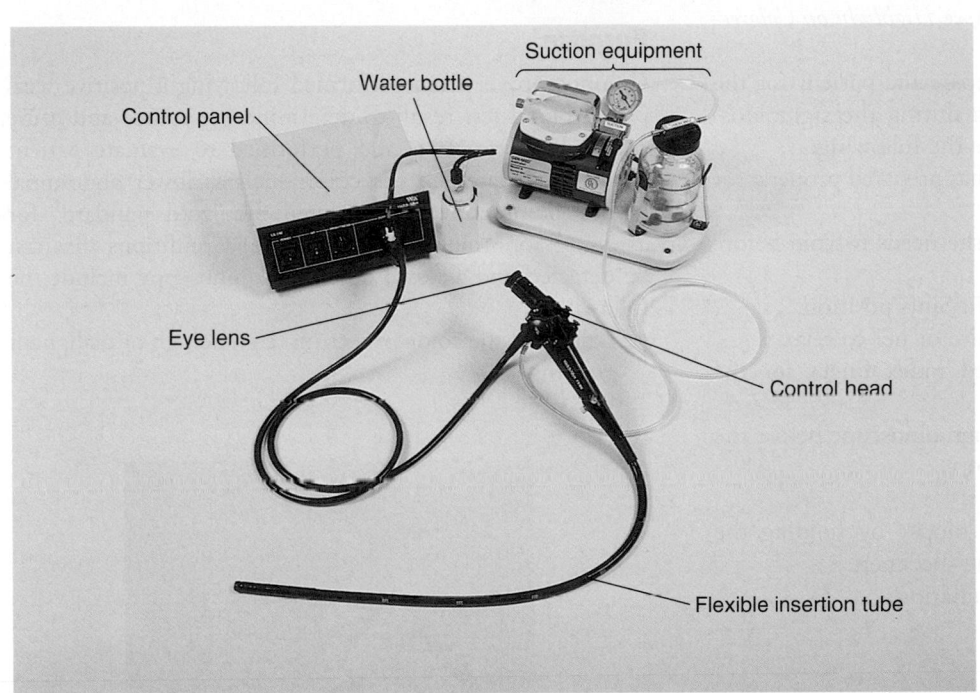

Figure 28-4 Flexible fiberoptic sigmoidoscope.

the presence of tenderness, hemorrhoids, polyps, and tumors. Any palpable abnormality is viewed directly when the endoscope is inserted. An **endoscope** is an instrument (e.g., sigmoidoscope, colonoscope) that consists of a tube and an optical system that is used for direct visual inspection of organs or cavities. The digital examination also helps relax the sphincter muscles of the anus and prepares the patient for the insertion of the endoscope.

Sigmoidoscope

A flexible fiberoptic sigmoidoscope consists of a control head and a long flexible insertion tube attached to a light source (Figure 28-4). The insertion tube is ½ inch (1.3 cm)

in diameter and 24 inches (60 cm) long, which allows the physician to view approximately one third of the colon, which includes the rectum and sigmoid colon.

The sigmoidoscope is composed of extremely thin fibers of bendable glass that transmit light and images of the colon back to the physician. The image, magnified ten times by the fiberoptic system, is viewed by the physician through the eye lens located in the handle of the sigmoidoscope. Alternatively, the sigmoidoscope may have a video camera attached to the distal end of the flexible insertion tube, which permits the physician to view images of the colon and rectum on a display screen (see Figure 28-3).

Procedure

When the sigmoidoscopy is performed, the patient is placed on his or her left side in the Sims position. The distal end of the sigmoidoscope is lubricated and inserted into the anus and rectum and then slowly advanced into the colon until it reaches the sigmoid colon. A small amount of air is usually blown, or **insufflated,** into the colon through tubing attached to the air control valve located on the head of the sigmoidoscope. The function of the air is to distend the lumen of the colon for better visualization. In addition, suction equipment can be used to remove secretions, such as mucus, blood, and liquid feces, which interfere with proper visualization of the intestinal mucosa. The physician then slowly withdraws the sigmoidoscope while carefully observing the mucosa of the colon for abnormalities.

If the physician discovers an abnormal lesion during the examination, a long thin instrument is passed through the lumen of the insertion tube to remove a specimen for **biopsy** (Figure 28-5). In addition, if a suspicious-looking polyp is discovered, the physician may remove it (polypectomy) or take a biopsy of it for analysis by the laboratory. Removal of a precancerous polyp prevents it from developing into colon cancer in the future (see *Highlight on Colorectal Cancer*).

The medical assistant must prepare the patient for the procedure and assist the physician during the sigmoidoscopy. These responsibilities include the following:

- Determine whether the patient has prepared properly for the sigmoidoscopy.
- Ask the patient whether he or she needs to void before the procedure.
- Position and drape the patient in Sims position.
- Reassure the patient and help him or her to relax.
- Lubricate the physician's gloved index finger for the digital examination.
- Lubricate the distal end of the sigmoidoscope before the physician inserts it (Figure 28-6).
- Assist with suction equipment.
- Assist with the collection of a biopsy by holding the specimen container to accept the specimen.
- Assist the patient after the examination.

- Prepare the biopsy specimen for transport to the laboratory.
- Clean the examining room.
- Sanitize and disinfect the sigmoidoscope.

COLONOSCOPY

A **colonoscopy** is the visual examination of the mucosa of the rectum and the entire length of the colon (sigmoid colon, descending colon, transverse colon, and ascending colon) using a flexible fiberoptic **colonoscope.** A colonoscope is basically a sigmoidoscope but with a longer insertion tube. The colonoscope has a video camera attached to the distal end of the flexible insertion tube. The camera transmits images of the colon to a video screen for viewing by the physician (see Figure 28-3).

Before a patient undergoes a colonoscopy, the physician explains the nature of the procedure and any risks to the patient and offers to answer questions. The medical assistant may be responsible for obtaining the patient's signature on a written consent to treatment form, which grants the physician permission to perform the procedure.

Purpose

Colonoscopy is often performed following a positive fecal occult blood test result to determine the source and cause of the bleeding. It is also performed to evaluate patient symptoms related to the colon such as lower abdominal pain. Colonoscopy is considered the "gold standard" for assessing abnormalities of the colon. Conditions that can be detected and assessed during a colonoscopy include the following:

- Lesions of the colon or rectum (e.g., benign or malignant growths)

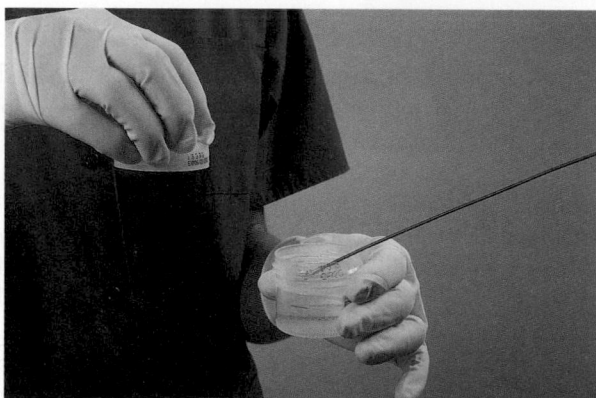

Figure 28-5 Collection of a specimen during a sigmoidoscopy.

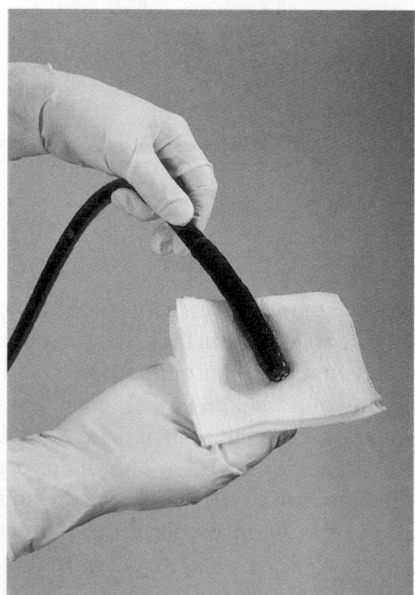

Figure 28-6 The distal end of the sigmoidoscope must be lubricated before insertion.

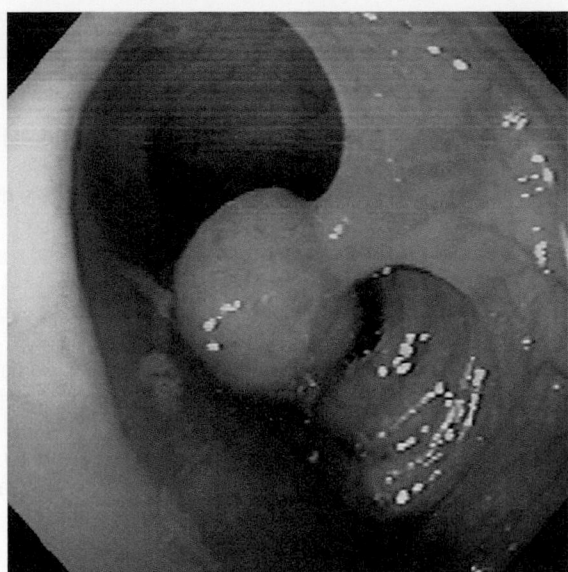

Figure 28-7 Colon polyp.

- Colorectal polyps (Figure 28-7)
- Hemorrhoids
- Fissures
- Infection and inflammation

Colonoscopy is particularly valuable for the early detection of symptomatic and asymptomatic colorectal cancer. Early detection of colorectal cancer leads to early diagnosis and treatment, which increases the chance of survival for patients with this disease.

Patient Preparation for Colonoscopy

A colonoscopy is usually performed in a hospital on an outpatient basis or in a large medical clinic. The rectum and the entire colon must be flushed out completely so that it is empty and free of fecal material; this is known as a *full bowel prep*. This is one of the most important parts of the colonoscopy. Fecal material can interfere with good visualization of the wall of the colon, making it difficult for the physician to detect abnormalities.

The medical assistant may be responsible for providing the patient with instructions on preparing the colon. The patient should be encouraged to follow the instructions exactly. If the patient does not prepare properly, the colonoscopy is usually cancelled and must be rescheduled, which requires the patient to go through the bowel preparation procedure again. The patient preparation instructions may vary from one facility to another. General patient preparation recommendations for a colonoscopy are outlined in Table 28-3, along with patient instructions following the procedure.

Procedure

A sedative is administered intravenously before the colonoscopy. The sedative causes the patient to become relaxed, sleepy, and less aware of what is taking place. Some patients do not remember the procedure at all afterward.

The procedure itself is similar to a sigmoidoscopy. The patient is placed on his or her left side in Sims position. The physician performs a digital rectal examination before inserting the colonoscope. The colonoscope is advanced all the way through the entire colon (approximately 4 to 5 feet) until it reaches the cecum. Air is inserted into the colon to distend it for better visualization. Suction is used to remove secretions such as mucus, blood, and liquid feces that interfere with proper visualization. The physician then slowly withdraws the colonoscope while carefully observing the mucosa of the colon for abnormalities.

If the physician discovers an abnormal lesion, a long thin instrument is passed through the lumen of the insertion tube to remove a specimen for biopsy. In addition, if a suspicious-looking polyp is discovered, the physician may remove it (polypectomy) or take a biopsy of it for analysis by the laboratory. Removal of a precancerous polyp prevents it from developing into colon cancer in the future.

Following the procedure, the patient may experience some bloating, abdominal cramping, and flatulence. If a polyp has been removed or if a biopsy has been performed, the patient may exhibit traces of blood in the stool for 1 to 2 days.

Male Reproductive Health

INTRODUCTION TO MALE REPRODUCTIVE HEALTH

Two important areas related to male reproductive health are prostate screening and testicular self-examination. Preventive examinations and tests can assist in the detection of prostate and testicular cancers. Both of these areas are described in the following section.

PROSTATE CANCER

According to the American Cancer Society, prostate cancer is the second most common cause of cancer deaths in men, lung cancer being the most common. Every year, approximately 200,000 men are diagnosed with prostate cancer, and approximately 27,000 die from this disease. The incidence of prostate cancer increases after age 50. Prostate cancer is found more often in African American men and men with a family history of prostate cancer.

The prostate gland surrounds the urethra and is located just below the bladder and in front of the rectum (Figure 28-8). It is approximately the size and shape of a walnut, and its function is to secrete fluid that transports sperm.

In the early stages, prostate cancer often causes no symptoms. Symptoms that occur when the cancer is more developed include the following:

- Difficulty in urinating
- Weak or interrupted urinary flow
- Pain or burning during urination
- Frequent urination, especially at night

Table 28-3 Patient Preparation for Colonoscopy

It is important to follow the patient preparation requirements as carefully as possible to ensure accurate results. The following preparation is required for a colonoscopy:

Beginning 5 days before the procedure	Discontinue taking iron, aspirin, and aspirin products. Iron can alter the color of the wall of the colon, and aspirin may cause bleeding if a polyp is removed from the colon.
Beginning 2 days before the procedure	Discontinue taking nonsteroidal antiinflammatory drugs such as ibuprofen and naproxen to minimize the risk of bleeding if a polyp is removed.
Medication restrictions	The physician will advise the patient of any other medication restrictions that need to be followed.
Beginning 1 day before the procedure and continuing until your examination is completed	a. Do not consume any solid food or milk products. b. Consume only gelatin (Jell-O) or popsicles (except purple or red, which could be mistaken for blood in the colon). c. Drink only clear liquids (water, apple juice, sport drinks [e.g., Gatorade], soft drinks, clear broth). Do not drink alcohol. d. Coffee or tea is permitted with no milk or cream.
Bowel preparation	Take a laxative on the afternoon (between 2 PM and 4 PM) before the procedure. The laxative is often in a powdered form (e.g., Colyte) and comes in a package that is attached to a plastic gallon container. Read the package instructions for preparing the laxative solution. The gallon container is filled with drinking water and mixed with the powdered laxative. After preparing the laxative solution, store it in the refrigerator. Most patients find it easier to drink the solution if it is chilled. a. Begin the bowel preparation by drinking one 8-ounce glass of the liquid laxative solution every 10 to 15 minutes until 2 quarts (eight 8-ounce glasses) have been consumed. It is best to drink the solution quickly rather than slowly sipping it. b. After drinking the first few glasses, you may experience nausea and a bloated feeling. This is temporary and will disappear once you start having bowel movements. If this occurs, you can slow down the drinking process or stop for 30 minutes and then resume drinking the solution every 15 minutes. c. Your first bowel movement should occur approximately 1 hour after you begin drinking the solution. You will need to have a bowel movement about 10 to 15 times. If your bowel movement is clear to pale yellow in color after drinking the first 2 quarts of the solution, you can stop drinking the solution. If your stool is not clear, continue drinking the solution every 15 minutes until your bowel movement is clear.
After midnight on the night before the examination	a. Do not eat or drink anything, including water. b. If medications need to be taken (as approved by the physician), take them with only a sip of water.
Transportation	Arrange to have someone drive you home following the procedure. You will be sedated during the procedure and cannot drive yourself, nor can you use public transportation.
Following the procedure	You may experience some bloating, abdominal cramping, and flatulence. If you had a polyp removed or a biopsy taken, it is normal to experience traces of blood in the stool for 1 to 2 days. Contact the office if you experience significant rectal bleeding, faintness, dizziness, shortness of breath, or heart palpitations.

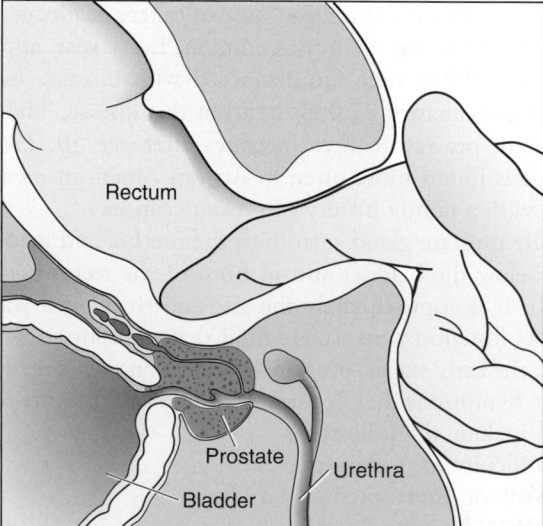

Figure 28-8 Digital rectal examination.

- Blood in the urine
- Pain in the lower back, pelvis, or upper thighs

PROSTATE CANCER SCREENING

The primary screening tests for prostate cancer are the digital rectal examination (DRE) and the prostate-specific antigen (PSA) test.

Digital Rectal Examination

The digital rectal examination (DRE) is a quick and simple procedure that causes only momentary discomfort. During the examination, the physician inserts a lubricated gloved finger into the patient's rectum. Because the prostate gland is located in front of the rectum, the physician is able to palpate the surface of the prostate gland through the rectal wall (see Figure 28-8). The physician palpates the gland to determine whether it is enlarged or has an abnormal consistency. Normally, the prostate gland should feel soft, whereas malignant tissue is firm and hard. The sensitivity of the DRE is limited, however, because the physician can palpate only the posterior and lateral aspects of the prostate gland.

Prostate-Specific Antigen Test

The prostate-specific antigen (PSA) test is a screening test that measures the amount of PSA in the blood. PSA is a protein normally produced by the cells of the membrane that covers the prostate gland. The normal range for PSA is 0 to 4 ng/mL of blood. The PSA level may become elevated in men who have a benign or malignant growth in the prostate. A PSA level of 4 to 10 ng/mL is considered slightly elevated; levels between 10 and 20 ng/mL are considered moderately elevated; and a value greater than 20 ng/mL is considered highly elevated. The higher the PSA level, the more likely that cancer is present. Other conditions (other than prostate cancer) that can cause an elevated PSA level include benign prostatic hyperplasia (BPH) and prostatitis.

The PSA level may normally increase after vigorous exercise, such as jogging or biking. The medical assistant should instruct the patient to engage only in normal activity for 2 days before having blood drawn for a PSA test. The patient also should be instructed not to have sexual intercourse for 2 days before the test because it can change the PSA level.

If the DRE is abnormal and/or the PSA test is elevated, further testing may be performed to determine whether prostate cancer is present. To make this assessment, one or more of the following tests may be performed: transrectal ultrasound (TRUS), biopsy of the prostate gland, bone scan, and computed tomography (CT) scan.

Recommendations for Prostate Screening

Screening refers to the process of testing an individual to detect a disease in that individual who is not yet experiencing symptoms of that disease. For certain types of cancer (e.g., colorectal cancer, cervical cancer), screening allows the cancer to be discovered early, when it is more treatable, which increases the patient's survival rate.

The DRE and PSA screening tests for prostate cancer have certain limitations. Abnormal results from both of these tests do not necessarily indicate that cancer is present. In addition, normal results from these tests do not mean that cancer is *not* present. An elevated PSA test may lead to a biopsy and the detection of cancer in an individual, which can pose a dilemma. Many prostate cancers are slow growing and do not result in the death of an individual, particularly if the man is older or in poor health. Because it is sometimes difficult to determine the aggressiveness of the cancer, these individuals may still be treated with surgery or radiation, which can seriously affect a man's quality of life.

The American Cancer Society (ACS) believes that available evidence does not currently support routine testing for prostate cancer. The ACS recommends that health care providers discuss the potential benefits and limitations of prostate screening with men older than 50 years of age.

Following this discussion, the PSA test and the DRE should be offered annually to men 50 years and older who are at average risk for prostate cancer and have at least a 10-year life expectancy. Those men who indicate a preference for testing should be tested. The ACS recommendation provides men with knowledge of the advantages and disadvantages of early detection and treatment of prostate cancer, which then allows them to share in the decision of whether or not to be tested.

What Would You Do? What Would You *Not* Do?

Case Study 2

Peter Bota, a 62-year-old retired Caucasian male, came to the medical office 1 week ago for a physical examination. The physician performed a DRE but did not palpate anything abnormal. At that visit, Mr. Bota's blood was drawn for a PSA test, and the results came back as slightly elevated (8 ng/mL). Mr. Bota has returned to the office and is waiting to talk with the physician about his test results and possible follow-up testing. Mr. Bota is extremely worried that he has cancer and wants to know the symptoms of prostate cancer. He also wants to know whether he did anything to cause prostate cancer. He says he does not smoke and drinks very little and that he walks his dog twice a day for exercise. ■

TESTICULAR SELF-EXAMINATION

The purpose of testicular self-examination (TSE) is early detection of testicular cancer. In the past 40 years, testicular cancer among young Caucasian men has more than doubled. Although testicular cancer can develop at any age, it is most common in males 15 to 34 years old. If detected early, it has a very high cure rate. Most cases of testicular cancer are detected by men themselves, either by accident or when performing a TSE. Certain risk factors increase a man's chance of getting testicular cancer, including the following:

- History of cryptorchidism (undescended testicles)
- Family history of testicular cancer
- Cancer of the other testicle
- Caucasian race (testicular cancer is five times more common in Caucasian men than in African American men)

TSE should be performed monthly, starting at 15 years of age. A good idea is for the patient to choose an easy-to-remember date each month, such as the first day of the month. The best time to perform the examination is after taking a warm bath or shower. Heat allows the scrotal skin to relax and become soft, making it easier to palpate the underlying testicular tissues.

The most common sign of testicular cancer is a small, hard, painless lump (about the size of a pea) located on the front or side of the testicle. Any abnormality of the testicles should be reported to the physician immediately. It does not mean that the patient has cancer, however; the

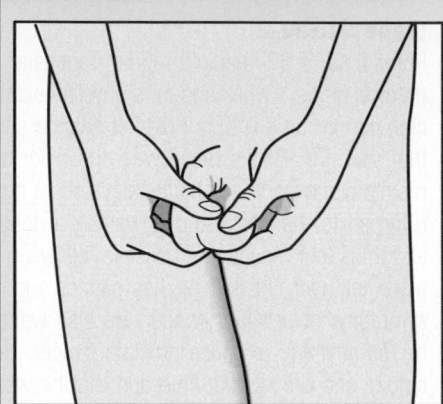

TESTICULAR SELF-EXAMINATION

1
Take a warm bath or shower.

2
Stand in front of a mirror. Look for any swelling of the skin of the scrotum.

3
Place the index and middle fingers of both hands on the underside of one testicle and the thumbs on top of the testicle.

4
Apply a small amount of pressure and gently roll the testicle between the thumb and fingers of both hands, feeling for lumps, swelling, or any change in the size, shape, or consistency of the testicle. A normal testicle should feel smooth, egg-shaped and rather firm. It is also normal for one testicle to be larger or hang lower than the other testicle.

5
Find the epididymis so that you do not confuse it with a lump. The epididymis is a soft tubular cord, located behind the testicle, that functions in storing and carrying sperm.
(Note: Tenderness in the area of the epididymis is considered normal.)

6
Repeat the examination outlined above on the other testicle.

7
Report any of the following abnormalities to the physician: any unusual lump, a feeling of heaviness in the scrotum, a dull ache in the lower abdomen or groin, enlargement of one of the testicles, tenderness or pain in a testicle, or any change in the way the testicle feels.

Figure 28-9 Testicular self-examination.

physician must make that determination. Figure 28-9 outlines the procedure for a TSE.

Radiology and Diagnostic Imaging
INTRODUCTION TO RADIOLOGY

Radiology is the branch of medicine that deals with the use of radiation and other imaging techniques (such as ultrasound, computed tomography [CT] scans, magnetic resonance imaging [MRI], and nuclear medicine) in the diagnosis and treatment of disease. A **radiologist** is a physician who specializes in the diagnosis and treatment of disease using radiation and other imaging techniques.

Wilhelm Konrad Roentgen, a German physicist, discovered x-rays on November 8, 1895, while working with a cathode ray tube. He noticed that these rays could pass through solid materials, such as paper, wood, and human skin. Because he did not know what they were, he named them *x-rays*. The rays have since been renamed *roentgen rays* after their discoverer; however, they are better known as "x-rays."

X-rays are high-energy electromagnetic waves that are invisible and have a short wavelength that enables them to penetrate solid materials. X-rays are used to visualize internal structures and serve as a diagnostic aid in determining the presence of disease. They are especially useful for detecting abnormal conditions associated with the skeletal system such as fractures. X-rays also are used therapeutically in the treatment of disease conditions, such as malignant neoplasms.

X-rays can be taken using the conventional film method or digitally with the use of a computer. The conventional film method is described in this section, and the digital method is described later in this chapter. When conventional radiographs are taken, radiographic film is loaded into a device known as an *x-ray cassette*. The cassette is placed behind the part being examined, and a shadow or image of the internal body structure photographed is produced on the film. After the x-ray has been taken, the film must be processed. A radiologic technician takes the cassette into a dark room and develops the image using an x-ray processor. **Radiograph** is the term for the permanent record of the picture produced on the radiographic film.

An orthopedic medical office may have its own radiograph machine, but more often radiographs are taken in a hospital by radiology personnel or a large medical clinic. Some radiographs, such as a chest x-ray, require no advance preparation, whereas others, such as a lower gastrointestinal (GI) study, require a great deal of special preparation. Medical assistants are usually responsible for patient instruction in the type of preparation necessary for a particular radiographic examination and for ensuring that the patient understands the importance of the preparation. If the patient does not prepare properly, the radiograph may be of poor quality, and the procedure may need to be rescheduled. This section provides an introduction to the study of radiographs, with a focus on the patient preparation necessary for common radiographs.

CONTRAST MEDIA

Radiography relies on differences in density between various body structures to produce shadows of varying intensity on the radiographic film. There is a difference in density between bone and flesh (bone is denser than flesh). Bone absorbs more x-rays and does not allow them to reach the radiographic film. This leaves that part of the film unexposed and causes white areas to appear on the processed film. If the x-rays penetrate an organ or structure, a black area appears on the film. Because the lungs contain air, x-rays are able to penetrate them easily. As a result, the lungs appear black on the processed film. The ribs absorb the x-rays and appear as white shadows on the film (Figure 28-10). A structure, such as lung tissue, that permits the passage of x-rays is **radiolucent.** A structure, such as bone, that obstructs the passage of x-rays and causes an image to be cast on the film is **radiopaque.**

In many cases, the natural densities of two adjacent organs or structures are similar. In this instance, a **contrast medium** (also known as a *contrast agent*) must be used to make a particular structure visible on the radiograph. Contrast media are usually radiopaque chemical compounds that cause the body tissue or organ to absorb more radiation. This absorption provides a contrast in density between the tissue or organ and the surrounding area. The tissue or organ becomes visible and appears white on the processed radiograph. Substances used as contrast media must be able to be ingested or injected into the body tissues or organs without causing harm to the patient. Contrast media are administered to the patient through various routes. Some are administered orally; others are injected into a vein or are delivered through an IV line or an enema.

Barium sulfate and inorganic iodine compounds are commonly used radiopaque contrast media. Barium sulfate is a chalky compound that is water-insoluble and does not allow penetration by x-rays. It is frequently used for examination of the GI tract because barium is not absorbed into the body through the GI tract and does not alter its normal function. Iodine salts are radiopaque and are combined with other compounds for radiographic examination of structures such as the urinary tract and blood vessels. Iodine contrast media consist of clear liquids and are usually injected. Iodine sometimes may produce an allergic reaction, and before administration, patients should be asked whether they have an allergy to iodine. Patients with known allergies may be given an iodine sensitivity test as a precautionary measure.

FLUOROSCOPY

A **fluoroscope** is an instrument used to view internal organs and structures of the body directly on a display screen. Examination of a patient with a fluoroscope is known as **fluoroscopy.** A radiopaque medium is often used with fluoroscopy to outline various parts of the body. The patient is positioned between the radiographic tube and a fluorescent screen composed of zinc cadmium sulfide crystals. When the x-rays pass through the body and strike the crystals, visible light is emitted so that the radiologist can view (on a screen) the action of body organs or structures, such as the stomach and intestines. During fluoroscopy, the radiologist can take radiographs that permit the study of the structure in detail and serve as a permanent record.

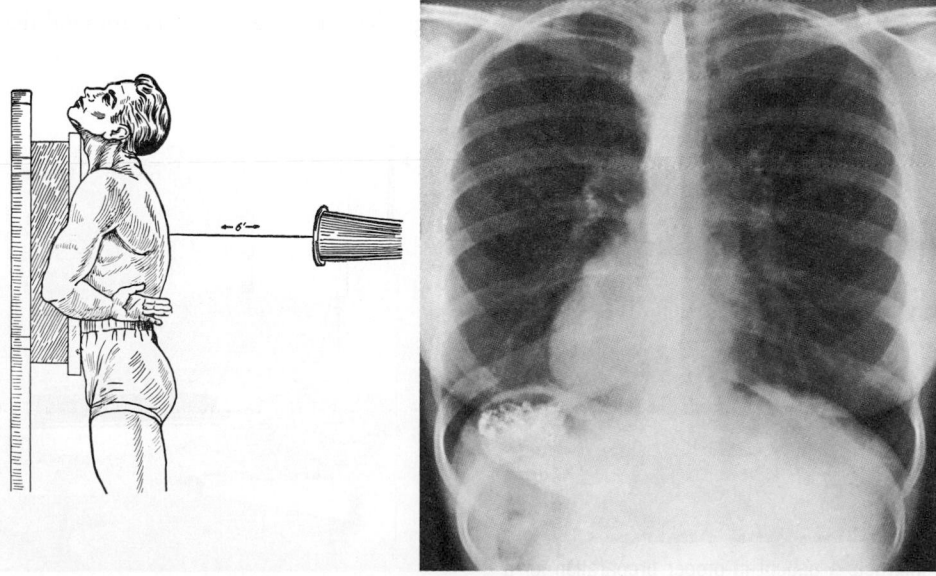

Figure 28-10 Posteroanterior view of the chest. Position of patient and radiograph.

POSITIONING THE PATIENT

The position of the patient is determined by the purpose of the examination and the area examined. The patient is generally positioned so that several different views can be taken to provide a complete three-dimensional picture of the part examined. Articles such as jewelry and hairpins must be removed so the image on the radiograph is not obscured. To prevent blurring of the image on the film, patients must maintain the position in which they are placed and not move during the radiographic examination. Blurring prevents good visualization of the part and may warrant retaking of the radiograph.

SPECIFIC RADIOGRAPHIC EXAMINATIONS

The medical assistant should understand the purpose of commonly performed radiographic examinations and should be able to instruct a patient on the proper preparation for each (Figure 28-11). Frequently performed radiographic examinations and the special advance preparation necessary for each are described. The preparation may vary, depending on the medical office.

Mammography

Mammography is a radiographic examination of the breasts used to detect many forms of breast disease, such as benign breast masses, breast calcifications, fibrocystic breast disease, and particularly breast cancer. It also is used to monitor the effects of surgery and radiation therapy on breast tumors.

Mammography uses low doses of x-rays that pass through the breast and create an image on a film. On the radiograph, an abnormal area appears noticeably different from normal breast tissue. Mammography can be used to detect a breast tumor when the growth is less than 1 cm in diameter (about the size of a pea) and before it is clinically palpable. A malignant lump can be removed at an early stage; this usually results in conservative treatment with less disfigurement and a high survival rate. With early diagnosis and treatment, breast cancer survival rates for women can reach as high as 94%.

No specific preparation is necessary for mammography. The patient should not wear any lotions, powders, or deodorants because they may contain small amounts of metal that can be seen on the radiograph and may interfere with interpretation. For the mammogram, the patient must remove clothing from the waist up; the patient should be told to wear a two-piece outfit so that the procedure is easier and more comfortable.

A radiology technician generally performs the mammogram. The patient's breast is positioned on the mammography machine, and pressure is applied with a plastic compression paddle that flattens the breast (Figure 28-12). Compression of the breasts is necessary to obtain a clear radiograph and to lower the radiation dosage as much as possible. During the procedure, the patient must hold her breath and remain still momentarily because any type of motion, even breathing, can blur the image and make a repeat radiograph necessary.

Two radiographs are taken of each breast—one from above and one from the side. A radiologist then checks the mammogram (Figure 28-13) and occasionally orders additional images to obtain a more complete view of the breast tissue. After the procedure, the radiologist studies the mammogram for any signs of breast cancer or other breast problems and sends a written report of the findings to the patient's physician.

Bone Density Scan

A bone density scan is an enhanced form of x-ray technology that measures the bone mineral density of the human

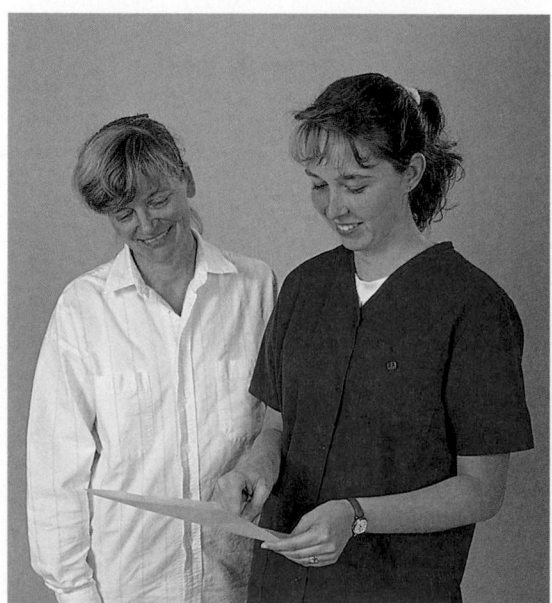

Figure 28-11 Megan instructs a patient in proper preparation for a radiographic examination.

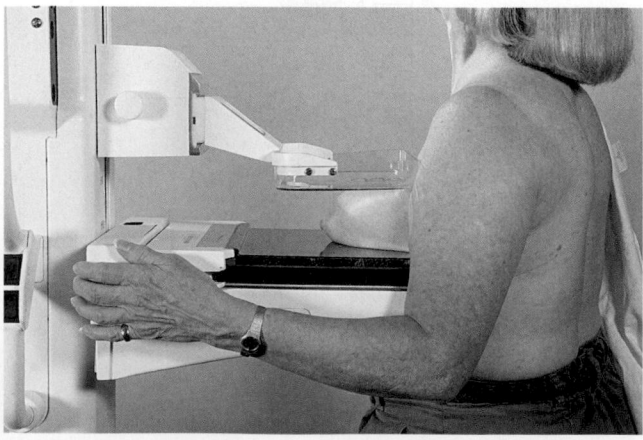

Figure 28-12 Patient positioning for mammography.

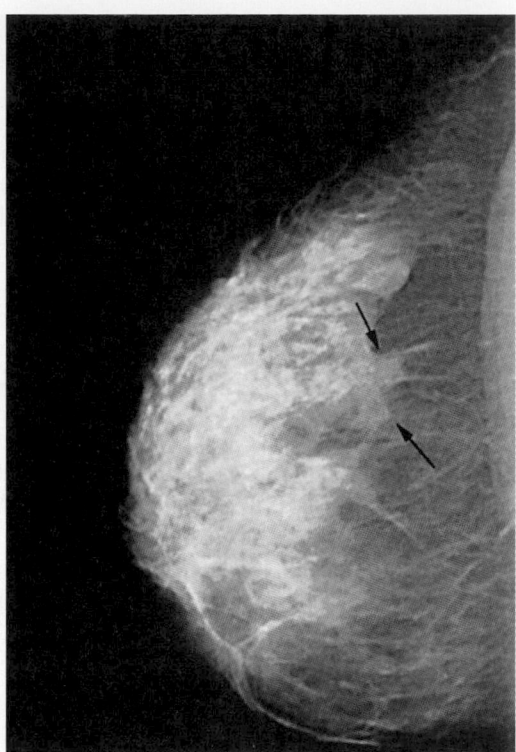

Figure 28-13 Mammogram. Arrows indicate suspicious area of increased density that needs further evaluation.

skeleton to detect bone loss. As individuals age, their bones may become less dense, causing them to become brittle and weak. This may lead to a bone fracture. Factors that cause bones to lose density include osteoporosis, thyroid and parathyroid conditions, and certain medications (e.g., corticosteroids). Postmenopausal women are at particular risk for osteoporosis; therefore, it is recommended that women above the age of 65 have a bone density scan every 2 years. *Osteoporosis* is a condition in which a gradual loss of calcium causes the bones to become thinner, more fragile, and more likely to break.

DEXA (dual energy x-ray absorptiometry) scanning is the most widely used bone density testing method. DEXA (pronounced "dexa") uses x-rays to determine the amount of bone in the human skeleton. During a DEXA scan, bone density measurements are taken at different parts of the body. The bone density measurements indicate if the patient has lost bone density. They also assist in detecting the presence of osteoporosis and can be used to predict the patient's risk of bone fracture. Patients on medication therapy for osteoporosis (e.g., Fosamax, Boniva) may also undergo DEXA to determine if the therapy is working.

The patient should be instructed to abstain from taking a calcium supplement or osteoporosis medication on the morning of the examination. These substances interfere with obtaining an accurate measurement of bone density. To perform the examination, the patient is positioned on an x-ray table and is instructed to remain as still as possible during the test. The radiologic technician then scans one or more areas of bone with the DEXA equipment. Areas that are typically scanned include the lower spine and hips.

Test results are in the form of two scores (a T score and a Z score), which are sent to the patient's physician. These scores assist the physician in diagnosing and treating the patient. The *T score* is derived by comparing the patient's measurements with those of healthy young normal adults with peak bone mass of the same gender and ethnic group as the patient. A score above −1 is considered normal. A score between −1 and −2.5 is classified as *osteopenia* or low bone mass. A score below −2.5 is defined as osteoporosis. The T score is used to estimate the patient's risk of developing a fracture. The *Z score* is derived by comparing the patient's measurements with an established database of normal individuals of the same age, gender, and ethnic group as the patient. An unusually high or low Z score may indicate the need for further testing.

Gastrointestinal Series

Upper Gastrointestinal Radiography

An upper GI (UGI) is an examination of the upper digestive tract using fluoroscopy and radiography. The examination is helpful in the diagnosis of disorders of the esophagus, stomach, duodenum, and small intestine (e.g., gastroesophageal reflux disease [GERD]), hiatal hernia, peptic ulcer, benign and malignant tumors). The procedure may be ordered when the patient complains of difficulty in swallowing, vomiting, abdominal pain, gastric reflux (burping up food [GERD]), severe indigestion, and blood in the stool.

Proper patient preparation is important for this procedure. The patient's stomach must be empty at the beginning of the study, so food does not obscure the radiographic image. To prepare for the examination, the patient must eat a light evening meal and then not eat or drink anything, including water and medications, after midnight on the day before the examination. Food and fluid in the GI tract have a degree of density and could cause confusing shadows on the radiograph.

The stomach varies little in density from the structures around it, and to make it show up on a radiograph, a contrast medium must be used. The patient drinks a suspension of barium mixed with water and flavoring, which resembles a milkshake and has a chalky taste. Before drinking the barium, the patient may be asked to drink a carbonated beverage that consists of baking soda granules. This solution puts air into the stomach, causing it to expand. The combination of air and barium allows the radiologist to view the stomach in greater detail.

As the patient swallows the barium mixture, the radiologist observes its passage down the esophagus and into the stomach and duodenum with fluoroscopy. The barium coats the lining of the gastrointestinal tract, making it visible on the screen of the fluoroscope. Radiographs are taken periodically during the examination to allow a detailed study of the upper GI tract and to provide a permanent record. The patient's position is changed at various times

---

PATIENT TEACHING   **Mammography**

Answer questions patients may have about mammography.

What is the purpose of mammography?

Mammography is a safe, low-dose radiographic examination used to screen for abnormal changes in the breasts. Mammography allows the physician to detect small lumps in the breast long before they can be felt. Although most breast lumps are not cancerous, breast cancer can be removed at an early stage when detected early, which usually results in treatment that is less deforming and has a much higher survival rate.

Who should have a mammogram?

The American Cancer Society recommends women 40 years old and older have an annual mammogram because the risk of breast cancer increases after this age. Women with a family history of, or other risk factors for, breast cancer should follow the advice of the physician regarding mammography; age guidelines do not apply because these women undergo examination on a more frequent basis.

What occurs during the mammography procedure?

During mammography, the breast is positioned on a special machine and is flattened with a compression paddle. Breast compression may be uncomfortable for some women. The discomfort can be reduced with avoidance of caffeine several days before the procedure and by scheduling the mammography the week after a menstrual period, when the breasts are less tender. Each breast is radiographed from above and from the side. A radiologist studies the resulting mammogram to detect any abnormalities. The results are reported to the physician.

Does mammography take the place of breast self-examination?

Mammography is not a substitute for breast self-examination. Women should continue to examine their breasts once a month and undergo a periodic breast examination by a physician. Most breast lumps are detected by women themselves.

- Encourage the patient to have a mammogram according to the schedule recommended by the American Cancer Society.
- Instruct the patient in the procedure for a breast self-examination.
- Provide the patient with educational materials on breast self-examination and mammography. ■

---

so that the upper digestive tract can be visualized from different profiles. If the radiologist wants to observe the passage of barium through the small and large intestines, the patient must wait at the facility and return to the radiology examination room several times for additional radiographs. After the procedure, the radiologist prepares an upper GI report of the findings, which is sent to the patient's physician.

The medical assistant should explain to the patient that the barium suspension will appear in the stool for 1 to 3 days following the procedure and will cause the stool to have a whitish color. The barium mixture may cause constipation and the need for a laxative. To help prevent constipation, the patient should be instructed to increase fiber and fluid intake for several days following the procedure.

Lower Gastrointestinal Radiography

A lower GI involves filling the colon with a barium sulfate mixture with a catheter (tube) inserted into the rectum through the anus. Because of this, the procedure is sometimes called a *barium enema*. The examination uses fluoroscopy and radiography to observe and obtain permanent pictures of the colon and rectum (Figure 28-14). A lower GI assists in diagnosis of disorders of the colon, such as polyps, cancerous tumors, diverticulosis, and the extent of inflammatory bowel disease (e.g., ulcerative colitis, Crohn disease). The colon must be thoroughly cleansed in advance to remove gas and fecal material. Gas has a certain degree of density and shows up as confusing shadows on the radiograph. If fecal material appears on the film, the image of the colon is obscured.

Instructions for cleansing the colon may vary from one medical office to another, but in general the patient is instructed to consume only clear liquids the day before the examination, such as water, plain coffee and tea, clear broth, and strained fruit juice. A laxative should be taken on the day before the scheduled examination; an **enema** also may be necessary. An **enema** is an injection of fluid into the rectum to aid in the elimination of feces from the colon. The patient should not drink anything (except water) after midnight on the day before the examination. On the morning of the examination, the patient may be required to perform a warm water cleansing enema until the returns are clear.

The patient should report at the scheduled time and is instructed to relax on one side while the rectal catheter is inserted. As the barium enters the colon, the radiologist watches it on the fluoroscopic screen and periodically takes radiographs. The patient has a sensation of fullness and the urge to defecate as the barium enters the colon. The catheter usually has a balloon on the tip of it to prevent the barium from coming back out. The patient is moved into various positions to allow the barium to fill the colon completely and to obtain better visualization of the colon. The patient is allowed to evacuate the barium, and another radiograph is taken to finish the radiographic examination. After the procedure, the radiologist prepares a lower GI report of the findings, which is sent to the patient's physician.

A *double-contrast barium enema radiographic study* is similar to a lower GI study; however (in addition to the barium), it also employs the use of air that is inserted into

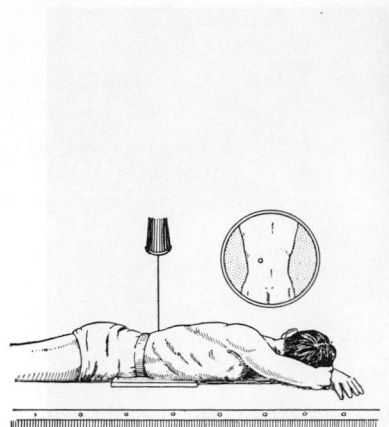

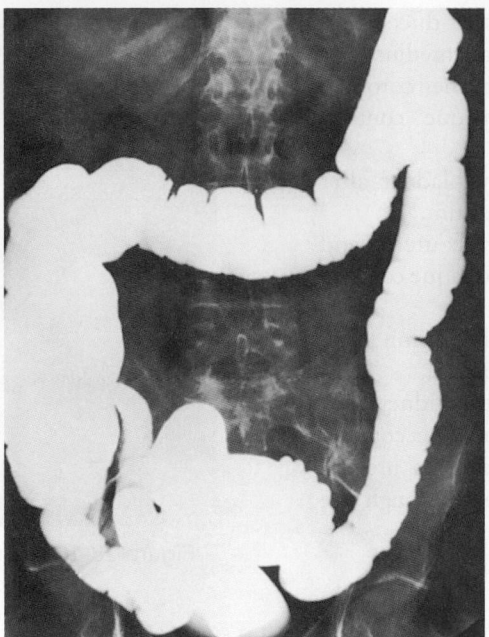

Figure 28-14 Lower GI. Colon is distended with barium. Positioning of patient and radiograph.

the colon through the same catheter as the barium. The air distends the wall of the colon and allows the radiologist to view the colon in greater detail, making it easier to detect polyps and small cancerous tumors.

Intravenous Pyelography

An intravenous pyelogram (IVP) is a radiograph of the kidneys, ureters, and bladder (Figure 28-15). An IVP is used to assist in the diagnosis of kidney stones, blockage or narrowing of the urinary tract, and growths within or near the urinary system.

The patient should consume only clear liquids starting at 4:00 PM the day before the examination. The evening before the examination, the patient must take a laxative such as magnesium citrate and/or Dulcolax tablets to remove gas and fecal material from the intestines. Removal of gas and fecal material permits proper visualization of the urinary tract. Starting at midnight the day before the examination, the patient should not eat, drink, smoke, or chew gum. Unless the patient is allergic to iodine, a contrast medium consisting of iodine is used and is administered intravenously to the patient. As the iodine enters the bloodstream, the patient may feel warm and flushed and have a metallic or salty taste in the mouth. This reaction is normal and lasts for only a few minutes. If the patient is allergic to iodine, a different type of contrast medium must be used. After the procedure, the radiologist prepares an IVP report of the findings, which is sent to the patient's physician.

Other Types of Radiographs

Other types of radiographs that the medical assistant may encounter include the following:

Angiocardiogram: Radiograph of the heart in which valves and vessels are examined with radiography and

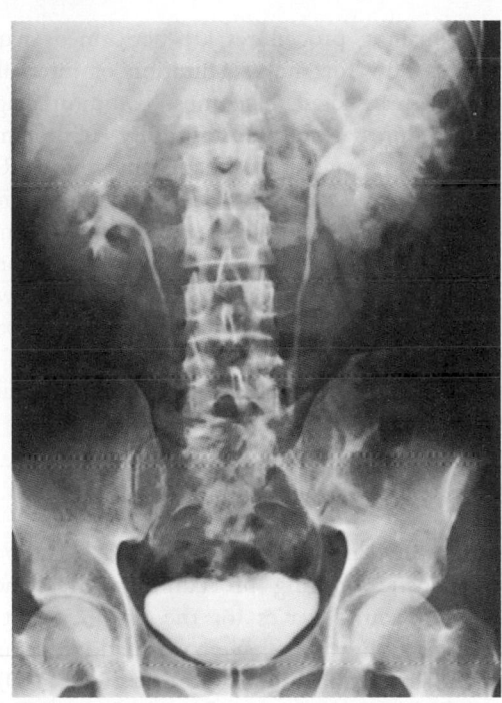

Figure 28-15 Intravenous pyelogram obtained 15 minutes after intravenous injection of a suitable contrast agent.

fluoroscopy after introduction of a radiopaque contrast medium.

Bronchogram: Radiograph of the lungs after introduction of a radiopaque contrast medium.

Cerebral angiogram: Radiograph of the major arteries of the brain after injection of a radiopaque contrast medium.

Chest radiograph: Radiograph of the chest that does not use a contrast medium.

Cholangiogram: Radiograph of the bile ducts after administration of a radiopaque contrast medium.

Coronary angiogram: Radiograph of the coronary arteries after injection of a radiopaque contrast medium.

Cystogram: Radiograph of the urinary bladder after injection of a radiopaque contrast medium.

Hysterosalpingogram: Radiograph of the uterus and fallopian tubes after injection of a radiopaque contrast medium.

Myelogram: Radiograph of the spinal column after injection of a radiopaque contrast medium.

Retrograde pyelogram: Radiograph of the kidneys and urinary tract after injection of radiopaque contrast medium directly into the ureter through a ureteral catheter. The dye flows to the kidneys through the ureters.

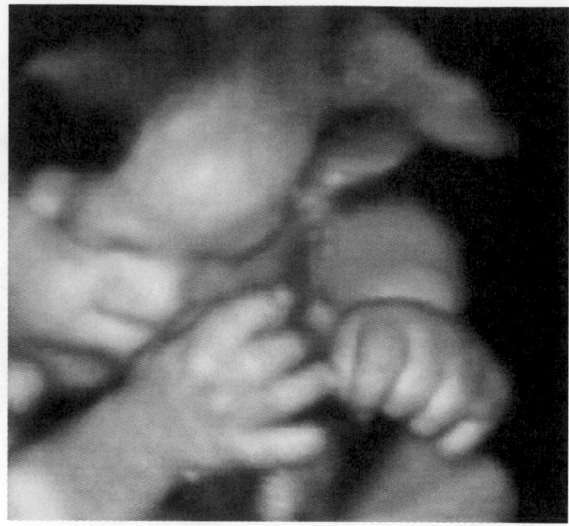

Figure 28-16 3-D ultrasound of a third-trimester fetus.

INTRODUCTION TO DIAGNOSTIC IMAGING

Diagnostic imaging procedures are performed frequently because they allow for the visualization of internal body structures in great detail. The most common diagnostic imaging procedures are **ultrasonography** (US), computed tomography (CT), magnetic resonance imaging (MRI), and nuclear medicine. Diagnostic imaging procedures are usually performed in a hospital or a large clinic. The medical assistant, however, may need to relay information to a patient scheduled for such a procedure, including what to expect during the procedure and any patient preparation that may be required. The medical assistant should have a basic knowledge of diagnostic imaging procedures and the preparation necessary for each.

ULTRASONOGRAPHY

Ultrasonography, also called "ultrasound," is the oldest of the diagnostic imaging procedures. Ultrasound uses high-frequency sound waves for the study of soft tissue structures. Recent advances have been made in technology in ultrasound. These include three-dimensional (3-D) ultrasound, in which sound waves are formatted into 3-D images (Figure 28-16). Four-dimensional (4-D) ultrasound is another new technology that consists of 3-D ultrasound, but in motion.

Ultrasound is frequently used in the diagnosis of conditions of the abdominal and pelvic organs, particularly the liver, gallbladder, spleen, pancreas, kidneys, uterus, ovaries, and abdominal aorta. Some examples of conditions that can be detected using ultrasound include breast cysts, gallstones, and kidney stones.

An ultrasound examination of the heart is called an **echocardiogram** and is used to determine the size, shape, and position of the heart and the movement of the heart valves and chambers. Ultrasonography is also used for guiding a needle or other device during a minimally invasive procedure such as amniocentesis, a needle biopsy, cortisone injection into a joint, and needle aspiration of fluid in a joint.

Ultrasonography offers many advantages as a diagnostic imaging procedure. It shows movement, allows continuous viewing of a structure, uses sound waves rather than radiation, and is less expensive than other imaging procedures. Ultrasound does have some minor limitations. Because sound waves are unable to penetrate bone and air- or gas-filled cavities such as the lungs, stomach, and intestines, ultrasound cannot be used in the evaluation of these structures. In addition, ultrasound may be difficult to use with obese patients because adipose tissue can interfere with sound wave transmission.

Before performing an ultrasound examination, a warm ultrasound gel must first be spread on the area to be examined. The purpose of the gel is to increase conductivity of the sound waves between the skin and the transducer. During the ultrasound examination, the examiner places a probe containing a transducer firmly on the patient's skin and moves it over the body areas to be examined. The transducer generates sound waves that are directed into the patient's tissues. The sound waves are reflected back to the transducer, similar to an echo. These sound waves are then transmitted to the ultrasound machine through a cable, where a computer converts them into an image. The size, shape, and consistency of the image are displayed on a video display screen; this image is known as a **sonogram** (Figure 28-17). The patient is often permitted to view the sonogram on the screen of the monitor as the procedure is performed. Selected images can be permanently recorded on paper, film, videotape, or a computerized storage medium. A radiologist reviews and interprets the images and prepares an ultrasound report that is sent to the patient's physician.

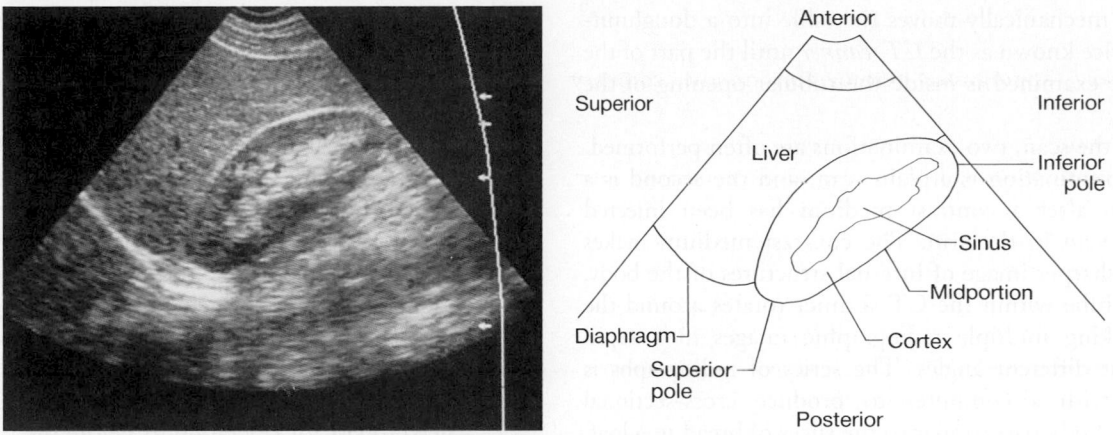

Figure 28-17 Sonogram of the right kidney.

Although ultrasound is commonly used for a wide variety of noninvasive imaging procedures, individuals are most familiar with its use in obstetrics. Obstetric ultrasound is most frequently used to determine the gestational age of a fetus and to confirm the due date; to detect congenital abnormalities, ectopic pregnancy, and multiple pregnancy; and to determine the fetus's position and size late in pregnancy. If the fetus is old enough and is positioned correctly, it also may be possible to determine its gender. Because the ultrasound machine is a compact unit, most obstetricians perform this procedure in their medical offices. Ultrasound is also used by gynecologists to evaluate and treat infertility problems.

Doppler ultrasound is a special application of ultrasound. It measures the direction and speed of blood as it flows through blood vessels, such as major arteries and veins in the abdomen, arms, legs, and neck. Doppler ultrasound images can assist the physician in diagnosing blood flow blockages, narrowing of blood vessels due to atherosclerosis, and congenital malformations.

Patient Preparation

The medical assistant should tell the patient what to expect during an ultrasound examination and instruct the patient in the preparation required for the procedure, as follows:

1. Ultrasound is a safe and painless procedure that takes approximately 15 to 45 minutes to complete, depending on the body part examined.
2. The patient may need to prepare for the procedure, depending on the part of the body examined. An ultrasound of the gallbladder, liver, spleen, and pancreas necessitates that the patient fast for 8 to 12 hours. For an obstetric ultrasound, the patient needs to have a full bladder. The patient should be instructed to consume approximately 32 ounces of fluid about 1 hour before the procedure.
3. The patient must remain still when requested during the procedure because movement can interfere with accurate results. In addition, the patient may be asked

to change positions so that the organs can be seen at different angles.

COMPUTED TOMOGRAPHY

Computed tomography (also known as a *CT* scan) is an advanced radiographic examination that uses only a minimal amount of radiation. It produces a series of cross-sectional images of a body part, permitting the imaging of structures that cannot be visualized with conventional radiographic procedures. A CT scan allows the radiologist to view the bones and organs of the head and body in fine detail and has been used most successfully in diagnostic studies of the brain, abdomen, and pelvis. CT scans are used primarily to detect and evaluate tumors and other abnormalities and to monitor the effects of surgery, radiation therapy, or chemotherapy on tumors.

The scan is conducted by a skilled diagnostic imaging technician. The patient is positioned on a special motorized table (Figure 28-18). From an adjoining room, the

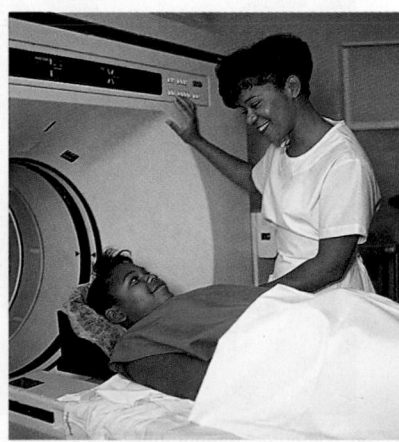

Figure 28-18 Positioning patient for computed tomography (CT) scan.

technician mechanically moves the table into a doughnut-shaped device known as the *CT scanner* until the part of the body to be examined is inside the tubular opening of the scanner.

During the scan, two examinations are often performed. The first examination is a plain scan, and the second is a repeat scan after a contrast medium has been injected through a vein in the arm. The contrast medium makes possible a sharper image of internal structures of the body. The x-ray tube within the CT scanner rotates around the patient, taking multiple radiographic images in a rapid sequence at different angles. The series of radiographs is processed with a computer to produce cross-sectional images of a body part similar to the slices of bread in a loaf. These images are permanently recorded on film or stored digitally on electronic media for evaluation by a radiologist (Figure 28-19). The radiologist reviews and interprets the images and prepares a CT report, which is sent to the patient's physician.

Patient Preparation

The medical assistant should tell the patient what to expect during the CT scan and should instruct the patient on the preparation required for the procedure, as follows:

1. Before the procedure, the patient must remove all radiopaque objects, such as dentures, eyeglasses, and jewelry, because they interfere with a clear image of the body part examined.

2. If a contrast medium is to be used, the patient may need to fast for several hours before the procedure. It is important to ask the patient whether he or she is allergic to radiographic contrast media to avoid an adverse reaction.

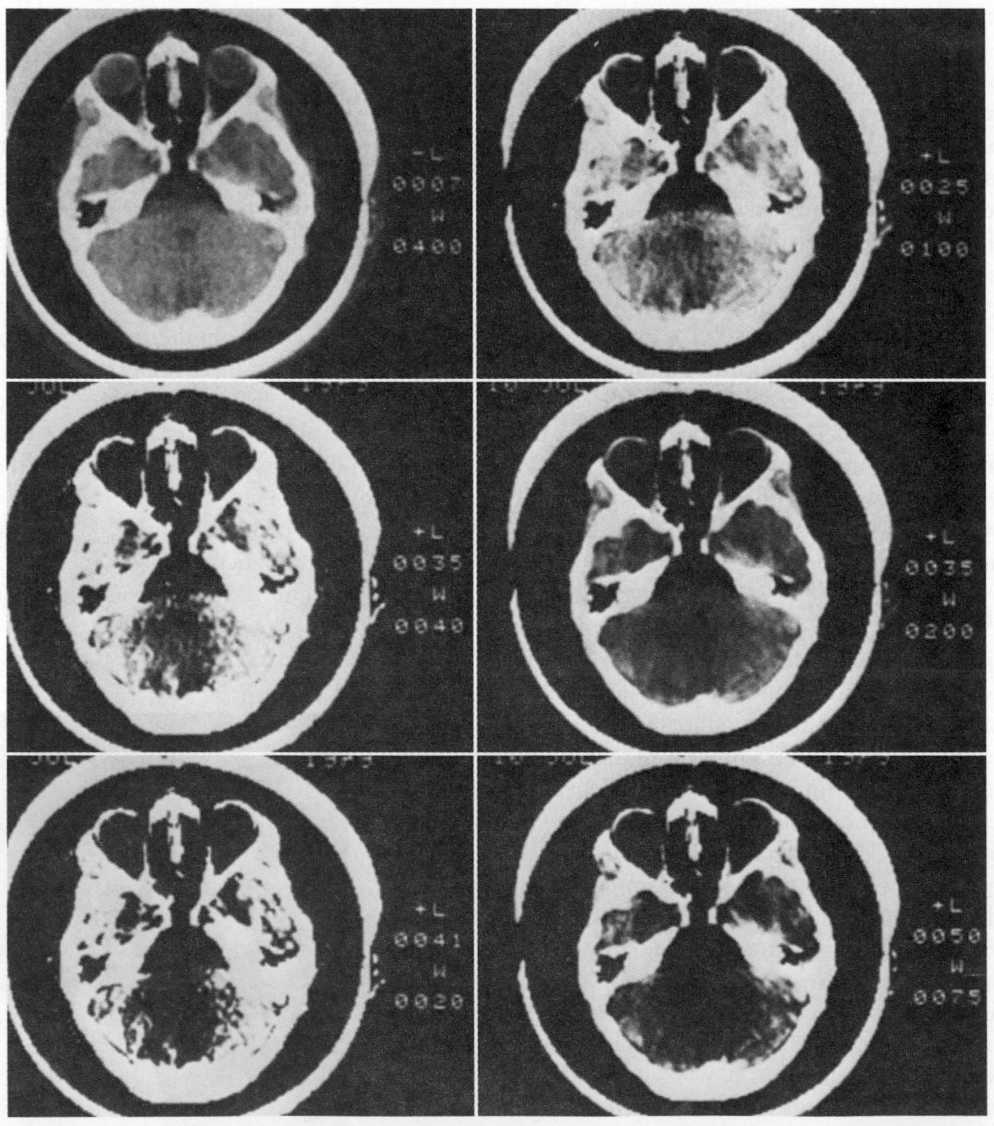

Figure 28-19 The computed tomography (CT) scanner takes multiple cross-sectional radiographic images. The images shown here are cross-sectional pictures of the head used to evaluate the orbits and sinuses.

3. The patient should lie motionless and breathe normally during the procedure. When a radiograph is being taken, the patient is usually asked to hold his or her breath so that the radiograph is not blurred. The patient hears mechanical clicking and whirring sounds from the scanner as pictures are taken.

4. Depending on the body part being examined, the procedure takes from 10 minutes to an hour to complete.

MAGNETIC RESONANCE IMAGING

MRI is used for imaging tissues of high fat and water content that cannot be seen with other radiologic techniques. MRI assists in the diagnosis of intracranial and spinal lesions and cardiovascular and soft tissue abnormalities, such as herniated discs and joint diseases. MRI allows the examiner to see through bone and view fluid-filled soft tissue in great detail.

MRI is a safe and painless procedure in which a strong magnetic field and ordinary radio waves produce computer-processed images of internal body structures. Because MRI does not involve radiation, the U.S. Food and Drug Administration has classified the MRI machine as a low-risk device.

The patient lies on a table inside the bore of the cylindrical MRI machine while a diagnostic imaging technician in an adjoining room monitors the procedure (Figure 28-20). Because of the closed space, some patients may have difficulty with claustrophobia. The physician may order a sedative for these patients. Open MRI machines are less confining than traditional MRI machines; however, they are a newer technology and may not be available at some facilities.

The high-resolution, three-dimensional images that are obtained with MRI are permanently recorded on film or stored digitally on electronic media for evaluation by a radiologist. The radiologist reviews and interprets the images and prepares an MRI report, which is sent to the patient's physician.

Patient Preparation

The medical assistant should tell the patient what to expect during the MRI and instruct the patient in the preparation required for the procedure, as follows:

1. MRI is a safe and painless procedure with a usual completion time between 20 minutes and 1½ hours.

2. No special preparation is necessary for the MRI examination. The patient may eat or drink before the examination and take any prescribed medication. The patient should wear loose, comfortable clothing, such as a jogging suit, for the procedure.

3. Because the procedure involves a strong magnet, the patient should remove any metal or magnetic-sensitive objects, such as hairpins, eyeglasses, hearing aids, watches, rings, and credit cards. Avoid wearing cosmetics, as certain types of cosmetic preparations contain small amounts of metal. Individuals with a pacemaker or inner ear implant may not be able to undergo an MRI.

4. A contrast medium may be used for the procedure. It improves the resolution of the image by increasing the brightness in various parts of the body.

5. The patient must remain completely still for 15- to 20-minute intervals during the procedure. The patient hears a metallic clacking sound like a muffled drumbeat during the procedure. Earplugs or headphones are available for use if the patient desires.

NUCLEAR MEDICINE

Nuclear medicine is an advanced diagnostic imaging procedure in which a tiny bit of radioactive material is introduced into the patient. The radiation is introduced into the body by a diagnostic imaging technician using one of the following methods: intravenously, by ingestion, or by inhalation. The technologist positions the patient on a scanning table that works in association with a specialized piece of equipment known as a *gamma camera*. The gamma camera is positioned above or below the scanning table and is able

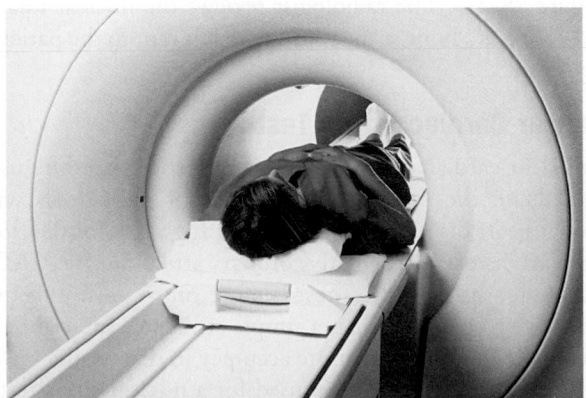

Figure 28-20 Magnetic resonance imaging (MRI). The patient lies on a table inside the bore of the cylindrical MRI machine while MRI technicians in an adjoining room monitor the procedure.

What Would You Do? What Would You *Not* Do?

Case Study 3

Michael Wendl is an 18-year-old high school varsity football player. For the past 3 months, he has had pain and swelling in his left shoulder. The physician schedules an MRI to assist in determining the cause of the problem. Michael has had several radiographs over the past 2 years and is worried about the radiation exposure to his body. He wants to know how much radiation will be involved with the procedure. Michael has problems with claustrophobia and wants to know whether he can play a game on his iPhone during the procedure to distract him. He also wants to know whether he is allowed to eat anything before the procedure. ∎

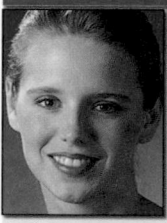

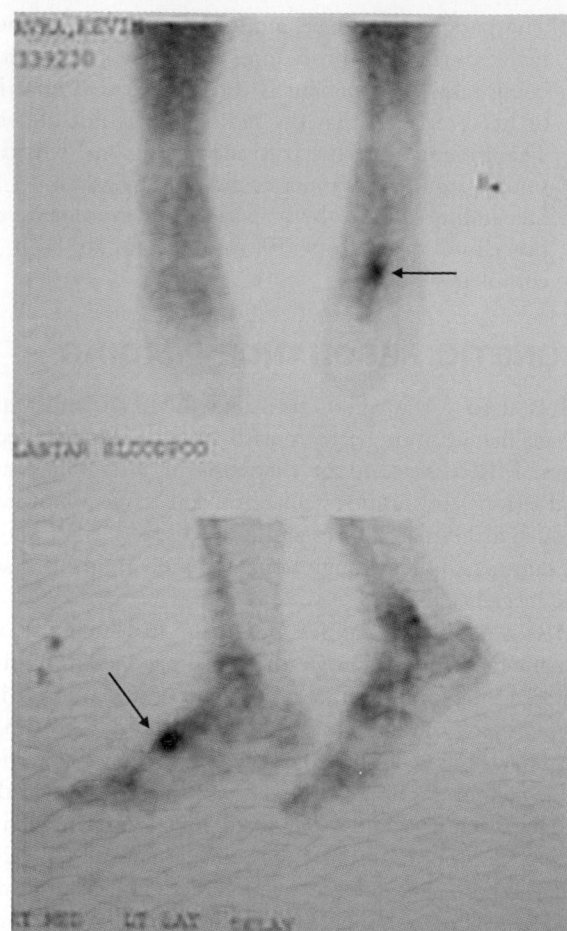

Figure 28-21 Bone scan of the foot. *Arrows* show the hot spot that indicates a stress fracture.

to detect the radiation being given off by the body part that has been targeted by the radiation. This is accomplished through the use of scintillation crystals. These crystals convert the radiation being given off by the body into light. This light is converted into electrical impulses, which are interpreted by a computer program contained within the gamma camera. The resulting information is displayed as still images or functional animations of body parts and organs. Because it can show the actual function of organs, nuclear medicine provides more detailed information for certain conditions than is provided by other diagnostic imaging examinations (e.g., CT scan, MRI).

The radioactive material used in nuclear medicine is known as a *radiopharmaceutical* (or radionuclide). Examples of commonly used radiopharmaceuticals include technetium-99 m, iodine-123 and iodine-131, and thallium-201. Most radiopharmaceuticals are chemically bound to a complex known as a *tracer.* A tracer is designed to be attracted to specific areas of the body or, in some cases, to types of diseased tissue.

The most common nuclear medicine procedures include bone scans and nuclear cardiac stress tests, which are described in more detail in the next section. Other types of nuclear medicine procedures that may be performed include gallbladder procedures, thyroid studies, brain scans, lung scans, and liver procedures.

Bone Scans

Bone scans are performed to detect small fractures (e.g., stress fractures) or lesions that may not be visible on other diagnostic imaging examinations. When a bone scan is performed, the patient is injected with a radiopharmaceutical. The patient must then wait at the facility for a predetermined period of time, based on the area being examined. The purpose of the waiting period is to allow the radiopharmaceutical to be absorbed sufficiently so that an accurate diagnosis can be made. The gamma camera detects the radiation given off by the small fracture, and it shows up as a "hot" spot on the nuclear images (Figure 28-21). The radiologist reviews the nuclear images and prepares a bone scan report, which is sent to the patient's physician.

Nuclear Cardiac Stress Test

A nuclear cardiac stress test is a diagnostic procedure used to evaluate the cardiovascular health of individuals with known heart disease or individuals at high risk for developing heart disease, particularly coronary artery disease (CAD). Although a nuclear stress test is more time-consuming and expensive to perform than a simple stress test (described in Chapter 27), it provides more accuracy in diagnosing CAD.

The radiopharmaceutical used for a nuclear stress test is usually technetium-99mTc sestamibi (trade name is Cardiolite), which is administered intravenously and targets the heart. Nuclear images included in the stress test are taken by the gamma camera during two phases: a *resting phase* and a *stress phase* (which is a functional study). The resting phase is performed with the heart at a normal rate, whereas the stress phase is performed immediately after the patient exercises at his or her maximal (target) heart rate. The two sets of nuclear images—the resting images and the images taken under cardiac stress—are then compared with each other. These images assist the radiologist in determining which parts of the heart are healthy and functioning normally. The images also identify areas of the heart that exhibit decreased blood flow during exercise, meaning that a portion of the heart muscle is not receiving enough oxygen. A decreased oxygen supply to a portion of the heart is known as *cardiac ischemia* and is typically due to the presence of coronary artery disease. The radiologist reviews and interprets the images and prepares a nuclear cardiac stress test report, which is sent to the patient's physician.

A PET (positron emission tomography) scan is a special type of nuclear imaging procedure. PET uses a special camera and computer to construct a 3-D image of the area being scanned. This procedure is particularly useful in diagnosing conditions of the brain and heart, such as brain cancer and heart disease.

Guidelines

Specific guidelines that may be required for nuclear medicine examinations are as follows:

1. Depending on the type of nuclear medicine examination being performed, the patient may be required to be in a fasting state or to abstain from consuming certain foods or substances such as caffeine for a period of time. The medical assistant should check with the facility performing the examination, so that proper dietary instructions can be relayed to the patient.

2. Nuclear medicine examinations are time-consuming because most examinations require multiple scans. The interval between scans is determined by the part being examined and the type of equipment and radiopharmaceutical being used. There may be a delay between administration of the radiopharmaceutical and when the patient is actually placed on the scanning table. Follow-up images that may be done later the same day or, in some cases, the following morning also may be needed. Because of this, the medical assistant must inform the patient of the amount of time required for the examination, so that arrangements can be made with work and home schedules if needed.

3. Because most nuclear medicine examinations require that the patient lie still on a table for a prolonged time, the patient should be advised to wear comfortable clothing to the examination. If a nuclear medicine examination requires exercise as a component of the test, the patient should be instructed to wear appropriate exercise clothing, including athletic shoes.

DIGITAL RADIOLOGY

Modern advances in digital imaging technology have made inroads into the field of radiology. The result is the transformation of film-based radiology into a system of computer-displayed and stored digital images. To assist in understanding digital radiology, this transformation can be compared with the replacement of film cameras with digital cameras.

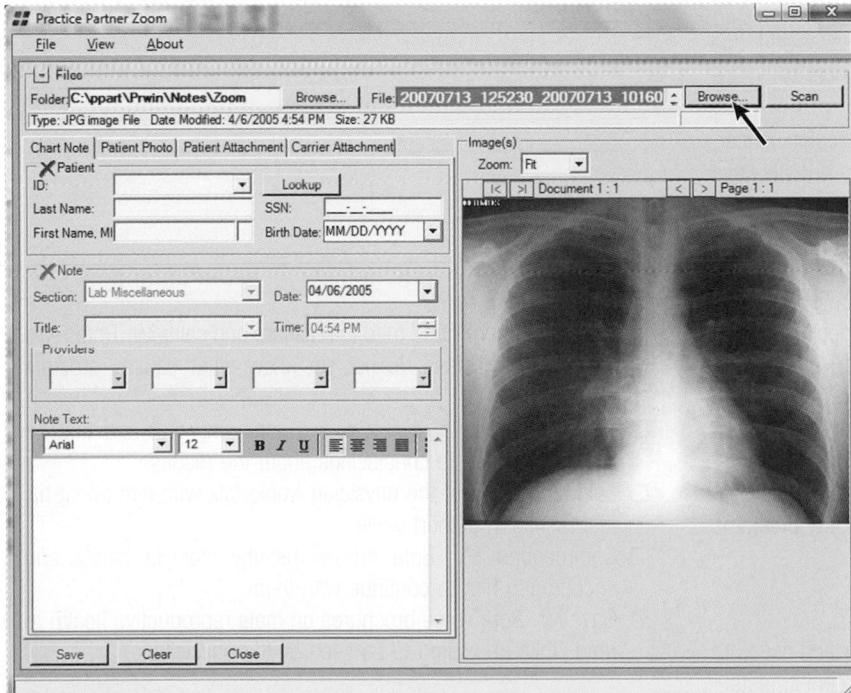

Figure 28-22 Digital image of a chest x-ray.

Images can be taken and viewed immediately, and then sent electronically to a network of computers. These images can also be saved on a CD or DVD and given to the patient to take to his or her physician for review.

Digital radiology allows for increased efficiency and cost savings and better patient care. Higher-quality images and the ability to transfer these digital images electronically are two important benefits that affect the patient directly. As a result of this digital revolution, the medical assistant may be required to use the medical office computer to access, display (Figure 28-22), and permanently save images taken by the facilities providing digital imaging services.

MEDICAL PRACTICE *and the* LAW

Colon procedures can be embarrassing for the patient. Many colon procedures can be diagnostic for cancer. This combination makes these procedures very stressful for the patient. Professionalism, compassion, and a caring attitude can alleviate many fears. Many invasive procedures require written informed consent.

While assisting with a sigmoidoscopy, assist the patient and maintain proper positioning as comfortable as possible. Be aware of the patient's condition, and inform the physician if the patient is not tolerating the procedure well.

Radiology and diagnostic imaging involve high-technology equipment and procedures that can be frightening and uncomfortable to the patient. Be aware of the patient's reactions, and provide assistance and comfort whenever possible. Be specific in providing the patient with instructions to ensure the best imaging results.

Procedures that involve injectable contrast media or that are invasive usually require written informed consent. Check office policy for procedures that require signed consent forms.

With procedures that use radiation, federal laws regulate usage and exposure testing and record keeping. The acronym ALARA (As Low As Reasonably Achievable) reminds workers to minimize exposure to themselves and patients. Ask female patients whether they may be pregnant before beginning any radiologic procedure. ∎

What Would You Do? What Would You *Not* Do? RESPONSES

Case Study 1
Page 656

What Did Megan Do?
❏ Relayed to Mrs. Bernard that this is not the most fun test to perform, but that if colon cancer is detected early, the cure rate is very high.
❏ Explained to Mrs. Bernard that colon cancer increases after age 50, and that an individual can develop colon cancer without a family history of it.
❏ Told Mrs. Bernard that during the early stages of colon cancer, no symptoms occur, so it is possible to feel fine but still have a problem.
❏ Explained to Mrs. Bernard in greater detail the reason for not eating red meat or taking aspirin during the testing period.
❏ Told Mrs. Bernard that disposable gloves could be given to her to take home to wear when she collected the specimens.
❏ Explained to Mrs. Bernard that the physician talks with patients every day about these types of things, and it is important to talk with him about all aspects of her health so that she receives the best care possible.
❏ Told Mrs. Bernard that the office would call her in 3 days to see whether she has any questions or is having any problems with the test.

What Did Megan Not Do?
❏ Did not tell Mrs. Bernard that she is getting older and needs to be more concerned about performing health screening tests.

What Would You Do?/What Would You *Not* Do?
Review Megan's response and place a checkmark next to the information you included in your response. List additional information you included in your response.

_____
_____
_____
_____
_____
_____
_____

Case Study 2
Page 667

What Did Megan Do?
❏ Listened patiently and tried to reassure and calm Mr. Bota. Told him that physicians do not yet know what causes prostate cancer.
❏ Explained that the PSA test is a screening test and that he should not jump to conclusions about the results.
❏ Told Mr. Bota that the physician would talk with him about his test results in a short while.
❏ Commended Mr. Bota on his healthy lifestyle habits and encouraged him to continue with them.
❏ Gave Mr. Bota some brochures on male reproductive health to read while he waited to be seen by the physician.

What Would You Do? What Would You *Not* Do? RESPONSES—cont'd

What Did Megan Not *Do?*

❏ Did not tell Mr. Bota that there was nothing to worry about.

What Would You Do?/What Would You Not *Do?*

Review Megan's response and place a checkmark next to the information you included in your response. List additional information you included in your response.

_____

_____

_____

_____

_____

Case Study 3
Page 677

What Did Megan Do?

❏ Explained to Michael that an MRI does not use radiation, so he would not be exposed to any radiation during the procedure.

❏ Told Michael that he would not be able to play a game on his iPhone during the procedure. Explained that the MRI works with a strong magnet that might damage the iPhone and also interfere with a good image of the shoulder. Told Michael that he would need to lie still during the procedure.

❏ Told Michael the physician would be informed of his problem with claustrophobia. Explained that the physician may want to give him something to help him relax during the procedure.

❏ Told Michael that it was fine to eat before the procedure.

What Did Megan Not Do?

❏ Did not overlook or minimize Michael's concern about claustrophobia.

What Would You Do?/What Would You Not *Do?*

Review Megan's response and place a checkmark next to the information you included in your response. List additional information you included in your response.

_____

_____

_____

_____

_____

_____

⟳ TERMINOLOGY REVIEW

Medical Term	Word Parts	Definition
Biopsy	*bi/o-:* life *-opsy:* to view	The surgical removal and examination of tissue from the living body. Biopsies generally are performed to determine whether a tumor is benign or malignant.
Colonoscope	*colon/o-:* colon *-scope:* instrument used for visual examination	An endoscope that is specially designed for passage through the anus to permit visualization of the rectum and the entire length of the colon.
Colonoscopy	*colon/o-:* colon *-scopy:* visual examination	The visualization of the rectum and the entire colon using a colonoscope.
Contrast medium		A substance used to make a particular structure visible on a radiograph.
Echocardiogram	*ech/o-:* sound *cardi/o-:* heart *-gram:* record	An ultrasound examination of the heart.
Endoscope	*endo-:* within *-scope:* instrument used for visual examination	An instrument that consists of a tube and an optical system that is used for direct visual inspection of organs or cavities.
Enema		An injection of fluid into the rectum to aid in the elimination of feces from the colon.
Fluoroscope	*fluor/o-:* fluorescence *-scope:* instrument used for visual examination	An instrument used to view internal organs and structures directly.
Fluoroscopy	*fluor/o-:* fluorescence *-scopy:* visual examination	Examination of a patient with a fluoroscope.
Insufflate		To blow a powder, vapor, or gas (e.g., air) into a body cavity.

Continued

TERMINOLOGY REVIEW—cont'd

Medical Term	Word Parts	Definition
Melena		The darkening of the stool caused by the presence of blood in an amount of 50 mL or greater.
Occult blood		Blood in such a small amount that it is not detectable by the unaided eye.
Peroxidase	*-oxia:* oxygen *-ase:* enzyme	(As it pertains to the guaiac slide test) A substance that is able to transfer oxygen from hydrogen peroxide to oxidize guaiac, causing the guaiac to turn blue.
Radiograph	*radi/o-:* radiation *-graph:* instrument used to record, x-ray film	A permanent record of a picture of an internal body organ or structure produced on radiographic film.
Radiography	*radi/o-:* radiation *-graphy:* process of recording, x-ray filming	The taking of permanent records (radiographs) of internal body organs and structures by passing x-rays through the body to act on a specially sensitized film.
Radiologist	*radi/o-:* radiation *-ologist:* one who studies and practices (specialist)	A physician who specializes in the diagnosis and treatment of disease using radiation and other imaging techniques.
Radiology	*radi/o-:* radiation *-ology:* study of	The branch of medicine that deals with the use of radiation and other imaging techniques (such as ultrasound, CT scans, MRIs, and nuclear medicine) in the diagnosis and treatment of disease.
Radiolucent	*radi/o-:* radiation *-lucent:* transparent	Describing a structure that permits the passage of x-rays.
Radiopaque	*radi/o-:* radiation *-opaque:* opaque	Describing a structure that obstructs the passage of x-rays.
Sigmoidoscope	*sigmoid/o-:* sigmoid (colon) *-scope:* instrument used for visual examination	An endoscope that is specially designed for passage through the anus to permit visualization of the rectum and sigmoid colon.
Sigmoidoscopy	*sigmoid/o-:* sigmoid (colon) *-scopy:* visual examination	The visual examination of the rectum and sigmoid colon using a sigmoidoscope.
Sonogram	*son/o-:* sound *-gram:* record	The record obtained with ultrasonography.
Ultrasonography	*ultra-:* beyond, excess *sono-:* sound *-graphy:* process of recording	The use of high-frequency sound waves to produce an image of an organ or tissue.

ON THE WEB

For information on colorectal cancer:

American Cancer Society: www.cancer.org

National Cancer Institute: www.cancer.gov

Prevent Cancer Foundation: www.preventcancer.org

Colon Cancer Alliance: www.ccalliance.org

Oncology Channel: www.oncologychannel.com

For information on prostate cancer:

Prostate Health: www.prostatehealth.com

Prostate Information: www.prostateinfo.com

Prostate.com: www.prostate.com

Prostate Cancer Foundation: www.prostatecancerfoundation.org

Prostatitis Foundation: www.prostatitis.org

Male Health: www.malehealthcenter.com

For information on radiography and diagnostic imaging:

BrighamRAD: www.brighamrad.harvard.edu

Society for Computer Applications in Radiology: www.scarnet.org

Whole Brain Atlas: www.med.harvard.edu/AANLIB/home.html

Radiology Information: www.radiologyinfo.org

For information on breast cancer:

American Cancer Society: www.cancer.org

Breast Cancer Treatment: AboutBreastCancerinfo.com

Breast Cancer: Cancercenter.com

Breast Cancer org: Breastcancer.org

Breast Cancer Site: www.thebreastcancersite.com

National Breast Cancer Foundation: www.nationalbreastcancer.org

Breast Cancer.Net: www.breastcancer.net

Breast Cancer Basics: breastcancer.about.com

 Check out the Evolve site at http://evolve.elsevier.com/Bonewit/today/ to actively Prepare for your Certification, and to access additional interactive activities and exercises to help you study and prepare for success.

29

Introduction to the Clinical Laboratory

KEY TERMS

analyte
calibration
clinical diagnosis
control
fasting
homeostasis (hoe-mee-oh-STAY-sis)
in vivo (in-VEE-voe)
laboratory test

nonwaived test
plasma (PLAZ-ma)
product insert
profile
qualitative test
quality control
quantitative test
reagent

reference range
routine test
serum (SERE-um)
specimen (SPES-i-men)
test system
waived test

INTRODUCTION TO THE CLINICAL LABORATORY

Clinical laboratory test results are often used along with a thorough health history and physical examination to obtain essential data needed by the physician for the accurate diagnosis and management of a patient's condition. Clinical **laboratory tests** provide objective and quantitative information regarding the status of body conditions and functions. When the body is healthy, its systems function normally, and a state of equilibrium of the internal environment is said to exist; this is termed **homeostasis.** When the body is in a state of homeostasis, the physical and chemical characteristics of body substances (e.g., fluids, secretions, excretions) are within an acceptable range known as the **reference range.**

When a pathologic condition exists, biologic changes occur within the body, altering the normal physiology or functioning of the body and resulting in an imbalance. These changes cause the patient to experience symptoms of that particular pathologic condition. Iron-deficiency anemia usually causes the patient to experience weakness, fatigue, pallor, irritability, and, in some cases, shortness of breath on exertion. In addition, these changes in the body's biologic processes may cause an alteration in the characteristics of body substances, such as an alteration in the chemical content of the blood or urine, an alteration in the antibody level, or an alteration in cell counts or cellular morphology.

Physical and chemical alterations of body substances become evident through abnormal values or results on laboratory tests—in other words, values outside the accepted reference range or limit for that particular test. Just as certain pathologic conditions cause specific symptoms to occur, certain pathologic conditions cause values outside of the reference range to occur for specific laboratory tests. Iron-deficiency anemia causes an alteration in normal red blood cell morphology and a decreased hemoglobin level.

An important realization is that a value outside of the reference range for a particular test may be seen with more than one pathologic condition. A decrease in the hemoglobin level is found with hyperthyroidism, cirrhosis of the liver, and autoimmune diseases. In this regard, the physician cannot rely solely on laboratory test results to make a diagnosis, but rather must rely also on the combination of data obtained from the health history, the physical examination, and diagnostic and laboratory test results.

LABORATORY TESTS

A **laboratory test** is defined as the clinical analysis and study of materials, fluids, or tissues obtained from patients to assist in the diagnosis and treatment of disease. Laboratory tests can be classified by function into one of the following categories: hematology, clinical chemistry, immunology and blood banking, urinalysis, microbiology, parasitology, cytology, and histology. Use of these classifications makes it easier to refer to laboratory tests.

The number of laboratory tests ordered for a patient varies depending on the physician's clinical findings. A clinical diagnosis of streptococcal sore throat usually requires only a strep test for confirmation. Many diseases cause more than one alteration in the physical and chemical characteristics of body substances, however, and a series of laboratory tests is often necessary to establish the pattern of abnormalities characteristic of a particular disease.

The medical assistant should realize that not all pathologic conditions necessitate the use of laboratory test results for arrival at a diagnosis; the information obtained from the patient's clinical signs and symptoms can be sufficient for a diagnosis of some conditions. In these instances, the physician is so certain of the clinical diagnosis that therapy can be instituted without laboratory confirmation. Most physicians diagnose acute purulent otitis media with the information obtained from patient symptoms (earache, fever, feeling of fullness in the ear) and from an otoscopic examination of the tympanic membrane (the tympanic membrane is red

and bulging). Information obtained through the clinical signs and symptoms is sufficiently specific to otitis media to allow the physician to make a diagnosis and to prescribe treatment.

The medical assistant must acquire knowledge and skill in basic clinical laboratory methods and techniques. It is important that the medical assistant have knowledge of the laboratory tests that are performed most often, including the purpose of these tests, the reference range for each test, any advance patient preparation or special instructions, and any substances that might interfere with accurate test results, such as food or medication.

The medical assistant frequently works with this information when instructing a patient in advance preparation for a laboratory test; collecting, handling, and storing specimens; performing laboratory tests; and receiving and filing laboratory reports. It is essential that the medical assistant understand the value of laboratory tests and alert the physician to any abnormal results as soon as the test is performed or the laboratory report is received.

This chapter serves as an introduction to the clinical laboratory by providing an overview of methods and general guidelines to follow and by focusing on the relationship between the medical office and an outside laboratory. Specific information for collection, handling, storing, and testing of biologic specimens is presented in subsequent chapters.

PURPOSE OF LABORATORY TESTING

The most frequent use of laboratory test results is to assist in the diagnosis of a patient's condition. Laboratory test results also have many other significant medical uses. A summary of the purpose and function of laboratory testing follows:

1. Laboratory tests are most frequently ordered by the physician *to assist in the diagnosis of pathologic conditions.* Along with the health history and the physical examination, laboratory test results provide the physician with essential data needed to arrive at a diagnosis and prescribe treatment. After obtaining the health history and performing the physical examination, the physician may order laboratory tests for these reasons:
   - *To confirm a clinical diagnosis.* A **clinical diagnosis** is defined as a tentative diagnosis of a patient's condition obtained through the evaluation of the health history and the physical examination, without the benefit of laboratory or diagnostic tests.
   - The patient's signs and symptoms may provide a strong clinical diagnosis of a particular condition, and the physician may order laboratory tests simply to confirm that diagnosis. For example, the patient may have the typical signs and symptoms of diabetes mellitus, which would provide the physician with a fairly certain clinical diagnosis. In this instance, an oral glucose tolerance test (OGTT)

may be ordered to confirm the diagnosis and to institute therapy.

- *To assist in the differential diagnosis of a patient's condition.* Two or more diseases may have similar signs and symptoms; the physician orders laboratory tests to assist in the differential diagnosis of the patient's condition. A diagnosis of streptococcal sore throat must be made with a laboratory test to differentiate it from other pathologic conditions with similar signs and symptoms, such as pharyngitis.

- *To obtain information regarding a patient's condition* when not enough concrete evidence exists to support a clinical diagnosis. The patient sometimes may have vague signs and symptoms, and laboratory tests are ordered to obtain information on what may be causing the patient's problem. For example, the patient may have nonspecific abdominal pain, and the physical examination may not yield enough information to support a clinical diagnosis. In this case, the physician may order a series of laboratory and diagnostic tests to assist in pinpointing the cause of the patient's problems.

2. *To evaluate the patient's progress and to regulate treatment.* When a diagnosis has been made, laboratory testing may be performed to evaluate the patient's progress and to regulate treatment. On the basis of the laboratory results, the therapy may need to be adjusted or further treatment prescribed. A patient undergoing iron therapy for iron-deficiency anemia should have a complete blood count (CBC) performed every month to assess the response to treatment and to ensure that the condition is improving. Another example is a patient who has had a cardiac valve replaced and is taking warfarin (Coumadin), an anticoagulant used to inhibit blood clotting. The patient must have a prothrombin time test at regular intervals to assess the clotting ability of the blood. On the basis of the test results, the medication may need to be adjusted to ensure the dosage is at a safe level. A patient with diabetes who measures his or her blood glucose level each day to regulate insulin dosage provides another example of laboratory tests used to regulate treatment.

3. *To establish a baseline level.* On the basis of such factors as age, gender, race, and geographic location, individuals have different normal levels within the established reference range for a particular test. In this respect, laboratory tests also can serve to establish each patient's baseline level with which future results can be compared. A patient who is going to receive warfarin (Coumadin) therapy should have a blood specimen drawn for a prothrombin time test before administration of this anticoagulant. The results serve as a baseline recording for that particular patient against which future prothrombin time test results can be compared.

4. *To prevent or reduce the severity of disease.* Laboratory tests also can help to prevent or reduce the severity of disease through early detection of abnormal findings. Certain conditions, such as high cholesterol, anemia, and diabetes, are relatively common disorders and sometimes may exist without symptoms in a patient, especially early in the development of the disease. Laboratory tests known as **routine tests** are performed on a routine basis on apparently healthy patients (usually as part of a general physical examination) to assist in the early detection of disease. These tests are relatively easy to perform and present a minimal hazard to the patient. The most commonly used routine tests are urinalysis, CBC, and routine blood chemistries.

5. *To comply with state laws.* Another reason for a laboratory test is its requirement by state law. The statutes of most states require a gonorrhea and syphilis test to be performed on pregnant women. The purpose of these tests is to protect the mother and fetus from harm by screening for the presence of these sexually transmitted diseases.

TYPES OF CLINICAL LABORATORIES

The medical office may use an outside laboratory for testing, or the office may contain its own laboratory, known as a *physician's office laboratory* (POL), in which the medical assistant performs various tests. Most medical offices use a combination of the two to fulfill the physician's need for test results.

Physician's Office Laboratory

Generally, laboratory tests that are CLIA-waived and commonly required, such as glucose determination and urinalysis, are performed in the POL (Figure 29-1). CLIA (Clinical

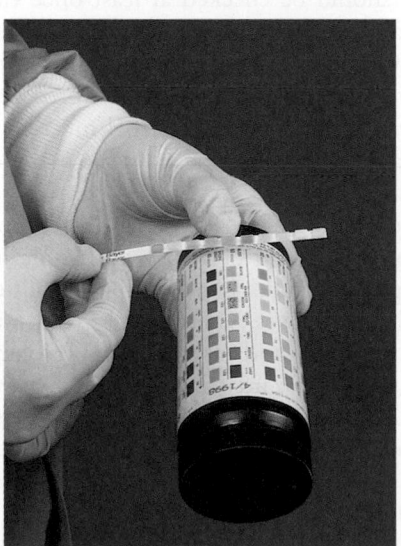

Figure 29-1 Urinalysis is frequently performed in a physician's office laboratory (POL).

Laboratories Improvement Amendments) consists of regulations developed in 1988 by the federal government to improve the quality of laboratory testing in the United States. A **waived test** is a laboratory test that has been determined by CLIA to be a simple procedure that is easy to perform and has a low risk of erroneous test results. CLIA regulations are described in greater detail later in this chapter.

Most physicians consider it too expensive in terms of equipment, supplies, and medical laboratory personnel to perform laboratory tests that are any more complex than waived tests in the medical office. These tests are usually performed at an outside laboratory. Outside laboratories use highly sophisticated automated equipment to perform the tests, providing the medical offices with fast and reliable test results.

Physical Structure of the POL

The physical structure of the POL should meet certain requirements to provide a safe and effective working environment for performing laboratory tests and storing laboratory equipment and supplies. The POL should be a separate room or work area in the medical office. Laboratory work counters should be large enough to provide ample space for testing specimens. Cabinets should be available for storing equipment and supplies. The medical assistant should check the supply inventory periodically and reorder supplies as needed. A refrigerator should be available in the POL for storing specimens that require refrigeration, such as blood tubes and urine awaiting pickup by a courier from an outside laboratory. In addition, certain testing components, such as controls and testing reagents, may require refrigeration. The temperature of the refrigerator must be maintained at between 36° F (2° C) and 46° F (8° C) to retard alterations in the physical and chemical compositions of specimens and to prevent deterioration of testing components that require refrigeration. The temperature of the refrigerator should be checked at least once each day and recorded on a refrigerator temperature log sheet. As specified by the Occupational Safety and Health Administration (OSHA) Standard, food must not be stored in the laboratory refrigerator, and a warning label must be attached to the refrigerator to alert employees to the presence of potentially infectious materials.

Equipment and supplies necessary to comply with the OSHA Standard should be readily accessible in the POL. These supplies include handwashing facilities, alcohol-based hand rubs, gloves, safety goggles and masks, safety-engineered syringes and needles, and biohazard sharps containers and biohazard trash bags. An eyewash station (Figure 29-2) is also recommended in the event of an exposure incident to the mucous membranes of the eyes, nose, or mouth.

The temperature of the room should be maintained within a range that is conducive to performing laboratory tests and storing testing materials that require room temperature storage. Temperatures outside of this range can

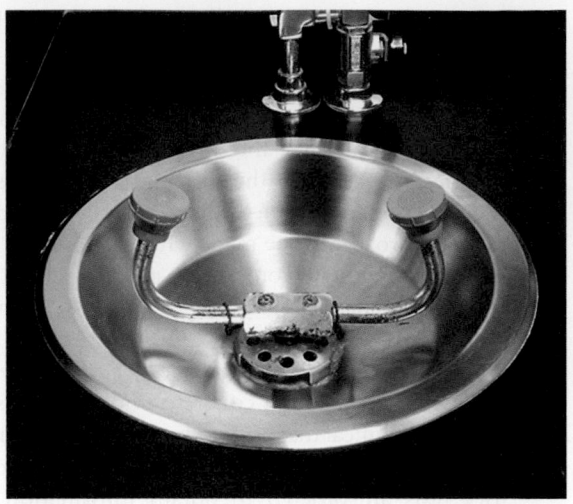

Figure 29-2 Eyewash station.

cause deterioration of testing materials, such as controls and testing reagents. Some automated analyzers are able to operate only within a specific temperature range. When a specimen is tested, a chemical reaction occurs between the specimen and the testing reagents to produce the test results. With some analyzers, the chemical reaction can occur only within a certain temperature range. If the temperature is outside of the required range, the analyzer cannot perform the test, resulting in an error message that appears on the screen of the analyzer. The temperature range required for the storage of testing materials and for performing tests is stated in the instructions accompanying them. It is usually a room temperature that falls between 59° F (15° C) and 86° F (30° C).

Adequate lighting is essential to assist in the proper collection, handling, and testing of specimens. Good lighting is also needed for the proper interpretation of test results that use a visual color comparison method to determine test results, such as the dipstick method of urinalysis.

The medical assistant is responsible for making sure the POL is clean and free of clutter. Biohazard sharps containers and trash bags should be replaced as needed. A disinfectant should be readily available for disinfecting the laboratory work counters each day. The medical assistant should know how to care for each piece of laboratory equipment; this information is indicated in the operating manual that accompanies the equipment.

Outside Laboratories

Outside laboratories include hospital and privately owned independent laboratories, which employ individuals specifically trained in clinical laboratory techniques and methods such as medical laboratory technologists and technicians. Because the medical assistant usually works closely with an outside laboratory, a basic knowledge of the relationship between the medical office and the outside laboratory (as described in this section) is important. If the specimen is collected at the medical office, the laboratory usually

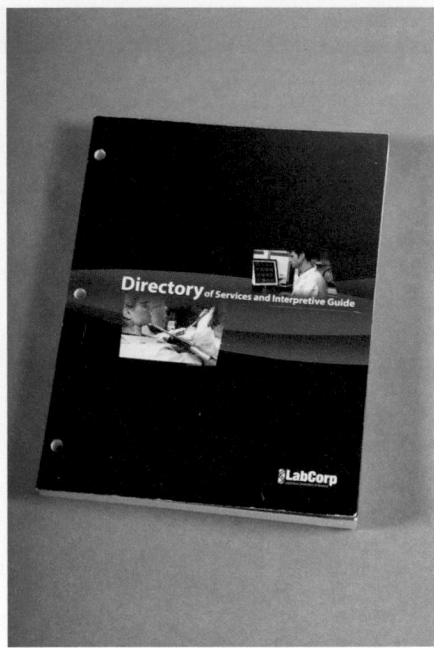

Figure 29-3 Laboratory directory.

provides the medical office with the supplies and forms necessary to collect the specimen and prepare it for transport to the laboratory. The medical assistant is responsible for checking these supplies periodically and for reordering them from the laboratory as needed.

Laboratory Directory

The outside laboratory provides the medical office with a laboratory directory (Figure 29-3), which serves as a valuable reference source for the proper collection and handling of specimens for transport to the outside laboratory. The laboratory may also maintain a website that includes a test menu of the specimen collection and handling requirements for each test performed by that laboratory. This allows the medical assistant to access this information easily and quickly using one or more of the following: a search box, an alphabetical index, or drop-down lists. If, after referring to the laboratory directory (or laboratory website), the medical assistant has a question regarding any aspect of the collection and handling of the specimen that is not clear, the laboratory should be contacted before proceeding.

Laboratory directories vary in organization, depending on the laboratory. The following information is generally included in the directory for each test performed by the laboratory:
- Name and CPT code of the test
- Reference range
- Amount and type of specimen required
- Supplies necessary for collection of the specimen (e.g., blood tubes)
- Techniques to be used for collection of the specimen
- Special instructions
- Patient preparation
- Proper handling and storage of the specimen
- Instructions for transporting the specimen
- Causes for rejection of the specimen by the laboratory
- Uses and limitations of the test
- Methodology used to perform the test

Table 29-1 is a (modified) table of representative tests included in a laboratory directory to provide an overall

Table 29-1 Representative Tests from a (Modified) Laboratory Directory

This table presents a modified table of representative tests included in a laboratory directory to provide you with an overall understanding of the components of a laboratory directory. The components presented in this modified directory include the name and CPT code of the test, reference range, amount and type of specimen required, supplies necessary for the collection of the specimen, techniques to use for collection of the specimen, patient preparation, proper handling and storage of the specimen, and causes for rejection of the specimen. This modified table does *not* include special instructions, instructions for transporting the specimen, uses and limitations of the test, and methodology used to perform the test. (*NOTE:* Refer to Figure 29-8 for an example of a laboratory test exactly as it is presented in a laboratory directory.)

Test and CPT Code	Specimen Requirements	Reference Range
ALT (alanine aminotransferase) CPT Code: 84460	2 mL serum in SST or transfer tube Centrifuge and separate serum within 45 minutes after collection. Refrigerate or store at RT.	45 U/L or less
AST (aspartate aminotransferase) CPT Code: 84450	2 mL serum in SST or transfer tube Centrifuge and separate serum from cells within 45 minutes after collection. Refrigerate or store at RT.	40 U/L or less
Bilirubin, total CPT Code: 82247	2 mL serum in SST or transfer tube Centrifuge and separate serum from cells within 45 minutes after collection. Refrigerate. Protect from light.	0.1-1.2 mg/dL
Blood group (ABO) and Rh Type CPT Codes: 86900, 86901	5 mL lavender-top tube A separate lavender-top tube is required for this test. Refrigerate or store at RT.	

Continued

Table 29-1 Representative Tests from a (Modified) Laboratory Directory—cont'd

BUN (blood urea nitrogen) CPT Code: 84520	2 mL serum in SST or transfer tube Centrifuge and separate serum within 45 minutes after collection. Refrigerate serum.	7-25 mg/dL
Calcium, serum CPT Code: 82310	2 mL serum in SST or transfer tube Centrifuge and separate serum from cells within 45 minutes after collection. Refrigerate or store at RT.	0-6 months: 8.9-11 mg/dL 7 months-adult: 8.5-10.6 mg/dL
CBC with differential CPT Code: 85025	5 mL lavender-top tube Gently invert tube 8-10 times immediately after drawing. Refrigerate or store at RT.	Values given with report
CK (creatine kinase) CPT Code: 82550	3 mL serum in SST or transfer tube Avoid exercise before venipuncture. Centrifuge and separate serum from cells within 45 minutes after collection. Refrigerate or store at RT.	Male: 17-148 U/L Female: 10-70 U/L
CRP (C-reactive protein) CPT Code: 86140	1 mL serum in SST or transfer tube Avoid hemolysis. Centrifuge and separate serum from cells within 45 minutes after collection. Refrigerate or store at RT.	0.0-4.9 mg/L
Glucose, plasma CPT Code: 82947	5 mL gray-top tube Patient should be fasting for 12 to 14 hours. Gently invert tube 8-10 times immediately after drawing. Refrigerate or store at RT.	65-99 mg/dL
LD (lactic acid dehydrogenase) CPT Code: 83615	3 mL serum in SST or transfer tube Hemolysis invalidates results. Centrifuge and separate serum from cells within 45 minutes after collection. Refrigerate or store at RT.	100-250 IU/L
PT/INR (prothrombin time) CPT Code: 85610	5-mL light blue–top tube Gently invert tube 3-4 times immediately after drawing. Clotting and hemolysis invalidate results. Store at RT.	PT/INR: 0.8-1.2 Patients on anticoagulant therapy: PT/INR: 2.0-3.0
RPR (rapid plasma reagin) CPT Code: 86592	1 mL serum in SST or transfer tube Centrifuge and separate serum from cells within 45 minutes after collection. Refrigerate.	Nonreactive
Sedimentation rate CPT Code: 85652	5 mL lavender-top tube Gently invert tube 8-10 times immediately after drawing. Refrigerate.	Male: 0-15 mm/hr Over 50 years: 0-20 mm/hr Female: 0-20 mm/hr Over 50 years: 0-30 mm/hr
Triiodothyronine (T₃) CPT Code: 84480	1 mL serum in SST or transfer tube Centrifuge and separate serum from cells within 45 minutes after collection. Refrigerate.	83-200 mg/dL
Thyroxine (T₄) CPT Code: 84436	2 mL serum in SST or transfer tube Centrifuge and separate serum from cells within 45 minutes after collection. Refrigerate.	4.5-12.0 μg/dL
Triglycerides CPT Code: 84478	2 mL serum in SST or transfer tube Patient should be fasting 12-14 hr. Centrifuge and separate serum from cells within 45 minutes after collection. Refrigerate or store at RT.	Less than 150 mg/dL
Urinalysis, routine CPT Code: 81003	Random sample in urine transport tube First morning specimen preferred (10 mL) Refrigerate.	Values given with report

SST, Serum separator tube.

understanding of the information included in a laboratory directory. The information presented in this modified directory includes all of the categories listed above with the exception of the following: special instructions, instructions for transporting the specimen, uses and limitations of the test, and methodology used to perform the test. (*Note:* Refer to Figure 29-8 for an example of a laboratory test exactly as it is presented in a laboratory directory.)

Collection and Testing Categories

Collection and testing of a specimen can be categorized as follows:

1. The specimen is collected and tested at the medical office.
2. The specimen is collected at the medical office and transferred to an outside laboratory for testing.
3. The patient is given a laboratory request to have the specimen collected and tested at an outside laboratory.

The medical assistant's responsibilities depend on which of these methods is used in the medical office. For example, a specimen collected at the medical office and transferred to an outside laboratory for testing involves a series of individual steps different from the steps followed when it is collected and tested at the medical office. The following clinical laboratory methods are presented in the remainder of this chapter to provide the student with the information needed to function competently in all three modes just described as follows:

1. Completing laboratory request forms and reviewing laboratory reports
2. Informing the patient of any necessary advance preparation or special instructions
3. Collecting, handling, and transporting specimens
4. Performing CLIA-waived tests in the medical office
5. Practicing quality control and laboratory safety

LABORATORY REQUESTS

Purpose

A laboratory request is a printed form that contains a list of the most frequently ordered laboratory tests (Figure 29-4). A laboratory request is required when the specimen is collected at the medical office and transferred to an outside laboratory for testing, or when the specimen is to be collected and tested at an outside laboratory, in which case the request is given to the patient at the medical office to take to the laboratory. The request provides the outside laboratory with essential information necessary for accurate testing, reporting of results, and billing. Organizational formats for the request forms vary, depending on the laboratory. In general, most outside laboratories find it more convenient and economical to provide the medical office with one form for designating all tests, with the possible exception of the Pap test, in which case a separate form, known as a *cytology request,* is provided.

Parts of Laboratory Request Form

The request form can be completed manually by the medical assistant by writing in all information required, or it may be completed on a computer screen by entering the information using a keyboard. Specific information that is required on the laboratory request form follows.

1. *Physician's name and address.* The physician's name and address should be clearly indicated on the laboratory request form to facilitate the reporting of test results to the physician. Laboratory request forms are usually prenumbered with the physician's account number, which assists in identification, reporting, and billing of laboratory tests.
2. *Patient's name and address.* The patient's name and address must be documented on the form as requested by the laboratory; for example, the laboratory may want the patient's name designated with the last name first, middle initial, and then first name. The patient's address is needed for billing purposes and must include the city, state, and zip code.
3. *Patient's age and gender.* The reference ranges for some tests vary depending on the patient's age and gender. The reference range for hemoglobin concentration varies according to gender (12 to 16 g/dL for a woman; 14 to 18 g/dL for a man).
4. *Date and time of collection of the specimen.* The date of the specimen collection indicates to the laboratory the number of days that have passed since the collection, providing the laboratory with information regarding the freshness of the specimen. A time lapse that is too long between collection and testing of a specimen may affect the accuracy of some test results. The time of collection is significant with respect to certain laboratory tests. The reference range for serum cortisol varies depending on whether the specimen is collected in the morning or in the afternoon.
5. *Laboratory tests desired.* The tests desired by the physician are usually indicated by marking a box adjacent to those tests (and their corresponding CPT code), as illustrated in Figure 29-3. A space designated as "additional tests" or "other tests" is provided on the laboratory request form for specifying the CPT code of a test that is desired but not listed on the request form. As previously indicated, the laboratory request form includes only the tests most frequently ordered. The laboratory directory contains a complete listing of all tests performed by the laboratory.
6. *Profiles.* Laboratory tests termed *profiles* may be ordered by the physician. A **profile** (also known as a *panel*) consists of an array of laboratory tests that have been determined to be the most sensitive and specific means of identifying a disease state or evaluating a particular organ or organ system. The profiles performed by an outside laboratory and the tests included in each are listed in the laboratory directory. A profile may be specific in nature, that is, all

LABORATORY REQUISITION
Biomedical Laboratories, Inc.
100 Main Street
Athens, Georgia 45760

☐ Fax	Send additional copy of report to:
☐ Call	Client Number/Physician's Name	Phone/Fax number
☐ Mail	Physician's Address	City, State, Zip

| Patient's Name (Last) | (First) | (MI) | Sex | Date of Birth MO DAY YEAR | Collection Time : AM PM | Fasting YES NO | Collection Date MO DAY YEAR |

| NPI/UPIN | Physician's ID # | Patient's SS # | Patient's ID # | Urine hrs/vol hrs_____ vol_____ |

PATIENT

Physician's Name (Last, First)	Physician's Signature	Patient's Address	Phone
Medicare # (Include prefix/suffix) ☐ Primary ☐ Secondary	City	State	ZIP
Medicaid # State	Physician's Provider #

RESP. PARTY

Name of Responsible Party (if different from patient)

Address of Responsible Party (if different from patient)   APT #

City   State   ZIP

Diagnosis/Signs/Symptoms in ICD-9 Format (Highest Specificity)
REQUIRED

INSURANCE

| Patient's Relationship to Responsible Party | ■ 1–Self | ■ 2–Spouse | ■ 3–Child | ■ 4–Other |

| Performance Lab ☐ | Carrier | Group # | Employee # | Mem |

Insurance Company Name	Plan	Carrier Code
Subscriber/Member #	Location	Group #
Insurance Address	Physician's Provider #
City	State ZIP
Employer's Name or Number	Insured SS # (If not patient)	Worker's Comp ☐ Yes ☐ No

I hereby authorize the release of medical information related to the service subscribed herein and authorize payment directed to LabCorp.
X _____   _____
             Patient's Signature   Date

MEDICARE ADVANCE BENEFICIARY NOTICE
I have read the ABN on the reverse. If Medicare denies payment, I agree to pay for the identified test(s).
X _____   _____
             Patient's Signature   Date

NOTE: WHEN ORDERING TESTS FOR WHICH MEDICARE OR MEDICAID REIMBURSEMENT WILL BE SOUGHT, PHYSICIANS SHOULD ONLY ORDER TESTS THAT ARE MEDICALLY NECESSARY FOR THE DIAGNOSIS OR TREATMENT OF THE PATIENT. COMPONENTS OF THE ORGAN OR DISEASE PANELS/COMBINATIONS PRINTED BELOW ARE SHOWN ON THE REVERSE SIDE AND MAY ALSO BE ORDERED INDIVIDUALLY BELOW. COMPONENTS MAY BE BILLED SEPARATELY PER CARRIER POLICY.

PROFILES (See reverse for components)

80049	Basic Metabolic Profile	(SST)
80054	Comp Metabolic Profile	(SST)
80051	Electrolyte Profile	(SST)
80058	Hepatic Profile	(SST)
80059	Hepatitis Profile	(SST)
80061	Lipid Profile	(SST)
80091	Thyroid Profile	(SST)
80055	Prenatal Profile	(RED)(LAV)
80072	Rheumatoid Profile	(SST)

HEMATOLOGY

85025	CBC w Diff	(LAV)
85027	CBC w/o Diff	(LAV)
85014	Hematocrit	(LAV)
85018	Hemoglobin	(LAV)
85595	Platelet Count	(LAV)
85041	RBC Count	(LAV)
85048	WBC Count	(LAV)
85007	WBC Differential	(LAV)
89190	Nasal Smear, Eosin	(Nasal Smear)
85060	Pathologist Consult–Peripheral Smear	(LAV)

ALPHABETICAL/COMBINATION TESTS

86900 86901	ABO and Rh	(LAV)
82040	Albumin	(SST)
84075	Alkaline Phosphatase	(SST)
84460	ALT (SGPT)	(SST)
82150	Amylase, Serum	(SST)
86038	Antinuclear Antibodies	(SST)
84450	AST (SGOT)	(SST)
82607 82746	B₁₂ and Folate	(SST)
82250	Bilirubin, Total	(SST)

ALPHABETICAL TESTS CON'T

84520	BUN	(SST)
82310	Calcium	(SST)
80156	Carbamazepine (Tegretol®)	(SER)
82378	CEA	(SST)
82465	Cholesterol, Total	(SST)
82565	Creatinine	(SST)
80162	Digoxin	(SER)
82670	Estradiol	(SST)
82728	Ferritin, Serum	(SST)
82985	Fructosamine	(SST)
83001	FSH	(SST)
83001 83002	FSH and LH	(SST)
82977	GGT	(SST)
82947	Glucose, Plasma	(GRY)
82947	Glucose, Serum	(SST)
82950	Glucose, 2-hr. PP	(SST)
83036	Glycohemoglobin, Total	(LAV)
84703	hCG, Beta Subunit, Qual	(SST)
84702	hCG, Beta Subunit, Quant	(SST)
83718	HDL Cholesterol	(SST)
86677	Helicobacter pylori, IgG	(SST)
86706	Hep B Surface Antibody	(SST)
87340	Hep B Surface Antigen	(SST)
86803	Hep C Antibody	(SST)
83036	Hemoglobin A₁C	(LAV)
86701	HIV Antibodies	(SST)
83540	Iron, Total	(SST)
83540 83550	Iron and IBC	(SST)
83615	LDH	(SST)

ALPHABETICAL TESTS CON'T

83002	LH	(SST)
83690	Lipase	(SER)
80178	Lithium (Eskalith®)	(SER)
83735	Magnesium, Serum	(SST)
80184	Phenobarbital (Luminal®)	(SER)
80185	Phenytoin (Dilantin®)	(SER)
84132	Potassium	(SST)
84146	Prolactin, Serum	(SST)
84153	Prostate-Specific Antigen	(SST)
84066	Prostatic Acid Phos	(SST)
84155	Protein, Total	(SST)
85610	Prothrombin Time (PT)	(BLU)
85610 85730	PT and PTT Activated	(BLU)
85730	PTT Activated	(BLU)
86431	Rheumatoid Arthritis Factor	(SST)
86592	RPR	(SST)
86762	Rubella Antibodies, IgG	(SST)
85651	Sed Rate	(LAV)
84295	Sodium	(SST)
84403	Testosterone	(SST)
80198	Theophylline	(SER)
84436	Thyroxine (T₄)	(SST)
84478	Triglycerides	(SST)
84480	Triiodothyronine (T₃)	(SST)
84443	TSH, High Sensitivity	(SST)
84550	Uric Acid	(SST)
81003	Urinalysis Microscopic on Positives	(URN)
81001	Urinalysis with Microscopic	(URN)
80164	Valproic Acid (Depakene®)	(SER)

MICROBIOLOGY   See Reverse Side

■ ENDOCERVICAL   ■ THROAT   ■ URINE
■ STOOL   ■ URETHRAL   INDICATE SOURCE

87070	Aerobic Bacterial Culture	(Bact Trnspt)
87490 87590	Chlamydia/GC DNA Probe w/ Confirmation on Positives	(Probe Trnspt)
87490 87590	Chlamydia/GC DNA Probe Without Confirmation	(Probe Trnspt)
87490	Chlamydia DNA Probe	(Probe Trnspt)
87081	Genital, Beta-Hemolytic Strep Cult, Group B	(Bact Trnspt)
87070	Genital Culture, Routine	(Bact Trnspt)
87070	Lower Respiratory Culture	(Steril Trnspt)
87590	N. gonorrhoeae DNA Probe	(Probe Trnspt)
87015 87211	Ova and Parasites	(O & P Kit)
87081 X2 87045	Stool Culture	(Fecal Trnspt)
87081	Throat, Beta-Hemolytic Strep Cult, Group A	(Bact Trnspt)
87060	Upper Respiratory Culture, Routine	(Bact Trnspt)
87086	Urine Culture, Routine	(Urn Cul Trnspt)

Clinical Information/Comments

OTHER TESTS/INDIVIDUAL COMPONENTS

TEST #	TEST NAMES

| LAB USE ONLY | STAT ☐ 998074 | VENIPUNCTURE ☐ 998085 | TRAVEL ☐ 998096 | NON LABCORP ☐ 998239 | VERBAL ORDER ☐ 998250 | CHART ORDER ☐ 998261 | HANDWRITTEN ☐ 998272 | 24 HR TUV ☐ 998283 | PST/PSC # |

| CONTAINERS RECEIVED | SST SPUN | USST UNSPUN | SER SERUM TRNSPT | FRZ FRZ TRNS | RED RED | LAV LAVENDER | SLD SLIDE | BLU LT. BLUE | GRY GREY | GRN GREEN | RYB RYL BLU | YEL ACD | PLS PLASMA | URN URINE | 24U 24 HR URINE | TA-U TART. ACID | FL FLUID | OT OTHER | BACT TRNSP | O & P KIT | PROBE TRNSP | URN CULT TRNSP | STERIL TRNSP | FECAL TRNSP | VIRAL TRNSP |

300-0384

Figure 29-4 Laboratory request form.

tests included relate to a specific organ of the body or a particular disease state. A specific profile is usually ordered when the physician does not have a definite clinical diagnosis but has a good idea of the patient's condition or what organ or organs are involved in the patient's condition. The physician orders a profile of the condition or organ in question. An example of a profile used to identify a disease state is the rheumatoid profile, which is used to assist in the diagnosis of rheumatoid arthritis. An example of a profile used to evaluate an organ is the hepatic function profile, which is used to assess liver function and to assist in the diagnosis of a pathologic condition that affects the liver.

A profile also may be general in nature. A general metabolic profile contains numerous routine laboratory tests and is used primarily in a routine health

screen of a patient. General metabolic profiles are used to detect any changes in the body's biologic processes that may be present, although the patient may not have had any symptoms to indicate that these changes have occurred. General metabolic profiles also are used when the patient's symptoms are so vague that the physician does not have enough concrete evidence to support a clinical diagnosis of a specific organ or disease state. An example of a general profile is the comprehensive metabolic profile; refer to Table 29-3 for a list of the tests included in this profile.

The medical assistant should have knowledge of the names of common profiles and the tests generally contained in each, which are listed in Table 29-2. The tests contained in each profile may vary slightly from one laboratory to another.

Table 29-2 Laboratory Profiles

Profile	Tests Included	Use
Comprehensive metabolic profile	Albumin, ALP, ALT, AST, Bilirubin (Total), BUN, Calcium, Carbon Dioxide, Chloride, Creatinine, Glucose, Inorganic Phosphorus, Potassium, Protein (Total), Sodium, Triglycerides	General health screen that provides information on kidneys, liver, acid-base balance, blood glucose level, and blood proteins. Used to evaluate organ function and to check for conditions such as diabetes, liver disease, and kidney disease. Routinely ordered as part of blood workup for physical examination or medical examination (particularly when patient's symptoms are vague). Abnormal test results are usually followed up with more specific tests before a diagnosis is made.
Electrolyte profile	Carbon Dioxide, Chloride, Potassium, Sodium	Screen for electrolyte or acid-base imbalance and monitor effect of treatment on disease or condition that causes electrolyte imbalance. This profile also is used to evaluate patient taking medication that can cause electrolyte imbalance.
Hepatic profile	Albumin, ALP, ALT, AST, Bilirubin (Direct), Bilirubin (Total), Protein (Total)	Detection of pathologic conditions affecting the liver. This test is often ordered when symptoms indicating a liver condition occur, such as jaundice, dark urine, light-colored bowel movements, or pain or swelling in the abdomen. This profile may be ordered when an individual has been exposed to hepatitis, has a family history of liver disease, has excessive alcohol consumption, or is taking medication that can result in liver damage.
Hepatitis profile	Hepatitis A Antibody, IgM; Hepatitis B Core Antibody, Total; Hepatitis B Surface Antigen; Hepatitis C Antibody	Detection of viral hepatitis.
Lipid profile	Total Cholesterol, LDL Cholesterol, HDL Cholesterol, Triglycerides, VLDL Cholesterol (Calculation), Total Cholesterol/HDL Ratio (Calculation)	Determine risk of coronary artery disease.

Continued

Table 29-2 Laboratory Profiles—cont'd

Profile	Tests Included	Use
Prenatal profile	ABO Grouping and Rh Typing CBC W/Diff and W/Plt Hepatitis B Surface Antigen Red Cell Antibody Screen Rubella Antibody Screen Syphilis Serology (RPR)	Establish baseline recordings and screenings of prenatal patients for disease or potential problems.
Renal function profile	Albumin BUN Calcium Carbon Dioxide Chloride Creatinine Glucose Phosphorus Potassium Sodium	Detection of kidney problems. This profile shows how well the kidneys are functioning to remove excess fluid and waste. When a problem is detected, diagnostic imaging tests may be used for further evaluation and diagnosis.
Rheumatoid profile	ANA CRP Rheumatoid Factor Sedimentation Rate Streptolysin O Uric Acid	Assist in diagnosis of rheumatoid arthritis and help distinguish it from other forms of arthritis and conditions with similar symptoms. This profile also is used to evaluate severity of rheumatoid arthritis, to monitor the condition and its complications, and to assess response to treatment.
Thyroid function profile	FTI Thyroxine (T_4) Triiodothyronine (T_3) Uptake	Detection of conditions affecting the thyroid gland.

ALP, Alkaline phosphatase; *ALT,* alanine aminotransferase; *ANA,* antinuclear antibody; *AST,* aspartate aminotransferase; *BUN,* blood urea nitrogen; *CBC,* complete blood count; *CRP,* C-reactive protein; *FTI,* free thyroxine index; *HDL,* high-density lipoprotein; *LDL,* low-density lipoprotein; *VLDL,* very-low-density lipoprotein.

7. *Source of the specimen.* Certain tests require that the source of the specimen (e.g., throat, wound, ear, eye, urine, vagina) be recorded on the laboratory request form. This is done for identification of the origin of the specimen for the laboratory, because this information is not available by looking at the specimen. In many instances, the source dictates the test method used by the laboratory to evaluate the specimen for the presence of a possible pathogen. The test method used to detect the presence of *Streptococcus* in a specimen obtained from the throat would be different from that used to detect *Candida albicans* in a vaginal specimen.

8. *Physician's clinical diagnosis (in International Classification of Diseases [ICD-9] format).* The clinical diagnosis assists the laboratory in correlating clinical laboratory data with the needs of the physician. In some instances, further testing is performed by the laboratory if one test method proves inconclusive with respect to providing the physician with the information necessary to confirm or reject the clinical diagnosis. Another function of the clinical diagnosis is to assure laboratory personnel that the test results are within the framework of the diagnosis. When the results of a test disagree with the physician's clinical diagnosis, the laboratory repeats

the test on the same or another specimen. The clinical diagnosis also alerts laboratory personnel to the possibility of the presence of a potentially dangerous pathogen, such as the hepatitis virus. In addition, this information is necessary for third-party billing by the laboratory. If the laboratory bills an insurance company for these tests, the ICD-9 code for the clinical diagnosis needs to be on the insurance form. The processing of insurance forms is facilitated by having the information at hand and not having to contact the medical office to obtain it.

9. *Medications.* Certain medications may interfere with the accuracy and validity of test results. The laboratory should be notified on the request form of any medications taken by the patient.

10. *STAT.* Sometimes the physician wants the laboratory test results reported as soon as possible. In this case, "STAT" should be clearly indicated in bold letters (or the appropriate STAT box checked) on the laboratory request form. Requests that are marked STAT are performed as soon as possible after receipt by the laboratory, and the results are telephoned or faxed to the physician as soon as they are available.

After the specimen has been collected, the completed request form must be placed with the specimen for transport to the outside laboratory. The medical assistant should realize the significance of this simple but important step. Numerous possible tests can be performed on one particular specimen, and without the request form, the laboratory does not have the information it needs to carry out the physician's orders, causing delays in completing the tests and reporting results.

What Would You Do? What Would You *Not* Do?

Case Study 1

Three days ago, Hildy McNicle was given a laboratory requisition at the medical office to have blood drawn and tested at an outside medical laboratory. Hildy calls the medical office and says she is a little confused. She called the laboratory for her test results, and they would not give them to her. They told her to call the medical office. She does not understand this because her blood was collected and tested at the laboratory, and it would seem logical to her that they would give her the test results, especially because she is paying the laboratory to perform the tests. The test results have come back with abnormal values, and the physician is at a medical convention and will not return until tomorrow. ■

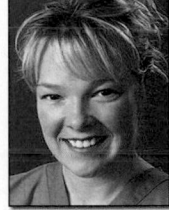

Putting it All into Practice

My name is Korey McGrew, and I am employed by a group of physicians in a family practice medical office. Some of my duties include showing patients to examining rooms, taking the patient's vital signs, administering medications, transcription, filing, and many other duties that medical assistants perform. I have found that being a medical assistant has been challenging and rewarding, and I wish you the best of luck in reaching your goals.

When I first started working as a practicing medical assistant, I had a challenging venipuncture experience. The patient was a kind and personable 64 year old man with hardening of the arteries. I tried to obtain the blood specimen from his arm but was not successful. The patient was calm and was not bothered at all by the unsuccessful stick. He said that it was hard to draw blood on him and to go ahead and try again. I decided to try taking blood from a vein on the back of his hand with a butterfly setup. To my relief, I obtained the blood specimen. I think that I was more nervous about this experience than the patient was. It is important to remain calm on the outside around patients even if you are nervous on the inside. ■

LABORATORY REPORTS

Laboratory report forms are used to relay the results of laboratory tests to the physician (Figure 29-5). The report is usually generated by a computer. It may consist of a pre-printed form with the test results printed in the appropriate spaces on the form by a computer (as illustrated in Figure 29-5), or the entire report may be generated by the computer (Figure 29-6). The report includes the following information:

1. Name, address, and telephone number of the laboratory
2. Physician's name and address
3. Patient's name, age, and gender
4. Patient accession number
5. Date the specimen was received by the laboratory
6. Date the results were reported by the laboratory
7. Names of the tests performed
8. Results of the tests
9. Reference range for each test performed

A patient accession number or laboratory number is assigned to each specimen received by the laboratory. Its purpose is to provide positive identification of each specimen within the laboratory and to allow easy access to the patient's laboratory records should a test result need to be located again. If the physician desires to have the laboratory test repeated, the accession number listed on the original report form must be included on the laboratory request form.

The **reference range** is also commonly referred to as a *reference interval* and a *reference value*. A reference range is defined as a certain established and acceptable parameter within which the laboratory test results of a healthy individual are expected to fall. The reference range is used to interpret laboratory test results for a particular patient. A range, rather than a single value, is necessary for laboratory test results because of individual differences among a general population caused by factors such as age, gender, race, and geographic location. In addition, no test can be so accurate that a single value is possible. The reference range for each test varies slightly from one laboratory to another, depending on the test method, equipment, and reagents used to perform the test. In this regard, it is essential that the medical assistant compare the test results with reference ranges supplied by the laboratory performing the test, rather than with a reference source such as a medical laboratory textbook.

Laboratory reports are delivered to the medical office using one or more of the following methods: faxed, mailed, hand-delivered by a laboratory courier, or sent electronically from the laboratory computer to the medical office computer. Abnormal results that pose a threat to the patient's health and laboratory reports marked STAT are telephoned or faxed to the medical office as soon as the tests are completed, and a complete written report follows immediately thereafter. The laboratory usually supplies the medical office with telephone reporting pads to transcribe results from the telephone report to reduce errors.

The medical assistant may be responsible for reviewing laboratory reports as they are received. The medical assistant should compare the patient's test results with the reference ranges supplied by the laboratory and notify the physician of any abnormal test results. Most laboratory computer systems automatically flag abnormal results on the laboratory report. The physician carefully reviews each laboratory report received by the office, and the data obtained are correlated with information obtained from the health history and physical examination. The physician indicates that he or she is finished with the report usually by placing his or

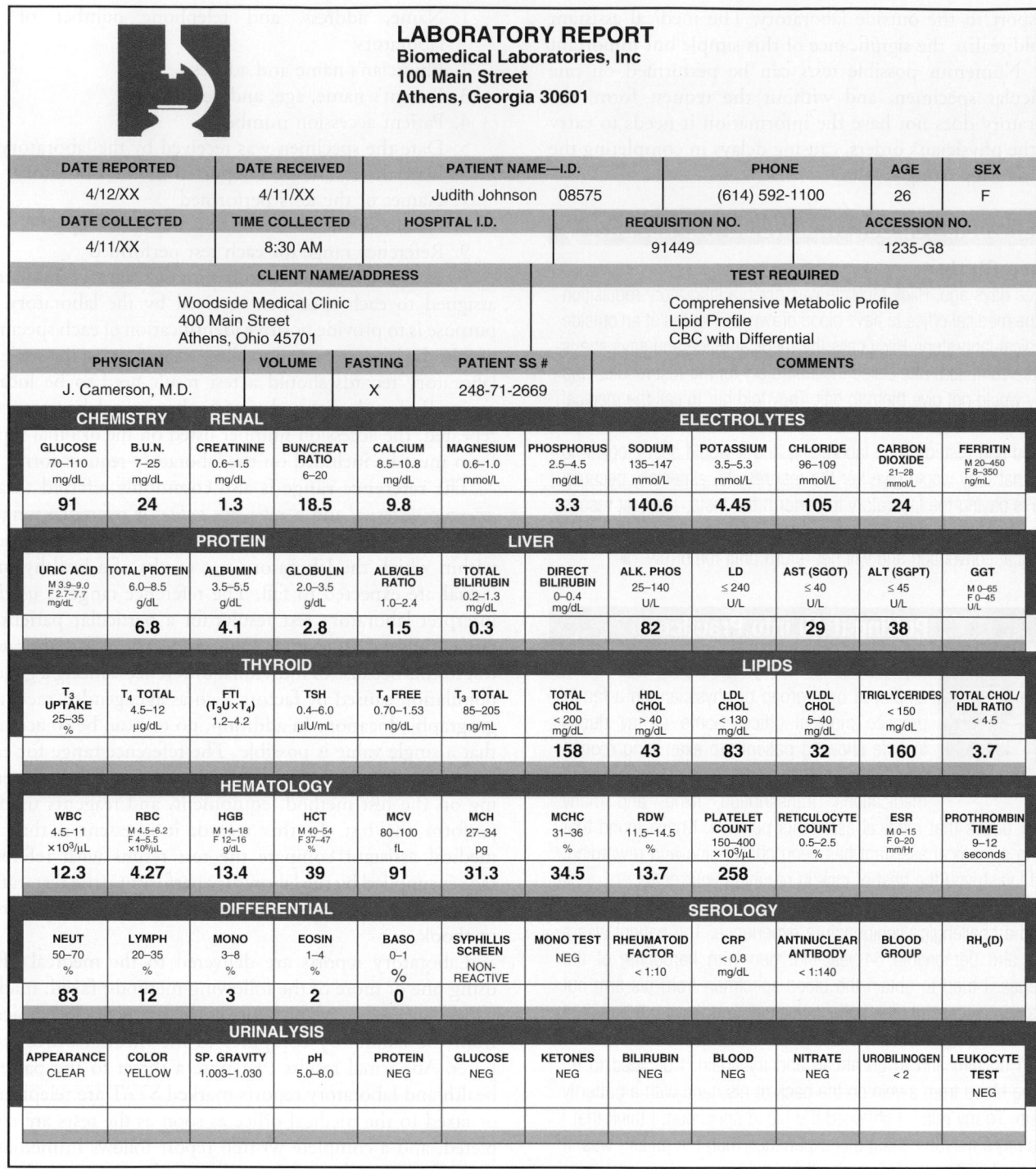

LABORATORY REPORT
Biomedical Laboratories, Inc
100 Main Street
Athens, Georgia 30601

DATE REPORTED	DATE RECEIVED	PATIENT NAME—I.D.		PHONE	AGE	SEX
4/12/XX	4/11/XX	Judith Johnson 08575		(614) 592-1100	26	F

DATE COLLECTED	TIME COLLECTED	HOSPITAL I.D.	REQUISITION NO.	ACCESSION NO.
4/11/XX	8:30 AM		91449	1235-G8

CLIENT NAME/ADDRESS	TEST REQUIRED
Woodside Medical Clinic 400 Main Street Athens, Ohio 45701	Comprehensive Metabolic Profile Lipid Profile CBC with Differential

PHYSICIAN	VOLUME	FASTING	PATIENT SS #	COMMENTS
J. Camerson, M.D.		X	248-71-2669	

CHEMISTRY   RENAL · ELECTROLYTES

GLUCOSE 70–110 mg/dL	B.U.N. 7–25 mg/dL	CREATININE 0.6–1.5 mg/dL	BUN/CREAT RATIO 6–20	CALCIUM 8.5–10.8 mg/dL	MAGNESIUM 0.6–1.0 mmol/L	PHOSPHORUS 2.5–4.5 mg/dL	SODIUM 135–147 mmol/L	POTASSIUM 3.5–5.3 mmol/L	CHLORIDE 96–109 mmol/L	CARBON DIOXIDE 21–28 mmol/L	FERRITIN M 20–450 F 8–350 ng/mL
91	24	1.3	18.5	9.8		3.3	140.6	4.45	105	24	

PROTEIN · LIVER

URIC ACID M 3.9–9.0 F 2.7–7.7 mg/dL	TOTAL PROTEIN 6.0–8.5 g/dL	ALBUMIN 3.5–5.5 g/dL	GLOBULIN 2.0–3.5 g/dL	ALB/GLB RATIO 1.0–2.4	TOTAL BILIRUBIN 0.2–1.3 mg/dL	DIRECT BILIRUBIN 0–0.4 mg/dL	ALK. PHOS 25–140 U/L	LD ≤ 240 U/L	AST (SGOT) ≤ 40 U/L	ALT (SGPT) ≤ 45 U/L	GGT M 0–65 F 0–45 U/L
	6.8	4.1	2.8	1.5	0.3		82		29	38	

THYROID · LIPIDS

T₃ UPTAKE 25–35 %	T₄ TOTAL 4.5–12 µg/dL	FTI (T₃U×T₄) 1.2–4.2	TSH 0.4–6.0 µIU/mL	T₄ FREE 0.70–1.53 ng/dL	T₃ TOTAL 85–205 ng/mL	TOTAL CHOL < 200 mg/dL	HDL CHOL > 40 mg/dL	LDL CHOL < 130 mg/dL	VLDL CHOL 5–40 mg/dL	TRIGLYCERIDES < 150 mg/dL	TOTAL CHOL/ HDL RATIO < 4.5
						158	43	83	32	160	3.7

HEMATOLOGY

WBC 4.5–11 ×10³/µL	RBC M 4.5–6.2 F 4–5.5 ×10⁶/µL	HGB M 14–18 F 12–16 g/dL	HCT M 40–54 F 37–47 %	MCV 80–100 fL	MCH 27–34 pg	MCHC 31–36 %	RDW 11.5–14.5 %	PLATELET COUNT 150–400 ×10³/µL	RETICULOCYTE COUNT 0.5–2.5 %	ESR M 0–15 F 0–20 mm/Hr	PROTHROMBIN TIME 9–12 seconds
12.3	4.27	13.4	39	91	31.3	34.5	13.7	258			

DIFFERENTIAL · SEROLOGY

NEUT 50–70 %	LYMPH 20–35 %	MONO 3–8 %	EOSIN 1–4 %	BASO 0–1 %	SYPHILLIS SCREEN NON- REACTIVE	MONO TEST NEG	RHEUMATOID FACTOR < 1:10	CRP < 0.8 mg/dL	ANTINUCLEAR ANTIBODY < 1:140	BLOOD GROUP	RHₑ(D)
83	12	3	2	0							

URINALYSIS

APPEARANCE CLEAR	COLOR YELLOW	SP. GRAVITY 1.003–1.030	pH 5.0–8.0	PROTEIN NEG	GLUCOSE NEG	KETONES NEG	BILIRUBIN NEG	BLOOD NEG	NITRATE NEG	UROBILINOGEN < 2	LEUKOCYTE TEST NEG

Figure 29-5 Laboratory report form.

her signature on it. The medical assistant is then responsible for filing the laboratory report in the patient's chart, according to the medical office policy.

LABORATORY DOCUMENTS AND THE EMR

Many medical offices communicate with outside laboratories electronically using a computer system that interfaces with the computer system in the outside laboratory. This provides distinct advantages for the medical office using an electronic medical record (EMR). Laboratory requisition forms can be completed on a request form displayed on the computer screen using fill-in boxes, drop-down lists, and check-boxes. Depending on the medical office policy, the form can then be transmitted electronically to the medical laboratory or printed out and placed with the specimen for transport to the laboratory.

Once the patient's tests have been completed, the laboratory test results are sent electronically to the medical office.

Family Practice Health Care Center
3477 Arrowhead Ave
Phoenix, Arizona 78351
(942) 871-3746

ID#	SEX	PATIENT DEMOGRAPHICS	RESULTS PROVIDED BY
3368	F	Leah Percival	Medical Center Laboratory
		2973 Flint Dr.	
DOB		Phoenix, AZ 78366	**ORDERING PROVIDER**
4/28/78			Thomas Murphy, MD

AGE	ACCESSION #	LAB RECEIVED ON	LAB REPORTED ON
34	3380837630	12/07/20XX 11:00:53	12/05/20XX 14:08:00

LAB ID	SPECIMEN ID	COLLECTION DATE/TIME	FASTING
4739	30180906	12/04/20XX 2:53:00	NO

NAME	VALUE	REFERENCE RANGE	UNITS	FLAG
CBC WITH DIFFERENTIAL/PLATELET				
-WBC	4.6	4.0-10.5	x10e3/uL	
-RBC	3.57	4.10-5.60	x10E3/uL	L
-Hemoglobin	11.2	12.5-17.0	g/dL	L
-Hematocrit	32.9	36.0-50.0	%	L
-MCV	92	80-98	fL	
-MCH	31.4	27.0-34.0	pg	
-MCHC	34.0	32.0-36.0	g/dL	
-RDW	15.6	11.7-15.0	%	H
-Platelets	308	140-415	x10E3/uL	
-Neutrophils	73	40-74	%	
-Lymphs	14	14-46	%	
-Monocytes	11	4-13	%	
-Eos	1	0-7	%	
-Basos	1	0-3	%	
-Neutrophils (Absolute)	3.4	1.8-7.8	x10E3/uL	
-Lymphs (Absolute)	0.6	0.7-4.5	x10E3/uL	L

Figure 29-6 Computer-generated laboratory report.

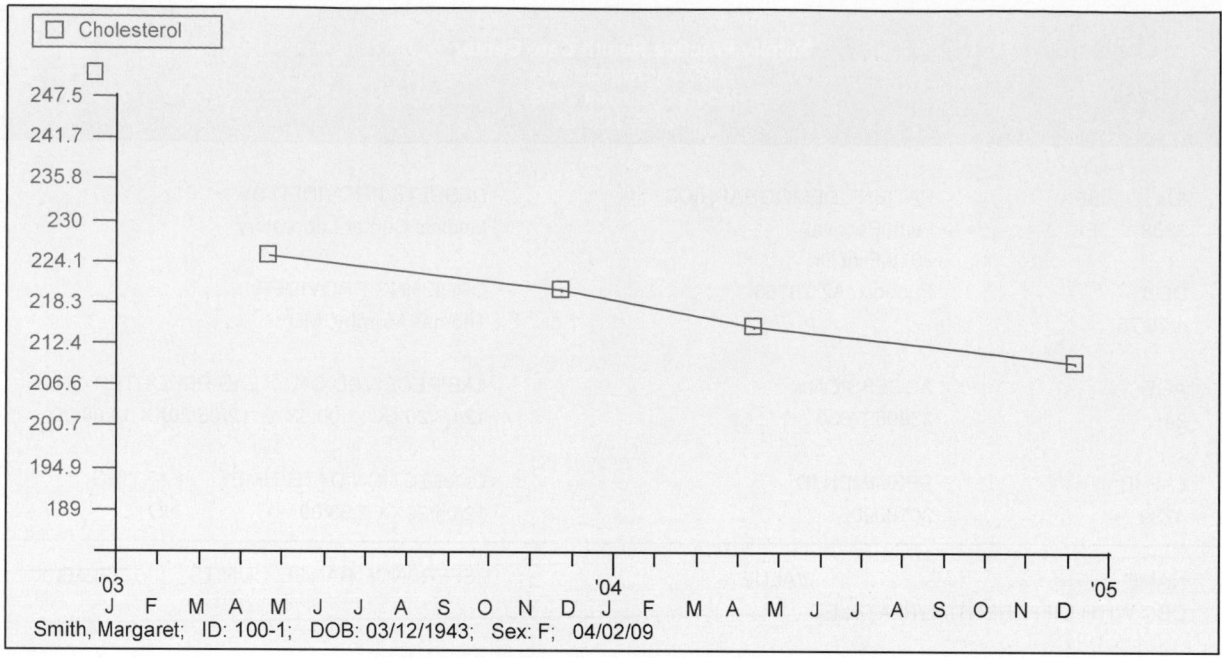

Figure 29-7 Cholesterol flow sheet generated by a computer.

The laboratory report is placed in the physician's "electronic review box" for his or her review and electronic signature. Abnormal values are often highlighted on the report as shown in Figure 29-6. If a critical result appears on the laboratory report, an urgent message is e-mailed to the physician. After the physician reviews the laboratory report and places his or her electronic signature on the report, the report is electronically filed in the patient's EMR.

Other advantages of the laboratory component of an EMR include the ability to quickly view laboratory results in chronological order. In addition, results of a laboratory test performed on a routine basis (e.g., glucose testing, cholesterol testing) can be accessed by the computer and plotted on a flow sheet (Figure 29-7). This permits an abnormal trend to be identified early, so that appropriate action can be taken.

If an EMR medical office is not networked through computers with an outside laboratory, the laboratory reports received by the office must be scanned into the computer and electronically filed in the patient's EMR. A scanned report has some limitations. The computer can display the report, but the data on the report cannot be accessed or manipulated. Because of this, laboratory data cannot be used for many of the functions previously described. For example, the data on a scanned report cannot be accessed and incorporated into a flow sheet for trend analysis.

PATIENT PREPARATION AND INSTRUCTIONS

Factors such as food consumption, medication, activity, and time of day affect the laboratory results of certain tests. For some laboratory tests, advance patient preparation is necessary to obtain a high-quality specimen suitable for testing, which leads to accurate results and assists the physician in

accurate diagnosis and treatment. The quality of laboratory test results can be only as good as the quality of the specimen obtained from the patient. A specimen obtained from a patient who has not prepared properly may invalidate the test results and necessitate calling the patient back to collect the specimen again.

The medical assistant is usually responsible for instructing the patient about the nature of the laboratory test and any advance preparation that might be necessary. A complete and thorough explanation of the information should be relayed clearly to the patient. The patient should be informed of the name of the test, how to prepare for the test, how the test is performed, and how and when to expect the test results. The medical assistant should make sure to explain the reason for the advance preparation, so the patient will be more likely to comply with the preparation necessary. It should be emphasized to the patient that the preparation is essential to obtain accurate test results and to avoid having to collect the specimen again.

After the instructions have been explained, the medical assistant needs to verify that the patient completely understands them and should offer to answer any questions. It also is advisable to provide the patient with a written information sheet (Figure 29-8) to serve as a reference, should the patient forget some of the information after leaving the medical office. Some specimen collections may require that the patient remain at the collection site for a specified time; an example of this is the OGTT, which requires several hours for the collection of multiple, timed specimens. The patient should be told in advance of the time requirement, so that any necessary arrangements can be made with an employer or babysitter.

Sometimes the patient collects the specimen at home. The medical assistant is responsible for explaining detailed

ORAL GLUCOSE TOLERANCE TEST

PATIENT INFORMATION SHEET

General Information

Your physician has requested that you have an oral glucose tolerance test (OGTT). This test is performed to see how well your body processes glucose (sugar). Glucose is the primary source of energy for your body. The OGTT is primarily used to assist in diagnosis of diabetes. Your test is scheduled in the early morning because you will need to perform an overnight fast. The test generally lasts for a period of 3 hours.

Patient Preparation

It is very important that you prepare properly to ensure accurate test results. Patient preparation for this test includes the following:

1. For 3 days prior to the test you should consume a high-carbohydrate diet consisting of at least 150 grams of carbohydrate per day. Foods that are high in carbohydrate include bread, pasta, cereal, potatoes, rice, and crackers.
2. Do NOT drink or eat anything except water for 12 to 14 hours before the test.
3. Your physician will discuss what medications (if any) to discontinue before the test.

Testing Procedure

When you arrive at the testing facility, your blood will be drawn. You will then be given a glucose (sugar) solution to drink. Some people have a brief period of nausea after consuming the glucose solution. Your blood will be collected at intervals over a period of several hours.

During the testing procedure, you may experience some normal side effects such as weakness, a feeling of faintness, or perspiration. They are caused by a decrease in your body's glucose level as insulin is secreted in response to the glucose solution. These side effects are temporary and will only last for a short period of time. To ensure accurate test results, you need to adhere to the following during the testing procedure:

1. Sit quietly and do not leave the testing facility.
2. Do not eat or drink anything except water.
3. Do not smoke or chew gum during the procedure.

Following the Procedure:

After the procedure you can eat and drink as usual and resume your normal activities. An appointment will be scheduled for you to discuss the test results with your physician.

Figure 29-8 Oral glucose tolerance test patient instruction sheet.

instructions to the patient on proper techniques for collection of the specimen. For example, if a first-voided morning urine specimen is necessary for the laboratory test, the medical assistant needs to provide the patient with the appropriate specimen container and to instruct the patient on proper collection, handling, and storage of the specimen until it reaches the medical office.

The specific type of preparation necessary for a particular test depends on the test ordered and the method used to run it. If the medical office uses an outside laboratory, the patient preparation necessary for each test can be found in the laboratory directory. If the test is performed in the medical office, the medical assistant should consult the manufacturer's instructions that accompany the test to obtain specific information regarding patient preparation. Advance patient preparation usually consists of fasting, diet modification (e.g., low-fat diet), or medication restrictions.

Fasting

Some blood specimens require the patient to fast before collection. The composition of blood is altered by the consumption of food because digested food is absorbed into the circulatory system, changing the results of certain laboratory tests. Food intake causes blood glucose and triglyceride laboratory tests to yield falsely high results. Any individual test (e.g., fasting blood glucose [FBG], OGTT) or profile including these tests (e.g., comprehensive

Case Study 2

Hans Volkman is leaving the medical office after being seen by the physician. The physician gave him a laboratory requisition for a complete blood count and a lipid profile. Hans notices that the clinical diagnosis on the form indicates iron-deficiency anemia and wants to know why the physician did not prescribe any medication for him if he thought he had anemia. Hans says that he told the physician his father had a heart attack at age 53 years and asked whether he would order a cholesterol test. He says the physician must have forgotten because the test was not marked on the laboratory form. Hans has been instructed to fast for the laboratory tests. He says that he stops every morning at the Coffee Cup restaurant and has coffee with cream and sugar, orange juice, and two doughnuts. He would like to know whether he could just have the coffee before the tests. Hans says he has a hard time functioning in the morning without coffee. ∎

specimen, and 4 to 24 hours before the collection of a blood specimen.

If the patient cannot be taken off medication, this information should be recorded on the laboratory request form for specimens transported to an outside laboratory for testing. This alerts the laboratory personnel to the presence of the medication. If the medication taken by the patient interferes with the method normally used to perform the test, the laboratory may be able to use an alternative method to obtain valid results. If the test is being performed in the medical office, the medical assistant should consult the manufacturer's instructions that accompany the test for the names of medications that interfere with test results.

The physician determines the need for a patient to discontinue medication before specimen collection. The medical assistant is responsible for ensuring that the patient understands any instructions regarding restrictions on medication and for recording medications the patient is taking on the laboratory request form.

metabolic profile, lipid profile) requires the patient to fast before the specimen is collected.

Fasting involves abstaining from food and fluids (except water) for a specified amount of time before the collection of the specimen (usually 12 to 14 hours). Fasting specimens are usually collected in the morning to allow food from the previous evening meal to be completely digested and absorbed. In addition, collection of the specimen in the morning causes the least amount of inconvenience to the patient in terms of abstaining from food and fluid.

The medical assistant must give detailed instructions to the patient, ensuring that the patient understands that fasting includes abstaining from food and fluid. The patient should be told, however, that it is permissible—in fact advisable—to drink water because dehydration caused by water abstinence can alter certain test results.

The medical assistant should indicate a specific time to the patient for initiation of the fast. If the specimen is to be collected in the morning, the patient should be instructed to begin fasting at 6:00 PM on the previous evening. The patient also must be told the time to report for collection of the specimen.

Medication Restrictions

Many medications affect the physical and chemical characteristics of body substances; medications taken by the patient may lead to inaccurate test results. Antibiotic therapy administered before collection of a throat specimen for strep testing may cause a falsely negative test result. The physician may ask the patient to avoid taking medication for a period of time before the collection of the specimen if discontinuing the medication would not cause any health threat or serious discomfort to the patient. Because medication is more likely to interfere with test results on urine than on blood, the patient is recommended to discontinue medication 48 to 72 hours before the collection of a urine

Case Study 3

Kathleen O'Leary is scheduled for a follow-up appointment today at the office. She was seen last week with fatigue, shortness of breath, weight loss, increased urination, and blurred vision. Kathleen was given a laboratory requisition to have blood drawn at an outside medical laboratory. The physician ordered a complete blood count with differential and a comprehensive metabolic profile. When the charts are prepared for the day, Kathleen's laboratory results are not in her chart. Kathleen is contacted by phone; she says she knows she should have gone to the laboratory to have her blood drawn, but she is afraid of needles and panics at the sight of blood. She says that the last time she had her blood drawn she started feeling hot and light-headed and had to lie down on a table and was embarrassed. Kathleen says she also is worried the laboratory results might show something is wrong with her. She is thinking of not coming for her appointment today and hopes that she starts feeling better on her own. ∎

COLLECTING, HANDLING, AND TRANSPORTING SPECIMENS

Clinical laboratory tests are performed on specimens obtained from the body. A **specimen** is a small sample or part taken from the body to represent the nature of the whole. Most laboratory tests are performed on specimens that are easily obtained from the body, such as blood, urine, feces, sputum, cervical and vaginal scrapings of cells, or samples of secretions or discharge from various parts of the body (e.g., nose, throat, wound, ear, eye, vagina, urethra), for microbiologic analysis. Other examples of specimens analyzed in the laboratory but more difficult to obtain from the body include gastric juices, cerebrospinal fluid, pleural fluid, peritoneal fluid, synovial fluid, and tissue specimens for biopsy. The source of the specimen may not be indicative of the pathologic condition in question, for example, triiodothyronine and thyroxine tests are performed on blood serum but are used to detect a condition that affects the thyroid gland.

The medical assistant is responsible for the collection of most specimens obtained from patients in the medical office; of these, blood and urine constitute the largest percentage of specimens collected. Certain specimens, such as a sample of vaginal or urethral discharge, cerebrospinal fluid, or a tissue specimen, must be collected by the physician; in these cases, the medical assistant assists with the collection.

The most important goal of specimen collection and handling is to provide the laboratory with a sample that is as biologically representative as possible of the body substance collected. If the specimen is collected or handled improperly, the **in vivo** characteristics of the specimen may be adversely affected, which may cause inaccurate and unreliable test results; this may interfere with the accurate diagnosis and treatment of the patient's condition.

Guidelines for Specimen Collection

Specific guidelines that should be used regarding specimen collection and handling follow. *Review and follow the Occupational Safety and Health Administration (OSHA) Bloodborne Pathogens Standards* during specimen collection (see Chapter 17).

1. *Review the requirements for collection and handling of the specimen,* which include the collection supplies necessary, the type of specimen to be collected (e.g., **serum, plasma,** whole blood, clotted blood, urine), the amount necessary for laboratory analysis, the techniques to follow to collect the specimen, and proper handling and storage of the specimen. The medical assistant must refer to the appropriate reference source to determine the collection and handling requirements for each test ordered by the physician. If the specimen is transported to an outside laboratory, this information is indicated in the laboratory directory. Figure 29-9 shows an example of the collection and handling requirements for a triglycerides test exactly as it is presented in a laboratory directory. The collection and handling requirements necessary for specimens tested in the medical office are listed in the manufacturer's instructions that accompany the test system. A **test system** is defined as a setup that includes all of the test components required to perform a laboratory test such as testing devices, controls, and testing reagents.

2. *Assemble the equipment and supplies.* Use only the appropriate specimen containers as specified by the laboratory directory or manufacturer's instructions accompanying a test system. Substituting containers may not yield the proper type of specimen required or may affect the test results, as shown by the following examples. If serum is required and a tube containing an anticoagulant is used (instead of a tube without an anticoagulant), the blood separates into plasma and cells, rather than serum and cells, and the wrong type of blood specimen is obtained, which necessitates another specimen from the patient. Collection of a microbiologic specimen that may contain anaerobic pathogens with supplies meant for aerobic pathogens results in death of the anaerobic pathogen.

The specimen container should be sterile to prevent contamination of the specimen. Many specimens, especially microbiologic ones, are adversely affected by contaminants, such as extraneous microorganisms, which may affect the accuracy of the test results.

The medical assistant should check each container before use to ensure it is not broken, chipped, cracked, or otherwise damaged. Damaged containers are unsuitable for specimen collection and should be discarded. Some containers such as blood tubes have an expiration date (Figure 29-10). The medical assistant should make sure to check the expiration date on these containers to avoid using an outdated container.

3. *Label each specimen container.* The medical assistant should label each tube and specimen container. An unlabeled specimen is a cause for rejection of the specimen by an outside laboratory. Two *unique identifiers* should be used to label the specimen. A unique identifier is information that clearly identifies a specific patient, such as the patient's name and date of birth. A specimen can be labeled by attaching a computerized bar code label to the specimen (Figure 29-11, *A*). Laboratory instruments that do the testing are able to read the bar codes and automatically record results on a laboratory report for a particular patient using the demographic information supplied by the bar code. A specimen can also be labeled by handwriting the information on the label, which should include the patient's name and date of birth, the date and time of collection, the medical assistant's initials, and any other information required by the laboratory, such as the source of the specimen (Figure 29-11, *B*). The information should be printed legibly, and the medical assistant should be certain that the information is accurate to avoid a mixup of specimens. The medical assistant must also complete a laboratory request form to accompany the specimen, as described earlier in this chapter. (*NOTE:* The medical assistant should follow the medical office policy as to when the tubes should be labeled. Some offices prefer that the tubes be labeled *before* the specimen is drawn; other offices want the tubes to be labeled *after* the specimen is drawn.)

4. *Identify the patient.* Proper patient identification is essential to avoid collecting a specimen on the wrong patient by mistake. After greeting the patient, the medical assistant should ask the patient to state his or her full name and date of birth. This information

Triglycerides

CPT code:	84478
Type of specimen:	Serum
Amount:	2 ml
Collection supplies:	SST or transfer tube
Collection techniques:	Let stand for 30 minutes. Separate serum from cells within 45 minutes of collection.
Patient preparation:	Patient should fast for 12 to 14 hours prior to collection.
Handling and storage:	Refrigerate or store at room temperature. Stable at room temperature for up to 7 days.
Causes for rejection:	Nonfasting specimen, improper labeling of tube

Reference range:		
	Desirable:	Less than 150 mg/dL
	Borderline high:	150-199 mg/dL
	High:	200-499 mg/dL
	Very high:	500 mg/dL or greater

Use:

Measurement of triglyceride levels assists with the diagnosis and treatment of diabetes mellitus, nephrosis, liver obstruction, and pancreatitis. In association with HDL cholesterol and total cholesterol, a triglyceride determination assists in the assessment of the risk for developing coronary artery disease. Elevated levels may occur with liver disease, nephritic syndrome, hypothyroidism, increased alcohol consumption, poorly controlled diabetes, and pancreatitis.

Limitations:

- Women on estrogens (high estrogen contraceptives can increase blood triglyceride levels).

- An increase in the triglyceride level may occur during pregnancy.

Methodology:

Enzymatic

Figure 29-9 Collection and handling requirements for a triglyceride test from a laboratory directory.

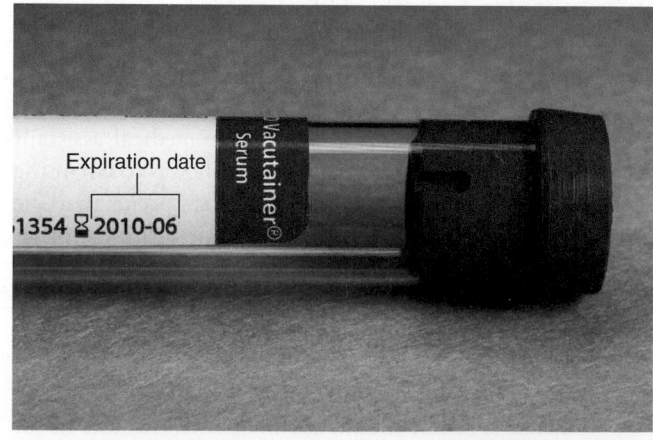

Figure 29-10 Blood tube showing expiration date.

should be compared with the demographic data indicated in the patient's chart. The patient should *not* be asked whether he or she is a certain patient. For example, the patient should not be asked, "Are you Brad Thompson?" The patient may not hear the medical assistant correctly or may not be paying attention and may answer in the affirmative even if he is not that patient. A specimen that is not identified correctly could lead to an inaccurate patient diagnosis and the wrong treatment.

5. *Determine whether the patient has prepared properly.* If the patient was required to prepare before the specimen was collected, determine whether this was done properly. Improper preparation may lead to inaccurate test results. If a test that requires fasting, such as

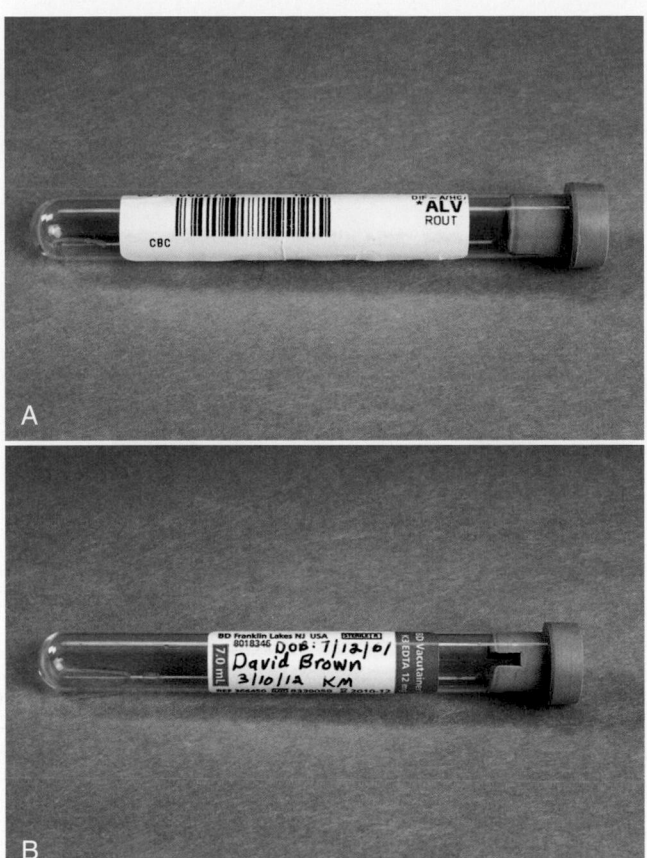

Figure 29-11 **A,** Computerized bar code label. **B,** Hand-labeled blood tube.

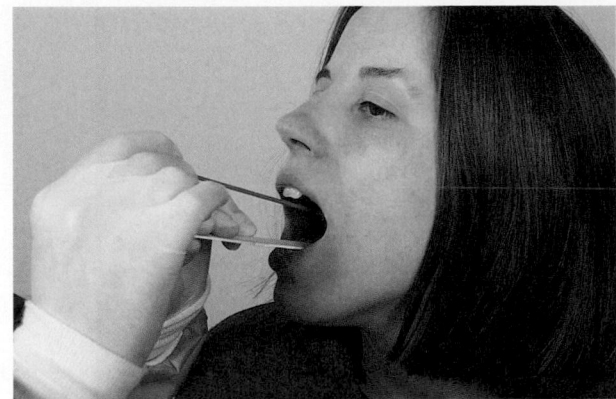

Figure 29-12 Medical and surgical asepsis must be used when collecting a specimen.

an FBG, is performed on a nonfasting specimen, the results are altered; in this case, they are falsely high. If the patient has not prepared properly, inform the physician; the physician may want the patient to prepare properly and return, or the physician may tell the medical assistant to go ahead with the collection but to alert the laboratory to the situation by marking the information on the laboratory request. In the example just given, "nonfasting specimen" would be written on the request form.

6. *Explain the procedure.* An explanation of the collection procedure helps relax and reassure the patient and gains the patient's confidence and cooperation, especially the first time the patient has a specimen collected.

7. *Collection of the specimen* involves a set of specific techniques for each type of specimen obtained. The information in this section is presented in general terms. Specific procedures for the collection of biologic specimens are included in this text in Chapters 30 through 34 (Urinalysis, Phlebotomy, Hematology, Blood Chemistry and Immunology, and Medical Microbiology).

   Specimen collection involves a combination of medical and surgical aseptic techniques. Certain parts of the collection materials, such as needles, swabs, and the insides of specimen containers, must remain

sterile. If a culture medium is used to collect a microbiologic specimen, the medical assistant must ensure that the lid of the container is removed only when the specimen is placed on the culture medium. Unnecessary removal of the lid results in contamination of the culture medium with extraneous microorganisms, which interferes with accurate test results. During the collection and handling of the specimen, the medical assistant must be careful to use medical and surgical asepsis to prevent contamination of the specimen, the patient, or the self (Figure 29-12).

The medical assistant must collect the specimen using proper technique. The proper type of specimen must be collected as designated in the laboratory directory or by the instructions that accompany the test system. The collection procedure should be followed exactly to ensure a high-quality and reliable specimen. For example, collection of a random urine specimen when a clean-catch midstream specimen is required may affect the accuracy of the test results.

The medical assistant must be sure to collect the amount of specimen necessary for the test, which varies depending on the type of test being performed and the number of laboratory tests ordered on the specimen. If the medical assistant fails to collect the specified amount of a specimen that is being transported to an outside laboratory, the laboratory may not be able to perform the test, and the laboratory request is returned marked "quantity not sufficient" (QNS). This situation warrants calling the patient back for collection of another specimen.

8. *Process the specimen.* The specimen may need to be processed after collection. For example, when collecting a serum specimen using a serum separator tube (SST), the medical assistant must allow the tube to stand for 45 minutes and then centrifuge the specimen to separate the serum from the cells (with a gel barrier), as shown in Figure 29-13.

9. *Properly handle and store the specimen* to preserve its in vivo physical and chemical characteristics. Some specimens, such as microbiologic specimens, are more

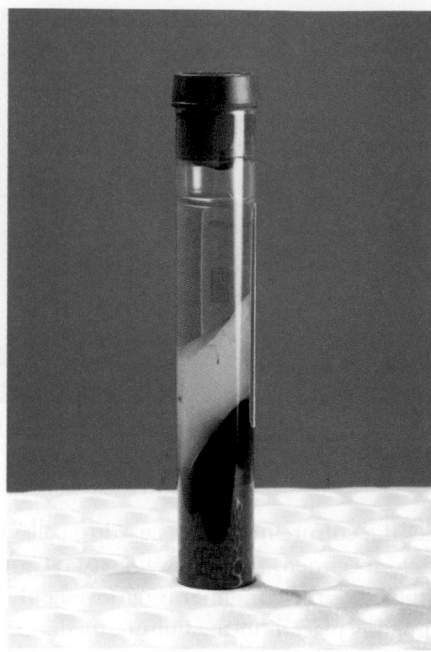

Figure 29-13 Serum specimen in a serum separator tube (SST) that has been centrifuged.

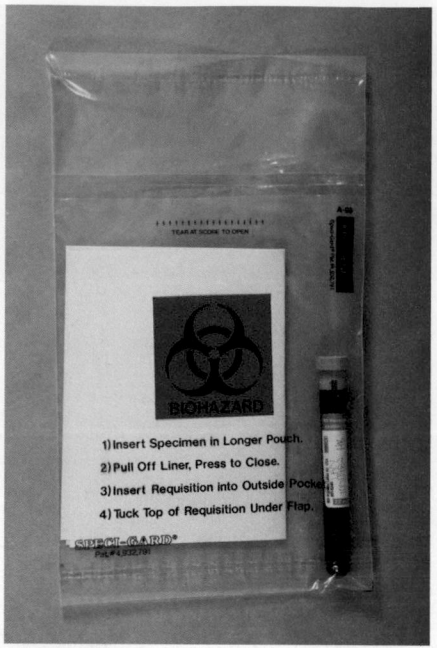

Figure 29-14 Biohazard specimen bag containing a specimen and laboratory request form.

sensitive to environmental influences and must be handled with special care. Whenever possible, laboratory tests are best performed on fresh specimens (for most specimens, within 1 hour after collection) because they yield the most reliable test results. When this is not possible, the specimen must be stored; storage may be required until it can be tested at the medical office or picked up by a laboratory courier from an outside laboratory. If the specimen is being picked up by a laboratory courier, the OSHA standard requires that it be placed in a biohazard specimen bag (Figure 29-14) to protect the courier from the possibility of an exposure incident. General guidelines for handling and storing biologic specimens most frequently collected in the medical office are presented in Table 29-3.

CLINICAL LABORATORY IMPROVEMENT AMENDMENTS

Purpose of CLIA 1988

In 1988, Congress passed the Clinical Laboratory Improvement Amendments (CLIA 1988), which established standards for improving the quality of laboratory testing in the United States. CLIA 1988 consists of federal regulations governing all facilities that perform laboratory tests for health assessment or for the diagnosis, prevention, or treatment of disease. CLIA 1988 includes facilities not previously covered under federal legislation, such as medical offices, health departments, and nursing homes. Regulations for implementing CLIA were developed by the Department of Health and Human Services (HHS). The Centers

for Medicare and Medicaid Services (CMS) is a division of HHS and is responsible for implementing and monitoring compliance with the CLIA regulations. In addition to CLIA regulations, a clinical laboratory must be in compliance with all other federal, state, and local laboratory legislation.

Categories of Laboratory Testing

CLIA regulations establish the following three categories of laboratory testing on the basis of the complexity of the testing methods.

1. Waived Tests

A **waived test** is a laboratory test that has been determined by HHS to meet the CLIA criteria for being a simple procedure that is easy to perform and has a low risk of erroneous test results. Waived tests include tests that have been approved by the Food and Drug Administration (FDA) for use by patients at home (e.g., blood glucose testing). Physician's office laboratories (POLs) that perform only waived tests must apply for a certificate of waiver (CW) from CMS, which exempts them from many of the CLIA oversight requirements. The CW must be renewed every 2 years.

POLs holding a CW are still expected to adhere to good laboratory practices. The manufacturer's most *current* instructions that accompany the test system must be followed exactly; these include the following:

- Proper storage of the test system
- Adhering to expiration dates
- Proper collection and handling of the specimen
- Performing quality control procedures
- Properly testing the specimen

Table 29-3 Handling and Storage of Biologic Specimens*

Specimen	Handling	Storage
Blood	**All Blood Specimens** Prevent hemolysis. Collect specimen in tube at room temperature.	**For Most Blood Specimens** Refrigerate at a temperature between 36° F (2° C) and 46° F (8° C) to retard alterations in physical and chemical composition of the specimen. (NOTE: Many blood specimens are stable at room temperature for up to 24 hours.) Plasma and serum may be frozen; however, whole blood should not be frozen because this would cause hemolysis.
	Serum Separate serum from cells within 45 min after collection.	
	Plasma Mix anticoagulant gently but thoroughly with blood specimen immediately after collection.	
Urine	Avoid contamination of inside of specimen container. Do not leave specimen standing out for longer than 1 hr after collection.	If urine specimen cannot be tested within 1 hr after collection, refrigerate it at a temperature between 36° F (2° C) and 46° F (8° C), or add an appropriate preservative.
Microbiologic specimens	Avoid contamination of swab used to collect specimen. Avoid contamination of inside of microbiologic specimen container. Protect yourself from contamination from microbiologic specimen. Protect anaerobic specimens from exposure to air.	Transport specimen immediately after collection. If not possible, place specimen in transport medium or inoculate it on appropriate culture medium, and (for most specimens) place it in refrigerator at a temperature between 36° F (2° C) and 46° F (8° C) to prevent drying and death of specimen or overgrowth of specimen with extraneous microorganisms.
Stool	Collect specimen in clean container. For detection of ova and parasites, keep stool warm.	For most accurate test results, deliver specimen to laboratory immediately. If transportation of specimen is delayed, mix stool with appropriate preservative or place it in transport medium.

*For all specimens: Do not expose to extreme temperature changes.

- Interpreting test results
- Recording test results

2. Moderate-Complexity Tests

A moderate-complexity test is a **nonwaived test** that is subject to the CLIA 1988 regulations. Moderate-complexity tests account for 75% of the estimated 7 to 10 billion laboratory tests performed in the United States each year. Most of these tests are performed in outside laboratories which include hospital and independent laboratories. Some medical offices perform moderate-complexity tests known as *provider-performed microscopy* (PPM) procedures, which involve the examination of a specimen under the microscope. An example of a PPM procedure is the microscopic analysis of urine sediment. Other moderate-complexity tests that are occasionally performed in the medical office include urine and throat cultures and hematology and blood chemistry tests performed on nonwaived automated blood analyzers. Examples of these "benchtop" analyzers include the QBC hematology analyzer (Becton-Dickinson, Franklin Lakes, NJ), the Cell-Dyn hematology analyzer (Abbott Laboratories, Abbott Park, Ill), the Ac*T hematology analyzer (Beckman Coulter, Brea, Calif), and the ATAT blood chemistry analyzer (GMI Inc., Ramsey, Minn).

3. High-Complexity Tests

A high-complexity test is a nonwaived test that is subject to the CLIA 1988 regulations. High-complexity tests include all procedures related to cytogenetics, histopathology, histocompatibility, and cytology (includes Pap testing). These tests are not performed in medical offices; most are performed in laboratories already subject to federal regulations.

Requirements for Moderate-Complexity and High-Complexity Testing

Laboratories that perform nonwaived tests (moderate- and high-complexity tests) must meet CLIA regulations and are subject to unannounced inspections every 2 years by CMS. Major components of the CLIA 1988 regulations include the following:

1. *Patient test management.* A system must be established to maintain optimal integrity and identification of patient specimens throughout the testing process. This system must also ensure accurate reporting of results.
2. *Quality control.* To ensure accurate and reliable test results, each laboratory performing nonwaived tests must establish and follow written quality control

procedures that monitor and evaluate the quality of each testing process. These include:

- *Developing a laboratory procedures manual.* The manual must include a clearly written procedure for each nonwaived test that is performed by the facility, following the manufacturer's instructions. The manual must be readily available and followed by laboratory personnel.
- *Performing calibration procedures at least every 6 months* (or more frequently if indicated in the test system's operating manual) and documenting results in a quality control log. The calibration verification must be checked at a minimum of three levels that are within the reportable range of the test.
- *Following the manufacturer's instructions for performing controls,* but at a minimum, performing two levels of controls daily and documenting results in a quality-control log. In addition, control procedures must be performed in the following situations: when there is a complete change of reagents, when major preventive maintenance is performed on an analyzer, or when any critical change occurs that may influence test performance.
- *Performing and documenting actions taken when problems or errors are identified*
- *Documenting all quality control activities*

3. *Quality assessment.* Each laboratory must establish and follow written policies and procedures to monitor and evaluate the overall quality of the total testing process to ensure the accuracy and reliability of patient test results.

4. *Proficiency testing.* Proficiency testing (PT) is a form of external quality control used to verify the accuracy and reliability of laboratory testing. Laboratory specimens are prepared by a CMS-approved proficiency testing agency. Three times a year, the POL must test a shipment of these unknown specimens using the same procedure as for testing a patient's specimen. The results are forwarded to the PT agency for evaluation. The PT agency grades the results using the CLIA grading criteria and sends the laboratory score to the POL, indicating how accurately it performed the testing.

5. *Personnel requirements.* CLIA regulations specify qualifications and responsibilities for personnel for laboratory directors, technical consultants, clinical consultants, and testing personnel. These regulations list specific education and training qualifications for the various positions and define responsibilities for persons who fill these positions. Personnel requirements are most stringent for high-complexity testing.

CLIA-WAIVED LABORATORY TESTING

Testing a laboratory specimen involves performing a series of steps to determine the presence or measurement of a

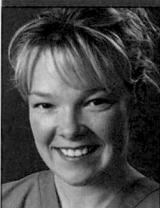

Memories *from* Externship

Korey McGrew: One of my most difficult situations as a medical-assisting student was taking the temperature of a patient who went through seizures. I was scared because I was only a student, and I had never been in a situation like that before. I knew I had to act immediately, and luckily one of the Certified Medical Assistants (CMA [AAMA]) was nearby. We immediately put the patient on the floor and moved things away from him to keep him from hurting himself. We then notified the physician, who was with a patient in another examining room. The seizure lasted only about 4 minutes, and the patient was fine. The CMA (AAMA) told me that the patient had a history of seizures and that I was not to be alarmed. That surely was a difficult but valuable learning experience for me. ∎

specific substance in the specimen. Most POLs only perform tests that are CLIA-waived, and the medical assistant is usually responsible for performing these tests. Because of this, the remainder of this chapter focuses on guidelines that should be followed when CLIA-waived tests are performed.

Approximately 1600 CLIA-waived tests are commercially available that test for 76 different analytes. An **analyte** is a substance that is being identified or measured in a laboratory test, such as glucose, hemoglobin, and group A strep. The number of waived tests is expected to increase as new technology becomes available. To help the medical office keep current with new CLIA-waived tests, the HHS maintains the following website: www.cms.hhs.gov/clia. The FDA also maintains a website that provides information on all commercially available CLIA-waived test systems, categorized by analyte and the name of the test system. This website can be accessed at www.fda.gov/MedicalDevices/DeviceRegulationandGuidance/IVDRegulatoryAssistance/ucm124103.htm.

CLIA-waived tests that are performed most frequently in the medical office include the following:

- Blood glucose determination (using an FDA-approved blood glucose monitor)
- Dipstick urinalysis
- Fecal occult blood testing
- Urine pregnancy tests with visual color comparisons
- Group A rapid streptococcus testing
- Hemoglobin testing (using a CLIA-waived analyzer)
- Cholesterol testing (using a CLIA-waived analyzer)
- Triglyceride testing (using a CLIA-waived analyzer)
- Prothrombin time testing (using a CLIA-waived analyzer)
- Spun microhematocrit

CLIA-Waived Testing Kits

A laboratory testing kit consists of a box packaged with the devices and supplies needed to perform a laboratory test and generate test results. Each kit contains enough testing materials to perform a specific number of tests as indicated on the box label. Most of these tests are screening tests, and a positive result may indicate the need for further testing. Examples of CLIA-waived testing kits (Figure 29-15) include the Hemoccult fecal occult blood test (SmithKline Diagnostics, Inc., Palo Alto, Calif), the QuickVue HCG urine pregnancy test, and the QuickVue In-Line Strep A test (Quidel Corp., San Diego, Calif).

Each testing kit comes with a **product insert** (also known as a *package insert*). Information included in the product insert is outlined in Table 29-4. The medical assistant should read the entire product insert before performing the test and should follow the instructions *exactly* to ensure accurate and reliable test results. Of particular importance are the quality control procedures that must be carefully followed when working with a testing kit. This area is discussed in greater detail later in this section. The testing kit may include a quick reference card, which is a condensed version of the steps in the testing procedure and can be used as a guide when performing the test. Because the quick reference card is only a synopsis of the testing procedure, it should never be substituted for the product insert when learning about the test and how to perform it.

Testing kits have specific stability and storage requirements that must be carefully followed. Before a testing kit is used, its expiration date must be checked. If the testing kit is outdated, the testing components may no longer

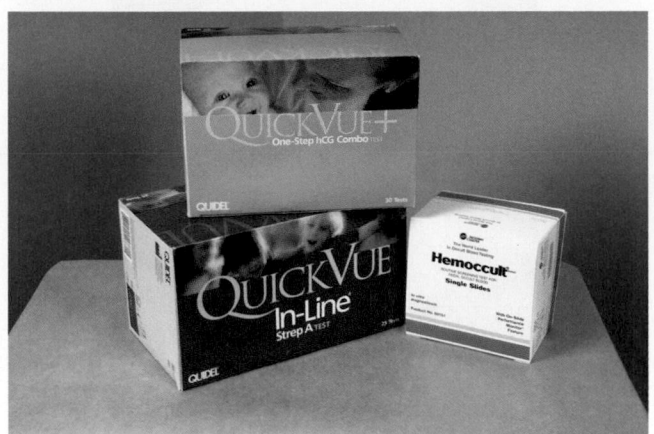

Figure 29-15 CLIA-waived testing kits.

Table 29-4 Information Included in the Product Insert of a Testing Kit

Section	Information Included
Intended Use	A description of the purpose of the test and the reason for performing the test.
Summary and Explanation	Provides a brief overview of the condition being detected by the test, including the symptoms, prevalence, and complications of the condition.
Principles of the Procedure	A detailed explanation of how the test works to detect the substance in the patient's specimen.
Precautions and Warnings	Outlines precautions that must be taken when running the test to ensure accurate and reliable test results. Also includes guidelines for safe handling, use, and disposal of chemical reagents included in the testing kit.
Reagents and Materials Provided	A list of the collection devices, controls, reagents, and other supplies included in the testing kit. Describes each component in detail, including the number of tests in the kit and the types and amounts of reagents and supplies.
Materials Not Provided	A list of the materials needed to perform the test, but not included in the testing kit.
Storage and Stability	A description of the proper storage requirements of the testing kit such as temperature range. Also identifies how long each testing component is stable for both unopened and opened components.
Specimen Collection and Handling	Type of specimen required and procedures that must be followed when collecting, handling, and storing the specimen to ensure a high-quality and reliable specimen. Also includes safety precautions to take when handling the specimen.
Test Procedure	Presents a step-by-step procedure that must be followed to test the specimen. Diagrams and illustrations of the procedural steps are often included in this section.
Interpretation and Reading Results	Guidelines for reading and interpreting the test results. If a color change is involved in reading the results, a color comparison chart or color diagram is included with the testing kit. Also explains the action to take if the test results are invalid.
Quality Control	An explanation of the quality control procedures that must be performed to ensure accurate and reliable test results. Includes instructions for performing control procedures. Also includes information on how often and when controls should be run and the expected results. Describes what should be done if the controls do not produce expected results.
Limitations of the Procedure	A test system works only within certain prescribed conditions and situations. Identifies conditions or situations that might prevent the test from performing correctly and influence the test results, such as medications or the presence of certain medical conditions. Also identifies any supplemental testing needed to confirm a waived test.
Expected Values	Identifies the test result(s) that should be expected by the user.
Performance Characteristics	Presents the results of research studies that have been conducted to evaluate test performance.

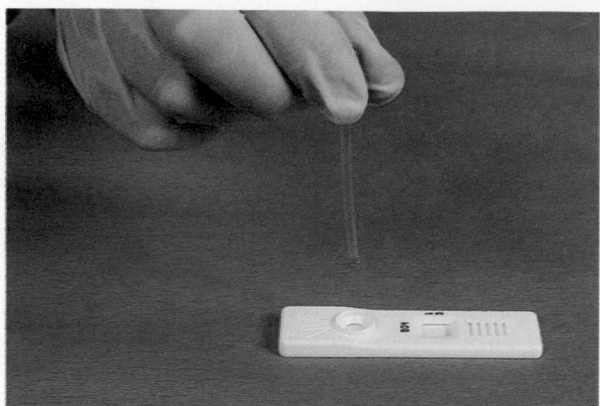

Figure 29-16 Unitized testing device.

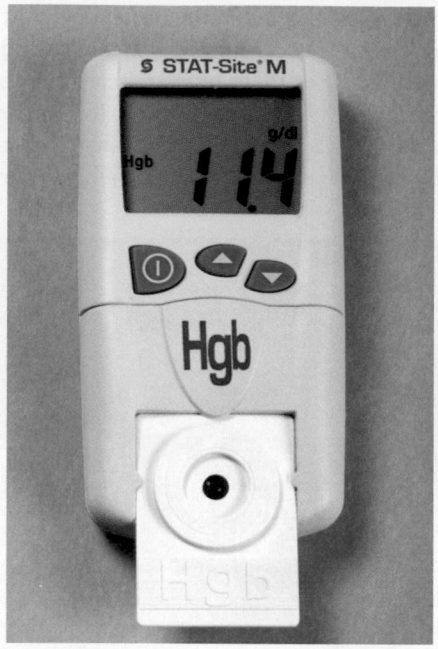

Figure 29-17 Digital readout of results on an automated analyzer.

be stable; expired components must not be used, to prevent inaccurate test results. Light, heat, and moisture can alter the effectiveness of a testing kit and cause premature expiration of the kit. The medical assistant should make sure to store testing kits according to the information in the product insert; this information is also indicated on the package label. Most testing kits are stored at room temperature.

Testing kits often use a *unitized testing device* to perform the test. A unitized testing device consists of a self-contained device, such as a cassette, to which a specimen is added directly and in which all of the steps of the testing procedure occur (Figure 29-16). A unitized device is used to perform one laboratory test (e.g., urine pregnancy testing) and is discarded after testing.

Many of the testing devices included in testing kits rely on a color change for interpretation of results. A color chart or color diagram is provided with the kit for making a visual comparison and interpreting results. When test results are recorded, the brand name of the testing kit should be specified. Some offices also require that the lot number of the testing kit be included with the recording.

CLIA-Waived Automated Analyzers

CLIA-waived automated analyzers have been developed for performing laboratory tests in the medical office; they are continually growing in number and are being modified as new technology becomes available. These analyzers consist of compact or handheld devices that permit the processing of a specimen in a short time with accurate test results. **Reagent** strips or test cassettes are often used with CLIA-waived analyzers. Test results are obtained through a direct (digital display or printed) readout (Figure 29-17).

The ease of operating automated systems should not lead to a false sense of security because these systems have limitations that must be recognized—the most critical one being the failure of the equipment. One of the most important aspects of use of an automated system is the ability to recognize signs that indicate the system is malfunctioning, because malfunctioning may lead to inaccurate test results.

The manufacturer of each automated system provides an operating manual (and sometimes an instructional video) with the instrument that includes information needed to collect and handle the specimen, perform quality control procedures, and test the specimen. In addition, the manufacturer typically has personnel available for on-site training and service. It is important that the medical assistant become completely familiar with all aspects of the automated systems used to perform laboratory tests in his or her medical office. Quality control procedures are of particular importance to ensure that the analyzer is functioning properly, and that the test results are reliable and accurate. Additional information on quality control procedures is presented later in this section.

When an automated analyzer is purchased, the testing components (e.g., controls, testing reagents) are usually purchased separately. The medical assistant is responsible for checking the supplies periodically and reordering them as needed. Each testing component comes with a product insert, which indicates the proper storage and stability requirements. Most testing components are stored at room temperature. If a testing component needs to be stored in the refrigerator, it must be allowed to come to room temperature before it is used. Unopened controls are stable until the expiration date marked on the container. Once opened, some controls are stable only for a certain period of time (e.g., 30 days). For these controls, the medical assistant must write the date the control was opened *and* the date it should be discarded (expiration date) on the label of the control.

Some examples of brand names of CLIA-waived automated analyzers (Figure 29-18) include Cholestech LDX (Cholestech Corp., Hayward, Calif), STAT-Site Hemoglobin Meter (Stanbio Laboratory, Boerne, Tex), CoaguChek system

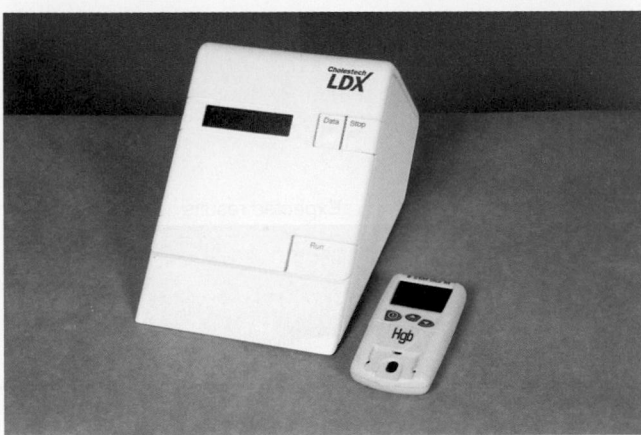

Figure 29-18 Clinical Laboratories Improvement Amendments (CLIA)–waived automated analyzers. Blood cholesterol analyzer *(left)* and hemoglobin analyzer *(right)*.

and Accu-Chek (Roche Diagnostics, Branchburg, NJ), A1C Now (Bayer Corporation, Morrisville, NJ), and Clinitek urine analyzer (Siemens Corporation, New York City, NY).

QUALITY CONTROL

The ultimate goal in the clinical laboratory is to ensure that the laboratory test accurately measures what it is supposed to measure; this involves practicing and maintaining a quality control program. **Quality control (QC)** may be defined as the application of methods and means to ensure that test results are reliable and valid, and errors that may interfere with obtaining accurate test results are detected and eliminated. Practicing quality control methods ensures that test results represent the true status of the patient's condition and body functions and provide the physician with reliable information for making a diagnosis and prescribing treatment.

Quality control is an ongoing process that encompasses every aspect of patient preparation and specimen collection, handling, transport, and testing. The quality control methods that should be used to obtain precision and accuracy when using a CLIA-waived test system are presented here.

1. Storage and Handling of Test Systems

a. Store the test system according to the manufacturer's instructions. Improper storage can cause deterioration of the testing components. Most test systems need to be stored at room temperature in a cool, dry area away from sources of heat and sunlight. Some testing components (e.g., controls, testing reagents) may need to be stored in the refrigerator.

b. Allow time for refrigerated testing components to reach room temperature before using them. It usually takes 15 to 30 minutes for a testing component to reach room temperature.

c. Controls often need to be shaken gently to mix them.

d. Do not transfer testing components from one testing kit to another.

e. Make sure environmental conditions are appropriate for running the test as specified in the manufacturer's instructions.

2. Stability of Testing Components

a. Check the expiration date of each component in the test system before using it. Do not use a test component if it is past its expiration date.

b. Unopened controls are stable until the expiration date marked on the container. Once opened, some controls are stable only for a certain period of time (e.g., 30 days). For these controls, the date the control is opened *and* the date it should be discarded (expiration date) must be written on the label of the control after it is opened. An opened control is stable until it reaches the expiration date stamped on the container or the expiration date indicated by the medical assistant on the container, whichever comes first.

c. Discard outdated testing components as soon as they reach their expiration dates.

3. Calibration

Calibration is a mechanism used to check the precision and accuracy of a test system, such as an automated analyzer, to determine if the system is providing accurate results. A calibration check detects errors caused by laboratory equipment that is not working properly. Calibration is typically performed using a calibration device, often called a *standard*. The calibration device may come in the form of a calibration strip or cassette. The device is inserted into the analyzer (Figure 29-19, *A*), and the calibration results are displayed on the LCD screen of the analyzer or printed out by the analyzer. The calibration results are then compared with the expected results provided in the product insert or on the calibration device (Figure 29-19, *B*). Calibration guidelines include the following:

a. Perform the calibration procedure by following the manufacturer's instructions. Instructions include information on the type of calibration device to use, how to perform the calibration procedure, and what action should be taken if the procedure does not perform as expected.

b. Document calibration results in a quality control log. This is a CLIA recommendation (not a requirement) for CLIA-waived test systems.

c. If the calibration procedure does not perform as expected, patient testing should not be conducted until the problem is identified and resolved.

d. The frequency of performing a calibration check is indicated in the manufacturer's instructions. At a minimum, a calibration check should be performed when a new lot number of testing reagents is put into use.

4. Controls

A **control** is a solution that is used to monitor a test system to ensure the reliability and accuracy of test results. Controls come with a product insert, which lists the expected ranges

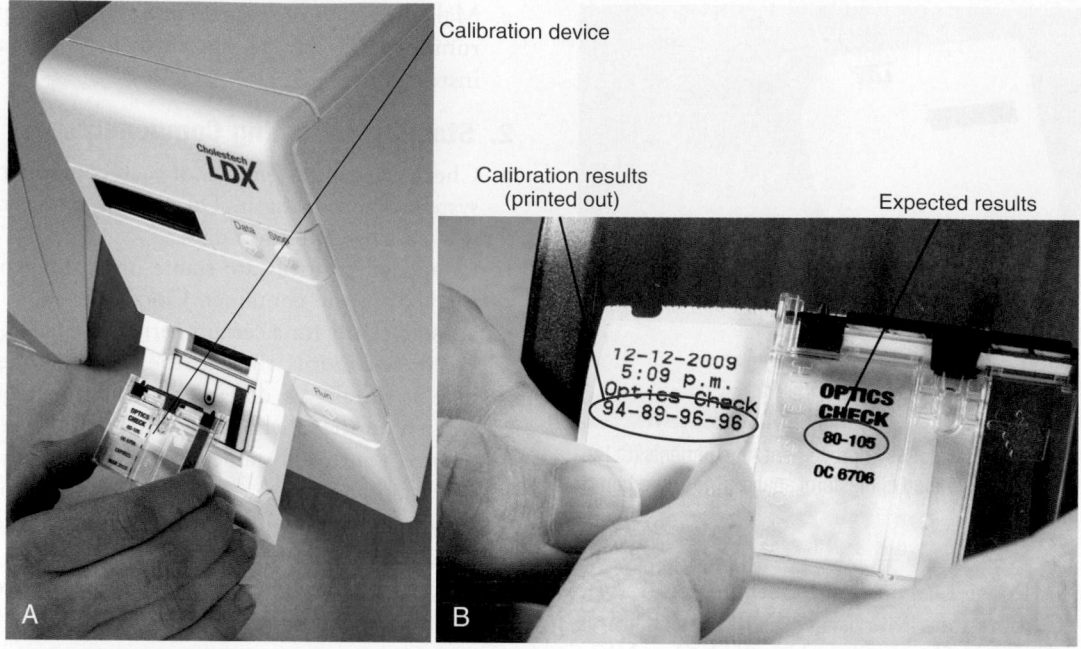

Figure 29-19 **A,** Calibrating an automated analyzer using a calibration device. **B,** Calibration results are compared with expected results on the calibration device.

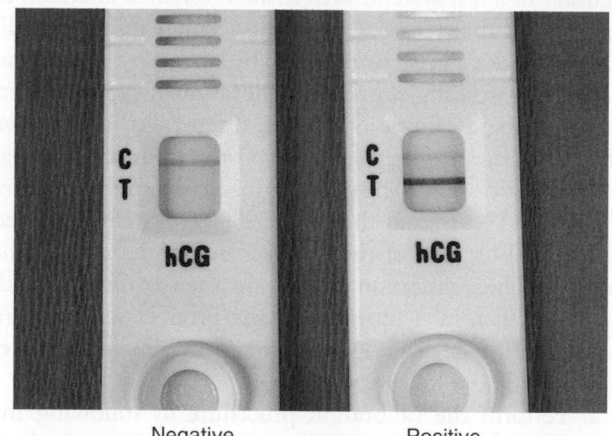

Figure 29-20 Internal control. The blue line next to the letter *C* indicates that the internal control has reacted as expected.

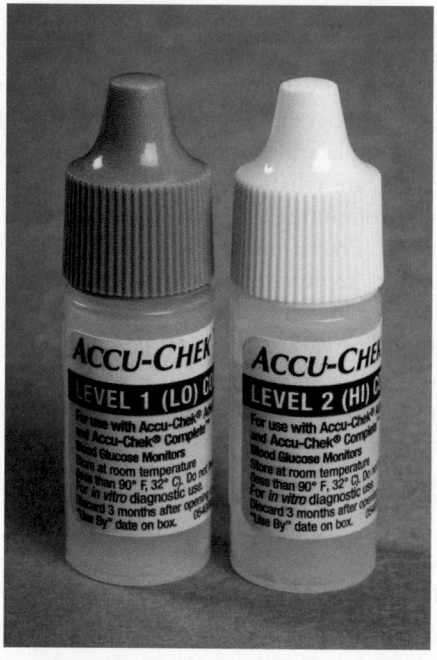

Figure 29-21 External controls. Low or level 1 control *(left)* and high or level 2 control *(right).*

for control results. There are two categories of controls, which include *external controls* and *internal controls.*

Internal control: An internal control is built into some test systems (Figure 29-20). It evaluates whether certain aspects of the testing procedure are working properly. An internal control is performed at the same time that the testing procedure is performed. It checks for one or more of the following: whether a sufficient amount of the specimen was added, whether a sufficient amount of testing reagent was added, or whether the testing reagent migrated through the test device properly. If the internal control does not perform as expected, the test result is invalid and the specimen must be retested.

External controls: External controls are used to determine if the testing reagents are performing properly and to detect any errors in technique of the individual performing the

test. External controls consist of commercially available solutions with known values. They may be included with the test system or may need to be purchased separately. Generally, two levels of controls must be performed on a test system. A *low-level control* (also known as a *Level 1 control*) produces results that fall below the reference range for the test; a *high-level control* (also known as a *Level 2 control*) produces results that fall above the reference range for the test (Figure 29-21). The control procedure is performed in a manner similar to the procedure for performing the test on a specimen collected from a patient. Instead of adding the patient specimen to the testing device, however, the control is added to it. Control results are compared with expected results provided in the product insert. Failure of a control to produce expected results may be due to the following: deterioration of testing components due to improper storage or components past their expiration date, improper environmental testing conditions, or errors in technique used to perform the procedure. External control guidelines include the following:

1. Perform control procedures by following the instructions in the product insert. These instructions include information on how to perform the control procedure, and what action should be taken if the controls do not perform as expected.

2. Document control results in a quality control log (Figure 29-22). This is a CLIA recommendation (not a requirement) for CLIA-waived test systems.

3. If the controls do not perform as expected, patient testing should not be conducted until the problem is identified and resolved. Factors that can cause abnormal control results include outdated controls or testing reagents, improper storage of testing components, and an error in the technique used to perform the procedure.

4. The frequency of performing external controls is indicated in the product insert. At a minimum, they should be performed on each new lot number of testing reagents and thereafter on a regular basis, such as monthly.

QUALITY CONTROL LOG
BLOOD GLUCOSE TEST

Name of meter: *Accu-Check Advantage*

Controls

TEST STRIPS:

Lot number: _522677_

Exp date: _4/30/20XX_

Code number _635_

LOW LEVEL CONTROL:

Lot number _63330_

Exp date _11/29/20XX_

Expected range: _18 – 64_

HIGH LEVEL CONTROL:

Lot number _63330_

Exp date _11/29/20XX_

Expected range: _270 – 324_

Date	Low level control	Accept	Reject	High level control	Accept	Reject	Technician
9/20/XX	61	X		315	X		K. Mcgrew, CMA (AAMA)
9/21/XX	53	X		310	X		K. Mcgrew, CMA (AAMA)
9/22/XX	50	X		302	X		K. Mcgrew, CMA (AAMA)
9/23/XX	48	X		300	X		K. Mcgrew, CMA (AAMA)
9/24/XX	51	X		305	X		K. Mcgrew, CMA (AAMA)

Figure 29-22 Quality control log sheet for blood glucose testing.

5. Collecting and Handling Specimens

a. Use the appropriate collection devices to collect the specimen. Do not substitute other devices.

b. Follow the manufacturer's instructions exactly for collecting and handling the specimen.

c. If a specimen (e.g., urine) cannot be tested immediately, information is provided in the manufacturer's instructions on proper storage of the specimen until it can be tested.

6. Testing the Specimen

a. If more than one patient is being tested at a time, label each testing device with the patient's name to prevent mixup of specimens.

b. Follow the procedure in the manufacturer's instructions *exactly* for testing the specimen. Specific requirements may include the following:

- Adding the proper amounts of reagents
- Adding reagents in the proper order
- Adhering to proper time intervals for various steps in the procedure
- Reading results within the proper time frame

7. Interpreting and Reading Test Results

Testing kits often rely on a color change for the interpretation of test results. The color change is compared with a color chart or a color diagram (Figure 29-23) included with the testing kit. Test results derived from an automated analyzer do not need to be interpreted and are printed out or displayed on the LCD screen of the analyzer. The following guidelines should be followed when test results from a testing kit are interpreted:

a. Interpret the results according to instructions outlined in the product insert that accompanies the testing kit.

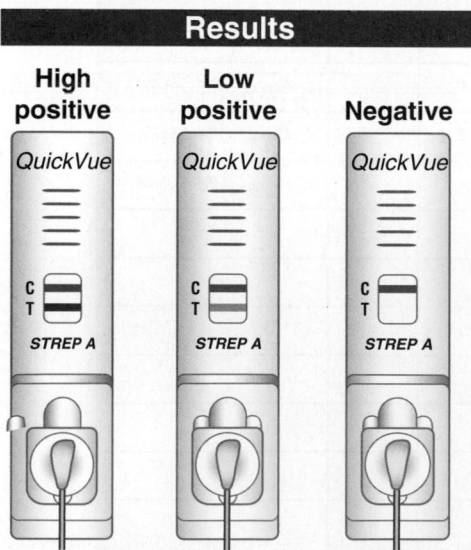

Figure 29-23 Color diagram used to interpret test results.

b. Test results are usually interpreted as positive, negative, or invalid. Invalid results may be due to an improperly collected specimen or an error in technique in performing the testing procedure.

c. If a test is invalid, retest a new sample with new testing materials. If the second test is invalid, contact the manufacturer.

CATEGORIES OF TEST RESULTS

Laboratory test results are categorized as qualitative or quantitative results.

Qualitative Test Results

Qualitative test results indicate whether or not a substance is present in the specimen being tested; they also provide an approximate indication of the amount of substance present. Interpretation of qualitative results usually involves the use of a color comparison chart or a color diagram. Results are recorded in terms of 1+, 2+, or 3+; trace, small, moderate, or large; negative or positive; or reactive or nonreactive. Testing kits usually provide qualitative test results.

Quantitative Test Results

Quantitative test results indicate the exact amount of a chemical substance that is present in the body; results are reported in measurable units (e.g., mg/dL). No interpretation is required to read quantitative results. Automated analyzers provide quantitative test results, with the results being printed out or displayed on the LCD screen of the analyzer.

RECORDING TEST RESULTS

The medical assistant is responsible for recording laboratory test results. Careful recording is essential to avoid errors, which could affect the patient's diagnosis. It is usually unnecessary to chart results from laboratory reports returned from outside laboratories because the report itself is filed in the patient's record. In case of a STAT request or critical findings, the test results may be telephoned to the medical office, requiring the medical assistant to record results on a report form.

Results of laboratory tests performed by the medical assistant in the POL should be charted in the medical record and must include the date and time, name of the test, and test results. Quantitative test results should be recorded using the units of measurement of the test system (e.g., mg/dL). Qualitative test results should be recorded using words or abbreviations (e.g., positive, negative) and not symbols (e.g., +, −), because symbols can be accidentally changed or misinterpreted. The office may also maintain a log of the tests performed in the POL, which includes the patient's name, date and time, name of the test, the test results, and the name and credentials of the individual performing the test (Figure 29-24).

QUALITY CONTROL LOG

BLOOD GLUCOSE TEST

ACCU-CHECK TEST STRIPS

Lot number: _____522677_____

Exp date: _____4/30/20XX_____

Code number _____635_____

Date	Patient name	Patinet ID	Glucose results (in mg/dL0	Technician
9/20/XX	Thomas Jeffers	1341	98	K. Mcgrew, CMA (AAMA)
9/20/XX	Diana Woods	3744	74	K. Mcgrew, CMA (AAMA)
9/21/XX	Lauren Campbell	6497	115	K. Mcgrew, CMA (AAMA)
9/21/XX	Jason Coates	5310	78	K. Mcgrew, CMA (AAMA)
9/21/XX	Chloe Pearson	2333	85	K. Mcgrew, CMA (AAMA)
9/22/XX	Kathleen Dobson	1466	65	K. Mcgrew, CMA (AAMA)
9/22/XX	Larry Wilson	5399	102	K. Mcgrew, CMA (AAMA)
9/23/XX	Samantha Byran	2512	92	K. Mcgrew, CMA (AAMA)
9/24/XX	Abbey Paulson	1788	88	K. Mcgrew, CMA (AAMA)
9/24/XX	Michael Williams	3903	105	K. Mcgrew, CMA (AAMA)

Figure 29-24 Patient log of laboratory tests.

LABORATORY SAFETY

Laboratory safety is an important aspect of clinical laboratory testing in the medical office. Many of the laboratory tests performed in the medical office involve the use of hazardous chemical reagents, the handling of specimens that may contain pathogens, and the use of laboratory equipment. Practicing good technique in testing laboratory specimens and recognizing potential hazards help to reduce accidents in the laboratory. Some areas specifically related to laboratory safety in the medical office are described here.

Careful handling and storing of glassware to prevent breakage should be performed as follows:

1. Carefully arrange glassware in storage cabinets to prevent breakage.
2. Carefully remove glassware from storage cabinets.
3. If glassware does break, dispose of it in a puncture-resistant container to protect trash handlers from the shards.

The medical assistant should handle all chemical reagents carefully by adhering to the following instructions:

1. Ensure that all reagent containers are clearly and properly labeled.
2. If a label is loose, reattach it immediately.
3. Recap reagent containers immediately after use to prevent spills.

Laboratory specimens should be handled carefully as follows:

1. Follow the OSHA Bloodborne Pathogens Standard in collecting and handling laboratory specimens.

2. Wash hands immediately if some of the material contained in the specimen is accidentally touched.

3. Avoid hand-to-mouth contact, such as eating, drinking, or applying makeup, while working with specimens.

4. Immediately clean up any specimen spilled on the worktable, and cleanse the table with a disinfectant.

5. Properly dispose of all contaminated needles, syringes, specimen containers, and infectious waste used in specimen collection and testing.

6. Cover any break in the skin, such as a cut or scratch, with a bandage.

7. Ensure that all specimen containers are tightly capped to prevent leakage.

8. Do not store food in refrigerators where testing supplies or specimens are stored.

9. Handle all laboratory equipment and supplies properly and with care, as indicated by the manufacturer. For example, wait until the centrifuge comes to a complete stop before opening it.

MEDICAL PRACTICE and the LAW

Laboratory procedures must be performed with precision to obtain accurate test results. Pay particular attention to each step in the procedure. Inaccurate laboratory results may cause the physician to incorrectly diagnose a patient's condition, which could lead to the wrong treatment. This situation can result in a lawsuit.

Certain federal regulations, including those from the Clinical Laboratories Improvement Amendments (CLIA) and the Occupational Safety and Health Administration (OSHA), govern laboratory testing. These regulations help ensure standardization of laboratory tests and safe handling of reagents, blood, and body fluids to prevent contamination of specimens and infection of health care workers. Know and follow all regulations. Failure to do so could result in legal liability. ■

What Would You Do? What Would You Not Do? RESPONSES

Case Study 1
Page 695

What Did Korey Do?
❑ Told Hildy that the laboratory cannot release test results. Explained that they are experts in performing tests but do not have the medical knowledge to know their meanings.
❑ Told Hildy that the physician needed to give her the test results. Explained that the physician was out of town today but that an appointment could be made for her for tomorrow to discuss the results with the physician.

What Did Korey Not Do?
❑ Did not give Hildy the test results.
❑ Did not alarm Hildy that something might be wrong.

What Would You Do?/What Would You Not Do?
Review Korey's response and place a checkmark next to the information you included in your response. List additional information you included in your response.

_____
_____
_____
_____
_____
_____

Case Study 2
Page 700

What Did Korey Do?
❑ Told Hans that the term clinical diagnosis means what the physician "thinks" is wrong before the laboratory tests are performed.
❑ Explained that when the test results are returned, the physician would be able to make a diagnosis, and then he would determine what treatment is needed.
❑ Told Hans that a lipid profile includes several tests, and one of those tests is a cholesterol test. Explained that the tests in a lipid profile all help to determine whether someone is at risk for heart disease.
❑ Told Hans that he could not have any coffee until after his blood was drawn because it would affect the test results. Told him that his test could be scheduled first thing in the morning if that would help.

What Did Korey Not Do?
❑ Did not tell Hans he could have a cup of coffee before the laboratory tests.
❑ Did not tell Hans that he should not be eating doughnuts if he is concerned about his heart.

What Would You Do?/What Would You Not Do?
Review Korey's response and place a checkmark next to the information you included in your response. List additional information you included in your response.

_____
_____
_____

What Would You Do? What Would You *Not* Do? RESPONSES—cont'd

Case Study 3
Page 700

What Did Korey Do?

❐ Stressed to Kathleen that if the laboratory test results are abnormal, it is better to know, so the physician can help make her better.

❐ Told Kathleen that many patients feel the same way about having blood drawn, so she is not alone. Relayed to her that her fear is normal, and she has no reason to be embarrassed.

❐ Told Kathleen that she should tell the laboratory about her last experience so they can make it easier for her. Explained that they would probably put her in a reclining position to draw her blood so that she would not get light-headed.

❐ Gave Kathleen some suggestions on how to relax during the venipuncture. Told her to turn her head when the blood was drawn.

❐ Asked Kathleen whether she had any additional symptoms.

❐ Checked with the physician to see whether he wanted to keep her appointment for today or have her appointment rescheduled after the laboratory work is completed.

What Did Korey Not Do?

❐ Did not ignore or minimize Kathleen's concerns and fears.

❐ Did not tell Kathleen that her test results would probably be fine.

What Would You Do?/What Would You *Not* Do?

Review Korey's response and place a checkmark next to the information you included in your response. List additional information you included in your response.

_____

_____

_____

_____

_____

_____

TERMINOLOGY REVIEW

Medical Term	Word Parts	Definition
Analyte		A substance that is being identified or measured in a laboratory test.
Calibration		A mechanism to check the precision and accuracy of a test system, such as an automated analyzer, to determine if the system is providing accurate results. Calibration is typically performed using a calibration device, often called a *standard.*
Clinical diagnosis		A tentative diagnosis of a patient's condition obtained through evaluation of the health history and the physical examination, without the benefit of laboratory or diagnostic tests.
Control		A solution that is used to monitor a test system to ensure the reliability and accuracy of test results.
Fasting		Abstaining from food or fluids (except water) for a specified amount of time before the collection of a specimen.
Homeostasis		The state in which body systems are functioning normally, and the internal environment of the body is in equilibrium; the body is in a healthy state.
In vivo		Occurring in the living body or organism.
Laboratory test		The clinical analysis and study of materials, fluids, or tissues obtained from patients to assist in diagnosis and treatment of disease.
Nonwaived test		A complex laboratory test that does not meet the CLIA criteria for waiver and is subject to the CLIA regulations.
Plasma		The liquid part of the blood, consisting of a clear, yellowish fluid that comprises approximately 55% of the total blood volume.
Product insert		A printed document supplied by the manufacturer with a laboratory test product that contains information on the proper storage and use of the product.
Profile		An array of laboratory tests for identifying a disease state or evaluating a particular organ or organ system.
Qualitative test		A test that indicates whether or not a substance is present in the specimen being tested and also provides an approximate indication of the amount of the substance present.

Continued

↻ TERMINOLOGY REVIEW—cont'd

Medical Term	Word Parts	Definition
Quality control		The application of methods to ensure that test results are reliable and valid and that errors are detected and eliminated.
Quantitative test		A test that indicates the exact amount of a chemical substance that is present in the body, with the results being reported in measurable units.
Reagent		A substance that produces a reaction with a patient specimen that allows detection or measurement of the substance by the test system.
Reference range		A certain established and acceptable parameter or reference range within which the laboratory test results of a healthy individual are expected to fall. (Also known as reference value and reference interval.)
Routine test		A laboratory test performed routinely on apparently healthy patients to assist in the early detection of disease.
Serum		The clear, straw-colored part of the blood (plasma) that remains after the solid elements and the clotting factor fibrinogen have been separated out of it.
Specimen		A small sample of something taken to show the nature of the whole.
Test system		A setup that includes all of the test components required to perform a laboratory test such as testing devices, controls, and testing reagents.
Waived test		A laboratory test that meets the CLIA criteria for being a simple procedure that is easy to perform and has a low risk of erroneous test results. Waived tests include tests that have been FDA-approved for use by patients at home.

🍃 ON THE WEB

For information on aging:

National Institute on Aging: www.nia.nih.gov

Administration on Aging: www.aoa.gov

American Association of Retired Persons: www.aarp.org

Social Security Administration: www.ssa.gov

Centers for Medicare and Medicaid Services: www.cms.hhs.gov

Growth House: www.growthhouse.org

The AGS Foundation for Health in Aging: www.healthinaging.org

The Institute for Geriatric Social Work: www.bu.edu/igsw

Geriatrics at Your Fingertips: www.geriatricsatyourfingertips.org

Family Caregiver Alliance: www.caregiver.org

Medicare: www.medicare.gov

Aging Statistics: www.agingstats.gov

Alzheimer's Foundation of America: www.alzfdn.org

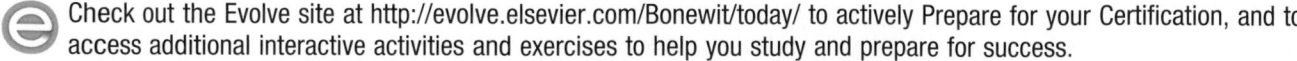 Check out the Evolve site at http://evolve.elsevier.com/Bonewit/today/ to actively Prepare for your Certification, and to access additional interactive activities and exercises to help you study and prepare for success.

30

Urinalysis

polyuria
uria
NYPRIARALLALKBARAWLA
suprapubic aspiration
urgency
urinary incontinence
[inkon-ti-nen(b)]

LEARNING OBJECTIVES

Urinary System
1. List conditions that may cause polyuria and oliguria.
2. Define the terms used to describe symptoms of the urinary system.

Collection of Urine
3. Explain why a first-voided morning specimen is often preferred for urinalysis.
4. Explain the purpose of collecting a clean-catch midstream specimen.
5. Explain the purpose of a 24-hour urine collection.
6. List changes that may occur if urine is allowed to remain standing for longer than 1 hour.

Analysis of Urine
7. List factors that may cause urine to have an unusual color or become cloudy.
8. Identify the various tests that are included in the physical and chemical examination of urine.
9. List the structures that may be found in a microscopic examination of urine.

Urine Pregnancy Testing
10. Explain the basis for urine pregnancy tests.
11. List the guidelines that must be followed in a urine pregnancy test to ensure accurate test results.

PROCEDURES

Instruct a patient in the procedure for collecting a clean-catch midstream urine specimen.

Assess the color and appearance of a urine specimen.
Perform a chemical assessment of a urine specimen.
Prepare a urine specimen for microscopic analysis by the physician.

Perform a urine pregnancy test.

CHAPTER OUTLINE

anuria (ah-NOOR-ee-ah)
bilirubinuria (bill-ih-roo-bin-YUR-ee-ah)
bladder catheterization
diuresis (di-ah-REE-sis)
dysuria (dis-YUR-ee-ah)
frequency
glycosuria (glie-koe-SOO-ree-ah)
hematuria (hem-ah-TOOR-ee-ah)
ketonuria (kee-toe-NOO-ree-ah)
ketosis (kee-TOE-sis)

micturition (mik-tur-ISH-un)
nephron (NEF-ron)
nocturia (nok-TOOR-ee-ah)
nocturnal enuresis (nok-TOOR-nal
   en-YUR-ee-sas)
oliguria (oh-lig-YUR-ee-ah)
pH (PEE-AYCH)
polyuria (pol-ee-YUR-ee-ah)
proteinuria (proe-teen-YUR-ee-ah)
pyuria (pi-YUR-ee-ah)

renal threshold (REE-nul-THRESH-hold)
retention
specific gravity
supernatant (soo-per-NAY-tent)
suprapubic aspiration
urgency
urinalysis (yur-in-AL-ih-sis)
urinary incontinence
void (VOYD)

COMPOSITION OF URINE

A physiologic change in the body caused by disease can create a disturbance in one or more of the functions of the kidney. Detection of such a disturbance can be made with the examination of urine and other body fluids such as blood.

Urine is composed of 95% water and 5% organic and inorganic waste products. Organic waste products consist of urea, uric acid, ammonia, and creatinine. Urea is present in the greatest amounts and is derived from the breakdown of proteins. Inorganic waste products include chloride, sodium, potassium, calcium, magnesium, phosphate, and sulfate.

A normal adult excretes approximately 750 to 2000 mL of urine per day. This amount varies according to the amount of fluid consumed and the amount of fluid lost through other means, such as perspiration, feces, and water vapor from the lungs. An excessive increase in urine output is known as **polyuria,** with the urine volume exceeding 2000 mL in 24 hours. Polyuria may be caused by the excessive intake of fluids or the intake of fluids that contain caffeine (e.g., coffee, tea, cola), which is a mild diuretic. Certain drugs, such as diuretics, and the pathologic conditions of diabetes mellitus, diabetes insipidus, and renal disease also may result in polyuria. Decreased or scanty urine output is known as **oliguria.** In the case of oliguria, the urine volume is less than 400 mL in 24 hours. Oliguria may occur with decreased fluid intake, dehydration, profuse perspiration, vomiting, diarrhea, or kidney disease. The normal act of voiding urine is known as **micturition.**

Terms Related to the Urinary System

The medical assistant should have a thorough knowledge of the following terms used to describe symptoms associated with the urinary system:

Anuria Failure of the kidneys to produce urine
Diuresis Secretion and passage of large amounts of urine
Dysuria Difficult or painful urination
Frequency The condition of having to urinate often
Hematuria Blood present in the urine
Nocturia Excessive (voluntary) urination during the night

Nocturnal enuresis Inability of an individual to control urination at night during sleep (bedwetting)
Oliguria Decreased output of urine
Polyuria Increased output of urine
Pyuria Pus present in the urine
Retention The inability to empty the bladder. The urine is being produced normally but is not being voided
Urgency The immediate need to urinate
Urinary incontinence The inability to retain urine

COLLECTION OF URINE

The advantage of urine testing is that urine is readily available and obtaining it does not require an invasive procedure or the use of special equipment. For accurate test results, however, the medical assistant must adhere to proper urine collection procedures to obtain the proper specimen as ordered by the physician.

Guidelines for Urine Collection

The guidelines listed should be followed in collection of a urine specimen:

1. The medical assistant must obtain an adequate volume of urine as necessary for the type of test (usually 30 to 50 mL of urine).
2. Each specimen must be labeled properly with the patient's name and date of birth, the date and time of collection, and the type of specimen (i.e., urine) to avoid any mix-ups in specimens.
3. Any medication the patient is taking should be recorded on the laboratory requisition and in the patient's chart, because some medications may interfere with the accuracy of the test results.
4. If possible, the collection of a urine specimen should be avoided in women during menstruation and for several days thereafter because the specimen may become contaminated with blood. This results in a false-positive test result for blood in the urine.
5. The medical assistant should take into consideration that voiding may be difficult for patients under stress and anxiety. In these instances, understanding and patience should be conveyed to the patient.

6. A urine specimen may be difficult to obtain from a child, even with the assistance of a parent. In this case, the physician should be informed because another collection method may be used, such as a urine collection bag, suprapubic aspiration, or catheterization of the patient.

Urine Specimen Collection Methods

The type of test to be performed often dictates the method used to collect the urine specimen. A first-voided morning specimen is recommended for pregnancy testing, and a clean-catch midstream specimen is necessary for identification of the presence of a urinary tract infection (UTI).

Most offices use disposable plastic urine specimen containers. These containers are available in different sizes and come with lids to prevent spillage and to reduce bacterial and other types of contamination.

What Would You Do? What Would You *Not* Do?

Case Study 1

Yusuke Urameshi is at the office with fever and chills, frequency, and painful and difficult urination. The physician suspects that Mr. Urameshi has prostatitis and orders a clean-catch urine specimen for a complete urinalysis, including a microscopic examination of the sediment. Mr. Urameshi tries to collect the specimen but is able to collect only 5 mL of urine. He says that he is worried about what is wrong with him and he thinks his nervousness is making it hard to get a specimen. Mr. Urameshi says that it is probably just as well because he did not understand how to cleanse himself, and he is not sure that he did it right. ■

Random Specimen

Urine testing in the medical office is often performed on freshly voided, random specimens. The medical assistant instructs the patient to **void** into a clean, dry, wide-mouthed container, and the urine is tested immediately at the medical office.

First-Voided Morning Specimen

In many cases, a first-voided morning specimen may be desired for testing because it contains the greatest concentration of dissolved substances, and a small amount of an abnormal substance that is present would be more easily detected. The patient should be instructed to collect the first specimen of the morning after rising and to preserve the specimen by refrigerating it until it is brought to the medical office. It is important to provide the patient with a specimen container to prevent the patient's use of a container from home that might harbor contaminants and affect the test results.

Clean-Catch Midstream Specimen

The urinary bladder and most of the urethra are normally free of microorganisms, whereas the distal urethra and the urinary meatus normally harbor microorganisms. If the urine is being cultured and examined for bacteria, a clean-catch midstream specimen is necessary to prevent contamination of the specimen with these normally present microorganisms. Only microorganisms that may be causing the patient's condition are desired in the urine specimen. A clean-catch midstream collection may be ordered for the detection of a UTI and the evaluation of the effectiveness of drug therapy in a patient undergoing treatment for such an infection.

The purpose of the clean-catch midstream collection is the removal of microorganisms from the urinary meatus and the distal urethra. This is accomplished by instructing the patient to thoroughly cleanse the area surrounding the meatus and to void a small amount of urine into the toilet, which flushes out microorganisms in the distal urethra. The urine specimen is collected in a sterile container using medically aseptic techniques. A properly collected specimen reduces the possibility of having to do a bladder catheterization or a suprapubic aspiration of the bladder. **Bladder catheterization** involves the passing of a sterile tube (the catheter) through the urethra and into the bladder to remove urine. **Suprapubic aspiration** involves the passing of a sterile needle through the abdominal wall into the bladder to remove urine. Both of these procedures must be performed using sterile technique.

Guidelines

Guidelines that should be followed when collecting a clean-catch midstream specimen are listed:

1. A clean-catch midstream specimen is collected by the patient at the medical office. The medical assistant must provide complete instructions for collection of this specimen. Failure to instruct the patient adequately may necessitate a return to the medical office for the collection of another specimen because of bacterial contamination. Patient instructions for obtaining a clean-catch midstream specimen are presented in Procedure 30-1.

2. The medical assistant must label the container with the patient's name and date of birth, the date, the time of collection, and the type of specimen (clean-catch midstream specimen).

3. For reliable test results, the specimen should be tested immediately and should not be allowed to stand. If this is not possible, the specimen should be refrigerated, or a preservative should be added.

4. If the specimen is to be tested at an outside laboratory, completion of a laboratory requisition to accompany it is necessary. A urinalysis laboratory request form is shown in Figure 30-1.

5. The procedure is completed by sanitizing the hands and recording the procedure in the patient's chart. The information to be charted for specimens tested at the medical office includes the date and time, the type of specimen collected, and the laboratory test results. If the specimen is being transported to an outside laboratory for testing, record the date and

NAME:	ADDRESS:	UR- **183900**
		ICDA
		REQUESTING PHYSICIAN
	DATE:	PHYSICIAN HAS SEEN-INITIAL

	ROUTINE URINALYSIS - 001				MICROSCOPIC - 022			QUANTITATIVE	
	APPEARANCE COLOR			WBC'S	/HPF	024	SULKOWITCH	
023	SPECIFIC GRAVITY			RBC'S	/HPF	026	BILE	
004	PH			CASTS (Hyaline)	/LPF		PHENYLPYRUVIC ACID	
	PROTEIN			CASTS (Granular)	/LPF	027	PHENESTIX	
	GLUCOSE			CASTS (Cellular)	/LPF	028	UROBILINOGEN	
007	KETONES (ACETONE)			CASTS (Waxy)	/LPF	029	PORPHOBILINOGEN	
3	OCCULT BLOOD			EPITHELIAL CELLS	/LPF	030	PORPHYRIN	
	BILE			BACTERIA		031	BENCE-JONES	
	UROBILINOGEN			MUCUS		025	TOTAL PROTEIN 24HR. SPECIMEN	
	LEUKOCYTE			CRYSTALS			TOTAL VOLUME REQUIRED:	
COMMENTS				AMORPHOUS				
URINALYSIS				OTHER:			SIGNATURE:	
DMH-0067 (Rev. 3/83)			33	**F P N**			DATE:	

DMH-MedR-1065-A

Figure 30-1 Urinalysis laboratory request form.

time, the type of specimen collected, and the date the specimen was transported to the laboratory.

Twenty-Four–Hour Urine Specimen

A 24-hour urine specimen is used for quantitative measurement of specific urinary components. With collection of urine over a 24-hour period, greater accuracy of measurement exists than with a random specimen. This is because body metabolism, exercise, and hydration can affect the excretion rate of substances in the urine. In addition, at certain times during a 24-hour period, increased excretion of substances (e.g., electrolytes, hormones, proteins, urobilinogen) is seen, and at other times decreased excretion is seen. Examples of substances measured in a 24-hour specimen include calcium, cortisol, lead, potassium, protein, and urea nitrogen. A 24-hour specimen is often used in the diagnosis of the cause of kidney stone formation and in the control and prevention of new stone formation. It may also be used to perform a creatinine clearance test, which provides the physician with information on kidney function.

A large wide-mouthed container (3000 mL) is used to store the urine collected over the 24-hour period. To prevent changes in the quality of the urine specimen, the specimen must be kept refrigerated or placed in an ice chest. Some containers also contain a chemical preservative (in the form of crystals, tablets, or a liquid) to assist in maintaining the quality of the specimen. Examples of urine preservatives include hydrochloric acid, boric acid, acetic acid, and toluene. A hazardous chemical warning label should be attached to a specimen container with a preservative, and the patient should be instructed not to discard or touch the preservative in the container.

The patient is also provided with a container in which to collect each urine specimen. A female patient may be given a urine "hat," which is placed over the commode under the toilet seat; a male patient is often provided with a collection cup. After collection, the urine is poured into the large specimen container. This method makes collection easier and safer for the patient. If the patient voids urine directly into a specimen container that holds a preservative, the preservative could splash onto the patient's skin, resulting in a chemical burn.

The medical assistant should provide the patient with verbal and written instructions for collection of the urine specimen. The patient should be advised to drink a normal amount of fluid during the collection period and to avoid alcohol intake for 24 hours before and during the collection period. The patient should be instructed to choose a 24-hour period when he or she will be at home, so that the urine will not have to be transported. The test should not be performed when the patient is menstruating. Certain medications, such as thiazides, phosphorus-binding antacids, allopurinol, and vitamin C, could alter the test results. The physician may want the patient to discontinue these medications for 1 week before the test.

PROCEDURE 30-1 Clean-Catch Midstream Specimen Collection Instructions

Outcome Instruct a patient in the procedure for collecting a clean-catch midstream urine specimen.

Equipment/Supplies

- Sterile specimen container and label
- Personal antiseptic towelettes

- Tissues

1. Procedural Step. Sanitize your hands. Greet the patient and introduce yourself. Identify the patient and explain the procedure.

2. Procedural Step. Assemble equipment. Label the specimen container with the patient's name and date of birth, the date, the type of specimen (clean-catch midstream), and your initials.

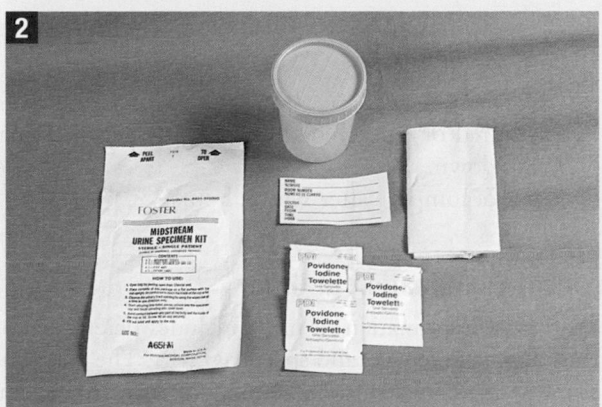

Assemble the equipment.

3. Procedural Step. Instruct a female patient on collection of the specimen as follows:

a. Wash the hands, open the package of towelettes, and place them on their wrapper.

b. Remove the lid from the specimen container and place it on a paper towel with the opening of the lid facing upward. Do not touch the inside of the lid or the inside of the specimen container.

c. Pull undergarments down and sit on the toilet. Expose the urinary meatus by spreading apart the labia with one hand.

d. Cleanse each side of the urinary meatus with an antiseptic towelette using a front-to-back motion (from pubis to anus). Use a separate antiseptic towelette for each side of the meatus. After use, discard each towelette in the toilet.
Principle. Cleansing removes microorganisms from the urinary meatus. A front-to-back motion must be used for cleansing to avoid drawing microorgan-

isms from the anal region into the area that is being cleansed.

e. Cleanse directly across the meatus (front to back) with a third antiseptic towelette.

f. Continue to hold the labia apart, and void a small amount of urine into the toilet.
Principle. Voiding a small amount flushes microorganisms out of the distal urethra.

g. Without stopping the urine flow, collect the next amount of urine by voiding into the sterile container. Do not touch the inside of the container. Fill the specimen container about half full with urine.
Principle. Touching the inside of the container contaminates it with microorganisms that normally reside on the skin.

h. Void the last amount of urine into the toilet. This means that the first and last portions of the urine flow are not included in the specimen. Replace the lid of the specimen container.

i. Wipe the area dry with a tissue, and discard it in the toilet. Flush the toilet and wash the hands.

4. Procedural Step. *Instruct a male patient as follows:*

a. Wash the hands, open the towelettes, remove the lid from the specimen container, and remove undergarments.

b. Stand in front of the toilet. Retract the foreskin of the penis (if uncircumcised).

c. Cleanse the area around the meatus (glans penis) and the urethral opening (meatal orifice) by wiping each side of the meatus with a separate antiseptic towelette.

d. Cleanse directly across the meatus with a third antiseptic towelette. After use, discard each towelette in the toilet.

e. Void a small amount of urine into the toilet.

f. Collect the next amount of urine by voiding into the sterile container without touching the inside of the container with the hands or penis. Fill the container about half full with urine.

g. Void the last amount of urine into the toilet and replace the lid on the container.

Continued

PROCEDURE 30-1

h. Wipe the area dry with a tissue, and discard it in the toilet. Flush the toilet and wash the hands.

5. Procedural Step. Provide the patient with instructions about what to do with the specimen after it has been collected (e.g., placing it in a designated area, directly handing it to the medical assistant).

6. Procedural Step. Record the procedure in the patient's chart. Include the date and time and the type of specimen collected (clean-catch midstream collection).

7. Procedural Step. Test the specimen at the office or prepare the specimen for transport to an outside laboratory for testing. If the specimen is to be transported to an outside laboratory, do the following:

a. Place the specimen container in a biohazard specimen bag.

b. Place the laboratory request in the outside pocket of the specimen bag.

c. Properly preserve the specimen while awaiting pickup by a laboratory courier by placing it in a refrigerator.

d. Chart the date the specimen was transported to the laboratory and the tests requested.

CHARTING EXAMPLE

Date	
3/24/XX	10:15 a.m. Clean-catch midstream collected by pt. Sent to Medical Center Laboratory for C & S on 3/24/XX. —L. Proffitt, CMA (AAMA)

ANALYSIS OF URINE

Urinalysis is the analysis of urine and is the laboratory test most commonly performed in the medical office because a urine specimen is readily obtainable and can be easily tested. Urinalysis consists of *physical, chemical,* and *microscopic examinations.* Deviation from normal in any of the three areas assists the physician in the diagnosis and treatment of pathologic conditions, not only of the urinary system, but also of other body systems. Urinalysis may be performed as a screening measure as part of a general physical examination or to assist in the diagnosis of a pathologic condition. It also may assist in the evaluation of effectiveness of therapy after treatment has been initiated for a pathologic condition.

Urinalysis should be performed on a fresh or preserved specimen. If a specimen cannot be examined within 1 hour of voiding, it should be preserved at once in the refrigerator in a closed container and later returned to room temperature and mixed before testing. Chemical additives also are used to preserve urine specimens but generally are used only with specimens that require prolonged storage, such as specimens that must be shipped a long distance, because the chemical preservative sometimes interferes with the chemicals used to perform the urine test.

If the urine is allowed to stand at room temperature for longer than 1 hour, some of the following changes may occur:

1. Bacteria in the environment that get into the urine specimen work on the urea present in the urine, converting it to ammonia. Because ammonia is alkaline, an acid urine becomes alkaline, increasing the pH. In addition, an alkaline pH may result in a false-positive result on the protein test.
2. Bacteria multiply rapidly in the urine, resulting in a cloudy specimen and an increase in the nitrite.
3. If glucose is present in the specimen, it decreases in amount because microorganisms use the glucose as a source of food.

4. If any red or white blood cells are present, they may break down.
5. Casts decompose after several hours.

Physical Examination of Urine

The physical examination of urine includes determination of the color, appearance, and specific gravity. The color and appearance of the urine specimen may be evaluated during preparation for another testing procedure, such as chemical testing of the urine, or before centrifugation of the specimen in preparation for microscopic analysis. For an accurate evaluation of the color and appearance, the urine specimen must be collected in a clear plastic container.

Color

The normal color of urine ranges from almost colorless to dark yellow. Dilute urine tends to be lighter yellow in color, whereas concentrated urine is a darker yellow. The first-voided morning specimen is usually the most concentrated because consumption of fluids is decreased during the night. Urine becomes more dilute as the day progresses and more fluids are consumed.

The color of the urine is the result of the presence of a yellow pigment known as *urochrome,* produced by the breakdown of hemoglobin. It is common for the color of urine to vary among different shades of yellow within the course of a day. Classifications that can be used to describe the color of urine include light yellow, yellow, dark yellow, light amber, amber, and dark amber (Figure 30-2).

The color of the urine specimen assists in determining additional tests that may be necessary. Abnormal colors may be caused by the presence of hemoglobin or blood (resulting in a red or reddish color), bile pigments (resulting in a yellow-brown or greenish color), and fat droplets or pus (resulting in a milky color). Some foods and medications also may cause the urine to change to an abnormal color. Phenazopyridine (Pyridium), a urinary

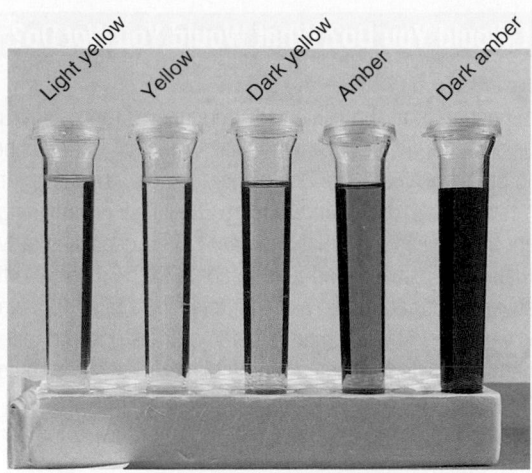

Figure 30-2 Color of urine.

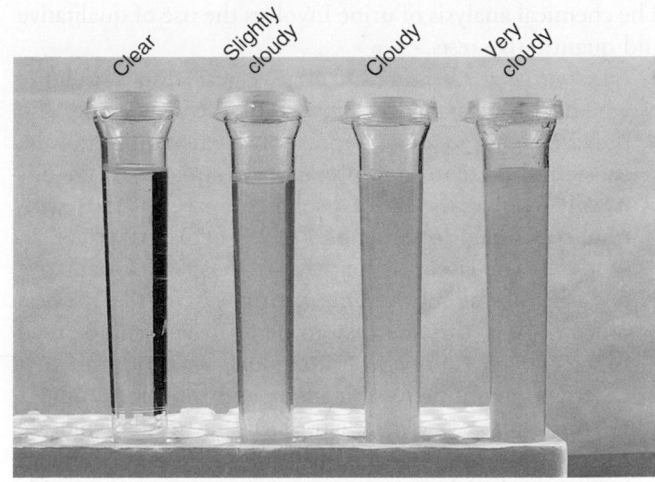

Figure 30-3 Appearance of urine.

tract analgesic, causes the urine to change to an orange to red color.

Appearance

Evaluation of the appearance of urine is usually performed at the same time as the color evaluation. Fresh urine is usually clear, or transparent, but becomes cloudy on standing out too long. Cloudiness in a freshly voided specimen may be the result of the presence of bacteria, pus, blood, fat, yeast, sperm, mucous threads, or fecal contaminants. A microscopic examination of the urine sediment should be performed on all cloudy specimens to determine the cause of the cloudiness. Cloudiness resulting from bacteria may be caused by a UTI.

Classifications used to describe the appearance of urine include clear, slightly cloudy, cloudy, and very cloudy (Figure 30-3). The medical assistant should develop skill in recognizing the varying degrees of urine clarity.

Odor

Freshly voided urine normally should have a slightly aromatic odor. Urine that has been standing for a long time develops an ammonia odor from the breakdown of urea by bacteria in the specimen. The urine of a patient with diabetes mellitus may have a fruity odor from the presence of ketone. The urine of a patient with a UTI is usually foul-smelling, and the odor becomes worse on standing. Certain foods, such as asparagus, can cause the urine to have a musty smell. Although urine may have many characteristic odors, as a rule the odor of urine is not generally used in the diagnosis of a patient's condition.

Specific Gravity

The **specific gravity** of urine measures the weight of the urine compared with the weight of an equal volume of distilled water. Specific gravity indicates the amount of dissolved substance present in the urine, providing information on the ability of the kidneys to dilute or concentrate the urine. Specific gravity is decreased in conditions in which the kidneys cannot concentrate the urine, such as chronic renal insufficiency, diabetes insipidus, and malignant hypertension. The specific gravity is increased in patients with adrenal insufficiency, congestive heart failure, hepatic disease, diabetes mellitus with glycosuria, and conditions that cause dehydration, such as fever, vomiting, and diarrhea.

The normal specific gravity of urine ranges from 1.003 to 1.030 but is usually between 1.010 and 1.025 (the specific gravity of distilled water is 1.000). Specific gravity varies greatly with fluid intake and the state of hydration of an individual. Dilute urine contains fewer dissolved substances and has a lower specific gravity. Concentrated urine has a higher specific gravity because of the increased amount of dissolved substances. A urine specimen is generally more concentrated in the morning and becomes more dilute after fluid consumption.

In the medical office, specific gravity is most commonly measured using a reagent strip. This involves a color comparison determination with a reagent strip that contains a reagent area for specific gravity. The reagent strip is dipped into the urine specimen, and the results are compared with a color chart (see Procedure 30-2).

Chemical Examination of Urine

The chemical examination of urine is used to assist in the evaluation and diagnosis of kidney function, urinary tract infection, carbohydrate metabolism (diabetes mellitus), and liver function. Substances present in excessive (abnormal) amounts in the blood are usually removed by the urine. For example, glucose is normally present in the blood, but if it exceeds a certain level or threshold, the excess amount is excreted in the urine. Chemical testing of urine is an indirect means of detecting abnormal amounts of chemicals in the body, indicating a pathologic condition. The chemical examination of urine also can be used to detect the presence of substances that, in the absence of disease, do not normally appear in the urine, such as blood and nitrite.

Chemical tests that are routinely performed during a urinalysis include testing for pH, glucose, protein, and ketone. Other chemical tests that may be performed include testing for blood, bilirubin, urobilinogen, nitrite, and leukocytes.

The chemical analysis of urine involves the use of qualitative and quantitative tests.

- *Qualitative test results.* Qualitative test results indicate whether a substance is present in the urine and also provide an approximate indication of the amount of the substance present. Interpretation of qualitative results usually involves the use of a color comparison chart, with results recorded in terms of 1+, 2+, or 3+; trace, small, moderate, or large; or negative or positive. Qualitative tests are useful for screening purposes in the medical office because they are easy to perform and can be used to screen large numbers of individuals—a procedure that otherwise might be too expensive and time consuming.
- *Quantitative test results.* Quantitative test results indicate the exact amount of a chemical substance that is present in the body; the results are reported in measurable units (e.g., mg/dL). Obtaining a quantitative test result on a urine specimen usually involves the use of more complex equipment and testing procedures than are found in the medical office; they also are more time-consuming to run.

Urine Testing Kits

Commercially prepared urine testing kits are most frequently used in the medical office for the chemical testing of urine. These kits are usually preferred because they contain premeasured reagents, the procedure is easy to follow, and they provide an immediate answer. Most of the test results are qualitative, and a positive result may indicate the need for further testing. Most of the tests are manufactured in the form of reagent strips, and they rely on a color change for interpretation of results. A color chart is provided with the kit for making a visual comparison.

For accurate and reliable test results, the medical assistant should carefully read and follow the instructions that accompany each kit. Test strips that contain more than one reagent may require different time intervals for reading results. Certain medications that the patient is taking also may interfere with the test results. These medications are listed in the manufacturer's instructions accompanying the test.

Before a test is used, its expiration date must be checked. If the test is outdated, it must not be used to prevent inaccurate test results. Test material must not be used if a color change has occurred, or if the *tested* strip gives off a color that does not match the shades on the color chart. Light, heat, and moisture can alter the effectiveness of the strips; care must be taken to store the test materials in a cool, dry area. Most test materials are packaged in light-resistant containers to protect them from light. The test materials must never be transferred from their original container to another because the other container may harbor traces of moisture, dirt, or chemicals that could affect the test results.

pH

The **pH** is the unit that indicates the acidity or alkalinity of a solution. The pH scale ranges from 0.0 to 14.0. The

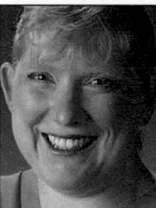

Putting it All into Practice

My name is Linda Proffitt, and I work for a urologist and his wife, who is a pediatrician. I work primarily in the urology practice and only occasionally in pediatrics. I am responsible for having the charts ready when the patients are seen and for doing their urinalysis. Another one of my responsibilities is to assist with special procedures, such as catheter insertions, male and female dilations, ultrasound examinations of the bladder, and prostate examinations.

When I first started working in the urology office, I had to learn to assist with transrectal ultrasounds of the prostate in case the US technician was sick. When she retired, I inherited the position, whether I wanted it or not. At first I dreaded doing the procedures and would be so nervous that I would get the shakes and forget the order in which things were supposed to be done. My physician was understanding and would help by talking me through it. I think the main reason I was so nervous was that sometimes patients have trouble and we have to administer oxygen and run IVs. One time, a patient had a reaction to the pain medication we gave before the procedure.

Time, practice, and confidence in myself have improved my nerves, even with the occasional emergency situation. ■

lower the number, the greater the acidity; the higher the number, the greater the alkalinity. A pH reading of 7.0 is neutral; a reading below 7.0 indicates acidity; and a reading above 7.0 indicates alkalinity.

The kidneys help regulate the acid-base balance of the body. For an accurate pH reading of the urine, the measurement should be performed on freshly voided urine. If the urine is allowed to remain standing, it becomes more alkaline as urea is converted to ammonia by bacterial action.

Although the pH of urine can normally range from 4.6 to 8.0, the pH of a freshly voided specimen of a patient on a normal diet is usually acidic and has a pH reading of about 6.0. An abnormally high pH reading on a fresh specimen (i.e., an alkaline urine) may indicate a bacterial infection of the urinary tract.

Highlight on Drug Testing in the Workplace

Statistics

Statistics suggest that the problem of drug abuse is growing in the workplace. On any one day, 8.9 to 16 million employees are estimated to be working under the influence of drugs. The effects of on-the-job drug use extend into every segment of the population and touch every business and industry. The Occupational Safety and Health Administration (OSHA) estimates that 65% of all work-related accidents can be traced to substance abuse. The Metropolitan Insurance Company states that drug abuse costs industry $85 billion annually because of absenteeism, lowered productivity, and higher health care costs.

Testing Programs

Because of these economic and safety factors, businesses across the United States are adopting a less permissive attitude toward drug use and are beginning compulsory drug testing in the workplace. Approximately one third of U.S. employers have implemented drug-testing programs in the workplace. These employers include utility companies, transportation operations, sports associations, and governmental agencies. Currently, many companies test blue-collar and white-collar employees for drug use. Companies with drug-testing programs report a significant reduction in employee accidents, fewer sick days, and healthier employees.

A comprehensive drug-testing program includes the detection of drug use in the workplace, policies to discourage further abuse, and the referral of employees for treatment and rehabilitation. Drug testing may be performed for one or more of the following purposes: (1) pre-employment drug screening, (2) testing for probable cause after unexplained behavior or incident (e.g., an accident on the job), and (3) random sample testing of the workforce to detect use of controlled substances by employees on the job.

Testing Methods

Blood testing is the best means for determining precise information concerning the amount of drug used and when the drug was taken. Blood tests are costly, however, and are time-consuming to perform. Urine drug testing offers the next best alternative; it is noninvasive and technically easier and cheaper to perform. Current urine screening tests target the most common drugs of abuse: amphetamines, barbiturates, benzodiazepines, cocaine, marijuana, opiates, PCP, methaqualone, and methadone.

Chain of Custody

The usual procedure for urine drug testing involves screening the specimen and confirming positive results with more specific urine tests. The specimen may be collected at the workplace, at the medical office, or at an outside laboratory. To help ensure reliable and valid drug-testing results, a security system or "chain of custody" must be followed in the collection and handling of the specimen. This typically includes ensuring the identification of the individual undergoing drug testing, taking precautions to avoid falsifying or tampering with specimens, properly labeling the urine specimen, sealing the sample in the specimen container after collection, and immediately sending it to the laboratory for analysis or refrigerating it at once for any delay in transport. Urine drug-testing kits are available for testing the specimen in the medical office. These kits provide immediate results and take only a few minutes to perform.

Disadvantages

The main disadvantage of urine drug testing is that a positive test result indicates only the presence of a drug in the urine; it does not provide any information regarding when the drug was taken. Drugs that are detected in the urine may or *may not* still be present in the blood, where they can affect an individual's behavior and impair performance. A positive urine test result does not reveal whether an individual is impaired by drugs. In addition, the initial urine screening tests are sometimes unreliable; unless positive results are confirmed with a more specific test, an individual may be unjustly accused of drug use. These factors and the violation of an individual's right to privacy are the main areas of dispute for individuals who oppose drug testing in the workplace.

Intervention

Companies with drug-testing programs have various options when results are positive, such as recommendations for drug treatment programs or disciplinary action. Many companies have established in-house employee assistance programs that include counseling and drug withdrawal therapy for employees who desire help. Most companies prefer to help current employees with rehabilitation instead of discharging them and hiring and training new employees. Studies show a 35% to 60% recovery rate for employees enrolled in drug treatment programs. ■

Glucose

Normally, no glucose should be detectable in the urine. Glucose in the blood is filtered through the nephrons and is reabsorbed into the body. If the glucose concentration in the blood becomes too high, the kidney is unable to reabsorb all of it back into the blood, the renal threshold is exceeded, and glucose is spilled into the urine—a condition known as **glycosuria.** (The **renal threshold** is the concentration at which a substance in the blood that is not normally excreted by the kidney begins to appear in the urine.) The renal threshold for glucose is generally 160 to 180 mg/ dL (100 mL of blood), but this number may vary among individuals. Diabetes mellitus is the most common cause of glycosuria. Some individuals have a low renal threshold, and glucose may appear in their urine after the consumption of a large quantity of foods containing sugar. This condition is known as *alimentary glycosuria.*

Protein

The presence of protein in the urine is known as **proteinuria.** Protein in the urine usually indicates a pathologic condition if found in several samples over time. A temporary increase in urine protein may be caused by stress or strenuous exercise. Some of the conditions that may cause proteinuria include glomerular filtration problems, renal disease, and bacterial infection of the urinary tract. If proteinuria occurs, the physician usually requests an examination of the sediment to determine, through visual observation, what is causing protein to be in the urine.

Ketone

Three types of ketone bodies exist: beta-hydroxybutyric acid, acetoacetic acid, and acetone. *Ketones* are the normal products of fat metabolism and can be used by muscle tissue as a source of energy. When more than normal amounts of fat are metabolized by the body, the muscles cannot handle all of the ketones that result. Large amounts of ketone accumulate in the tissues and body fluids; this condition is known as **ketosis.** The body rids itself of these excess ketones by excreting them in the urine. **Ketonuria** is the term that refers to the presence of ketone bodies in the urine. Conditions that may lead to ketonuria include uncontrolled diabetes mellitus, starvation, and a diet composed almost entirely of fat.

Bilirubin

The average life span of a red blood cell is 120 days. When a red blood cell breaks down, one of the substances released from the breakdown of hemoglobin is a vivid yellow pigment known as *bilirubin.* Normally, bilirubin is transported to the liver and excreted into the bile, and it eventually leaves the body through the intestines in the feces. Certain liver conditions, such as gallstones, hepatitis, and cirrhosis, may result in the presence of bilirubin in the urine, or **bilirubinuria.** The urine becomes yellow-brown or greenish, and a yellow foam appears when the urine is shaken.

Urobilinogen

Normally, bilirubin is excreted by the liver into the intestinal tract. Bacteria present in the intestines convert it to urobilinogen. Approximately 50% of the urobilinogen is reabsorbed into the body for reexcretion by the liver. Small amounts may appear in the urine, but most of the urobilinogen is excreted in the feces. An increase in the production of bilirubin increases the amount of urobilinogen excreted in the urine. Conditions such as excessive hemolysis of red blood cells, infectious hepatitis, cirrhosis, congestive heart failure, and infectious mononucleosis may increase the level of urobilinogen in the urine.

Blood

Blood is considered an abnormal constituent of urine, unless it is present as a contaminant during menstruation. The condition in which blood is found in the urine is termed *hematuria.* Hematuria may be the result of injury or disorders such as cystitis, tumors of the bladder, urethritis, kidney stones, and certain kidney disorders.

Nitrite

Nitrite in the urine indicates the presence of a pathogen in the (normally sterile) urinary tract, which results in a UTI. The pathogen possesses the ability to convert nitrate, which normally occurs in the urine, to nitrite, which is normally absent. The nitrite test must be performed with urine that has been in the bladder for at least 4 to 6 hours to ensure that bacteria have converted nitrate to nitrite. Therefore, use of a first-voided morning specimen is recommended. The test should *not* be performed on specimens that have been left standing out because a false-positive result may occur from bacterial contamination from the environment. The nitrite test is a screening test and is usually followed by a quantitative culture and identification of the invading pathogen.

Leukocytes

The presence of leukocytes in the urine is known as *leukocyturia* and accompanies inflammation of the kidneys and the lower urinary tract. Examples of specific conditions include acute and chronic pyelonephritis, cystitis, and urethritis. Reagent strips are available that contain a reagent area that permits the chemical detection of intact and lysed leukocytes in the urine. The advantage of detecting lysed leukocytes is that these cells cannot be observed during a microscopic examination of urine sediment and would otherwise remain undetected. The recommended urine specimen, particularly for women, is a clean-catch midstream collection to prevent contamination of the specimen with leukocytes from vaginal secretions leading to false-positive test results.

Reagent Strips

In the medical office, reagent strips are the most commonly used diagnostic urine testing kit. Reagent strips consist of disposable plastic strips on which separate reagent areas are affixed for testing specific chemical constituents that may be present in the urine during pathologic conditions. The results provide the physician with information to assist in diagnosis of the following:

- Conditions affecting kidney function (e.g., kidney stones)
- Urinary tract infection
- Conditions affecting carbohydrate metabolism (e.g., diabetes mellitus)
- Conditions affecting liver function (e.g., hepatitis)

Test results also provide the physician with information related to the status of the patient's acid-base balance and urine concentration. Reagent strips are considered qualitative tests, and a positive result necessitates further testing. The number and type of reagent areas included on the reagent strip depend on the particular brand of reagent strips. Multistix 10 SG (Bayer Corporation, Tarrytown, NY) contains 10 reagent areas for testing pH, protein, glucose, ketone, bilirubin, blood, urobilinogen, nitrite, specific gravity, and leukocytes. The reagent strip urine testing procedure presented in this chapter (Procedure 30-2) is specifically for Multistix 10 SG; however, this procedure can be followed for the chemical testing of urine with most reagent strips. In all instances, the medical assistant should read the manufacturer's instructions before performing the test.

Guidelines for Reagent Strip Urine Testing

Testing urine with reagent strips is a relatively easy procedure to perform. Specific guidelines must be followed, however, to obtain accurate test results.

1. *Type of specimen.* The best results are obtained with a freshly voided and thoroughly mixed urine specimen. If the medical assistant is unable to test the specimen within 1 hour of voiding, the specimen should be refrigerated immediately and then allowed to return to room temperature before testing.

2. *Type of collection.* Most reagent strips are designed to be used with a random specimen collection; however, clean-catch midstream and first-voided morning specimens are suggested for specific tests. The nitrite test results are optimized with a first-voided morning specimen, whereas a clean-catch midstream collection is recommended for the leukocyte test.

3. *Specimen container.* The specimen container used must be thoroughly clean and free from any detergent or disinfectant residue because cleansing agents contain oxidants that react with the chemicals on the reagent strip, leading to inaccurate test results. The container should be large enough to allow for complete immersion of all reagent strip areas.

4. *Time intervals.* Read the test results at the exact time intervals specified on the color chart. Do not read any test results after 2 minutes.

5. *Interpretation of results.* Of particular importance is the comparison of the reagent strip with the color chart. The reagent strip must be compared with the color chart in good lighting to obtain a good visual match of the color reactions with the color chart provided with the test kit.

6. *Storage of reagent strips.* The reagents on the strips are sensitive to light, heat, and moisture, and the bottle containing the strips must be stored in a cool, dry area away from direct sunlight, with the cap tightly closed to maintain reactivity of the reagent. The bottle may contain a desiccant that should not be removed because its purpose is to promote dryness by absorbing moisture. The bottle of reagent strips must be stored at a temperature between 59° F (15° C) and 86° F (30° C). The strips should not be stored in the refrigerator or freezer. A tan-to-brown discoloration or darkening on the reagent areas indicates deterioration of the chemical reagent strips, in which case the strips should not be used because the test results would be inaccurate.

Quality Control Testing

Quality control testing should be used in a chemical examination of urine with a reagent strip. Quality control testing

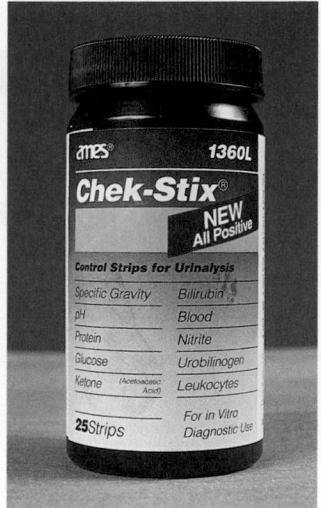

Figure 30-4 Chek-Stix control strips.

ensures the reliability of test results by (1) determining whether the reagent strips are reacting properly, and (2) confirming that the test is being properly performed and accurately interpreted.

To check the reliability of Multistix reagent strips, the Chek-Stix control (Bayer Corporation) should be used. Each Chek-Stix control consists of a firm plastic strip to which are affixed synthetic ingredients (Figure 30-4). The control strip is reconstituted by immersing it in distilled water for 30 minutes, which allows the ingredients on the strip to dissolve in the water. After reconstitution, the resulting solution is tested in the same manner as a urine specimen. The values to be expected are outlined in the product insert that accompanies the control strips. The results of the control test should be recorded in a quality control log. If the expected values are not obtained, the cause of the problem must be determined and corrected. Factors that can cause a problem include outdated reagent strips, improper storage of the strips, and an error in testing technique. The quality control test should be performed when each bottle of strips is opened for the first time, or when a question of reliability arises regarding the testing strips.

Urine Analyzer

Urine analyzers are used to perform an automatic chemical examination of urine with reagent strips. They offer the advantage of the ability to perform the chemical analysis quickly and to interpret results automatically. These analyzers are used most often in medical offices that perform moderate-volume to large-volume urine testing.

The Clinitek Analyzer (Bayer Corporation) is an example of a urine analyzer that automatically reads Multistix SG and other (Bayer) urinalysis reagent strips (Figure 30-5, *A*). The results are printed out, and abnormal results are flagged to call attention to them (Figure 30-5, *B*). Different models are available; some can be used to perform a color and appearance analysis and a microscopic examination of the urine.

PROCEDURE 30-2

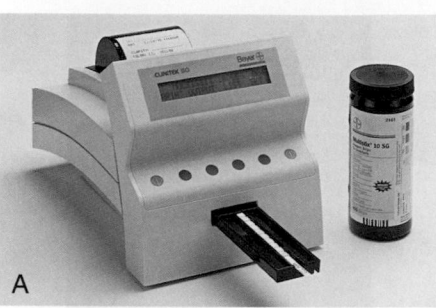

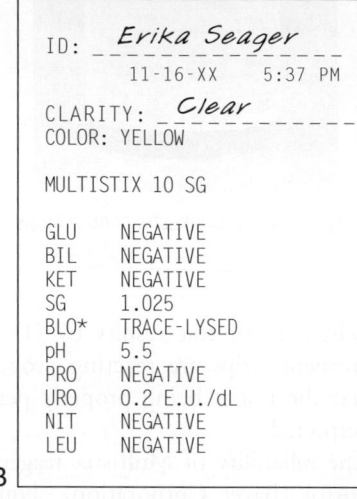

```
ID: ___Erika Seager___
        11-16-XX    5:37 PM
CLARITY: ___Clear___
COLOR: YELLOW

MULTISTIX 10 SG

GLU   NEGATIVE
BIL   NEGATIVE
KET   NEGATIVE
SG    1.025
BLO*  TRACE-LYSED
pH    5.5
PRO   NEGATIVE
URO   0.2 E.U./dL
NIT   NEGATIVE
LEU   NEGATIVE
```

Figure 30-5 **A,** Clinitek Urine Analyzer. **B,** Clinitek printout.

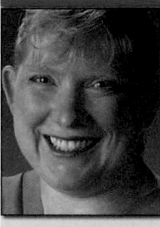

---

see DVD

PROCEDURE 30-2   Chemical Testing of Urine with the Multistix 10 SG Reagent Strip

Outcome Perform a chemical assessment of a urine specimen.

Equipment/Supplies

- Disposable gloves
- Multistix 10 SG reagent strips
- Urine container
- Timer
- Laboratory report form

1. **Procedural Step.** Perform the quality control testing procedure if using a new bottle of testing strips.
   Principle. Performing the quality control procedure ensures the reliability of test results.

2. **Procedural Step.** Obtain a freshly voided urine specimen from the patient with a clean container. The specimen should be uncentrifuged and at room temperature.
   Principle. The best results are obtained with a freshly voided specimen. The container should be clean because contaminants could affect the results. Uncentrifuged specimens ensure a homogeneous sample.

3. **Procedural Step.** Sanitize your hands.

4. **Procedural Step.** Assemble the equipment. Check the expiration date of the reagent strips.
   Principle. Outdated reagent strips may lead to inaccurate test results.

5. **Procedural Step.** Apply gloves. Remove a reagent strip from its plastic container, and recap the container immediately. Do not touch the test areas with your fingers or lay the strip on the table. It is permissible, however, to lay the reagent strip on a clean, dry paper towel.
   Principle. Recapping the container is necessary to prevent exposing the strips to environmental moisture, light, and heat, which cause altered reagent reactivity. Contamination of test areas by the hands or table surface may affect the accuracy of test results.

6. **Procedural Step.** Thoroughly mix the urine specimen and remove the lid from the container. Using the dominant hand, completely immerse the reagent strip in the urine specimen, and remove it immediately. While removing, run the edge of the strip against the rim of the urine container to remove excess urine.

PROCEDURE 30-2   Chemical Testing of Urine with the Multistix 10 SG Reagent Strip—cont'd

Principle. The strip should be completely immersed to ensure that all test areas are moistened for accurate test results. Prolonged immersion of the reagent strip and failure to remove excess urine may cause the reagents to dissolve and leach onto adjacent test areas, affecting the accuracy of the test results.

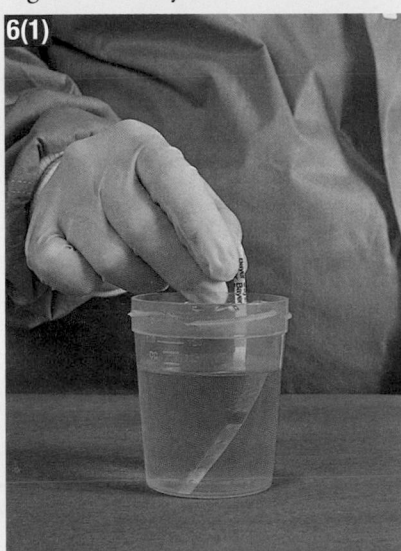

Completely immerse the reagent strip in the urine.

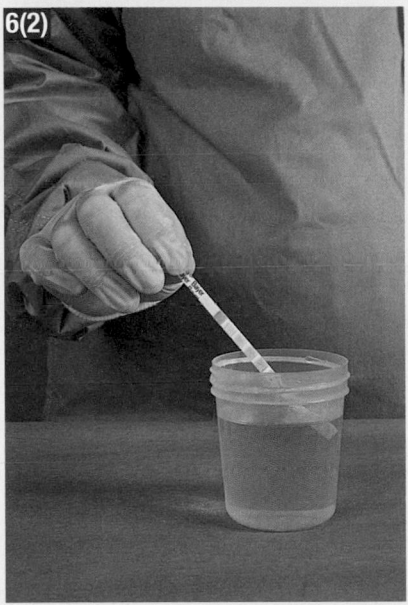

Run the edge of the strip against the urine container.

7. Procedural Step. With the nondominant hand, start the timer, pick up the reagent strip container, and rotate it to the color chart. Hold the reagent strip in a horizontal position and place it as close as possible to the corresponding color blocks on the color chart. Do not lay the strip directly on the color chart because this will result in soiling of the chart by the urine. Read the results carefully and at the exact reading times, starting with the shortest time specified on the color chart and as indicated here:

Glucose, 30 seconds	Bilirubin, 30 seconds
Ketone, 40 seconds	Specific gravity, 45 seconds
Blood, 60 seconds	pH, 60 seconds
Protein, 60 seconds	Urobilinogen, 60 seconds
Nitrite, 60 seconds	Leukocytes, 2 minutes

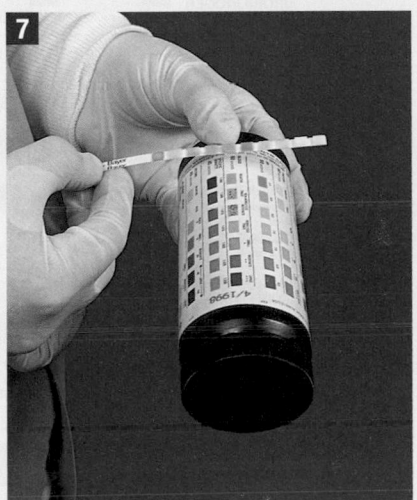

Hold the strip horizontally and read the results.

Principle. Holding the strip in a horizontal position avoids soiling your gloves with urine and prevents reagents from running over into adjacent testing areas, causing inaccurate test results. The strip must be read at the proper time interval to avoid dissolving out reagents, leading to inaccurate test results.

8. Procedural Step. Dispose of the strip in a regular waste container.

9. Procedural Step. Remove gloves, and sanitize your hands.

10. Procedural Step. Chart the results. Results should be charted by following the interpretation guide provided above each color block on the color chart. Most offices use a preprinted reporting form to make it easier to record results. The recording should include the date and time, the brand name of the test used (Multistix 10 SG), and the results.

Continued

PROCEDURE 30-2   Chemical Testing of Urine with the Multistix 10 SG Reagent Strip—cont'd

2161

Multistix® 10 SG

Reagent Strips for Urinalysis
For In Vitro Diagnostic Use

READ PRODUCT INSERT BEFORE USE.
IMPORTANT: Do not expose to direct sunlight.
Do not use after 4/01.

COLOR CHART

Bayer

TESTS AND READING TIME

Test							
LEUKOCYTES 2 minutes	NEGATIVE		TRACE	SMALL +	MODERATE ++	LARGE +++	
NITRITE 60 seconds	NEGATIVE		POSITIVE	POSITIVE	(Any degree of uniform pink color is positive)		
UROBILINOGEN 60 seconds	NORMAL 0.2	NORMAL 1	mg/dL 2	4	8	(1 mg = approx. 1EU)	
PROTEIN 60 seconds	NEGATIVE	TRACE	mg/dL 30 +	100 ++	300 +++	2000 or more ++++	
pH 60 seconds	5.0	6.0	6.5	7.0	7.5	8.0	8.5
BLOOD 60 seconds	NEGATIVE	NON-HEMOLYZED TRACE	NON-HEMOLYZED MODERATE	HEMOLYZED TRACE	SMALL +	MODERATE ++	LARGE +++
SPECIFIC GRAVITY 45 seconds	1.000	1.005	1.010	1.015	1.020	1.025	1.030
KETONE 40 seconds	NEGATIVE	mg/dL	TRACE 5	SMALL 15	MODERATE 40	LARGE 80	LARGE 160
BILIRUBIN 30 seconds	NEGATIVE		SMALL +	MODERATE ++	LARGE +++		
GLUCOSE 30 seconds	NEGATIVE	g/dL (%) mg/dL	1/10 (tr.) 100	1/4 250	1/2 500	1 1000	2 or more 2000 or more

Do not use this chart for interpreting test results.

©1999 Bayer Corporation, Diagnostics Division, Tarrytown, NY 10591   Rev. 4/99 0401123

CHARTING EXAMPLE

Multistix® 10 SG Reagent Strips for Urinalysis

PATIENT	Annette Ross						
DATE	3/22/XX				TIME	9:45 a.m.	
LEUKOCYTES	NEGATIVE ☑		TRACE ☐	SMALL + ☐	MODERATE ++ ☐	LARGE +++ ☐	
NITRITE	NEGATIVE ☑		POSITIVE ☐	POSITIVE ☐	(Any degree of uniform pink color is found)		
UROBILINOGEN	NORMAL 0.2 ☑	NORMAL 1 ☐	mg/dL 2 ☐	4 ☐	8 ☐	(1mg = approx. 1 BU)	
PROTEIN	NEGATIVE ☐	TRACE ☑	mg/dL 30 * ☐	100 ++ ☐	300 +++ ☐	2000 OR MORE ☐	
pH	5.0 ☑	6.0 ☐	6.5 ☐	7.0 ☐	7.5 ☐	8.0 ☐	8.5 ☐
BLOOD	NEGATIVE ☑	NON-HEMOLYZED TRACE	NON-HEMOLYZED MODERATE	HEMOLYZED TRACE ☐	SMALL + ☐	MODERATE ++ ☐	LARGE +++ ☐
SPECIFIC GRAVITY	1.000 ☐	1.006 ☐	1.010 ☐	1.015 ☑	1.020 ☐	1.025 ☐	1.030 ☐
KETONE	NEGATIVE ☑	mg/dL	TRACE 5 ☐	SMALL 15 ☐	MODERATE 40 ☐	LARGE 80 ☐	LARGE 160 ☐
BILIRUBIN	NEGATIVE ☑		SMALL + ☐	MODERATE ++ ☐	LARGE +++ ☐		
GLUCOSE	NEGATIVE ☑	g/L (%) mg/dL	1/10 tr.) 100 ☐	1/6 250 ☐	1/2 500 ☐	1 1000 ☐	2 or more 2000 or more ☐

Microscopic Examination of Urine

Urine sediment is the solid material contained in the urine. A microscopic examination of the urine sediment performed by the physician helps clarify results of the physical and chemical examinations. A first-voided morning specimen is generally preferred because it is more concentrated and contains more dissolved substances; small amounts of abnormal substances are more likely to be detected. Use of a fresh specimen is important because changes occur in a specimen left standing out, as was previously discussed. These changes affect the reliability of the test results. The medical assistant is responsible for preparing the urine specimen for microscopic examination by the physician, as pre a microscopic examination of urine are described next.

Red Blood Cells

Red blood cells appear as round, colorless, biconcave discs that are highly refractile (Table 30-1). The presence of 0 to 5 per high-power field (HPF) is considered normal. More than this amount may indicate bleeding somewhere along the urinary tract. Table 30-1 lists the possible causes of an abnormal number of red blood cells in the urine. Concentrated urine causes the red blood cells to become shrunken or *crenated,* whereas dilute urine causes them to swell and become rounded, which may cause them to hemolyze. If the red blood cells have hemolyzed, they cannot be seen under the microscope. The presence of blood in the urine still can be identified, however, with a reagent strip, such as Multistix, which is designed to detect free hemoglobin.

Table 30-1 Structures in Urine Sediment

Structure	Possible Causes	Microscopic Appearance
Red blood cells	Inflammatory diseases Acute glomerulonephritis Pyelonephritis Hypertension Renal infarction Trauma Stones Tumor Bleeding diseases Use of anticoagulants	 Red blood cells
White blood cells	Pyelonephritis Cystitis Urethritis Prostatitis Transplant rejection (manifested by lymphocytes in urine) Tissue injury accompanied by severe inflammation (manifested by monocytes in urine) Inflammation, immune mechanisms, and other host defense mechanisms (manifested by histiocytes in urine)	 White blood cells
Squamous epithelial cells	Vaginal contamination	 Squamous epithelial cells
Renal tubular epithelial cells	Acute tubular necrosis Glomerulonephritis Acute infection Renal toxicity Viral infection	 Renal tubular epithelial cells

Continued

Table 30-1 Structures in Urine Sediment—cont'd

Structure	Possible Causes	Microscopic Appearance
Hyaline casts	Normal urine Strenuous exercise Acute glomerulonephritis Acute pyelonephritis Malignant hypertension Chronic renal disease	 *Hyaline cast
Amorphous urate	Nonpathologic	 *Amorphous urate crystals
Uric acid	Usually nonpathologic; in large numbers, may indicate gout	 *Uric acid crystals
Calcium oxalate	Usually nonpathologic; may be associated with stone formation	 †Calcium oxalate crystals
Bacteria	More than 100,000 bacteria per mL indicates urinary tract infection 10,000-100,000 bacteria per mL indicates that tests should be repeated Less than 10,000 bacteria per mL may signify urine in which any bacteria are due to urethral organisms or contamination Bacteria accompanied by white blood cells or white blood cell or mixed casts may indicate acute pyelonephritis	 *Bacteria (small rod structures)
Yeast	May indicate contamination by yeasts from skin or hair May indicate diabetes mellitus or urinary tract infection *Candida albicans* may occur in patients with diabetes mellitus or in the contaminated urine of female patients with candidal vaginitis	 *Candida albicans* (yeast)

Table 30-1 Structures in Urine Sediment—cont'd

Structure	Possible Causes	Microscopic Appearance
Parasites and parasitic ova	Usually indicate fecal or vaginal contamination and should be reported *Trichomonas* may be found in patients with urethritis and in contaminated urine of women with *Trichomonas* vaginitis Pinworm is a common contaminant and should be reported	 **Trichomonas* (parasite)
Spermatozoa	Nonpathologic	 *Spermatozoa
Urinary artifacts Hair (a) Pollen grains Bubbles Oil droplets Fibers (b) Powder (c) Dust Mucous threads (d) Glass particles	Nonpathologic May result from improper urine collection, improper slide preparation, or outside contamination	 (a) †Hair (b) *Fiber (c) *Powder (d) ‡Mucous threads

Text courtesy Boehringer Mannheim Diagnostics, Indianapolis, Ind.
*Photomicrographs courtesy Bayer Corporation, Diagnostics Division, Elkhart, Ind.
†Photomicrograph from Lehman CA: *Saunders manual of clinical laboratory science,* Philadelphia, 1998, Saunders.
‡Photomicrograph from Stepp CA, Woods M: *Laboratory procedures for medical office personnel,* Philadelphia, 1998, Saunders.

White Blood Cells

White blood cells are round and granular and have a nucleus (see Table 30-1). They are approximately 1.5 times as large as a red blood cell. The presence of 0 to 8 per HPF is considered normal. More than this amount may indicate inflammation of the genitourinary tract. Table 30-1 lists the possible causes of an abnormal number of white blood cells in the urine.

Epithelial Cells

Most structures that make up the urinary system are composed of several layers of epithelial cells. The outer layer is constantly sloughed off and replaced by the cells underneath it. *Squamous epithelial cells* are large, clear, flat cells with an irregular shape. They contain a small nucleus and come from the urethra, bladder, and vagina. Squamous epithelial cells are normally present in small amounts in the urine. *Renal epithelial cells* are round and contain a large nucleus. They come from the deeper layers of the urinary tract, and their presence in the urine is considered abnormal. Table 30-1 lists the types of epithelial cells and possible causes of the presence of abnormal amounts in the urine.

Casts

Casts are cylindrical structures formed in the lumen of the tubules that make up the nephron. Materials in the tubules harden, are flushed out, and appear in the urine in the form of casts. Various types of casts may be present in the urine. Their presence generally indicates a diseased condition.

Casts are named according to what they contain. *Hyaline casts* are pale, colorless cylinders with rounded edges that vary in size (see Table 30-1). *Granular casts* are hyaline casts that contain granules and are described as "coarsely granular" or "finely granular," depending on the size of the granules. *Fatty casts* are hyaline casts that contain fat droplets. *Waxy casts* are light yellow and have serrated edges; their name is derived from the fact that they appear to be made of wax. *Cellular casts* contain organized structures and are named according to what they contain. Examples include red blood cell casts, which are hyaline casts containing red

blood cells; white blood cell casts, which are hyaline casts containing white blood cells; epithelial casts, which are hyaline casts containing epithelial cells; and bacterial casts, which are hyaline casts containing bacteria.

Crystals

A variety of crystals may be found in the urine. The type and number vary with the pH of the urine. Abnormal crystals include leucine, tyrosine, cystine, and cholesterol. Crystals that commonly appear in acid urine include amorphous urates, uric acid, and calcium oxalate (see Table 30-1). Crystals that commonly appear in alkaline urine include amorphous phosphate, triple phosphate, calcium phosphate, and ammonium urate crystals.

Miscellaneous Structures

Mucous threads are normally present in small amounts in the urine. They appear as long, wavy, threadlike structures with pointed ends.

Bacteria should not normally exist in the urinary tract. The presence of more than a few bacteria may indicate either contamination of the specimen during collection or a UTI. Bacteria are small structures that may be rod-shaped or round.

Yeast cells are smooth, refractile bodies with an oval shape. A distinguishing feature of yeast cells is small buds that project from the cells involved with reproduction. Yeast cells in the urine of female patients are usually a vaginal contaminant caused by the yeast *Candida albicans* and produce the vaginal infection known as *candidiasis*. They also may be present in the urine of patients with diabetes mellitus.

Parasites may be present in the urine sediment as a contaminant from fecal or vaginal material. *Trichomonas vaginalis* is a parasite that causes trichomoniasis vaginitis.

Spermatozoa may be present in the urine of a man or woman after intercourse. The spermatozoa have round heads and long, slender, hairlike tails.

Table 30-1 lists the miscellaneous structures that may be present in the urine and the significance when found.

PATIENT TEACHING | Urinary Tract Infections

Answer questions patients may have about UTIs.

What is a UTI?

UTI is a general term for the presence of bacteria in any portion of the urinary tract. UTIs, particularly those involving the bladder (cystitis) and urethra (urethritis), are common and treatable. A UTI is usually treated with an antibiotic. Use of all of the antibiotic for the full number of days prescribed by the physician is important, even if the symptoms disappear. If the medication is stopped too soon, the infection may recur and may be more difficult to treat than the original infection.

What are the symptoms of a UTI?

The symptoms of a simple UTI (cystitis) commonly include the frequent need to urinate, urgency (meaning the immediate need

to urinate), a burning sensation during urination, and sometimes blood in the urine. Symptoms of a more complicated UTI involving the kidneys (pyelonephritis) include the above symptoms as well as lower abdominal discomfort, low back pain, fever, cloudy or foul-smelling urine, and blood in the urine.

Why do women have UTIs more frequently than men?

Women are more prone than men to the type of UTI called *cystitis* because the urethra of a woman is much shorter than that of a man, which makes travel up the urethra and into the bladder easier for bacteria. The most common source of infection is bacteria *(Escherichia coli)*. This organism is normally found in the large intestine but can travel from the anal area to

PATIENT TEACHING | **Urinary Tract Infections—cont'd**

the urinary bladder, often as the result of poor hygienic practices. Cystitis occurs if *E. coli* organisms are able to overcome the body's natural defenses when the bacteria reach the urinary bladder and set up an infection.

What can women do to prevent a UTI?

Women prone to development of UTIs should practice the following prevention measures:

- Practice good hygienic measures by always cleaning the genital area from front to back after a bowel movement.
- Avoid possible irritants, such as bubble baths, perfumed soaps, feminine hygiene sprays, and the use of strong powders and bleaches for washing underclothes.
- Avoid clothing that traps moisture and encourages the growth of microorganisms, such as tight, constricting clothing; nylon panties; and panty hose.

- Avoid activities that can contribute to irritation of the urinary meatus, such as prolonged bicycling, motorcycling, horseback riding, and travel that involves prolonged sitting.
- Urinate as soon as possible when you feel the urge. Holding urine in the bladder gives the bacteria more time to grow, which can cause more infection. The more often you urinate, the more quickly the bacteria are removed from the bladder.
- Seek prompt treatment if you experience any of the symptoms of a UTI.

Encourage the patient with a UTI to drink plenty of water to help flush the bacteria out of the urinary tract.

Emphasize to the patient the importance of taking all of the antibiotic for the duration of time prescribed by the physician.

Emphasize the importance of practicing preventive measures to prevent the occurrence of UTIs.

Provide the patient with educational materials on UTIs. ∎

PROCEDURE 30-3 Prepare a Urine Specimen for Microscopic Examination: Kova Method

Outcome Prepare a urine specimen for microscopic analysis by the physician.

Equipment/Supplies

- Disposable gloves
- Urine specimen (first-voided morning specimen)
- Kova urine centrifuge tube
- Kova cap
- Kova pipet

- Kova slide
- Kova stain
- Test tube rack
- Urine centrifuge
- Mechanical stage microscope

Preparing the Specimen

1. Procedural Step. Sanitize the hands, and assemble the equipment.

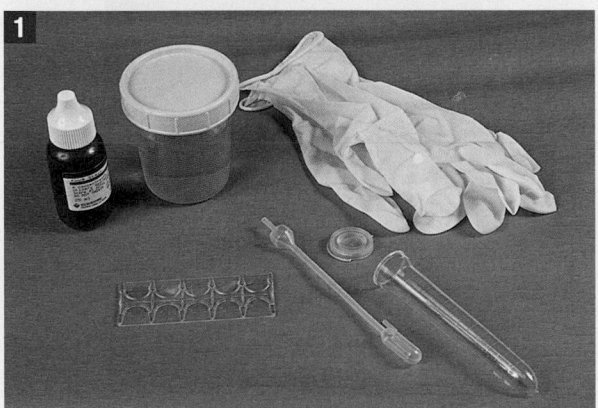

Assemble the equipment.

2. Procedural Step. Apply gloves. Mix the urine specimen with the Kova pipet.

Principle. The specimen must be well mixed to ensure accurate test results.

3. Procedural Step. Pour the urine specimen into the urine centrifuge tube. Fill it to the 12-mL graduation mark, and cap the tube.

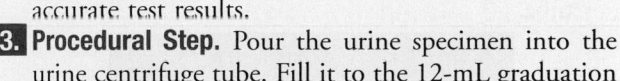
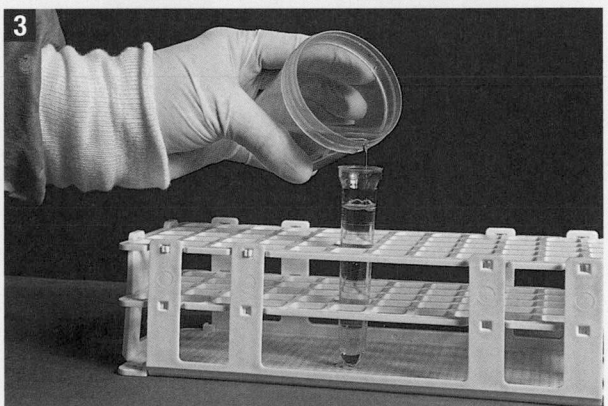

Pour the specimen into the urine tube.

Continued

4. Procedural Step. Centrifuge the tube for 5 minutes at approximately 1500 revolutions per minute (rpm). *Principle.* Centrifuging the specimen causes the solid elements in the urine to settle to the bottom of the tube.

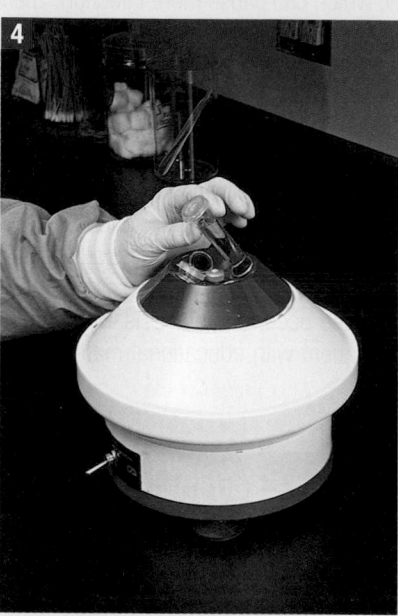

Centrifuge the specimen.

5. Procedural Step. Remove the urine tube from the centrifuge; do not disturb or dislodge the sediment.

6. Procedural Step. Remove the cap. Insert the Kova pipet into the urine tube, and push it to the bottom of the tube until it seats firmly. Ensure that the clip on the bulb is hooked over the outside edge of the tube.

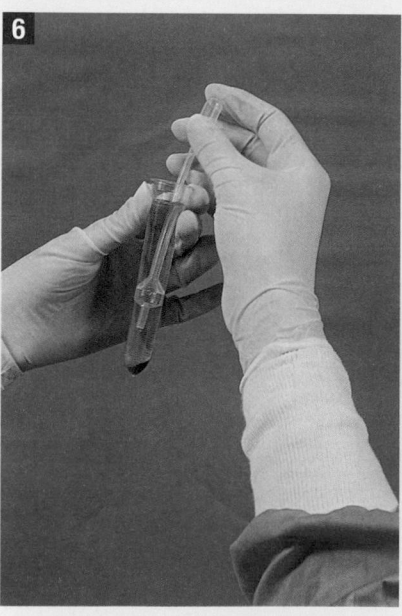

Insert the pipet until it seats firmly.

7. Procedural Step. Decant the specimen by inverting the tube and pouring off the **supernatant** fluid. Approximately 1 mL of sediment is retained in the bottom of the tube.

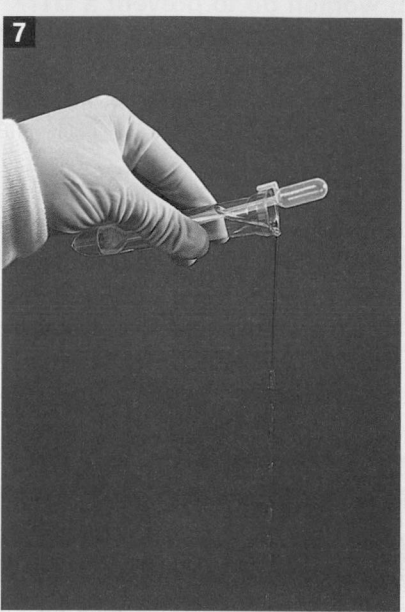

Pour the supernatant fluid.

8. Procedural Step. Remove the pipet from the tube. Add 1 drop of Kova stain to the tube. Place the pipet back in the tube, and mix the sediment and stain together vigorously with the pipet. Ensure that the sediment and the stain are well mixed. Place the urine tube in a test tube rack.

Principle. Kova stain improves the detail of the sediment for better visualization of structures under the microscope.

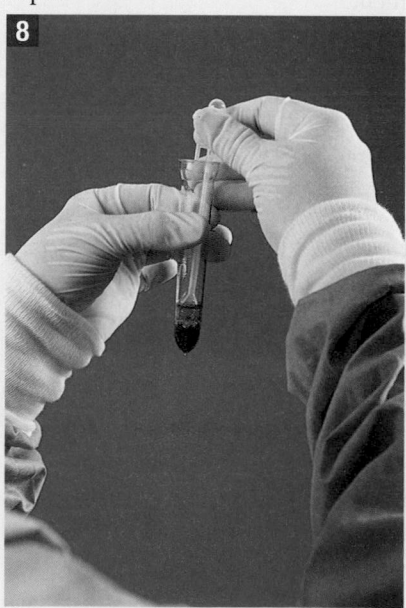

Mix the sediment and stain.

PROCEDURE 30-3   **Prepare a Urine Specimen for Microscopic Examination: Kova Method—cont'd**

9. **Procedural Step.** Transfer a sample of the sediment to the Kova slide as follows:
   a. Place the Kova slide on a flat surface with the open "envelope" areas facing upward.
   b. Squeeze the bulb of the pipet to draw a sample of the sediment into the tip of the pipet.
   c. Place the tip of the pipet so that it just touches the notched corner edge of the slide.
   d. Gently squeeze the bulb to allow the specimen to fill the well. Do not overfill or underfill the well.
   e. Place the pipet in the urine tube.

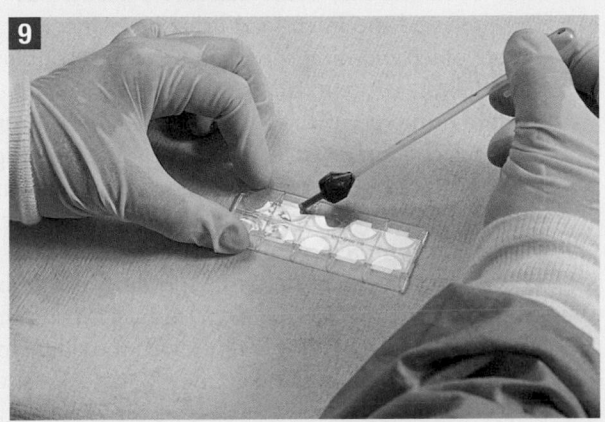

Fill the well with the specimen.

10. **Procedural Step.** Allow the specimen to sit for 1 minute to permit the sediment to settle in the well. *Principle.* Allowing the sediment to settle prevents structures from moving when the slide is viewed under the microscope.

11. **Procedural Step.** Place the slide on the stage of the microscope. Focus the specimen for the physician under the microscope by following the procedure presented in Procedure 34-1: Using the Microscope.

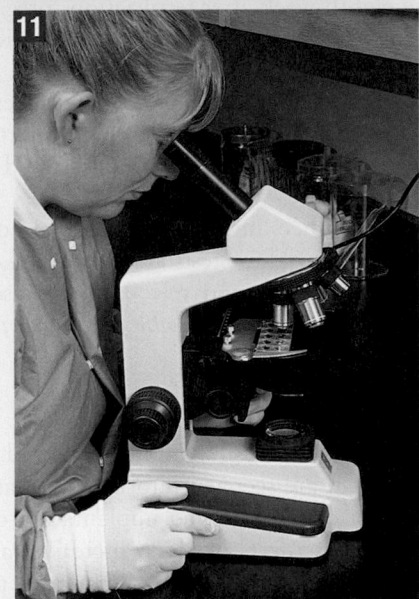

Examine the specimen.

12. **Procedural Step.** When the physician is finished examining the urine sediment, remove the slide from the stage.

13. **Procedural Step.** Dispose of the plastic slide and pipet in a regular waste container. Rinse the remaining urine down the sink. Cap the empty plastic urine tube, and dispose of it in a regular waste container.

14. **Procedural Step.** Remove gloves, and sanitize your hands.

LAB REPORT		
Date	Time	Name
3/18/XX	10:00 a.m.	Tanya Howe
	MICROSCOPIC	
	WBCs	20 /HPF
	RBCs	3 /HPF
	CASTS (Hyaline)	0 /LPF
	CASTS (Granular)	0 /LPF
	CASTS (Cellular)	0 /LPF
	CASTS (Waxy)	0 /LPF
	EPITHELIAL CELLS	0 /LPF
	BACTERIA	Freq
	MUCUS	Occ
	CRYSTALS	0 WBCs
		——— T. Bach, MD

URINE PREGNANCY TESTING

The diagnosis of pregnancy can be accomplished several ways. By the eighth week after fertilization, pregnancy can be confirmed with the medical history and physical examination. The physician may desire an earlier diagnosis, however, with a pregnancy test to initiate early prenatal care. A pregnancy test also may be necessary before certain medications are ordered or procedures are performed that may cause injury to a fetus.

In the medical office, immunologic tests are often used for pregnancy testing. These tests are performed on a concentrated urine specimen and rely on the presence of a hormone known as *human chorionic gonadotropin* (HCG) for a positive reaction.

Human Chorionic Gonadotropin

HCG is produced by the developing fertilized egg, and small amounts of it are secreted into the urine and blood. Immediately after conception and implantation of the fertilized egg, the plasma level of HCG increases rapidly and can be used to detect pregnancy with a serum pregnancy test as early as 6 days before the first missed menstrual period. The highest plasma levels of HCG occur at about 8 weeks after conception. After this time, the production of HCG declines and remains at a lower level for the duration of the pregnancy. Within 72 hours of delivery, HCG disappears entirely from the plasma. As a result, pregnancy tests are more sensitive during the first trimester and may show a negative reaction when the level of HCG begins to decline during the second and third trimesters.

Immunoassay Tests

Immunoassay tests are used in the medical office for the detection of pregnancy. These tests are convenient to perform and provide immediate test results. Positive and negative reactions are evidenced by a specific visible reaction that is observed and interpreted by the individual performing the test.

Immunoassay tests are commercially available in testing kits that contain the required reagents and supplies to perform the test. Each kit can be used to perform a specific number of tests, ranging from 25 to 50. The instructions in the product insert accompanying the testing kit should be followed exactly to prevent inaccurate test results. When performed correctly, most urine pregnancy tests are 99% accurate with low occurrences of false-positive test results.

Immunoassay tests provide for the rapid, qualitative detection of HCG in a urine specimen; brand names include QuickVue One-Step (Quidel, San Diego, Calif), OSOM (Genzyme Diagnostics, Cambridge, Mass), and Clearview (Inverness Medical, Princeton, NJ). Early prediction pregnancy tests may be able to detect pregnancy as early as 2 to 3 days before a first missed menstrual period. Urine pregnancy tests performed this early, however, may show a false-negative result and should be repeated later to confirm the results. Accurate results are much more probable if the urine is tested 1 week after a missed period.

Immunoassay tests take approximately 5 minutes to perform, and the test results are easily observed as a color change. Specific instructions for interpreting the test results are included in the product insert. The procedure for performing an immunoassay test with QuickVue (Quidel) is outlined in Procedure 30-4.

Guidelines for Urine Pregnancy Testing

Specific guidelines must be followed in a urine pregnancy test to ensure accurate test results:

1. Use clean, preferably disposable, urine containers to collect the specimen. Traces of detergent in the specimen container may cause inaccurate test results.
2. The preferred specimen for a urine pregnancy test is a first-voided morning specimen because it contains the highest concentration of HCG; however, a random urine specimen can also be used. If the urine specimen cannot be tested immediately after voiding, it should be preserved in the refrigerator. A patient who collects the specimen at home should be given instructions on preserving the specimen.
3. The specific gravity of the urine specimen should be determined before the test is performed. A specific gravity of less than 1.007 is considered too dilute for pregnancy testing because it may lead to a false-negative test result.
4. The urine specimen should be at room temperature before the procedure is performed.
5. The urine pregnancy testing kit should be stored according to the information in the product insert. Most testing kits are stored at a room temperature between 59° F (15° C) and 86° F (30° C) and away from direct sunlight.
6. Testing kits past their expiration dates should not be used.
7. If more than one patient is being tested at a time, label each testing device with the patient's name to prevent mix-up of specimens.
8. Most urine pregnancy testing kits include a built-in internal control to evaluate whether certain aspects of the testing procedure are working properly. The internal control is performed at the same time that the testing procedure is performed. The urine pregnancy internal control determines whether a sufficient amount of the specimen was added to the testing cassette, and if the correct procedural technique was followed. If the internal control does not perform as expected, the test result is invalid and the specimen must be retested. It is recommended that the internal control be documented in a quality control log for the first pregnancy test run each day.
9. It is recommended that a positive and a negative external control be performed with each new lot of shipment of urine pregnancy testing kits, and then monthly thereafter. External controls are used to

determine if the testing reagents are performing properly and to detect any errors in technique of the individual performing the test. External controls consist of commercially available solutions and may be included with the test system or may need to be purchased separately. The control procedure is performed in a similar manner to the procedure for performing the test on a specimen collected from a patient. Instead of adding the patient specimen to the testing device, however, the control is added to it. The positive control should produce a positive result, and the negative control should produce a negative result. The results should be documented in a quality control log (Figure 30-6). Failure of an external control to produce expected results may be due to the following: deterioration of testing components due to improper storage, improper environmental testing conditions, or errors in technique used to perform the procedure.

10. Conditions other than a normal pregnancy that can result in a positive result include ectopic pregnancy and molar pregnancy.

SERUM PREGNANCY TEST

The radioimmunoassay (RIA) for HCG is a quantitative test used to detect HCG in the serum of the blood. This test can detect pregnancy earlier and with greater accuracy than a urine pregnancy test. A serum pregnancy test can usually detect pregnancy at approximately the eighth day after fertilization, which is 6 days before the first missed menstrual period. This test uses a radioisotope technique and is capable of detecting minute amounts of HCG in the blood. This test is generally used to diagnose abnormalities, such as ectopic pregnancy; to follow the course of early pregnancy when abnormalities of embryonic development are suspected; and to provide an early diagnosis of pregnancy in individuals at high risk, such as patients with diabetes.

QUALITY CONTROL LOG

URINE PREGNANCY TEST

	Date	Name of test	Control lot #	Control expiration date	External positive control	External negative control	Technician
1	3/25 20XX	Quick Vue One Step HCG	140400	3/16/XX	+	−	L. Proffit CMA (AAMA)
2	4/22 20XX	Quick Vue One Step HCG	140400	3/16/XX	+	−	L. Proffit CMA (AAMA)
3	5/27 20XX	Quick Vue One Step HCG	140400	3/16/XX	+	−	L. Proffit CMA (AAMA)
4							
5							
6							
7							
8							
9							
10							

Figure 30-6   Quality control log for urine pregnancy testing.

What Would You Do? What Would You *Not* Do?

Case Study 3
Rita Lavelle is 8½ months pregnant and is at the clinic for a pre-natal appointment. Lately, she has been having difficulty obtaining a urine specimen at the medical office because of her enlarged abdomen. At her last appointment, the office provided her with a urine specimen container so that she could obtain her specimen more easily at home. Rita brings in a first-voided urine specimen in a glass jar. She says her dog chewed up the specimen container from the office, so she used an empty peanut butter jar. The urine

testing results from her specimen show that her glucose level is normal, but her protein level is 4+. Until this time, her urine test results all have been normal. Rita is concerned about her baby. She says that she was cleaning her bathroom cabinet yesterday and came across a pregnancy test; just for the fun of it, she decided to run the test. The results were negative, and now she is worried that something is wrong. Rita says that she has not been sleeping as well at night, and that she has noticed more Braxton-Hicks contractions, but the baby has been kicking and moving as usual. ■

PROCEDURE 30-4   Performing a Urine Pregnancy Test

Outcome Perform a urine pregnancy test.

Equipment/Supplies
- Disposable gloves
- Urine pregnancy testing kit (QuickVue by Quidel)
- Urine specimen (first-voided morning specimen)

1. Procedural Step. Sanitize the hands, and assemble the equipment. Check the expiration date on the urine pregnancy testing kit. It should not be used if the expiration date has passed. When a new testing kit is opened (and thereafter on a monthly basis), external positive and negative controls should be performed according to the instructions in the product insert accompanying the controls. Document the control results in a quality control log. If the controls do not perform as expected, patient testing should not be conducted until the problem is identified and resolved.
Principle. An expired pregnancy test may produce inaccurate test results. Running positive and negative external controls ensures that the test results are valid and reliable. Factors that can cause abnormal control results include outdated controls or testing reagents, improper storage of testing components, and an error in the technique used to perform the procedure.

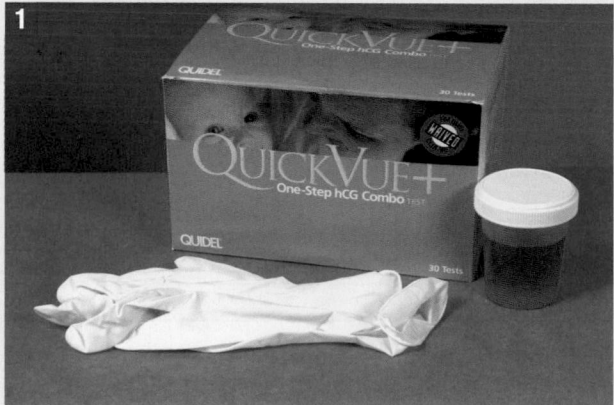
Assemble the equipment.

2. Procedural Step. Apply gloves. Rotate the urine specimen cup to mix the urine. Inspect the foil pouch containing the cassette. If it is torn or punctured, discard the test and obtain another one from the testing kit.

Remove the test cassette from its foil pouch, and place it on a clean, dry, level surface.
Principle. The foil pouch should not be opened until it is time to perform the test.
3. Procedural Step. Add 3 drops of urine to the round sample well on the test cassette with a disposable pipet supplied with the kit. The test cassette should not be handled or moved again until the test is ready for interpretation. Dispose of the pipet in a regular waste container.

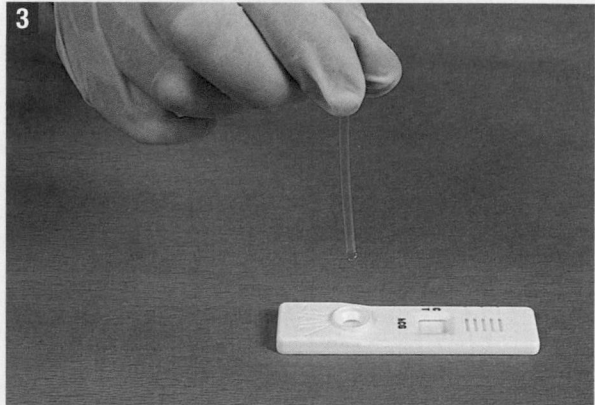
Add 3 drops of urine to the test well.

4. Procedural Step. Wait 3 minutes, and read the results by observing the test result window.
5. Procedural Step. Interpret the test results as follows:
Negative: The appearance of the blue procedural control line next to the letter *C* only and no pink to purple test line next to the letter *T* in the test result window. In addition, the background of the test window should be clear and not interfere with the ability to read the test results. (*NOTE:* If the test result is negative and pregnancy is suspected, another specimen should be collected and tested 48 to 72 hours later.)

PROCEDURE 30-4 Performing a Urine Pregnancy Test—cont'd

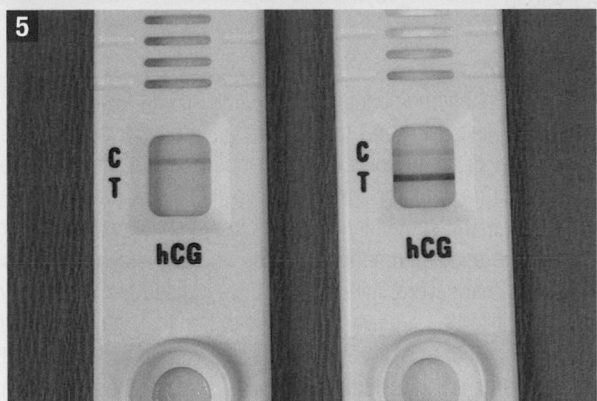

Negative	Positive

Interpret the results.

Positive: The appearance of any pink to purple line next to the letter *T* along with a blue procedural control line next to the letter *C* in the test result window. In addition, the background of the test window should be clear and should not interfere with the ability to read test results.

Invalid result: If no blue procedural control line appears within 3 minutes, or if the background of the test window interferes with reading the results, the test result is invalid, and the specimen must be retested with a new cassette.

Principle. The blue procedural control line is a positive internal quality control indicator designating that a sufficient urine sample was added to the cassette well and that the test is working properly. A background in the test window that is clear and does not interfere with reading the test results is a negative internal quality control indicator and also indicates that the test is working properly.

6. **Procedural Step.** Dispose of the test cassette in a regular waste container. Remove gloves, and sanitize your hands.

7. **Procedural Step.** Chart the results. Include the date and time of the patient's last menstrual period (LMP), the name of the test, and the results recorded as either positive or negative.

CHARTING EXAMPLE

Date	
3/25/XX	10:30 a.m. LMP: 2/20/XX.
	QuickVue preg test: Positive. _____
	_____ L. Proffitt, CMA (AAMA)

MEDICAL PRACTICE and the LAW

In collection and analysis of patient urine, meticulous attention should be paid to patient instructions, such as cleansing and collecting first morning, midstream, or 24-hour specimens. Patients are often embarrassed to have someone else see their urine, so handle urine specimens in a professional, matter-of-fact manner, with universal precautions to protect yourself. As with all diagnostic procedures, care must be taken to perform the test correctly and treat results confidentially.

Civil versus Criminal Law
Civil law involves a conflict with another person, and if found guilty by a preponderance of evidence (greater than 50%), the loser may lose money or property. Malpractice is a type of civil law. Civil law is divided into *torts,* or wrongs, and *contracts,* or promises. Malpractice is a tort, and nonpayment for services is a contract.

Criminal law involves a conflict with society as a whole (local, state, or federal law). If found guilty beyond a reasonable doubt, the loser may lose money, property, freedom (jail), or life (execution). Violation by the physician of licensure laws and failure to report child abuse are criminal suits. ■

What Would You Do? What Would You *Not* Do? RESPONSES

Case Study 1
Page 719

What Did Linda Do?
❐ Took some time to try to calm and relax Mr. Urameshi. Reassured him that the physician would do everything he could to make him better.
❐ Offered Mr. Urameshi something to drink and told him it might help him obtain a specimen.
❐ Went over the directions again with Mr. Urameshi.

❐ Asked Mr. Urameshi if he would try again to obtain a specimen.

What Did Linda Not Do?
❐ Did not tell Mr. Urameshi that he was not trying hard enough.

What Would You Do?/What Would You Not Do?
Review Linda's response and place a checkmark next to the information you included in your response. List additional information you included in your response.

Continued

PROCEDURE 30-4

What Would You Do? What Would You *Not* Do? RESPONSES—cont'd

_____
_____
_____
_____
_____
_____

Case Study 2
Page 724

What Did Linda Do?
- ❏ Asked Nora whether she takes all of the antibiotic she is prescribed when she has a UTI.
- ❏ Explained to Nora in terms she can understand why women seem to be more prone to development of UTIs.
- ❏ Explained to Nora what she could do to help prevent UTIs. Gave her a patient education brochure on UTIs to take home.
- ❏ Told Nora that the physician is not legally or ethically permitted to call in a prescription for her without seeing her. Also explained that it is in the best interests of her health care to be seen by the physician.

What Did Linda Not Do?
- ❏ Did not tell Nora that she could not test her urine at home.

What Would You Do?/What Would You Not Do?
Review Linda's response and place a checkmark next to the information you included in your response. List additional information you included in your response.

_____
_____
_____
_____
_____
_____

Case Study 3
Page 740

What Did Linda Do?
- ❏ Told Rita that some peanut butter residue might have been left in the jar she used and might have affected the test results. Asked her to try to collect another specimen at the office so that the urine could be tested again.
- ❏ Told Rita that if something happens to the specimen container again, she should come to the office and get another one.
- ❏ Told Rita that several things could have caused her pregnancy test result to be negative. Explained to her that the test could have been outdated or not stored properly. Also explained that as a pregnancy gets farther along, less of the hormone that causes the test to be positive is secreted, so negative test results at the end of a pregnancy are not unusual.
- ❏ Reassured Rita that many women have trouble sleeping during the last month of pregnancy and that it is normal to have more Braxton-Hicks contractions as she gets closer to delivery.
- ❏ Told Rita that Linda would inform the physician of her symptoms so that he could discuss them in more detail with her.

What Did Linda Not Do?
- ❏ Did not criticize Rita for collecting her specimen in a peanut butter jar.
- ❏ Did not ignore or minimize Rita's concerns.

What Would You Do?/What Would You Not Do?
Review Linda's response and place a checkmark next to the information you included in your response. List additional information you included in your response.

_____
_____
_____
_____
_____
_____

⟲ TERMINOLOGY REVIEW

Medical Term	Word Parts	Definition
Anuria	*an-:* without, absence of *ur/o-:* urine *-ia:* condition of disease or abnormal state	Failure of the kidneys to produce urine.
Bilirubinuria	*bilirubino/o:* bilirubin *ur/o-:* urine *-ia:* condition of disease or abnormal state	The presence of bilirubin in the urine.
Bladder catheterization		The passing of a sterile catheter through the urethra and into the bladder to remove urine.
Diuresis		Secretion and passage of large amounts of urine.
Dysuria	*dys-:* difficult, labored, painful *ur/o-:* urine *-ia:* condition of disease or abnormal state	Difficult or painful urination.

TERMINOLOGY REVIEW—cont'd

Medical Term	Word Parts	Definition
Frequency		The condition of having to urinate often.
Glycosuria	*glyc/o-:* sugar *ur/o-:* urine *-ia:* condition of disease or abnormal state	The presence of glucose in the urine.
Hematuria	*hemato/o-:* blood *ur/o-:* urine *-ia:* condition of disease or abnormal state	Blood present in the urine.
Ketonuria	*keton/o-:* ketone *ur/o-:* urine *-ia:* condition of disease or abnormal state	The presence of ketone bodies in the urine.
Ketosis	*keton/o-:* ketone *-osis:* abnormal condition	An accumulation of large amounts of ketone bodies in the tissues and body fluids.
Micturition		The act of voiding urine.
Nephron		The functional unit of the kidney.
Nocturia	*noct/i-:* night *ur/o-:* urine *-ia:* condition of disease or abnormal state	Excessive (voluntary) urination during the night.
Nocturnal enuresis		Inability of an individual to control urination at night during sleep (bedwetting).
Oliguria	*olig/o-:* scanty, few *ur/o-:* urine *-ia:* condition of disease or abnormal state	Decreased or scanty output of urine.
pH		The unit that describes the acidity or alkalinity of a solution.
Polyuria	*poly-:* many *ur/o-:* urine *-ia:* condition of disease or abnormal state	Increased output of urine.
Proteinuria	*protein-:* protein *ur/o-:* urine *-ia:* condition of disease or abnormal state	The presence of protein in the urine.
Pyuria	*py/o-:* pus *ur/o-:* urine *-ia:* condition of disease or abnormal state	The presence of pus in the urine.
Renal threshold		The concentration at which a substance in the blood that is not normally excreted by the kidneys begins to appear in the urine.
Retention		The inability to empty the bladder. The urine is being produced normally but is not being voided.
Specific gravity		The weight of a substance compared with the weight of an equal volume of a substance known as the standard. In urinalysis, the *specific gravity* refers to the measurement of the amount of dissolved substances present in the urine compared with the same amount of distilled water.
Supernatant	*super:* over, above	The clear liquid that remains at the top after a precipitate settles.
Suprapubic aspiration	*supra-:* above *pub/o-:* pubis *-ic:* pertaining to	The passing of a sterile needle through the abdominal wall into the bladder to remove urine.
Urgency		The immediate need to urinate.
Urinalysis	*urin/o-:* urine	The physical, chemical, and microscopic analyses of urine.
Urinary incontinence		The inability to retain urine.
Void		To empty the bladder.

ON THE WEB

For information on kidney disease:

National Kidney Foundation: www.kidney.org

National Institute of Diabetes and Digestive and Kidney Diseases: www.niddk.nih.gov

For information on drug abuse:

National Institute on Drug Abuse: www.nida.nih.gov

American Council for Drug Education: www.acde.org

Research Institute on Addictions: www.ria.buffalo.edu

Alcohol and Drug Free Workplace: www.dol.gov/workingpartners

Alcohol and Drug Abuse: www.alcoholanddrugabuse.com

DARE: www.dare.com

Dependency Free: www.dependencyfree.com

 Check out the Evolve site at http://evolve.elsevier.com/Bonewit/today/ to actively Prepare for your Certification, and to access additional interactive activities and exercises to help you study and prepare for success.

31

Phlebotomy

LEARNING OBJECTIVES

Venipuncture

1. List and describe the general guidelines that should be followed when performing a venipuncture.
2. Explain how each of the following blood specimens is obtained:
   Clotted blood
   Serum
   Whole blood
   Plasma
3. List the layers the blood separates into when an anticoagulant is added to the specimen.
4. List the layers the blood separates into when an anticoagulant is not added to the specimen.
5. List the OSHA safety precautions that must be followed during venipuncture and when separating serum or plasma from whole blood.
6. State the additive content of each of the following vacuum tubes, and list the types of blood specimens that can be obtained from each: red, lavender, gray, light blue, green, royal blue.
7. Identify and explain the order of draw for the vacuum tube and butterfly methods of venipuncture.
8. List and describe the guidelines for use of evacuated tubes.
9. Identify possible problems during a venipuncture.
10. List four ways to prevent a blood specimen from becoming hemolyzed.
11. Explain how the serum separator tube functions in the collection of a serum specimen.

Skin Puncture

12. Explain when a skin puncture would be preferred over a venipuncture.
13. Describe each of the following skin puncture devices: disposable semiautomatic lancet and reusable semiautomatic lancet.
14. List and describe the guidelines for performing a finger puncture.

PROCEDURES

Perform a venipuncture using the vacuum tube method.
Perform a venipuncture using the butterfly method.

Obtain a capillary blood specimen using a disposable semiautomatic lancet.
Obtain a capillary blood specimen using a reusable semiautomatic lancet.

CHAPTER OUTLINE

KEY TERMS

antecubital space (an-tih-KYOO-bih-tul
   SPAYS)
anticoagulant (an-tih-koe-AG-yoo-lent)
buffy coat
evacuated tube
hematoma (hee-mah-TOE-mah)

hemoconcentration
   (hee-moe-kon-sen-TRAY-shun)
hemolysis (hee-MOL-ih-sis)
osteochondritis (OS-tee-oh-kon-DRY-tis)
osteomyelitis (OS-tee-oh-mie-LIE-tis)
phlebotomist (fleh-BOT-oe-mist)

phlebotomy (fleh-BOT-oe-mee)
plasma
serum
venipuncture (VEN-ih-punk-chur)
venous reflux (VEEN-us-REE-fluks)
venous stasis (VEEN-us-STAE-sis)

INTRODUCTION TO PHLEBOTOMY

The purpose of phlebotomy is to collect a blood specimen for laboratory analysis. The word *phlebotomy* is derived from the Greek words for "vein" *(phlebos)* and "incision" *(otomy)* and literally means making an incision into a vein. As used in the clinical laboratory sciences, **phlebotomy** is defined generally as the collection of blood. An individual who collects a blood sample is a **phlebotomist.**

Some blood specimens are tested in the medical office, and others are picked up and taken to an outside laboratory for testing. The latter specimens need to be placed in a biohazard specimen bag along with a laboratory request (Figure 31-1), so that laboratory personnel know what type of test the physician desires. The medical assistant may be responsible for completing the laboratory request form either on the computer or manually. The request form includes the physician's name and address; the patient's name, address, age, and gender; the date and time of collection of the specimen; the International Classification of Diseases (ICD) code of the clinical diagnosis;

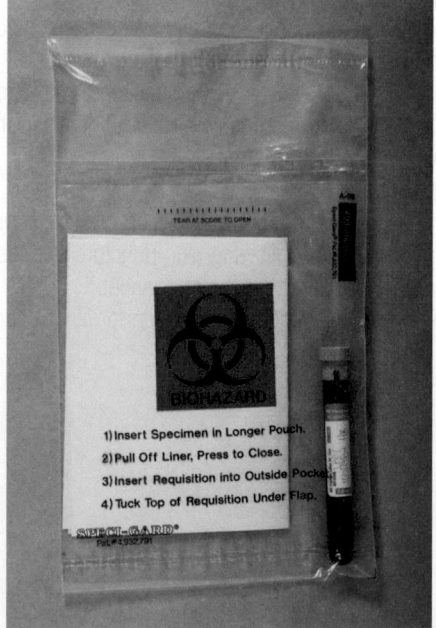

Figure 31-1 Specimen in a biohazard specimen bag along with the laboratory request form.

and a mark next to the type of test or tests to be performed.

Phlebotomy encompasses three major areas of blood collection:

- Arterial puncture
- Venipuncture
- Skin puncture

An arterial puncture is typically performed in a hospital to assess the oxygen level, carbon dioxide level, and acid-base balance of arterial blood; medical assistants do not perform arterial punctures. In the medical office, medical assistants perform venipunctures and skin punctures. This chapter focuses on these two ways to obtain blood.

VENIPUNCTURE

Venipuncture means the puncturing of a vein for the removal of a venous blood sample. In the medical office, a venipuncture is performed when a large blood specimen is needed for testing. Venipuncture can be performed by the following two methods:

- Vacuum tube method
- Butterfly method

The vacuum tube method is the fastest and most convenient of the three methods and is used most often. This method relies on the use of an **evacuated tube,** which is a closed glass or plastic tube that contains a vacuum. The butterfly method is used for difficult draws, such as when a vein is small or sclerosed (hardened). This chapter presents the theory and procedure for both methods.

GENERAL GUIDELINES FOR VENIPUNCTURE

General guidelines that are common to both methods of venipuncture include any advance preparation, reviewing specimen collection and handling requirements, identification of the patient, reassuring the patient, assembling equipment and supplies, positioning the patient, applying the tourniquet, selecting a site for the venipuncture, obtaining the type of blood specimen required, and following the Occupational Safety and Health Administration (OSHA) Bloodborne Pathogens Standard.

Patient Preparation for Venipuncture

The patient should be given instructions an appropriate number of days before the specimen collection on any advance preparation that is required. Although most tests require no preparation, some tests require fasting or the avoidance of certain medications. *Fasting* involves abstaining from food or fluids (except water) for a specified amount of time before the collection of a specimen. If the medical assistant is unsure whether a laboratory test requires advance patient preparation, an appropriate reference source should be consulted. If the specimen is being tested at an outside

laboratory, references consist of a laboratory directory and the laboratory's technical support staff. If the specimen is being tested at the medical office, references include the manufacturer's operating manual and/or product inserts included with blood analyzers and testing kits.

When a laboratory test requires advance preparation, before performing the venipuncture, verify that the patient has prepared properly. If the patient has not properly prepared, do not collect the specimen unless directed otherwise by the physician. If the venipuncture is to be rescheduled, carefully review the preparation requirements with the patient.

Review Collection and Handling Requirements

The medical assistant must review the requirements for collecting and handling the blood specimen. These include the collection supplies necessary, the type of specimen to be collected (e.g., **serum, plasma,** whole blood, clotted blood), the amount necessary for laboratory analysis, the techniques to follow to collect the specimen, and the proper handling and storage of the specimen. The medical assistant must refer to the appropriate reference source to determine the collection and handling requirements for each test ordered by the physician. If the specimen is transported to an outside laboratory, this information is indicated in the laboratory directory. Figure 31-2 shows an example of the collection and handling requirements for a complete blood count (CBC) as it is presented in a laboratory directory. The collection and handling requirements necessary for specimens tested in the medical office are listed in the manufacturer's instructions that accompany the test system.

Identification of the Patient

It cannot be emphasized enough how important it is to identify the patient using two forms of identification (e.g., name and date of birth) before performing a venipuncture. Proper patient identification is essential to avoid collecting a specimen on the wrong patient by mistake. After greeting the patient, the medical assistant should ask the patient to state his or her full name and date of birth. This information should be compared with the demographic data indicated in the patient's chart. The patient should *not* be asked whether he or she is a certain patient. For example, the patient should not be asked: "Are you Brad Thompson?" The patient may not hear the medical assistant correctly or may not be paying attention and may answer in the affirmative even if he is not that patient. If the patient is not properly identified, this, in turn, could lead to incorrect labeling of the specimen. A specimen that is not identified correctly could lead to an inaccurate patient diagnosis and the wrong treatment.

Assemble the Equipment and Supplies

Use only the appropriate blood tubes as specified by the laboratory directory or manufacturer's instructions accompanying a test system. Substituting blood tubes may not

CBC (with differential and platelet count)

CPT Code: 85025

Tests included: WBC, RBC, hemoglobin, hematocrit, platelet count, differential, and red blood cell indices (MCV, MCH, MCHC, and RDW). If abnormal cells are observed on a manual differential or if the automated differential results meet specific flagging criteria, a full manual differential will be performed.

Type of specimen: Whole blood

Amount: 7 ml

Collection supplies: 7-ml lavender (EDTA) stoppered tube

Collection techniques: Red-stoppered and SST tubes should be collected before the lavender-stoppered tube. Completely fill tube to the exhaustion of the vacuum to ensure a proper blood to anticoagulant ratio. Gently invert tube 8-10 times immediately after drawing to mix the anticoagulant with the blood.

Patient preparation: None

Handling and storage: Store at room temperature for up to 24 hours following collection. Store in refrigerator for up to 48 hours following collection.

Causes for rejection: Hemolyzed or clotted specimen, under-filled tube, improper labeling of tube. Specimen collected in any tube other than an EDTA (lavender-stoppered) tube or a specimen that is more than 48 hours old.

Reference range: Values given with report

Use:
The CBC is used as a screening test to assess the overall health of an individual and to detect a wide range of hematologic conditions such as anemia, leukemia, and inflammatory processes. The CBC is also used to assist in managing medication and chemotherapeutic decisions.

Limitations:
- A manual differential can identify cells that may be misidentified by an automated analyzer
- Red blood cell indices are not a substitute for the direct examination of a blood smear

Methodology: Automated cell counter and microscopy

Figure 31-2 Collection and handling requirements for a complete blood count (CBC) from a laboratory directory.

yield the proper type of specimen required or may affect the test results, as shown by the following examples. If serum is required and a tube containing an anticoagulant is used (instead of a tube without an anticoagulant), the blood separates into plasma and cells, rather than serum and cells, and the wrong type of blood specimen is obtained, which necessitates obtaining another specimen from the patient.

The medical assistant should check each blood tube before use to ensure that it is not broken, chipped, cracked, or otherwise damaged. Damaged blood tubes are unsuitable for specimen collection and should be discarded. Blood tubes have an expiration date (Figure 31-3). The medical assistant should make sure to check the expiration date on the tube to avoid using an outdated blood tube.

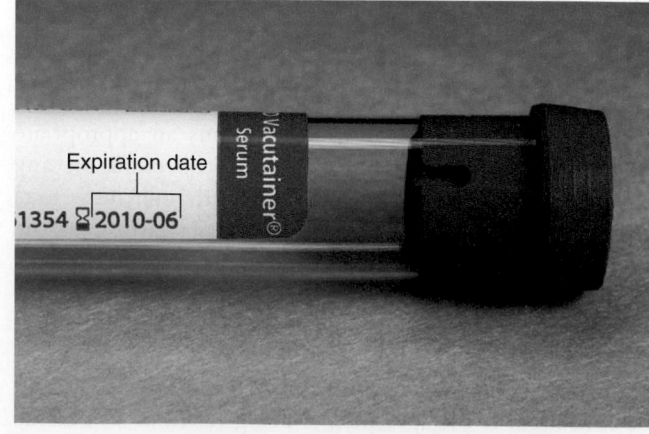

Figure 31-3 Blood tube showing expiration date.

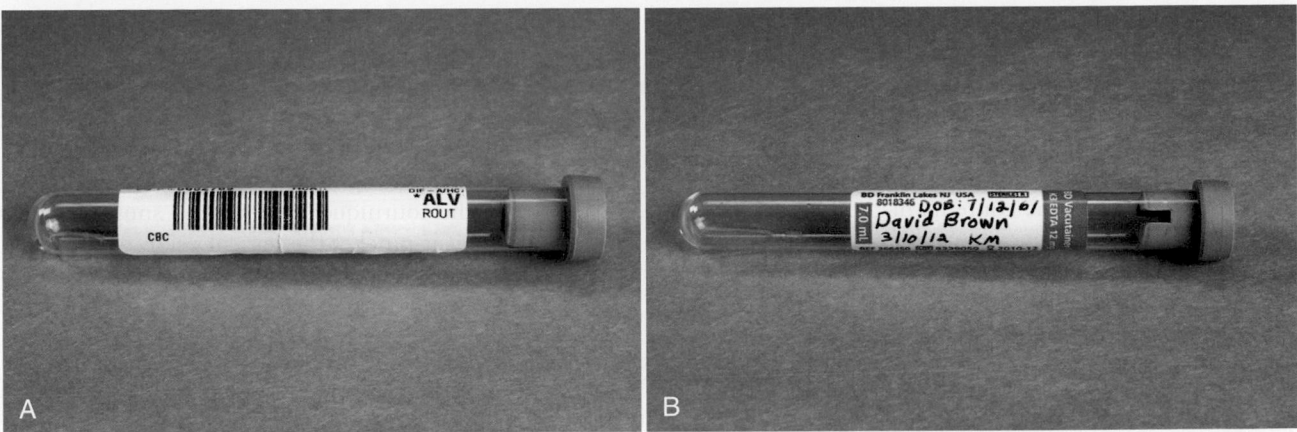

Figure 31-4 **A,** Computerized bar code label. **B,** Hand-labeled blood tube.

The medical assistant must be sure to label each blood tube. An unlabeled specimen is a cause for rejection of the specimen by an outside laboratory. Two *unique identifiers* should be used to label the specimen. A unique identifier is information that clearly identifies a specific patient, such as the patient's name and date of birth. A specimen can be labeled by attaching a computerized bar code label to the specimen (Figure 31-4, *A*). The bar code label includes (at least) two unique patient identifiers. A specimen can also be labeled by handwriting the information on the label, which should include the patient's name and date of birth (two unique identifiers), the date and time of collection, the medical assistant's initials, and any other information required by the laboratory (Figure 31-4, *B*). The information should be printed legibly, and the medical assistant should be certain that the information is accurate to avoid a mix-up of specimens. The medical assistant must also complete a laboratory request form to accompany the blood specimen. (*NOTE:* The medical assistant should follow the medical office policy as to when the tubes should be labeled. Some offices prefer the tubes be labeled *before* the specimen is drawn; other offices want the tubes to be labeled right *after* the specimen is obtained.)

Reassuring the Patient

Venipuncture is often a frightening experience for the patient. For many patients, the anticipation of the procedure is worse than the actual drawing of the blood. The medical assistant should take time to explain the procedure to the patient in an unhurried and confident manner. This helps to alleviate the patient's fears, which relaxes the patient's veins. Relaxed veins make venipuncture easier to perform and result in less pain for the patient.

Instruct the patient to remain still during the procedure. Explain to the patient that a small amount of pain is associated with a venipuncture, but it is brief. Never tell the patient that the venipuncture will not hurt. Just before inserting the needle, tell the patient that he or she will "feel a small stick." This prevents startling the patient, which could cause the patient to move. Movement causes pain for the patient, and it may damage the venipuncture site.

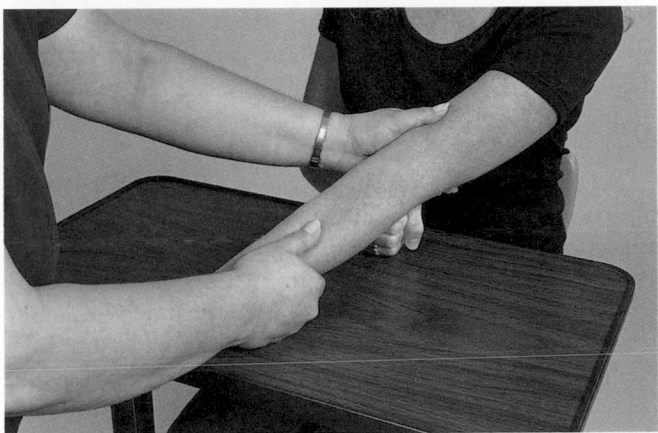

Figure 31-5 Patient position for obtaining a blood specimen from the antecubital veins.

Patient Position for Venipuncture

The patient position for venipuncture is especially important to the successful collection of a blood specimen. Proper positioning allows easy access to the vein and is more comfortable for the patient. The patient position depends on the vein to be used. The most common site for venipuncture is the **antecubital space,** and the information presented next refers to this site.

The patient should be seated comfortably in a chair. The arm should be extended downward to form a straight line from the shoulder to the wrist with the palm facing up; the arm should not bend at the elbow. The arm should be well supported on the armrest by a rolled towel or by having the patient place the fist of the other hand under the elbow (Figure 31-5).

A venipuncture should never be performed with the patient sitting on a stool or standing. The patient may faint and injure himself or herself. If the patient appears nervous or has fainted in the past from a venipuncture, it is best to place the patient in a semireclining position (semi-Fowler position) on the examining table. A pillow or a cushion should be placed under the patient's arm to support the arm in a straight line from the shoulder to the wrist.

Although unusual, it is possible for blood to flow from the evacuated tube back into the patient's vein during the procedure. This condition is known as **venous reflux.** Venous reflux could cause the patient to have an adverse reaction to a tube additive, particularly if the additive in the tube is ethylenediaminetetraacetic acid (EDTA). Venous reflux can occur only if the contents of the evacuated tube are in contact with the tube stopper while the specimen is being drawn. Venous reflux is prevented by keeping the patient's arm in a downward position so that the evacuated tube remains below the venipuncture site and fills from the bottom up.

Application of the Tourniquet

An important step in the venipuncture procedure is the application of the tourniquet. The tourniquet makes the patient's veins stand out so that they are easier to palpate. The tourniquet acts as a "dam," which causes the venous blood to slow down and pool in the veins in front of the tourniquet. This pooling of blood makes the veins more prominent so that they are more visible and can be palpated.

When applying a tourniquet, it is important to obtain the correct tourniquet tension. The tourniquet should be applied with enough tension to slow the venous flow without affecting the arterial flow. A tourniquet that is too tight obstructs both venous blood flow and arterial flow, which may result in a specimen that produces inaccurate test results. A tourniquet that is too loose fails to cause the veins to stand out enough to be palpated. A correctly applied tourniquet should fit snugly and not pinch the patient's skin.

Guidelines for Applying the Tourniquet

The following guidelines help to ensure successful application of the tourniquet:

1. Do not apply the tourniquet over sores or burned skin.
2. Place the tourniquet 3 to 4 inches above the bend in the elbow. This allows adequate room for cleansing the site and performing the venipuncture without the tourniquet getting in the way.
3. Apply the tourniquet so that it is snug, but not so tight that it pinches the patient's skin or is otherwise painful to the patient.
4. When applying the tourniquet, ask the patient to clench his or her fist. This pushes blood from the lower arm into the veins and makes them easier to palpate. You can ask the patient to clench and unclench the fist a few times; however, vigorous pumping should be avoided because it could lead to hemoconcentration, which could produce inaccurate test results.
5. Never leave the tourniquet on for longer than 1 minute because this would be uncomfortable for the patient. In addition, prolonged application of the tourniquet causes the venous blood to stagnate, or pool in one place too long—a condition known as **venous stasis.** When venous stasis occurs, the plasma portion of the blood filters into the tissues, causing hemoconcentration. **Hemoconcentration** is an increase in the concentration of nonfilterable blood components in the blood vessels, such as red blood cells, enzymes, iron, and calcium, as a result of a decrease in the fluid content of the blood. This can result in inaccurate results for a variety of laboratory tests.
6. Ideally, you should remove the tourniquet as soon as a good blood flow is established; however, this may not be practical when you are first learning the venipuncture procedure. Removing the tourniquet may cause the needle to move such that no more blood

Putting it All into Practice

My name is Dori Glover, and I work in a very busy, fast-paced family practice office for two physicians. I love my job. The physicians are great, with very different styles; the pace is fast; and the time flies by. I am constantly challenged, learning new things, meeting and helping people, and being a part of a team that works well together.

While performing a venipuncture for a routine blood chemistry profile (a procedure I have performed many times), I accidentally stuck myself. I could see the blood inside my glove, and I could see the patient's blood clinging to the point of the needle—my heart sank. I placed the needle and holder in the sharps container and tried to keep my cool and not alarm the patient. I mentally assessed the patient. He was an older man from a rural community, but I know you cannot always judge a book by its cover.

I excused myself and immediately proceeded to wash my hands thoroughly with soap and water and rinse, rinse, rinse! I then notified the physician. The physician questioned the patient regarding operations he had had in the previous year. He had undergone bypass surgery and had received 2 units of blood. Although blood is effectively screened, I thought about that one-in-a-zillion chance that it could have been contaminated. Thankfully, I had received the hepatitis B immunization series, but there was still concern regarding hepatitis C and, of course, HIV.

The patient was gracious and complied with our request to be tested for hepatitis and HIV. The physician and I discussed the situation, and we determined the risk to be low, but he nonetheless offered me the option of getting the HIV postexposure prophylactic treatment. This treatment is very toxic and is not something you want to receive needlessly. I declined and proceeded to wait in agony for the patient's test results. The word *relief* hardly describes how I felt when the patient's laboratory results came back negative!

This incident confirmed the importance of getting the hepatitis B immunization and paying attention to good technique when performing procedures involving blood. ■

can be obtained, and the blood has to be redrawn. When you are learning the venipuncture procedure, it is better to wait until just before the needle is removed to remove the tourniquet.

7. *Always* remove the tourniquet before removing the needle from the patient's arm. If the needle is removed first, the pressure of the tourniquet causes blood to be forced out of the puncture site and into the surrounding tissue, resulting in a hematoma. A **hematoma** is defined as a swelling or mass of coagulated blood caused by a break in a blood vessel.

8. After use, wipe a tourniquet thoroughly with a disinfectant such as alcohol. Disposable tourniquets are available that are thrown away after one use.

Types of Tourniquets
The most common tourniquets are the *rubber* tourniquet and the *Velcro-closure* tourniquet. The type of tourniquet used is a matter of individual preference.

Rubber Tourniquet
The rubber tourniquet consists of a flat, soft band of rubber approximately 1 inch (2.5 cm) wide and 15 to 18 inches (38 to 45 cm) long. Rubber tourniquets are commercially available in latex or nonlatex rubber. They offer the advantage of being easily removable with one hand. The technique for applying a rubber tourniquet is described next and is illustrated in Figure 31-6.

Procedure: Rubber Tourniquet
1. Hold each end of the tourniquet with one hand. Position the tourniquet 3 to 4 inches (7.5 to 10 cm) above the bend in the elbow, making sure that the tourniquet lies flat against the patient's skin. Pull the ends away from each other to create tension (see Figure 31-6, *A*).
2. Bring the ends of the tourniquet toward each other and cross one over the other at the point of your grasp, with enough tension so that the tourniquet is snug but is not pinching the patient's skin (see Figure 31-6, *B*).
3. Tuck a portion of the top length into the bottom length, forming a loop between the tourniquet and the patient's arm. This allows for a one-handed release of the tourniquet when pulled on one end. Make sure the flaps are directed upward so that they do not dangle into the working area (see Figure 31-6, *C*).

Velcro-Closure Tourniquet
The Velcro-closure tourniquet consists of a band of rubber or elastic material with Velcro attached at the ends. This type of tourniquet is easier to apply and is more comfortable for the patient than the rubber tourniquet. The disadvantage of the Velcro-closure tourniquet is that it is more difficult to remove with one hand than the rubber tourniquet. In addition, this type of tourniquet may not fit around the arms of extremely obese patients. The technique for applying a Velcro-closure tourniquet is described next and is illustrated in Figure 31-7.

Procedure: Velcro-Closure Tourniquet
1. Hold each end of the tourniquet with one hand. Position the tourniquet 3 to 4 inches (7.5 to 10 cm) above the bend in the elbow.
2. Wrap the tourniquet around the arm, and secure it with the Velcro fastener. The tourniquet should be applied with enough tension so that it is snug but is not pinching the patient's skin.

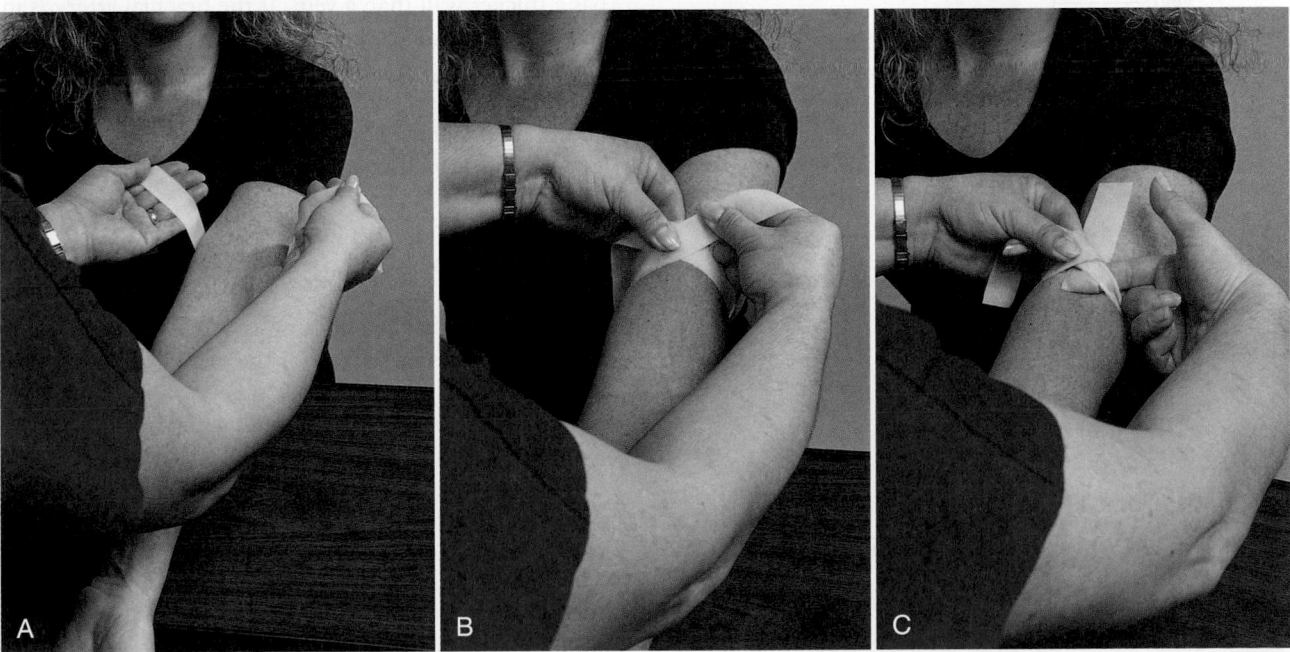

Figure 31-6 Application of a rubber tourniquet. **A,** Create tension by pulling the ends of the tourniquet away from each other. **B,** With tension, cross one flap over the other at the point of your grasp. **C,** Form a loop by tucking a portion of the top length into the bottom length.

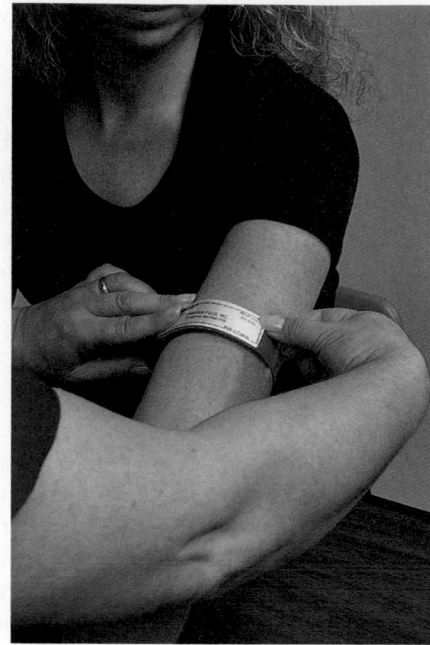

Figure 31-7 Application of a Velcro-closure tourniquet.

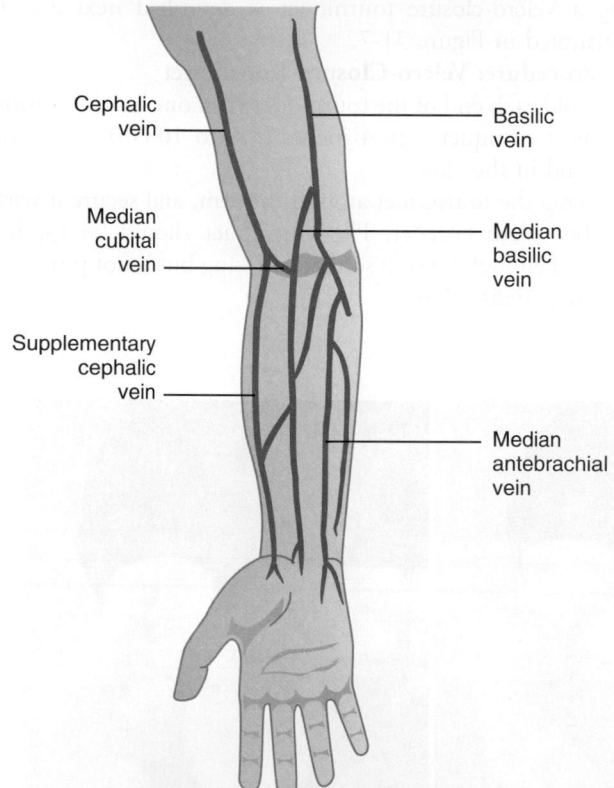

Cephalic vein

Basilic vein

Median cubital vein

Median basilic vein

Supplementary cephalic vein

Median antebrachial vein

Figure 31-8 Antecubital veins.

Site Selection for Venipuncture

For most patients, the best site to use is the veins in the antecubital space (Figure 31-8). If the patient has large, visible antecubital veins, drawing blood is easy. If the patient has small veins or veins that cannot be palpated, obtaining a blood specimen can be quite a challenge, even for the most experienced medical assistant.

The antecubital space is the surface of the arm in front of the elbow. The antecubital veins generally have a wide lumen and are close to the surface of the skin, which makes them easily accessible. In addition, these veins typically have thick walls, making them less likely to collapse. Using the antecubital space spares the patient unnecessary pain because the skin is less sensitive there than at other sites, such as the back of the hand. The medical assistant should not be misled by the presence in some patients of many small, very blue "spidery" veins that lie close to the surface of the skin. These veins are not suitable for performing a venipuncture. The antecubital veins lie beneath these veins.

The best vein to use in the antecubital space is the *median cubital*. The median cubital is a prominent vein in the middle of the antecubital space and does not roll (see Figure 31-8). At times, however, the median cubital vein cannot be used, for example, when it lies deep in the tissues and cannot be palpated or is scarred from repeated venipunctures.

The *cephalic* and *basilic* veins are located on opposite sides of the antecubital space and provide an alternative site when the median cubital vein is unavailable. The cephalic vein is located on the thumb side of the antecubital space, and the basilic vein is located on the little finger side of the antecubital space. The disadvantage of these "side" veins is that they tend to roll or move away from the needle, escaping puncture. To prevent rolling, firm pressure should be applied below and to the side of the vein to stabilize it as the needle is inserted.

The brachial artery also is located in the antecubital space, but it lies deeper in the tissues. This is the artery that is used to measure blood pressure. Before performing a venipuncture, palpate for the presence of this artery. In contrast to a vein, an artery pulsates, is more elastic, and has a thicker wall than a vein. If the brachial artery is inadvertently punctured, the patient feels more than the usual amount of pain, and the blood is bright red and comes out in pulsing movements. If this situation occurs, the tourniquet should be removed and then the needle. Pressure with a gauze pad should be applied for 4 to 5 minutes.

Guidelines for Site Selection

Specific guidelines should be followed to facilitate the selection of a good vein:
1. Ensure that the lighting is adequate. Good lighting facilitates inspection of the veins.
2. Ensure that the veins "stand out" as much as possible. Before locating a venipuncture site, always apply the tourniquet, and have the patient make a fist. This combination makes the veins more prominent.
3. Examine the antecubital veins of both arms. The best site to perform a venipuncture varies with each individual. The patient may have larger veins in one arm than in the other. It is advisable to ask the patient whether he or she has had a venipuncture before. Most adults have had previous venipunctures and know which of their veins are best to use and

which should be avoided. Listen to and evaluate information offered by the patient.

4. Use inspection and particularly palpation to select a vein. A vein does not have to be seen to be a good selection. If you cannot see a vein, palpation alone can be used to locate it. A vein feels like an elastic tube that "gives" under the pressure of the fingertips.

5. Always palpate for the median cubital vein (middle vein) first. It usually is bigger, is anchored better, bruises less, and poses the smallest risk of injuring underlying structures (e.g., nerves and arteries) than the other veins. Because of this, if the patient's median cubital vein cannot be seen but still can be palpated, it should be used as the first choice when selecting a vein. If the median cubital vein is good in both arms, select the one that appears the fullest. The cephalic vein located on the thumb side is the next best vein choice because it does not roll and bruise as easily as the basilic vein. The basilic vein, located on the little finger side of the antecubital space, is the least desirable venipuncture site in the antecubital space. Branches of the median nerve may lie close to this vein in some individuals. In addition, the basilic vein lies in close proximity to the brachial artery. Both of these conditions pose a risk of injury to underlying structures when blood is drawn from the basilic vein.

6. Thoroughly assess the patient's veins. To assess a vein as a possible site for venipuncture, place one or two fingertips (index and middle fingers) over it and press lightly, then release pressure. Do not use your thumb to palpate the vein because it is not as sensitive as the index finger. To be suitable for a venipuncture, the vein should feel round, firm, elastic, and engorged. When you depress and release an engorged vein, it should spring back in a rounded, filled state.

7. Determine the size, depth, and direction of the vein. When a suitable vein has been located, it should be palpated thoroughly and carefully to determine the direction of the vein and to estimate the size and depth of the vein. Palpate and trace the path of the vein several times by rolling your index finger back and forth over the vein to determine its size. Inspect and palpate the vein for problems. Some veins that appear suitable at first sight feel small, hard, bumpy, or flat when palpated.

8. Map the location of the site. After locating an acceptable vein, mentally "map" the location of the puncture site on the patient's arm with "skin marks." This technique is particularly helpful if the vein cannot be seen, but only palpated. The puncture site may be located on or next to a skin mark, such as a freckle, a small wrinkle, or a pigmented area.

9. Do not leave the tourniquet on for longer than 1 minute. When first learning the venipuncture procedure, you may need to perform numerous assessments of the patient's arms to locate the best vein. After each assessment, remove the tourniquet for approximately 2 minutes to allow normal circulation of the blood to occur. This prevents patient discomfort and hemoconcentration, which can lead to inaccurate results for a variety of laboratory tests.

10. If a good vein cannot be found, the following techniques can be employed to make the veins more prominent:
    o Remove the tourniquet, and have the patient dangle the arm over the side of the chair for 1 to 2 minutes.
    o Tap the vein site sharply a few times with your index finger and second finger.
    o Gently massage the arm from the wrist to the elbow.
    o Apply a warm, moist washcloth to the area for 5 minutes.

Alternative Venipuncture Sites

If it is impossible to locate a suitable vein in the antecubital space, alternative sites are available, including the inner forearm, the wrist area above the thumb, and the back of the hand (Figure 31-9). These alternative veins are smaller and have thinner walls than the antecubital veins and should be used for venipuncture only when all possibilities for obtaining the blood specimen at the antecubital site have been considered. If the medical assistant is able to palpate a small vein in the antecubital space, it may be possible to obtain blood there using the butterfly method of venipuncture.

The hand veins, in particular, should be used only as a last resort. The veins of the hand have a tendency to roll because they are not supported by much tissue and are close to the surface of the skin. This makes them more difficult to stick. In addition, an abundant supply of nerves is present in the hands, which makes this procedure more uncomfortable for the patient. Hand veins tend to have thin walls, which makes them more susceptible to collapsing, bruising, and phlebitis. In some patients, however, especially the obese and the elderly, the hand veins may be the only accessible site.

Types of Blood Specimens

The type of blood specimen required depends on the type of test to be performed. Serum is required for most blood chemistry studies, whereas whole blood is required for a complete blood count. The various types of blood specimens that the medical assistant would be required to obtain through the venipuncture procedure are as follows:

1. *Clotted blood.* Clotted blood is obtained from a tube that does not contain an anticoagulant. A tube without an anticoagulant causes the blood cells to clot.
2. *Serum.* Serum is obtained from clotted blood by allowing the specimen to stand and then centrifuging it. Centrifuging a blood specimen that does not contain an anticoagulant causes the blood to separate into the following layers (Figure 31-10, *A*):

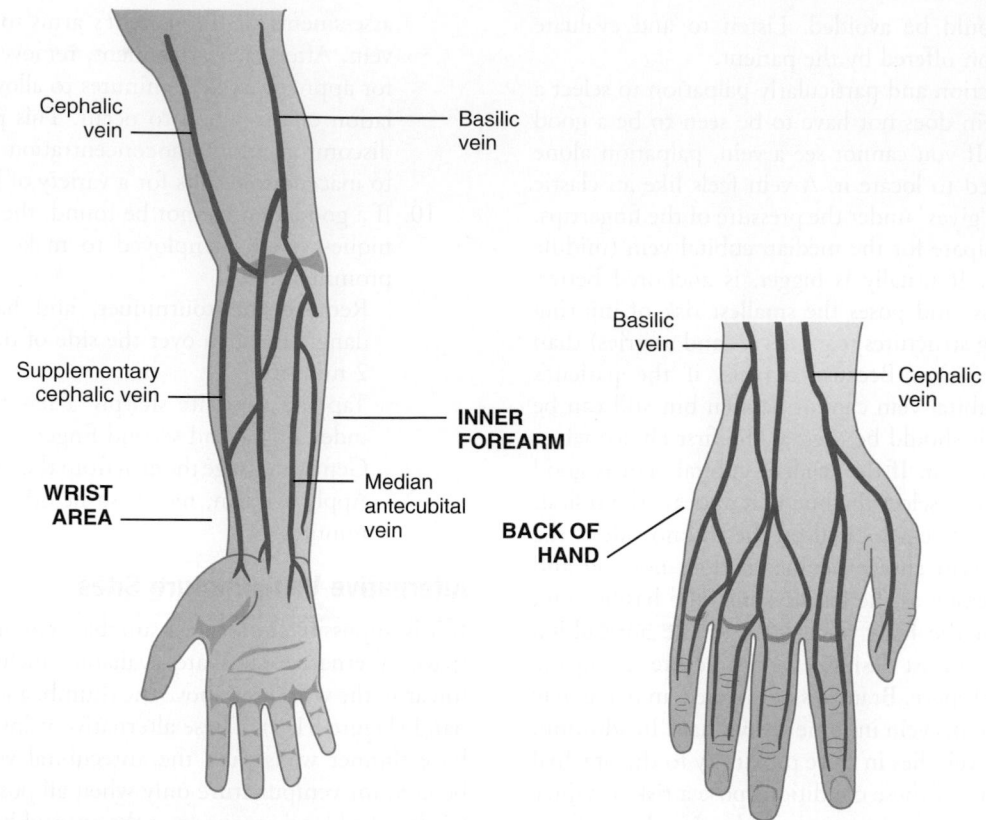

Figure 31-9 Alternative venipuncture sites: the inner forearm, the wrist area above the thumb, and the back of the hand.

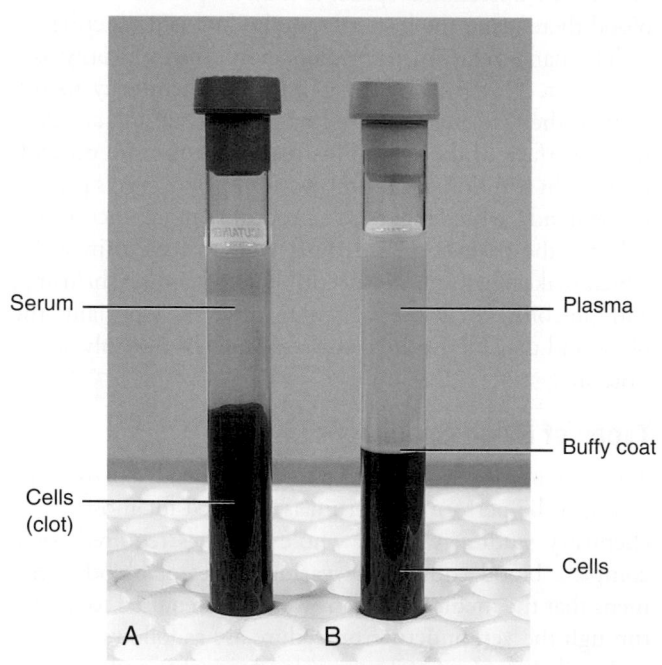

Figure 31-10 Layers into which the blood separates when there is no anticoagulant (**A**) and when an anticoagulant is present (**B**).

- Top layer—serum
- Bottom layer—clotted blood cells

3. *Whole blood.* Whole blood is obtained by using a tube that contains an **anticoagulant.** An anticoagulant is a substance that inhibits blood clotting. It is important to mix the anticoagulant with the blood by gently inverting the tube back and forth 8 to 10 times after collection.

4. *Plasma.* Plasma is obtained from whole blood that has been centrifuged. Centrifuging a blood specimen that contains an anticoagulant causes the blood to separate into the following layers (Figure 31-10, *B*):
   - Top layer—plasma
   - Middle layer—**buffy coat** (contains white blood cells and platelets)
   - Bottom layer—red blood cells

OSHA Safety Precautions

The OSHA Bloodborne Pathogens Standard presented in Chapter 17 must be carefully followed during the venipuncture procedure to avoid exposure to bloodborne pathogens. The following OSHA requirements apply specifically to the venipuncture procedure and to separation of serum from whole blood (see later):

1. Wear gloves when it is reasonably anticipated that you will have hand contact with blood.
2. Avoid hand-to-mouth contact, such as eating, drinking, or applying makeup, while working with blood specimens.
3. Wear a face shield or mask in combination with an eye protection device whenever splashes, spray, splatter, or droplets of blood may be generated.
4. Perform all procedures involving blood in a manner so as to minimize splashing, spraying, splattering, and generating droplets of blood.

5. Bandage cuts and other lesions on the hands before gloving.

6. Sanitize hands as soon as possible after removing gloves.

7. If your hands or other skin surfaces come in contact with blood, wash the area as soon as possible with soap and water.

8. If your mucous membranes (e.g., eyes, nose, mouth) come in contact with blood, flush them with water as soon as possible.

9. Do not bend, break, or shear contaminated venipuncture needles.

10. Do not recap a contaminated venipuncture needle.

11. Locate the sharps container as close as possible to the area of use. Immediately after use, place the contaminated venipuncture needle (and plastic holder) in the biohazard sharps container.

12. Place blood specimens in containers that prevent leakage during collection, handling, processing, storage, transport, and shipping.

13. Handle all laboratory equipment and supplies properly and with care as indicated by the manufacturer. For example, wait until the centrifuge comes to a complete stop before opening it.

14. Do not store food in refrigerators where testing supplies or specimens are stored.

15. If you are exposed to blood, report the incident immediately to your physician-employer.

VACUUM TUBE METHOD OF VENIPUNCTURE

The vacuum tube method is frequently used to collect venous blood specimens. This method is considered ideal for collecting blood from normal healthy antecubital veins that are adequate in size to withstand the pressure of the vacuum in the evacuated tube. Procedure 31-1 outlines the venipuncture vacuum tube method. The vacuum tube system consists of a collection needle, a plastic holder, and an evacuated tube (Figure 31-11). One commercially available vacuum tube system is the Vacutainer System (Becton Dickinson, Franklin Lakes, NJ).

Needle

The needle used with the vacuum tube method consists of a double-pointed stainless steel needle with a threaded hub near its center (Figure 31-12). The needle is coated with silicon, enabling it to penetrate the skin smoothly. The threaded hub of the needle screws into the plastic holder. Vacuum tube needles are packaged in sealed twist-apart plastic containers. The needle gauge and length are printed on the paper seal on the container (see Figure 31-12). A needle should not be used if the seal has been broken.

The double-pointed needle consists of an anterior needle and a posterior needle. The *anterior needle* is longer and has a beveled point designed to facilitate entry into the skin and the vein. The *posterior needle* is shorter, and its purpose is to pierce the rubber stopper of the evacuated tube. The

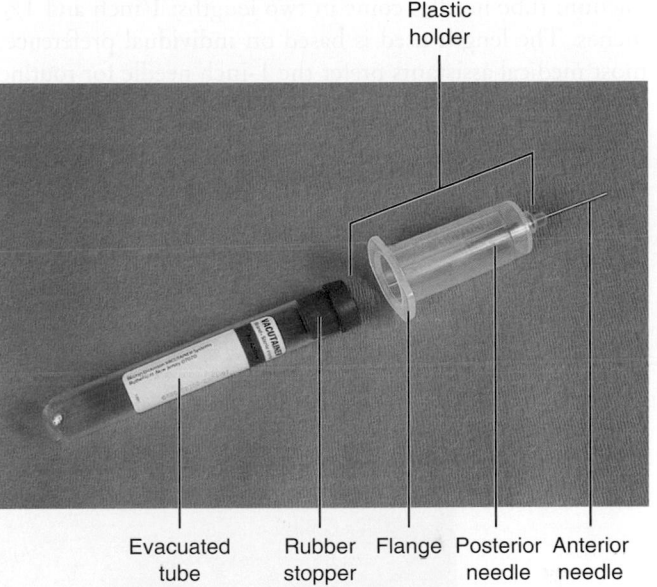

Figure 31-11 Vacuum tube system.

Labels: Plastic holder; Evacuated tube; Rubber stopper; Flange; Posterior needle; Anterior needle

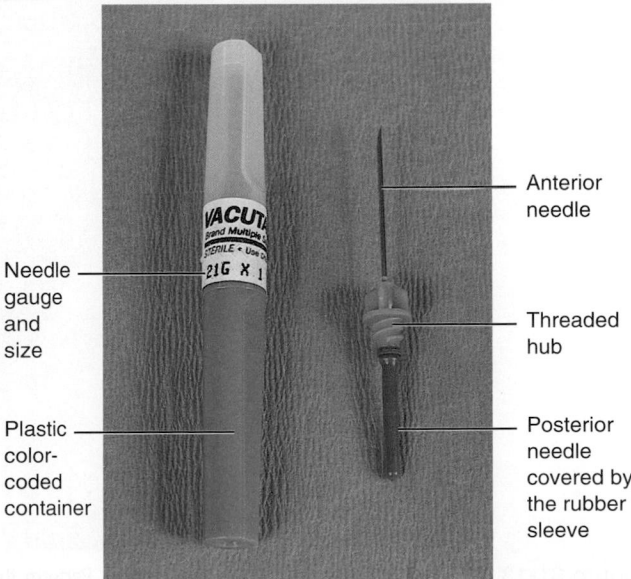

Figure 31-12 Vacuum tube needle in its container showing the gauge and size of the needle. The gauge of this needle is 21 G, and the size is 1 inch.

Labels: Anterior needle; Needle gauge and size; Threaded hub; Plastic color-coded container; Posterior needle covered by the rubber sleeve posterior needle has a rubber sleeve that functions as a valve. Pushing the tube stopper of an evacuated tube onto the posterior needle compresses this rubber sleeve and exposes the opening of the needle, allowing blood to enter the tube. When a tube is removed, the sleeve slides back over the needle opening and stops the flow of blood.

Vacuum tube needles are available in sizes 20 G to 22 G, with 21 G needles used most often for a routine venipuncture. A 22 G needle is recommended for children and adults with smaller veins, and a 20 G needle is sometimes used when a large-volume tube is used to collect a blood specimen. Manufacturers often color-code the needle guard and hub of venipuncture needles by gauge for easier identification; for example, Becton Dickinson uses the following color-coding system: yellow for 20 G needles, green for 21 G needles (see Figure 31-12), and black for 22 G needles. Vacuum tube needles come in two lengths: 1 inch and 1½ inches. The length used is based on individual preference; most medical assistants prefer the 1-inch needle for routine

venipunctures. A 1-inch needle is less intimidating to the patient and tends to offer greater control because it allows the medical assistant to rest the fourth and fifth fingers on the patient's arm for stability. A 1½-inch needle allows more room for stabilizing the vein.

Safety-Engineered Venipuncture Devices

OSHA stipulates requirements to reduce needlestick and other sharps injuries among health care workers. As discussed in Chapter 17, employers are required to evaluate and implement commercially available safer medical devices that reduce occupational exposure to the lowest extent feasible.

Safer medical devices include safety-engineered venipuncture devices. These devices incorporate a built-in safety feature to reduce the risk of a needlestick injury. Figure 31-13 illustrates a safety-engineered venipuncture device and the method for using it.

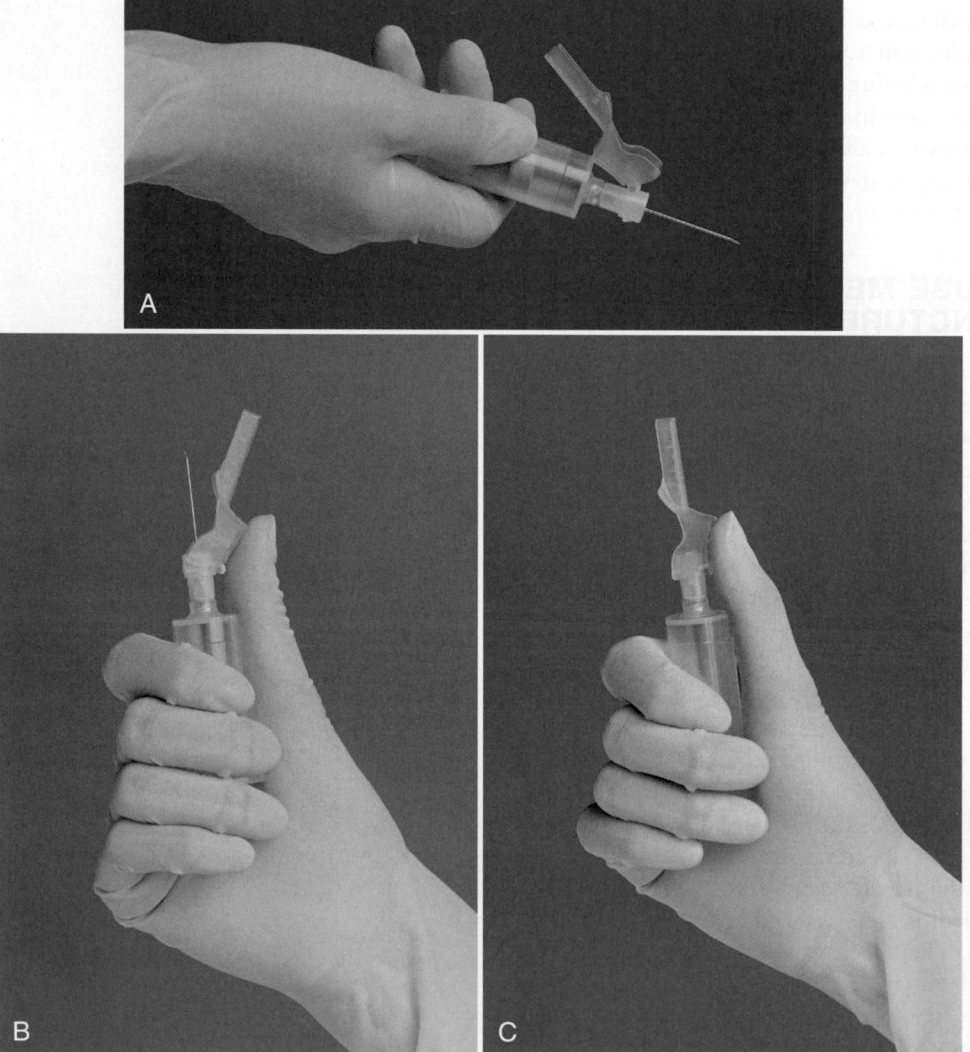

Figure 31-13 Safety-engineered venipuncture device. **A,** Perform the venipuncture with the shield in a downward position. **B,** After performing the venipuncture, push the shield forward. **C,** Continue pushing until the needle tip is fully covered by the shield. Discard the needle and holder in a biohazard sharps container.

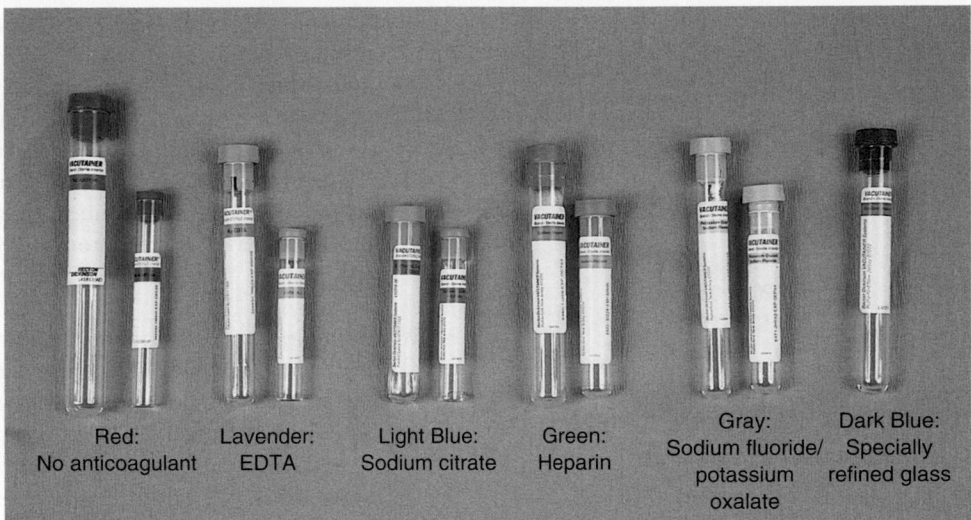

Figure 31-14 Vacutainer evacuated tubes. The stoppers of the evacuated tubes are color-coded for ease in identifying the additive content. The lavender-, light blue-, green-, gray-, and royal blue–stoppered tubes contain an anticoagulant and are used to obtain whole blood or plasma. The red-stoppered tube contains no additive and is used to obtain clotted blood or serum.

Plastic Holder

The plastic holder consists of a plastic cylinder with two openings. The small opening is used to secure the double-pointed needle, and the large opening is used to hold the evacuated tube. The large opening has a plastic extension known as the *flange.* The flange assists in the insertion and removal of evacuated tubes and prevents the plastic holder from rolling when it is placed on a flat surface.

The plastic holder has an indentation about ½ inch from the hub of the needle. This marks the point at which the posterior needle starts to enter the rubber stopper of the tube. If a tube stopper is inserted past this point before the vein is entered, the tube fills with air, which prevents blood from entering the tube.

Evacuated Tubes

Evacuated tubes consist of a glass or plastic tube with either a rubber stopper or a *Hemogard closure* stopper. The tube contains a premeasured vacuum that creates suction to pull the blood specimen into the tube. Evacuated tubes use a color-coded stopper system for ease in identifying the additive (or no additive) content of the tube. The additive content of evacuated tubes is described in the next section and is illustrated in Figures 31-14 and 31-15. A tube additive must not alter the blood components or affect the laboratory test to be performed.

The color of the tube stopper used depends on the type of test to be performed. The medical assistant must determine the correct stopper color to use for each collection. The color-coded stoppered tubes must not be substituted for one another because inaccurate test results could occur. If a CBC has been ordered by the physician, a lavender-stoppered tube must be used and a different color–stoppered tube cannot be substituted for it.

Evacuated tubes are available in varying capacities that range between 2 mL and 10 mL (see Figure 31-14). The

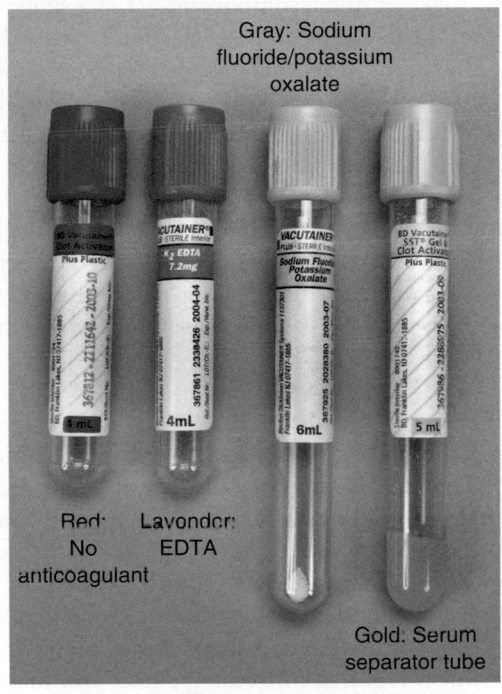

Figure 31-15 Hemogard tubes.

capacity of the tube used depends on the amount of the specimen required for the test. If the medical assistant is working with an outside laboratory, information on the amount of specimen required for a laboratory test and the stopper color of the tube required is indicated in the laboratory directory. If the test is being performed in the medical office, this information is indicated in the instructions accompanying the blood analyzer or testing kit.

Information regarding additive content, expiration date, and tube capacity is on the label of each package of evacuated tubes (Figure 31-16). In addition, evacuated tubes have a label affixed to them indicating the additive content, expiration date, and tube capacity, as well as a fill indicator

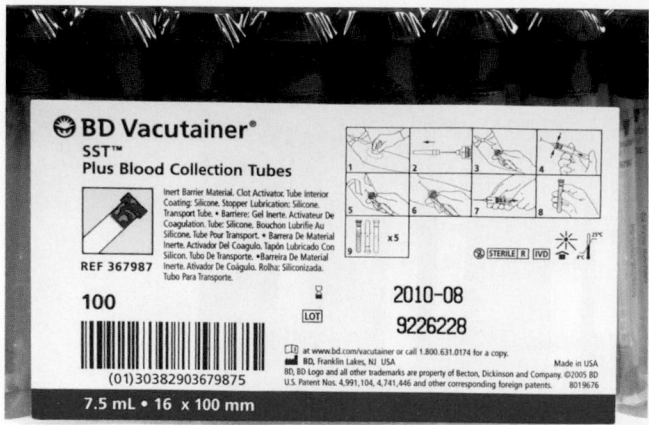

Figure 31-16 Evacuated tube package label.

to indicate when the vacuum has been exhausted and the tube is full.

A Hemogard closure stopper consists of a special rubber stopper and a plastic closure that overhangs the outside of the tube. Together, these components act as a single unit to reduce the likelihood of coming in contact with the contents of the tube. After collecting a blood specimen, the medical assistant may need to gain access to the blood in the tube for testing it or for further processing, such as in separating serum from whole blood. A conventional rubber stopper–evacuated tube "pops" as the top is removed, which may result in splattering of blood. The design of the Hemogard stopper works to prevent splattering of blood when the top is removed. The color coding of Hemogard closure stoppers is similar to that of rubber-stopped tubes (see Figure 31-15).

Additive Content of Evacuated Tubes

Evacuated tubes use a color-coded system for ease in identifying the additive content of each type of tube (see Figures 31-14 and 31-15). The most frequently used evacuated tubes in the medical office are classified here according to the color of the stopper and the additive content:

1. **Red.** Red-stoppered tubes do not contain an anticoagulant and are used to obtain clotted blood or serum. Serum is required for serologic tests and most blood chemistries.
2. **Red/gray-speckled tube (often called a "tiger top" tube).** The tube has a gold stopper if Hemogard tubes are used. These tubes are used to obtain serum. These tubes do not contain an anticoagulant; however, they do contain an additive known as a clot activator. A *clot activator* consists of a substance that makes the red blood cells in the tube clot more quickly to yield serum. Red/gray and gold–stoppered tubes also contain a gel that separates the cells from the serum when the tube is centrifuged. A tube with a clot activator must be inverted five times after it is drawn to mix the clot activator with the blood specimen.
3. **Lavender.** Lavender-stoppered tubes contain the anticoagulant *ethylenediaminetetraacetic acid* (EDTA) and are used to obtain whole blood or plasma. The most

common use is to collect a blood specimen for a complete blood count (CBC).
4. **Light blue.** Light blue–stoppered tubes contain the anticoagulant sodium citrate and are used to obtain whole blood or plasma; the most common use is for coagulation tests, such as prothrombin time.
5. **Green.** Green-stoppered tubes contain the anticoagulant heparin and are commonly used to collect blood specimens to perform blood gas determinations and pH assays.
6. **Gray.** Gray-stoppered tubes contain sodium fluoride (a preservative) and potassium oxalate (an anticoagulant) and are used to obtain whole blood or plasma; the most common use is to collect blood specimens to perform an oral glucose tolerance test (OGTT).
7. **Royal blue.** Royal blue–stoppered tubes contain either EDTA or no additive at all. These tubes are made of a specially refined glass and rubber stopper and are used for the detection of trace elements, such as lead, zinc, arsenic, and copper, which are contracted through occupational or environmental exposure.

Order of Draw for Multiple Tubes

When the vacuum tube system is used, and when multiple tubes of blood are to be drawn, the following order of draw (Table 31-1) is recommended by the *Clinical Laboratory Standards Institute (CLSI):*

1. **Blood culture tube:** Yellow-stoppered glass tube that contains the anticoagulant sodium polyanethol sulfonate (SPS), which is used for blood cultures and other tests that require sterile specimens.
   Rationale: To prevent contamination of the specimen by other tubes, which may lead to inaccurate test results.
2. **Coagulation tube:** Light blue–stoppered tube for coagulation tests.
   Rationale: To prevent additives from other tubes from getting into the tube.
   Note: The tubing of the butterfly setup contains 0.3 to 0.5 mL of air. If a light blue–stoppered tube is the first or only tube to be drawn, a 5-mL red-stoppered tube must be drawn first and discarded. This is because some of the tube's vacuum is exhausted by the air in the tubing (rather than blood), resulting in underfilling of the tube. If the light blue–stoppered tube is filled first, the underfilled tube results in an incorrect anticoagulant-to-blood ratio. An incorrect ratio when performing a coagulation test leads to inaccurate coagulation test results. It is also important to completely fill coagulation tubes to the exhaustion of the vacuum; failure to do so leads to erroneous coagulation test results.
3. **Serum tubes:** Tubes with or without a clot activator, and tubes with or without a gel barrier (e.g., red-stoppered tube; red/gray- or gold-stoppered tubes)
   Rationale: To prevent contamination of serum tubes by tubes with an anticoagulant.

Table 31-1 Order of Draw for Collection of Multiple Evacuated Tubes

Order of Draw by Color of Stopper	Additive or Anticoagulant	Number of Inversions after Collection
Yellow	Sterile blood culture tube that contains SPS (sodium polyanethol sulfonate)	8 to 10 inversions
Light blue	Sodium citrate	3 to 4 inversions
Red	Glass: no additive Plastic: clot activator	No inversions 5 inversions
Red/Gray	Serum separator gel and clot activator	5 inversions
Gold		
Green	Heparin	
Light green/gray	Plasma separator gel and lithium heparin	8 to 10 inversions
Light green		
Lavender	EDTA	8 to 10 inversions
Royal blue	EDTA No additive	8 to 10 inversions No inversions
Gray	Sodium fluoride/potassium oxalate	8 to 10 inversions

EDTA, Ethylenediaminetetraacetic acid; *SPS,* sodium polyanethol sulfonate.

4. **Anticoagulant tubes** in this order of stopper color: green, lavender, royal blue (that contains EDTA), and gray

   Rationale: To prevent cross-contamination between different types of anticoagulants, which may lead to inaccurate test results.

Evacuated Tube Guidelines

Certain guidelines should be followed when using evacuated tubes, as follows:

1. Select the proper evacuated tubes according to the tests to be performed and the amount of specimen required.
2. Check to ensure that the tube is not cracked. A cracked tube no longer has a vacuum.
3. Check the expiration date on each tube. Outdated tubes may no longer contain a vacuum, and, as a result, they would not be able to draw blood into the tube.
4. Make sure each tube is properly labeled. Proper labeling avoids mixing up specimens. Advances in specimen identification include the use of computer bar codes to identify specimens. Laboratory instruments that do the testing are able to read the bar codes and automatically record results onto the laboratory report form for a particular patient using the identification number supplied by the bar code. Along with the bar code, additional printed information is included on a bar code label (Figure 31-17). It is important to attach the correct bar code label to the blood tube. Inspect the label for printed information indicating the color-stopper tube (e.g., LV for lavender) or type of tube (e.g., SST for serum separator tube) to which the label must be attached. For example, the bar code label illustrated in Figure 31-17 must be placed on a lavender (LV) tube that is being collected to perform a CBC.
5. Before using tubes that contain powdered additives (e.g., gray-stoppered tube), gently tap the tube just below the stopper so that all of the additive is dislodged from the stopper. If an additive remains trapped in the stopper, erroneous test results may occur.

What Would You Do? What Would You *Not* Do?

Case Study 2

Buzz Braydon had a heart attack 4 weeks ago and is taking the anticoagulant warfarin (Coumadin). He is at the office for a checkup and to have his prothrombin time tested. Blood is collected from a small vein in Buzz's left arm using the butterfly method. After the specimen is collected, Buzz wants to know why a red-stoppered tube was used to draw blood from him and then thrown away. Buzz says that he is going on vacation in North Carolina for 2 weeks. He says that they explained to him at the hospital why he should have his blood tested every week, but he's not sure where to go to get his blood tested while he's on vacation. Buzz wants to know if, as long as he takes his medication exactly as he should, it would be all right to skip his weekly prothrombin test during that time. ■

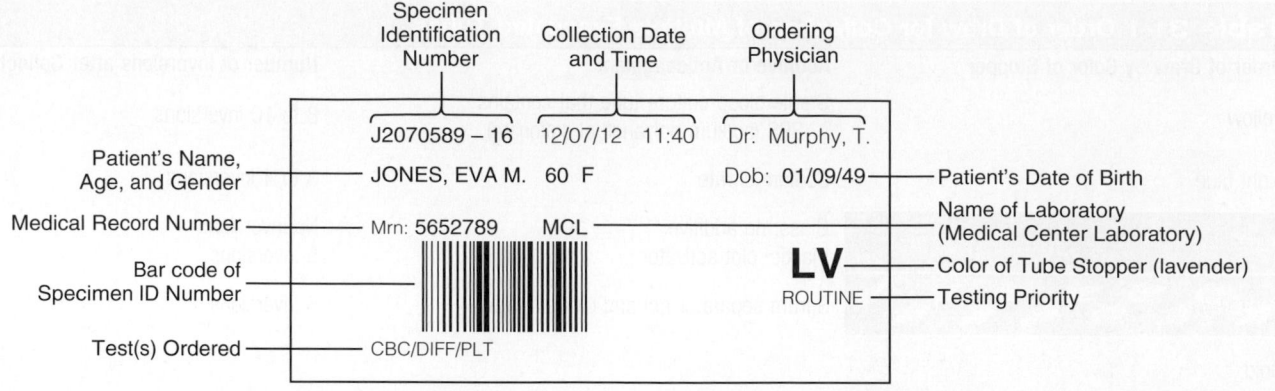

Figure 31-17 Information included on a laboratory specimen bar code label.

6. Take precautions to avoid premature loss of the tube's vacuum. Premature loss of vacuum can occur from the following:
   - Dropping the tube
   - Pushing the posterior needle through the tube stopper before puncturing the vein
   - Partially pulling the needle out of the vein after penetrating the patient's vein
7. Use a continuous, steady motion to make the puncture. Performing the puncture with a slow, timid motion or a rapid, jabbing motion is painful for the patient. In addition, a rapid motion could cause the needle to go completely through the vein, resulting in failure to obtain blood and possibly a hematoma.
8. When multiple tubes are to be drawn, follow the proper *order of draw.* This prevents contamination of nonadditive tubes by additive tubes and cross-contamination between different types of additive tubes, which could lead to inaccurate test results.
9. Fill evacuated tubes until the vacuum is exhausted, as evidenced by cessation of blood flow into the tube. The tube is almost, but not quite, full when the vacuum is exhausted. If the evacuated tube is removed before the vacuum is exhausted, a rush of air enters the tube, damaging the red blood cells. A

tube that contains an anticoagulant must be filled completely to ensure the proper ratio of anticoagulant to the blood specimen.
10. Remove the last tube from the plastic holder before removing the needle from the patient's vein. This prevents blood from dripping out of the tip of the needle after it is withdrawn from the patient's skin.
11. Mix tubes that contain a clot activator or an anticoagulant immediately after drawing by gently inverting them. Gentle inversion provides adequate mixing without causing **hemolysis,** or breakdown of blood cells. One inversion consists of one complete turn of the wrist (180 degrees) and then back again. Tubes with a clot activator should be inverted five times, and tubes with an anticoagulant (with the exception of sodium citrate tubes) should be inverted 8 to 10 times. Tubes containing sodium citrate (light-blue stopper) should be gently inverted 3 to 4 times. (see Table 31-1). Inadequate mixing or not mixing tubes with an anticoagulant immediately after drawing them may result in clotting of the blood, leading to inaccurate test results.
12. After the venipuncture, the top of the stopper may contain residual blood. Take precautions by following the OSHA Standard when handling these tubes.

 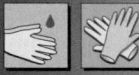

PROCEDURE 31-1 Venipuncture—Vacuum Tube Method

Outcome Perform a venipuncture using the vacuum tube method.

Equipment/Supplies
- Disposable gloves
- Tourniquet
- Antiseptic wipe
- Double-pointed needle
- Plastic holder
- Evacuated tubes with labels
- Sterile 2 × 2 gauze pad
- Adhesive bandage
- Biohazard sharps container
- Biohazard specimen bag
- Laboratory request form

1. Procedural Step. Review the requirements for collecting and handling the blood specimen as ordered by the physician. Sanitize your hands.

2. Procedural Step. Greet the patient and introduce yourself. Identify the patient by asking the patient to state his or her full name and date of birth. Compare

PROCEDURE 31-1 Venipuncture—Vacuum Tube Method—cont'd

this information with the demographic data in the patient's chart. If the patient was required to prepare for the test (e.g., fasting, medication restriction), determine whether he or she has prepared properly. If the patient has not followed the patient preparation requirements, notify the physician for instructions on handling this situation.

Principle. It is important to confirm that you have the correct patient to avoid collecting a specimen on the wrong patient. The patient must prepare properly to obtain a high-quality specimen that would lead to accurate test results.

3. Procedural Step. Assemble the equipment. Select the proper evacuated tubes for the tests to be performed. Check the expiration date on the tubes. Label each tube using one of the following methods: (a) attaching a computer bar code label to each tube to be drawn and labeling it with your initials, or (b) manually labeling each tube with the patient's name and date of birth, the date, and your initials. If the specimen is to be tested at an outside laboratory, complete a laboratory request form. (*NOTE:* Follow the medical office policy as to when the tubes should be labeled. Some offices prefer that tubes be labeled *before* the specimen is drawn; other offices want the tubes to be labeled right *after* the specimen is drawn.)

Principle. Outdated tubes may no longer contain a vacuum, and, as a result, they may not be able to draw blood into the tube. Proper labeling of blood specimens avoids a mix-up of specimens.

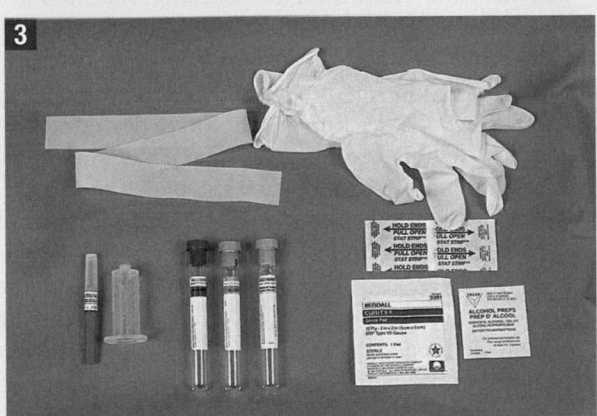

Assemble the equipment.

4. Procedural Step. Prepare the vacuum tube system. Remove the cap from the posterior needle using a twisting and pulling motion. Insert the posterior needle into the small opening on the plastic holder. Screw the plastic holder onto the Luer adapter, and tighten it securely.

Principle. An unsecured needle can fall out of its plastic holder.

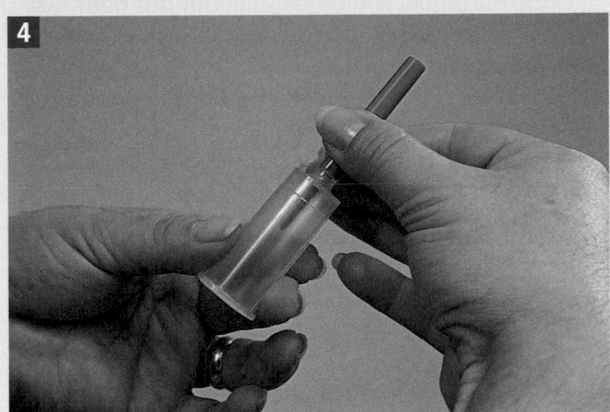

Insert the posterior needle into the plastic holder.

5. Procedural Step. Open the sterile gauze packet, and lay it flat to allow the gauze pad to rest on the inside of its wrapper. Position the evacuated tubes in the correct order of draw. If the evacuated tube contains a powdered additive, tap the tube just below the stopper to release any additive adhering to the stopper.

Principle. If an additive remains trapped in the stopper, erroneous test results may occur.

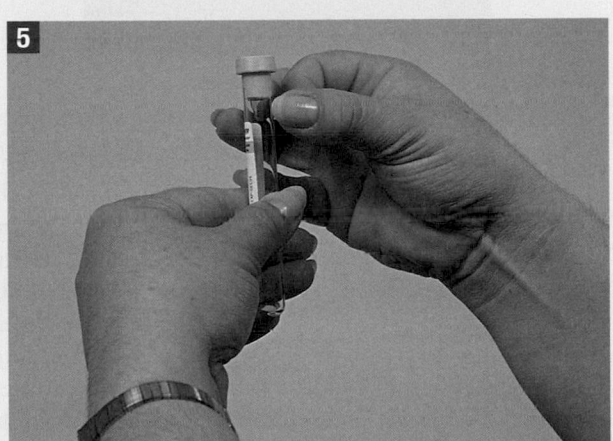

Tap tubes with powdered additives.

6. Procedural Step. Place the first tube loosely in the plastic holder.

7. Procedural Step. Explain the procedure to the patient, and reassure the patient. Perform a preliminary assessment of both arms to determine the best vein to use. It also is helpful to ask the patient which arm has been used in the past to obtain blood.

Principle. Venipuncture is often a frightening experience for the patient, and reassurance should be offered to reduce apprehension.

Continued

8. Procedural Step. Apply the tourniquet. Position the tourniquet 3 to 4 inches above the bend in the elbow. The tourniquet should be snug but not tight. Ask the patient to clench the fist of the arm to which the tourniquet has been applied.

Principle. The combined effect of the pressure of the tourniquet and the clenched fist should cause the antecubital veins to stand out so that accurate selection of a puncture site can be made.

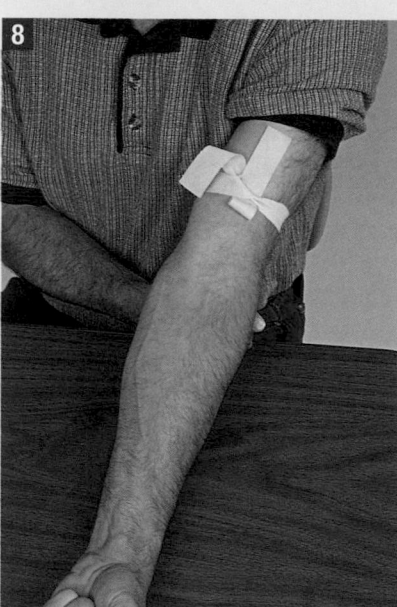

Apply the tourniquet.

9. Procedural Step. With a tourniquet in place, thoroughly assess the veins of first one arm and then the other to determine the best vein to use.

10. Procedural Step. Position the patient's arm. The arm with the vein selected for the venipuncture should be extended and placed in a straight line from the shoulder to the wrist with the antecubital veins facing anteriorly. The arm should be supported on the armrest by a rolled towel or by having the patient place the fist of the other hand under the elbow.

Principle. This position allows easy access to the antecubital veins.

11. Procedural Step. Thoroughly palpate the selected vein. Gently palpate the vein with the fingertips to determine the direction of the vein and to estimate its size and depth. Never leave the tourniquet on an arm for longer than 1 minute at a time. (*NOTE:* If you need to perform several assessments to locate the best vein, the tourniquet must be removed and reapplied after a 2-minute waiting period.)

Principle. Leaving the tourniquet on for longer than 1 minute is uncomfortable for the patient and may alter the test results.

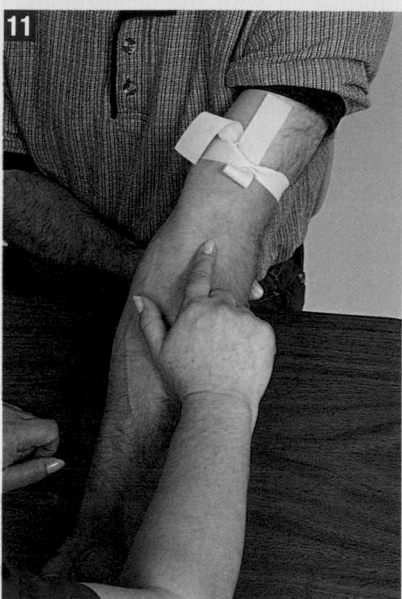

Palpate the vein.

12. Procedural Step. Remove the tourniquet and cleanse the site with an antiseptic wipe. Cleansing should be done in a circular motion, starting from the inside and moving away from the puncture site. Allow the site to air-dry; after cleansing, do not touch the area, wipe the area with gauze, or fan the area with your hand. Place the remaining supplies within comfortable reach of your nondominant hand.

Principle. Using a circular motion helps carry foreign particles away from the puncture site. The site must be allowed to air-dry to allow the alcohol enough time to destroy microorganisms on the patient's skin. Residual alcohol entering the blood specimen can cause hemolysis, leading to inaccurate test results. In addition, residual alcohol causes the patient to experience a stinging sensation when the puncture is made. Touching or fanning the area causes contamination of the puncture site, and the cleansing process must be repeated. Items used during the procedure should be positioned so that you do not have to reach over the patient and possibly move the needle, resulting in pain, injury, or both.

13. Procedural Step. Reapply the tourniquet. Apply gloves. If you are using a needle with a safety shield, rotate the shield backward toward the holder (refer to Figure 31-13, *A*). Remove the cap from the needle using a twisting and pulling motion. Hold the vacuum tube system by placing the thumb of the dominant hand on top of the plastic holder and the pads of the first three fingers underneath the holder and evacuated tube. The needle should be positioned with the bevel facing up. Position the evacuated tube so that the label is facing down.

PROCEDURE 31-1   Venipuncture—Vacuum Tube Method—cont'd

Principle. Gloves provide a barrier against blood-borne pathogens. Positioning the needle with the bevel up allows easier entry into the skin and the vein, resulting in less pain for the patient. With the label facing down, you would be able to observe the blood as it fills the tube, which allows you to know when the tube is full.

14. **Procedural Step.** Anchor the vein. Grasp the patient's arm with the nondominant hand. Your thumb should be placed 1 to 2 inches below and to the side of the puncture site. Using your thumb, draw the skin taut over the vein in the direction of the patient's hand.

    Principle. The thumb helps hold the skin taut for easier entry and helps stabilize the vein to be punctured. Placing the thumb to the side keeps it out of the way of the vacuum tube setup, so that you can maintain a 15-degree angle when entering the vein.

15. **Procedural Step.** Position the needle at a 15-degree angle to the arm. Rest the backs of the fingers on the patient's forearm. Ensure that the needle points in the same direction as the vein to be entered. The needle should be positioned so that it enters the vein approximately $\frac{1}{8}$ inch below the place where the vein is to be entered.

    Principle. An angle of less than 15 degrees may cause the needle to enter above the vein, preventing puncture. An angle of more than 15 degrees may cause the needle to go through the vein by puncturing the posterior wall. This could result in a hematoma.

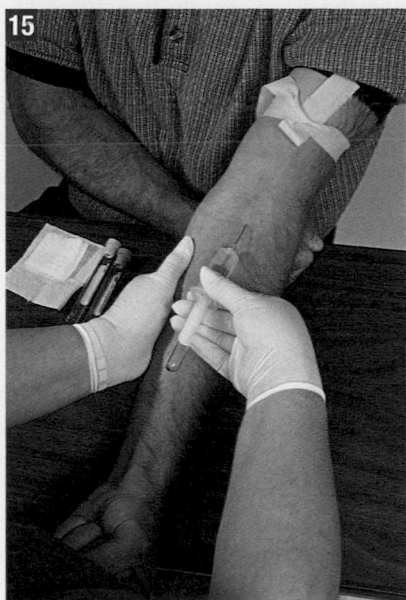

Position the needle.

16. **Procedural Step.** Tell the patient that he or she will "feel a small stick," and with one continuous steady motion, enter the skin and then the vein. You will feel

a sensation of resistance followed by a "release" as the vein is entered. When the "release" is felt, you have entered the vein and should not advance the needle any farther.

Principle. Using one continuous steady motion helps to prevent tissue damage.

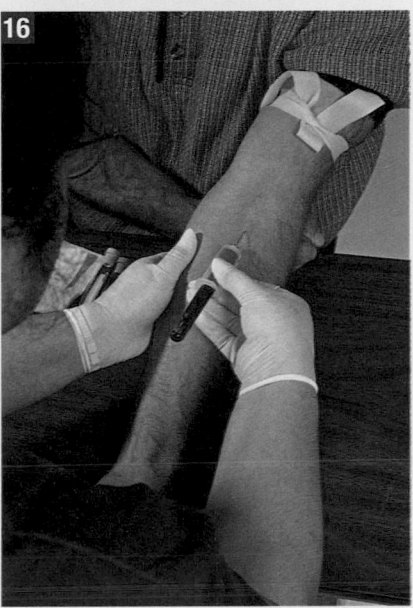

Make the puncture.

17. **Procedural Step.** Stabilize the vacuum tube setup by firmly grasping the holder between the thumb and the underlying fingers to prevent the needle from moving. Do *not* change hands during the procedure.

    Principle. Stabilizing the holder helps prevent the needle from moving when a tube is inserted or removed. Changing hands may cause the needle to move, which is painful for the patient.

18. **Procedural Step.** With the nondominant hand, place the first two fingers on the underside of the flange on the plastic holder, and with the thumb, slowly push the tube forward to the end of the holder. This allows the posterior needle to puncture the rubber stopper. Blood begins flowing into the tube if the (anterior) needle is in a vein.

    Principle. Not using the flange may cause the needle to advance forward and go completely through the vein, resulting in failure to obtain blood; internal bleeding also may occur, resulting in a hematoma.

19. **Procedural Step.** Allow the evacuated tube to fill to the exhaustion of the vacuum, as indicated by cessation of the blood flow into the tube. The suction of the evacuated tube automatically draws the blood into the tube.

    Principle. If the evacuated tube is removed before the vacuum is exhausted, a rush of air enters the tube, damaging the red blood cells. Also, a tube containing

Continued

PROCEDURE 31-1   Venipuncture—Vacuum Tube Method—cont'd

an additive, such as an anticoagulant, must be filled completely to ensure accurate test results.

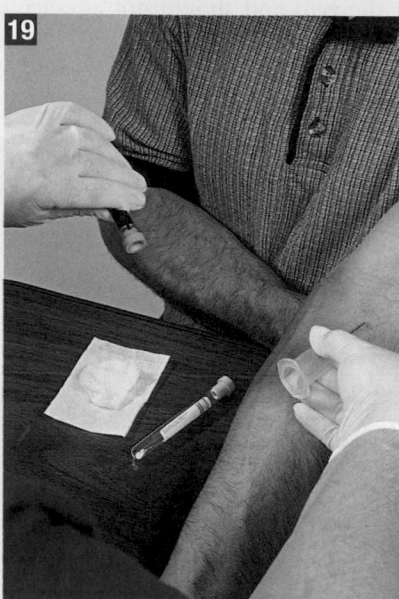

Invert tubes with additives back and forth 8 to 10 times.

20. **Procedural Step.** Remove the tube from the holder by grasping the tube with the fingers, placing the thumb or index finger against the flange, and pulling the tube off the posterior needle. Do not change the position of the needle in the vein. If the tube contains a clot activator, gently invert the tube back and forth 5 times before laying it down. If the tube contains an anticoagulant, gently invert the tube 8 to 10 times.

    Principle. The rubber sheath covers the point of the needle, stopping the flow of blood until the next tube is inserted. Not using the flange to remove the tube can cause the needle to come out of the vein prematurely, resulting in blood being forced out of the puncture site. A tube containing an anticoagulant must be inverted immediately to prevent the blood from clotting. Careful mixing of the blood with a clot activator or an anticoagulant prevents hemolysis.

21. **Procedural Step.** Using the flange, carefully insert the next tube into the holder. Continue in this manner until the last tube has been filled.

22. **Procedural Step.** Remove the tension from the tourniquet by pulling upward on one of the flaps of the tourniquet. Ask the patient to unclench the fist.

    Principle. The tourniquet tension must be removed before the needle. Otherwise, the pressure on the vein from the tourniquet could cause internal and external bleeding around the puncture site.

23. **Procedural Step.** Remove the last tube from the holder. Immediately invert the tube back and forth 5

times if it contains a clot activator and 8 to 10 times if it contains an anticoagulant.

Principle. Removing the last tube prevents blood from dripping out of the tip of the needle after it is removed from the patient's arm.

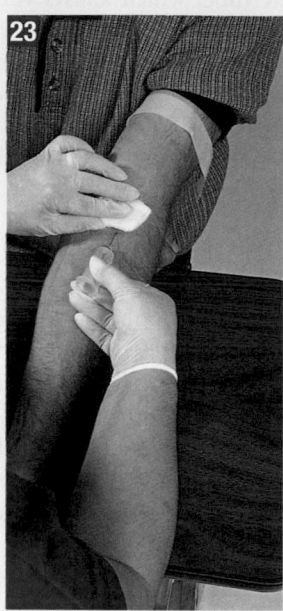

Remove the tourniquet and withdraw the needle.

24. **Procedural Step.** Place a sterile gauze pad slightly above the puncture site, and carefully withdraw the needle at the same angle as for penetration. Immediately move the gauze over the puncture site, and apply firm pressure. (Do not apply any pressure to the puncture site until the needle is completely removed.) If you are using a needle with a safety shield, push the shield forward with your thumb until you hear an audible click, which indicates the shield has locked into place. Do not push the shield forward by pressing it against a hard surface. (See Figure 31-13, *B, C*.)

    Principle. Placing the gauze pad above the puncture helps prevent tissue movement as the needle is withdrawn and reduces patient discomfort. Careful withdrawal prevents further tissue damage.

25. **Procedural Step.** Immediately discard the plastic holder and attached needle in a biohazard sharps container. Do not remove the needle from the holder; the holder must be discarded and not reused.

    Principle. Immediate disposal of the needle and holder unit is required by the OSHA Standard to prevent a needlestick injury; even if a safety shield has been activated to encase the anterior needle, a needlestick injury can still occur from the posterior needle, which is only covered with a rubber sleeve. Plastic

PROCEDURE 31-1 Venipuncture—Vacuum Tube Method—cont'd

holders are often contaminated with blood and must not be reused.

26. **Procedural Step.** Continue to apply pressure with the gauze pad. Cooperative patients can be asked to assist by applying pressure with the gauze pad for 1 to 2 minutes. The arm can be elevated to facilitate clot formation. Do not allow the patient to bend the arm at the elbow because this increases blood loss from the puncture site.

    Principle. Applying pressure reduces the leakage of blood from the puncture site externally or internally. Internal leakage of blood into the tissues could result in a hematoma.

27. **Procedural Step.** Stay with the patient until the bleeding has stopped. Remove the gauze, and inspect the puncture site to ensure that the opening is sealed with a clot. Apply an adhesive bandage to the puncture site. As an alternative, the gauze pad can be folded into quarters and taped on the puncture site to be used as a pressure bandage. Instruct the patient not to pick up anything heavy for about an hour. (*NOTE:* If swelling or discoloration occurs, apply an ice pack to the site after bandaging it.)

    Principle. Lifting a heavy object causes pressure on the puncture site, which could result in bleeding.

28. **Procedural Step.** Place the tubes in an upright position in a test tube rack. Remove the gloves, and sanitize your hands.

29. **Procedural Step.** Chart the procedure. Include the date and time, which arm and vein were used, unusual patient reaction, and your initials.

30. **Procedural Step.** If needed, process the specimen (e.g., centrifuging the specimen to separate serum from the cells). Test the specimen or prepare the specimen for transport to an outside laboratory for testing according to the medical office policy. If the specimen is to be transported to an outside laboratory, do the following:

    a. Place the specimen tube in a biohazard specimen bag.

    b. Place the laboratory request in the outside pocket of the specimen bag.

    c. Properly handle and store the specimen while awaiting pickup by a laboratory courier.

    d. Chart the date the specimen was transported to the laboratory in the patient's record.

    Principle. The biohazard bag protects the laboratory courier from the possibility of an exposure incident. The outside laboratory must have the completed request form to know which laboratory tests have been ordered by the physician. The specimen must be handled and stored properly to maintain the in vivo characteristics of the specimen.

CHARTING EXAMPLE	
Date	
4/5/XX	9:00 a.m. Venous blood specimen collected from (L) arm. Picked up by Medical Center Laboratory on 4/5/XX. ———————
	——————— D. Glover, CMA (AAMA)

BUTTERFLY METHOD OF VENIPUNCTURE

The butterfly method of venipuncture is also called the *winged infusion method.* This is because a winged infusion set is used to perform the procedure. The term *butterfly* is derived from the plastic "wings" located between the needle and the tubing of the winged infusion set (Figure 31-18).

The butterfly method is used to collect blood from patients who are difficult to stick by conventional methods because it provides better control when making the puncture, and less pressure is exerted on the vein wall from the evacuated tube. The butterfly method is recommended for adults with small antecubital veins and children, who typically have small antecubital veins. The butterfly method also is used when the antecubital veins are unavailable and veins in the forearm, wrist area, or back of the hand are used, as may occur with elderly and obese patients. These alternative veins are usually smaller and sometimes have a thin wall

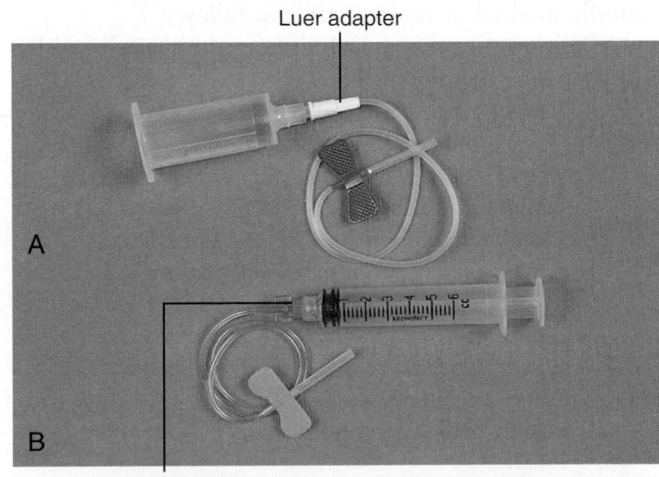

Figure 31-18 Winged infusion set. **A,** Luer adapter with evacuated tube. **B,** Hub adapter with syringe.

(e.g., hand veins), making them more likely to collapse when using the vacuum tube method of venipuncture. With the vacuum tube method, the "sucking action" exerted on the vein when the pressure in the vacuum is released causes the vein to collapse, blocking the flow of blood into the tube. The butterfly method results in less pressure on the vein wall because the pressure exerted by the evacuated tube must travel through a length of tubing before reaching the vein. Because the pressure against the vein wall is minimized, the vein is less likely to collapse with the butterfly method. Procedure 31-2 describes the venipuncture procedure using the butterfly method.

The gauge of the winged infusion needle used to collect a blood specimen ranges from 21 G to 23 G, and the length of the needle ranges from $\frac{1}{2}$ to $\frac{3}{4}$ inch. The needle is short and sharp, making it easier to stick difficult veins. For extremely small veins, a 23 G needle should be used to prevent rupture of the vein by a larger needle. In this case, it is preferable to use smaller-volume tubes (e.g., 2-mL evacuated tubes) because large evacuated tubes may put too much vacuum pressure on the vein, causing it to collapse. Manufacturers often color-code the wings of the infusion setup by gauge for easier identification; for example, Becton Dickinson uses the following color coding system: green for 21 G needles and light blue for 23 G needles (see Figure 31-18).

The winged infusion needle is attached to a 7- or 12-inch length of tubing and a *Luer adapter,* which is attached to a (posterior) needle with a rubber sleeve. A plastic holder is screwed onto the Luer adapter, which allows it to be used with evacuated tubes (see Figure 31-18, *A*). Winged infusion sets also are available with a hub adapter that allows them to be used with a syringe (see Figure 31-18, *B*). Safety needles are available with a shield that covers the contaminated needle after it is withdrawn from the patient's vein (Figure 31-19).

Guidelines for the Butterfly Method

Certain guidelines should be followed when performing the butterfly method of venipuncture, as follows:

1. Position the patient according to the site selected for the venipuncture as follows:
   - **Antecubital, wrist, and forearm veins.** Position the arm in a straight line from the shoulder to the wrist as described in the vacuum tube method of venipuncture.
   - **Hand veins.** Position the patient's hand on the armrest, and ask the patient to make a loose fist or to grasp a rolled towel. This combination causes the hand veins to stand out so that accurate selection of a puncture site can be made. Locate a suitable vein between the knuckles and the wrist bones. Hand veins are usually visible and easy to locate.
2. Position the tourniquet according to the venipuncture site as follows: If the veins of the forearm or wrist are used, apply the tourniquet to the forearm, approximately 3 inches above the puncture site. For hand

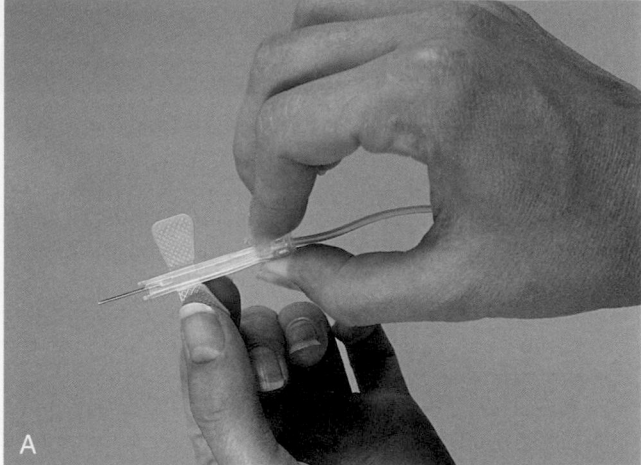
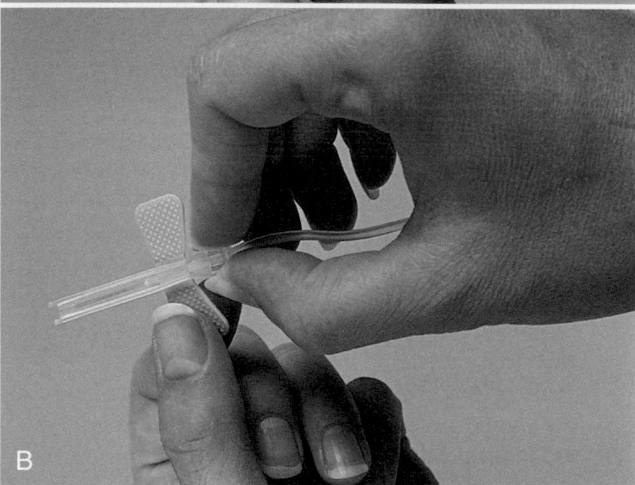

Figure 31-19 Butterfly safety needle. The safety needle has a shield that covers the contaminated needle after it is withdrawn from the patient's vein. **A,** The medical assistant has covered one half of the needle with the shield. **B,** The needle is completely covered with the shield.

veins, position the tourniquet on the arm just above the wrist bone (Figure 31-20).
3. Grasp the needle by compressing the plastic wings together. Insert the needle with the bevel facing up at a 15-degree angle to the skin. When the vein has been entered, decrease the angle to 5 degrees.
4. After decreasing the needle angle to 5 degrees, slowly thread the needle inside the vein an additional $\frac{1}{4}$ inch. This anchors or seats the needle in the center of the vein and allows the medical assistant to use both hands to change tubes.
5. To prevent venous reflux, keep the evacuated tube and holder in a downward position as in the vacuum tube venipuncture procedure. This technique ensures that the blood fills from the bottom up and not near the rubber stopper.
6. When multiple tubes are to be drawn, follow the proper order of draw. The order of draw for the butterfly method is identical to that for the vacuum tube method (previously presented). Following this order of draw prevents contamination of nonadditive tubes and cross-contamination of additive tubes.

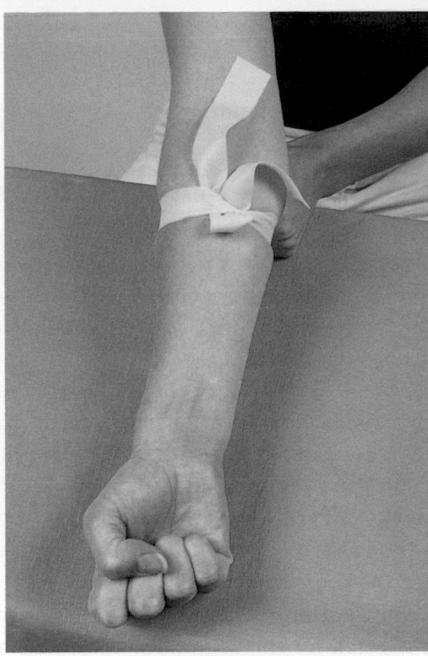
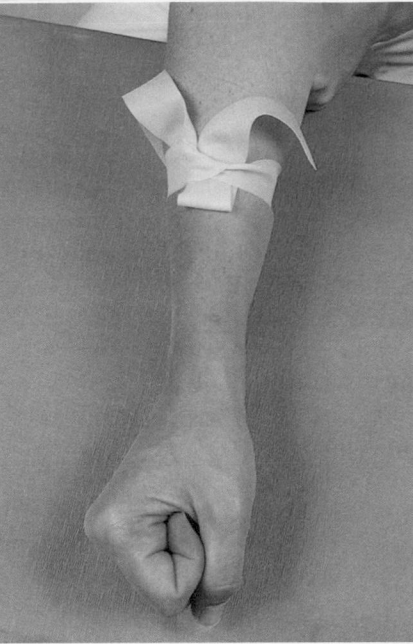
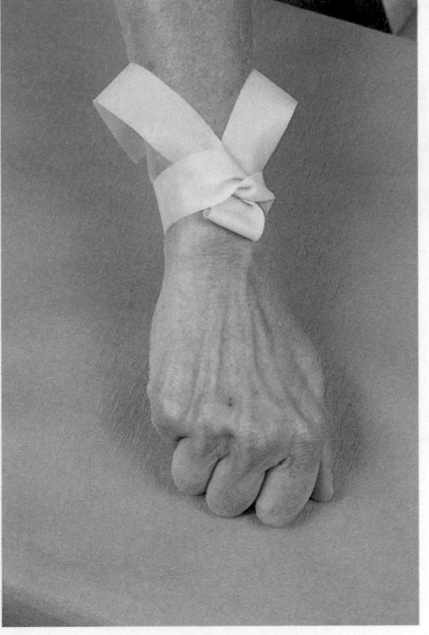

A. Forearm site	B. Wrist site	C. Hand

Figure 31-20 Application of the tourniquet for alternative venipuncture sites.

PROCEDURE 31-2 Venipuncture—Butterfly Method

Outcome Perform a venipuncture using the butterfly method.

Equipment/Supplies

- Disposable gloves
- Tourniquet
- Antiseptic wipe
- Winged infusion set with a Luer adapter
- Plastic holder
- Evacuated tubes with labels

- Sterile 2 × 2 gauze pad
- Adhesive bandage
- Biohazard sharps container
- Biohazard specimen bag
- Laboratory request form

1. **Procedural Step.** Review the requirements for collecting and handling the blood specimen as ordered by the physician. Sanitize your hands.

2. **Procedural Step.** Greet the patient and introduce yourself. Identify the patient by asking the patient to state his or her full name and date of birth. Compare this information with the demographic data in the patient's chart. If the patient was required to prepare for the test (e.g., fasting, medication restriction), determine whether he or she has prepared properly. If the patient has not followed the patient preparation requirements, notify the physician for instructions on handling this situation.
   Principle. It is important to confirm that you have the correct patient to avoid collecting a specimen on the wrong patient. The patient must prepare properly to obtain a high-quality specimen that would lead to accurate test results.

3. **Procedural Step.** Assemble the equipment. Select the proper evacuated tubes for the tests to be performed. Check the expiration date on the tubes. Label each tube using one of the following methods: (a) attaching a computer bar code label to each tube and labeling it with your initials, or (b) manually labeling each tube with the patient's name and date of birth, the date, and your

initials. If the specimen is to be tested at an outside laboratory, complete a laboratory request form. (*NOTE:* Follow the medical office policy as to when the tubes should be labeled. Some offices prefer that tubes be labeled *before* the specimen is drawn; other offices want the tubes to be labeled right *after* the specimen is drawn.)
Principle. Outdated tubes may no longer contain a vacuum, and, as a result, they may not be able to draw blood into the tube. Proper labeling of blood specimens avoids the mix-up of specimens.

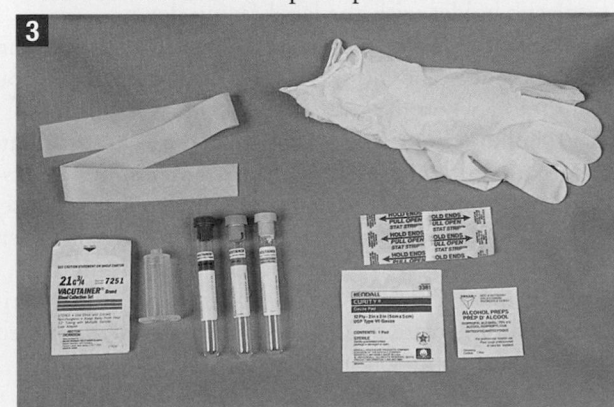

Assemble the equipment.

Continued

4. Procedural Step. Prepare the winged infusion set. Remove the winged infusion set from its package. Extend the tubing to its full length, and stretch it slightly to prevent it from recoiling. Insert the posterior needle into the small opening on the plastic holder. Screw the plastic holder onto the Luer adapter, and tighten it securely.

Principle. Extending the tubing straightens it to permit a free flow of blood in the tubing. An unsecured needle can fall out of its plastic holder.

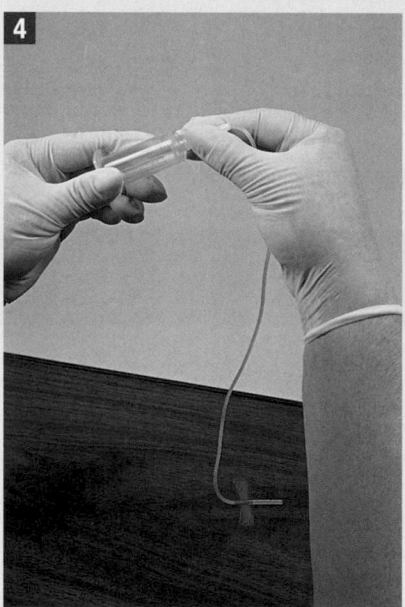

Screw the Luer adapter into the holder.

5. Procedural Step. Open the sterile gauze packet, and lay it flat to allow the gauze pad to rest on the inside of its wrapper. Position the evacuated tubes in the correct order of draw. If the evacuated tube contains a powdered additive, tap the tube just below the stopper to release any additive adhering to the stopper.

Principle. If an additive remains trapped in the stopper, erroneous test results may occur.

6. Procedural Step. Place the first tube loosely in the plastic holder with the label facing down.

Principle. With the label facing down, you can observe the blood as it fills the tube, which allows you to know when the tube is full.

7. Procedural Step. Explain the procedure to the patient, and reassure the patient. Perform a preliminary assessment of both arms to determine the best vein to use. It also is helpful to ask the patient which arm has been used in the past to obtain blood.

Principle. Venipuncture is often a frightening experience for the patient, and reassurance should be offered to reduce apprehension.

8. Procedural Step. Apply the tourniquet. Position the tourniquet 3 to 4 inches above the bend in the elbow. The tourniquet should be snug but not tight. Ask the patient to clench the fist of the arm to which the tourniquet has been applied.

Principle. The combined effect of the pressure of the tourniquet and the clenched fist should cause the antecubital veins to stand out so that accurate selection of a puncture site can be made.

9. Procedural Step. With a tourniquet in place, thoroughly assess the veins of first one arm and then the other to determine the best vein to use.

10. Procedural Step. Position the patient's arm. The arm with the vein selected for the venipuncture should be extended and placed in a straight line from the shoulder to the wrist with the antecubital veins facing anteriorly. The arm should be supported on the armrest by a rolled towel or by having the patient place the fist of the other hand under the elbow.

Principle. This position allows easy access to the antecubital veins.

11. Procedural Step. Thoroughly palpate the selected vein. Gently palpate the vein with the fingertips to determine the direction of the vein and to estimate its size and depth. Never leave the tourniquet on an arm for longer than 1 minute at a time. (*NOTE:* If you need to perform several assessments to locate the best vein, the tourniquet must be removed and reapplied after a 2-minute waiting period.)

Principle. Leaving the tourniquet on for longer than 1 minute is uncomfortable for the patient and may alter the test results.

12. Procedural Step. Remove the tourniquet and cleanse the site with an antiseptic. Cleansing should be done in a circular motion, starting from the inside and moving away from the puncture site. Allow the site to air-dry, and after cleansing, do not touch the area, wipe the area with gauze, or fan the area with your hand. Place your remaining supplies within comfortable reach.

Principle. Using a circular motion helps carry foreign particles away from the puncture site. The site must be allowed to air-dry to allow the alcohol enough time to destroy microorganisms on the patient's skin. Residual alcohol entering the blood specimen can cause hemolysis, leading to inaccurate test results. In addition, residual alcohol causes the patient to experience a stinging sensation when the puncture is made. Touching or fanning the area causes contamination of the puncture site, and the cleansing process must be repeated. Items used during the procedure should be positioned so that you do not have to reach over the patient and possibly move the needle, resulting in patient pain, injury, or both.

13. **Procedural Step.** Reapply the tourniquet. Apply gloves. With the dominant hand, grasp the winged infusion set by pressing the butterfly tips together. Remove the protective sheath from the needle of the infusion set. The needle should be positioned with the bevel facing up.

Principle. Gloves provide a barrier against blood-borne pathogens. Positioning the needle with the bevel up allows easier entry into the skin and the vein, resulting in less pain for the patient.

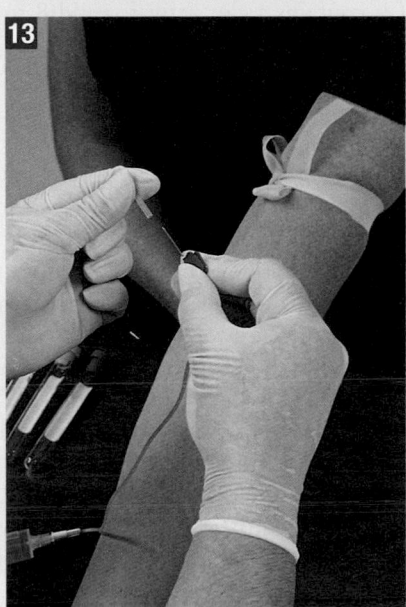

Remove the protective shield from the needle.

14. **Procedural Step.** Anchor the vein. Grasp the patient's arm with the nondominant hand. The thumb should be placed 1 to 2 inches below and to the side of the puncture site. Using the thumb, draw the skin taut over the vein in the direction of the patient's hand.

Principle. The thumb helps hold the skin taut for easier entry and helps stabilize the vein to be punctured. Placing the thumb to the side keeps it out of the way of the winged infusion setup so that you can maintain a 15-degree angle when entering the vein.

15. **Procedural Step.** Position the needle at a 15-degree angle to the arm. Rest the backs of the fingertips on the patient's skin. Make sure the needle points in the same direction as the vein to be entered. The needle should be positioned so that it enters the vein approximately $\frac{1}{8}$ inch below the place where the vein is to be entered.

Principle. An angle of less than 15 degrees may cause the needle to enter above the vein, preventing puncture. An angle of more than 15 degrees may cause the needle to go through the vein by puncturing the posterior wall. This could result in a hematoma.

16. **Procedural Step.** Tell the patient that he or she will "feel a small stick," and with one continuous steady

motion, enter the skin and then the vein. You will feel a sensation of resistance followed by a "release" as the vein is entered. After penetrating the vein, decrease the angle of the needle to 5 degrees. If the needle is in the vein, a flash of blood appears at the top of the tubing.

Principle. Using one continuous motion reduces tissue damage.

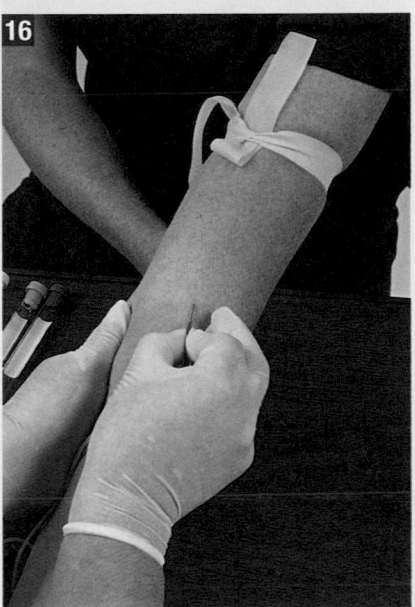

Make the puncture.

17. **Procedural Step.** Seat the needle by threading it forward an additional $\frac{1}{4}$ inch inside the center of the vein so that it does not twist out of the vein, even if you let go of it. Open the butterfly wings and securely rest the wings flat against the skin. Ensure that the needle does not move.

Principle. Seating the needle anchors the needle in the center of the vein and allows the use of both hands for changing tubes. Moving the needle is painful for the patient.

18. **Procedural Step.** Keep the tube and holder in a downward position so that the tube fills from the bottom up and not near the rubber stopper. Slowly push the tube forward to the end of the holder. This allows the needle to puncture the rubber stopper. Blood begins to flow into the tube. Allow the evacuated tube to fill to the exhaustion of the vacuum, as indicated by cessation of the blood flow into the tube. The suction of the evacuated tube automatically draws the blood into the tube.

Principle. The tube must fill from the bottom up to prevent venous reflux. If the evacuated tube is removed before the vacuum is exhausted, a rush of air enters the tube, damaging the red blood cells. Also, a tube containing an anticoagulant must be filled completely to ensure accurate test results.

Continued

PROCEDURE 31-2

PROCEDURE 31-2 **Venipuncture—Butterfly Method—cont'd**

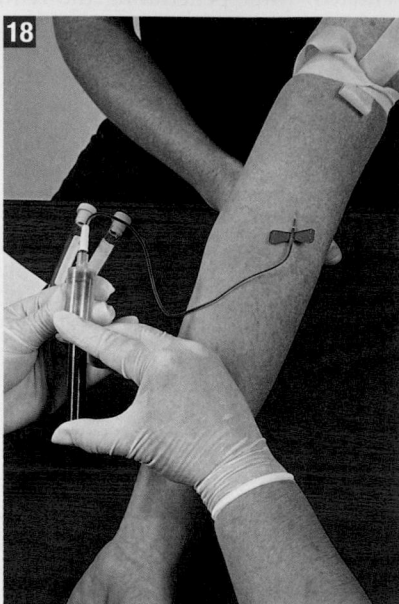

Fill the tubes in a downward position.

19. Procedural Step. Remove the tube from the plastic holder. If the tube contains a clot activator, gently invert the tube back and forth 5 times before laying it down. If the tube contains an anticoagulant, gently invert the tube 8 to 10 times.

Principle. The rubber sheath covers the point of the needle, stopping the flow of blood until the next tube is inserted. A tube containing an anticoagulant must be inverted before laying it down to prevent the blood from clotting. Careful mixing of the blood with a clot activator or an anticoagulant prevents hemolysis.

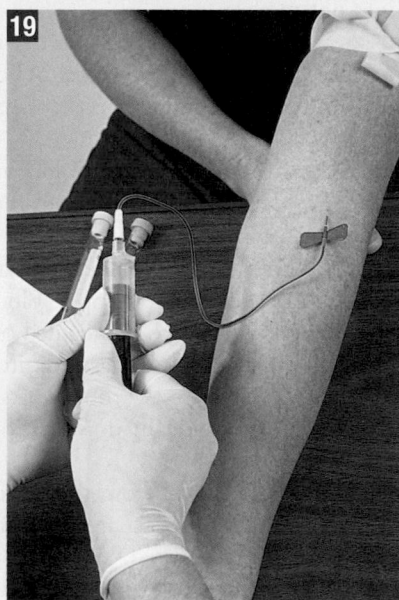

Remove the tube from the holder.

20. Procedural Step. Using the flange, carefully insert the next tube into the holder. Continue in this manner until the last tube has been filled.

21. Procedural Step. Remove the tension from the tourniquet by pulling upward on one of the flaps of the tourniquet. Ask the patient to unclench the fist.

Principle. The tourniquet tension must be removed before the needle. Otherwise, pressure on the vein from the tourniquet could cause internal and external bleeding around the puncture.

22. Procedural Step. Remove the last tube from the holder. Immediately invert the tube back and forth 5 times if it contains a clot activator and 8 to 10 times if it contains an anticoagulant.

Principle. Removing the last tube from the holder prevents blood from dripping out of the tip of the needle after it is removed from the patient's arm.

23. Procedural Step. Place a sterile gauze pad slightly above the puncture site. Grasp the setup just below the wings, and slowly withdraw the needle at the same angle as for penetration. Immediately move the gauze over the puncture site, and apply firm pressure. (*NOTE:* Do not apply pressure to the puncture site until the needle is completely removed.) Cooperative patients can be asked to assist by applying pressure with the gauze pad. If you are using a butterfly needle with a safety shield, grasp the base of the shield with the thumb and index fingers of one hand and, with the other hand, grasp either wing. Slide the wing back into the rear slot of the safety shield until you hear an audible click, which indicates the shield has locked into place (see Figure 31-18, *A, B*).

Principle. Placing the gauze pad above the puncture site helps prevent tissue movement as the needle is withdrawn and reduces patient discomfort. Careful withdrawal prevents further tissue damage.

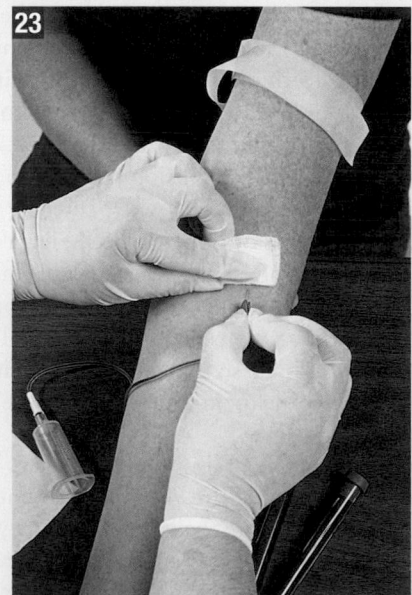

Release the tourniquet and remove the needle.

PROCEDURE 31-2 Venipuncture—Butterfly Method—cont'd

24. Procedural Step. Immediately discard the winged infusion set and attached plastic holder. Holding onto the plastic holder, first drop the needle into a biohazard sharps container followed by the tubing and holder. Do not remove the plastic holder from the setup; the plastic holder must be discarded and not reused.

Principle. Proper disposal is required by the OSHA Standard to prevent a needlestick injury; even if a safety shield has been activated to encase the butterfly needle, a needlestick injury can still result from the posterior needle, which is covered with only a rubber sleeve. Plastic holders are often contaminated with blood and must not be reused.

25. Procedural Step. Continue to apply pressure with the gauze pad. The arm can be elevated to facilitate clot formation. Do not allow the patient to bend the arm at the elbow because this increases blood loss from the puncture site.

Principle. Applying pressure reduces the leakage of blood from the puncture site externally or internally. Internal leakage into the tissues could result in a hematoma.

26. Procedural Step. Stay with the patient until the bleeding has stopped. Remove pressure, and inspect the puncture site to ensure that the opening is sealed with a clot. Apply an adhesive bandage to the puncture site. As an alternative, the gauze pad can be folded into quarters and taped onto the puncture site to be used as a pressure bandage. Instruct the patient not to pick up anything heavy for about an hour. (*NOTE:* If swelling or discoloration occurs, apply an ice pack to the site after bandaging it.)

Principle. Lifting a heavy object causes pressure on the puncture site, which could result in bleeding.

27. Procedural Step. Place the tubes in an upright position in a test tube rack. Remove the gloves, and sanitize your hands.

28. Procedural Step. Chart the procedure. Include the date and time, which arm and vein were used, unusual patient reactions, and your initials.

29. Procedural Step. If needed, process the specimen (e.g., centrifuging the specimen to separate serum from the cells). Test the specimen or prepare the specimen for transport to an outside laboratory for testing according to the medical office policy. If the specimen is to be transported to an outside laboratory, do the following:

a. Place the specimen tube in a biohazard specimen bag.

b. Place the laboratory request in the outside pocket of the specimen bag.

c. Properly handle and store the specimen while awaiting pickup by a laboratory courier.

d. Chart the date the specimen was transported to the laboratory in the patient's record.

Principle. The biohazard bag protects the laboratory courier from the possibility of an exposure incident. The outside laboratory must have the completed request form to know which laboratory tests have been ordered by the physician. The specimen must be handled and stored properly to maintain the in vivo characteristics of the specimen.

CHARTING EXAMPLE

Date	
4/10/XX	10:30 a.m. Venous blood specimen collected from Ⓛ arm. Picked up by Medical Center Laboratory on 4/10/XX. ———— ———— D. Glover, CMA (AAMA)

Memories *from* Externship

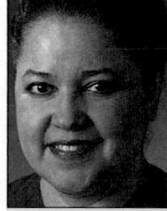

Dori Glover: One of the most terrifying things for me as a student was learning venipuncture. Even though I would practice during classroom laboratory hours and felt comfortable with it, it still scared me to know I would have to draw on a real person one day. When the day arrived to draw on my laboratory partner, I became sick to my stomach. In the end, we both got through it just fine and walked away without hurting each other. I spent days trying to prepare myself for that first experience, but after it was over, I felt more confident and relaxed that I could do this. At my externship site, I was able to perform several venipunctures a day, which raised my confidence level. Today venipuncture is my favorite responsibility of all. I would draw blood all day if I could. I know I could even draw with my eyes closed, but never would, of course! ■

What Would You Do? What Would You *Not* Do?

Case Study 3

Maud Gabriel is at the office complaining of persistent headaches and abdominal pain over the past 3 months. The physician gives Mrs. Gabriel a laboratory requisition to have her blood drawn and tested at an outside laboratory. Mrs. Gabriel says that her daughter who lives with her works as a phlebotomist at the local hospital. Mrs. Gabriel wants to know whether her daughter can draw her blood at home and then drop it off at the laboratory. She says that the last time she had her blood drawn, they had to stick her two times and then she got a big bruise on her arm afterward. She says the laboratory technician kept digging around in her arm to find the vein and that it was quite painful. ■

PROBLEMS ENCOUNTERED WITH VENIPUNCTURE

Sometimes the medical assistant encounters problems when attempting to draw blood from a patient. The appropriate response depends on the type of problem.

Failure to Obtain Blood

Periodically, even individuals highly skilled at performing venipuncture have difficulty obtaining blood. Although large and prominent veins make it easier to collect the blood specimen, conditions often exist that make the procedure more difficult.

It is often difficult to draw blood from obese patients who have small, superficial veins and whose veins suitable for venipuncture are buried in adipose tissue. Elderly patients with arteriosclerosis may have veins that are thick and hard, making them difficult to puncture. Other patients have veins that are small or have a thin wall, making the veins likely to collapse. After two unsuccessful attempts at venipuncture, the medical assistant should seek assistance in obtaining the blood specimen.

Factors that result in failure to obtain blood after the needle has been inserted include not inserting the needle far enough, preventing it from entering the vein (Figure 31-21); insertion of the needle too far, causing it to go through the vein; and the bevel opening becoming lodged against the wall of the vein. In these instances, most authorities recommend removal of the needle, rather than trying to probe the vein. Probing is often uncomfortable for the patient and can affect the integrity of the blood specimen, leading to inaccurate test results. Occasionally, an evacuated tube loses its vacuum because of a manufacturing defect or through improper handling of the tube. If suspected, this problem can be corrected by removing the defective tube and inserting another vacuum tube.

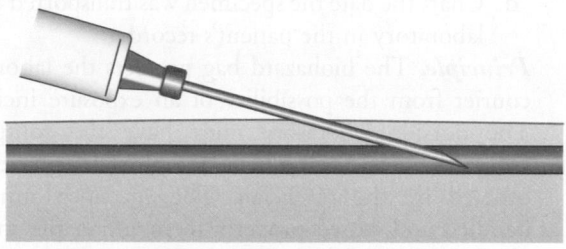

A. Correct insertion of the needle into the vein.

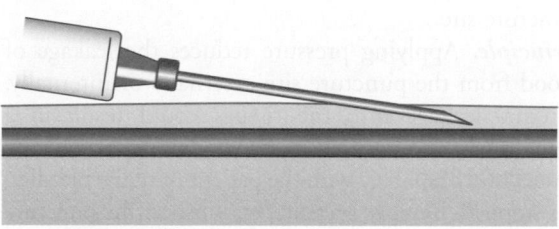

B. Improper angle of insertion (<15 degrees), causing the needle to enter above the vein.

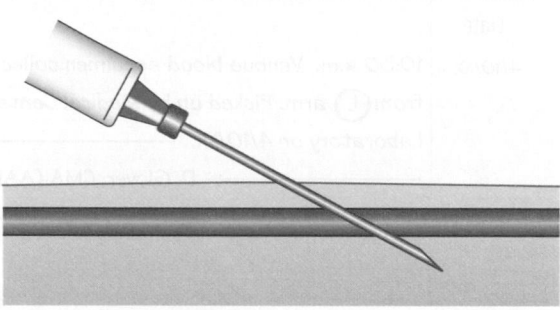

C. Improper angle of insertion (>15 degrees), causing the needle to go through the vein.

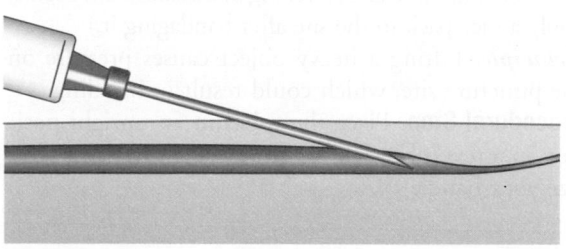

D. Collapsed vein (most likely to occur in persons with small veins).

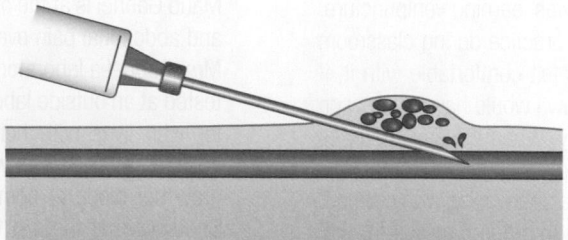

E. The beveled opening is partially within and partially outside of the vein, causing a hematoma.

Figure 31-21 Problems encountered with venipuncture.

Inappropriate Puncture Sites

If a patient complains of pain or soreness in a potential venipuncture site, this area should be avoided. In addition, any skin areas that are scarred, bruised, burned, or adjacent to areas of infection should not be used. A venipuncture should not be performed on an arm with edema or an arm on the same side as a mastectomy. Swelling makes is more difficult to locate a vein and results in a longer time for healing of the puncture site to occur. Other sites to avoid include an arm that has a cast applied to it and an arm on the same side as a radical mastectomy.

Scarred and Sclerosed Veins

An individual who has had many venipunctures over a period of years often develops scar tissue in the wall of the vein. Elderly patients may have veins that have become thickened from arteriosclerosis. In both cases, the veins feel stiff and hard when palpated. A scarred or sclerosed vein is difficult to stick, and the blood return may be poor owing to a narrowed lumen; it is recommended that another vein be used for the venipuncture. If this is impossible, the needle should be inserted with careful pressure to avoid going completely through the vein.

Rolling Veins

The median cubital vein, located in the center of the antecubital space, is considered the best vein for a venipuncture. Sometimes it is impossible to use this vein, however, such as when it lies deep in the tissues and cannot be palpated or is scarred from repeated venipunctures. The veins on either side of the median cubital (cephalic or basilic) can be used, but they have a tendency to "roll," or move away from the needle, escaping puncture. To prevent rolling, firm pressure should be applied below and to the side of the vein to stabilize it as the needle is inserted.

Collapsing Veins

Veins are most likely to collapse in individuals who have small veins or veins with thin walls. This is particularly true when the vacuum tube method is used. The "sucking action" exerted on the vein when the pressure in the vacuum is released causes the vein to collapse, blocking the flow of blood into the tube (see Figure 31-21). The typical result observed is that a small amount of blood enters the tube and then stops. Because better control and less pressure on the vein is possible, the butterfly or syringe method of venipuncture is recommended to obtain the specimen in patients with small veins.

Premature Needle Withdrawal

Patient movement or improper venipuncture technique can cause the needle to come out of the vein prematurely. Because of the pressure exerted by the tourniquet, blood may be forced out of the puncture site, and immediate action is required to prevent a hematoma. The tourniquet should be removed at once, a gauze pad placed on the puncture site, and pressure applied until the bleeding has stopped.

Hematoma

A hematoma is caused by blood leaking from the puncture site of the vein and into the surrounding tissues, resulting in a bruise. A hematoma is caused by a needle that is inserted too far and goes through the vein, a bevel opening that is partially in the vein and partially out of the vein (see Figure 31-21), and insufficient pressure applied to the puncture site after removing the needle. The first sign of a hematoma is a sudden swelling around the puncture site. If this occurs when the needle is in the patient's vein, first the tourniquet and then the needle should be removed immediately, and pressure should be applied to the puncture site until the bleeding stops.

Hemolysis

The blood specimen should be handled carefully at all times. Blood cells are fragile, and rough handling may cause hemolysis, or breakdown of the blood cells. Hemolyzed blood specimens produce inaccurate test results. To prevent hemolysis, these guidelines should be followed:

1. Store the vacuum tubes at room temperature because chilled tubes can result in hemolysis.
2. Allow the alcohol to air-dry completely before performing the venipuncture. Alcohol entering a blood specimen can cause hemolysis.
3. Use an appropriate-gauge needle to collect the specimen. Using a small-gauge needle (e.g., 25 G) can cause the blood cells to rupture as they pass through the lumen of the needle.
4. Practice good technique in collecting the specimen; excessive trauma to the blood vessel can result in hemolysis.
5. Always handle the blood tube carefully; do not shake it or handle it roughly.

Fainting

Occasionally, a patient experiences dizziness or fainting during or after a venipuncture. Should this occur, the most immediate concern is to protect the patient from injury, for example, by preventing the patient from falling. The patient should be placed in a position that promotes blood flow to the brain, and the physician should be notified for further treatment; see the box *Highlight on Vasovagal Syncope (Fainting)*.

OBTAINING A SERUM SPECIMEN

Serum

Serum is plasma from which the clotting factor fibrinogen has been removed.

Serum is normally clear in appearance and light yellow to yellow in color. Serum contains many dissolved

Highlight on Vasovagal Syncope (Fainting)

Most people experience no change in their sense of well-being when they have blood taken. A very small percentage of individuals experience a type of fainting, however, known as *vasovagal syncope.*

Cause and Symptoms

Vasovagal syncope is caused by unpleasant physical or emotional stimuli, such as pain, fright, and the sight of blood. A sudden pooling of blood occurs, which results in a sudden decrease in blood pressure. This momentarily deprives the brain of blood, causing a temporary loss of consciousness, usually lasting only 1 to 2 minutes. Vasovagal syncope usually occurs when an individual is in an upright position, as in standing or sitting. Before fainting, the patient usually experiences some warning signals, such as sudden light-headedness, nausea, weakness, yawning, paleness, blurred vision, a feeling of warmth, and sweating followed by drooping eyelids; a weak, rapid pulse; and finally unconsciousness.

Treatment

A person who is about to faint should be placed in a position that facilitates blood flow to the brain and told to breathe deeply. The preferred position is lying down (supine) with the legs elevated and the collar and clothing loosened. This position may not always be possible, such as when a patient is seated and the venipuncture needle has already been inserted. In this case, the tourniquet and then the needle should be removed, and the patient's head should be lowered between the legs. An individual who has fainted should be protected from injury by falling and should be placed in a position that facilitates blood flow to the brain, as just described.

Prevention

Fainting during or after venipuncture is more likely in the following individuals: patients having a venipuncture for the first time, young patients, thin patients, patients with a low diastolic or high systolic blood pressure, patients with a history of fainting, nervous and apprehensive patients, and patients who are very quiet or very talkative. Fainting often can be prevented by identifying and closely observing individuals who are more likely to faint (as described). Talking to the patient often helps relax the patient and divert attention from the venipuncture procedure. If a patient has a history of fainting, he or she should be in a semi-Fowler position for the venipuncture procedure because people rarely faint in this position. Other factors that contribute to fainting and that should be avoided include fatigue, lack of sleep, hunger, and environmental factors, such as a noisy, crowded, or overheated room. ■

---

substances, such as glucose, cholesterol, sodium, potassium, chloride, antibodies, hormones, and enzymes. As a result, many laboratory tests require a serum specimen to determine whether these substances are within normal limits and to detect substances that should not normally be in the serum, and that, if present, indicate a pathologic condition.

Tube Selection

A tube without an anticoagulant (e.g., red-stoppered or SST) must be used to collect the blood specimen, to allow the specimen to separate into serum and clotted blood cells. Because the amount of serum recovered is only a portion of the specimen, a blood specimen must be drawn that is 2.5 times the amount required for the test. If 2 mL of serum is required, a 5-mL tube of blood must be collected; if 3 mL of serum is required, an 8-mL tube is collected, and if 4 mL of serum is required, a 10-mL tube is collected.

Preparation of the Specimen

After the blood specimen has been collected, the red-stoppered tube or SST must be allowed to stand upright at room temperature for 30 to 45 minutes before being centrifuged. This allows clot formation of the blood cells, which yields more serum from the specimen. If the specimen is centrifuged too soon after collection of the blood specimen, the clotting factors do not have an opportunity to settle down into the cell layer to form a whole blood clot. The result of this is the formation of a *fibrin clot*

in the serum layer. A fibrin clot is a spongy substance that occupies space, interfering with adequate serum collection (Figure 31-22). The blood specimen should not be allowed to stand for longer than 1 hour, however, because leaching of substances from the cell layer into the serum may occur. This leaching of substances changes the integrity of the serum, leading to inaccurate test results.

Removal of Serum

After the blood cells have clotted by allowing the specimen to stand, the specimen is centrifuged for 10 minutes. If a red-stoppered tube has been used to collect the specimen, the serum is removed from the clot using a pipet and is placed in a separate transfer tube. It is important that proper technique be employed in removing the serum, to avoid disturbing the cell layer of the clot and drawing red blood cells into the serum layer. If cells do enter the serum, the entire specimen must be recentrifuged.

When the serum has been removed from the blood specimen, the medical assistant should hold the specimen in the transfer tube up to good light. The serum specimen should be inspected for the presence of intact red blood cells or hemolyzed blood; in both cases, the specimen has a reddish appearance. A specimen that has a reddish appearance must be recentrifuged. If the specimen contains intact red blood cells, they settle to the bottom of the tube, and the serum can be removed. If the blood is hemolyzed, recentrifugation would not make the red color disappear because the red blood cells have ruptured and released hemoglobin into the

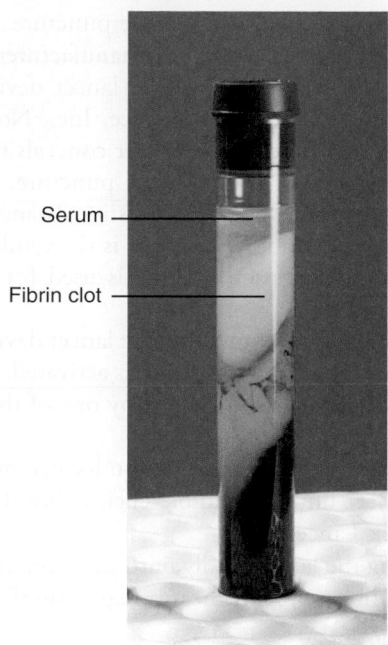

Figure 31-22 A fibrin clot may interfere with adequate collection of serum.

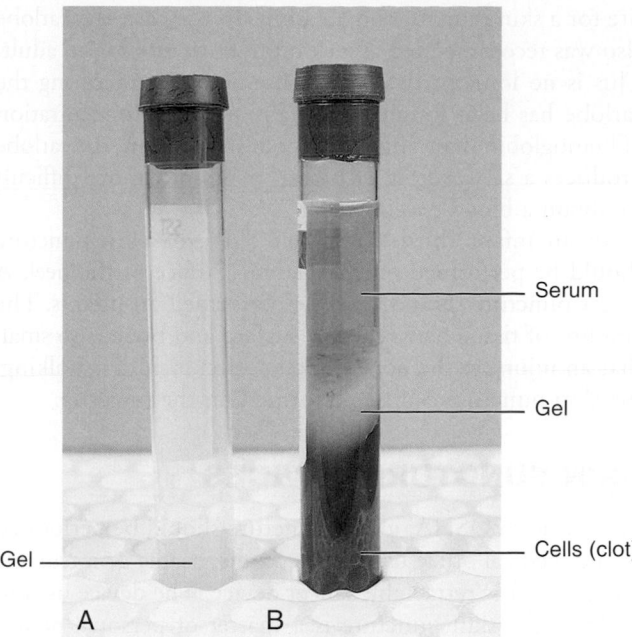

Figure 31-23 Serum separator tubes. **A,** An unused tube that contains the thixotropic gel in the bottom of the tube. **B,** A tube that has been used to collect a blood specimen. During centrifugation, the gel temporarily becomes fluid and moves to the dividing point between the serum and blood cells in a fibrin clot.

serum. Hemolyzed serum is unsuitable for laboratory tests because the results would be inaccurate; another blood specimen must be collected.

Serum Separator Tubes

A serum separator tube (SST), which is also known as a gel barrier tube, is an evacuated tube specially designed to facilitate the collection of a serum specimen. The SST tube is identified by a red/gray stopper (or gold stopper if using Hemogard tubes) and is used for collection and separation of blood. The serum separator tube contains a thixotropic gel, which is in a solid state at the bottom of the unused tube (Figure 31-23, *A*).

The blood specimen is collected and processed following the appropriate venipuncture method. The specimen must be allowed to stand in an upright position for 30 to 45 minutes for proper clot formation of the blood cells and centrifuged as previously described. During centrifugation, the gel temporarily becomes fluid and moves to the dividing point between the serum and clotted cells, where it re-forms into a solid gel, serving as a physical and chemical barrier between the serum and the clot (Figure 31-23, *B*). It is important to centrifuge the specimen for the proper length of time (i.e., 10 minutes). Centrifuging the specimen for less than 10 minutes can result in an incomplete gel barrier between the serum and the clot.

The serum can be transported or stored in the separator tube; the medical assistant must inspect the tube carefully to ensure that the gel barrier is firmly attached to the glass wall. If a complete barrier has not formed, the serum specimen must be removed and placed in a properly labeled transfer tube to prevent leaching of substances from the cell

layer into the serum, affecting the accuracy of the test results.

SKIN PUNCTURE

A skin puncture is used to obtain a capillary blood specimen and is also called a *capillary puncture.* Laboratory testing of a capillary blood specimen is usually performed at the medical office. Examples of such tests are hemoglobin, hematocrit, blood glucose, mononucleosis, and prothrombin time.

A skin puncture is performed when a test requires only a small blood specimen. Skin puncture is the method preferred for obtaining blood from infants and young children. Collecting blood in this age group by venipuncture is often difficult and may damage veins and surrounding tissues. In addition, infants and young children have such a small blood volume that removing large quantities of blood may cause anemia. A skin puncture also might be performed as a last resort on an adult when a blood specimen is needed and there are no acceptable veins. Before collecting a capillary blood specimen, the medical assistant must (1) select a puncture site, (2) select the skin puncture device, and (3) obtain the proper microcollection device to collect the specimen.

PUNCTURE SITES

The puncture site varies depending on the age of the patient. The fingertip of the third or fourth finger is the preferred site for a skin puncture on an adult. In the past, the earlobe also was recommended as a skin puncture site for an adult. This is no longer true. Blood obtained by puncturing the earlobe has been found to contain a higher concentration of hemoglobin than fingertip blood. In addition, the earlobe produces a slower flow of blood, making it more difficult to obtain a blood specimen.

In an infant (birth to 1 year old), the skin puncture should be performed on the plantar surface of the heel. A finger puncture should *never* be performed on infants. The amount of tissue between skin surface and bone is so small that an injury to the bone is likely. After a child is walking, the skin puncture can be performed on the fingertip.

SKIN PUNCTURE DEVICES

According to OSHA, a skin puncture should be performed in the medical office using either a disposable or a reusable semiautomatic retractable lancet device. The device used to perform the skin puncture is a matter of personal preference, and the technique for performing the puncture depends on the device that is used. A description of skin puncture devices is presented next, and procedures for using them are presented at the end of this section.

Regardless of the skin puncture device, the puncture must not penetrate deeper than 3.1 mm on adults and 2.0 mm on infants (plantar surface of the heel) and children. If the puncture is deeper than this, the bone may be penetrated, which could result in the painful and serious conditions of osteochondritis or osteomyelitis. **Osteochondritis** is inflammation of bone and cartilage, and **osteomyelitis** is inflammation of the bone or bone marrow caused by bacterial infection. To avoid these complications, skin puncture devices are used with a spring-loaded blade (available in different lengths) to control the depth of puncture. The blade length used to perform a skin puncture is based on the sizes of the patient's fingers and the amount of blood specimen required. Adults with thin fingers and children require a shorter blade to avoid penetrating the bone. A longer blade must be used to obtain enough blood to fill a microcollection device, whereas a shorter blade can be used if only a drop of blood is needed.

OSHA does not recommend the use of lancets that are not retractable. A lancet that is not retractable increases the possibility that the medical assistant will stick himself or herself accidentally, resulting in an exposure incident. A disadvantage of a lancet that is spring-loaded and does not retract automatically is that some patients may become apprehensive and flinch when they see the point of the lancet. Children might pull their hands out of the medical assistant's grasp.

Disposable Semiautomatic Lancet

A disposable semiautomatic retractable lancet consists of a spring-loaded plastic holder with a metal blade inside the holder. Disposable lancets are available in different lengths

of blades to control the depth of the puncture. The plastic holder may be color-coded by the manufacturer for ease in identifying the blade length of the lancet device, such as Surgilance Safety Lancets (Surgilance, Inc., Norcross, Ga) (Figure 31-24, *A*). The plastic holder conceals the blade so the patient cannot see it during the puncture, as with the CoaguChek Lancet (Roche Diagnostics, Branchburg, NJ) (Figure 31-24, *B*). Another example is the Quikheel Infant Lancet (Becton Dickinson), which is used for heel punctures on infants.

To perform the skin puncture, the lancet device is placed on the patient's skin, and the device is activated. Depending on the brand, this is accomplished by one of the following methods:

- Depressing an activation button located on the top of the lancet until an audible click is heard (e.g., CoaguChek Lancet)
- Pushing the lancet firmly onto the puncture site until an audible click is heard (e.g., Surgilance Safety Lancet)

When the device is activated, the spring forces the blade into the skin and retracts the blade into the holder. The concealed blade and automatic puncture tend to result in less patient apprehension. After the puncture, the entire lancet device is discarded in a biohazard sharps container. Procedure 31-3 describes the skin puncture procedure using a disposable semiautomatic lancet.

Reusable Semiautomatic Lancet

A wide variety of reusable semiautomatic lancets are commercially available; however, not all are appropriate for use in the medical office. Some of these devices are suitable for use only by an individual patient to perform home blood glucose monitoring. When used by more than one patient in the medical office, they have been associated with the transmission of hepatitis B. The safest reusable device is one in which the part that becomes contaminated is retractable and can be disposed of easily. This type of device reduces the risk of a sharps injury and infection from a contaminated sharp. An example of a reusable lancet that is safe to use in the medical office is the Glucolet II (Bayer Corporation, Morristown, NJ).

The Glucolet II consists of a plastic spring-loaded lancet holder and a retractable lancet/endcap (Figure 31-24, *C*). The lancet holder is reusable, whereas the lancet/endcap is retractable and disposable and is meant for only one use. To perform the puncture, the lancet/endcap is placed on the patient's skin, and a release button is depressed. The spring forces the blade into the skin and retracts the blade into the endcap. After the procedure, the lancet/endcap is discarded in a biohazard sharps container.

MICROCOLLECTION DEVICES

After the skin has been punctured, a capillary blood specimen must be collected. The blood specimen can be

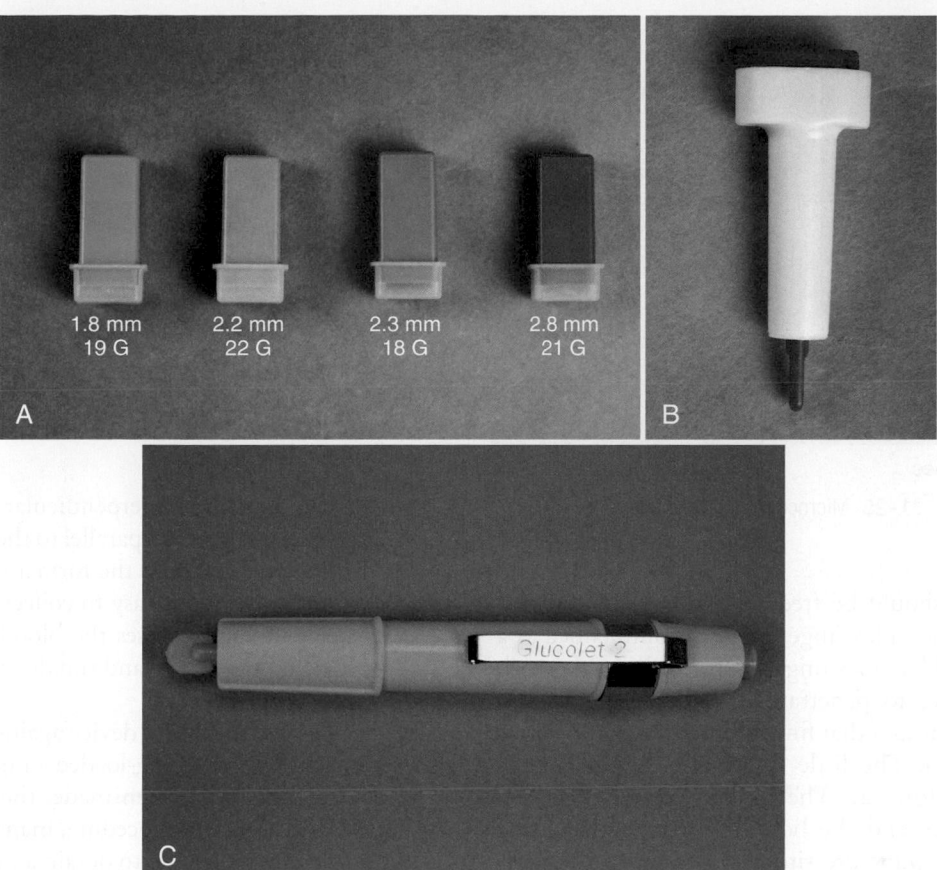

Figure 31-24 **A,** Surgilance color-coded lancet devices. **B,** CoaguChek Lancet device. **C,** Glucolet 2.

collected directly onto a reagent strip, such as occurs with blood glucose monitors. It also can be collected in a small container known as a *microcollection device*. The device depends on the laboratory equipment running the test. Common microcollection devices are capillary tubes and microcollection tubes.

Capillary Tubes

A capillary tube consists of a disposable glass or plastic tube (Figure 31-25, *A*). Depending on the size of the tube, it can hold 5 to 75 μl of blood. In the medical office, a capillary tube is used to collect a blood specimen for a hematocrit determination. This procedure is presented in Chapter 32.

Microcollection Tubes

A microcollection tube consists of a small plastic tube with a removable blood collector tip. The tip is designed to collect capillary blood from a skin puncture, which results in a relatively large blood specimen. After the specimen has been collected, the collector tip is removed, discarded, and replaced by a plastic plug. Microcollection tubes are available with or without anticoagulants. The plugs are color-coded and correspond to the color-coded evacuated tube system used in venipuncture. One such device is the Microtainer (Becton Dickinson) (Figure 31-25, *B*).

GUIDELINES FOR PERFORMING A FINGER PUNCTURE

1. If a laboratory test requires advance preparation, before you perform the finger puncture, verify that the patient has prepared properly. If this is not the case, do not collect the specimen unless directed otherwise by the physician. If the finger puncture is to be rescheduled, carefully review the preparation requirements with the patient.

2. The patient should be seated comfortably in a chair. The arm should be firmly supported and extended with the palmar surface of the hand facing up. Never perform a skin puncture with the patient sitting on a stool or standing. The patient may faint and injure himself or herself.

3. Instruct the patient to remain still during the procedure. Explain to the patient that the procedure should be relatively quick and only slightly uncomfortable. Just before making the puncture, tell the patient that he or she will "feel a small stick." This prevents startling the patient, which could cause the patient to move.

4. Use the lateral part of the tip of the third or fourth finger (middle or ring finger) of the nondominant hand for the puncture site. The capillary beds in these fingers are large, and the skin is easy to penetrate. The

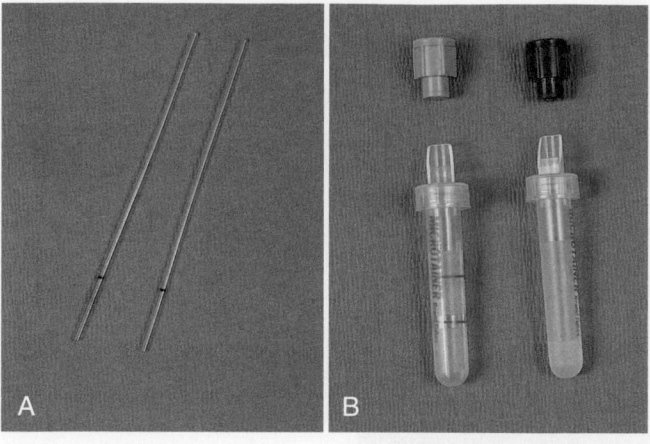

Capillary tubes   Microcollection tubes

Figure 31-25 Microcollection devices.

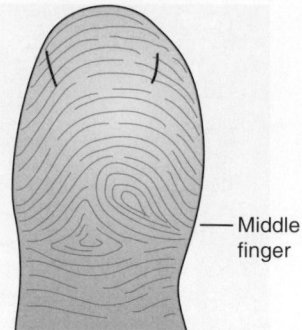

Figure 31-26 Recommended sites for a finger puncture.

puncture site should be free of lesions, scars, bruises, and edema. The index finger is not recommended as a puncture site. The index finger is more calloused, which makes it harder to penetrate than the other fingers. Also, the patient uses that finger more and would notice the pain longer. The little finger also should not be used as a puncture site. The amount of tissue between the skin surface and the bone is so small that using this finger as a puncture site could result in injury to the bone.

5. After selecting the puncture site, warm the site to increase the blood flow to the capillary bed. Warming the site can be accomplished by gently massaging the finger 5 or 6 times from base to tip, or by placing the hand in warm water for a few minutes (105° F [40° C]). Warming the site promotes bleeding after an effective puncture.

6. Cleanse the site with an antiseptic wipe, and allow it to dry thoroughly. The site must be dry to allow a round drop of blood to form on the finger. Otherwise, the drop would leach out onto the skin of the patient's finger and be difficult to collect. In addition, alcohol entering the capillary specimen contaminates it, leading to inaccurate test results. Alcohol also causes the patient to experience a stinging sensation when the puncture is made.

7. Firmly grasp the finger in front of the most distal knuckle joint. Apply enough pressure to cause the fingertip to become hard and red so that adequate penetration and depth of puncture will occur.

8. Make the puncture in the fleshy portion of the fingertip, slightly to the side of center. To prevent injury to the bone, do not puncture the side or very tip of the finger. The blade of the lancet should be positioned so

that the puncture is perpendicular to the lines of the fingerprint rather than parallel to the fingerprint (Figure 31-26). This facilitates the formation of a well-formed drop of blood that is easy to collect. A puncture that is not perpendicular causes the blood flow to follow the lines of the fingerprint and run down the finger, making it difficult to collect.

9. Firmly press the lancet device against the puncture site, and activate the spring-loaded puncturing device. If a good puncture has been made, the blood flows freely. When learning this procedure, many individuals do not apply enough pressure to obtain a puncture that is deep enough. If this occurs, a poor blood flow results, and the patient has to be punctured again. A deep puncture hurts no more than a superficial one and provides a much better blood flow.

10. Wipe away the first drop of blood with a gauze pad. The first drop of blood is diluted with alcohol and tissue fluid and is not a suitable specimen for testing. Using the first drop of blood may lead to inaccurate test results.

11. Allow a large drop of blood to form by applying continual gentle pressure near the puncture site. Collect the blood specimen using a reagent strip or the appropriate microcollection device. If the required amount of blood is not obtained, you can gently massage the tissue surrounding the puncture site to promote blood flow. Do not squeeze or massage excessively because doing so causes dilution of the blood specimen with tissue fluids, which can affect the accuracy of the test results.

12. Check the puncture site to make sure the bleeding has stopped. Apply an adhesive bandage, if needed. A bandage is not recommended for children younger than 2 years old. The bandage may irritate the skin of a young child, and the child might put the bandage in his or her mouth, aspirate it, and choke.

PROCEDURE 31-3   Skin Puncture—Disposable Semiautomatic Lancet Device

Outcome Obtain a capillary blood specimen.

Equipment/Supplies

- Disposable gloves
- Antiseptic wipe
- CoaguChek lancet

- Sterile 2 × 2 gauze pad
- Adhesive bandage
- Biohazard sharps container

1. **Procedural Step.** Sanitize your hands.
2. **Procedural Step.** Greet the patient and introduce yourself. Identify the patient by asking the patient to state his or her full name and date of birth. Compare this information with the demographic data in the patient's chart. If the patient was required to prepare for the test (e.g., fasting, medication restriction), determine whether he or she has prepared properly. If the patient has not followed the patient preparation requirements, notify the physician for instructions on handling this situation.
3. **Procedural Step.** Assemble the equipment. Open the sterile gauze packet and lay it flat to allow the gauze pad to rest on the inside of its wrapper.

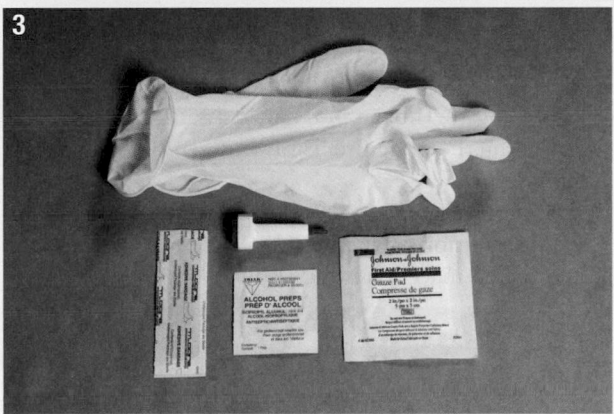

Assemble the equipment.

4. **Procedural Step.** Explain the procedure to the patient, and reassure the patient.
   Principle. Reassurance should be offered to reduce apprehension.
5. **Procedural Step.** Seat the patient comfortably in a chair. The patient's arm should be firmly supported and extended with the palmar surface of the hand facing up.
6. **Procedural Step.** Select an appropriate puncture site. Use the lateral part of the tip of the third or fourth finger of the nondominant hand to make the puncture. If the patient's finger is cold, you can warm it by gently massaging the finger 5 or 6 times from base to tip, or by placing the hand in warm water for a few minutes.

Principle. Warming the site increases the blood flow to the area and promotes bleeding from the puncture site.

7. **Procedural Step.** Cleanse the site with an antiseptic wipe. Allow the site to air-dry, and after cleansing it, do not touch the area, wipe the area with gauze, or fan the area with your hand.
   Principle. The site must be allowed to air-dry to allow enough time for the alcohol to destroy microorganisms on the patient's skin. If the site is dry, a round drop of blood forms on the finger, making it easy to collect the specimen. If the site is not dry, the blood leaches out and runs down the finger, making it difficult to collect. Residual alcohol entering the blood specimen can cause hemolysis, leading to inaccurate test results. In addition, residual alcohol causes the patient to experience a stinging sensation when the puncture is made. Touching or fanning the area causes contamination, and the cleansing process has to be repeated.
8. **Procedural Step.** Apply gloves. Using a twisting motion, remove the plastic post from the lancet.
   Principle. Gloves provide a barrier precaution against bloodborne pathogens.
9. **Procedural Step.** Without touching the puncture site, firmly grasp the patient's finger in front of the most distal knuckle joint. Apply enough pressure to cause the fingertip to become hard and red. Position the blade of the lancet perpendicular to the lines of the fingerprint on the fleshy portion of the fingertip, slightly to the side of center.

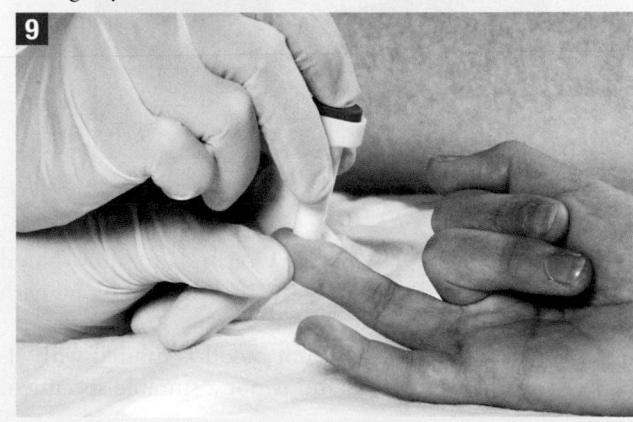

Make the puncture.

Continued

PROCEDURE 31-3

Principle. The site must be grasped with enough pressure so that adequate penetration and depth of puncture can occur. Punctures that are not perpendicular cause the blood to run down the finger, making it difficult to collect. Puncturing the side or tip of the finger may cause the lancet to penetrate the bone.

10. **Procedural Step.** Firmly depress the activation button, without moving the lancet or finger, until an audible click is heard. Pressing the activation button causes the lancet to puncture the skin and then retract into its plastic casing. A well-made puncture results in a free-flowing wound that needs only slight pressure to make it bleed.

    Principle. Moving the lancet or finger before the process is complete can result in an inadequate puncture and poor blood flow.

11. **Procedural Step.** Immediately dispose of the lancet device in a biohazard sharps container.

    Principle. Proper disposal of contaminated sharps is required by the OSHA Standard to prevent exposure to bloodborne pathogens.

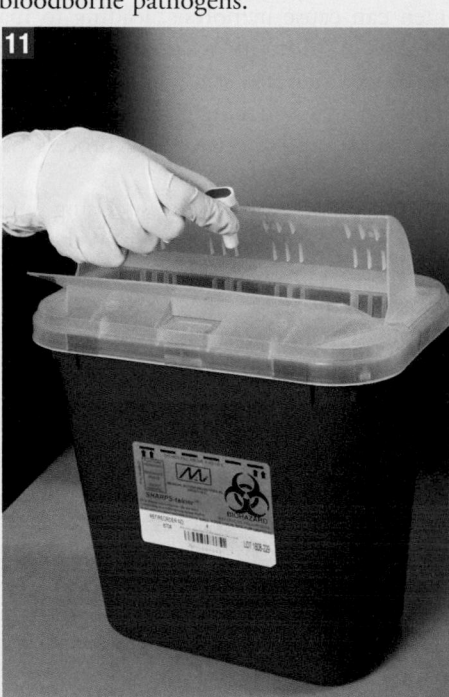

Discard the lancet.

12. **Procedural Step.** Wait a few seconds to allow blood flow to begin. Wipe away the first drop of blood with a gauze pad.

    Principle. The first drop of blood is diluted with alcohol and tissue fluid and is not a suitable specimen.

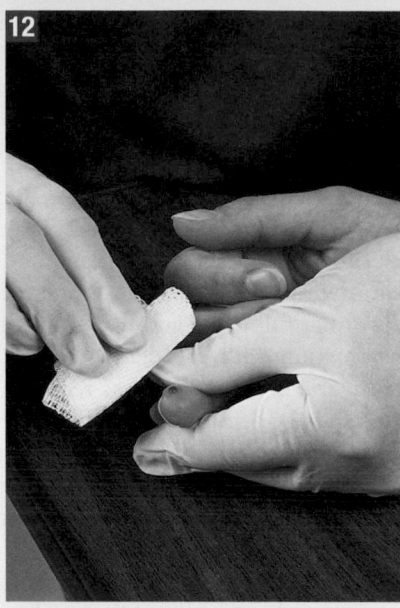

Wipe away the first drop of blood.

13. **Procedural Step.** Use the second drop of blood for the test. Allow a large well-rounded drop of blood to form by holding the hand in a downward position and applying gentle continuous pressure without squeezing the finger. You can massage the tissue surrounding the puncture firmly but gently to encourage blood flow.

    Principle. Squeezing or massaging the site excessively causes dilution of the blood sample with tissue fluid, leading to inaccurate test results.

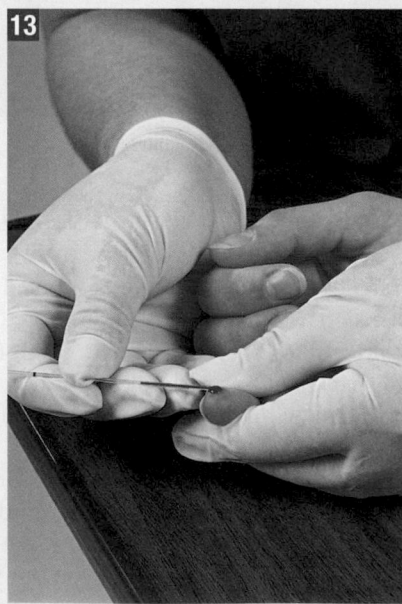

Collect the specimen.

PROCEDURE 31-3 Skin Puncture—Disposable Semiautomatic Lancet Device

14. Procedural Step. Collect the blood specimen on a test strip or in the appropriate microcollection device.

15. Procedural Step. Have the patient hold a gauze pad over the puncture and apply pressure until the bleeding stops. As a safety precaution, remain with the patient until the bleeding stops. If needed, apply an adhesive bandage.

16. Procedural Step. Test the blood specimen by following the manufacturer's instructions that accompany the blood analyzer or testing kit.

17. Procedural Step. Remove the gloves, and sanitize your hands.

MEDICAL PRACTICE and the LAW

Phlebotomy is an invasive procedure that can harm the patient if performed incorrectly. Sharps and medical waste contaminated with blood must be disposed of according to federal regulations. Laboratory tests involving blood must be performed correctly for accurate results. Incorrect results can lead to inaccurate diagnosis and treatment. Currently, performing HIV testing requires the patient's written consent. If the patient has questions regarding HIV, refer him or her to the physician for discussion. Never give out laboratory results without checking with the physician. Medical assistants are usually given permission by the physician to relay negative laboratory test results; however, abnormal laboratory results should be relayed by the physician. The medical assistant does not have the medical knowledge to answer the questions the patient may have when the results are abnormal. HIV results (negative or positive) should be given only by the physician. Never speculate to the patient or coworkers about the results of any test. All test results must remain confidential.

Use appropriate personal protective equipment to prevent the transmission of bloodborne pathogens to protect yourself, your coworkers, and your patients. ■

What Would You Do? What Would You Not Do? RESPONSES

Case Study 1
Page 755

What Did Dori Do?
❑ Told Angela that it was fine to have her friend there while she gets her blood drawn.
❑ Told Angela that she could not have the blood drawn out of her left arm because a good vein could not be located in that arm.
❑ Told Angela that using the hand veins is always the last choice when drawing blood. Explained that there are a lot of nerve endings in the hand, which makes it hurt more.
❑ Explained to Angela that there will just be a small stick and that it will heal quickly, and there should be no reason it would affect her softball game this evening.
❑ Tried to relax and reassure Angela before the venipuncture. Carefully explained the procedure to her because it was her first one.
❑ Because Angela was nervous, took precautions to prevent her from fainting by placing her in a semi-Fowler position on the examining table.
❑ Had Angela's friend stand near the head of the table to help calm her down.

What Did Dori Not Do?
❑ Did not try to draw Angela's blood from her left arm or hand.
❑ Did not ignore the fact that Angela was nervous about the venipuncture.

What Would You Do?/What Would You Not Do?
Review Dori's response and place a checkmark next to the information you included in your response. List additional information you included in your response.

_____
_____
_____
_____
_____
_____

Case Study 2
Page 759

What Did Dori Do?
❑ Told Buzz that when a butterfly setup is used, the air in the tubing alters the test results. Explained that the red tube is used to get rid of the air, and because it is not needed for testing, it is thrown away.

Continued

What Would You Do? What Would You *Not* Do? RESPONSES—cont'd

❏ Stressed to Buzz how important it is to have his blood tested every week to ensure there is not too much or too little of the Coumadin in his body. Explained to him again what might occur if his Coumadin were at the wrong level.

❏ Told Buzz that the office would help him locate a medical laboratory where he will be vacationing, so he can have his test done.

❏ Made sure that Buzz had a laboratory requisition so that he could have his test done while he was on vacation.

What Did Dori Not Do?

❏ Did not tell Buzz that it would be all right to skip his prothrombin test during his vacation.

What Would You Do?/What Would You *Not* Do?

Review Dori's response and place a checkmark next to the information you included in your response. List additional information you included in your response.

_____
_____
_____
_____
_____
_____

Case Study 3
Page 771

What Did Dori Do?

❏ Told Mrs. Gabriel that the laboratory can accept only specimens drawn at the laboratory or at the medical office.

❏ Told Mrs. Gabriel that if it would make her feel more comfortable, the laboratory could drop off the blood-drawing supplies at the office, and her blood could be drawn tomorrow at the office.

❏ Informed the physician about Mrs. Gabriel's experience at the laboratory.

What Did Dori Not Do?

❏ Did not tell Mrs. Gabriel that probing a vein could cause the test results to be inaccurate.

What Would You Do?/What Would You *Not* Do?

Review Dori's response and place a checkmark next to the information you included in your response. List additional information you included in your response.

_____
_____
_____
_____

TERMINOLOGY REVIEW

Medical Term	Word Parts	Definition
Antecubital space	*ante-:* before	The surface of the arm in front of the elbow.
Anticoagulant	*anti-:* against	A substance that inhibits blood clotting.
Buffy coat		A thin, light-colored layer of white blood cells and platelets that lies between a top layer of plasma and a bottom layer of red blood cells when an anticoagulant has been added to a blood specimen.
Evacuated tube		A closed glass or plastic tube that contains a premeasured vacuum.
Hematoma	*hemat/o-:* blood *-oma:* tumor or swelling	A swelling or mass of coagulated blood caused by a break in a blood vessel.
Hemoconcentration	*hem/o-:* blood	An increase in the concentration of the nonfilterable blood components in the blood vessels, such as red blood cells, enzymes, iron, and calcium, as a result of a decrease in the fluid content of the blood.
Hemolysis	*hem/o-:* blood *-lysis:* breakdown	The breakdown of blood cells.
Osteochondritis	*oste/o-:* bone *myel/o-:* bone marrow *-itis:* inflammation	Inflammation of bone and cartilage.

TERMINOLOGY REVIEW—cont'd

Medical Term	Word Parts	Definition
Osteomyelitis	*oste/o-:* bone *myel/o-:* bone marrow *-itis:* inflammation	Inflammation of the bone or bone marrow as a result of bacterial infection.
Phlebotomist	*phleb/o-:* vein *tomist:* specialist	A health care professional trained in the collection of blood specimens.
Phlebotomy	*phleb/o-:* vein *-otomy:* incision	Incision of a vein for the removal of blood; the collection of blood.
Plasma		The liquid part of the blood consisting of a clear, straw-colored fluid that comprises approximately 55% of the blood volume.
Serum		Plasma from which the clotting factor fibrinogen has been removed.
Venipuncture	*ven/o-:* vein	Puncturing of a vein.
Venous reflux	*ven/o-:* vein *-ous:* pertaining to	The backflow of blood (from an evacuated tube) into the patient's vein.
Venous stasis	*ven/o-:* vein *stasis:* control, stop	The temporary cessation or slowing of the venous blood flow.

ON THE WEB

For information on phlebotomy:

Clinical Laboratory Standards Institute: www.clsi.org

Lab Explorer: www.labexplorer.com

American Society for Clinical Laboratory Science (ASCLS): www.ascls.org

American Society for Clinical Pathology (ASCP): www.ascp.org

American Society of Phlebotomy Technicians (ASPT): www.aspt.org

Becton Dickinson: www.bd.com

National Phlebotomy Association (NPA): www.nationalphlebotomy.org

The Safety Lady: www.safetylady.com

My Blood Draw: www.myblooddraw.com

Phlebotomy Pages: www.phlebotomypages.com

 Check out the Evolve site at http://evolve.elsevier.com/Bonewit/today/ to actively Prepare for your Certification, and to access additional interactive activities and exercises to help you study and prepare for success.

32

Hematology

KEY TERMS

anemia (ah-NEE-mee-ah)
anticoagulant (an-tih-koe-AG-yoo-lent)
hematology (hee-mah-TOL-oe-jee)

hemoglobin (HEE-moe-gloe-bin)
leukocytosis (loo-koe-sie-TOE-sis)

leukopenia (loo-koe-PEE-nee-ah)
polycythemia (pol-ee-sie-THEE-mee-ah)

INTRODUCTION TO HEMATOLOGY

Hematology is the study of blood, including the morphologic appearance and function of blood cells and diseases of the blood and blood-forming tissues. Before beginning a study of this chapter, it is suggested that you review the components and function of blood presented in Chapter 12.

Laboratory analysis in hematology is concerned with the examination of blood for the purpose of detecting pathologic conditions. It includes performing blood cell counts, evaluating the clotting ability of the blood, and identifying cell types. These tests are valuable tools that allow the physician to determine whether each blood component falls within its reference range.

Examples of hematologic tests include hemoglobin, hematocrit, white blood cell count, red blood cell count, differential white blood cell count, prothrombin time, erythrocyte sedimentation rate, and platelet count. Certain hematologic laboratory tests may be performed in the medical office. Advances in CLIA-waived automated blood analyzers designed for use in the medical office have made this possible. Automated blood analyzers perform laboratory tests with accurate test results in a short time. Each automated analyzer is accompanied by a detailed operating manual that explains its operation, test parameters, care, and maintenance.

The most frequently performed hematologic laboratory test is the *complete blood count* (CBC). A CBC is routinely performed on new patients and on patients with a pathologic condition. The test results provide valuable information to assist the physician in making a diagnosis, evaluating the patient's progress, and regulating treatment. The tests included in a CBC are as follows:

- White blood cell (WBC) count
- Red blood cell (RBC) count
- Platelet count
- Hemoglobin (Hgb)
- Hematocrit (Hct)
- Differential white blood cell count (Diff)
- Red blood cell indices

An example of a laboratory report indicating the results of a CBC is presented in Figure 32-1.

HEMOGLOBIN DETERMINATION

Hemoglobin (Hgb) is a major component of red blood cells. Hemoglobin transports oxygen to the tissue cells of the body and is responsible for the color of the red blood cell.

The hemoglobin determination is used to measure indirectly the oxygen-carrying capacity of the blood. The reference range for an adult female is 12 to 16 g/dL, and the reference range for an adult male is 14 to 18 g/dL. A hemoglobin determination is performed as an individual test or as part of the CBC. A hemoglobin determination is often performed as a routine test on individuals, such as children

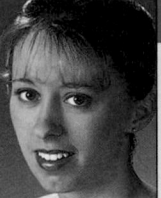

younger than 2 years of age and pregnant women, who are at risk for developing anemia.

A decreased hemoglobin level occurs with **anemia** (especially iron-deficiency anemia), hyperthyroidism, cirrhosis of the liver, severe hemorrhaging, hemolytic reactions, and certain systemic diseases, such as leukemia and Hodgkin disease. Increased levels of hemoglobin are present with **polycythemia,** chronic obstructive pulmonary disease, and congestive heart failure.

The hemoglobin determination can be performed on capillary or venous blood. Hemoglobin can be measured in the medical office using a hemoglobin analyzer. A hemoglobin analyzer permits processing of the specimen in a short time with accurate and reliable test results, allowing the physician to evaluate the condition while the patient is still at the medical office. Examples of CLIA-waived hemoglobin analyzers often used in the medical office include the Hemoglobin Hb 201+ Analyzer (HemoCue, Inc., Lake Forest, Calif.) and the Stat-Site Hgb Meter (Stanbio Laboratory, Boerne, Tex.) (Figure 32-2).

One of the primary advantages of using a hemoglobin analyzer is that it requires only a finger puncture to perform the test rather than a venous blood specimen collected through a venipuncture. The manufacturer of each hemoglobin analyzer provides an operating manual (and sometimes an instructional video) with the instrument that includes information needed to perform quality control procedures, precautions to take when running the test, and information on storage and stability of the testing devices (e.g., testing cards or cuvettes) and control reagents, collection of the specimen, and the procedure for testing the specimen. It is important that the medical assistant become completely familiar with all aspects of the hemoglobin analyzer. Quality control procedures are of particular importance to ensure that the analyzer is functioning properly, and that test results are reliable and accurate. (Refer to Chapter 29, Quality Control, to review quality control guidelines for laboratory testing.)

Family Practice Health Care Center
3477 Arrowhead Ave
Phoenix, Arizona 78351
(942) 871-3746

LAB REPORT

ID#	SEX	PATIENT DEMOGRAPHICS	RESULTS PROVIDED BY
3569	M	Laurence F. Dodds	Medical Center Laboratory
		1073 Longview Dr.	
DOB		Brighton, Arizona 78351	ORDERING PROVIDER
06/17/1989			Thomas Murphy, MD

AGE	ACCESSION #	LAB RECEIVED ON	LAB REPORTED ON
20	33972405	12/07/2012 11:00:53	12/05/2012 14:08:00

LAB ID	SPECIMEN ID	COLLECTION DATE/TIME	FASTING
5701	82540339	12/04/2012 2:53:00	NO

NAME	VALUE	REFERENCE RANGE	UNITS	FLAG
CBC WITH DIFFERENTIAL/PLATELET				
-WBC	4.6	4.0-10.5	x10E3/uL	
-RBC	3.57	4.10-5.60	x10E3/uL	L
-Hemoglobin	11.2	12.5-17.0	g/dL	L
-Hematocrit	32.9	36.0-50.0	%	L
-MCV	92	80-98	fL	
-MCH	31.4	27.0-34.0	pg	
-MCHC	34.0	32.0-36.0	g/dL	
-RDW	15.6	11.7-15.0	%	H
-Platelets	308	140-415	x10E3/uL	
-Neutrophils	73	40-74	%	
-Lymphocytes	14	14-46	%	
-Monocytes	11	4-13	%	
-Eosinophils	1	0-7	%	
-Basophils	1	0-3	%	

Figure 32-1 Computer-generated laboratory report for a complete blood count (CBC).

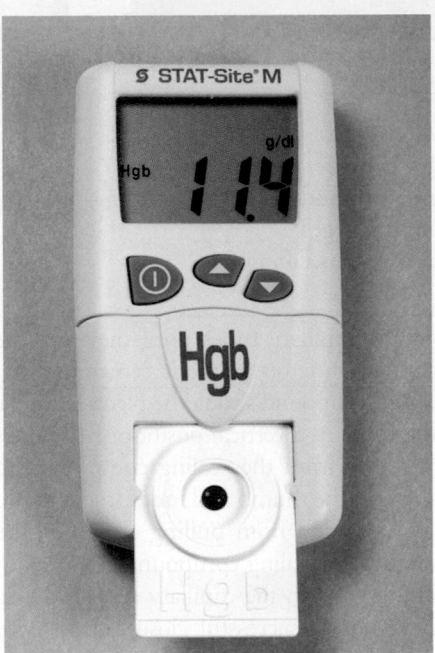

Figure 32-2 CLIA-waived hemoglobin analyzer.

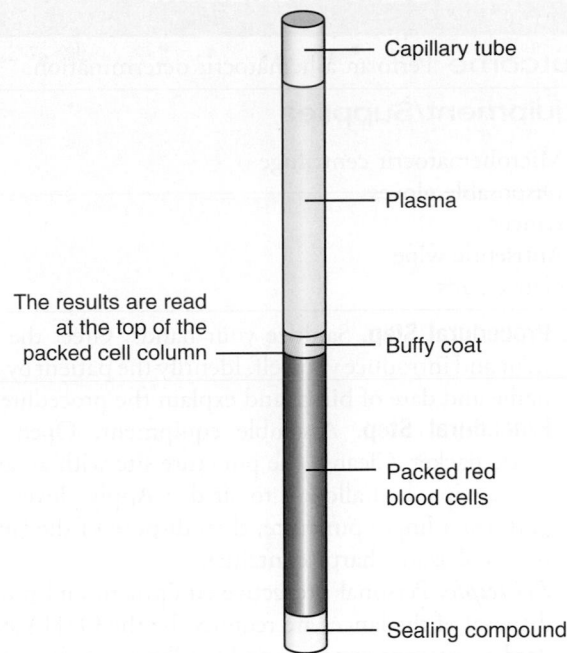

Figure 32-3 Hematocrit test results. The blood cells are separated from the plasma by centrifuging an anticoagulated blood specimen, and the results are read at the top of the packed cell column.

The medical assistant must follow the hemoglobin procedure *exactly* as presented in the operating manual. The basic procedure for performing a hemoglobin test involves placing a testing device in the analyzer. A skin puncture is performed on a finger, and a drop of the patient's blood is placed on the testing device. After a countdown period in which the analyzer determines the hemoglobin test results, the hemoglobin results are displayed on the LCD screen of the analyzer. The medical assistant should record the results in the patient's chart, including the date and time, the name of the test (hemoglobin), and the results measured in g/dL.

HEMATOCRIT

The hematocrit (Hct) is a simple, reliable, and informative test that is frequently performed in the medical office. The word *hematocrit* means "to separate blood." The solid or cellular elements are separated from the plasma by centrifuging an anticoagulated blood specimen. The heavier red blood cells become packed and settle to the bottom of a tube. The top layer contains the clear, straw-colored plasma. Between the plasma and the packed red blood cells is a small, thin, yellowish-gray layer known as the *buffy coat,* which contains the platelets and white blood cells (Figure 32-3).

The purpose of the hematocrit is to measure the percentage volume of packed red blood cells in whole blood. The normal hematocrit range for a woman is 37% to 47%; for a man, 40% to 54%. A low hematocrit reading may indicate anemia, and a high reading may indicate polycythemia. The hematocrit, in conjunction with other hematologic tests, is an aid to the physician in the diagnosis of a patient's condition. The hematocrit also is used as a screening measure for the early detection of anemia and is often included in a general physical examination.

The *microhematocrit method* is used most often in the medical office to perform a hematocrit determination. Through capillary action, blood is drawn directly from a free-flowing skin puncture into a disposable capillary tube lined with an **anticoagulant**. An anticoagulated blood specimen collected by venipuncture also can be used; through capillary action, the blood specimen is drawn into the capillary tube from the evacuated collection tube. After the specimen is collected, one end of the capillary tube is sealed with a commercially prepared sealing compound (e.g., Cha-Seal [Chase Scientific, Langley, Wash.], Seal-Ease [Becton Dickinson, Franklin Lakes, NJ]). The capillary tube is then placed in a microhematocrit centrifuge. The centrifuge spins the blood at an extremely high speed; only 3 to 5 minutes are required to pack the red blood cells. The results are read at the top of the packed cell column. Procedure 32-1 describes how to perform a hematocrit determination.

What Would You Do? What Would You *Not* Do?

Case Study 1

Theodore Pascal is at the office for a general physical examination. The physician orders a routine urinalysis and a hemoglobin determination be done on Theodore at the office. Theodore wants to know whether the physician thinks there is something wrong with him. He also wants to know the purpose of the blood test and how it is done. When Theodore realizes that a hemoglobin determination involves a finger-stick, he says that he does not like having his finger stuck and wants to know whether the blood can be taken out of his earlobe instead. ■

Outcome Perform a hematocrit determination.

Equipment/Supplies

- Microhematocrit centrifuge
- Disposable gloves
- Lancet
- Antiseptic wipe
- Gauze pads

- Capillary tubes
- Sealing compound
- Adhesive bandage
- Biohazard sharps container

1. **Procedural Step.** Sanitize your hands. Greet the patient and introduce yourself. Identify the patient by full name and date of birth, and explain the procedure.

2. **Procedural Step.** Assemble equipment. Open the gauze packet. Cleanse the puncture site with an antiseptic wipe, and allow it to air-dry. Apply gloves and perform a finger puncture, then dispose of the lancet in a biohazard sharps container.

   Principle. Personal protective equipment and proper disposal of the lancet are required by the OSHA standard to prevent exposure to bloodborne pathogens.

3. **Procedural Step.** Wipe away the first drop of blood with a gauze pad. Fill the first capillary tube by holding one end of it horizontally, but slightly downward, next to the free-flowing puncture. Keep the tip of the capillary tube in the blood, but do not allow it to press against the patient's skin. Calibrated tubes are filled to the calibration line; uncalibrated tubes are filled approximately three quarters (within 10 to 20 mm of the end of the tube). The blood is drawn into the tube through capillary action. Fill a second tube using the method just described. Place a gauze pad over the puncture site and apply pressure.

   Principle. Not keeping the tip of the capillary tube in the blood can cause air bubbles in the stem of the tube, which leads to inaccurate test results. Allowing the capillary tube to press against the skin closes the opening of the capillary tubes and does not allow blood to enter. The type of tube (calibrated or uncalibrated) is based on the method used to read the test results. The hematocrit should be performed in duplicate to ensure accurate and reliable test results.

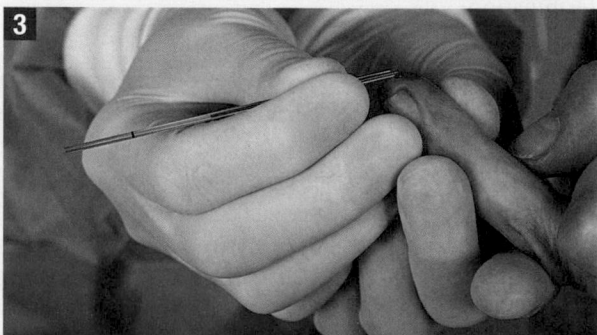

Fill the capillary tube.

4. **Procedural Step.** Push the dry end of the tube (end opposite the filling end that does not contain blood) down into the sealing compound. This seals the end of the capillary tube. The sealing compound can be used to hold the capillary tubes until they are ready to be placed in the microhematocrit centrifuge. To do this, the sealing compound should be placed on a flat surface with the tubes in a vertical position. Before removing a capillary tube from the sealing compound, rotate the tube between the thumb and index finger to prevent the sealing compound from pulling out when the tube is lifted out of the sealing compound.

   Principle. Blood in the capillary tube at the end being sealed prevents a successful closure, which may cause leakage of the blood specimen, leading to inaccurate test results. Capillary tubes must be sealed properly to prevent leakage of the blood specimen during centrifugation.

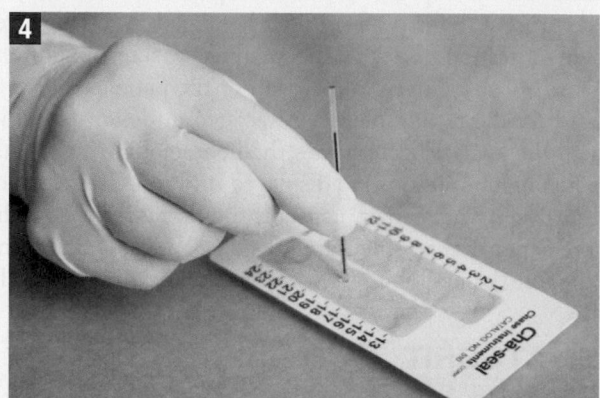

Seal one end of the tube.

5. **Procedural Step.** Check the patient's puncture site for bleeding and apply an adhesive bandage, if needed.

6. **Procedural Step.** Place the capillary tubes in the microhematocrit centrifuge with the sealed end facing out. Balance one tube with the other capillary tube placed on the opposite side of the centrifuge.

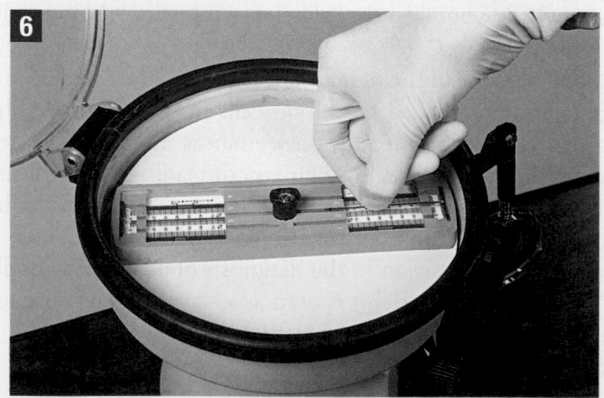

Place the tube in the centrifuge.

PROCEDURE 32-1   Hematocrit

Principle. Placing the sealed end toward the outside prevents the blood specimen from spinning out of the capillary tube when the centrifuge is in operation.

7. **Procedural Step.** Place the cover on the centrifuge, and lock it securely. Centrifuge the blood specimen for 3 to 5 minutes at a speed of 10,000 rpm.

   Principle. Centrifuging the blood specimen causes the red blood cells to become packed and to settle on the bottom of the tube.

8. **Procedural Step.** Allow the centrifuge to come to a complete stop. Read the results, as follows:

   Calibrated tube. If a capillary tube with a calibration line was used, read the results using the special graphic reading device that is part of the centrifuge. Adjust the capillary tube so that the bottom of the red blood cell column (just above the sealing compound) is placed on the 0 line. With a magnifying glass, read the results at the top of the packed red blood cell column, and you will see a percentage on the reading device.

   Uncalibrated tube. If an uncalibrated tube was used, you must use a microhematocrit reader card to determine the results; place the top of the plasma column on the 100% mark and the bottom of the cell column on the 0 line. Read the results on the scale, which corresponds to the top of the packed cell column.

   In both cases, the buffy coat should not be included in the reading. The answer represents the percentage

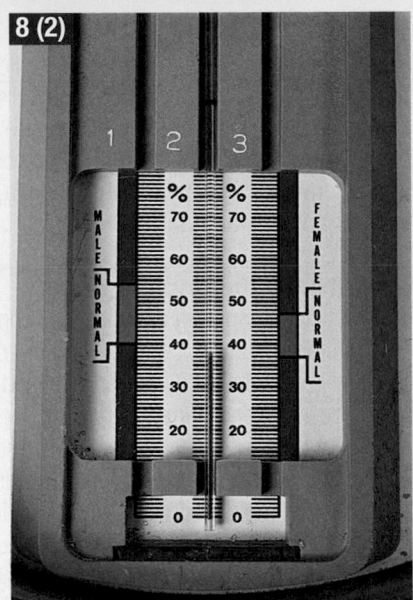

Read the results.

of blood volume occupied by the red blood cells. (The hematocrit determination on this reading device is 38.)

   Principle. Stopping the centrifuge with your hands can injure you and can damage the machine.

9. **Procedural Step.** Read the second tube in the manner just described; the results of the tubes should agree within 4 percentage points. If not, the hematocrit procedure must be repeated. If they are within 4 percentage points, the two values are averaged to derive the test results.

10. **Procedural Step.** Properly dispose of the capillary tubes in a biohazard sharps container. Remove gloves and sanitize your hands. Chart the results. Include the date and time and the hematocrit results.

11. **Procedural Step.** Return the equipment to its proper storage place. Store the sealing compound at room temperature. Exposing it to a temperature above 80° F adversely affects its consistency.

Reference Range for Hematocrit

Female: 37% to 47%
Male: 40% to 54%

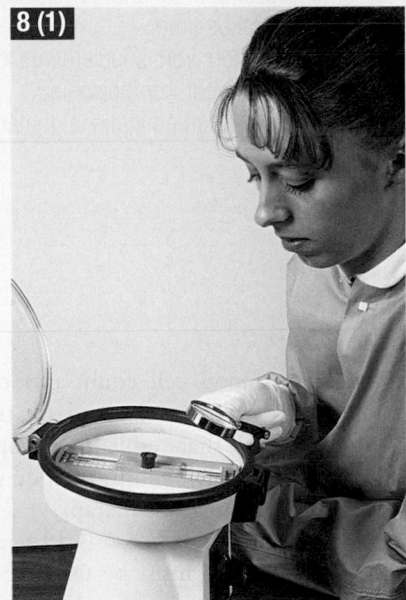

Align the bottom of the red cell column with the 0 line.

CHARTING EXAMPLE	
Date	
5/5/XX	11:15 a.m. Hct: 38%. ————————
	———————— L. Sharpe, CMA (AAMA)

PROCEDURE 32-1

PATIENT TEACHING   Iron-Deficiency Anemia

Answer questions patients have about iron-deficiency anemia.

What is anemia?

Anemia is a shortage of red blood cells or hemoglobin. Hemoglobin, the part of the blood that gives red blood cells their color, carries oxygen to all the cells in the body. There are many types of anemia, of which iron-deficiency anemia is the most common. Other types of anemia include pernicious anemia, sickle cell anemia, hemolytic anemia, and aplastic anemia.

What causes iron-deficiency anemia?

In general, iron-deficiency anemia is caused by conditions that deplete the iron stored in the body; it can result from an increased need for iron by the body or an increased loss of iron from the body. Iron-deficiency anemia may occur in children younger than 2 years old if their diet does not include enough iron to meet the demands of rapid growth. This is especially true in children whose main source of nutrition during these years is breast milk or bottle milk, because milk contains very little iron. Adolescent girls are prone to iron-deficiency anemia because of growth spurts during puberty and blood loss through menstruation. In adults, the most common cause of anemia is chronic blood loss, such as from a bleeding ulcer or bleeding hemorrhoids and heavy menstrual bleeding. Pregnant women also are at increased risk because of the demands of the growing fetus.

What can be done for individuals at risk for iron-deficiency anemia?

Individuals prone to developing iron-deficiency anemia are encouraged to increase foods in their diet that contain iron, such as beef, liver, spinach, eggs, and iron-fortified breads and cereals. As a preventive measure, the physician usually prescribes vitamin supplements for individuals who are at increased risk for developing iron-deficiency anemia, such as pregnant women, infants, and young children. Infant formulas and cereals that have been supplemented with iron are also available.

What are the symptoms of anemia?

All types of anemia have the same general symptoms. Often these symptoms do not develop right away; when they do develop, feeling tired and run down may be the only sign of anemia. Other symptoms that may occur, particularly as the anemia becomes worse, are paleness of the skin, fingernail beds, and mucous membranes; shortness of breath, especially during physical activity; dizziness; headache; irritability; and inability to concentrate. These symptoms result from the diminished ability of the blood to carry oxygen to the cells of the body. Blood tests are necessary to diagnose anemia and to determine the specific type of anemia present.

How is iron-deficiency anemia treated?

The most important part of treating anemia is to determine its cause, such as not enough iron consumed in the diet or chronic blood loss, and to correct that condition. The physician usually prescribes an iron supplement to replace the iron that has been depleted from the body. It is generally prescribed in oral form, but it is given through an injection in special situations. An oral iron supplement causes the stool to turn a black, tarlike color. This is normal and should not be a cause for concern. Also, an effort should be made to consume foods high in iron content.

- For patients who have had a vitamin supplement prescribed to *prevent* iron-deficiency anemia, such as children younger than 2 years old and pregnant women: Emphasize to the patient the importance of taking the vitamin supplement every day to prevent the development of iron-deficiency anemia.
- For patients who have had an iron supplement prescribed to treat iron-deficiency anemia: Emphasize to the patient the importance of taking the iron supplement for the period of time prescribed by the physician, because replacement of iron takes time.
- Instruct patients to keep iron supplements out of the reach of children to prevent iron poisoning.
- Provide patients with written educational materials about anemia. ■

WHITE BLOOD CELL COUNT

The white blood cell (WBC) count is used by the physician to assist in the diagnosis and prognosis of disease. The white blood cell count is an approximate measurement of the number of white blood cells in the circulating blood. The reference range for a white blood cell count is 4500 to 11,000 white blood cells per cubic millimeter of blood, which is expressed as 4.5 to 11 $(\times 10^3/mm^3)$ on laboratory reports. An increase in the white blood cell count, or leukocytosis, is most commonly seen in acute infection such as appendicitis, chickenpox, diphtheria, infectious mononucleosis, meningitis, and rheumatic fever. Normal elevation of the white blood cell count can occur with pregnancy, strenuous exercise, stress, and treatment with corticosteroids. Conditions that result in leukopenia, or a decrease in the white blood cell count, include viral infections, chemotherapy, and radiation therapy.

If performed in the medical office, a (CLIA-nonwaived) automated blood cell counter must be used to obtain the WBC count, which is a moderately complex test. Blood cell counters also are able to perform a red blood cell count, platelet count, hemoglobin, hematocrit, and differential white blood cell count, as well as calculation of red blood cell indices. Examples of nonwaived blood cell counters include the QBC Autoread (Becton Dickinson), the

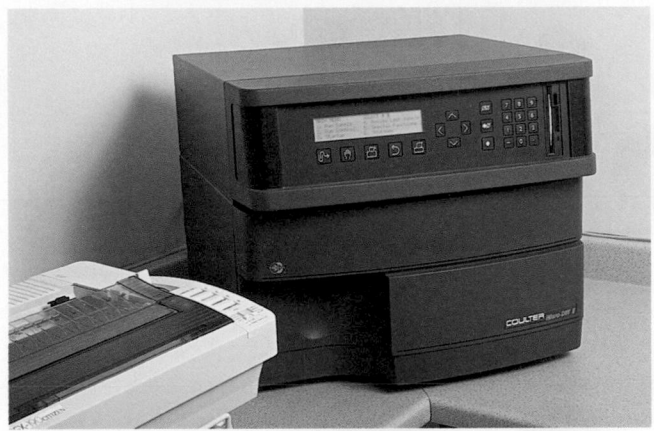

Figure 32-4 Coulter blood cell counter.

Cell-Dyn (Abbott, Santa Clara, Calif.), and the Coulter (Coulter Company, Brea, Calif.) (Figure 32-4).

RED BLOOD CELL COUNT

The red blood cell (RBC) count is a measurement of the number of red blood cells in whole blood. The range for the red blood cell count in a healthy woman is 4 to 5.5 million red blood cells per cubic millimeter of blood, expressed on laboratory reports as 4 to 5.5 ($\times10^6$/mm^3). The range for a healthy man is 4.5 to 6.2 million red blood cells per cubic millimeter of blood, expressed on a laboratory report as 4.5 to 6.2 ($\times10^6$/mm^3). In the medical office, the red blood cell count is performed using a blood cell counter.

Conditions that cause a decrease in the red blood cell count include anemia, Hodgkin disease, and leukemia; conditions that cause an increase in red blood cells include polycythemia, dehydration, and pulmonary fibrosis.

RED BLOOD CELL INDICES

The red blood cell (RBC) indices are measurements that are reported as part of the CBC (complete blood count) test. RBC indices provide the physician with information about the size and hemoglobin content of a patient's red blood cells. The RBC indices include the MCV (mean corpuscular volume), MCH (mean corpuscular hemoglobin), MCHC (mean cell hemoglobin concentration), and the RDW (red cell distribution width). The RBC indices are obtained from calculations performed on certain test results included in a CBC, specifically, the RBC count, hemoglobin, and hematocrit. The calculation is automatically performed by the blood cell analyzer that performs the CBC.

A decrease in the number of red blood cells or in the amount of hemoglobin is known as anemia. More than 400 types of anemia have been identified, but many of them are rare conditions. Each of the various forms of anemia (e.g., iron-deficiency anemia, pernicious anemia) may alter one or more of the RBC indices in a particular way. This information is used by the physician to assist in the diagnosis of the type of anemia a patient has and in determination of its cause.

WHITE BLOOD CELL DIFFERENTIAL COUNT

There are five types of white blood cells, or leukocytes, each having a certain size, shape, appearance, and function (Figure 32-5). The purpose of the differential cell count is to identify and count the five types of white blood cells in a representative blood sample. An increase or decrease in one or more types may occur in pathologic conditions; this assists the physician in making a diagnosis.

The differential cell count can be performed automatically or manually. The automatic method is faster and more convenient; however, the manual method allows for closer inspection of abnormal white blood cells. If a differential cell count is performed on an automated analyzer at an outside laboratory and abnormalities are flagged by the analyzer, the laboratory will then perform a differential cell count by using the manual method.

Automatic Method

The automatic method involves the use of a blood cell counter, such as the Coulter cell counter (see Figure 32-4). The specimen requirement is an ethylenediaminetetraacetic acid (EDTA)–anticoagulated blood specimen, which is obtained through venipuncture using a lavender-stoppered tube. The blood cell counter automatically performs the differential cell count, and the results are printed on a laboratory report.

Manual Method

If a physician orders a manual differential cell count on a blood specimen, the medical assistant must prepare two blood smears at the medical office for transport to the outside laboratory. The preparation of a blood smear is outlined in Procedure 32-2. Fresh whole blood is preferred for blood smears; however, a satisfactory smear can be made from an EDTA-anticoagulated blood specimen, provided that the smear is made within 24 hours after collection.

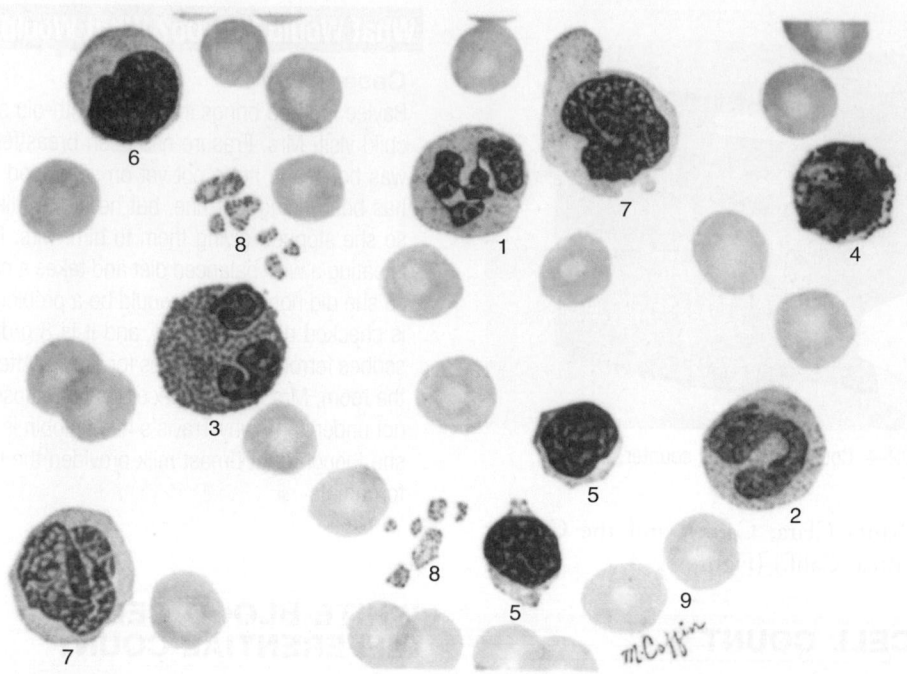

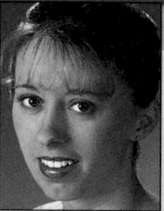

Figure 32-5 Types of human blood cells. *1* to *7*, White blood cells (leukocytes) stained as they are in the laboratory to show the many types. They play the active role in immune response or in defense against disease. *1*, Neutrophil; *2*, neutrophilic band; *3*, eosinophil; *4*, basophil; *5*, lymphocyte; *6*, (large) lymphocyte; *7*, monocyte; *8*, platelets (thrombocytes), which are responsible for clotting; and *9*, red blood cells (erythrocytes), which carry oxygen.

Other anticoagulants should not be used because they could alter the morphology and staining reaction of the white blood cells. After preparing the blood smear, the medical assistant places the slides in a protective slide container for transport to an outside laboratory.

The blood smear is evaluated at the laboratory by medical laboratory personnel. Because white blood cells are clear and colorless, they must be stained with an appropriate dye (usually Wright stain) before a differential count is performed. The nucleus, the cytoplasm, and any granules in the cytoplasm take on the characteristic color of their cell type; this aids in proper identification. A minimum of 100 white blood cells is identified on the blood smear using a microscope, and each is assigned to its appropriate category (neutrophil, eosinophil, basophil, lymphocyte, or monocyte). The number of each type of leukocyte is recorded as a percentage and reflects the overall distribution of white blood cells in the patient's bloodstream. During the manual evaluation of the blood smear, the laboratory technologist will also examine the slide for abnormalities in the morphology of the red blood cells, including their size, shape, and structure.

Reference Range

The healthy adult reference range for each type of white blood cell making up the total number of leukocytes is listed here:

> Neutrophils: 50% to 70%
> Eosinophils: 1% to 4%
> Basophils: 0% to 1%
> Lymphocytes: 20% to 35%
> Monocytes: 3% to 8%

Memories *from* Externship

Latisha Sharpe: During my externship experience, I had a female patient who drank too much the night before and had been vomiting for 3 hours before coming to the physician's office. Although this incident was self-inflicted, I still found myself feeling deeply sorry for the patient. She was so weak she could not hold her head up, so I stayed with her and held her head up while she was vomiting. I stayed with her throughout this time, and my sympathy for her really made a difference. No matter what the situation is, I always let the patient know that I care. ■

What Would You Do? What Would You *Not* Do?

Case Study 3

Marjorie Merrick comes to the office for a follow-up visit to discuss her laboratory results with the physician. Marjorie is in perimenopause and has been having problems with heavy menstrual periods, hot flashes, insomnia, fatigue, and shortness of breath. Marjorie's laboratory tests indicate that she has iron-deficiency anemia. The physician orders an injection of iron dextran, Z-track technique, and instructs Marjorie to take an iron supplement every day and to return in 3 months for a recheck. Marjorie says she has heard that an iron injection can stain the skin and wants to know whether that is true. She says she has a friend who has anemia, and he has to go in every week for a vitamin B_{12} shot. Marjorie wants to know whether she will have to do that, too. Marjorie signed up to donate blood this week at her church's Red Cross blood drive. She wants to know whether it is all right for her to donate. ■

Outcome Prepare a blood smear for a differential white blood cell count.

Equipment/Supplies

- Disposable gloves
- Supplies to perform a finger puncture or venipuncture
- Lavender-stoppered evacuated tube
- Slides with a frosted edge
- Slide container
- Biohazard specimen bag
- Laboratory request form
- Biohazard sharps container

1. **Procedural Step.** Sanitize your hands. Greet the patient and introduce yourself. Identify the patient by full name and date of birth, and explain the procedure.

2. **Procedural Step.** Assemble the equipment. Using a pencil, label two slides on the frosted edge with the patient's name and date of birth, and the date.
   Principle. Laboratories request the preparation of two blood smears as a means of quality control.

3. **Procedural Step.** Open the gauze packet. Cleanse the puncture site with an antiseptic wipe. Apply gloves, obtain a blood sample from the patient, and place a drop of fresh whole blood on each slide as follows:
   From a venipuncture. You can obtain the blood specimen from the fresh whole blood left in the needle immediately after performing a venipuncture for a CBC (using a lavender-stoppered tube) as follows: After withdrawing the needle from the patient's arm, deposit the drops of blood remaining in the needle onto the middle of each slide, approximately ¼ inch from the slide's frosted edge. The lavender tube can be used to help push the blood out of the needle. The drop of blood should be approximately 1 to 2 mm in diameter, which is about the size of the head of a matchstick. Immediately discard the venipuncture needle and attached holder in a biohazard sharps container.
   From a skin puncture. Perform a finger puncture, and wipe away the first drop of blood. Place a drop of blood from the patient's finger in the middle of each slide, approximately ¼ inch from the slide's frosted edge, by touching the slide to the drop of blood. Do not allow the patient's finger to touch the slide.
   Principle. If the patient's finger touches the slide, it will spread out the blood specimen, producing an uneven smear. In addition, moisture or oil from the patient's finger could interfere with the smear.

4. **Procedural Step.** Make the blood smear as follows:
   a. Hold a second "spreader" slide between the thumb and index finger of the dominant hand. Position a nondominant finger (or fingers) at the end of the

   slide (end opposite the frosted edge). Position the spreader slide in front of the drop of blood and at a 30-degree angle to the first slide.

   b. Move the spreader slide until it touches the drop of blood. The blood distributes itself along the edge of the spreader by capillary action.

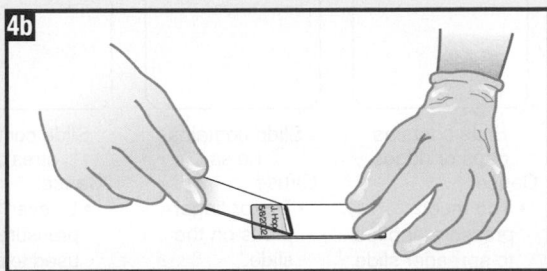

Move the spreader into the drop of blood.

   c. Using a smooth, continuous motion, with a light, but firm pressure, spread the blood thinly and evenly across the surface of the first slide, ending the motion by lifting the spreader slide off the specimen in a smooth, low arc. The smear should be approximately 1½ inches long. The blood smear is thickest at the beginning and gradually thins to a very fine "feathered" edge.

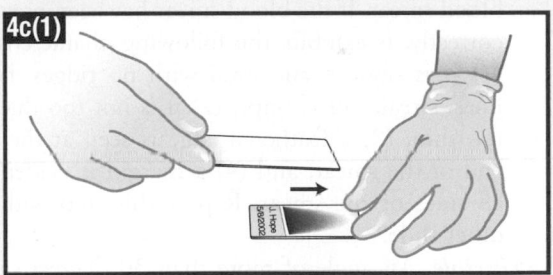

Spread the blood across the slide.

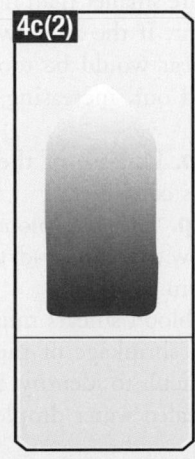

Properly prepared blood smear.

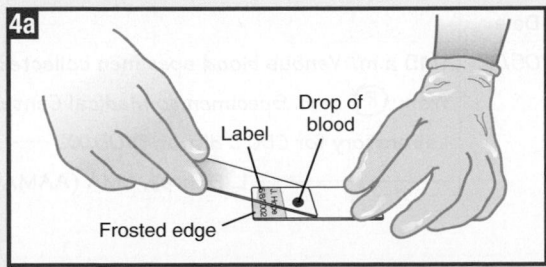

Hold the spreader slide in front of the drop of blood.

Continued

PROCEDURE 32-2   Preparation of a Blood Smear for a Differential Cell Count—cont'd

4c(3)

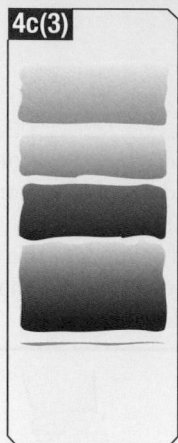 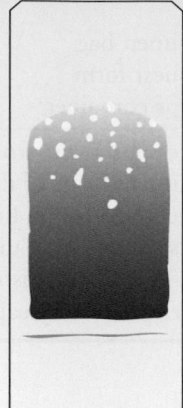 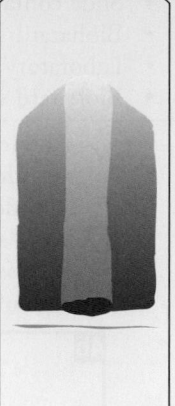 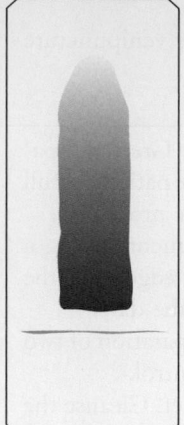 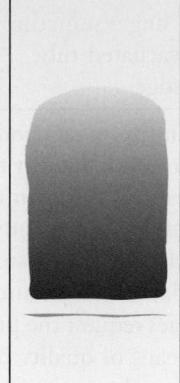 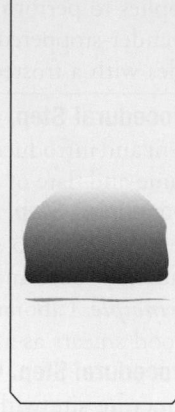

Slide contains gaps or ridges	Slide contains holes	Slide contains streaks	Slide is too thin	Slide is too thick	The length of the smear is too short
Cause: • Too much pressure applied to spreader slide • Uneven pressure used to push spreader slide	Cause: • Dirt or finger-prints on the slide • Fat globules or lipids in the specimen • Blood is contaminated with powder from glove	Cause: • Uneven pressure used to push spreader slide • Drop of blood started to dry out	Cause: • Blood drop is too small • Angle of less than 30 degrees is used	Cause: • Blood drop is too large • Angle of less than 30 degrees is used	Cause: • Blood drop is too small • Angle of more than 30 degrees is used • Spreader slide is pushed too quickly and not far enough along the slide

Improperly prepared blood smears.

d. Repeat the above procedure to prepare the second blood smear. If the blood smear has been prepared correctly, it exhibits the following characteristics: (1) It is smooth and even with no ridges, holes, lines, streaks, or clumps; (2) it is not too thick or too thin; (3) a feathered edge is seen at the thin end of the smear; and (4) a margin is evident on all sides of the smear. Repeat this step with the other slide.

Principle. An angle of more than 30 degrees causes the smear to be too thick; the cells overlap, do not stain well, and are smaller than normal, making them difficult to count. If the angle were smaller than 30 degrees, the smear would be too thin, and the cells would be spread out, increasing the time needed to count them.

5. **Procedural Step.** Dispose of the spreader slide in a biohazard sharps container.

6. **Procedural Step.** Lay the blood smears on a flat surface, and allow them to air-dry. Never blow on the slides to dry them.

Principle. The blood smears must be dried immediately to prevent shrinkage of the blood cells, which makes them difficult to identify. Blowing on the slide might cause exhaled water droplets to make holes in the smears.

7. **Procedural Step.** Once the slides are completely dry, place them in a protective slide container. Prepare the blood tube and slides for transport to the laboratory. Place the lavender-stoppered tube and slide container in a biohazard specimen bag and seal the bag.

8. **Procedural Step.** Remove your gloves, and sanitize your hands. Complete a laboratory request form. Place a copy of the laboratory request in the outside pocket of the specimen bag.

9. **Procedural Step.** Chart the procedure. Include the date and time, the type of collection and the date the specimen was transported to the laboratory. File a copy of the laboratory request in the patient's chart. Place the specimen bag in the appropriate location for pickup by a courier.

CHARTING EXAMPLE

Date	
5/05/XX	11:15 a.m. Venous blood specimen collected from Ⓡ arm. Specimen to Medical Center Laboratory for CBC c̄ diff on 5/05/XX. ——— ———————— L. Sharpe, CMA (AAMA)

PT/INR

The PT/INR test is a combination of a PT (prothrombin time) test and a mathematical calculation performed on the PT test to arrive at a standardized value known as an *INR* (International Normalized Ratio). The PT test result measures how long it takes an individual's blood to form a clot. PT test results are measured in seconds. The reference range for a PT for an adult is 10 to 20 seconds; this means that the blood of a healthy adult should clot within 10 to 20 seconds.

A variety of testing reagents can be used to measure PT. Each of these reagents works in a slightly different way to assess the clotting ability of the blood. Because of this, a PT result obtained when one reagent is used at a particular laboratory cannot be compared with a PT result that has been tested using a different reagent at another laboratory. To account for these differences, the coagulation analyzer running a PT test performs a mathematical calculation on the PT results to convert the results to a standardized ratio. This ratio, known as an *INR,* is obtained by comparing the patient's PT results with those of a normal (control) sample. The INR allows a patient's PT test results to be compared regardless of the testing reagent or laboratory used to run the test.

The PT/INR result is expressed as a number, and because the value is a ratio, the result does not have a unit of measurement attached to it. A healthy individual with a normal clotting ability should have a PT/INR result that falls between 0.8 and 1.2. The higher the number, the longer it takes for the blood to clot. For example, an individual with a PT/INR of 3.0 would have blood that takes longer to clot than an individual with a PT/INR of 1.0. The risk of spontaneous bleeding begins to rise dramatically as the INR reaches a level of 4.0 or higher.

Purpose

The PT/INR test is most commonly performed on patients undergoing long-term warfarin therapy. Brand names for warfarin include Coumadin and Jantoven. Warfarin is an anticoagulant, which inhibits the formation of blood clots in the body. An anticoagulant works by interfering with the blood clotting mechanism in the body; thus, the blood takes longer to clot. The PT/INR test measures the effect that warfarin has on the clotting ability of a patient's blood.

Warfarin is prescribed for patients who are likely to form clots. The most common conditions for which warfarin is prescribed include heart attack, stroke, and thrombophlebitis (also known as *deep vein thrombosis,* or DVT). Patients who experience recurrent atrial fibrillation are often placed on warfarin therapy. Atrial fibrillation is an irregular heartbeat, which can cause blood to pool in the heart; the pooled blood may cause a blood clot to form, which can travel to the brain, resulting in a stroke. Patients who have had a heart valve replaced with a mechanical valve are also placed on long-term warfarin therapy because of the increased risk that a clot may form on the mechanical valve, causing heart blockage. A PT/INR test also may be ordered for patients who are exhibiting signs and symptoms of a coagulation disorder, such as unexplained nosebleeds, excessive bleeding from the gums, easy bruising, heavy menstrual periods, and unexplained blood in the stool or urine.

The physician determines the ideal PT/INR range for a patient on long-term warfarin therapy, which depends on the condition being treated. The usual desired PT/INR range for a patient on warfarin therapy following a stroke or heart attack, or for a patient with recurring atrial fibrillation, is between 2.0 and 3.0. The PT/INR for a patient with a mechanical valve replacement has a higher range, which falls between 2.5 and 3.5. The goal of warfarin therapy is to increase the clotting time to a level that prevents the formation of blood clots without causing excessive bleeding or bruising.

To ensure that a patient remains in his or her ideal PT/INR range and thereby minimize complications of warfarin therapy, the patient must undergo periodic PT/INR testing. The frequency of testing depends on several factors, which include the stability of the patient's previous test results and the occurrence of conditions that may cause the test results to fall outside of the patient's desired range. When a patient is first placed on warfarin therapy, a PT/INR test is performed once or twice a week to assess the patient's response to the warfarin. Based on the PT/INR results, the dosage is adjusted so that the patient's results become stable and consistently fall within his or her ideal PT/INR range. Once the test results become stabilized, a patient on long-term warfarin therapy should have a PT/INR test performed every 2 to 4 weeks. If the PT/INR result is outside of the patient's predetermined ideal range, the physician adjusts the patient's warfarin dosage to bring the patient back into the range that is optimal for that patient. For example, if the PT/INR of a stroke patient on warfarin therapy is 3.6, which is higher than the desired range (2.0 to 3.0) for such a patient, the physician will lower the patient's warfarin dosage until the patient returns to a value that is within his or her desired range.

Collection of the Specimen

The medical assistant may be responsible for collecting the specimen for a PT/INR test that is to be transported to an outside laboratory for testing. The PT/INR test requires only a small (4 to 5 mL) tube of blood. The blood must be collected in a tube containing sodium citrate, which is a light blue–stoppered tube (Figure 32-6). The sodium citrate prevents the specimen from clotting without affecting the test results.

As described in Chapter 31, when the butterfly method is used to collect the specimen, a red-stoppered discard tube must first be drawn, followed by collection in the light blue tube. If a light blue–stoppered tube is the first or only tube to be drawn, a 5-mL red-stoppered tube must be drawn first and discarded. This is because some of the tube's vacuum is exhausted by the air in the butterfly tubing setup (rather than blood), resulting in underfilling of the tube. A butterfly setup with 7-inch tubing contains 0.3 mL of air, and a setup with 12 inches of tubing contains 0.5 mL of

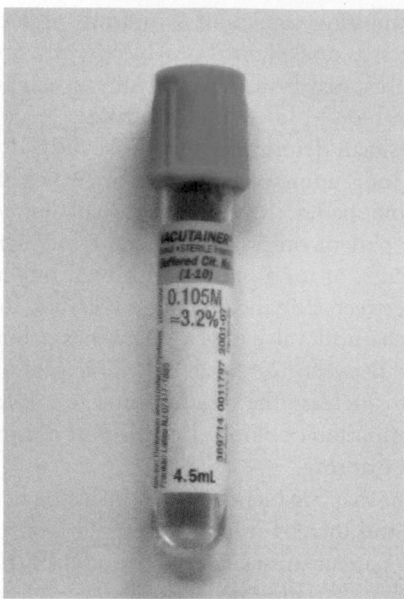

Figure 32-6 Light blue–stoppered tube used to collect a specimen for a PT/INR test.

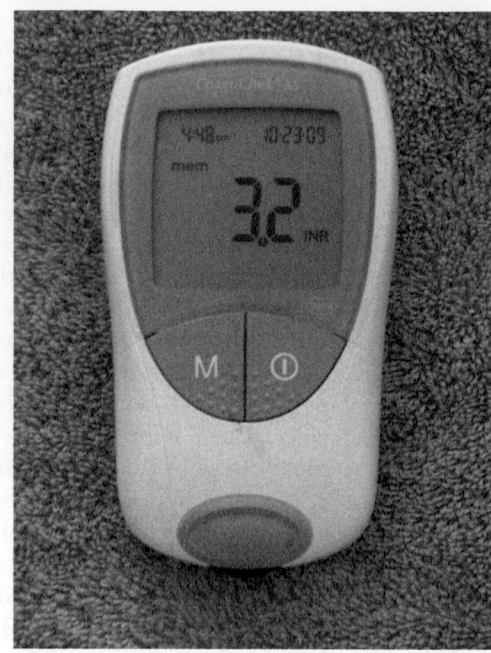

Figure 32-7 PT/INR analyzer.

air. If the light blue–stoppered tube is filled first, the underfilled tube results in an incorrect anticoagulant-to-blood ratio. An incorrect ratio when performing a PT/INR test leads to inaccurate test results.

When collecting a specimen for a PT/INR, it is very important to fill the tube to the exhaustion of the vacuum. Failure to do so results in an underfilled tube and, as described above, leads to inaccurate test results. Most light blue–stoppered tubes have a fill indicator, so the medical assistant can determine if the tube has been completely filled. Once the tube has been drawn, it should be immediately and gently inverted 3 to 4 times to mix the anticoagulant with the blood. The tube should then be placed in a biohazard specimen bag, along with a laboratory request for pickup by a laboratory courier.

Performing a PT/INR Test

CLIA-waived handheld coagulation analyzers are commercially available for performing a PT/INR test in the medical office. Brand names include HemoSense INRatio 2 (Inverness Medical Innovations, Inc., Waltham, Mass) and CoaguChek System (Roche Diagnostics, Branchburg, NJ) (Figure 32-7). One of the primary advantages of these coagulation analyzers is that they require only a finger puncture to perform the test, rather than a venous blood specimen collected through a venipuncture. The manufacturer of each coagulation analyzer provides an operating manual (and sometimes an instructional video) with the instrument that includes information needed to perform quality control procedures, precautions to take when running the test, and information on storage and stability of the testing strips, collection of the specimen, and the procedure for testing the specimen. It is important that the medical assistant become completely familiar with

all aspects of the coagulation analyzer used to perform a PT/INR test. Quality control procedures are of particular importance to ensure that the analyzer is functioning properly and that the test results are reliable and accurate. (Refer to Chapter 29, Quality Control, to review quality control guidelines for laboratory testing.)

The medical assistant must follow the PT/INR procedure *exactly* as presented in the operating manual. The basic procedure for performing a PT/INR test involves placing a testing strip in the analyzer. A skin puncture is performed on a finger, and a drop of the patient's blood is placed on the strip. After a countdown period in which the analyzer determines the PT test results and calculates the INR, the PT/INR results are displayed on the LCD screen of the analyzer. The medical assistant should record the results in the patient's chart, including the date and time, the name of the test (PT/INR), and the ratio value.

PT/INR Home Testing

The health insurance company of a patient on long-term warfarin therapy may provide the patient with a coagulation analyzer to test his or her blood at home (Figure 32-8). Home testing provides the patient with the convenience of not having to make periodic visits to a laboratory or medical office to have a PT/INR test performed. In addition, the patient is able to test his or her blood without a laboratory order from the physician. This provides a distinct advantage because patients are able to check their PT/INR immediately when conditions occur that might indicate a problem, such as nosebleeds, bleeding gums, or unexplained bruising. In these situations, treatment can be instituted immediately to prevent the problem from getting worse. Other factors that can affect the PT/INR results and cause them to be outside of the patient's ideal range include the following: a

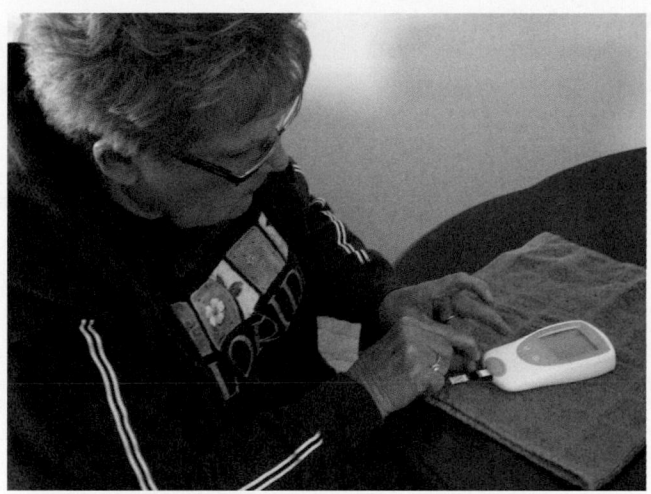
Figure 32-8 Patient performing a PT/INR test at home.

change in diet; use of prescription or over-the-counter medications that interact with warfarin; vitamins and herbal preparations; a change in the level of exercise; illness; smoking; and alcohol consumption. It is important that the patient keep his or her physician informed of any factors that may alter the body's response to warfarin.

MEDICAL PRACTICE *and the* LAW

Any blood specimen can contain bloodborne pathogens, such as hepatitis B and HIV. If spraying or splashing of blood is a possibility, use personal protective equipment, including gloves, mask, and goggles.

Laboratory test results are confidential. Giving out results without the patient's permission can result in an invasion of privacy lawsuit. Usually only the physician gives these results, so he or she can explain their meaning to the patient. ∎

What Would You Do? What Would You *Not* Do? RESPONSES

Case Study 1
Page 787

What Did Latisha Do?
❑ Told Theodore that the physician was running some routine screening tests on him to make sure he is in good health. Explained that all patients have these tests run as part of a physical examination.
❑ Told Theodore that it was not possible to get the specimen from the earlobe. Explained that the earlobe is not recommended as a good site from which to obtain blood.
❑ Reassured Theodore that the finger-stick would be made on the least sensitive part of his finger. Told him that it would hurt for just a second, and then it would be all over and it would heal quickly.
❑ Told Theodore that the purpose of the blood test is early detection of anemia. Explained that if anemia is present, it can be caught early and treated before symptoms develop.

What Did Latisha Not Do?
❑ Did not collect the specimen from Theodore's earlobe.
❑ Did not tell Theodore that he is healthy and does not have anything wrong with him.

What Would You Do?/What Would You Not Do?
Review Latisha's response and place a checkmark next to the information you included in your response. List additional information you included in your response.

_____
_____
_____
_____
_____

Case Study 2
Page 791

What Did Latisha Do?
❑ Commended Mrs. Frasure on eating nutritiously.
❑ Told Mrs. Frasure that breast milk does not contain very much iron. Explained that because of this, it is important to give Travis his liquid vitamins, which have iron in them.
❑ Reassured Mrs. Frasure that breastfeeding does provide very good nutrition for Travis.
❑ Explained to Mrs. Frasure that the iron supplement may cause Travis's stool to be a dark, tarlike color, and she should not be alarmed because this is normal.

What Did Latisha Not Do?
❑ Did not criticize Mrs. Frasure for not giving Travis his vitamins or make her feel it was her fault that his hemoglobin was low.

What Would You Do?/What Would You Not Do?
Review Latisha's response and place a checkmark next to the information you included in your response. List additional information you included in your response.

_____
_____
_____
_____
_____
_____

Continued

What Would You Do? What Would You *Not* Do? RESPONSES—cont'd

Case Study 3
Page 792

What Did Latisha Do?

❑ Told Marjorie that the iron injection can stain the skin but that it would be given in a special way to prevent that from happening.

❑ Told Marjorie that vitamin B12 injections are given for pernicious anemia and that her type of anemia is iron-deficiency anemia.

❑ Gave Marjorie a patient education brochure on iron-deficiency anemia to take home with her.

❑ Told Marjorie that the Red Cross requires that a blood donor's hemoglobin level be within the normal range. Explained that she could not donate this time, but that when her hemoglobin is back to normal, she will be able to donate.

❑ Explained to Marjorie that the iron supplement may cause her stool to be a dark, tarlike color, and she should not be alarmed because this is normal.

What Did Latisha Not Do?

❑ Did not tell Marjorie that her friend has pernicious anemia because there is no way of knowing this.

What Would You Do?/What Would You Not *Do?*

Review Latisha's response and place a checkmark next to the information you included in your response. List additional information you included in your response.

_____

_____

_____

_____

_____

_____

TERMINOLOGY REVIEW

Medical Term	Word Parts	Definition
Anemia	*an-:* without or absence of *-emia:* blood condition	A condition in which there is a decrease in the erythrocytes or amount of hemoglobin in the blood.
Anticoagulant	*anti-:* against *-coagulant:* clotting	A substance that inhibits blood clotting.
Hematology	*hemat/o-:* blood *-ology:* study of	The study of blood and blood-forming tissues.
Hemoglobin	*hem/o-:* blood *-globin:* protein	The protein- and iron-containing pigment of erythrocytes that transports oxygen in the body.
Leukocytosis	*leuk/o-:* white *cyt/o:* cell *-osis:* abnormal condition (means increased when used with blood cell word parts)	An abnormal increase in the number of white blood cells (greater than 11,000 per cubic millimeter of blood).
Leukopenia	*leuk/o-:* white *-penia:* abnormal reduction in number	An abnormal decrease in the number of white blood cells (less than 4500 per cubic millimeter of blood).
Polycythemia	*poly-:* many *cyt/o:* cell *hem/o:* blood *-ia:* condition of diseased or abnormal state	A disorder in which there is an increase in the red blood cell mass.

ON THE WEB

For information on anemia:

National Anemia Action Council: www.anemia.org

Anemia Education: www.anemia.com

For information on leukemia:

The Leukemia and Lymphoma Society: www.leukemia.org

Leukemia Research Foundation: www.leukemia-research.org

Leukemia: www.oncologychannel.com

For information on clotting disorders:

Clotting Disorders: www.coagulation-factors.com

National Alliance for Thrombosis and Thrombophilia: www.stoptheclot.org

Clot Care Online Resource: www.clotcare.com

 Check out the Evolve site at http://evolve.elsevier.com/Bonewit/today/ to actively Prepare for your Certification, and to access additional interactive activities and exercises to help you study and prepare for success.

33

Blood Chemistry and Immunology

LEARNING OBJECTIVES

Blood Chemistry

1. Explain the purpose of a blood chemistry test.
2. Explain the functions of glucose and insulin in the body.
3. State the patient preparation for a fasting blood glucose test.
4. Identify the normal range for a fasting blood glucose test.
5. State the purpose of each of the following tests: fasting blood glucose test, 2-hour postprandial glucose test, and oral glucose tolerance test.
6. Describe the procedure for a 2-hour postprandial blood glucose test.
7. Identify the patient preparation required for an oral glucose tolerance test.
8. State the restrictions that must be followed by the patient during an oral glucose tolerance test.
9. List three advantages of self-monitoring of blood glucose by diabetic patients.
10. Explain the purpose of the hemoglobin A_{1c} test.
11. State the hemoglobin A_{1c} level for an individual without diabetes.
12. State the recommended blood glucose level and hemoglobin A_{1c} percentage for an individual with diabetes.
13. Explain the storage requirements for blood glucose test strips.
14. Describe the functions of LDL cholesterol and HDL cholesterol in the body.
15. State the desirable ranges for each of the following tests: total cholesterol, LDL cholesterol, and HDL cholesterol.
16. State the patient preparation for a triglyceride test.

Immunology

17. Explain the purpose of each of the following immunologic tests: hepatitis tests, HIV tests, syphilis tests, mononucleosis test, rheumatoid factor, antistreptolysin test, C-reactive protein, cold agglutinins, ABO and Rh blood typing, and Rh antibody titer.
18. List the symptoms of infectious mononucleosis.

PROCEDURES

Perform a fasting blood glucose test using a glucose monitor.

Instruct a patient on how to measure blood glucose using a glucose monitor.

Perform blood chemistry testing using an automated blood chemistry analyzer and operating manual.

Demonstrate the proper care and maintenance of a glucose monitor.

Perform a rapid mononucleosis test.

CHAPTER OUTLINE

INTRODUCTION TO BLOOD CHEMISTRY AND IMMUNOLOGY
BLOOD CHEMISTRY
Collection of a Blood Chemistry Specimen
Automated Blood Chemistry Analyzers
Quality Control
Blood Glucose
Blood Glucose Testing

Tests for Management of Diabetes
Self-Monitoring of Blood Glucose
Hemoglobin A_{1c} Test
Glucose Meters
Reagent Test Strips
Calibration Procedure
Control Procedure
Care and Maintenance

KEY TERMS

agglutination (ah-gloo-ti-NAY-shun)
analyte
antibody (AN-ti-bod-ee)
antigen (AN-ti-jen)
blood antigen

glycogen (GLIE-koe-jen)
glycosylation
HDL cholesterol
hemoglobin A1c
hyperglycemia (hie-per-glie-SEE-me-ah)

hypoglycemia (hie-poe-glie-SEE-me-ah)
LDL cholesterol
lipoprotein (lie-poe-PROE-teen)

INTRODUCTION TO BLOOD CHEMISTRY AND IMMUNOLOGY

CLIA-waived blood chemistry and immunologic laboratory tests are often performed in the medical office. Advances in CLIA-waived automated blood analyzers and testing kits designed specifically for use in the medical office have made this possible. Automated blood analyzers perform laboratory tests in a short time with accurate test results.

This chapter is divided into two units. The first presents blood chemistry laboratory tests, and the second presents immunologic tests. The material in this chapter about blood testing is intended to serve only as a basic guide for the medical assistant and should be supplemented by much well-supervised practice in a classroom laboratory, the medical office, or both.

BLOOD CHEMISTRY

Blood chemistry testing involves the quantitative measurement of chemical substances in the blood. These chemicals are dissolved in the liquid portion (plasma) of the blood. Numerous types of blood chemistry tests are available; the type of test (or tests) the physician orders depends on the clinical diagnosis. Examples of common blood chemistry tests include alanine aminotransferase (ALT), alkaline phosphatase (ALP), aspartate aminotransferase (AST), blood urea nitrogen (BUN), calcium, chloride, cholesterol, creatinine, globulin, glucose, lactate dehydrogenase (LD), phosphorus, potassium, sodium, total bilirubin, total protein, total thyroxine, triglycerides, and uric acid levels. The blood chemistry tests that are most frequently performed are described in greater detail in this chapter.

COLLECTION OF A BLOOD CHEMISTRY SPECIMEN

Most blood chemistry tests performed at an outside laboratory require a serum specimen for analysis (Figure 33-1). If the specimen is collected at the medical office, the medical assistant will need to perform a venipuncture using a serum separator tube (SST) or a red-stoppered tube. An example of a blood chemistry profile frequently ordered on patients in the medical office is a *comprehensive metabolic profile* (CMP).

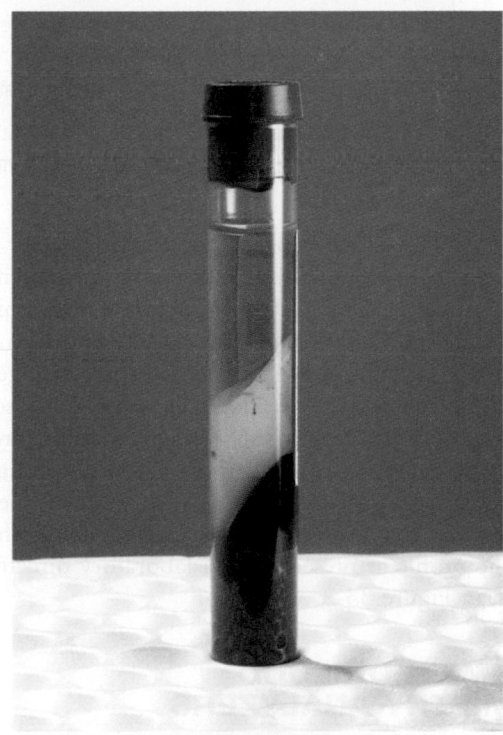

Figure 33-1 Most blood chemistry tests are performed on a serum specimen collected in a serum separator tube (SST).

Comprehensive Metabolic Profile

CPT Code:　　　　　80053

Tests included: albumin, albumin/globulin ratio (calculated), alkaline phosphatase, ALT, AST, BUN/creatinine ratio (calculated), calcium, carbon dioxide, chloride, creatinine, globulin, glucose, potassium, sodium, total bilirubin, total protein.

Type of specimen:　　Serum

Amount:　　　　　　4 mL

Collection supplies:　SST (send entire tube)

Collection techniques: Let SST stand for 30 minutes. Centrifuge SST within 45 minutes of collection to separate serum from cells with gel barrier.

Patient preparation:　Patient should fast for 12 to 14 hours prior to collection.

Handling and storage: Refrigerate or store at room temperature. Stable at room temperature for 24 hours and stable in the refrigerator for 72 hours.

Causes for rejection:　Nonfasting specimen, hemolysis, improper labeling of tube

Reference range:　　Values given with report.

Use:
The CMP is used as a screening test to assess the overall health of an individual. It is used to detect any changes in the body's biologic processes that may be present, although the patient may not have had any symptoms to indicate these changes have occurred. Also see uses of individual tests.

Limitations:　　　　See individual tests for limitations.

Methodology:　　　See individual tests for methodologies.

Figure 33-2 Specimen collection and handling requirements for a comprehensive metabolic profile as presented in a laboratory directory.

A CMP contains numerous blood chemistry tests and is used primarily in routine health screening of a patient. It is frequently used to detect any changes in the body's biologic processes that may be present, although the patient may not have had any symptoms to indicate that these changes have occurred. A comprehensive metabolic profile is also used when the patient's symptoms are so vague that the physician does not have enough concrete evidence to support a clinical diagnosis of a specific organ or disease state. Specimen collection and handling requirements for a comprehensive metabolic profile as presented in a laboratory directory are outlined in Figure 33-2.

AUTOMATED BLOOD CHEMISTRY ANALYZERS

Automated blood chemistry analyzers are used to perform blood chemistry testing. A blood chemistry analyzer consists of a reflectance photometer that quantitatively measures the amount of chemical substances, or analytes, in the blood. An **analyte** is defined as a substance that is being identified or measured in a laboratory test. Specifically, a reflectance photometer measures light intensity to determine the exact amount of an analyte in a specimen.

Most physicians consider it too expensive in terms of equipment, supplies, and medical laboratory personnel to perform blood chemistry tests that are any more complex than waived tests in the medical office. These tests are usually performed at an outside laboratory. However, if moderately complex blood chemistry tests are performed in the medical office, a "benchtop" blood chemistry analyzer is typically used to run them; examples of these nonwaived "benchtop" analyzers include the ATAC lab system (Clinical Data, Inc., Newton, Mass) (Figure 33-3) and the Reflotron Chemistry Analyzer (Roche Diagnostics, Branchburg, NJ). Examples of CLIA-waived blood chemistry analyzers that are more commonly used to run blood chemistry tests in the medical office include the Accu-Check Advantage blood glucose meter (Roche Diagnostics), A₁c Now (Bayer Corporation, Morrisville, NJ), and the Cholestech LDX cholesterol system (Cholestech Corporation, Hayward, Calif).

The manufacturer of each blood chemistry analyzer provides an operating manual (and sometimes an instructional video) with the instrument that includes information needed to collect and handle the specimen, perform quality control procedures, and test the specimen. The manufacturer also has personnel available for on-site training and service. Because most medical offices use CLIA-waived blood chemistry analyzers (rather than nonwaived analyzers), the remainder of this chapter focuses on CLIA-waived blood chemistry analyzers used in the medical office.

It is important that the medical assistant become completely familiar with all aspects of the CLIA-waived analyzer

used to perform blood chemistry testing in his or her medical office. Medical offices running CLIA-waived tests are required to follow the manufacturer's instructions *exactly* for each testing procedure. Instructions include information on the quality control procedures that must be performed when running the test. Quality control procedures are of particular importance to ensure that the analyzer is functioning properly, and that the test results are reliable and accurate. Additional information on quality control procedures is presented below (also refer to the quality control section in Chapter 29).

Quality Control

The ultimate goal when performing blood chemistry testing is to ensure that the test accurately measures what it is supposed to measure; this involves practicing and maintaining a quality control program. Quality control consists of methods and means to ensure that test results are reliable and valid. Two important quality control measures must be performed routinely when a blood chemistry analyzer is used: calibration of the instrument and running controls.

Calibration

Calibration is a mechanism used to check the precision and accuracy of a blood chemistry analyzer, to determine if the system is providing accurate results. A calibration check detects errors caused by laboratory equipment that is not working properly. Calibration is typically performed using a calibration device, often called a *standard*. The calibration device may come in the form of a calibration strip or cassette. The device is inserted into the analyzer (Figure 33-4, *A*) and the calibration results are displayed on the LCD screen of the analyzer. The calibration results

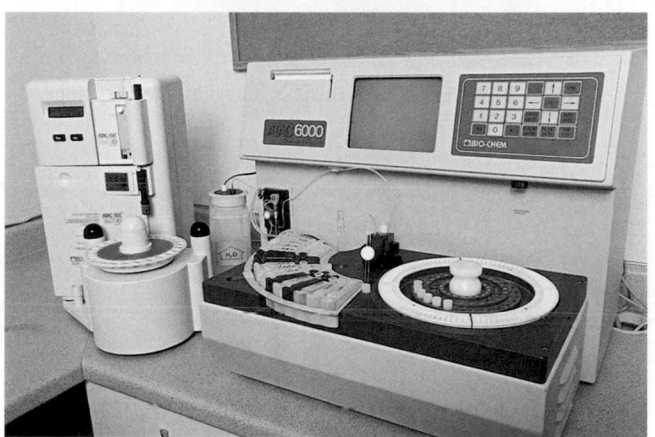

Figure 33-3 Blood chemistry analyzer.

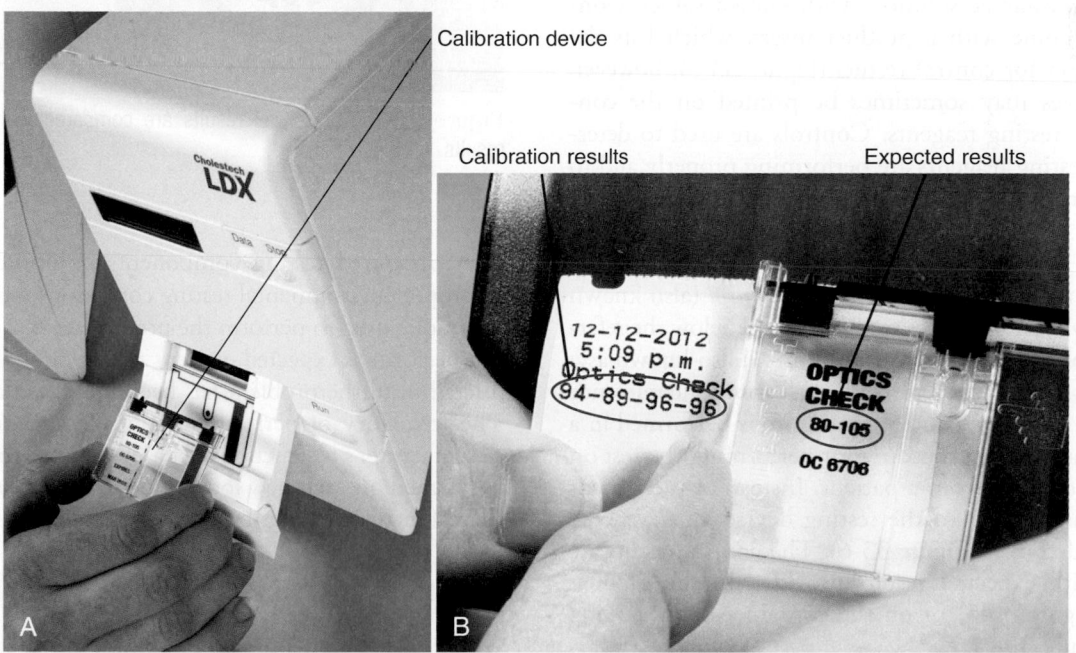

Figure 33-4 **A,** Calibrating a blood chemistry analyzer using a calibration device. **B,** The calibration results are compared with the expected results on the calibration device.

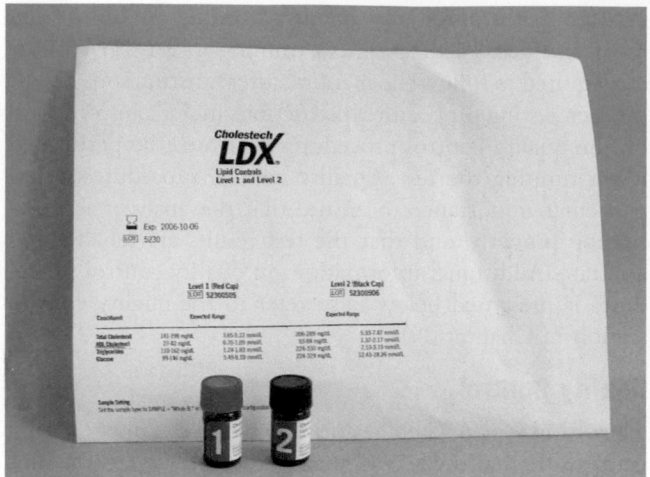

Figure 33-5 Controls come with a product insert, which lists the expected ranges for control results.

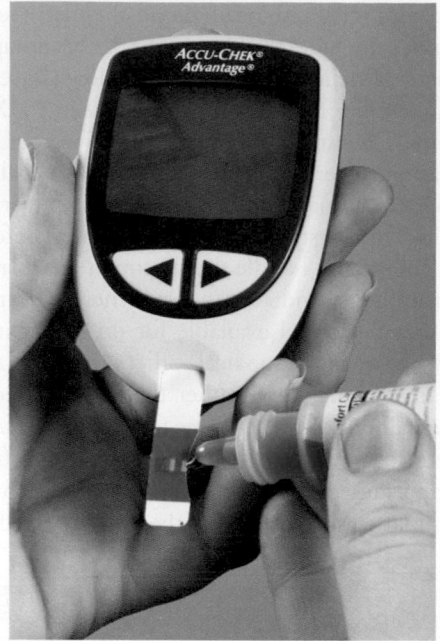

Figure 33-6 The control solution is added to a testing strip.

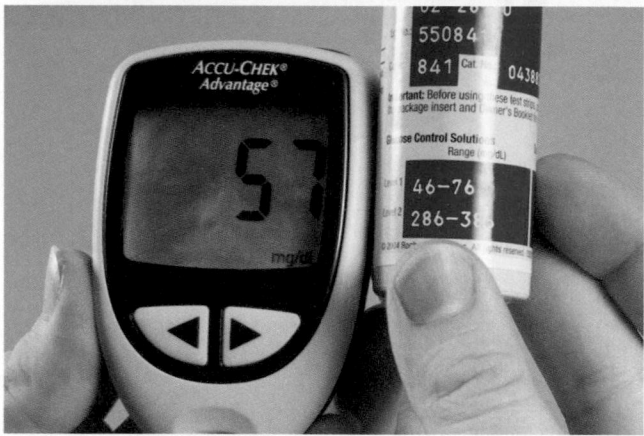

Figure 33-7 The control results are compared with the expected results.

are then compared with the expected results provided in the product insert or on the calibration device (Figure 33-4, *B*). If the calibration procedure does not perform as expected, patient testing should not be conducted until the problem has been identified and resolved. The frequency of performing a calibration check is indicated in the manufacturer's instructions. At a minimum, a calibration check should be performed when a new lot number of testing reagents is put into use.

Controls

A blood chemistry control consists of a solution that is used to monitor a blood chemistry analyzer to ensure the reliability and accuracy of the test results. Controls consist of commercially available solutions with known values. Controls usually come with a product insert, which lists the expected ranges for control results (Figure 33-5); however, expected ranges may sometimes be printed on the containers of the testing reagents. Controls are used to determine if the testing reagents are performing properly and to detect any errors in technique by the individual performing the test.

Generally, two levels of controls must be performed on a blood chemistry analyzer. A *low-level control* (also known as a *Level 1 control*) produces results that fall below the reference range for the test; a *high-level control* (also known as a *Level 2 control*) produces results that fall above the reference range for the test. The control procedure is performed in a similar manner to the procedure for performing the test on a specimen collected from a patient. Instead of the patient specimen being added to the testing device, however, the control is added to it (Figure 33-6). The control results are compared with expected results provided in the product insert (see Figure 33-5) or on the container of the testing reagents (Figure 33-7).

Failure of a control to produce expected results may be due to the following: deterioration of testing components

due to expired testing components or improper storage, improper environmental testing conditions, or errors in the technique used to perform the procedure. If the controls do not perform as expected, patient testing should not be conducted until the problem has been identified and resolved. The frequency of performing controls is indicated in the manufacturer's instructions. At a minimum, they should be performed on each new lot number of testing reagents, and thereafter on a regular basis, such as monthly.

BLOOD GLUCOSE

Glucose is the end product of carbohydrate metabolism; it is the chief source of energy for the body. Energy is needed to perform normal functions and to maintain body temperature. The body maintains a constant blood glucose level to ensure a continuous source of energy for the body. Ingested glucose that is not needed for energy can be stored for later use in the form of glycogen in muscle and liver tissue. When no more tissue storage is possible, excess glycogen is converted to triglycerides (a form of fat) and is stored as adipose tissue.

Insulin is a hormone secreted by the beta cells of the pancreas that is required for normal use of glucose in the body. Insulin enables glucose to enter the body's cells and be converted to energy. Insulin also is needed for the proper storage of glycogen in liver and muscle cells.

Blood Glucose Testing

Measuring the amount of glucose in a blood specimen is one of the most commonly performed blood chemistry tests. It is used to detect abnormalities in carbohydrate metabolism such as those that occur in prediabetes, diabetes, gestational diabetes, **hypoglycemia,** and liver and adrenocortical dysfunction. Blood glucose is measured by several different testing methods, which include the fasting blood glucose, the 2-hour postprandial blood sugar test, and the oral glucose tolerance test. Each of these methods serves a specific role in diagnosing and evaluating abnormalities in carbohydrate metabolism, and each is described in greater detail here.

Fasting Blood Glucose Test

Blood glucose is usually measured when the patient is in a fasting state. This type of test, termed a *fasting blood glucose* (FBG), involves collecting a fasting blood sample and measuring the amount of glucose in it. The patient should not have anything to eat or drink except water for 12 hours preceding the test. Certain medications, such as oral contraceptives, salicylates, diuretics, and steroids, may affect the test results; the physician may place the patient on medication restrictions for a specific period before the test—usually 3 days. The patient should be scheduled for the test in the morning to minimize the inconvenience of abstaining from food and fluid.

An FBG is often performed on patients diagnosed with diabetes to evaluate their progress and regulate treatment, and on other patients as a routine screening test to detect prediabetes and diabetes. *Prediabetes* is the term used to describe the condition in which glucose levels are higher than normal, but not high enough to be classified as diabetes. An individual with prediabetes has an increased risk of developing type 2 diabetes. The American Diabetes Association (ADA) recommends the following guidelines for interpretation of FBG test results:

70-99 mg/dL	Normal
100-125 mg/dL	Prediabetes (also termed *impaired fasting glucose*)
126 mg/dL or above	Diabetes (confirm by repeating the FBG test on another day)

Two-Hour Postprandial Blood Glucose Test

The 2-hour postprandial blood glucose (2-hour PPBG) test is used to screen for diabetes and to monitor the effects of insulin dosage in patients with diabetes. The patient is required to fast, beginning at midnight preceding the test and continuing until breakfast. For breakfast, the patient must consume a prescribed meal that contains 100 g of carbohydrate, which consists of orange juice, cereal with sugar, toast, and milk. An alternative to this is the consumption of a 100-g test-load glucose solution. A blood specimen is collected from the patient exactly 2 hours after consumption of the meal or glucose solution.

In a nondiabetic patient, the glucose level returns to the fasting level within $1\frac{1}{2}$ to 2 hours of glucose consumption, whereas the glucose level in a diabetic patient does not return to the fasting level. A postprandial glucose level of 140 g/dL or higher suggests diabetes and warrants further testing, such as the oral glucose tolerance test.

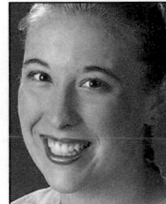

Putting It All into Practice

My name is Michelle Villers, and I work for a physician in an internal medicine medical office. My primary job responsibility includes running the laboratory at the office. I mainly draw blood and perform blood chemistry tests. I also work up patients, run electrocardiograms, apply Holter monitors, and perform pulmonary function tests.

When performing a venipuncture, you need to make sure all the necessary equipment is on hand and ready. Sometimes you may have a tube that has no vacuum in it. In cases like these, it is always better to have a couple of spare tubes on hand. I recently had an experience in which one of my tubes had no vacuum. Luckily, I had a few extra tubes within arm's reach, so I did not have to interrupt the procedure to get a new one. I have learned that you can never be too prepared. ■

Oral Glucose Tolerance Test

The oral glucose tolerance test (OGTT) provides more detailed information about the ability of the body to metabolize glucose by assessing the insulin response to a glucose load. The OGTT is used to assist in the diagnosis of prediabetes, diabetes, gestational diabetes, hypoglycemia, and liver and adrenocortical dysfunction. It provides a more thorough analysis of glucose use than is provided by the FBG or the 2-hour PPBG test.

Testing Requirements

The patient is usually required to consume a high-carbohydrate diet, consisting of 150 g of carbohydrate per day, for 3 days before the oral glucose tolerance test. The patient must be in a fasting state when the test begins. On the morning of the test, a blood specimen is drawn from the patient for an FBG. If the FBG indicates **hyperglycemia,** the physician should be notified because this situation is a contraindication for the administration of a large test load of glucose.

After the FBG has been performed, the patient is instructed to drink a solution containing 75 g of glucose. At regular intervals thereafter a blood specimen is taken to determine the patient's ability to handle the increased amount of glucose. Each blood specimen must be labeled carefully with the exact time of collection. The patient is permitted to eat and drink normally after completion of the test.

It is important that the patient adhere to certain restrictions during the test to ensure accurate results. Because food and fluid affect blood glucose levels, the patient must not eat or drink anything except water during the test. Smoking is not permitted during the test because tobacco is a stimulant that increases the blood glucose level. The patient should remain at the testing site so that he or she is present when needed for collection of blood specimens and to minimize activity. Activity affects the test results by using up glucose; the patient should remain relatively inactive during the test. Sitting and reading is an activity that would be recommended.

What Would You Do? What Would You *Not* Do?

Case Study 1
Crystal Louellen is at the medical office for an oral glucose tolerance test. She says that she tried not to eat anything, but she started shaking, so she stopped at McDonald's on the way over and got a sausage biscuit and orange juice. Crystal gets quite upset when she learns that she has to come back again to have her test run. She said that she hired a babysitter to watch her four preschool-age children. She demands to know why this test takes so long and why she can't have anything to eat before the test. Crystal wants to know if she can bring her children next time, so she doesn't have to hire a babysitter. Crystal says that she's a "nicotine" addict, and when she's not needed for testing, she could take the kids outside to play. She says that way the kids won't bother anyone and she can have a cigarette at the same time. ■

Side Effects

During the test, the patient may experience some normal side effects, including weakness, a feeling of faintness, and perspiration. These are considered normal reactions of the body to a decrease in the glucose level as insulin is secreted in response to the glucose load. The patient should be reassured that this is a temporary condition. Serious symptoms of severe hypoglycemia should be reported immediately to the physician; these may include headache; pale, cold, and clammy skin; irrational speech or behavior; profuse perspiration; and fainting.

Interpretation of Results

As glucose is absorbed into the bloodstream, the blood glucose level of a nondiabetic individual increases to a peak level of 160 to 180 mg/dL approximately 30 to 60 minutes after the glucose solution is consumed. The pancreas secretes insulin to compensate for this rise, and the blood glucose returns to the fasting level within 2 hours of ingestion of the glucose solution.

The individual with diabetes does not exhibit the normal use of glucose just described. This is because individuals with diabetes are unable to remove glucose from the bloodstream at the same rate as nondiabetic individuals. The blood glucose peaks at a much higher level. In addition, blood glucose levels are above normal throughout the test because of the lack of insulin.

Two hours after the glucose solution is consumed, the test results are interpreted as follows, according to guidelines set forth by the American Diabetes Association (ADA):

139 and below	Normal
140-199 mg/dL	Prediabetes (also known as *impaired glucose tolerance*)
200 mg/dL or above	Diabetes (confirm by repeating the OGTT test on another day)

Hypoglycemia

Hypoglycemia is a condition in which the glucose in the blood is abnormally low (FBG below 70 mg/dL). During the OGTT, patients with this condition exhibit an abnormally low blood glucose level, beginning at the 2-hour interval and continuing for 4 or 5 hours. Hypoglycemia results from removal of glucose from the blood at an excessive rate, or from decreased secretion of glucose into the blood, which can be caused by an overdose of insulin, Addison disease, bacterial sepsis, carcinoma of the pancreas, hepatic necrosis, or hypothyroidism.

TESTS FOR MANAGEMENT OF DIABETES

It is important for individuals with diabetes to manage their condition effectively. This is best accomplished by keeping blood glucose levels as close to normal as possible. Diabetic patients who maintain good blood glucose control generally experience fewer symptoms and delay or prevent long-term complications of the disease; these results can lead to a longer life.

Two testing methods are used for the management of diabetes—self-monitoring of blood glucose and the hemoglobin A_{1c} test. Self-monitoring of blood glucose, which is performed by diabetic patients at home, measures day-to-day fluctuations in blood glucose levels. The hemoglobin A_{1c} test must be ordered by the physician and provides an average or overall picture of the patient's blood glucose levels over time. These testing methods assist the patient and the physician in determining whether the diabetes management plan is working or whether it needs to be adjusted.

Self-Monitoring of Blood Glucose

Individuals with diabetes cannot usually tell by the way they feel whether or not their blood glucose levels are within normal range. The only way for them to know for certain is by self-monitoring of blood glucose (SMBG). SMBG not only provides diabetic patients with feedback for maintaining normal blood glucose levels, it also assists them in anticipating and treating day-to-day, or even hour-to-hour, fluctuations in glucose levels brought on by food, exercise, stress, and infection.

Diabetic patients who take insulin (insulin-dependent) must monitor their blood glucose levels each day. Based on the results of SMBG, decisions can be made regarding insulin and dietary adjustments that may be necessary to maintain normal glucose levels and to avoid the extremes of hypoglycemia and hyperglycemia (see Chapter 35). Satisfactory control of the blood glucose level on a day-to-day basis through SMBG reduces symptoms of the disease and helps delay or prevent long-term complications that can occur with diabetes.

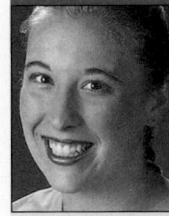

Memories *from* Externship

Michelle Villers: During my externship experience, I was assigned to a four-physician pediatric practice. The office was constantly busy with screaming children. As if I were not nervous enough, I was asked to assist in the removal of sutures. When I walked into the room with the physician, beads of sweat began to form on my forehead. A child was lying on the examining table—a little boy no more than 7 years old. He was there to have sutures removed from a recent surgery. The sutures had been tied very well, and it was difficult for the physician to cut them. The little boy lay there with tears streaming down his cheeks. I reassured him and talked to him, and his tears began to subside. "A few more minutes and it will be all over," I told him. And within those next few minutes, the physician cut the last suture. The little boy eagerly hopped down off the examining table and gave me a big hug. I learned that day how a little reassurance can make everyone involved feel better. ■

PATIENT TEACHING   Diabetes

Answer questions patients have about diabetes.

What is diabetes?

Diabetes is a lifelong condition that occurs when the body is not able to use glucose for energy because of a problem with insulin. Diabetes develops when the body produces little or no insulin, or when the body cannot use the insulin it does produce (known as *insulin resistance*). According to the American Diabetes Association, almost 24 million Americans have diabetes; of these, nearly 6 million are not yet diagnosed and are unaware that they have diabetes. An additional 57 million people have prediabetes. Prediabetes is a condition in which the glucose levels of an individual are higher than normal, but not high enough to be classified as diabetes. An individual with prediabetes has an increased risk of developing type 2 diabetes.

The cause of diabetes is not completely understood, but it seems that the predisposition to develop diabetes is inherited. Diabetes increases the risk of developing serious complications, including heart disease, blindness (retinopathy), nerve damage (neuropathy), kidney damage (nephropathy), and poor circulation, which can result in amputation of a limb.

What is the function of insulin?

Insulin is a hormone produced and secreted by the beta cells of the pancreas. The pancreas is a gland located just behind the stomach and is about the size of a hand. Insulin is required for the normal use of glucose in the body. Through the process of digestion, carbohydrates are broken down into glucose. Shortly after a meal containing carbohydrates is consumed, glucose levels in the blood begin to increase. This sends a message to the pancreas to secrete insulin. Insulin "unlocks" the cells of the body and allows glucose to enter the cells. Inside the cells, glucose is converted into energy. Glucose is the main source of energy for the body and is needed to carry out normal body functions and to assist in maintaining body temperature.

What are the symptoms of diabetes?

Individuals with diabetes produce little or no insulin or cannot use the insulin they do produce. Without insulin, glucose cannot get into the cells of the body, and it builds up in the bloodstream, resulting in a high blood glucose level, known as *hyperglycemia.* Although blood glucose levels are increased, the body is unable to use the glucose for energy. This results in increased hunger, weight loss, and fatigue. The body attempts to get rid of the excess glucose by expelling it in the urine. To be excreted, the glucose must be diluted in large amounts of water. This results in increased urination and increased thirst to replace the water being lost. A summary of the symptoms of diabetes follows:

- Increased urination
- Excessive thirst
- Weight loss
- Constant hunger
- Nausea and vomiting
- Abdominal pain
- Fatigue
- Blurred vision

What is the difference between type 1 diabetes and type 2 diabetes?

Two main categories of diabetes have been identified: type 1 diabetes and type 2 diabetes. Type 2 diabetes is the most common form of diabetes. Approximately 90% of individuals with diabetes have type 2 diabetes.

Continued

Type 1 Diabetes

Type 1 diabetes can occur at any age but is most apt to begin in childhood, adolescence, or early adulthood (before age 30). Type 1 diabetes is an autoimmune disease in which the body produces antibodies that attack and gradually destroy the insulin-producing beta cells of the pancreas. This results in an inability of the body to produce any insulin at all, or it may produce very little insulin. The symptoms are usually severe and occur rapidly—typically over weeks or months. Individuals with type 1 diabetes almost always require insulin therapy. The insulin is administered subcutaneously using an insulin syringe/needle or an insulin pen. An insulin pen is an insulin injection device that contains a needle and holds a vial of insulin. Insulin also can be administered through an insulin pump, which is a small, battery-operated device about the size of a cell phone that is clipped to a belt or carried in a pocket (see illustration). The pump is connected to plastic tubing that continuously delivers insulin into the subcutaneous tissue of the abdomen. An insulin pump also can be programmed to deliver varying doses of insulin as a patient's need for insulin changes during the day (e.g., before exercise or meals).

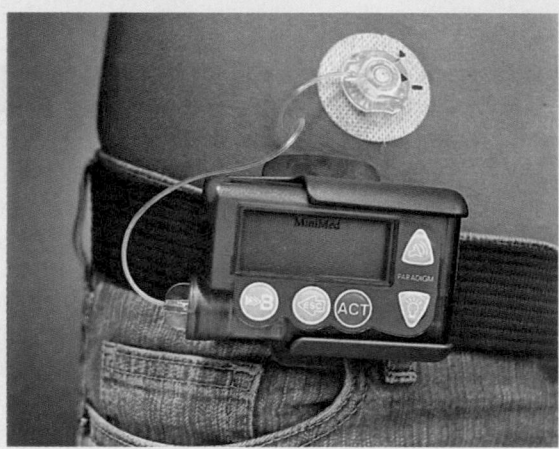

Insulin pump.

Type 2 Diabetes

Type 2 diabetes can affect people at any age, but the chance of developing it increases with age, and it is more likely to occur in individuals who are 40 years of age or older. The biggest risk factor for developing type 2 diabetes is excess body weight. As a result of the recent increase in childhood obesity combined with a sedentary lifestyle, type 2 diabetes is starting to appear in younger age groups. Individuals with type 2 diabetes do not produce enough insulin or are not able to use the insulin they do produce (insulin resistance), resulting in high blood glucose levels. Type 2 diabetes almost always has a slow onset with mild symptoms that appear gradually over a long time (often years). Some individuals have no symptoms at all (except for high blood glucose levels). Because of this, they may be unaware that they have diabetes until a complication from prolonged hyperglycemia occurs, such as a vision problem or foot pain. Type 2 diabetes is first treated by dietary adjustments, weight reduction, and exercise. These changes sometimes can restore insulin sensitivity, even if the weight loss is modest. Approximately 20% of cases of type 2 diabetes can be managed by lifestyle changes alone. The next step, if necessary, is treatment with oral hypoglycemics, which are medications taken by mouth that stimulate the release of insulin from the pancreas,

help the body use its own insulin better, or both. If this treatment is ineffective, insulin therapy becomes necessary to maintain normal or near-normal glucose levels.

What factors increase the risk of developing type 2 diabetes?

The cause of type 2 diabetes is unknown, although certain factors, known as *risk factors,* make a person more prone to developing type 2 diabetes. The more risk factors present, the more likely it is that an individual will develop type 2 diabetes. Some of these factors can be controlled, and others cannot.

Risk Factors That Can Be Controlled

1. **Weight.** The risk factor that contributes most to the development of type 2 diabetes is excess body weight. Approximately 80% of individuals with type 2 diabetes are overweight. Being overweight (body mass index of 25 or greater) makes it harder for the body to use insulin. A research study by the Diabetes Prevention Program showed that people who followed a low-fat, low-calorie diet; lost a moderate amount of weight; and engaged in regular physical activity (five times a week for 30 minutes) sharply reduced their chances of developing type 2 diabetes.
2. **Smoking.** Smoking makes it harder for the body to control the blood glucose level.
3. **Lack of physical activity.** Regular exercise helps the body to use insulin normally, whereas a sedentary lifestyle contributes to insulin resistance.
4. **High blood pressure, abnormal lipid profile, or both.** The following factors contribute to insulin resistance: blood pressure greater than 130/80 mm Hg, HDL cholesterol of 35 mg/dL or less, and triglyceride level of 250 mg/dL or greater. Decreasing blood pressure also can reduce the risk of cardiovascular complications.

Risk Factors That Cannot Be Controlled

1. **Family history.** The risk of developing type 2 diabetes is increased if a close relative (parent, brother, sister) has diabetes.
2. **Gestational diabetes or giving birth to a large infant.** Women who have diabetes during pregnancy or gave birth to an infant weighing more than 9 lb are at greater risk for developing type 2 diabetes.
3. **Age.** Type 2 diabetes is more common in people 40 years and older, but it is increasing among young people who are overweight and inactive.
4. **Ethnic group.** The following ethnic groups are more likely to develop type 2 diabetes: African Americans, Latinos, Hispanics, Native Americans, Asian Americans, and Pacific Islanders.

Can diabetes be cured?

There is no cure for diabetes, but the outlook for individuals with this condition is improving. This is primarily due to better patient education, advances in blood glucose monitoring, and newer methods of insulin delivery that help simplify management of the disease. Today, most individuals with diabetes under good control have life expectancies comparable with those of individuals without diabetes. ■

Case Study 2

Dave Felden has recently been diagnosed with type 1 diabetes and is taking insulin. He has come to the office for an FBG. A finger-stick will be performed to collect the specimen, and a glucose meter will be used to test the specimen. Dave has been performing this test on himself at home now for 2 weeks and wants to know whether he can stick his own finger. Dave says that he's been having a few problems giving himself his insulin injections. He says that he has been getting some very large air bubbles in his syringe when he draws up the insulin. He says he's been having trouble getting them out and wants to know how important that is. Dave says he is on a limited income and wants to know whether he could use his needle and syringe for more than one injection. He also wants to know whether he should throw his used needle and syringes in the regular trash. ■

Frequency of Testing

The frequency of blood glucose testing depends on numerous factors, including the severity of the diabetes, diet, activity level, and special conditions such as pregnancy. Ideally, the blood glucose level for an insulin-dependent diabetic patient should be measured 4 times a day: in the morning (after an 8-hour fast), before lunch, before dinner, and at bedtime. The FBG test result (obtained in the morning) is the best overall indicator of control, and the other determinations provide guidance for adjusting insulin dosage, diet, and exercise.

Test Results

Blood glucose levels are measured using a glucose meter, and the results are displayed in mg/dL. Table 33-1 lists recommended blood glucose levels for patients with diabetes based on when the testing is performed. Diabetic patients should be instructed to maintain a cumulative record of their daily SMBG test results for periodic review by the physician. This record assists the physician in making decisions regarding the patient's diabetes management plan.

Advantages

Research shows that SMBG is the most effective way for a diabetic patient to maintain a normal blood glucose level and delay or prevent long-term complications associated with diabetes. High blood glucose levels (greater than 180 mg/dL) for a long time can cause progressive damage to the body organs, resulting in blindness, kidney disease, nerve damage, and circulation problems. Because of the

Table 33-1 Recommended Blood Glucose Levels for Patients with Diabetes

Time of Day	Recommended Blood Glucose Level (mg/dL)
Before meals	80-120
1-2 hr after meals	100-180
At bedtime	100-140

From Bonewit-West K: *Clinical procedures for medical assistants*, ed 8, St Louis, 2011, Saunders.

necessity of performing a skin puncture and the fact that the patient must assume responsibility in self-management decisions, the medical assistant may need to reinforce the advantages of self-monitoring of blood glucose, as follows:

1. **Convenience of testing.** The patient is able to test his or her blood at any time of the day without a laboratory order from the physician. This provides a distinct advantage because patients are able to check their blood glucose level when a side effect common to diabetes occurs, such as hypoglycemia. In these situations, treatment can be instituted immediately to prevent the problem from getting worse.

2. **Greater involvement in self-management decisions.** The patient is able to become more involved in self-management decisions regarding insulin dosage, meal planning, and physical activity. Initially some patients lack confidence in making insulin and dietary adjustments based on the blood glucose test results. The medical assistant should provide encouragement and stress the benefits to be derived in terms of improved regulation of the blood glucose level.

3. **Reliable decision making regarding insulin dosage.** More reliable decisions regarding insulin needs can be made during situations that affect the blood glucose level, such as illness, emotional stress, increased physical activity, or suspected hypoglycemia.

4. **Delay in or prevention of long-term complications.** The medical assistant should emphasize to patients how important it is to perform daily SMBG testing to increase their chances of staying healthy. As previously discussed, diabetic patients who maintain good blood glucose control generally experience fewer symptoms and a delay in or prevention of long-term complications of the disease.

Hemoglobin A$_{1c}$ Test

The hemoglobin A$_{1c}$ test (HbA$_{1c}$ test or A$_{1c}$ test) provides valuable information for determining whether a diabetic patient's blood glucose level is under control. The A$_{1c}$ test supplies the physician with an assessment of the average amount of glucose in the blood over a 3-month period.

When an individual consumes food containing glucose, the glucose is absorbed from the digestive tract and into the circulatory system. Glucose (sugar) has a "sticky" quality to it and thus has a tendency to stick to protein in the body. One of the proteins it attaches to is the protein included in hemoglobin. Hemoglobin is found in red blood cells and functions in transporting oxygen in the body. The process of glucose attaching to hemoglobin is known as **glycosylation.**

When glucose attaches or glycosylates to the protein in hemoglobin, it forms a compound known as **hemoglobin A$_{1c}$.** Glycosylation occurs in all individuals—hemoglobin A$_{1c}$ is formed in diabetic patients and healthy individuals. The amount of glucose that attaches to hemoglobin is proportional to the amount of glucose in the blood; the more glucose in the blood, the more hemoglobin becomes glycated and the higher the A$_{1c}$ level. Individuals with undiagnosed or poorly controlled diabetes have a higher than normal blood glucose level, and more hemoglobin A_{1c} forms in these individuals. The percentage of hemoglobin A_{1c} in the blood can be measured by the A_{1c} laboratory test. The attachment of the glucose to the hemoglobin is permanent for the life of the red blood cell (90 to 120 days); the A_{1c} test result is able to provide an overall picture of the patient's blood glucose level for the past 3 months. CLIA-waived analyzers are available for performing a hemoglobin A_{1c} test in the medical office; an example is the A1c Now (Bayer Corporation).

Interpretation of Results

The normal A_{1c} level for an individual without diabetes is 4% to 6%. Patients with diabetes usually have a higher A_{1c} level than this. The American Diabetes Association (ADA) strongly recommends that patients with diabetes maintain an A_{1c} level of less than 7%. Table 33-2 shows the correlation between hemoglobin A_{1c} percentages and average blood glucose levels. A change in a patient's diabetes management plan is almost always required if the A_{1c} test result is greater than 8%.

Patients who keep their hemoglobin A_{1c} levels close to 7% have a much better chance of delaying or preventing diabetic complications than do patients with A_{1c} levels that are 8% or greater. Studies show that for every 1 percentage point drop in the A_{1c} value, a 35% reduction in risk for diabetes-related complications occurs.

The physician orders an A_{1c} test when a patient is first diagnosed with diabetes to determine how elevated the blood glucose level has been before the condition was diagnosed. The test is usually ordered several times after a diabetes management plan has been prescribed to verify that blood glucose control is being achieved. The A_{1c} test is ordered periodically for patients already diagnosed with diabetes to evaluate the effectiveness of their diabetes management plan. For stable diabetic patients under good control, the test is typically ordered at least twice a year (every 6 months). The test is usually ordered on a more frequent basis for patients who have difficulty maintaining control of their blood glucose levels. The A_{1c} test also is ordered when the physician makes an adjustment to a patient's diabetic management plan to assess the effectiveness of the change in treatment.

GLUCOSE METERS

In the medical office, a CLIA-waived glucose meter is often used to measure the blood glucose level quantitatively. The test most frequently performed using the glucose meter is the FBG, although some offices also perform the OGTT and the 2-hour postprandial test. By measuring the blood glucose concentration in the medical office, better patient care can be provided. On-site testing eliminates the time required for an outside laboratory to provide the results, allowing the physician to make decisions immediately regarding diagnosis, treatment, and follow-up care. Procedure 33-1 describes how to measure blood glucose using the Accu-Chek Advantage glucose meter.

Table 33-2 Comparison of Hemoglobin A_{1c} Percentages with Average Blood Glucose Levels

Hemoglobin A_{1c} (%)	Average Daily Blood Glucose Level (mg/dL)
4	65
5	100
6	135
7	170
8	205
9	240
10	275
11	310
12	345

From Bonewit-West K: *Clinical procedures for medical assistants,* ed 8, St Louis, 2011, Saunders.

Reagent Test Strips

A reagent test strip must be used with the glucose meter; it consists of a plastic strip with a reaction pad. The pad contains chemicals that react with the glucose in whole blood to determine the blood glucose level in mg/dL. Through an electronic signal, the glucose results are displayed as a digital readout. The manufacturer's instructions accompanying the glucose meter must be followed exactly to ensure accurate and reliable test results.

It is important to store the container of test strips properly to prevent their deterioration, which affects the test results. The chemical reagents on the strips are sensitive to heat, light, and moisture and must be stored in a cool, dry area at room temperature (less than 90° F [32° C]) with the cap tightly closed. Strips that are discolored or that have darkened should be discarded to prevent inaccurate test results. The container of test strips includes a desiccant. Its purpose is to promote dryness by absorbing moisture.

Calibration Procedure

A calibration procedure may be required for a glucose meter. Because the Accu-Chek Advantage glucose meter is presented in Procedure 33-1, the calibration method discussed here relates specifically to this meter.

The calibration procedure is a coding procedure that is performed to ensure accurate and reliable test results; most glucose meters require this calibration procedure. The coding procedure must be performed each time a new container of test strips is opened. It is performed to compensate for variables that occur in the manufacturing process, which cause one batch of test strips to be a little different from another batch. The coding procedure programs the electronics of the glucose meter to match the reactivity of the container of strips that are in current use.

The coding procedure for the Accu-Chek Advantage is performed using a plastic code key that accompanies each container of Accu-Chek Advantage test strips (Figure 33-8). Accu-Chek requires lot-specific calibration, meaning that the calibration procedure needs to be performed only once per container of test strips. This is possible because the Accu-Chek glucose meter has a built-in memory system that enables it to retain a point of reference after it has been

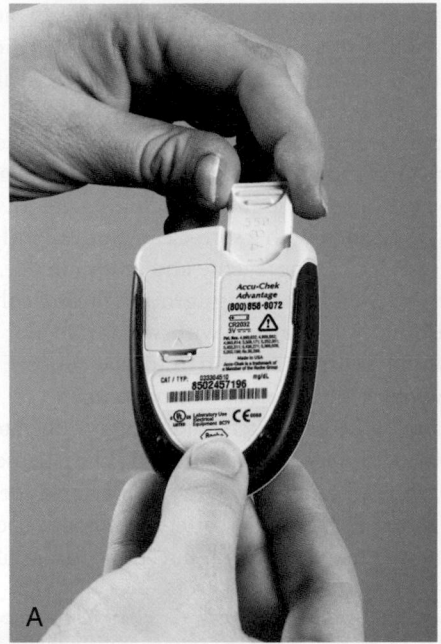
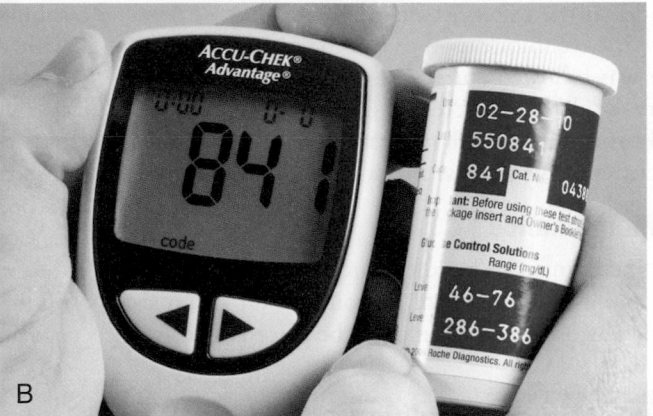

Figure 33-8 Accu-Chek Advantage code key calibration procedure. **A,** The code key is inserted into the monitor. **B,** The code number must match the code number of the vial of test strips.

calibrated. This reference point is retained until the glucose meter is reprogrammed for a new container of test strips. The coding procedure delineated next should be followed when a new container of Accu-Chek test strips is opened:

1. Ensure that the meter is turned off.
2. Turn the meter over so that the back of the meter is facing you.
3. Remove the old code key, if one is installed, and discard it in a waste container.
4. Insert a new code key by sliding it into the code key slot until it snaps into place (see Figure 33-8, *A*).
5. Turn the meter on. A three-digit code number appears on the display screen. This number must match the code number of the vial of test strips (see Figure 33-8, *B*). If it does not, repeat steps 1 through 3.

Control Procedure

A control test should be run to ensure that test results are reliable and valid, and that errors that might interfere with test results are detected and eliminated. A control check is performed on the Accu-Chek Advantage using commercially available glucose control solutions. Two levels of controls (high and low) (Figure 33-9) should be used.

The control solution is effective for 3 months from the date it is opened. When the control solution is opened, the medical assistant must write the date on the container label. The control solution can then be used for 3 months from that date (which should also be written on the container) or until the manufacturer's expiration date (stamped on the container) is reached, whichever comes first. The control solution is sensitive to heat, light, and moisture and must be stored with the cap tightly closed in a cool, dry area at room temperature between 36° F (2° C) and 86° F (30° C).

A control test should be performed under the following circumstances:

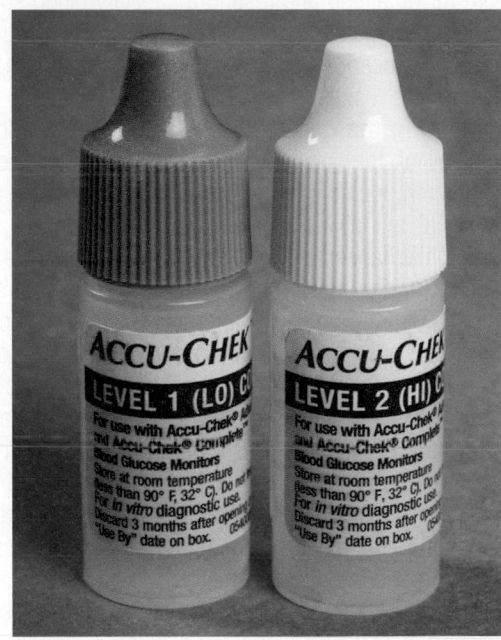

Figure 33-9 Glucose controls.

1. When the meter is new
2. Daily, before the meter is used for the first time
3. When a new container of test strips is opened
4. If the cap is left off the vial of test strips for any length of time
5. If the meter is dropped
6. If the test result does not agree with the way the patient feels
7. If a test has been repeated, and the blood glucose result is still lower or higher than expected

If Level 1 or Level 2 control results are not within the acceptable range, the following should be performed:

1. Check the expiration date of the test strips and control solutions to make sure they are not outdated.
2. Determine whether the test strips and control solutions were stored at room temperature.
3. Make sure the container lids were tight on the test strips container and the control solution containers.
4. Check to make sure the code on the meter matches the code on the test strip vial.
5. Review the technique used to run the control to make sure it was followed correctly.

Any errors should be corrected, and the control should be run again. If the results are still not within acceptable range, the manufacturer of the glucose meter should be contacted.

Care and Maintenance

The glucose meter must be handled carefully. It is a delicate instrument, and a severe physical jar could result in a malfunction. The glucose meter should not be placed in an area of high humidity, such as a bathroom. In addition, the meter should not be exposed to severe variations in environmental temperature, such as would occur if it is left in a closed vehicle on a hot or cold day.

Proper cleaning of the glucose meter is essential for its accurate and reliable operation. On a regular basis, the exterior of the glucose meter, including the display screen, should be cleaned with a soft, clean cloth slightly dampened with a mild cleaning agent, and it should be dried thoroughly. Acceptable cleaning agents include alcohol and mild dishwashing liquid mixed with water. Do not allow water or cleaning solution to run into the glucose meter; this could damage the internal components.

Because glucose meters are battery operated, periodic replacement of the battery is required. The glucose meter alerts the user to low battery voltage by displaying a special notation on the screen. The type of battery required is specified in the operating manual, along with directions for installation.

The medical assistant may need to instruct the patient in the procedure for obtaining and testing a capillary blood specimen for blood glucose measurement. Properly educating the patient to perform the procedure is the most important factor in obtaining accurate test results.

1. **Obtaining the capillary blood specimen.** Inform the patient of the sites available for obtaining the blood specimen, including the fingers and the side of the hand that has no calluses. Most patients prefer to use an automatic lancet to perform the skin puncture. Using such a device makes the puncture less painful, and the preset puncture depth generally ensures a successful stick. For a finger puncture, instruct the patient to obtain the blood specimen from the lateral side of the fingertip because this area contains fewer nerve endings, and less pain results. If the patient's hands are cold, tell him or her to rub them together or place them in warm water, which improves blood flow to the area. Instruct the patient in the proper procedure for obtaining enough blood to ensure accurate test results.
2. **Performing the blood glucose test.** The patient performs the test with a test strip using a glucose meter.

Instruct the patient in the proper procedure for performing the test, making sure he or she understands that accurate test results assist in achieving greater glucose control. Patients also should be given detailed instructions on proper care and maintenance of the glucose meter.

3. **Recording results.** Instruct the patient to record each test result in a log book between office visits to provide a permanent record. In addition, most glucose meters are equipped with a memory system that stores test results for later retrieval. Keeping track of these factors helps explain a shift in the blood glucose level and provides the basis for sound self-management decisions. The following information should be included with each recording:
- Date and time
- Number of hours since the patient last ate
- Time of the last insulin injection or oral hypoglycemic medication
- Any feeling of physical or emotional stress
- Amount of exercise the patient has had

PROCEDURE 33-1 **Blood Glucose Measurement Using the Accu-Chek Advantage Glucose Meter**

Outcome Perform a fasting blood glucose (FBG) test.

Equipment/Supplies

- Disposable gloves
- Accu-Chek Advantage glucose meter
- Accu-Chek Advantage test strips
- Code key
- Control solutions
- Lancet
- Antiseptic wipe
- Gauze pad
- Biohazard sharps container

PROCEDURE 33-1 Blood Glucose Measurement Using the Accu-Chek Advantage Glucose Meter—cont'd

1. Procedural Step. Sanitize your hands. Assemble the equipment. Check the expiration date on the container of test strips. Check to make sure the environmental temperature falls between 57° F (14° C) and 104° F (40° C).

Principle. Outdated test strips can cause inaccurate test results. If the temperature is outside of the required range, the meter cannot perform the test, causing an error message to appear on the screen of the analyzer.

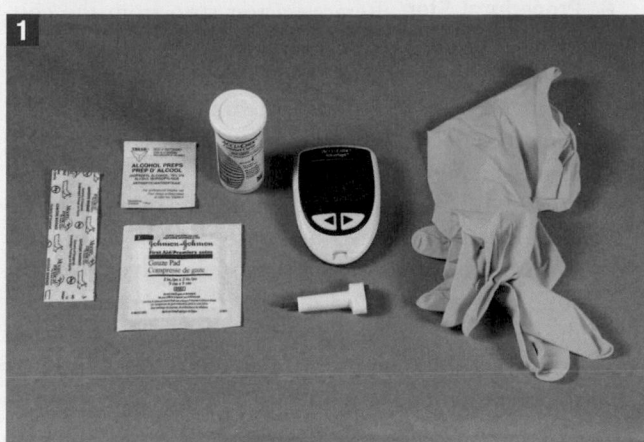

Assemble the equipment.

2. Procedural Step. If necessary, calibrate the glucose meter using the code key that accompanies the container of test strips.

a. Ensure that the meter is turned off.

b. Turn the meter over so that the back of the meter is facing you.

c. Insert the code key into the slot on the back of the meter.

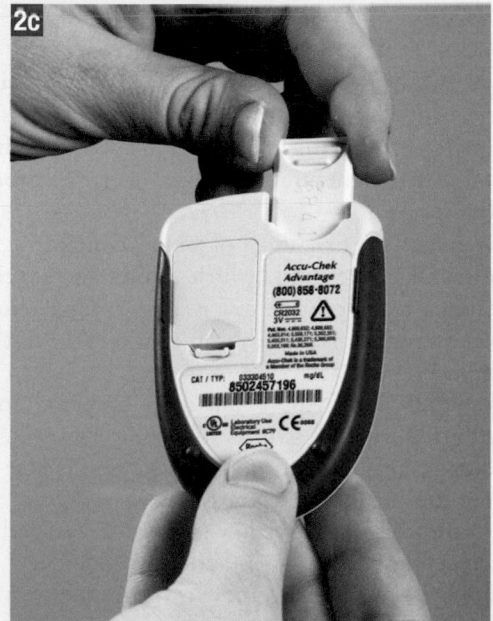

Insert the code key.

d. Push on the code key until it snaps into place.

e. Turn on the meter.

f. A three-digit code number appears on the display screen. The number must match the code number on the container of test strips.

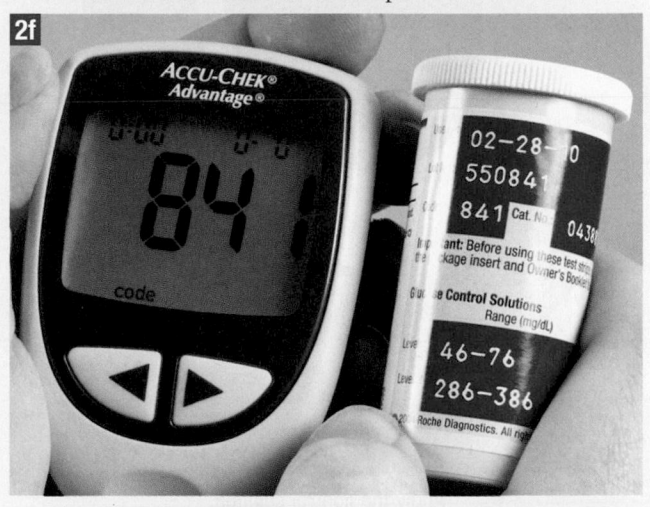

Check the code number.

Principle. Calibrating with the code key compensates for variables that occur in the manufacturing process of the test strips and must be performed before strips from a new container are used.

3. Procedural Step. Run a Level 1 (low) and Level 2 (high) control check on the glucose meter using Accu-Chek Advantage control solutions as follows:

a. Check the expiration date on the control solutions. (*NOTE:* The expiration date for the test strips was checked previously and therefore does not need to be checked again.)

b. Remove a test strip from the container and immediately recap the container.

c. Gently insert the end of the test strip with the silver-colored bars into the test strip guide with the yellow target area facing up. This automatically turns on the meter.

d. Check to make sure the code number matches the number displayed on the container of strips.

e. When the strip is inserted correctly, a blood drop symbol flashes on the display screen, indicating that it is ready to accept the control solution.

f. Roll the Level 1 low control solution between the palms of your hands to mix it.

g. Press and release the right arrow button once to select the Level 1 control.

h. Hold the control solution at an angle to the edge of the yellow target area of the test strip. Squeeze the container, and touch and hold a drop of control solution to the edge (not the top) of the yellow target area. Promptly replace the cap for the control solution.

Continued

PROCEDURE 33-1   Blood Glucose Measurement Using the Accu-Chek Advantage Glucose Meter—cont'd

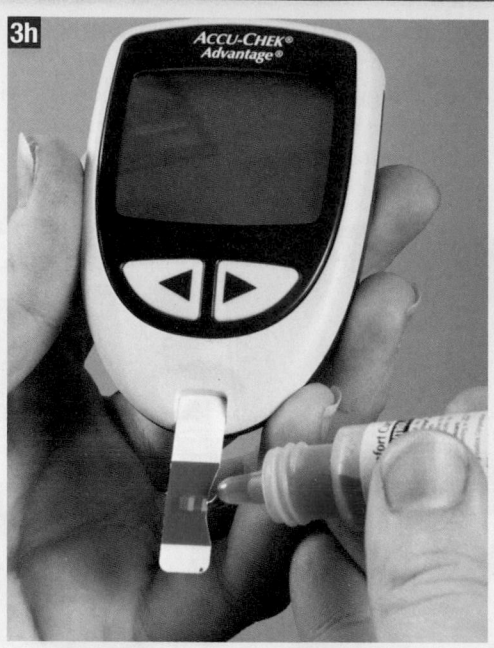

Apply the control solution.

i.   After a short time, the control result is displayed on the screen of the glucose meter.

j. If the low control result is within the acceptable range, the result will alternate with the word "OK" on the display screen. The result will also fall within the expected range listed on the test strip container.

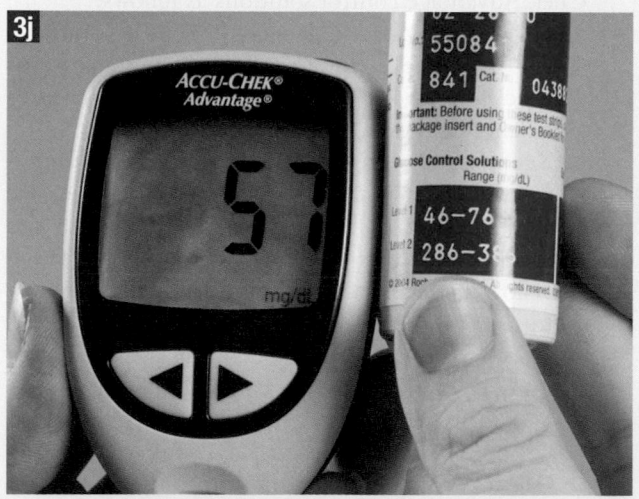

Control results should fall within the expected range.

k.   Repeat the control procedure outlined above using a Level 2 high control.

l.   Record the control results in the Quality Control log.

Principle. Running a low and a high control check ensures that the test results are reliable and valid. Gloves do not need to be worn because the control consists of a glucose solution.

4. **Procedural Step.** Sanitize your hands. Greet and introduce yourself. Identify the patient by full name and date of birth. Explain the procedure.

5. **Procedural Step.** Ask the patient whether he or she has had anything to eat or drink (besides water) for the past 12 hours.
    Principle. Consumption of food or fluid increases the blood glucose level, leading to inaccurate interpretation of FBG test results.

6. **Procedural Step.** Remove a test strip from the container. Promptly replace the lid of the container to prevent the strips from being exposed to moisture.
    Principle. The reagent pads are moisture sensitive and could be affected by environmental moisture, leading to inaccurate test results.

7. **Procedural Step.** Gently insert the end of the test strip with the silver-colored bars into the test strip guide with the yellow target area facing up. Check that the code number displayed matches the code number on the vial of test strips that you are using. When the test strip symbol flashes on the display, the meter is ready to accept a blood specimen.
    Principle. When the strip is correctly inserted, a blood drop symbol flashes on the display.

8. **Procedural Step.** Open the gauze packet. Cleanse the puncture site with an antiseptic wipe, and allow it to air-dry. Apply gloves, and perform a finger puncture. Dispose of the lancet in a biohazard sharps container.
    Principle. The antiseptic must be allowed to dry to prevent it from reacting with the chemicals on the reagent pad, which would lead to inaccurate test results. Gloves provide a barrier against bloodborne pathogens.

9. **Procedural Step.** After the puncture has been made, wipe away the first drop of blood with a gauze pad. Place the hand in a dependent position (palm facing down), and gently massage the finger around the puncture site until a large drop of blood forms.
    Principle. The first drop of blood contains a large amount of tissue fluid, which dilutes the specimen and leads to inaccurate test results. A large drop of blood is needed to cover the target area of the test strip completely.

10. **Procedural Step.** Apply the drop of blood to the Comfort Curve test strip as follows:
    a.   Touch and hold a drop of blood to the edge (not the top) of the yellow target area.
    b.   Completely fill the yellow target area. You will hear a beeping sound when sufficient blood has been applied. If any yellow mesh is visible after you have applied the initial drop of blood, a second drop of blood may be applied to the target area within 15

PROCEDURE 33-1 **Blood Glucose Measurement Using the Accu-Chek Advantage Glucose Meter—cont'd**

seconds of the first drop. If more than 15 seconds has passed, the test result may be erroneous, and you should discard the test strip and repeat the test.

Principle. The entire yellow target area must be completely covered with blood to ensure accurate and reliable test results.

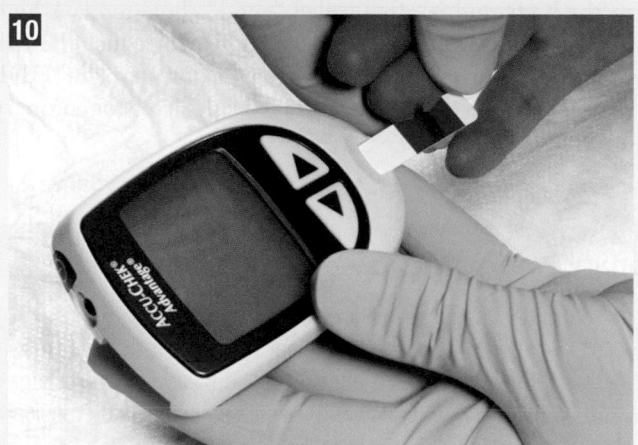

Apply a drop of blood.

11. Procedural Step. Have the patient hold a gauze pad over the puncture site and apply pressure until the bleeding stops.

12. Procedural Step. When the blood is correctly applied to the strip, an hourglass flashes on the screen while the meter analyzes the blood specimen. After a short time, the glucose value is displayed in milligrams per deciliter (mg/dL). If the glucose value is higher or lower than expected, or if the screen displays something other than the glucose value, see the Troubleshooting Guide section of the operator's manual to obtain instructions for correcting the problem. (The glucose result indicated on this glucose meter is 98 mg/dL.)

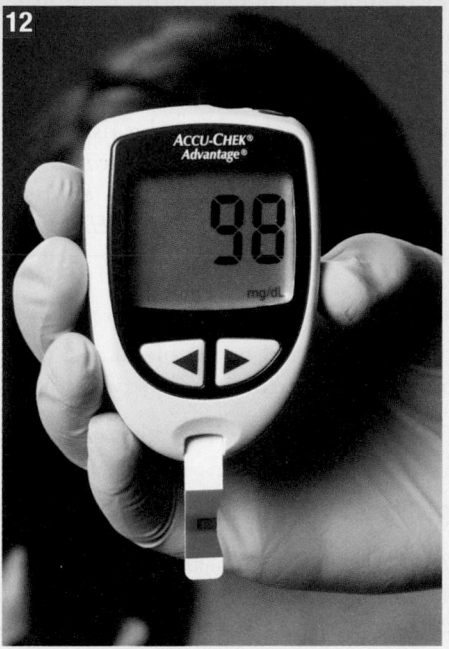

Read the glucose results.

13. Procedural Step. Remove the test strip from the meter, and discard it in a biohazard waste container. Turn the meter off.

14. Procedural Step. Check the puncture site and apply an adhesive bandage to the patient's finger if needed.

15. Procedural Step. Remove your gloves, and sanitize your hands. Chart the results. Include the date and time, the type of glucose test (e.g., FBG), the glucose test results, and when the patient last ate. If the patient has diabetes, also record the time of his or her last insulin injection or last consumption of oral hypoglycemic medication.

16. Procedural Step. Properly store the glucose meter according to the manufacturer's instructions.

CHARTING EXAMPLE

Date	
5/18/XX	8:30 a.m. FBS: 98 mg/dL. Pt last ate on
	5/17 @ 7:00 p.m. ————————————
	——————————— M. Villers, CMA (AAMA)

CHOLESTEROL

Cholesterol is a white, waxy, fatlike substance (lipid) that is essential for normal functioning of the body. It is an important component of all cell membranes in the body and is used in the production of essential hormones and bile. Most of the cholesterol circulating in the blood is manufactured by the liver; however, a portion of it comes from an individual's diet and is known as *dietary cholesterol*. Dietary cholesterol is found only in animal products, such as organ meats, egg yolk, and dairy products.

High blood cholesterol means an excessive amount of cholesterol is present in the blood. An individual's cholesterol level is determined by his or her genetic makeup and by the amounts of dietary cholesterol, saturated fat, and *trans* fat consumed. High blood cholesterol may cause fatty deposits, or plaque, to build up on the walls of the arteries, a condition known as *atherosclerosis.* As the atherosclerosis progresses, the arteries become more occluded, which eventually could lead to a heart attack or stroke. Because of this, high blood cholesterol is considered a risk factor for coronary artery disease (see *Highlight on Heart Disease with a Focus on Coronary Artery Disease*), and efforts should be made to reduce the cholesterol level (see *Highlight on Lowering Cholesterol*).

HDL and LDL Cholesterol

Cholesterol is transported in the blood as a complex molecule known as a **lipoprotein.** Two types of lipoproteins contain cholesterol: low-density lipoprotein (LDL) and high-density lipoprotein (HDL).

LDL picks up cholesterol from ingested fats and the liver and delivers it to blood vessels and muscles, where it is deposited in the cells. **LDL cholesterol** is often referred to as "bad" cholesterol because an excess amount of it in the blood can cause plaque to build up on the arterial walls, resulting in atherosclerosis. *HDL* removes excess cholesterol from the cells and carries it to the liver to be excreted. Because HDL removes excess cholesterol from the walls of the blood vessels, it is protective and beneficial to the body and is often called "good" cholesterol. A high **HDL cholesterol** level has been shown to reduce the risk of coronary artery disease, whereas a low level of HDL cholesterol (less than 40 mg/dL) is a risk factor for coronary artery disease.

Highlight on Heart Disease with a Focus on Coronary Artery Disease

Heart disease is a general term used to refer to a variety of medical conditions that affect the heart. The primary forms of heart disease include coronary artery disease (CAD), high blood pressure, heart attacks, strokes, congestive heart failure, congenital heart disease, and rheumatic heart disease. These various forms of heart disease are interrelated and have elements in common—for example, atherosclerosis can lead to a stroke or heart attack.

Heart disease is the number one killer of adults in the United States today. Because of the national focus on heart disease and cholesterol reduction, since 1985 a decline in heart attacks by 25% has been reported, as well as a decline in strokes by nearly 40%; however, heart disease is likely to remain the number one cause of death until more Americans adopt a more heart-healthy lifestyle.

Coronary Artery Disease

The most common symptom of coronary artery disease is chest pain, which is known as *angina pectoris.* Angina pectoris is a symptom, or a set of symptoms, rather than a disease. Angina pectoris occurs when the muscle tissue of the heart does not receive enough oxygenated blood, resulting in discomfort or pain under the sternum.

Cause

For most patients, the cause of angina is atherosclerosis of the coronary arteries. *Atherosclerosis* of the coronary arteries is a condition in which fibrous plaques of fatty deposits and cholesterol build up on the inner walls of the coronary arteries. This causes narrowing and partial blockage of the lumen of these arteries, along with hardening of the arterial wall. CAD results in a reduction of oxygenated blood flow to the heart muscle. Despite the narrowing, enough oxygen may still reach the heart muscle for normal needs. More oxygen is needed, however, when situations occur that increase the workload of the heart, such as physical activity, emotional stress, a heavy meal, and exposure to cold weather. If the coronary arteries cannot deliver enough oxygen to the heart muscle during these times of increased need, angina pectoris may result. Severe and prolonged anginal pain generally suggests a myocardial infarction (heart attack) caused by complete blockage of the coronary arteries and requires immediate medical attention.

CAD Risk Factors

Not everyone is equal when it comes to CAD. Some individuals have a much higher risk of developing it than others. The following are risk factors for CAD:

- High total blood cholesterol (greater than 200 mg/dL confirmed by repeated measurement)
- High blood pressure
- Cigarette smoking (more than 10 cigarettes per day)
- Family history of premature CAD (definite heart attack or sudden death in a parent or sibling before age 55 years)
- Diabetes
- History of blood vessel disease
- Obesity and overweight
- Low HDL cholesterol (less than 40 mg/dL confirmed by repeated measurement)
- Elevated triglyceride level (greater than 150 mg/dL)
- Being a man older than 45 years
- Being a woman older than 55 years or postmenopausal

Some of these risk factors can be modified; others, such as age, gender, and a family history of CAD, cannot be modified or controlled. The three major risk factors for CAD are high total blood cholesterol, high blood pressure, and cigarette smoking, all of which are modifiable.

Each person's overall risk of CAD must be assessed individually by the physician, based on the type and number of risk factors present. A 47-year-old man with a cholesterol level of 220 mg/dL who smokes a pack of cigarettes a day and is overweight is at greater risk than a 28-year-old man who is within a normal weight range, does not smoke, and exercises regularly but has a cholesterol level of 250 mg/dL. ■

Highlight on Lowering Cholesterol

Research has shown, beyond doubt, that high total blood cholesterol is a major risk factor for coronary artery disease, and the higher the cholesterol, the greater the risk. The National Institutes of Health (NIH) has established guidelines on safe levels of blood cholesterol. The NIH recommends that adults not exceed 200 mg/dL of blood cholesterol.

The National Cholesterol Educational Program (NCEP) was established in 1985 by the federal government to reduce the prevalence of elevated blood cholesterol levels in the United States by educating the public about the health risks associated with high blood cholesterol and to make recommendations for helping individuals reduce their cholesterol levels. It has been shown that for every 1% that an individual lowers his or her total blood cholesterol, the risk of coronary artery disease is reduced by 2%. Taking the following measures can help individuals reduce their level of "bad" LDL cholesterol and increase their level of "good" HDL cholesterol.

Diet

Dietary therapy is the first line of treatment for high blood cholesterol. The NCEP recommends that all individuals (older than 2 years of age) reduce dietary cholesterol, *trans* fat, and saturated fats. Many foods high in fat tend to be high in cholesterol. Nutrition labels on packaged products provide information on the cholesterol and fat content of a food.

Dietary Cholesterol

The body manufactures all the cholesterol it needs for normal functioning, and dietary intake of cholesterol (in foods) serves only to increase the blood cholesterol. According to the NCEP, dietary cholesterol should be limited to 300 mg daily, which is slightly more than the amount of cholesterol in one egg (270 mg). Cholesterol is found only in animal foods and shellfish. Egg yolks, dairy products, and organ meats such as liver and kidneys are especially high in cholesterol.

Saturated Fat

The intake of saturated fat is the most important dietary factor leading to high blood cholesterol, even more so than consuming dietary cholesterol. In general, the more saturated a fat is, the harder and more solid it is at room temperature. The main source of saturated fat is animal products, including meat fat, poultry skin, and the fat in dairy products (butter, cream, ice cream, cheese, whole milk). Unsaturated fats have little or no effect on the blood cholesterol level; they include olive oil, canola oil, peanut oil, and sunflower, safflower, and corn oils. The NCEP recommends that no more than 30% of the calories consumed each day come from fat, with no more than 10% of calories coming from saturated fat and the remaining 20% from unsaturated fat.

Soluble Fiber

Soluble fiber has been shown to lower the cholesterol level by keeping the cholesterol consumed from being absorbed by the body. Examples of foods high in soluble fiber are bran, oats, and beans.

Weight Reduction

It is estimated that one in four Americans is overweight. It is recommended that these individuals follow a sensible eating plan along with an exercise program to reach and maintain desirable weight. Losing weight reduces total cholesterol and triglyceride levels. Overweight and obese people are at very high risk for heart disease because their hearts have to work harder to pump blood through the body.

Exercise

An aerobic exercise program is especially beneficial for weight control because it improves cardiovascular fitness and lowers blood cholesterol level. People who exercise regularly generally have higher HDL cholesterol levels and lower triglyceride levels in their blood. The American Heart Association recommends that healthy individuals perform any moderate- to vigorous-intensity aerobic activity for at least 30 minutes on most days of the week at 50% to 85% of their maximum heart rate. These activities can include brisk walking, jogging, hiking, bicycling, swimming, and stair climbing.

Smoking Cessation

Smoking is one of the three main risk factors for coronary artery disease. By quitting smoking, an individual may be able to strengthen the heart and lower the cholesterol level. Also, non-smokers tend to have higher HDL levels in their blood. A variety of smoking cessation programs are usually available in the community. Some people have succeeded by using nicotine patches, which help them adjust gradually to lower levels of nicotine.

Generally, the cholesterol level begins to decrease 2 to 3 weeks after a cholesterol-lowering diet and other cholesterol-lowering measures are begun. Over time, it is possible to reduce the total cholesterol level by 30 to 55 mg/dL or even more through these lifestyle changes. If the blood cholesterol level cannot be lowered to an acceptable level, the physician may prescribe cholesterol-lowering medications along with continuation of the aforementioned measures. ■

Cholesterol Testing

All adults older than 20 years of age should have a cholesterol test at least once every 5 years. Initial testing includes a *total cholesterol* determination, which is a combined measurement of LDL cholesterol and HDL cholesterol in the blood. To obtain a fuller picture of a patient's cholesterol status, physicians typically also order an HDL cholesterol determination, which measures only the HDL cholesterol in the blood. Cholesterol tests are considered screening tests, and elevated results usually require confirmation through repeat testing before a diagnosis of high blood cholesterol is made.

Interpretation of Results

Cholesterol test results are interpreted as follows: Total cholesterol levels less than 200 mg/dL are desirable. Levels between 200 and 239 mg/dL are borderline high, and levels of 240 mg/dL and greater are high. Based on confirmed testing, individuals in the high category are clearly at increased risk for coronary artery disease, and individuals in the borderline high category are at increased risk if they have other risk factors, such as being overweight or smoking. According to the American Heart Association, an HDL cholesterol level less than 40 mg/dL for men and less than 50 mg/dL for women is considered a risk factor for coronary artery disease. An HDL cholesterol level between 40 and 50 mg/dL for men and between 50 and 60 mg/dL for women is desirable, whereas an HDL cholesterol level greater than 60 mg/dL is considered optimal and provides some protection against heart disease.

Although the primary use of cholesterol testing is to screen for the presence of high blood cholesterol related to coronary artery disease, this test also is used as a secondary aid in the study of thyroid and liver function.

Patient Preparation

Because total cholesterol and HDL cholesterol determinations are not affected significantly by food consumption, the patient usually is not required to fast before collection of the blood specimen. Some physicians prefer the patient to be in a fasting state, however.

If the total cholesterol level is 200 mg/dL or greater, the physician usually orders a *lipid profile,* which includes total cholesterol, HDL cholesterol, LDL cholesterol, and triglycerides. (The LDL cholesterol level is usually determined as a calculation from the triglyceride and HDL cholesterol levels.) Because triglyceride levels are affected by the consumption of food, the patient must be instructed to fast for at least 12 hours before the blood specimen is collected. An elevated triglyceride level (150 mg/dL or higher) is considered a risk factor for coronary artery disease, particularly when the LDL cholesterol is high and the HDL cholesterol is low.

Although the primary use of cholesterol testing is to screen for the presence of high blood cholesterol related to coronary artery disease, this test also is used as a secondary aid in the study of thyroid and liver function.

CLIA-Waived Cholesterol Analyzers

CLIA-waived analyzers are available for performing cholesterol testing in the medical office; an example is the Cholestech LDX cholesterol system (Cholestech Corporation) (Figure 33-10).

The manufacturer of each cholesterol analyzer provides an operating manual (and sometimes an instructional video) with the instrument that includes information needed to

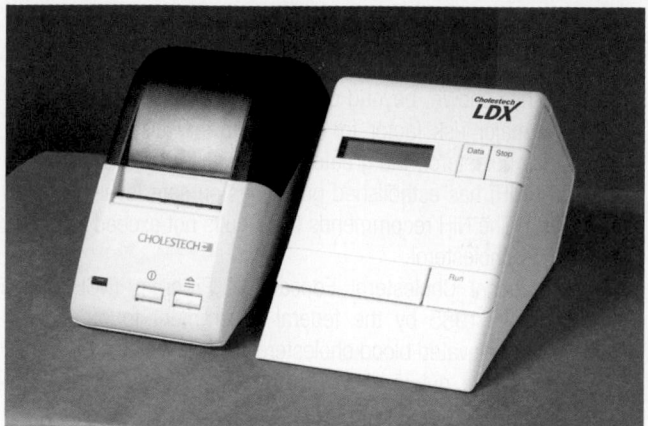

Figure 33-10 Cholestech LDX cholesterol system.

What Would You Do? What Would You *Not* Do?

Case Study 3

Karen Scrimshaw is at the office. She is 20 years old and is mildly obese. Karen had her cholesterol tested at a health fair, and it was 325. The physician orders a CBC, lipid profile, and thyroid profile on Karen and instructs her to return in 1 week for a follow-up visit to discuss the test results. Karen is very concerned about her cholesterol. She says that she had a candy bar and some potato chips before going to the health fair and wants to know whether that could have caused her cholesterol to be so high. She also wants to know the accuracy of machines that are used at health fairs. Karen says that if she has to go on cholesterol medication, it would be hard to decide between Lipitor and Zocor. She says she has seen them advertised on television, and they both seem pretty good to her. ■

collect and handle the specimen, perform quality control procedures, and test the specimen. The manufacturer may also have personnel available for on-site training.

It is important that the medical assistant become completely familiar with all aspects of the CLIA-waived analyzer used to perform cholesterol testing in his or her medical office. Medical offices running CLIA-waived tests are required to follow the manufacturer's instructions *exactly* for each testing procedure. These instructions include the quality control procedures that must be performed when the test is run. Quality control procedures are of particular importance to ensure that the analyzer is functioning properly, and that the test results are reliable and accurate.

TRIGLYCERIDES

Triglycerides are the chemical form in which most fat exists in food, as well as in the body. Triglycerides are derived from two sources. The first is synthesis by the body. Ingested glucose that is not needed for energy can be stored in the form of **glycogen** in muscle and liver tissue for later use. When no more tissue storage is possible, most of the excess glycogen is synthesized by the body into triglycerides (a form of fat) and stored as adipose tissue. Excess protein not needed by the body is also converted to triglycerides and stored as adipose tissue. The second source of triglycerides is food. Excess triglycerides consumed by eating foods containing fat are also stored as adipose tissue.

Some of the triglycerides in the body are not stored as fat, but remain in the bloodstream, specifically in the plasma. Most triglycerides in the bloodstream are carried by a lipoprotein known as very-low-density lipoprotein (VLDL). In normal amounts, triglycerides are essential to good health. Triglycerides carried by the blood serve as a major source of energy for the body. An excess of blood triglycerides, however, places an individual at increased risk for coronary artery disease, particularly when the LDL cholesterol is high and the HDL cholesterol is low. Triglyceride levels in the blood are usually measured as part of a lipid profile and are interpreted as follows:

Normal | Less than 150 mg/dL
Borderline high | 150 to 199 mg/dL
High | 200 to 499 mg/dL
Very high | 500 mg/dL or higher

Conditions that result in elevated blood triglyceride levels include obesity, type 2 diabetes, being physically inactive, excessive alcohol consumption, smoking, hypothyroidism, kidney disease, and liver disease.

BLOOD UREA NITROGEN

The blood urea nitrogen (BUN) is a kidney function test. Urea is the end product of protein metabolism and is normally present in the blood. Certain kidney diseases may interfere with the ability of the body to excrete the urea properly, causing an increased level of urea in the blood.

IMMUNOLOGY

Immunology is the scientific study of antigen and antibody reactions. An **antigen** is a substance that is capable of stimulating the formation of antibodies in an individual. Antigens may consist of protein, glycoprotein, complex polysaccharides, or nucleic acid. Specific examples of antigens include bacteria and viruses, bacterial toxins, allergens, and **blood antigens**. An **antibody** is a substance that is capable of combining with an antigen, resulting in an antigen-antibody reaction.

Laboratory testing in immunology deals with studying antigen-antibody reactions to assess the presence of a substance (e.g., ABO blood typing) or to assist in the diagnosis of disease (e.g., mononucleosis testing). Immunologic tests are often used for the early diagnosis of disease and are used to follow the course of the disease.

IMMUNOLOGIC TESTS

Specific examples of immunologic tests are described next.

Hepatitis Tests

Hepatitis testing is performed to detect viral hepatitis. There are five types of viral hepatitis—A, B, C, D, and E—which are described in detail in Chapter 17. Hepatitis testing not only detects the presence of viral hepatitis, it also determines the type of hepatitis present.

HIV Tests

The enzyme immunoassay (EIA) test and the enzyme-linked immunosorbent assay (ELISA) test are used as screening tests for the presence of HIV. Newer rapid screening HIV testing kits are also commercially available; brand names include Uni-Gold Recombigen HIV (Trinity Biotech Plc, Bray County Wicklow, Ireland), Clearview HIV (Inverness Medical Innovations, Inc., Waltham, Mass), and the OraQuick Rapid HIV test (OraSure Technologies, Bethlehem, Pa). Because of the possibility of a false-positive result, a second screening test is always performed if a blood specimen tests positive. If the second test also is positive, a more specific test, such as the Western blot test, is performed to confirm the test results. An individual who tests positive for HIV is seropositive.

A negative HIV test result is not conclusive for the absence of HIV infection. If an individual has recently been infected with HIV, the antibodies may not have had time to develop. It generally takes 2 to 12 weeks (but possibly as long as 6 months) for the HIV antibodies to appear in the blood.

Syphilis Tests

Syphilis is a sexually transmitted disease (STD) caused by the microorganism *Treponema pallidum*. The most common tests used to detect the presence of syphilis are the Venereal Disease Research Laboratories (VDRL) test and the rapid plasma reagin (RPR) test. Test results are reported as nonreactive, weakly reactive, or reactive. Weakly reactive and reactive results are considered positive for the presence of syphilis antibodies. These tests are screening tests, and a positive result warrants more specific testing to arrive at a diagnosis of syphilis.

Mononucleosis Test

The mononucleosis test ("mono test") is used to detect the presence of infectious mononucleosis. The theory and procedure for this test are discussed in detail in this chapter.

Rheumatoid Factor

Rheumatoid arthritis is a chronic inflammatory disease that affects the joints of the body. The blood of patients with rheumatoid arthritis contains a type of antibody called *rheumatoid factor* (RF). This test detects the presence of rheumatoid factor antibodies and assists in the diagnosis of rheumatoid arthritis.

Antistreptolysin O Test

The antistreptolysin O (ASO) test is used to detect ASO antibodies in the serum. It is the most widely used immunologic test for the detection of conditions resulting from streptococcal infections and diseases that occur secondary to a streptococcal infection. This test is useful in assisting in the diagnosis of rheumatic fever, glomerulonephritis, bacterial endocarditis, and scarlet fever.

C-Reactive Protein

During inflammation and tissue destruction, an abnormal protein called *C-reactive protein* (CRP) appears in the blood. Patients with inflammatory conditions or disorders accompanied by tissue destruction have positive results to this test. Because of this, the CRP test is used to assist in diagnosing or charting the progress of rheumatoid arthritis, acute rheumatic fever, widespread malignancy, and bacterial infections.

Cold Agglutinins

The cold agglutinins test is used to detect the presence of antibodies called *cold agglutinins*. This test is performed by incubating the patient's serum with erythrocytes at cold temperatures. If cold agglutinins are present, this causes **agglutination** of the erythrocytes. Cold agglutinins are found in patients with infectious mononucleosis, mycoplasmal pneumonia, chronic parasitic infections, and lymphoma.

ABO and Rh Blood Typing

Blood typing is performed to determine an individual's ABO and Rh blood type. Knowledge of blood type helps to prevent transfusion and transplant reactions and to identify problems such as hemolytic disease of the newborn.

Rh Antibody Titer

The Rh antibody titer test detects the amount of circulating Rh antibodies in the blood. These antibodies can occur in a pregnant woman who is Rh-negative and is carrying an Rh-positive fetus. This test is most frequently used to detect the presence of an Rh incompatibility problem with a mother and her unborn child.

RAPID MONONUCLEOSIS TESTING

Infectious mononucleosis is an acute infectious disease caused by the Epstein-Barr virus (EBV). Infectious mononucleosis most frequently affects children and young adults. It is transmitted through saliva by direct oral contact, and because of this, it is often called the "kissing disease." Symptoms of infectious mononucleosis include mental and physical fatigue, fever, sore throat, severe weakness, headache, and swollen lymph nodes.

The (CLIA-waived) rapid mono test is often performed in the medical office and is used to assist in the diagnosis of infectious mononucleosis. Rapid mono tests are easy to perform and provide reliable results in a short time. Patients with infectious mononucleosis produce an antibody called *heterophile antibody,* usually by 6 to 10 days into the illness. Rapid mono tests detect this antibody. The presence of the heterophile antibody along with patient symptoms can provide the basis for the diagnosis of infectious mononucleosis.

Figure 33-11 illustrates the QuickVue+ mononucleosis test setup (Quidel Corporation, San Diego, Calif), and Figure 33-12 outlines the procedure for performing a rapid mono test using the QuickVue+ mononucleosis test. Figure 33-13 is an illustration of positive and negative test results for the QuickVue+ mononucleosis test.

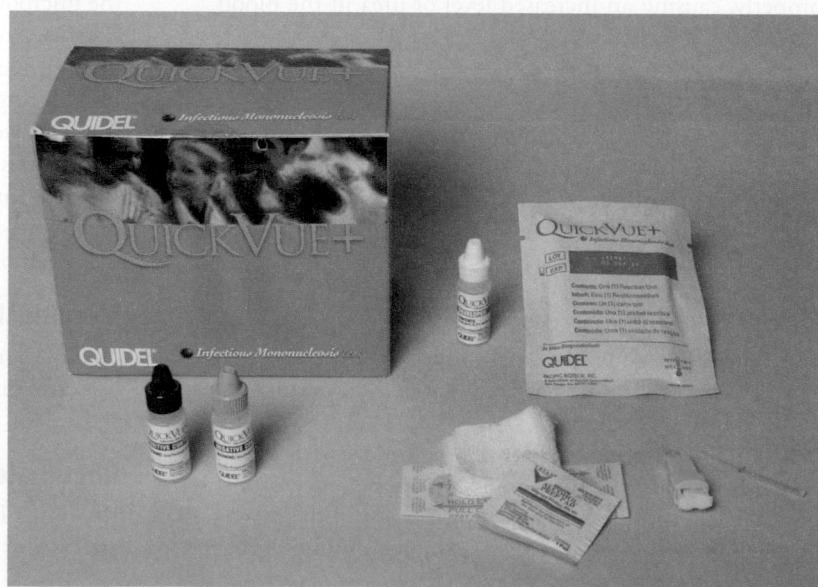

Figure 33-11 QuickVue+ mononucleosis test setup.

QuickVue+ Infectious Mononucleosis Test

FOR INFORMATIONAL USE ONLY ■ FOR INFORMATIONAL USE ONLY ■ FOR INFORMATIONAL USE ONLY

Not to be used for performing assay. Refer to most current package insert accompanying your test kit.

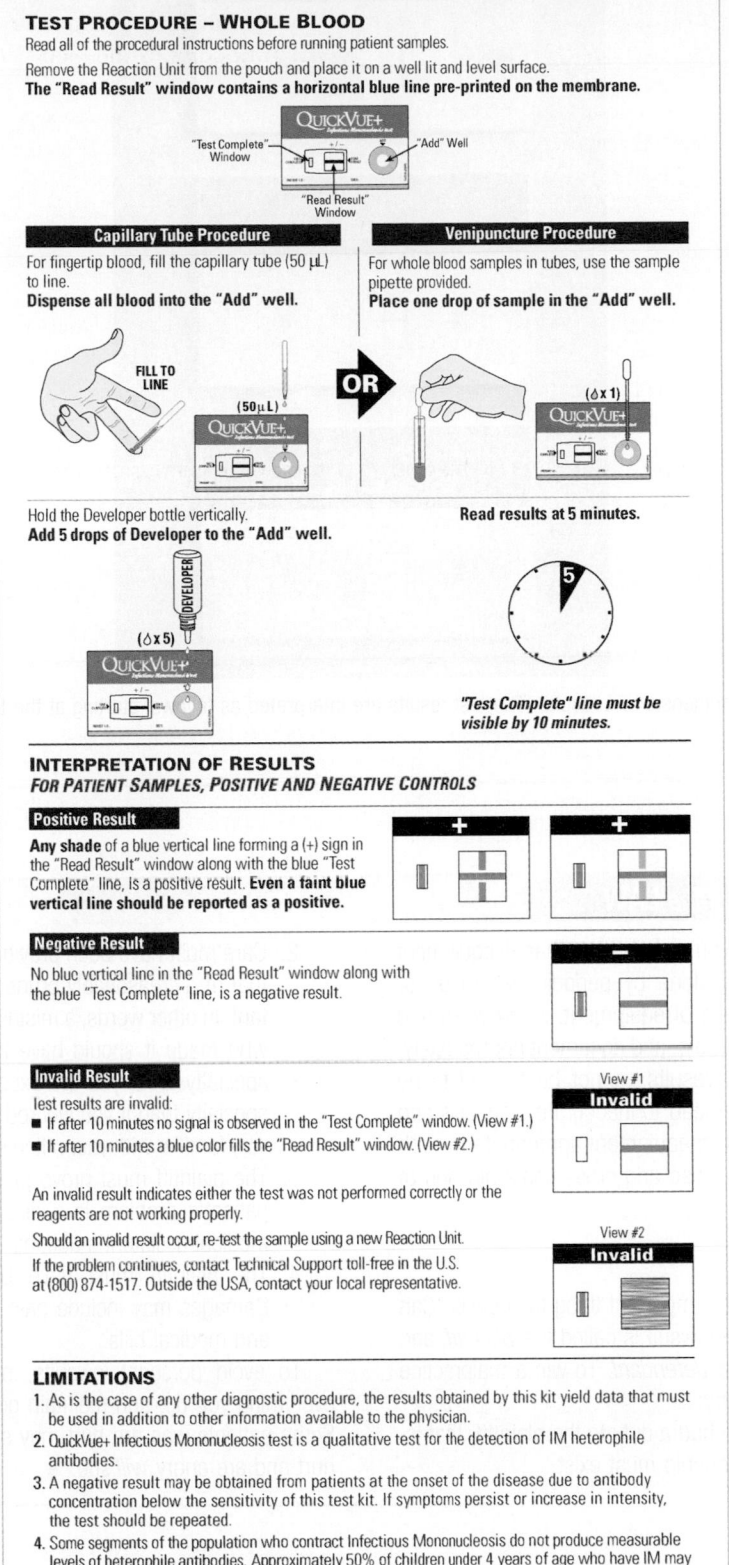

TEST PROCEDURE – WHOLE BLOOD

Read all of the procedural instructions before running patient samples.

Remove the Reaction Unit from the pouch and place it on a well lit and level surface.

The "Read Result" window contains a horizontal blue line pre-printed on the membrane.

Capillary Tube Procedure	Venipuncture Procedure
For fingertip blood, fill the capillary tube (50 μL) to line. **Dispense all blood into the "Add" well.**	For whole blood samples in tubes, use the sample pipette provided. **Place one drop of sample in the "Add" well.**

Hold the Developer bottle vertically.
Add 5 drops of Developer to the "Add" well.

Read results at 5 minutes.

"Test Complete" line must be visible by 10 minutes.

INTERPRETATION OF RESULTS
FOR PATIENT SAMPLES, POSITIVE AND NEGATIVE CONTROLS

Positive Result

Any shade of a blue vertical line forming a (+) sign in the "Read Result" window along with the blue "Test Complete" line, is a positive result. **Even a faint blue vertical line should be reported as a positive.**

Negative Result

No blue vertical line in the "Read Result" window along with the blue "Test Complete" line, is a negative result.

Invalid Result

Test results are invalid:
■ If after 10 minutes no signal is observed in the "Test Complete" window. (View #1.)
■ If after 10 minutes a blue color fills the "Read Result" window. (View #2.)

An invalid result indicates either the test was not performed correctly or the reagents are not working properly.

Should an invalid result occur, re-test the sample using a new Reaction Unit.

If the problem continues, contact Technical Support toll-free in the U.S. at (800) 874-1517. Outside the USA, contact your local representative.

LIMITATIONS

1. As is the case of any other diagnostic procedure, the results obtained by this kit yield data that must be used in addition to other information available to the physician.
2. QuickVue+ Infectious Mononucleosis test is a qualitative test for the detection of IM heterophile antibodies.
3. A negative result may be obtained from patients at the onset of the disease due to antibody concentration below the sensitivity of this test kit. If symptoms persist or increase in intensity, the test should be repeated.
4. Some segments of the population who contract Infectious Mononucleosis do not produce measurable levels of heterophile antibodies. Approximately 50% of children under 4 years of age who have IM may test as IM heterophile antibody negative.[4]

Figure 33-12 Procedure for performing the QuickVue+ mononucleosis test.

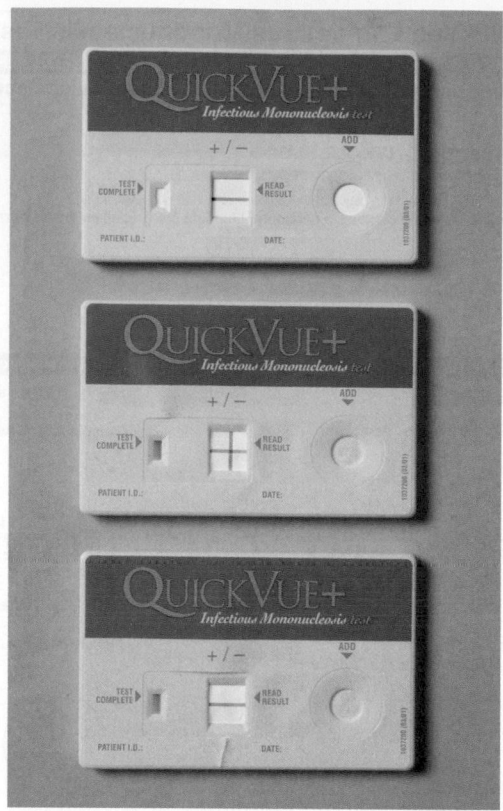

Figure 33-13 QuickVue+ mononucleosis test results. The test results are interpreted as follows, starting at the top of the illustration: invalid, positive, and negative.

MEDICAL PRACTICE *and the* LAW

When running laboratory tests, you must ensure that all equipment is functioning properly. This is done by periodic calibration or running of controls on each piece of equipment. Know when and how often to calibrate or run controls, and document appropriately. Without these quality controls, results cannot be trusted to be accurate. Inaccurate results can lead to inaccurate diagnosis and treatment. Use personal protective equipment appropriate to each test to avoid transmission of disease and cross-contamination of specimens.

Who Can Sue?

Anyone can sue for anything. The important thing to know is "Can they win?" The person filing the lawsuit is called the *plaintiff,* and the one being sued is called the *defendant.* To win a malpractice lawsuit, four things are necessary:

1. The defendant must have had a duty to the plaintiff, that is, a physician-patient relationship must exist.

2. Care must have been provided that was not consistent with that of a "reasonably prudent" physician or medical assistant. In other words, a mistake was made, and the individual who made it should have known better. If you work in a specialty area, you are expected to know more about that specialty than if you worked in a general practice office. Be very familiar with your office's policy and procedures manual.

3. The plaintiff must prove proximate cause. This means the patient's problem is a direct cause of the physician's or medical assistant's actions.

4. The plaintiff must have been injured by the mistake. Damages may include pain and suffering, loss of income, and medical bills.

To avoid personal lawsuits, practice good care, document everything you do, and maintain good relationships with patients. Some patients who are hurt may sue, but most patients who are hurt and are angry *will* sue. ■

What Would You Do? What Would You *Not* Do? RESPONSES

Case Study 1
Page 806

What Did Michelle Do?

❏ Apologized to Crystal for the inconvenience. Explained to her that it takes 3 to 4 hours to run an oral glucose tolerance test because several specimens must be collected over time to see how her body handles sugar.

❏ Explained to Crystal that eating and smoking cause the test results to be inaccurate. Told her that she could eat and smoke as soon as the test was over.

❏ Told Crystal that she needs to sit quietly during the test, so it would not be possible for her to bring her children.

❏ Informed the physician of Crystal's situation to see whether he had any suggestions.

What Did Michelle Not Do?

❏ Did not become defensive or intimidated by Crystal's behavior.

❏ Did not tell Crystal that the staff would watch Crystal's children during the test.

❏ Did not tell Crystal that it was not a good idea for her to smoke around her children.

What Would You Do?/What Would You Not Do?

Review Michelle's response and place a checkmark next to the information you included in your response. List additional information you included in your response.

_____

_____

_____

_____

_____

Case Study 2
Page 809

What Did Michelle Do?

❏ Told Dave that it would be fine for him to perform his own finger-stick.

❏ Made sure that his finger was cleansed with an antiseptic wipe and that he wiped away the first drop of blood.

❏ Explained to Dave that the air bubbles take up space that the insulin should occupy, and that if he does not get rid of them, he will not get his full dose of insulin.

❏ Demonstrated how to remove air bubbles, and had Dave practice it at the office.

❏ Told Dave he must not reuse his needle and syringe. Explained that a used needle could cause him to get an infection. Asked Dave whether he had checked to see if his insurance would cover the cost of the needles and syringes.

❏ Told Dave that he should put his used needles and syringes in a thick plastic container such as an empty detergent container.

After the container is full, he should close it tightly with a screw lid, then it can be thrown out with his regular trash. Explained that this will protect his family and the trash handlers from getting stuck while disposing of the trash.

What Did Michelle Not Do?

❏ Did not tell Dave he didn't need to worry about the air bubbles in the syringe.

What Would You Do?/What Would You Not Do?

Review Michelle's response and place a checkmark next to the information you included in your response. List additional information you included in your response.

_____

_____

_____

_____

_____

_____

Case Study 3
Page 818

What Did Michelle Do?

❏ Tried to calm and reassure Karen.

❏ Explained to Karen that the cholesterol results are not affected by food, so eating before the health fair should not have affected her results.

❏ Told Karen that before a cholesterol analyzer is used, it is usually checked to ensure that it is working properly.

❏ Reassured Karen that the physician was checking her cholesterol again and was running some additional tests to determine whether she is having any problems.

❏ Told Karen that if she must take medication, the physician will determine what drug is best for her.

What Did Michelle Not Do?

❏ Did not tell Karen that her cholesterol is extremely high.

❏ Did not tell Karen that she should be more careful about what she eats because she is overweight.

❏ Did not tell Karen that there was no way to know whether the cholesterol analyzer used at the health fair was calibrated and had controls run on it.

What Would You Do?/What Would You Not Do?

Review Michelle's response and place a checkmark next to the information you included in your response. List additional information you included in your response.

_____

_____

_____

_____

_____

☞ TERMINOLOGY REVIEW

Medical Term	Word Parts	Definition
Agglutination (as it pertains to blood)		Clumping of blood cells.
Analyte		A substance that is being identified or measured in a laboratory test.
Antibody	*anti-:* against	A substance that is capable of combining with an antigen, resulting in an antigen-antibody reaction.
Antigen	*anti-:* against *-gen:* substance or agent that produces or causes	A substance capable of stimulating the formation of antibodies.
Blood antigen	*anti-:* against *-gen:* substance or agent that produces or causes	A protein present on the surface of red blood cells that determines a person's blood type.
Glycogen	*glyco-:* sugar *-gen:* substance or agent that produces or causes	The form in which carbohydrate is stored in the body.
Glycosylation	*glyco-:* sugar	The process of glucose attaching to hemoglobin.
HDL cholesterol		A lipoprotein, consisting of protein and cholesterol, that removes excess cholesterol from the cells.
Hemoglobin A_{1c}	*hemo-:* blood	Compound formed when glucose attaches or glycosylates to the protein in hemoglobin.
Hyperglycemia	*hyper-:* above, excessive *glyc/o:* sugar *-emia:* blood condition	An abnormally high level of glucose in the blood.
Hypoglycemia	*hypo-:* below, deficient *glyc/o:* sugar *-emia:* blood condition	An abnormally low level of glucose in the blood.
LDL cholesterol		A lipoprotein, consisting of protein and cholesterol, that picks up cholesterol and delivers it to the cells.
Lipoprotein	*lipo-:* fat	A complex molecule consisting of protein and a lipid fraction such as cholesterol. Lipoproteins function in transporting lipids in the blood.

☞ ON THE WEB

For information on diabetes:

American Diabetes Association: www.diabetes.org

Joslin Diabetes Center: www.joslin.org

National Diabetes Education Initiative: www.ndei.org

The National Institute of Diabetes: www.niddk.nih.gov

 Check out the Evolve site at http://evolve.elsevier.com/Bonewit/today/ to actively Prepare for your Certification, and to access additional interactive activities and exercises to help you study and prepare for success.

34

Medical Microbiology

LEARNING OBJECTIVES	PROCEDURES
Microorganisms and Disease	
1. List and explain the stages of an infectious disease.	
2. List and describe the three classifications of bacteria based on shape.	
3. Give examples of infectious diseases caused by the following types of cocci: Staphylococci Streptococci Diplococci	
4. State examples of infectious diseases caused by bacilli, spirilla, and viruses.	
Microscope	
5. Explain the function of each of the following parts of a compound microscope: base, arm, stage, light source, substage condenser, iris diaphragm, body tube, coarse adjustment, and fine adjustment.	Use a microscope. Properly handle and care for a microscope.
6. Identify the function of each of the following microscope lenses: low-power, high-power, and oil-immersion.	
7. List the guidelines for proper care of the microscope.	
Microbiologic Specimen Collection	
8. Explain the purpose of obtaining a specimen, and identify body areas from which a specimen can be taken for microbiologic examination.	Collect a throat specimen.
9. List ways to prevent contamination of a specimen by extraneous microorganisms.	
10. Explain the precautions a medical assistant should take to prevent infection from a pathogenic specimen.	
Microbiologic Tests	
11. Explain the importance of the early diagnosis of streptococcal pharyngitis.	Perform a streptococcus test using a rapid strep test.
12. Explain the purpose of and describe the procedure for a sensitivity test.	
13. Explain the purpose of a microbiologic smear.	
14. Explain the purpose of Gram staining.	
15. Identify infectious diseases caused by gram-positive bacteria and gram-negative bacteria.	
16. Give examples of methods to prevent and control infectious diseases in the community.	

KEY TERMS

bacilli (bah-SILL-ie)
cocci (KOK-sie)
contagious (kon-TAE-jus)
culture
culture medium
false-negative
false-positive
immunization (im-yoo-ni-ZAY-shun)

incubate (IN-kyoo-bate)
incubation period
infectious disease
inoculate (in-NOK-yoo-late)
microbiology (mie-kroe-bie-OL-oe-jee)
mucous membrane (MYOO-kus MEM-brain)
normal flora
resistance

sequela (SEK-kwe-lah)
smear
specimen (SPESS-ih-men)
spirilla (spa-RILL-ah)

INTRODUCTION TO MICROBIOLOGY

Microbiology is the scientific study of microorganisms and their activities. As described in Chapter 17, microorganisms are tiny living plants and animals that cannot be seen by the naked eye, but must be viewed under a microscope. Anton van Leeuwenhoek (1632-1723) designed a magnifying glass strong enough for viewing microorganisms. He was the first individual to observe and describe protozoa and bacteria (Figure 34-1). Leeuwenhoek's magnifying glass was the precursor of modern microscopes used today to study microorganisms. A microscope allows the observer to see individual microbial cells and to differentiate and identify microorganisms.

For the most part, microbiology deals with unicellular, or one-celled, microscopic organisms. All of the life processes necessary to sustain the microbe are performed by one cell. Among them are the ingestion of food substances and their use for energy, growth, reproduction, and excretion.

Microorganisms are *ubiquitous;* they are found almost everywhere—in the air, in food and water, in the soil, and in association with plants, animals, and human life. Although vast numbers of microorganisms exist, only a relatively small number are pathogenic and able to cause disease.

When a pathogen infects a host, it often produces a set of symptoms peculiar to that disease. Scarlet fever is characterized by a sore throat, swelling of the lymph nodes in the neck, a red and swollen tongue, and a bright red rash covering the body. These symptoms aid the physician in

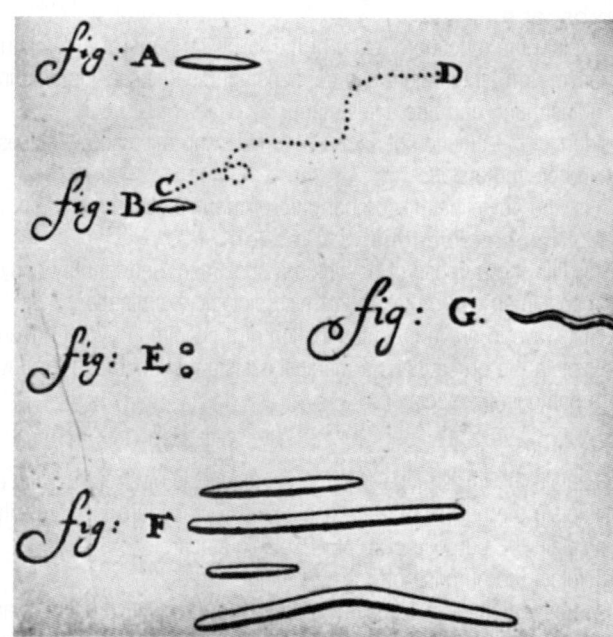

Figure 34-1 Bacteria drawn by van Leeuwenhoek in 1684.

diagnosing the disease. The medical assistant must be alert to all symptoms that the patient describes and must relay this information to the physician through careful and concise charting of these symptoms in the patient's medical record.

If the physician is not able to diagnose the disease from the patient's clinical signs and symptoms, laboratory tests may be used to help the physician identify the pathogen.

Identification of the pathogen leads to proper treatment of the disease. Categories of laboratory tests used to identify a pathogen include the following:

- Microbial culture
- Biochemical tests
- Microscopy
- DNA testing (also known as PCR testing)

Although most laboratory tests used to identify a pathogen are performed at an outside laboratory, the medical assistant is frequently responsible for collection of the specimen that will be transported to the outside laboratory.

This chapter provides an introduction to microbiology, including a description of proper microbiologic collection and handling techniques that must be followed to ensure a high-quality specimen. Identification of a pathogen using microbial culturing, biochemical testing, and microscopy is also discussed in this chapter. DNA testing to detect pathogens (e.g., chlamydia and gonorrhea) was previously described in Chapter 23. Before undertaking this study, the medical assistant should review Chapter 17, which discusses introductory concepts that are basic to this chapter.

NORMAL FLORA

Every individual has a **normal flora,** which consists of the harmless microorganisms that normally reside in many parts of the body but do not cause disease. The surface of the skin, the **mucous membrane** of the gastrointestinal tract, and parts of the respiratory and genitourinary tracts all have an abundant normal flora. Some microorganisms that make up the normal flora are beneficial to the body, such as those that inhabit the intestinal tract that feed on other potentially harmful microscopic organisms. Other examples are microorganisms found in the intestinal tract that synthesize vitamin K, an essential vitamin needed by the body for proper blood clotting. In rare instances, if the opportunity arises (e.g., lowered body **resistance**), certain microorganisms of the normal flora can become pathogenic and cause disease.

INFECTION

Invasion of the body by pathogenic microorganisms is known as *infection.* Under conditions favorable to the pathogens, they grow and multiply, resulting in an **infectious disease** (also known as a communicable disease) that produces harmful effects on the host. Not all pathogens that enter a host are able to cause disease, however. When a pathogen enters the body, it attempts to invade the tissues so that it can grow and multiply. The body tries to stop the invasion with its second line of natural defense mechanisms,* which includes inflammation, phagocytosis by

---

*The first line of natural defense mechanisms, which work to prevent the entrance of pathogens into the body (e.g., coughing, sneezing), is described in Chapter 17.

white blood cells, and the production of antibodies. These defense mechanisms work to destroy the pathogen and remove it from the body. If the body is successful, the pathogens are destroyed, and the individual experiences no adverse effects. If the pathogen is able to overcome the body's natural defense mechanisms, an infectious disease results.

Many infectious diseases are **contagious,** meaning that the pathogen that causes the disease can be spread from one person to another directly or indirectly. Frequently, *droplet infection* is the mode of transmission of a contagious disease. *Droplet infection* refers to an infection that is indirectly transmitted by tiny contaminated droplets of moisture expelled from the upper respiratory tract of an infected individual. When an individual exhales (as during breathing, talking, coughing, or sneezing), a fine spray of moisture droplets is emitted by that individual from the upper respiratory tract. If the individual has a contagious disease that is transmitted by droplet infection, the pathogens are carried into the air by these tiny moisture droplets. Another individual may inhale these contaminated droplets and become infected with the disease. To help prevent the spread of droplet infections, contagious individuals should cover their mouths and noses while coughing or sneezing. See Figure 17-1 for examples of other means of pathogen transmission.

Stages of an Infectious Disease

When a pathogen becomes established in the host, a series of events generally ensues. The stages of an infectious disease are as follows:

1. The *infection* is the invasion and multiplication of pathogenic microorganisms in the body.
2. The *incubation period* is the interval of time between the invasion by a pathogenic microorganism and the appearance of the first symptoms of the disease. Depending on the type of disease, the **incubation period** may range from a few days to several months. During this time, the pathogen is growing and multiplying.
3. The *prodromal period* is a short period in which the first symptoms that indicate an approaching disease occur. Headache and a feeling of illness are common prodromal symptoms.
4. The *acute period* is when the disease is at its peak and symptoms are fully developed. Fever is a common symptom of many infectious diseases.
5. The *decline period* is when symptoms of the disease begin to subside.
6. The *convalescent period* is the stage in which the patient regains strength and returns to a state of good health.

MICROORGANISMS AND DISEASE

The groups of microorganisms known to contain species capable of causing human disease include bacteria, viruses, protozoa, fungi (including yeasts), and animal parasites. Bacteria and viruses are most frequently responsible for causing human diseases and are discussed next.

Bacteria

Bacteria are microscopic single-celled organisms. Of the 1700 species known to dwell in humans, only approximately 100 produce human disease. The discovery of antibiotics has helped immensely in combating and controlling bacterial infections. Antibiotics are not effective against viral infections, however.

Bacteria can be classified according to their shape into three basic groups (Figure 34-2). Round bacteria are known as **cocci.** Cocci can be categorized further as diplococci, streptococci, or staphylococci, depending on their pattern of growth. Rod-shaped bacteria are **bacilli.** Spiral and curve-shaped bacteria are **spirilla,** and they include spirochetes and vibrios.

Cocci

Staphylococci are round bacteria that grow in grapelike clusters (Figure 34-3, *A*). The species *Staphylococcus epidermidis* is widely distributed and is normally present on the surface of the skin and the mucous membranes of the mouth, nose, throat, and intestines. *S. epidermidis* is usually nonpathogenic; however, a cut, abrasion, or other break in the skin can allow invasion of the tissues by the organism, resulting in a mild infection.

Staphylococcus aureus is commonly associated with pathologic conditions such as boils, carbuncles, pimples, impetigo, abscesses, *Staphylococcus* food poisoning, and wound infections. Infections caused by staphylococci usually cause much pus formation (suppuration) and are termed *pyogenic* infections.

Streptococci are round bacteria that grow in chains (Figure 34-3, *B*). Before the advent of antibiotics, streptococcal infections were a major cause of human death. Diseases caused by streptococci include streptococcal sore throat ("strep throat"), scarlet fever, rheumatic fever, pneumonia, puerperal sepsis, erysipelas, and skin conditions such as carbuncles and impetigo.

Diplococci are round bacteria that grow in pairs. Pneumonia, gonorrhea, and meningitis are infectious diseases caused by diplococci.

What Would You Do? What Would You *Not* Do?

Case Study 1

Paula Hutchinson brings her 8-year-old daughter Caitlin to the medical office. Caitlin has had a fever, sore throat, and difficulty eating for the past 2 days. The physician orders a rapid strep test. Caitlin refuses to open her mouth so that the specimen can be collected. She says that she doesn't want that "swab thing" in her mouth because she's afraid it will make her throw up. Paula wants to know why the strep test must be run. She says that Caitlin's throat is very red with white patches and wants to know why the physician doesn't just prescribe an antibiotic for her without running the test. ■

Bacilli

Bacilli are rod-shaped bacteria that are frequently found in the soil and air (Figure 34-3, *C*). Some bacilli are able to form spores, a characteristic that enables them to resist adverse conditions such as heat and disinfectants. Diseases caused by bacilli include botulism, tetanus, gas gangrene, gastroenteritis produced by *Salmonella* food poisoning, typhoid fever, pertussis (whooping cough), bacillary dysentery, diphtheria, tuberculosis, leprosy, and plague.

Escherichia coli is a species of bacillus that is found among the normal flora of the large intestine in enormous numbers (Figure 34-3, *D*). It is normally a harmless bacterium; however, if it enters the urinary tract as a result of lowered resistance, poor hygiene practices, or both, it may cause a urinary tract infection.

Spirilla

Spirilla are spiral or curve-shaped bacteria. *Treponema pallidum,* a spirochete, is the causative agent of syphilis (Figure 34-3, *E*). This microorganism cannot be grown in commonly available culture media; the diagnosis of syphilis is generally made using serologic tests. A serologic test is

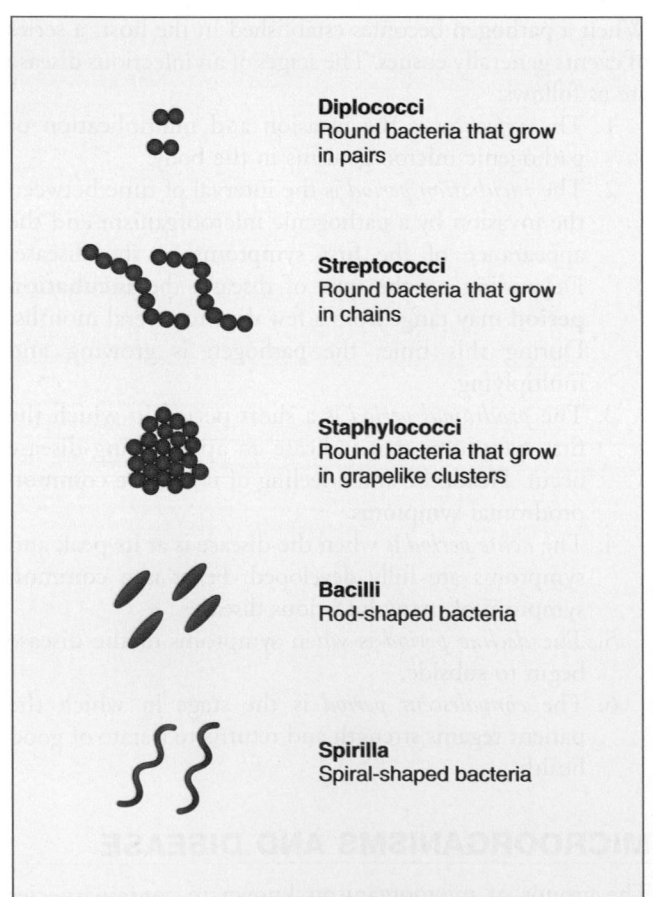

Diplococci
Round bacteria that grow in pairs

Streptococci
Round bacteria that grow in chains

Staphylococci
Round bacteria that grow in grapelike clusters

Bacilli
Rod-shaped bacteria

Spirilla
Spiral-shaped bacteria

Figure 34-2 **Classification of bacteria based on shape.**

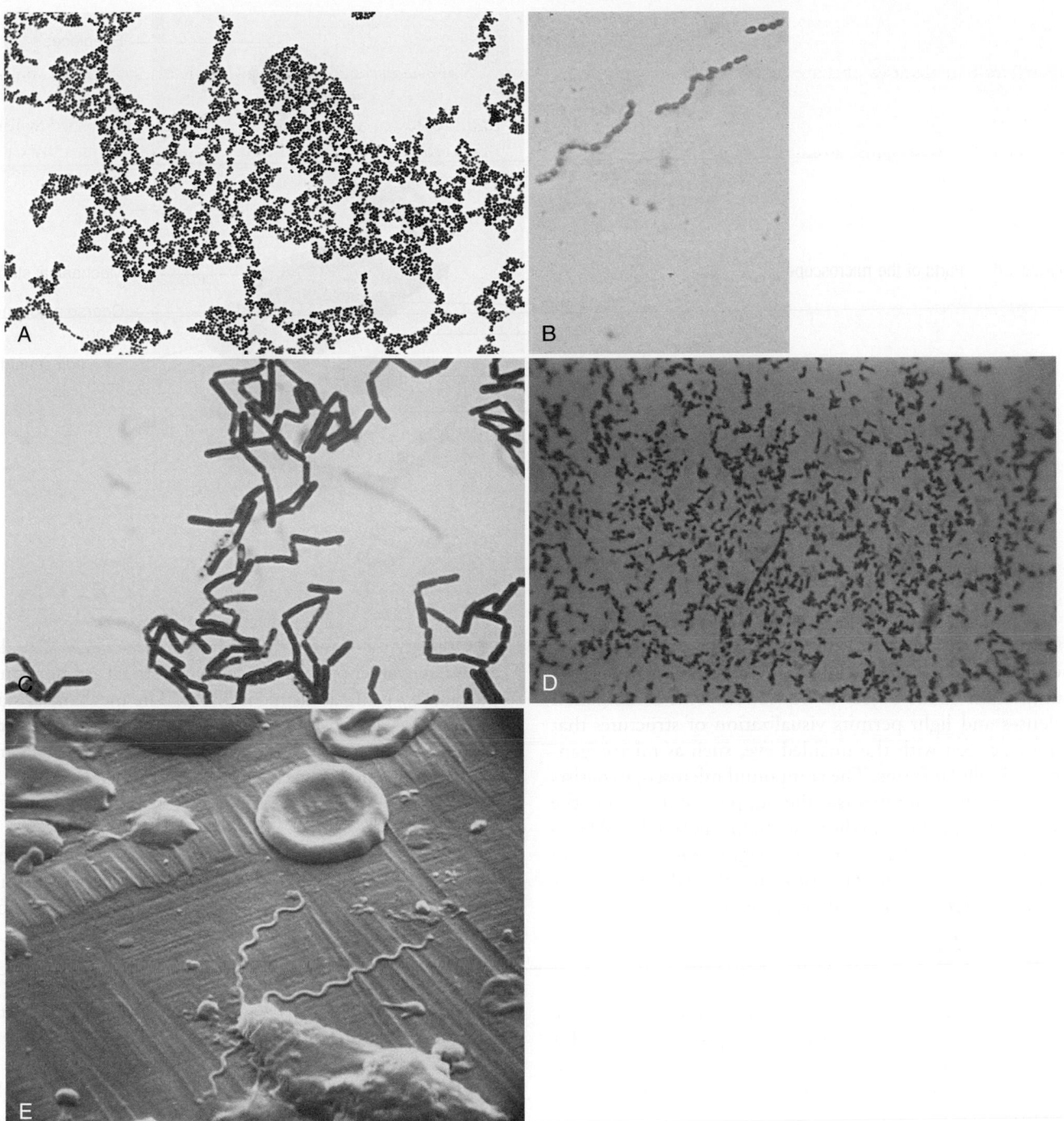

Figure 34-3 Types of bacteria. **A,** Staphylococci. **B,** Streptococci. **C,** Bacilli. **D,** *Escherichia coli.* **E,** Spirilla.

performed on the serum of the blood. Cholera is caused by another type of spirillum, *Vibrio cholerae.* **Immunization** and proper methods of sanitation and water purification have all but eliminated cholera in the United States.

Viruses

Viruses are the smallest living organisms. They are so small that an electron microscope must be used to view them. Viruses infect plants, animals, and humans and use nutrients inside the host's cells for their metabolic and reproductive needs. Infectious diseases caused by viruses include influenza, chickenpox, rubeola (measles), rubella (German measles), mumps, poliomyelitis, smallpox, rabies, herpes simplex, herpes zoster, yellow fever, hepatitis, and most infectious diseases of the upper respiratory tract, including the common cold.

MICROSCOPE

Many kinds of microscopes are available, but the type used most often for office laboratory work is the *compound microscope.* The compound microscope consists of a two-lens

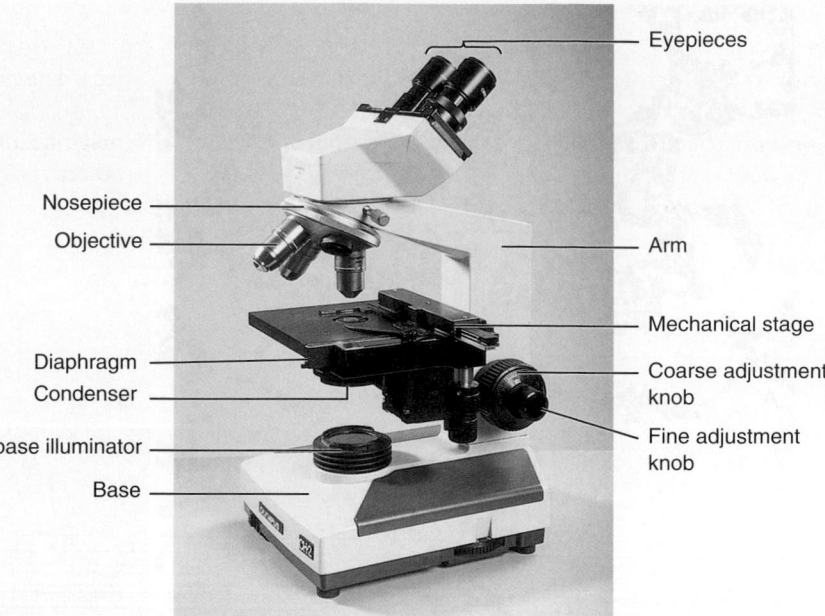

Figure 34-4 Parts of the microscope.

system, and the magnification of one system is increased by the other. A source of bright light is required for proper illumination of the object to be viewed. This combination of lenses and light permits visualization of structures that cannot be seen with the unaided eye, such as microorganisms and cellular forms. The compound microscope consists of two main components—the support system and the optical system. The medical assistant should be able to identify the parts of a microscope (Figure 34-4) and should be able to use and care for it properly. Procedure 34-1 outlines the correct use and care of a microscope.

Support System

Frame
The working parts of the microscope are supported by a sturdy frame consisting of a *base* for support and an *arm* for carrying it without damaging the delicate parts. The arm also is needed to support the magnifying and adjusting systems.

Stage
The *stage* of a microscope is the flat, horizontal platform on which the microscope slide is placed. It is located directly over the condenser and beneath the objective lenses. The stage has a small round opening in the center that permits light from below to pass through the object being viewed and up into the lenses above. The slide should be placed on the stage; the object to be viewed is positioned over this opening so that it is satisfactorily illuminated by the light source below. Standard microscope stages have metal clips attached to the stage to hold the glass slide securely in place. With this type of stage, the slide must be moved by hand for examination of various areas on it.

Other types of microscopes have a *mechanical stage* that allows movement of the slide in a vertical or horizontal position by using adjustment knobs. The mechanical stage provides precise positioning of the slide, which is essential for performing certain procedures, such as differential white blood counts and inspection of Gram-stained smears.

Light Source
The light source is at the base of the microscope and consists of a built-in illuminator, along with a switch for turning it on and off. The light is directed to the condenser above it and then through the object to be viewed.

Condenser
Compound microscopes have a lens system between the light source and object, known as the *substage condenser*. A popular condenser is the *Abbe condenser,* which consists of two lenses used to illuminate objects with transmitted light. The condenser collects and concentrates the light rays and directs them up, bringing them to a focus on the object so that it is well illuminated.

Diaphragm
The amount of light focused on the object also can be controlled by the *diaphragm,* located beneath or inside the condenser. The diaphragm consists of a series of horizontally arranged interlocking plates with a central opening, or *aperture.* The diaphragm has a lever that is used to increase or decrease the amount of light admitted by increasing or decreasing the aperture.

Appropriate intensity of light is essential for proper viewing of the specimens, especially at a higher magnification. A general rule is that as the desired magnification increases, the more intense the light must be. Increased light intensity is required for good visualization of a specimen with the oil-immersion objective. With the low-power objective, the light must be diminished to produce the appropriate contrast for specimen detail and to reduce glare. The degree of illumination also is influenced by the density of the object; stained structures (e.g., a Gram-stained smear of bacteria) usually require more light than do unstained specimens.

Adjustment Knobs

Two adjustment knobs are used to bring the specimen into focus: the coarse adjustment knob and the fine adjustment knob. The *coarse adjustment* is used first to obtain an approximate focus quickly. The *fine adjustment* is then used to obtain the precise focusing necessary to produce a sharp, clear image. On some microscope models, the adjustment knobs are mounted as two separate knobs; on others, they are placed together with the smaller fine adjustment knob extending from a larger coarse adjustment wheel.

Optical System

Compound microscopes have a two-lens magnification system. *Magnification* is defined as the ratio of the apparent size of an object viewed through the microscope to the actual size of the object.

Eyepiece

The first lens system is the eyepiece, or ocular lens, located at the top of the body tube and marked 10×, meaning that it magnifies 10 times. Microscopes that have one eyepiece only are called *monocular* microscopes, and microscopes with two eyepieces are called *binocular*. A binocular microscope is recommended for medical office laboratory work because it causes less eye fatigue than the monocular type. The binocular eyepieces can be adjusted to the individual by moving the eyepieces apart or together as needed.

Objective Lenses

The second lens system consists of three objective lenses located on the revolving *nosepiece,* each with a different degree of magnification. The metal shafts of the objective lenses differ in length and are identified by power of magnification. The short objective is known as the *low-power objective* and has a magnification of 10×. The *high-power objective* is known as the "high-dry objective" because it does not require the use of immersion oil; it has a magnification of 40×. The *oil-immersion objective* has the highest power of magnification, which is 100×.

The degree of magnification is engraved onto the metal shaft of each objective. In addition, some microscope manufacturers identify each objective lens by colored rings that encircle the metal shaft of the objective. Yellow is used for low power, blue for high power, and white for oil immersion. If the objective is not color-coded, it can be identified by the length of the metal shaft; the low-power objective is the shortest, and the oil-immersion objective is the longest.

The objective lens magnifies the specimen, and the ocular lens magnifies the image produced by the objective lens. The *total magnification* of each objective is determined by multiplying the ocular magnification by the objective magnification. The total magnification of the low-power objective is 100 times (100×) the actual size of the object being viewed (10 × 10). The total magnification of the high-power objective is 400× (10 × 40), and that of the oil-immersion magnification is 1000× (10 × 100).

Focus

Depending on the type of microscope, two ways may be used to focus on a specimen. Some microscopes are equipped with a *barrel focus.* With this type of microscope, the body tube (or barrel) moves, while the stage remains stationary during focusing. Other microscopes focus on the specimen using *stage focus.* With this type of microscope, the stage moves while the body tube remains stationary during focusing.

Low and High Power

The low-power objective is used for the initial focusing and light adjustment of the microscope. The low-power objective also is used for the initial observation and scanning requirements needed for most microscopic work. Urine sediment is first examined using the low-power objective to scan the specimen for the presence of casts.

The high-power objective is used for a more thorough study, such as observing cells in greater detail. The *working distance,* defined as the distance between the tip of the lens and the slide, is short when using this objective. Because of this, care must be taken in focusing the high-power objective to prevent it from striking and breaking the slide or damaging the lens.

Most compound microscopes are *parfocal.* This means that when the specimen is focused with the low-power objective, the nosepiece can be rotated to the high-power objective and focused simply with the fine adjustment knob.

Oil Immersion

The oil-immersion objective provides the highest magnification and is used to view very small structures or the detail of larger structures, such as microorganisms and blood cells. The oil-immersion objective has a very short working distance, and when it is in use, the lens nearly rests on the microscope slide itself. A special grade of oil, known as *immersion oil,* must be used with this lens. Oil has the advantage of not drying out when exposed to air for a long time. A drop of oil is placed on the slide and resides between the oil-immersion objective and the slide. The oil provides a path for the light to travel on between the slide and the lens and prevents the scattering of light rays, which permits clear viewing of very small structures. The oil also improves the resolution of the objective lens, that is, its ability to provide sharp detail, which is particularly necessary at high magnifications. Procedures that require oil immersion include differential white blood cell counts and examination of Gram-stained smears.

Care of the Microscope

The microscope is a delicate instrument and must be handled carefully. These guidelines should be followed to care for the microscope properly:

1. Always carry the microscope with two hands. Place one hand firmly on the arm and the other hand under the base for support. Place the microscope down gently to prevent jarring it, which could damage delicate parts.
2. Always handle the microscope in such a way that your fingers do not touch the lenses to avoid leaving fingerprints on them. When using a microscope, avoid wearing mascara because it is difficult to remove from the ocular lens.
3. When it is not in use, keep the microscope covered with its plastic dust cover and stored in a case or cupboard. Store it with the nosepiece rotated to the low-power objective and as close as possible to the stage.
4. Periodically clean the microscope by washing the enameled surfaces with mild soap and water and

drying them thoroughly with a soft cloth. Never use alcohol on the enameled surfaces because it might remove the finish.

5. After each use, wipe the metal stage clean with gauze or tissue. If immersion oil comes in contact with the stage, remove it with a piece of gauze that is slightly moistened with xylene.
6. The ocular, objectives, and condenser consist of hand-ground optical lenses, which must be kept spotlessly clean by using clean, dry lens paper. Optical glass is softer than ordinary glass; to prevent scratching the lens, do not use tissues or gauze. If the lenses are especially dirty, use a commercial lens cleaner or xylene in the cleaning process. Apply a small amount of cleaner to the lens paper, followed by thorough drying and polishing with a clean piece of lens paper.
7. Keep the light source free of dust, lint, and dirt by periodic polishing with lens paper.
8. A malfunctioning microscope should be repaired only by a qualified service person. Attempting to fix the microscope yourself may result in further damage.

PROCEDURE 34-1   Using the Microscope

Outcome Use a microscope.

Equipment/Supplies

- Microscope
- Lens paper
- Specimen slide
- Tissue or gauze

- Immersion oil
- Xylene
- Soft cloth

1. Procedural Step. Clean the ocular and objective lenses with lens paper.

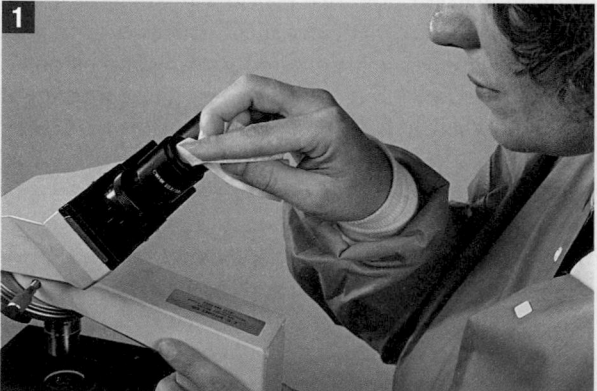

Clean the lens.

2. Procedural Step. Turn on the light source.

3. Procedural Step. Rotate the nosepiece to the low-power objective (10×), clicking it into place. Use the coarse adjustment knob to provide sufficient working space for placing the slide on the stage and to avoid damaging the objective lens as follows:

 a. **Barrel focus:** Raise the objective all the way up using the coarse adjustment knob.

 b. **Stage focus:** Lower the stage all the way down using the coarse adjustment knob.

4. Procedural Step. Place the slide on the stage specimen side up, and make sure it is secure.

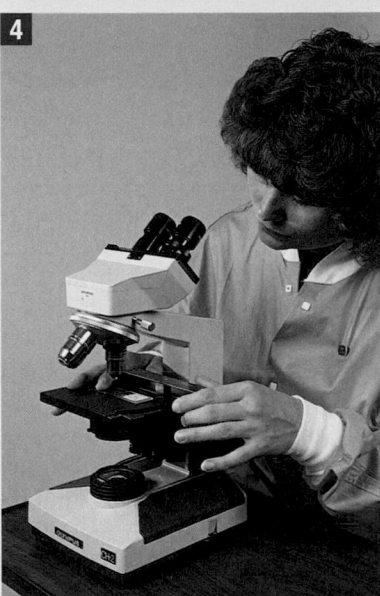

Place the slide on the stage.

5. Procedural Step. Position the low-power objective until it almost touches the slide using the coarse adjustment knob. Be sure to observe this step to prevent the objective from striking the slide.

6. Procedural Step. Look through the ocular. If a monocular microscope is being used, keep both eyes open to prevent eyestrain. With a binocular microscope, adjust the two oculars to the width between your eyes until a single circular field of vision is obtained.

7. Procedural Step. Bring the specimen into coarse focus as follows:

a. **Barrel focus:** Slowly raise the objective using the coarse adjustment knob.

b. **Stage focus:** Slowly lower the stage using the coarse adjustment knob.

Observe the specimen through the ocular until it comes into focus.

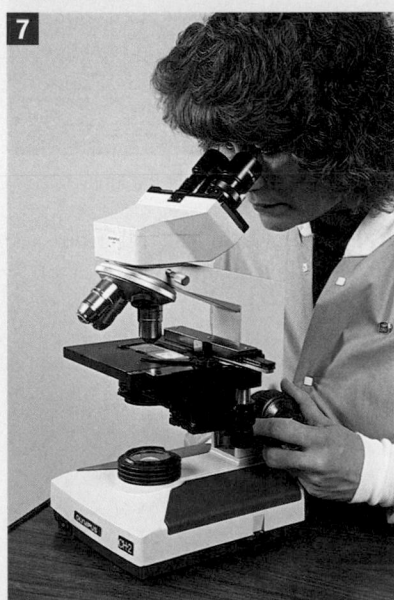

Focus the specimen.

8. Procedural Step. Use the fine adjustment knob to bring the specimen into a sharp, clear focus.

9. Procedural Step. Adjust the light as needed, using the iris diaphragm to provide maximal focus and contrast.

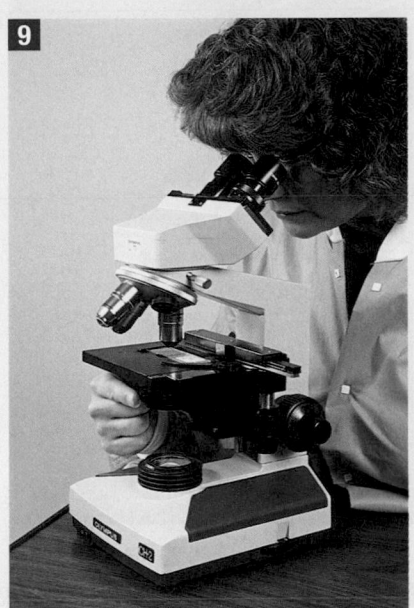

Adjust the light.

10. Procedural Step. Rotate the nosepiece to the high-power objective, making sure it clicks into place. Proper focusing with the low-power objective ensures that the objective does not hit the slide during this operation. Use the fine adjustment knob to bring the specimen into a precise focus. Do not use the coarse adjustment to focus the high-power objective to prevent the objective from moving too far and striking the slide.

11. Procedural Step. Examine the specimen as required by the test or procedure being performed.

12. Procedural Step. Turn off the light after use, and remove the slide from the stage.

13. Procedural Step. Clean the stage with a tissue or gauze.

14. Procedural Step. Properly care for and store the microscope.

Using the Oil-Immersion Objective

1. Procedural Step. Rotate the nosepiece to the oil-immersion objective. Do not click it into place, but move it to one side.

2. Procedural Step. Place a drop of immersion oil on the slide directly over the center opening in the stage.

Continued

PROCEDURE 34-1

PROCEDURE **34-1** **Using the Microscope—cont'd**

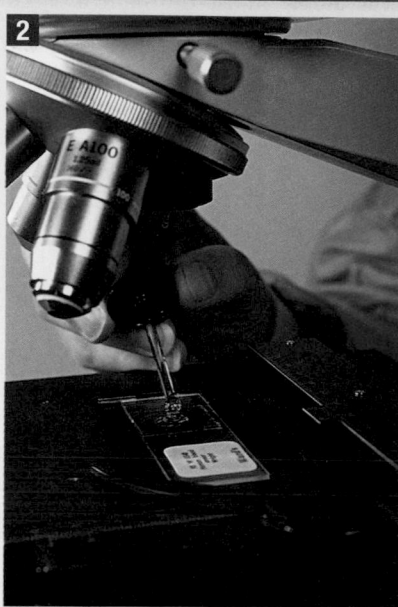

Place a drop of oil on the slide.

3. **Procedural Step.** Move the oil-immersion objective into place until a click is heard. Ensure that the objective does not touch the stage or slide.

4. **Procedural Step.** Using the coarse adjustment, slowly position the oil-immersion objective until the tip of the lens touches the oil but does not come in contact with the slide. A "pop" of light is observed. Be sure to observe carefully this step of the procedure.

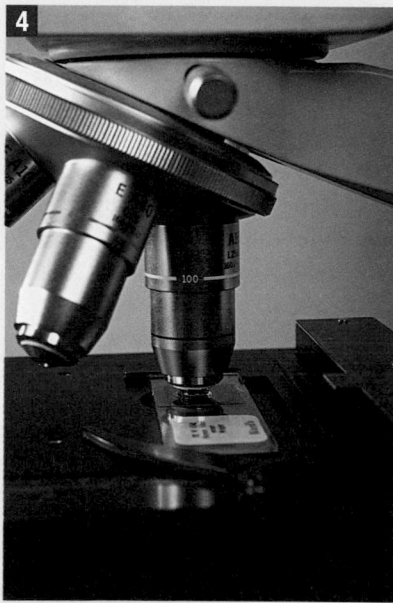

Move the lens until it just touches the oil.

5. **Procedural Step.** Look through the eyepiece, and focus slowly using the coarse adjustment until the object is visible.

6. **Procedural Step.** Use the fine adjustment to bring the object into sharp focus to view fine details.

7. **Procedural Step.** Adjust the light as needed, using the iris diaphragm to provide maximal focus and contrast. Increased light intensity is required for good visualization of the specimen with the oil-immersion objective.

8. **Procedural Step.** Examine the specimen as required by the test or procedure being performed.

9. **Procedural Step.** Turn off the light after use. Remove the slide from the stage, being careful not to get oil on the high-power objective or the stage.

10. **Procedural Step.** Using a piece of clean, dry lens paper, gently clean the oil-immersion objective. The lens must be cleaned immediately after use to prevent oil from drying on the lens surface. In addition, the oil may seep into the lens and perhaps loosen it.

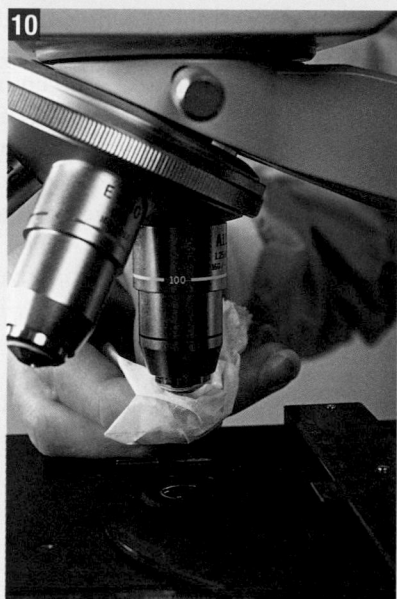

Clean the oil from the lens.

11. **Procedural Step.** Clean the oil from the slide by immersing it in xylene and wiping it off with a soft cloth.

MICROBIOLOGIC SPECIMEN COLLECTION

If the physician suspects that a particular disease is caused by a pathogen, he or she may want to obtain a specimen for microbiologic examination. This examination identifies the pathogen causing the disease and aids in diagnosis. If a urinary tract infection is suspected, a urine specimen is obtained for bacterial examination. In this instance, a clean-catch midstream collection is required to obtain a specimen that excludes the normal flora of the urethra and urinary meatus.

A **specimen** is a small sample or part taken from the body to represent the whole. The medical assistant is often responsible for collecting specimens from certain areas of the body, such as the throat, nose, and wounds. The medical assistant may be responsible for assisting the physician in the collection of specimens from other areas, such as the cervix, vagina, urethra, and rectum. In most instances, a sterile swab is used to collect the specimen. A *swab* is a small piece of cotton wrapped around the end of a slender wooden or plastic stick. It is passed across a body surface or opening to obtain a specimen for microbiologic analysis.

To prevent inaccurate test results, good techniques of medical and surgical asepsis must be practiced when a specimen is obtained. The medical assistant must be careful not to contaminate the specimen with *extraneous microorganisms*. These are undesirable microorganisms that can enter the specimen in various ways; they grow and multiply and possibly obscure and prevent identification of pathogens that might be present. To prevent extraneous microorganisms (i.e., normal flora) from contaminating the specimen, all supplies used to obtain the specimen (e.g., swabs, specimen containers) must be sterile. In addition, the specimen should not contain microorganisms from areas surrounding the collection site. When obtaining a throat specimen, the swab should not be allowed to touch the inside of the mouth.

The OSHA Bloodborne Pathogens Standard presented in Chapter 17 should be carefully followed when performing microbiologic procedures. Specifically, the medical assistant must wear gloves when it is reasonably anticipated that hand contact might occur with blood or other potentially infectious materials. Eating, drinking, smoking, and applying makeup are strictly forbidden when one is working with microorganisms because pathogens can be transmitted to the medical assistant through hand-to-mouth contact. In addition, labels for specimen containers should not be licked, and any break in the skin, such as a cut or scratch, must be covered with a bandage. If the medical assistant accidentally touches some of the material in the specimen, the area of contact should be washed immediately and thoroughly with soap and water. If the specimen comes in contact with the worktable, the table should be cleaned immediately with soap and water, followed by a suitable disinfectant, such as phenol. The worktable also should be cleaned with a disinfectant at the end of each day.

After collection, the specimen must be placed in its proper container with the lid securely fastened. The container must be clearly labeled with the patient's name and date of birth, the date, the source of the specimen, the medical assistant's initials, and any other required information. Procedure 34-2 outlines the procedure for collecting a specimen for a throat culture.

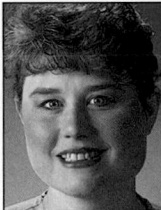

Putting It All into Practice

My name is **Natalie Moorehead,** and I work for a physician who specializes in family practice. Working as a medical assistant, one can encounter many challenges. One experience that I had involved a 4-year-old boy. The patient came into the office with a very sore throat and a high fever. He did not think that his office visit had gone too badly until he found out that the physician had ordered a rapid strep test to check for strep throat. That's when he decided he did not care for me, my tongue depressor, or my swab. He decided to protest by keeping his mouth tightly shut. Rather than forcing the procedure on the child, I took my time and kept my patience. I managed to convince the child that even though the procedure was uncomfortable and tasted bad, it was the only way we would know if he was really sick or not. I also explained that the test was the only way the doctor would know what kind of medicine to prescribe so he could get well and feel like playing again. It took a while, but we got our specimen, and the patient received the right antibiotic that he needed to get better. ∎

Handling and Transporting Microbiologic Specimens

After the microbiologic specimen has been collected, care should be taken in handling and transporting it. Delay in processing the specimen may cause the death of pathogens or overgrowth of the specimen by microorganisms that are part of the normal flora usually collected along with the pathogen from the specimen site. If the specimen is to be analyzed in the medical office, it should be examined under the microscope or cultured immediately. Otherwise, it should be preserved (if possible) with the method used by the medical office.

Specimens transported to an outside medical laboratory by a courier service are usually placed in a transport medium. The transport medium prevents drying of the specimen and preserves it in its original state until it reaches its destination. Transport media are discussed in greater detail in the section on "Collection and Transport Systems."

Outside laboratories provide the medical office with specific instructions on the care and handling of specimens being transported to them. These specimens must be accompanied by a laboratory request that designates the physician's name and address; the patient's name, age, and gender; the date and time of collection; the type of microbiologic examination requested; the source of the specimen (e.g., throat, wound, urine); and the physician's clinical diagnosis. The form usually includes a space to indicate whether the patient is receiving antibiotic therapy. Antibiotics may suppress the growth of bacteria, a factor that could produce **false-negative** results.

Wound Specimens

Wound specimens are collected using many of the techniques described previously. In many cases, two swabs are used to collect the specimen. The specimen is obtained by inserting the swab into the area of the wound that contains the most drainage and gently rotating the swab from side to side to allow it to absorb completely any microorganisms present. The swab is placed in the specimen container, and the process is repeated using a second swab. To obtain accurate and reliable test results, it is important to collect a specimen from within the wound, rather than from the surface.

Collection and Transport Systems

Microbiologic collection and transport systems are available to facilitate the collection of a specimen to be transported to an outside laboratory for analysis; examples include Culturette (Becton Dickinson, Franklin Lakes, NJ) and Starswab II (Starplex Scientific, Beverly, Mass) (Figure 34-5). These systems consist of a sterile swab and a plastic tube that contains a transport medium. The transport medium prevents drying of the specimen and preserves it in its original state until it reaches its destination. The collection and transport system comes packaged in a peel-apart envelope and should be stored at room temperature. The procedure for the use of a microbiologic collection and transport system is outlined next.

1. Sanitize your hands, and apply gloves.
2. Check the expiration date on the peel-apart envelope.
3. Peel back the package, and remove the cap from the collection tube. Remove the cap/swab unit from the peel-apart package. The cap is permanently attached to the sterile swab.
4. Using aseptic technique, collect the specimen. Do not allow the swab to touch any area other than the collection site.
5. Insert the swab into the collection tube.

6. Push the cap/swab in as far as it will go to immerse the swab completely in the transport medium. Make sure the cap is tightly in place.
7. Remove gloves, and sanitize your hands.
8. Label the tube with the patient's name and date of birth, the date, the source of the specimen (e.g., throat, wound), and your initials. Place the tube in a biohazard specimen transport bag. Place the laboratory request in the outside pocket of the bag.
9. Complete a laboratory request form.
10. Place the collection tube in a biohazard specimen bag with the laboratory requisition form in the outside pocket.
11. Chart the procedure.
12. Transport the specimen to the laboratory within 24 hours.

What Would You Do? What Would You *Not* Do?

Case Study 2

Hollie Dolley, age 18, is at the medical office complaining of fatigue, fever, headache, and a terrible sore throat. She just enrolled in a medical assisting program and has been really worried about doing well in her classes. Hollie says that she stays up until midnight every night studying, and she works 30 hours at a drugstore on the weekends. The physician orders a rapid mononucleosis test on Hollie, and it is positive. Hollie says she has never felt so awful in her whole life and wants to know whether she is going to die from this. She says it hurts really bad to swallow and she cannot eat. Hollie says that she has heard one gets mono from kissing, and she does not have a boyfriend, so she doesn't understand how she could possibly have mono. Hollie wants to know why the physician did not prescribe an antibiotic for her so that she could get well sooner and not have to miss any of her classes. ■

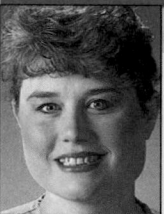

Memories *from* Externship

Natalie Moorehead: Terrified and excited at the same time to be experiencing my first externship, I found myself in a busy pediatric office. After a few days of watching and learning, I prepared to work up an infant for a well-child examination. Before entering the room, I was told by a staff member that the HIV status of the infant's mother was questionable. Alarmed at first as to how I would feel in this situation, I immediately remembered all the precautions we had talked about in class. As I took the infant from the mother to weigh and measure him, I have to admit many thoughts ran through my mind, but again I was calmed because of all the information we had received in school regarding OSHA precautions. Faced with that situation today, after practicing wisely and safely for 5 years, I would not think twice about it because I know from my education and experience that these types of situations can be handled without alarm ■

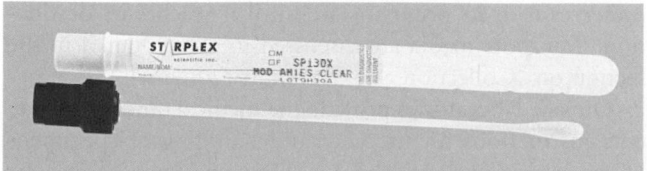

Figure 34-5 Starswab II Culture Collection and Transport System.

PROCEDURE 34-2 Collecting a Throat Specimen

Outcome Collect a throat specimen for a rapid strep test.

A throat specimen is obtained by using a sterile swab. It is commonly collected to aid in the diagnosis of infections such as streptococcal sore throat, pharyngitis, and tonsillitis. Less frequently, it is used to diagnose whooping cough and diphtheria. These latter diseases are not prevalent today because of the availability of immunizations against them. This procedure outlines the steps necessary to obtain a throat specimen to perform a rapid streptococcus test, which is discussed later in the chapter.

Equipment/Supplies

- Disposable gloves
- Tongue depressor
- Sterile swab
- Waste container

1. **Procedural Step.** Sanitize your hands, and assemble the equipment.
2. **Procedural Step.** Greet the patient and introduce yourself. Identify the patient by full name and date of birth and explain the procedure.
3. **Procedural Step.** Position the patient, and adjust the light to provide clear visualization of the throat.
   Principle. The throat must be clearly visible so that the medical assistant is able to determine the proper area for obtaining the specimen.
4. **Procedural Step.** Apply gloves. Remove the sterile swab from its peel-apart package, being careful not to contaminate it.
   Principle. Contamination of the swab may lead to inaccurate test results.

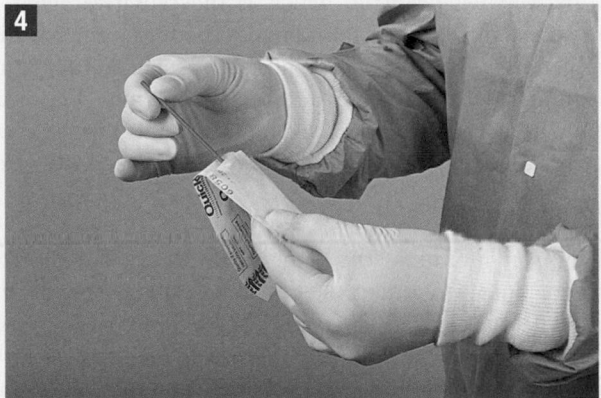
Remove the swab.

5. **Procedural Step.** Depress the tongue with the tongue depressor.
   Principle. The tongue depressor holds the tongue down and facilitates access to the throat.
6. **Procedural Step.** Place the swab at the back of the throat (posterior pharynx), and firmly rub it over any lesions or white or inflamed areas of the mucous membrane of the tonsillar area and posterior pharyngeal wall. Rotate the swab constantly as you collect the specimen, making sure there is good contact with the tonsillar area. Do not allow the swab to touch any areas other than the throat, such as the inside of the mouth.

Principle. The swab should be rubbed over suspicious-looking areas where pathogens are likely to be found. A rotating motion is used to deposit the maximal amount of material possible on the swab. Touching it to any areas other than the throat contaminates the specimen with extraneous microorganisms.

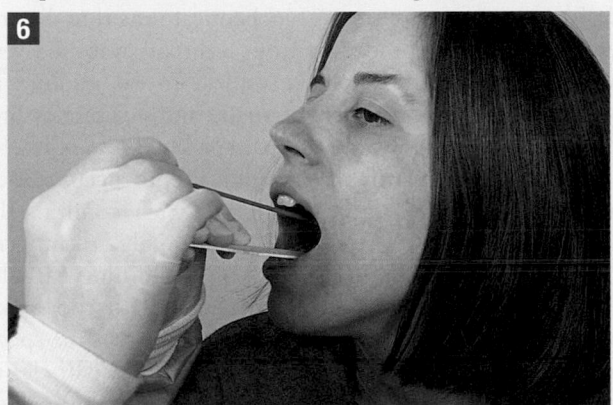
Collect the specimen.

7. **Procedural Step.** Keeping the patient's tongue depressed, withdraw the swab, and remove the tongue depressor from the patient's mouth.
8. **Procedural Step.** Properly dispose of the tongue depressor in a regular waste container to prevent transmission of microorganisms.
9. **Procedural Step.** Process the swab according to the directions accompanying the rapid strep test.
10. **Procedural Step.** Remove gloves, and sanitize your hands. Chart the test results.

CHARTING EXAMPLE

Date	
9/20/XX	10:30 a.m. Throat specimen collected.
	QuickVue Strep Test: Positive. ————
	———— N. Moorehead, CMA (AAMA)

PROCEDURE 34-2

STREPTOCOCCUS TESTING

The most common streptococcal condition is streptococcal sore throat, or *streptococcal pharyngitis,* which primarily affects children and young adults. The causative agent of streptococcal pharyngitis is a group A beta-hemolytic streptococcus known as *Streptococcus pyogenes.*

Streptococcal pharyngitis is a potentially serious condition because some patients develop a poststreptococcal sequela. A **sequela** is a morbid secondary condition that occurs as a result of a less serious primary infection. A few patients with streptococcal pharyngitis (primary infection) develop rheumatic fever; the rheumatic fever is considered a poststreptococcal sequela. Owing to the risk of a sequela, early diagnosis and treatment with antibiotics of streptococcal pharyngitis are important. In the medical office, commercially available tests are often used for identification of group A beta-hemolytic streptococci.

Rapid Streptococcus Tests

Rapid streptococcus tests are biochemical tests that directly detect group A streptococcus from a throat swab in a very short time. Most tests require only 4 to 10 minutes to process; diagnosis can often be made and antibiotics prescribed, if necessary, before the patient leaves the office.

The most frequently used rapid streptococcus test is the direct antigen identification test, which confirms the presence of group A streptococcus through an antigen-antibody reaction. The test works by combining particles sensitized to the streptococcus antibody with the throat specimen. If group A streptococcal antigen is in the specimen, it combines with the antibody-sensitized particles to produce a color change that can be observed with the unaided eye. Rapid streptococcus tests also include a control that determines whether the test results are accurate and reliable.

The advantage of the direct antigen identification test is that it provides the physician with immediate test results rather than requiring an overnight culture. Specific instructions are included with every commercially available antigen identification test; examples of these tests include QTest Strep (Becton Dickinson, Franklin Lakes, NJ), Clearview Strep A (Wampole Laboratories, Princeton, NJ), and QuickVue In-Line Strep A (Quidel, San Diego, Calif) (Figure 34-6).

SENSITIVITY TESTING

The physician may request not only that the laboratory identify the infecting pathogen, but also that a sensitivity test be performed on it to determine the best antibiotic to treat the condition. The test is always performed on a pure rather than a mixed culture. A sensitivity test determines the susceptibility of pathogenic bacteria to various antibiotics; only the growth of the infectious pathogen is desired on the culture.

The most common method for sensitivity testing is the *disc-diffusion method* (Figure 34-7). Commercially prepared discs impregnated with known concentrations of various antibiotics are dropped on the surface of a solid culture medium in a Petri plate inoculated with the pathogen. The culture is incubated, allowing the antibiotics to diffuse into the culture medium. If the pathogen is susceptible or sensitive to an antibiotic, a clear zone without bacterial growth surrounds the disc. This indicates that the antibiotic was effective in destroying the pathogen. If the pathogen is unaffected by or resistant to the antibiotic, no clear zone is seen around the disc, indicating that the antibiotic was unable to kill the pathogen. Sensitivity testing enables the physician to decide which antibiotics would most likely be effective against the infectious disease in question.

MICROSCOPIC EXAMINATION OF MICROORGANISMS

Microorganisms can be examined under a microscope in the fixed state or in the living state. Examination in the fixed state involves the preparation of a smear through heat fixation, followed by a staining process such as Gram stain (see later). Most microorganisms are examined in the fixed state because it is easier to examine them when they are stained.

Some microorganisms require examination in the living state, however, owing to special circumstances, such as their inability to be readily stained or difficulty in culturing them. The living state also allows visualization of the movement of motile microorganisms. This is especially helpful in the identification of certain motile microorganisms, such as *Trichomonas vaginalis,* which is the causative agent of the vaginal infection trichomoniasis. To observe the motility of microorganisms, they first must be suspended in a liquid medium so that they are free to move about. The most common method of examining microorganisms in the living state is the wet mount method, which is described next.

Wet Mount Method

In the wet mount method, the medical assistant places a drop of fluid containing the organism on a glass slide and covers it with a cover slip (Figure 34-8). The cover slip may be ringed with petroleum jelly to provide a seal between the slide and the cover slip. The purpose is to reduce the rate of evaporation through air currents that lead to drying and possible death of the specimen.

The slide is placed under the microscope for examination by the physician using the high-power objective. For satisfactory visualization, the intensity of the light must be diminished by partially closing the diaphragm of the microscope. The slide and coverslip should be properly disposed of in a biohazard sharps container.

Smears

A **smear** consists of material spread on a slide for microscopic examination. It can be prepared directly from the specimen collected on the swab, or the specimen can be grown first on a culture medium and a smear then prepared. Most smears must be stained before they can be viewed

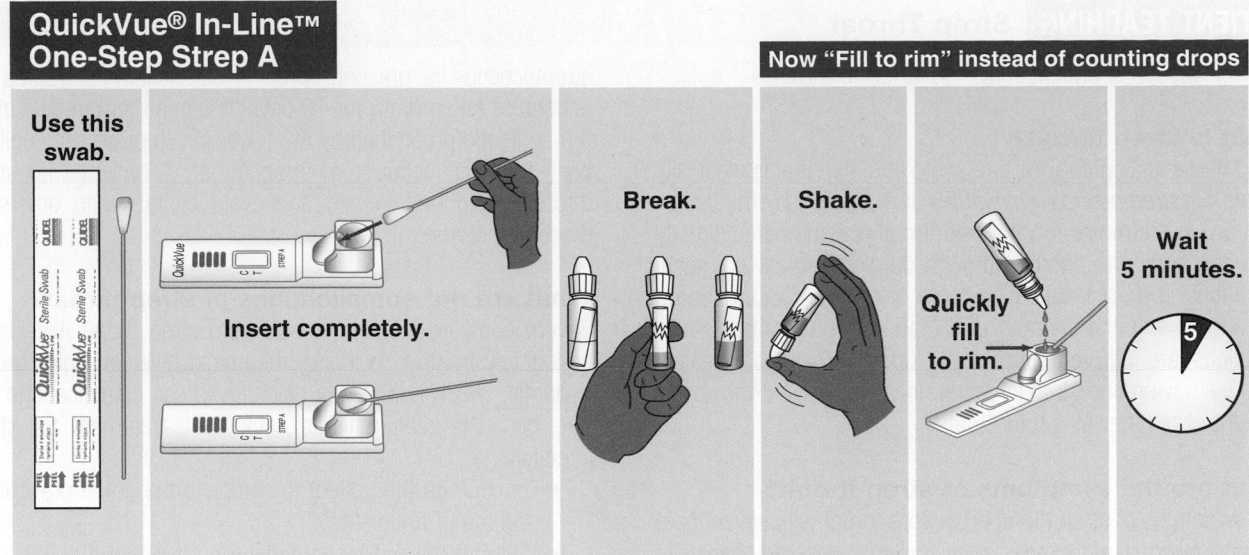

Figure 34-6 Procedure for performing the QuickVue In-Line one-step strep A test.

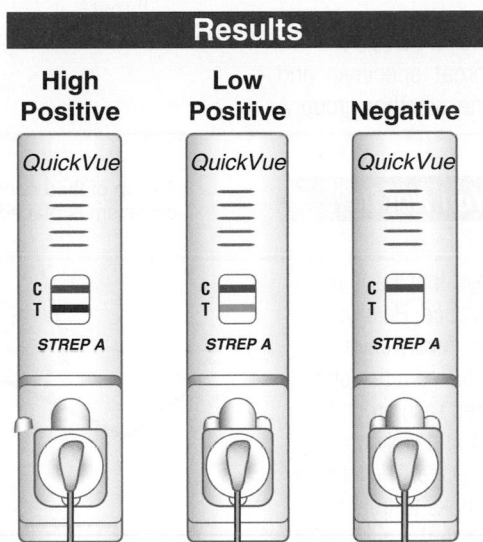

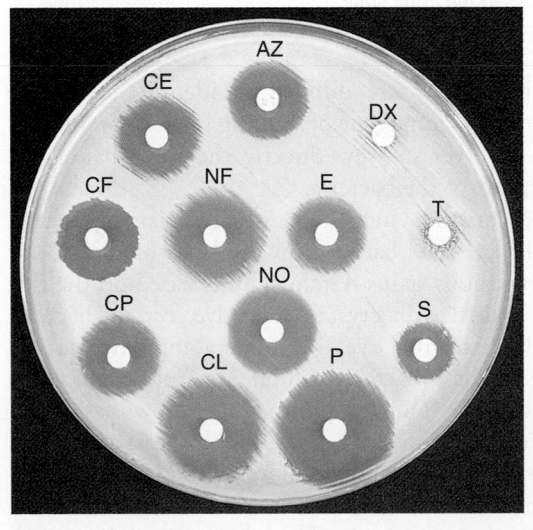

AZ:	Azithromycin
CE:	Cephalothin
CF:	Ciprofloxacin
CL:	Clarithromycin
CP:	Ciprozil
DX:	Doxycycline
E:	Erythromycin
NF:	Nitrofurantoin
NO:	Norfloxacin
P:	Penicillin
S:	Sulfisoxazole
T:	Tetracycline

Figure 34-7 Sensitivity testing.

Answer questions patients have about strep throat.

What is strep throat?
Strep throat is a contagious and acute infection that is medically known as *streptococcal pharyngitis.* It is caused by the bacterium group A streptococcus. Strep throat is transmitted directly from one person to another through droplets of saliva or nasal secretions. It most frequently occurs in children 5 to 10 years old and during the months of October through April. Strep infections are different from most other infectious diseases because having one strep infection does not prevent the development of another at a future date.

What are the symptoms of strep throat?
The symptoms of strep throat are a sore throat with severe pain on swallowing, a bright red pharynx (called "beefy red pharynx"), fever, white patches on the tonsils, swollen glands in the neck, muscular aches and pains, and a feeling of tiredness.

How is strep throat diagnosed and treated?
Strep throat is diagnosed by taking a throat specimen and running a laboratory test on it to determine whether group A

streptococcus is present. Strep throat usually is treated by antibiotics taken orally for 10 days. It is important to take all of the antibiotic prescribed by the physician to prevent complications that can occur from strep throat. A patient with strep throat should rest in bed and avoid contact with others to prevent spreading it.

What are the complications of strep throat?
Severe complications can result from strep throat if it is not adequately treated, including rheumatic fever and glomerulonephritis, which is a kidney disorder. These complications are rare because most patients seek early treatment for strep infections.
- Encourage the patient to complete the entire prescribed course of antibiotics.
- Instruct the patient to notify the physician if new symptoms develop.
- Provide the patient with educational materials about strep throat.

Case Study 3
John Seimer calls the medical office. He says that he is not a patient at the office but would like some assistance. He says that for the past 3 days he has had a headache, fever, chills, and aching muscles. He says that a week ago he pulled a tick off his lower leg, and several days later he found a red rash around the tick bite. He says that he went on the Internet and looked up his symptoms, and he is sure that he has Lyme disease. The Internet site recommended taking doxycycline for 3 weeks to treat Lyme disease. John says that he does not like to go to the doctor and has not been to see a doctor for over 10 years. He wants to know whether the doctor could call in a prescription for doxycycline for him. He says that he has health insurance and the doctor could bill him for an appointment, just as long as he does not have to come in. ■

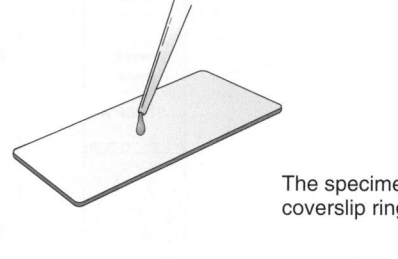

A drop of fluid containing the organism is placed on a glass slide.

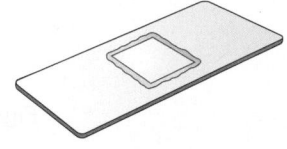

The specimen is covered with a coverslip ringed with petroleum jelly.

Figure 34-8 Wet mount method of slide preparation for examining microorganisms in the living state.

---

under the microscope, using one of many staining techniques. Bacteria contained in a smear are colorless and usually are difficult to identify under the microscope unless some type of staining is used.

Smears are often helpful when time is a factor because a smear can be prepared immediately from the specimen. This procedure gives the physician a preliminary clue to the causative agent while other, more time-consuming tests are being performed.

Gram Stain

Gram stain is often used in combination with other tests to help in the diagnosis and treatment of infectious diseases. As already discussed, bacteria contained in a smear are

colorless and usually are difficult to identify under the microscope unless some type of staining is used. Gram stain allows the observer to view directly the size, shape, and growth patterns of the bacteria.

In 1883, Christian Gram, a Danish physician, discovered a way to differentiate bacteria on the basis of their color reactions to various stains. Gram stain is based on the fact that when treated with crystal violet dye, certain bacteria permanently retain this dye after undergoing a decolorization process. These bacteria exhibit a purple color when viewed under the microscope and are known as *gram-positive* bacteria (Figure 34-9, *A*). Other bacteria are unable to retain this dye after being decolorized and become colorless. They must be counterstained with a red dye to become visible under the microscope. These bacteria exhibit a pink

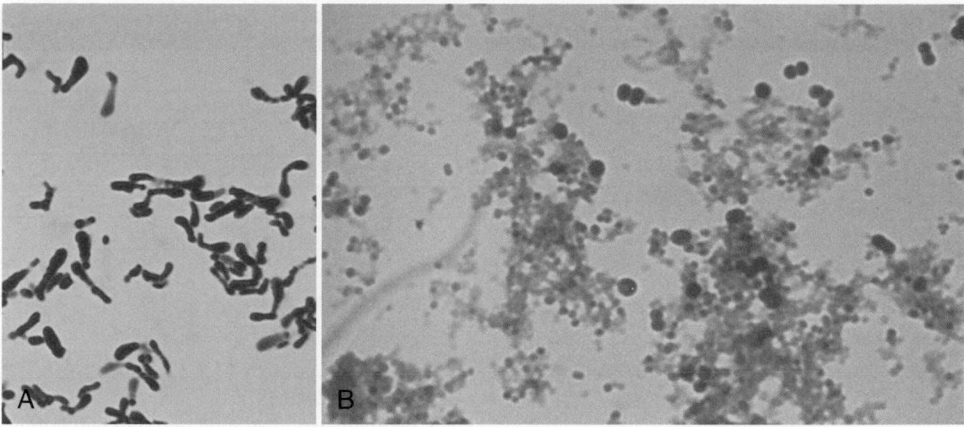

Figure 34-9 Gram-positive and gram-negative bacteria. **A,** Diphtheria is caused by a gram-positive bacillus. **B,** Gonorrhea is caused by a gram-negative diplococcus.

or red color and are known as *gram-negative* bacteria (Figure 34-9, *B*). These staining characteristics are due to differences in the chemical composition of the bacterial cell walls.

Gram stain allows for the division of most bacteria into two groups—gram-positive and gram-negative. Infectious diseases caused by gram-positive bacteria include streptococcal sore throat, scarlet fever, rheumatic fever, diphtheria, lobar pneumonia, tetanus, and botulism. Infectious diseases caused by gram-negative bacteria include whooping cough, gonorrhea, meningitis, bacillary dysentery, cholera, typhoid fever, and plague.

Bacteria that are Gram-stained also are observed for their characteristic shape and fall into one of the following categories: gram-positive rods, gram-negative rods, gram-positive cocci, or gram-negative cocci. The causative agent of gonorrhea is a gram-negative diplococcus.

PREVENTION AND CONTROL OF INFECTIOUS DISEASES

Individuals in the community can help prevent and control infectious diseases by practicing good techniques of medical asepsis, by obtaining proper nutrition and rest, and by using good hygienic measures. In addition, infected individuals should contact their physicians in an effort to ensure early diagnosis and treatment of the infectious disease. Immunizations are available to prevent a wide range of infectious diseases. The medical assistant has a responsibility to help educate community members about practices that reduce the transmission of pathogens and help control and prevent infectious diseases.

MEDICAL PRACTICE *and the* LAW

This chapter addresses the collection and identification of microorganisms that cause infections. You must maintain standard precautions whenever handling potentially infectious material to protect yourself, your co-workers, and your patients. Microbiology is an exact science—one stray microorganism can contaminate the entire specimen. Sanitize hands thoroughly, and apply new gloves between handling of specimens to avoid cross-contamination. If specimen contamination occurs, immediately discard the specimen and collect a new one. Be precise in your labeling—a mislabeled specimen can cause unnecessary concern, treatment, or both for the patient.

Maintain confidentiality of information. Certain infectious diseases must be reported to the Centers for Disease Control and Prevention (CDC) or the local board of health. Otherwise, do not give information to anyone other than the patient or legal guardian. ■

What Would You Do? What Would You *Not* Do? RESPONSES

Case Study 1
Page 828

What Did Natalie Do?
❏ Told Paula that it is important that the physician find out whether Caitlin has strep throat because strep can sometimes develop into a more serious infection. Explained that if Caitlin does have strep throat, the doctor would want to prescribe the best antibiotic to treat the infection.

❏ Talked with Caitlin about the reason for the test. Explained that it will help the doctor find the best way to treat her so that she starts feeling better as soon as possible.
❏ Reassured Caitlin that the procedure would be very quick and it would be over before she knew it.
❏ Told Caitlin that after the specimen was obtained, she could choose a prize from the treasure box.

Continued

What Would You Do? What Would You *Not* Do? RESPONSES—cont'd

What Did Natalie Not Do?
❑ Did not force the collection swab into Caitlin's mouth.

What Would You Do?/What Would You Not Do?
Review Natalie's response and place a checkmark next to the information you included in your response. List additional information you included in your response.

_____
_____
_____
_____
_____

Case Study 2
Page 836

What Did Natalie Do?
❑ Told Hollie that mononucleosis is usually transmitted by kissing, but it sometimes can be transmitted by coughs and sneezes from an infected person.
❑ Sympathized with Hollie and told her that it probably feels like she is going to die, but she should start to feel better as her body begins to fight off the disease.
❑ Explained to Hollie that mononucleosis is caused by a virus and that antibiotics do not work against viruses.
❑ Told Hollie to try drinking cold fluids or sucking on a Popsicle until she feels more like eating.

What Did Natalie Not Do?
❑ Did not ignore or minimize Hollie's concerns.

What Would You Do?/What Would You Not Do?
Review Natalie's response and place a checkmark next to the information you included in your response. List additional information you included in your response.

_____
_____
_____
_____
_____
_____

Case Study 3
Page 840

What Did Natalie Do?
❑ Sympathized with John and told him that a lot of people do not like coming to see the doctor. Told him that the doctor could not legally or ethically prescribe medication for him without seeing him.
❑ Told John that the office could not bill him for an appointment that he did not have.
❑ Asked John whether he wanted to make an appointment to see the doctor.

What Did Natalie Not Do?
❑ Did not tell John he should not be diagnosing himself with information he found on the Internet.

What Would You Do?/What Would You Not Do?
Review Natalie's response and place a checkmark next to the information you included in your response. List additional information you included in your response.

_____
_____
_____
_____
_____

TERMINOLOGY REVIEW

Medical Term	Word Parts	Definition
Bacilli (sing. *bacillus*)		Bacteria that have a rod shape.
Cocci (sing. *coccus*)	-*cocci*: berry-shaped	Bacteria that have a round shape.
Contagious		Capable of being transmitted directly or indirectly from one person to another.
Culture		The propagation of a mass of microorganisms in a laboratory culture medium.
Culture medium		A mixture of nutrients on which microorganisms are grown in the laboratory.
False-negative		A test result denoting that a condition is absent when it is actually present.
False-positive		A test result denoting that a condition is present when it is actually absent.
Immunization	-*immuno*: immune	The process of becoming protected from a disease through vaccination.
Incubate		In microbiology, the act of placing a culture in a chamber (incubator) that provides optimal growth requirements for the multiplication of the organisms, such as the proper temperature, humidity, and darkness.
Incubation period		The interval of time between the invasion by a pathogenic microorganism and the appearance of first symptoms of the disease.

TERMINOLOGY REVIEW—cont'd

Medical Term	Word Parts	Definition
Infectious disease		A disease caused by a pathogen that produces harmful effects on its host (also known as a *communicable disease*).
Inoculate		To introduce microorganisms into a culture medium for growth and multiplication.
Microbiology	*micro-:* small *bi/o:* life *-ology:* study of	The scientific study of microorganisms and their activities.
Mucous membrane		A membrane lining body passages or cavities that open to the outside.
Normal flora		Harmless, nonpathogenic microorganisms that normally reside in many parts of the body but do not cause disease.
Resistance		The natural ability of an organism to remain unaffected by harmful substances in its environment.
Sequela		A morbid (secondary) condition occurring as a result of a less serious primary infection.
Smear		Material spread on a slide for microscopic examination.
Specimen		A small sample or part taken from the body to show the nature of the whole.
Spirilla (sing. *spirillum*)		Bacteria that have a spiral or curved shape.

ON THE WEB

For information on disease and infection control:

American Society for Microbiology: www.asm.org

Association for Professionals in Infection Control and Epidemiology: www.apic.org

Centers for Disease Control and Prevention: www.cdc.gov

World Health Organization (WHO): www.who.int/en

Infection Control Today: www.infectioncontroltoday.com

Infectious Diseases Society of America (IDSA): www.idsociety.org

National Multiple Sclerosis Society: www.nmss.org

Cystic Fibrosis Foundation (CFF): www.cff.org

Disease Information: www.disease.com

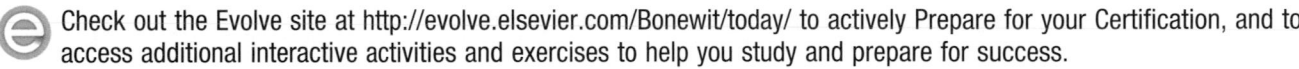

Check out the Evolve site at http://evolve.elsevier.com/Bonewit/today/ to actively Prepare for your Certification, and to access additional interactive activities and exercises to help you study and prepare for success.

35

Emergency Medical Procedures

LEARNING OBJECTIVES

First Aid
1. State the purpose of first aid.
2. Explain the purpose of the emergency medical services (EMS) system.
3. List the OSHA standards for administering first aid.
4. List the guidelines that should be followed when providing emergency care.

Common Emergency Situations
5. List and describe conditions that cause respiratory distress.
6. List the symptoms of a heart attack and a stroke.
7. Explain the causes of each of the following types of shock: cardiogenic, neurogenic, anaphylactic, and psychogenic.
8. Identify and describe the three classifications of external bleeding.
9. Explain the difference between an open wound and a closed wound.
10. Describe the characteristics of each of the following fractures: impacted, greenstick, transverse, oblique, comminuted, and spiral.
11. Identify the characteristics of each of the following burns: superficial, partial-thickness, and full-thickness.
12. Explain the difference between a partial seizure and a generalized seizure.
13. List examples of each of the following types of poisoning: ingested, inhaled, absorbed, and injected.
14. Identify factors that place an individual at higher risk for developing heat-related and cold-related injuries.
15. Describe the differences between type 1 and type 2 diabetes mellitus.
16. Explain the causes of insulin shock and diabetic coma.
17. Identify the symptoms and describe emergency care for each of the following conditions: respiratory distress, heart attack, stroke, shock, bleeding, wounds, musculoskeletal injuries, burns, seizures, poisoning, heat and cold exposure, and diabetic emergencies.

PROCEDURES

Respond to common emergency situations.

CHAPTER OUTLINE

burn	fracture (FRAK-shur)	splint
crash cart	hypothermia (hie-poe-THER-mee-ah)	sprain
crepitus (KREP-it-us)	poison	strain
dislocation	pressure point	wound
emergency medical services (EMS) system	seizure (SEE-zhur)	
first aid	shock	

INTRODUCTION TO EMERGENCY MEDICAL PROCEDURES

Medical emergencies often arise inside and outside of the workplace that can result in sudden loss of life or permanent disability. If an emergency situation occurs in the medical office, the physician provides immediate medical care for the patient. Some medical offices maintain a crash cart for this purpose. In these situations, the medical assistant may be required to assist the physician in providing emergency medical care.

The medical assistant may need to administer first aid for medical emergencies that occur outside of the medical office environment. **First aid** is defined as the immediate care administered before complete medical care can be obtained to an individual who is injured or suddenly becomes ill. The medical assistant is most likely to administer first aid to a family member or friend. The purposes of first aid are to save a life, reduce pain and suffering, prevent further injury, reduce the incidence of permanent disability, and increase the opportunity for an early recovery.

This chapter focuses on common emergency situations that the medical assistant may encounter and the first aid required for each. It is not intended, however, as a substitute for thorough first aid instruction through the American Red Cross, National Safety Council, or American Heart Association.

OFFICE CRASH CART

A **crash cart** is a specially equipped cart for holding and transporting medications, equipment, and supplies needed to perform lifesaving procedures in an emergency. A growing number of physicians are incorporating crash carts into their medical offices. Patients who are injured or suddenly become ill might be brought to the medical office for emergency medical care. In addition, a patient might develop a sudden illness at the medical office that requires emergency medical care. Examples of these situations include life-threatening cardiac dysrhythmias, shock, cardiac arrest, poisoning, and traumatic injury.

The items on an office crash cart vary widely among medical offices depending on the extent of the emergency medical care that is likely to be administered. This is directly related to the time it takes for emergency medical personnel to arrive and the location of the nearest hospital. The medical assistant may be responsible for regularly checking the crash cart to replenish supplies and to check the expiration dates on medications.

EMERGENCY MEDICAL SERVICES SYSTEM

The **emergency medical services (EMS) system** is a network of community resources, equipment, and emergency medical technicians (EMTs) that provides emergency care to victims of injury or sudden illness. An *EMT* is a professional provider of prehospital emergency care, which includes care at the scene and during transportation to the hospital. An EMT-basic (EMT-B) has received formal training and is certified to provide basic life support measures. An *EMT-paramedic* (EMT-P) is qualified to provide advanced life support care, including advanced airway maintenance, starting intravenous drips, administration of medication, cardiac monitoring and interpretation, and cardiac defibrillation.

Activating EMS is often the most important step in an emergency. Rapid arrival of EMTs increases the patient's chances of surviving a life-threatening emergency. In most urban and in some rural areas in the United States, the medical assistant can activate the local EMS by dialing 911 on the telephone. Other areas have a local seven-digit number, in which case it is important to keep the number at hand.

When calling local EMS, the medical assistant speaks with an *emergency medical dispatcher* (EMD). An EMD has had formal training in handling emergency situations over the phone. The responsibility of the EMD is to answer the emergency call, listen to the caller, obtain critical information, determine what help is needed, and send the appropriate personnel and equipment. The EMD also is responsible for relaying instructions to the caller about providing emergency care until the EMTs arrive.

These guidelines should be followed when calling EMS:
- Speak clearly and calmly to the EMD. Identify the problem as accurately and concisely as possible so that proper equipment and personnel can be sent. The EMD needs to know the number of victims, the condition of the victim or victims, and the emergency care that has already been administered.
- The EMD will ask you for your phone number and address. In responding, relay to the dispatcher the exact

location of the victim, including the correct street name and house number and (if applicable) the building name, floor, and room number. With the 911 enhanced emergency system, the address automatically appears on a monitor; however, there is a chance that the address will not show up on the monitor. In addition, the emergency may not be happening in the same location as the caller. If possible, have someone meet the ambulance personnel and direct them to the scene.

- Do not hang up until the EMD gives you permission to do so. The dispatcher may need additional information or may give you instructions on treating the patient until EMTs arrive.

FIRST AID KIT

The medical assistant should acquire and maintain a first aid kit. A first aid kit contains basic supplies to provide emergency care to individuals who have been injured or become suddenly ill (Figure 35-1). It is recommended that a first aid kit be kept at home and in the car.

First aid kits are available at most drug stores. It also is possible to make your own. Along with the items shown in Figure 35-1, the first aid kit should include the phone numbers of the local emergency medical service, the poison

control center, and the police and fire departments. It is important to check the first aid kit regularly and replace supplies as needed.

OSHA SAFETY PRECAUTIONS

To avoid exposure to bloodborne pathogens and other potentially infectious materials, the OSHA Bloodborne Pathogens Standard presented in Chapter 17 should be followed when performing first aid. The following guidelines help reduce or eliminate the risk of infection:

1. Make sure that your first aid kit contains personal protective equipment, such as gloves, a face shield and mask, and a pocket mask.
2. Wear gloves when it is reasonably anticipated that your hands will come into contact with the following: blood and other potentially infectious materials, mucous membranes, nonintact skin, and contaminated articles or surfaces.
3. Perform all first aid procedures involving blood or other potentially infectious materials in a manner that minimizes splashing, spraying, spattering, and generation of droplets of these substances.
4. Wear protective clothing and gloves to cover cuts or other lesions of the skin.

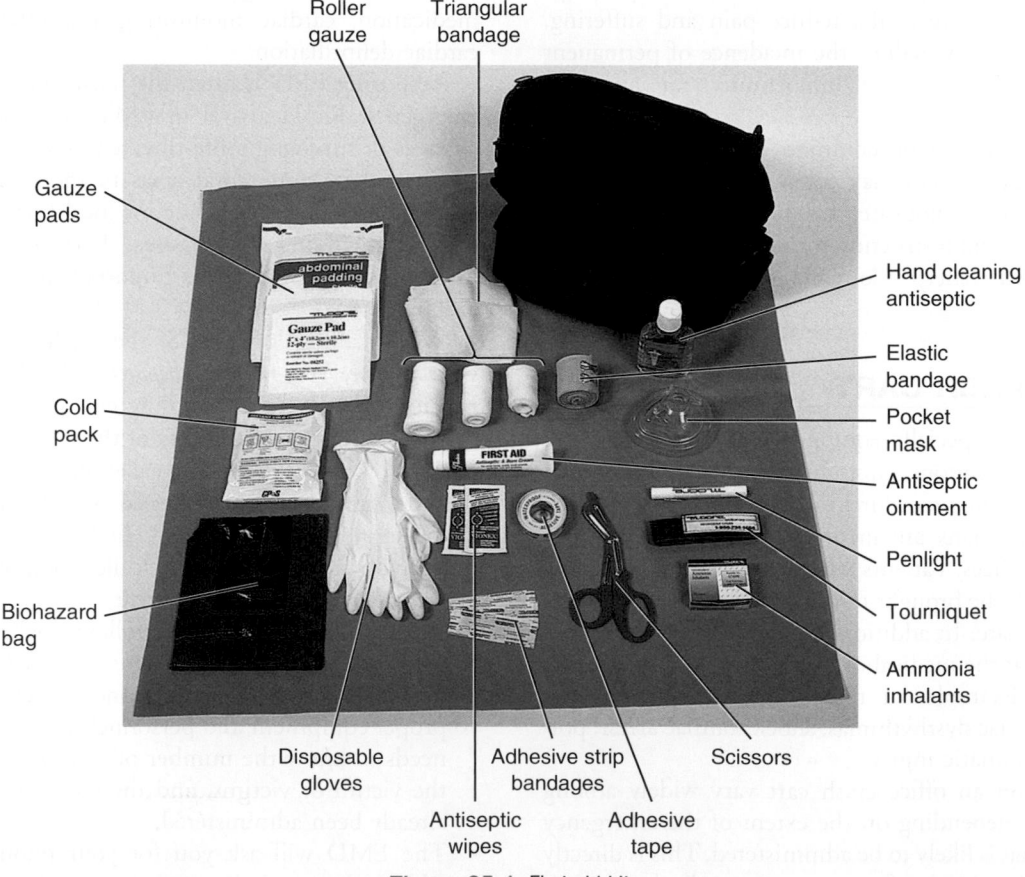

Figure 35-1 First aid kit.

5. Sanitize your hands as soon as possible after removing gloves.
6. Avoid touching objects that may be contaminated with blood or other potentially infectious materials.
7. If your hands or other skin surfaces come in contact with blood or other potentially infectious materials, wash the area as soon as possible with soap and water.
8. If your mucous membranes (in eyes, nose, and mouth) come in contact with blood or other potentially infectious materials, flush them with water as soon as possible.
9. Avoid eating, drinking, and touching your mouth, eyes, and nose while providing emergency care or before you sanitize your hands.
10. If you are exposed to blood or other potentially infectious materials, report the incident as soon as possible to your physician so that postexposure procedures can be instituted.

GUIDELINES FOR PROVIDING EMERGENCY CARE

The remainder of this chapter presents specific emergency situations that may be encountered by the medical assistant and the emergency care required for each. These guidelines should be followed when providing emergency care:

1. Remain calm, and speak in a normal tone of voice. These measures help calm and reassure the patient.
2. Make sure that the scene is safe before approaching the patient. It is important that you protect yourself from harm in an emergency situation.
3. Before administering emergency care to a conscious patient, you must first have permission or consent. To obtain consent, you must inform the patient who you are, your level of training, and what you are going to do to help. *Never* administer care to a conscious patient who refuses it. When a life-threatening condition exists, and the patient is unconscious or otherwise unable to give consent, consent is assumed or implied. Under law, it is implied that if the patient could give consent to care, he or she would.
4. Follow the OSHA standards when providing emergency care to reduce or eliminate exposure to bloodborne pathogens or other potentially infectious materials.
5. Know how to activate your local EMS system. Activating the EMS is often the most important step you can take to help a patient who has experienced an injury or sudden illness.
6. Do not move the patient unnecessarily. Unnecessary movement can result in further injury or can be life-threatening to a patient with a serious condition.
7. Obtain information as to what happened from the patient, family members, co-workers, or bystanders.
8. Look for a medical alert tag on the patient's wrist or neck. A medical alert tag provides information on a medical condition the patient may have.

9. Continue caring for the patient until more highly trained personnel arrive. On the arrival of emergency medical personnel or a physician, relay the condition in which you found the patient and the emergency care that has been administered.

Highlight on Good Samaritan Laws

In most states, Good Samaritan laws have been enacted to provide immunity to individuals, such as the medical assistant who administers first aid at the scene of an emergency. These laws were enacted to encourage individuals to help others in an emergency. They assume that an individual would do her or his best to save a life or prevent further injury.

The legal immunity provided by Good Samaritan laws protects an individual from being sued and found financially responsible for a patient's injury. The individual is immune from liability (except for "gross negligence") if he or she acts in good faith and uses a reasonable level of skill that does not exceed the scope of the individual's training.

Good Samaritan laws do not mean that an individual cannot be sued for administering first aid. An individual is not protected from liability if he or she is grossly careless or reckless in handling the situation. Because the components of Good Samaritan laws vary from state to state, the medical assistant must become familiar with the laws that govern his or her state. ■

Respiratory Distress

Respiratory distress indicates that the patient is breathing but is having great difficulty in doing so. Respiratory distress sometimes may lead to respiratory arrest. It is important that the medical assistant be alert for the signs and symptoms of respiratory distress, which may include noisy breathing, such as gasping for air or rasping, gurgling, or whistling sounds; breathing that is unusually fast or slow; and breathing that is painful. The general care for respiratory distress is to place the patient in a comfortable position that facilitates breathing. Most patients prefer a sitting or semireclining position. Remain calm, and reassure the patient to help reduce anxiety. Calming the patient may help the patient breathe easier. If the patient's condition worsens or does not resolve within a few minutes, activate the local EMS. Examples of conditions that frequently cause respiratory distress are described next.

Asthma
Asthma is a condition characterized by wheezing, coughing, and dyspnea. During an asthmatic attack, the bronchioles constrict and become clogged with mucus, which accounts for many of the symptoms of asthma.

Asthma may occur at any age, but it is more common in children and young adults. If the condition is not treated, it can lead to serious complications, such as permanent lung damage. It is frequently, but not always, associated with a family history of allergies. Any of the common allergens, such as house dust, pollens, molds, or animal danders, may trigger an asthmatic attack. Asthmatic attacks also may be caused by nonspecific factors, such as air pollutants, tobacco smoke, chemical fumes, vigorous exercise, respiratory infections, exposure to cold, and emotional stress. Normally, an individual with asthma easily controls attacks with medications. These medications stop the muscle spasms and open the airway, making breathing easier.

Some patients may develop a severe prolonged asthmatic attack that is life-threatening, which is known as *status asthmaticus*. These patients can move only a small amount of air. Because so little air is being moved, the typical breathing sounds associated with asthma may not be audible. The patient may have a bluish discoloration of the skin and extremely labored breathing. Status asthmaticus is a true emergency and requires immediate transportation of the patient to an emergency care facility by the fastest way possible.

Emphysema

Emphysema is a progressive lung disorder in which the terminal bronchioles that lead into the alveoli become plugged with mucus. Because of this problem, the alveoli become damaged, resulting in less surface area to diffuse oxygen into the blood. Eventually, this condition results in loss of elasticity of the alveoli, causing inhaled air to become trapped in the lungs. This makes breathing difficult, particularly during exhalation.

Emphysema usually develops over many years and is found most frequently in heavy smokers. It also occurs in patients with chronic bronchitis and in elderly patients whose lungs have lost their natural elasticity. Chronic emphysema is one of the major causes of death in the United States. As the lungs progressively become less efficient, breathing becomes more and more difficult. Patients with advanced cases may go into respiratory or cardiac arrest.

Hyperventilation

Hyperventilation literally means "overbreathing." Hyperventilation is a manner of breathing in which the respirations become rapid and deep, causing an individual to exhale too much carbon dioxide. Low carbon dioxide levels in the body account for many of the symptoms of hyperventilation. Hyperventilation is often the result of fear or anxiety and is more likely to occur in individuals who are tense and nervous. It also is caused by serious organic conditions, such as diabetic coma, pneumonia, pulmonary edema, pulmonary embolism, head injury, high fever, and aspirin poisoning.

In addition to rapid and deep respirations, the signs and symptoms of hyperventilation include dizziness, faintness, and light-headedness; visual disturbances; chest pain; tachycardia; palpitations; fullness in the throat; and numbness and tingling of the fingers, toes, and the area around the mouth. Despite their rapid breathing efforts, patients complain that they cannot get enough air. They often think they are having a heart attack.

Treatment for hyperventilation caused by emotional factors is as follows: Calm and reassure the patient, and encourage him or her to slow the respirations, allowing the carbon dioxide level to return to normal. In the past, breathing into a paper bag was advocated as a remedy for hyperventilation. More recent studies no longer recommend this practice because it could be harmful if an underlying medical condition exists, or if the patient is not actually hyperventilating. If the medical assistant suspects that hyperventilation has been caused by an organic problem, EMS should be activated immediately.

Heart Attack

A heart attack, also known as a *myocardial infarction* (MI), is caused by partial or complete obstruction of one or both of the coronary arteries or their branches. In most cases, the severity of the attack depends on the size of the obstructed artery and the amount of myocardial tissue nourished by that artery. If a small branch of a coronary artery is obstructed, myocardial damage and symptoms may be mild, whereas the damage is usually extensive and the symptoms intense if a coronary artery is completely blocked.

The principal symptom of a heart attack is chest pain or discomfort. Patients describe the chest pain as squeezing or crushing pressure, severe indigestion or burning, heaviness, or aching. Chest discomfort can range in severity from feeling only mildly uncomfortable to being intense and accompanied by a feeling of suffocation and doom. The pain is usually felt behind the sternum and may radiate to the neck, throat, or jaw, or to both shoulders and both arms. The pain associated with a heart attack is prolonged and usually is not relieved by resting or taking nitroglycerin. Other signs and symptoms of a heart attack include shortness of breath, profuse perspiration, nausea, and fainting.

If the medical assistant suspects that the patient is having a heart attack, EMS should be activated immediately. Meanwhile, loosen tight clothing and have the patient rest in a comfortable position that facilitates breathing. If cardiac arrest occurs, the medical assistant should begin CPR immediately.

Stroke

A stroke, also called a *cerebrovascular accident* (CVA), results when an artery to the brain is blocked or ruptures, causing an interruption of blood flow to the brain. The signs and symptoms of a stroke include sudden weakness or numbness of the face, arm, or leg on one side of the body; difficulty in speaking; dimmed vision or loss of vision in one eye; double vision; dizziness; confusion; severe headache; and loss of consciousness.

If the medical assistant suspects that the patient is having a stroke, EMS should be activated immediately. Meanwhile, loosen tight clothing and have the patient rest in a comfortable position. If respiratory arrest, cardiac arrest, or both occur, begin rescue breathing cardiopulmonary resuscitation (CPR) as required.

Shock

For the body to function properly, adequate blood flow must be maintained to all of the vital organs. This is accomplished by the three important cardiovascular functions, as follows:

- Adequate pumping action of the heart
- Sufficient blood circulating in the blood vessels
- Blood vessels being able to respond to blood flow

When an individual experiences a severe injury or illness, one or more of these cardiovascular functions may be affected, which can lead to shock.

Shock is defined as the failure of the cardiovascular system to deliver enough blood to all of the body's vital organs. Shock accompanies different types of emergency situations, such as hemorrhaging, a myocardial infarction, and severe allergic reaction. The five major types of shock are categorized according to cause: hypovolemic, cardiogenic, neurogenic, anaphylactic, and psychogenic. Each type of shock is described in this section. If not treated, most types of shock become life-threatening. This is because shock is progressive—when it reaches a certain point, it becomes irreversible, and the patient's life cannot be saved.

The signs and symptoms of shock are caused by the failure of the vital organs to receive enough oxygen and nutrients. The organs most affected are the heart, brain, and lungs, which can be irreparably damaged in 4 to 6 minutes. The general signs and symptoms of shock are weakness, restlessness, anxiety, disorientation, pallor, cold and clammy skin, rapid breathing, and rapid pulse.

If not treated, these symptoms can progress rapidly to a significant drop in blood pressure, cyanosis, loss of consciousness, and death. The signs and symptoms of shock may be subtle or pronounced. In addition, no single sign or symptom determines accurately the presence or severity of the shock. Because of this, it is crucial to consider the nature of the illness or injury in determining whether the patient is a possible victim of shock. If a patient has a traumatic injury to the abdomen, shock should be considered a possibility, even if the patient's signs and symptoms do not suggest shock.

Shock (with the exception of psychogenic shock) requires immediate medical care. The medical assistant should activate EMS without delay so that proper medical care can be obtained as soon as possible.

Hypovolemic Shock

Hypovolemic shock is caused by loss of blood or other body fluids. Conditions that result in this type of shock include external and internal hemorrhaging; plasma loss from severe burns; and severe dehydration from vomiting, diarrhea, or profuse perspiration. The first priority in hypovolemic shock is to control bleeding. A patient in hypovolemic shock must have the volume of fluid that was lost replaced and must be transported to an emergency care facility immediately.

Cardiogenic Shock

Cardiogenic shock is caused by the failure of the heart to pump blood adequately to all of the body's vital organs. This type of shock occurs when the heart has been injured or damaged. Cardiogenic shock is most frequently seen with myocardial infarction. Other causes include dysrhythmias, severe congestive heart failure, acute valvular damage, and pulmonary embolism. When a patient develops cardiogenic shock, it is difficult to reverse and has a high fatality rate (80% to 90%).

Neurogenic Shock

Neurogenic shock occurs when the nervous system is unable to control the diameter of the blood vessels. In normal situations, the nervous system instructs the blood vessels to constrict or dilate, which controls blood pressure. In neurogenic shock, that control is lost, and the blood vessels dilate, causing the blood to pool in peripheral areas of the body away from vital organs.

This type of shock is most often seen with brain and spinal injuries. The blood vessels become dilated, and not enough blood is present in the circulatory system to fill the dilated vessels, which causes the blood pressure to drop significantly.

Anaphylactic Shock

Anaphylactic shock is a life-threatening reaction of the body to a substance to which an individual is highly allergic. Allergens that are most apt to result in anaphylaxis are drugs (e.g., penicillin), insect venoms, foods, and allergen extracts used in hyposensitization injections.

An anaphylactic reaction causes the release of large amounts of histamine, resulting in dilation of the blood vessels throughout the entire body and a decrease in blood pressure. The symptoms of anaphylactic shock begin with sneezing, hives, itching, angioedema, erythema, and disorientation and progress to difficulty in breathing, dizziness, fainting, and loss of consciousness. Medical care should be obtained immediately because most fatalities occur within the first 2 hours.

The emergency care for anaphylactic shock is the administration of epinephrine. Because time is a factor, individuals known to have a severe allergy carry an anaphylactic emergency treatment kit that contains injectable epinephrine (Figure 35-2) and oral antihistamines. With the kit, treatment for a severe allergic reaction can be started immediately.

Psychogenic Shock

Psychogenic shock is the least serious type of shock. It is caused by unpleasant physical or emotional stimuli, such as pain, fright, and the sight of blood. With psychogenic shock, sudden dilation of the blood vessels causes blood to pool in the abdomen and extremities. This temporarily deprives the brain of blood, causing a temporary loss of consciousness (fainting), usually lasting 1 to 2 minutes. Fainting generally occurs when an individual is in an upright

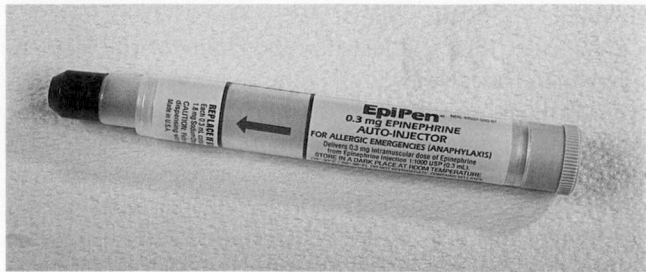

Figure 35-2 Anaphylactic emergency epinephrine injector.

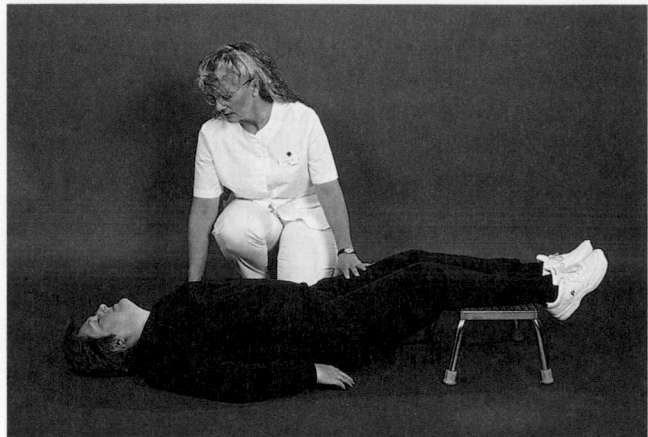

Figure 35-3 Prevention and treatment of fainting.

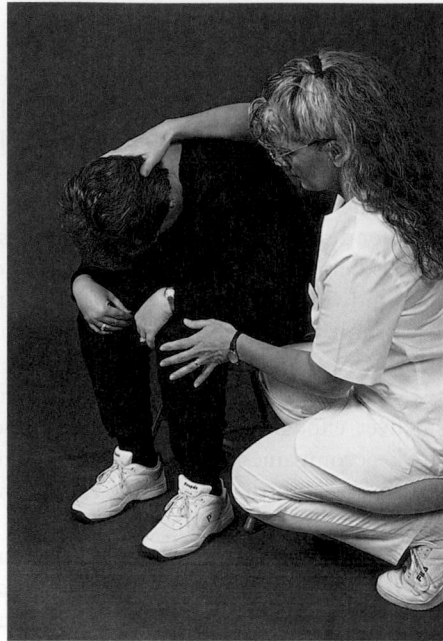

Figure 35-4 Prevention of fainting.

position. Before fainting, the patient usually experiences some warning signals such as sudden light-headedness, pallor, nausea, weakness, yawning, blurred vision, a feeling of warmth, and sweating.

An individual who is about to faint should be placed in a position that facilitates blood flow to the brain and told to breathe deeply. The preferred position is to move the patient into a supine position with the legs elevated approximately 12 inches and the collar and clothing loosened (Figure 35-3). This position is not always possible, such as when a patient is seated; in this case, the patient's head should be lowered between the legs (Figure 35-4). A patient who has fainted should be placed in the supine position with the legs elevated. It is recommended that a patient who has fainted should contact her or his physician for further evaluation.

Bleeding

Bleeding, or hemorrhaging, is the escape of blood from a severed blood vessel. Bleeding can range from very minor to very serious, leading to shock and death. The amount of blood that can be lost before bleeding becomes life-threatening varies according to each individual. In general, loss of 25% to 40% of an individual's total blood volume can be fatal. This equates to approximately 2 to 4 pints of blood for the average adult.

External Bleeding

External bleeding is bleeding that can be seen coming from a wound. Common examples of external bleeding include bleeding from open fractures, lacerations, and the nose. Individuals with serious external bleeding exhibit the following symptoms: obvious bleeding, restlessness, cold and clammy skin, thirst, increased and thready pulse, rapid and shallow respirations, a drop in blood pressure (a late symptom), and decreasing levels of consciousness. Three types of external bleeding can be classified according to the type of blood vessel that has been injured: capillary, venous, and arterial.

Capillary Bleeding

Capillary bleeding, the most common type of external bleeding, consists of a slow oozing of bright red blood. This type of bleeding occurs with minor cuts, scratches, and abrasions.

Venous Bleeding

Venous bleeding occurs when a vein has been punctured or severed. This type of bleeding is characterized by a slow and steady flow of dark red blood.

Arterial Bleeding

Arterial bleeding, the most serious type of external bleeding, occurs when an artery is punctured or severed. It is the least common type of bleeding because arteries are situated deeper in the body and are protected by bone. Arterial bleeding is characterized by bright red blood that spurts. The arteries most frequently involved in accidents are the carotid, brachial, radial, and femoral arteries.

Emergency Care for External Bleeding
The most effective way to control bleeding is to apply direct pressure to the bleeding site. The pressure functions by slowing down or stopping the flow of blood. The amount of pressure required depends on the type of bleeding.

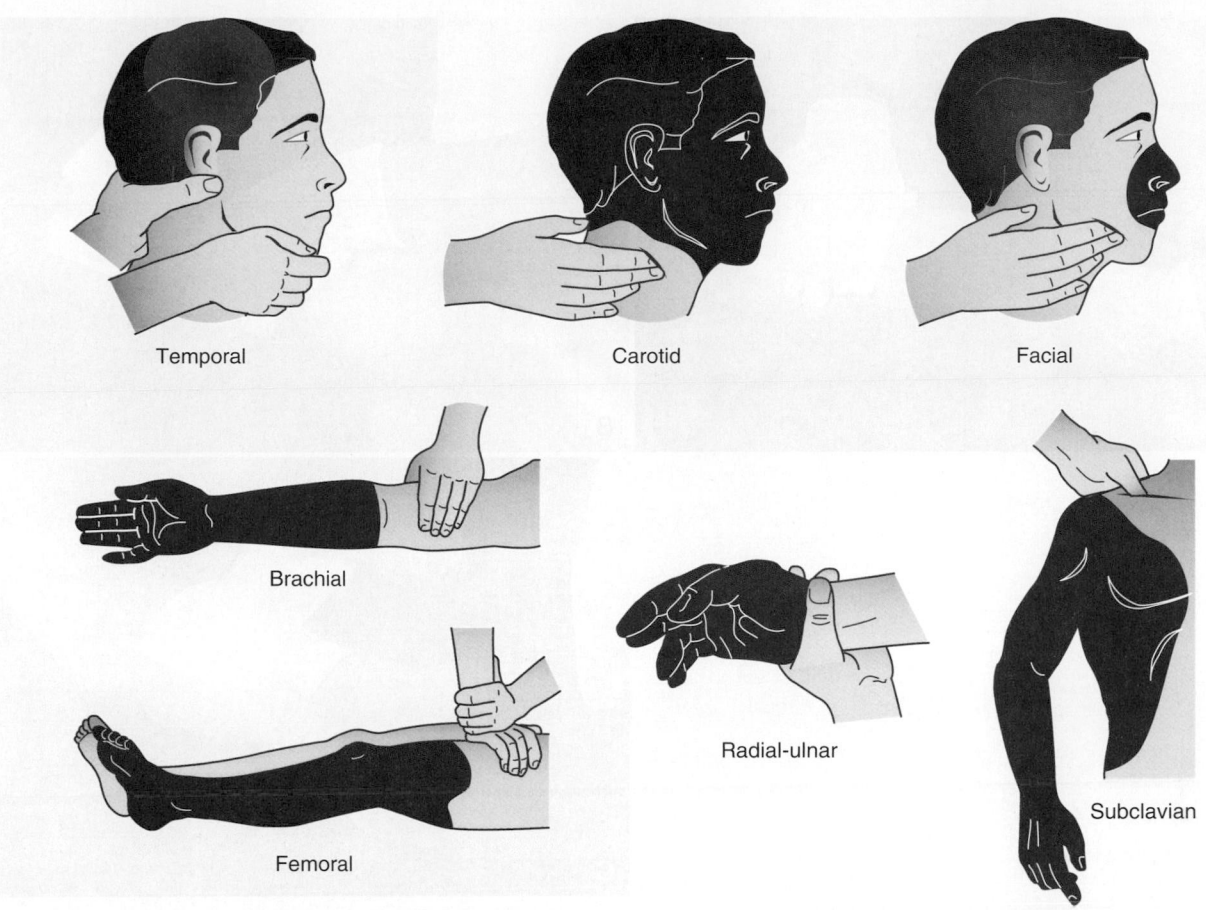

Figure 35-5 Locations of pressure points. Shaded areas show the regions in which bleeding may be controlled by pressure at the points indicated.

A small amount of pressure is usually sufficient to control capillary bleeding, whereas significant pressure is often required to control arterial bleeding.

If bleeding cannot be controlled with direct pressure, a pressure point can be used. A **pressure point** is a site on the body where an artery lies close to the surface of the skin and can be compressed against an underlying bone. Figure 35-5 illustrates pressure points. Using a pressure point helps slow or stop the flow of blood from the wound. The pressure points used most often are found on the brachial and femoral arteries. The brachial artery is located on the inside of the upper arm midway between the elbow and the shoulder. Squeezing the brachial artery helps control severe bleeding in the arm. The femoral artery is located in the groin, and squeezing helps control severe bleeding in the leg.

The specific steps for controlling bleeding are as follows:

1. Apply direct pressure to the wound with a clean covering such as a large, thick gauze dressing (Figure 35-6, *A*). If gauze is unavailable, a clean material such as a sanitary napkin, washcloth, handkerchief, or sock can be used. If the wound is located on an extremity, elevate the limb while continuing to apply direct pressure.
2. Apply additional dressings if needed. If the dressing soaks through, apply another dressing over the first one, and continue to apply pressure (Figure 35-6, *B*).

(Never remove a dressing after it has been applied because this could result in more bleeding.) If bleeding cannot be controlled with direct pressure, apply pressure to the appropriate pressure point while continuing to apply direct local pressure.

3. Apply a pressure bandage. When bleeding has been controlled, apply a bandage snugly over the dressing to maintain pressure on the wound (Figure 35-6, *C*).
4. Transport the patient to an emergency care facility, or, if the case is serious enough, activate the local emergency medical services.

Nosebleeds

A nosebleed, or epistaxis, is a common form of external bleeding that usually is not serious but is more of a nuisance. Nosebleeds are usually caused by an upper respiratory infection but can result from a direct blow from a blunt object, hypertension, strenuous activity, and exposure to high altitudes.

Emergency Care for a Nosebleed

1. Position the patient in a sitting position with the head tilted forward. This prevents the blood from running down the back of the throat, which may result in nausea.
2. Apply direct pressure by pinching the nostrils together (Figure 35-7, *A*). Do not release the pressure too soon because the bleeding may resume. Adequate clot

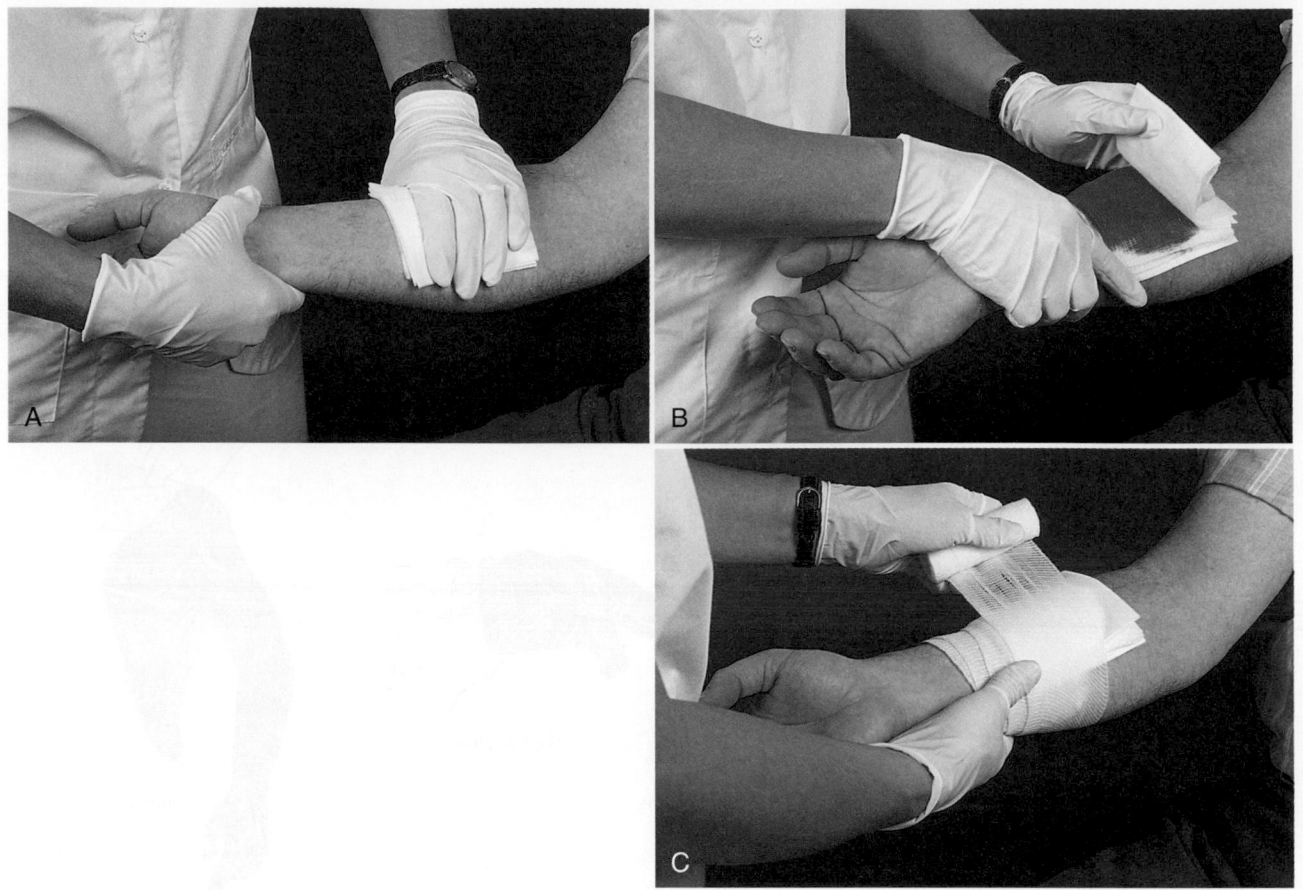

Figure 35-6 Control of bleeding. **A,** Apply direct pressure to the wound with a large, thick gauze dressing. **B,** If blood soaks through the dressing, apply another dressing over the first one, and continue to apply pressure. **C,** When bleeding has been controlled, apply a pressure bandage.

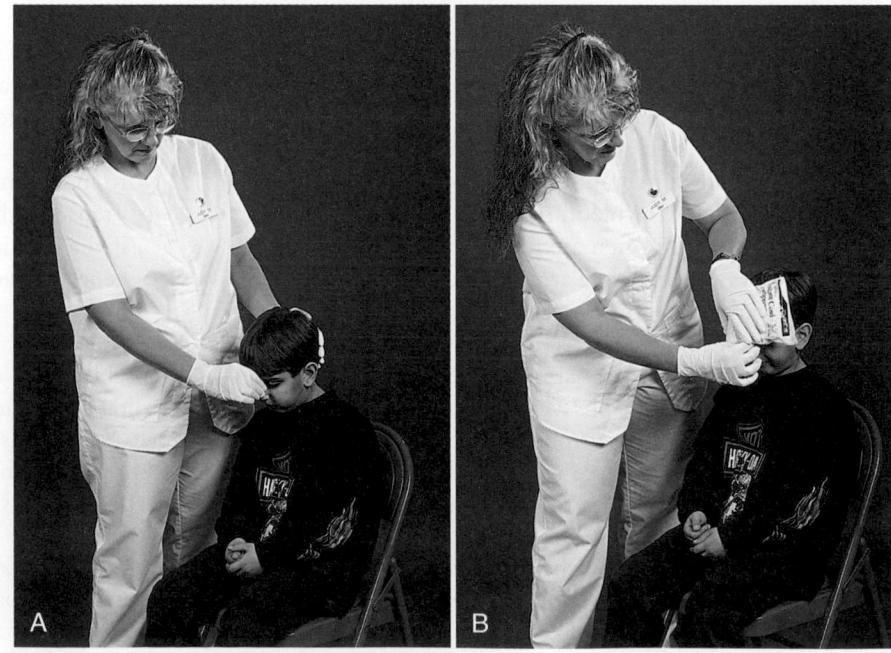

Figure 35-7 Care of a nosebleed. **A,** Apply direct pressure by pinching the nostrils together. **B,** An ice pack can be applied to the bridge of the nose to help control the bleeding.

formation usually takes about 15 minutes. An ice pack can be applied to the bridge of the nose to help control the bleeding (Figure 35-7, *B*). If these measures do not control the bleeding, apply pressure on the upper lip, just below the nose.

3. After the bleeding has stopped, tell the patient not to blow the nose for several hours because this could loosen the clot, causing the bleeding to start again.

4. If bleeding cannot be controlled, transport the patient to an emergency care facility for further treatment.

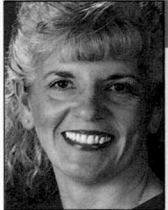

Putting It All into Practice

My name is Judy Markins, and I work at a large clinic in the family medicine department with 12 physicians. We also have 6 to 10 physicians who do their internships and residency programs with us.

One day as I was performing my usual morning duties of getting the office ready for that day's patients, the office door opened. There stood a mother with her very ill child. I immediately took them back to a room. When I took the boy's temperature, it was 104° F. I asked the mother if she had been giving him any type of fever reducer. She said she had, but that it was not helping. Under the direction of our physician, I immediately started trying to reduce the fever. The fever started to come down, and the look of relief on the mother's face was beyond words. That was one of the many days that reinforced how satisfied I am with my career choice. ■

Internal Bleeding

Internal bleeding is bleeding that flows into a body cavity or an organ, or between tissues. It may be minor, as in the case of a contusion, or it may be very serious, such as with a severe, blunt blow to the abdomen.

Severe internal bleeding is a life-threatening emergency. Because no obvious blood flow occurs, the nature of the injury and the signs and symptoms of bleeding must be used to recognize internal bleeding. Signs and symptoms include bruises, pain, tenderness, or swelling at the site of the injury; rapid weak pulse; cold, clammy skin; nausea and vomiting; excessive thirst; a drop in blood pressure; and a decreased level of consciousness.

If a patient is suspected to have internal bleeding, the local EMS should be activated immediately. Until emergency medical personnel arrive, the patient should be kept quiet and treated for shock.

Wounds

A **wound** is a break in the continuity of an external or internal surface, caused by physical means. Wounds may be open or closed.

Open Wounds

An open wound is a break in the skin surface or mucous membrane that exposes the underlying tissues. Because the skin is broken, hemorrhaging and wound contamination are primary concerns with open wounds. Open wounds include incisions, lacerations, punctures, and abrasions (Figure 35-8). An individual with an open wound should

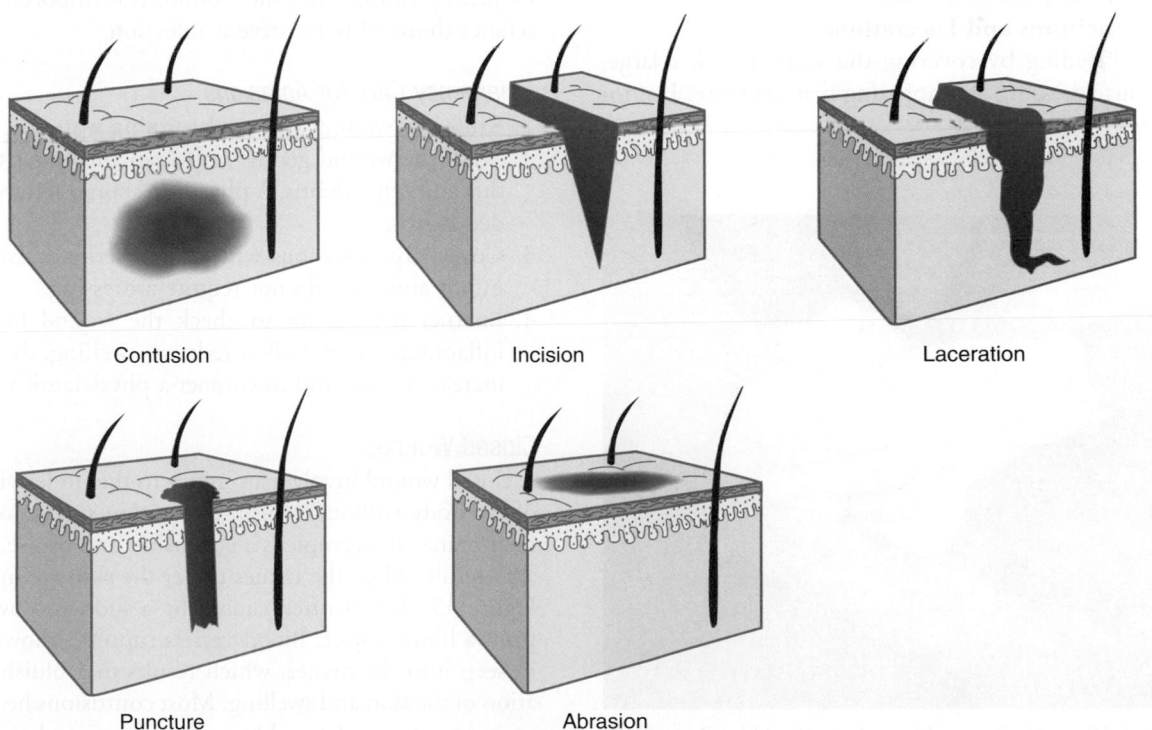

Contusion   Incision   Laceration

Puncture   Abrasion

Figure 35-8 Types of wounds.

receive prompt medical attention by a physician if any of the following occur: spurting blood; bleeding that cannot be controlled; a break in the skin that is deeper than just the outer skin layers; embedded debris or an embedded object in the wound; involvement of nerves, muscles, or tendons; and occurrence on the mouth, tongue, face, genitals, or other area where scarring would be apparent.

Incisions and Lacerations

An incision is a clean, smooth cut caused by a sharp cutting instrument, such as a knife, a razor, or a piece of glass. Deep incisions are accompanied by profuse bleeding; in addition, damage to muscles, tendons, and nerves may occur. Because the edges of the wound are smooth and straight, incisions usually heal better than lacerations.

A laceration is a wound in which the tissues are torn apart, rather than cut, leaving ragged and irregular edges. Lacerations are caused by dull knives, large objects that have been driven into the skin, and heavy machinery. Deep lacerations result in profuse bleeding, and a scar often results from jagged tearing of the tissues.

Emergency Care for Incisions and Lacerations

Minor Incisions and Lacerations
1. Assess the length, depth, and location of the wound.
2. Control bleeding by covering the wound with a dressing and applying firm pressure.
3. Clean the wound with soap and water to remove dirt and other debris (Figure 35-9).
4. Cover the wound with a dry, sterile dressing. Instruct the patient to check the wound for redness, swelling, discharge, or an increase in pain, and to contact a physician if any of these problems occur.

Serious Incisions and Lacerations
1. Control bleeding by covering the wound with a large, thick gauze dressing and applying firm pressure. Do not

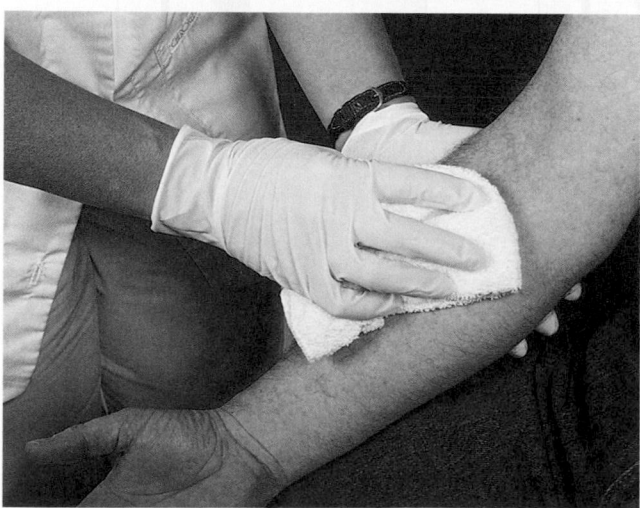

Figure 35-9 Minor incisions and lacerations should be cleaned with soap and water to remove dirt and other debris.

clean or probe the wound because this may result in more bleeding.
2. Transport the individual to a physician, or, if the wound is serious enough, activate the local EMS.

Punctures

A puncture is a wound made by a sharp, pointed object piercing the skin layers and sometimes the underlying structures. Objects that cause a puncture wound include a nail, splinter, needle, wire, knife, bullet, and animal bite. A puncture wound has a very small external skin opening, and for this reason bleeding is usually minor. A tetanus booster may be administered because the tetanus bacteria grow best in a warm, anaerobic environment, as would be found in a puncture wound.

Emergency Care for Puncture Wounds
1. Allow the wound to bleed freely for a few minutes to help wash out bacteria.
2. Clean the wound with soap and water.
3. Apply a dry, sterile dressing to prevent contamination.
4. Transport the individual to a physician so that medical care can be provided to prevent infection and to ensure that the patient's tetanus toxoid immunization is up to date.

Abrasions

An abrasion, or scrape, is a wound in which the outer layers of the skin are scraped or rubbed off. Blood may ooze from ruptured capillaries; however, the bleeding usually is not severe. Abrasions are caused by falls, resulting in floor burns and skinned knees and elbows. Dirt and other debris are frequently rubbed into the wound; it is important to clean scrapes thoroughly to prevent infection.

Emergency Care for Abrasions
1. Rinse the wound with cold running water.
2. Wash the wound gently with soap and water to remove dirt and other debris. A physician should remove embedded debris.
3. Cover large abrasions with a dry, sterile dressing. Small minor abrasions do not require a dressing.
4. Instruct the patient to check the wound for signs of inflammation, including redness, swelling, discharge, or increased pain, and to contact a physician if they occur.

Closed Wounds

A closed wound involves an injury to the underlying tissues of the body without a break in the skin surface or mucous membrane; an example is a contusion or a bruise. A contusion results when the tissues under the skin are injured (see Figure 35-8); it is often caused by a sudden blow or force from a blunt object. Blood vessels rupture, allowing blood to seep into the tissues, which results in a bluish discoloration of the skin and swelling. Most contusions heal without special treatment, but cold compresses may reduce bleeding, reduce swelling and discoloration, and relieve pain. After several days, the color of the contusion turns greenish or yellow, owing to oxidation of blood pigments. Contusions commonly occur with injuries such as fractures, sprains, strains, and black eyes. These injuries, along with the corresponding emergency care, are discussed next.

Musculoskeletal Injuries

The musculoskeletal system comprises all of the bones, muscles, tendons, and ligaments of the body. Injuries that affect the musculoskeletal system include fractures, dislocations, sprains, and strains.

Fracture

A **fracture** is any break in a bone. The break may range in severity from a simple chip or a crack to a complete break or shattering of the bone. Fractures can occur anywhere on the surface of the bone, including across the surface of a joint such as the wrist or ankle. Fractures result from a direct blow, a fall, bone disease, or a twisting force as may occur in a sports injury. Although fractures often cause severe pain, they are seldom life-threatening.

The two basic types of fracture are closed fractures and open fractures (Figure 35-10). A *closed fracture,* the most common type, occurs when there is a break in a bone but no break in the skin over the fracture site. An *open fracture* involves a break in the bone along with penetration of the overlying skin surface. Open fractures are more serious owing to the risk of blood loss and contamination leading to infection.

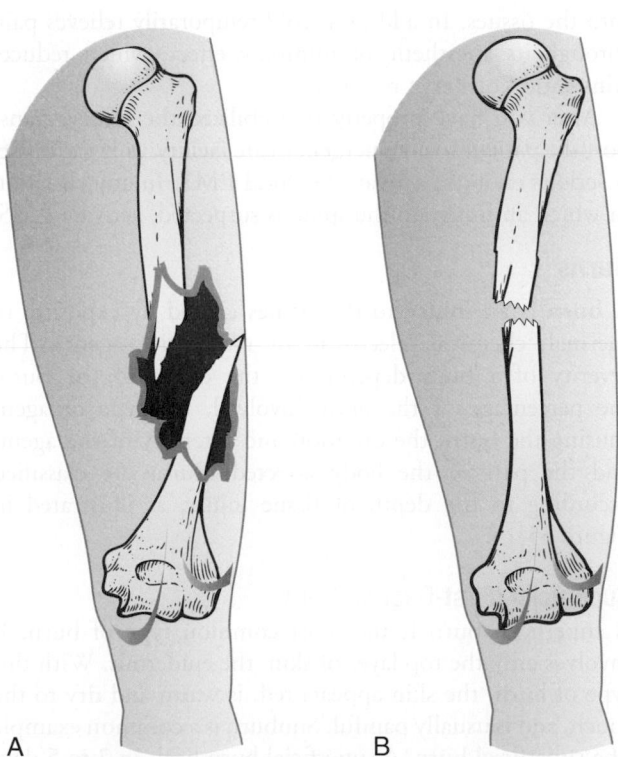

Figure 35-10 Fractures. **A,** Open fracture. **B,** Closed fracture.

The signs and symptoms of a fracture include pain and tenderness, deformity, swelling and discoloration, loss of function of the body part, and numbness or tingling. The patient usually guards the injured part and may relay to you that he or she heard the bone break or snap or felt a grating sensation. This grating sensation, known as **crepitus,** is caused by the bone fragments rubbing against each other.

Fractures also can be classified according to the nature of the break: impacted, greenstick, transverse, oblique, comminuted, and spiral. Figure 35-11 illustrates and describes these types of fracture.

Dislocation

A **dislocation** is an injury in which one end of a bone making up a joint is separated or displaced from its normal position. A dislocation is caused by a violent pulling or pushing force that tears the ligaments. Dislocations usually result from falls, sports injuries, and motor vehicle accidents. Signs and symptoms of a dislocation include significant deformity of the joint, pain and swelling, and loss of function.

Sprain

A **sprain** is the tearing of ligaments at a joint. Sprains may result from a fall, a sports injury, or a motor vehicle accident. The joints most often sprained are the ankle, knee, wrist, and fingers. Signs and symptoms of a sprain include pain, swelling, and discoloration. Sprains can vary in seriousness from mild to severe, depending on the amount of damage to the ligaments.

Strain

A **strain** is the stretching and tearing of muscles or tendons. Strains are most likely to occur when an individual lifts a heavy object or overworks a muscle, as during exercise. The muscles most commonly strained are those of the neck, back, thigh, and calf. Signs and symptoms of a strain are pain and swelling. Strains do not usually cause the intense symptoms associated with fractures, dislocations, and sprains.

Emergency Care for a Fracture

It is often difficult to determine whether a patient has a fracture, a dislocation, or a sprain because the symptoms of these injuries are similar. Because of this, any serious musculoskeletal injury to an extremity should be treated as though it were a fracture.

The primary goal of emergency care for a fracture is to immobilize the body part. Immobilization reduces pain and prevents further damage. A **splint** is any item that immobilizes a body part. In an emergency situation, items such as a length of wood, cardboard, or rolled newspapers or magazines can be used for splinting. The splint should be padded with a soft material such as a rolled-up towel.

The body part should be splinted in the position in which you found it. Severely angulated fractures may have to be straightened before splinting, however. If you attempt

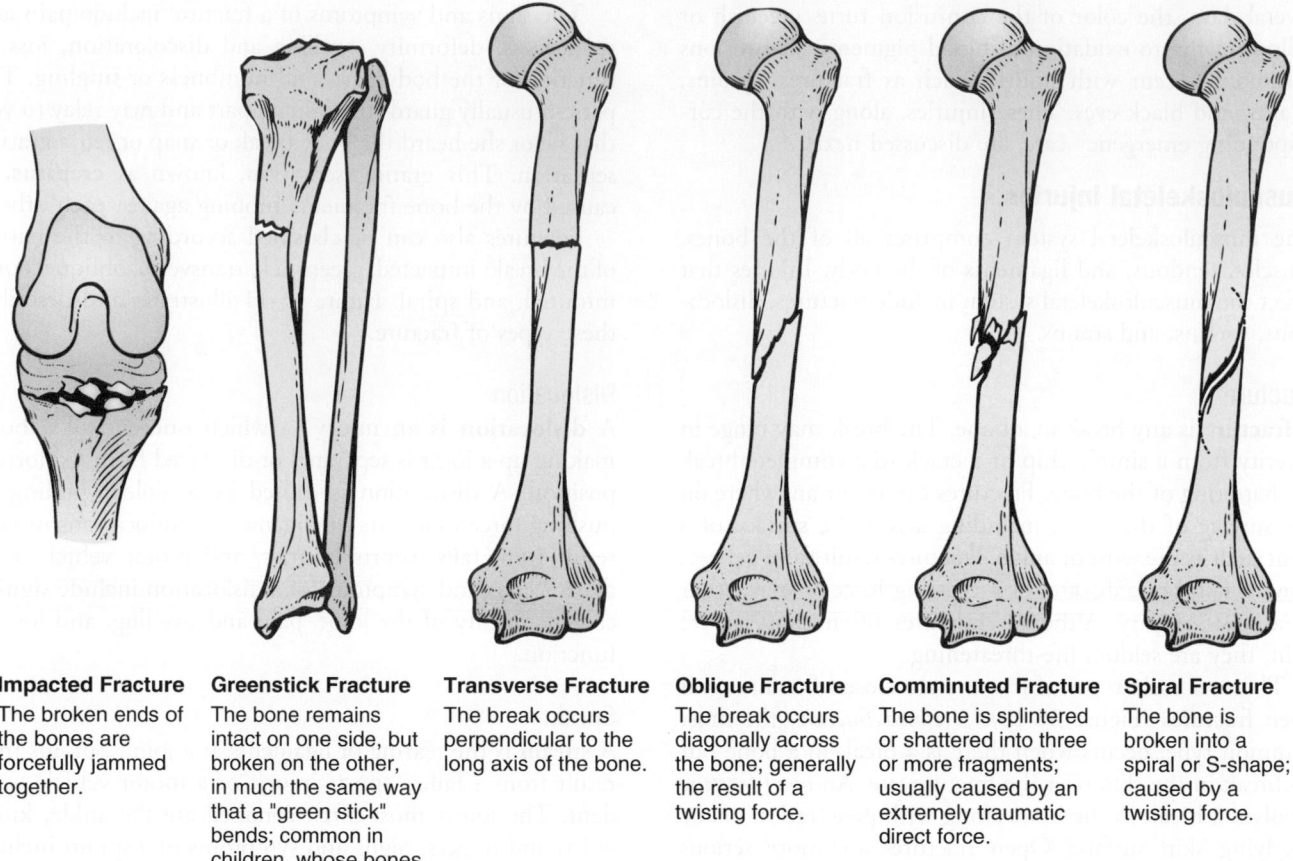

Impacted Fracture	**Greenstick Fracture**	**Transverse Fracture**	**Oblique Fracture**	**Comminuted Fracture**	**Spiral Fracture**
The broken ends of the bones are forcefully jammed together.	The bone remains intact on one side, but broken on the other, in much the same way that a "green stick" bends; common in children, whose bones are more flexible than those of adults.	The break occurs perpendicular to the long axis of the bone.	The break occurs diagonally across the bone; generally the result of a twisting force.	The bone is splintered or shattered into three or more fragments; usually caused by an extremely traumatic direct force.	The bone is broken into a spiral or S-shape; caused by a twisting force.

Figure 35-11 Types of fractures.

to straighten an angulated fracture, be careful not to force the affected part. A dislocated bone end can become "locked" and would have to be realigned at the hospital. If you straighten an angulated bone and encounter pain, stop and splint it in the position in which you found it. The splint also should immobilize the area above and below the injury. When splinting an injury to the wrist, the hand and forearm also should be immobilized (Figure 35-12, *A*). When splinting an injury to the shaft of the bone, the joints above and below the injury should be immobilized. When splinting the forearm, the elbow joint and the wrist joint should be immobilized.

The splint should be held in place with a roller gauze bandage or other suitable material, such as neckties, scarves, or strips of cloth (Figure 35-12, *B*). The splint should be applied snugly, but not so tightly that it interferes with proper circulation. After applying the splint, check the pulse below the splint to ensure the splint has not been applied too tightly. If you cannot detect a pulse, immediately loosen the splint until you can feel the pulse (Figure 35-12, *C*).

Whenever possible, elevate an injured extremity after it has been immobilized to reduce swelling (Figure 35-12, *D*). An ice pack also can be applied to the injured part. Cold limits the accumulation of fluid in the body tissues by constricting blood vessels and reducing leakage of fluid

into the tissues. In addition, cold temporarily relieves pain through its anesthetic or numbing effect, which reduces stimulation of nerve receptors.

After you have properly immobilized the injury, transport the patient to an emergency care facility, or if the injury is serious enough, activate the local EMS. In any situation in which an injury to the spine is suspected, activate EMS.

Burns

A **burn** is an injury to the tissues caused by exposure to thermal, chemical, electrical, or radioactive agents. The severity of a burn depends on the depth of the burn, the percentage of the body involved, the type of agent causing the burn, the duration and intensity of the agent, and the part of the body affected. Burns are classified according to the depth of tissue injury, as illustrated in Figure 35-13.

Superficial (First-Degree) Burn

A superficial burn is the most common type of burn. It involves only the top layer of skin, the epidermis. With this type of burn, the skin appears red, is warm and dry to the touch, and is usually painful. Sunburn is a common example of a superficial burn. A superficial burn heals in 2 to 5 days of its own accord and does not cause scarring.

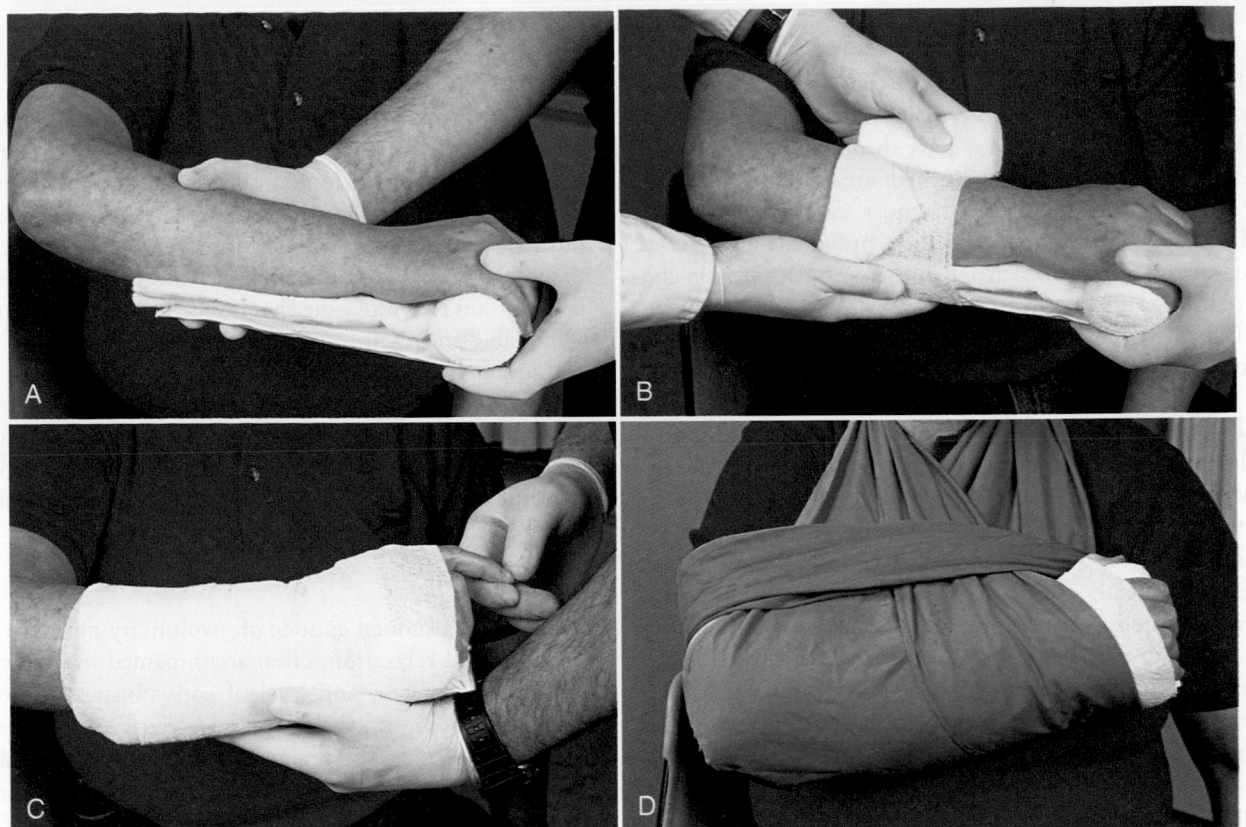

Figure 35-12 Emergency care of a fracture. **A,** The splint should immobilize the area above and below the injury. **B,** The splint is held in place with a roller gauze bandage. **C,** After the splint is applied, the pulse below the splint should be checked to ensure that the splint has not been applied too tightly. **D,** A sling can be used to elevate the extremity to reduce swelling.

		APPEARANCE	SENSATION	COURSE
EPIDERMIS Sweat duct Capillary	SUPERFICIAL BURN	Mild to severe erythema; skin blanches with pressure	Painful Hyperesthetic Tingling Pain eased by cooling	Discomfort lasts about 48 hours Desquamation (peeling) in 3-7 days
Sebaceous gland Nerve endings DERMIS Hair follicle	PARTIAL-THICKNESS BURN	Large, thick-walled blisters covering extensive area (vesiculation) Edema; mottled red base; broken epidermis; wet, shiny, weeping surface	Painful Sensitive to cold air	Superficial partial-thickness burn heals in 14-21 days Deep partial-thickness burn requires 21-28 days for healing Healing rate varies with burn depth and presence or absence of infection
Sweat gland Fat Blood vessels SUBCUTANEOUS TISSUE	FULL-THICKNESS BURN	Variable (e.g., deep red, black, white, brown) Dry surface Edema Fat exposed Tissue disrupted	Little pain Insensate	Full-thickness dead skin suppurates and liquefies after 2-3 weeks Spontaneous healing impossible Requires removal of eschar and subsequent split- or full-thickness skin grafting Hypertrophic scarring and wound contractures likely to develop without preventive measures

Figure 35-13 Types of burns.

Partial-Thickness (Second-Degree) Burn

A partial-thickness burn involves the epidermis and extends into the dermis but does not pass through the dermis to the underlying tissues. The burned area usually appears red, mottled, and blistered. In most cases, the blisters should not be broken because they provide a protective barrier against infection. Partial-thickness burns are usually very painful, and the area often swells. This type of burn usually heals within 3 to 4 weeks and may result in some scarring.

Full-Thickness (Third-Degree) Burn

A full-thickness burn completely destroys the epidermis and the dermis and extends into the underlying tissues, such as fat, muscle, bone, and nerves. The affected area appears charred black, brown, and cherry red, with the damaged tissues underneath often pearly white. The patient may experience intense pain; however, if damage to the nerve endings is substantial, the patient may feel no pain at all. During the healing process, dense scars typically result. Infection is a major concern, and the patient must be carefully monitored.

Thermal Burns

Thermal burns usually occur in the home, often as a result of fire, scalding water, or coming into contact with a hot object such as a stove or curling iron.

Emergency Care for Major Thermal Burns

1. Stop the burning process to prevent further injury. If the individual is on fire, wrap him or her in a blanket, rug, or heavy coat and push him or her to the ground to help smother the flames. If a covering is unavailable, shout at the individual to drop to the ground and roll around to smother the flames.
2. Cool the burn, using large amounts of cool water from a faucet or garden hose. Do not use ice or ice water because this may result in further tissue damage; it also causes heat loss from the body. If the burn covers a large surface area (greater than 20%), do not use water. The loss of a large amount of skin surface places the patient at risk for hypothermia (generalized body cooling). With large surface area burns, you may cool the most painful areas, but not an area greater than 20% of the body (i.e., two arms, one leg).
3. Activate the local EMS.
4. Cover the patient with a clean, nonfuzzy material such as a tablecloth or sheet. The cover maintains warmth, reduces pain, and reduces the risk of contamination. Do not apply any type of ointment, antiseptic, or other substance to the burned area.

Emergency Care for Minor Thermal Burns

1. Immerse the affected area in cold water for 2 to 5 minutes. Be careful not to break any blisters because they provide a protective barrier against infection.
2. Cover the burn with a dry sterile dressing.

Chemical Burns

Chemical burns occur in the workplace and at home. The severity of the burn depends on the type and strength of the chemical and the duration of exposure to the chemical. The main difference between a chemical burn and a thermal burn is that the chemical continues to burn the patient's tissues as long as it is on the skin. Because of this factor, it is important to remove the chemical from the skin as quickly as possible and then to activate the local EMS.

Liquid chemical burns should be treated by flooding the area with large amounts of cool running water until emergency personnel arrive. If a solid substance such as lime has been spilled on the patient, it should be brushed off before flooding the area with water. This is because a dry chemical may be activated by contact with water.

Seizures

A **seizure** is a sudden episode of involuntary muscular contractions and relaxation, often accompanied by changes in sensation, behavior, and level of consciousness. A seizure results when the normal electrical activity of the brain is disturbed, causing the brain cells to become irritated and overactive. Specific conditions that trigger a seizure include epilepsy, encephalitis, a recent or old head injury, high fever in infants and young children, drug and alcohol abuse or withdrawal, eclampsia associated with toxemia of pregnancy, diabetic conditions, and heatstroke.

Seizures are classified as partial or generalized according to the location of the abnormal electrical activity in the brain. *Partial seizures* are the most common type, occurring in approximately 80% of individuals who have seizures. With a partial seizure, the abnormal electrical activity is localized into specific areas of the brain; only the brain functions in those areas are affected.

Partial seizures are further classified as simple or complex, depending on whether the patient's level of consciousness is affected. The symptoms of a *simple partial seizure* include twitching or jerking in just one part of the body. This type of seizure lasts less than 1 minute, and the patient remains awake and alert during the seizure. With a *complex partial seizure,* the patient's level of consciousness is affected, and the patient has little or no memory of the seizure afterward. Symptoms of this type of seizure include abnormal behavior such as confusion, a glassy stare, aimless wandering, lip smacking or chewing, and fidgeting with clothing, which lasts from a few seconds to a minute or two. A simple and a complex partial seizure can progress to a generalized seizure.

With a *generalized seizure,* the abnormal electrical activity spreads through the entire brain. The best-known type of generalized seizure is a *tonic-clonic seizure* (formerly known as a "grand mal seizure"). With this type of seizure, the patient exhibits tonic-clonic activity followed by a postictal state. During the tonic phase, the patient suddenly loses consciousness and exhibits rigid muscular contractions, which result in odd posturing of the body. Respirations are inhibited, which may cause cyanosis around the mouth and lips. The patient may lose control of the bladder or bowels, resulting in involuntary urination and defecation. The tonic phase lasts 30 seconds, followed by the clonic phase. During the clonic phase, the patient's body jerks about violently. The patient's jaw muscles contract, which may cause the patient to bite the tongue or lips. The final phase of the seizure is the postictal state, lasting 10 to 30 minutes, in which the patient exhibits a depressed level of consciousness, is disoriented, and often has a headache. The patient generally has little or no memory of the seizure and feels confused and exhausted for several hours after the seizure.

In some instances of seizures, particularly in patients with epilepsy, an aura precedes the seizure. An *aura* is a sensation perceived by the patient that something is about to happen; examples include a strange taste, smell, or sound; a twitch; or a feeling of dizziness or anxiety. An aura provides the patient with a warning signal that a seizure is about to begin.

Although seizures are frightening to observe, they usually are not as bad as they look. Most patients fully recover within a few minutes after the seizure begins. An exception to this is *status epilepticus,* in which seizures are prolonged or come in rapid succession without full recovery of consciousness between them. Status epilepticus is a potentially life-threatening situation that requires immediate medical care.

Emergency Care for Seizures

The most important criterion in caring for a patient in a seizure is to protect the patient from harm. Remove hazards from the immediate area to protect the patient from injury sustained by striking a surrounding object. Do not restrain the patient. Loosen restrictive clothing that may interfere with breathing, such as collars, neckties, scarves, and jewelry. The seizure will occur no matter what you do; restraining the patient could seriously injure the patient's muscles, bones, or joints. Do not insert anything into the patient's mouth during the seizure because this could damage the teeth or mouth or interfere with breathing. In addition, it could trigger the gag reflex, causing the patient to vomit and possibly aspirate the vomitus into the lungs. If the patient vomits, roll him or her onto one side so that the vomitus can drain from the mouth.

If you are uncertain as to the cause of the seizure, or if you suspect that the patient is having status epilepticus, activate your local EMS immediately. Otherwise, transport the patient to an emergency medical care facility for further evaluation and treatment after the seizure is over.

Poisoning

A **poison** is any substance that causes illness, injury, or death if it enters the body. Most poisoning episodes occur in the home, are accidental, and occur in children younger than 5 years of age. Poisoning usually involves common substances, such as cleaning agents, medications, and

pesticides. For most poisonous substances, the reaction is more serious in children and the elderly than in adults. A poison can enter the body in four ways: ingestion, inhalation, absorption, or injection.

Poison control centers are valuable resources that are easily accessible to medical personnel and the community. More than 500 regional poison control centers have been established across the United States; most are located in the emergency departments of large hospitals. These centers are staffed by personnel who have access to information about almost all poisonous substances. Most centers are staffed 24 hours a day, and calls are toll-free. In addition, a National Poison Control Hotline number (1-800-222-1222) can be called 24 hours a day.

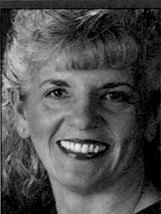

Memories *from* Externship

Judy Markins: As it turned out, one of my most terrible moments during my externship was a great learning experience. I was drawing blood (which was not my favorite procedure) and missed the vein—not once, but twice. You could see the sweat under my gloves. My stomach was in my throat, and I did not want to try again. Thank goodness my patient was understanding, and I had an excellent externship supervisor. She insisted that I try again, encouraging me that I could do it and suggesting some techniques that she had learned from her many years of experience. I got the blood specimen, along with some new-found confidence.

In most situations, someone can help you if you have questions. Use your resources when you need to. Be honest, know your procedure, and have confidence in yourself. ■

What Would You Do? What Would You *Not* Do?

Case Study 1
Beth Eaton calls the office. She says that she thinks her 3-year-old daughter, Olivia, has eaten some chewable vitamins. Beth was taking a shower, and when she came out, Olivia was holding an empty vitamin bottle and saying "Good candy." Beth says she does not know how Olivia got the child-proof top off. She thinks the bottle was about a third of the way full. Beth says that Olivia is complaining that her tummy hurts. Beth says she has syrup of ipecac and wants to know whether she should give some to Olivia. ■

Ingested Poisons

Poisons that are ingested enter the body by being swallowed. Ingestion is the most common route of entry for poisons. Examples of poisons that are often ingested include cleaning products, pesticides, contaminated food, petroleum products (e.g., gasoline, kerosene), and poisonous plants. Abuse of drugs, alcohol, or both also can result in poisoning from an accidental or intentional overdose. Signs and symptoms of poisoning by ingestion are based on the specific substance that has been consumed but often include strange odors, burns or stains around the mouth, nausea, vomiting, abdominal pain, diarrhea, difficulty in breathing, profuse perspiration, excessive salivation, dilated or constricted pupils, unconsciousness, and convulsions.

Emergency Care for Poisoning by Ingestion

1. Acquire as much information as possible about the type of poison, the amount ingested, and when it was ingested.
2. Call your poison control center or local EMS. *Never* induce vomiting unless directed to do so by a medical authority. Vomiting is often contraindicated—when an individual is unconscious, has swallowed a petroleum product, or has swallowed a corrosive poison such as a strong acid or base. Corrosive poisons may cause more injury to the esophagus, throat, and mouth if they are vomited back up. If it is available, you may be directed by the poison control center to administer activated charcoal. Activated charcoal is used to absorb the poison that remains in the stomach and prevents absorption by the intestine.
3. If the individual vomits, collect some of the vomitus for transport with the patient to the hospital for analysis by a toxicologist, if necessary. In addition, bring along containers of any substances ingested, such as empty medication bottles and household cleaner containers, because the label of the container often lists the ingredients in the product.

Inhaled Poisons

A poison that is inhaled is breathed into the body in the form of gas, vapor, or spray. The most commonly inhaled poison is carbon monoxide, such as from car exhausts, malfunctioning furnaces, and fires. Other inhaled poisons include carbon dioxide from wells and sewers and fumes from household products such as glues, paints, insect sprays, and cleaners (e.g., ammonia, chlorine). Signs and symptoms of inhaled poisoning often include severe headache; nausea and vomiting; coughing or wheezing; shortness of breath; chest pain or tightness; facial burns; burning of the mouth, nose, eyes, throat, or chest; cyanosis; confusion; dizziness; and unconsciousness.

Emergency Care for Inhaled Poisons

1. Determine whether it is safe to approach the patient. Toxic gases and fumes also can be dangerous to individuals helping the patient.
2. Remove the individual from the source of the poison and into fresh air as quickly as possible.
3. Call your poison control center or local EMS.
4. If oxygen is available, you may be directed to administer it under the supervision of a physician. Oxygen is the primary antidote for carbon monoxide poisoning.

Absorbed Poisons

A poison that is absorbed enters the body through the skin. Examples of absorbed poisons include fertilizers and pesticides used for lawn and garden care. Signs and symptoms of absorbed poisoning include irritation, burning and itching, burning of the skin or eyes, headache, and abnormal pulse or respiration or both.

Emergency Care for Absorbed Poisons

1. Remove the patient from the source of the poison. Avoid contact with the toxic substance.
2. Call your poison control center or local EMS. In most cases, you will be instructed to flood the area that has been exposed to the poison with water. Dry chemicals should be brushed from the skin before flooding with water.

What Would You Do? What Would You Not Do?

Case Study 2

Anita Alland calls the office and says that her son, Garon, was stung by a yellow jacket about an hour ago while mowing the grass. She says that his entire arm and back are red and swollen, and that he has a lot of redness and swelling around his eyes. Garon is itching all over and seems fuzzy-headed. Anita says she has never seen anyone do this after being stung. She says she had Garon take a cold shower to see if it would help. After the shower, he started feeling faint and dizzy, and now he is having trouble breathing. Anita wants to know whether she can bring him to the office so that he can be seen by the physician. ■

Injected Poisons

An injected poison enters the body through bites, through stings, or by a needle. Examples of injected poisons include the venom of insects, spiders, snakes, and marine creatures such as jellyfish and the bite of rabid animals. The poison also may be a drug that is self-administered with a hypodermic needle, such as heroin. General signs and symptoms of injected poisoning include an altered state of awareness; evidence of stings, bites, or puncture marks on the skin; mottled skin; localized pain or itching; burning, swelling, or blistering at the site; difficulty in breathing; abnormal pulse rate; nausea and vomiting; and anaphylactic shock.

Insect Stings

It is estimated that 1 of every 125 Americans is allergic to insect stings. Approximately 40 people in the United States die every year from a severe allergic reaction to insect stings. The incidence of deaths is low because most people know they need to obtain medical attention immediately if an allergic reaction begins.

Almost all of the insects whose venom can cause allergic reactions belong to a group called *Hymenoptera*, which includes honeybees and bumblebees, wasps, yellow jackets, and hornets. When a honeybee stings, its stinger remains embedded in the victim's skin, causing the bee to die as it tries to tear itself away. Wasps, yellow jackets, and hornets are more aggressive than bees and can sting repeatedly. Hornets are the most aggressive of the group and may sting even when not provoked. Yellow jackets are close behind in aggressiveness, and wasps usually sting only if someone interferes with them near their nest.

If an insect sting does not cause an allergic reaction within 30 minutes, chances are excellent that no problem will occur. A normal reaction to an insect sting includes localized pain, redness, swelling, and itching lasting 1 to 2 days. Any generalized reaction not arising directly from the area of the sting is almost certain to be an allergic reaction, which begins with symptoms such as sneezing, hives, itching, angioedema, erythema, and disorientation and progresses to difficulty in breathing, dizziness, faintness, and loss of consciousness.

Medical care should be sought immediately because these are the symptoms of an anaphylactic reaction, and most fatalities occur within 2 hours of the sting. Because time is a factor, individuals known to have a severe allergy to insect stings carry an anaphylactic emergency treatment kit containing injectable epinephrine and oral antihistamines (see Figure 35-2). With this kit, treatment for a severe allergic reaction can be started immediately.

Emergency Care for Insect Stings

1. Remove the stinger and attached venom sac. Scrape the stinger off the patient's skin with your fingernail or a plastic card such as a credit card (Figure 35-14). Do not use tweezers or forceps because squeezing the venom sac may cause more venom to be injected into the patient's tissues.
2. Wash the site with soap and water.
3. Apply a cold pack to the affected area to reduce pain and swelling.
4. Observe the patient for signs of an anaphylactic reaction.

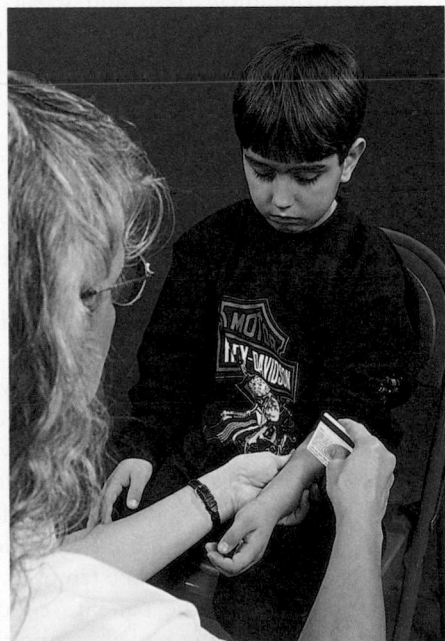

Figure 35-14 Removing a honeybee stinger and venom sac using the edge of a credit card.

Spider Bites

Although spiders are numerous throughout the United States, most do not cause injuries or serious complications. Only two spiders have bites that cause serious or life-threatening reactions: the black widow spider and the brown recluse spider. Both of these spiders prefer dark, out-of-the-way places such as in woodpiles, in brush piles, under rocks, and in dark garages and attics. Because of this, bites usually occur on the hands and arms of individuals reaching into places where the spiders are hiding. Often the individual does not know that he or she has been bitten until he or she begins to feel ill or notices swelling and a bite mark on the skin.

The black widow spider is approximately 1 inch long and is black with a distinctive bright-red hourglass shape on its abdomen. The venom injected when this spider bites an individual is toxic to the central nervous system. Signs and symptoms of a black widow bite include swelling and a dull pain at the injection site; nausea and vomiting; a rigid, boardlike abdomen; fever; rash; and difficulty in breathing or swallowing. Although the symptoms are severe, they are not usually fatal. An antivenin is available; however, because of its undesirable and frequent side effects, it generally is administered only to individuals with severe bites and to those who may have a heightened reaction, such as elderly individuals and children younger than 5 years old.

The brown recluse spider is light brown with a dark-brown violin-shaped mark on its back. The bite of a brown recluse causes severe local effects, including tenderness, redness, and swelling at the injection site. Systemic effects, such as difficulty in breathing or swallowing, seldom occur.

Emergency Care for Spider Bites

1. Wash the wound.
2. Apply a cold pack to the affected area to reduce pain and swelling.
3. Obtain medical help immediately if you suspect the individual has been bitten by a black widow spider or a brown recluse spider, or if a severe reaction begins to occur.

Snakebites

Snakebites kill very few people in the United States. Every year, approximately 45,000 persons are bitten by a snake; however, only 7000 of these bites involve a poisonous snake, and fewer than 15 of the individuals die. Species of poisonous snakes in the United States include rattlesnakes, copperheads, cottonmouths (water moccasins), and coral snakes. Individuals, zoos, or laboratories may own other poisonous species, however. Rattlesnakes account for most snakebites and nearly all fatalities from snakebites. Most snakebites occur near the home, as opposed to in the wild. Because it is often difficult to identify a snake, any unidentified snake should be considered poisonous. General signs and symptoms of a bite from a poisonous snake include puncture marks on the skin, pain and swelling at the puncture site, rapid pulse, nausea, vomiting, unconsciousness, and convulsions.

Emergency Care for Snakebites

1. Wash the bite area gently with soap and water.
2. Immobilize the injured part, and position it below the level of the heart.
3. Call emergency personnel. Do not apply ice to a snakebite. Do not apply a tourniquet, and do not cut or suction the wound.
4. If the snake is dead, inform emergency personnel of its location so that it can be transported to the hospital for identification.

Animal Bites

Bites and other injuries from animals range in severity from minor to serious and fatal. Most people who are bitten by animals do not report the bite to a physician. Because of this factor, the incidence of animal bites in the United States each year is unknown but has been estimated at approximately 1 to 2 million for dog bites and 400,000 for cat bites.

The most serious type of bite is one from an animal with rabies. Rabies is a viral infection transmitted through the saliva of an infected animal. If the condition is not treated, rabies is generally fatal. Certain animals tend to have a higher incidence of rabies than others. These include skunks, bats, raccoons, cats, dogs, cattle, and foxes. Hamsters, gerbils, guinea pigs, chipmunks, rats, mice, gophers, and rabbits are rarely infected with the rabies virus.

An individual who has been bitten by an animal that has rabies or is suspected of having rabies must obtain medical care. To prevent rabies, a rabies vaccine, which produces antibodies to fight the rabies virus, is administered to the individual.

Emergency Care for Animal Bites

Minor animal bites. Wash the wound with soap and water. Apply an antibiotic ointment and a dry sterile dressing. Transport the individual to a physician so that medical care can be provided to prevent infection and to ensure that the patient's tetanus toxoid immunization is up-to-date.

Serious bites. If the wound is bleeding heavily, first control the bleeding with direct pressure. Do not clean the wound because this may result in more bleeding. Transport the patient to a physician, or if the bite is serious enough, call the local EMS.

All animal bites. If you suspect that the animal has rabies, relay this information to the appropriate authorities, such as medical personnel, the police, or animal control personnel. If possible, try to remember what the animal looked like and the area in which you last saw it.

Heat and Cold Exposure

Exposure to excessive environmental heat or cold can result in injury to the body ranging in severity from minor to life-threatening. Heat-related injuries are most apt to occur on very hot days that are accompanied by high humidity with little or no air movement. The three conditions caused by overexposure to heat are heat cramps, heat exhaustion, and heatstroke.

The two major types of cold-related injury are frostbite and hypothermia. Although cold-related injuries are most apt to occur in the winter months, they can occur at other times of the year, such as when an individual is exposed to cold water in a near-drowning incident.

Certain individuals are at higher risk for developing heat-related and cold-related injuries, as follows:
- Elderly individuals
- Young children, particularly infants
- Individuals who work or exercise outdoors
- Individuals with medical conditions that cause poor blood circulation, such as diabetes mellitus and cardiovascular disease
- Individuals who have had heat-related or cold-related injuries in the past
- Individuals under the influence of drugs or alcohol

Heat Cramps

Heat cramps are the least serious of the three types of heat-related injury. Heat cramps are most apt to occur when an individual is exercising or working in a hot environment and fails to replace lost fluids and electrolytes. Lost electrolytes can be replaced with a commercial sports drink (e.g., Gatorade).

Signs and symptoms of heat cramps include painful muscle spasms, particularly of the legs, calves, and abdomen; hot, sweaty skin; weakness; and a rapid pulse. These symptoms are a warning that an individual is having a problem with the heat. If the problem is ignored, heat cramps may progress to a more serious condition, such as heat exhaustion or heatstroke.

Treatment of heat cramps consists of removal of the patient to a cool environment, rest, and replacement of fluids and electrolytes. If the patient's condition does not improve, he or she should be transported to an emergency care facility for further treatment.

Heat Exhaustion

Heat exhaustion is the most common heat-related injury. It occurs most often in individuals involved in vigorous physical activity on a hot and humid day, such as athletes and construction workers. It also can occur in people who are wearing too much clothing on a hot and humid day. Signs and symptoms of heat exhaustion are similar to those of influenza: cold and clammy skin that is pale or gray, profuse sweating, headache, nausea, dizziness, weakness, and diarrhea.

Treatment of heat exhaustion consists of removal of the patient to a cool environment, replacement of fluids and electrolytes, application of a cold compress to the forehead, and rest (Figure 35-15). Tight clothing should be loosened, and excessive layers of clothing should be removed. In most cases, these measures improve the patient's condition in approximately 30 minutes. If the patient's condition does not improve, however, he or she should be transported to an emergency care facility.

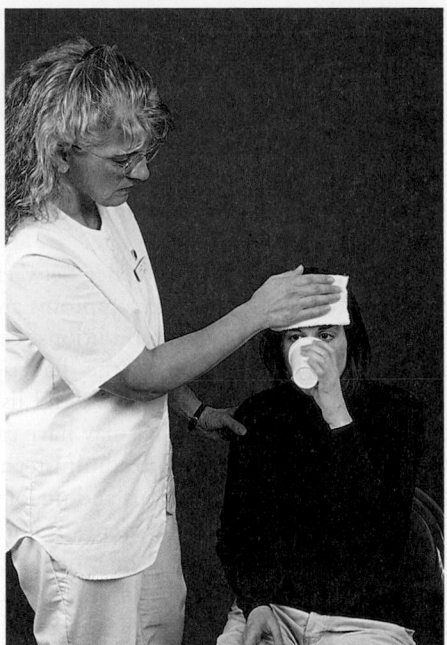

Figure 35-15 Treatment of heat exhaustion consists of moving the patient to a cool environment, replacing fluids and electrolytes, and applying a cold compress to the forehead; the patient should then rest.

Heatstroke

Heatstroke is the least common, but most serious, of the three heat-related injuries. Heatstroke is most apt to occur in elderly people during a heat wave and in athletes who overexert in a hot and humid environment. Heatstroke can occur in a very short time, as when a child has been left to wait in a closed car on a hot day.

During heatstroke, the body becomes so overheated that the heat-regulating mechanism breaks down and is unable to cool the body. The body temperature increases to a dangerous level, causing destruction of tissues. Signs and symptoms of heatstroke include a body temperature of 105° F (40° C) or greater; red, hot, dry skin; a rapid, weak pulse; dizziness and weakness; rapid, shallow breathing; decreased levels of consciousness; and seizures.

Heatstroke is a life-threatening emergency that requires immediate transport of the patient to an emergency care facility by the fastest way possible. If not treated, heatstroke is always fatal. During transport, every attempt should be made to lower the body temperature, such as setting the air conditioner to its maximal capacity; covering the victim with cool, wet sheets; and fanning the victim.

Frostbite

Frostbite is the localized freezing of body tissue as a result of exposure to cold. The severity of frostbite depends on the environmental temperature, the duration of exposure, and the wind-chill factor. Frostbite most commonly affects the hands, fingers, feet, toes, ears, nose, and cheeks. Although frostbite is not life-threatening, it can cause severe tissue damage that may require amputation of the affected body part. Signs and symptoms of frostbite include loss of feeling

Case Study 3

David Brently has come to the medical office. He is a member of Kiwanis, and this year it was his turn to deliver Easter candy and flowers to patients at the local hospital and nursing home while wearing a bunny costume. It is a very warm day, and David says that he got really hot and sweaty in his costume and then started feeling dizzy and nauseous. He got a little worried and decided to drive himself to the medical office. David says he cannot get his costume off because the zipper is stuck. He does not want to cut it off because that would ruin it and Kiwanis would not be able to use it next year. He is hoping the physician can fix him up well enough so that he can drive home. David says he is sure his wife can get the costume off without damaging it. ■

in the affected area; cold and waxy skin; and white, yellow, or blue discoloration of the skin.

Treatment of frostbite requires rewarming of the affected body part to prevent permanent damage. This is best accomplished in an emergency care facility because improper rewarming can result in further tissue damage. To transport the patient, loosely wrap warm clothing or blankets around the affected body part. The frozen area also can be placed in contact with another body part that is warm. It is important to handle the affected area gently. Do not rub or massage the affected area because this can damage frozen tissue further.

Hypothermia

Hypothermia is a life-threatening emergency in which the temperature of the entire body falls to a dangerously low level. Hypothermia can occur rapidly, such as when an individual falls through the ice on a frozen lake. It also can occur slowly when an individual is exposed to a cold environment for a long time, such as when a hiker is lost in the woods.

When the core body temperature decreases too much, the body loses its ability to regulate its temperature and to generate body heat. Signs and symptoms of hypothermia include shivering, numbness, drowsiness, apathy, a glassy stare, and decreased levels of consciousness.

Treatment of hypothermia should focus on preventing further heat loss. Remove the patient from the cold, or, if this is impossible, wrap him or her in blankets. Do not attempt to rewarm the patient such as through immersion in warm water. Rapid rewarming can result in serious respiratory and cardiac problems. The patient should be transported immediately to an emergency care facility.

Diabetic Emergencies

Glucose is the end product of carbohydrate metabolism. It serves as the chief source of energy to perform normal body functions and to assist in maintaining body temperature. The body maintains a constant blood glucose level to ensure a continuous source of energy for the body. Glucose that is not needed for energy can be stored in the form of glycogen in muscle and liver tissue for later use. When no more tissue storage is possible, excess glucose is converted to fat and stored as adipose tissue.

Insulin, a hormone secreted by the beta cells of the pancreas, is required for normal use of glucose in the body. Insulin enables glucose to enter the body's cells and be converted to energy. Insulin also is needed for proper storage of glycogen in liver and muscle cells.

Diabetes mellitus is a disease in which the body is unable to use glucose for energy because of a lack of insulin in the body. There are two types of diabetes—a severe form, usually appearing in childhood, known as *type 1 diabetes,* and a mild form, usually appearing in adulthood, known as *type 2 diabetes.* Most individuals with diabetes (90%) have type 2 diabetes. No cure for diabetes mellitus is known, but significant advances have been made in controlling the disease through a combination of drug therapy, diet therapy, and activity. The goal for the diabetic patient is to balance food intake and level of activity with the body's insulin.

A diabetic patient can experience two types of emergency: *hypoglycemia,* commonly referred to as "insulin shock," and *diabetic ketoacidosis,* commonly known as "diabetic coma." Insulin shock (hypoglycemia) occurs when there is too much insulin in the body and not enough glucose. Insulin shock can be caused by administration of too much insulin, skipping meals, and unexpected or unusual exercise. Symptoms of insulin shock include normal or rapid respirations; pale, cold, and clammy skin; sweating; dizziness and headache; full, rapid pulse; normal or high blood pressure; extreme hunger; aggressive or unusual behavior; fainting; and seizure or coma. The onset of insulin shock occurs rapidly, usually over 5 to 20 minutes, after the blood glucose level begins to decrease. Because the brain requires a constant supply of glucose for proper functioning, permanent brain damage or death can result from severe hypoglycemia.

Diabetic coma (diabetic ketoacidosis) occurs when there is not enough insulin in the body. This causes the blood glucose level to increase, resulting in hyperglycemia. When glucose cannot be used for energy, fat is broken down. This results in a buildup of acid waste products in the blood, known as *ketoacidosis.* The combined effect of the hyperglycemia and the ketoacidosis causes the following symptoms: polyuria; excessive thirst and hunger; vomiting; abdominal pain; dry, warm skin; rapid, deep sighing respirations; a sweet or fruity (acetone) odor to the breath; and a rapid, weak pulse.

If the condition is not treated, diabetic coma can progress to dehydration, hypotension, coma, and death. In contrast to insulin shock, however, the onset of diabetic coma is gradual, usually developing over 12 to 48 hours. Diabetic coma can be caused by illness and infection, overeating, forgetting to administer an insulin injection, or administering an insufficient amount of insulin.

Most individuals with diabetes have a thorough knowledge of their disease and manage it effectively. Because of this, diabetic emergencies are most apt to occur when there is an unusual upset in the insulin/glucose balance in the body, such as might be caused by illness or infection. An emergency situation also may arise in an individual who has diabetes but in whom the condition has not yet been diagnosed.

It may be difficult to tell the difference between insulin shock and diabetic coma because the symptoms are similar. Often a patient with either of these conditions seems to be intoxicated. If he or she is conscious, the diabetic patient usually knows what the trouble is; you should listen carefully to the patient to determine what may have caused the problem (e.g., not eating, forgetting to administer an insulin injection). If the patient is unconscious and unable to communicate, you should observe the patient's respirations. A patient in insulin shock has normal or rapid respirations, whereas a patient in diabetic coma has deep, labored respirations. Most diabetic patients carry an emergency medical identification, such as a medical alert bracelet or necklace and a wallet card (Figure 35-16), to alert others to their condition when they cannot.

Emergency Care in Diabetes
Insulin Shock (Hypoglycemia)
A patient in insulin shock needs sugar immediately. For a conscious patient, glucose should be administered by mouth

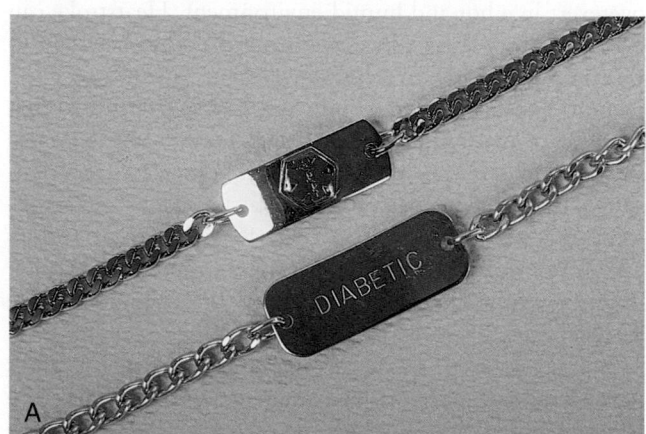

A

| ALERT | **I HAVE TYPE I DIABETES**
If I appear to be intoxicated or am unconscious, I may be having a reaction to diabetes or its treatment.

EMERGENCY TREATMENT
If I am able to swallow, please give me a beverage that contains sugar, such as orange juice, cola or even sugar in water. Then please send me to the nearest hospital **IMMEDIATELY.** |

B

Figure 35-16 Diabetic medical identification. **A,** Diabetic medical alert bracelet. **B,** Diabetic wallet card.

in the form of fruit juice (e.g., orange juice), nondiet soft drinks, candy, honey, or table sugar dissolved in water (Figure 35-17). Improvement is usually rapid after the glucose has been consumed. If the patient is unconscious, do not give anything by mouth because it may be aspirated into the lungs. Instead, provide the fastest possible transportation of the patient to an emergency care facility.

Diabetic Coma (Diabetic Ketoacidosis)

A patient in diabetic coma needs insulin and must be transported as soon as possible to an emergency care facility.

Doubtful Situations

If you are ever in doubt as to whether a patient is developing insulin shock or diabetic coma, give sugar, even though the final diagnosis may be diabetic coma. This is because insulin shock develops much more rapidly than diabetic coma and can quickly cause permanent brain damage or death. If you give sugar to a patient in diabetic coma, there is little risk of making the condition worse because a patient can withstand a high blood glucose level longer than he or she can tolerate a low blood glucose level.

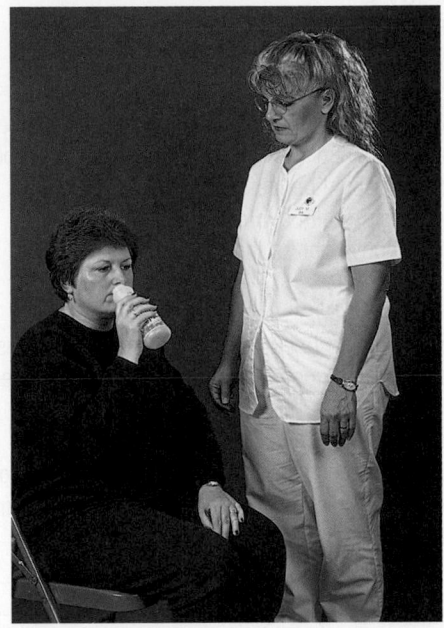

Figure 35-17 Orange juice is administered to a diabetic patient showing signs and symptoms of insulin shock.

MEDICAL PRACTICE and the LAW

Emergency medicine is one of the most litigious (lawsuit-prone) areas of health care. Owing to the nature of emergencies, there is little time to plan your actions, and one misstep could cause damage. Keep in mind that your actions would be compared in court with those of a "reasonably prudent medical assistant with similar education and experience." Do not perform procedures you are not comfortable performing.

Whenever possible, obtain written consent for all procedures. In a life-or-death situation, this usually is not possible. In this case, you are held accountable to try to save the life of the patient, even without consent.

Patients or families often become hysterical during emergencies. As a health care professional, you are expected to keep a cool head and calm the patient and family while attending to the emergency situation.

If you are out of the office and encounter an emergency situation, many states have a "Good Samaritan" law that protects you from legal action if you perform only procedures with which you are familiar, such as emergency first aid or CPR. ■

What Would You Do? What Would You *Not* Do? RESPONSES

Case Study 1
Page 859

What Did Judy Do?
❏ Gave Beth the National Poison Control hotline number (1-800-222-1222) and told her to call it immediately. Explained that was the fastest way to obtain information on what to do.
❏ Told Beth not to give the syrup of ipecac to Olivia unless she was told to do so by the poison control center.
❏ Told Beth to have the vitamin bottle in her hand when she calls. Told her that the poison control center would want to know information from the label and would especially want to know whether the vitamins contained iron.
❏ Told Beth to call the office back if she needs any more help after talking with the poison control center.

What Did Judy Not Do?
❏ Did not tell Beth she should give Olivia syrup of ipecac, because some poisons can cause additional problems if they are brought back up.

What Would You Do?/What Would You Not Do?
Review Judy's response and place a checkmark next to the information you included in your response. List additional information you included in your response.

_____
_____
_____
_____
_____

Continued

Case Study 2
Page 860

What Did Judy Do?

❑ Told Anita that Garon needs to get to the hospital as soon as possible. Explained that he is having a very serious allergic reaction that could be life-threatening.

❑ Told her to stay calm and call 911 immediately.

❑ Notified the physician of the situation.

What Did Judy Not Do?

❑ Did not tell her to bring Garon to the office because he may need special life-support equipment available at the hospital.

What Would You Do?/What Would You Not *Do?*

Review Judy's response and place a checkmark next to the information you included in your response. List additional information you included in your response.

_____
_____
_____
_____
_____
_____

Case Study 3
Page 863

What Did Judy Do?

❑ Took David to an examining room that was cool and gave him a glass of water.

❑ Told David she needed to get his costume off as soon as possible. Explained that if his condition gets worse, it could become life-threatening.

❑ Helped David out of the costume and gave him another glass of water.

What Did Judy Not Do?

❑ Did not let David keep the costume on.

What Would You Do?/What Would You Not *Do?*

Review Judy's response and place a checkmark next to the information you included in your response. List additional information you included in your response.

_____
_____
_____
_____
_____
_____

↻ TERMINOLOGY REVIEW

Medical Term	Word Parts	Definition
Burn		An injury to the tissues caused by exposure to thermal, chemical, electrical, or radioactive agents.
Crash cart		A specially equipped cart for holding and transporting medications, equipment, and supplies needed for lifesaving procedures in an emergency.
Crepitus		A grating sensation caused by fractured bone fragments rubbing against each other.
Dislocation	*dis-:* to undo, free from	An injury in which one end of a bone making up a joint is separated or displaced from its normal anatomic position.
Emergency medical services (EMS) system		A network of community resources, equipment, and personnel that provides care to victims of injury or sudden illness.
First aid		The immediate care administered before complete medical care can be provided to an individual who is injured or suddenly becomes ill.
Fracture		Any break in a bone.
Hypothermia	*hypo-:* below, deficient *therm/o:* heat *-ia:* condition of diseased or abnormal state	A life-threatening condition in which the temperature of the entire body falls to a dangerously low level.
Poison		Any substance that causes illness, injury, or death if it enters the body.
Pressure point		A site on the body where an artery lies close to the surface of the skin and can be compressed against an underlying bone to control bleeding.
Seizure		A sudden episode of involuntary muscular contractions and relaxation, often accompanied by changes in sensation, behavior, and level of consciousness.
Shock		The failure of the cardiovascular system to deliver enough blood to all of the vital organs of the body.
Splint		Any device that immobilizes a body part.
Sprain		Trauma to a joint that causes tearing of ligaments.
Strain		A stretching or tearing of muscles or tendons caused by trauma.
Wound		A break in the continuity of an external or internal surface, caused by physical means.

ON THE WEB

For information on emergency medicine:

American Red Cross: www.redcross.org

Federal Emergency Management Agency: www.fema.gov

 Check out the Evolve site at http://evolve.elsevier.com/Bonewit/today/ to actively Prepare for your Certification, and to access additional interactive activities and exercises to help you study and prepare for success.

 Check out the Evolve site at http://evolve.elsevier.com/Bonewit/today/ to actively Prepare for your Certification, and to access additional interactive activities and exercises to help you study and prepare for success

36

The Medical Record

LEARNING OBJECTIVES

Components of the Medical Record

1. List and describe the functions served by the medical record.
2. Identify the information contained in each of the following medical office administrative documents: patient registration record, NPP form, and correspondence.
3. Identify the information contained in each of the following medical office clinical documents: health history report, physical examination report, progress notes, medication record, consultation report, and home health care report.
4. State the purpose of a laboratory report and describe the information included in each of the following categories of laboratory reports: hematology, clinical chemistry, immunology, urinalysis, microbiology, parasitology, cytology, and histology.
5. List and describe the information included in each of the following diagnostic procedure documents: electrocardiogram report, Holter monitor report, sigmoidoscopy report, colonoscopy report, spirometry report, radiology report, and diagnostic imaging report.
6. State the purpose of each of the following therapeutic services: physical therapy, occupational therapy, and speech therapy.
7. Identify the information contained in each of the following hospital documents: history and physical report, operative report, discharge summary report, pathology report, and emergency department report.

Consent Documents

8. Identify the information contained in each of the following consent documents: consent to treatment form and release of medical information form.

Types of Medical Records

9. Explain the difference between a PPR and an EMR.
10. List the general functions of electronic medical record (EMR) software.

PROCEDURES

Prepare a medical record for a new patient.

Obtain patient consent for treatment on a consent to treatment form.
Assist a patient in completing a release of medical information form.
Release information according to a completed release of medical information form.

LEARNING OBJECTIVES

Medical Record Formats

11. Describe the organization of a source-oriented medical record and a problem-oriented medical record.
12. List and define the four subcategories included in the progress notes of a problem-oriented record (POR).

Health History

13. List and describe the seven sections of the health history.
14. List the guidelines that should be followed in recording the chief complaint.

Charting

15. List and describe the guidelines to follow to ensure accurate and concise charting.
16. List and describe the types of progress notes that are charted by the medical assistant.
17. List examples of subjective symptoms and objective symptoms.
18. List and describe common symptoms.

PROCEDURES

Identify the parts of a source-oriented medical record and a problem-oriented medical record.

Assist the patient in completing a health history form.

Chart the following:
  Procedures
  Administration of medication
  Specimen collection
  Laboratory tests
  Progress notes
  Instructions given to the patient
Obtain and record patient symptoms.

CHAPTER OUTLINE

INTRODUCTION TO THE MEDICAL RECORD
Components of the Medical Record
Medical Office Administrative Documents
Patient Registration Record
NPP Acknowledgment Form
Correspondence
Medical Office Clinical Documents
Health History Report
Physical Examination Report
Progress Notes
Medication Record
Consultation Report
Home Health Care Report
Laboratory Documents
Diagnostic Procedure Documents
Electrocardiogram Report
Holter Monitor Report
Sigmoidoscopy Report
Colonoscopy Report
Spirometry Report
Radiology Report
Diagnostic Imaging Report
Therapeutic Service Documents
Physical Therapy
Occupational Therapy

Speech Therapy
Hospital Documents
History and Physical Report
Operative Report
Discharge Summary Report
Pathology Report
Emergency Department Report
Consent Documents
Consent to Treatment Form
Release of Medical Information Form
Types of Medical Records
Electronic Medical Record
Medical Record Formats
Source-Oriented Record
Problem-Oriented Record
Preparing a Medical Record for a New Patient
Medical Record Supplies
Taking a Health History
Components of the Health History
Charting in the Medical Record
Charting Guidelines
Charting Progress Notes
Charting Patient Symptoms
Other Activities That Need to Be Charted

KEY TERMS

attending physician
charting
consultation report
diagnosis (dye-ag-NOE-sis)
diagnostic procedure
discharge summary report
electronic medical record (EMR)
familial (fah-MIL-yul)
health history report

home health care
informed consent
inpatient
medical impressions
medical record
medical record format
objective symptom
paper-based patient record (PPR)
patient

physical examination
physical examination report
problem
prognosis (prog-NOE-sis)
reverse chronological order
SOAP
subjective symptom
symptom (SIMP-tum)

INTRODUCTION TO THE MEDICAL RECORD

Medical records are a crucial part of a medical practice. A **medical record** is a written record of the important information regarding a patient, including the care of that individual and the progress of his or her condition. A **patient** is defined as an individual receiving medical care.

The patient's medical record serves many important functions. The physician uses the information in the medical record as a basis for decisions regarding the patient's care and treatment. The medical record documents the results of treatment and the patient's progress. The medical record provides an efficient and effective method by which information can be communicated to authorized personnel in the medical office.

The medical record also serves as a legal document. The law requires that a record be maintained to document the care and treatment being received by a patient. If something goes wrong, good documentation works to protect the physician and the medical staff legally. Incomplete records could be used as evidence in court to show that a patient did not receive the quality of care that meets generally accepted standards.

The medical assistant must always keep in mind that the information contained in a patient's medical record is strictly confidential and must not be read by or discussed with anyone except the physician or medical staff involved with the care of the patient (see Highlight on the HIPAA Privacy Rule).

COMPONENTS OF THE MEDICAL RECORDS

A medical record consists of numerous documents. Each document in the medical record has a specific function or purpose. Most of these documents are preprinted forms or computer templates that contain specific information entered by a physician or other health professionals. A large variety of forms or templates are available; the type of form or template used is based on the specific requirements of each medical office.

Medical record documents can be classified into categories. Each of these categories is outlined in the box on page 872 along with the specific documents included in each.

It is important that the medical assistant be familiar with each type of document in the medical record. A description of the function or purpose of each type of medical record document follows (by category), along with the specific information that each contains.

Highlight on the HIPAA Privacy Rule

What Is the HIPAA privacy rule?
The acronym *HIPAA* stands for the *Health Insurance Portability and Accountability Act.* HIPAA is a federal law consisting of several components, one of which contains provisions to protect a patient's privacy, known as the *HIPAA Privacy Rule.*

The HIPAA Privacy Rule went into effect on April 14, 2003. The primary purpose of this rule is to provide patients with better control over the use and disclosure of their health information. All health care providers, health plans, and health care clearinghouses (e.g., billing services) that use, store, maintain, or transmit health information must comply with this rule.

What is included in the HIPAA privacy rule?
The HIPAA Privacy Rule is outlined here as it relates to the medical office:

1. The medical office must develop a written document known as a *Notice of Privacy Practices* (NPP). The NPP must explain to patients how their protected health information (PHI) will be used and protected by the medical office. *Protected health information* includes health information in any form (written, electronic, or oral) that contains patient-identifiable information (e.g., name, social security number, telephone number). The medical office must make a reasonable effort to provide an NPP to each patient and to obtain a signed acknowledgment from the patient that he or she has received an NPP.

2. A patient's written consent is not required for the use or disclosure of PHI for the following:
   - Medical treatment: *Examples:*
     (1) Patient referral to a specialist
     (2) Emergency care provided at a hospital
     (3) Tests on a patient performed by the laboratory
   - Payment: *Examples:*
     (1) Determination of eligibility for insurance benefits
     (2) Review of services provided for medical necessity
     (3) Utilization review activities
   - Health care operations: *Examples:*
     (1) Quality assessment activities
     (2) Contacting patients with information about care or treatment
     (3) Employee review activities
     (4) Training of health care students

3. Patients have the right to access their medical records and to request changes to the records if they believe them to be inaccurate.

4. To prevent unnecessary or inappropriate access to PHI, the medical office must make an effort to limit the use of, disclosure of, and requests for PHI to the minimum necessary to accomplish the intended purpose (e.g., a request from an insurance company for procedures performed on a patient). This requirement does not apply, however, to the

Continued

Highlight on the HIPAA Privacy Rule—cont'd

use of PHI for the routine practice of medicine within the medical office.

5. Patients have a right to request an accounting of the transfer of their information for purposes other than treatment, payment, or health care operations.

6. Business associates to whom the medical office may disclose PHI must respect the HIPAA Privacy Rule. The medical office must execute a written agreement with each business associate to handle PHI in accordance with HIPAA. Business associates may include the following organizations and firms:
   - Medical laboratories
   - Transcription services
   - Law firms
   - Accounting firms
   - Software and hardware consultants
   - Billing services

7. The medical office must implement for all employees a basic training program on privacy and security of PHI.

8. The medical office is required to put in place appropriate administrative, physical, and technical security safeguards to protect the privacy of PHI from accidental use or disclosure or violation of the above-listed requirements.

What if a medical office does *not* comply with the HIPAA privacy rule?

There are severe penalties if a medical office fails to comply with the HIPAA Privacy Rule, which can include civil and criminal penalties.

Where Can More Information on the HIPAA Privacy Rule Be Found?

The following websites contain current information on HIPAA:
   www.cms.gov/hipaageninfo
   www.hhs.gov/ocr/privacy

Categories of Medical Record Documents

Medical Office Administrative Documents
- Patient registration record
- NPP acknowledgment form
- Correspondence

Medical Office Clinical Documents
- Health history report
- Physical examination report
- Progress notes
- Medication record
- Consultation report
- Home health care report

Laboratory Documents
- Hematology report
- Clinical chemistry report
- Immunology report
- Urinalysis report
- Microbiology report
- Parasitology report
- Cytology report
- Histology report

Diagnostic Procedure Documents
- Electrocardiogram report
- Holter monitor report

- Sigmoidoscopy report
- Colonoscopy report
- Spirometry report
- Radiology report
- Diagnostic imaging report

Therapeutic Service Documents
- Physical therapy report
- Occupational therapy report
- Speech therapy report

Hospital Documents
- History and physical report
- Operative report
- Discharge summary report
- Pathology report
- Emergency department report

Consent Documents
- Consent to treatment form
- Release of medical information form

MEDICAL OFFICE ADMINISTRATIVE DOCUMENTS

Administrative documents contain information necessary for the efficient (record-keeping) management of the medical office. Medical office administrative documents include the patient registration record and patient-related correspondence.

Patient Registration Record

The patient registration record (Figure 36-1) consists of demographic and billing information. All new patients must complete a patient registration record form. After the patient completes the registration record, the medical assistant enters the information into a computer. This allows the demographic and billing information to be used for numerous computerized functions, such as scheduling appointments, posting patient transactions, and processing patient statements and insurance claims. With a paper-based patient record (PPR), the original patient registration record is then usually placed in the front of the patient's medical record. With an electronic medical record (EMR), the original registration record is usually shredded.

PATIENT INFORMATION **CONFIDENTIAL**

File no. 10140
Date 11-21-XX

(PLEASE PRINT)

Name Carol (First) H (Middle) Jones (Last) Birth date 1-20-68 Home phone 740-555-1248

Address 743 Evergreen Terrace City Springfield State OH ZIP 12345

Check appropriate box: ☐ Minor ☐ Single ☒ Married ☐ Divorced ☐ Widowed ☐ Separated Gender: ☐ Male ☒ Female

Employer Rockford, Inc. Work phone 740-555-1234

Business Address 1 Rockford Place City Shelbyville State OH ZIP 21346

Spouse or parent's name John Jones Employer Self-emp. Work phone 740-555-8654

If patient is a student, name of school/college N/A City State

Whom may we thank for referring you? Henry Peterson, MD

Person to contact in case of emergency John Jones Phone 740-555-1248

RESPONSIBLE PARTY

Name of person responsible for this account Carol Jones Relationship to patient Self

Address 743 Evergreen Terrace City Springfield State OH ZIP 12345 Home phone 740-555-1248

Employer Rockford, Inc. Work phone 740-555-1234

Is this person currently a patient in our office? ☒ Yes ☐ No

INSURANCE INFORMATION

Name of insured Carol Jones Relationship to patient Self

Birth date 1-20-68 Social Security number 123-45-6789 Date Employed 5-1-93

Name of Employer Rockford, Inc. Work phone 740-555-1234

Address of Employer 1 Rockford Place City Shelbyville State OH ZIP 21346

Insurance company Anthem BC/BS Group number 51045

Insurance company address 521 Anthem Drive City New Haberville State OH ZIP 21436

DO YOU HAVE ANY ADDITIONAL INSURANCE? ☐ YES ☒ NO **IF YES, COMPLETE THE FOLLOWING:**

Name of insured Relationship to patient

Birth date Social Security number Date Employed

Name of Employer Work phone

Address of Employer City State ZIP

Insurance company Group number

Insurance company address City State ZIP

X Carol Jones

SIGNATURE OF PATIENT OR PARENT IF MINOR

Figure 36-1 Patient registration record.

Demographic Information

Demographic information required on a patient registration form includes the following:

- Full name
- Address
- Telephone number (home and work)
- Date of birth
- Gender
- Marital status
- Employer

Billing Information

Billing information is required to bill charges to the patient or an insurance company. Billing information required on a patient registration form includes the following:

- Name of responsible party (person responsible for the account)
- Social security number
- Address of responsible party
- Name of insured (policyholder)
- Insurance company
- Policy number and group number

NPP Acknowledgment Form

A Notice of Privacy Practices (NPP) is a written document that explains to patients how their protected health information will be used and protected by the medical office. The patient must sign a form acknowledging that he or she has received the NPP. The NPP form is then filed in the patient's chart.

Correspondence

Correspondence is an important part of the medical record. Correspondence regarding a patient may be received from various individuals or facilities, such as the patient's insurance company, the patient's attorney, and the patient himself or herself. Insurance correspondence includes such documents as a precertification authorization for a hospital admission and a request for additional information from the insurance company. Correspondence also includes copies of letters concerning the patient that are sent out of the office; examples are a copy of a letter referring the patient to a specialist and a copy of a collection letter sent to the patient.

MEDICAL OFFICE CLINICAL DOCUMENTS

Medical office clinical documents include a variety of records and reports that assist the physician in the care and treatment of the patient. Common medical office clinical documents are listed and described next.

Health History Report

A **health history report** is a collection of subjective data about the patient. Most of this information is obtained by having the patient complete a preprinted form that is then

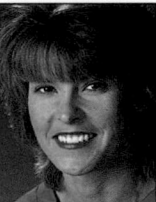

Putting It All into Practice

My name is Dawn Bennett, and I work for an orthopedic surgeon. I work in the front area of the office as an administrative supervisor in billing and collections.

Working in billing and collections is very challenging and sometimes stressful. It can even be embarrassing. We are a new practice, and when we opened, there was no collection system. When it came time to review our accounts, we realized that, like every other business, we needed a collection system. We immediately jumped in and took charge.

The primary physician at our office is from New York, and we were unfamiliar with his family members. One day he walked into our office with a very puzzled look. I asked him what was wrong. He replied, "You guys are doing a great job with our collection rate. I asked you to be stern, but thoughtful, when sending out patient collection letters, but did you have to send one to my mother-in-law?!" Needless to say, we fixed the error immediately. This incident prompted us to restructure our collection system, and we added a comment screen to our computer system on all of our patients' accounts. Going into a medical office that already has a system in place may be easier, but you can learn a lot more by setting up an office system yourself. ∎

reviewed for completeness by the medical assistant. Some of the information included in the health history is obtained by the physician or medical assistant by interviewing the patient.

Along with the physical examination and laboratory and diagnostic tests, the health history is used for the following reasons: to determine the patient's general state of health, to arrive at a diagnosis and to prescribe treatment, and to document any change in a patient's illness after treatment has been instituted. The term **diagnosis** refers to the scientific method of determining and identifying a patient's condition.

A thorough history of personal health is obtained for each new patient, and subsequent office visits provide additional information regarding changes in the patient's condition or treatment. A complete discussion of the health history report is presented later in this chapter.

Physical Examination Report

A **physical examination** is an assessment of each part of the patient's body. The purpose of the physical examination is to provide objective data about the patient, which assists the physician in determining the patient's state of health. (The physical examination is described in detail in Chapter 20.)

The **physical examination report** is a summary of the physician's findings from the assessment of each part of the patient's body and includes the following:
- General appearance
- Head and neck
- Eyes
- Ears
- Nose
- Mouth and pharynx
- Arms and hands
- Chest and lungs
- Heart
- Breasts
- Abdomen
- Genitalia and rectum
- Legs and feet

Progress Notes

Progress notes involve updating the medical record with new information each time the patient visits or telephones the medical office. Progress notes serve to document the patient's health status from one visit to the next. It is important that the date and time be included with each progress note, along with the signature and credentials of the individual making the entry. A thorough discussion of charting progress notes is presented later in this chapter.

Medication Record

A medication record consists of detailed information related to a patient's medications. The record may include one or more of the following categories: prescription medications, over-the-counter (OTC) medications, and medications administered at the medical office. Most medical offices use one form to record prescription and OTC medications and another form to record medications administered to the patient at the medical office.

Prescription and Over-the-Counter Medication Record Form

A medication record form for recording the patient's prescription and OTC medications includes the following:
- Patient's name and date of birth
- Drug allergies
- Date the patient began taking the medication

- Name of the medication
- Dosage
- Frequency of administration of the medication
- Route of administration
- Refills (prescription medications only)
- Date the patient stopped taking the medication

Medication Administration Record Form

A form for recording medications administered to the patient at the medical office (Figure 36-2) includes the following:
- Patient's name and date of birth
- Drug allergies
- Name of the medication
- Dosage administered
- Route of administration
- Injection site
- Date of administration
- Manufacturer, lot number, and expiration date of the medication
- Signature and credentials of the individual administering the medication

Consultation Report

A **consultation report** is a narrative report of a clinical opinion about a patient's condition by a practitioner other than the primary physician, known as a *consultant* (Figure 36-3). The consultant is usually a specialist in a certain field of medicine (e.g., cardiology, endocrinology, urology). The consultant's opinion of the patient's condition is based on a review of the patient's record and an examination of the patient. The consultation report must include the following:
- Documentation that the consultant reviewed the patient's health history
- Documentation that the consultant examined the patient
- A report of the consultant's impressions
- Any care or treatment provided by the consultant
- A report of the consultant's recommendations

Home Health Care Report

Home health care is the provision of medical and nonmedical care in a patient's home or place of residence. The purpose of home health care is to minimize the effect of disease or disability by promoting, maintaining, and restoring the patient's health. There is a growing preference for home health care over equivalent health care options. Research shows that familiar surroundings contribute positively to a patient's emotional and physical well-being.

Home health care must be ordered by the patient's physician and is provided by skilled professionals. Home health care professionals include nurses, home health aides, dietitians, physical therapists, occupational therapists, speech therapists, and social workers. Examples of specialized services available through home health care include cardiac home care, intravenous (IV) therapy, respiratory therapy, pain management, diabetes management, rehabilitation,

MEDICATION ADMINISTRATION RECORD

PATIENT NAME _Kristen Antle_   BIRTH DATE _1/9/1984_

ALLERGIES _Ø_

SITE ABBREVIATIONS:

RD: Right deltoid   RDG: Right dorsogluteal   RVL: Right vastus lateralis
LD: Left deltoid   LDG: Left dorsogluteal   LVL: Left vastus lateralis

MEDICATION AND DOSAGE	ROUTE	DATE	MANUFACTURER	LOT#	EXP DATE	SITE	ADMIN BY
Rocephin 500 mg	IM	2/5/XX	Roche	1053	10/5/XX	RDG	D. Bennett, CMA (AAMA)
Depo-Provera 150 mg	IM	8/14/XX	Pharmacia & Upjohn	68FUF	12/5/XX	LDG	D. Bennett, CMA (AAMA)
Fluzone 0.5 mL	IM	11/4/XX	Aventis Pasteur	OF1120	6/10/XX	RD	D. Bennett, CMA (AAMA)
Depo-Provera 150 mg	IM	11/4/XX	Pharmacia & Upjohn	87FUF	12/7/XX	RDG	D. Bennett, CMA (AAMA)

Figure 36-2 Medication record.

and maternal-child care. Home health care providers must periodically provide a summary report (Figure 36-4) to the patient's physician that includes the following:

- Observations and evaluations
- Type of care or service provided
- Instructions given to the patient on medications
- Safety measures recommended for the home
- Diet
- Activities permitted

LABORATORY DOCUMENTS

A laboratory report is a report of the analysis or examination of body specimens. Its purpose is to relay the results of laboratory tests to the physician to assist in diagnosing and treating disease. The specific categories of laboratory tests include hematology, clinical chemistry, immunology, urinalysis, microbiology, parasitology, cytology, and histology. A thorough discussion of laboratory documents is presented in Chapter 29.

DIAGNOSTIC PROCEDURE DOCUMENTS

A diagnostic procedure report consists of a narrative description and interpretation of a diagnostic procedure. A **diagnostic procedure** is a type of procedure performed to assist in

the diagnosis, management, or treatment of a patient's condition. The procedure may be performed by a physician, the medical assistant, or a technician specially trained in the procedure. A physician is responsible for interpreting the results of the diagnostic procedure and completing the written report. Examples of diagnostic procedure reports follow.

Electrocardiogram Report

An electrocardiogram (ECG) report is a narrative description of a cardiologist's interpretation of an ECG, including the implications for the patient. The graphic tracing is usually included with the report.

Holter Monitor Report

A Holter monitor report is a narrative description of the interpretation of a 24-hour ambulatory ECG, including the evaluator's impressions. Portions of the graphic tracing are usually included with the report.

Sigmoidoscopy Report

A sigmoidoscopy report is a narrative description of the interpretation of a sigmoidoscopic examination, including the practitioner's impressions.

Colonoscopy Report

A colonoscopy report is a narrative description of a colonoscopic examination, including the practitioner's impressions.

HAROLD B. COOPER, M.D.
6000 MAIN STREET
VENTURA, CA 93003

June 15, 20XX

John F. Millstone, M.D.
5302 Main Street
Ventura, CA 93003

Dear Dr. Millstone:

RE: Elaine J. Silverman

This 69-year-old woman was seen at your request. The patient was admitted to the hospital yesterday because of chills, fever, and abdominal and back pain.

REVIEW OF HEALTH HISTORY: The history has been reviewed. A prominent feature of the history is the presence of intermittent, severe, shaking chills for four days with associated left lower back pain, left lower quadrant abdominal pain, and fever to as high as 103 or 104 degrees. The patient has had hypertension for a number of years and has been managed quite well with Aldomet 250 mg twice a day.

PHYSICAL EXAMINATION: On examination her temperature at this time is 100.6 degrees. The pulse is 110 and regular. Blood pressure is 190/100. The patient has partial bilateral iridectomies, the result of previous cataract surgery. Otherwise, the head and neck are not remarkable. Lung fields are clear throughout. The heart reveals a regular tachycardia, and heart sounds are of good quality. No murmurs are heard, and there is no gallop rhythm present. The abdomen is soft. There is no spasm or guarding. A well-healed surgical scar is present in the right flank area. There is considerable tenderness in the left lower quadrant of the left mid abdomen, but as noted, there is no spasm or guarding present. Bowel sounds are present. Peristaltic rushes are noted, and the bowel sounds are slightly high pitched. The extremities are unremarkable.

IMPRESSIONS: I believe the patient has acute diverticulitis. She may have some irritation of the left ureter in view of the findings on the urinalysis. She appears to be responding to therapy at this time in that her temperature is coming down and there has been a slight reduction in the leukocytosis from yesterday.

RECOMMENDATIONS: I agree with the present program of therapy, and the only suggestion would be to possibly increase the dose of gentamicin to 60 mg q8h, rather than the 40 mg q8h that she is now receiving.

Thank you for asking me to see this patient in consultation.

Sincerely,

Harold B. Cooper

Harold B. Cooper, M.D.

mtf

Figure 36-3 Consultation report.

Form 3514/2 (if 2-part set) or
Form 3514/3 (if 3-part set)

BRIGGS, Des Moines, IA 50306 (800) 247-2343
PRINTED IN U.S.A.

Home Health Agency — Visit Report

| Date of Visit | 11/21/XX | Start: 7 | Mileage Finish: 9 |

Patient's Name Clarence Castor

BP: (L): 160/82   (R): 160/82   T: 97.7

P: (A): 78   (R): 76   Wt.: 151   R: 18

Pt. Instruction: Continue O₂ as needed

Financial:		Med. A:	Med. B:
GH:	VA:	Pvt:	Other: Hospice
Area:		Diagnosis: Lung cancer	
Procedures:			Age: 74

Comments/Observations: (Physical, mental, emotional, activity level, Environ., S/S, Treatments & Effects, Procedures, Med. Effects, Other)

Pt complaining of some difficulty breathing and swelling of his feet. Pt was given Proventil Atrovent neb tx

and started on oxygen at 2 liters per nasal cannula. Tx was discussed with Dr. Shay.

Plan: Monitor vitals every 2 hrs.

Supplies Used: O₂ @ 2 liters

Signature: D. Talley, RN

Next Visit: 11/22/XX	RN ✓	PT	HHA	MSW	Other
Freq. of Visits: daily	✓				
Travel Time:			Service Time:		

Supervisory Visit:

Form 3514 © BRIGGS, Des Moines, IA 50306 (800) 247-2343 PRINTED IN U.S.A.

Figure 36-4 Home health care report.

Spirometry Report

A spirometry report is a narrative and graphic description of the interpretation of a patient's breathing capacity using a spirometer.

Radiology Report

A radiology report is a narrative description of a diagnostic or therapeutic radiologic procedure (Figure 36-5). A radiologist examines the radiograph and provides a written report, which includes a detailed interpretation of the radiograph and his or her impressions. The patient's physician receives a copy of the radiology report; the actual radiographic film or digital images are kept on file in the hospital's radiology department but are available for review by the patient's physician.

Diagnostic Imaging Report

A diagnostic imaging report is a narrative description of a diagnostic imaging procedure (Figure 36-6). The report includes a detailed interpretation of the diagnostic image, along with the practitioner's impressions. Examples of common diagnostic imaging procedures include ultrasonography, computed tomography (CT) scan, and magnetic resonance imaging (MRI). The diagnostic computer image is kept on file at the hospital but is available for review by the patient's physician.

THERAPEUTIC SERVICE DOCUMENTS

A therapeutic service report documents the assessments and treatments designed to restore a patient's ability to function. Examples of therapeutic services that the physician may order follow.

Physical Therapy

Physical therapy involves the use of therapeutic exercise, thermal modalities, cold, hydrotherapy, electrical stimulation, massage, and other physical agents to restore function and promote healing after an illness or injury. A physical therapist might help a football player with a knee injury to regain normal functioning of the knee or assist a patient recovering from a stroke to use his or her legs to walk again. Figure 36-7 shows an example of a physical therapy report.

Occupational Therapy

Occupational therapy helps a patient learn new skills to adapt to a physically, developmentally, emotionally, or mentally disabling condition. This enables the patient to perform activities of daily living and to achieve as much independence as possible. An occupational therapist might help an individual with a physical disability learn how to get dressed and how to prepare meals.

COLLEGE HOSPITAL
4567 BROAD AVENUE
WOODLAND HILLS, MD 21532

RADIOLOGY REPORT

Examination Date:	June 14, 20XX	Patient:	Rose Baker
Date Reported:	June 14, 20XX	X-ray No.:	43200
Physician:	Harold B. Cooper	Age:	19
Examination:	PA Chest, Abdomen	Hospital No.:	80-32-11

FINDINGS

PA CHEST: Upright PA view of chest shows the lung fields are clear, without evidence of an active process. Heart size is normal. There is no evidence of pneumoperitoneum.

IMPRESSION: NEGATIVE CHEST

ABDOMEN: Flat and upright views of the abdomen show a normal gas pattern without evidence of obstruction or ileus. There are no calcifications or abnormal masses noted.

IMPRESSION: NEGATIVE STUDY

RADIOLOGIST: *Marian B. Skinner*

Marian B. Skinner, MD

Figure 36-5 Radiology report.

Speech Therapy

Speech therapy refers to treatment for the correction of a speech impairment resulting from birth, disease, injury, or previous medical treatment.

HOSPITAL DOCUMENTS

Hospital documents are prepared by the physician responsible for the care of a patient while at the hospital; this physician is known as the **attending physician.** The attending physician may be the patient's regular physician or a different physician. An example of the latter is a physician attending a patient at an urgent care center or in the emergency department of a hospital.

Hospital documents are dictated by the attending physician and transcribed at the hospital. The original document is filed in the patient's hospital medical record, and a copy is sent to the patient's regular physician. Hospital documents assist the patient's physician in reviewing the patient's hospital visit and in providing follow-up care.

History and Physical Report

The term **inpatient** refers to a patient who has been admitted to the hospital for at least one overnight stay. A health history must be obtained and a physical examination performed on all inpatients. There is one exception to this: If a patient history and physical examination are performed at the medical office within 1 week before admission, a copy of these documents may be used. In the event that a reliable health history cannot be obtained from the patient, it must be obtained from the person best able to relay the facts.

The history and physical report is a physician's narrative report of the patient's history and physical examination, along with the physician's medical impressions (Figure 36-8). The purpose of the history is to document the patient's current complaints and symptoms, whereas the purpose of the physical examination is to assess the patient's current health status. **Medical impressions,** or simply *impressions,* are conclusions drawn from an interpretation of data. In this case, the physician interprets the data from the health history and physical examination and draws conclusions as to the patient's state of health. Other terms for impressions include *provisional diagnosis* and *tentative diagnosis.*

Operative Report

An operative report (Figure 36-9) must be completed for all patients who have had a surgical procedure. This report describes the surgical procedure and must be completed and signed by the surgeon who performed the operation. The operative report must include the following:
• Patient identification information
• Date and location of the surgery

Text continued on p. 884

DIAGNOSTIC IMAGING REPORT

Mt. Carmel Hospital,
Columbus, OH 43201

DATE REQUESTED	DATE TO BE DONE	TODAY'S DATE	DATE OF BIRTH
6/6/20XX	6/10/20XX	6/10/20XX	8/19/1943

☐ WHEELCHAIR   ☐ PORTABLE   ☒ AMBULATORY   ☐ CART

PATIENT:	INSURANCE:
Vera Ruth	Industrial

SEX	ROOM NO.	RESPONSIBLE PERSON OR EMPLOYER	RADIOLOGIST
F	OP	J.B. Warren, Inc.	Richard W. Adams, MD

CLINICAL INFORMATION AND PROVISIONAL DIAGNOSIS

Back injury

ATTENDING PHYSICIAN
Christopher Robb, MD

NURSE

EXAMINATION REQUESTED (PINPOINT AREA OF CONCERN IF POSSIBLE)
CT LUMBAR SPINE

TECHNIQUE:

CT of the lumbar spine without contrast was performed from L-3 through S-1.

FINDINGS:

The L3-4 level appears satisfactory without evidence of osseous proliferation or disc protrusion.

At the L4-5 level there is some increased density at the disc level, which may be more prominent on the left. This is partially obscured due to facet artifact crossing obliquely.

There does appear to be some retention of epidural fat plane. This, however, may represent left-sided disc bulge or protrusion with the appropriate corresponding clinical appearance. Osseous variation at this level is not identified.

At the L5-S1 level, significant variation is not apparent.

IMPRESSION:

Variation at the L4-5 level on the left, which may represent annular disc bulge or perhaps protrusion on the left. However, confirmation with myelography and/or Ampaque enhanced computed tomography of the lumbar spine should be suggested prior to any surgical intervention.

Richard W. Adams, MD

Richard W. Adams, MD

Figure 36-6 Diagnostic imaging (CT scan) report.

PHYSICAL THERAPY EVALUATION

OBJECTIVE DATA TESTS AND SCALES PRINTED ON REVERSE.

DATE OF SERVICE ___9_ / _23_ / _XX_

HOMEBOUND REASON: ❑ Needs assistance for all activities ❑ Residual weakness
❑ Requires assistance to ambulate   ❑ Confusion, unable to go out of home alone
❑ Unable to safely leave home unassisted ❑ Severe SOB, SOB upon exertion
❑ Dependent upon adaptive device(s)   ❑ Medical restrictions
❑ Other (specify)_____

SOC DATE ___9_ / _23_ / _XX_
(If Initial Evaluation, complete Physical Therapy Care Plan)

PERTINENT BACKGROUND INFORMATION

OTHER DISCIPLINES PROVIDING CARE: ❑ SN ❑ OT ❑ ST ❑ MSW ❑ Aide

MEDICAL HISTORY

❑ Hypertension   ❑ Cancer
❑ Cardiac   ❑ Infection
❑ Diabetes   ❑ Immunosuppressed
❑ Respiratory   ❑ Open wound
❑ Osteoporosis   ❑ Falls with injury
❑ Fractures   ❑ Falls without injury
❑ Other (specify)_____

REASON FOR EVALUATION (Diagnosis/Problem)

Hx Ⓛ knee pain x 5 yrs; little relief c̄ PT
_____
_____
_____
_____
_____

LIVING SITUATION

☒ Capable ❑ Able ❑ Willing caregiver available
❑ Limited caregiver support (ability/willingness)
❑ No caregiver available

HOME SAFETY BARRIERS:
❑ Clutter ❑ Throw rugs ❑ Bath bench/equipment ❑ Needs grab bar
❑ Needs railings ❑ Steps (number/condition)_____
❑ Other (specify)_____
_____

PRIOR LEVEL OF FUNCTION

ADLs:
☒ Independent ❑ Needed assistance ❑ Unable
Equipment used:_____

IN-HOME MOBILITY (gait or wheelchair/scooter):
☒ Independent ❑ Needed assistance ❑ Unable
Equipment used:_____

COMMUNITY MOBILITY (gait or wheelchair/scooter):
❑ Independent ❑ Needed assistance ❑ Unable
Equipment used:_____

BEHAVIOR/MENTAL STATUS

☒ Alert ❑ Oriented ❑ Cooperative ❑ Confused ❑ Memory deficits
❑ Impaired judgement ❑ Other (specify)_____
_____

VITAL SIGNS/CURRENT STATUS

Blood Pressure:_____
Temperature:_____
Pulse:_____
Respirations:_____
O_2 saturation _____% (when ordered): ❑ at rest ❑ with activity
Skin:_____
Edema:_____
Vision: _____glasses_____
Sensation:_____
Communication:_____

PAIN

INTENSITY: 0 1 2 3 4 ⑤ 6 7 8 9 10
LOCATION: _____
AGGRAVATING FACTORS: _____
_____
_____
RELIEVING FACTORS: _____
_____
_____
BEST PAIN GETS: ___2___   **WORST PAIN GETS:** ___8___
ACCEPTABLE LEVEL OF PAIN: _____
CURRENT LEVEL OF PAIN: _____
IMPACT ON THERAPY POC? ❑ None ❑ (describe)_____
_____
_____

Hearing:_____
Posture:_____
Endurance:_____

PATIENT NAME – Last, First, Middle Initial
Johnson, Thomas, J.

ID#

Form 3507P © BRIGGS, Des Moines, IA 50306 (800) 247-2343 www.BriggsCorp.com
305   PRINTED IN U.S.A.

PHYSICAL THERAPY EVALUATION
❑ Continued on Reverse

Figure 36-7 Physical therapy report.

Continued

PHYSICAL THERAPY EVALUATION (Cont'd.)

MUSCLE STRENGTH/FUNCTIONAL ROM EVAL

AREA		STRENGTH		ACTION	ROM	
		Right	Left		Right	Left
UPPER EXTREM.	Shoulder	5	5	Flex/Extend		5
		5	5	Abd./Add.		5
		5	5	Int. Rot./Ext. Rot.		5
	Elbow	5	5	Flex/Extend		5
	Forearm	5	5	Sup./Pron.		5
	Wrist	5	5	Flex/Extend		5
	Fingers	5	5	Flex/Extend		5
LOWER EXTREM.	Hip	5	2 (knee pain)	Flex/Extend		3 (10° to 70°)
		5	3	Abd./Add.		3
		5	3	Int. Rot./Ext. Rot.		4
	Knee	5	2+→3-	Flex/Extend		3
	Ankle	5	3	Plant./Dors.		4
	Foot	5	3	Inver./Ever.		4
SPINE	AREA	STRENGTH		ACTION	ROM	

FUNCTIONAL INDEPENDENCE/BALANCE EVAL

	TASKS	ASSIST SCORE	ASSISTIVE DEVICES/COMMENTS
BED MOBILITY	Roll/Turn	Not assessed	2° surgery
	Sit/Supine	2	Assist to (L) LE
	Scoot/Bridge	2	Uses overhead trapeze
TRANSFERS	Sit/Stand	2	
	Bed/Wheelchair	2	
	Toilet	2	
	Floor	Not assessed	
	Auto	Not assessed	
BALANCE	Static Sitting	5	
	Dynamic Sitting	5	
	Static Standing	3	
	Dynamic Standing	3	
W/C SKILLS	Propulsion	N/A	
	Pressure Reliefs	N/A	
	Foot Rests	N/A	
	Locks	N/A	

MANUAL MUSCLE TEST (MMT) MUSCLE STRENGTH

GRADE	DESCRIPTION
5	Normal functional strength - against gravity - full resistance.
4	Good strength - against gravity with some resistance.
3	Fair strength - against gravity - no resistance - safety compromise.
2	Poor strength - unable to move against gravity.
1	Trace strength - slight muscle contraction - no motion.
0	Zero - no active muscle contraction.

FUNCTIONAL RANGE OF MOTION (ROM) SCALE

GRADE	DESCRIPTION	GRADE	DESCRIPTION
5	100% active functional motion.	2	25% active functional motion.
4	75% active functional motion.	1	Less than 25%.
3	50% active functional motion.		

FUNCTIONAL INDEPENDENCE SCALE (bed mobility, transfers, balance, W/C skills)

GRADE	DESCRIPTION
5	Independent - physically able and independent.
4	Verbal cue (VC) only needed.
3	Stand-by assist (SBA) - 100% patient/client effort.
2	Minimum assist (Min A) - 75% patient/client effort.
1	Maximum assist (Max A) - 25% - 50% patient/client effort.
0	Totally dependent - total care/support.

GAIT

ASSISTANCE: ☐ Independent ☐ SBA ☒ Min. assist ☐ Mod. assist ☐ Max. assist ☐ Unable

SURFACES: ☐ Level ☐ Uneven ☐ Stairs (number/condition)_____ **DISTANCE/TIME:**_____

WEIGHT BEARING STATUS: ☐ FWB ☐ WBAT ☒ PWB ☐ TDWB ☐ NWB

ASSISTIVE DEVICE(S): ☐ Cane ☐ Quad Cane ☐ Crutches ☐ Hemi Walker ☒ Walker ☐ Wheeled Walker
☐ Other (specify)_____

QUALITY/DEVIATIONS/POSTURES: _____

SUMMARY

Instruction provided: ☐ Safety ☐ Exercise ☐ Other (describe)_____

Equipment needed (describe) __Walker_____

☐ PT Evaluation only. No further indications for PT services.

☐ Orders for PT evaluation only. Needs additional PT services. See PT Care Plan for recommendations.

☐ Need to obtain orders.

☐ Orders for PT services with specific treatments, frequency and duration. See PT Care Plan/485.

DISCHARGE DISCUSSED WITH: ☒ Patient/Family

☐ Care Manager ☐ Physician ☐ Other (specify)_____

CARE COORDINATION: ☐ Physician ☐ SN ☐ PT ☐ OT ☐ ST ☐ MSW

☐ Aide ☐ Other (specify)_____

APPROXIMATE NEXT VISIT DATE_____/_____/_____

PLAN FOR NEXT VISIT_____

PATIENT SIGNATURE (if applicable) _Thomas Johnson J._____

THERAPIST'S SIGNATURE/TITLE_ _Michael Howe, MD_____

DATE _9_/_23_/_XX_ **TIME IN**_____ **TIME OUT**_____

Figure 36-7, cont'd

HISTORY AND PHYSICAL
ST. MERCY HOSPITAL

Patient Name: Carol Jacobs   Room #: 215

Physician: Charles Thomas, MD   Hospital #: 5422

Admission Date: 12/14/XX

CHIEF COMPLAINT: Chest pain

HISTORY OF PRESENT ILLNESS: Patient is an 85-year-old female complaining of chest pain. Patient was found to have abnormal cardiac enzymes in the Emergency Room consistent with acute myocardial infarction. Patient denied any pain radiating; however, she did complain of left-sided chest pain and lower back pain. Patient did not admit to any shortness of breath, nausea, or diaphoresis.

MEDICATIONS: Lasix, Darvocet-N 100, Lisinopril, Lopressor, Glynase, Relafen, Cytotec, and Micro K.

ALLERGIES: No drug allergies known.

PAST MEDICAL HISTORY: Significant for congestive heart failure, chronic obstructive pulmonary disease, diabetes mellitus type 2, coronary atherosclerosis, hypertension, and osteoporosis.

SOCIAL HISTORY: Not a drinker and not a smoker. Patient resides in a nursing home.

PHYSICAL EXAMINATION:

General: Patient is in acute distress. She is obese.

HEENT: She has 2 centimeters jugular venous distention. Pupils are equal and reactive to light and accommodation. No evidence of scleral or conjunctival icterus.

Chest: +2 bibasilar rales.

Heart: Regular rate and rhythm. +2/6 systolic ejection murmur in the left sternal border.

Abdomen: Soft, nontender, no splenomegaly and no hepatomegaly and positive bowel sounds.

Extremities: No evidence of edema or deep venous thrombosis.

Neurological: Cranial nerves II through XII grossly intact.

IMPRESSIONS: Congestive heart failure
Rule out myocardial infarction

Charles Thomas, MD

Charles Thomas, MD

Figure 36-8 Hospital history and physical examination report.

OPERATIVE REPORT
ST. MARY'S HOSPITAL

Name: _Natalie Boyer_

Hospital #: _291734_   Room #: _OP_

Surgeon: _Paul Cain, M.D._   Date of Surgery: _1/6/XX_

Anesthesiologist: _John Adams, M.D._   Anesthesia: _General_

PRE-OP DIAGNOSIS: Abnormal Pap test with history of cervical carcinoma.

POST-OP DIAGNOSIS: Same and awaiting path report.

OPERATION: D&C, laser cone of the cervix.

PROCEDURE: The patient to the operating room, lithotomy position, perineum and vagina were prepped, and moist sterile drape was used. Laser precautions all in place. Bimanual examination revealed a uterus enlarged with a second-degree uterine prolapse. The cervix was dilated. Uterus sounded to around 9 cm. The endocervical canal was dilated and D&C was performed with tissue recovered and submitted to Pathology. The cervix was stained with iodine, and the nonstaining area was identified. The laser was brought in, 50 watts of current were used to remove laser cone, and we submitted that to Pathology. We then vaporized beyond the margins of the cone, 3-4 mm to a depth of 4-5 mm. Hemostasis was adequate. We placed 0 Vicryl figure-of-eight sutures at the 3 and the 9 o'clock positions in the cervix, and then we put Monsel solution on the cervix. Hemostasis adequate. Sponge and needle counts correct times two. The patient tolerated the procedure well, and she returned to the recovery room in stable condition. She will be discharged home when awake and stable on Cipro 250 mg twice a day for a week, Darvocet-N 100, #20 as needed for pain. If she continues to have abnormal Pap tests, we will probably want to do a vaginal hysterectomy.

SURGEON: _Paul Cain, MD_

Paul Cain, MD

Figure 36-9 Operative report.

- Names of primary surgeon and assistants
- Preoperative diagnosis
- Name of the surgical procedure
- Full description of the findings at surgery (normal and abnormal)
- Description of the technique and procedures used during surgery
- Ligatures and sutures used
- Numbers of packs, drains, and sponges used
- Description of any specimens removed
- Condition of the patient at the completion of surgery
- Postoperative diagnosis
- Instructions for follow-up care

Discharge Summary Report

The **discharge summary report** is a brief (usually one-page) summary of the significant events of a patient's hospitalization (Figure 36-10). The report must be completed and signed by the attending physician. The discharge summary report includes a concise account of the patient's illness, course of treatment, and response to treatment, as well as the condition of the patient at the time of discharge from the hospital. The purpose of this report is to document information needed by the patient's physician to provide for the continuity of future care. It also is used to respond to authorized requests for information regarding the patient's hospitalization. The discharge summary report must include the following:

- Patient identification information
- Dates of hospitalization
- Reason for the hospitalization (provisional diagnosis)
- Brief health history
- Significant findings from examinations and tests
- Course of treatment
- Response to treatment
- Condition of the patient at discharge
- Discharge diagnosis (final diagnosis)
- Prognosis

DISCHARGE SUMMARY

Brennan, Susan
97-32-11
June 18, 20XX

ADMISSION DATE: June 14, 20XX   DISCHARGE DATE: June 16, 20XX

HISTORY OF PRESENT ILLNESS:
This 19-year-old female, nulligravida, was admitted to the hospital on June 14, 20XX, with fever of 102°, left lower quadrant pain, vaginal discharge, constipation, and a tender left adnexal mass. Her past history and family history were unremarkable. Present pain had started two to three weeks prior to admission. Her periods were irregular, with latest period starting on May 30, 20XX, and lasting for six days. She had taken contraceptive pills in the past but had stopped because she was not sexually active.

PHYSICAL EXAMINATION:
She appeared well developed and well nourished, and in mild distress. The only positive physical findings were limited to the abdomen and pelvis. Her abdomen was mildly distended, and it was tender, especially in the left lower quadrant. At pelvic examination, her cervix was tender on motion, and the uterus was of normal size, retroverted, and somewhat fixed. There was a tender cystic mass about 4-5 cm in the left adnexa. Rectal examination was negative.

PROVISIONAL DIAGNOSIS:
1. Probable pelvic inflammatory disease (PID).
2. Rule out ectopic pregnancy.

LABORATORY DATA ON ADMISSION:
Hgb 10.8, Hct 36.5, WBC 8,100 with 80 segs and 18 lymphs. Sedimentation rate 100 mm in one hour. Sickle cell prep+ (turned out to be a trait). Urinalysis normal. Electrolytes normal. SMA-12 normal. Chest x-ray negative, 2-hour UCG negative.

HOSPITAL COURSE AND TREATMENT:
Initially, she was given cephalothin 2 gm IV q6h, and kanamycin 0.5 gm IM bid. Over the next two days the patient's condition improved. Her pain decreased and her temperature came down to normal in the morning and spiked to 101° in the evening. Repeat CBC showed Hgb 9.8, Hct 33.5. The pregnancy test was negative. She was discharged on June 16, 20XX in good condition. She will be seen in the office in one week.

DISCHARGE DIAGNOSIS:
Pelvic inflammatory disease.

Harold B. Cooper, MD
Harold B. Cooper, MD

Figure 36-10 Discharge summary report.

- Discharge instructions
- Recommendations and arrangements for follow-up care

Pathology Report

A pathology report consists of a macroscopic (gross) and a microscopic description of tissue removed from a patient during surgery or a diagnostic procedure. The macroscopic description includes information about the size, shape, and appearance of the specimen as it appears to the naked eye.

The report also includes a diagnosis of the patient's condition (Figure 36-11). A pathologist is required to examine the tissue specimen, complete the report, and sign it.

Emergency Department Report

The emergency department report is a record of the significant information obtained during an emergency department visit (Figure 36-12). The report is prepared and signed by the emergency department physician, and a copy is sent

COLLEGE HOSPITAL
4567 BROAD AVENUE
WOODLAND HILLS, MD 21532

PATHOLOGY REPORT

Date:	June 20, 20XX	Pathology No.:	430211
Patient:	Molly Ramsdale	Room No.:	1308
Physician:	Harold B. Cooper, M.D.		
Specimen Submitted:	Tumor, right axilla		

FINDINGS

GROSS DESCRIPTION: Specimen A consists of an oval mass of yellow fibroadipose tissue measuring 4 x 3 x 2 cm. On cut section, there are some small, soft, pliable areas of gray apparent lymph node alternating with adipose tissue. A frozen section consultation at time of surgery was delivered as NO EVIDENCE OF MALIGNANCY on frozen section, to await permanent section for final diagnosis. Majority of the specimen will be submitted for microscopic examination.

Specimen B consists of an oval mass of yellow soft tissue measuring 2.5 x 2.5 x 1.5 cm. On cut section, there is a thin rim of pink to tan-brown lymphatic tissue and the mid portion appears to be adipose tissue. A pathological consultation at time of surgery was delivered as no suspicious areas noted and to await permanent sections for final diagnosis. The entire specimen will be submitted for microscopic examination.

MICROSCOPIC DESCRIPTION: Specimen A sections show fibroadipose tissue and nine fragments of lymph nodes. The lymph nodes show areas with prominent germinal centers and moderate sinus histiocytosis. There appears to be some increased vascularity and reactive endothelial cells seen. There is no evidence of malignancy.

Specimen B sections show adipose tissue and 5 lymph node fragments. These 5 portions of lymph nodes show reactive changes including sinus histiocytosis. There is no evidence of malignancy.

DIAGNOSIS: A & B: TUMOR, RIGHT AXILLA: SHOWING 14 LYMPH NODE FRAGMENTS WITH REACTIVE CHANGES AND NO EVIDENCE OF MALIGNANCY.

Stanley T. Nason, MD

_____
Stanley T. Nason, MD

Figure 36-11 Pathology report.

EMERGENCY DEPARTMENT REPORT
CAMDEN CLARK HOSPITAL

Name: John Larimer   DOB: 2/2/68

ER Physician: John Parsons, MD   Date: 7/7/XX

ER Number: 07398

Physician: James Woods, MD

NATURE OF ILLNESS/INJURY: This 40-year-old male presents to the Emergency Department complaining of a laceration of the sole of his right foot. Patient cut his foot on a rock 2 days ago and thinks he might have an infection now. Patient also complains of coughing over the past several days.

PHYSICAL EXAMINATION: Temperature 97.4, Pulse 76, Respirations 20, Blood Pressure 120/70. Patient is alert and oriented and is in no acute distress. ENT is normal. Lungs show diffuse rhonchi without crackles or wheezing. Heart has a regular rate and rhythm. Right great toe with marked tenderness with edema and erythema and heat.

DIAGNOSIS: Asthmatic Bronchitis
        Cellulitis, right foot first MTP

TREATMENT: PCMX scrub to right foot. Bacitracin dressing. Tetanus Diphtheria 0.5 cc IM. Biaxin 500 mg bid x 10 days. Guaifenesin with codeine 2 tsp q4h prn. Entex LA,1 bid prn. Debridement of skin flap.

PATIENT INSTRUCTIONS: Patient to follow up with family doctor in 7 days. Discussed bronchospasms with the patient.

James Woods, MD
_____
James Woods, MD

Figure 36-12 Emergency department report.

to the patient's family physician for the purpose of providing follow-up care. The emergency department report includes the following:

- Date of service
- Patient identification information
- Nature of the illness or injury
- Laboratory or diagnostic test results
- Procedures performed
- Treatment rendered
- Diagnosis
- Condition of the patient at discharge
- Instructions regarding follow-up care

CONSENT DOCUMENTS

Consent forms are legal documents required to perform certain procedures or to release information contained in the patient's medical record.

Consent to Treatment Form

Completion of a consent to treatment form (Procedure 36-1) is required for all surgical operations and nonroutine therapeutic and diagnostic procedures (e.g., sigmoidoscopy)

performed in the medical office. The form must be signed by the patient or his or her legally authorized representative and must provide written evidence that the patient agrees to the procedure or procedures listed on the form (Figure 36-13).

For the patient's consent to be valid, it must be informed consent. **Informed consent** means that the patient has received the following information before giving consent:

- The nature of the patient's condition
- The nature and purpose of the recommended procedure
- An explanation of risks involved with the procedure
- Alternative treatments or procedures available
- The likely outcome (**prognosis**) of the procedure
- The risks of declining or delaying the procedure

The explanation must be given in terms the patient can understand, and the patient should be given an opportunity to ask questions regarding the information.

The consent to treatment form should not be signed until the patient has been provided with all necessary information related to the procedure. The patient's signature must be witnessed; this is usually the responsibility of the medical assistant. *Witnessing a signature* means only that the

Figure 36-13 Consent to treatment form.

medical assistant verified the patient's identity and watched the patient sign the form; it *does not* mean that the medical assistant is attesting to the accuracy of the information provided.

The consent to treatment form outlines the details of the discussion with the patient and includes the following information:
• The patient's full name
• Name of the procedure to be performed
• Name of the surgeon
• A statement indicating that the patient agrees to receive the procedure
• Acknowledgment that a disclosure of information has been made
• Acknowledgment that all questions were answered in a satisfactory manner
• A statement that no guarantee as to the outcome has been made
• Signature of the patient or his or her legal representative
• Signature of the witness

Release of Medical Information Form

As previously explained in the box entitled *Highlight on the HIPAA Privacy Rule,* a patient's written consent is not required for the use or disclosure of protected health information (PHI) for the purpose of medical treatment, payment, and health care operations (TPO). If a request for protected health information is required for purposes that are not part of TPO, however, a detailed form must be completed, known as a *release of medical information form* (Figure 36-14). If a patient is moving to another state and wants to transfer his or her medical record to a new physician, a release of medical information form must be completed.

The release of medical information form must be signed by the patient authorizing the disclosure of his or her PHI (Procedure 36-2). If the patient is a minor, the form must be signed by the parent or legal guardian of the minor. The release of medical information form must stipulate the following:
• The patient's full name and address
• Name of the medical practice releasing the information
• Name of the individual or facility to receive the information
• Specific information to be released
• The purpose of or the need for the information
• Method of release of the information
• Signature of the patient or his or her legal representative

RELEASE OF MEDICAL INFORMATION

All information contained in the medical record is confidential, and the release of information is closely controlled. A properly completed and signed authorization form is required for the release of the following information.

PATIENT INFORMATION

Patient Name _____

Address _____ Social Security # _____

City _____ State _____ ZIP _____ Birth date _____/_____/_____

Phone (Home) _____ Work _____

RELEASE FROM:

Name _____

Address _____

City _____ State _____ ZIP _____

RELEASE TO:

Name _____

Address _____

City _____ State _____ ZIP _____

INFORMATION TO BE RELEASED:

1. GENERAL RELEASE:

____Entire Medical Record (excluding protected information)

____Hospital Records only (specify)_____

____Lab Results only (specify) _____

____X-ray Reports only (specify) _____

____Other Records (specify) _____

2. INFORMATION PROTECTED BY STATE/FEDERAL LAW:
If indicated below, I hereby authorize the disclosure and release of information regarding:

____Drug Abuse Diagnosis/Treatment

____Alcoholism Diagnosis/Treatment

____Mental Health Diagnosis/Treatment

____Sexually Transmitted Disease

PURPOSE/NEED FOR INFORMATION:

____Taking records to another doctor

____Moving

____Legal purposes

____Insurance purposes

____Worker's Compensation

____Other/Explain:_____

METHOD OF RELEASE:

____ US Mail

____ Fax

____ Telephone

____ To Patient

PATIENT AUTHORIZATION TO RELEASE INFORMATION:

Authorization is valid for 60 days only from the date of my signature. I reserve the right to revoke this authorization at any time prior to 60 days (except for action that has already been taken) by notifying the medical office in writing.

I understand that my records are protected under HIPAA (Health Insurance Portability and Accountability Act) Standards for Privacy of Individually Identifiable Information (45 CFR Parts 160 and 164) unless otherwise permitted by federal law. Any information released or received shall not be further relayed to any other facility or person without my written authorization. I also understand that such information will not be given, sold, transferred, or in any way relayed to any other person or party not specified above without my further written authorization.

I hereby grant authorization to release the information listed above. I certify that this request has been made voluntarily and that the information given above is accurate to the best of my knowledge.

_____   _____

Signature of Patient/Legally Responsible Party   Date

_____   _____

Witness Signature   Date

OFFICE USE ONLY

Information indicated above released on _____
                                        Date

Explanation of information released: _____

_____

Signature and credentials of individual releasing information: _____

Figure 36-14 Release of medical information form.

- Date that the consent was signed
- Expiration date of the consent form

Mailed or Faxed Requests for Release of Medical Information

Most medical offices require that the patient come to the office to sign the release of medical information form; however, this may not always be possible. An example is a patient who has moved away and is requesting the transfer of his or her medical records to a new physician. In this instance, a completed and signed release of medical information form may be mailed or faxed to the medical office. The procedure for processing this type of request is outlined at the end of Procedure 36-2.

PROCEDURE 36-1 Completion of a Consent to Treatment Form

Outcome Complete a consent to treatment form.

Equipment/Supplies

- Consent to treatment form

1. **Procedural Step.** Type or print all required information on the consent to treatment form in the spaces provided (e.g., patient's full name, name of the procedure to be performed).
2. **Procedural Step.** Ensure that the physician has had a discussion to give the patient complete information about the procedure to be performed.
   Principle. For the patient's consent to be valid, it must be informed consent.
3. **Procedural Step.** Greet the patient and introduce yourself. Identify the patient by his or her full name and date of birth. Explain to the patient the purpose of the consent form.
4. **Procedural Step.** Give the consent form to the patient and ask him or her to read it. Ask the patient whether he or she has any questions.

5. **Procedural Step.** Ask the patient to sign the consent form. Witness the patient's signature by signing your name in the appropriate space on the form. Include today's date.
   Principle. Witnessing a signature means only that the medical assistant verified the identity of the patient and watched the patient sign the form; it does not mean that the medical assistant is attesting to the accuracy of the information provided.

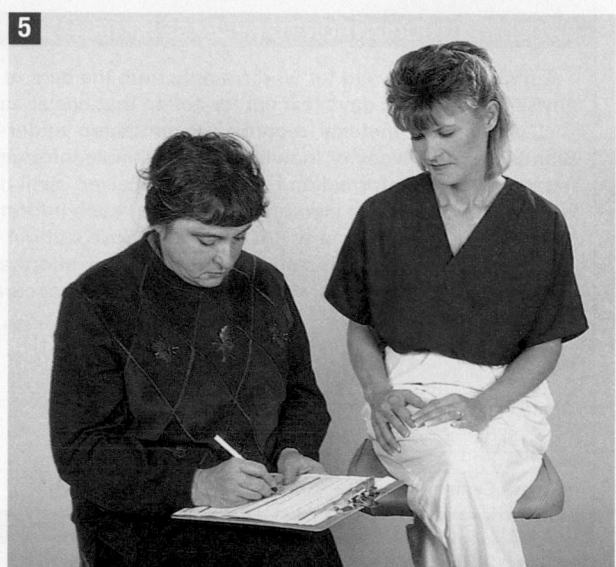

Ask the patient to sign the consent form.

6. **Procedural Step.** Provide the patient with a copy of the completed consent form for his or her files.
7. **Procedural Step.** File the original consent to treatment form in the patient's medical record.
   Principle. Maintaining the form provides legal documentation that the patient gave permission for treatment.

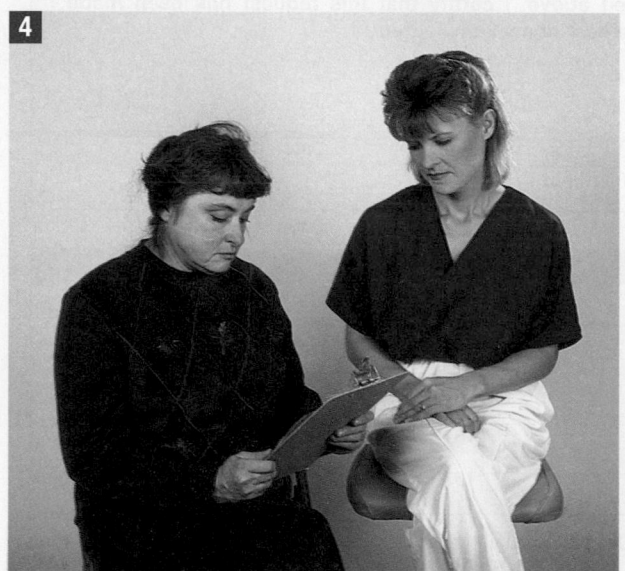

Ask the patient to read the consent form.

PROCEDURE 36-2   Release of Medical Information

Outcome

1. Assist a patient in the completion of a release of medical information form.
2. Release medical information according to a completed release of medical information form.

Equipment/Supplies

- Release of medical information form

1. Procedural Step. Greet the patient and introduce yourself. Identify the patient by his or her full name and date of birth. Explain the purpose of the release of medical information form. (*NOTE:* If you do not recognize the patient, ask him or her to provide photo identification such as a driver's license.)

2. Procedural Step. Provide the patient with a release of medical information form, and ask the patient to complete the form. Provide assistance if needed.
Principle. Information from a patient's medical record can be released only on written authorization of the patient (except when permitted by law).

3. Procedural Step. Check to ensure that all information requested on the form has been completed by the patient.

4. Procedural Step. Ask the patient to sign the form. Witness the patient's signature by signing your name in the appropriate space on the form. Include today's date. If required by your medical office policy, ask the physician to initial the completed release of medical information form.
Principle. For information to be released, the form must be signed by the patient authorizing the disclosure of medical information.

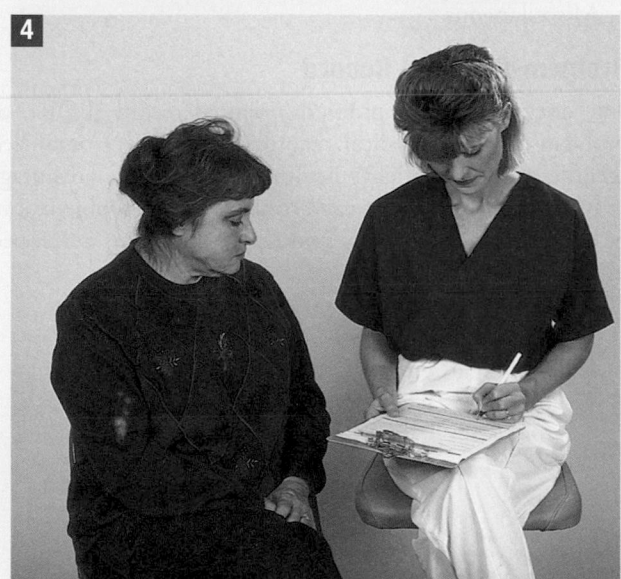

Witness the patient's signature.

Procedural Step. Provide the patient with a copy of the release of medical information form for his or her files.

5. Procedural Step. Copy the information requested on the form. Release only the information requested. Include a copy of the completed release form with the medical information.

6. Procedural Step. Document what information is being released and the date of its release on the appropriate space on the release of information form. Sign the release of information form with your name and credentials verifying you were the individual releasing the information.

7. Procedural Step. File the original document and the release of medical information form in the patient's medical record.
Principle. Maintaining the release form provides legal documentation that the patient gave permission for the release of his or her medical information.

8. Procedural Step. Send the medical information to the appropriate site according to your medical office policy.

Mailed or Faxed Requests for Release of Medical Information

These steps should be followed when a completed release of medical information form has been mailed or faxed to the medical office:

1. Procedural Step. Check the expiration date on the release of medical information form. If the authorization is outdated, a new release form needs to be completed.

2. Procedural Step. Verify the authenticity of the signature on the form. This can be accomplished by comparing the patient's signature on the form with the patient's signature in his or her medical record. If you have any doubt as to the authenticity of the signature, do not release the records.

3. Procedural Step. Copy the information requested on the form. Release only the information requested. Include a copy of the completed release form with the medical information.

4. Procedural Step. Document what information is being released and the date of its release. Sign the document with your name and credentials.

5. Procedural Step. File the original document and the release of medical information form in the patient's medical record.

6. Procedural Step. Send the medical information according to your medical office policy.

TYPES OF MEDICAL RECORDS

Medical offices may rely on the use of paper medical records, known as **paper-based patient records (PPRs).** Although most of the medical record is paper based, some patient data are maintained on the computer; these include patient registration information and patient charges and payments. As technology advances, more and more offices are converting to an **electronic medical record (EMR)** for maintaining patient health information. With an electronic medical record, the entire record is stored in a database on the computer, including the health history report and physical examination report, progress notes, laboratory and diagnostic reports, and hospital reports. The electronic medical record is discussed further in the next section and in Chapters 38 and 41, whereas the remainder of this chapter focuses on the paper-based patient record.

Electronic Medical Record

The electronic medical record is a computerized record of the important health information regarding a patient, including the care of that individual and the progress of the patient's condition. Making the transition to an EMR is a major undertaking for a medical office. Medical offices are gradually moving toward the EMR. Approximately 51% of the medical offices in the United States have converted to an EMR and this percentage is expected to increase over time. The biggest deterrent is the financial and time investment required for a medical office to make the conversion to the EMR.

EMR software allows for the creation, storage, organization, editing, and retrieval of medical records on a computer. The EMR software is usually linked to the practice management software. This allows the EMR to communicate with the practice management software and facilitates certain administrative tasks such as billing and insurance. Refer to Chapter 38 for a detailed discussion of the electronic medical record.

MEDICAL RECORD FORMATS

The way a medical record is organized is known as its *format.* The two main types of **medical record formats** are the *source-oriented record* and the *problem-oriented record.* Each of these formats is described.

Source-Oriented Record

The source-oriented format is used most often in the medical office for organizing a medical record. The documents in a source-oriented record are organized into sections based on the department, facility, or other source that generated the information (e.g., laboratory, hospital, consultant). Because documents from each source are filed together, it is easy to compare information from laboratory and diagnostic test results, assessments, and treatments.

Each section in a source-oriented record is separated from the other sections by a chart divider. Attached to each divider is a color-coded tab labeled with the title of its section (Figure 36-15). Within each of these sections, the documents are arranged according to date. Most offices use reverse chronological order to arrange the documents. **Reverse chronological order** means that the most recent document is placed on top or in front of the others, and thus the oldest document is on the bottom or at the end of that section.

The titles that identify each section vary depending on the medical office's preference; however, typical examples include the following:

- History and physical
- Progress notes
- Medications
- Laboratory reports
- ECG
- X-ray reports
- Consultations
- Rehabilitation therapy
- Home health care
- Hospital reports
- Insurance
- Consents
- Correspondence
- Miscellaneous

Problem-Oriented Record

The documents in a problem-oriented record (POR), or problem-oriented medical record (POMR), are organized according to the patient's health problems. The advantage of using the POR is that each of the patient's problems can be defined and followed individually. The POR is developed in four stages:

1. Establishing a *database*
2. Compiling a *problem list*
3. Devising a *plan* of action for each problem
4. Following each problem with *progress notes*

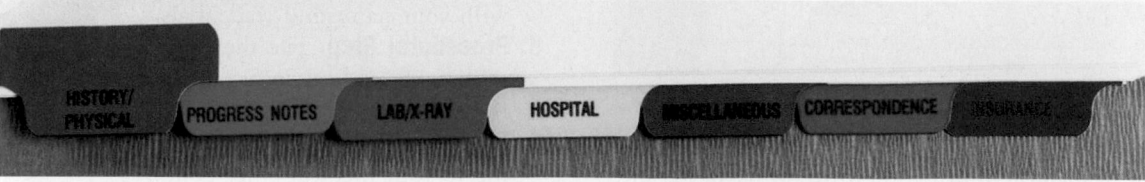

Figure 36-15 Chart dividers in a source-oriented record.

What Would You Do? What Would You *Not* Do?

Case Study 2

Tessa Walsh, her husband, and their two children are moving to another state. They will be leaving in 2 days. Tessa calls the office to have their medical records transferred to their new physician. Tessa's daughter has type 1 diabetes, so it is important that this be done as soon as possible. Tessa is quite annoyed to learn that she has to come in and sign a special form. She says that their medical records belong to them. Tessa says that the whole family has been coming there for the past 8 years and is well known by the physician and staff. She says that they have been good patients, have followed the physician's advice, and have always paid their bills on time. Tessa thinks that verbal permission should be enough. She's extremely busy packing and taking care of other moving details and doesn't have a minute to spare. ■

Database

The first step in developing a POR is to establish a database. The database consists of a collection of subjective and objective data. These data include the health history report, the physical examination report, and results of baseline laboratory and diagnostic tests. The information in the database is used to identify and compile a problem list.

Problem List

The problem list is developed shortly after the database is completed and consists of a list of all of the patient's problems (Figure 36-16). A **problem** is defined as any patient condition that requires observation, diagnosis, management, or patient education. This includes not only medical problems but also psychological and social problems. The problem list is a crucial part of the POR and is always located in the front of the medical record.

The problem list should be thought of as a table of contents for the record. Each problem in the list is numbered and titled. The problem title is stated as a diagnosis, a physiologic finding, a symptom, or an abnormal test result. All subsequent data (plans and progress notes) added to the medical record are cross-referenced to these numbered problems.

The problem list is modified as needed. If a new problem is identified, it is added to the list and dated accordingly. When a problem is resolved, it is marked as such, and the date is recorded.

Plan

After examining the problem list, the physician develops the third section of the POR. This involves devising a plan of action for further evaluation and treatment of each problem. Each plan begins with a heading that identifies the number of the problem, followed by the plan of action for the problem. This may include plans for laboratory and diagnostic tests, medical or surgical treatment, therapy, and patient education.

Progress Notes

The last stage in the development of the POR is the follow-up for each problem, or the progress notes (Figure 36-17). The progress notes begin with the number of the problem and include the following four categories:

1. *Subjective data:* Subjective data obtained from the patient

2. *Objective data:* Objective data obtained by observation, physical examination, and laboratory and diagnostic tests
3. *Assessment:* The physician's interpretation of the current condition based on analysis of the subjective and objective data
4. *Plan:* Proposed treatment for the patient

The acronym for this process is **SOAP,** and the writing of progress notes in this format is called *soaping.* Some physicians who use the source-oriented format have found it advantageous to record progress notes in SOAP format. This structured type of note increases the physician's ability to deal with each problem clearly and to analyze data in an orderly, systematic manner.

PREPARING A MEDICAL RECORD FOR A NEW PATIENT

When a patient comes to the medical office for his or her first visit, a medical record must be prepared for that patient (Procedure 36-3). The method used to prepare the record depends on the following criteria: the format used to organize the record, the filing system, and the type of storage equipment. Most medical offices use the source-oriented format to organize their medical records, the alphabetic filing system to arrange the records, and shelf filing units to store the medical records. Methods used to prepare a medical record are described in the following sections and are based on these criteria.

Medical Record Supplies

Certain supplies are required to prepare a medical record. These supplies are categorized and described next.

File Folders

A file folder is a protective cover made of a heavy material such as manila card stock. A file folder is used to hold medical record documents in an organized format. Flexible metal fasteners are typically used to hold documents in the folder. Folders are available with fasteners located on the top or left side of the folder.

Folders are available with tabs. A tab is a projection extending from a folder that is used to identify its contents.

PATIENT RECORD

Name	Morani, Betty			ALLERGIES/SENSITIVITY		
Number		Blood Type:	A+	Codeine, Sulfa		

Prob. No.	Date	PROBLEM DESCRIPTION	Date Resolved	Index	Prob. No.	Date	PROBLEM DESCRIPTION	Date Resolved	Index
1	10/XX	Hypertension - essential		✓					
2	10/XX	Diabetes mellitus (mild)		✓					
3	1/XX	L. Retinopathy	see below						
4	4/20XX	Atherosclerosis with cerebral vascular insuffic.							
5	4/20XX	Hearing loss							
6	1/20XX	HBP Non-compliance	2/XX						
3	1/20XX	Bilat. Grade II Retinopathy							

Prob. No.	CONTINUING MEDICATIONS	Start	Stop	Prob. No.	CONTINUING MEDICATIONS	Start	Stop
1	Sinoserp 1 mg. b.i.d.	10/XX	10/XX				
2	Orinase 0.5 gm. daily	10/XX	10/XX				
1	Hydrodiuril 50 mg. A.M.	10/XX					
2	1500 cal. diet low Na hi K	2/20XX					

Periodic Health Examination	Dates	1/04	4/2006						

Figure 36-16 POR problem list.

The tab is located on either the side or the top of the folder. A folder with a tab extending across its entire side or top is called a *full cut tab*.

In the medical office, a file folder with a full cut side tab is typically used to prepare a new patient's chart. There are indentations at intervals along the full cut tab to indicate the placement of adhesive labels. This ensures that the labels on all medical records are affixed at the same place on the file folders.

Folder Labels

Labels to identify the medical record are commercially available on $8\frac{1}{2} \times 11$-inch sheets for use with a computer and printer. The types of labels most commonly used in the medical office include name labels, alphabetic color-coded labels, color-coded year labels, and miscellaneous chart labels.

Chart Dividers

Chart dividers are used to identify each section of the medical record by subject (see Figure 36-15). Chart dividers consist of a heavy material such as manila card stock. Attached to each divider is a color-coded tab labeled with a subject title; the most frequently used subject titles are illustrated in the accompanying box, along with the documents typically filed under each title.

PROBLEM ORIENTED - PROGRESS NOTES

Date	Time	Problem Number	FORMAT: Problem Number and TITLE: S = Subjective O = Objective A = Assessment P = Plan
11/15/XX	9:30 AM	1	S: Mother states that her child has had a runny nose and her throat has been sore for 2 days.
			O: Vital signs: T 98.8 P 96 R 24
			Weight: 42 lb.
			General: alert and active. HEENT: sclera clear. TMs negative. Positive clear rhinorrhea. Pharynx benign. Heart: regular without murmur.
			Lungs: clear to auscultation and percussion. Abdomen: negative tenderness. Positive bowel × 4. GU: negative. Neuro: good tone.
			A: Upper respiratory tract infection.
			P: 1. A prescription for Rondec DM, 1/2 tsp q6h prn cough and congestion.
			2. Instructed mother to contact office if child does not improve.

NAME–Last	First	Middle	Attending Physician	Record No.	Room/Bed
Michaels	Jessica	L	Frank Edwards, MD	1	24

Form 653/2S © BRIGGS, Des Moines, IA 50306 (800) 247-2343 www.BriggsCorp.com
R404   PRINTED IN U.S.A.

PROBLEM ORIENTED - PROGRESS NOTES

Figure 36-17 POR SOAP progress notes.

Continued

PROBLEM ORIENTED - PROGRESS NOTES

Date	Time	Problem Number	FORMAT: Problem Number and TITLE: S = Subjective O = Objective A = Assessment P = Plan

NAME–Last	First	Middle	Attending Physician	Record No.	Room/Bed
Michaels	Jessica	L	Frank Edwards, MD	1	24

PROBLEM ORIENTED - PROGRESS NOTES

Figure 36-17, cont'd

PROCEDURE 36-3

Outcome Prepare a medical record.
The following procedure outlines the method for preparing a medical record for a new patient using the following organization: a source-oriented format stored in shelf files using a color-coded alphabetic filing system.

Equipment/Supplies

- Patient registration form
- Notice of Privacy Practices (NPP)
- NPP acknowledgment form
- File folder with a full cut side tab
- Metal fasteners
- Name labels
- Color-coded alphabetic bar labels
- Miscellaneous chart labels
- Set of chart dividers
- Blank preprinted forms
- Two-hole punch

1. **Procedural Step.** Greet the patient when he or she arrives at the medical office. Introduce yourself and identify the patient. Verify that the patient is a new patient.
2. **Procedural Step.** Ask the patient to do the following:
   a. Complete a patient registration form.
   b. Read a Notice of Privacy Practices (NPP).
   c. Sign an NPP acknowledgment form.
3. **Procedural Step.** When the patient returns the completed forms, check the patient registration form for accuracy, and make sure that you can read the patient's handwriting. If you have any questions regarding the information on the form, ask the patient for clarification. If required by the medical office policy, ask the patient for his or her insurance card and make a copy of it.
   Principle. A copy of the patient's insurance card is used for third-party billing.
4. **Procedural Step.** Enter into the computer the data on the completed registration record.
5. **Procedural Step.** Assemble supplies needed to prepare the medical record. Enter the patient's full name into the computer for printing on a name label while following these guidelines:
   a. Enter the patient's name in transposed order as follows: last name, first name, middle name (or initial).
   b. Enter the patient's name two or three spaces from the left edge of the label and one line down from the top of the label.
   c. Ensure that the patient's name is spelled correctly.
   Principle. Following these guidelines facilitates the accurate and efficient filing of the patient's medical record.
6. **Procedural Step.** Determine the first two letters of the patient's last name and select the appropriate alphabetic color-coded labels. Attach the color-coded labels to the (full cut) side tab. The labels should be affixed to the folder using the label placement indentations on the tab.
   Principle. Using the label placement indentations ensures that all labels on medical records are affixed at the same place.
7. **Procedural Step.** Affix the name label immediately above the first color-coded alphabetic label.

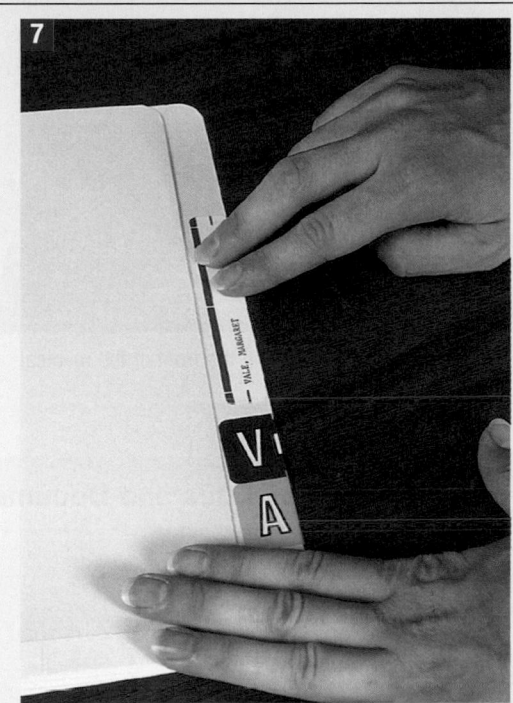

Affix the name label.

8. **Procedural Step.** Attach any additional chart labels, such as a year label and miscellaneous chart labels (e.g., allergy, insurance), to the folder according to the office policy.
9. **Procedural Step.** Insert the chart dividers onto the metal fasteners of the file folder.

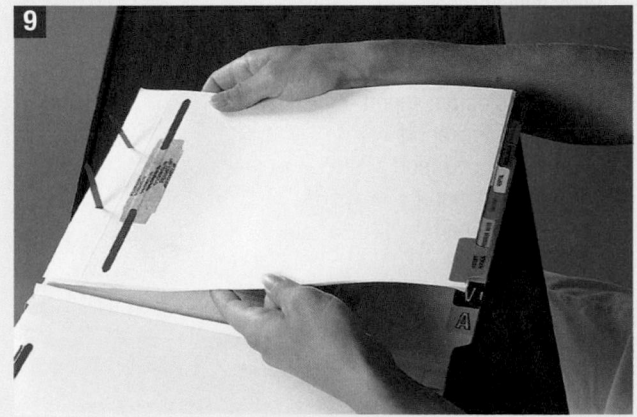

Insert the chart dividers into the metal fasteners.

Continued

PROCEDURE 36-3   Preparing a Medical Record—cont'd

10. Procedural Step. Place the original patient registration form in the front of the medical record. Place the signed NPP acknowledgment form and the copy of the patient's insurance card in the appropriate section of the record.

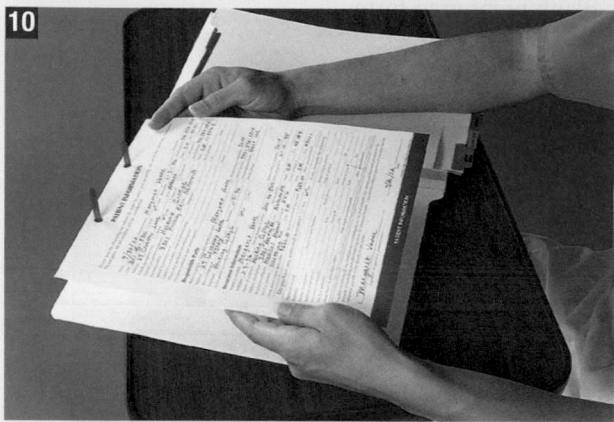

Place the patient registration form in the front of the medical record.

11. Procedural Step. Label preprinted forms to be placed in the record with required information such as the patient's name and date. These forms typically include the medical history form, the physical examination form, progress note sheets, and a medication record form. If the forms are not prepunched, the medical assistant must use a two-hole punch to insert two holes into the top or side of the form.

12. Procedural Step. Insert each form under its proper chart divider. Refer to the box below for a list of chart divider subject titles and documents typically filed under each title.

13. Procedural Step. Check the medical record to ensure that it has been prepared properly.

Chart Divider Subject Titles and Documents Typically Filed under Each Title

History and Physical
- Health history
- Physical examination report

Progress Notes
- Progress notes
- Medication record

Laboratory/X-ray
- Hematology report
- Clinical chemistry report
- Immunology report
- Urinalysis report
- Microbiology report
- Parasitology report
- Cytology report
- Histology report
- Electrocardiogram report
- Holter monitor report
- Sigmoidoscopy report
- Colonoscopy report
- Spirometry report
- Radiology report
- Diagnostic imaging report

Hospital
- History and physical report
- Operative report
- Pathology report
- Discharge summary report
- Emergency department report

Correspondence
- Consultation report
- Letter from patient
- Letter from patient's attorney
- Referral letter

Insurance
- Copy of patient's insurance card
- Precertification authorization for hospital admission
- Request for additional information from insurance company

Miscellaneous
- Consent to treatment form
- Release of medical information form
- Home health care report
- Physical therapy report
- Occupational therapy report
- Speech therapy report

TAKING A HEALTH HISTORY

The health history is a collection of subjective health data obtained by interviewing the patient and by having the patient complete a preprinted health history form that is then reviewed for completeness by the medical assistant. A thorough history is taken for each new patient, and subsequent office visits (in the form of progress notes) provide information regarding changes in the patient's illness or treatment. A quiet, comfortable room that allows for privacy encourages the patient to communicate honestly and openly. Showing genuine interest in and concern for the patient reduces apprehension and facilitates the collection of data.

In an office with an EMR, the patient may complete a health history paper-and-pencil form, and the medical assistant then enters the data into the computer. An alternative is for the medical assistant to enter the information directly into the computer while asking the patient questions related to his or her health status. Although not yet in widespread use, computer-guided questionnaires are available for some patients to complete their own health histories. The medical office must provide a private area for the patient to complete the questionnaire, and the medical assistant must be available to answer questions.

Components of the Health History

The health history is taken before the physical examination is performed, providing the physician the opportunity to compare findings. The health history consists of seven parts or sections.

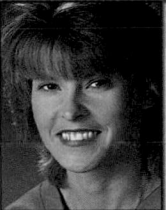

Memories from Externship

Dawn Bennett: During my externship as a medical assisting student, I was placed in a family practice clinic. I was very nervous my first day, wondering how in the world I would be able to remember everything I had learned in school. My first patients were an elderly couple. The wife was there for some test results for cancer. I looked at the results, and they were positive. After the physician relayed the results, the husband broke down. He had just lost his granddaughter to a heart attack and his son-in-law to a stroke. You could tell that he just could not bear losing his wife too.

One week later, the elderly man's wife was placed in a nursing home. He came into our office for an appointment. As I was working him up, he was telling me stories about himself and his wife when they were first married. He looked so sad. I sat with him for a few minutes after completing his workup and gave his stories my full attention. As I was leaving the room, a smile came across his face, and he thanked me for listening to him. I realized that working in a physician's office is more than just knowing what I learned in school. Compassion and showing patients you really do care about them are just as important. I felt good about myself that day. ∎

Case Study 3

Brett Oberlin is 21 years old and lives at home. He commutes to a local college and is a junior majoring in art education. His mother and father have come to the medical office and ask to see his medical record. The physician is attending a medical conference and will not return for another 4 days. Mr. and Mrs. Oberlin found some medications in Brett's room and looked them up on the Internet. They found out that they are used to treat HIV infection. Brett would not talk to them about the medications and told them he is an adult and it is none of their business. Mr. and Mrs. Oberlin are very concerned about Brett. They also are worried about other members of the family being exposed to HIV. They say that because they are supporting him, they should be allowed to see his record. ∎

Identification Data

The identification data section is included at the beginning of the health history form to obtain basic demographic data on the patient (Figure 36-18, *A*). The patient completes the identification data section.

Chief Complaint

The chief complaint (CC) identifies the patient's reason for seeking care—that is, the symptom that is causing the patient the most trouble. The CC is used as a foundation for the more detailed information obtained for the present illness and review of systems sections of the health history. The medical assistant is usually responsible for obtaining the CC from the patient and recording it in the patient's chart. In most offices, this information is recorded on a preprinted, lined form (see Figure 36-18, *F*). Certain guidelines must be followed in obtaining and recording the CC, as follows:

- An open-ended question should be used to elicit the CC from the patient: What seems to be the problem? How can we help you today? What can we do for you today?
- The CC should be limited to one or two symptoms and should refer to a specific, rather than vague, symptom.
- The CC should be recorded concisely and briefly, using the patient's own words as much as possible.
- The duration of the symptom (onset) should be included in the CC.
- The medical assistant should avoid using names of diseases or diagnostic terms to record the CC.

Recording Chief Complaints

Following are correct and incorrect examples of recording chief complaints.

Correct Examples
- Burning during urination that has lasted for 2 days
- Pain in the shoulder that started 2 weeks ago
- Shortness of breath for the past month

Incorrect Examples
- Has not felt well for the past 2 weeks (This statement refers to a vague, rather than a specific, complaint.)

PATIENT HEALTH HISTORY

A

IDENTIFICATION DATA   Please print the following information.

Name _____

Address _____

_____

Telephone _____

Home number _____ Work number

Today's date _____

____ Male ____ Female

____ Married ____ Separated ____ Divorced ____ Widowed ____ Single

Date of Birth _____

B

PAST HISTORY

Have you ever had the following: (Circle "no" or "yes", leave blank if uncertain)

Measles _____ no yes	Heart Disease _____ no yes	Diabetes _____ no yes	Hemorrhoids _____ no yes
Mumps _____ no yes	Arthritis _____ no yes	Cancer _____ no yes	Asthma _____ no yes
Chickenpox _____ no yes	Sexually Transmitted no yes Disease	Polio _____ no yes	Allergies _____ no yes
Whooping Cough ___ no yes	Anemia _____ no yes	Glaucoma _____ no yes	Eczema _____ no yes
Scarlet Fever _____ no yes	Bladder Infections ___ no yes	Hernia _____ no yes	AIDS or HIV+ _____ no yes
Diphtheria _____ no yes	Epilepsy _____ no yes	Blood or Plasma ___ no yes Transfusions	Infectious Mono ___ no yes
Pneumonia _____ no yes	Migraine Headaches ___ no yes	Back Trouble _____ no yes	Bronchitis _____ no yes
Rheumatic Fever ___ no yes	Tuberculosis _____ no yes	High Blood _____ no yes Pressure	Mitral Valve Prolapse no yes
Stroke _____ no yes	Ulcer _____ no yes	Thyroid Disease ___ no yes	Any other disease ___ no yes
Hepatitis _____ no yes	Kidney Disease _____ no yes	Bleeding Tendency _ no yes	Please list: _____

MAJOR HOSPITALIZATIONS: If you have ever been hospitalized for any major medical illness or operation, write in your most recent hospitalizations below.

Hospitalizations	Year	Operation or illness	Name of hospital	City and state
1st Hospitalization				
2nd Hospitalization				
3rd Hospitalization				
4th Hospitalization				

TESTS AND IMMUNIZATIONS: Mark an X next to those that you have had.

Tests:

☐ TB Test
☐ Rectal/Hemoccult
☐ Sigmoidoscopy
☐ Colonoscopy

☐ Electrocardiogram
☐ Chest x-ray
☐ Mammogram
☐ Pap Test

Immunizations:

☐ Influenza
☐ Hepatitis B
☐ Tetanus
☐ MMR
☐ Polio

ALLERGIES: List all allergies (foods, drugs, environment). ☐ None

_____

_____

_____

CURRENT MEDICATIONS: List the following that you are currently taking: Prescription medications, over-the-counter (OTC) medications, vitamin supplements, and herbal supplements. ☐ None

Medication	Frequency

ACCIDENTS/ INJURIES: Describe all serious accidents, severe injuries, head injury, or fractures. Include the date each occurred. ☐ None

Accident/Injury: Date:

_____

_____

_____

_____

Figure 36-18 Health history form.

C   FAMILY HISTORY

For each member of your family, follow the purple or blue line across the page and check boxes for:
1. His or her present state of health
2. Any illnesses he or she has had

	Good Health	Poor Health	Deceased	If deceased, write in age and cause of death.	Allergies or Asthma	Diabetes	Heart Disease	Stroke	Cancer	High Blood Pressure	Glaucoma	Arthritis	Ulcer	Kidney Disease	Mental Health Problems	Alcohol/Drug Abuse	Obesity	High Cholesterol	Thyroid Disease
Father:																			
Mother:																			
Brothers/Sisters:																			

D   SOCIAL HISTORY

EDUCATION _____ High school _____ College _____ Postgraduate

Occupation _____ Years _____

Previous occupations _____ Years _____

_____ Years _____

Have you ever been exposed to any of the following in your environment?

☐ Excess dust (coal, lime, rock)   ☐ Cleaning fluids/solvents   ☐ Radiation   ☐ Other toxic materials

☐ Sand   ☐ Hair spray   ☐ Insecticides

☐ Chemicals   ☐ Smoke or auto exhaust fumes   ☐ Paints

Please answer the follwing questions by placing an X in the box in front of the word Yes or No, except where you are asked for specific information. This information is obviously highly confidential and will be released to other healthcare professionals or insurance carriers ONLY with your consent.

DIET:

Do you eat a good breakfast? ☐ Yes ☐ No

Do you snack between meals (soft drinks, chips, candy bars)? ☐ Yes ☐ No

Do you eat fresh fruits and vegetables each day? ☐ Yes ☐ No

Do you eat whole grain breads and cereals? ☐ Yes ☐ No

Is your diet high in fat content? ☐ Yes ☐ No

Is your diet high in cholesterol content? ☐ Yes ☐ No

Is your diet high in salt content? ☐ Yes ☐ No

Are you allergic to any foods? ☐ Yes ☐ No

How many glasses of water do you drink each day? _____

How would you describe your overall eating habits? ☐ Excellent ☐ Good ☐ Fair ☐ Poor

PERSONAL HISTORY:

Do you find it hard to make decisions? ☐ Yes ☐ No

Do you find it hard to concentrate or remember? ☐ Yes ☐ No

Do you feel depressed? ☐ Yes ☐ No

Do you have difficulty relaxing? ☐ Yes ☐ No

Do you have a tendency to worry a lot? ☐ Yes ☐ No

Have you gained or lost much weight recently? ☐ Yes ☐ No

Do you lose your temper often? ☐ Yes ☐ No

Are you disturbed by any work or family problems? ☐ Yes ☐ No

Are you having sexual difficulties? ☐ Yes ☐ No

Have you ever considered committing suicide? ☐ Yes ☐ No

Have you ever desired or sought psychiatric help? ☐ Yes ☐ No

EXERCISE:

Do you exercise on a regular basis? ☐ Yes ☐ No

Does your job require strenuous, sustained physical work? ☐ Yes ☐ No

SLEEP PATTERNS:

Do you seem to feel exhausted or fatigued most of the time? ☐ Yes ☐ No

Do you have difficulty either falling asleep or staying asleep? ☐ Yes ☐ No

USE OF TOBACCO/ALCOHOL/CAFFEINE/DRUGS: Amt:

How much do you smoke per day? ☐ Cigarettes __

☐ Don't smoke ☐ Cigars/pipes __

Do you take two or more alcoholic drinks per day? ☐ Yes ☐ No

Do you drink six or more cups of coffee or tea per day? ☐ Yes ☐ No

Are you a regular user of sleeping pills, marijuana, tranquilizers, pain killers, etc? ☐ Yes ☐ No

Have you ever used heroin, cocaine, LSD, PCP, etc? ☐ Yes ☐ No

List any country outside the USA you have visited in the past six months. _____

When did you have your last physical examination? _____

Figure 36-18, cont'd

Continued

Patient's Name_____

E REVIEW OF SYSTEMS

HEAD AND NECK
_____ Frequent headaches
_____ Neck pain
_____ Neck lumps or swelling

EYES
_____ Wears glasses
_____ Blurry vision
_____ Eyesight worsening
_____ Sees double
_____ Sees halo
_____ Eye pain or itching
_____ Watery eyes
_____ Eye trouble

EARS
_____ Hearing difficulties
_____ Earaches
_____ Running ears
_____ Buzzing in ears
_____ Motion sickness

MOUTH
_____ Dental problems
_____ Swellings on gums or jaws
_____ Sore tongue
_____ Taste changes

NOSE AND THROAT
_____ Congested nose
_____ Running nose
_____ Sneezing spells
_____ Head colds
_____ Nosebleeds
_____ Sore throat
_____ Enlarged tonsils
_____ Hoarse voice

RESPIRATORY
_____ Wheezes or gasps
_____ Coughing spells
_____ Coughs up phlegm
_____ Coughed up blood
_____ Chest colds
_____ Excessive sweating,
       night sweats

CARDIOVASCULAR
_____ High blood pressure
_____ Racing heart
_____ Chest pains
_____ Dizzy spells
_____ Shortness of breath
_____ Shortness of breath at night
_____ More pillows to breathe
_____ Swollen feet or ankles
_____ Leg cramps
_____ Heart murmur

DIGESTIVE
_____ Heartburn
_____ Bloated stomach
_____ Belching
_____ Stomach pains
_____ Nausea
_____ Vomited blood
_____ Difficulty swallowing
_____ Constipation
_____ Loose bowels
_____ Black stools
_____ Gray stools
_____ Pain in rectum
_____ Rectal bleeding

URINARY
_____ Night frequency
_____ Day frequency
_____ Wets pants or bed
_____ Burning on urination
_____ Brown, black, or bloody urine
_____ Difficulty starting urine
_____ Urgency

MALE GENITAL
_____ Weak urine stream
_____ Prostate trouble
_____ Burning or discharge
_____ Lumps on testicles
_____ Painful testicles

FEMALE GENITAL
_/_/_ Last menstrual period
_/_/_ Last Pap test
_____ Postmenopausal or hysterectomy
_____ Noticed vaginal bleeding
_____ Abnormal LMP
_____ Heavy bleeding during periods
_____ Bleeding between periods
_____ Bleeding after intercourse
_____ Recent vaginal itching/discharge
_____ No monthly breast exam
_____ Lump or pain in breasts
_____ Complications with birth control

OBSTETRIC HISTORY
_____ Gravida
_____ Para
_____ Preterm
_____ Miscarriages
_____ Stillbirths
_____ Has had an abortion

MUSCULOSKELETAL
_____ Aching muscles
_____ Swollen joints
_____ Back or shoulder pains
_____ Painful feet
_____ Disability

SKIN
_____ Skin problems
_____ Itching or burning skin
_____ Bleeds easily
_____ Bruises easily

NEUROLOGICAL
_____ Faintness
_____ Numbness
_____ Convulsions
_____ Change in handwriting
_____ Trembles

F PROGRESS NOTES

Date	

Figure 36-18, cont'd

- Ear pain and fever (The duration of the symptoms is not listed.)
- Pain on urination indicative of a urinary tract infection (Names of diseases should not be used to record the chief complaint; the duration of the symptom is not listed.)

Present Illness

The present illness (PI) is an expansion of the chief complaint and includes a full description of the patient's current illness from the time of its onset. The medical assistant is often responsible for completing this section of the health history, which is recorded on the same form as the chief complaint (see Figure 36-18, *F*). To complete this section of the health history, the medical assistant asks the patient questions to obtain a detailed description of the symptom causing the greatest problem. Much skill and practice in asking the proper questions are required to elicit detailed information. A general guide for obtaining further information on symptoms is presented in Procedure 36-4, and a more thorough study for analyzing a symptom is included in the *Study Guide for Students*.

Past History

The past medical history is a review of the patient's past medical status (see Figure 36-18, *B*). Obtaining information on past medical care assists the physician in providing optimal care for the current problem. Most medical offices ask the patient to complete this section of the health history through a checklist type of form. The medical assistant should assist the patient with this section as necessary by offering to answer any questions regarding the information required. The past history includes the following areas:

- Major illnesses
- Childhood diseases
- Unusual infections
- Accidents and injuries
- Hospitalizations and operations
- Previous medical tests
- Immunizations
- Allergies
- Current medications

Family History

The family history is a review of the health status of the patient's blood relatives (see Figure 36-18, *C*). This section of the health history focuses on diseases that tend to be familial. A **familial** disease is one that occurs in or affects blood relatives more frequently than would be expected by chance. Examples of familial diseases include hypertension, heart disease, allergies, and diabetes mellitus. The patient usually completes this section of the health history and is asked to provide the following information about each blood relative:

- State of health
- Presence of any significant disease
- If deceased, cause of death

Social History

The social history section of the health history includes information on the patient's lifestyle, such as health habits and living environment (see Figure 36-18, *D*). The social history is important because the patient's lifestyle may have an impact on his or her condition and may influence the course of treatment chosen by the physician. The social history also provides the physician with information regarding the effect that the illness may have on the patient's daily living pattern. If it is necessary for the individual to make a major lifestyle adjustment (e.g., stop smoking, reduce working hours), the physician may recommend support services to assist in this transition. This section of the history is usually completed by the patient and includes the following areas:

- Education
- Occupation (past and present)
- Living environment
- Diet
- Personal history
- Exercise

Review of Systems

A review of systems (ROS) is a systematic review of each body system to detect any symptoms that have not yet been revealed. The importance of the ROS is that it assists in identifying symptoms that might otherwise remain undetected. The physician usually completes the ROS by asking a series of detailed and direct questions related to each body system; the results of this section of the health history assist the physician in a preliminary assessment of the type and extent of physical examination required. Figure 36-18, *E* shows an example of an ROS form.

CHARTING IN THE MEDICAL RECORD

Charting is the process of making written entries about a patient in the medical record and is performed by medical office personnel who are directly involved with the health care of the patient. The medical record is considered a legal document; the information must be charted as completely and accurately as possible. Developing good charting skills requires a thorough knowledge of charting guidelines combined with much repeated practice. To provide guidance in attaining this important skill, PPR charting guidelines are presented in this section, followed by examples of proper charting entries. With an EMR, the medical assistant enters charting information into a computer using free-text entry, drop-down lists, and check-boxes.

Charting Guidelines

To ensure accurate and concise charting, specific guidelines must be followed. These are listed and described as follows:

1. *Check the name on the chart before making an entry to ensure you have the correct chart.* If the medical assistant records in the wrong patient's chart by mistake, information such as a procedure that was performed on a patient may be excluded from the correct patient's

record. As previously stated, from a legal standpoint, a procedure not documented was not performed.

2. *Use black ink to make entries in the patient's chart.* Black ink must be used to provide a permanent record. In addition, entries made in black ink are easier to reproduce when a record must be duplicated for insurance company purposes and patient referral.

3. *Write in legible handwriting.* For the medical record to be meaningful to others, the medical assistant must chart information legibly. If the medical assistant's cursive script is not legible, the information should be printed.

4. *Chart information accurately, using clear and concise phrases.*
   - The medical assistant should be brief but thorough and should avoid vagueness and duplication of information.
   - It is not necessary to include the patient's name in the entry because the entire medical record centers on one patient; it is assumed the information refers to that patient.

- Each phrase should begin with a capital letter and end with a period.
- Each new entry should begin on a separate line and be dated with the month, day, year, and time (either AM/PM or military time).
- Standard abbreviations, medical terms, and symbols can be used to help save time and space. It is *crucial* that the medical assistant first check the office policy to determine the abbreviations, medical terms, and symbols that are commonly used in that office. Using commonly accepted terminology avoids confusing others who read the chart. A list of abbreviations and symbols commonly used in medical offices is presented in Table 36-1.
- *Spell correctly.* Correct spelling is essential for accuracy in charting. If you are in doubt about the spelling of a word, consult a dictionary.

5. *Chart immediately after performing a procedure.* When a procedure has been performed, it should be charted without delay. If a time lapse occurs between performing the procedure and charting it, the medical

Table 36-1 Abbreviations and Symbols Commonly Used in the Medical Office

Abbreviations Used to Chart Symptoms and Procedures

$\overline{aa}$	of each	/d	per day
Ab	abortion	d/c	discontinue
abd	abdomen	D&I	dry and intact
abs	absent	dil	dilute
ac	before meals	disch	discharge
ad lib	as desired	DNKA	did not keep appointment
admin	administer	DOB	date of birth
am or a.m.	before noon	DOI	date of injury
amt	amount	DRE	digital rectal examination
AP	apical pulse	DSD	dry, sterile dressing
approx	approximately	DTaP	diphtheria and tetanus toxoids and acellular pertussis vaccine
appt	appointment	D&V	diarrhea and vomiting
ASA	acetylsalicylic acid (aspirin)	DVA	distance visual acuity
ASAP	as soon as possible	ea	each
BA	backache	ED	emergency department
b/c	because	EDD	expected date of delivery
BC	birth control	Fe	iron
bid	twice a day	flex sig	flexible sigmoidoscopy
BM	bowel movement	freq	frequent
BP	blood pressure	F/U	follow-up
BPM	beats per minute	Fx	fracture
BS	blood sugar	GYN	gynecology
BSE	breast self-examination	h or hr	hour
$\overline{c}$	with	H/A	headache
caps	capsules	HBP	high blood pressure
cath	catheter, catheterize	HC	head circumference
CC	chief complaint	Hep B	hepatitis B vaccine
chemo	chemotherapy	Hg	mercury
CMA (AAMA)	certified medical assistant (American Association of Medical Assistants)	H_2O	water
		HR	heart rate
c/o	complains of	HRT	hormone replacement therapy
CS	cesarean section	hs	at bedtime
Cx	cervix	ht	height
d	day	ID	intradermal

IM	intramuscular	quad	quadriplegic
IPV	inactivated polio vaccine	R	respiration
IV	intravenous	RE	rectal examination
lab	laboratory	reg	regular
lac	laceration	rehab	rehabilitation
lat	lateral	RMA	registered medical assistant
lax	laxative	Rx	prescription
LB	lower back	$\overline{s}$	without
LBP	lower back pain	SC or SQ	subcutaneous
liq	liquid	S/E	side effects
LMP	last menstrual period	sec	second
med, meds	medication, medications	sigmoid	sigmoidoscopy
min	minute	sl	slight
MMR	measles, mumps, and rubella	sm	small
mod	moderate	SOB	shortness of breath
N/A	not applicable	sol	solution
NB	newborn	spec	specimen
N/C	no complaints	STAT	immediately
neg	negative	surg	surgery
NH	nursing home	T	temperature
NICU	newborn intensive care unit	tab, tabs	tablet, tablets
NKA	no known allergies	temp	temperature
NKDA	no known drug allergies	ther	therapy
NMP	normal menstrual period	tid	three times a day
noct	nocturnal	TLC	total lung capacity, tender loving care
NS	normal saline	TPR	temperature, pulse, and respiration
N&V	nausea and vomiting	tr	trace
NVA	near visual acuity	TSE	testicular self-examination
NVD	nausea, vomiting, and diarrhea	vag	vagina, vaginal
OB	obstetrics	VE	vaginal examination
occ	occasionally	vit	vitamin
oint	ointment	VO	verbal order
op	operation	VS	vital signs
OR	operating room	wk	week
OT	occupational therapy	WNL	within normal limits
OTC	over-the-counter (nonprescription medication)	WO	written order
		w/o	without
OV	office visit	wt	weight
P	pulse	W/U	workup
Pap	Pap test	**Abbreviations Used to Chart Body Parts and Locations**	
path	pathology	abd	abdomen
pc	after meals	AD	right ear
peds	pediatrics	AS	left ear
PEN	penicillin	AU	In each ear, both ears
per	by or through	EENT	eye, ear, nose, and throat
pharm	pharmacy	GI	gastrointestinal
pm or p.m.	afternoon	GU	genitourinary
PMS	premenstrual syndrome	Ⓛ or lt	left
po or PO	by mouth	Ⓛ A	left arm
pos	positive	Ⓛ L	left leg
postop	postoperative (after surgery)	LLQ	lower left quadrant
preop	preoperative (before surgery)	LRQ	lower right quadrant
prep	preparation	LUQ	left upper quadrant
prn	as needed	OD	right eye
PT	physical therapy, prothrombin time	OS	left eye
Pt or pt	patient	OU	in each eye, both eyes
qd	every day	Ⓡ or rt	right
qh	every hour	Ⓡ A	right arm
q(2,3,4)h	every (2, 3, 4) hours	Ⓡ L	right leg
qid	four times a day	RLQ	right lower quadrant
qn	every night	RUQ	right upper quadrant
QNS	quantity not sufficient	**Abbreviations Used to Chart Measurement**	
qod	every other day	C	Celsius
QS	quantity sufficient		

Continued

Table 36-1 Abbreviations and Symbols Commonly Used in the Medical Office—cont'd

cc	cubic centimeter	Echo	echocardiogram
cm	centimeter	EEG	electroencephalogram
dL	deciliter	FOBT	fecal occult blood test
F	Fahrenheit	IVP	intravenous pyelogram
g	gram	LP	lumbar puncture
kg	kilogram	MRI	magnetic resonance imaging
L	liter	NST	nonstress test
lb	pound	PFT	pulmonary function test
m	meter	TRUS	transrectal ultrasound
mcg	microgram	US	ultrasound
mg	milligram	***Laboratory Tests***	
mL or ml	milliliter	ABG	arterial blood gas
mm	millimeter	BG	blood glucose
oz	ounce	Bx	biopsy
pt	pint	CBC	complete blood count
qt	quart	C&S	culture and sensitivity
ss	one half	diff	differential
T	tablespoon	ESR	erythrocyte sedimentation rate
tsp	teaspoon	FBG	fasting blood glucose
Miscellaneous Abbreviations		FBS	fasting blood sugar
Patient Examination		GCT	glucose challenge test
Dx	diagnosis	GTT	glucose tolerance test
H/O	history of	Hct	hematocrit
H&P	history and physical	Hgb	hemoglobin
Hx	history	OGTT	oral glucose tolerance test
MHx	medical history	PET	positron emission tomography
PE or Px	physical examination	PPBS	postprandial blood sugar
prog	prognosis	PSA	prostate-specific antigen
Sx	symptoms	PT	prothrombin time
Tx	treatment	RBC	red blood cell
Conditions		RBS	random blood sugar
BPH	benign prostatic hyperplasia	SG	specific gravity
CA	cancer	trig	triglycerides
CAD	coronary artery disease	UA	urinalysis
CHF	congestive heart failure	U/C	urine culture
COPD	chronic obstructive pulmonary disease	WBC	white blood cell
CRC	colorectal cancer	**Symbols**	
CVA	cerebrovascular accident	∅	none, no
DM	diabetes mellitus	✓	check
DVT	deep vein thrombosis	>	greater than
Fe def	iron deficiency	<	less than
GC	gonorrhea	↑	increase
GDM	gestational diabetes mellitus	↓	decrease
HTN	hypertension	♀	female
IBS	irritable bowel syndrome	♂	male
MI	myocardial infarction	°	degree
MS	multiple sclerosis	@	at
OA	osteoarthritis	·	times
OM	otitis media	x̄	except
PID	pelvic inflammatory disease	p̄	after
RA	rheumatoid arthritis	#	number
RF	rheumatic fever	1°	primary
STD	sexually transmitted disease	2°	secondary
TB	tuberculosis	+	positive
URI	upper respiratory infection	−	negative
USI	urinary stress incontinence	Ⓡ	rectal temperature
UTI	urinary tract infection	Ⓐ	axillary temperature
Diagnostic Procedures		"	inches
CT, CAT	computed axial tomography	'	feet
CXR	chest x-ray		
ECG	electrocardiogram		

assistant may not remember certain aspects of the procedure, such as the results of the treatment or the patient's reaction.

6. Procedures should never be charted in advance. The individual performing the procedure should be the one to chart it; in other words, never chart for someone else.

7. *Each charting entry should be signed by the person making it.* The signature should include the medical assistant's first initial, full last name, and title (e.g., D. Bennett, CMA [AAMA]). The following title abbreviations are often used for medical assistants:

    CMA (AAMA): certified medical assistant
    RMA: registered medical assistant
    MA: medical assistant
    SMA: student medical assistant

8. *Never erase or obliterate an entry.* If an error is made in charting, the medical assistant must never erase or obliterate it. Should the physician or medical staff be involved in litigation, erased or obliterated entries tend to reduce credibility. If incorrect information is charted, the medical assistant should draw a single line through the incorrect information, permitting it to remain legible. The word *error* is then written above the incorrect data, including the date and the medical assistant's first initial, last name, and credentials. Some medical offices may request that the reason for the change also be recorded. The correct information is then inserted next to the error (Figure 36-19).

The medical assistant should always take the time to chart properly in the patient's medical record. Good charting helps coordinate efforts in the medical office and leads to high-quality health care.

Charting Progress Notes

After completion of the initial health history, a system is needed to update the medical record with new information each time the patient visits the medical office. Most offices use progress notes to fulfill this function. Progress notes document the patient's health status and the care and treatment being received by the patient in chronological order.

Progress notes provide effective communication among medical office personnel and serve as a legal document.

The medical assistant is frequently responsible for charting progress notes in the medical record. They are usually charted on special preprinted lined sheets known as *progress note sheets.* These sheets have a column for the date and a column for charting information (see Figure 36-18, *F*). Types of progress notes that are often charted by the medical assistant are presented next, along with a charting example of each.

Charting Patient Symptoms

The medical assistant takes patient symptoms during office visits and telephone conversations. Information conveyed during a telephone conversation helps the medical assistant determine whether the patient needs to be seen and the immediacy of the situation.

A **symptom** is any change in the body or its functioning that indicates the presence of disease. Symptoms can be classified as subjective or objective. A **subjective symptom** is one that is felt by the patient and cannot be observed by another person. Pain, pruritus, vertigo, and nausea are examples of subjective symptoms. An **objective symptom** is one that can be observed by another person and by the patient. Rash, coughing, and cyanosis are objective symptoms. The medical assistant should have a thorough knowledge of common symptoms and should be able to recognize them. Table 36-2 lists and describes common symptoms.

Taking patient symptoms during an office visit consists of the following:

1. Obtaining a chief complaint (see earlier discussion)
2. Obtaining additional information about the chief complaint

If the patient complains of pain in the abdomen that has lasted for 2 days (chief complaint), additional information is needed to describe the pain, including its type, specific location, onset, intensity, precipitating factors, and duration. The procedure for taking patient symptoms during an office visit is outlined in Procedure 36-4. Additional skills and practice on taking patient symptoms are included in Chapter 36 of the *Study Guide for Students.*

Table 36-2 Common Symptoms	
Symptom	**Definition**
Integumentary System	
Diaphoresis	Excessive perspiration.
Flushing	A red appearance to the skin, which generally affects the face and neck. A flushed appearance is commonly present with a fever.
Jaundice	A yellow appearance to the skin, first evident in the whites of the eyes.
Rash	An eruption on the skin.
Circulatory System	
Bradycardia	An abnormally slow pulse rate.
Dehydration	A decrease in the amount of water in the body. The patient has a flushed appearance, dry skin, and decreased output of urine.
Edema	The retention of fluid in the tissues, resulting in swelling. Skin over the area is tight. Edema is most easily observed in the extremities.
Tachycardia	An abnormally fast pulse rate.

Continued

Table 36-2 Common Symptoms—cont'd

Symptom	Definition
Gastrointestinal System	
Anorexia	A loss of appetite and a lack of interest in food.
Constipation	A condition in which the stool becomes hard and dry, resulting in difficult passage from the rectum. The consistency of the stool, rather than the frequency of defecation, is used as a guide in determining the presence of constipation. (Frequency of bowel movements varies with the individual; some people have a bowel movement only every 2 to 3 days but are not constipated.) Other symptoms of constipation include headache, nausea, and general malaise.
Diarrhea	The passage of an increased number of loose, watery stools. The fecal material moves rapidly through the intestinal tract, resulting in decreased absorption by the body of water, electrolytes, and nutrients. Other symptoms usually associated with diarrhea are intestinal cramping and general weakness.
Flatulence	The presence of excessive gas in the stomach or intestines.
Nausea and vomiting	Nausea is a sensation of discomfort in the stomach with a feeling that vomiting may occur. Vomiting is the ejection of the stomach contents through the mouth, also known as *emesis*. The ejected content is known as *vomitus*.
Respiratory System	
Cough	An involuntary and forceful exhalation of air followed by a deep inhalation. A cough may be productive (meaning a discharge is produced) or nonproductive (no discharge is present).
Cyanosis	A bluish discoloration of the skin due to lack of oxygen.
Dyspnea	Labored or difficult breathing.
Epistaxis	Hemorrhaging from the nose (nosebleed).
Nervous System	
Chills	A feeling of coldness accompanied by shivering. Chills are generally present with a fever.
Convulsions	Involuntary contractions of the muscles.
Fever or pyrexia	A body temperature that is higher than normal.
Headache	A feeling of pain or aching in the head. It is a common symptom that accompanies many illnesses. Tension, fatigue, and eyestrain can result in a headache.
Malaise	A vague sense of body discomfort, weakness, and fatigue, often marking the onset of a disease and continuing through the course of the illness.
Pain	Irritation of pain receptors, resulting in a feeling of distress or suffering. Pain is an important indication that a part of the body is not working properly.
Pruritus	Severe itching.
Vertigo	A feeling of dizziness or light-headedness.

PROCEDURE 36-4 Obtaining and Recording Patient Symptoms

Outcome Obtain and record patient symptoms.

Equipment/Supplies

- Medical record of the patient to be interviewed
- Black ink pen

1. **Procedural Step.** Assemble the equipment. Ensure that you have the correct patient's record and a black ink pen for charting patient symptoms.
   Principle. Black ink must be used to provide a permanent record.
2. **Procedural Step.** Go to the waiting room and ask the patient to come back.
3. **Procedural Step.** Escort the patient to a quiet, comfortable room, such as an examination room, that allows for privacy.
   Principle. Patient symptoms should be taken in a room that encourages communication.
4. **Procedural Step.** In a calm and friendly manner, greet the patient and introduce yourself. Identify the patient by his or her full name and date of birth.

   Principle. A warm introduction sets a positive tone for the remainder of the interview.
5. **Procedural Step.** Ask the patient to be seated. You should seat yourself so that you face the patient at a distance of 3 to 4 feet.
   Principle. This type of seating arrangement facilitates open communication.
6. **Procedural Step.** Use good communication skills to interact with the patient. These include the following:
   a. Use the patient's name of choice.
   b. Show genuine interest and concern for the patient.
   c. Maintain appropriate eye contact.
   d. Use terminology the patient can understand.
   e. Listen carefully and attentively to the patient.
   f. Pay attention to the patient's nonverbal messages.

PROCEDURE 36-4   Obtaining and Recording Patient Symptoms—cont'd

g. Avoid judgmental comments.

h. Avoid rushing the patient.

7. Procedural Step. Locate the progress note sheet in the patient's medical record. Chart the date and time and the abbreviation for chief complaint (CC).

8. Procedural Step. Use an open-ended question to elicit the chief complaint, such as "What seems to be the problem?"

Principle. An open-ended question allows the patient to verbalize freely.

9. Procedural Step. Chart the chief complaint while following the charting guidelines outlined on pages 903 to 907. In addition, these guidelines should be followed:

a. Limit the chief complaint to one or two symptoms, and refer to a specific rather than a vague symptom.

b. Chart the chief complaint concisely and briefly, using the patient's own words as much as possible.

c. Include the duration of the symptom (onset) in the chief complaint.

d. Avoid using names of diseases or diagnostic terms to record the chief complaint.

10. Procedural Step. Obtain additional information regarding the chief complaint using *what, when,* and *where* questions. While following proper charting guidelines, chart this information after the chief complaint.

What Questions:

• What exactly have you been experiencing?

• Does the symptom occur suddenly or gradually?

• Does anything make it worse?

Where Question:

• Where is the symptom located?

When Questions:

• When did the symptom first occur?

• How long does it last?

• Does anything cause it to occur?

Principle. This information provides a complete description of the chief complaint.

11. Procedural Step. Thank the patient and proceed to the next step in the patient workup. (This usually includes measuring vital signs and height and weight and preparing the patient as needed for the physical examination [see Chapters 19 and 20].)

12. Procedural Step. Inform the patient that the physician will be with him or her soon.

13. Procedural Step. Place the patient's medical record where it can be reviewed by the physician (as designated by the medical office policy).

Principle. The physician will want to review the patient's medical record before examining the patient.

CHARTING EXAMPLE

Date	
6/30/XX	3:15 p.m. CC: Intense pain in the (L) ear for the past 2 days. Pt states pain is sharp and continuous. Pt noted sl yellow discharge from (L) ear. Fever of 101° F began last night about 9 p.m. Took Tylenol 2 tabs @ 8 a.m. —————— D. Bennett, CMA (AAMA)

Other Activities That Need to Be Charted

Procedures

The medical assistant frequently charts procedures performed on the patient, including vital signs, weight and height, visual acuity, and ear irrigations. Procedures should be charted immediately after they are performed; from a legal standpoint, a procedure that is not documented was not performed. In general, the following information should be included: the date and time, the type of procedure, the outcome, and the patient reaction. The specific information to be charted is included with each procedure presented in this text.

CHARTING EXAMPLE

Date	
6/30/XX	9:15 a.m. Irrigated (R) ear c̄ 200 mL of normal saline @ 98.6° F. Mod amt of cerumen in returned solution. Pt states can hear better. ——— D. Bennett, CMA (AAMA)

Procedure.

	error 10/15/XX ——— D. Bennett, CMA (AAMA)	
10/15/XX	9:30 a.m. Tubersol Mantoux test: 9mm induration. —————— 12 ——— D. Bennett, CMA (AAMA)	

Figure 36-19 Proper method for correcting an error in a patient's medical record.

Administration of Medication

Charting medications administered to the patient is an important responsibility in the medical office. The recording should include the date and time, the name of the medication, the lot number (if required), the dosage given, the route of administration, the injection site used (for parenteral medication), and any significant observations or patient reactions.

> **CHARTING EXAMPLE**
>
> | Date | |
> |---|---|
> | 6/30/XX | 10:15 a.m. Bicillin 900,00 units IM, ⓛ |
> | | dorsogluteal. ——— D. Bennett, CMA (AAMA) |

Administration of medication.

Specimen Collection

Each time a specimen is collected from a patient, the medical assistant should chart the date and time of the collection, the type of specimen, and the area of the body from which the specimen was obtained. If the specimen is to be sent to an outside laboratory for testing, this information also should be charted, including the tests requested, the date the specimen was sent, and where it was sent. In this way, the physician would know that the specimen was collected and sent to the laboratory when test results are not back yet.

> **CHARTING EXAMPLE**
>
> | Date | |
> |---|---|
> | 6/30/XX | 1:30 p.m. Venous blood spec collected from Ⓡ |
> | | arm. Sent to Ross Lab for CBC and diff on |
> | | 6/30/XX. ——— D. Bennett, CMA (AAMA) |
> | Date | |
> | 6/30/XX | 2:00 p.m. Throat spec collected. Sent to |
> | | Ross Lab for C&S on 6/30/XX.——— |
> | | ——— D. Bennett, CMA (AAMA) |

Specimen collection.

Diagnostic Procedures and Laboratory Tests

Diagnostic procedures and laboratory tests ordered for a patient should always be charted in the medical record. If the patient does not undergo the test, documented proof exists that the test was ordered. Charting diagnostic procedures and laboratory tests protects the physician legally and refreshes the physician's memory of the procedures and tests being run on the patient when results are not yet back from the testing facility. Information to include in the charting entry consists of the date and time, the type of procedure or test ordered, the scheduling date, and where it is being performed.

> **CHARTING EXAMPLE**
>
> | Date | |
> |---|---|
> | 6/30/XX | 10:15 a.m. Mammography scheduled for |
> | | 7/5/XX at Grant Hospital. ——— |
> | | ——— D. Bennett, CMA (AAMA) |
> | Date | |
> | 6/30/XX | 11:30 a.m. Pt given lab request for GTT at |
> | | Ross Lab. ——— D. Bennett, CMA (AAMA) |

Diagnostic/laboratory tests.

Results of Laboratory Tests

It is usually unnecessary to chart results from laboratory reports returned from outside laboratories because the report itself is filed in the patient's record. In case of a STAT request or critical findings, the test results may be telephoned to the medical office, requiring the medical assistant to record the results on a report form. Careful recording is essential to avoid errors, which could affect the patient's diagnosis. Results of laboratory tests performed by the medical assistant in the office should be charted in the medical record and must include the date and time, name of the test, and test results.

> **CHARTING EXAMPLE**
>
> | Date | |
> |---|---|
> | 6/30/XX | 8:00 a.m.   FBS: 82 mg/dL.——— |
> | | ——— D. Bennett, CMA (AAMA) |
> | Date | |
> | 6/30/XX | 4:15 p.m.   Quick Vue+ Mono Test: neg.——— |
> | | ——— D. Bennett, CMA (AAMA) |

Laboratory test results.

Patient Instructions

It often is necessary to relay instructions to a patient regarding medical care (e.g., wound care, cast care, care of sutures). The medical assistant should chart this information, taking care to include the date and time and the type of instructions relayed to the patient. Many medical offices have printed instruction sheets that are given to the patient. The patient is asked to sign a form, which is filed in the patient's record, indicating that he or she has read and understands the instructions (Figure 36-20). The form also should be signed by the medical assistant, who functions as a signature witness. This protects the physician legally in the event that the patient fails to follow the instructions and causes further harm or damage to a body part.

Other areas that the medical assistant is responsible for charting in the medical record include missed or canceled appointments, telephone calls from patients, medication refills, and changes in medication or dosage by the physician.

CHARTING EXAMPLE

Date	
6/30/XX	9:30 a.m. Instructions provided for BSE. Pt given a BSE educational brochure. ———— ———————— D. Bennett, CMA (AAMA)
Date	
6/30/XX	10:00 a.m. Explained wound care. Written instructions provided. Signed copy in chart. To return in 2 days for suture removal. ——— ———————— D. Bennett, CMA (AAMA)
Date	
6/30/XX	10:25 a.m. Provided instructions for applying a heating pad to the lower back. ———— ———————— D. Bennett, CMA (AAMA)

Patient instructions.

CHARTING EXAMPLE

Date	
6/30/XX	11:15 a.m. Phoned office. States that swelling in the Ⓡ ankle is almost gone. ———————— D. Bennett, CMA (AAMA)
Date	
6/30/XX	1:15 p.m. Missed appointment scheduled for 6/30/XX @ 1:00 p.m. ———— ———————— D. Bennett, CMA (AAMA)

Telephone call and missed appointment.

PATIENT INSTRUCTIONS FOR WOUND CARE

Name of patient: _____

Follow the instructions indicated below for care of your wound:

1. Use ice bag and elevate to reduce swelling and pain. Elevate higher than your heart.
2. You may take aspirin/Tylenol for pain.
3. Keep the dressing clean and dry.
4. Replace the dressing within _____ days.
5. Discard the dressing within _____ days.
6. Cleanse the wound daily as instructed.
7. Stitches should be removed in _____ days.
8. Despite the greatest of care, any wound can become infected. If your wound becomes red or swollen, shows pus or red streaks, or feels more sore instead of less sore, contact the physician **immediately.**

I have received and understand the above instructions:

Patient (or representative): _____

Relationship to patient: _____

Witness: _____   Time and date: _____

Figure 36-20 Instruction sheet for patients.

MEDICAL PRACTICE *and the* LAW

Documentation can be a deciding factor in a legal case. Everything you do for a patient should be documented in a factual manner in the medical record, or "chart." When a legal issue arises, often several years pass before it comes to trial. If you are involved, you will be asked detailed questions as to your actions on a particular day for a particular patient. Few people have accurate memories for that long. Juries give more credibility to documentation performed at the time of the action than to a memory of years ago.

Ethically, you owe the patient thorough documentation to provide optimal continuity of care. Remember that all patient information is confidential.

Proper charting is a crucial skill for a medical assistant to master. Although proper documentation would not prevent a lawsuit, it might determine the outcome. Pay particular attention to the rules for consents and charting guidelines outlined in this chapter, and follow them to the letter. ■

What Would You Do? What Would You *Not* Do? RESPONSES

Case Study 1
Page 874

What Did Dawn Do?
- ❏ Listened carefully to Mrs. Celeste and relayed concern through both verbal and nonverbal behavior.
- ❏ Reassured Mrs. Celeste that her information would be kept completely confidential. Explained to Mrs. Celeste that health care professionals are required by law to keep all patient information confidential.
- ❏ Told Mrs. Celeste how important it is to chart information that relates to her health. Explained that the physician must have accurate data to diagnose and treat her. Stressed that certain medications can be harmful to a patient if consumed with alcohol.
- ❏ Gave Mrs. Celeste information (including brochures) on community agencies that could help her. Explained that these agencies are required to maintain confidentiality and encouraged her to contact them.

What Did Dawn Not Do?
- ❏ Did not tell Mrs. Celeste to go to a different physician to ensure that her information remained private.
- ❏ Did not tell Mrs. Celeste that she needed to stop drinking before it affected her health.

What Would You Do/What Would You Not Do?
Review Dawn's response and place a checkmark next to the information you included in your response. List the additional information you included in your response.

_____
_____
_____
_____
_____
_____

Case Study 2
Page 893

What Did Dawn Do?
- ❏ Reassured Tessa that she and her family have been good patients and apologized for the inconvenience.
- ❏ Told Tessa that it is against the law to transfer medical records without the patient's written authorization. Explained that the reason for the law is to safeguard a patient's privacy.
- ❏ Asked Tessa if she has a fax machine because the forms could be faxed to her for signing and then faxed back to the office. If not, explained that Tessa and her husband would need to come to the office to sign release forms.

What Did Dawn Not Do?
- ❏ Did not get defensive about Tessa being so annoyed.
- ❏ Did not send their medical records to the new physician without the signed release forms.

What Would You Do/What Would You Not Do?
Review Dawn's response and place a checkmark next to the information you included in your response. List the additional information you included in your response.

_____
_____
_____
_____
_____
_____

Case Study 3
Page 899

What Did Dawn Do?
- ❏ Listened to and empathized with Mr. and Mrs. Oberlin's concerns.
- ❏ Told Mr. and Mrs. Oberlin that because Brett is of adult age, it would be against the law to let them see his medical record without his written authorization. Explained that the law is there to protect a patient's right to privacy, and just as it protects Brett's right, the law also protects their right, so that no one can obtain information from their medical records without their authorization.
- ❏ Suggested that they talk with Brett again regarding the situation.

What Did Dawn Not Do?
- ❏ Did not give them any information from Brett's medical record.

What Would You Do/What Would You Not Do?
Review Dawn's response and place a checkmark next to the information you included in your response. List the additional information you included in your response.

_____
_____
_____
_____
_____
_____

TERMINOLOGY REVIEW

Medical Term	Word Parts	Definition
Attending physician		The physician responsible for the care of a hospitalized patient.
Charting		The process of making written entries about a patient in the medical record.
Consultation report		A narrative report of an opinion about a patient's condition by a practitioner other than the attending physician.
Diagnosis	*dia-:* through, complete *-gnosis:* knowledge	The scientific method of determining and identifying a patient's condition.
Diagnostic procedure	*dia-:* through, complete *gnos/o:* knowledge *-ic:* pertaining to	A procedure performed to assist in the diagnosis, management, or treatment of a patient's condition.
Discharge summary report		A brief summary of the significant events of a patient's hospitalization.
Electronic medical record (EMR)		A medical record that is stored on a computer.
Familial	*famil:* family *-al:* pertaining to	Occurring in or affecting members of a family more frequently than would be expected by chance.
Health history report		A collection of subjective data about a patient.
Home health care		The provision of medical and nonmedical care in a patient's home or place of residence.
Informed consent		Consent given by a patient for a medical procedure after he or she has been informed of the nature of his or her condition and the purpose of the procedure, and has been given an explanation of risks involved with the procedure, alternative treatments or procedures available, the likely outcome of the procedure, and the risks involved with declining or delaying the procedure.
Inpatient		A patient who has been admitted to a hospital for at least one overnight stay.
Medical impressions		Conclusions drawn by the physician from an interpretation of data. Other terms for impressions include *provisional diagnosis* and *tentative diagnosis.*
Medical record		A written record of important information regarding a patient, including the care of that individual and the progress of the patient's condition.
Medical record format		The way a medical record is organized. The two main types of medical record formats are the source-oriented record and the problem-oriented record.
Objective symptom		A symptom that can be observed by an examiner.
Paper-based patient record (PPR)		A medical record in paper form.
Patient		An individual receiving medical care.
Physical examination		An assessment of each part of the patient's body to obtain objective data about the patient that assists the physician in determining the patient's state of health.
Physical examination report		A report of the objective findings from the physician's assessment of each body system.
Problem		Any condition that requires further observation, diagnosis, management, or patient education.
Prognosis	*pro-:* before *-gnosis:* knowledge	The probable course and outcome of a disease and the prospects for a patient's recovery.
Reverse chronological order		Arranging documents with the most recent document on top or in the front, which means that the oldest document is on the bottom or at the back of a section or file.
SOAP format		A method of organization for recording progress notes. The SOAP format includes the following categories: subjective data, objective data, assessment, and plan.
Subjective symptom		A symptom that is felt by the patient but is not observable by an examiner.
Symptom		Any change in the body or its functioning that indicates the presence of disease.

ON THE WEB

For information on the medical record:

American Health Information Management Association: www.ahima.org

Privacy Rights Clearinghouse: www.privacyrights.org

Getting Medical Records: www.genetichealth.com

Electronic Medical Record: www.openclinical.org

For information on communication assistance:

Toll-Free Directory: inter800.com

U.S. Postal Service ZIP Code Access: www.usps.com/zip4

United Parcel Service: www.ups.com

Federal Express: www.fedex.com

Check out the Evolve site at http://evolve.elsevier.com/Bonewit/today/ to actively Prepare for your Certification, and to access additional interactive activities and exercises to help you study and prepare for success.

37

Patient Reception

INTRODUCTION TO PATIENT RECEPTION

The medical assistant may be responsible for opening the office, preparing for patients, and processing patients as they arrive for appointments. It is important to be sure that all parts of the office are prepared for patients because there is little time to pick up or arrange facilities once patient appointments begin. There are several forms that new patients must fill out, and the patient signature must be kept on file as permission to provide treatment, bill insurance, and verify that the patient has been given an opportunity to read the office's Notice of Privacy Practices. At the end of the day, the medical assistant must prepare for the next day and close the medical office.

PREPARING FOR PATIENTS

Opening the Medical Office

Office staff need to arrive at the medical office early enough to make sure the office is prepared for the patients. The medical assistant is often responsible for opening the office (Procedure 37-1). Several activities must be performed immediately:
- Disarming the alarm system (if the office has one)
- Turning on the lights
- Unlocking the door through which patients enter
- Unlocking file cabinets, medical record files, and medication cabinets
- Turning on all of the office equipment that will be used during the day, such as computers and copy machines

Depending on the way the medical office is organized, there may be several other tasks that should be completed before the first patient arrives.

Checking for Messages and/or Faxes

Someone must review messages and prepare the telephone system for the day's activities. The telephone message must be switched from the night and weekend message to the telephone system used during the day. Usually the night and weekend message states that the office is closed, gives an emergency telephone number, or directs the caller to leave a message if the matter is not urgent. During the day, the medical assistant may answer the telephone directly or the caller may have to select an option from a menu before being connected to a member of the office staff.

If the medical office uses an answering service, the medical assistant must call the service to indicate that the office is open. The medical assistant must also obtain any messages that have come in within the past hour or nonurgent messages left during the night. For calls relating to illness, the answering service would have contacted the physician on call overnight.

After checking the message mailbox or answering machine, the medical assistant usually checks for faxes that have arrived overnight and routes the messages and faxes to the appropriate person.

A separate mailbox or answering machine may be used for prescription refill requests. If this is the case, the medical assistant should retrieve the messages from this mailbox before the physician arrives.

Preparing for the Day's Activities

It is helpful to take a minute at the beginning of the day to organize the day's tasks. This includes reviewing the appointment schedule and noting deviations from the routine schedule, such as physicians who are out of the office for all or part of the day. If the medical office uses a manual day sheet, it must be dated and prepared for use. (This is discussed in detail in Chapter 44.) Reminders about the day's activities may be stored using an electronic task system and/or a physical **tickler file.** A tickler file is a set of 43 file folders, one for each month (for a total of 12 folders) and an additional set of 31 folders for the days of the current month. Written notes, bills to be paid, receipts, or other items are filed in these folders to "tickle" the memory at the time when they must be handled. (Tickler files are also discussed in Chapter 41.)

The medical assistant usually counts the cash in the cash drawer, a fixed amount of money used to make change when patients pay in cash. The cash drawer (change fund) is usually kept locked except when the medical assistant is actually sitting at the reception desk.

Making Sure Patient Charts Are Prepared

Patient charts are usually pulled the evening before the next appointment day or are prepared in the morning before the patients arrive. Even if the office uses an electronic medical record, some providers will want to be able to consult a patient's old paper medical record. The charts must be arranged for each physician in order of the arrival of the patient. A separate appointment schedule is usually prepared for each physician. A charge slip may be created for each person before the visit, or the entire billing and charging system may be electronic. Some offices also print other sheets, for example, a list of medications for the patient to review and update.

Copies of the appointment schedule(s) are printed and placed at designated locations. The medical assistant usually places a schedule in each physician's office, at the reception desk, and at the medical assistant's desk. The schedule may be printed the evening before in case of a power outage or server problem, but it is usually updated with new appointments in the early morning so a new schedule should be printed just before patients start arriving.

Charts or other forms for the day are usually kept at the front desk. Some physicians prefer to have all medical records for their scheduled patients on their private desk when they start to see patients.

Checking the Office and Waiting Room

The waiting room, reception area, and examination and treatment rooms all need to be checked for the following: cleanliness, neatness, correct temperature, and appropriate reading material. The medical assistant should make sure that the cleaning service has cleaned all parts of the office and emptied the trash. The medical assistant may need to turn on a television, radio, and/or DVD player in the patient waiting room. Magazines should be stored neatly and replaced with current issues as needed. If there are toys in the waiting room, they should be cleaned regularly and stored neatly. Holders in the waiting room that contain information brochures for patients should be restocked and arranged neatly (Figure 37-1).

Checking Equipment and Supplies

The medical assistant should perform a visual safety check of the medical office daily. This includes removing any hazards that might block hallways or exits and making sure that all equipment is performing correctly. It is helpful to fill the paper trays of the copier, printer, and fax machine every morning.

The reception area and examination rooms should be tidied and restocked daily, either in the morning or at closing and sometimes again at a specified time during the day. Biohazard waste containers should be checked, and waste discarded properly if necessary. The medical assistant

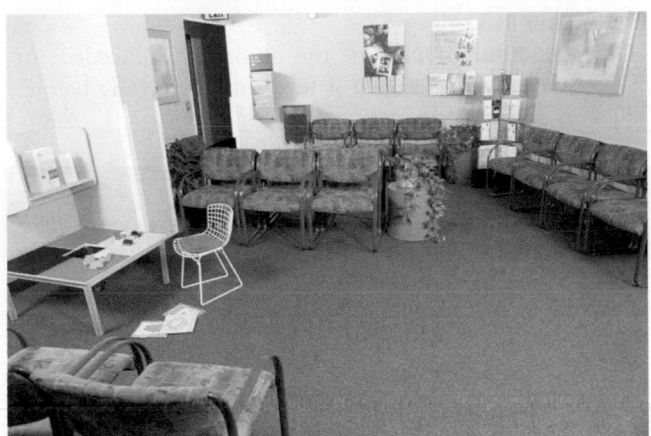

Figure 37-1 The waiting area should be kept tidy for patients.

may need to turn on or set up equipment used for clinical procedures, run controls in the laboratory, and/or remove items from a battery charger. It may also be necessary to unload the autoclave and put away items that were sterilized the evening before.

Closing the Medical Office

At the end of the day, the activities of the morning are reversed. Many medical offices run the autoclave in the afternoon so that items can dry overnight. Medical records for the following day may be created for new patients and removed from the files for established patients. This is often done in the afternoon because it leaves more time in the morning. Before leaving the office, the medical assistant must perform the following tasks (Procedure 37-2):

- Prepare the bank deposit and balance the cash drawer. At the end of the day, the money in the cash drawer must be balanced against cash receipts. Any amount above the usual change fund is added to the bank deposit (see Chapter 44).
- Make a backup copy of the main computer hard drive if the office does not subscribe to an online computer backup service.
- Check the fax machine for faxes that have come in during the day.
- Turn off computers, printers, copiers, and other equipment (with the exception of the fax machine).
- Change the telephone to the night message or call the answering service to tell them the office is closing.
- Lock the door through which patients enter.
- Lock file cabinets, medical record files, and medication cabinets.
- Make sure the coffee machine or other kitchen equipment is turned off.
- Unplug equipment, such as a toaster, that might be a fire hazard.
- Turn off the lights.
- The last person to leave the medical office makes sure the door is locked and sets the alarm system.

PROCEDURE **37-1** Opening the Medical Office

Outcome Open the medical office.

Equipment/Supplies

- Medical office

1. **Procedural Step.** Enter the office and disarm any alarm system immediately.
2. **Procedural Step.** Turn on the lights.
3. **Procedural Step.** Adjust heat or air conditioning to a comfortable setting.
4. **Procedural Step.** Unlock the door through which patients and visitors will enter the office.

Principle. Medical office staff usually enter the office through a different door than patients and visitors.
5. **Procedural Step.** Turn on machines that will be used all day, including computers, printers, and copier.
6. **Procedural Step.** Set the telephone system to the day setting and get messages from the electronic mailbox, telephone answering machine, or answering service.

Continued

PROCEDURE **37-1**   Opening the Medical Office—cont'd

Principle. Callers to a business expect calls to be picked up as soon as the business opens. An important telephone message may need attention.

7. Procedural Step. Listen to any messages in order, writing down the pertinent information for each message on a message pad. (See Chapter 39, Procedure 39-2, Taking a Telephone Message.) Fill in the information, including the name of the caller, business affiliation (if any), date, time of the call, telephone number including area code, and information the caller wishes to leave about the reason for the call. Place your initials on the message in case there are questions.

Principle. Complete information is necessary to return a call.

8. Procedural Step. Arrange the messages in order of importance. Deal with any urgent calls at once, then work through other calls. Pull medical records for calls from patients and place the messages in the appropriate locations for various office staff to review.

9. Procedural Step. Review the day's activities and note any special tasks that must be completed that day.

10. Procedural Step. Count the money in the cash drawer and record the amount.

11. Procedural Step. Check the office for safety hazards including frayed wires, items blocking corridors or walkways, and other hazards.

12. Procedural Step. Straighten up the waiting room, including reading material; clean children's toys as needed; turn on radio, television, and/or DVD player; and restock patient information brochures.

13. Procedural Step. Print appointment lists as needed and make sure all patient medical records have been pulled and arranged in order. Print or stamp today's date on the progress notes and place the medical records in the designated location. If an electronic medical record system is used, be sure any necessary paperwork has been printed.

14. Procedural Step. If it is office policy, prepare charge slips and clip to each patient's medical record or paperwork.

15. Procedural Step. Check biohazard waste containers and discard properly.

16. Procedural Step. Check examination rooms to be sure they are clean and contain all needed supplies and equipment.

17. Procedural Step. Run the autoclave as needed, or empty the autoclave if it was run the evening before.

PROCEDURE **37-2**   Closing the Medical Office

Outcome Close the medical office.

Equipment/Supplies

- Medical office

1. Procedural Step. Make sure examination rooms are clean and contain all necessary supplies.

2. Procedural Step. Run the autoclave if needed.

Principle. If the autoclave is run at the end of the day, supplies can dry overnight.

3. Procedural Step. Print a patient schedule for the next day, and pull paper medical records. Print charge slips and clip to each patient's medical record if it is office policy.

4. Procedural Step. Make sure all cabinets or rooms containing medical records are locked.

5. Procedural Step. Balance the cash drawer and prepare the bank deposit. Lock the cash drawer or place the change fund in the office safe. If possible, make the bank deposit at the end of the day.

Principle. It is best to leave as little money in the office as possible. The change fund should be kept under lock and key.

6. Procedural Step. Make sure the night system for the telephones is activated. Switch the message on the electronic telephone system or answering machine, and call the answering service as needed.

7. Procedural Step. Turn off all machines throughout the medical office that are used only during the day. Exceptions include the fax machine and telephone system. Unplug machines such as the coffee maker or toaster oven that might pose a fire hazard.

Principle. Machines that generate heat such as coffee makers can pose a fire hazard. Unplugging these machines is also an extra reminder to make sure they do not remain on overnight.

8. Procedural Step. Lock the door through which patients and visitors enter the medical office.

9. Procedural Step. Turn the heat or air conditioning to the night setting.

10. Procedural Step. Turn off the lights.

11. Procedural Step. Arm the security system and make sure the door is securely locked as you leave the medical office.

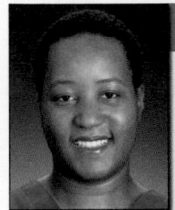

Putting It All into Practice

My name is Keisha White, and I work in a small office with two internists. We are the primary care providers for most of our patients. I am responsible for opening the office every day, and I usually arrive at about 8:00 am. I leave before the office closes every day except Friday. Gerri, another medical assistant, is responsible for closing the office. We had an alarm system put in about 5 years ago, so as soon as I enter the office, I go to the keypad and enter the code so that the alarm won't go off. Then I have a look around as I turn on the lights. Sometimes the air seems a little stale, so I either open a window or turn up the air conditioning, depending on how hot it is outside. After I turn on the copier and the computers, I call the answering service to tell them that I have arrived. I take down any messages and handle them. Then I make sure the telephones are set so that patients can call. Next I turn on the lights in the patient waiting area, make sure everything is tidy, and unlock the door for patients. We like to have music in the waiting room, so I make sure there are six CDs in the player and turn it on. I usually change the selection every day because we get tired of hearing the same music all the time. We have shifted over to an electronic medical record, but we haven't finished scanning in all our old records.. Gerri pulls the old medical records for the next day before she leaves in the afternoon. Once the computers are warmed up, I check the electronic calendar to see if there is anything special to do that day, and I print appointment schedules. We keep one schedule at the front desk, and I put one on each physician's desk. When each patient arrives, we print a charge slip for the physician. Then we call the patient to escort him or her to the examination room. The first appointment is scheduled for 8:30, so I really have to keep moving in order to be ready for the day. ■

PATIENT CHECK-IN

It is important to acknowledge each person who enters the office as soon as possible to prevent that person from feeling awkward. The medical assistant or a receptionist usually sits at the reception desk. This person should greet everyone who enters the office. If a sign-in sheet is used, it is recommended that this sign-in sheet have adhesive peel-off strips for each line so that the medical assistant can remove the patient's name immediately after check-in.

Maintaining Confidentiality

Many offices have a sliding glass window. This prevents people in the waiting room from hearing telephone conversations or other discussions in the reception area. In some facilities, the medical assistant sits behind a reception desk that is recessed but open (Figure 37-2). Because patients standing near the desk can hear any conversation behind the desk, these offices usually have a separate room for scheduling appointments. When a patient is at the desk, the medical assistant should not carry on a telephone conversation with another patient. Only one patient should be at the desk or window at a time. The medical assistant can instruct other patients and/or family members to have a seat in the waiting room.

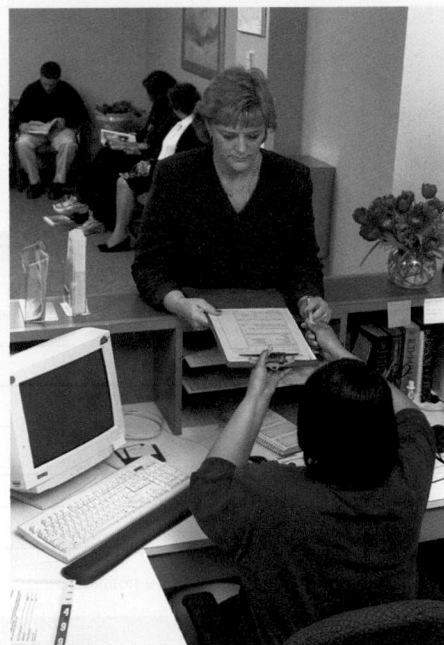

Figure 37-2 If an open desk is used for reception, the waiting room should be large enough to prevent other patients from overhearing the conversation at the desk.

If it is necessary to discuss sensitive or personal information, the patient should be taken to a private area.

New Patients

The office must obtain several types of information about new patients. Personal and insurance information is either obtained when the appointment is made or at the first visit.

The patient is usually asked to sign a statement that allows the office to release information to the insurance company for billing purposes. This consent may be part of the patient information form or may be a separate sheet. If the office accepts payments directly from the insurance company (called accepting **assignment of benefits**), the patient must also sign a form authorizing this. The assignment of benefits statement is usually included with the consent to release information to insurance companies. Figure 37-3 shows an example of a new patient information form. By signing the bottom section, the patient authorizes the physician or medical practice to release information to the insurance company and authorizes the insurance company to pay the medical practice directly. In addition, the patient has agreed to be responsible for charges not covered by insurance. The medical office may also use a more extensive form authorizing the release of protected health information. This form is optional, but it does allow the office to obtain consent to leave voicemail messages at the patient's home and mail laboratory reports or appointment reminders (Figure 37-4).

Acknowledgement of Receipt of HIPAA Privacy Practices

The Health Insurance Portability and Accountability Act (HIPAA) requires that patients sign a form acknowledging

REGISTRATION
(PLEASE PRINT)

Home Phone: _____   Today's Date: _____

PATIENT INFORMATION

Name_____ Soc. Sec.#_____
          Last Name   First Name   Initial

Address_____

City_____ State _____ Zip _____

Single ___ Married ___ Widowed ___ Separated ___ Divorced ___ Sex M___ F___ Age ___ Birthdate _____

Patient Employed by_____ Occupation _____

Business Address _____ Business Phone _____

By whom were you referred?_____

In case of emergency who should be notified? _____ Phone _____
                                   Last Name   Relationship to Patient

PRIMARY INSURANCE

Person Responsible for Account _____
                               Last Name   First Name   Initial

Relation to Patient _____ Birthdate _____ Soc. Sec.# _____

Address (if different from patient's) _____ Phone _____

City_____ State _____ Zip _____

Person Responsible Employed by_____ Occupation _____

Business Address _____ Business Phone _____

Insurance Company_____

Contract # _____ Group # _____ Subscriber # _____

Name of other dependents covered under this plan _____

ADDITIONAL INSURANCE

Is patient covered by additional insurance? _____ Yes _____ No

Subscriber Name _____ Relationship to Patient _____ Birthdate _____

Address (if different from patient's) _____ Phone _____

City_____ State _____ Zip _____

Subscriber Employed by_____ Business Phone _____

Insurance Company _____

Contract #_____ Group # _____ Subscriber # _____

Name of other dependents covered under this plan _____

ASSIGNMENT AND RELEASE

I, the undersigned, certify that I (or my dependent) have insurance coverage with _____
                                                    Name of Insurance Company(ies)

and assign directly to Dr. _____ insurance benefits, if any, otherwise payable to me for services rendered. I understand that I am financially responsible for all charges whether or not paid by insurance. I hereby authorize the doctor to release all information necessary to secure the payment of benefits. I authorize the use of this signature on all insurance submissions.

_____   _____   _____
     Responsible Party Signature   Relationship   Date

ORDER# 58-8426 • © 1996 BIBBERO SYSTEMS, INC. • PETALUMA, CALIFORNIA • TO REORDER CALL TOLL FREE: (800) 242-9330

Figure 37-3 New patient information form.

Patient Consent for Use and Disclosure of Protected Health Information

I hereby give my consent for [**Practice Name**] to use and disclose protected health information (PHI) about me to carry out treatment, payment and health care operations. (The *Notice of Privacy Practices* describes such uses and disclosures more completely.)

I have the right to review the *Notice of Privacy Practices* before signing this consent. I understand that the *Notice of Privacy Practices* can be revised at any time, and I can obtain a copy of any revision upon written request.

I authorize [**Practice Name**] to call my home or other alternative location and leave a message on voice mail or in person in reference to any items related to treatment, payment and health care operations. This includes appointment reminders, questions about insurance and any calls pertaining to my clinical care, including laboratory test results, among others.

I authorize [**Practice Name**] to mail to my home or other alternative location any items that assist in my care such as appointment reminder cards and patient statements as long as they are marked "Personal and Confidential."

I have the right to request that [**Practice Name**] restrict how it uses or discloses my PHI to carry out treatment, payment and health care operations. The practice is not required to agree to my requested restrictions, but if it does, it is bound by this agreement.

By signing this form, I am consenting to allow [**Practice Name**] to use and disclose my PHI as required in the course of treatment and obtaining payment for services to me.

I may revoke my consent in writing except to the extent that the practice has already made disclosures in reliance upon my prior consent.

_____   _____   _____
Patient or Legal Guardian's Signature   Date   Relationship to Patient

_____   _____
Print Patient's Name   Print Name of Legal Guardian (if any)

Figure 37-4 The office may use an optional consent for disclosure of personal health information.

that they were given the opportunity to read or were given a copy of the office Notice of Privacy Practices (Figure 37-5). The Notice of Privacy Practices itself is usually very detailed.

Patient History Form

Most offices also have a history form for the patient to fill out before being seen by the physician (see Chapter 36). It may be mailed to the new patient before the first appointment, or the patient may fill it out in the waiting room. The medical assistant goes over this form with the patient in the examination room to be sure that all of the relevant information has been included. Medical information should not be discussed at the front desk.

Verifying Insurance and Obtaining Authorizations

After a new patient has filled out the patient information sheet, the medical assistant should ask for his or her insurance

What Would You Do? What Would You *Not* Do?

Case Study 1

Angela Harris is a 62-year-old new patient. When she comes to the reception desk to check in, she gives Keisha the completed patient history form that had been mailed to her. Keisha hands her a Notice of Privacy Practices and a clipboard and pen. She asks her to fill out a new patient information form and sign the form acknowledging the receipt of the Notice of Privacy Practices. Ms. Harris seems reluctant to take the clipboard. She says, "I'm sorry, I don't have my reading glasses with me. I didn't know I would need them. Besides, I gave you all that information on the telephone, didn't I?" ∎

Acknowledgement of Receipt of the Notice of Privacy Practices

Please Review Carefully

The Notice of Privacy Practices tells you how [**Practice Name**] uses and discloses information about you. Not all situations will be described. We are required to give you a notice of our privacy practices for the information we collect and keep about you. We reserve the right to revise this notice, and you can obtain a copy of any revision upon written request.

I, _____ , have been given a copy of the **Notice of Privacy Practices.**

_____   _____   _____
Patient or Legal Guardian's Signature   Date   Relationship to Patient

_____   _____
Print Patient's Name   Print Name of Legal Guardian (if any)

_____   _____
Signature of Witness (If signed with an "X" or mark)   Date

Effective Date: April 14, 2003

Figure 37-5 The Health Insurance Portability and Accountability Act (HIPAA) requires new patients to sign a form acknowledging receipt of a medical office's Notice of Privacy Practices.

card. After making a photocopy of both sides or scanning the card, the copy is stored with the patient's medical record. It verifies the information given by the patient and sometimes gives additional information needed for billing. An insurance card scanner at the front desk may be used to read both sides of the insurance card and scan it into the computer. Information from the card can be transferred to the practice management software, and an image of the card can be saved to the patient's electronic medical record.

It may also be office policy to verify a patient's identity at every visit by asking for photo ID or two other forms of identification and retaining photocopies. Medical identity theft has become a more common problem in the past decade. It can result in incorrect information in the medical record as well as fraudulent charges to insurance companies.

Some types of insurance require authorization every time the patient visits the primary care physician. Patients with Medicaid must usually have their coverage verified and/or must receive prior authorization for each visit. **Medicaid** is an insurance program established by the federal government that pays for low-income patients' medical needs. Each state administers Medicaid, and the program has a different name in each state. The cost is split between the state and the federal government. In some states, some patients on Medicaid receive new identification cards each month; in other states, patients' insurance coverage can be verified by telephone, fax, or an electronic card reader. An electronic card reader is a small machine in the physician's office that is connected via telephone to the insurance company's database and can verify insurance benefits while the patient is

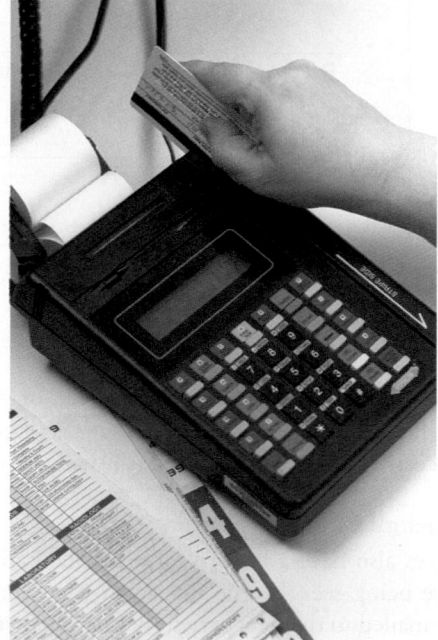

Figure 37-6 Card reader used to validate insurance coverage for Medicaid and other insurance plans.

in the office. Many offices use a card reader that can read not only the patient's insurance card, but also several types of credit cards (Figure 37-6).

For other types of insurance, it may be necessary to call the patient's insurance company to obtain authorization for treatment (especially if the patient needs minor surgery or a special treatment). This may be done when the patient makes the appointment, when the patient checks in, or after the first visit, when the physician has identified what treatment is necessary and how many visits are anticipated.

Each office has its own procedure for verifying insurance. In general, if there is a question whether the patient has insurance coverage, or whether the service will be covered, the medical assistant should contact the insurance company before the service is provided (Procedure 37-3).

Verifying a Managed Care Referral

If the patient has been referred by another physician through a managed care plan, it is important to validate that the patient has a completed referral form from the primary care physician. This may be a paper form. Sometimes the referring physician has sent it in advance, but the patient may bring it personally to the visit. For most managed care plans, it will be possible to access the referral using the Internet. If there is no valid referral, the insurance company may not pay for the visit.

The referral will state how many visits are allowed (how many will be paid for by the managed care plan) and the problem for which the patient is being referred. Depending on the patient's insurance or managed care plan, the patient may also be required to sign a statement promising to pay any charges that the insurance does not cover.

Managed care plans usually do not allow physicians who accept referrals to bill for excess charges to the patient (a practice known as *balance billing*). Medicare also does not allow balance billing from providers who agree to accept Medicare patients. The medical office is allowed to bill for services that the patient's insurance plan does not cover.

If the patient has not yet obtained a referral authorization, or if it is uncertain that the insurance will cover the services, the patient must be informed before any service is provided that he or she will be responsible for payment of the bill.

Established Patients

If the patient has been seen in the office before, it is necessary to verify that the billing information is still correct. When checking a patient in, the medical assistant should verify the patient's address and telephone number. Patients who have moved may assume that the office is aware of the change, so it is recommended to ask, "Is your address still…?" and "Is your telephone number still…?" The patient should also be asked for his or her insurance card. If any information has changed, the new card should be photocopied and the updated information should be entered into the computer billing system and into the medical record, whether paper or electronic. As stated previously, established patients may also be asked to verify their identity using a photo ID if they are not personally known to the person checking them in.

Accepting Copayments

A **copayment** is a fixed amount of money that the patient is required to pay each time he or she receives medical

treatment. The amount of the copayment is usually printed on the patient's insurance card. If there is any question about the amount of the copayment, it may be easily determined by checking the patient's eligibility on the website of his or her insurance company. Many offices collect the copayment before the visit because it is a fixed fee, although this can also be done at the end of the visit. The amount paid is entered on the patient's charge slip or entered directly into the computer. A receipt should be given to the patient at the time the copayment is made. It may be generated by the computer when the payment is entered. Most offices use a numbered receipt system for handwritten receipts so that payments are accounted for.

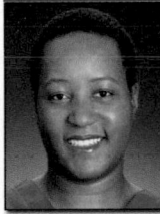

PROCEDURE 37-3   Obtaining New Patient Information

Outcome Obtain information from a new patient, obtain consents, and validate insurance coverage.

Equipment/Supplies

- Clipboard
- Pen
- New patient information form containing consent to treatment and assignment of benefits consents
- Notice of Privacy Practices
- Receipt of Notice of Privacy Practices form
- Consent for release of protected health information (optional)

- Photocopier
- Insurance card reader (optional)
- Telephone
- Medical record
- Computer
- Scanner

1. **Procedural Step.** Place a new patient information form on a clipboard with a pen, and ask a new patient to complete the form and return it to you.
   Principle. Complete information about the patient facilitates the billing and insurance process.

2. **Procedural Step.** Make sure the form is complete and the patient or authorized representative has signed the form as needed.
   Principle. The patient must consent in writing to treatment, to allowing the office to bill the insurance company, and to allowing the insurance company to pay the physician.

3. **Procedural Step.** Ask to see the insurance card of the patient or other insured person.

4. **Procedural Step.** Photocopy both sides of the insurance card and place the copy in the patient's medical record.
   Principle. The insurance card contains information about the patient's copayment amount, as well as the address and telephone number of the insurance company.

5. **Procedural Step.** Confirm patient eligibility for insurance coverage using a card reader, computer, or telephone if required by the patient's insurance, and confirm that there is a complete referral form if necessary. If the visit will not be completely covered by insurance, discuss the patient's financial responsibility. If personal information is discussed, take the patient to a private area.
   Principle. The patient has a right to know what his or her financial obligation will be before receiving service.

6. **Procedural Step.** Ask to see a+ photo ID or two other forms of identification if it is office policy.
   Principle. Verifying patient identity may be part of the office's plan to prevent identity theft.

7. **Procedural Step.** Give the patient a copy of the Notice of Privacy Practices and ask the patient to sign the form acknowledging the receipt of the Notice of Privacy Practices. Sign the form as a witness to the patient's signature.
   Principle. HIPAA requires that the patient acknowledge the receipt of the Notice of Privacy Practices in writing.

8. **Procedural Step.** Ask the patient to read and sign any consent for release of protected health information used by the office.
   Principle. A general consent for release of personal health information enables the office to obtain written consent to leave messages on the patient's answering machine, to send laboratory results to the patient's home address, and so on.

9. **Procedural Step.** Insert any new forms into the medical record and place it with the charge slip to indicate that the patient is ready to be examined. Ask the patient to have a seat and tell him or her the approximate waiting time for the examination.
   Principle. When the paperwork is complete, it will help the patient feel more in control to know how long he or she can expect to wait before the examination.

10. **Procedural Step.** Transfer the information from the new patient information form to the patient's computer account, or validate that information obtained by telephone is correct.
    Principle. Billing is almost always performed using the computer.

11. **Procedural Step.** Scan the new patient information form, insurance card, and other consent forms if it is office policy (usually if the office uses an electronic medical record).
    Principle. If the office stores a patient's medical record electronically in addition to billing records, all new paper forms must be scanned into the computer.

Indicating That the Patient Is in the Waiting Room

After the patient has been checked in at the front desk, the charge slip and the medical record or information printed from the electronic record are placed in the designated space for patients who are ready to be seen. If a computerized record is used, copies of the most recent progress notes, copies of recent lab work, and/or a form for patients to complete updating medical history and current medications may be printed at the time of the visit.

ORIENTING PATIENTS TO THE MEDICAL OFFICE

Information for New or Prospective Patients

The medical assistant may be responsible for informing new patients and prospective patients about the medical office and its policies and procedures (Procedure 37-4). The medical assistant should be familiar with all of the following information:

- A brief description of the physicians, how long each has been in practice, each physician's credentials, and whether each physician is accepting new patients.
- Specialties of the physicians in the practice, types of patients seen, and basic philosophy of the physician(s).
- Information about languages spoken by staff, whether the physician practices alternative therapies (e.g., acupuncture), or whether the physician insists that patients stop smoking.
- Location of the main office and satellite offices, directions to each office, and a description of available parking and access to public transportation, if applicable.
- The types of insurance that the practice accepts, whether the patient's insurance will be accepted, and whether payment is required at each visit.
- How to make appointments and the policy regarding canceling appointments. Patients are normally asked to give 24 hours' notice if possible for a cancellation.
- The telephone procedure and whether the physician has **call-in times** (when the physician takes telephone calls).
- What hospital(s) each physician is affiliated with; some patients might also want to know whether the physician makes nursing home visits.
- How medication refills are handled.

A physician might not be accepting new patients for a few reasons:

- A physician may have so many patients that he or she cannot in all fairness accept new patients. If the patient load decreases, the physician may begin again to accept new patients.
- The physician may be returning from a maternity, family, or personal disability leave and be working a reduced schedule.
- The physician may be easing back before retiring.

The medical assistant should also be able to tell prospective patients how much time to allow for a first (new patient) visit. Most physicians see new patients only on certain days and at certain times. Medical assistants should be sure to remind new patients to bring all of their medications to the initial appointment, as well as a written list of concerns.

What Would You Do? What Would You *Not* Do?

Case Study 3

Donna Pohl calls the office to ask about the medical practice. An acquaintance has recommended Dr. Sylvia Lawrence. She says that she prefers a female physician. She asks for information about her and her specialty. Dr. Lawrence specializes in general internal medicine. At the current time the doctor is pregnant, and her due date is 1 month away. Although Dr. Lawrence is still seeing established patients, she has instructed Keisha not to make any appointments for her with new patients for the next 4 months. The other physician in the practice, Dr. William Rudner, also specializes in general internal medicine. ■

Patient Informational Materials

An increasing number of practices today have a website that contains the previously mentioned information. There are also often photographs of the office and office staff. Pages on the website usually include information about the practice as well as directions to the main facility and any satellite facilities. There may be a section related to health and wellness with information about specific medical conditions, especially those related to the specialty of the practice. Maintaining the website is usually not the responsibility of the medical assistant, but he or she can remind the office administrator if certain information needs to be updated. Photographs of patients should be used only if the patient has signed a release form. The Web address of the practice website can be added to the business cards of the practice physicians.

In addition to a practice website, there is usually information about each physician available on the website of the hospital(s) where the physician has privileges as well as the website of any large group with which the medical practice is affiliated. Most of these websites have a "find a doctor" feature for all their physicians, and these usually link to an information page about each physician. These links may need updating if the physician obtains new credentials or if the physician starts or stops accepting new patients.

Patient informational booklets are another very successful marketing and public relations tool, but they must be kept up to date. A patient information booklet should include all the information listed section above that describes information to give to new patients. Patients appreciate having something in writing to which they can refer. A patient informational booklet should be given to a new patient at the first visit and should be on display for established patients to request if they want one.

PROCEDURE 37-4 Explaining Office Policies and Procedures

Outcome Orient a new or prospective patient to the medical office.

Equipment/Supplies

- Patient information booklet (if available)
- Map
- List of points to cover

1. **Procedural Step.** Offer to give or send the patient a patient information booklet if one is available.
   Principle. A patient information booklet provides a handy resource to answer questions about a medical practice.

2. **Procedural Step.** Identify the name, credentials, and specialties of physicians who are accepting patients in the medical office.
   Principle. Some physicians may not currently be accepting patients.

3. **Procedural Step.** Offer information as required about languages spoken by staff in the medical office and additional services or specialized complementary practices.

4. **Procedural Step.** Identify the location of the office and/or satellite offices and give directions as needed. Identify where the patient can park if necessary.

5. **Procedural Step.** Tell the patient if the office accepts his or her medical insurance plan and discuss expectations for payment of the patient's bill.

Principle. The patient has a right to know what his or her financial obligation will be before receiving service.

6. **Procedural Step.** Describe how far in advance to make appointments and the office policy on canceling appointments.
   Principle. Most offices reserve the right to charge the patient if the appointment is not cancelled at least 24 hours in advance.

7. **Procedural Step.** Tell the patient when and how to contact the office, and notify the patient if the physician has specific call-in times (times when he or she takes telephone calls.)

8. **Procedural Step.** Explain how prescriptions and prescription refills are handled as needed.

9. **Procedural Step.** Identify the hospital(s) with which each physician is affiliated. Answer any questions about other services (e.g., nursing home visits) that each physician may provide.

MEDICAL PRACTICE *and the* **LAW**

One function of the medical office that has been affected by the Health Insurance Portability and Accountability Act (HIPAA) is patient check-in. The Privacy Rule is not specific about sign-in lists, but medical offices need to take all possible measures to protect patient privacy. Not all offices use sign-in sheets, but if they are used, they should have adhesive peel-off strips for each line so that patients who come later cannot read the names of patients who arrived earlier. The Privacy Rule does permit incidental disclosures of certain information as long as the health care facility has reasonable safeguards to protect against disclosure of protected health information. Silent wireless paging systems are available but are usually too expensive for medical offices. Generally, it is considered acceptable to have patients say their names at the reception desk and to call patients by name from the waiting room unless patients have asked specifically for the staff not to do this. In some offices, however, patients may check in at the window by signing a sheet with a map of the waiting room that indicates their seat location. They do not have to say their names out loud, and they can be located without having their names called.

It is important to protect information on paper and computer screens at the information desk from being seen by others. The computer screen should be turned so that it cannot be read from the patient side of the reception desk. If medical assistants leave the reception desk for any reason, they should log off from their computer account. In addition, all patient records and information should be stored so that names and other information are not visible to patients who approach the desk. A shredder is usually available at the front desk so that any information that will not be filed in the patient's medical record can be destroyed.

The Red Flags Rule of the Federal Trade Commission has been enforced since August 2009. It requires businesses considered "creditors" to set up a written identity theft detection program that identifies red flags of identity theft and provides a program to respond when red flags are detected. Medical offices that bill patients for an account balance or deductible after insurance has paid would usually be considered "creditors" who must comply with the Red Flags Rule. If patients must pay before service is provided or if accounts are covered by Medicaid or another program in which the patient has no responsibility for the fees, the office would not be considered a creditor. ∎

What Would You Do? What Would You *Not* Do? RESPONSES

Case Study 1
Page 921

What Did Keisha Do?
❐ Checked to see if there were other patients in the waiting room. Because there were, she took Ms. Harris to a private area.
❐ Asked Ms. Harris for each piece of information on the new patient information form and filled it in for her.
❐ Read each statement at the bottom of the form out loud and showed Ms. Harris where to sign the form.
❐ Explained that Ms. Harris could read the Notice of Privacy Practices at a later time when she had her glasses, but Keisha asked her to sign the form acknowledging receipt of the Notice of Privacy Practices.

What Did Keisha Not Do?
❐ Did not tell the patient that she should have realized she might need her reading glasses.
❐ Did not tell the patient to sign any of the consents without reading them to her.
❐ Did not ask for protected health information where another patient could hear the conversation.

What Would You Do/What Would You **Not** *Do?*
Review Keisha's response and place a checkmark next to the information you included in your response. List the additional information you included in your response.

_____
_____
_____
_____
_____
_____
_____

Case Study 2
Page 923

What Did Keisha Do?
❐ Looked up the policy number for Mr. Ritano in the computer and handed it to him in writing so that he could write it on the form.
❐ Attempted to call the insurance company to verify his coverage.
❐ Explained that she needed to take a photocopy of his insurance card and asked him to bring it in as soon as possible.
❐ Accepted his check for $10.00 for his copayment.
❐ Explained that if it turned out that his insurance did not cover this visit or if he needed an authorization or referral, he would be responsible to pay the charges for the visit.
❐ Gave him an estimate of the cost of the visit.
❐ Allowed him to reschedule if he wanted to wait until he had his insurance card.

What Did Keisha Not Do?
❐ Did not refuse to let Mr. Ritano see the physician until he brought his insurance card.
❐ Did not make negative comments about forgetting the insurance card or imply that she didn't believe he had insurance.

❐ Did not discuss his protected health information in front of other patients.
❐ Did not talk to other staff members about the forgotten insurance card to other staff members unless he stated he would bring the card when she did not expect to be in the office.

What Would You Do/What Would You **Not** *Do?*
Review Keisha's response and place a checkmark next to the information you included in your response. List the additional information you included in your response.

_____
_____
_____
_____
_____
_____
_____

Case Study 3
Page 925

What Did Keisha Do?
❐ Explained that Dr. Sylvia Lawrence would be out on leave and could not accept appointments for 4 months.
❐ Offered to make an appointment with Dr. Lawrence after the 4-month period.
❐ Offered to make an appointment with Dr. William Rudner as soon as he had one available.
❐ Listened sympathetically if Ms. Pohl was displeased about not being able to be seen more promptly by a female physician.
❐ Responded calmly and in a normal speaking voice if the patient became irritated or upset.
❐ Made a recommendation about another female physician only if specifically instructed to do so by Dr. Lawrence.

What Did Keisha Not Do?
❐ Did not agree to make an appointment with Dr. Sylvia Lawrence before the end of the 4-month period just this once.
❐ Did not become defensive or imply that Ms. Pohl's preference for a female physician was silly.
❐ Did not become irritated or upset with Ms. Pohl.
❐ Did not talk about the telephone conversation later to other office staff.

What Would You Do/What Would You **Not** *Do?*
Review Keisha's response and place a checkmark next to the information you included in your response. List the additional information you included in your response.

_____
_____
_____
_____
_____
_____
_____

TERMINOLOGY REVIEW

Medical Term	Word Parts	Definition
Assignment of benefits		Authorization given by the patient to allow the insurance company to make payments directly to the health care provider instead of to the patient.
Call-in times		Blocks of time when a physician accepts telephone calls from patients.
Copayment		A fixed amount of money that the patient is responsible to pay at each visit.
Medicaid		A federal and state insurance program for low-income patients. The Medicaid program has a different name in each state.
Tickler file		A chronological file containing reminders of things to be done.

ON THE WEB

For information on HIPAA:

U.S. Department of Health and Human Services, Office for Civil Rights—HIPAA: www.hhs.gov/ocr/hipaa

Sample Notice of Privacy Practices at Medicare.gov: www.medicare.gov/privacypractices.asp

For information on the Red Flags Rule:

Federal Trade Commission: www.ftc.gov/bcp/edu/microsites/redflagsrule/index.shtml

 Check out the Evolve site at http://evolve.elsevier.com/Bonewit/today/ to actively Prepare for your Certification, and to access additional interactive activities and exercises to help you study and prepare for success.

38

Medical Office Computerization

LEARNING OBJECTIVES

Computer Concepts

1. Explain the difference between data and a program.
2. Explain the purpose of each of the following parts of the data processing cycle: input, processing, and output.
3. List examples of input and output devices.
4. Explain the difference between software and hardware.
5. Explain the function of an operating system.
6. State the function of application software.
7. List and state the function of the following components of the main computer unit: mainboard, CPU, main computer memory, hard drive, optical disc drive, and power supply.
8. Describe the care and maintenance of the main computer unit.
9. Describe the function, care, maintenance, and ergonomics of the computer monitor.
10. List and describe the function of the special keys on a computer keyboard.
11. Describe the care, maintenance, and ergonomics of a computer keyboard.
12. Identify the guidelines to follow in the care and maintenance of a printer.
13. List and describe the storage devices used with microcomputer systems.
14. Describe the method of organization that a hard disk uses to store and retrieve information.

Medical Office Computerization

15. Explain why it is important to have a foundation in computer concepts before engaging in hands-on computer operations.
16. List and explain the advantages and disadvantages of medical office computerization.
17. List and describe measures that can be taken to promote the efficient running of a computerized medical office.
18. Explain the purpose of a medical practice management software program.
19. Explain the function performed by each of the following parts of the medical office computer system: patient registration, appointments, posting transactions, patient billing, insurance billing, reports, file maintenance, and electronic medical record.

Electronic Medical Record

20. List the general functions of electronic medical record (EMR) software.
21. Explain the advantages and disadvantages of EMRs.
22. Describe the processes required to produce or convert each administrative and clinical document in a medical record into a digital format.
23. Discuss concepts of networking and electronic transfer of information.
24. List the procedures performed by the physician and medical assistant using an EMR.

Computer Maintenance and Security

25. Describe the methods used to maintain security of the medical office computer system.
26. List and describe methods used to back up computer data in the medical office.
27. State the various types of system maintenance that should be performed on a computer system.
28. List the various types of service agreements available for a computer system.

INTRODUCTION TO MEDICAL OFFICE COMPUTERIZATION

The computer is the most frequently used piece of equipment in today's medical office. It may be used to schedule appointments, process patient statements and insurance claims, order supplies, maintain computerized medical records, prescribe medications, receive e-mail, and/or create reports, to mention only a few common functions. The medical assistant must be very familiar with the computer system used in his or her office and the programs (e.g., medical practice management program, electronic medical record [EMR] program) being run on that computer system.

This chapter presents an overview of the parts of the medical office computer system, as well as important information about maintenance and data storage.

COMPUTER CONCEPTS

A **computer** is a device consisting of electronic components that has the ability to process data according to a program in order to produce a desired result. The primary advantage of using a computer to perform administrative procedures in the medical office is that these tasks are performed with greater speed and accuracy than with other types of devices (e.g., typewriter, pegboard system, calculator). In addition, computers are versatile: Rather than performing only one function (e.g., typing, posting a payment, math calculations), a computer can perform many different types of tasks.

Computers are useful tools because they can perform the same tasks repeatedly while maintaining the same level of efficiency. It should always be remembered, however, that the computer does not have a mind of its own. You are always in charge, and the computer will never do anything without your direction.

Most medical offices use **microcomputers** (also known as *personal computers* or *desktop computers*) linked together to form a **network,** a collection of computers that can share data and resources (Box 38-1). The number of computers in a network varies based on the size of the medical practice and the type and number of tasks performed on the computer. For example, a two-physician medical office using a practice management program typically has four to eight networked computers. A small network is called a *local area network* (LAN). In a larger system, the computers in a medical office may be linked to a hospital and possibly other offices. A *wide area network* (WAN), such as the Internet, is a collection of connected LANs. Networks for large systems usually contain one or more **servers,** large computers that store data and manage tasks for the computers on the network.

This section on computer concepts has been designed to provide you with the theoretical foundation necessary to effectively use computers in the medical office. Because the microcomputer is typically used in the medical office, this

section focuses on the theory and techniques of microcomputer systems.

BOX 38-1   Types of Microcomputers

Desktop Computer

A desktop computer, named because it can fit on and under a desk, usually consists of a plastic case containing the CPU (central processing unit), storage devices (e.g., hard disk, DVD/CD-ROM discs), other personal computer (PC) components (e.g., video card, sound card), a monitor, a keyboard, and a mouse.

Workstation

A workstation designates a desktop computer that is more powerful than a typical desktop computer and is normally devoted to one task. The term may also be used to indicate an area for a single worker in an office or laboratory setting.

Laptop Computer

A laptop computer (also called a *notebook*) usually weighs less than 5 lb and contains the processor, screen, other PC components, storage devices, and a means to input data, all contained in one portable unit.

Tablet Computer

A tablet computer is a complete computer with a touch screen contained in one portable unit. This may be a modified laptop that folds so that the screen faces out.

DATA PROCESSING CYCLE

As previously described, computers function by processing data. **Data processing** is the term applied to changing raw facts or data into an organized, recognizable form. To fully comprehend data processing, it is important to have a thorough understanding of the terms *data* and *program.* **Data** is a general term used to describe the raw, unorganized facts presented to the computer for processing. Patients' names, addresses, and telephone numbers are examples of data frequently entered into the computer in the medical office.

A **program** is defined as a set of instructions organized in a logical step-by-step sequence that tells the computer how to perform a specific function. As in cooking, when a recipe is required to tell you how to mix ingredients, a computer requires a program to tell it how to process data.

Computers process data in a logical three-part sequence known as the *data processing cycle* (Figure 38-1). The data processing cycle includes the following phases: input, processing, and output. Each phase of the data processing cycle involves a specific activity, which is described as follows.

The terms *input* and *output* have slightly different meanings depending on how they are used. When referring to the data processing cycle, they are used from the

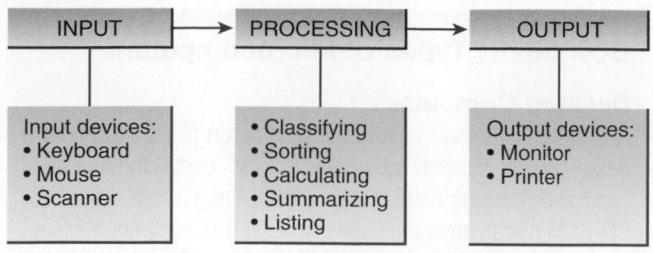

Figure 38-1 Data processing cycle.

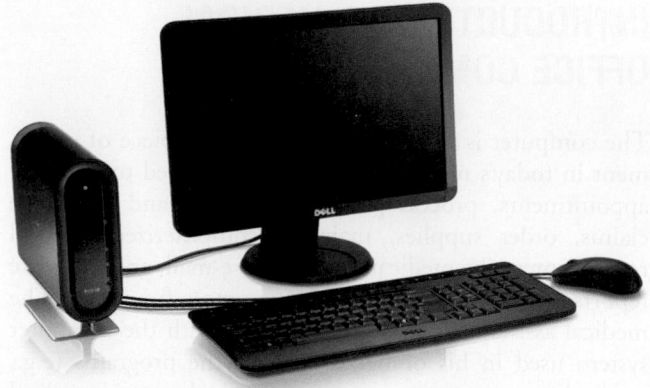

Figure 38-2 Computer system.

"computer's point of view" as verbs to describe the transfer of information. Input and output are also used as nouns to describe the data that have been entered into the computer (input) and the information that has been generated by the computer (output). As these terms appear throughout this chapter, you will become familiar with their different meanings.

Input

The **input** of data is the transfer of data to the computer for processing. Input includes both the entering of data into the computer and the conversion of it into an electronic form that can be understood by the computer. Because computers cannot understand the "written word" in the form used in communication by humans, the data must first be translated into an electronic code that can then be processed by the computer. Once the computer is finished working on the "electronic" data, the result must be converted back into a form that can be understood by the user. A **user** is defined as the individual using the computer.

Data must be entered into the computer through an **input device** (see Figure 38-1). The most common examples of input devices are the computer keyboard and the mouse, which are usually used together. They convert data into the electronic code that can be understood and processed very quickly by the computer. Other examples of input devices include a scanner and a microphone.

Processing

The **processing** of data is the computer's handling and arranging of the electronic data according to a program; in other words, the data undergo some type of manipulation or change to produce useful information. Depending on the result, the processing phase may include one or more of the following: classifying, sorting, calculating, summarizing, or listing of the data (see Figure 38-1).

Output

The final phase of the data processing sequence is the output of the processed data. **Output** is the transfer of usable information back to the user. Because the computer works with an electronic code, an output device must be used to communicate with the user. The **output device** converts the electronic code into a form that can be understood by the user. The most common output devices are the monitor and the printer (see Figure 38-1).

COMPONENTS OF THE COMPUTER SYSTEM

All of the components making up the computer are collectively known as the **computer system** (Figure 38-2). Computer systems include two major divisions: software and hardware.

Software

Software is a general term for the programs or instructions that tell a computer what to do. Software tells the computer how to perform specific tasks in a series of step-by-step instructions organized in a logical sequence. Two categories of software exist: system software and application software. System software assists the computer in carrying out its tasks, whereas application software assists the user in carrying out his or her computer tasks. Each software category is described in more detail next.

System Software

System software is made up of a group of special programs that control or maintain the operations of a computer. The most important type of system software is the **operating system.** The operating system is installed on the hard disk of the computer and is automatically loaded into the computer's main memory (RAM) when the computer is turned on. An example of an operating system frequently used in the medical office is Windows (Microsoft Corporation). The operating system performs "housekeeping" chores required by the computer system to operate itself. The most important function performed by an operating system is to serve as an intermediary to tell the hardware how to run an application program. Hence, application programs are useless without an operating system.

Application Software

Software designed to allow a user to accomplish a specific task is known as **application software,** also known as an *application program* or *software program.* Application software constitutes the greatest proportion of the software available for use with a computer.

Highlight on Operating Systems

Almost all of today's medical office computers run on a Windows operating system. The Windows operating system was designed in the 1980s to mimic the Apple Macintosh operating system (Mac OS) designed for Macintosh computers. An operating system allows interactions between the computer and the user, between the computer and peripheral equipment, and between computer and computer. The interaction may occur using a direct connection, a wireless network, a telephone line, and the Internet. Each time a new operating system is developed, it allows for more complex computer system interactions.

Windows and the Mac OS are based on the concept of the graphical user interface (GUI, pronounced "gooey"). The theory behind this type of operating system is that it operates the way people think—it is intuitive. When the computer is turned on, a desktop appears. The desktop is the computer analogy of all the items needed to open and view programs and files, to perform operations, and to create and store files.

An individual item, such as a patient record, a daily appointment list, or a medical record, is called a *file*. A file is a set of computer data that has been saved to disk. Files are collected in folders, indicated by an icon of a file folder. Folders can be displayed individually either within a window or on the desktop. When a folder is opened, it appears as a window, and all the files that reside in the folder are in the window. Files can be moved from one folder to another, just as they might be at a desk with papers, folders, and files.

Arranged on the desktop screen are icons. Icons are small graphics that provide a link to files, folders, or applications. With a Windows operating system, these icons include a small computer (My Computer), a recycle bin, and icons for application programs. At the bottom left of the screen is a start button. One click on the start button causes a list of options to rise from it. Many of the options have small arrows pointing to the right; highlighting one of these items causes submenus to appear. By clicking again, an application can be opened. ■

The medical practice management program contains features of four types of application programs: word processing, spreadsheets, telecommunications, and database management. In more detail, these application programs are as follows:

Word processing. Word processing software allows the user to enter, edit, format, and file (store) text. Microsoft Word is an example of a commercially available word processing application program. A medical practice management program can produce letters, statements, receipts, and insurance forms using data from its database.

Spreadsheet. A spreadsheet is an electronic ledger designed to perform mathematic calculations quickly. Spreadsheet programs are used to produce financial reports and to analyze and process statistics. An example of a commercially available spreadsheet application program is Microsoft Excel. A medical practice management program can generate financial reports for the office and revise the data quickly in the same way as a spreadsheet application program.

Telecommunications. A telecommunications application provides the means for one computer to "talk" with another computer. Electronic communication between computers greatly reduces the time it takes to send information. A medical practice management program uses a telecommunications application for the electronic submission of insurance claims. In addition, telecommunications software is used to send letters and messages as electronic mail (e-mail).

Database management. Database management is the storing and retrieving of data in and from a database. Database management allows the user to store large amounts of data on a storage device (e.g., hard disk).

The data can then be easily retrieved and manipulated. An example of a commercially available database management software program is Microsoft Access. A medical practice management program performs the majority of the administrative procedures in the medical office using the data in its database. Database management increases efficiency in recordkeeping and eliminates numerous time-consuming repetitive tasks. The database for a medical practice consists of patient records, patient transactions, diagnosis codes, procedure codes, insurance carriers, and so on. This information is stored on the hard disk of the computer or server for later retrieval and use as needed. A database also provides the ability to add new information, modify existing information, and delete unneeded information. The most significant aspect of a database is that the computer can cross-reference all of the information stored in its database. The medical practice database can be thought of as a large pool of information that the computer can access in a multitude of ways according to the task being performed.

Documentation

In the context of computer systems, **documentation** is a written set of instructions designed to assist the user in understanding how to operate an application program. Clear, concise, and easy-to-understand documentation makes it much easier to learn and use the program. Documentation includes the following: (1) the program user manual, which contains complete instructions for learning and using the program; (2) online help screens displayed on the computer monitor; and (3) reference cards containing frequently needed details for quick reference. It is important to learn to seek out and rely on the documentation that comes with the medical practice management program you are using. This results in more efficient operation of the computer system and less frustration in solving computer problems when they arise.

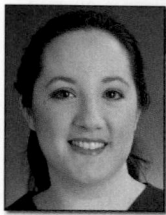

Putting It All into Practice

My name is Emma Hayes, and I am a certified medical assistant. Since I graduated, I have been working at the main office of an internal medicine practice. Our office manager is very interested in computers, and we have been using integrated practice management and EMR software for the past 4 years. When a new patient calls for an appointment, we obtain all his or her personal and insurance information and enter it into the computer during that first conversation. When patients first come to the office, we have them sit at a computer terminal in a private room next to the waiting room and enter their medical history. If the patient is not comfortable with the computer, we have the patient complete a paper form, and then I enter the data from the form into the computer. We have a scanner at the front desk to scan the patients' insurance cards and all the forms they sign at the first visit. We keep a folder for our patients with forms that they have signed, but everything is also available in electronic form.

One of the things our patients really like is that our physicians send all prescriptions to the pharmacy electronically. At the first visit, we ask patients for the name, address, and telephone number of the pharmacy they want to use. Some patients like to get their prescriptions by mail order, and we can also indicate that. I also ask the patient what medications he or she taking and enter them into the computer. After that, the physician can go to the patient's EMR, enter the information about the medication he wants to prescribe, and automatically send the prescription directly to the patient's pharmacy. The EMR program checks for drug interactions with all the medications that the patient is taking. Our physicians believe that this saves time and is actually more accurate, because the pharmacist doesn't have to read their handwritten prescriptions. ∎

Hardware

Hardware is the term for the physical equipment making up the computer system—that is, the tangible computer parts. Although a computer system may include a variety of hardware, the following hardware devices are necessary to perform administrative procedures in the medical office: main computer unit, monitor, computer keyboard and mouse, and printer.

MAIN COMPUTER UNIT

The main computer unit, or simply the main unit, consists of a hard plastic case that is usually rectangular in shape. The main unit houses all the components that make the

computer work and consists of the following components: mainboard, central processing unit (CPU), main computer memory (RAM), video card, sound card, power supply, and storage devices. The components of the main computer unit are discussed next.

Mainboard

The **mainboard** (also known as the "motherboard") is the primary circuit board of the main computer unit. Each of the other components of the main computer unit either sits on the mainboard itself (e.g., CPU) or is connected to it in some way (e.g., hard disk). Electrical circuits the width of human hairs are etched onto the mainboard; the electrical impulses that carry messages to and from the computer travel through these circuits. The mainboard provides a means for all of the components making up the main unit to communicate with one another and can be thought of as the nervous system of the computer.

Central Processing Unit

The **central processing unit (CPU)** is the functional core or "brain" of the computer and is the most complex computer component. The CPU interprets and executes the instructions that operate the computer. The CPU consists of a microprocessor chip, and therefore the CPU is often referred to as a *microprocessor*. The CPU resides on the mainboard housed in the main unit of the computer. More so than any other computer component, the CPU determines how fast a computer can process information. The speed of the CPU is expressed in gigahertz (abbreviated GHz), and the higher the value, the faster the computer. For example, a computer with a 3-GHz microprocessor chip can process information approximately twice as fast as a computer with a 1.5-GHz chip. The power of the CPU is determined by the number of bits it contains. A **bit** is the smallest amount of computer storage. Modern computers usually have at least 32-bit microprocessors, and 64-bit microprocessors are commonly found in servers and more powerful computers. Examples of manufacturers of these microprocessor chips are Intel and AMD.

Main Computer Memory

Main computer memory (or simply *main memory*) consists of computer chips mounted on a small board that connects the mainboard. Main memory is responsible for temporarily storing information until ready for use by the CPU. Main memory can be likened to a holding tank for the CPU in which items are placed for immediate access and for use when needed for processing. Among those items commonly held in main memory are the operating system, the application program in current use, data waiting to be processed, and information ready for output.

In a microcomputer, main computer memory has a special name: **random-access memory (RAM).**

RAM is the acronym for random-access memory and, as you have just learned, is the main memory of a microcomputer. It is called *random access* because the computer can get to any part of the information stored in its memory directly, rather than having to look through all the rest of its stored information. This is in contrast to **sequential-access memory,** in which all stored data must be searched sequentially from beginning to end to locate the desired information. Much less time is involved in locating information using random access, and it is one of the factors that allows computers to perform tasks very quickly.

As previously described, the purpose of RAM is to temporarily store items until they are needed by the computer. When you first turn on the computer, RAM is empty; therefore you must first place the items you want to work with in RAM. A copy of the application program is transferred into RAM from the hard disk (by using the mouse to click on the appropriate program icon on the desktop of the computer). Data are transferred into RAM through an input device, such as a keyboard. To run the application program, a copy of the operating system needs to be transferred from the hard disk into RAM; this is accomplished automatically by the computer when you turn on the computer. Once these items are in RAM, they are easily accessible and can be quickly retrieved when needed by the CPU for processing. After the data have been processed according to the instructions in the program, the resulting usable information is then placed back in RAM for temporary storage.

One very important aspect of RAM is that it provides only *temporary* storage, not permanent storage. When the computer is turned off, all of the items stored in RAM are "dumped out"; in other words, RAM will be empty when the computer is turned back on and therefore ready to accept more storage items. Because of this, you *must be sure* to permanently store information that you do not want to lose before turning off the computer. In the medical office, this information is either stored on the hard disk of the computer or on the server by way of the network. Other common storage devices include Universal Serial Bus (USB) flash drives and optical disc drives, which are described later in this chapter.

Storage Capacity

Storage capacity (the amount of information that can be stored) is measured in units of storage known as **bytes.** One byte, usually 8 bits, is approximately equal to one character, such as a letter or number. Stating the capacity of RAM in bytes, however, results in astronomically high numbers. Therefore it is more convenient to use larger units, such as kilobytes, megabytes, gigabytes, and terabytes. A **kilobyte (KB)** is equal to 1024 bytes, which is usually rounded off to 1000 bytes. A **megabyte (MB)** is equal to a little more than 1 million bytes; in terms of kilobytes, 1 MB is equal to 1000 KB. An even larger measure than a megabyte is a **gigabyte (GB);** 1 GB is equal to 1 billion bytes or 1000 MB. The largest measure in current use is a **terabyte (TB);** 1 TB is equal to 1 trillion bytes or 1000 GB.

As you would imagine, the larger the capacity of RAM, the more information it can hold at one time. For example, a computer with 2 GB of RAM has the ability to hold more than 2 billion bytes. Most microcomputers now come with a main memory of 2 GB or more.

The capacity of a computer's memory (RAM) correlates directly with the level of complexity of the programs it can run. A program takes up a certain amount of space in RAM. A small and simple application program that performs a limited number of tasks occupies much less space in RAM than a large, complex, and powerful program that performs numerous complicated tasks, such as a medical practice management program. The capacity of RAM is an important criterion to consider when working with or purchasing a computer or an application program. A computer with less than the required memory for a particular program would not have enough storage space to hold that program. Hence, that program could not be run on that particular computer. The packaging of the application program is labeled with information on *computer system requirements.* System requirements tell you what requirements your computer system must have (e.g., type of operating system, microprocessor speed, amount of memory, hard disk space) in order to run the program. Storage devices will be discussed later in the chapter.

Other Personal Computer Components

Sound Card and Video Card

The **video card** (also known as a *graphics card*) connects to the mainboard through a video card slot. A video card converts video output into electronic signals. These electronic signals are then sent to the monitor, where they are converted into text and images that are displayed on the screen of the monitor. The **sound card** is a small circuit board that is connected to the mainboard. A sound card converts audio output into electronic signals. The electronic signals are then sent to speakers that convert them into sound, such as sound effects, music, and narration.

Power Supply

The power supply provides the power needed by the computer to run itself.

Care and Maintenance of the Main Computer Unit

The main computer unit should be placed on a flat, stable surface, such as a computer desk. This prevents excessive vibration during operation, which could loosen the electronic circuit boards. If the main unit is found in a tower, it is designed to be placed in a vertical position. Information on proper positioning is always indicated in the instruction manual accompanying the computer. Laptops should also be placed on a flat, stable surface if possible, and they should be lifted by the base, not the screen.

Computers operate best in a moderately cool temperature environment. Extreme heat and inadequate ventilation increase the chance of malfunction. As a precautionary measure, the main unit should not be placed near a window or other areas that receive direct sunlight. In addition, to prevent overheating, the ventilation slots on the main unit should not be obstructed.

The primary cause of improper functioning of the computer is exposure to environmental contaminants, such as dust, dirt, and smoke. For this reason, rooms with computers should be kept clean with no smoking permitted. The casing of the main unit should be periodically wiped with a slightly damp, lint-free cloth to remove dust and dirt. Aerosol sprays, solvents, and abrasives should never be used to clean the casing because they can damage the finish. The interior of the main computer unit should be cleaned occasionally according to the instructions outlined in the computer's user manual.

Liquids should be kept away from the computer. A liquid spilled into the main unit can cause irreparable damage to the electronic circuit boards. In addition, an electrical short may occur and could result in a fire or small explosion.

The main unit is attached by cables to the other computer components (e.g., monitor, keyboard, printer). The cables should be checked on a regular basis to be sure that they are secure. A loose or disengaged cable can result in temporary malfunctioning of the computer system.

COMPUTER MONITOR

A computer monitor is a piece of electrical equipment that displays images generated by a computer. The monitor permits the user to view both input, or more specifically, the data entered into the computer, and output, or the information produced by the computer as a result of processing.

Viewing the input displayed on the monitor allows the user to check the data for accuracy as it is entered. As an output device, the monitor is often used to review information that needs to be viewed briefly and for which a printed copy (hard copy) is not necessary. For example, if a patient calls your office to inquire when his next appointment is scheduled, you can quickly call up this information, view it on the display screen, and relay it to the patient.

Types of Monitors

Modern liquid-crystal display (LCD) flat panel monitors (Figure 38-3) are small, lightweight, and compact and therefore take up much less desk space than traditional monitors (cathode-ray tube [CRT] monitors) which were bulkier because they used a cathode ray tube. LCD monitors consume very little power and are therefore very energy efficient. An LCD monitor creates a visual image on the screen by manipulating light within a layer of liquid crystal cells. With an LCD monitor, it is sometimes difficult to view the image on the screen from an angle

Screen Size

Screen size refers to the measurement of a computer screen in inches from one corner of the screen diagonally across to the opposite corner. The typical desktop monitor used in a medical office has a screen size from 17 to 20 inches across measured diagonally, with the range of available screen sizes

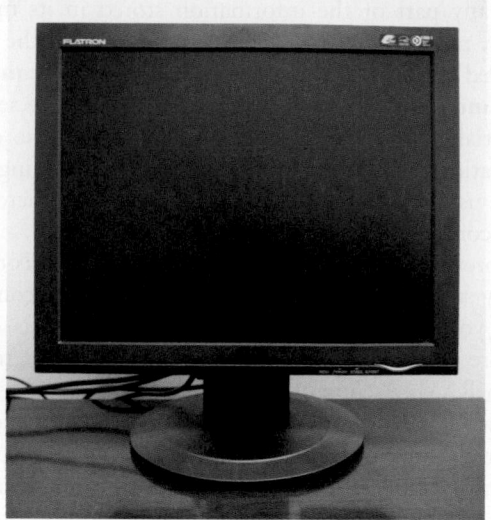

Figure 38-3 Liquid-crystal display (LCD) flat panel monitor.

being 14 to 23 inches. This is much larger than the screen of a laptop computer, which is limited to the size of the laptop unit.

Monitor Resolution

An important area of consideration when working with a computer system is the resolution of the monitor. The term **resolution** refers to the sharpness of the image displayed on the screen. A computer monitor with a high resolution produces a sharp image with crisp, clear, easy-to-read characters, which helps prevent eyestrain and headaches. High resolutions also allow the computer to display a larger work area.

Resolution is measured in units called *picture elements* or *pixels*. **Pixels** are "dot" locations on the screen that can be lit up as needed to display characters and other images. The more dots present, the sharper the image. A monitor with a resolution of 1280 × 1024 can display 1280 pixels horizontally and 1024 pixels vertically on the screen. The larger the monitor, the more pixels that can be displayed. Most monitors display 90 to 100 pixels per square inch.

Monitor Controls

Controls to operate and adjust the display screen are located on either the front or the side of the monitor. One control is a push-button *on/off button*. When the monitor is turned on, an indicator light comes on, denoting the monitor is receiving power and ready for use.

Other controls typically found on a computer monitor menu include a menu to adjust contrast, brightness, vertical and horizontal size, and position.

Monitor Ergonomics

The monitor should be placed directly in front of the user and at an arm's length distance when sitting back in a chair. This position provides the most comfortable viewing distance. The monitor should be positioned so that the top of the monitor is approximately 2 to 3 inches above eye level.

This position helps to prevent back and neck tension. It is known that eye muscles must work harder to focus on near objects. Therefore when working on the computer for a prolonged period of time, occasionally focus your eyes on a distant object (more than 20 feet away) to prevent eyestrain. It is also important to blink frequently while you work to lubricate and moisten the eyes to prevent them from drying out.

To avoid glare, the monitor should be positioned so that the screen does not reflect bright light, which could decrease visibility and also result in eyestrain. For example, positioning the monitor directly in front of a bright window causes a distracting reflection on the screen. Subdued overhead lighting is considered best for computer use because it causes the least amount of glare. Glare filters are available to help reduce unavoidable reflections, such as from bright overhead fluorescent lights. Privacy filters reduce glare and also increase privacy of screen information by blurring or blacking out the screen image to anyone who is not directly in front of it.

Monitor Care and Maintenance

The monitor should rest on a flat, stable surface, such as a computer desk.

Monitors collect dust and dirt, and therefore must be properly maintained. The screen should be cleaned regularly. To clean an LCD monitor, first turn the monitor off. Wipe it gently with a soft, lint free cloth. Do not use paper towels or tissues because they can scratch the screen. If the dry cloth does not remove all soil, do not press harder because the screen can be damaged. If necessary, use distilled water on a soft cloth or commercial wipes or cleaners for LCD screens. Do not use cleaners that contain chemicals like ethyl alcohol or acetone, because these can discolor the screen. The cleaner should not be applied directly to the screen or sprayed on the screen as it may run down into the inside of the case and damage the electrical circuits. Keeping the screen clean helps prevent distracting reflections. If the office still uses older CRT monitors (easily recognizable because they are more than six inches deep from front to back), a commercial glass cleaner can be used to clean them with a soft cloth.

The outside casing of the monitor should periodically be wiped with a damp, lint-free cloth to remove dust and dirt. Aerosol sprays, solvents, and abrasives should not be used to clean the casing because they can damage the finish.

COMPUTER KEYBOARD

The computer keyboard is the most common input device. It contains keys that are pressed to enter data and instructions into the computer. Different brands of computer keyboards vary in size, shape, and layout, but all contain the same basic elements (Figure 38-4).

Computer keyboards include all the keys normally found on a typewriter keyboard. The composition of the keyboard is alphanumeric—that is, it consists of both alphabetic and

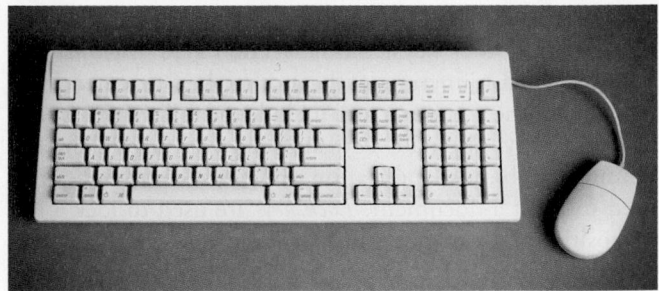

Figure 38-4 Computer keyboard.

numeric keys. The keys are located in the same place as on the standard typewriter keyboard and are used for the same purpose. Computer keyboards produce both uppercase and lowercase letters and have the standard typewriter "QWERTY" layout, named for the first row of letters. Many desktop computer keyboards also have a numeric keypad on the right side of the keyboard, which is used for entering numbers quickly.

As previously explained, computers can work only with electronic data. When a key is pressed on a computer keyboard, an electronic code is generated, which is passed along to the computer for processing. At the same time, the electronic code is sent to the video card, which then allows that computer to display the input as words and symbols on the monitor.

The keyboard of a desktop computer is either attached by a cable to the main computer unit or is wireless and transmits signals to a receiver that is connected to the computer through a USB port. The user positions the keyboard of a desktop computer according to his or her preference and comfort. The keyboard is usually built into a laptop computer, whereas tablet devices and handheld devices often use a touchscreen keyboard.

Special Keys

The most significant difference between a computer keyboard and a typewriter keyboard is the presence of additional keys known as **special keys.** Special keys issue commands to the computer to perform specific functions on the information displayed on the screen. Pressing a special key does not cause a character to be typed on the screen, nor does the command appear on printed copy. Instead these keys allow the user to perform such tasks as saving text, printing text, capitalizing text, deleting and inserting text, and moving the cursor.

An example of a special key that functions in the same manner regardless of the type of computer or program being used is the enter key. The enter key (also called the *return key*) is the most frequently used special key. Pressing the enter key tells the computer to act on the instructions that have been given to it. In simple terms, it gives the computer permission to go ahead with a function. For example, if you have given the computer the print command, the enter key can be pressed to tell the computer to go ahead with this instruction.

Special keys can be divided into categories and include modifier keys, lock keys, and navigation keys. *Modifier keys* are used in conjunction with another key to enter commands into the computer and include the following: control key, shift key, alternate key, and the command key. For example, with most application programs, control-P can be used to print a document. *Lock keys* are used to lock a key in position and include the following: caps lock, numeric lock, and scroll lock. *Navigation keys* are used to control the movement of the cursor on the screen and include the following: arrow keys, home and end keys, page scroll key, enter key, backspace key, insert key, delete key, and tab key.

Most keyboards have *function keys* that can be programmed to perform certain tasks that will assist the user, such as saving text or printing a document. The number of such keys varies but is now usually 12 or more. Function keys are usually located above the top row of alphanumeric keys on the keyboard. These keys are usually preprogrammed by the application software package that makes use of them, but some computers permit these keys to be user programmed directly from the keyboard.

Mouse

After the keyboard, the mouse is the second most commonly used input device. A mouse is a pointing device that fits comfortably under the palm of your hand. The mouse is used to move the pointer on the screen to an object on the screen, such as a menu item, an icon, or a line of text. The mouse must then be "clicked" to perform a certain action associated with that object. The mouse may be wireless or connected directly to the computer.

Keyboard Ergonomics

To prevent muscle fatigue of the upper extremities, the computer keyboard should be placed at a level that is lower than that of a conventional desk or table. The feet should be flat on the floor and the hands should rest comfortably at the keyboard with the shoulders relaxed and the elbows flexed at a 90-degree angle or tilted slightly upward. An adjustable chair with good back support is recommended to attain the proper typing height for each individual working with the computer (Figure 38-5).

For entering data, a light touch should be used and the hands and fingers should be kept as relaxed as possible. If using a mouse, position it at the same height as the keyboard. Be sure to allow adequate workspace to use both the keyboard and mouse comfortably. These measures help to prevent strain on the wrists and hands.

An adequate working space should be available to position the material being entered into the computer. The material should be placed so that it can be viewed easily either by placing it lying flat on the work surface or being held vertically in a copy holder.

Keyboard Care and Maintenance

With extended use, a residue may build up on the surface of the keyboard. This residue, often referred to as *grime,* should be cleaned with an antiseptic wipe or a slightly damp, lint-free cloth. Aerosol sprays should never be used to clean the keyboard because liquid may drip down into the keyboard, damaging its electrical components. The keyboard interior can be "dusted" by using a compressed inert gas that comes in a pressurized can and is available from computer supply stores. Alternatively, a vacuum cleaner with a small brush attachment may be used to clean the keyboard interior.

The following steps should be followed when cleaning the computer keyboard:
1. Shut down the computer.
2. Disconnect the keyboard cable.
3. Hold the keyboard upside down and shake it to remove any dust, dirt, or crumbs that may be stuck in the keyboard.

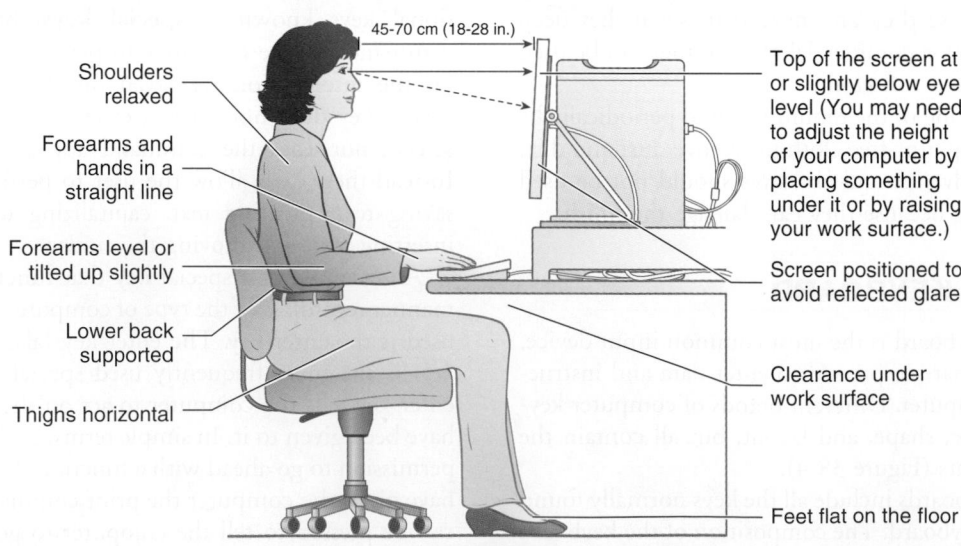

Figure 38-5 Keyboard ergonomics.

4. Clean the keyboard using a can of compressed air following the manufacturer's instructions. Use the can in an upright position. Do not tilt or shake the can.

5. Clean the top and side of the keys with an antiseptic wipe or a damp, lint-free cloth to remove grime. A cotton swab moistened with alcohol can be used to clean between the keys.

6. Allow the keyboard to dry completely (about 30 minutes) before reconnecting it to the computer.

Because of their electronic components, computer keyboards can be damaged if liquids spill into them, particularly those that are sweet or sticky, such as soft drinks. Therefore it is best not to place beverages close to the keyboard. If a liquid is accidentally spilled into the keyboard, the computer should immediately be turned off. If the liquid spilled is thin and clear, such as water, unplug the keyboard, turn it upside down and shake it gently to get as much liquid out as possible. Keep the keyboard inverted to allow additional liquid to drain out, and use a paper towel or cloth to wipe off the top of the keyboard. Let the keyboard dry in an inverted position for 24 hours at room temperature. If after these steps have been taken the keyboard does not work, it should be replaced. A greasy, sweet, or sticky liquid such as a soft drink spilled into the keyboard often causes permanent damage and the keyboard must be replaced.

PRINTER

A printer is an output device capable of printing text and graphics on paper. Printers convert processed data from a combination of electronic impulses into a printed form called **hard copy.** In the medical office, a hard copy of the computer input is frequently required; examples include patient reminders, patient receipts, prescriptions, patient statements, and office reports.

Some printers can also double as fax machines and photocopiers, but this is practical only when there is a small volume of work. A printer can be dedicated to one computer or can be networked to a number of computers.

The printers most commonly used in the medical office are inkjet and laser printers.

Inkjet Printer

An inkjet printer (Figure 38-6) uses droplets of ink to form text characters and graphics. This type of printer contains nozzles that spray tiny drops of ink onto the paper to create an image. Inkjet printers are lightweight and inexpensive and can produce text and graphics in both black and white and color on a variety of paper types.

Printing speed refers to the number of pages per minute (ppm) generated by the printer. Printing speed for an inkjet printer ranges from 8 to 36 ppm. Pages that contain text print at a faster rate than pages that are in color or contain graphics.

Although the initial cost of an inkjet printer is low, operating costs are higher than those of a laser printer. The

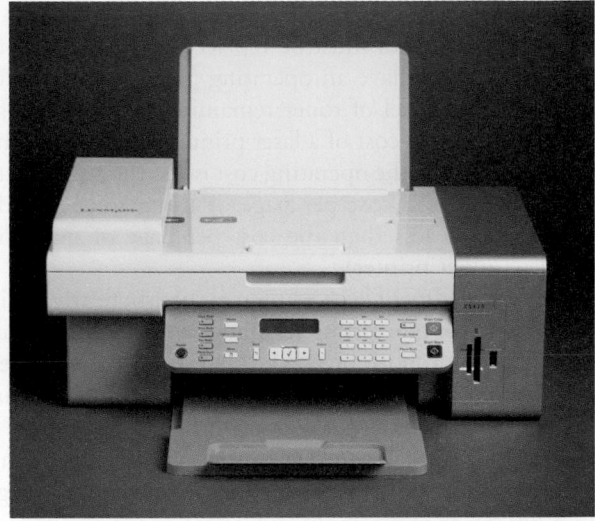

Figure 38-6 Inkjet printer.

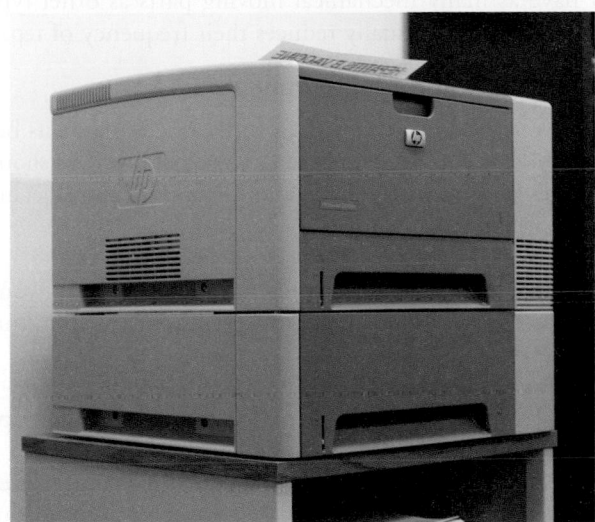

Figure 38-7 Laser printer.

ink used by an inkjet printer is contained in cartridges, which are expensive and must be replaced frequently. Most inkjet printers have at least two ink cartridges—one containing black ink, and one or more containing colored ink.

Laser Printer

The most significant feature of a laser printer (Figure 38-7) is that it has a "computer of its own" to direct its functioning. Laser printers use a micro-thin beam of light (laser beam), electric charges, and a toner powder to produce each page of text. Under direction of the printer's computer, the laser beam is bounced off a series of mirrors onto a positively charged rotating drum. The pulses of the beam correspond to the characters making up the document being printed. The areas where the laser beam hits the drum become neutral, which enables the toner powder to stick to them and form characters. Finally, the characters are transferred from the rotating drum to paper with the use of pressure and heat to solidify the toner powder on the paper. This process is similar to that of a photocopy machine.

The toner powder used with a laser printer is housed in a plastic cartridge and must be replaced when it runs out. Most laser printers have an operating panel on the printer that displays the level of toner remaining in the cartridge. Although the initial cost of a laser printer is more than that of an inkjet printer, the operating cost is less than an inkjet's. This is because the cost per page of using toner powder (laser printer) is less than the cost per page of using ink cartridges (inkjet printer).

The print quality of laser printers is superb, nearly attaining the quality of typesetting seen in textbooks. Laser printers are available in both black-and-white and color models. Other advantages of laser printers include their fast printing speed and quiet mode of operation. The printing speed of laser printers is faster than that of inkjet printers. Depending on the model of laser printer, the printing speed ranges from 12 to 35 or more ppm. Text prints at a faster rate and color and graphics print at a slower rate. Laser printers do not have as many mechanical moving parts as other types of printers, which usually reduces their frequency of repair.

Printer Care and Maintenance

Proper maintenance keeps the printer operating at its best and prolongs its life. Some general guidelines that should be followed to properly care for and maintain an inkjet and a laser printer are as follows:

1. Place the printer on a flat, stable surface.
2. Avoid placing the printer in a location that would expose it to direct sunlight, excessive heat, moisture, or dust.
3. Sufficient room should be left around the printer to allow for easy access for such tasks as adding paper and replacing ink or toner cartridges.
4. Add paper when needed, following the manufacturer's instructions. Inkjet and laser printers use individual sheets of paper stored in a tray in the printer's casing.
5. Replace ink cartridges in inkjet printers and toner cartridges in laser printers as required, following the manufacturer's instructions.
6. After turning off the printer, wait at least 5 seconds before turning it back on. Rapid switching of the power off and on can damage the printer.
7. The printer should be cleaned regularly to remove accumulated dust and dirt. The outside case should be cleaned with a soft clean cloth dampened with a mild detergent solution. Never use strong detergents or solvents on the casing because they could damage the finish. Clean the platen glass, inside of the document cover, and document feeder with a lint-free cloth moistened with water to prevent streaks. The inside of the printer should be cleaned according to the instructions in the printer's user manual.

STORAGE DEVICES

A **storage device** consists of a storage medium that permanently stores information for later retrieval by the computer. A storage device retains its information after the power has been removed and is used to store both programs and data. Examples of storage devices available for microcomputer systems include hard disks, CDs, DVDs, and USB flash drives, which are discussed on the following pages.

Storage capacity varies widely based on the type of storage device and usually is related to the cost of the device. For example, a flash drive can hold from 4 to over 100 GB, whereas a typical hard disk has a storage capacity of at least 250 GB.

Hard Disks

A **hard disk** derives its name from the fact that it consists of thin, rigid platters made of metal or glass (Figure 38-8). The composition of a hard disk is designed to maximize its important functions: the storage and retrieval of information. To accommodate the storage of information, hard disks are coated with a magnetically sensitive material. Data are stored on the disk as magnetic particles.

To store and retrieve the information on the disk as quickly as possible, a method or organization that divides the disk into designated areas similar to the division of a piece of property into housing lots is used. The disk surface is divided into a set of concentric circles; each of these circles is called a *track* (Figure 38-9). Data are stored on these tracks in the form of magnetized particles. Tracks are further divided into *sectors* that resemble the wedge-shaped pieces of a pie (see Figure 38-9). Through a process called *formatting,* the tracks and sectors are numerically marked to facilitate the location of information stored on the disk.

The following example provides a comparison of how the arrangement of tracks and sectors and formatting assist in locating information stored on the disk. Let's say that a friend invites you to her house at 102 Sunnyside Drive in Greenfield Village. You arrive at Greenfield Village and first locate the proper street and then you look for the house number. But just think how difficult and time consuming it would be to locate your friend's house without a street name or a house number. Comparing this example to the organization of hard disks, tracks and sectors are

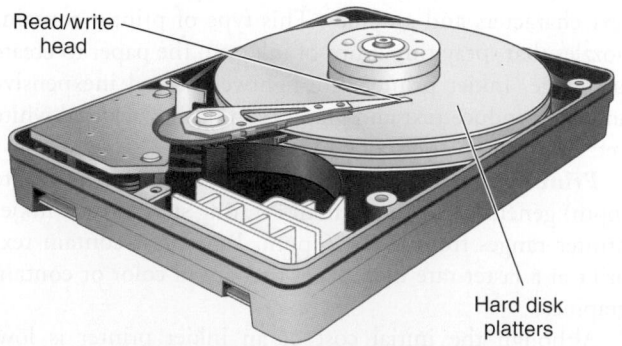

Figure 38-8 Hard disk drive.

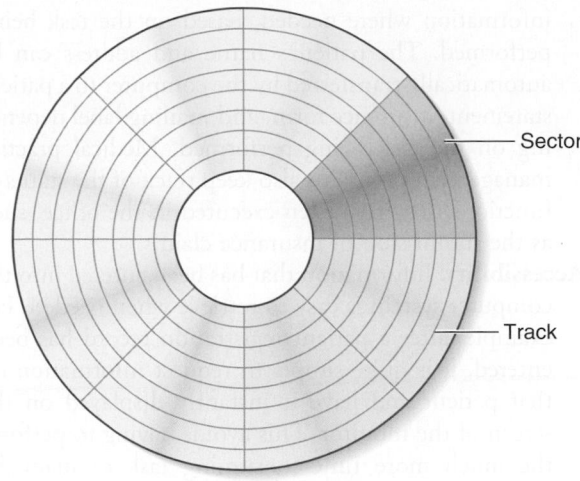

Figure 38-9 Tracks and sectors.

comparable to the division of Greenfield Village into streets and housing lots, and the formatting process (which numerically marks each track and sector) is comparable to the street names and house numbers.

Hard Disk Drive

Information is stored on a hard disk and retrieved from a hard disk within a device known as a *hard disk drive.* A hard disk drive is a mechanical device that rotates a hard disk at a high rate of speed. A read/write head mounted on an arm (see Figure 38-8) floats on a layer of air above the spinning disk and has instant access to all the tracks and sectors on the disk. All computers have an internal hard disk drive, meaning it is located inside the main computer unit. Because a hard disk is very sensitive to dirt, dust, and smoke, the entire disk unit is encased in a permanently sealed, airtight container to protect it from these contaminants. The entire disk unit (consisting of the hard disks and read/write heads) makes up the hard disk drive.

Hard disks come in a variety of storage sizes beginning at about 250 GB and ranging up to 1 TB or more depending on the computer.

Optical Discs

Optical discs are storage devices that store data using laser technology. They have replaced floppy disks, which were once commonly used storage devices for microcomputers. Optical discs are used to store system software, application software, data, photographs, music, and movies. An optical disc consists of a flat, round portable disc made of metal, plastic, and lacquer. It is usually $4\frac{3}{4}$ inches in diameter and less than $\frac{1}{20}$ inch thick.

An optical disc may be *read only,* which means that data can only be read (retrieved) from the disc; data cannot be written (saved) on the disc. An example of a read-only disc is a CD-ROM. The data on a CD-ROM are stored as microscopic pits along a spiral groove that runs along the surface of the disc. Data are read from a CD-ROM with a beam of laser light known as a *laser diode.*

Application software may come on a CD-ROM, and it is installed onto a computer's hard drive to operate. CD-ROMs hold about 650 MB of information. Sometimes the CD must be in the CD-ROM optical disc drive to successfully run the program.

Optical discs may also be *read/write,* which means that data can be read from the disc and written onto the disc. Writing on an optical disc is often termed "burning" a disc. An example of a read/write disc is a CD-RW (compact disc rewritable).

A DVD (digital versatile disc or digital video disc) uses another type of optical disc technology. This type of disc can hold about six times as much information as a CD-ROM, and therefore it has become popular as a means of storing music and movies, both of which require large amounts of storage space.

An **optical disc drive** uses a laser to read an optical disc or write onto an optical disc. Today's computers include one or more optical disc drives that can read and write both CD-ROM discs and DVD discs. The optical disc drives are installed in drive bays on the main computer unit. For an optical disc drive to be used, a button is pushed to slide out a tray; the optical disc is then inserted into the tray (label-side up), and the same button is pushed to close the tray.

USB Flash Drive

A USB flash drive is a portable storage device that consists of a small circuit board in a plastic case. Other terms for a flash drive include a *jump drive* and a *thumb drive.* A flash drive stores information using flash memory, which is a type of electrical computer memory. For a flash drive to be used, it must be inserted into a USB port on the main unit. A USB flash drive has a storage capacity that usually ranges from 4 GB to 100 GB, although some flash drives have considerably more memory.

MEDICAL OFFICE COMPUTERIZATION

Medical office computerization is the use of the computer to perform medical office administrative procedures. With the advent of the microcomputer, medical offices now use a computer to perform administrative procedures that were previously performed manually. This, in turn, has increased the demand for qualified individuals trained in medical office computerization not only to perform the administrative tasks on the computer, but also to instruct other staff members in computer operations.

Prerequisite Computer Concepts

Before beginning to work with a medical practice management program, it is important to first acquire a thorough knowledge of computer concepts. Just as medical terminology is a necessary prerequisite to clinical procedure courses, a knowledge of computer concepts is necessary to effectively operate a computer system in the front office.

The benefits of understanding computer concepts include increased confidence and ease when working on the computer and the ability to understand the computer terminology presented in the program user manual. Furthermore, a computer concepts base helps you to communicate with computer software specialists, such as the technical support staff for your medical practice management program. Working with technical support is often necessary when first learning the medical practice management program or when a problem is encountered with the program. To help you acquire this foundation, the beginning of this chapter provides a presentation of computer concepts.

Impact of Medical Office Computerization

Almost all medical offices use computers to perform at least some functions. Although there are distinct advantages to using a computer, it should be realized that there are also some disadvantages that can lead to difficulties. It is important to be aware of these problem areas so that steps can be taken to either prevent them altogether or be better prepared for them if they occur. Adequate preparation will result in the least amount of disruption to the efficient running of a computerized front office. The following discussion outlines both advantages and disadvantages of medical management computerization.

Advantages of Computerization

The advantages of computerizing the front office include the following:

Speed and productivity. One of the principal advantages of a computer is that it can process a large amount of data quickly. For example, if your physician asks you to compile a list of all patients with a diagnosis of hypertension, accomplishing this task by hand would require considerable time and effort. However, with a computer an inquiry search can be performed in which the computer searches all the patient files and automatically generates a list of patients with hypertension. Billing and health insurance requirements have placed a tremendous burden on the medical office of today. In addition, the completion of insurance claims becomes ever more complicated. Therefore a large portion of front office responsibility is often devoted to preparing and submitting patient statements and insurance claims. Because they can prepare and process items in a short period of time, computers provide much assistance in this area. In addition, faster computer processing of these items often leads to better collections for the medical office.

Efficiency. Computers are particularly good at performing repetitive tasks in which information is used over and over again but in a different format. For example, once a patient's name and address have been entered into the computer's database, they can be used on a number of different forms without having to reenter them. The computer automatically transfers this information where needed, based on the task being performed. The patient's name and address can be automatically transferred by the computer to a patient statement, insurance form, and mailing label depending on the task being performed. Medical practice management programs also keep track of the status of functions that have been executed in the office, such as the submission of insurance claims.

Accessibility. Information that has been entered into the computer system is easy to retrieve when needed. For example, after a patient registration record has been entered, it is quite simple to request information on that patient and have it instantly displayed on the screen of the monitor. This avoids having to perform the much more time-consuming task of manually hunting through a filing system to locate the patient's chart.

Audit trail. The computer can keep track of data entry. When new information is entered or existing information is changed, a log is created to record the time and date of the entry, as well as the name of the computer operator. This log is stored and can be retrieved by the practice manager to detect irregularities. If an error was made, the program lists the name of the operator and date the information was entered.

Reduced costs. After the initial cost of purchasing the hardware and software, computerization of the front office helps to decrease operating costs by reducing the amount of time required to perform front office procedures.

Disadvantages of Computerization

The disadvantages presented by computers in the medical office include the following:

Initial cost and maintenance. The combined expense of initially purchasing hardware and software can easily fall into thousands of dollars. In addition, an office must periodically upgrade its computer system and software or even purchase an entirely new system altogether, leading to further expenses.

Time investment. Because medical management programs perform highly sophisticated tasks, it takes considerable time to learn a program and use it with ease. Most software vendors provide on-site training of staff for a newly purchased program, as well as technical support when problems are encountered with the program. Even with all of this assistance, however, learning a medical management program, an electronic record program, or even an updated version of either can easily take a month or more. During this time, the medical assistant may experience much frustration when difficulty is encountered in executing a task. However, once the initial training period has been completed, most individuals agree that the time and patience expended are worth the outcome.

Start-up tasks. Certain tasks must be performed before a medical practice management program or EMR becomes operational, or in other words, before a new program can be used in its intended manner. Examples of start-up tasks include (1) entering background information that the program will use, such as diagnosis and procedure codes or customized menus, and (2) entering patient information such as demographic information and/or health history. In implementing an EMR, a decision must be made about how much of the old medical record to enter into the new electronic record. The start-up data need to be entered only once. Later, additional information can be added as needed, and the length of input time is greatly diminished.

Computer System Malfunctions

Even the best hardware and software systems can and will occasionally fail, and one or more of the front office procedures will come to an abrupt halt. Some problems have no explanations, whereas others are directly related to a specific event, such as operator error, a software bug, or a hardware malfunction. In order to minimize computer down time, most medical offices are connected to some kind of network or server that stores information and provides backup systems.

Measures to Promote Efficient Computer Operation

The challenges presented by computerizing the front office can for the most part be overcome by implementing the following preventative measures. Measures work to reduce computer frustration and promote the efficient running of a computerized medical office:

Selection of hardware and software. Hardware and software should be selected from experienced and established vendors. Some medical offices use a consultant to assist with this process.

Qualified personnel. Individuals working on the computer should be well trained in computer concepts and hands-on computer operation. This can be accomplished by employing office staff who have graduated from a formal educational program or by having the front office staff attend computer workshops and seminars. Untrained staff can adversely affect the efficient operation of a computer system.

Proper care and maintenance of the computer system. Proper care and maintenance of the computer system are undoubtedly directly related to reliable operation of the system. The beginning of this chapter presents the proper care and maintenance for each component in the computer system. Make sure you thoroughly review this information before working with a computer system. In addition to providing many years of reliable service, a well-cared-for system is much less likely to malfunction.

MEDICAL PRACTICE MANAGEMENT PROGRAM

A **medical practice management program** provides instructions to the computer for performing front office procedures. Almost all offices use some type of practice management program, and many have already incorporated or are in the process of incorporating an EMR that works together with the practice management program.

Practice management programs consist of a number of areas of specialization. Each area of specialization is known as a *system,* and each system performs procedures related to its particular area of specialization. Practice management programs include the following: patient registration system, appointment system, posting transactions system, patient billing system, insurance billing system, reports system, and file maintenance system. Each system is described in detail next.

Patient Registration System

The patient registration system is used to set up a registration record for each patient in the medical practice. The patient registration record includes demographic and medical insurance information, such as the patient's name and address, telephone number, gender, date of birth, and Social Security number and the patient's insurance carrier, policy number, and group number. This system is also used to review and update information on existing registration records. For example, if the patient's address changes, this system is used to delete the old address and enter the new address. Information entered into the patient registration system is used for a number of procedures, such as preparing a new patient's chart, posting transactions, and processing patient statements and insurance claims.

Appointment System

The appointment system handles all procedures related to appointment scheduling. These include making an appointment, canceling an appointment, rescheduling an appointment, finding an appointment, printing an appointment log, and printing a patient reminder card. Occasionally a medical office prefers to use an appointment book for patient scheduling rather than or in addition to the computer. Even though the computer is faster, some medical offices prefer to have a written record of appointments rather than storing this information in the computer system. They reason that in the event of a computer breakdown, a written record of appointments is still accessible.

Computerized appointment scheduling accomplishes three important goals. First, it is easier to change an appointment on a computer than with pencil and paper. With a computer, the patient's name can simply be deleted and the space in the schedule template left open. Second, at the beginning of the day the day's schedule can be printed out and does not have to be generated manually from the appointment book. Third, if a patient needs to make regular weekly or monthly visits, a time of day and day of week can be chosen and the computer will automatically record the patient's name in that time slot for as many visits as are needed.

Posting Transactions System

When a patient has been seen by the physician, the medical assistant must post the charges of the office visit and any payments made by the patient. The posting transactions system is responsible for performing this task. Using the posting transactions system, the medical assistant enters the services and procedures provided to the patient from the charge slip. The charge slip lists all of the services and procedures that were performed during the visit. The computer has codes for all services and procedures in its database and knows how much should be charged for each service and procedure. Diagnosis codes are also found in the database, and one code is selected for each charge that is posted.

In addition, the posting transactions system also permits the medical assistant to post payments made by the patient (e.g., copayment) or a third-party payer. A receipt of the charges and/or payments can be printed for the patient immediately.

Patient Billing System

One of the most important tasks required for the effective functioning of a medical office is to ensure prompt payment of patient bills. The function of the patient billing system is to prepare bills and print billing statements. When patient charges, payments, and adjustments are posted, this information is stored in the computer and is available when needed by the patient billing system. This system is responsible for searching the medical practice database to obtain the information necessary to generate bills for patients with outstanding balances. If the billing is done off site, this system prepares the information for electronic transmission to the billing facility.

Insurance Billing System

The function of the insurance billing system is to prepare and generate insurance claims. As procedures and diagnoses are entered into the computer during posting transactions, they are stored in the medical practice database. Later, this information is available when needed to prepare insurance claims. From the information stored in the database, the computer can automatically fill out every portion of the insurance claim form.

Insurance claims can be submitted to insurance companies either by mailing paper claim forms or sending them electronically. Medical practices must submit insurance claims electronically unless they meet certain requirements related to the size of the practice. With electronic filing, the insurance claim is sent using a computer protocol called *electronic data interchange.* Issues of data security in electronic transactions and their effect on patient confidentiality have been the biggest barriers to more rapid implementation of electronic claim submission. With electronic

claim filing comes electronic payment, which means that insurance companies transfer payment electronically into the medical practice's bank account rather than issuing paper checks.

Reports System

The function of the reports system is to generate a variety of reports for the medical practice. The information contained in the reports is accessed by the computer from the medical practice database. These reports allow the physician to review and analyze many business and practice activities.

File Maintenance System

Before a medical practice management program becomes operational—in other words, before you can start performing front office procedures on the computer—a number of start-up tasks must be performed. These tasks are performed using the file maintenance system and are required in order to customize the practice management program to meet the specific requirements of a medical office. Start-up tasks include the following: entering practice information, assigning user passwords, entering provider information, entering diagnosis and procedure codes, entering names of insurance carriers, entering place of service information, and entering information about referring physicians into the computer system.

Fortunately, most offices are already computerized, and these start-up tasks have previously been performed. However, if an office is just opening, or if an office purchases a new practice management program, start-up tasks will be required. Once a practice management program is operational, the file maintenance system continues to be used to add additional information as required and to review, edit, and delete information previously entered into the system.

ELECTRONIC MEDICAL RECORD

If the office uses an EMR, it usually interfaces with the practice management functions so that demographic information and appointment information can be accessed at the same time as the medical record. It is usually possible to move directly from the daily appointment schedule into any patient's medical record.

The Centers for Medicare and Medicaid Services (CMS) has begun to offer incentives to hospitals and health care providers who demonstrate meaningful use of an electronic health record. After 2015 the electronic health record will be required for eligible hospitals and health care providers or reimbursements will be affected.

An **electronic medical record (EMR)** or *electronic health record* (EHR) is a computerized record of the important health information regarding a patient including the care of that individual and the progress of the patient's condition. Making the transition to an EMR is a major undertaking for a medical office. Medical offices are slowly moving toward the EMR. Approximately 25% of the medical offices in the United States have converted to an EMR, and the percentage is expected to gradually increase over time. The biggest deterrent is the financial and time investment required for a medical office to make the conversion to the EMR.

EMR software allows for the creation, storage, organization, editing, and retrieval of medical records on a computer. The EMR software is usually linked to the practice management software. This allows the EMR to communicate with the practice management software and facilitates certain administrative tasks, such as billing and insurance.

As previously discussed in Chapter 36, a medical record consists of numerous documents. Each document in the medical record has a specific function. In a paper-based patient record (PPR), some of these documents consist of preprinted forms that contain specific information entered by a physician or other health professional (e.g., patient registration form, health history form, laboratory report form). With an EMR, the preprinted forms of a PPR are displayed on a computer screen, and each form (known as a *template*) is filled out in much the same way as a paper form. A familiar example of an on-screen form is the form an individual completes when purchasing an item on the Internet; in this case, the form includes spaces (known as *fields*) for the individual to enter shipping and billing information.

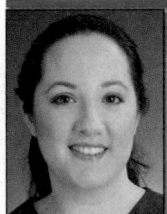

Memories *from* Externship

Emma Hayes: When I did my externship, it was the first time I really realized how much a modern medical office relies on its computer system. At that time, the office where I was placed was using a computer program to schedule appointments and manage the patient billing, but they were using a traditional paper medical record. There were four computers in the office, and they were networked together with two laser printers. The night before, we printed a list of patients scheduled for the next day, and we used that list to pull the medical records. In the evening, we also backed up all the computer files from that day. We were using a magnetic tape drive at that time to make a copy of all the files from the financial management software and appointment program. Individuals who did word processing or used a spreadsheet program had to back up their own files. I think that there wouldn't be enough storage space for most offices to do backups this way today. One day, the office computer system was not working, and we couldn't look anything up. It was very frustrating because we didn't know how much the patient's copayment was and we couldn't enter information about the visit. We did have the paper charge slips that the physicians had filled out, and by the next day everything was working again. I think it would be even more difficult now because we are using an electronic medical record as well. ■

Advantages of the Electronic Medical Record

The incorporation of an EMR in the medical office typically leads to better-quality patient care through improved communication, faster access to data, and clearer and better documentation. These advantages are accomplished in the following ways:

Speed and productivity. One of the principal advantages of an EMR is that the computer can retrieve requested documents from a patient's record very quickly. This avoids having to perform the much more time-consuming task of manually hunting through the record to locate this information. In addition, documents received from outside facilities, such as laboratory reports, can be stored very quickly in the EMR. EMRs do not need to be filed as with a paper-based medical record. This saves considerable time and frees up the office space required to store paper records. Paper costs are also reduced, and time is saved in not having to look for lost charts.

Efficiency. EMR software facilitates the entry of data into the patient's medical record. To assist in entering data, EMR programs use point-and-click technology, such as check-boxes and drop-down lists. A familiar example of this is the drop-down list of states often used when an individual must indicate his or her state on an online address form. EMR programs also have the capability to print customized patient education instructions and handouts. For example, if a patient has been diagnosed with strep throat, patient education on strep throat can be printed and given to the patient. One of the principle advantages of an EMR is the ability to generate prescriptions, which is described in detail later in this chapter.

Accessibility. The EMR provides ready access to the patient's medical record. A patient's EMR is available at any EMR computer workstation, allowing more than one person to view the chart at the same time. The EMR is also readily accessible if a patient telephones the office. This avoids having to find the patient's record and call the patient back.

Disadvantages of the Electronic Medical Record

The disadvantages presented by the EMR in the medical office include the following:

Initial cost. An initial investment is required for the purchase of hardware and EMR software. Because computer access is required to use an EMR, the office must have a sufficient number of desktop computers, laptop computers, or tablet computers to accommodate the number of health care providers in the medical office. The combined expense of the hardware and software can easily fall into thousands of dollars. In addition, an office must periodically upgrade the EMR software, leading to further expenses.

Time investment. It takes considerable time to learn an EMR program and use it with ease. Most software vendors provide on-site training of staff for a newly purchased program, as well as technical support when problems are encountered with the program. Even with all of this assistance, however, learning an EMR program and using it with ease can take up to several months or more.

Operational tasks. Certain tasks must be performed before an EMR program becomes operational. To be effective, older records are usually incorporated into a patient's EMR.

This can be accomplished by manually scanning all or some of the records into a digital format using an input device known as a *scanner*. An application program known as an *optical character recognition* (OCR) program can also assist in this process. Once the record has been scanned into the computer, the OCR program converts typed text into text that can be manipulated by the computer. An OCR program can also convert a handwritten document into text, but it has a difficult time converting illegible handwriting into text.

Once a document has been scanned into the computer, the medical assistant must follow the medical office policy on what to do with the paper document. Most offices shred the paper documents, but some offices may want to keep certain documents such as consent to treatment forms. If all or part of the old record is not scanned, the office may continue to use the old paper medical record along with the EMR.

Electronic Medical Record Documents

The documents included in an EMR come from many locations and sources. These documents fall into two categories: administrative documents and clinical documents. The type of administrative and clinical documents included in an EMR are identical to those included in a paper-based record (refer to Chapter 36 for a review of paper-based record documents). The difference is that the EMR documents are in a digital format rather than a paper format. These documents are described here in terms of the processes that are necessary to produce them in a digital format or convert them into a digital format.

What Would You Do? What Would You *Not* Do?

Case Study 1

Olivia Young has moved to the community and has come to the medical office for a new patient appointment for her chronic asthma. Olivia is leaving the office and is quite upset. She says that she doesn't like having computers in the examining rooms—that it's not natural. She feels like the physician and medical assistant are ignoring her and interacting more with the computer than with her. Olivia says it's like there's a barrier between her and the doctor. She says that the medical office she used to go to didn't have computers in the examination rooms and the doctor really paid attention to her and listened to what she had to say. She says she's thinking of looking for another doctor so that she doesn't have to play second fiddle to a computer. ■

Electronic Medical Record Administrative Documents

Administrative documents in the EMR contain information necessary for efficient management of the medical office. They include the patient registration record and patient-related correspondence.

Patient registration record. The patient registration record consists of demographic and billing information. In most EMR medical offices, the patient completes a paper-and-pencil patient registration form. The medical assistant then enters the data into a form on the screen of the computer and then (if office policy dictates) shreds the paper form. In some offices, the patient may be asked to enter this information directly into the computer. A private area must be provided for this task, and the medical assistant must be available to answer any patient questions related to this task.

NPP acknowledgement form. A Notice of Privacy Practices (NPP) is a written document that explains to patients how their protected health information will be used and protected by the medical office. The patient must sign a form acknowledging that he or she has received the NPP. Most medical offices give the patient a paper consent form to sign, and then the form is scanned into the computer and filed in the patient's EMR.

Correspondence. Correspondence regarding a patient may be received from a number of individuals or facilities. Examples include the patient's insurance company, the patient's attorney, or the patient himself or herself. If the correspondence is transmitted electronically to the medical office, it will already be in a digital format and can be transferred to the patient's EMR. An example of this is a letter from an insurance company sent as an attachment to an e-mail. If the correspondence is received in a paper format, the medical assistant must first convert the correspondence into a digital format by scanning it into the computer (Figure 38-10). The medical assistant then transfers the correspondence to the patient's EMR and (if office policy dictates) then shreds the paper document. Correspondence also includes copies of letters concerning the patient that are sent out of the office; examples are a copy of a letter referring the patient to a specialist and a copy of a collection letter sent to the patient. Because this correspondence is generated by the office in an electronic format through word processing, it can easily be transferred to the patient's EMR.

Electronic Medical Record Clinical Documents

Clinical documents in the EMR include a variety of records and reports that assist the physician in the care and treatment of the patient. Common EMR clinical documents are listed and described next.

Health history report. A health history report is a collection of subjective data about the patient. In an office with an EMR, the patient may complete a health history paper-and-pencil form, and the medical assistant then

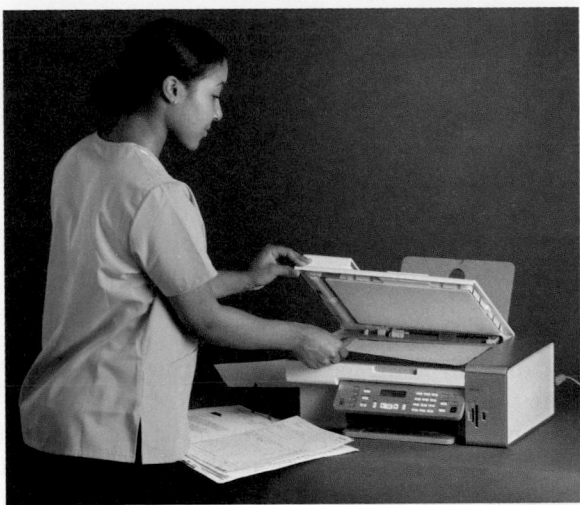

Figure 38-10 Medical assistant scanning information into the computer.

enters the data into the computer and (if office policy dictates) then shreds the paper form. An alternative is for the medical assistant to enter the information directly into the computer while asking the patient questions related to his or her health status. Although not yet in widespread use, computer-guided questionnaires are available for some patients to complete their own health histories. The medical office must provide a private area for the patient to complete the questionnaire, and the medical assistant must be available to answer questions.

Physical examination report. A physical examination is an assessment by the physician of each part of the patient's body. With an EMR, the physician can use free-text entry (often facilitated by voice-recognition software), drop-down lists, and check-boxes on an on-screen form to record findings. The EMR program uses this information to generate the physical examination report. This means that by the end of the examination, the physical examination report is complete and the physician does not need to dictate his or her findings at a later time. This alleviates the need for transcribing the physician's dictation into a written report.

Progress notes. Progress notes update the medical record with new information each time the patient visits or telephones the medical office. With an EMR the physician or medical assistant enters this information directly into the computer using free-text entry, drop-down lists, and check-boxes.

Medication record. A medication record consists of detailed information related to the patient's medications. The medical assistant enters this information into a digital form on the screen of the monitor using free-text entry, drop-down lists, fill-in boxes, and check-boxes.

EMR software includes a prescription program, which greatly reduces the amount of time needed to prescribe and refill medication. The prescription program generates and prints a prescription(s) on a regular sheet of 8½ by 11-inch paper, which is then signed by the physician

and given to the patient. The program can also transmit the prescription electronically (by e-fax or e-mail) to the patient's pharmacy. Both of these features eliminate the need of the pharmacist to decipher the physician's handwriting. If the medical office uses a paper medical record, physicians may still have the ability to send prescriptions directly to the patient's pharmacy using a handheld device, such as a smartphone.

To use an EMR, the physician first selects the medication. The program displays a list of the available dosage strengths and preparation forms (e.g., tablets, oral solution, parenteral solution, suppository) for that medication. The physician highlights the dosage strength and preparation desired and enters the information into the computer. Next, the physician selects additional information related to the prescription, such as dosage frequency and number of refills, using fill-in boxes, drop-down lists, and check-boxes. The program automatically checks the prescription against any drug allergies the patient may have. It also checks for potential interactions with other medications being taken by the patient. Once the physician has entered the prescription into the computer, the medication is recorded in the patient's medication list. The prescription is then printed out, signed by the physician, and given to the patient or sent by fax or electronically to the pharmacy. The prescription program usually provides access to extensive and current product information on all FDA-approved medications.

The EMR prescription program usually has the capability to compare the prescription with the formulary or list of drugs covered by the patient's insurance plan. If the prescription is not in the patient's formulary, the physician is advised of alternative drugs that are covered by the patient's insurance plan.

What Would You Do? What Would You *Not* Do?

Case Study 2
Kacy Ervin comes to the medical office and is diagnosed with strep throat. The physician gives her a prescription for an antibiotic, instructions for taking the medication, and patient information on strep throat printed on two regular sheets of paper that have been generated by the computer. The next day Kacy calls the office to say that she drove to her pharmacy on the way home from the doctor's appointment. When she pulled the papers out of her purse from the doctor's office, she found a sheet of paper with information about her prescription that was signed by the physician, but could not find the prescription form to give to the pharmacist. She says she must have lost the prescription and wants to know if the office could call in the prescription to her pharmacy. ∎

The EMR prescription program also has the capability to quickly refill a prescription and print a list of prescriptions being taken by the patient. The patient can use this list to keep track of the medications he or she is taking.

Consultation report. A consultation report is a narrative report of a clinical opinion about a patient's condition from someone other than the primary physician. If the consultation report is received by the office as an electronic letter, the medical assistant transfers it to the patient's EMR. If the correspondence is received in a paper format, the medical assistant is responsible for scanning the report into the computer and transferring it to the patient's EMR and (if office policy dictates) then shredding the paper document.

Home health care report. Home health care is the provision of medical and nonmedical care in a patient's home or place of residence. The purpose of home health care is to minimize the effect of disease or disability by promoting, maintaining, and restoring the patient's health. Currently, most home health care reports are in a paper format and must be scanned into the computer and transferred to the patient's EMR, and (if office policy dictates) then the paper report is shredded. As technology advances, the outside facility providing the service will be able to complete this report on a computer and transmit it electronically to the medical office for inclusion in the EMR.

Laboratory documents. A laboratory document is a report of the analysis or examination of body specimens. Many medical offices already communicate with outside laboratories electronically using a computer system that interfaces with the computer of the outside laboratory. This provides distinct advantages for the medical office using an EMR. Laboratory requisition forms can be completed on a request form displayed on the computer screen using fill-in boxes, drop-down lists, and checkboxes. The form can then be transmitted electronically to the medical laboratory. Once the patient's tests have been completed, the laboratory test results can be sent electronically to the medical office. The EMR program receives this electronic information, which is available in the appropriate patient's EMR. At the same time, a copy of the laboratory report is placed in the physician's "electronic review bin" for his or her review and electronic signature. Abnormal values are highlighted on the report; for example, a high value may be highlighted in red and a low value in green. If a critical result appears on the laboratory report, an urgent message is e-mailed to the physician.

Other advantages of the EMR include the ability to quickly view laboratory results in a chronological order. In addition, the results of a laboratory test performed on a routine basis (e.g., blood glucose) can be accessed by the computer and graphed. This permits an abnormal trend to be identified early so that appropriate action can be taken.

If the medical office is not networked through computers with an outside laboratory, the laboratory reports received by the office must be scanned into the computer and filed in the patient's EMR, and (if office policy dictates) then the paper report is shredded. A scanned report has some limitations. The computer can display the report, but the data on the report cannot be accessed or manipulated. Because of this, the laboratory data cannot be used for many of the functions available with an electronic report. For example, the data on a scanned report cannot be accessed and incorporated into a graph for trend analysis.

Diagnostic procedure documents. A diagnostic procedure report consists of a narrative description and interpretation of a diagnostic procedure. Diagnostic procedure reports completed by an outside facility may be sent electronically to the medical office. This makes it easy to store the report in the patient's EMR. If the report is in the form of a paper report, the medical assistant must first convert it to a digital format by scanning it into the computer. The medical assistant must then transfer the report to the patient's EMR and (if office policy dictates) shred the paper report.

The image of the diagnostic procedure (e.g., x-ray study, computed tomography [CT] scan, magnetic resonance imaging [MRI] scan, electrocardiogram [ECG]) can also be stored in the EMR as a digital image. A **digital image** is a picture stored in the computer in the form of pixels. EMR software can then display the digital image on the screen of the computer. If the diagnostic procedure is performed at an outside facility (e.g., an x-ray department of a hospital), the outside facility must have the capability to produce and transmit digital images. If the procedure is performed in the medical office (e.g., ECG, spirometry), the diagnostic equipment must be linked with the office's computer system. This enables a digital image of the result to be sent from the diagnostic equipment to the computer.

Therapeutic service documents. A therapeutic service report documents the assessments and treatments designed to restore a patient's ability to function. Such reports include physical therapy reports, occupational therapy reports, and speech therapy reports. Currently, most of these reports are in a paper format and must be scanned into the computer and transferred to the patient's EMR, and (if office policy dictates) then the paper report is shredded. As technology advances, the outside facility providing the service will be able to complete this report on a computer and transmit it electronically to the medical office for inclusion in the EMR.

Hospital documents. Hospital documents are prepared by the physician responsible for the care of a patient while at the hospital. These reports include a history and physical report, operative reports, discharge summary report, pathology report, and emergency department report. If a hospital document is received by the office in an electronic format, the medical assistant can file it in the patient's EMR without any further processing. If the report is received in a paper format, however, the medical assistant must first scan the document into the computer and file it in the patient's EMR. The medical assistant must then (if office policy dictates) shred the paper report.

Consent forms. Consent forms are legal documents required for performance of certain procedures or release of information contained in the patient's medical record. Most medical offices give the patient a paper consent form to sign, and then the form is scanned into the computer and filed in the patient's EMR.

ELECTRONIC INFORMATION TRANSFER

One of the major developments of the past 25 years has been the significant increase in the use of the Internet to transfer data over great distances. The first network of computers sharing information by telephone lines was set up in 1969, but the Internet as we know it first became available to commercial users and the general public in the 1990s. In the medical office, electronic data sharing is primarily used for e-mail, transfer of billing and insurance information, banking, and e-prescribing, in addition to local network capabilities that allow for communication of data within the office itself or between different facilities of the same organization.

Internet

The **Internet** is a global system of interconnected computer networks that use the Internet protocol (TCP/IP) to transmit and exchange data. Individual computers or LANs are connected to the Internet by **routers,** various types of wired or wireless devices to connect networks. Various technologies exist to link a computer or LAN to the Internet, but some are considerably faster than others. Modern systems usually use a **broadband** router, which handles a wide range of frequencies. **Digital subscriber line (DSL)** technologies allow for continuous digital connection over the telephone line, which can still be used for voice calls. This type of connection provides very fast transmission. Telephone companies are also providing fiberoptic cables with a glass core that transmit electronic information as light impulses. A method of transmitting electronic information that does not use a telephone line is a cable modem. This type of modem hooks up to a cable television connection. For a business such as the medical office, speed and reliability are major concerns when selecting a means of electronic transmission. Connection to the Internet allows a medical office to access the World Wide Web, send and receive e-mail, and transfer data electronically.

The **World Wide Web** is a series of documents, or webpages, that can be accessed by a software application called a **Web browser,** such as Internet Explorer or Firefox. To access resources, the user inputs a type of "Web address"—a uniform resource locator **(URL)**—that identifies the specific page to be located. Many medical offices and other medical facilities maintain websites with information for prospective and current patients.

E-mail

E-mail (electronic mail) is a method of composing, sending, receiving, and storing messages that are sent over the Internet. Files, such as documents, spreadsheets, and images, can be attached. Security and confidentiality are issues when using e-mail. The medical assistant should assume that an e-mail message may be read by someone else (e.g., a member of the recipient's family). It is also likely that the organization for which the medical assistant works may have access to e-mail messages, even if they have been deleted. In the medical office, e-mail should not be used for private messages or information.

Clinical Messaging

Most EMRs incorporate some type of clinical messaging system, which can be thought of as e-mail within the EMR. It allows secure communications among health care providers to link directly to clinical and laboratory data regarding patients (Figure 38-11). When there is an interface with patient insurance information, the physician can often identify which specific medications a patient's insurance will cover.

Electronic Transmission of Billing and Insurance Information

Insurance and billing information is often transmitted electronically via telephone lines to billing departments, billing affiliates, and/or insurance companies. The HIPAA Security Rule sets standards to safeguard the transmission of patient health information electronically, and each medical office must comply with these standards. This includes maintaining secure networks and using an encryption system, to maintain data security. **Encryption** refers to a process by which electronic information is changed into an unreadable form that requires the original encryption software to reverse the process. Effective January 1, 2012, covered healthcare entities are required to adhere to new standards for electronic transmission (Version 5010). This will facilitate the transition to a revised diagnostic coding system (International Classification of Diseases, 10th Revision, Clinical Modification [ICD-10 CM]) which is scheduled to occur in 2014.

E-Prescribing

Traditionally patients have been given written prescriptions, and prescription refills have often been handled either by telephone or by fax. The last 10 years have seen a significant increase in the transmission of prescriptions directly to pharmacies both by fax and electronically. This is usually accomplished either by a stand-alone program or as a function of an EMR. The computer program used by the physician and/or the pharmacy usually can access drug information; information about the patient's history, allergies, and so on; information about the patient's insurance coverage for specific medications; and information about drug interactions. Because the patient's entire medication history is usually available through a national database, it can be an effective way to identify patients who see multiple physicians for the same complaint in an effort to obtain certain medications.

The CMS has begun providing incentives for e-prescribing and will begin to impose penalties in 2012 for those physicians who have not begun to use this method.

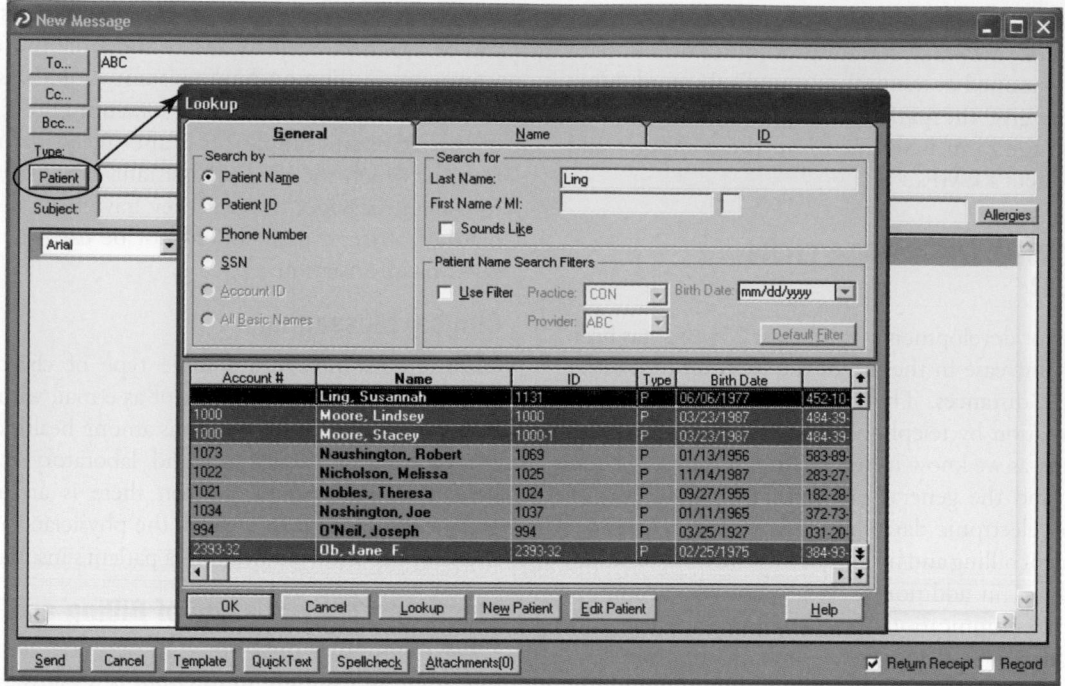

Figure 38-11 Clinical messaging is more secure than ordinary e-mail because it is part of the electronic medical record system. An individual record can be attached to a clinical message.

The e-prescribing of controlled substances will also become a reality once e-prescribing clearinghouses have updated their systems to comply with DEA regulations of 2010 defining how controlled substances can legally be e-prescribed, and state laws have been updated to allow this service. This is expected to take at least 1 or 2 years.

MEDICAL ASSISTANT'S USE OF THE ELECTRONIC MEDICAL RECORD

EMR programs include an index that allows the medical assistant to access the various areas of information in the EMR program. The medical assistant must first select the patient who is being seen and enter information about the visit (Figure 38-12). Once the medical assistant begins working with the patient, there is a mechanism within the EMR program to select an activity or topic. The selection may be made through a set of tabs on the screen or through a drop-down list. Selecting a tab such as *Medical History* moves the user to a screen containing information about the patient's medical history and the ability to move to other screens with more specific information. The EMR combines areas where data can be entered (e.g., blood pressure) and lists from which the user chooses an option (e.g., sitting, standing, lying).

Functions Performed by the Medical Assistant

The following functions are typically performed by the medical assistant using an EMR:
- Access the daily schedule
- Select a patient

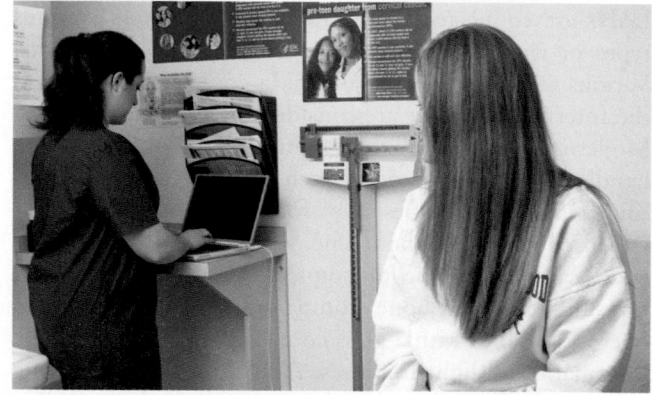

Figure 38-12 Medical assistant taking patient symptoms using a computer and an electronic medical record program.

- Enter the time that the patient has checked in
- Enter the examination room number (Figure 38-13)
- Enter the patient's chief complaint
- Enter or review the patient history
- Enter or review patient allergies
- Enter or review the patient's current medications
- Enter vital signs
- Enter measurements such as height and weight
- Enter results of tests, such as vision screening or hearing screening
- Enter results of laboratory tests performed at the office (e.g., urinalysis, hemoglobin, strep testing) (Figure 38-14)

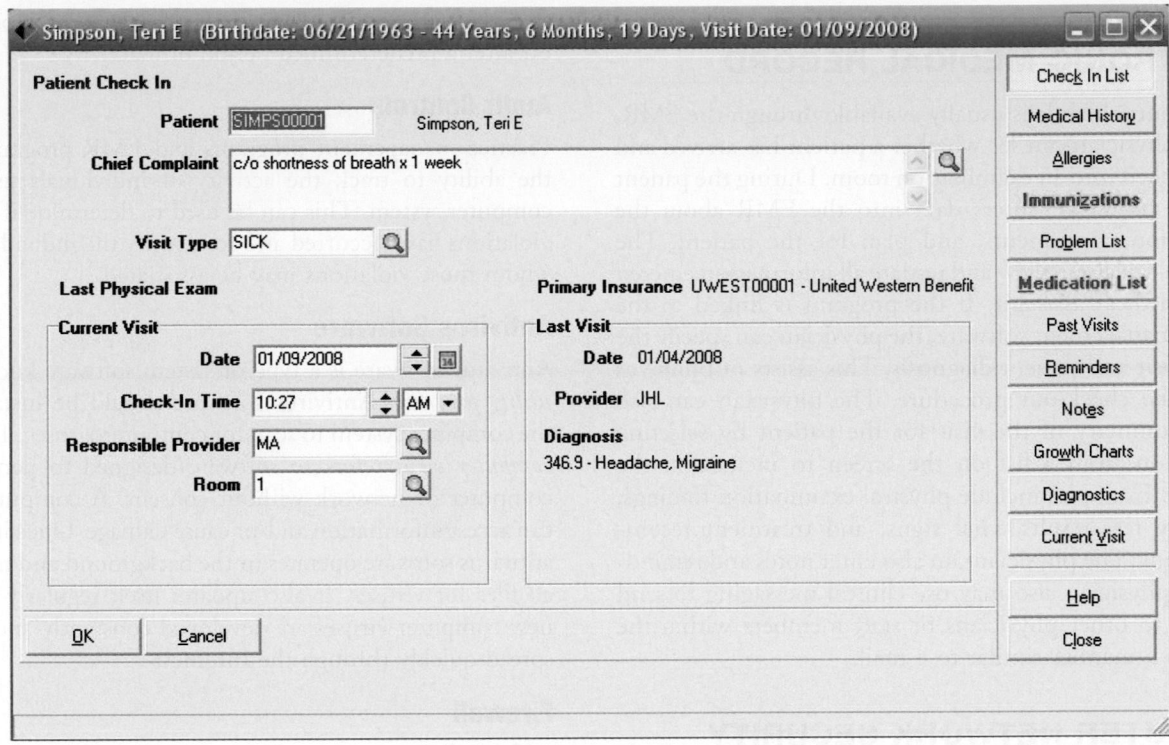

Figure 38-13 Electronic medical record screen.

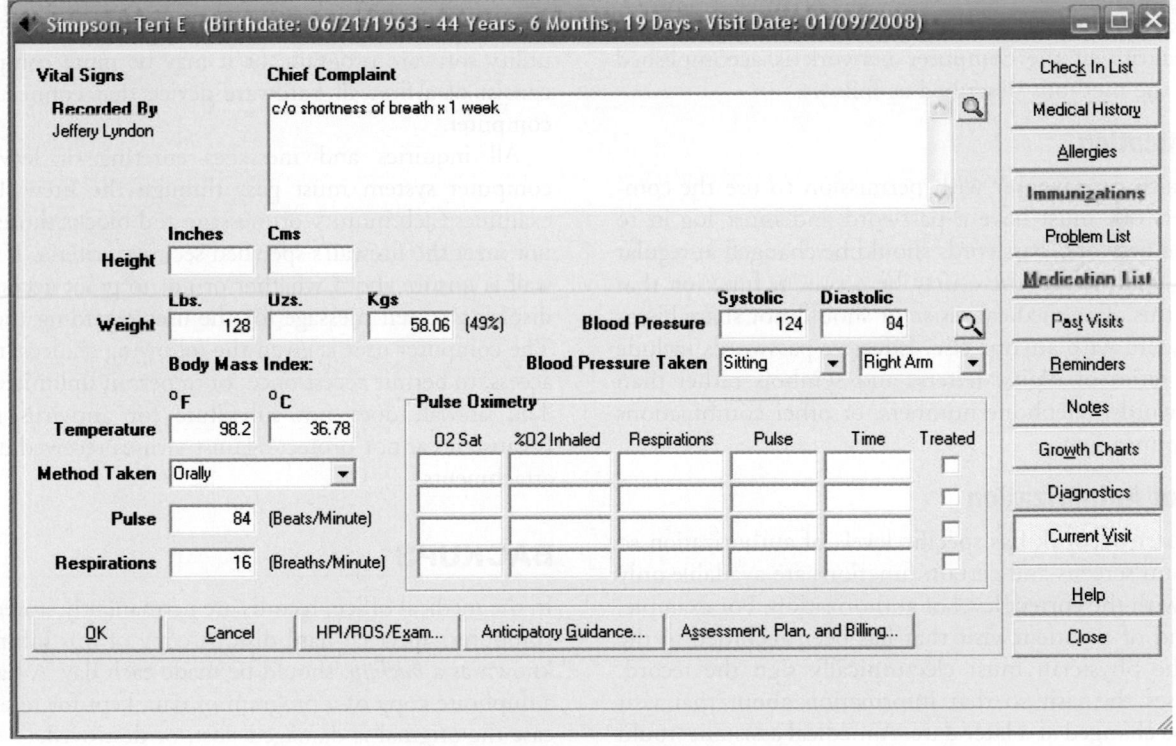

Figure 38-14 Electronic medical record screen.

PHYSICIAN'S USE OF THE ELECTRONIC MEDICAL RECORD

The patient schedule is usually available through the EMR, and the physician can see whether a patient has arrived and been checked into an examination room. During the patient visit, the physician enters data into the EMR about the examination, assessments, and plan for the patient. The physician can also review and update all information entered by the medical assistant. If the program is linked to the practice management software, the physician can specify the type of visit and patient diagnosis. This assists in billing as part of the check-out procedure. The physician can also print a summary of the visit for the patient by selecting information from a list on the screen to include in the summary. Examples include physical examination findings, laboratory test results, vital signs, and treatment recommendations. The physician can also enter notes and reminders. The physician also may use clinical messaging to send messages to other physicians or staff members within the system in a manner similar to e-mail.

COMPUTER NETWORK SECURITY

Because all HIPAA regulations apply to the EMR, the medical office must provide secure access to patient demographic and health information stored in the computer's database. If there is a centralized system used in several office locations, there may be more extensive security controls. Security of the computer network is accomplished through the methods described as follows.

Authentication

Each health care worker with permission to use the computer network must have a password and must log in to access the network. Passwords should be changed at regular intervals, and in fact there may be a system function that requires this. The medical assistant should not share his or her password with anyone else. Effective passwords include random series of digits, letters, and symbols rather than English words, telephone numbers, or other combinations that have meaning.

Levels of Authorization

A computer network has specific levels of authorization so that certain screens and certain functions are available only to users with the correct level of authorization. For example, at the end of a patient visit that has been recorded in the EMR, the physician must electronically sign the record. This closes the visit so that information about that visit cannot be changed at a later date. A medical assistant would not be authorized to perform this function.

Automatic Logoff

All users should log out of the computer network when their workstations are unattended. If the user forgets to do this, the software has a feature that automatically logs a user off after a predetermined period of inactivity.

Audit Controls

Practice management programs and EMR programs have the ability to track the activity of individuals using the computer system. This can be used to determine if security violations have occurred and to identify the individual with whom those violations may be associated.

Antivirus Software

Antivirus software is a type of system software known as a *utility program.* Antivirus software should be installed on the computer system to scan for computer viruses. The term *computer virus* refers to software designed to penetrate a computer or network without consent. A computer virus can access information and/or cause damage. Once installed, antivirus software operates in the background and monitors all files for viruses. It also updates itself regularly because new computer viruses are developed constantly and can be spread quickly through the Internet.

Firewall

A **firewall** is a system that protects a computer network from unauthorized access by users on its own network or another network, such as the Internet. A firewall takes its name from a wall in a building that is made of a material that will prevent a fire from spreading from one part of a building to another. A firewall may be in the form of a utility software program, or it may be more complex and consist of a firewall hardware device that connects to the computer.

All inquiries and messages entering or leaving the computer system must pass through the firewall, which examines each inquiry or message and blocks those that do not meet the firewall's specified security criteria. If the firewall is unsure about whether or not to grant access, it will display a screen message for the user regarding the access. The computer user is given the following choices: to refuse access, to permit access once, or to permit unlimited access. The firewall does not substitute for antivirus software because it cannot protect against viruses received as e-mail attachments.

BACKUPS

In the medical office, records are permanently stored on the computer's internal hard disk. A copy of this information, known as a *backup,* should be made each day. A **backup** is a duplicate copy of a program or data kept for reference in case the original is damaged, lost, or destroyed.

Many medical offices contract with an online backup service that provides secure backups of all files used in the office for a monthly fee. These backups may be performed every few hours or at scheduled times. The information is encrypted using methods similar to those used by banks and financial institutions. Although this service may seem expensive, it ensures that data will not be lost or destroyed.

Large health care facilities may be able to back up information from individual computers using their own network system. These backups usually occur automatically, although it may be necessary for a staff member to initiate the backup.

Using external hard drives, CD-RWs, and DVD-RWs to create physical backup copies is also possible. When a physical copy is used for backup, it should be stored in a safe place that is physically remote from the computer system. Many small offices accomplish this by having the physician or medical assistant take the backup home. Another option is to store the backup in a fireproof safe in the medical office.

SYSTEM MAINTENANCE

The medical office must assign an individual to be responsible for system maintenance. System maintenance involves setting up and overseeing the computer system. System maintenance consists of three aspects:

1. Disk cleanup
2. Disk defragmentation
3. System administration

What Would You Do? What Would You *Not* Do?

Case Study 3
John Gurnsey comes to the medical office for a checkup for his psoriasis and clinical depression. John says he likes the computer system used in the office but worries about the security of his medical record. He says that he doesn't want any of his friends or co-workers to know that he has psoriasis or that he is on an antidepressant. John wants to know how the office protects his medical record from people like computer hackers. He says that since there is a computer in every room, how is a patient who has been left alone in a room prevented from looking up patient records on the computer? John says that viruses keep getting into his computer at home and that data on his hard drive have been destroyed three different times. He wants to know if this ever happens at the medical office. ∎

Disk Cleanup

Unneeded files stored on the hard drive slow down system performance and should be removed periodically. This is especially important if the Internet is being used frequently by the medical office. In addition, outgoing e-mail messages

and incoming messages that have been read and deleted continue to reside in the system and should be eliminated. Disk cleanup is accomplished through a utility program that may come with the computer or can be purchased separately. Disk cleanup frees up significant amounts of hard drive space and can significantly improve system performance.

Disk Defragmentation

Disk defragmentation rearranges information on the hard disk so that files and programs are stored closer together. This allows the computer to locate information on the hard disk in a shorter period of time, which results in improved system performance. Disk defragmentation can take a long time, particularly with a hard disk that has a large storage capacity, such as those being used in a medical office. To avoid interfering with the office routine, disk defragmentation is usually performed at night or on a weekend.

System Administration

The system administrator is the person designated to maintain the computer system, especially a large network system. He or she is responsible for overall system/network function. The system administrator is usually a computer specialist. Small offices often use a consultant, sometimes from the company that provided the practice management software. Practices with several sites, health maintenance organizations, and community health centers often have an information technology (IT) specialist, or even an IT department, that handles both administration of the current system and planning for future computer needs.

SERVICE AGREEMENTS

The medical assistant is usually responsible for maintaining the service agreements for the office's computer systems. These agreements include maintenance agreements for the hardware, system support agreements for the software, and training of personnel on the software.

The medical assistant should designate an area in the medical office for the storage of the user manuals that come with the hardware and software. Examples of user manuals include the computer manuals, printer and scanner manuals, and application program manuals. One individual in the office should be designated to be responsible for all the computers. This person is responsible for being the liaison with any companies providing service for the hardware and software, such as maintenance, software upgrades, and software consultations.

MEDICAL PRACTICE *and the* LAW

As more patient information is stored on computers, shared on computer networks that often can be accessed from a doctor's home, and sent electronically to third-party payers, security and privacy have become national priorities. Several legal and regulatory measures can have an impact on health care organizations and the way they maintain security of electronically recorded and stored patient information. These include federal regulations, as well as guidelines from professional organizations and accrediting agencies, such as the Joint Commission. The most comprehensive regulation is provided by the Health Insurance Portability and Accountability Act of 1996 (HIPAA).

The Transaction and Code Set Rule prescribes electronic data interchange standards for structuring information that must be used for Medicare and Medicaid insurance claims.

The Security Rule complements the Privacy Rule by setting standards to maintain security of personal health information that is transmitted electronically. It identifies administrative, physical, and technical security safeguards for electronic protected health information (EPHI).

In addition, within a medical office, each individual who uses the computer should have a unique password, which should be changed on a regular basis. The password is a set of alphanumeric characters that allows the user to log onto (enter) the computer system or specific parts of it. Individuals should not share their passwords with others.

Each individual should have access to only the types of information and applications that fall within his or her scope of work and responsibility. System security should be designed in such a way that each security level permits access to only the applications and databases each individual needs to perform his or her tasks. Each specific application should know which individuals are authorized to use it.

If a practice uses a service bureau to prepare documents, at the end of the contractual period all documents, on paper or electronic media, should be returned to the practice. ■

What Would You Do? What Would You *Not* Do? RESPONSES

Case Study 1
Page 946

What Did Emma Do?
❑ Listened carefully to what Olivia was saying and agreed that sometimes patients feel like the computer seems to place a barrier between the patient and the doctor.
❑ Reassured Olivia that the doctor and staff always pay attention and listen very closely to what she has to relay about her health.
❑ Explained that the staff is still getting used to the computer system and that it takes more of their attention now than it will when everyone becomes familiar with the system.
❑ Stressed to Olivia that computerized medical records provide better patient care through improved communication, faster access to data, and clearer and better documentation.
❑ Relayed Olivia's concern at the next medical office staff meeting.

What Did Emma Not Do?
❑ Did not minimize or ignore Olivia's concerns.
❑ Did not tell Olivia that she is outdated and needs to adjust to the twenty-first century.

What Would You Do/What Would You Not *Do?*
Review Emma's response and place a checkmark next to the information you included in your response. List the additional information you included in your response.

_____
_____
_____
_____
_____
_____
_____

Case Study 2
Page 947

What Did Emma Do?
❑ Explained that the physician sent the prescription to the pharmacy by computer and instructed Kacy simply to stop by the pharmacy to pick it up.
❑ Reassured Kacy that many patients are confused about this until they get used to the new system.

What Did Emma Not Do?
❑ Did not imply that Kacy should have realized that the physician was using an e-prescription.
❑ Did not promise to call the pharmacy to make sure they had received the prescription.

What Would You Do/What Would You Not *Do?*
Review Emma's response and place a checkmark next to the information you included in your response. List the additional information you included in your response.

_____
_____
_____
_____
_____
_____
_____

Case Study 3
Page 953

What Did Emma Do?
❑ Reassured John that it is a legitimate concern to want to make sure his medical information is kept confidential.

What Would You Do? What Would You *Not* Do? RESPONSES—cont'd

❏ Explained to John that something called a "firewall" protects the office computers from unauthorized access by computer hackers.

❏ Told John that each staff member has to enter a password to log onto the computer and that a patient would not have a password and would not be able to log onto the computer.

❏ Explained to John that the office places a lot of emphasis on maintaining security of the computer system and preventing loss of data. Told John that the office has antivirus software running all the time to protect the computer from viruses and that the office also has a backup system so that even if data were lost, there would be a backup of the data.

What Did Emma Not Do?
❏ Did not minimize John's concerns.

❏ Did not criticize John for not having an antivirus program on his home computer.

What Would You Do/What Would You *Not* Do?
Review Emma's response and place a checkmark next to the information you included in your response. List the additional information you included in your response.

_____
_____
_____
_____
_____
_____
_____

TERMINOLOGY REVIEW

Medical Term	Word Parts	Definition
Application software		Software designed to accomplish a specific task (e.g., word processing); also called *application program* and *software program.*
Backup		A duplicate copy of a program or data kept for reference in case the original is damaged, lost, or destroyed.
Bit		The smallest unit of computer storage capacity.
Broadband		A method of transmitting electronic data that handles a wide range of frequencies.
Byte		A unit of computer storage capacity, usually eight bits. One byte is approximately equal to one character.
Computer		An electronic machine that has the ability to process data according to a program in order to produce a desired result.
Computer system		All of the hardware and software components making up the computer.
CPU (central processing unit)		The "brain" of the computer housed in the main unit that interprets and executes the instructions that operate the computer. The CPU consists of the control unit and the arithmetic logic unit (ALU).
Data		Raw, unorganized facts about subject matter presented to the computer for processing.
Data processing		The changing of raw facts or data into usable information following a three-part sequence: input, processing, output.
Digital image		A picture stored in the computer in the form of pixels.
Digital subscriber line (DSL)		Technology that allows digital signals to be transmitted over telephone lines at high speed even if the telephone line is also being used for voice transmission.
Documentation		A written set of instructions accompanying an application program, designed to assist the user in understanding how to operate the program. Examples include the user manual, help screens, and reference cards.
Electronic medical record (EMR)		A computerized record of the important health information regarding a patient including the care of that individual and the progress of the patient's condition.
E-mail		A method of composing, sending, receiving, and storing messages that are sent over the Internet.
Encryption	*crypt-*: secret	A process by which electronic information is changed into an unreadable form that requires the original encryption software to reverse the process.

Continued

TERMINOLOGY REVIEW—cont'd

Medical Term	Word Parts	Definition
Firewall		A system that protects a computer network from unauthorized access by users on its own network or another network, such as the Internet.
Gigabyte (GB)		A unit of computer storage capacity. One gigabyte is equal to a little more than 1 billion bytes or 1000 megabytes.
Hard disk		A storage device consisting of one or more rigid, nonflexible platters coated with a magnetically sensitive material and encased in a permanently sealed, airtight container.
Hard copy		Printed output from a computer.
Hardware		The physical devices making up a computer system (e.g., main computer unit, keyboard, monitor, printer).
Input		1. (noun) Data that have been entered into the computer. 2. (verb) The transfer of data to the computer for processing.
Input device		A device for entering data into the computer (e.g., keyboard, mouse, scanner).
Internet		A global system of interconnected computer networks that use the Internet protocol (TCP/IP) to transmit and exchange data.
Kilobyte (KB)		A unit of computer storage capacity. One kilobyte is equal to 1024 bytes (characters).
Main computer memory		The part of the CPU that is responsible for temporarily storing information until it is needed for processing by the computer. Main memory in a microcomputer is known as *RAM*.
Mainboard		The primary circuit board of the main computer unit, which allows all of the computer components to communicate with one another.
Medical practice management program		A program that provides instructions to the computer for performing medical practice management procedures.
Megabyte (MB)		A unit of computer storage capacity. One megabyte is equal to a little more than 1 million bytes or 1000 kilobytes.
Microcomputer	*micro-*: small	A small general-purpose computer that relies on a tiny microprocessor chip to perform its processing functions.
Network		A group of computers that share data and resources.
Operating system		A type of system software that performs tasks required by the computer to operate itself.
Optical disc		A storage device consisting of a flat, round portable disk that stores data using laser technology.
Optical disc drive		A device installed in a drive bay on the main computer unit that uses a laser to read an optical disc or write onto (burn) an optical disc.
Output		1. (noun) Information that has been generated by the computer. 2. (verb) The transfer of processed data back to the user.
Output device		A device that transfers processed data to the user (e.g., computer monitor, printer).
Pixels		Dot locations on a computer screen that can be lit up as needed to display images.
Printing speed		The number of pages per minute (ppm) generated by a printer.
Processing		The manipulation and reorganization of data according to the instructions in a program.
Program		A set of instructions organized in a logical step-by-step sequence, which tells the computer how to perform a specific function.
RAM (random-access memory)		The main computer memory of a microcomputer, which is used to temporarily store items until needed by the computer for processing. Also known as *main computer memory*.
Resolution		The number of horizontal and vertical pixels in a display device, such as a computer screen.
Router		A wired or wireless device used to form or connect networks.
Sequential-access memory		Computer memory in which all stored data must be searched sequentially from beginning to end to locate the desired information.
Server		A large computer that stores data and manages tasks for other computers on a network.

⟲ TERMINOLOGY REVIEW—cont'd

Medical Term	Word Parts	Definition
Software		A general term for the programs or instructions that tell a computer what to do.
Sound card		A circuit board connected to the mainboard that converts computer audio output into electronic signals. The electronic signals are then sent to speakers that convert them into sound.
Special keys		Keys that issue commands to the computer to perform specific functions on the information displayed on the screen.
Storage capacity		The maximum amount of information that a device can hold, measured in bytes.
Storage device		A device that permanently stores information for later retrieval by the computer.
System software		A group of programs that control or maintain the operations of a computer.
Terabyte (TB)		A unit of computer storage. One terabyte is equivalent to a little more than a trillion bytes or 1000 gigabytes.
URL		The characters and/or words used to access a specific website or file on the World Wide Web.
User		The individual using the computer.
Video card		A circuit board connected to the mainboard that converts computer video output into electronic signals. The electronic signals are then sent to the monitor, where they are converted into text and images that can be viewed by the user.
Web browser		A software program used to access the World Wide Web.
World Wide Web		A series of interlinked websites or files accessed via the Internet.

◈ ON THE WEB

For information on medical office computerization:

American Health Information Management Association (AHIMA): www.ahima.org

Computer Security Institute: www.gocsi.com

Department of Health and Human Services HIPAA website: www.hhs.gov/ocr/hipaa

Microsoft Windows: www.microsoft.com/windows

Microsoft Office: www.microsoft.com/office

 Check out the Evolve site at http://evolve.elsevier.com/Bonewit/today/ to actively Prepare for your Certification, and to access additional interactive activities and exercises to help you study and prepare for success.

39

Telephone Techniques

LEARNING OBJECTIVES

1. Describe the importance of effective telephone courtesy and a pleasing telephone personality for the medical assistant.
2. Explain the use of multiline telephones, cell phones, smartphones, and pagers in the medical office.
3. Differentiate between incoming telephone calls the medical assistant can handle and other incoming calls.
4. Describe the correct procedure for screening incoming calls.
5. Describe the correct procedure for taking messages and transcribing messages recorded on an answering machine or voicemail.

6. Identify the correct steps to respond to a telephone call regarding an emergency or urgent medical problem.
7. Describe how to deal with problem calls.
8. Explain how the medical assistant should make outgoing telephone calls.

PROCEDURES

Perform telephone screening.
Take a telephone message.
Take requests for medication or prescription refills.

Call a patient for follow-up

CHAPTER OUTLINE

INTRODUCTION TO TELEPHONE TECHNIQUES
Using the Telephone Effectively
Telephone Courtesy
Telephone Personality
Effective Telephone Communication
Telephone Technology
Multiline Phones
Answering Machines and Voicemail
Cell Phones and Smartphones
Pagers

Incoming Calls
Centralized or Electronic Routing
Managing Incoming Calls
Urgent or Emergency Calls
Dealing with Problem Calls
Outgoing Calls
Local Calls
Appointment Reminders
Long-Distance Calls
Conference Calls

KEY TERMS

enunciation (ee-nun-see-AY-shun)
pager

personal digital assistant (PDA)
smartphone

voicemail

INTRODUCTION TO TELEPHONE TECHNIQUES

Contact with a patient takes many forms. In addition to face-to-face contact, medical assistants often speak to patients and other callers over the telephone. The telephone is often the first contact between the medical office and a patient. In addition, the telephone is used throughout the day to make and receive referrals, request laboratory results, call in prescriptions for patients, and respond to patient questions.

Managing the phone is one of the most important jobs in the office. It is the first chance the medical assistant has to project a positive attitude and image to a patient. One never has a second chance to make a first impression.

USING THE TELEPHONE EFFECTIVELY

Telephone Courtesy

The telephone in a medical office should always be answered promptly. Some offices have a policy that every phone call should be answered within three rings. The medical assistant identifies the office, gives his or her name, then finds out who is calling. If the call will be transferred, the staff member needs to know who will be on the other end of the call.

The medical assistant should always speak before putting someone on hold. It is not courteous to place a call to hold immediately before speaking to the caller. The caller cannot even be sure that they have reached the correct telephone number. It is far more polite to obtain the caller's name and purpose for calling before putting the caller on hold. It is helpful to keep a written record of each caller's name, with the number of the line where he or she is holding. A physician should not be placed on hold if it can be avoided. The medical assistant should check back about every 30 seconds or so with a person who is on hold. This reassures the caller that the medical assistant is aware of the call. The medical assistant should also try to give an idea of how long it will take before the call will be answered.

When handling a call, the medical assistant should not chew gum or eat. Paying close attention during the telephone call is also important. A caller can tell if the medical assistant is distracted.

Telephone Personality

In addition to words, many nonverbal cues are given in the quality of a medical assistant's voice on the telephone. The "telephone personality" is important. It is important to stay focused on the call and smile. The medical assistant should use the same volume as when speaking in person and speak naturally. An artificial telephone voice may be perceived as cold and "fake."

All words should be spoken clearly so that they are easy to understand. **Enunciation** is the act of speaking so that the message can be easily understood. It may be necessary to speak a little more slowly on the telephone, and it is very important to avoid mumbling. It may be helpful for a medical assistant to record a telephone greeting and analyze the quality of his or her voice and the personality that is projected.

Qualities such as interest, friendliness, concern, and understanding are clearly communicated over the telephone. So too are boredom, anxiety, and indifference.

Effective Telephone Communication

When speaking on the telephone, the medical assistant should try to complete the call without interruption. If it is necessary to put someone on hold, the medical assistant should give a reason and apologize to the caller when the call is resumed. Information and materials should be readily available to handle calls and take messages. These include message slips, a pen, the office appointment book or computer appointment screen, and a list of frequently used telephone numbers. A desk clock, computer clock, or wristwatch should be visible to note the time when taking messages.

The medical assistant begins the conversation by identifying the practice—for example, "Primary Care Associates, Channa speaking." If the caller asks a question or asks for a staff member without identifying himself or herself, the medical assistant asks politely for the caller's name: "With whom am I speaking?" or "May I ask who is calling?" Using complete sentences is important because the medical assistant does not want to sound abrupt or rude.

The medical assistant should sit with the back supported and the head in a neutral position (not forward or to one side). The feet should be flat on the floor or supported on a foot stool. Figure 39-1 shows proper body position for answering the telephone. If the receiver is tucked between the head and shoulder, it places strain on the shoulder muscles and may change the voice quality, so this should be avoided. A headset, which consists of an earpiece that fits over the ear and a mouthpiece in front of the mouth, allows for good body posture and leaves the hands free. This is

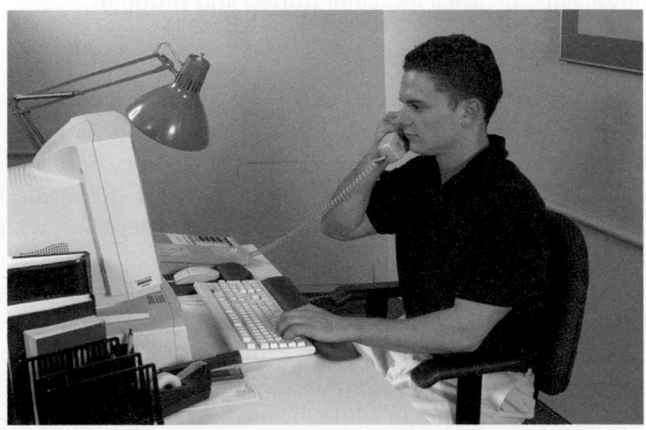

Figure 39-1 Good posture when answering the telephone improves voice quality and prevents muscle strain.

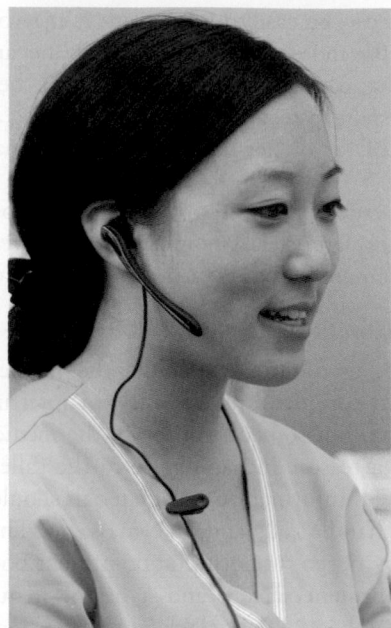

Figure 39-2 A telephone headset leaves the hands free and facilitates good body posture.

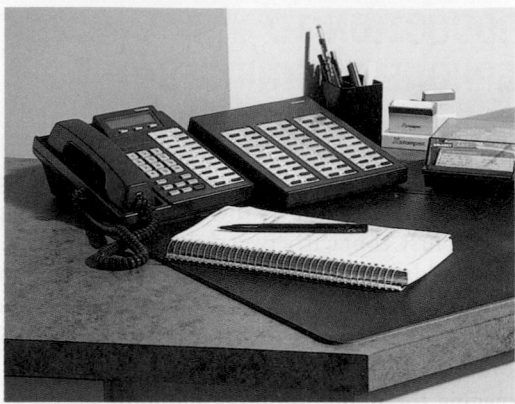

Figure 39-3 A multiline telephone is commonly used in a medical office.

recommended if the medical assistant spends a lot of time on the telephone. Figure 39-2 shows such a headset.

The medical assistant should be clear with callers who leave messages about when they can expect their calls to be returned. Many physicians have specific times when they return nonurgent telephone calls, such as late morning, lunch time, or the end of the day.

One should avoid cutting into a person's replies, even if he or she rambles on and repeats information. When the medical assistant gets the chance to speak, he or she should try to give a focused answer that lets the caller know what can be done and what the medical assistant is going to do.

TELEPHONE TECHNOLOGY

Advances in telephone technology have given medical offices many options to maintain contact with patients, physicians, pharmacies, laboratories, and hospitals.

Multiline Phones

Most offices have a multiline phone, with several extensions. It is important for the medical assistant to learn how to determine which line is ringing, how to place calls on hold, and how to transfer calls to all parts of the medical office. Figure 39-3 illustrates a multiline telephone with many extensions.

A flashing light usually identifies a line that is ringing; it flashes at a different rate on a line where a person is on hold. The medical assistant answers a call by pressing the button on the telephone that corresponds to the line that is ringing. If a second call comes in while the medical assistant is speaking to a caller, the medical assistant should tell the first caller that he or she needs to place the caller on hold, then he or

she presses the hold button. The medical assistant answers the second call, identifies the caller, and usually places that caller on hold before returning to the first caller and apologizing for the interruption. The calls are then handled in order.

If the caller asks to be connected to another extension or person, the medical assistant should first obtain the caller's name. To transfer a call, the medical assistant may need to press another button and/or dial an extension number, depending on the type of telephone system. Knowing the caller's name allows the medical assistant to announce the caller when the call is connected, and it is also helpful if the call is disconnected for some reason.

While a caller is on hold, the light on that line will flash. If the light continues to flash, the medical assistant should pick up that line about every 30 seconds and ask if the person would like to continue holding or leave a message. Sometimes transfers do not go through or the call is not picked up.

Special Features

Multiline telephone systems come with many other features, including speed dialing, call forwarding, call park, and caller ID.

Speed dialing allows storage of frequently called telephone numbers in the telephone system's memory. These numbers can be called by pressing a button or a one- or two-digit code.

Call forwarding allows forwarding of incoming calls to another telephone number. This service is turned on and off by dialing a sequence of numbers and activity keys.

Call park allows a call to be placed on hold and retrieved from another telephone.

Caller ID identifies the caller's telephone number before the telephone is answered. This feature may be available on some, but not all, telephones within a telephone system.

The medical assistant must learn how to use these and other features of the telephone system efficiently.

Answering Machines and Voicemail

Physicians have always needed to be available at all times. Most physicians' offices still use an answering service for getting messages to physicians during hours when the office is normally closed. This is an independent company that answers telephones for a number of clients. Some offices also have an answering machine or voicemail system, which has a message with a number to call outside of office hours and gives people the option to leave a nonurgent message. **Voicemail** is a method for message delivery, storage, and retrieval that is built into the telephone system. It is usually attached to each individual extension. Answering services and answering machines are activated whenever the office is closed, including during lunch break if no one is assigned to take phone calls during that time. The answering service should be notified if the office is closed, although they usually pick up phones after a predetermined number of rings.

Increasingly, physicians' offices are going to voicemail systems. Voicemail is a system provided by the office's telephone carrier that allows for messages to be left in a number of "mailboxes" for different people. Each physician might have his or her own voicemail box, as well as each medical assistant, the business manager, and so on.

The message will have a number to call for urgent messages outside of office hours but will also offer the caller the option of leaving a message in any voicemail box. Each box has a two- to four-number extension. Many voicemail systems have a directory by which people can find voicemail box numbers by using their touch-tone phone to type in some or all of the letters of the last name of the person with whom they would like to speak.

Even if an office has a voicemail system, most medical offices will still need to have a contract with an answering service. The answering service provides a medical office with coverage outside of normal business hours. The service either answers all of the office's telephone calls or takes calls that are forwarded to it by individuals who listen to the voicemail system message and press the appropriate message code for an urgent message. The answering service must be informed how to deal with urgent calls.

Cell Phones and Smartphones

Cell phones allow two individuals to speak to each other as they would using regular telephones, but the cell phone uses radio signals instead of telephone wires. A **smartphone** is a device that adds computer capabilities to the cell phone, with a drug reference, address book, and other tools; an Internet connection; the ability to send and receive e-mails; and sometimes even access to the electronic medical record system used by the health care facility. This type of handheld computer was formerly called a **personal digital assistant (PDA),** but today almost all PDAs are smartphones. Many physicians use cell phones or smartphones to remain in contact with the medical office when they are in other locations. The physicians' cell phone numbers should never

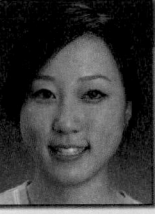

Putting It All into Practice

My name is Channa Eng, and I am a certified medical assistant. I work for an internal medical practice with two physicians and two nurse practitioners in an urban area. We have many Asian and Hispanic patients. I don't speak much Spanish, but I do speak Cambodian and some Vietnamese. Another medical assistant speaks Spanish, and we both help with translating telephone calls from patients who have difficulty in English. When patients call our office, they get three choices right away. They can hear the message in English, Spanish, or Cambodian. Most patients like this because they can hear the instructions in a language they are comfortable with. On Tuesdays and Thursdays, I spend most of the day on the telephone making appointments and responding to patients with medical problems. I don't usually sit at the front desk. Instead, we have a telephone room with three telephones. When it is very busy, there are usually two of us. I can tell if a patient wants a routine appointment or has medical questions depending on which line the call comes in on. When patients are sick, I have to ask a lot of questions to find out how urgent their problem is. Last year I worked with the office manager to revise our procedure manual, so I am very familiar with what questions to ask. My goal is to handle each call as quickly and efficiently as possible while still making the patients feel that their needs were met. Every time I take a message, I put it on the corner of my desk, and a file clerk takes it to get the patient's medical record. In our office we think that telephone conversations are very important. We try very hard to answer all telephone calls promptly and to avoid putting patients on hold. ∎

be given to patients, but they should be available to office staff so that physicians can be contacted as needed.

Pagers

Pagers are used in areas with unreliable cell phone service and sometimes in large institutions such as hospitals. A **pager** (also called a *beeper*) is like a radio that is always tuned in to a single station. When it "hears" its unique access code signal, it lights up, beeps, or vibrates to indicate that a message is being received. Some pagers are also linked to voicemail. Pagers used by physicians or other health professionals are either numeric or alphanumeric. A numeric pager's message is a telephone number (e.g., the answering service, the office, the emergency department, home, a colleague). The physician then returns the call to the number on the display. An alphanumeric pager displays an entire message, so the physician can return a phone call or act on the information that is relayed to the pager. Some pagers also include e-mail so that a return message can be sent. If the physicians use pagers, the office staff should have the pager numbers for each physician in the practice.

A simple type of pager may also be used for patients in ambulatory care areas of hospitals or clinics. It is similar to pagers used in restaurants and lights up and/or vibrates to notify patients when it is their turn. Patients can leave the waiting area and be notified when to return. This type of pager provides patient confidentiality because it eliminates the need to call the patient by name.

Highlight on Analog versus Digital Technology

Until the middle of the 1980s, telephone service used only analog technology, which translates the audio signals from a telephone into electronic pulses. These pulses are usually transmitted along wires that link all telephones together physically. In cordless telephones analog signals are transmitted from the telephone base to the receiver using radio waves. The advantage of analog technology was, and still is, high sound quality with minimal distortion. Analog telephones are also relatively inexpensive. The disadvantage is that analog signals can carry only a limited amount of information. Also, analog signals cannot be encrypted, so the information being transmitted is not secure, especially when a cordless telephone or cell phone is used.

Digital technology converts analog signals from a microphone in the telephone into binary code (consisting of 0s and 1s). The message is transmitted to the receiver through wires or radio signals, where it is converted back into its original signal. Because of the conversion, quality of the signal may be lost, although modern digital equipment has improved in this area. Digital technology is also more expensive. The main advantage of digital technology for the medical office is the ability to transfer electronic data securely using telephone lines. Both voice and computer transmissions can be encrypted in such a way that they cannot be intercepted and decoded. The encryption key is necessary at the receiving end in order to decode the information.

Digital and analog equipment cannot be connected together without using an adapter. Modern multiline telephone systems are digital. If an analog telephone, modem, or fax machine is connected to a digital system without using a digital-to-analog adapter, it can draw too much current and damage itself or even the entire telephone system. ∎

INCOMING CALLS

An incoming telephone call sounds like a routine event. But breaking down the process, it becomes clear that a number of different elements go into answering a routine call.

Centralized or Electronic Routing

Many offices use an electronic routing system to direct calls. At each extension, the telephone may be answered or the call will go to voicemail, and the caller can leave a message for office staff members who are not available. By offering the caller several options (e.g., scheduling an appointment, speaking with the medical assistant, discussing a billing question), the electronic routing system directs the call to the appropriate part of the office, saving the expense of a staff person who would otherwise be answering the call. It

also keeps patients from being put on hold, which some people appreciate.

However, other patients find electronic routing of messages confusing and frustrating, especially if the person they need to speak with is not available and does not return calls promptly.

If electronic routing is used, the message should be kept up to date and should be as clear and concise as possible.

In other offices, incoming calls are answered directly by the medical assistant. Although the personal touch is appreciated by many patients, when several calls come in at the same time, some callers end up on hold. If the office has several staff members, many of the calls end up being transferred anyway.

Managing Incoming Calls

Performing Telephone Screening

The first step in handling telephone calls is to find out how urgent the call is and what is necessary to handle the call.

Most calls are routine and can be taken in the order in which they come. In most cases a new call is placed on hold while the previous call is handled. However, there are some exceptions:

- Calls from other physicians are put through at once.
- Emergency calls are treated as urgent and receive top priority. They will be discussed in detail later in this chapter.
- If the caller is a relative of the physician, the medical assistant either puts the caller through or speaks to the physician via intercom to determine how to handle the call.

When answering calls, it is polite to obtain the caller's name and ask permission to place the caller on hold. This gives the caller the opportunity to identify the call as urgent.

After the caller's name has been obtained, the caller usually states the reason for the call or asks for a staff member or department. When the caller asks for a staff member by name, the medical assistant usually transfers the call. If that staff member is with a patient, the medical assistant may offer to take a message or transfer the call to voicemail. Often the caller asks for the physician. Most physicians do not take calls while they are seeing patients. Additional questions may show that the medical assistant can handle the call, or it may be necessary to take a message for the physician (Procedure 39-1).

Calls the Medical Assistant Usually Handles

The medical assistant usually handles four kinds of calls.

1. *Requests to schedule appointments*—The medical assistant will usually schedule appointments and tests, either in the office or at an outside laboratory or the hospital. This topic is discussed in the next chapter.
2. *Billing inquiries*—The medical assistant may handle inquiries about a patient bill or insurance. For this type of call, the medical assistant refers to the patient account in the computer and gives the caller the information requested. If the caller's question is

complicated, the call may be referred to a billing specialist or the office manager.

3. *Receiving diagnostic test and lab results*—The medical assistant can also take calls regarding diagnostic test and lab results. Many lab results today are sent to physicians' offices by fax or directly on the computer system. But if a laboratory calls in test results, the medical assistant needs to have a blank laboratory slip so that the results can be filled in, along with the patient's name and the date the tests were taken. After taking the results, the medical assistant pulls the patient's medical record, clips the results to the front, and places the medical record where the physician can review it. Taking all results accurately is very important.

4. *Requests for information*—Finally, the medical assistant can handle calls requesting information, such as directions to get to the office, office hours, and the office's medical specialty.

Taking Messages

The medical assistant usually takes messages using a message form. Some forms are pressure sensitive so that a copy is created with the original message. The originals stay in the message book and form a telephone log. If the message form does not create a copy, it is helpful to keep a separate telephone log for future reference. In some offices a form is used that has a space for the physician to write orders or desired follow-up on the bottom of the form. The medical assistant should not write in this space when taking the message. If telephone messages are filed in the patient's medical record after the physician or other recipient has responded to the message, a form with a peel-off backing is preferable.

When taking a message about a patient, the message should include the following information:

- Date and time
- Name of the physician or staff member
- Patient's full name and date of birth (or age)
- Name of the caller (if not the patient)
- Message or question that indicates clearly what the patient wants (e.g., prescription, laboratory results, medical advice)

- Additional information to clarify the message, such as symptoms, medication and pharmacy information, and actions that have already been taken
- If the patient is ill or requests medication, any medication allergies should be noted
- Telephone number
- Initials of the person taking the message

When a medical assistant transcribes messages from an answering machine or from voicemail, the same message form should be used. The time the call was recorded should be used. The medical assistant may need to play the message more than once in order to record all information (Procedure 39-2).

Taking Messages Using the Computer

The medical assistant may work in a facility where telephone messages are taken using the computer, either using a stand-alone computer messaging program or using the clinical messaging feature within the electronic medical record. Built-in message templates facilitate taking the message during the telephone call and forwarding the message to one or more recipients. When this feature is part of the electronic medical record, the patient's medical record can be attached to the message, and the transmission is secure. This can be very useful for questions about lab results and requests to renew prescriptions.

Patients Requesting Test Results

When a patient calls requesting test results, the medical assistant should find out when and where the test was done and take a message for the physician. After the call, the medical assistant should locate the medical record, be sure the results of the laboratory or diagnostic test in question are in the record, and leave the message and medical record for the physician. It may be office policy to use a sticky paper flag to identify the report in the medical record. Some offices choose to send patients letters about laboratory results, which cuts down on the number of telephone calls requesting information, especially for routine tests. After reviewing the laboratory or diagnostic test results, the physician may instruct the medical assistant to call the patient back to give the results, to schedule follow-up testing, and/ or to ask the patient to schedule an appointment to discuss the results.

Patients Reporting Satisfactory or Unsatisfactory Progress

Physicians often tell a patient to call and check at a specified interval after a visit, to report on how a condition is resolving after treatment. If the patient reports satisfactory progress, the medical assistant should take a brief message, clip it to the chart, and leave it for the physician. An unsatisfactory report should generate a more complete message, and the chart should be pulled and the message clipped to it so that the physician can call the patient. When a patient gives a progress report on the telephone, either the original message should be filed in the patient record or the medical assistant should document the telephone conversation in the record.

Requests for Medication or Prescription Refills

Often patients or pharmacies call with requests to have prescriptions refilled or renewed. When the pharmacy calls, it is important to get the patient's name and date of birth, name of the medication, dosage, and amount of medication prescribed. When the patient calls, it is important to get the name of the medication, dosage, and how often the patient takes it. In addition, it is important to determine how the patient wants to receive the medication (from the pharmacy or by mail order). It is helpful to verify the information in the patient's medical record when an electronic medical record is used. Otherwise the message should include the name, telephone number, and location of the pharmacy or mail order company. It is more common for a physician to prescribe using a computer program, but if this is not the case, a written prescription should be sent to the patient if mail order is specified. If the medication is an antibiotic or a controlled substance used for pain relief, the medical assistant should ask about symptoms that would require a refill. The medical assistant should tell patients to check with the pharmacy the next day unless they hear from the physician or office. A message to request medication is also clipped to the patient's medical record. Physicians often follow up directly with the pharmacy, especially if they are using an electronic prescription routing service, but in some offices the physician writes the prescribing information on the bottom of the message for the medical assistant to call in to the pharmacy. When medical assistants call in prescriptions, they should always note this in the progress notes and/or medication record (Procedure 39-3).

Calls for Referrals or Requesting Laboratory or Diagnostic Tests

A patient may call to say he or she needs a referral (because of a particular insurance company's policy) to see a specialist outside the medical group or to have a laboratory test or diagnostic procedure done.

The medical assistant takes the necessary information (what type of referral, for what, to whom) on a message form for the physician. If a referral is appropriate—or necessary because of an insurance company or health maintenance organization policy—the medical assistant may complete a paper or electronic form. If the patient is asking for a laboratory test, such as a throat culture, the medical assistant should fill out the laboratory form for the patient to pick up or should enter the information into the computer, after verifying with the physician that the requested test is appropriate. The physician may ask the medical assistant to call the patient and schedule an appointment before authorizing the referral.

Patients with Medical Questions

For patients with medical questions, the medical assistant takes a message for a physician or refers the call to another staff member designated by the office to handle such calls. The office should have written guidelines to follow if a medical assistant screens medical questions. The medical assistant should follow the written guidelines closely and take a message for the physician about any concern or question that falls outside the preset guidelines.

Calls from Other Physicians

Calls from other physicians are usually put through right away, even if the physician is examining a patient. If the medical assistant has to find the physician, this may be given as a reason to place the caller on hold briefly, but the medical assistant should locate the physician as quickly as possible and explain which physician is calling. The physician may ask the medical assistant to transfer the call to another extension to avoid talking in front of a patient.

Calls from Salespeople

Often a sales representative from a pharmaceutical company or equipment company calls before visiting the physician's office. Salespeople are usually seen by the office manager, who gives the information to the physician. Drug representatives sometimes drop by, but if they hope to talk to the physician they usually must call and ask for an appointment. Physicians usually schedule sales representatives during lunch. The physician has to agree to see the representative before a medical assistant makes an appointment.

Urgent or Emergency Calls

If a patient calls with a medical problem, the medical assistant asks questions to determine how urgent the problem is. After obtaining the caller's name and telephone number and identifying who has the problem (the patient's name, age or date of birth, and relationship to the caller), the medical assistant should obtain the patient's symptoms and current condition. In most offices there is a guide to telephone screening in the office procedure manual. This helps the medical assistant identify which questions to ask in order to determine how urgent the problem is. In the next chapter, there is a more complete discussion on the kind of appointment to offer a patient based on the symptoms the patient reports.

If the medical assistant determines that the call represents an urgent problem or emergency, he or she should follow office policy. The call should be referred to a physician if one is in the office; in a group practice, one physician may be assigned at all times to take urgent calls. If there is no physician in the office, a nurse practitioner or physician's assistant may be assigned to take urgent calls. If no licensed professional is present in the office, the medical assistant must advise the caller or contact the on-call physician. The following are the guidelines for dealing with such a call:

1. If the emergency is serious or life-threatening, the caller should be instructed to call an ambulance by dialing 911. This activates the emergency medical services (EMS) system. If the caller is a child or seems upset or confused, the medical assistant can offer to call an ambulance for the caller.

2. If the emergency is a case of poisoning, the caller should be instructed to call the local poison control center. The telephone number of the poison control center (1-800-222-1222) should be placed next to every telephone in the medical office. Even if it is a case of poisoning, if the patient is unconscious or not breathing, the caller should be instructed to call an ambulance.

3. If the patient has a problem that requires treatment in an emergency department but is conscious and able to walk (e.g., a fractured arm), the caller should be instructed to take the patient to the nearest emergency department or call an ambulance. If the patient is alone, an ambulance should be called.

4. If the patient's problem is usually treated in the office, the patient should be given an appointment for that day.

5. If the condition of the patient is not life-threatening and/or the medical assistant is unsure how urgent the problem is, the physician should be contacted for instructions either by cell phone or pager. If there is any doubt about how serious the patient's condition is, it is safer to instruct the patient to call an ambulance and/or go to the hospital emergency department.

Whenever an urgent call is handled, the medical assistant should fill out a message form to be sure that the information has been written down. Either the message form or the instructions given to the patient should later be documented in the medical record. If a patient has been instructed to go to the emergency department, the physician should be notified promptly.

Dealing with Problem Calls

The Caller Who Refuses to Give Information

When callers ask for a physician and refuse to identify themselves, it is probably because they want to speak to the physician but suspect that if they give a name, they will be asked to leave a message. The medical assistant should explain politely that the physician is not available and offer to take a message. If the caller still refuses to give information, the medical assistant can instruct the caller to write a letter to the physician and mark it "personal."

Complaints

The medical assistant should listen carefully to callers with complaints, avoid getting defensive or angry, and ask for specific information. It is important to remain calm so that a professional demeanor is maintained. The medical assistant should state clearly what he or she can and will do. It may be necessary to refer the matter to the office manager or the physician, but the medical assistant should get as much information as possible at the initial contact.

It is important to avoid hanging up on an angry caller. It is usually possible to calm a caller down as long as the medical assistant does not raise his or her voice and does not become defensive. The caller should be told a specific time when he or she can expect to hear back from someone in the office.

Patients with Special Problems

If a patient calls who is confused or has difficulty with English, the medical assistant should listen carefully and try as hard as possible to understand. The medical assistant may speak more slowly than usual but should not speak more loudly. If it is impossible to communicate, even using simple language, the medical assistant should try to at least obtain the caller's name and telephone number. Then it may be possible to find out from the medical record if the patient speaks a different language or if there is an emergency contact number. If the person seems confused, the medical assistant should ask if there is another person with whom he or she can speak because this may be a medical emergency. The medical assistant may need to ask for guidance from the physician or office manager.

PROCEDURE 39-1 **Performing Telephone Screening**

Outcome Screen incoming telephone calls.

Equipment/Supplies

- Telephone
- Message pad
- Pen or pencil

- Appointment book or computer terminal
- Clock or watch

1. **Procedural Step.** Answer every telephone call within the first three rings.
   Principle. Callers become annoyed when their calls are not answered promptly.

2. **Procedural Step.** Identify the medical office and give your name. Each practice will have a preferred way for all employees to answer the telephone. Example: "Primary Care Associates, this is Channa speaking." Do not rush through the greeting. The caller needs to hear this first sentence clearly.
   Principle. Callers need to know what business they have reached and with whom they are speaking. Otherwise they will have to ask if this is Primary Care Associates.

3. **Procedural Step.** Listen carefully to what the caller says, and decide as soon as possible whether this is a call you can handle, whether you need to take a message, or whether the call should be transferred to someone else in the office.
   Principle. The caller does not want to have to repeat all the details if the call must be transferred. If you need to take a message, begin writing.

4. **Procedural Step.** Ask for the caller's name. "May I ask who is calling?"
   Principle. You will need the caller's name to address the caller by name, to take a message, or to identify the caller before transferring the call.

5. **Procedural Step.** If you can handle the call, such as a call for an appointment, do so promptly.

6. **Procedural Step.** If you need to take a message, see Procedure 39-2, Taking a Telephone Message.

7. **Procedural Step.** If you need to transfer the call to someone else in the office, place the caller on hold, noting the caller's name and the extension. Tell the person you are transferring the call to who is calling and what extension the call is on.
   Principle. It is a courtesy to tell the person you transfer a call to who is calling; he or she must be able to locate the call if more than one line has a call on hold.

8. **Procedural Step.** If the caller describes symptoms that require immediate care, ask questions to assess the problem, following guidelines in the office procedure manual. If there is a physician or other licensed professional in the office, transfer the call immediately. Otherwise, assess the urgency of the problem and follow up according to office guidelines. If the patient's health is at risk, instruct the caller to call 911.
   Principle. Patients expect correct medical advice from a health care facility when they have urgent medical problems.

9. **Procedural Step.** If your telephone has more than two lines, it is helpful to keep a list of the names of callers and extensions. When a call is on hold, the light for that telephone line blinks. If you have transferred a call but the call remains on hold, within 30 to 45 seconds you should determine if the caller is still holding; if so, you should try to transfer the call again or take a message.
   Principle. Sometimes a transfer does not go through or the call is not picked up. The caller has no way to get back in contact with you to leave a message or ask to speak to someone else.

10. **Procedural Step.** If the telephone rings for another call, ask if you may put the caller you are speaking to on hold and wait for the caller to agree. After pressing the hold button, answer the other call and explain that you are speaking to a caller on another line. Give the second caller the option to hold and wait for you or take their number and offer to call back as soon as you are finished.
    Principle. In general calls are handled in the order they are received. By asking for permission to put the caller on hold, you give the caller a chance to tell you if it is an emergency. Some callers prefer to hold; others prefer to be called back. Time passes slowly when a caller is on hold, and the caller may become tired of waiting and wish to leave a message.

11. **Procedural Step.** At the end of the call, repeat any information you have discussed (such as the date and time of an appointment). End the call politely by thanking the caller (if appropriate) and saying goodbye.
    Principle. Confirmation helps avoid misunderstandings. Thanking the caller and closing the conversation demonstrates telephone courtesy.

PROCEDURE 39-2 Taking a Telephone Message

Outcome Take a telephone message.

Equipment/Supplies

- Telephone
- Computer
- Message pad

- Pen or pencil
- Clock or watch

1. **Procedural Step.** If you determine that the person to whom a telephone caller wants to speak is not available, offer to take a message.
   Principle. A message is a way of communicating to a person who is not available to speak on the telephone.
2. **Procedural Step.** Give the caller a reason why the person cannot take the call. Acceptable reasons are as follows: busy with a patient, not at his or her desk, not in the office, on another line. Generally physicians do not take calls except possibly during specified hours. Patients who ask for the physician are told that the physician is not in the office or that the physician is busy with patients.
   Principle. Most callers are willing to leave a message if they understand why their call is not being answered.
3. **Procedural Step.** Fill in the information on the message form or in the computer messaging program, including

the name of the caller, business affiliation (if any), date, time of the call, telephone number including area code, and information the caller wishes to leave about the reason for the call. Place your initials on the message in case there are questions. If there is a section at the bottom for a response to the message, leave that area blank.
   Principle. Complete information is necessary for a call to be returned.
4. **Procedural Step.** Verify the information. If possible, give a time when the call might be returned. If the message recipient does not have a scheduled time to return messages, say, "I will give him (or her) the message."
   Principle. Callers like to know when to expect a return call.

4

MESSAGE FROM								
For Dr. *Lawler*	Name of Caller *Anne Richards*	Ref. to pt. *mother*	Patient *Janice*	Pt. Age *4*	Pt. Temp. *101°*	Message Date *10/13/XX*	Message Time *9:00* AM PM	Urgent ☐ Yes ☐ No

Message: *Child has been on antibiotic for two days – still has fever. Should she come in again?*   Allergies *Ø*

Respond to Phone # *814-322-6510*	Best Time to Call *any* AM PM	Pharmacy Name / # *West Side* *814-754-9817*	Patient's Chart Attached ☒ Yes ☐ No	Patient's chart #	Initials *KJ*

DOCTOR - STAFF RESPONSE

Doctor's / Staff Orders / Follow-up Action

	Call Back ☐ Yes ☐ No	Chart. Mes. ☐ Yes ☐ No	Follow-up Date / /	Follow-up Completed-Date/Time / / AM PM	Response By:

Product # 78-9156-Pkg, #78-9157-Pads, Bibbero Systems, Inc., Petaluma, CA. To order, call toll free 800-BIBBERO (800 242-2376) OR FAX 800-242-9330.

Fill in the information on the message form.

---

5. **Procedural Step.** End the call politely.
6. **Procedural Step.** If the call is from a patient or concerns a patient, pull the medical record and clip the message to it or attach the medical record in a clinical messaging computer program.
   Principle. This ensures that information about the patient is available and the action taken on the call can be documented if necessary.
7. **Procedural Step.** Place the message (with the patient record, if needed) where the person for whom it is

intended expects to find messages. This may be on a desk or in a mailbox. If a computer messaging program was used, send the message to the intended recipient(s) using clinical messaging or e-mail.
8. **Procedural Step.** Perform follow-up according to office procedure.
   Principle. This ensures that important issues do not fall through the cracks.

PROCEDURE 39-3   Taking Requests for Medication or Prescription Refills

Outcome Take a message requesting medication or a prescription refill.

Equipment/Supplies

- Telephone
- Computer
- Message pad
- Pen or pencil
- Medical record
- Clock or watch

1. **Procedural Step.** Identify the caller and telephone number.
2. **Procedural Step.** Identify if the caller is a patient or a pharmacy.
3. **Procedural Step.** If the caller is a patient, take the information about the medication requested, dose, and number of times a day the patient takes the medication. Write down or enter into the computer the name and telephone number of the patient's preferred pharmacy or mail order supplier.
4. **Procedural Step.** If the caller is a pharmacy, usually the medical assistant takes a message, including the name and address of the patient, the medication requested, and the dosage and amount of medication to be prescribed. Inform the pharmacy when the physician is likely to approve the refill so that the pharmacy can tell the patient.
   Principle. Usually physicians have specific times when they review and respond to messages.
5. **Procedural Step.** End the call politely.

6. **Procedural Step.** Follow usual procedures to attach the patient's medical record to the message (either manually or electronically) and place the message where the physician can review it, or send the message electronically. If the physician responds directly to pharmacy calls, put the pharmacist on hold, pull the patient's medical record, and give it to the physician before transferring the call.
   Principle. The physician will need to review information about the patient before agreeing to refill or prescribe medication.
7. **Procedural Step.** Usually the physician fills the prescription directly by computer, indicates on the message slip whether the prescription may be refilled, or writes a new prescription on the message slip. The medical assistant can then call the pharmacy with the information. Read the prescription from the message slip exactly as the physician has written it.
   Principle. The medical assistant functions as an agent of the physician in this case. He or she must give the exact information the physician has indicated.

7

MESSAGE FROM								
For Dr. Hughes	Name of Caller	Ref. to pt.	Patient Roland Aiken	Pt. Age 40+	Pt. Temp.	Message Date 10/13/XX	Message Time 3:00 PM	Urgent ☐ Yes ☒ No

Message: needs more Aldactazide (25mg tabs) — takes T daily   Allergies Ø

| Respond to Phone # 814-798-2010 | Best Time to Call AM PM | Pharmacy Name/# Westside 814-754-9817 | Patient's Chart Attached ☒ Yes ☐ No | Patient's chart # | Initials KJ |

DOCTOR - STAFF RESPONSE

Doctor's / Staff Orders / Follow-up Action
OK - call to pharmacy JH
#30
12 refills
Sig: T po qam

| Call Back ☐ Yes ☐ No | Chart. Mes. ☐ Yes ☐ No | Follow-up Date / / | Follow-up Completed-Date/Time / / | AM PM | Response By |

Product # 78-9156-Pkg, #78-9157-Pads, Bibbero Systems, Inc., Petaluma, CA. To order, call toll free 800-BIBBERO (800 242-2376) OR FAX 800-242-9330.

The physician may write prescription information on the message form.

8. **Procedural Step.** Document the refill or prescription in the patient's medical record. In some offices the message itself is filed in the medical record, and in others the medical assistant writes the information in the progress notes of the medical record.
   Principle. Any treatment of the patient must be documented in the medical record as part of the continuous record of care given. See Chapter 26 for specifics on documenting medications.

CHARTING EXAMPLE

Date	
10/13/XX	4:30 p.m. Prescription called to Westside Pharmacy for Aldactazide 25 mg tabs, #30, Sig: i po q am, 12 refills. —————— K. Anderson, CMA (AAMA)

OUTGOING CALLS

More calls come into the office than go out. But there are certainly enough outgoing calls. Medical assistants make many of them. Outgoing calls a medical assistant may make include calls to patients, suppliers, insurance companies, other medical offices, laboratories, pharmacies, and hospitals. In some systems it is necessary to dial the number 9 before the telephone number in order to get an outside line. Local telephone books are still provided by the telephone service provider, although it is also possible to look up telephone numbers using the Internet.

Local Calls

Calls to patients, whether the matter is medical or financial, should not be made from the front desk unless a privacy window is closed. The medical assistant must prepare information and supplies before making the call. If the medical assistant is calling a patient, the patient's medical record should be at hand with any notes from the physician. If the call is picked up by an answering machine, it is permissible to leave your name, practice name, and telephone number for the patient to call back. Because the patient's family members may have access to the answering machine or voicemail, no medical information should be included in the message (Procedure 39-4).

It may be necessary to call a patient about an overdue account. The medical assistant should not call the patient at work for this type of call or discuss billing information with anyone other than the person responsible for the bill.

For calls to laboratories, hospitals, or suppliers, the medical assistant should be sure to have organized the information necessary to complete the call before dialing the telephone number.

What Would You Do? What Would You Not Do?

Case Study 3
The physician asks Channa to schedule an appointment for Andrew Page, a 35-year-old man whose recent lipid profile shows an elevated cholesterol and triglyceride level. This is a change from previous laboratory work. The physician says to tell the patient that he wants to discuss the recent blood work in person. When Channa calls the patient, his wife answers the telephone. Channa identifies herself and the medical office and asks to leave a message for Mr. Page to return her call. Mrs. Page says, "He's away on a business trip until Thursday. What is this about? Is it really important?" ∎

If the medical assistant places a call for one of the office's physicians, the physician must be ready to talk before the call is placed. As soon as the physician being called is located, the medical assistant connects the physician placing the call.

Medical assistants and other office staff should not make or receive personal calls using the office telephone system except for emergencies, both to avoid tying up the telephone and because telephone calls take time away from work. The medical assistant can check messages and make outgoing calls during breaks or at lunchtime using a pay phone or personal cell phone. Although permission may be given to make an urgent call using the office telephone, a personal long-distance call is never appropriate.

Appointment Reminders

Medical assistants may be asked to place reminder telephone calls to patients 24 to 48 hours before their scheduled appointments. The HIPAA Privacy Rule allows health care providers to call patients and leave messages regarding their care as long as the patient has not requested confidential communication. It is recommended to limit the information left in a message to the minimum required to confirm the appointment.

Medical offices have begun to use computer programs that interface with scheduling programs and call patients automatically 24 to 48 hours before a scheduled appointment. They provide a recorded message about the appointment and will leave a message if no one answers the telephone. It may be possible to confirm or cancel the appointment after receipt of the message. The patient is instructed to call the office with any questions and sometimes to confirm or cancel the appointment if a message has been left.

Long-Distance Calls

Long-distance calls are almost always dialed directly. The telephone number for a long-distance call can be obtained from directory assistance (411). The medical assistant should know what kind of calling plan the office has because the time of a call can make a difference in the rate for long-distance calls. When calling distant locations, it is important to be aware of the different time zones. To make international calls, the medical assistant should dial 1, then the country code, then the telephone number. In order to prevent unauthorized long-distance calls, most offices have a code that must be used to access the long-distance system. Long-distance services may also be limited to one or two extensions.

Conference Calls

Some phone systems allow conference calls among three or more parties, such as a physician and other individuals who are being called at different telephone numbers. If the telephone system allows this, the medical assistant should learn how to set up such calls for the physicians.

PROCEDURE 39-4   Telephoning a Patient for Follow-Up

Outcome Place an outgoing telephone call to a patient for follow-up.

Equipment/Supplies

- Telephone
- Scratch paper
- Pen or pencil

- Material necessary to place the call, such as a telephone book, instructions from physician, and/or patient medical record

1. **Procedural Step.** Organize all materials that may be necessary during the telephone call. Schedule calls during business hours.
   Principle. Preparation allows calls to be made more efficiently.

2. **Procedural Step.** Write the telephone number on a piece of paper. Include the area code and a country code, if necessary.
   Principle. It may be difficult to remember the number, especially if you do not reach the number on the first attempt.

3. **Procedural Step.** Place the call. When it is answered, ask for your party. Identify yourself with your practice name and your name ("This is Channa from Primary Care Associates").

4. **Procedural Step.** If you reach an answering machine, identify yourself with your practice name and your

name and ask the intended recipient to call you back. Leave your telephone number with area code.
   Principle. Unless it is an appointment reminder, the subject of the telephone call should not be left on an answering machine to protect patient confidentiality.

5. **Procedural Step.** If you are speaking to the patient, give the information requested by the physician. This may be an instruction to make an appointment or may include laboratory results. Do not give more information than the physician has authorized.
   Principle. As an agent of the physician, you have limited authorization to provide information.

6. **Procedural Step.** If the patient has additional questions, offer to take a message for the physician.

7. **Procedural Step.** Close the call politely. Repeat instructions if any were given.

Memories *from* Externship

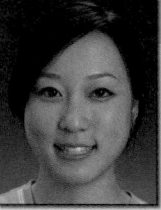

Channa Eng: I was terrified of the telephone when I first started my externship. It was a busy clinic, and I started out in adult medicine. In the morning, I sat at the front desk to check patients in, take copayments, and answer the telephone. I was always afraid that I wouldn't know what to say. We got the callers who wanted to speak to someone in person, so you never knew what to expect. My supervisor told me to answer each call with the name of the clinic and my own name, and then ask how I could help the caller. If I didn't know how to handle the call, I was supposed to put the caller on hold and ask Mary Lynn, the other medical assistant, for guidance. One call that I remember particularly was from an older woman who seemed lonely and confused. She asked for her physician, but she was willing to leave

a message when I told her that the physician didn't take calls while he was seeing patients. She said that she couldn't remember if she was supposed to take her blood pressure medication once a day or twice a day and she wasn't sure if it was one pill or two pills. She told me that her daughter set up her pills in a pill container every week but she had forgotten if she should take them both in the morning or one in the morning and one at night. I told her to get the bottle of medication and read the label to me. From the label we determined that she was supposed to take two pills every morning. She thanked me, and I indicated on the message form that we had clarified the problem. After the call, Mary Lynn complimented me for being so helpful and for handling the call by myself. After that I began to feel more confident about taking telephone calls. ■

MEDICAL PRACTICE *and the* LAW

Recognizing and Responding to Medical Emergencies

When a telephone call concerns a life-threatening or serious emergency, the medical assistant becomes legally responsible to provide appropriate assistance, even if the medical office is not equipped to provide the actual care needed. Once the medical assistant has identified an emergency, he or she must maintain contact with the caller, help the caller get assistance, and follow up to be sure that care was received.

Good Samaritan laws generally do not apply to the medical office because people expect to receive medical care and/or medical advice from physicians and medical offices.

The most desirable response is to refer an emergency or urgent call to a physician or other licensed health care provider in the office (nurse practitioner, physician's assistant, or licensed nurse). However, if no licensed professional is able to take the call, the medical assistant should assist the caller. The medical assistant should assess the situation and instruct the caller to arrange transportation to an emergency department if the patient's health will be harmed by delayed treatment.

The following guidelines describe an appropriate response to an emergency call:

- Medical assistants should always ask if they may put the caller on hold and wait for a response. This gives the caller an opportunity to state that the call is truly urgent or an emergency.
- Every medical office should keep an updated procedure manual near the telephone. The manual should list specific urgent problems and situations, specific questions to ask, and responses to the caller's questions. A list of emergency numbers should be placed near all telephones; these include the numbers for the EMS system (usually 911); the number for the poison control center; and the pager numbers or cell phone numbers for all the physicians in the practice.
- Medical assistants should write down a caller's name and telephone number as early in the call as possible, in case the call is interrupted. Keeping a telephone log provides documentation of how calls were handled.

- If the medical assistant believes delay in treatment poses a threat to the health of the ill or injured person, the caller should be instructed to call an ambulance. If the caller is a child or seems too confused or anxious to make the call, the medical assistant can call 911. The location of the emergency should be determined before the call is made. It is preferable to use a different line to place a call to an ambulance so that contact can be maintained with the caller.

After a caller has been instructed to call an ambulance, there are several steps that follow. The medical assistant should notify the physician (if this has not already been done) and call the emergency department at the local hospital to inform them that one of the practice's patients will be coming in. If the injured or ill person is a patient of the practice, this should be noted in the patient's medical record. If the injured or ill person is not a patient of the practice, an incident report should always be completed. See Chapter 48 to learn how to fill out an incident report. ∎

What Would You Do? What Would You *Not* Do? RESPONSES

Case Study 1
Page 963

What Did Channa Do?
- Spoke politely, and told Mrs. Weston that she needed to pick up the other call.
- Gave Mrs. Weston the choice of being placed on hold or being called back.
- Assured Mrs. Weston that she would get back to the telephone call with her as soon as possible.
- Kept her voice calm and friendly.

What Did Channa Not Do?
- Did not let the second telephone call ring more than three times.
- Did not promise Mrs. Weston that she would put the other call on hold immediately.
- Did not try to rush through the call with Mrs. Weston without making sure that she was clear about the appointment date and time.

What Would You Do/What Would You Not Do?
Review Channa's response and place a checkmark next to the information you included in your response. List the additional information you included in your response.

_____
_____
_____

_____
_____
_____

Case Study 2
Page 964

What Did Channa Do?
- Told Mrs. Woodward to get the bottle of pills, which has a record of the dose and the pharmacy telephone number.
- Told Mrs. Woodward she would place her on hold; instructed Mrs. Woodward to stay on the line after finding the medication bottle.
- Gave Mrs. Woodward the option of calling back when she had found the bottle of pills.
- If Mrs. Woodward seemed confused or distressed, Channa could verify the medication dose from the patient's medical record and look up the telephone number of the pharmacy.
- Remained calm and friendly.
- Made sure to follow up and complete the message.

What Did Channa Not Do?
- Did not become impatient or tell Mrs. Woodward that she should know she needed her bottle of medication ready when she called to ask for a refill.
- Did not pass on the message without confirming that Mrs. Woodward had asked for the correct dose of medication.
- Did not pass on the message without a pharmacy telephone number.

Continued

What Would You Do? What Would You *Not* Do? RESPONSES—cont'd

What Would You Do/What Would You Not *Do?*

Review Channa's response and place a checkmark next to the information you included in your response. List the additional information you included in your response.

_____

_____

_____

_____

_____

_____

Case Study 3
Page 969

What Did Channa Do?

❑ Reassured Mrs. Page that it was not an urgent matter, but said she hoped Mr. Page would return her call after his trip.

❑ Told Mrs. Page politely that she could not discuss the matter with anyone but Mr. Page.

What Did Channa Not Do?

❑ Did not tell Mrs. Page exactly why she was calling her husband.

❑ Did not tell Mrs. Page that the matter was not important.

❑ Did not ask Mrs. Page to contact her husband before he returned from his business trip.

❑ Did not tell Mrs. Page that the physician could give her more information about the matter.

What Would You Do/What Would You Not *Do?*

Review Channa's response and place a checkmark next to the information you included in your response. List the additional information you included in your response.

_____

_____

_____

_____

_____

_____

_____

TERMINOLOGY REVIEW

Medical Term	Word Parts	Definition
Enunciation		The act of speaking clearly and concisely.
Pager		An electronic device that notifies the recipient to receive a message or return a telephone call.
Personal digital assistant (PDA)		A portable handheld computing device with access to various reference tools, such as a drug reference, calculator, and address book.
Smartphone		A cell phone with computer capabilities.
Voicemail		A method for delivery, storage, and retrieval of telephone messages that is built into the telephone system.

ON THE WEB

For information on the Health Insurance Portability and Accountability Act (HIPAA) and appointment reminders:

U. S. Department of Health and Human Services:

http://www.hhs.gov/ocr/privacy/hipaa/faq/smaller_providers_and_businesses/286.html

For information on poison control centers:

American Association of Poison Control Centers: www.aapcc.org

For information on time zones:

The Official U.S. Time: www.time.gov

 Check out the Evolve site at http://evolve.elsevier.com/Bonewit/today/ to actively Prepare for your Certification, and to access additional interactive activities and exercises to help you study and prepare for success.

40

Scheduling Appointments

LEARNING OBJECTIVES	PROCEDURES
Methods of Scheduling	
1. Describe how scheduling appointments efficiently meets the needs of both physicians and patients.	
2. Describe the correct use of appointment books and computer scheduling to make appointments.	
3. Explain why the medical office must retain an updated copy of the daily appointment schedule.	
Types of Scheduling	
4. Describe several types of scheduling, including stream scheduling, wave scheduling, modified wave scheduling, double booking, open booking, and patient self-scheduling.	
5. Identify types of patient appointments that may be clustered in the appointment schedule.	
Setting up the Appointment Schedule	
6. Identify factors to be considered when setting up the appointment schedule.	Set up the appointment schedule.
7. Explain how to set up the appointment schedule.	
Making an Appointment	
8. Differentiate between the information needed to make an appointment for a new patient and an established patient.	Make an appointment.
9. Differentiate among medical conditions that require emergency care, urgent care, and routine care.	
10. Describe how to schedule appointments for individuals who are not patients.	
Managing the Appointment Schedule	
11. Describe the method for changing or canceling appointments.	Manage the appointment schedule.
12. Describe how to update the schedule on the day of the appointment and document changes.	
13. Identify three methods to remind patients to make or keep appointments.	
14. Describe how to store appointment books and daily schedules.	
Scheduling Diagnostic Tests, Procedures, and Admissions	
15. Identify how to schedule inpatient and outpatient diagnostic tests and procedures.	Schedule inpatient and outpatient diagnostic tests or procedures.
16. Identify how to schedule hospital admissions and surgery.	Schedule inpatient or outpatient surgery.

KEY TERMS

blocked	modified wave scheduling	referral
clustering	new patient	single booking
double booking	no-show	stream scheduling
established patient	patient self-scheduling	time-specified scheduling
fixed appointment scheduling	preadmission testing (PAT)	triage (TREE-ahzh)
hospice	preauthorization	wave scheduling
matrix (MAY-trix)	(pree-awe-thur-eye-ZAY-shun)	

INTRODUCTION TO APPOINTMENT SCHEDULING

Scheduling appointments is one of the most important administrative responsibilities performed in the medical office. Until the 1970s, people went to a medical office expecting to wait as long as an hour or more. Most physicians liked to see a full waiting room; it reassured them that their practice was healthy.

In the twenty-first century, people have little tolerance for waiting in a medical office. Lifestyles have changed and people have busy lives. Many have to take personal time away from work to go to the medical office, and they feel that their time is as valuable as the physician's time.

Scheduling appointments correctly and efficiently is crucial to the smooth operation of the medical office. Many factors must be taken into consideration when scheduling appointments. The patient who has made an appointment weeks or even months in advance wants to be seen within 15 to 20 minutes after arriving at the medical office. The physician wants a smooth flow of patients during the time scheduled for seeing patients. Patients who are ill or have accidents want to be able to see their physician on the day of the illness or injury. They prefer to be given a specific time, even if it is later in the day, rather than come into the office and wait for an open moment.

GUIDELINES FOR APPOINTMENT SCHEDULING

The most important criteria the medical assistant must take into consideration when scheduling appointments are exhibiting good interpersonal skills and reducing the amount of time a patient has to wait to see the physician. To meet these criteria, the medical assistant should follow seven guidelines:

1. Maintain the confidentiality of the patient. For example, do not discuss protected health information within hearing distance of other patients.
2. Speak clearly and do not appear rushed. Make sure the tone of your voice is friendly and courteous.
3. Concentrate only on the person to whom you are speaking.
4. Obtain all of the necessary information from the patient. Make sure the information is both correct and complete.
5. Repeat the information relayed to you by the patient. This avoids errors.

6. Schedule the proper amount of time for the type of appointment you are scheduling. For example, a new patient requires more time than an established patient.
7. Document all of the necessary information correctly in the appointment book or in the computer appointment scheduling system.

METHODS OF SCHEDULING

Two methods are used to schedule appointments. Appointments can be scheduled manually, using an appointment book. They can also be scheduled electronically using a computer. These methods are described in more detail next.

Appointment Book Scheduling

Appointment books are usually spiral-bound, so they will lie flat when opened (Figure 40-1). Each physician in the practice may have a separate book, or one book may serve the needs of two or more physicians. Appointment books are available in the following formats: pages for a single day, pages that display a week when open (over two pages), or pages with two or three physicians' schedules for a single day. The pages are further divided into time intervals. The pages are typically divided into 10- or 15-minute intervals. The medical assistant should choose the appointment book format that meets the needs of the practice.

The appointment book is usually maintained in pencil so that information can be changed if needed (e.g., when rescheduling a patient's appointment). In preparing for a day's visits, a typed or hand-printed list of patients, known as a *daily appointment schedule,* must be created. This list or the appointment book itself (if kept in ink) must be retained as a permanent record. The daily appointment schedule is discussed in more detail later in the chapter.

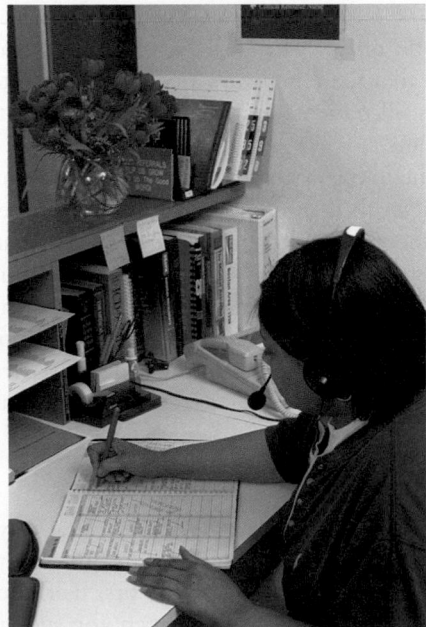

Figure 40-1 Medical assistant with appointment book.

Computer Scheduling

Using a computer to schedule appointments offers advantages. The computer allows the medical assistant to designate appointment intervals. The appointment interval can be adjusted to 10, 15, or 20 minutes depending on the needs of the practice. The computer makes it easy to add, delete, or change appointments; set up repeating appointments; and set up a recall system. A recall system identifies patients that need to be contacted when it is time for them to schedule another appointment.

The medical assistant enters the patient's appointment into a data entry screen. This screen requires the entry of the same information as an appointment book. The computer also allows the medical assistant to print out a daily appointment schedule of patients to be seen that day (Figure 40-2).

DAILY APPOINTMENT SCHEDULE

Each day the list of the patients to be seen that day, called a *daily appointment schedule,* serves several functions. It is used as a guide for pulling the patients' medical records for that day. It also is used as an office reference sheet of patients with appointments on that day. Usually the daily appointment schedule contains the patients' names and telephone numbers and the reasons for their visits (e.g., new patient, physical examination, recheck).

If the medical office uses an appointment book, the daily appointment schedule must be typed or hand-printed by the medical assistant. More commonly, a computer is used to schedule appointments, and the list is printed out in hardcopy form or viewed by staff directly on the computer. According to Health Insurance Portability and Accountability Act (HIPAA) requirements, the daily appointment schedule should never be posted in an office area accessible to patients. This list may be updated and reprinted if there are changes or additions, or changes can be made in dark-blue or black ink. The office must keep an updated record either on paper or electronically to verify tax returns and insurance claims.

TYPES OF SCHEDULING

Several methods are available to schedule appointments in the medical office. They include time-specified scheduling, wave scheduling, modified wave scheduling, double booking, and open booking. Many offices allow established patients to request appointments or schedule appointments using the Internet. In addition, appointments may be clustered or categorized depending on the type of patient or type of examination or treatment. The method an office uses to schedule appointments is based on the needs of the practice and physician preference.

Time-Specified (Stream) Scheduling

Time-specified scheduling, also known as **stream scheduling,** involves scheduling appointments at a specific

Western Medical Center

Richard Warner, MD
Schedule for May 30, 2010

Time	Name	Reason	Home Phone	Work Phone
9:00 AM	ROBERT RICIGLIANO	Physical exam	(490) 459-2811	(490) 459-6217
9:10 AM	*			
9:20 AM	*			
9:30 AM	JUNE ST. JAMES	BP & ECG	(490) 459-5807	(490) 459-9222
9:40 AM	*			
9:50 AM	DARLA SISSLE	Influenza vaccine	(490) 220-1156	
10:00 AM	Catch-up			
10:10 AM	*			
10:20 AM	LLOYD RIDLON	Recheck	(490) 459-4242	(490) 459-0419
10:30 AM	ESTELLE JORDAN	New patient	(490) 459-8249	(490) 459-1062
10:40 AM	*			
10:50 AM	*			
11:00 AM	MARIA SANTOS	Physical exam	(490) 459-0022	
11:10 AM	*			
11:20 AM	THOMAS MAXWELL	Recheck	(490) 459-4123	(490) 459-9201
11:30 AM	*			
11:40 AM	ROBIN SOTO	Well baby	(490) 459-1349	
11:50 AM	*			
12:00 PM	LUNCH			
12:10 PM	*			
12:20 PM	*			
12:30 PM	*			
12:40 PM	*			
12:50 PM	*			
1:00 PM	LUCILLE MORENA	Chem screen	(490) 459-6677	(490) 459-1566
1:10 PM	*			
1:20 PM	*			
1:30 PM	*			

Figure 40-2 Computer appointment schedule.

time. Most offices use this method for scheduling appointments. The goal of time-specified appointments is to minimize the waiting time for the patient and at the same time to keep a steady flow of patients moving through the office (like a stream of water). The amount of time allotted for a time-specified appointment depends on the reason for the visit. In general, the following times are allotted:

- New patient: 30 to 45 minutes
- Complete physical examination: 30 to 45 minutes
- Established patient: 10 to 20 minutes

When using the time-specified method, the medical assistant needs to make sure to allow time in the schedule to accommodate urgent visits, such as ill or injured patients. There are two other terms that may be used for this type of scheduling: **fixed appointment scheduling** and **single booking.**

Wave Scheduling

With **wave scheduling,** three or four patients are scheduled every half-hour and are seen in the order in which they arrive at the office. The goal is for patients to arrive in "waves" so that there is always a patient waiting to be seen. Sometimes, ill patients are seen before those with routine appointments.

This scheduling system assumes that some patients will need to be worked into the schedule. Sometimes patients become uncomfortable when they realize that another patient was given the same appointment time, but a simple explanation can usually reassure the patient. The medical assistant might say, "We schedule all our patients on the hour, and then they are seen in the order they arrive. There is always a patient to be seen, and we find that waiting time is often shorter."

Modified Wave Scheduling

The wave system can be changed in several ways. This is called **modified wave scheduling.** The office may schedule patients at specific times during the first half of each hour, and keep the second half-hour open for special circumstances. This may include working in patients, seeing

Time	Single Booking	Time	Wave Scheduling	Time	Modified Wave Scheduling
9:00	Robert Ricigliano	9:00	Robert Ricigliano	9:00	Robert Ricigliano
	(490) 459-1111		(490) 459-1111		(490) 459-1111
9:10	*Physical exam*		*Physical exam*		*Physical exam*
			June St. James *Re* √		
9:20			(490) 459-1000		
			Robin Soto		
9:30	June St. James *Re* √		(490) 297-1349	9:30	June St. James *Re* √
	(490) 459-1000		*Well-child visit*		(490) 459-1000
9:40	Robin Soto				Robin Soto
	(490) 297-1349				(490) 297-1349
9:50	*Well-child visit*				*Well-child visit*

Figure 40-3 Comparison of single booking, wave scheduling, and modified wave scheduling.

patients who arrived late, or finishing up with patients from the first half-hour.

Another modification to the wave system is to schedule one appointment that is expected to take longer (e.g., physical examination) on the hour and to schedule three or four follow-up appointments on the half-hour (Figure 40-3).

Double Booking

When two patients are given the same appointment time, the practice is called **double booking.** Double booking means that two patients are scheduled into a single time slot. Double booking may be used when a patient can be fitted in around a patient undergoing a diagnostic procedure such as an electrocardiogram (ECG). It is also used when a patient with an injury or acute illness must be added to an already-full schedule.

Open Booking

Sometimes patients are not given a specific appointment time but are told to come in during a time range, such as between 9:00 AM and 11:00 AM. The patients are then seen in the order in which they arrive. In an open-booking system, patients with an injury or an acute illness are usually seen ahead of patients with less significant complaints.

Sometimes medical offices and clinics have walk-in hours designated for acute conditions before regular office hours. In this situation, patients are seen in the order of arrival.

Open booking works best when there is a constant stream of patients or when a practice is not busy. Because patient flow is unpredictable, patients often have to wait a long time.

Patient Appointment Requests and Self-Scheduling

Many medical practices allow patients to request routine appointments from the practice website. Office staff usually schedules the appointment, making every effort to accommodate the patient's request. After the appointment is made, staff notifies the patient either electronically or by a letter. Some practices even give patients limited access to their appointment scheduling software so that patients can schedule their own appointments if a desired time is available. This is called **patient self-scheduling.**

Clustering or Categorization

Clustering involves scheduling patients with similar problems or conditions into groups. Each group is seen on a certain day or within a certain time block during the day. This scheduling method is also called *categorization.* Examples of conditions that can easily be clustered into a day or portion of a day are:
- Physical examinations
- Prenatal patients in an OB/GYN practice
- Diagnostic procedures

Multiple Offices

Some physicians see patients in more than one office. Appointments may be scheduled in each office or through a central system. In this case, it is important to clarify which office the patient wants to visit. It may be necessary to transport the medical record from office to office if an electronic medical record system is not in place.

SETTING UP THE APPOINTMENT SCHEDULE

Appointments are usually scheduled up to 6 months in advance. Before scheduling can begin, the appointment book or computer software must be set up to indicate the times when the physician will see patients. Times when the physician is not available to see patients must be **blocked** out. The appointment schedule showing only available times for appointments is sometimes called the appointment **matrix** (Procedure 40-1).

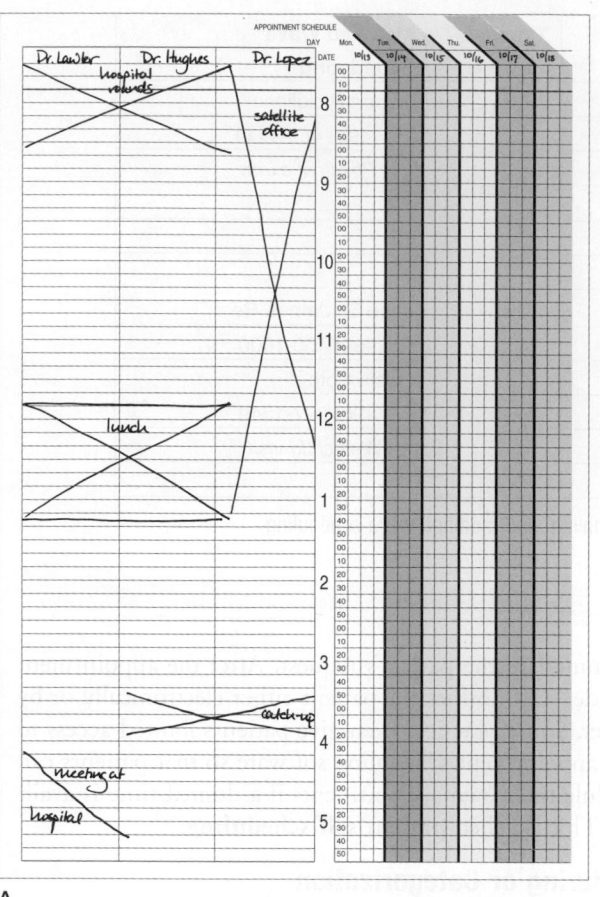

A

Time	Dr. Warner	Dr. Gomez
8:30 AM		
8:40 AM		
8:50 AM		
9:00 AM		
9:10 AM		
9:20 AM		
9:30 AM		
9:40 AM		
9:50 AM		
10:00 AM		
10:10 AM	Catch-up	
10:20 AM		
10:30 AM		
10:40 AM		Catch-up
10:50 AM		
11:00 AM		
11:10 AM		
11:20 AM		
11:30 AM		
11:40 AM		
11:50 AM	Lunch meeting – Memorial Hospital	
12:00 PM		
12:10 PM		
12:20 PM		
12:30 PM		Lunch
12:40 PM		
12:50 PM		
1:00 PM		
1:10 PM		
1:20 PM		
1:30 PM		

B

Figure 40-4 **A,** Appointment schedule from appointment book. **B,** Computer appointment schedule.

How the times are blocked out depends on the scheduling method used by the office. If the office uses an appointment book, the times are blocked out by drawing lines through the blocked times. If a computer is used to schedule appointments, the times are blocked out by setting aside blocks of time. Various types of color-coding are used in a computer scheduling program, but blocked times are different colors than open appointment times (Figure 40-4).

The appointment schedule must take three variables into consideration: the scheduling system, the physician's preferences and needs, and the facilities and equipment requirements. Each of these is discussed later.

Appointment Intervals

Appointments are usually scheduled at intervals of 10 minutes, 15 minutes, or 20 minutes in either a manual or a computer system. An appointment may be scheduled for more than one block, depending on the type of appointment. For example, if a 10-minute interval is used, an established patient coming to have his blood pressure checked might be scheduled for one 10-minute interval and a new patient might be scheduled for three 10-minute intervals. In this case, a 10-minute interval uses one line and a new patient uses three lines in the appointment book or on the computer schedule. If a 15-minute interval is used, all appointments are scheduled in multiples of 15 minutes. In general, more time must be allotted for new patients, physical examinations, and special procedures than for routine follow-up visits.

Physician's Preferences and Needs

The second variable influencing the appointment schedule is the physician's preferences and needs. Physicians may prefer to do physical examinations and/or procedures at specific times as well as a certain number of either during a day. The appointment slots for those times would need to indicate the type of visit (such as a physical). If there are multiple physicians, their preferences may vary and certain rooms may need to be shared.

At times during the day the physician is not able to see patients, and therefore these times must be blocked out on the schedule. Time must be blocked out when the physician has another obligation, such as hospital rounds and nursing-home visits. Time may also need to be blocked out for lunch, pharmaceutical representatives, and catch-up. Days are also blocked out of the schedule for vacation, days off, attendance at conferences, giving lectures, and other professional activities. Protocols for each physician should be kept available for those setting up the appointment schedule.

Facilities and Equipment Requirements

The third variable affecting the appointment schedule is the availability of facilities and equipment. The appointment schedule must be set up so that examination rooms and rooms with equipment required for certain procedures are available to all physicians who are seeing patients.

For optimal use of resources, one or more physicians should be available to see patients whenever the office is open. Physicians like to have at least two examination rooms available for seeing patients, preferably side by side. This improves efficiency and time management for examining patients.

PROCEDURE 40-1 Setting up the Appointment Schedule

Outcome Set up an appointment schedule.

Equipment/Supplies

- Appointment book or computer program
- Pen
- Physician schedule
- Office calendar

1. **Procedural Step.** Block times when the office is not open to see patients. This includes times before office hours begin, lunch and/or breaks, afternoons or days when the office is closed, and holidays when the office will be closed. Some offices set up the appointment schedule 6 months in advance, whereas others do it for a year in advance. In an appointment book, draw an X through times when the office is closed. If the office uses a computer program, set up times when the office is open and set the appointment interval (10, 15, or 20 minutes).

   Principle. In an effective appointment schedule, only available appointment times are blank.

2. **Procedural Step.** Block times when each individual physician is *not* available to see patients, including lunch and hospital rounds. In addition, block days when each physician will be away from the office for vacations, conferences, or other anticipated absences. If the physician has regular meetings or other regular commitments (such as nursing home visits), mark these also. In an appointment book, draw an X through the times when the physician is not available. If the office uses a computer program, schedule the meeting, vacation, or other anticipated absence like an appointment, using color-coding to show that the times are unavailable.

3. **Procedural Step.** For each physician, mark times when the physician does certain types of examinations, procedures (e.g., physical examinations, obstetric visits), or surgery. In an appointment book these are often highlighted with a marker or given a written title at the beginning of the time block. In a computer program these times may be set up as if for a separate physician (e.g., Dr. Gomez and Dr. Gomez—OB visits), or a color-coding system can be used.

4. **Procedural Step.** Depending on office policy, block out as much time as is anticipated for same-day appointments, catch-up time, and unexpected needs. Depending on the practice, catch-up time may be 15 minutes in the morning and afternoon for each doctor, and time

for same-day appointments may be an hour or longer for all physicians or one particular physician on a rotating basis. These times can be marked in various ways as long as office staff understand that they must be saved until the scheduled day.

Example: On this day, the office will be open from 9 to 5, but Dr. Warner will be available to see patients only from 9 to 1 because he plans to attend a conference in the afternoon. The appointment interval is 15 minutes. Dr. Warner likes to have 15 minutes set aside for catch-up time at 10:30 in the morning.

Block times when the physician is not available using a colored background.

GUIDELINES FOR SCHEDULING

When scheduling an appointment, the medical assistant needs to obtain the proper information from the patient, document it accurately, and confirm it with the patient. The procedure for scheduling appointments varies depending on whether the patient is an established patient or a new patient.

Established Patients

For insurance billing, an **established patient** is defined as a patient who has received services from the physician or another physician of the same specialty in the same group practice within the past 3 years. If the patient is seen by another physician in the group who has a different specialty, this does not make the patient an established patient for that physician. For example, a patient has been treated for several years by a family practice physician who refers the patient to an orthopedic surgeon within the group. The patient is a new patient for the orthopedic surgeon. If the patient is seen by a different family practice physician for an urgent care appointment, the patient is an established patient for that physician. Patients who have not been seen within the past 3 years are typically treated as new patients, although their old medical records will be found if possible.

If an established patient is scheduling a return appointment, the physician usually specifies a time period on the patient's charge slip for the return visit (e.g., 1 week, 2 weeks, 1 month, 6 months). The appointment should be scheduled as close as possible to the date specified by the physician. The appointment must also be scheduled for the length of time preferred by the physician, which is usually 10 to 15 minutes. Before locating available appointment times to offer the patient, the medical assistant should ask what day of the week and what time of day are convenient for the patient. For an established patient, it is necessary to obtain the patient's name, date of birth, and physician. If an appointment book is being used, it may be easier to ask the patient for a home and work telephone number than to look up this information. When a computer system is used, telephone numbers appear in the appointment window when the correct patient is selected.

If the patient is at the office, the medical assistant should complete an appointment reminder card and give it to the patient. The medical assistant enters the patient's name, the name of the physician, and the date and time of the new appointment on the card.

If the patient has submitted an appointment request electronically, the medical assistant should attempt to accommodate the patient's wishes when scheduling the appointment or make the appointment as close to the time requested as possible. The patient should receive an e-mail or letter verifying the date and time of the appointment.

Special Situations

Some situations require special attention when scheduling an appointment for an established patient. The most common situation is when a patient visits the medical office and the physician orders laboratory tests to be performed at a medical laboratory. The physician will want to review the results of these tests before the patient comes in for a return visit. When scheduling the patient's return visit, the medical assistant must be sure to allow enough time for the patient to have these tests performed and the results to be returned to the office.

Patients who must undergo a laboratory test at the medical office that requires fasting (e.g., fasting blood sugar) should be scheduled early in the morning and provided with written instructions. This provides the least amount of inconvenience for the patient who must abstain from food and fluids until the specimen has been collected.

Sometimes the patient needs to be scheduled for an appointment for a date later than can be accommodated by the appointment schedule. In this situation, the medical assistant can either tell the patient the date when he or she can request the appointment, or the patient's name can be put on a recall list. When the patient's name comes up, the medical assistant either schedules the appointment and notifies the patient or sends a letter reminding the patient to schedule the appointment.

New Patients

Specific information needs to be obtained when scheduling an appointment for a **new patient.** This includes the patient's full name and daytime telephone number and the reason for the visit or type of visit (e.g., sick visit, physical examination, diagnostic procedure). The medical assistant should ask the patient if he or she has been referred by another physician and determine if the patient's insurance requires preauthorization (precertification). The process for verifying that insurance requirements have been met will be discussed later in the chapter.

Most offices schedule new patients for 30 to 45 minutes. The medical assistant should set aside the correct amount of time for the appointment depending on the physician's preference.

The medical assistant may need to relay directions to the office location to the patient. Some offices mail the health history form to new patients and instruct them to bring the completed form to the first appointment. An office brochure containing information about the practice may also be mailed to the patient or given to the patient at the first appointment.

When the patient has been referred by another physician, the patient should be given an appointment as soon as possible, especially if the patient has urgent symptoms or if the patient's primary physician's office is calling to make the appointment (Procedure 40-2).

Same-Day Appointments

The following problems are usually treated in the medical office and are usually scheduled the same day as the patient calls. The medical assistant should be familiar with office policy because each office varies in the degree of complexity of care it offers.

- Wounds without fracture or dislocation
- Sprains and strains
- Nausea, vomiting, or diarrhea that has persisted for more than 2 or 3 days
- High fever (over 101° F for children and over 102° or 103° F for adults)
- Sudden illness or severe pain without bleeding, fainting, or loss of consciousness
- Sore throat, especially with fever
- Burning, frequency, or urgency associated with urination, especially if accompanied by fever or blood in the urine
- Vaginal bleeding in a pregnant woman (who may also be sent to the emergency department)

If a patient's primary physician's schedule is booked, patients with these types of conditions may need to be scheduled with a practitioner who has a more flexible schedule. In many multipractitioner offices, a period of time is blocked off in one physician's schedule to accommodate same-day appointments.

What Would You Do? What Would You *Not* Do?

Case Study 1

Sandra Meyers has been sitting in the waiting room for several minutes. She arrived at the office at 10:50 AM for an appointment scheduled at 11:00 AM. At 11:15 AM she approaches the front desk and asks how long she will have to wait to see the physician. On this day the physician is running about 25 minutes behind schedule, and there are still two patients ahead of Sandra. She appears to be upset, and she says that she needs to be back in her office by 12:30 PM to prepare for an important afternoon meeting. ■

Urgent Care and Emergencies

The majority of appointments are made well in advance of the date a patient will see the physician, but there are times when urgent or emergency situations occur. A patient calling the office with an emergency presents a challenging situation for the medical assistant. It is important to give a caller a chance to tell you that it is an urgent situation before putting the call on hold. A life-threatening or serious medical problem should be immediately referred to the physician. The physician will make the decision about the appropriate course of action to take. If the physician is not present, the caller should be referred to emergency medical services, usually activated by calling 911 (Box 40-1). The office procedure manual should be used when responding to emergencies.

Walk-in Patients

Sometimes patients come to the office without an appointment and ask to be seen. If the patient is experiencing an emergency or urgent problem, the physician may ask the medical assistant to work the patient into the schedule. In routine situations, however, the patient is asked to return at a later date and offered an appointment. In these situations the medical assistant should tactfully inform the patient of the medical office policy with respect to scheduling appointments.

Individuals Who Are Not Patients

The physician may see various individuals who are not patients during office hours. Time should be blocked from the schedule to accommodate these appointments. Many offices have a specific time slot, often during the lunch hour, to schedule representatives of pharmaceutical companies or representatives of companies with medical equipment or computer equipment that the office may be thinking of purchasing. There is usually a maximum of one or two appointments set aside for each physician for this type of appointment each day. Some physicians may have only one day a week for this type of appointment.

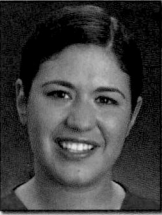

Putting It All into Practice

My name is Elaine Wyatt, and I am a certified medical assistant. My primary responsibility is to schedule routine and urgent care appointments, although sometimes I sit at the front desk and check patients in. I work in an office with five internists and two nurse practitioners. Calls from patients who select "make an appointment" from our telephone menu will end up with me or another medical assistant, or the receptionist may transfer a call to me. I also check patients out after they have been seen and make follow-up appointments using our computer system. Sometimes the telephone is ringing off the hook, and I really have to concentrate to keep track of each call. Our office has a procedure manual with guidelines for handling urgent calls,

and we try very hard to give patients appointments the same day if they are sick. We leave several open appointments for this, but even if we have to double book, we will fit them in because our physicians want to be sure that everyone receives the care they need. All of our physicians and nurse practitioners are accepting new patients, and we always ask new patients to arrive at the office about 15 minutes early to fill out a patient history form. Usually our appointment system works pretty well and patients do not have to wait more than 10 or 15 minutes—at least, that is our goal. There are days, of course, when the physicians get behind, but through trial and error, we have developed a system that works pretty well for us. ■

PROCEDURE 40-2   Making an Appointment

Outcome Make an appointment for a patient.

Equipment/Supplies

- Appointment book or computer program
- Pencil

1. **Procedural Step.** Obtain information from the patient: which physician to book the appointment with, the purpose of the appointment, and any scheduling preference. Referrals are usually offered the first available appointment. If you do not recognize the patient's name, ask if the patient has been seen before. New patients may be encouraged to choose a physician who has joined the practice recently and is not as busy as the more established physicians. Established patients are usually booked with their primary physician, but if it is an urgent problem they may accept an appointment with another provider in the practice.

2. **Procedural Step.** Offer the patient a date and time for the appointment. Keep locating appointments until an acceptable date and time have been found. The more urgent the appointment, the more the patient must adapt to the office schedule.

3. **Procedural Step.** For a new patient, obtain the patient's demographic data (e.g., address, telephone number, date of birth), the name of the patient's insurance company, the name of the insured, the patient's insurance group number and ID number, a prior authorization (precertification) number, or other information related to insurance. Be sure to discuss the cost of the visit or procedure if the patient does not have insurance. Inform the patient if a referral form from the primary physician is necessary. Enter this information directly into the computer as you obtain it from the patient.

Principle. Before making an appointment for a new patient, it is important to be sure that the patient can pay the bill. Information about insurance and referral provides a basis to inform the patient what his or her personal financial liability is likely to be.

4. **Procedural Step.** For an established patient, obtain the information to make the appointment. This includes the patient's name, date of birth, reason for the visit, and daytime telephone number.

5. **Procedural Step.** If using an appointment book, enter the information in pencil and block out the correct amount of time. If using a computer program, enter the patient's name, the correct amount of time for the appointment, and the reason for the visit.

6. **Procedural Step.** Repeat the information to the patient before ending the call. Offer a new patient directions to the office.

Example: The appointment schedule shows a 30-minute appointment for the new patient Estelle Jordan, a 20-minute appointment to evaluate headaches for the established patient Maria Santos, and a 10-minute appointment for Thomas Maxwell (also an established patient).

6				
10:30 AM	ESTELLE JORDAN	New Patient	(490) 459-8249	(490) 459-1062
10:40 AM	*			
10:50 AM	*			
11:00 AM	MARIA SANTOS	Headaches	(490) 459-0022	
11:10 AM	*			
11:20 AM	THOMAS MAXWELL	Recheck	(490) 459-4123	(490) 459-9201
11:30 AM	*			

Schedule appointment times for the correct amount of time.

BOX 40-1   Medical Conditions Referred to Emergency Medical Services (911)

1. Conditions that may result in damage to body structures. This is especially important for problems that can cause a significant decrease in oxygen to the body because of breathing or circulation disorders:
   - Breathing problems or respiratory arrest
   - Severe chest pain or cardiac arrest
   - Bleeding that cannot be controlled
   - Large open wounds
   - Any condition that raises the suspicion of internal bleeding
   - Potential poisoning or overdose

   - Bleeding in, or injury to, a pregnant woman
2. Conditions that result in very low blood pressure:
   - Shock
   - Serious burns
   - Severe bleeding
3. Conditions that result in a change in the level of consciousness (loss of consciousness, disorientation, confusion, loss of alertness)
4. Fractures or large wounds that require the equipment found in an emergency department

Highlight on Triage

Triage is the process of sorting patients according to their need for care. When a disaster occurs, health care workers choose which patients to treat first, depending both on the severity of their injuries and the likelihood the person will survive.

Victims are sorted into three groups—hence the word *triage,* from a French word meaning "sort." Some victims' injuries are minor and can wait for treatment; some victims have injuries so severe that they will probably not survive no matter what effort is put into their treatment; and some have severe injuries but will probably survive if prompt treatment is given.

This system has been adapted to office and appointment scheduling to decide if a patient can wait for the next available appointment, if the patient should be seen immediately, or if the patient should be sent to the emergency department. Triage in the medical office setting is rarely a case of life or death, and the term *triage* is usually reserved for screening performed by licensed health care personnel with the education needed to assess the medical needs of ill patients.

The medical assistant does screen calls and make decisions on the basis of guidelines established by the physicians where he or she works. The medical assistant must remember that if there is any question about a patient needing immediate care, either the telephone call should be referred to a qualified person in the office or the patient should be directed to an emergency department or other facility where care can be obtained. The medical assistant should be familiar with the policies of his or her employer and work within them, both to avoid injuring the patient and to protect against liability in a potential lawsuit. ■

What Would You Do? What Would You *Not* Do?

Case Study 2

On a winter afternoon, there is only one physician in the office. He must leave promptly at 3:45 because he is scheduled to give a lecture to medical students at a nearby hospital shortly after 4:00. The physician has been running behind because two extra patients have been worked into the schedule. At 2:30, in addition to three patients in the waiting room, he still has four established patients scheduled, as well as one new patient scheduled for 3:15, the last appointment of the day. ■

MANAGING THE APPOINTMENT SCHEDULE

Changing Appointments

The most frequent modification required in the appointment schedule is to change an appointment from one time slot to another. The way in which this is done is based on the method used by the medical office to schedule appointments. If the manual method is used, the original appointment is erased and the information is written into the new time slot. If a computer is used to schedule appointments, the original appointment is deleted and then inserted into the new time slot. Usually the computer program has a feature that does this with one operation.

Occasionally an entire block of patients has to be rescheduled. This occurs when the physician is unexpectedly absent or delayed during office hours. The absence or delay may be the result of an emergency, being delayed at the hospital, or personal illness. Every effort must be made to accommodate scheduled patients by giving them a new appointment as quickly as possible. If there are patients in the office when a physician is severely delayed or must leave, it is important to tell patients how long they can expect to wait. The patients should be given the option of waiting or rescheduling their appointments.

If the physician is running seriously behind schedule, patients often become impatient. Some may wish to reschedule, and this should be done willingly. Usually the physician is willing to stay late to finish the day's appointments, but if the physician must leave at a particular time, appointments set for late in the day may need to be rescheduled.

No-shows are patients who simply do not show up for their appointment. No-shows and cancellations on the day of the appointment should be noted on the official appointment schedule. The information should also be documented in the patient's medical record. This provides a permanent record if the patient's condition becomes worse and the patient claims that the physician would not see him or her.

Most offices have a policy of reviewing records of patients after three consecutively missed appointments. If the patient is not motivated to adhere to the treatment plan, the physician may wish to terminate the relationship with the patient (Procedure 40-3).

Late Patients

The office should have a policy regarding late patients. Traffic problems or other incidents can delay even the most punctual person, and usually the office attempts to work the patient into the schedule. If a patient telephones to say that he will be unexpectedly delayed, either the schedule can be adjusted or the patient can be offered a new appointment. Patients who habitually arrive late can cause delays in the appointment schedule. They may be given the last appointment of the day when the physician is most likely to be running late. In some practices habitual latecomers are told that their appointment time is 15 to 30 minutes earlier than the appointment is actually scheduled.

Appointment Reminders

Patients who make appointments while in the office are usually given an appointment reminder card. Appointment cards help patients remember the exact date and time of their next appointment.

Most offices also send reminder letters and/or call patients 1 or 2 days before the appointment. The medical

PROCEDURE 40-3

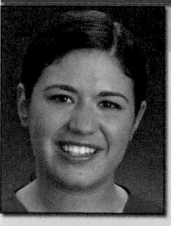
Elaine Wyatt: The office where I did my externship was always very busy. I remember one afternoon when one of the physicians had to leave suddenly. She was expected to be gone about 2 hours. I was told to call the list of afternoon patients and tell them that the physician had been called away from the office and would be delayed about 2 hours. If the patient wanted to reschedule, I had to put him or her on hold and transfer the call to the appointment scheduler. If the patient wanted to be seen that day, I had to give him or her a time from the revised list. I was surprised that about half of the patients were completely willing to reschedule, so there did end up being enough appointment times for the patients who still wanted to be seen. The major problems occurred when we could not reach the patients by telephone. There were about five of them, and they all came. Two of them were during the 2-hour delay, and both of them decided to reschedule. The other three had appointments after the physician returned. We managed to fit them in close to their original appointment time, and they never even knew that the physician had been out of the office unexpectedly. ∎

assistant uses the information that was documented when the appointment was made (manually or by computer) to call each patient scheduled for an appointment (see Chapter 39). The office may use a computer-generated appointment reminder system. The computer may also be used to generate letters or e-mails reminding patients to make appointments for periodic routine examinations such as a physical examination or a mammogram.

Storing Appointment Books and Daily Schedules

In some offices, the appointment book is maintained in ink and used as the office record of appointments. The official book or all daily schedules are updated as described earlier in this chapter and should be stored in a secure area. When computer appointment schedules are used as official schedules, backups should be made according to the guidelines in Chapter 38.

PROCEDURE 40-3   Managing the Appointment Schedule

Outcomes

1. Review the daily appointment schedule.
2. Cancel a patient appointment.
3. Change a patient appointment.
4. Indicate a missed appointment.
5. Document cancellations and missed appointments on the day of the appointment.

Equipment/Supplies

- Appointment book or computer program
- Printed appointment schedule
- Red pen

1. **Procedural Step.** Review the daily appointment schedule and be sure that all medical records and other necessary paperwork have been prepared.
2. **Procedural Step.** Check patients in as they arrive. Depending on office procedure, you may check them in using the electronic medical record and/or a paper appointment schedule.
3. **Procedural Step.** If a patient calls to cancel an appointment, locate the appointment on the appointment schedule, in the appointment book, and/or in the computer appointment program. Ask whether the patient wants to reschedule the appointment.
   Principle. The patient may have a schedule conflict with the original appointment.
4. **Procedural Step.** To cancel an appointment without rescheduling, erase the appointment in the appointment book or delete the appointment in the computer program. To cancel an appointment on the day of the appointment, draw a line through the appointment

on the official paper schedule in ink and note that the appointment was canceled. If the patient wants to reschedule, erase the appointment in a manual appointment book, but leave the appointment in the computer schedule.
   Principle. The official schedule is a legal document so changes to a paper schedule must be made in ink.
5. **Procedural Step.** If the patient cancels an appointment and declines or postpones making a new appointment, document the cancellation in the patient's medical record.
   Principle. Documentation of cancelled or missed appointments makes it readily apparent if this behavior is a common pattern for the patient.
6. **Procedural Step.** If the patient wants to change or reschedule an appointment, find an acceptable time to reschedule.
7. **Procedural Step.** Enter the patient's name and contact information into the new time in the appointment

PROCEDURE 40-3 Managing the Appointment Schedule—cont'd

book. Change the appointment in the computer program by finding the appointment at the originally scheduled date and time and changing to the new date and time.

Principle. By changing the appointment in the computer (instead of deleting), it is not necessary to re-enter the appointment information.

8. **Procedural Step.** Repeat the information to the patient before ending the call, or fill out an appointment card if the patient is present in the office.

9. **Procedural Step.** If the patient misses an appointment without canceling, draw a line in ink through the appointment on the daily appointment sheet and label the appointment "No Show." If the official schedule is maintained in the computer, indicate that

the appointment was not kept by marking the appointment as a missed appointment or no-show or adding a comment that the patient did not keep the appointment, depending on the computer program.

Principle. Computer scheduling programs often give the opportunity to track no-show or missed appointments. If it becomes a pattern for an individual patient, it is easy to identify the problem.

10. **Procedural Step.** It may be office policy to telephone the patient to determine why the appointment was missed and offer another appointment.

11. **Procedural Step.** Document the missed appointment in the medical record, and indicate whether the patient has rescheduled.

9

Western Medical Center

Richard Warner, MD
Schedule for May 30, 2010

Time	Name	Reason	Home Phone	Work Phone
9:00 AM	ROBERT RICIGLIANO	Physical exam	(490) 459-2811	(490) 459-6217
9:10 AM	*			
9:20 AM	* NO SHOW			
9:30 AM	JUNE ST. JAMES	BP & ECG	(490) 459-5807	(490) 459-9222
9:40 AM	*			
9:50 AM	DARLA SISSLE	Influenza vaccine	(490) 220-1156	
10:00 AM	Catch-up			
10:10 AM	*			

Draw a single line in ink through appointments that the patient fails to keep.

SCHEDULING REFERRAL APPOINTMENTS, DIAGNOSTIC TESTS, PROCEDURES, AND ADMISSIONS

Referrals

A **referral** is an authorization for a visit to another physician, usually a specialist. A referral is made by the patient's primary care physician. It may be necessary to obtain **preauthorization** (official permission from the patient's insurance company) before the patient can see the specialist. The physician determines the type and amount of service needed, but the medical assistant usually obtains the necessary insurance authorization (see Chapter 46).

After obtaining all necessary information and insurance authorization, the medical assistant either instructs the patient to make the appointment or calls to make the

appointment for the patient. Some managed care plans require the referring provider's office to make the appointment. If the medical assistant calls from the office, the patient may be able to obtain an earlier appointment, but it is important to verify the date and time with the patient. Figure 40-5 is an example of an approved electronic request for referral to a medical specialist.

For a referral to a community resource, the medical assistant must know the patient's name, address, and telephone number, as well as the particular resource needed, the diagnosis, and the reason for the service. Community services include home health care and **hospice** care (a range of services provided to an individual with a terminal illness). Most community agencies do an intake evaluation of the patient, but others depend on the primary care or other physician and staff to tell them what resources the patient needs.

SH9999999 Detail Approved			Mary Patient SH123456789		
			Request Information		
Patient	MARY PATIENT	Requesting provider	RICHARD WARNER (1234567890 NPI)	Contact info	(490) 555-6464
Diagnosis	I145.10 RT BUNDLE BRANCH BLOCK	Servicing provider	THOMAS HIGHT (2345678901 NPI)	Contact info	(490) 222-3232
Requested service	Specialist consult			Units	1 visit approved
Procedure code				Procedure date	
Start date	4/5/XX	End date	9/5/XX	Delay reason	
Level of service		Related causes		Release of information	Signed statement/ claims
Remarks	Transaction approved				
Procedures and Services					
Status			Reason	Follow-up	Description
Approved (Transaction approved)					Consult
Additional Information					
Additional information requested			Identification code	Description	
No paper work at this time					

Edit   Cancel

Figure 40-5 Approved electronic request for referral to a specialist.

Scheduling Diagnostic Procedures and Hospital Admissions

It is often easier for a physician's office to schedule a diagnostic procedure or laboratory test for a patient than to have the patient schedule it. Hospital admissions are always scheduled by the physician's office. Scheduling procedures and admissions can be performed while the patient is at the office or when the patient is at home. If the patient is at home, the details of the appointment and any special patient instructions must be mailed to the patient and confirmed with a follow-up telephone call.

Scheduling a Diagnostic Procedure

Before scheduling a diagnostic procedure for a patient with an outside facility, the medical assistant should compile all of the information that needs to be relayed to the facility. This includes the patient's name and telephone number, the type of procedure being performed, the reason for the procedure, the time frame within which the procedure must be performed, the physician NPI number and contact information, and insurance information including any preauthorization number.

After an appointment has been made, the medical assistant must contact the patient to relay when and where the procedure will be performed. The medical assistant may also need to provide directions to the facility. Patients are often required to prepare for a diagnostic procedure. For example, a patient undergoing a colonoscopy needs to perform procedures at home to cleanse the colon of gas and fecal material. These instructions must be relayed to the patient by the medical assistant. If written instructions are available, they should be given or sent to the patient. The medical assistant should document in the patient chart the type of verbal and written instructions provided to the patient. After the procedure, the medical assistant should document when and how the patient was notified of the results of the diagnostic procedure. Precise documentation in patient charts is necessary to avoid later claims of malpractice or abandonment (Procedure 40-4).

Scheduling an Inpatient Admission

The medical assistant has several tasks that must be performed when a patient is admitted to the hospital. The medical assistant must contact the patient's insurance

Case Study 3

Anna Greene, a 17-year-old girl, came to see the physician for a physical examination. On the basis of her history and physical examination, the physician has ordered her to have an echocardiogram (ultrasound of the heart). Anna's mother says that the physician did not really explain why Anna needs this test, and she expresses concern that her insurance will not cover the total cost of the test. She appears to be reluctant to allow the test to be scheduled and says that she will call and schedule it herself in a few days. ■

company to obtain preauthorization. The next step is to call the hospital's admitting department to schedule the admission.

The medical assistant must provide the admitting department with the patient's name, address, date of birth, admitting diagnosis, and insurance information and preauthorization number. A patient must be seen by his or her physician within the first 24 hours after admission. Because of this, the hospital may ask when the physician is coming to see the patient. In addition, admitting orders must be sent (electronically or by mail) or faxed before the patient is admitted to the hospital.

The procedure for admitting a patient to the hospital is modified somewhat if the patient is first seen in the emergency department and then admitted to the hospital. In this situation, the hospital obtains the information from the patient and then contacts the physician to obtain admitting orders (Procedure 40-5).

Scheduling Surgery

Scheduling a surgery is similar to scheduling a diagnostic procedure; however, more information is necessary to schedule a patient for surgery. In addition to the patient's name, date of birth, and telephone number, the medical assistant must also know the type of surgery to be performed, the time frame within which the surgery is to be performed, who the surgeon and any assistant surgeons will be, who the anesthesiologist will be, and the name of the hospital or outpatient center at which the surgery will be performed.

Before scheduling the surgery, the medical assistant must call the patient's insurance company and obtain preauthorization (prior approval by the insurance company). The preauthorization number must be relayed when scheduling

surgery. This number facilitates payment by the insurance company for the procedure. The patient's insurance may require the patient to undergo the surgery at specific hospitals or outpatient facilities.

Before a patient undergoes a surgical procedure, **preadmission testing (PAT)** is performed. PAT includes blood tests, an ECG, and a chest x-ray examination. The purposes of PAT are to obtain data about the patient's health before surgery, to be sure that the patient can tolerate the proposed surgical procedure and anesthesia, and to obtain baseline data for comparison during and after the surgical procedure. The medical assistant helps the patient to schedule this testing.

In some communities the hospital performs the PAT, whereas in other communities the PAT is performed in the medical office. If performed in the medical office, the PAT is done either at the surgeon's office or at the office of the patient's primary care physician.

A patient may also need to be scheduled to donate one or more units of his or her own blood. This blood would then be available if a patient needs a transfusion during or after surgery.

Giving a Patient Instructions before Surgery

The medical assistant is often responsible for providing the patient with specific instructions before the surgery. The office usually gives the patient a set of written instructions so that the patient will remember everything. If the patient is receiving a general anesthetic, he or she must fast for a period of time before the surgery. Fasting requires that the patient have nothing to eat or drink for approximately 12 hours before the surgery. If the patient takes medication for hypertension or heart problems, the surgeon may allow the patient to take his or her morning medication with a sip of water. Other examples of preparation that may be required before a surgical operation include washing with an antibiotic soap and taking antibiotics for 1 to 2 days. Patients should be instructed not to bring valuables with them to the hospital. If they are having outpatient surgery, they need to have someone available to drive them home after the surgery.

Documenting an Appointment for Surgery

It is important for the medical assistant to carefully document all information relayed to the patient regarding the surgery. Other information that should be documented includes the interactions with the surgical team members, patient, and facilities.

PROCEDURE 40-4   Scheduling Inpatient or Outpatient Diagnostic Tests or Procedures

Outcome Schedule an inpatient or outpatient diagnostic test or procedure.

Equipment/Supplies

- The patient's medical record and insurance information
- Name of the test or procedure to be scheduled
- Telephone

- Telephone number of the facility and name of the appropriate department with which to schedule the test or procedure

---

1. **Procedural Step.** Assemble necessary information about the patient, including the patient's demographic and insurance information.

2. **Procedural Step.** From the patient's medical record and/or a diagnostic test or procedure requisition filled out by the physician, determine the facility and department to call for scheduling. If the office uses a computerized system, be sure the test, procedure, or hospital admission has been ordered in the computer.
   Principle. Any admission, diagnostic test, or diagnostic procedure must have a valid physician order. For insurance reimbursement, a facility that participates in the patient's insurance plan must be used.

3. **Procedural Step.** Determine the time frame for scheduling and, if possible, discuss with the patient preferred days and times.

4. **Procedural Step.** Obtain preauthorization from the patient's insurance, if necessary.
   Principle. The patient's medical condition must justify the service requested. Failure to obtain preauthorization required by the insurance company will result in denial of the patient's insurance claim.

5. **Procedural Step.** Call the department of the facility where the procedure will be performed.

6. **Procedural Step.** Provide the patient's name and demographic and insurance information as needed and a preauthorization number if needed. Identify the test or procedure to be scheduled, and set up a specific day and time.

7. **Procedural Step.** Inform the patient of the date and time for the test or procedure and provide verbal and written instructions, including preparation for the test, special instructions, and dietary restrictions.
   Principle. The patient must know how to prepare for the test or procedure. Written instructions reinforce verbal explanations.

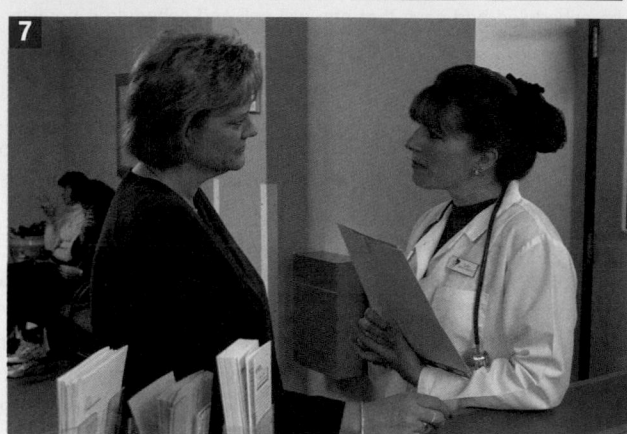

Go over any instructions with the patient before the test.

8. **Procedural Step.** Send a computer or paper requisition to the facility, or give a paper requisition to the patient to take to the test.

9. **Procedural Step.** Document the scheduled diagnostic test or procedure and instructions given to the patient in the patient's medical record.

CHARTING EXAMPLE

Date	
9/22/XX	3:45 p.m. Barium swallow scheduled at Memorial Hospital for 9/28/XX at 9:15 a.m. Pt. instructed to remain NPO after midnight and given directions to Memorial Hospital x-ray department. Pt. verbalizes understanding that she cannot eat or drink anything (including water) after midnight. ——————— ——————— Elaine Wyatt, CMA (AAMA)

PROCEDURE 40-5 Scheduling Inpatient or Outpatient Admissions

Outcome Schedule an inpatient or outpatient admission for a patient.

Equipment/Supplies

- The patient's medical record and insurance information
- Name of the procedure to be scheduled or reason for the hospital admission
- Telephone
- Telephone number of the facility and the admitting department

1. **Procedural Step.** Assemble necessary information about the patient, including the patient's demographic and insurance information.

2. **Procedural Step.** From the patient's medical record and/or directions from the physician, determine the reason for the inpatient or outpatient admission.

   Principle. Any admission must have a valid physician order. For insurance reimbursement, a facility that participates in the patient's insurance plan must be used.

3. **Procedural Step.** Determine the time frame for the admission. If it is for an elective procedure or surgery, discuss with the patient preferred days and times.

4. **Procedural Step.** Obtain preauthorization from the patient's insurance company.

   Principle. The patient's medical condition must justify the service requested. Failure to obtain preauthorization required by the insurance company will result in denial of the patient's insurance claim.

5. **Procedural Step.** Call the admissions department to schedule the admission.

   Principle. The patient must be entered into the facility's computer system with all demographic and insurance information for an inpatient or outpatient hospital admission.

6. **Procedural Step.** Provide all necessary information including demographic and insurance information about the patient, preauthorization number (if any), diagnosis or reason for the admission, and date of the admission.

7. **Procedural Step.** For an inpatient admission, provide admitting orders as needed or fill out admitting orders according to the patient's medical record and fax to the department or nursing floor.

8. **Procedural Step.** If the patient is to be admitted to the hospital directly from the physician's office, assist the patient to notify a family member, prepare a patient transfer form, obtain consent forms to release information, and make arrangements for the patient to be transported to the hospital.

9. **Procedural Step.** If the patient is to be admitted for a procedure or surgery in the future, inform the patient of the date and time for the test or procedure and provide verbal and written instructions, including preparation, special instructions, and dietary restrictions.

   Principle. The patient must know how to prepare for the procedure or surgery. Written instructions reinforce verbal explanations.

10. **Procedural Step.** Document the admission or scheduled procedure or diagnostic test and instructions given to the patient in the patient's medical record. For a hospital admission, identify any documents sent with the patient.

CHARTING EXAMPLE

Date	
6/15/XX	1:30 p.m. Patient to be admitted to Memorial
	Hospital. Room 802 by ambulance for
	shortness of breath and dyspnea. Admitting
	orders and copy of medical record will be sent
	with the patient. Patient's son notified and
	states he will meet his mother at the hospital.
	— Elaine Wyatt, CMA (AAMA)

MEDICAL PRACTICE and the LAW

If a patient consistently breaks appointments or fails to keep appointments, it is impossible for the physician to monitor a patient's health status adequately. The physician may want to terminate the physician-patient relationship. It is recommended that the patient be sent a letter informing him or her of the date that care will be terminated, giving the patient at least a month to arrange for other medical care, and offering to help find alternative care. This protects the physician if the patient initiates a lawsuit for abandonment. Without proper notification, the patient may still consider himself or herself the physician's patient, even if he or she does not follow the physician's treatment plan or keep scheduled appointments. In order to be sure that the patient has received the letter, it should be sent certified mail with return receipt requested, and copies of all correspondence should be retained. ■

PROCEDURE 40-5

What Would You Do? What Would You *Not* Do? RESPONSES

Case Study 1
Page 981

What Did Elaine Do?
❑ Listened to Sandra's concerns without interrupting.
❑ Apologized for the delay and agreed that it is difficult to wait when you have other obligations.
❑ Informed Sandra that the physician was running behind schedule and that there were two patients ahead of her. Gave her a realistic estimate of when she would be taken to an examination room.
❑ Offered to reschedule the appointment if Sandra said that she really could not wait to see the physician that day.

What Did Elaine Not Do?
❑ Did not tell Sandra that she would be taken to an examination room in just a minute.
❑ Did not give a long explanation about why the physician was delayed.
❑ Did not give exaggerated or made-up excuses to imply that this was a one-time crisis.
❑ Did not become defensive or interrupt Sandra.

What Would You Do/What Would You Not Do?
Review Elaine's response and place a checkmark next to the information you included in your response. List the additional information you included in your response.

_____
_____
_____
_____
_____
_____

Case Study 2
Page 983

What Did Elaine Do?
❑ Asked the physician if it would be a good idea to reschedule the new patient or some of the other patients for another appointment in the next few days.
❑ If instructed to do so, called patients, explained that the physician was going to have to leave the office early, and asked if they would be willing to reschedule.
❑ If instructed to do so, explained to the patients in the waiting room that the physician was delayed and asked if they would like to reschedule.
❑ Evaluated all patients carefully to be sure that everything was prepared to make their examinations go smoothly.

What Did Elaine Not Do?
❑ Did not reschedule patients without discussing it with the physician.

❑ Did not tell the patients specific information about the physician's commitments.

What Would You Do/What Would You Not Do?
Review Elaine's response and place a checkmark next to the information you included in your response. List the additional information you included in your response.

_____
_____
_____
_____
_____
_____

Case Study 3
Page 987

What Did Elaine Do?
❑ Made a general statement that the physician thought the test was important, and it would help the physician to provide the best care for Anna.
❑ Asked Mrs. Greene and Anna to wait to see if the physician could give them more information about the reason for and need for the test.
❑ Offered to call the insurance company to determine whether Mrs. Greene's insurance would cover the cost of the test.
❑ Explained that the office preferred to schedule this type of test to be sure that the testing facility had all necessary information from the physician.
❑ Documented the interaction with the patient in detail.

What Did Elaine Not Do?
❑ Did not give a reason for the test unless authorized by the physician.
❑ Did not imply that the mother cared more about the money than her daughter.
❑ Did not say that the physician knows what he is doing.
❑ Did not insist on scheduling the test even if Mrs. Greene did not agree to it.

What Would You Do/What Would You Not Do?
Review Elaine's response and place a checkmark next to the information you included in your response. List the additional information you included in your response.

_____
_____
_____
_____
_____
_____
_____

TERMINOLOGY REVIEW

Medical Term	Word Parts	Definition
Blocked		Times in the appointment schedule when physicians are not available to see patients.
Clustering		Scheduling similar types of patients or examinations on the same day or part of the day.
Double booking		Scheduling two patients for the same appointment time.
Established patient		A patient who has been seen by one of the physicians in the practice within the past 3 years.
Fixed appointment scheduling		An appointment scheduling method in which each patient is given a different, specific appointment time. Also called *stream scheduling, time-specified scheduling,* or *single booking.*
Hospice		Palliative service provided for patients whose life expectancy is less than 6 months. Services may be provided in the patient's home, a nursing home, or a special hospice facility.
Matrix		A rectangular or linear arrangement of numbers or information.
Modified wave scheduling		An appointment system that has some fixed appointments and some appointment times during which patients are seen in order of arrival.
New patient		For billing purposes, a patient who has not received services during the previous 3 years from any physician in a medical practice.
No-show		A patient who does not keep a scheduled appointment.
Patient self-scheduling		The practice of allowing patients to have access to the computer scheduling program so that they can schedule their own appointments.
Preadmission testing (PAT)		A series of diagnostic tests done before surgery to establish the patient's health status and identify any potential problems that may occur during surgery.
Preauthorization		Permission from a patient's insurance company for a test, procedure, or surgery.
Referral		The directing of a patient to a medical specialist by a primary care physician.
Single booking		An appointment scheduling method in which each patient is given a different, specific appointment time. Also called *stream scheduling* or *fixed appointment scheduling.*
Stream scheduling		An appointment scheduling method in which each patient is given a different, specific appointment time. Also called *fixed appointment scheduling, time-specified scheduling,* or *single booking.*
Time-specified scheduling		An appointment scheduling method in which each patient is given a different, specific appointment time. Also called *stream scheduling, fixed appointment scheduling,* or *single booking.*
Triage		The process of separating patients by the urgency of their need for care.
Wave scheduling		A method of scheduling appointments in which several patients are given the same appointment time and are seen in the order in which they arrive.

ON THE WEB

For information on Health Insurance Portability and Accountability Act (HIPAA) regulations:

U.S. Department of Health and Human Services, Office for Civil Rights—HIPAA: www.hhs.gov/ocr/hipaa

Center for Medicare and Medicaid Services HIPAA website: www.cms.hhs.gov/HIPAAGenInfo

For information on open access (same-day appointment scheduling):

American Academy of Family Physicians: http://www.aafp.org/online/en/home/practicemgt/quality/qitools/
pracredesign/practredesignresource/samedaysched.html

 Check out the Evolve site at http://evolve.elsevier.com/Bonewit/today/ to actively Prepare for your Certification, and to access additional interactive activities and exercises to help you study and prepare for success.

41

Medical Record Management

INTRODUCTION TO MEDICAL RECORDS

A medical record (also known as a *patient chart*) contains the important information related to an individual patient in written or electronic form. It includes the care given to that patient and the progress of the patient's condition. **Medical record management** is the process of controlling and handling medical records from the time a record is created until it is placed in permanent storage or destroyed. In addition to recording the care given to patients, both paper-based records and electronic medical records (EMRs) may also be used to review quality of care and for recording statistical information.

It is impossible for a physician or other professional to remember every detail of care, such as the results of a physical examination or doses of particular medications. Many people in the primary care physician's office have contact with a patient, as well as consulting professionals, laboratories, and hospitals. It is important that each interaction be recorded in the patient's medical record. This provides an ongoing record of both the patient's state of health and the service provided by the medical office.

Medical records are also legal documents, if there are questions about the care given. If a patient sues a physician, the court will require documentary evidence, such as a medical record, to be presented in court. The court will take the position that whatever is documented in the record is the care that was given. If something is not documented, officially it never happened. To protect the legal interests of the physician's office, it is therefore important to keep complete medical records.

PAPER-BASED MEDICAL RECORDS

Many medical offices still rely on paper-based medical records to document care. A manila file folder is created for each patient, containing all documents related to the care of that patient. These records are maintained in files to be available each time the patient is seen at the office. After the transition to an EMR, the old paper record may be destroyed if the entire record has been scanned. In some offices, most of the paper record is scanned into the new electronic record system, and the old record is placed in storage. In most offices, however, only baseline data and very recent information are entered into the new electronic record, because large charts are time-consuming to scan, and too much information tends to overwhelm the system. For at least 2 to 3 years after the transition to an EMR, the old paper chart is made available to the physician for each patient visit.

ELECTRONIC MEDICAL RECORDS

In many medical offices, part or all of the medical record is maintained on computer. This is usually called an electronic health record (EHR) or **electronic medical record (EMR).**

There is a growing movement to develop **health information exchanges (HIEs)** so that electronic data can be shared among institutions in a given area. Currently each EMR system uses its own standards and is not necessarily able to share data with other systems. A **Nationwide Health Information Network (NHIN)** is being developed through the Office of the National Coordinator for Health Information Technology (ONC) to allow for the national exchange of health care information.

When a medical office uses an EMR, information is entered directly into the computer system via a keyboard, mouse, screen display, and/or voice recognition systems. Computer terminals may be located in each examination room or at selected areas within the office. As an alternative, staff may rely on portable devices such as laptops, tablets, or personal digital assistants (PDAs). Entry of information is necessary whenever care is provided or information is obtained from the patient. The EMR is usually linked to the computer appointment system and often to the billing systems.

An electronic medical record offers a number of advantages:

- Medical information is always legible.
- Information is easy to retrieve.
- Medical offices can be linked to laboratories, hospitals, and insurance companies. Access to laboratory data and test results is also easy and quick.
- The EMR can be linked to medical information such as information about medications or treatment protocols for specific medical conditions.
- Less time is spent filing.
- Less storage space is required.

The change from a paper system to an electronic system often seems overwhelming. In addition to the important issues related to data security (and hence patient confidentiality), there are several other challenges to overcome:

- Cost of computer hardware, software maintenance, and staff training
- Orienting new or temporary staff to the EMR system
- Difficulty in adding older records to an EMR system
- Difficulty preventing unauthorized alterations and authenticating digital signatures
- Structuring data so that they can be transferred among different digital systems
- Incorporating updates to the software and medical codes as well as meeting new standards for electronic data transfer (see Chapter 46)

Some facilities print a full or partial record for office visits and then enter new information during the visit or immediately after the patient has been seen. Old records may be gradually scanned into the system, but until this process is complete, established patients often have an old paper record in addition to the new electronic record. Even with high-quality scanning systems, handwritten originals may not be legible after scanning.

Despite the problems of change, many hospitals have made or are in the process of making the transition to a paperless system for maintaining patient records. This encourages physicians who are affiliated with those hospitals to do the same. The number of physician offices using electronic records continues to increase. The current challenge is to include implementation of standards to allow for interchange of data among different systems. This will improve patient care by making all health care data for an individual available to any practitioner treating that patient.

EQUIPMENT AND SUPPLIES

Storage Equipment

Paper medical records may be kept in various types of file cabinets or on open shelves. The choice of equipment depends on the following: the number of people who need to access the medical records, the office layout, and the amount of floor space available. Usually the records are stored with the files side to side. The files may take up part or all of a room. In a rotary system, the medical assistant can move sections of shelving to access other shelves behind. Large offices may even use an automated system, which stores more records and brings the record to the medical assistant.

File Cabinets

Cabinets or shelves used to store medical records should always be of heavy construction, with proper weighting on the bottom so that they will not tip over, especially if the drawers or shelves pull out. File cabinets should have a locking system. Lateral drawer file cabinets are more common than vertical file cabinets for medical records, although vertical file cabinets may be used for storing other types of information. Lateral drawer file cabinets have drawers that open from the long side, resembling a chest of drawers.

Shelf Filing Units

Shelf filing units consist of shelves arranged horizontally similar to bookshelves. Shelf units are often used to store medical records because the records can be accessed without having to open and close drawers. Adjustable metal shelf dividers that interlock at the back of the shelves come with the units. Their function is to keep the records in an upright position, thus preventing the records from slumping or sliding under one another.

File folders with side tabs (described later in this chapter) must be used with shelf units to permit the patient's name to be visible on the shelf. A record is placed on the shelf with the bottom edges of the folder down and the side tabs facing outward. This means that the record is accessed from the side, rather than the top, as with drawer filing cabinets.

Shelf files are preferred because they allow easier access to records, and a number of people can have access to the

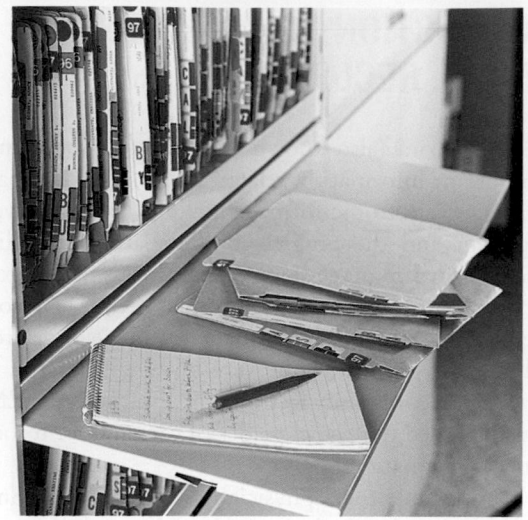

Figure 41-1 The pull-down front of a shelf storage unit may function as a work space.

shelves at the same time. For example, a medical assistant may need to retrieve the medical records of patients to be seen that day, while at the same time another medical assistant may need to look up information for an insurance company or to document a patient telephone call.

Shelf units are available in two styles: open-shelf units or pull-down front units. As the name suggests, open-shelf units are open to the environment and cannot be closed. They must be in a room that can be locked separately from other parts of the office. The pull-down front units have lids that can be pulled over the front of the shelves and locked. This protects the records from environmental factors and allows each part of the file to be locked (Figure 41-1). It must always be possible to lock either the entire medical record room or individual shelving units.

Filing Supplies

File Folders

A file folder is a protective cover used to hold medical record documents in an organized format. Usually file folders are made of manila card stock. Flexible metal fasteners at the top of the inside of the folder hold documents in place. Although the folders expand as the number of documents increase, it is recommended that the folder be broken down into two folders after attaining a width of ¾ inch.

Folders are available with tabs. A **tab** is a projection of a folder that extends beyond the top or side edge of the folder. Folders for a file cabinet with drawers have tabs on the top, whereas folders for shelf units have tabs at the side of the file folder. In the medical office with shelf filing cabinets, a folder with a full-cut side tab is used. Indentations at intervals along the tab indicate the placement of adhesive labels. This ensures that all the labels on all the medical records are affixed at the same place on the file folders (Figure 41-2).

Putting It All into Practice

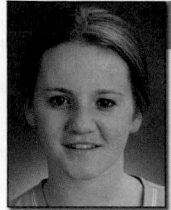

My name is Ellen McDonald, and I am a certified medical assistant. I have been working for a group practice specializing in internal medicine and cardiology for about a year. Although our office uses a computer-based billing and appointment system, our patient medical records are still in paper-based format. We file our records alphabetically. We are changing to an electronic system this year, but we will be using the paper system during the transition. There is always a big stack of reports, correspondence, and other paperwork to be filed. We are not allowed to file any report unless the physician has seen it. In addition, our physicians dictate their progress notes, which are sent electronically to a transcription service. Every day we print the dictation that the transcription service has returned to us electronically, and we stamp them for the physicians to initial after they read them and make any corrections. I am responsible for making sure the files of medical records are kept in good order. In addition

to pulling records and putting them away, I sometimes have to look for a misplaced record. If I can't find a patient's medical record, I begin to look for it. First I check the stacks of records for patients who will be seen that day or the next day. Sometimes a medical record gets caught on another record, so it is important to check through the stacks thoroughly. Next I check the computer to find out when the patient was last seen. I check on and behind the desks of the physician the patient last saw, as well as the billing desk. I also check through the files looking for a record that has been misfiled. We use color-coded labels, so it is usually easy to see when a record is out of place. These measures are usually enough to find the record, although sometimes it may take as long as a week before the record turns up. One time we looked for a record for 3 weeks before we found it. Whenever I am filing, I am very careful, because I remember how much work it is to find a record that has been misfiled. ■

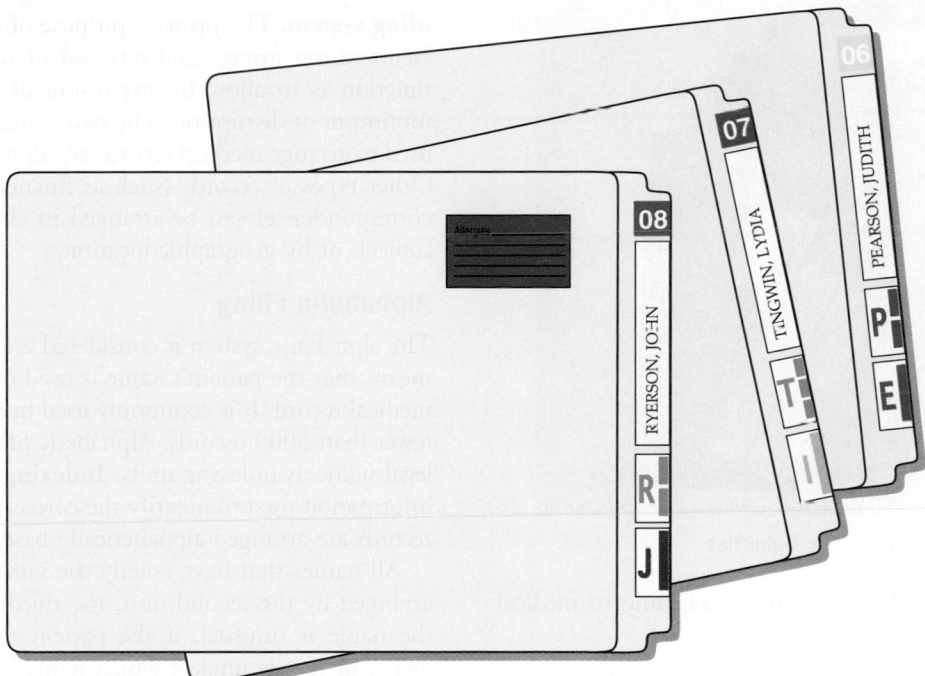

Figure 41-2 File folders for shelf units have a full-cut side tab. Color labels are affixed in the same position on each folder.

Folder Labels

Labels are used to identify the medical record and are commercially available in rolls or continuous folded strips. Most offices use pressure-sensitive self-adhesive labels. The labels for an alphabetic system assign colors to letters in either the first third or first half of the alphabet, and the remaining letters are assigned the same colors along with some type of distinguishing mark, such as one or two white stripes. If the office uses a numeric filing system, each digit from zero to nine is assigned a specific color. Color-coded year labels are often used to identify the last year a patient was seen at the office. The current year label is placed on a new record and

updated the first time a patient has an office visit each year. This allows the records of patients who have not been seen for some time to be removed from the active files and placed in inactive storage.

Chart Dividers

Chart dividers are used to identify each section of the medical record by subject. Chart dividers are made of a heavy material such as manila card stock. Each divider has a tab for identification. Common categories include Progress Notes, History/Physical, Lab Reports, Diagnostic Testing, Hospital Reports, Immunizations/Medications,

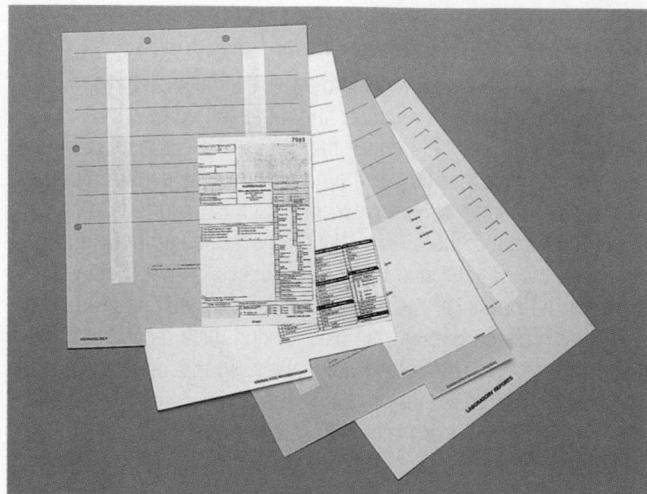

Figure 41-3 Laboratory reports are often mounted one above another so that the most recent is visible on top.

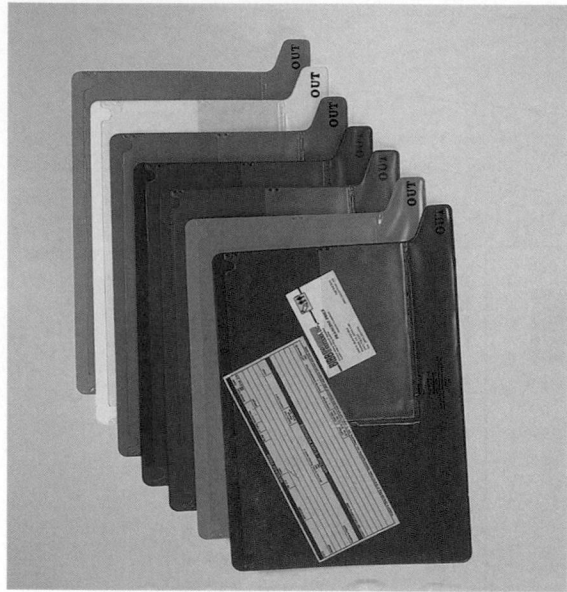

Figure 41-4 Outguides.

and Correspondence, but this varies according to medical office requirements.

Mounting Sheets

Laboratory reports, copies of prescriptions, and telephone messages are often filed on mounting sheets with adhesive strips. Usually several items can be filed on the same sheet. The medical assistant files the first item at the bottom, with each succeeding item shingled up the mounting sheet. With this system the most recent item is always on top. Figure 41-3 shows this type of mounting sheet.

Other Supplies

Outguides, shown in Figure 41-4, are placed in the file to mark the place where a folder has been removed. Each guide has a pocket for a card indicating who removed the record and/or items that accumulate while the record is out of its storage area. Another type of outguide is made of heavy

cardboard and has lines to write the name of the individual removing the record.

A **sorter** is a device that facilitates placing documents in alphabetic or numeric order. It has pockets or dividers for each letter or number.

What Would You Do? What would You *Not* Do?

Case Study 1
A patient has come to the office to request that a copy of her medical record be sent to another physician. She says that her name is Anna Soubrette and her birth date is April 25, 1952. She says that she has not been seen for 4 years, but her current physician had asked about various medications she had taken for a heart problem in the past. Ellen looks the patient up on the computer under Soubrette, but she does not find the patient listed. ∎

FILING SYSTEMS

The way in which records are arranged is referred to as a **filing system.** The primary purpose of a filing system is to facilitate the storage and retrieval of records; a secondary function is to allow for expansion of the records with a minimum of disruption. The two systems most commonly used to arrange medical records are alphabetic and numeric. Other types of records (such as financial records or office correspondence) can be arranged in chronologic order, by subject, or by geographic location.

Alphabetic Filing

The alphabetic system is considered a direct system, which means that the patient's name is used directly to locate the medical record. It is commonly used in medical offices with fewer than 5000 records. Alphabetic filing uses parts of the legal name as indexing units. **Indexing units** are pieces of information used to identify the correct filing location. The records are arranged alphabetically based on the first unit.

All names that have exactly the same first unit are then arranged by the second unit, the third unit, and so on. If the name is unusual, if the patient uses more than one name, or if it is unclear which name is the last name, the record may be cross-indexed. To **cross-index** means to file under one unit and to file a guide or card referring to the primary filing location under another unit.

It is important to follow rules when filing alphabetically. One resource for guidelines is ARMA International, an association for records and information management personnel. The medical assistant must always clarify the procedures followed by any given medical office (Procedure 41-1).

Rule 1: Individual Names

In a patient's name, the **surname** (last name) is the first indexing unit, the given name (first name) is the second unit, and the middle name or middle initial is the third unit. A name with only two units is filed before a name with three units. ("Nothing" always comes before "something".) A unit with only an initial is filed before a unit with a full name beginning with that initial. Business names are indexed in the order of the names in the business (excluding *a*, *an*, and *the*). Examples are as follows:

Name	Unit 1	Unit 2	Unit 3
Mary Ann Stede	Stede	Mary	Ann
Alan Stone	Stone	Alan	
Alan C. Stone	Stone	Alan	C.
Alan Charles Stone	Stone	Alan	Charles
Stoneham Medical Supply	Stoneham	Medical	Supply
Peter H. Stones	Stones	Peter	H.

Rule 2: Prefixes

If the last name has a prefix, such as Mc, Mac, Van, de, Des, or D', the prefix is considered part of the last name. Therefore it begins the first indexing unit. Traditionally these prefixes were lowercase, but today they may be uppercase or lowercase. The prefixes Mc and Mac are usually filed in regular order. In some medical offices, however, they may all be filed as Mc, often as a separate group from other names beginning with "M." Examples are as follows:

Name	Unit 1	Unit 2	Unit 3
Lyndon A. De Larosa	Delarosa	Lyndon	A.
Stephen P. Dennis	Dennis	Stephen	P.
Mary Ann d'Entremont	Dentremont	Mary	Ann
Joanne McCarthy	Mccarthy	Joanne	
John Vanderbilt	Vanderbilt	John	
Joel P. van Twisk	Vantwisk	Joel	P.

Rule 3: Abbreviations and Nicknames

It is recommended that abbreviated first and last names be filed as written. If the patient commonly uses an abbreviated first name, the abbreviation is used as an indexing unit. If a nickname is used on the record, it is indexed as if it were the legal name (often it is). If an abbreviation is part of the last name (such as St.), it is part of the first indexing unit. (In some offices, abbreviations such as St. are filed as though they were written out.) Acronyms or initials in business names are indexed as one unit. Examples are as follows:

Name	Unit 1	Unit 2	Unit 3
Dottie A. Settland	Settland	Dottie	A.
SSI Transport Service	SSI	Transport	Service
Alex M. St. Croix	Stcroix	Alex	M.
E. V. Thomas	Thomas	E.	V.
Bill van der Post	Vanderpost	Bill	
Wm. T. Vanderpost	Vanderpost	Wm.	T.

Rule 4: Hyphenation

Hyphenated names are indexed as one unit, whether first names, last names, or names of children using both parents' last names. Examples are as follows:

Name	Unit 1	Unit 2	Unit 3
Eustace F. Brightfellow	Brightfellow	Eustace	F.
Claire Bryant-Litson	Bryantlitson	Claire	
Ann Marie Smith	Smith	Ann	Marie
Annabelle Smith	Smith	Annabelle	
Ann-Marie Smith	Smith	Annmarie	

Rule 5: Titles and Seniority Terms

Disregard titles unless the complete name is not given or unless they are necessary to distinguish between two individuals with the exact same name. Seniority terms, such as Jr., may be indexed as the last unit. Numeric seniority terms are indexed in numeric order before alphabetic terms. If a male child has exactly the same name as his father, he is called "Jr." until his father dies. He is a "III" if his father is a "Jr." In this case, he has the exact same name as his father and his grandfather. If he is named exactly for his grandfather, who is still living, but not for his father, he is called "II." Examples are as follows:

Name	Unit 1	Unit 2	Unit 3
Samuel Molson Jr.	Molson	Samuel	Jr.
Samuel Molson Sr.	Molson	Samuel	Sr.
Dr. Patricia A. Moy	Moy	Patricia	A.

Rule 6: Names of Married Women

A married woman may take her husband's surname, but she retains her own first and middle names. She may also retain her original name or use both her original name and her husband's name. If two last names are used, they may or may not be hyphenated. It may be necessary to cross-index the name to prevent confusion.

A woman's married name may take several forms. The examples assume that Helen Ann Thurman marries James M. Walker.

- She may keep her own first and middle names, and take her husband's surname (Helen Ann Walker).
- She may keep her own first name, use her family's surname as a middle name (her maiden name), and take her husband's surname (Helen Thurman Walker).
- She may keep her own first and middle name and use a hyphenated last name consisting of her original name and her husband's surname (Helen Ann Thurman-Walker).
- She may keep her own first name, middle name, and her original (family) surname (Helen Ann Thurman).

Sometimes the hyphenated surname is used only for the couple's children, with the woman using one of the other options. It would not be correct to use the husband's first name as a filing unit of a married woman unless her given name is unknown. Examples are as follows:

Name	Unit 1	Unit 2	Unit 3
Mrs. Arlene Sandra Trim	Trim	Arlene	Sandra
Mrs. Joan Walker Trim	Trim	Joan	Walker
Mrs. John (Sandra A.) Trim	Trim	Sandra	A.
Mrs. Ann Walker	Walker	Ann	
Mrs. Ann R. Walker	Walker	Ann	R.
Mrs. Diane A. Walker-Trim	Walkertrim	Diane	A.

Rule 7: Companies and Businesses

The names of companies and businesses are indexed in the same order as written. These are not used for medical records, but the medical assistant may use an alphabetic file for telephone numbers. Disregard punctuation, such as commas, apostrophes, or hyphens. Disregard articles such as *a, an,* and *the.* When indexing an **acronym** (a word formed using the first letters of all the words in a name, such as NYNEX), the acronym is indexed as one word. Examples are as follows:

Company Name	Unit 1	Unit 2	Unit 3
Edson's Pharmacy	Edsons	Pharmacy	
The Redline Supply Company	Redline	Supply	Company
Rent-A-Computer Service	Rentacomputer	Service	

Rule 8: Identical Names

If two names are exactly the same, index them first under the name, and then under the location, beginning with the city as the first unit, state as second unit, street as third unit, and street number from lowest to highest. This applies to names of patients and businesses.

Numeric Filing

In many practices, each new patient is assigned a number. This number is used to identify the patient and file the paper medical record (Procedure 41-2). The patient's number can be accessed with other data in the computer, usually from the name and date of birth, although the patient may also be given a plastic identification card with the medical ID number. A numeric system has two major advantages:

- It is easier to preserve confidentiality.
- In a large practice, it is easier to identify a patient by number when several patients have the same last name.

The main disadvantage of using a numeric system for medical record management is that it is an indirect system. This means a cross-referenced index must be maintained to link the patient's name with the record identification number. Computers can cross-reference information without difficulty, so the EMR is usually linked to a patient identification number.

Terminal Digit Filing Systems

The most common numeric filing system used in medical offices and hospitals uses a six-digit number with a hyphen between each group of two digits (e.g., 01-22-19). The filing system is called **terminal digit filing,** an indexing system that uses the final group of digits as the first indexing unit. A terminal digit filing system mixes up active and inactive records in the files, so the numbers of the newest (and usually most active) patients are not all located in the same section of the file shelves as they tend to be in a consecutive numeric system.

With terminal digit filing, the numbers are indexed by group, working back from the final to the first group. Within each group the numbers are arranged from lowest to highest. To file the record with the number 01-22-19, the medical assistant would first locate the position of charts that end in 19 (first indexing unit). Assuming that there would be several records that end in -19, the medical assistant would then locate the position of charts that end in -22-19. Finally, the medical assistant would file the record between 00-22-19 and 02-22-19.

Examples using two-digit groups are as follows:

Number	Unit 1	Unit 2	Unit 3
89-25-68	68	25	89
48-31-69	69	31	48
48-35-69	69	35	48

Another way to provide nonconsecutive filing is to assign each patient a combination of both letters and numbers. The records are then filed under the letters alphabetically, followed by the numbers.

Consecutive Filing Systems

In consecutive filing systems, numbers are arranged and filed from the lowest to the highest. In such a system, zeroes are assigned or assumed as the first unit. This type of filing system may be used in a small medical office. Examples are as follows:

Number	Unit 1	Unit 2	Unit 3	Unit 4	Unit 5	Unit 6
000642	0	0	0	6	4	2
000853	0	0	0	8	5	3

Subject Filing

Filing systems for documents (e.g., preprinted forms, invoices, purchase orders, service agreements) are often arranged according to subject. Within the subject category, documents may be arranged alphabetically or by date. In the medical office, subject filing is often used for insurance, bills, research, or other documents related to running the practice rather than the patient records.

Chronologic Filing

A tickler file, which is used to "tickle" the memory by serving as a reminder that a specific action must be taken on a specific date, is a type of chronologic system. It may consist of cards or folders or it may be electronic. A card or folder is used for each day of the month, with file guides for each of the 12 months and each day of the month. As each month passes, the day guides are added to items for the current months. A manual system may be useful to identify bills to pay or other activities related to paper documents, but a computer reminder system is often used for daily tasks and/or patient reminders.

Choosing a Filing System

It is important to consider several factors when choosing a filing system for paper medical records. Numeric systems are best for maintaining privacy, but they are more complex because of the need for cross-indexing. When the system is very large, it is easier to prevent confusion if each patient is given a unique number, because many patients may have similar names or even the same name. If several individuals will be filing paper records, a nonconsecutive system such as the terminal digit filing system will make it easier for more than one individual to work comfortably in the filing area.

PROCEDURE 41-1 Filing Patient Records: Alphabetic

Outcome File patient records correctly using an alphabetic filing system.

Equipment/Supplies

- Patient records with patient names
- Alphabetic sorter
- File cabinet or shelves
- Outguides
- Index cards

1. **Procedural Step.** Gather the records that are ready to be filed and remove any elastic bands or paper clips.
   Principle. Paper clips, elastic bands, and so on prevent the record from sliding easily into and out of the file.
2. **Procedural Step.** Check the records to be sure that no loose sheets of paper are present. If loose sheets are found, insert them in the record.
3. **Procedural Step.** Sort the records alphabetically by last name, using the alphabetic sorter if available.
4. **Procedural Step.** Find the correct location in the file for the first record, pull the outguide halfway out, slide the record in front of the outguide in the correct location in the file, and finish removing the outguide. If your office does not use outguides, use your hand to make a space between the record before and the record after the one you are filing.
5. **Procedural Step.** If there is an index card in the outguide showing who had the record from the outguide, remove it. Place the outguide with other unused outguides. Some offices keep index cards for the physicians in separate boxes so that new cards do not need to be

written; some offices cross out the name and reuse the index cards; some offices use slips of paper that are discarded after each use.

6. **Procedural Step.** File each record in the same way until all records have been filed.

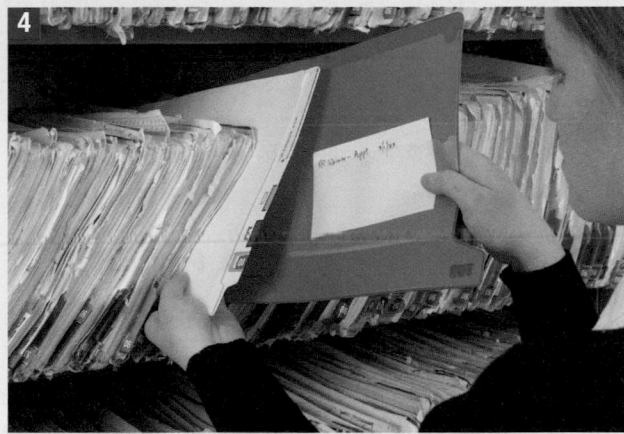
Slide the record in front of the outguide.

PROCEDURE 41-2 Filing Patient Records: Numeric

Outcome File patient records correctly using a terminal digit filing system.

Equipment/Supplies

- Patient records with terminal digit labels
- File cabinet or shelves
- Numeric sorter
- Outguides
- Index cards

1. **Procedural Step.** Gather the records that are ready to be filed and remove any elastic bands or paper clips.

Principle. Paper clips, elastic bands, and so on prevent the record from sliding easily into and out of the file.

Continued

2. **Procedural Step.** Check the records to be sure that no loose sheets of paper are present. If loose sheets are found, insert them in the record.

3. **Procedural Step.** Sort the records according to the terminal digit indexing units, using the sorter if available.

4. **Procedural Step.** Find the correct location in the file for the first record, based on the final group of numbers. Refine your search based on the middle group of numbers and then the first group of numbers. At the correct location for the record, pull the outguide halfway out, slide the record in front of the outguide, and finish removing the outguide. If your office does not use outguides, use your hand to make a space between the record before and the record after the one you are filing.

5. **Procedural Step.** If there is an index card in the outguide showing who had the record from the outguide, remove it. Place the outguide with other unused outguides. Some offices keep index cards for the physicians in separate boxes so that new cards do not need to be written; some offices cross out the name and reuse the index cards; some offices use slips of paper that are discarded after each use.

6. **Procedural Step.** File each record in the same way until all records have been filed.

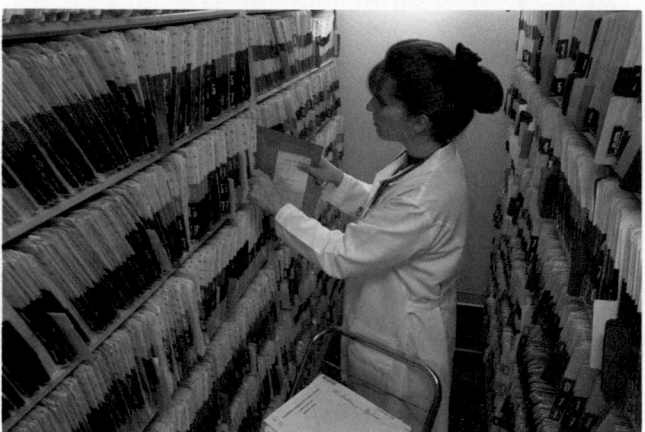

Figure 41-5 Placing an outguide.

RETRIEVING OR FILING A PAPER MEDICAL RECORD

Retrieving Patient Records

A patient record has to be removed from its proper location in the file whenever someone in the office wants to look at it (e.g., for an appointment, when a patient leaves a message).

The record is located using the filing guidelines of the particular office. Paper medical records needed for patients with appointments on a particular day are usually pulled the afternoon before the appointments, using the printed appointment list. Each time a record is taken from storage, an outguide is placed exactly where the record was removed, as illustrated in Figure 41-5.

The person removing the record fills in a card with the name or number on the record and the name of the person who will have the record. Although it seems cumbersome to fill in a card for every record removed, in the long run it is much less frustrating than searching the entire office for a record when the patient is in the waiting room.

Filing Records

Each day, several records need to be returned to the file. In most offices, records ready for filing are placed in one location.

Before filing records or documents, the medical assistant should be sure that the records are ready to file. To condition a record, the medical assistant takes several steps:

- All clips, pins, or other extraneous material should be removed.
- Any tears or broken punch holes should be repaired with tape.
- Any sticky notes or other loose papers should be either removed or filed in the record in the correct location.

A sorter is used to arrange the records so that they can be filed efficiently according to name or medical record number. It is important to locate the correct position to replace the record and remove the outguide. Any items to be filed in the pocket of the outguide should be filed in the record at this time.

Filing Reports and Correspondence

All reports, letters, and other materials that come into the office should be reviewed by the physician, initialed, and then filed in the patient record. A date stamp is often used to identify exactly when a report or letter was received. If the physician dictates progress notes, these must also be reviewed and initialed before filing. With the paper medical record, there is no end to the number of papers that the physician must review. Sometimes physicians even come into the office on the weekend to catch up with all their paperwork. Because of this, there is often a stack of material to be filed on Monday. The physician may indicate an action for the medical assistant to take on a message form or sticky note. These actions can range from arranging laboratory or diagnostic follow-up to notifying the patient of results of laboratory or diagnostic tests to calling a pharmacy with a prescription. The medical assistant must complete any follow-up before filing the report (or record) (Procedure 41-3).

Several steps facilitate filing reports or other items in the paper medical record:

- Each report or note to be filed should be initialed by the physician, and any required action should be completed.
- Reports should be sorted before filing according to name or medical record number.
- Once the correct record has been located, the report is filed at the front of the appropriate section. It may be necessary to remove a section of the record to insert the new item.
- The record should be reassembled before being replaced in the file.
- Reports for items that are not in their correct locations should be set aside. After all other reports have been filed, if time permits, the medical assistant can search for the missing records.

Measures to Ensure Accuracy or Locate Misplaced Records

Seven steps can ensure accuracy in filing or locating a misplaced record. A missing record creates multiple problems. Working carefully can help avoid lost records.

1. The medical assistant should work slowly and carefully when filing records.
2. It is recommended to use outguides to keep track of the record.

3. Medical records should be returned to storage after use and not just handed on to others in the medical office. If it is necessary to give a record to the physician, the outguide should be updated.
4. Physicians and other personnel should be discouraged from hoarding records. The medical assistant should encourage the physician(s) to finish all dictation each day, review laboratory reports, and sign off on them.
5. Records should be kept in orderly stacks when they are out of the files. This makes it easier to scan for one particular record.
6. If the medical assistant notices a misfiled record in the files, it should be removed and filed correctly without delay.
7. Hunting for "missing" records and being alert to find them in unexpected places are important. After all possible measures fail to locate a missing record, it may be necessary to create a second record for a patient until the record can be found.

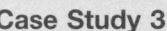

What Would You Do? What Would You *Not* Do?

Case Study 3

When Ellen is pulling medical records for the next day's appointments, she does not find the medical record for Alan DuBois under "Dubois." The file also has no outguide. Ellen remembers that the patient was seen within the past week or two. She also checks under "Bois," but the record is not filed there, either. ∎

PROCEDURE 41-3 Filing Reports

Outcome File reports, correspondence, and other material in a patient record.

Equipment/Supplies

- Medical records
- Assorted reports
- Letters or other material to be filed
- Hole punch
- Tape
- Stapler
- Sorter

1. Procedural Step. Assemble materials to be filed and necessary supplies to assist in the filing process.

2. Procedural Step. Remove extraneous materials, such as paper clips or pins; mend any tears with tape; and staple related pages together. Punch holes if necessary.
Principle. Preparation before filing allows all materials in the record to be maintained in good condition.

3. Procedural Step. Verify that each report is ready to be filed. In most offices the physician initials reports after he or she has seen them. If the initials are missing, the report should go back to him or her.
Principle. The physician must see each report that comes to the medical office. A procedure verifying that the physician has seen the report before filing prevents reports from being accidentally overlooked.

4. Procedural Step. Sort the reports using the sorter alphabetically or numerically, depending on the filing system. Sort by letters, numbers, or number groups first, then sort within each letter or number group.
Principle. Even in a small office, large numbers of reports need to be filed in patient records if a paper record system is used. It is more efficient to file in order, especially when patients have more than one report to be filed.

5. Procedural Step. Gather all reports for a particular patient, find the correct record, and insert the report(s) into the record in the correct location. In any section, reports are filed chronologically with the most recent reports at the front of the section. When several reports are shingled on a page, the oldest report goes at the

Continued

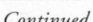

PROCEDURE 41-3   Filing Reports—cont'd

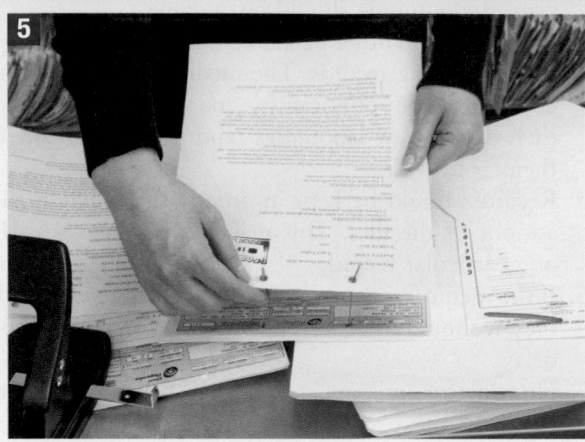

Insert the report(s) into the medical record.

bottom with newer reports progressing up the page and in front of the older reports. You may need to place a divider in the record if you are filing the first report in a given section.

Principle. The record usually contains several sections in a specific order. Reports need to be in the correct section to be easily located.

6. **Procedural Step.** Put the record back together if necessary and file with other medical records.

Principle. It is easier to file reports in the wrong record when several records are out.

7. **Procedural Step.** If the record is not in the file, place the report back in the sorter or in the pocket of the outguide.

Principle. It is more efficient to file reports in records you can find easily than to hunt for records just to file reports.

ELECTRONIC MEDICAL RECORD

The EMR is usually updated immediately by medical assistants, physicians, or other staff members who interact with patients. The physician may use voice recognition software to generate reports, or a transcription service may be used that links the transcribed reports directly into the patient's record. Use of the EMR greatly reduces the need for filing, although paper reports, correspondence, and consent forms are usually scanned into the record as soon as possible. The originals may be shredded or stored in a paper record depending on the office.

EMRs are password protected, and patient data are compartmentalized so that access can be limited to the information that any given staff member needs to view. A system administrator should authorize users and remove them from the system as appropriate. Data should be encrypted between the server and the user, and the infrastructure for access should be secure. The medical assistant should never allow other personnel to access patient information with his or her password.

STORING MEDICAL RECORDS

The storage area for paper medical records should be well-lighted and climate controlled. It is important to maintain the relative humidity at 48% to 52% to prevent deterioration of the records. Basement storage is not recommended unless the humidity is well controlled. The records should also be protected from dust, insects, rodents, fires, and floods. As discussed earlier, records should be secure when the office is closed so that unauthorized personnel do not have access to them. The Occupational Health and Safety Administration (OSHA) requires that main aisles leading out of a room or to a fire exit must be a minimum of 5 feet

wide, and secondary aisles, such as between shelving units, must be a minimum of 3 feet wide.

The shelf files should be full enough to allow the folders to stand upright but loose enough to allow folders to be easily stored and retrieved.

Active Records

Active records (records regarding patients who have been seen within the past 2 to 5 years) are stored in the medical office as described earlier. These records need to be readily available for daily use.

Inactive Records

Paper records of patients who have not been seen within a time period specified by the practice (**inactive records**) are usually kept in the office in closed storage. If there is not enough space in the office to store inactive records, they are sometimes stored in a storage room elsewhere in the office building, or in rented storage space. If a patient has not been seen for several years, a new medical record may be created. However, the old record may still need to be consulted.

At regular intervals inactive records are removed from the active record area. Most offices place a sticker for the current year on a patient's medical record at the first visit in a new year to show that the record is active for that year. This facilitates removal of inactive records after a specified interval.

Retention of Records

The length of time that a medical record must be retained is difficult to determine. Each state has a law limiting the time period for beginning a lawsuit for malpractice. This is known as the *statute of limitations* for medical malpractice. A state may also have a minimum requirement for retaining medical records. In the absence of state regulations, a

Memories *from* Externship

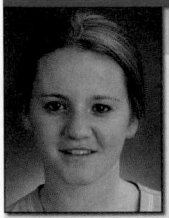

Ellen McDonald: I did my externship in a clinic affiliated with a large hospital that had made the transition from paper medical records to an EMR. When a patient checked in, we entered the data from the patient information sheet into the computer immediately, and we used a signature pad at the front desk to obtain electronic signatures from the patient for consent to treatment, authorization to disclose information for billing, and acknowledgement of receipt of HIPAA confidentiality information.

Each medical assistant had to log into the system in order to enter information in the medical record. Even as a student, I was given a password so that I could check patients in, enter vital signs, and enter other information. For example, the machine for electrocardiograms (ECGs) looked like a laptop computer attached to the ECG cables. It was also connected to the EMR. We entered patient information using a computer keyboard. I learned how to print the ECG as a hard copy, but the physician could also view the tracing on the computer.

When the clinic made the transition to the EMR, the records of active patients were scanned into the system, but they kept the paper records for inactive patients. I remember one time when a patient who had not been seen for about 6 years made an appointment. He was experiencing medical problems that he thought might be connected to earlier radiation therapy. I was instructed to create a new electronic record for him, and then I was sent to find the old record. Several rooms were full of paper medical records, arranged in order by clinic number. I found it confusing because I was not that familiar with the terminal digit method of filing, but one of the staff members helped me to find the record. After the appointment, I had to return the record to storage. ■

Highlight on Electronic Signatures

When talking about electronic signatures, it is important to distinguish between actual signatures that are captured electronically and an electronic entry specific to one individual that authenticates identity and can be linked to a specific date and time.

When a medical office uses an electronic medical record (EMR), the staff can use two ways to handle actual patient signatures. With the first method, the patient signs a paper consent form and the paper consent form is then scanned into the electronic record. With the second method, the patient reads the consent form, either in a paper version or on a computer screen, and then the patient signs an electronic signature pad that captures an image of the actual signature and inserts it into an electronic version of the form being signed.

Physicians and other staff in the medical office usually use an *electronic signature,* an electronic sound, symbol, or process added to an electronic record that indicates intent to sign. These processes are built into the software with safeguards to validate the time of the entry and the identity of the individual making the entry. Electronic signatures are also used for transmitting insurance claims and for validating entries to the EMR. Electronic signatures are valid in all states and are accepted by the Health Insurance Portability and Accountability Act (HIPAA), provided that the software being used validates identity, validates that the document was not altered later, and provides that the user cannot later repudiate the electronic signature.

The term *digital signature* is used for a form of encryption that binds electronic records to an "electronic fingerprint." Digital signatures require validation by private companies called *certification authorities.* The entire document is encrypted and decrypted using public and private keys (mathematic formulas). Digital signatures are used for transferring money and signing legal documents electronically. This level of security is currently not required for EMRs. ■

medical office can review retention guidelines established by the American Medical Association (AMA) in 1994. The AMA recommends that records be retained primarily based on the health needs of the patient, but at least as long as the state requires or the length of time of the statute of limitations for malpractice claims. For a minor, the time period should be considered to begin at the age of majority. Records of Medicare and Medicaid patients should be retained for at least 5 years after the last contact.

At the end of the retention period, the inactive medical record may be destroyed (by shredding or burning) or put in a final storage place to be kept permanently. The AMA recommends that the patient have an opportunity to claim the record before it is destroyed, if possible. Records that are closed (it is known that the patient will not return) may be transferred to microfilm or microfiche. They can also be copied using a laser beam and stored on laser disks. These options are expensive and time-consuming, but may be worthwhile for larger practices. Other records that should be kept indefinitely are insurance policies, licenses, and Drug Enforcement Administration (DEA) controlled-substance records. All tax records should also be kept for 7 years; after that, background records used to determine taxes can be destroyed, but copies of tax forms should be kept indefinitely.

Storing Computerized Records

EMRs should be backed up regularly and securely. The system manager is usually responsible for ensuring that the backup system is implemented according to plan. Backups may be done to network storage and/or storage devices, such as hard drives, DVDs, or other devices. It is important to maintain some kind of backup off-site in case of fire or disaster. Inactive electronic records can be transferred to separate storage if the system capacity becomes strained. The system administrator must also be sure that program updates are compatible with previously stored data.

MEDICAL PRACTICE and the LAW

Legal Implications of the Medical Record and Protected Health Information

The medical record is initiated by the medical office and belongs to the person or group who produced it. The physician or office owns the physical record whether its form is paper or electronic.

The information in the record belongs to the patient, however, and the patient controls access to the information. Any request to release copies of records must come from the patient or someone who is authorized to act for the patient.

The original record must never be released. If the original record is subpoenaed by a court, an employee of the office should travel with the record to safeguard it and be sure that no part is lost or tampered with. A copy of the record should be left at the office.

The office should have a form for patients to sign that gives permission to release the medical record or information about specific conditions that require separate consent forms (e.g., HIV or AIDS). The release must be signed by the patient or by a guardian if the patient is a minor.

When a patient begins a new relationship with a physician's office, the patient routinely signs a release form allowing the physician to send necessary information to an insurance company. One of the standards being developed under the Health Insurance Portability and Accountability Act legislation concerns a standard format for electronic signatures.

Another time that records are usually released is when a patient moves away or begins a relationship with another physician. Offices usually charge a copying fee, a handling fee, and postage, especially if the record is requested by a lawyer for litigation. The amount that can be charged may be regulated by state law.

Under the Health Information Technology for Economic and Clinical Health Act (HITECH), health care facilities using EMRs are required to keep track of every access of patient information through logs. If a patient's unsecured data are accessed without authority, the patient must be notified. The patient also has the right to an accounting of disclosures of private information to anyone outside the office within the previous 3 years. The patient can also request that an office not disclose certain information to a health plan or insurance company. Finally, only necessary information can be shared with other entities (if the information is shared for purposes other than treatment). In order to meet these requirements, all health care institutions using electronic medical records must keep extensive logs showing who accessed information and when. ∎

What Would You Do? What Would You *Not* Do? RESPONSES

Case Study 1
Page 996

What Did Ellen Do?
❑ Made every possible attempt to find the patient's record.
❑ Asked the patient if she could have been seen under another last name.
❑ Tried to locate the patient under her maiden name.
❑ Attempted to locate the patient in the computer using the birth date and/or the first name.
❑ Attempted to locate the record in the storage area for inactive patients under Soubrette.
❑ Even if Ellen was not able to locate the record, she asked Ms. Soubrette to fill out a release of information sheet, took her telephone number, and said she would contact her to let her know if she had been able to locate the record.
❑ Asked the office manager for other ideas to locate the record.

What Did Ellen Not Do?
❑ Did not tell the patient that she must have been thinking about a different practice.
❑ Did not assume that the record had been lost or destroyed.
❑ Did not tell the patient that after such a long time, the information probably would not be useful anyway.

What Would You Do/What Would You Not Do?
Review Ellen's response and place a checkmark next to the information you included in your response. List the additional information you included in your response.

_____
_____
_____
_____
_____
_____
_____

Case Study 2
Page 998

What Did Ellen Do?
❑ Explained that the office would be glad to send or provide a copy of the medical record to the new physician as soon as Ms. Bennett provided a physician name and address.
❑ Encouraged the patient to fill out a release of information sheet or to take a copy to mail back when she had selected a new physician.
❑ Explained that Ms. Bennett was in charge of the information in the medical record, but the original record belonged to her physician.
❑ Notified Ms. Bennett how long it would take to prepare a copy and if any copying fee would be required.

What Did Ellen Not Do?
❑ Did not allow the patient to take the original medical record.
❑ Did not promise to prepare a copy of the entire medical record that day.

What Would You Do? What Would You *Not* Do? RESPONSES—cont'd

What Would You Do/What Would You Not *Do?*

Review Ellen's response and place a checkmark next to the information you included in your response. List the additional information you included in your response.

_____

_____

_____

_____

_____

_____

Case Study 3
Page 1001

What Did Ellen Do?

❏ Looked up Allan DuBois in the computer to identify the date of his last appointment and who saw him.

❏ Checked the physician's office, as well as the billing desk.

❏ Looked behind furniture, especially in the physician's office.

❏ Asked other staff members if they had seen this medical record.

What Did Ellen Not Do?

❏ Did not give up looking for the record until she had made an extensive search.

❏ Did not accuse any staff member of hiding the medical record.

❏ Did not call the patient and change his appointment in case the record could not be located.

What Would You Do/What Would You Not *Do?*

Review Ellen's response and place a checkmark next to the information you included in your response. List the additional information you included in your response.

_____

_____

_____

_____

_____

_____

_____

⟳ TERMINOLOGY REVIEW

Medical Term	Word Parts	Definition
Acronym		A word formed from the first letters in a name.
Active record		The medical record of a patient who has been seen within a time frame specified by the office (usually 2 to 3 years).
Cross-index		To file under one unit and use a guide or card filed under another unit that refers to the primary filing location.
Electronic health record (EHR)		An individual patient's health record in digital format. Also called an *electronic medical record.*
Electronic medical record (EMR)		An individual's medical record in digital format. Also called an *electronic health record.*
Filing system		The way in which records are arranged. Common filing systems in the medical office include alphabetic, numeric, by subject, or chronologic.
Health information exchange (HIE)		The electronic exchange of health care–related data among different institutions.
Inactive record		The medical record of a patient who has not been seen within the past 2 to 3 years, or some other time frame specified by a given medical office.
Indexing units		Pieces of information used to identify a correct filing location.
Medical record management		Activities related to the creation, management, use, and disposition of patient medical records.
Nationwide Health Information Network (NHIN)		A set of standards, services, and policies to facilitate national HIE (health information exchange.)
Outguide		A cardboard or plastic card to insert in a file when a medical record is removed.
Sorter		A device that facilitates putting papers or records in alphabetic or numeric order.
Surname		Last name or family name of an individual; used as the first indexing unit in alphabetic filing.
Tab		A projection of a folder that extends beyond the top or side of the folder.
Terminal digit filing		A chronologic filing system that uses the last number or number group as the first indexing unit.

ON THE WEB

For information on record management:

American Health Information Management Association: www.ahima.org

ARMA International: www.arma.org

National Information Standards Organization: www.niso.org

Nationwide Health Information Network: www.hhs.gov/healthit/healthnetwork/background/

U.S. Department of Health and Human Services—Office of the National Coordinator for Health Information Technology (OCN): www.hhs.gov/healthit

 Check out the Evolve site at http://evolve.elsevier.com/Bonewit/today/ to actively Prepare for your Certification, and to access additional interactive activities and exercises to help you study and prepare for success.

42

Written Communications

Business Letters

1. Define the parts of a business letter.
2. Identify different formats for preparing business letters.
3. Explain how to format and compose a business letter.

Responding to Written Communication

4. Identify how to respond to written communication from businesses and patients.
5. Discuss the importance of using correct grammar and spelling in written communication.

Memoranda and Other Documents

6. Describe the process of creating memoranda.
7. Explain how to prepare and proofread documents and use proofreader's marks.

E-mail or Other Electronic Transmission

8. Compare the use and style of business letters and electronic communication, such as e-mail or clinical messaging.
9. Explain how to use e-mail and attachments for business communication.
10. Explain how to transmit information using a fax machine.

Photocopying Documents

11. Describe how to make copies of multiple-page documents.

Compose a business letter.

Send a fax.

Prepare copies of multiple-page documents.

CHAPTER OUTLINE

INTRODUCTION TO WRITTEN COMMUNICATION
Business Letters
Equipment and Supplies
Parts of a Business Letter
Format of Business Letters
Composing a Business Letter
Responding to Written Communication
Grammar and Punctuation
Parts of Speech
Sentence Structure
Comma Rules

Spelling and Proofreading
Spelling
Proofreading
Preparing Memoranda
Electronic Data Transmission
E-mail
Clinical Messaging
E-mail Attachments
Fax Transmissions
Photocopying

KEY TERMS

clinical messaging
collate (CALL-ate)
complimentary closing
duplex
e-mail
fax

full block style
grammar
left justified
letterhead
memo (memorandum)
modified block style

proofread
right justified
salutation
semiblock style
simplified letter style
template

INTRODUCTION TO WRITTEN COMMUNICATION

Until 20 years ago, almost all written communication between the medical office and other parties was managed by letters or forms and mailed through the U.S. Postal Service. Today, it is also common to transmit data electronically or by fax, and these data can be viewed and/or printed in written form. Regardless of how the written material is transmitted, however, written communication must still adhere to professional standards. The medical assistant is often responsible for preparing letters, memoranda, reports, and other types of written communication. To do this professionally requires thorough knowledge of grammar, spelling, format, and the technology that supports modern methods of producing written documents. In addition, the medical assistant must be familiar with the implications of Health Insurance Portability and Accountability Act (HIPAA) regulations regulating access to patient health information. These regulations were covered in detail in Chapter 3. The procedure for obtaining consent to release information from the medical record was discussed in Chapter 36.

BUSINESS LETTERS

Letters leaving the medical office—whether sent to a referring physician, an attorney, another business, or an insurance company—require proper formatting. Some letters may be dictated by the physician and transcribed by the medical assistant. He or she may also compose and send letters independently. The medical office may also use form letters and/or templates for routine matters. A **template** is a standard form to which additional data can be added as needed.

Equipment and Supplies

Business letters are usually created using a computer and printer. A word processing program is used to create the letter so that formatting can easily be adjusted and any necessary corrections can be made.

The medical office orders stationery and envelopes preprinted with the practice name, address, telephone number, and business logo. Individual physician names are also often included. A sheet of this type of stationery is called **letterhead.** Blank sheets of the paper of exactly the same type and weight must be purchased for letters that are longer than one page. Photocopies of letters printed on letterhead are often retained for office records in addition to the computer file used to create the letter.

Parts of a Business Letter

Heading

The heading includes the return address and the date line. The return address is composed of the name and address of the business sending the letter. If office letterhead is used, no return address needs to be added. The date line is the date the letter is mailed in month, day, year order. The month is written out in full on the date line. It is usually entered on the second or third line below the return address. On letterhead stationery, it is placed to fall a few spaces below the bottom of the letterhead.

Inside Address

The inside address includes the name and address of the party to whom the letter is being sent. Beginning with the inside address, information is single spaced with a blank space between sections. The inside address should be located in a position so that the body of the letter is centered top to bottom on the page. If the letter is long enough to require two pages, the inside address begins on the second or third space below the date line.

Salutation or Greeting

The **salutation** (the greeting that begins a letter) is found below the inside address. A business letter is formal, so the recipient's last name and title (e.g., Mr., Ms., Miss, Dr.) should be used. The salutation is punctuated with a colon. Correct examples include the following:

Dear Ms. Wilson:

Dear Dr. Taylor:

Dear Mrs. Porto:

Titles or initials indicating credentials (such as MD or RN) are not used after names. The following are *incorrect:*

Dear Amy,

Dear Amy Wilson:

Dear William Taylor, MD:

If the recipient's name is not known, it is permissible to use "Dear Sir," "Dear Madam," "Dear Sir or Madam," or "To Whom It May Concern." One line is left blank after the salutation.

Body of the Letter

The body of the letter contains the content, which should be presented clearly and concisely. A subject line may be used to begin this section. Within a paragraph the letter is single spaced, but a blank line should separate each new paragraph.

Complimentary Closing

The **complimentary closing** (or *complimentary close*) is a term for the words used as a polite ending to a letter just before the writer's signature. It is a sign of respect and can be adjusted depending on how well the letter's author and the party being addressed know each other. "Sincerely" is the standard close. A more formal closing is "Yours truly" or "Very truly yours." It is followed by a comma and separated from the body of the letter by a blank line.

Signature, Printed Signature, and Title

The signature is the actual written signature of the individual sending the letter. It is added after the letter has been printed. The signature line contains the printed signature of the individual sending the letter, with credentials (e.g., MD). It is entered four to five lines below the complimentary close to leave room for the written signature. A business title (e.g., Office Manager) is capitalized if used and entered on the line below the printed signature.

The medical assistant uses his or her own name and signature for a letter to a supplier or a letter to a patient responding to a billing question. Any letter dictated or composed by a physician will be signed by the physician.

End Notations

Various pieces of information may be given in notations at the bottom of the letter, generally with a blank line between each item. The order of the end notations may vary

according to the preference of the office. A reference notation notes the initials of the person who composed the letter (in uppercase) followed by the initials of the person who typed or keyed the letter (in lowercase). If the letter contains enclosures, such as a log of visits and/or billing records, this is noted in the enclosure notation, on the second line below the title. "Enclosure" or "Enc." may be used for one enclosure. "Enclosures" followed by the number in parentheses is used for more than one enclosure. This alerts the recipient to make sure that everything the sender intended to include actually accompanies the letter. A copy notation (distribution notation) identifies the recipient(s). The letter "c" is used, followed by a colon and the name(s) of those who are receiving copies. Figure 42-1 shows a business letter with the parts of the letter identified.

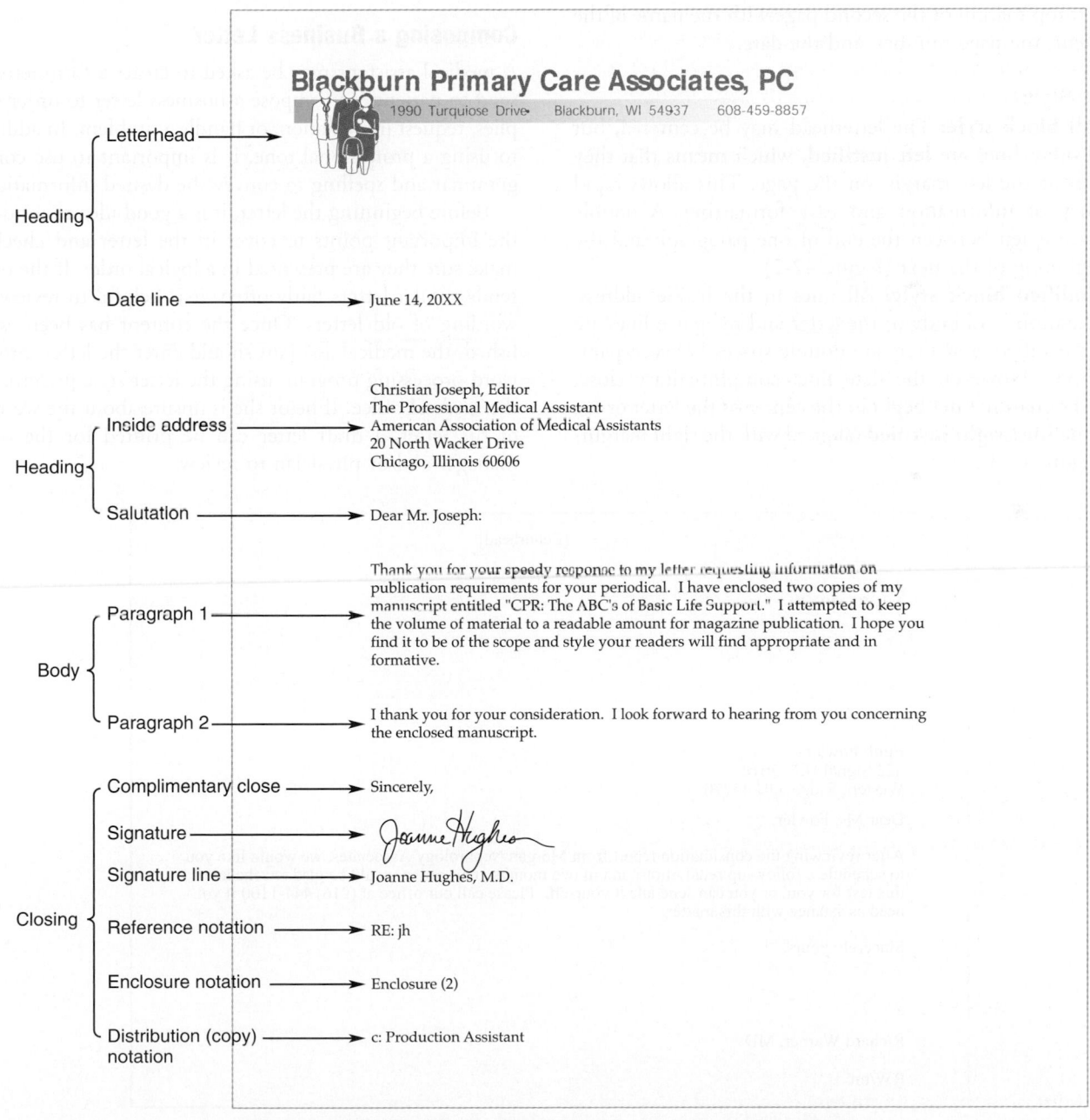

Blackburn Primary Care Associates, PC
1990 Turquoise Drive   Blackburn, WI 54937   608-459-8857

Letterhead

Heading

Date line → June 14, 20XX

Inside address →
Christian Joseph, Editor
The Professional Medical Assistant
American Association of Medical Assistants
20 North Wacker Drive
Chicago, Illinois 60606

Salutation → Dear Mr. Joseph:

Body

Paragraph 1 →
Thank you for your speedy response to my letter requesting information on publication requirements for your periodical. I have enclosed two copies of my manuscript entitled "CPR: The ABC's of Basic Life Support." I attempted to keep the volume of material to a readable amount for magazine publication. I hope you find it to be of the scope and style your readers will find appropriate and informative.

Paragraph 2 →
I thank you for your consideration. I look forward to hearing from you concerning the enclosed manuscript.

Complimentary close → Sincerely,

Signature → Joanne Hughes

Signature line → Joanne Hughes, M.D.

Reference notation → RE: jh

Enclosure notation → Enclosure (2)

Distribution (copy) notation → c: Production Assistant

Closing

Figure 42-1 Sample business letter with the parts of the letter identified.

Format of Business Letters

Setting up a Letter

When preparing letters using a word processing program, the first step is to set the margins. The top margin of the letter should be large enough to accommodate the letterhead (usually 2 to 2½ inches). The side margins may be 1 to 2 inches. Wider margins are used for a short letter. The body of the letter is single spaced.

In writing a business letter, a generally accepted font is Times New Roman 12 point. The entire letter should be created in the same font. The word processing program may include a letter wizard, which formats the letter automatically. It is also possible to use or create a letter template so that all letters from the office have the same format.

If the letter has two pages, a header should be placed at the left top margin of the second page with the name of the recipient, the page number, and the date.

Letter Styles

- **Full block style:** The letterhead may be centered, but all other lines are **left justified,** which means that they start at the left margin on the page. This allows rapid entry of information and easy formatting. A double space is left between the end of one paragraph and the beginning of the next (Figure 42-2).
- **Modified block style:** All lines in the inside address, salutation, and body of the letter and reference lines are left justified, and there are double spaces between paragraphs. However, the date line, complimentary close, and signature lines begin in the center of the letter or are sometimes **right justified** (aligned with the right margin) (Figure 42-3).

- **Semiblock style** (also called *modified block with indented paragraphs*): All lines in the inside address, salutation, and body of the letter and reference lines are left justified. Paragraphs are indented five to eight spaces, and there are double spaces between paragraphs. The date line, complimentary close, and signature lines begin in the center of the letter or are sometimes right justified. Semiblock style is the same as modified block style, except that the first sentence of each new paragraph is indented (Figure 42-4).
- **Simplified letter style:** This style resembles a memorandum. Instead of a salutation, a subject line typed all in capital letters is placed three lines below the inside address, and the complimentary close and signature lines are replaced by an all–capital-letter signature five lines below the letter's body (Figure 42-5).

Composing a Business Letter

A medical assistant may be asked to create a form letter to send to patients or compose a business letter to order supplies, request information, or handle a problem. In addition to using a professional tone, it is important to use correct grammar and spelling to convey the desired information.

Before beginning the letter, it is a good idea to jot down the important points to cover in the letter and check to make sure they are presented in a logical order. If the office sends similar letters fairly often, it is helpful to review the wording of old letters. Once the content has been established, the medical assistant should enter the letter into the word processing program using the letter style preferred by the medical office. If he or she is unsure about the wording of the letter, a draft letter can be printed for the office manager and/or physician to review.

[Letterhead]

July 21, 20XX

Edith Fowler
222 Signal Hill Drive
Western Ridge, OH 44770

Dear Ms. Fowler:

After reviewing the consultation report from Morgan Nephrology Associates, we would like you to schedule a follow-up renal ultrasound in two months. Our office would be glad to schedule this test for you, or you can schedule it yourself. Please call our office at (216) 444-1100 if you need assistance with this matter.

Sincerely yours,

Richard Warner, MD

RW/mt

Figure 42-2 Sample letter—full block style.

[Letterhead]

July 21, 20XX

Edith Fowler
222 Signal Hill Drive
Western Ridge, OH 44770

Dear Ms. Fowler:

After reviewing the consultation report from Morgan Nephrology Associates, we would like you
to schedule a follow-up renal ultrasound in two months. Our office would be glad to schedule
this test for you, or you can schedule it yourself. Please call our office at (216) 444-1100 if you
need assistance with this matter.

                                   Sincerely yours,

                                   Richard Warner, MD

RW/mt

Figure 42-3 Sample letter—modified block style.

[Letterhead]

July 21, 20XX

Edith Fowler
222 Signal Hill Drive
Western Ridge, OH 44770

Dear Ms. Fowler:

    After reviewing the consultation report from Morgan Nephrology Associates, we would
like you to schedule a follow-up renal ultrasound in two months. Our office would be glad to
schedule this test for you, or you can schedule it yourself. Please call our office at (216) 444-
1100 if you need assistance with this matter.

                                   Sincerely yours,

                                   Richard Warner, MD

RW/mt

Figure 42-4 Sample letter—semiblock style (also called *modified block with indented paragraphs*).

[Letterhead]

July 21, 20XX

Edith Fowler
222 Signal Hill Drive
Western Ridge, OH 44770

FOLLOW-UP RENAL ULTRASOUND

After reviewing the consultation report from Morgan Nephrology Associates, we would
like you to schedule a follow-up renal ultrasound in two months. Our office would be glad to
schedule this test for you, or you can schedule it yourself. Please call our office at (216) 444-
1100 if you need assistance with this matter.

RICHARD WARNER, MD

RW/mt

Figure 42-5 Sample letter—simplified style.

The letter should be proofread for accuracy, grammar, and spelling before the final version is printed. Because letters represent the medical practice, they must be as accurate and professional as possible (Procedure 42-1).

Responding to Written Communication

On a daily basis the medical office receives letters and/or e-mails that require follow-up. Unless letters are marked "personal" or "private," the medical assistant usually screens correspondence. He or she may respond personally to correspondence related to supply orders, billing questions, insurance-related questions, and requests for information about the practice. If an urgent response appears necessary, the telephone can be used, but in most cases the response will be in the same format as the original communication.

Correspondence relating to patient care is referred to the physician, and the medical assistant may clip the letter to the patient's medical record if a paper-based medical record system is used in the office. If the physician dictates a reply to a letter, the medical assistant may transcribe the letter or edit a letter dictated using voice recognition software.

Highlight on Letters to Inform Patients of Test Results

Although medical offices use many different methods to inform patients of results of laboratory and diagnostic test results, notifying patients by letter is a method that preserves patient confidentiality and provides consistent and reliable information to the patient about follow-up. Studies have shown that patients prefer to receive all results, whether or not they are normal.

Many medical practices use templates or form letters that allow the medical assistant or physician to fill in the appropriate values and add comments. The final letter may include the actual results or a general statement about the results (e.g., "All your blood test results are within normal limits.") Specific time frames for follow-up testing or instructions to make a follow-up appointment are also included.

If the practice uses an electronic medical record, test results can be tracked in the system to be sure that results have been received from the laboratory or testing facility. It is also possible to track that the patient has been notified and follow-up testing has been performed. The system can also post an alert when follow-up testing is overdue. If the office uses a paper-based medical record, a separate log book can be kept for laboratory and diagnostic tests to track receipt of results, review by physicians, and follow-up to patients.

As a means of managing physician time efficiently while maintaining the personal touch, the medical assistant may prepare the letter, enter the information about the laboratory results, and place the letter with the test results for the physician to verify accuracy, sign the letter, and add any comments. ■

PROCEDURE 42-1   Composing a Business Letter

Outcome Compose and key a business letter.

Equipment/Supplies

- Letterhead stationery
- Blank stationery
- Typewriter
- Computer and printer

1. **Procedural Step.** Assemble materials, determine the address of the recipient, and decide on a format for the letter.
2. **Procedural Step.** Formulate the content for the business letter. List and organize the essential content to be sure all necessary information is included.
3. **Procedural Step.** Insert the date on the second or third line below the letterhead. For block style, the date is at the left margin. For modified block style and semiblock style, the date begins at the center of the line.
4. **Procedural Step.** Place the inside address four to 10 lines below the date at the left margin. If using a computer, adjust the number of spaces below the date line after the letter has been keyed so that the body of the letter is centered on the page.
5. **Procedural Step.** Place the salutation on the second line below the inside address. The salutation should include a title and the person's last name (e.g., Dear Dr. Gordon, Dear Mrs. Wilson, Dear Rev. Meyers). It is followed by a colon.
   Principle. A business letter is more formal than personal correspondence.
6. **Procedural Step.** If desired, place a subject line on the second line below the salutation. A subject line begins with the Latin abbreviation "re" (meaning about) followed by a colon. The abbreviation is usually capitalized (e.g., RE: Annual meeting on Thursday, June 12, 2010).
   Principle. Although optional, a subject line helps the recipient identify the subject of the letter before reading it.
7. **Procedural Step.** Begin the body of the letter on the second line below the salutation (or subject line, if used). The body of the letter is single spaced and double-spaced between paragraphs. In block and modified block letter styles, the paragraphs begin at the left margin. If semiblock style is used, indent the first line of each paragraph five to eight spaces.
8. **Procedural Step.** The final paragraph of the letter should summarize the contents and/or most important ideas.
9. **Procedural Step.** Place the complimentary close on the second line below the final paragraph of the body of the letter. For the block letter style, the complimentary close begins at the left margin. For the modified block letter style, it begins at a tab directly below the date line. The complimentary close is followed by a comma.
10. **Procedural Step.** Drop down four lines and insert the first and last name of the sender followed by his or her credentials. Begin the typed signature directly under the complimentary close. Place a job title, if appropriate, on the next line.
    Principle. Typing the name under the handwritten signature facilitates a response because the signature may be difficult to read.
11. **Procedural Step.** If necessary, add a reference line, enclosure notation, and/or distribution notation, below the typed signature at the left margin. Double space between each notation. If you compose and key your own letter, a reference line is unnecessary. If you compose and key a letter for someone else, place your initials in lowercase letters. If you key a letter that was dictated by the person signing the letter, place his or her initials (uppercase) followed by your initials (lowercase) separated by a colon or slash. The enclosure notation may be written out or abbreviated "Enc." The number of enclosures is placed in parentheses if there is more than one. The distribution notation identifies individuals who receive a copy of the letter. The letter "c" followed by a colon is used with the name of the individual receiving a copy.
    Principle. The person who receives the letter is entitled to know who prepared the letter and who received copies. If the number of enclosures is indicated, it is easier to tell if all intended material is enclosed with the letter.
12. **Procedural Step.** If the letter is longer than one page, the second page should be printed or typed on stationery of the same quality and weight as the letterhead stationery, beginning 1 inch from the top. Include the name of the recipient, the date, and the page number in the top left corner. Space the letter so that at least two lines of the body of the letter continue to the second page.
13. **Procedural Step.** Spell-check the letter and proofread it carefully. If using a computer, print the letter.

Continued

PROCEDURE 42-1

Principle. A business letter should not contain errors. If errors are present, the credibility and professionalism of the sender may be doubted.

14. **Procedural Step.** Obtain the appropriate signature or sign the letter below the complimentary close.

15. **Procedural Step.** Make a photocopy of the letter for your files and for any individual who will receive a copy of the letter.

Principle. Copies of all business letters are retained in case there are questions or further correspondence is necessary.

16. **Procedural Step.** Prepare an envelope (see Chapter 43, Procedure 43-3) and place the letter in the designated area to be prepared for mailing. If the letter concerns a patient, a copy of the letter is filed in the patient's medical record. Other letters (e.g., letters to suppliers) are usually filed in folders by subject.

GRAMMAR AND PUNCTUATION

It is important to respond in a timely manner to written communication using proper grammar and spelling. **Grammar** is a term for the accepted rules to create meaningful sentences in a language.

Parts of Speech

In English, words are classified as one of eight different parts of speech, a set of categories that describe how words are used. Many words can be used in more than one way.

1. **Nouns:** A noun is the name of a person, place, or thing. It can also be a word used to identify a concept or idea. *Common nouns* refer to general things or categories (e.g., *tree, house*). *Proper nouns* are names of specific individuals or places (e.g., *John Stanton, Philadelphia*).

2. **Pronouns:** A pronoun is used in place of a noun. Examples include *I, me, you, he, she, it,* and *they.* Possessive pronouns show ownership (e.g., *mine, yours, hers, its*). None of the possessive pronouns are written with an apostrophe.

3. **Verbs:** A verb shows either action or a state of being. Every sentence requires a verb in order to be complete. Verbs that show a state of being are also called *linking verbs.* Action verbs include *talk, sing, help,* and *communicate.* Verbs that show a state of being include *is, are, feel,* and *seem.*

4. **Adjectives and articles:** An adjective modifies or qualifies a noun. It is a describing word. Examples include *white, pretty, little,* and *thin.* When two or more words are used together as an adjective to modify or qualify a noun, they are often connected by a hyphen (*a 20-year-old woman*). English has three articles: *a, an,* and *the.* They may be included as adjectives or sometimes a separate part of speech.

5. **Adverbs:** An adverb modifies a verb, adjective, or other adverb. Adverbs include words that question (*how? where?*) and words that end in *-ly* (*slowly, perfectly*).

6. **Prepositions:** A preposition shows the connection of a noun or pronoun to some other word, especially in relation to space, time, or possession. Examples include *on, in, of,* and *to.*

7. **Conjunctions:** A conjunction joins words, phrases, or clauses in a sentence. The common conjunctions include *and, but, or,* and *because.*

8. **Interjections:** An interjection is a word that expresses feelings. It is often followed by an exclamation point. Examples include *oh! yeah!* and *ouch!* Interjections are rarely used in correspondence or reports.

Sentence Structure

Sentences are composed of various combinations of independent and dependent clauses. A clause contains a subject (noun or pronoun) and a verb. If it can stand alone, it is

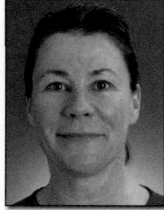

Putting It All into Practice

My name is Christine Walters, and I am a Registered Medical Assistant. I have been working for a nephrology practice for the past 3 years. This practice was started by two doctors about 15 years ago, and their office is in a building located next to the local hospital. About a year ago a third nephrologist joined the practice, and it is surprising how much more paperwork this has created. Because the physicians specialize in diseases of the kidney, our patients are usually referred by other physicians. This means that our physicians must communicate with the patient's primary care physician for almost every patient they see. Our physicians use handheld digital recorders that are connected to our computer network. One of the physicians prefers to have his reports formatted as a consultation report, which is sent with a cover letter to the referring physician. We use a template for the cover letter so that he doesn't have to dictate it each time. The other two physicians usually include their findings in a letter. I am responsible for preparing these letters and reports, but it really isn't difficult because they follow a fairly regular pattern. The physicians create the letters and reports using voice recognition software. I proofread and format each letter as needed, then print a final copy for mailing to the referring physician after it has been signed. It may take me up to 2 hours a day, and when the office is busy, sometimes I do get behind and I may even have to stay late to finish. I have been able to personalize the spell-checker on the computer I use, so even proofreading isn't that difficult. ■

Case Study 1

The physician asks Christine to send letters to obtain brochures with information about different types of electrocardiograph machines. He gives her the name of two manufacturers in which he is interested. The physician says, "I don't want to talk to anyone yet. I just want to see some brochures." ■

called an *independent clause.* If it requires an additional clause in order to be meaningful, it is called a *dependent* or *subordinate clause.* Sentence classifications are as follows:

1. **Simple sentence:** A sentence composed of one independent clause. Example: *The dog was very hungry.*

2. **Compound sentence:** A sentence composed of two independent clauses connected by a conjunction. A comma separates the two clauses. Example: *The dog returned from its walk, and it drank all the water in its bowl.*

3. **Complex sentence:** A sentence composed of one independent clause and one or more dependent clauses. If the dependent clause begins the sentence, it is followed by a comma. Example: *When it returned from its walk, the dog drank all the water in its bowl.* If the dependent clause comes after the independent clause, the dependent clause is not separated by a comma. Example: *The dog drank all the water in its bowl when it returned from its walk.*

Sentence Errors

1. **Sentence fragment:** A sentence fragment is a dependent clause used to stand alone as a sentence. In this case, an additional independent clause is necessary for meaning. *Sentence fragment:* When I arrive for my appointment. *Correct sentence:* When I arrive for my appointment, I will bring my insurance card.

2. **Run-on sentence:** A run-on sentence is a sentence in which two or more independent clauses are joined without a conjunction. *Run-on sentence:* My appointment is on Thursday I will bring my insurance card. *Correct sentence:* My appointment is on Thursday, and I will bring my insurance card.

3. **Comma splice:** A comma splice is the incorrect use of a comma to separate two sentences. The sentences should be separated by using a period and beginning a new sentence or by using a semicolon. It is also permitted to separate the sentences with a comma and a conjunction.

Comma Rules

1. Use a comma to separate the elements in a series of three or more things. The comma before the conjunction "and" is optional.
   Example: The patient complained of abdominal pain, difficulty breathing, and headache.
   Example: This 40-year-old, well-nourished, Caucasian woman was seen on 12/22/10.

2. Use a comma before a conjunction, such as "and," "but," or "for," when the conjunction connects two independent clauses. An independent clause could be used as a complete sentence.
   Example: The patient called an ambulance, and the ambulance brought her to Memorial Hospital.
   Example: We gave the patient furosemide intravenously, but after an hour her urine output was still poor.

3. Use a comma to set off introductory elements such as prepositional phrases or dependent clauses.
   Example: After the upper GI, the patient continued to experience epigastric pain.
   Example: Because we were planning surgery for next week, I did not want to prescribe any new medications.

4. Use a comma to set off information that could be omitted or placed in parentheses without changing the meaning of the sentence.
   Example: The patient, who was referred by Dr. Jenkins, is a 40-year-old woman in good health.
   Example: We will follow this patient closely in the clinic, which is open on Tuesdays and Thursdays.

5. Use a comma before quotation marks except at the end of the sentence where a period precedes the close quotation marks. Do not use a comma to introduce quoted elements introduced by the word *that.*
   Example: The patient said, "My incision burns like fire."
   Example: "My incision burns like fire," said the patient.
   Example: The patient states that her incision burns like fire.

6. Use a comma to avoid confusion.
   Example: For most the year is already finished.
   Example: For most, the year is already finished.

7. Use a comma between the city and the state, the date and the year, a name and a title, and in long numbers. No comma is necessary when only the month and year are used.
   Example: The patient was admitted to Memorial Hospital, Westford, Massachusetts in late July 2002.
   Example: On July 5, 2002 the patient was burned severely in a fire in Las Vegas, Nevada.

8. Use commas with terms like *not, however,* and *but* to express contrast.
   Example: The wound was large, but healing well.
   Example: I had not prescribed antibiotics for the patient before; however, she had obtained them from another physician.

9. Use a comma to separate appositives, nouns of direct address, titles that follow a person's name, and introductory words from the rest of the sentence.
   Example: We will make an appointment with Dr. Cannon, a gynecologist, sometime next week.
   Example: Doctor, there is something else I wanted to ask you.

10. Separate parenthetical expressions from the rest of the sentence using commas. These expressions include the following: *I believe, I am sure, on the contrary, indeed, of course, nevertheless, in my opinion,* and *in fact.*

Example: The report, I hope, will give you more information about multiple sclerosis.

Example: An inadequate supply of oxygen to the myocardium, for example, is caused by narrowing of the coronary arteries.

SPELLING AND PROOFREADING

Spelling

Although word processing programs usually provide a spell-check feature, the medical assistant must still proofread all documents for spelling. The spell-check function verifies the spelling of a given word but cannot confirm that it is the intended word or that it is used correctly in context. See Box 42-1 for a list of pairs of words that are commonly confused.

A tool to improve spelling is a personal list of words that cause difficulty. It is important to make an effort to learn these words, and remember to spell-check these words every time they are used. The medical office may purchase a medical dictionary program that can be installed on office computers for reference.

Proofreading

After preparing any letter or document, the medical assistant should spell-check or look up any unfamiliar words in order to spell them correctly. Abbreviations for medical conditions should be written out, but abbreviations for medication times, measurements, and vital signs are usually acceptable.

It is helpful to use medical spell-check software, which is available from several companies. An ordinary spell-check program can also be personalized over time by adding medical words and abbreviations that the program does not recognize; however, additions should always be checked for correctness. After the document or letter has been keyed, the medical assistant should print a copy, **proofread** it (read it carefully and make corrections), and then correct it and print out a final copy. If there is an unintelligible word, a space can be left and marked in pencil for the physician to fill in before the final copy is printed. Figure 42-6 is a list of proofreader's marks.

PREPARING MEMORANDA

A common way to communicate within the office is through the use of a **memo (memorandum)**, a document used within a company that is usually short and limited to one subject. Although a printed form can be used, it is not difficult to produce a template that can be used frequently in a given office. The title "Memorandum" or "Interoffice Memorandum" should appear at the top of the page.

Four headings commonly appear at the top of the memo:
TO:
FROM:
DATE:
SUBJECT:

The headings may be separated from the body of the memorandum by a line that extends from 2 inches to completely across the page. The message should be informative but succinct. The body of the memo is single spaced. A memo may be printed and circulated to all individuals included in the distribution list, or it may be sent as an e-mail attachment. If the memo is written to all staff members, a copy may be posted on a central bulletin board (Figure 42-7).

ELECTRONIC DATA TRANSMISSION

E-mail

E-mail (electronic mail) has become an accepted means of communication throughout the business world. **E-mail** is the exchange of information from one computer to another. As described in Chapter 38 a computer with an Internet

---

BOX 42-1   Confusing Pairs of Words

Nouns and Adjectives

affect (mood) and effect (result)

councilor (member of a council) and counselor (someone who gives guidance)

ileum (last part of the small intestine) and ilium (part of the pelvis)

principal (head of a school; most important) and principle (basis of a system of belief)

stationary (fixed in place) and stationery (paper and other writing materials)

Verbs, Adjectives, and Adverbs

accept (agree or believe in) and except (verb: exclude; adverb: left out)

adverse (unfavorable or bad) and averse (strongly disliking)

affect (to make a difference to) and effect (to bring about a difference)

complement (to contribute extra features) and compliment (to praise)

continual (happening frequently) and continuous (without interruption)

eminent (distinguished) and imminent (about to occur)

fewer (not as many) and less (not as much)

imply (to suggest) and infer (to deduce)

loose (to set free; not tight) and lose (to be unable to find)

precede (to go before) and proceed (to continue)

Pronouns

whose (shows possession) and who's (contraction of "who is")

your (shows possession) and you're (contraction of "you are")

its (shows possession) and it's (contraction of "it is")

their (shows possession) and there (shows location)

What Would You Do? What Would You *Not* Do?

Case Study 2

Christine is proofreading a letter created by voice recognition software related to the examination of a patient with hematuria (blood in the urine). She has no difficulty proofreading the patient's history and presenting symptoms, but in the section related to diagnostic testing, there is an abbreviation that is clearly incorrect. She also does not understand the sentence in which the unknown abbreviation occurs. She proofreads the rest of the report and then returns to the section that caused difficulty. She is still unable to make any sense of the abbreviation and the rest of the sentence. ∎

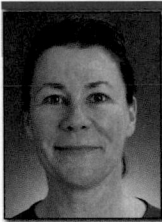

Memories *from* Externship

Christine Walters: I did my externship in the office of a family practitioner. I really enjoyed seeing patients of all ages because it gave me different kinds of experiences. In that office they used several different kinds of form letters. For example, their computer system kept a record of infants who were due for immunizations until the child was 2 years old. If the immunizations were more than 1 month overdue, the office sent a letter reminding the parents which immunizations were due and asking them to make an appointment. Twice while I was on my externship, they gave me a computer printout of the children who were overdue for immunizations to prepare letters for. First I had to check the computer system for each child to see if an appointment was scheduled in the next month. If there was an appointment, we didn't send a letter. Then I had to prepare a letter for each child still on the list. It was a form letter template, and I used the mail merge function in our word processing program to create a list of names and addresses and create the letters. When all the letters were prepared, I made copies for the medical records. I folded the letters and placed them in window envelopes so that the address was visible. I remember one patient's mother who kept apologizing for forgetting to make an appointment for her son. She said she had not been able to make the appointment when the child was in the office because she wasn't sure of her schedule, and then she just forgot about it. She thanked us for sending the reminder because she didn't want her son to get behind on his immunizations. ∎

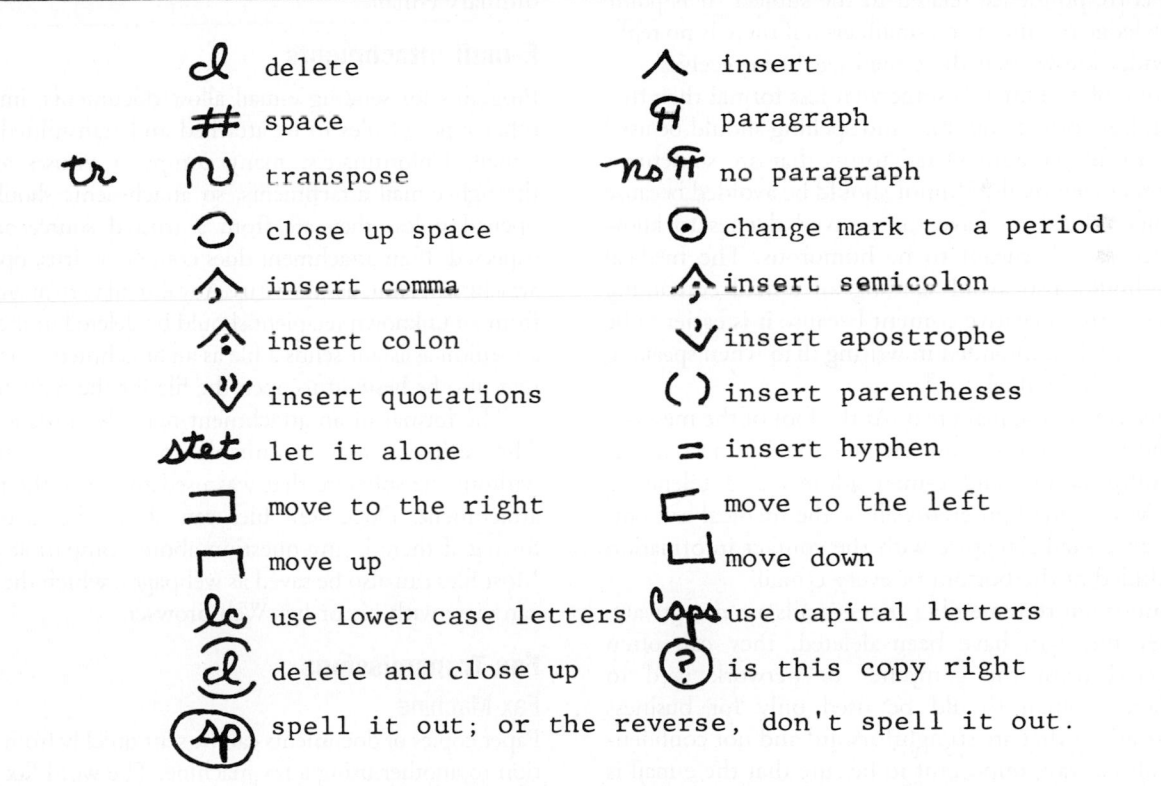

Figure 42-6 Standard proofreader's marks.

INTEROFFICE MEMORANDUM

TO:	All Staff
FROM:	Howard Lawler, MD
DATE:	6/18/XX
SUBJECT:	Introduction of new office manager

- -

It is my pleasure to announce that effective July 1, Diane Janes, CMA (AAMA), will join our staff as office manager. Ms. Janes has had extensive experience in a variety of medical settings. Most recently she has been employed as office manager in a family care practice in Minnesota. With the relocation of her family to Wisconsin, Ms. Janes has become available to join our practice. I hope that you will join me in welcoming Ms. Janes over lunch in the office on Friday, June 28.

Figure 42-7 A memo is used for communication within a business.

connection is used to send e-mail. Medical assistants usually use e-mail to communicate with business contacts, not patients. These may include other medical assistants, vendors, and insurance companies. It is usually faster and more efficient to send an e-mail for a short message.

An e-mail message should contain an informative subject line. Successive e-mails relating to the same subject are usually created as a reply so that the recipient can read the previous correspondence related to the subject. It is polite to acknowledge receipt of an e-mail, even if there is no reply, so the sender knows that the e-mail has been received.

The tone of an e-mail is somewhat less formal than that of a letter, but correct grammar and spelling should be used without any of the abbreviated forms that are sometimes used in personal e-mails. Humor should be avoided because the recipient does not have the nonverbal cues to know when a message is meant to be humorous. The medical assistant should also avoid sending an e-mail containing criticism or other negative content because it is easier to be more negative than intended in writing than when speaking directly to an individual.

E-mails usually use plain text. At the foot of the message, the medical assistant should include the business name, contact information, and e-mail address and telephone number. Most e-mail programs allow the medical assistant to create an e-mail signature with the contact information to be included at the bottom of every e-mail.

It is important to remember that e-mails are not private. Even after messages have been deleted, they can often be recovered from the computer or network used to create them. E-mail should be used only for business communications that are straightforward and not confidential. It is also always important to be sure that the e-mail is being sent to the correct recipient. It is a good policy to review the recipient name(s) before hitting the "send" button. The account should be set up so that sent messages are saved, but the medical assistant may also want to create printed copies of e-mails related to orders or billing problems.

Clinical Messaging

Clinical messaging (also called *clinical e-mail*) refers to electronic messages sent to other health professionals using the electronic medical record (EMR). It is considered as secure as the EMR itself, so it is often used to communicate information about patients to colleagues. The record of an individual patient can be attached to the message. The format and tone are the same as in an ordinary e-mail.

E-mail Attachments

Programs for sending e-mail allow documents, images, and other types of files to be attached and transmitted with the e-mail. Unfortunately, many computer viruses are spread through e-mail attachments, so attachments should not be opened unless they are from a trusted source and/or are expected. If an attachment does contain a virus, opening the attachment launches the virus. Any e-mail with an attachment from an unknown recipient should be deleted immediately. If a medical assistant sends a file as an attachment, the recipient may also be hesitant to open the file for the same reason.

The format of an attachment may also pose a problem. The recipient may be unable to open the attachment without the software that was used to create the file in the attachment. Document files can always be saved in text format if there is any question about compatible software. Most files can also be saved as webpages, which the recipient can view with his or her Web browser.

Fax Transmissions

Fax Machine

Paper copies of documents can be sent quickly from one location to another using a fax machine. The word **fax** is a short form of *facsimile* and is a method of sending images over telephone lines. The original document is fed into the fax machine, which encodes the images on the paper into signals to be sent over the phone. At the other end, a second fax machine prints black dots on a piece of paper that correspond to the information received. There should be a dedicated

PROCEDURE 42-2

What Would You Do? What Would You *Not* Do?

Case Study 3
An order for clinical supplies has been delivered to the office, and Christine is putting the supplies away. While checking the received items against the packing list, she notices that although there are 10 boxes of urine test strips listed, only nine boxes have been shipped. In addition, the packing slip states that only one package of five rolls of paper for the Clinitek machine was shipped, but five packages were ordered. As an experiment, the office has placed this order with an Internet supplier. No telephone number is given for the supplier on its home page. On the company's invoice (bill), which has arrived separately, the medical office has been charged for 10 boxes of urine test strips and one package of paper for the Clinitek machine. ∎

telephone line and telephone number for the fax machine, which is shown in Figure 42-8. The phone number for the fax machine should be listed next to each telephone so that any caller can be told how to fax information to the office.

Sending a Fax
The fax is useful for doing business (e.g., ordering supplies) and for sending out meeting agendas or receiving résumés when hiring. To protect confidentiality, fax transmissions of

patient health information should be made only when patient consent has been obtained or in an emergency situation when prompt information transfer is required. A cover sheet should be used for privacy, and the recipient should be notified by telephone when the fax is being sent so that he or she can remove it from the receiving fax machine promptly (Procedure 42-2). The cover sheet should contain a confidentiality statement similar to the one in Figure 42-9.

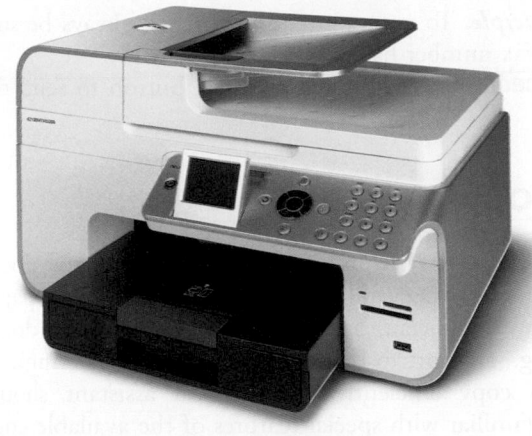

Figure 42-8 A fax machine allows transmission of images from one location to another using a telephone line.

CONFIDENTIALITY STATEMENT:

The documents accompanying this transmission may contain confidential information that is protected under the Privacy Act of 1974. It is being faxed to you after appropriate patient authorization or under circumstances that do not require patient authorization. This information is intended only for the use of the intended recipient(s). The authorized recipient(s) of this information is/are prohibited from disclosing this information to any other party unless permitted to do so by law or regulation.

If the reader of this message is not the intended recipient(s) or the employee or agent responsible for delivering the attached information to the intended recipient(s), please note that any dissemination, distribution, or copying of this information is strictly prohibited. **Anyone who receives this information in error should notify the sender immediately and arrange for the return or destruction of the transmitted information.**

Figure 42-9 A medical office should include a confidentiality statement on the cover sheet for fax transmissions.

PROCEDURE 42-2   Sending a Fax

Outcome Send a fax.

Equipment/Supplies

- Fax machine
- Cover sheet
- Document to be faxed

1. **Procedural Step.** Prepare the cover sheet including the name, address, and fax number of the recipient; fax number of the sender; and number of pages (including the cover sheet). If there is a message to the sender, include it on the bottom of the cover sheet.
2. **Procedural Step.** Organize all pages to be faxed with the cover sheet first.

Principle. Pages should be in order and all facing the same direction.
3. **Procedural Step.** Place pages in the fax machine, face up or face down as is correct for the machine being used.
4. **Procedural Step.** Enter the fax number. Include any extra digits as required, such as a "9" to obtain an outside line, a "1" for long-distance, and/or an area code if required.

Continued

PROCEDURE **42-2**   Sending a Fax—cont'd

Principle. Some areas of the country have introduced so-called overlay area codes requiring all telephone numbers to be dialed with an area code.

5. Procedural Step. Verify the fax number as it appears in the window or on the computer screen to be sure the number is correct.

Principle. To maintain confidentiality, always be sure the fax number has been entered correctly.

6. Procedural Step. Press the correct button to send the fax.

7. Procedural Step. If the fax contains patient health information, place a telephone call to the recipient so that the fax can be removed from the recipient's fax machine as soon as it is received.

8. Procedural Step. Check back to be sure the fax has been sent. Some machines print a confirmation for every fax, and some print a written report only if the fax does not go through.

9. Procedural Step. File the original document appropriately.

PHOTOCOPYING

It may be necessary to use a copy machine to copy documents of one or several pages (e.g., an article or paper written by a physician) or to make several copies of a document (e.g., a report to be discussed at a staff meeting). In order to copy efficiently, the medical assistant should become familiar with special features of the available copy machine. Before copying, staples should be removed from the document to be copied, the pages should be arranged in order, and the copy machine should be checked to be sure it has enough paper.

When several copies of a multiple-page document are needed, the machine should be preset to **collate** (arrange each copy in sequence) or sort the pages if the machine has this feature. Some machines will also staple documents.

For a machine that copies only single pages, the desired number of copies of each page must be copied, arranged in order, and stapled manually. The medical assistant should avoid distractions when copying and should be careful to copy each page correctly and place pages in the correct order (Procedure 42-3).

Another feature of many photocopiers is the ability to **duplex,** or store images from both sides of a page in memory to produce two-sided copies.

When copying a patient's medical record, the medical assistant must preserve the confidentiality of the information. Before beginning to make a copy, verify that the patient has signed an authorization for the release of information. After copying, it is important to double-check that no originals or copies were left at the machine. The medical assistant is responsible for shredding any spoiled copies.

PROCEDURE **42-3**   Preparing Copies of Multiple-Page Documents

Outcome Prepare copies of documents with multiple pages.

Equipment/Supplies

- Photocopy machine
- Paper
- Document to be copied
- Stapler
- Staples
- Staple remover

1. Procedural Step. Assemble all pages of the document or report. If it is stapled, remove all staples.

Principle. Staples may damage the glass or the feeder of the copier.

2. Procedural Step. Be sure that the copy machine is on and warmed up.

3. Procedural Step. If the report to be copied includes all or part of a patient's medical record, verify that there is a signed release of information.

4. Procedural Step. Place the originals in the machine according to the directions for the individual machine.

Principle. Depending on the size and complexity of the machine and the type of document to be copied, it may be necessary to copy one page at a time, or the machine may accept the entire document. The original

may have to be placed face down on the glass (single-sheet copying), or the document may be loaded face down or face up into a feeder.

5. Procedural Step. Set the size and number of copies, and, if the machine allows, press buttons so that copies will be collated and/or stapled.

6. Procedural Step. Press the "start" button.

7. Procedural Step. After the copies have been made, if necessary, arrange the pages in the correct order and staple.

8. Procedural Step. If the patient will be charged for copying sections of the medical record, verify the number of pages and submit to the person responsible for billing.

MEDICAL PRACTICE and the LAW

When a patient's protected health information (PHI) must be communicated in writing, it is always preferable to send the information in a letter instead of writing an e-mail or sending a fax. Although it is possible for a letter to be read by someone other than the addressee, the sender has made every reasonable effort to protect a patient's confidentiality as required by the Health Insurance Portability and Accountability Act (HIPAA).

If a medical office has a secure electronic messaging system with approved encryption, it may be acceptable to send e-mail messages containing PHI. It is also acceptable to send patient information using clinical messaging. Before any communication with patients via e-mail relating to PHI, the patient should be required to provide consent, recognizing that e-mail is not a secure form of communication. Care should be taken to ensure that an e-mail containing PHI is sent only to the intended recipient.

Fax transmissions should be used only if it is necessary to transmit information without the delay inherent in sending a letter. A cover sheet containing a confidentiality statement should be used, and the transmission should be confirmed by telephone if possible. Neither the sending nor the receiving fax machine should be located in an area that is accessible to unauthorized personnel (to prevent interception of incoming faxes). If a fax that contains PHI is received in error, the sender should be notified immediately and the fax should either be returned to the sender by mail or destroyed. ∎

What Would You Do? What Would You *Not* Do? RESPONSES

Case Study 1
Page 1015

What Did Christine Do?
☐ Looked up the two companies mentioned by the physician using the Internet to obtain the exact business names and addresses and model numbers of machines in which the physician might be interested.
☐ Also looked for other companies that might manufacture similar machines.
☐ Prepared letters to each company requesting information using the usual format for office letters.
☐ Used the salutation "Dear Sir or Madam."
☐ Proofread and signed the letters before mailing.
☐ Made a note to herself to follow up after a week.

What Did Christine Not Do?
☐ Did not ask the physician how to find the addresses.
☐ Did not initiate a contact that would result in a call by a salesperson.
☐ Did not send the letters out with an incomplete address or with errors.

What Would You Do/What Would You Not Do?
Review Christine's response and place a checkmark next to the information you included in your response. List the additional information you included in your response.

_____
_____
_____
_____
_____
_____
_____

Case Study 2
Page 1017

What Did Christine Do?
☐ Asked another medical assistant in the office if she knew what the abbreviation should be.

☐ Tried to look it up in a dictionary of abbreviations to make sense of the sentence.
☐ If still unable to identify an appropriate abbreviation, left a blank line in the letter and indicated on a sticky note that the physician should fill in the blank.
☐ After the letter was reviewed by the physician, corrected the letter and printed a new copy for the physician to sign.

What Did Christine Not Do?
☐ Did not leave the abbreviation if it did not make sense, hoping that the physician would not notice.
☐ Did not mail the letter without correcting and reprinting it.
☐ Did not interrupt the physician to ask about the confusing abbreviation and sentence.
☐ Did not complain to other office staff about the voice recognition software program.

What Would You Do/What Would You Not Do?
Review Christine's response and place a checkmark next to the information you included in your response. List the additional information you included in your response.

_____
_____
_____
_____
_____
_____

Case Study 3
Page 1019

What Did Christine Do?
☐ Used either office e-mail or the contact button on the website to send an e-mail about the missing box of test strips.
☐ Used the same professional tone in the e-mail that she would have used in a letter or telephone call.
☐ In the e-mail, included the order number, billing name and address, number of boxes of test strips ordered, and number of boxes of test strips received.

❏ In the e-mail, stated clearly that the company should send an additional box of test strips.

❏ Because the bill charged for only the one package of paper that was shipped, decided to order the other four packages of paper for the Clinitek machine from a more reliable company.

What Did Christine Not Do?

❏ Did not cross out the charge for 10 boxes and test strips and change it to nine boxes when approving the bill for payment without contacting the company.

❏ Did not ignore the missing box of strips when approving the bill for payment, assuming that the company would send another box automatically.

❏ Did not use casual, critical, or hostile language in the e-mail.

What Would You Do/What Would You Not Do?

Review Christine's response and place a checkmark next to the information you included in your response. List the additional information you included in your response.

_____

_____

_____

_____

_____

_____

_____

_____

TERMINOLOGY REVIEW

Medical Term	Word Parts	Definition
Clinical messaging		Communication among health professionals within the electronic medical record.
Collate		To assemble the pages of a document in numeric order.
Complimentary closing		Words used as a polite ending to a letter just before the writer's signature.
Duplex		To produce double-sided copies by storing images from both sides of the original in the memory of a photocopier.
E-mail		The exchange of information from one computer to another using telecommunication.
Fax		Transmission of scanned, printed material by telephone. A short form of the word *facsimile*.
Full block style		A letter format in which all parts of the letter are left justified.
Grammar		The study of accepted rules used to create meaning in a language.
Left justified		Lines of type that begin at the left margin of a document.
Letterhead		A sheet of stationery preprinted with information about a business, including name, address, telephone number, and other information.
Memo (memorandum)		A form of communication within a company that is usually short and limited to one subject.
Modified block style		A format for business letters in which the date line, complimentary close, and printed signature line are on a tab at the center or right justified and all other parts of the letter are left justified.
Proofread		To identify and correct errors in a document.
Right justified		Type that is aligned with the right margin of a document.
Salutation		The greeting that begins a letter.
Semiblock style		A letter format in which the date line, complimentary close, and printed signature line are on a tab at the center or right justified, all paragraphs are indented five to eight spaces, and the other parts of the letter are left justified.
Simplified letter style		A letter format in which all elements are left justified. The greeting is replaced by a subject line in all capital letters. The complimentary close and typed signature are replaced by a typed signature in all capital letters.
Template		A standard form to which additional information can be added as needed.

ON THE WEB

For information on improving written communication:

Grammar and Spelling—The Purdue Online Writing Lab (OWL): http://owl.english.purdue.edu/owl/section/1/5/

For information on patient confidentiality in written communication:

Centers for Medicare and Medicaid Services—HIPAA Privacy Rule: www.hhs.gov/ocr/hipaa

 Check out the Evolve site at http://evolve.elsevier.com/Bonewit/today/ to actively Prepare for your Certification, and to access additional interactive activities and exercises to help you study and prepare for success.

43

Mail

some scrambled/overlapping background text faintly visible at top

LEARNING OBJECTIVES

U.S. Mail

1. Identify the function of the U.S. Postal Service (USPS).
2. State the purpose of the ZIP and ZIP+4 systems.
3. Describe the use of the following USPS mail classifications: Express Mail, Priority Mail, First-Class Mail, Standard Mail, and classifications used for packages.
4. Correlate available insurance and delivery confirmation services to their appropriate use in the medical office.

Other Package Delivery Services

5. Compare and contrast the use of private package delivery services with the use of the USPS.

Processing Incoming Mail

6. List and describe the steps for processing incoming mail.

Preparing Envelopes for Mailing

7. List and describe the USPS addressing standards that must be followed to prepare mail.

8. List and describe the equipment used to prepare envelopes for mailing.
9. Compare and contrast postage meters and online postage services.

PROCEDURES

Process incoming mail.

Look up a ZIP code for automated processing.

Prepare envelopes for mailing.

CHAPTER OUTLINE

INTRODUCTION TO MAIL AND SHIPPING
U.S. Postal System
ZIP Code and Bar Code Systems
Classifications of Domestic Mail
Insurance and Delivery Confirmation Services
Other Package Delivery Services
Processing Incoming Mail
Opening Mail
Automated Mail Processing

Postal Addressing Standards
Letters and Large Envelopes
Complete Address
Address Format
Return Address
Outgoing Mail
Preparing Envelopes or Mailing Labels
Folding and Inserting Letters into Envelopes
Adding Postage

KEY TERMS

annotate (ANN-oh-tate)
barcode clear zone
metered mail

postage meter
postal bar code
ZIP code

ZIP+4 code

INTRODUCTION TO MAIL AND SHIPPING

Mail communication is an important aspect of the efficient operation of the medical office. Every day the medical assistant processes incoming mail to facilitate delivery to physicians and other employees in the medical office. Preparing outgoing mail is also important. Most of this chapter is devoted to the services and postal addressing standards of the U.S. Postal Service (USPS), which is used to send the bulk of outgoing mail.

U.S. POSTAL SYSTEM

The USPS is an independent agency with an official monopoly on the delivery of mail within the United States. It is financed primarily through the sale of postage and postage stamps. The postal service processes more than 563 million pieces of mail daily and is one of the largest employers in the United States. The USPS provides a variety of ways for mail to be transported from sender to receiver. The cost of these various services depends on the urgency with which mail must be received, as well as any special handling services provided.

ZIP Code and Bar Code Systems

In 1963 the USPS introduced the Zone Improvement Plan (ZIP) code system. This system enables the postal service to process mail more accurately, quickly, and economically with automated equipment. A **ZIP code** consists of a five-digit code that identifies the post office to which a piece of mail is to be delivered. In 1967 it became mandatory to use the ZIP code for second- and third-class bulk mailing.

The **ZIP+4 code,** which was introduced in 1983, consists of the original five-digit code followed by a hyphen and four additional digits. These digits identify a specific geographic segment within the five-digit delivery area, such as a city block, an office building, or a group of post office boxes. The plus-four code is required for certain presorted mailings. The USPS maintains a ZIP code lookup service that makes it easy to use the Internet to look up the ZIP+4 code for any address in the United States.

For bulk mailing, the ZIP code is translated into a postal bar code that is printed on the piece of mail by the sender. A computer program is used to add the bar code to pieces of mail, mailing labels, and mailing lists. For ordinary letters, the postal service may add the postal bar code because it makes the mail easier to sort. Unlike supermarket bar codes, which consist of wide and narrow bars, the **postal bar code** consists of long and short bars. Each individual digit in the ZIP code is represented by five bars, and a check digit is used after the ZIP code or ZIP+4 code. The postal bar code may be printed in the address block above or below the mailing address. When not included in the address block, the postal bar code is placed in the **barcode clear zone,** a blank rectangular area at the lower right of the card or envelope (Figure 43-1).

Classifications of Domestic Mail

Domestic mail includes mail that is collected and distributed within, among, and between the United States, its territories and possession, the military service, and the United Nations. Classifications are based on speed of

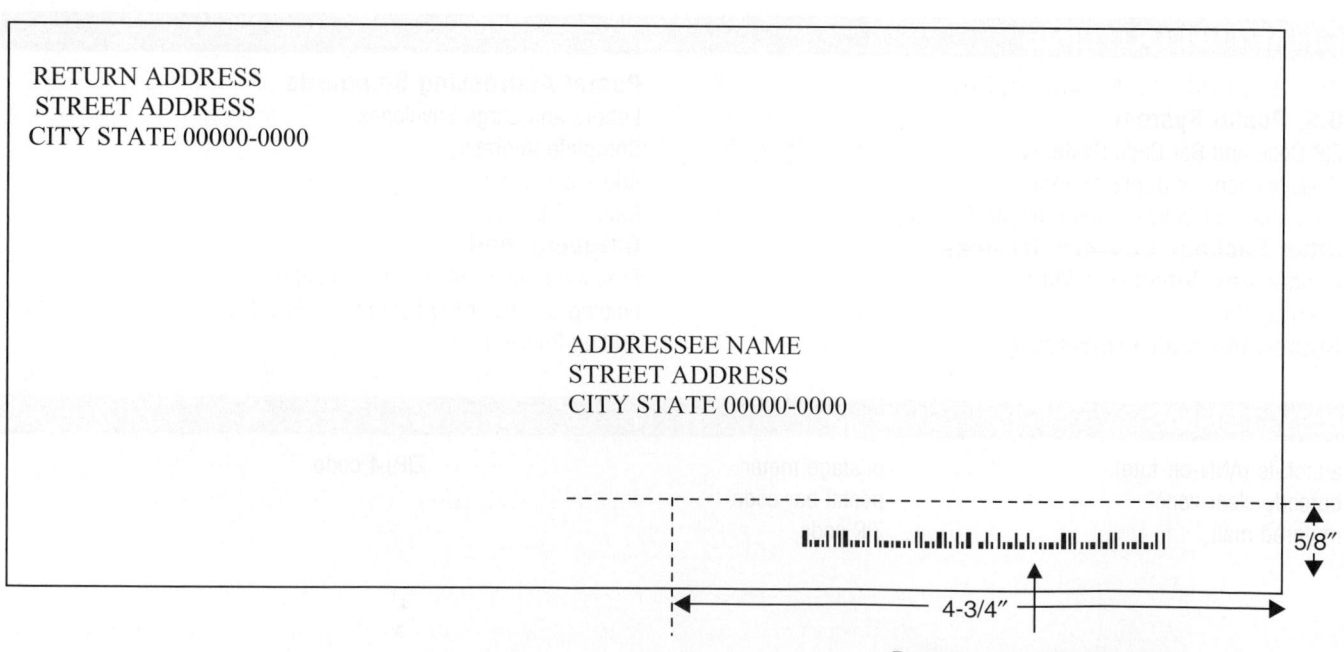

Figure 43-1 The postal bar code is a series of long and short lines that is either printed by the sender above or below the address or added by the post office in the barcode clear zone at the lower right of the envelope.

delivery, weight of individual pieces of mail, and number of pieces of mail in the mailing.

Express Mail

Express Mail received by the post office before 5 PM is delivered within 24 hours, and by noon to most major cities, including on weekends and holidays. It includes letters and packages weighing up to 70 pounds. Envelopes and packing materials are available from the post office. Medical offices may use Express Mail to send laboratory specimens to an outside laboratory for testing. The postage rates for Express Mail are considerably higher than other rates, but they do include insurance against loss or damage.

First-Class Mail

First-Class Mail is used for letters or other lightweight items up to 13 ounces. The postage is based on weight, with a base rate for one ounce and additional postage for each additional ounce. The medical office uses this mail classification to send letters, postcards, patient statements, and some insurance claim forms.

Sending an item First Class usually results in overnight service to local cities and second-day service nationwide. Delivery by the third day can be anticipated for some outlying areas. All First-Class Mail should be sealed, and it may not be opened for postal inspection without a federal search warrant.

Additional extra mailing services can be purchased for First-Class Mail, such as Certificates of Mailing, Certified Mail, Registered Mail, Collect on Delivery (COD), and Restricted Delivery. If the item that is being sent First Class is letter size, no additional designation is required on the letter. However, if the item is not letter size, it must be clearly marked "First Class."

Priority Mail

Priority Mail is used for mail weighing more than 13 ounces that is to be treated as First-Class Mail. It will be delivered anywhere in the United States within 2 to 3 days. The USPS has a set rate for items up to 1 pound, and flat rate envelopes and boxes are available. For an item over 1 pound in ordinary packaging, the rate depends on both the weight of the item and the distance it must be transported. For an additional charge Priority Mail can be combined with Insured Mail, Registered Mail, or Certified Mail or sent COD. Some examples of items that might be sent from the medical office using Priority Mail include copies of medical records.

Standard Mail

The Standard Mail classification is used by newspapers and periodical publishers to send newspapers, journals, magazines, and other periodicals. Periodical mailings must not be sealed, and handwritten messages are not permitted. Standard Mail is also used to send large mailings of newsletters and bulletins. The medical office usually does not obtain the special permit to send items at this rate, but it may receive newspapers, magazines for the waiting room, and medical journals. Standard Mail requires a minimum of 200 pieces or 50 pounds per mailing.

Parcel Post and Other Packages

If time is not a significant factor, packages may be sent using one of the ground mail classifications. Parcel Post is used to send merchandise and other items that weigh up to 70 pounds and measure up to 108 inches in length and girth. Instruction slips, packing slips, sales slips, or invoices can be enclosed in a package sent Parcel Post without additional postage. However, in order to send a letter with a package, the letter must be attached to the outside of the package and paid for at the First-Class rate. The medical office rarely sends items by Parcel Post, although it may receive supplies sent by this method. Media Mail is a special classification for packages containing books, sound recordings, film, manuscripts, and computer media but not advertising. Bound Printed Matter is a classification for packages containing permanently bound catalogs and other volumes containing advertising (e.g., telephone books).

Insurance and Delivery Confirmation Services

The USPS offers a number of extra mailing services. These services must be purchased in addition to the regular postage required to send an item. The medical assistant must understand these extra services, particularly those that are used most frequently in the medical office, such as Certified Mail and Return Receipt.

Certified Mail

Certified Mail is available for First-Class Mail and Priority Mail. It serves as legal evidence that an item was mailed by providing the sender with a mailing receipt. In addition, a record of delivery of the certified item is maintained for 2 years. A green certified mail sticker affixed to the envelope identifies the envelope as Certified Mail. The recipient must sign on delivery of a piece of Certified Mail. This service can also be combined with a Return Receipt for an additional fee (Figure 43-2).

Return Receipt

A Return Receipt provides the sender with proof of delivery of a piece of mail and the signature of the person receiving the mail. This may be done through a postcard signed by the recipient and returned to the sender or by an e-mail with an attachment containing the recipient's signature. The sender then has a copy of the signature of the person who signed for the piece of mail. This service can be combined with other services. It is often used with Certified Mail to establish proof of mailing, as well as proof of receipt (Figure 43-3).

Signature Confirmation

Signature Confirmation provides a record of the date and time an item was delivered, as well as the name of the person who signed for the item. A delivery record, including the signature of the recipient, is available by fax or mail on

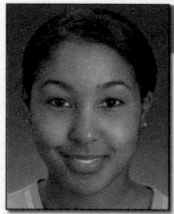

Putting It All into Practice

My name is Diane Waters, and I am a certified medical assistant. I have been working for a group practice with three general surgeons for the past 6 years. Our physicians usually have office hours three times a week, either in the morning or the afternoon. They usually operate two or three times a week, and they have to make hospital rounds every day. Two of them also work with residents at a large hospital located near our practice. In the past, each surgeon received an operative report and discharge summary for each patient he or she had operated on in hard copy. When I opened the mail, I had to date stamp each report, find the patient's medical record, and place it for the physician to review before it could be filed. A few years ago the hospital went to an electronic medical record. The operative reports and discharge summaries are now entered into the electronic medical record automatically, and the physicians review them online. That means that we get significantly less mail because not only those reports but also laboratory reports, pathology reports, and other types of reports no longer come to the office. Of course, we don't have as much filing, either. Our office still gets piles of journals, magazines, and other printed matter, however. Every day when I am sorting the mail, I have to separate the professional journals that our physicians want to read from magazines, catalogs, circulars, and other items that they would only look at if we found some item of special interest to them. One physician likes to look through this material if it comes with his name on it, but the others don't even want it to show up on their desks. ■

request. The medical office usually uses Return Receipt instead of Signature Confirmation for evidence of delivery because the return postcard or e-mail will be sent automatically.

Certificate of Mailing

A Certificate of Mailing provides evidence of the date and time an item was mailed, but there is no legal proof that the item was actually delivered to the recipient. A certificate of mailing might be used when proof of timely mailing is required, such as a tax return. No record is maintained at the post office, so the sender is responsible for keeping the form.

Restricted Delivery

If an item is strictly confidential, Restricted Delivery limits delivery to the addressee, the individual authorized in writing to sign for the addressee, or a parent or guardian. It is not generally necessary to use this service for letters from the medical office, but if a legal case is pending, it might be advisable.

Registered Mail

Registered Mail is available for First-Class and Priority Mail, to insure the contents up to $25,000.00. Registered Mail is used when the contents of the item mailed are valuable. The items are tracked, and the date and time of delivery or delivery attempts can be verified online. The cost depends on the value of the item being sent. The sender receives a receipt that is kept until the recipient receives the item. The

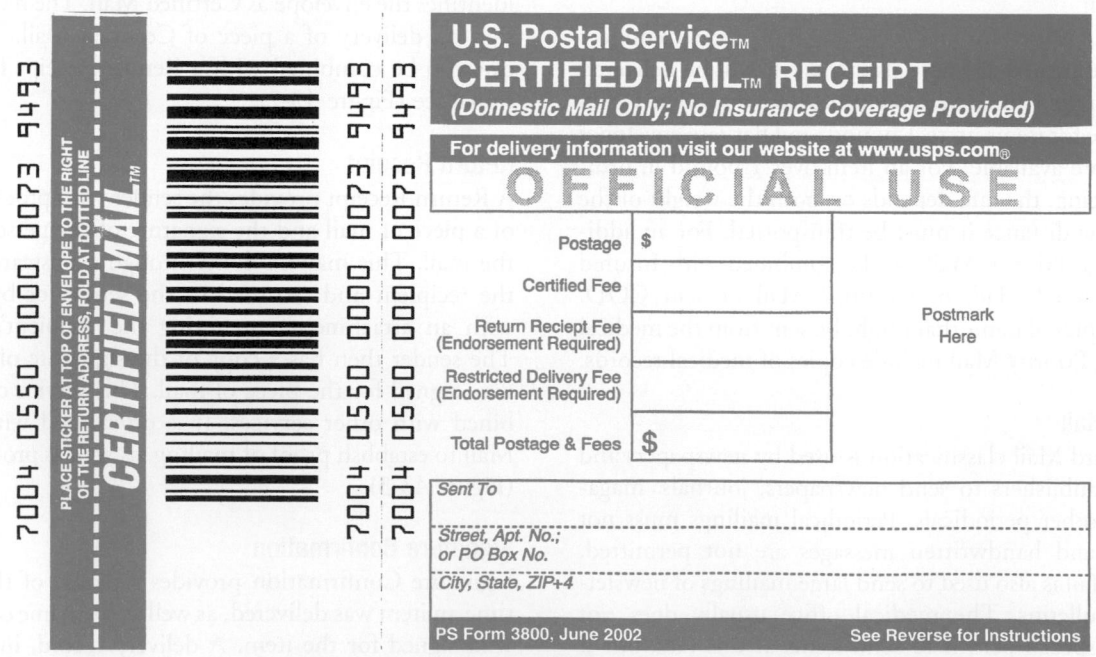

Figure 43-2 A receipt for Certified Mail form must be filled out by the sender and signed by the recipient.

UNITED STATES POSTAL SERVICE

|||||

First-Class Mail
Postage & Fees Paid
USPS
Permit No. G-10

• Sender: Please print your name, address, and ZIP+4 in this box •

SENDER: *COMPLETE THIS SECTION*

■ Complete items 1, 2, and 3. Also complete item 4 if Restricted Delivery is desired.
■ Print your name and address on the reverse so that we can return the card to you.
■ Attach this card to the back of the mailpiece, or on the front if space permits.

1. Article Addressed to:

2. Article Number
   (Transfer from service label)

COMPLETE THIS SECTION ON DELIVERY

A. Signature

X

☐ Agent
☐ Addressee

B. Received by (*Printed Name*)

C. Date of Delivery

D. Is delivery address different from item 1?   ☐ Yes
   If YES, enter delivery address below: ☐ No

3. Service Type
   ☐ Certified Mail   ☐ Express Mail
   ☐ Registered   ☐ Return Receipt for Merchandise
   ☐ Insured Mail   ☐ C.O.D.

4. Restricted Delivery? *(Extra Fee)*   ☐ Yes

PS Form **3811**, February 2004   Domestic Return Receipt   102595-02-M-1540

Figure 43-3 The sender must fill out a Return Receipt form.

recipient must sign a form acknowledging receipt. For an additional fee, the sender can receive a Return Receipt.

Insured Mail
Insurance can be purchased on the contents of mail up to $5000.00. The cost depends on the declared value of the contents. If the mail is lost or damaged, the sender presents the receipt to make a claim for reimbursement of the declared value.

Special Handling
Special Handling is used for unusual items that require special treatment, such as a shipment of live bees. Ordinary packages with breakable items can be marked "FRAGILE"

and do not require Special Handling provided they are packed with adequate packing material to protect the contents. This service is not usually used by the medical office.

Collect on Delivery
COD is a special mailing service that allows a sender to collect for merchandise and postage on delivery. The amount due is collected by the postal carrier and returned to the sender by a postal money order. This service is rarely used by the medical office.

Postal Money Orders
Postal money orders are a safe way to send money through the mail within the United States. They may be purchased

in an amount up to $1000.00. The sender is given a customer receipt. If the money order is lost or stolen, the sender presents the receipt to the post office for replacement. Some patients may pay bills with postal money orders.

OTHER PACKAGE DELIVERY SERVICES

Private carriers compete with the USPS to provide delivery service of letters and packages. Many companies use DHL, FedEx, or United Parcel Service (UPS) for next-day and 2-day delivery service. Larger packages that are not time sensitive can be shipped via UPS or FedEx Ground service. A shipping service company will pick items up from an office and offer continuous item tracking over the company's website. Each company also provides mailing envelopes and small boxes at no cost to the customer. Once an account has been established, shipping can be arranged and paid for using the Internet.

Private carriers often deliver packages to the medical office. Examples include business supplies and laboratory reagents requiring refrigeration. The medical office may use a private delivery service to send some laboratory specimens to a laboratory for testing if the specimen must go to a special laboratory or cannot wait for the regular laboratory pickup service.

What Would You Do? What Would You *Not* Do?

Case Study 1
Jerome Stone, a 68-year-old man who has had two laparoscopic surgeries in the past, has called the office and asked to have a copy of his medical record sent to his new surgeon in another state because he needs to have another surgery for the same condition. He tells Diane that the surgery is scheduled for the following week and asks if she can send the copy of the record immediately. He states that he can come into the office the following day to sign the form giving permission to release the record. He gives her the name, address, and telephone number of the new physician. ∎

PROCESSING INCOMING MAIL

Mail is delivered to the medical office in various ways. The postal carrier may deliver the mail directly to the office, or it may be placed in an outside mailbox. Some medical offices use a post office box. In this case the medical assistant must go to the post office to collect the mail each day. In a large clinic the mail may be delivered to a central mailroom, where it is sorted and distributed to each department or individual mailbox.

Once the mail is received by the medical office, it must be processed according to the preferences of individual physicians. One physician may want to see all the incoming mail, whereas another physician may want the medical assistant to screen the mail and remove circulars, patient and insurance payments, and magazines for the waiting room (Procedure 43-1).

Incoming mail should be sorted in the following way. If the mail is addressed to a particular physician, it goes into that physician's mailbox or pile. Mail from another physician's office that is not addressed to a particular physician should go into the box or pile of the managing partner, medical director, or office manager.

The medical assistant handles patient and insurance payments, mail from insurance companies, and catalogs from business and medical supply companies. Table 43-1 provides a guide for sorting incoming mail.

Opening Mail

Once the mail has been sorted, it must be opened. The medical assistant must know which mail he or she is to open and which is to go to the individual who must deal with it unopened. Some physicians like to open their own mail, whereas others like to have the mail opened, organized, and ready for them to read and respond to. Clearly, any mail marked "personal" or "confidential" should not be opened.

Table 43-1 Sorting Incoming Mail

Mail Category	Recipient
First-Class Mail	
Correspondence addressed to the physician marked "Confidential" or "Personal"	Physician
Correspondence from an attorney	Physician
Laboratory reports	Physician (attach laboratory report to patient's paper medical record)
Patient records	Physician
Patient payments	Medical assistant
Insurance payments	Medical assistant
Bills for office supplies and equipment	Medical assistant
Bank statements	Medical assistant
Letters from insurance companies	Medical assistant
Résumés for employment	Medical assistant
Periodicals, Circulars, Catalogs	
Professional journals	Physician
Medical conventions and seminars	Physician
Pharmaceutical advertising	Physician
Advertisements for equipment and supplies	Physician
Magazines for the waiting room	Medical assistant
Catalogs for equipment and supplies	Medical assistant
Drug Samples and Packages	
Overnight packages	Screen appropriately
Administrative and clinical office supplies	Medical assistant
Drug samples	Medical assistant (place in drug sample storage area)

If the physician or physicians prefer mail to be opened, the medical assistant should use a letter opener to open each piece carefully at the top edge. Each letter or report is stamped with the receipt date and then alphabetized by the patient's last name. The pages of each report should be stapled together, if they are not already that way. A letter or report containing patient information should be attached to the patient's medical record with a paper clip. Some offices use a cover sheet on the top of each report, on which the physician can check off the action he or she wishes to occur with regard to the report (e.g., file, respond, call the patient).

Non–patient-related items are stacked together to be dealt with by the medical assistant or another member of the staff. Medical journals addressed to a particular physician can be put in his or her mail pile; those addressed to the practice can be put into the medical library or staff lounge. If the office is large, each staff member may have a cubicle in a central location, as shown in Figure 43-4.

Some physicians may instruct the medical assistant to annotate letters. To **annotate** means to underline or highlight important words or phrases in the correspondence. This saves the physician time when reading and responding to the mail. The medical assistant may also be instructed to underline or highlight abnormal values on laboratory reports or diagnostic tests.

When a physician is on vacation, someone on the office staff is delegated to review his or her mail and refer any urgent mail to the physician by telephone or e-mail at the vacation location or to a covering physician. Arrange non-urgent mail by date received for the physician to review when he or she returns to the office.

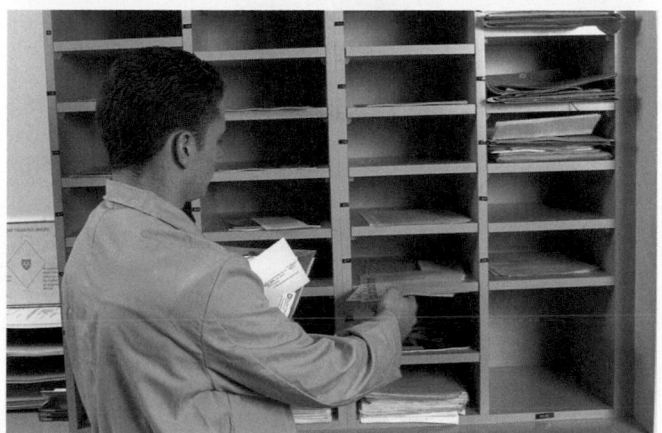
Figure 43-4   In a large office, each staff member may have a mailbox at a central location.

What Would You Do? What Would You *Not* Do?

Case Study 2

Diane is preparing an envelope in order to mail a letter that the physician has dictated to a colleague named Dr. Leonie. She uses the USPS website to look up the ZIP code. Although a five-digit ZIP code is displayed, it is accompanied by a message that says, "This address may be nondeliverable." ∎

PROCEDURE 43-1   Processing Incoming Mail

Outcome   Process incoming mail.

Equipment/Supplies

- Letter opener
- Date stamp
- Paper clips
- Stapler
- Pen or highlighter
- Transparent tape

1. **Procedural Step.** Assemble supplies in a work area large enough to make several piles of mail.
2. **Procedural Step.** Stack all the envelopes so that they face in the same direction. Place any envelopes marked "personal" or confidential" to the side.
   Principle. Letters marked "personal" or "confidential" should be opened only by the person to whom they are addressed.
3. **Procedural Step.** Tap the lower edge of the first envelope on the desk so that the contents fall to the bottom.
   Principle. Tapping the envelope prevents cutting the contents when the envelope is opened.
4. **Procedural Step.** Using a letter opener, open the envelope along its top edge.

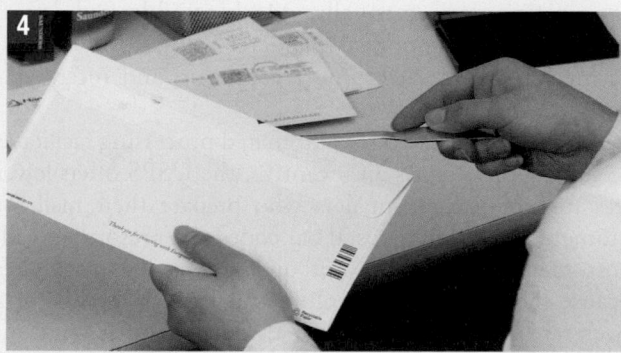
Use a letter opener to open the envelope.
Principle. Using a letter opener makes it easier to open the envelope neatly and preserves the return address should it be needed.

Continued

PROCEDURE 43-1 **Processing Incoming Mail—cont'd**

5. Procedural Step. Remove the contents of the envelope. Check to be sure the envelope is empty.

6. Procedural Step. Unfold and flatten letters. Date stamp each letter, preferably in the upper right-hand corner of the letter.
Principle. A date stamp provides a record of when the letter was received.

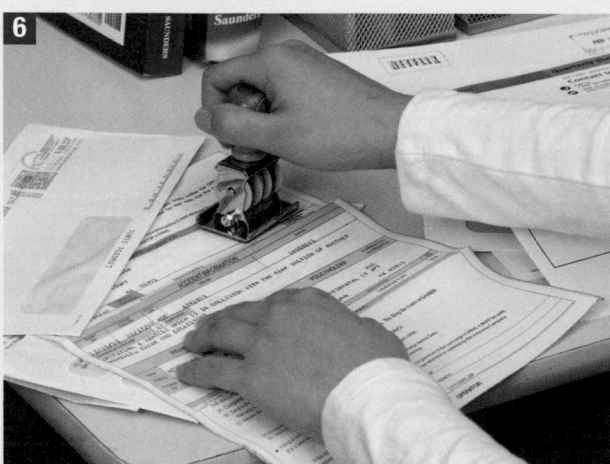

Date stamp each letter.

7. Procedural Step. Check to make sure that the letter contains an inside address. If not, staple the envelope to the letter. Discard the envelope if it is not needed, unless office policy states otherwise.

8. Procedural Step. Fasten enclosures to the letter with a paper clip. If a letter indicates an enclosure, but it is missing, write "No" next to the enclosure notation and circle or highlight it.

9. Procedural Step. Mend any torn paper with transparent tape to prevent further damage.

10. Procedural Step. If directed by the physician, annotate the correspondence by underlining or highlighting important words and phrases in the correspondence. Attach a sticky note indicating any action that should be taken in response to the correspondence.
Principle. Annotating saves the physician time in reading and responding to incoming mail.

11. Procedural Step. Follow the same steps to open each piece of mail as described earlier, and separate the pieces of mail into categories: urgent or very important, other letters, letters or reports containing patient information or results, medical journals, and circulars or advertising.

12. Procedural Step. Arrange letters and reports containing patient information in alphabetic order. If the office uses paper medical records, find the appropriate medical record, and attach each letter or report to the medical record with a paper clip.

13. Procedural Step. Arrange the mail for each physician with the most important mail on top and the least important on the bottom.

14. Procedural Step. Distribute each stack of mail to the appropriate individual.

AUTOMATED MAIL PROCESSING

Since the early 1980s the methods used to process the mail have evolved from manual and mechanized processing to automated processing. Automated equipment can read and sort mail more than six times faster than sorting mail manually. Machine-addressed letters are processed using optical character recognition (OCR), the mechanical or electronic recognition and interpretation of text.

Mail that is prepared for automated processing facilitates the sorting process. As an incentive, the USPS offers lower rates to high-volume mailers who prepare their mail for automation by adding postal bar codes and presorting mail. Most medical offices do not qualify for the lower rates because they are not high-volume mailers. To qualify for a lower rate on First-Class Mail, the mailer must send out 500 letters in one mailing.

POSTAL ADDRESSING STANDARDS

Specific addressing standards must be met to prepare a piece of mail so that it can be processed by automated equipment.

The medical assistant should be familiar with these standards and put them into practice to ensure the most efficient and timely delivery of outgoing mail.

Letters and Large Envelopes

To be mailed as a letter, an envelope must be $3\frac{1}{2}$ to $6\frac{1}{8}$ inches in height and 5 to $11\frac{1}{2}$ inches in length. The two most common sizes for business envelopes are the No. 10 envelope ($4\frac{1}{8} \times 9\frac{1}{2}$ inches) and the smaller No. $6\frac{3}{4}$ envelope ($3\frac{5}{8} \times 6\frac{1}{2}$ inches), but other sizes may be used. Square letters and letters that are too thick to pass through automated equipment require additional postage. The address may be printed directly on an envelope or on a label that will be attached to the envelope.

A large envelope requires more postage. It may be $6\frac{1}{8}$ to 12 inches in height and $11\frac{1}{2}$ to 15 inches in length. Large manila or white envelopes may be used to send patient medical records or other documents that have too many pages to fold.

Complete Address

The USPS defines a complete address as one that includes all elements necessary for OCR. To be complete, the address

Highlight on Automated Postal Equipment

Automated postal equipment can handle most letters and process them without human intervention. At a Processing and Distribution Center, packages and large pieces of mail are diverted from the stream of mail. All other mail enters the Advanced Facer-Canceller System (AFCS), which rotates the mail so that it faces in the proper direction to postmark and cancel the postage stamp. If a piece of mail has a printed address, it goes to the Multiline Optical Character Reader (MLOCR), which reads the delivery address, translates this information into a bar code, and prints the bar code in the lower right-hand corner of the envelope. If the MLOCR cannot read the address, the piece of mail is separated out of the stream to go to a more sensitive address reader or a postal worker. Once a bar code has been added to the piece of mail, it goes to a Delivery Barcode Sorter (DBCS), which reads and interprets the bar code and sorts it accordingly. Items for local delivery are retained, but other mail is shipped either by air or truck to a destination station, where it is passed through another Delivery Barcode Sorter. At the local destination station the mail is sorted right down to arranging the mail in the order of a carrier's delivery route. Automated equipment is continuously updated and improved by the U.S. Postal Service. ▪

block must include all of the following elements in correct order:

RECIPIENT LINE
DELIVERY ADDRESS LINE
CITY STATE and ZIP LINE

The post office recommends that the address be printed using all uppercase letters without punctuation except for the hyphen after the first five digits in the ZIP+4.

Recipient Line

The name of the intended recipient must appear on the recipient line, which is the first line of the address. The recipient may be either the name of an individual (e.g., Andrew Davis) or the name of a company (e.g., Riverside Laboratory).

Optional Attention Line

If the name of a company is listed on the recipient line and the mail needs to be directed to a specific individual within the company, an optional attention line containing the name of the recipient is placed above the recipient line.

Example:

GERALDINE KAUFMAN	attention line
BROADVIEW HEALTH CLINIC	recipient line
242 SOUTH STREET	
BLACKBURN WI 54937-0012	

Delivery Address Line

The delivery address specifies the street address, post office box, rural route, or highway contract and is located above the bottom line (city, state, and ZIP) (Box 43-1).

Examples:

100 MAIN ST	Street Address
PO BOX 277	Post Office Box
RR1 BOX 75	Rural Route
HC 55 BOX 32	Highway Contract

City, State, and ZIP Code Line

The city, state, and ZIP code should appear in that order on the bottom line of the address block. There should be at least one space between the city name and the state abbreviation. Two spaces are recommended between the state abbreviation and the ZIP code. The ZIP+4 code should be used if known (Procedure 43-2). The only punctuation in this line is the hyphen before the final 4 digits of the ZIP+4 code (Table 43-2).

Address Format

Address format refers to how the various address elements appear on an envelope. The following standards must be followed to format an envelope for automation:

1. The address must be machine-printed for OCR.
2. The automated character reader performs best with black ink on a white background.
3. The address should be printed using plain block letters. A typeface without serifs (cross strokes at the end of the main strokes of the letter), such as Helvetica or Arial, is preferred. Script and italic styles should be avoided because they cannot be read by the automated equipment.
4. All lines of the address should be formatted with a uniform left margin.
5. All letters in the address should be capitalized.
6. All lines of the address should be parallel to the bottom of the envelope.
7. No punctuation should be used in the address except the hyphen in the ZIP+4 code.
8. If a window envelope is used, the entire address must be visible through the window. At least $\frac{1}{8}$-inch clearance ($\frac{1}{4}$ inch is preferred) must be maintained between the address and the edges of the window to distinguish the address from the edge of the window. No other print should show through the window.
9. Delivery instructions (e.g., personal, confidential) must be placed immediately below the return address. Special services (e.g., registered, certified, insured) must be placed above the address and to the right of the return address below the area where stamps or postage will be affixed.
10. Address labels should be applied using methods and materials that prevent them from becoming

BOX 43-1 Specific Delivery Address Standards

1. Use common Postal Service standard abbreviations as much as possible.

AVE	Avenue
BLVD	Boulevard
CTR	Center
CIR	Circle
DR	Drive
EXT	Extension
HWY	Highway
IS	Island
JCT	Junction
LN	Lane
MTN	Mountain
PARK	Park
PKWY	Parkway
RIV	River
RD	Road
SQ	Square
ST	Street
TER	Terrace
VLG	Village
VLY	Valley

2. Use secondary address directional abbreviations (e.g., N, S, NE, SW).

3. Include secondary address locators, such as apartment numbers, suite numbers, and room numbers, at the end of the delivery address line. If an additional line is required for apartment or suite numbers, the secondary address locator should be placed on the line above the delivery address line.

APT	Apartment
BLDG	Building
STE	Suite
UNIT	Unit

Examples:

RECIPIENT LINE	RECIPIENT LINE
100 MAIN ST APT 54	STE 45
CITY STATE ZIP	2500 GRANDVIEW LEVINE BLVD
	CITY STATE ZIP

4. Dual addressing is not recommended. Dual addressing means that two delivery addresses (e.g., both a street address and a post office box) are included on the piece of mail. If dual addressing is used, the post office delivers according to the information on the delivery address line (i.e., the line immediately above the city, state, and ZIP).

Table 43-2 Two-Letter State and Territory Abbreviations

AL	Alabama	MT	Montana
AK	Alaska	NE	Nebraska
AZ	Arizona	NV	Nevada
AR	Arkansas	NH	New Hampshire
CA	California	NM	New Mexico
CO	Colorado	NY	New York
CT	Connecticut	NC	North Carolina
DE	Delaware	ND	North Dakota
DC	District of Columbia	OH	Ohio
FL	Florida	OK	Oklahoma
GA	Georgia	OR	Oregon
GU	Guam	PA	Pennsylvania
HI	Hawaii	PR	Puerto Rico
ID	Idaho	RI	Rhode Island
IL	Illinois	SC	South Carolina
IN	Indiana	SD	South Dakota
IA	Iowa	TN	Tennessee
KS	Kansas	TX	Texas
KY	Kentucky	UT	Utah
LA	Louisiana	VT	Vermont
ME	Maine	VI	Virgin Islands
MD	Maryland	VA	Virginia
MA	Massachusetts	WA	Washington
MI	Michigan	WV	West Virginia
MN	Minnesota	WI	Wisconsin
MS	Mississippi	WY	Wyoming
MO	Missouri		

damaged or removed during high-speed automated processing.

11. The address should be placed within an area that extends from $\frac{5}{8}$ inch to $2\frac{3}{4}$ inches from the bottom edge of the envelope with a $\frac{1}{2}$-inch margin on each side. This is called the *OCR read area* (Figure 43-5).

12. The barcode clear zone is the area on an envelope where a bar code is printed by the automated equipment. It represents an area that is $\frac{5}{8}$ inch high × $\frac{3}{4}$ inches long. It must remain free of all printing, markings, or colored borders.

Return Address

The return address identifies the location to which a piece of mail should be returned if it cannot be delivered. It must be located in the upper left corner of the envelope and must not extend into the OCR read area. The return address should include the following elements:

SENDER'S NAME (OPTIONAL)
SENDER'S DELIVERY ADDRESS
SENDER'S CITY, STATE, ZIP

Letterhead envelopes or envelopes preprinted with the return address are usually used.

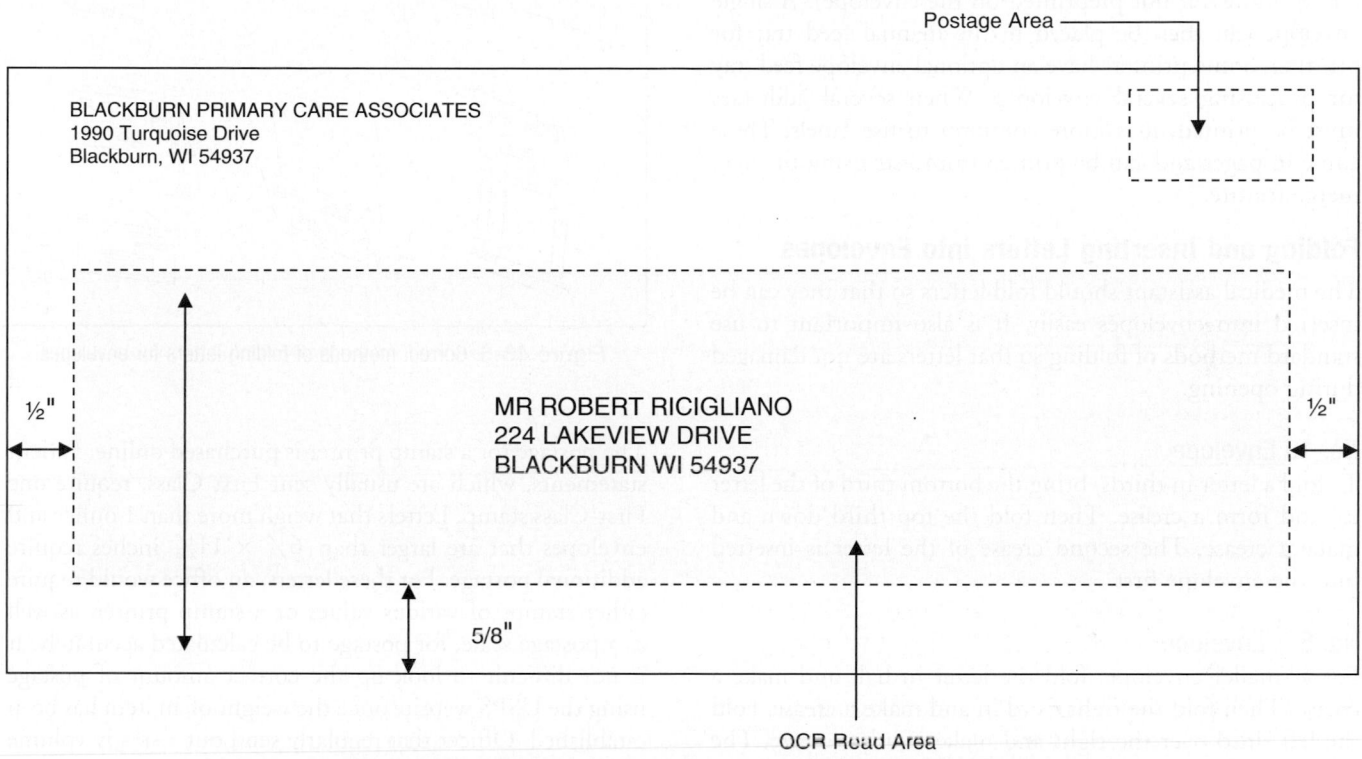

Figure 43-5 Envelope showing address in the optical character recognition *(OCR)* read area.

PROCEDURE 43-2   Looking up a ZIP Code

Outcome Find the correct ZIP+4 code for a given address.

Equipment/Supplies

- Computer with Internet access
- Pen and pencil

- Address with incorrect and/or incomplete ZIP code

1. **Procedural Step.** Open the computer's Web browser and enter the Web address for the USPS.
2. **Procedural Step.** From the USPS home page, click on the link labeled "Look Up a ZIP code."
3. **Procedural Step.** In the address popup window, enter the delivery address, city, and state abbreviation of the address for which a ZIP code is sought. (It is also possible to search for a ZIP code if only the city and state are known.)
4. **Procedural Step.** Copy the ZIP+4 code on a piece of paper to use in preparing a label or envelope or use the computer "copy" function to copy and paste into a computer file.

OUTGOING MAIL

The process of preparing items for mailing may include addressing envelopes, preparing mailing labels, folding letters or statements to place into envelopes, calculating and adding postage, and mailing items either in mailboxes or at the post office.

Preparing Envelopes or Mailing Labels

Most word processing programs have a feature that creates and prints an address (and return address if desired) on various sizes of envelope. The medical assistant selects the envelope function and enters the delivery address (and return address if not preprinted on the envelope). A single envelope can then be placed in the manual feed tray for printing. Some printers have an optional envelope feed tray for processing several envelopes. When several addresses must be printed, it is more common to use labels. These come in pages and can be printed from lists using the mail merge feature.

Folding and Inserting Letters into Envelopes

The medical assistant should fold letters so that they can be inserted into envelopes easily. It is also important to use standard methods of folding so that letters are not damaged during opening.

No. 10 Envelope

To fold a letter in thirds, bring the bottom third of the letter up and form a crease. Then fold the top third down and make a crease. The second crease of the letter is inserted into the envelope first.

No. 6¾ Envelope

For a smaller envelope, fold the letter in half and make a crease. Then fold the right third in and make a crease. Fold the left third over the right and make another crease. The final crease of the letter is inserted into the envelope first.

Window Envelope

A letter for a window envelope must be folded so that the delivery address is visible through the window. The bottom third of the envelope is folded up to make a crease. The top third of the envelope is then folded back from the previous crease so that the delivery address shows on the outside of the letter. Patient statements are often mailed in window envelopes, and the format of the statement must be adjusted to the specific envelopes that the office uses (Figure 43-6).

Adding Postage

The medical assistant may add postage using stamps or postage meters or by printing postage from the computer (Procedure 43-3).

Postage stamps can be purchased at the post office or by telephone or mail from the USPS. Stamps can also be printed from the computer using software and stamp labels.

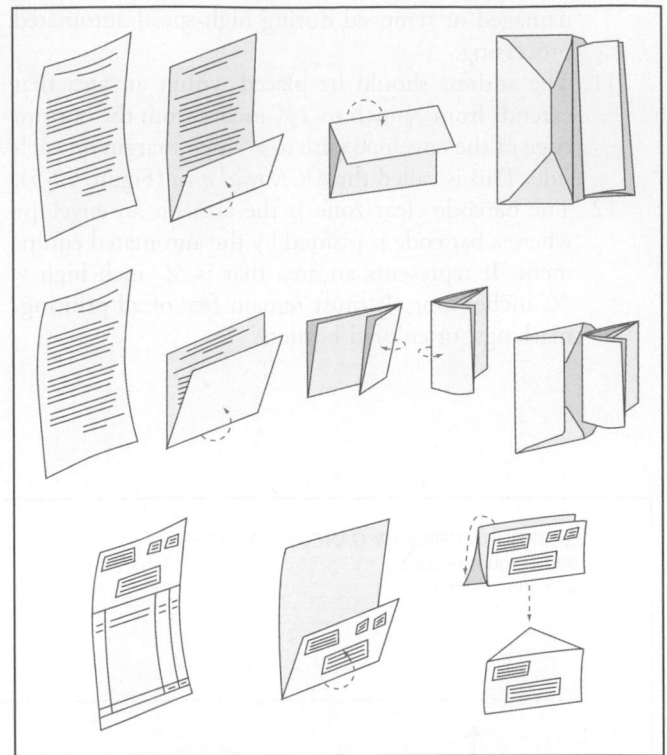

Figure 43-6 Correct methods of folding letters for envelopes.

The postage for a stamp printer is purchased online. Patient statements, which are usually sent First Class, require one First-Class stamp. Letters that weigh more than 1 ounce and envelopes that are larger than $6\frac{1}{8} \times 11\frac{1}{2}$ inches require additional postage. For these letters, an office would require either stamps of various values or a stamp printer, as well as a postage scale, for postage to be calculated accurately. It is not difficult to look up the correct amount of postage using the USPS website once the weight of an item has been established. Offices that regularly send out a steady volume of mail often use a mechanical postage meter or an online postage service.

Postage Meters

A **postage meter** is a machine that automatically stamps outgoing mail with the proper postage. Postage meters may be used for all classes of mail and for any denomination of postage. The postage can be printed directly onto an envelope or onto an adhesive tape strip that is affixed to an envelope or package. Mail that has been stamped by a postage meter is known as **metered mail.**

Postage meters cannot be purchased. Instead, they must be leased from one of the postal service's approved vendors. The amount of postage that can be stamped with the meter is predetermined and prepaid either on a regular basis, such as monthly, or when the amount remaining is getting low. Postage can be purchased by telephone or from the post office. In order to use a postage meter for bulk mailings, the medical office must apply for a bulk mailing permit and pay an annual fee.

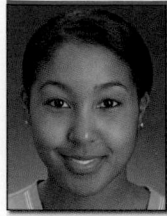
Many different types of postage meters are available, ranging from simple to complex models. The simplest model has only the ability to stamp the mail. More complex models, on the other hand, have security features and may automatically weigh the mail, fold and insert letters into envelopes, seal the envelopes, and catch envelopes in a stacker tray. Complex models typically consist of two separate components: the meter that adds the postage and a base that performs the other functions. A base that is compatible with the chosen model of postage meter can be purchased outright by the medical office.

Safety Precautions
Certain safety precautions should be followed when using a postage meter:
1. Read the operating guide carefully before operating the postage meter.
2. Do not touch any moving parts of the postage meter when it is in operation.
3. Make sure to keep loose clothing, jewelry, and long hair away from all moving parts of the postage meter.
4. Do not cover the ventilation slots on the machine to prevent overheating.
5. If a paper jam occurs, unplug the machine and make sure all machine mechanisms have come to a stop before clearing the jam.
6. Never attempt to disassemble the machine for repair. If service is required, contact the manufacturer's service representative.

Online Postage Services
The medical office may also subscribe to a service that allows the medical assistant to purchase, calculate, and print postage directly from the computer. These services usually allow the client to print stamps, print shipping labels, print postage directly on envelopes, and add special services (e.g., insurance, delivery confirmation, Return Receipt requested). The computer program can also check the accuracy of the address. Postal scales can be integrated with the computer software to calculate postage automatically. Online postage services offer increased versatility with respect to printing and personalizing labels, but if an office has a large volume of First-Class envelopes, a postage meter with envelope handling features may provide more efficient mail handling.

What Would You Do? What Would You *Not* Do?

Case Study 3
The medical office where Diane works has been using the same postage meter to prepare the mail for several years, and most of the staff is familiar with it. It usually works well when operated by someone who is familiar with it, but new staff members complain that it is "difficult." Diane is familiar with this postage meter and has used another model of postage meter, but she does not know anything specific about online postage services. At a staff meeting, the office manager suggests that it may be time to update the postage meter to a newer model. One of the physicians says that he has heard that the office could save money and handle the mail more efficiently using an online postage service. He asks Diane for her opinion. ■

PROCEDURE 43-3 Preparing Envelopes for Mailing

Outcome Address an envelope, and process envelopes to be mailed.

Equipment/Supplies

- Envelope
- Other items to be mailed
- Pen
- Typewriter

- Computer and printer
- Postal scale
- Postage meter (optional)
- Stamps

1. Procedural Step. Determine the exact address to be used to address the envelope. Addresses may be kept in a computer file or manually in an index card box or circular card file (e.g., Rolodex).

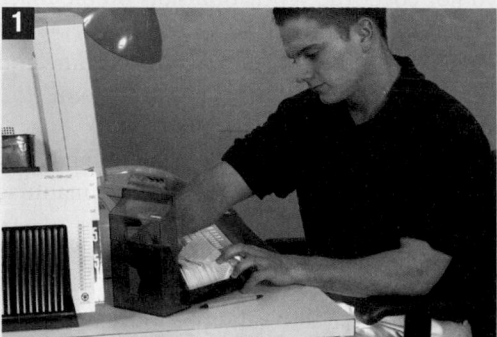

Look up the address in a rotary file.

2. Procedural Step. Select an envelope of the appropriate size. For business letters a No. 10 envelope is most commonly used. A large manila envelope may be used for documents containing several pages.

3. Procedural Step. Decide on a means to address the envelope (e.g., typewriter, computer, label printer). The address may be printed directly on the envelope or on a label. Avoid addressing ordinary correspondence by hand.
Principle. Standard business correspondence appears more professional if addressed using a typewriter or computer.

4. Procedural Step. Key the address in capital letters near the center of the envelope in the OCR read area with the name of the recipient on the first line, t the street address and apartment or suite on the second line, and the city, state, and nine-number ZIP code on the bottom line. If an additional line is needed for the apartment or suite, place it above the street address. Punctuation is not required except for a hyphen after the first five numbers of the ZIP+4 code. If using an envelope without letterhead, key the return address in the upper left corner using the same guidelines.
Principle. These are guidelines recommended by the USPS.

5. Procedural Step. Add any special notations, such as "Personal" or "Confidential," below the return address and above the address at the left side of the envelope.
Principle. Nothing must be placed below the address in order for post office equipment to read the envelope correctly.

6. Procedural Step. Add any mailing instructions or special services (e.g., "Certified") on the right side of the envelope above the address, leaving room for a postage label above.

7. Procedural Step. Place the item to be mailed in the envelope, folding it as needed, and seal the envelope (unless a postage meter with a sealer will be used).

8. Procedural Step. Weigh the piece of mail if it contains more than two sheets of paper or if an envelope larger than $6\frac{1}{8} \times 11\frac{1}{2}$ is used.
Principle. Large envelopes, rigid envelopes, and envelopes that are not rectangular require more postage than First-Class letters weighing less than 1 ounce.

9. Procedural Step. Calculate and apply the correct amount of postage. One First-Class stamp or equivalent is required for First-Class letters weighing less than 1 ounce. Postage for other items may be calculated from the USPS website, using a postage meter, or using an online postage service. If a postage meter is used, all envelopes to be mailed in one day may be processed together.

10. Procedural Step. Assemble all letters and other items to be mailed.

11. Procedural Step. Sort envelopes according to size.

12. Procedural Step. Separate any items with special mailing instructions that must be taken to the post office. If necessary, add instructions to the envelopes. If the office does not have a postal scale, include any letters that may need extra postage.

13. Procedural Step. Place items with postage in a mailbox, or request a pickup from the postal service.

14. Procedural Step. Take special items to the post office. This may include items that are to be sent Return Receipt, Certified Mail, Registered Mail, or Insured Mail and stamped items weighing more than 13 ounces.
Principle. Stamped mail and Priority Mail weighing more than 13 ounces will not be accepted from a mailbox even if proper postage is attached.

MEDICAL PRACTICE and the LAW

Certain hazardous and perishable items may be mailed through the USPS but are subject to specific packaging and labeling requirements.

- Diagnostic clinical specimens that are liquid or contained in liquid must be mailed in a sturdy, securely sealed watertight primary container cushioned in a secondary container. There must be enough cushioning to absorb all the material if the primary container were to break. If the material is or potentially may be infectious, both primary and secondary containers must be marked with the biohazard symbol.
- Noninfectious specimens (e.g., stool specimens for occult blood, newborn blood spots, slides for Pap tests, liquid Pap test bottles) may be mailed in a leakproof envelope or box without any special marking. In the case of a liquid sample, the outer packaging should be sufficient to absorb all material if the inner container were to leak.
- Sharps and regulated medical waste can be mailed only in approved shipping containers marked as containing regulated medical waste and bearing a properly prepared merchandise return service label held in the name of the authorized medical waste manufacturer. The container must be marked with the biohazard symbol, and there must be markings designating the normal upright position of the container. A shipping manifest (which should be provided by the medical waste company) must be affixed to the outside of the container.

What Would You Do? What Would You Not Do? RESPONSES

Case Study 1
Page 1028

What Did Diane Do?
☐ Asked Mr. Stone if he wanted her to send the form to sign for release of the medical record as an e-mail attachment.
☐ Informed Mr. Stone of the standard charge for copying a medical record and also whether he would be required to pay for postage.
☐ After receiving the consent form, took precautions to maintain privacy of Mr. Stone's record while photocopying it.
☐ Determined the best way to send the record so that it would arrive in time. Obtained authorization to send the record Express Mail or Priority Mail if it was not office policy to charge the patient for postage.

What Did Diane Not Do?
☐ Did not tell Mr. Stone that his request could not be granted because there wasn't enough time.
☐ Did not send the record until she had received the signed consent form to release the record.
☐ Did not criticize Mr. Stone for making an unreasonable request.
☐ Did not fail to follow up on this request.

What Would You Do/What Would You Not Do?
Review Diane's response and place a checkmark next to the information you included in your response. List the additional information you included in your response.

_____
_____
_____
_____
_____
_____

Case Study 2
Page 1029

What Did Diane Do?
☐ Searched for the correct (or complete) address of Dr. Leonie using other methods, such as looking up the address in the office's address file, looking at previous correspondence, looking up the address using the Internet, or calling Dr. Leonie's office.
☐ After locating the correct (or complete) address, looked up the ZIP code again until she obtained a complete ZIP+4 code.
☐ Finished preparing the envelope using the correct address and ZIP+4 code.

What Did Diane Not Do?
☐ Did not ask the physician to find Dr. Leonie's address for her.
☐ Did not send the letter using the five-digit ZIP she found from the first search.

What Would You Do/What Would You Not Do?
Review Diane's response and place a checkmark next to the information you included in your response. List the additional information you included in your response.

_____
_____
_____
_____
_____
_____

Continued

What Would You Do? What Would You *Not* Do? RESPONSES—cont'd

Case Study 3
Page 1035

What Did Diane Do?

❒ Stated that she was familiar with postage meters but that she did not know about online postage services.
❒ Gave her honest opinion about the ease of using the current postage meter.
❒ Offered to research the benefits and costs of an online postage service versus updating the postage meter.
❒ Offered to try to find out how much time it would take to orient staff to a new method of preparing the mail.

What Did Diane Not Do?

❒ Did not give a negative opinion of online postage services just because she did not want to cope with a system change.

❒ Did not automatically agree with the physician that changing to an online postage system would be a good idea.
❒ Did not say that the current postage meter worked very well if a person just took the time to try to understand it.

What Would You Do/What Would You Not Do?

Review Diane's response and place a checkmark next to the information you included in your response. List the additional information you included in your response.

_____
_____
_____
_____
_____
_____
_____

TERMINOLOGY REVIEW

Medical Term	Word Parts	Definition
Annotate		To underline or highlight important words and phrases in correspondence.
Barcode clear zone		The area on the lower right-hand corner of a card or letter that is left clear for the postal bar code to be printed.
Metered mail		Mail for which the postage has been applied using a postage meter.
Postage meter		A machine that automatically stamps a piece of mail with the correct postage.
Postal bar code		A series of vertical bars of two lengths, which represent the delivery address of a piece of mail. The bar code facilitates automated sorting of mail.
ZIP code		A five-digit code that identifies the post office to which a given piece of mail is to be delivered.
ZIP+4 code		A more detailed mailing code consisting of the original five-digit ZIP code followed by a hyphen and four additional digits. These digits identify a specific geographic segment within the delivery area.

ON THE WEB

For information on the U.S. Postal Service:

Calculate postage and look up ZIP codes: www.usps.com

Domestic mail manual: pe.usps.gov

Online postage: www.usps.com/business/online-postage.htm

Postage meters: www.usps.com/business/postage-meters.htm?

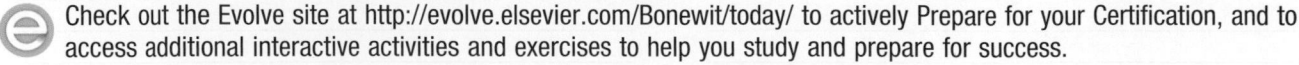 Check out the Evolve site at http://evolve.elsevier.com/Bonewit/today/ to actively Prepare for your Certification, and to access additional interactive activities and exercises to help you study and prepare for success.

$$44$$

Managing Practice Finances

1. Describe manual and computerized methods of maintaining patient accounts.
2. Differentiate between a simple charge slip and a charge slip with diagnosis and procedure codes (superbill).
3. Describe how a charge slip is completed.

Complete a patient charge slip.

4. Identify the information contained on a fee schedule, and describe how it is used.
5. Describe the information contained in a patient account ledger.
6. List the steps to post charges, payments, and/or adjustments to the patient account.

Post charges to the patient ledger.
Post payments and/or adjustments.

7. List the information recorded on a day sheet.

Record a patient's visit on the day sheet.

8. Describe the process to print patient ledgers and day sheets using a computerized billing system.

Use a computerized office billing system.

9. Identify various types of bank accounts.
10. Discuss the information printed on a check.
11. Describe various methods to write checks.

Write a check.

12. Describe how to balance a cash drawer.
13. Describe how a bank deposit is prepared and made.

Prepare a bank deposit.

14. Identify reasons why it is important to reconcile every bank statement.

Reconcile a bank statement.

15. Describe the components of accounts payable.
16. Describe how entries are made in the cash disbursement journal.
17. Describe how to maintain a petty cash fund.

Create and maintain a petty cash fund.

CHAPTER OUTLINE

INTRODUCTION TO DAILY FINANCIAL ACTIVITIES
Maintaining Patient Accounts
Components of a Patient Account
Charge Slip
Fee Schedule
Patient Account Ledger
Day Sheet
Printing Day Sheets and Other Reports

Banking Activities
Types of Accounts
Checks
Bank Deposits
Reconciling a Bank Statement
Other Financial Accounts
Accounts Payable or Record of Cash Disbursements
Petty Cash

KEY TERMS

ABA routing number
accounting
accounts payable
accounts receivable
accrual (ah-KREW-ul) basis of accounting
adjustment
assets
bookkeeping
cash basis of accounting

cashier's check
certified check
charge slip
credit
day sheet
debit
disbursements
fee schedule
invoice

ledger
liabilities
MICR line
payee (pay-EE)
petty cash
proof of posting
reconciling
superbill

INTRODUCTION TO DAILY FINANCIAL ACTIVITIES

A medical office is a business. The business of a medical office is providing medical services—one of the most important services in the entire economy. Because the medical office is a business, daily management of the practice's finances is key to the physicians' ability to provide the best services possible for patients. If the practice's bills are not paid and fees are not collected, the practice will cease to be a viable business and the patients will suffer.

Accounting is the term for systematic recording and reporting of financial transactions. The **cash basis of accounting,** which is generally used by medical offices, enters income when payment is received for services. This contrasts with the **accrual basis of accounting,** in which income is entered at the time of sale, even if payment has not yet been received. Companies that sell merchandise usually use the accrual basis of accounting. In both systems, expenses are entered when they are incurred, even if they have not yet been paid.

Bookkeeping refers to the process of keeping detailed records of financial transactions. Managing the daily finances is a task that often falls to a medical assistant. Professional accountants are usually responsible for general aspects of financial management, such as preparing detailed financial reports, financial planning, and preparing tax returns.

This chapter focuses on the parts of the daily financial activities involved in charging patients for the services provided each day, maintaining patient accounts and other **accounts receivable** (money owed to the practice), and managing the **accounts payable** (money the practice owes).

MAINTAINING PATIENT ACCOUNTS

Patient accounts make up the bulk of the medical practice's income. Some income might come from rental of space—for instance, to a particular laboratory for a specimen collection station or to a social worker, psychologist, or other specialist who consults for the practice. Other income may come from royalties—from a particular medical instrument that one or more of the physicians developed, for instance, or from a book written by the professionals in the practice. But the bulk of the practice's income will be earned on a daily basis from the charges for services to patients.

Patient accounts may be recorded manually or using a computer. Most medical offices use a computerized medical billing system, although they may maintain some manual records, such as a day sheet. A manual bookkeeping system uses the following:

- A daily journal, commonly called a day sheet, to record all transactions that occurred on that day.
- An accounts receivable ledger for each patient, to keep a record of transactions related to that patient.
- A cumulative record of financial activity for the month, both for the practice as a whole and for each individual physician; this information is recorded on the day sheet, and cumulative totals are carried forward throughout the month.

In a computerized billing system, the same types of records are maintained. When procedures are performed, charges for individual patients are entered into the medical computer billing program and automatically posted to the patient's account and the daily record of charges. In a similar way, payments made by the patient (or an insurance company) are posted to both the patient account and the daily record of charges. The computer program can access data to generate patient bills, insurance claims, and a variety of reports, including monthly statements, activity of individual physicians, and number of specific procedures billed.

Highlight on Bookkeeping Systems

The two most common systems for keeping records of accounts in the medical office are single-entry and double-entry systems. Historically, financial transactions were recorded in a book called a *ledger* with separate pages for individual accounts. In medical offices, separate cards began to be used for individual accounts (instead of pages of a book). These cards came to be called *ledger cards,* and in medical computer billing programs, a screen showing cumulative charges and payments for a single patient is called a *patient ledger.*

Single-entry bookkeeping system
The single-entry bookkeeping system is the simplest system. It requires at least three records:

1. A chronologic journal that keeps track of all charges and patient payments, such as a daily journal.

2. A journal that keeps track of payments made by the medical office, traditionally a checkbook but now usually an electronic check register.

3. A method to keep track of individual patient accounts; these used to be recorded on pages of a book, index cards, or ledger cards, but today they are usually accounts in a computerized billing program.

Although the single-entry system is simple, it lacks methods for cross-checking to prevent and/or detect errors.

Double-entry bookkeeping system
The double-entry system is the most complete type of bookkeeping system. However, it usually requires a trained bookkeeper or accountant in order to be used effectively.

Highlight on Bookkeeping Systems—cont'd

Every transaction is posted into two different records, as a credit in one and a debit in the other. A credit is a posting that is subtracted from the balance, and a debit is a posting that is added. Records of **assets**—money and property owned by the business and money owed to the business—are balanced against records of **liabilities**—money owed to others by the business.

A charge for service to a patient, for example, is a credit (added to the balance) in the records of assets because it increases the total assets; but it is a debit (subtracted from the balance) in the records of liabilities because it decreases the amount owed by the business.

The accounting principle

A common formulation of the accounting principle is as follows:

$$\text{Assets} = \text{Liabilities} + \text{Owner's equity}$$

where assets are property owned by the business, liabilities are debts, and owner's equity is the amount by which the owner's assets exceed liabilities.

When a double-entry bookkeeping system is used by a medical practice, the medical assistant is usually responsible only for keeping the daily journal and/or entering charges in the computer. The actual records of assets and liabilities are kept by an accountant. ■

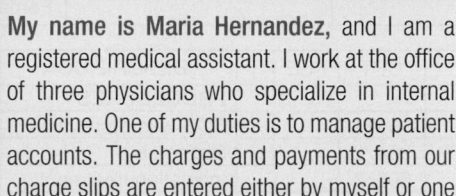

Putting It All into Practice

My name is Maria Hernandez, and I am a registered medical assistant. I work at the office of three physicians who specialize in internal medicine. One of my duties is to manage patient accounts. The charges and payments from our charge slips are entered either by myself or one of the other medical assistants, but I enter almost all of the payments we receive in the mail including checks from patients, as well as insurance payments. I am also responsible for paying the bills for the practice. We use two different computer programs, one for patient billing and another to manage our accounts payable and pay bills. We also use online banking, and we have set up automatic bill payment for those bills that occur every month including our mortgage, condominium fee, electricity, telephone, and answering service bills. We usually pay our other bills by check. The computer accounting program tracks all payments and prints checks. All of the physicians are authorized to sign checks under $500.00. If we purchase an item that costs more than $500.00, the check must be signed by any two physicians. When I was in school, I didn't appreciate what a big job it is to manage financial accounts. I really enjoy this part of my job now, and I have come to understand that it always saves time to work carefully and avoid mistakes. ■

COMPONENTS OF A PATIENT ACCOUNT

Four components are used to maintain a patient account, whether a manual or computer accounting system is used:

- Charge slip
- Fee schedule
- Patient account ledger
- Day sheet

Charge Slip

A **charge slip** is a means of keeping track of charges for services and payments made at the time of the patient visit. The charge slip is usually prepared before the patient visit and completed after the patient has been seen. In its simplest form, the charge slip contains the patient's name, the date of the service rendered, any procedures performed (including the visit itself), the total charges, and the amount the patient paid.

In traditional medical office manual accounting systems, a "one-write" or "write-it-once" system (also called a *pegboard system*) is used. All necessary forms are held in place on a metal or plastic board by a row of pegs across the left side. In this type of system, information from the top form is transferred to the forms below. Entering information once generates a charge slip and receipt, an entry on the patient's ledger card, and an entry on the daily journal (day sheet) (Figure 44-1).

Some offices continue to use a pegboard-mounted day sheet as a manual record of daily transactions. Pegboard charge slips and paper ledger cards are rarely used today because most offices use a medical computer billing program to keep track of individual patient accounts. The format of computer billing programs is based on the old pegboard system, however. A pegboard system may also be used to write checks and keep a check register.

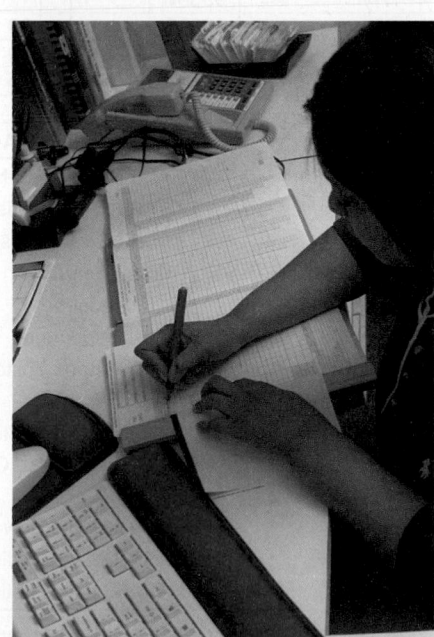

Figure 44-1 Medical assistant using a pegboard system.

When insurance companies began requiring numeric codes for procedures and diagnoses, a new type of charge slip was developed so that these codes could be identified at the time of service. A **superbill** (sometimes called a *billing encounter form*) is a form containing both diagnosis and procedure codes in addition to charges and payments.

Although simple charge slips are still sometimes used, most medical offices use a customized superbill as a charge slip. The top section of the form is filled out with patient information by using a printed label, filling it out manually, or printing the information on the form from the computer. Figure 44-2 shows an example of a completed superbill.

Western Medical Center
109 River Street
Western, OH 44770-0421
(490) 555-6464

Richard Warner, MD   NPI # 23456781XX
Maria Gomez, MD   NPI # 34567891XX
Tax ID 52-XX63777

Patient Name and Address	Birthdate	Subscriber Name	MD Name	Today's Date
DARLA SISSLE 10 MAPLE STREET WESTERN, OH 44770	2/17/52	DARLA SISSLE	WARNER	6/26/XX
	Account #	Insurance Company	Insurance Phone #	Time
	1015	SHHMO	(490) 565-2000	10:00 AM
Telephone No.	Insurance ID #	Group/Plan #	Sex
(490) 220-1156	21-58624	8300099	Male ☐ Female ☒

√	DESCRIPTION	CPT	FEE	√	DESCRIPTION	CPT	FEE	√	DESCRIPTION	CPT	FEE
	OFFICE VISIT				**IMMUNIZATIONS**				**PROCEDURES**		
	NEW PATIENT				Imm. admin, one	90471		√	ECG w/interpretation	93000	65--
	Problem Focused	99201			Imm. admin, each add'l	90472			Spirometry	94010	
	Exp. Prob. Focused	99202			Influenza < 3	90657			Inhalation treatment	94640	
	Detailed	99203			Influenza 3 and >	90658			Remove skin tag <15	11200	
	Comp/Mod MDM	99204			Medicare code	G0008			Cerumen removal	69210	
	Comp./High MDM	99205			Varicella	90716			Wart destruction < 14	17110	
	ESTABLISHED PATIENT				DTaP	90700			I & D abscess	10060	
	Minimal/Nurse Visit	99211			Td adult	90718					
	Problem Focused	99212			Rubella	90706					
√	Exp. Problem Focused	99213	65--		MMR	90707			**OTHER**		
	Detailed	99214			Hep B Child	90744					
	Comprehensive	99215			Hep B Adult	90746					
	Post-op Exam	99024	0.00		IPV	90713					
	WELL VISIT				**WELL VISIT**				**LABORATORY**		
	NEW PATIENT				ESTABLISHED PATIENT				Blood collection Vein	36415	
	Infant–1 year	99381			Infant–1 year	99391			Venipuncture, Medicare	G0001	
	1 yr–4 yr	99382			1 yr–4 yr	99392			Finger stick, glucose	82948	
	5 yr – 11 yr	99383			5 yr –11 yr	99393			Hemoccult, guaiac	82270	
	12 yr–17 yr	99384			12 yr–17 yr	99394			Strep, rapid	87880	
	18 yr –39 yr	99385			18 yr –39 yr	99395			UA, dipstick (manual)	81000	
	40 yr –64 yr	99386			40 yr –64 yr	99396			UA, automated	81003	
	65 yr and over	99387			65 yr and over	99397			Urine pregnancy	81025	

DIAGNOSTIC CODES (ICD-10-CM)

☐ R10.9 Abdominal Pain	☐ E11.9 Diabetes II–Non Ins	☐ H66.9_ Otitis Media	☐ Z23 Immunization Encounter
☐ E63.4 AllergicReaction	☐ K57.92 Diverticulitis	☐ J02.9 Pharyngitis	☐ Z00.12_ Well Child Check
☐ D64.9 Anemia	☐ K57.90 Diverticulosis	☐ M06.9 Rheumatoid Arthritis	☐ Z00.0_ Well Adult
☐ D51.0 Anemia, Pernicious	☐ R60.9 Edema	☐ R06.02 Short of Breath	☐ _____
■ I12.9 Angina Pectoris	☐ R51 Headache	☐ J32.9 Sinusitis	☐ _____
☐ I49.9 Arrhythmia, Cardiac	☐ R31.9 Hematuria	☐ L19.8 Skin Tag(s)	☐ _____
☐ I70.0 Atherosclerosis, Aorta	☐ B00.9 Herpes Zoster	☐ J02.0 Streptococcal Sore Throat	☐ _____
☐ J45.909 Asthma	☐ I10 Hypertension	☐ N39.0 Urinary Tract Infection	☐ _____
☐ M54.9 Back Pain	☐ E03.9 Hypothyroidism	**RETURN APPOINTMENT**	**BALANCE DUE**
☐ J20._ Bronchitis, Acute	☐ H61.2_ Impacted Cerumen	_____ Days	Total Charge $ 130.00
☐ J42 Bronchitis, Chronic	☐ J10.1 Influenza	_____ Weeks	Amount Paid $ 20.00
☐ R07.9 Chest Pain	☐ K58.9 Irritable Bowel Syndrome	_____ Months	Previous Bal $ 35.00
☐ J44.9 COPD	☐ M19.0 Osteoarthritis	_____ PRN	Adjustment $ 0.00
☐ E10.0 Diabetes I–Ins. Dep	☐ M19.0 Osteoarthritis		Balance Due $ 145.00

Figure 44-2 Completed charge slip (superbill) containing procedure and diagnosis codes.

When the patient is seen, the physician or other provider who sees the patient checks off the boxes next to the correct code for the type of visit (problem-focused, straightforward, detailed, low-complexity, comprehensive, moderately complex, and so forth), as well as any other procedures performed, and also fills in the patient's diagnosis.

Using the fee schedule, charges are added and any payments made by the patient are entered. The completed superbill is used to enter billing information into the computer. For this reason, it is extremely important to be sure that the superbill is filled out accurately.

Fee Schedule

A **fee schedule** is a list of charges for the various procedures a physician performs. Years ago, a physician had one set of fees that he or she charged patients for office visits, procedures, and/or treatments. Today, however, a medical practice may have to accept different amounts as payment for each service it performs, depending on which insurance provider is paying for the service. The reimbursement varies from a fixed percentage of the physician's charges to a set amount for a given service. Insurance is discussed in detail in Chapter 46.

The medical office usually has a basic fee schedule, listing the usual charges for office visits and procedures. The fee schedule is used to fill out charges on the charge slip or superbill. When a computer billing program is used, the amount charged for each procedure is linked to the procedure and usually comes up automatically when the correct procedure is selected. Most computer billing programs can link a patient's fees to his or her specific insurance fee schedules, such as Medicare and Medicaid (Procedure 44-1).

Patient Account Ledger

Each patient has his or her own account. It is important to verify that all information about the account is current

when the patient arrives at the office, because address information and insurance information can change between visits. A cumulative record of charges and payments is kept, usually using a computer program. It is also possible to keep account records manually. This record of charges and payments is called the patient account **ledger.** In a computer billing program, the patient account ledger is linked to the patient demographic and insurance information so that periodic bills and insurance claims can be generated. Information about services provided to an individual patient and payments received for that patient show up in chronologic order on the patient ledger (Figure 44-3).

After the charge slip has been completed, the charges are posted to the patient ledger (Procedure 44-2).

Posting Payments to the Patient Account

Payment for services performed can be received in four ways:

1. The patient pays at the time of service, in full, or in part (e.g., a copayment for managed care insurance). The office will accept cash and checks, and most offices also accept credit and debit cards.

Western Medical Center
PATIENT ACCOUNT LEDGER
April 20, 20XX

Date	POS	Description	Procedure	Provider	Amount
MILJU122		**Justin Miller**			
		Last Payment $15.00 on 4/11/20XX			
2/28/20XX	11		99213	RW	65.00
2/28/20XX	11	Carrier: SH was billed	CLAIM	RW	0.00
3/14/20XX	11		INSPAY	RW	−34.00
3/14/20XX	11		WROFF	RW	−16.00
3/20/20XX	11	Patient statement was billed	STATEMENT	RW	0.00
4/11/20XX	11		CHECK	RW	−15.00
				Patient Total	$0.00

Figure 44-3 Patient account ledger.

2. The patient may make a payment through the mail in response to a bill.

3. The patient may make an online payment using a credit or debit card through the medical practice website.

4. An insurance company may make a payment either by mail or, increasingly, by electronic transfer.

All payments must be posted to the account of the patient for whom they are made. Most computer programs have different codes for each method of payment. Cash and checks must match daily bank deposits. Payments using credit cards, online banking, or electronic transfer must later be matched to bank statements or online banking records.

Posting Adjustments to the Patient Account

A change to the patient account that is neither a charge for services nor a payment is called an **adjustment. Credit** (negative) adjustments are subtracted from the patient balance. Examples of credit adjustments include discounts for payment at the time of service, professional courtesy, and discounts given to insurance companies (also called *insurance write-offs*). Credit adjustments are usually discounts that are given in specific circumstances. (See Box 44-1 for common terminology used in accounting.)

Debit (positive) adjustments are added to the patient balance. Debit adjustments will be discussed in more detail in Chapter 47. When using a computer billing program, the medical assistant selects a code for each charge, payment, or adjustment. The correct mathematical operation is linked to the transaction code so that the computer automatically adds charges and debit adjustments (such as a returned check) to the patient balance and subtracts payments and credit adjustments (such as an insurance write-off). (Procedure 44-3).

Day Sheet

The **day sheet** keeps a running tally of the practice's income for that day and is a record of daily transactions. Even if a computer billing program is used, a manual day sheet may be kept as a control for data entry into the computer (Figure 44-4). A manual day sheet is also useful if the computer system is temporarily unavailable.

For each individual patient seen, the day sheet records the following:

1. Charges
2. Payments
3. Previous balance
4. Adjustments
5. New balance

A new sheet is used for each day. Each transaction is recorded on the day sheet in the order it occurs. This includes not only patient visits but also all checks received in the mail that day. Even though the checks pay all or part of a patient balance from a previous day, they are posted to the patient account on the day they are received and deposited. The day sheet usually includes a deposit slip that can

---

BOX 44-1 Common Terminology Used in Accounting

Account balance: The amount remaining in the account after all entries have been totaled.

Accounts receivable control: A summary of all unpaid accounts.

Adjustment: An entry to change an account balance that is not a charge for services or a payment, often a discount.

Credit: An entry that reduces an account balance, usually a payment.

Credit balance: The balance on an account when payments exceed charges.

Day sheet: The record of daily financial transactions (daily journal in a pegboard accounting system).

Debit: An entry that increases an account balance, usually a charge.

Disbursements: Money paid out.

Invoice: A bill or written statement describing a purchase or service and the amount due.

Journal: The original record of financial transactions that identifies the accounts to which they belong.

Ledger: A card, book, or computer database in which financial transactions are recorded.

Payables: Amounts owed to others.

Posting: Recording financial transactions or transferring information from one record to another.

Proof: Validation of calculations.

Receivables: Amounts of money owed by others.

ROA (received on account): Designation used for payments that reduce the amount owed but are not payment in full.

Trial balance: A method of checking the accuracy of calculations of accounts.

From Hunt SA: *Saunders fundamentals of medical assisting,* St Louis, 2007, Saunders.

---

be created as each payment is entered. At the end of the day, the day is closed (i.e., no further transactions are allowed for that day). (Procedure 44-4).

In addition, the day sheet has columns labeled "distribution" that can be used by the practice to itemize charges under several headings, commonly by the physician or other provider who generated the charge. However, these columns can also be used to track the type of procedure performed.

At the bottom of the day sheet is a section used to check for the correctness of the entries. In this area the daily totals are checked, as well as the monthly and year-to-date totals, which are carried forward from sheet to sheet. The process of calculating and comparing various figures on the day sheet is called **proof of posting.** The totals on a day sheet are often entered first in pencil. After the totals of each proof agree, a pen is used to rewrite all totals. Once the figures for the day are accepted, no changes are made to the day sheet. In a pegboard billing system, month-to-date and year-to-date running totals are calculated and carried

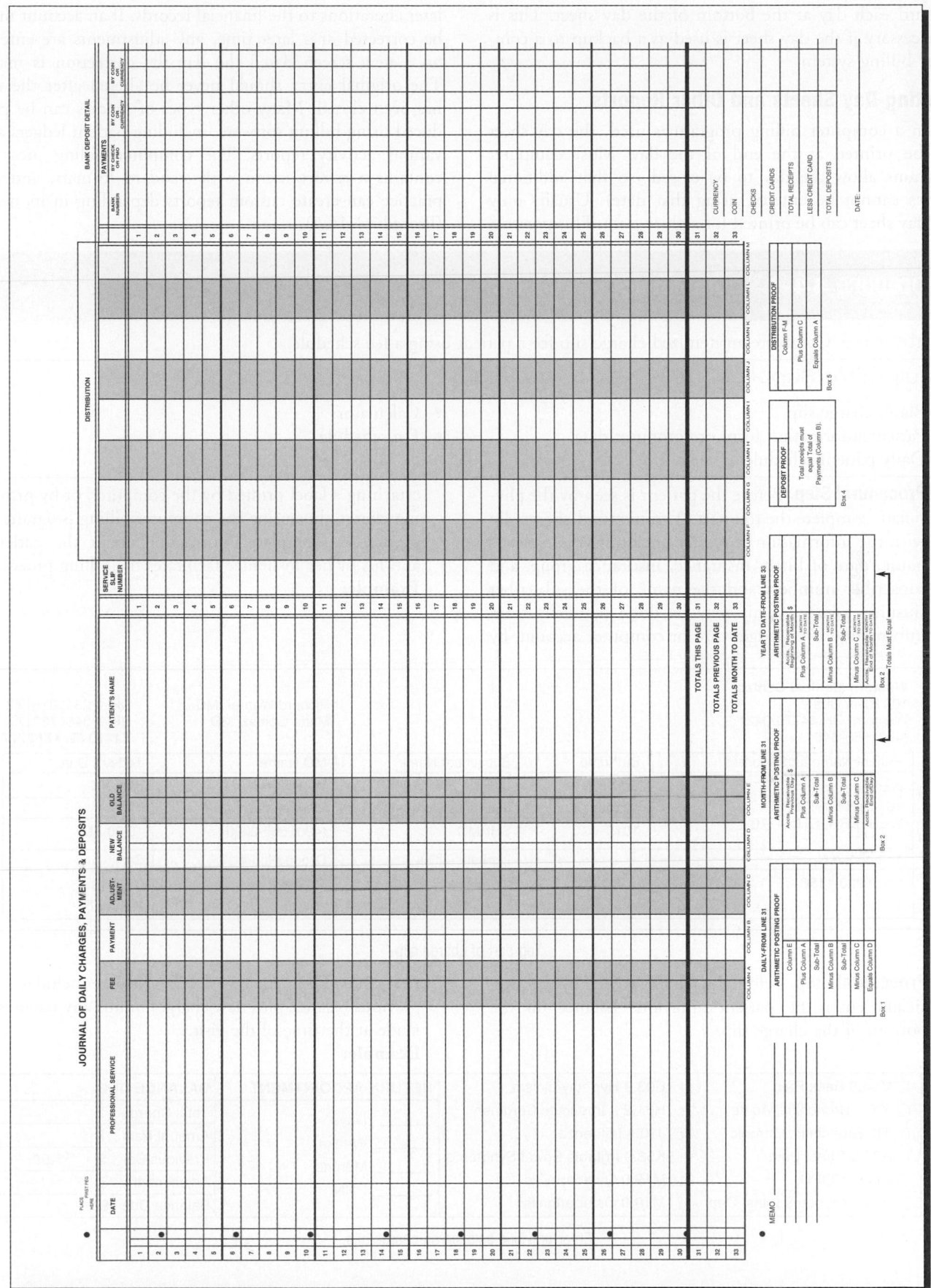

Figure 44-4 Day sheet.

forward each day at the bottom of the day sheet. This is unnecessary if the day sheet is used as a backup to a computer billing system.

Printing Day Sheets and Other Reports

When a computer billing program is used, the day sheet can be printed at the end of the day. Most computer programs allow the day to be closed (so that additional entries cannot be entered using that date). Usually only one day sheet can be printed for a given date. This prevents

later alterations to the financial records. If an account must be corrected at a later time, any adjustments are entered on a new screen dated the day the correction is made. The original entry should never be altered after the day has been closed. Many other types of reports can be produced using billing software, including patient ledgers and various activity reports. The computer billing program contains a report menu with standard formats, and the practice can create custom reports depending in its needs (Procedure 44-5).

PROCEDURE 44-1 Completing a Patient Charge Slip

Outcome Complete an itemized charge slip for a patient using a fee schedule.

Equipment/Supplies

- Blank charge slip
- Patient information form or computer data
- Daily patient schedule
- Calculator
- Fee schedule

1. Procedural Step. Before the patient is seen by the physician, complete the top part of an itemized charge slip with the information requested including the patient's name, date of birth, insurance, insurance group, and subscriber numbers and the name of the subscriber (insured person). This may be done manually from information on a ledger card or computer account, by

attaching a label printed by the computer, or by printing charge slips using the computer billing program. **Principle.** Complete information about the patient and his or her insurance facilitates the billing process.
Example:

Western Medical Center				
109 River Street Western, OH 44770-0421 (490) 555-6464			Richard Warner, MD Maria Gomez, MD	NPI # 23456781XX NPI # 34567891XX Tax ID 52-XX63777

Patient Name and Address	Birthdate	Subscriber Name	MD Name	Today's Date
DARLA SISSLE 10 MAPLE STREET WESTERN, OH 44770	2/17/52	DARLA SISSLE	WARNER	6/26/XX
	Account #	Insurance Company	Insurance Phone #	Time
	1015	SHHMO	(490) 565-2000	10:00 AM
Telephone No.		Insurance ID #	Group/Plan #	Sex
(490) 220-1156		21-58624	8300099	Male ☐ Female ☒

Top part of charge slip.

2. Procedural Step. Before the patient is seen by the physician, enter the patient's previous balance on the bottom of the charge slip.

Principle. The patient's account balance includes the previous balance plus new charges minus any payment made at the time of the visit.
Example:

		RETURN APPOINTMENT	BALANCE DUE	
☐ M54.9 Back Pain	☐ E03.9 Hypothyroidism		Total Charge $	
☐ J20._ Bronchitis, Acute	☐ H61.2_ Impacted Cerumen	_____ Days	Amount Paid $	
☐ J42 Bronchitis, Chronic	☐ J10.1 Influenza	_____ Weeks	Previous Bal $	35.00
☐ R07.9 Chest Pain	☐ K58.9 Irritable Bowel Syndrome	_____ Months	Adjustment $	
☐ J44.9 COPD	☐ M19.0 Osteoarthritis	_____ PRN	Balance Due $	
☐ E10.0 Diabetes I–Ins. Dep	☐ M19.0 Osteoarthritis			

Enter previous balance on charge slip.

3. Procedural Step. Using the fee schedule, fill in the charges on the charge slip by writing the fee for each service provided beside the line containing the correct code and procedure name (if the physician has not already done so).

Example:

3	√	DESCRIPTION	CPT	FEE	√	DESCRIPTION	CPT	FEE	√	DESCRIPTION	CPT	FEE
		OFFICE VISIT				**IMMUNIZATIONS**				**PROCEDURES**		
		NEW PATIENT				Imm. admin, one	90471		√	ECG w// interpretation	93000	65--
		Problem Focused	99201			Imm. admin, each add'l	90472			Spirometry	94010	
		Exp. Prob. Focused	99202			Influenza < 3	90657			Inhalation treatment	94640	
		Detailed	99203			Influenza 3 and >	90658			Remove skin tag < 15	11200	
		Comp/ Mod MDM	99204			Medicare code	G0008			Cerumen removal	69210	
		Comp./ High MDM	99205			Varicella	90716			Wart destruction < 14	17110	
		ESTABLISHED PATIENT				DTaP	90700			I & D abscess	10060	
		Minimal / Nurse Visit	99211			Td adult	90718					
		Problem Focused	99212			Rubella	90706					
	√	Exp. Problem Focused	99213	65--		MMR	90707			**OTHER**		
		Detailed	99214			Hep B Child	90744					
		Comprehensive	99215			Hep B Adult	90746					
		Post-op Exam	99024	0.00		IPV	90713					

Enter charges on charge slip.

4. Procedural Step. Complete the remainder of the charge slip by entering the total charges and payment made, and then calculate the new balance. The new balance is the sum of the total charges and previous balance minus any payment.

5. Procedural Step. Complete other information requested on the charge slip, such as the place of service and check number and/or method of payment.

Principle. The information on the charge slip must be complete and accurate because it will be used to post the charges and payment to the day sheet and patient ledger.

Example:

5			
☐ M54.9 Back Pain	☐ E03.9 Hypothyroidism	**RETURN APPOINTMENT**	**BALANCE DUE**
☐ J20._ Bronchitis, Acute	☐ H61.2_ Impacted Cerumen	_____ Days	Total Charge $ 130.00
☐ J42 Bronchitis, Chronic	☐ J10.1 Influenza	_____ Weeks	Amount Paid $ 20.00
☐ R07.9 Chest Pain	☒ K58.9 Irritable Bowel Syndrome	_____ Months	Previous Bal $ 35.00
☐ J44.9 COPD	☐ M19.0 Osteoarthritis	_____ PRN	Adjustment $ 0.00
☐ E10.0 Diabetes I–Ins. Dep	☐ M19.0 Osteoarthritis		Balance Due $ 145.00

Enter totals on charge slip.

Outcome Using the information from the completed charge slip, post patient charges to a patient account.

Equipment/Supplies

- Patient charge slip
- Patient ledger
- Fee schedule
- Pen or computer

1. Procedural Step. If using a manual system, post the charges from a completed patient charge slip on the patient ledger using one line for one day's services. Place the total charges for the services in the column labeled "charges." If using a computer program, post the first charge on the first line of the transaction entry screen. For most computer programs, entering the procedure code will prompt the computer to automatically generate the correct charge for the patient's insurance.

2. Procedural Step. If using a computer system, post each additional charge on a new line.

3. Procedural Step. If using a manual system, enter the total charge in the balance column. If using a computer system, save your work after all charges have been posted.

Example:

3	Charges:								
	Date	Procedure	Diag 1	Diag 2	Diag 3	Provider	POS	Units	Amount	Total
	3/21/XX	99213	I12.9			RW	11	1	65.00	65.00
	3/21/XX	93000	I12.9			RW	11	1	65.00	65.00

Transaction entry screen.

PROCEDURE 44-3

Outcome Post payments and/or adjustments to a patient account.

Equipment/Supplies

- Patient ledger card or computer
- Check or cash from the patient or payment from the insurance carrier
- Calculator
- Stamp with restrictive endorsement
- Stamp pad

1. **Procedural Step.** When a payment has been made, locate the patient account in the computer or select the patient ledger card.
   Principle. Both payments received at the patient visit and checks received in the mail must be entered to the correct patient account.
2. **Procedural Step.** Compare the amount of the payment against the total amount owed.
   Principle. The total amount owed will be the balance due and charges for new services.

3. **Procedural Step.** If using a manual system, post the payment from a completed patient charge slip on the patient ledger on the same line as the day's charges. If it is a check, record the number of the check. If using a computer program, post the patient payment on the same screen as the charges from the day's visit. Use the appropriate payment code for cash or check when entering the payment.

3 Charges:

Date	Procedure	Diag 1	Diag 2	Diag 3	Provider	POS	Units	Amount	Total
3/21/XX	99213	I12.9			RW	11	1	65.00	65.00
3/21/XX	93000	I12.9			RW	11	1	65.00	65.00

Payments and adjustments:

Date	Pay/Adj Code	Paid By:	Description	Amount	Check #
3/21/XX	Check	Darla Sissle	Patient Payment, Check	−20.00	144

Charges and payments entered into the computer.

4. **Procedural Step.** If posting an insurance payment, use a new line on a ledger card and a new transaction entry screen in a computer program.
   Principle. All payments are posted using the date of posting. In the case of insurance payments, this is not the same as the date of service.
5. **Procedural Step.** If using a computer program to post an insurance payment, use the code for an insurance payment.
6. **Procedural Step.** Enter the amount excluded by the insurance company as a credit adjustment. On a ledger card, enter in the adjustment column. If using

a computer program, use the code for write-off or insurance write-off, and the program will automatically deduct the amount.
Principle. The transaction code tells the computer whether to add or subtract the entry from the patient balance.
Example: The statement from the insurance company shows that the insurance company paid $57.00 on the claim for Michael Lee. It excluded $23.00, which must be entered as a credit adjustment or write-off. The patient's copayment is $20.00.

6

UNITED WESTERN BENEFIT
1220 SIXTH STREET
WESTERN RIDGE, OH 45770

FOR SERVICES PROVIDED BY: WESTERN MEDICAL CENTER

Name of Insured: Michael Lee

Patient/ Service	Service Date(s)	Total Charge	Excluded Amounts	Patient Copayment	Plan Paid Amount
Office Visit	11/24/20XX	$ 65.00	$ 15.00 EAC	$ 20.00	$ 30.00
Cerumen Removal	11/24/20XX	$ 35.00	$ 8.00 EAC		$ 27.00
Total		**$ 100.00**	**$ 23.00**	**$ 20.00**	**$ 57.00**

EAC: This amount exceeds the allowable charge for the service. The provider is prohibited by law from billing the patient for this amount.

Insurance explanation of benefits.

7. Procedural Step. Calculate the balance. (A computer program does all calculations.)
Example: The insurance payment of $75.00 has been entered as an insurance payment (INS). The excluded

amount has been entered on a second line as a write-off (WO). The computer program will calculate the patient balance.

	Payments and adjustments:				
Date	Pay/Adj Code	Paid By:	Description	Amount	Check #
12/15/XX	INSPAY	United Western Benefit	Insurance Payment	−57.00	
12/15/XX	INSWO		Insurance Adjustment	−23.00	

Insurance payment and insurance adjustment entered into the computer.

8. Procedural Step. Endorse a check using a stamp containing the practice name, the statement "For deposit only," and the number of the checking account.
Principle. This type of endorsement only allows the bank to deposit the check and prevents anyone

from cashing the check or using it in any other way.
9. Procedural Step. Place cash or a processed check in the designated drawer or money box for later deposit.

Outcome Post patient charges, payments, and adjustments on a day sheet.

Equipment/Supplies

- Day sheet or accounts receivable record
- Day sheet from the previous day
- Charge slips
- Ledger cards (optional)
- Checks
- Pencil
- Pen

1. Procedural Step. Prepare the day sheet by reviewing the appointment schedule. Place the day sheet on the pegboard and date the day sheet and deposit slip.
Principle. All day sheets and deposit slips must be dated.
2. Procedural Step. If using a complete pegboard accounting system, lay a bank of patient receipts on the pegs so that the top receipt lines up with the first line of the day sheet. If patients are given separate receipts or one copy of the charge slip as an itemized receipt, this step is not necessary.
3. Procedural Step. As each patient completes his or her appointment, enter information on the top blank line in ink including the name of the patient, the professional services provided (either abbreviations or procedure codes), the fee, payment, any adjustment, new balance, and old balance. If using a complete pegboard system, the charge slip and patient ledger card will be filled out at the same time as the entry is made on the day sheet. This happens automatically because the information is transferred from the charge slip to the patient ledger and day sheet when the top of the charge slip is completed. If using a computerized billing system, the charge slip is completed first and the information is then transferred to the day sheet and entered into the patient's computer account.

Principle. The day sheet is the journal of original entry, which is a running record of charges and payments made during the day.
4. Procedural Step. Complete the columns on the right side of the day sheet or accounts receivable record manually according to office policy by entering information tracked by the practice. This may include entering charges and payments for each physician in the practice, or it may include entering information about specific procedures performed.
Principle. This enables a practice to accumulate data about the financial activity of each physician or about specific procedures. If a computer billing program is used, this type of information can be tracked through the report features of the program.
5. Procedural Step. Record payments received in the mail on the day sheet and patient ledger when the mail is processed. Be sure to include insurance adjustments as needed.
Principle. Payments made at the completion of the visit are posted at the same time and using the same date as the charges. Payments made through the mail are posted using the date they are received.
6. Procedural Step. Record all payments on the deposit slip when they are received or processed. The deposit slip can be totaled at the end of the day and used as

the itemization for the deposit (see Procedure 44-7). A record can be made for the practice by filling out a duplicate deposit slip or by photocopying the deposit slip when it is complete.

Principle. It is more efficient to enter checks on the deposit slip when they are received.

Example: Two transactions on 11/24/20XX are as follows:

6

JOURNAL OF DAILY CHARGES, PAYMENTS, AND DEPOSITS

	DATE	PROFESSIONAL SERVICE	FEE		PAYMENT		ADJUST-MENT		NEW BALANCE		OLD BALANCE		PATIENT NAME
1	11/24/20XX	99213, 69210, ch # 282	100	00	20	00			80	00	0		Michael Lee
2	11/24/20XX	Ins pay, write-off			25	00	8	00	10	00	42	00	Sharon Smith

Entering charges and payments.

1. Michael Lee is seen as a patient for an office visit (99213) and removal of earwax (69210). He has no previous balance. He pays a copayment of $20.00 by check (no. 282). The charge is $65.00 for the office visit and $35.00 for the cerumen removal. His total charges are $100.00.

2. A payment from Sharon Smith's insurance company is received. The payment is for $25.00. The excluded amount (write-off) is $8.00. Her previous balance was $42.00. After the insurance payment and adjustment, she owes $10.00.

PROCEDURE **44-5**   **Utilize a Computerized Office Billing System**

Outcome Use a computerized office billing system to view and print reports such as a patient ledger and/or a day sheet.

Equipment/Supplies

- Computer
- Computer billing program

1. **Procedural Step.** Make sure the computer billing system is open, or open the computer billing program.
2. **Procedural Step.** To view or print a patient ledger, select the patient ledger function from the reports menu.

   Principle. The computer billing program can display all financial transactions for patients in a ledger format that displays charges, payments, and adjustments chronologically. The patient ledger format is modeled after the patient ledger cards that were used in the manual pegboard billing system. In the computer billing program, each patient has a ledger.
3. **Procedural Step.** Select the desired range of patients, range of dates, range of providers, or other criteria to create a report with the desired information. Use drop-down menus if they are provided. To select a single record, select the same name in both boxes of the range.

   Principle. Computer billing programs can select records to create reports using various filters. In the computer program, a range is a sorting device allowing records that meet specific criteria to be included in the report. Two values must be selected to delineate the range.
4. **Procedural Step.** If the report is several pages long, use arrows at the top of the screen to page through the report. Examine the patient ledger(s) for completeness.

Create a hard copy if desired by clicking the printer icon.

5. **Procedural Step.** To create a computer day sheet, select "day sheet" or "daily journal" from the reports menu. Some computer billing programs allow the day sheet to be created only once. The day sheet shows all transactions from a single day in chronologic order. If given a choice of type of day sheet, select a patient day sheet.
6. **Procedural Step.** Select the desired range, and preview the report. Usually the day sheet is viewed by date created.
7. **Procedural Step.** If the report is complete, a hard copy can be printed using the print icon.

   Principle. The day sheet represents the official record of charges and payments for a single day. Once accepted, it should not be altered, and corrections or additional transactions should be entered using a later date.
8. **Procedural Step.** Create additional reports as needed for your medical office. Medical computer billing programs allow a variety of analysis and activity reports to be created using the same type of process as discussed earlier.

   Principle. Analysis of financial activity is an important tool for practice managers to be sure that financial systems facilitate smooth operation of a medical practice.

What Would You Do? What Would You *Not* Do?

Case Study 2

When posting charges and payments for a new patient named Linda Harris, Maria notices that the physician has written in an amount for the patient's office visit that is $15.00 less than the usual charge for the service. The physician has also written an amount for a flu shot that was given that is $10.00 less than the usual charge. Maria notices that the patient has paid $75.00 on the account, which is about half the amount of the bill. In Maria's office the usual charge for every procedure is entered for every patient. On the rare occasions when charges are reduced, any reduction is posted as a write-off. ■

BANKING ACTIVITIES

If the medical practice is to pay its bills, including salaries for medical assistants and other employees, it must have money in the bank. Part of the responsibility of the individual who handles the office's financial management is maintaining the practice's bank accounts.

Types of Accounts

Businesses such as medical practices will generally have one or more of the following types of bank accounts—checking, savings, or money market accounts.

Checking Account

A checking account is an account in which the money held can be withdrawn by simply writing a check against the funds available. Many banks allow businesses to earn interest on their checking accounts as long as a certain amount of money remains in the account (the minimum balance). The minimum balance can range from as little as $500 to as much as $2500. Interest is the payment the bank makes to the owner of the money on deposit for the privilege of being able to use the depositor's money to make loans to other bank customers.

If the checking account balance falls below the minimum, the account does not earn interest and there is usually a monthly service charge and a charge for each check written against the account for the entire monthly reporting period in which the balance was below the minimum. Sometimes a bank will waive the minimum balance in the practice's checking account if the practice agrees to keep a higher minimum balance in either a savings account or a money market account.

Savings Account

A practice may want to keep cash that is not necessary to pay expenses in a savings account, which usually earns interest at a slightly higher rate than an interest-bearing checking account. A savings account does not have any check-writing privileges, but money can be withdrawn or transferred to the checking account if necessary.

Money Market Account

A money market account offers features of both savings and checking accounts. Money market accounts usually require a fairly high minimum balance (often $2500). However, they may earn interest at the money market rate—the rate at which major corporations lend to or borrow from one another for 10- to 30-day periods.

Money market accounts let the owner draw a specified number of checks per month without a processing fee. They often require checks to be for at least $500.

A medical practice might want to maintain a money market account in order to hold money for regular but infrequent expenses, such as quarterly, semiannual, or annual payments for malpractice insurance; licenses for physicians and other licensed professionals on the staff; or dues to the state, county, or local medical association or chamber of commerce.

Checks

Types of Checks

Checks are slips of paper used by a checking account owner to authorize payments to a third party **(payee)** for the amount of money written on the check. Paying by checks allows the medical practice to maintain a permanent record of the payments it makes for goods and services.

In addition to the checks from the practice's checkbook or money market account, the practice may have occasion to ask its bank to prepare a cashier's check to assure the payee (person or company being paid) that funds are available. A **cashier's check** is a check drawn on the bank itself rather than on an individual account. Because the bank assumes liability for payment of the check, a cashier's check is considered more reliable than the check of an individual or business. This might be the case if the office were purchasing a large piece of equipment for which the seller is unwilling to accept a simple business check. The bank may also guarantee a personal or business check by withdrawing the funds from the checking account at the time the check is issued. This is called a **certified check.**

Check Format

At the top of each check toward the right, under the check number, is a fractional number that identifies the bank on which the check is drawn. This ABA number, which is assigned by the American Bankers Association, designates the federal reserve bank zone, the state or territory, and the unique identification number for the bank on which the check is drawn. Across the bottom of checks is a set of numbers called the **MICR line,** written in magnetic ink. When checks are processed and "cleared" for payment from the issuing bank to the account of the individual making the deposit, this set of numbers is read by a magnetic ink character recognition (MICR) system. The MICR line contains the **ABA routing number** (the unique number of the bank), the account number, and the check number. Other information that is usually printed on a check includes the name and address of the account holder and the name of the bank.

Business Checkbook with Stubs

One type of business checkbook that is commonly used has three checks to a page with check stubs on the left on which to record the same information that is recorded on the check when it is written (Figure 44-5). The checks and matching stubs are preprinted in order. In addition, the stubs have room in which to write in the amount of deposits made; the stubs therefore act as a running checkbook ledger.

Computer-Generated Checks

A number of business accounting computer programs will generate checks and immediately post the payment to the accounts payable ledger. To use these systems, the practice will need to buy compatible blank checks for computer printing. The software can also generate the fractional bank number and MICR numbers, or they may be preprinted on the check forms.

Online Payment

Most medical offices pay bills online either as a single payment or every month. This is also popular with

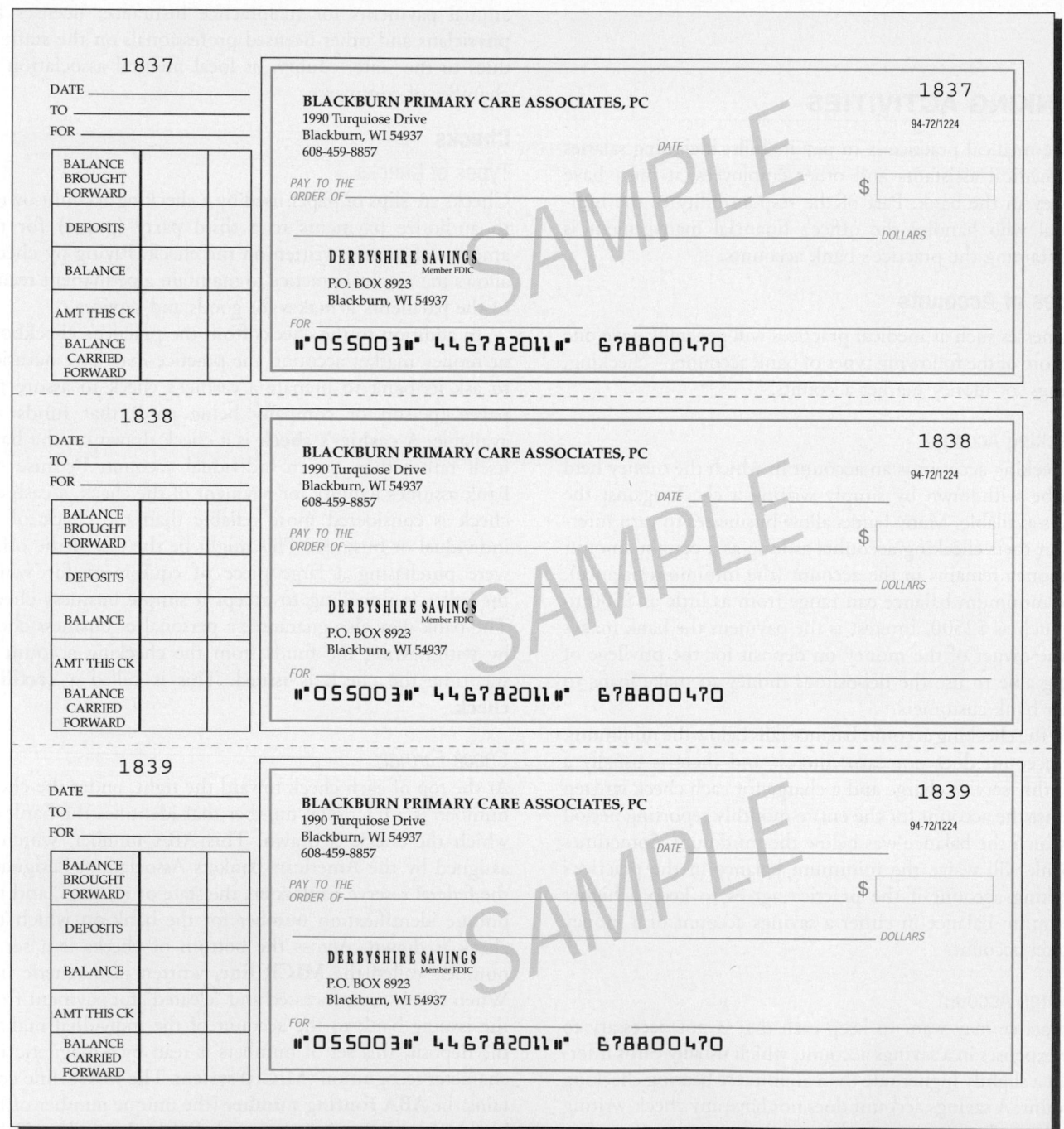

Figure 44-5 A business checkbook is often arranged with three checks per page and check stubs to record transactions.

suppliers, who create online accounts and accept payments directly using a pay-by-computer system.

Because some businesses still do not accept online payment, a medical practice will still need to write or print some checks. If an office handles its own payroll, it may encourage employees to use direct deposit instead of paper checks. Some practices may do all of their bill paying to regular suppliers, medical associations, liability insurance carriers, and other creditors online, and have their payroll checks written by an outside service provider, so checks are written only occasionally.

Preparing a Check

Checks are produced on watermarked paper to make it difficult for people to erase and then overwrite part of the check. The bank has the right to refuse to honor a check with erasures, overwrites, or other alterations. Minor corrections may be accepted if initialed by the person who signs the check. This protects the account holder from having people to whom checks are written cross out the amount and write in a larger amount. However, this also makes it important that checks be written carefully.

Most checks have at least one memo line—a line on which to write the purpose of the check. If the check is for payment of a bill or **invoice** (itemized bill), the invoice number or the account number for that particular vendor would go on the memo line.

If a mistake is made on a check, the medical assistant should write "void" on the check and check stub. The voided check should not be destroyed. It should be filed with bank statements and other account records so that it is available for the practice's auditors. When writing a check, the medical assistant should begin the amount in numbers immediately after the printed dollar sign and write the amount in words at the left side of the check. Legally, the amount in words is accepted as the amount for which the check is written if there is a discrepancy. After all of the checks for a particular period (week or month) have been written, they are attached to the supporting invoices and placed in a folder or envelope on the desk of the physician who is to sign the checks that week. In many practices, two physicians have check-signing privileges so that one can sign if the other is on vacation. Also, in some practices, checks exceeding a certain amount (e.g., $500, $1000) must be signed by two people; this is often a provision of that part of the practice's general liability insurance policy that covers employee theft (Procedure 44-6).

Bank Deposits

Balancing the Cash Drawer

As a first step to preparing the bank deposit at the end of the day, the cash drawer should be balanced. The office maintains a cash drawer or change fund so that patients can be given change for cash payments. The money should be in a drawer with compartments for bills of different denominations. The drawer may be moved to a safe at night depending on the office. A standard sum (such as $200.00)

in small bills is arranged in the drawer at the beginning of the day. At the end of the day, the money in the drawer should be counted, and the usual amount of cash on hand is returned to the drawer. Any additional cash should be removed, counted, checked against the receipts issued to patients, and added to the daily bank deposit. Usually the person who checks patients in has the key and is responsible for maintaining the cash drawer. Note that money from the cash drawer should not be used for petty cash. The office should maintain a separate petty cash fund, which is discussed later in the chapter.

Preparing a Bank Deposit

Every time a deposit is made at the bank, it must be recorded on a deposit slip. A deposit slip is an itemized listing of the cash or checks being deposited. Deposit slips used to itemize checks are found at the far right side of the day sheet (Figure 44-6). A deposit slip preprinted with the account number will be found in the back of the practice's checkbook. Deposit slips may also be created and printed using a computer accounting program. This allows for deposits to be entered in the computer records for the office's checking account. For making a deposit, the amount of the total cash being deposited is written on the cash line, with the total of the checks on the check line. An itemized listing of the checks being deposited must be included with the deposit. The numerator of the fractional bank number (e.g., 94-72) or the check number from the top right of the check should be entered on the deposit slip in the box to the left of the amount to identify each check (Figure 44-7; Procedure 44-7).

What Would You Do? What Would You *Not* Do?

Case Study 3

On January 4, Leonard Simpson pays $25.00 by check as a copayment at the time of an office visit. At the end of the day when Marla is preparing the daily deposit, she notices that the date on Mr. Simpson's check is January 4 of the previous year instead of the current year. ■

Highlight on Check Security Features

Because of the prevalence of color copiers, many security features are built into the paper used to print checks. The paper usually has a watermark that cannot be photocopied and/or invisible florescent fibers that can be viewed under black light. The paper should have erasure protection so that the background color fades if writing or printing is altered. The paper of the check may also have a chemical stain that reacts if chemicals are used to alter information. A word, such as "nonnegotiable" or "void," may appear if the check is passed through a photocopier or treated with chemicals. Various parts of the check usually have also been treated in a special way so that they will not be reproduced if the check is photocopied. The border and endorsement line usually include microprinting that will not be reproduced if the check is photocopied. ■

BANK DEPOSIT DETAIL

BANK NUMBER	PAYMENTS		
	BY CHECK OR PMO	BY COIN OR CURRENCY	CREDIT CARD
TOTALS			

CURRENCY

COIN

CHECKS

CREDIT CARDS

TOTAL RECEIPTS

LESS CREDIT CARD $

TOTAL DEPOSITS

DEPOSIT
DATE: _____   FIRM: _____

Figure 44-6 Bank deposit slip of the type found on the right side of a pegboard day sheet.

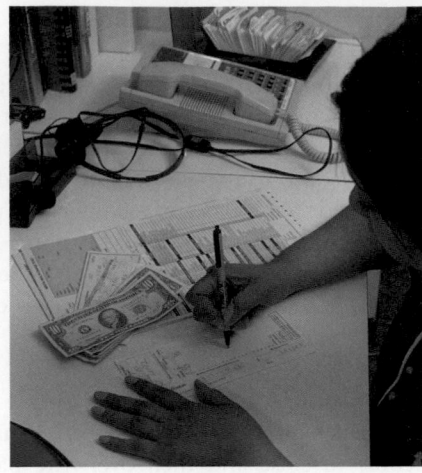

Figure 44-7 Medical assistant preparing a bank deposit.

Precautions for Accepting Checks

When a patient offers a check for payment at an office visit, the medical assistant should look at the check carefully to avoid accepting a phony check (see Highlight on Check Security Features). In addition, the medical assistant should make sure that the date and amount of the check are correct. A third-party check should never be accepted, even a payroll check. (Third-party checks are written to one party and later endorsed to another party.) If there is any problem with the check, it is very difficult to obtain reimbursement. Checks should only be accepted for the outstanding amount. If a patient needs cash, the medical assistant can direct him or her to the nearest ATM machine. A postal money order may have only one endorsement. If the patient presents a postal money order with more than one endorsement, the medical assistant should not accept it. A check with the notation "payment in full" written anywhere on the check should not be accepted unless the medical assistant is sure that the check covers the patient's entire outstanding balance. If a check is received in the mail with this notation, there are two options, and the medical assistant should follow office policy. The first option is to return the check to the patient with a letter explaining that the check cannot be accepted and requesting a new check. The other option is to write the following on the back of the check before endorsing it: "This check is deposited under protest, without prejudice, and with preservation of all rights of the payee against the drawer of this check pursuant to UCC § 1-207." The check should be endorsed under this disclaimer and can be deposited after both sides are photocopied. If the office accepts a check that claims to be "payment in full" without this disclaimer, the physician may forfeit the right to collect any balance due.

Endorsing Checks

Each check being deposited must have an endorsement on its back. An endorsement authorizes a bank to cash or deposit the check. Endorsements are of several types.

Blank Endorsement

A blank endorsement is a simple signature of the party to whom the check was written. Once a check has been signed, it can be cashed by anyone holding the check.

Special Endorsement

The special endorsement begins with a statement of the party to whom the check should be paid (usually using the words, "Pay to the order of …") followed by the signature of the party to whom the check was written.

Restrictive Endorsement

The restrictive endorsement begins with instructions that specify how the check can be paid out (e.g., "For deposit only"), followed by the signature of the party to whom the check was written. The bank must follow the instructions.

This type of endorsement can be entered on a check using a stamp approved by the bank that includes the words "for deposit only," the name of the physician or medical practice, and the bank account number. All checks received in the medical office should be stamped with the restrictive endorsement before deposit.

Making a Deposit

Deposits can be made in person or by using the night deposit box, usually located near the bank's front door. The night deposit box may require a key or personal identification number (PIN) code, which is supplied by the bank to customers who use it. (This prevents tampering or unauthorized use of the deposit slot.) Electronic technology now permits electronic readers to read the deposit bag's serial number, or there may be a radio frequency identification (RFID) tag in the deposit bag similar to the devices used for mass transit passes, parking passes, and inventory control.

Reconciling a Bank Statement

Reconciling a bank statement means making sure that the balance in the checkbook and the balance on the bank statement equal each other after adjusting for checks that were written but have not yet cleared through the bank and deposits recorded after the statement period ended.

Each month the bank will send the practice a statement of account activity, or the practice may access this statement online. The account balance at the end of the statement period will almost always be different from the account balance in the office's checking account ledger.

There are several reasons for this discrepancy. First, it usually takes about a week from the time the statement period ends until the office receives the statement, during which time more checks have been written. Second, checks written near the end of the statement period usually will not have cleared the account when the period ends. Third, some vendors and others do not promptly deposit or cash checks; thus some checks will not clear the account for a month or more. Fourth, bank charges are added to the statement for such things as checks returned for insufficient funds, per-check fees, and lockbox fees. Finally, interest may accrue on the balance during the month.

For these reasons, it is important to reconcile the bank statement with the office's checkbook to verify the arithmetic used by those who have written checks. Before reconciling, enter and subtract any bank fees in the office's checking account ledger and add any interest. The amount of all outstanding checks (checks that have not cleared the bank) should be totaled and subtracted from the "new balance" shown on the bank statement. The amount of any deposits made during the month that do not appear on the statement should be added to obtain a true balance. The figures may be taken from a paper statement or an online statement using a form such as the one shown in Figure 44-8. This true balance should match the balance in the office's checking account ledger (Procedure 44-8).

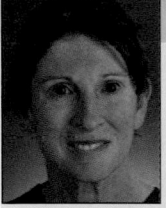

Outcome Write checks to pay bills for a medical office and record them in the checkbook or check register.

Equipment/Supplies

- Checks with check register or check stubs
- Monthly bills to be paid
- Pen

1. **Procedural Step.** Organize bills to be paid by opening envelopes and/or arranging invoices. Use a pen to prepare a check for each bill or invoice.
   Principle. This prevents alterations after the check has been written.

2. **Procedural Step.** Write the date on the line that says "Date."
   Principle. The date identifies when the check was written. Banks have specific policies that specify how long the check is valid.

3. **Procedural Step.** Write the name of the payee on the line of the check that says "Pay to the order of."

4. **Procedural Step.** Write the amount of the check in numbers in the box next to the dollar sign. When writing the numbers, use a decimal between the number of dollars and the number of cents.
   Example: $1568.42

5. **Procedural Step.** Write the amount of the check in words on the line below the name of the payee. Begin writing at the beginning of the line. When writing the words, remember that "and" is used only before the number of cents. Numbers such as 25 contain a hyphen when written in words (e.g., twenty-five). Write the number of cents as a fraction over 100. Draw a line from the end of the fraction to the word "dollars."
   Example:
   One thousand five hundred sixty-eight and 42/100————————DOLLARS
   Principle. Writing the amount in numbers, as well as words, helps prevent alteration of the amount of the check.

6. **Procedural Step.** Write the invoice number, account number, and/or purpose of the check on the line marked "for" or "memo."
   Principle. If the check is separated from the payment slip, this helps the payee identify what the check is for. It may also assist in record keeping after the check is returned by the bank.

7. **Procedural Step.** Record the date, check number (if not preprinted), payee, amount of the check, and reason the check was written on the check stub in the checkbook or in the check register.
   Principle. A record is kept of every check that is written.

8. **Procedural Step.** Subtract the amount of each check from the balance on the check stub or in the check register. If completing a check stub, enter and add any deposits since the previous check and add them to the previous balance. Then subtract the amount of the check and enter the new balance. Write the new balance on the stub of the check below in the box labeled "Balance carried forward."
   Principle. Keeping a running balance makes it possible to determine easily how much money is present in the checking account.
   Example:
   Completed check stub for a check to D&D Medical Supply.

8

1837

DATE 3/12/XX

TO D & D Med. Supply

FOR Invoice #JTS006

BALANCE BROUGHT FORWARD	4,482	21
DEPOSITS		
BALANCE	4,482	21
AMT. THIS CHECK	1,000	00
BALANCE CARRIED FORWARD	3,482	21

Filling out a check stub.

9. **Procedural Step.** If you make a mistake, draw a single line through the mistake, correct the error, and initial the correction.

10. **Procedural Step.** If the check cannot be used, write the word "Void" across the check and enter the word "Void" in the check register. Place the voided check in the folder where accounts payable records are kept.
    Principle. Keeping voided checks instead of destroying them facilitates accurate record keeping and provides proof that the check was voided.

11. **Procedural Step.** Prepare an envelope to mail the payment, or use a window envelope supplied by the vendor.

12. **Procedural Step.** Clip the prepared check to the envelope with the payment slip, and place it in the designated place for review and signature by the physician authorized to sign office checks.

PROCEDURE 44-7 Preparing a Bank Deposit

Outcome Prepare a bank deposit.

Equipment/Supplies

- Account deposit slip
- Deposit slip itemization record from the day sheet (optional)
- Cash and checks received as payments
- Calculator or adding machine
- Bank deposit envelope or bag

1. **Procedural Step.** Obtain an account deposit slip and place today's date on it. If the deposit slip from a day sheet is used, write the name of the medical practice and the bank account number at the top.
   Principle. The date, practice name, and account number must appear on the deposit slip so that the bank can credit the deposit correctly.
2. **Procedural Step.** Write the amount of currency and the amount in coins on the correct lines.
3. **Procedural Step.** Stamp each check with the restrictive endorsement, and write the amount of each check on the bank deposit detail with either the numerator of the fractional ABA number or the check number. If a deposit slip has been created as part of the day sheet, it can be used as itemization and clipped to the bank's deposit slip.
   Principle. A reference number for each check allows the bank to verify individual items if questions arise.
4. **Procedural Step.** Total all the checks and place that total on a deposit slip in the box for checks.
5. **Procedural Step.** Total the cash and total amount of checks for the total amount of the bank deposit. The

total amount of this deposit should be equal to the amount in the payments column on the day sheet or accounts receivable record for the given day.
6. **Procedural Step.** Make a copy of the deposit slip if a duplicate deposit record has not been made when creating the day sheet.
   Principle. The office should keep a copy of information regarding the checks and cash included in a deposit in case there are questions at a later date.
7. **Procedural Step.** Place the cash, checks, and deposit slip in a bank envelope or bank deposit bag and take or send it to the bank.
8. **Procedural Step.** Record the amount of the deposit on the accounts payable record and in the check register or on the check stub nearest to the date of deposit.
   Principle. This provides information on the amount of money in the checking account against which checks can be written.
9. **Procedural Step.** File the bank deposit receipt and copy of the bank deposit detail in a labeled file folder.
   Principle. All bank records must be saved for a period of time for tax and accounting purposes.

PROCEDURE 44-8 Reconciling a Bank Statement

Outcome Reconcile a bank statement.

Equipment/Supplies

- Monthly bank statement (paper or online)
- Checkbook and check stubs or check register
- Pen
- Calculator

1. **Procedural Step.** Open the current bank statement and locate the ending balance and the list of checks and deposits.
   Principle. Reconciling a bank account requires comparing the bank statement with the checkbook record of deposits and checks written for the same time period.
2. **Procedural Step.** Locate the same time period in the checkbook record of deposits and checks.
3. **Procedural Step.** Check the checkbook register against the bank statement and place a checkmark against each check and deposit that are recorded on the bank statement.

4. **Procedural Step.** Note those checks and deposits in your record that have not cleared the bank (i.e., do not appear on the statement).
   Principle. There are several days from the bank closing date on the statement until the statement is received in the office or practice. During that period, additional checks could be written and deposits made.
5. **Procedural Step.** Note any additional charges, such as service charges, ATM charges, or charges for returned checks. If there are additional charges, include them in the check register or on a check stub.
6. **Procedural Step.** Note any credits, such as interest. Include them in the check register or on a check stub and calculate the new balance.

Continued

PROCEDURE 44-8 Reconciling a Bank Statement—cont'd

Principle. To calculate the correct balance, it is necessary to include any charges or credits that do not already appear in the check ledger.

7. Procedural Step. Calculate the balance using a bank statement reconciliation form:

a. Start with the bank's ending balance.

b. Add any deposits listed on your check register but not listed on the bank statement to that ending balance.

c. Subtract any outstanding checks from that subtotal.

The balance on the bank statement should equal the current balance in the check register or on the last check stub.

8. Procedural Step. If the balances do not equal, recheck all calculations in the check ledger. If the check register still does not balance with the bank statement and you suspect an error, contact the bank.

THIS WORKSHEET IS PROVIDED TO HELP YOU BALANCE YOUR ACCOUNT

1. Go through your register and mark each check, withdrawal, Express ATM transaction, payment, deposit or other credit listed on this statement. Be sure that your register shows any interest paid into your account, and any service charges, automatic payments, or Express Transfers withdrawn from your account during this statement period.

2. Using the chart below, list any outstanding checks, Express ATM withdrawals, payments or any other withdrawals (including any from previous months) that are listed in your register but are not shown on this statement.

3. Balance your account by filling in the spaces below.

ITEMS OUTSTANDING	
NUMBER	**AMOUNT**
TOTAL	**$**

ENTER

The NEW BALANCE shown on this statement _____ $

ADD

Any deposits listed in your register $
or transfers into your account $
which are not shown on this $
statement. + $ _____

TOTAL

CALCULATE THE SUBTOTAL _____ $

SUBTRACT

The total outstanding checks and withdrawals from the chart at left _____ -$

CALCULATE THE ENDING BALANCE

This amount should be the same as the current balance shown in your check register _____ $

Figure 44-8 Bank statement reconciliation form.

OTHER FINANCIAL ACCOUNTS

In addition to taking money in, a practice pays money out. Some of this is done on a regular basis—for example, taking care of weekly or biweekly salaries, mortgage or rent, equipment leases, and utilities. Other payments are made in relation to specific invoices for materials or equipment.

Unless a bill is paid immediately when presented, it becomes part of the accounts payable (money owed by the business). A complete bookkeeping system notes each month any outstanding accounts payable, as well as the **disbursements** (payments) made during the month.

In addition, many offices keep a **petty cash** account, a small amount of cash available for everyday expenses. Again, petty cash must be recorded.

Accounts Payable or Record of Cash Disbursements

The record of cash disbursements is called the *cash disbursement journal*. In a one-write or pegboard system, cash disbursements are automatically recorded at the time each check is written out. In a computerized bookkeeping system, the cash disbursement journal is also automatically updated, or posted, when a check is drawn. In a single- or double-entry system, the cash disbursement journal must be separately maintained.

Each line of the cash disbursement journal has columns to record information about payments. Usually there are also columns to track expenses by categories. These features are also found in computer accounting programs.

Petty Cash

Petty cash is the cash kept on hand to pay for small, miscellaneous items, such as tips for a delivery, postage due, reimbursement to a staff member for parking at a meeting, or even a box of Girl Scout cookies for the office break room.

A check for a predetermined amount—usually $100 to $200—is drawn to cash to establish the petty cash account. It is important to keep each office account separate. Thus, cash should never be taken from any patient payment and put into petty cash. The petty cash account should always be funded via a check drawn on the practice's checking account.

A petty cash journal should be located near the cash box so that each disbursement can be recorded. Also, a pad of petty cash receipts should be available so that a receipt can be filled out each time a person receives money from the petty cash account. When the amount in the petty cash account falls below a predetermined amount (such as $20 or $30), a new check is drawn in the amount that will return the petty cash fund to the original starting balance (Figure 44-9).

Like any account, the petty cash account should be balanced on a regular basis. Staff members may need periodic reminders to fill out receipt forms every time they remove funds from petty cash (Procedure 44-9).

PROCEDURE 44-9   Creating and Maintaining a Petty Cash Fund

Outcome Create and maintain a petty cash fund.

Equipment/Supplies

- Bag or box with a lock
- Receipt slips
- Pen

- Petty cash log sheet
- Computer (optional)

---

1. **Procedural Step.** Set aside a predetermined amount, such as $100.00, in a secure location in a locked bag or box. The individual designated to be responsible for petty cash holds the key to the cash bag or box.
   Principle. The petty cash fund is used for incidentals, so the maximum amount is usually $100.00 or $200.00. The petty cash bag or box is kept locked to prevent pilfering.

2. **Procedural Step.** When a request is made for petty cash, the designated fund manager approves the request and fills out a receipt that includes the date, amount, and reason for the request. Filling in the amount may be delayed until the purchase has been made and change returned to the petty cash fund.
   Principle. Each purchase must be accounted for. The total amount of money in the petty cash fund should always balance against written receipts.

4. **Procedural Step.** The designated fund manager records the transaction in the petty cash log. This may be a paper log or a computer spreadsheet.
   Principle. The petty cash log summarizes all transactions.

5. **Procedural Step.** When the amount of cash falls below a predetermined level, a check is cashed to replenish the fund to its predetermined level. This is usually done weekly or monthly. The petty cash fund manager places the cash in the petty cash bag or box.

6. **Procedural Step.** The fund manager counts the money in the petty cash fund to verify that the fund contains the correct amount of cash. The old log and receipts are given to the accountant and a new log is started.
   Principle. The petty cash receipts and petty cash logs are retained for accounting purposes.

Petty Cash Log

Date	Description	Add Amount	Amount	Balance	Initials
10/1/20XX	Opening balance			$ 100.00	sh
10/4/20XX	Postage due		$ 0.52	$ 99.48	sh
10/4/20XX	Cab fare for Dr. Warner		$ 12.00	$ 87.48	sh
10/15/20XX	Coffee and creamer		$ 14.72	$ 72.76	sh
10/16/20XX	Refreshments for staff meeting		$ 22.83	$ 49.93	sh
10/17/20XX	Binder clips		$ 5.52	$ 44.41	sh
10/19/20XX	Flowers for Dr. Gomez		$ 22.75	$ 21.66	sh
10/26/20XX	Blank name tags		$ 12.95	$ 8.71	sh
10/31/20XX	Check to replenish petty cash	$ 91.29		$ 100.00	sh

Figure 44-9 Petty cash log created using MS Excel.

MEDICAL PRACTICE and the LAW

Medical offices are susceptible to embezzlement (stealing money or assets of a business) by employees. A questionnaire sent by the Medical Group Management Association in 2009-2010 found that 85% of responding practice managers reported being associated with a practice that had been the victim of employee theft or embezzlement. Medical assistants should be aware of measures that may be in place to reduce the incidence or impact of embezzlement. They should understand that measures to prevent fraud are also measures to ensure the financial health of the medical office as a business. These measures should not be interpreted as evidence that the employees are not trusted.

- Medical offices should check a candidate's references and job history carefully before hiring the candidate.
- The power to sign checks should be controlled, and all checks should be reviewed carefully. A signature stamp should not be allowed for signing checks.
- Job rotation should be encouraged, and employees should take earned vacations. Fraud is more easily spotted when different individuals handle financial transactions.

- Fidelity bonding is a type of insurance purchased by a business to provide reimbursement if embezzlement occurs. The medical office may purchase a blanket policy that covers all employees or a policy for specific individuals or positions within the office. This type of insurance may be part of the overall insurance plan for the medical office. Bonding deters illegal activity because bonding companies are known to prosecute perpetrators to the full extent of the law.
- Because cash is more difficult to keep track of than checks, receipts should be issued for all cash collected, using either a receipt book that makes a carbon copy or immediate entry into the computer billing program. Cash receipts should be accounted for on a daily basis.
- Employees should be encouraged to report any suspicious activity of other employees. Unfortunately, it is often a trusted employee with several years of service who has the best knowledge of the weaknesses of the financial systems of a medical office. ■

What Would You Do? What Would You Not Do? RESPONSES

Case Study 1
Page 1043

What Did Maria Do?
❑ Looked for the two missing charge slips at the front desk, in the physician's office, in the medical records of the two patients, and anywhere else that she thought they might be.
❑ Found out who had checked the two patients out and asked if that worker could remember what he or she had done with the missing charge slips.
❑ If Maria was unable to find the charge slips, she created new ones using the information from the day sheet.
❑ Verified that she had charged the patient for the correct services using the medical record and/or by checking with the physician who saw the two patients.
❑ Made a note of the numbers of the two missing charge slips so that they could be voided if they were found at a later time.

What Did Maria Not Do?
❑ Did not assume that the charge slips would turn up eventually and could be entered at that time.
❑ Did not leave the day "open" because she knew that two charge slips were missing.
❑ Did not assume that she knew what the charges should be based on the reason for each patient's visit.

What Would You Do/What Would You Not Do?
Review Maria's response and place a checkmark next to the information you included in your response. List the additional information you included in your response.

_____
_____
_____
_____
_____

What Would You Do? What Would You *Not* Do? RESPONSES—cont'd

Case Study 2
Page 1051

What Did Maria Do?
❑ Looked at the medical record and asked other staff members to determine why Linda Harris had been given a reduced rate. Possible reasons include a discount for cash payment or professional courtesy.
❑ If she could not determine the reason using other means, Maria asked the physician what the reason for the discount was.
❑ Entered the charges for Linda Harris into the computer at the usual rate. On a separate line she entered an adjustment of $25.00 ($15.00 for the office visit and $10.00 for the flu shot). She identified the reason for the adjustment (e.g., cash payment, professional courtesy) using the correct computer code.
❑ Also entered the amount of the patient's payment into the patient's account.

What Did Maria Not Do?
❑ Did not enter the charges as the amount indicated by the physician on the charge slip because that was not the office policy.
❑ Did not guess at the reason for the reduction in charges.
❑ Did not enter the usual charges into the patient account without making an adjustment.
❑ Did not tell the physician that she had written down the wrong charges for the patient.

What Would You Do/What Would You Not *Do?*
Review Maria's response and place a checkmark next to the information you included in your response. List the additional information you included in your response.

_____
_____
_____
_____
_____

Case Study 3
Page 1053

What Did Maria Do?
❑ Contacted Leonard Simpson by telephone to tell him that he had used the incorrect date on his check.
❑ Arrange to have Mr. Simpson either send or drop off a new check. When the new check arrived, Maria returned the check with the incorrect date to Mr. Simpson.
❑ Might also have arranged for Mr. Simpson to come to the office, change the date on the check, and initial the correction.
❑ Waited until the new check arrived to post the payment to Mr. Simpson's account and deposit the check.
❑ Corrected the charge slip and the day sheet to remove the payment from that day.

What Did Maria Not Do?
❑ Did not try to deposit the check with the incorrect date.
❑ Did not alter the date and put her own initials by the correction.
❑ Did not post the payment to Mr. Simpson's account until the new check arrived.

What Would You Do/What Would You Not *Do?*
Review Maria's response and place a checkmark next to the information you included in your response. List the additional information you included in your response.

_____
_____
_____
_____
_____

↻ TERMINOLOGY REVIEW

Medical Term	Word Parts	Definition
ABA routing number		A nine-digit number that identifies a bank; the number is printed at the beginning of the magnetic ink character recognition line at the bottom of a check. It also appears in fractional form at the top right of the check under the check number.
Accounting		Systematic recording and reporting of financial transactions.
Accounts payable		The outstanding bills of a business, such as a medical office.
Accounts receivable		Total amount owed to a business for goods and services.
Accrual basis of accounting		Accounting method in which income is entered at the time of sale or provision of service.
Adjustment		A change to a patient account that is neither a charge nor a payment.
Assets		In accounting, a combination of property owned and money owed to a business.
Bookkeeping		The process of keeping detailed records of financial transactions.

Continued

TERMINOLOGY REVIEW—cont'd

Medical Term	Word Parts	Definition
Cash basis of accounting		Accounting method in which income is entered when payment is received.
Cashier's check		A check drawn on a bank instead of an individual account.
Certified check		A check on an individual account that a bank assumes responsibility for, usually by withdrawing funds to cover the check from the checking account at the time the check is certified.
Charge slip		A form used to keep track of charges and payments at the time of a patient visit.
Credit		A posting that is subtracted from an account balance.
Day sheet		The record of daily transactions in the pegboard or "write-it-once system" and also in computer medical billing programs.
Debit		A posting that is added to an account balance.
Disbursements		Money paid out.
Fee schedule		List of charges (fees) for specific procedures that may be performed in a medical office.
Invoice		Itemized bill for goods or services.
Ledger		A book, card, or computer account used to record financial transactions.
Liabilities		In accounting, the amount owed by a business to creditors.
MICR line		A line of numbers containing the ABA transit routing number and the account number that appears at the bottom left of a check. These numbers are read by a magnetic ink character recognition (MICR) system.
Payee		The person to whom a check is made out.
Petty cash		A cash account kept in a business office to pay for incidentals, such as postage due and other small items.
Proof of posting		A process of calculation to verify that calculations on a day sheet are internally consistent and all totals are correct.
Reconciling		Making sure that two financial records agree, such as a bank statement and bank balance.
Superbill		An itemized charge slip usually also containing diagnosis codes and procedure codes required for insurance billing.

ON THE WEB

For information on Centers for Medicare and Medicaid Services (CMS):

Physician Center: www.cms.hhs.gov/center/physician.asp

Physician Fee Schedule for Medicare: www.cms.hhs.gov/PhysicianFeeSched

 Check out the Evolve site at http://evolve.elsevier.com/Bonewit/today/ to actively Prepare for your Certification, and to access additional interactive activities and exercises to help you study and prepare for success.

45

Medical Coding

LEARNING OBJECTIVES	PROCEDURES
1. Describe the history and rationale for using coding systems in medical care.	
Procedure Coding	
2. Describe the levels of HCPCS codes	
3. Describe the type of codes included in each section of the CPT manual (Level I HCPCS codes).	
4. Describe how to locate an accurate CPT code.	Perform CPT coding.
5. Identify when HCPCS Level II codes should be used.	
6. Describe how to locate an accurate HCPCS Level II code.	Perform HCPCS coding.
7. Perform procedural coding.	
Diagnostic Coding	
8. Describe the format and use of ICD-9-CM codes.	
9. Describe how to select an accurate code with the correct level of detail using ICD-9-CM codes.	
10. Describe the format and use of ICD-10-CM codes.	
11. Describe how to select an accurate code with the correct level of detail using ICD-10-CM codes.	
12. Perform diagnostic coding.	Perform ICD coding.

CHAPTER OUTLINE

INTRODUCTION TO CODING

Procedure Coding

Levels of Procedure Codes

CPT Manual

Sections of the CPT Manual

Looking up CPT Codes in the Index

Selecting a Specific CPT Code

Healthcare Common Procedure Coding System Level II Codes

Looking up HCPCS Level II Codes

Diagnosis Coding

History of Diagnosis Coding

ICD-9-CM Manual

Format of ICD-9-CM Codes

Using the Index (Volume 2)

Using the Tabular List (Volume 1)

ICD-10-CM Manual

Format of ICD-10-CM Codes

Using the Alphabetic Index

Using the Tabular List

KEY TERMS

established patient
inpatient
modifier
morphology (mor-FOL-o-jee)
NEC
neoplasm (NEE-oh-plazm)
new patient
NOS
outpatient
panel
sequela (seh-KWELL-a)
surgical package
upcoding

INTRODUCTION TO CODING

For hundreds of years, medical researchers have been interested in collecting statistics related to health and disease, including the number of individuals who contract certain diseases and the number of deaths caused by those diseases. To facilitate this undertaking, it was necessary for physicians to agree on a system to classify diseases and procedures. Lists of symptoms and diseases had existed in various countries for many years, but the first comprehensive disease classification system in the United States was published in 1869 by the American Medical Association (AMA) as the American Nomenclature of Disease. (The word *nomenclature* means what things are called; in essence, this book was a dictionary of diseases.)

Turning a classification system into a coding system requires systematic replacement of names with numbers or combinations of numbers and letters. This allows information to be standardized. Numbers or combinations of numbers and letters can be easily managed and manipulated by computers.

PROCEDURE CODING

Procedure codes are a means to classify the type of care given to patients. The three main reasons for developing what have come to be called *procedure codes* are:

1. To justify medical services to insurance companies by correlating procedures to diagnosis
2. To collect statistics about the outcome and effectiveness of treatments
3. To help physicians and hospitals set fees based on the amount of time and skill required to provide a specific service

In 1966 the AMA published the first edition of the *Current Procedural Terminology* (CPT) coding system. The original version focused primarily on surgical procedures and was one of many attempts to translate medical and surgical procedures into numeric codes.

Levels of Procedure Codes

The fourth edition of the CPT, first published in 1977, became the standard for insurance billing in the early 1980s, when it was used as the basis for a Medicare procedure coding system, the Healthcare Common Procedure Coding System (HCPCS), pronounced "hick-picks." Medicare, the government insurance program for the elderly and disabled, is administered by the Centers for Medicare and Medicaid Services (CMS). It will be discussed in detail in Chapter 46.

Level I Codes

The first level of HCPCS codes (95% to 98% of codes used for Medicare Part B) includes the current CPT codes. Level I codes are updated annually by the AMA, which publishes code books and electronic code sets.

Level II Codes

In addition, there are additional HCPCS codes for procedures, injections, and durable medical equipment covered by Medicare Part B that are not included in the CPT system. These are called *Level II codes*. HCPCS Level II code books are available from several publishers and can also be obtained electronically from the CMS. Each medical office must purchase updated versions of code books and/or computer files containing all codes used for insurance billing every year. In the past there were also local codes (Level III codes) used for Medicaid (the state-run insurance plan for low-income individuals), which varied from location to location. These have been phased out and are no longer in use.

CPT MANUAL

The CPT manual provides both a narrative description and a five-digit code for each procedure or service a physician or other licensed provider may perform for a patient. There must be documentation of a diagnosis in the medical record to support the need for any procedure performed for the patient and any procedure code used in billing the patient. Diagnosis coding will be discussed in the next section. In entering procedure codes on insurance claims in the outpatient setting, the five-digit code is sufficient for most procedures.

Sections of the CPT Manual

The CPT manual is used for most procedure coding. Its main part is divided into six sections, each of which defines the procedures and services provided for specific types of medical services. The six sections, and the range of codes for each, are as follows:

Evaluation and Management	99201 to 99499
Anesthesia	00100 to 01999, 99100 to 09140
Surgery	10021 to 69990
Radiology	70010 to 79999
Pathology and Laboratory	80047 to 89356
Medicine	90281 to 99199, 99500 to 99607

In each annual update of the CPT, new codes may be added for new procedures, old codes may be dropped for procedures no longer in use, and modifications may be made to current procedures. A darkened circle in front of a code indicates that the code is new. A darkened triangle in front of the code indicates that the description for the code has been changed or modified (Figure 45-1). The medical assistant must familiarize himself or herself with the important revisions each year when the new codes are published. In addition, codes must be updated in the office computer system and on office forms such as charge slips to be sure that insurance is billed correctly.

The main body of the CPT manual is organized by section, then subsection, subheading, and finally category,

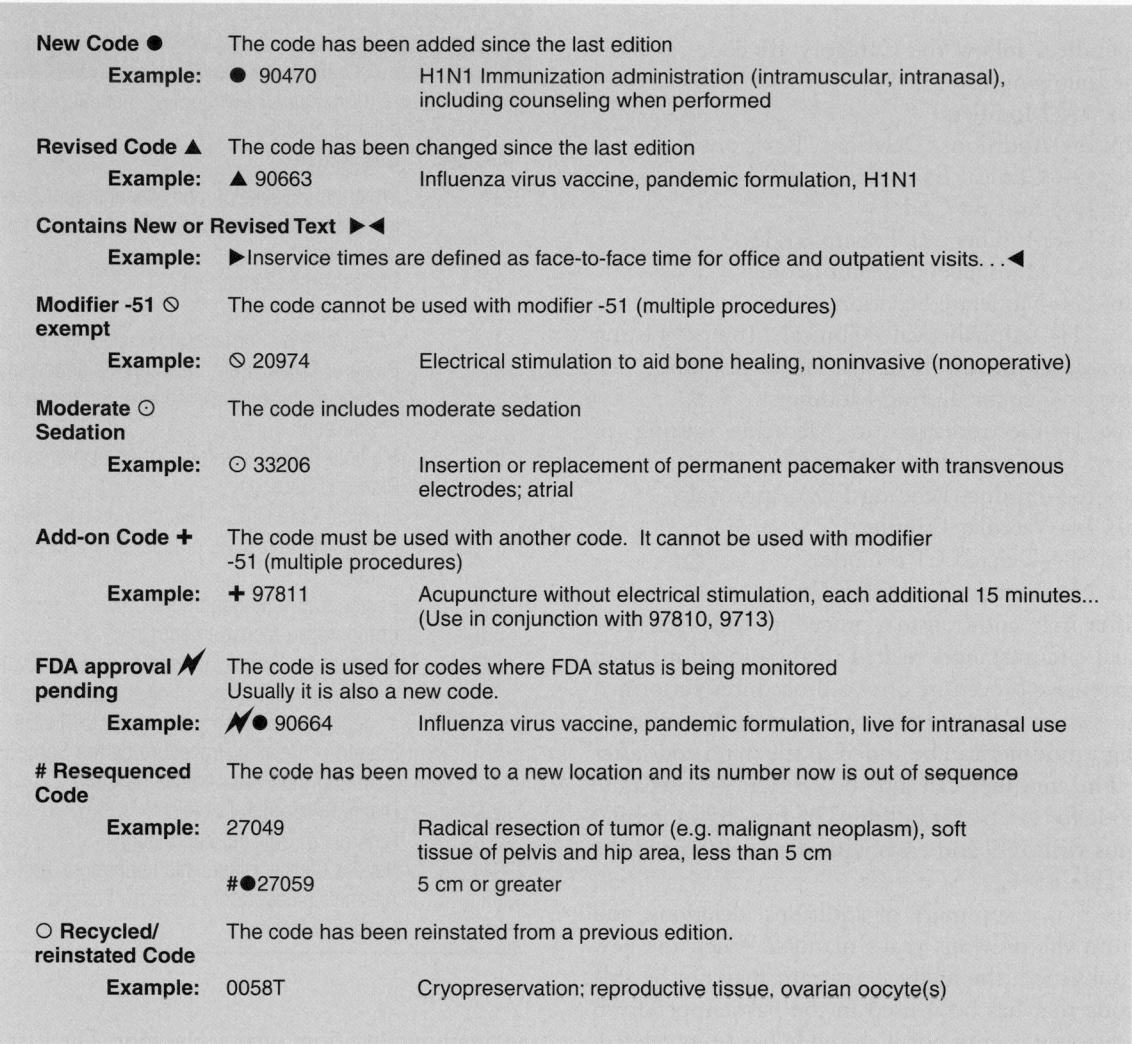

New Code ●	The code has been added since the last edition	
Example:	● 90470	H1N1 Immunization administration (intramuscular, intranasal), including counseling when performed
Revised Code ▲	The code has been changed since the last edition	
Example:	▲ 90663	Influenza virus vaccine, pandemic formulation, H1N1
Contains New or Revised Text ▶◀		
Example:	▶Inservice times are defined as face-to-face time for office and outpatient visits. . .◀	
Modifier -51 ⊘ exempt	The code cannot be used with modifier -51 (multiple procedures)	
Example:	⊘ 20974	Electrical stimulation to aid bone healing, noninvasive (nonoperative)
Moderate ⊙ Sedation	The code includes moderate sedation	
Example:	⊙ 33206	Insertion or replacement of permanent pacemaker with transvenous electrodes; atrial
Add-on Code +	The code must be used with another code. It cannot be used with modifier -51 (multiple procedures)	
Example:	+ 97811	Acupuncture without electrical stimulation, each additional 15 minutes... (Use in conjunction with 97810, 9713)
FDA approval 𝒩 pending	The code is used for codes where FDA status is being monitored Usually it is also a new code.	
Example:	𝒩● 90664	Influenza virus vaccine, pandemic formulation, live for intranasal use
# Resequenced Code	The code has been moved to a new location and its number now is out of sequence	
Example:	27049	Radical resection of tumor (e.g. malignant neoplasm), soft tissue of pelvis and hip area, less than 5 cm
	#●27059	5 cm or greater
○ Recycled/ reinstated Code	The code has been reinstated from a previous edition.	
Example:	0058T	Cryopreservation; reproductive tissue, ovarian oocyte(s)

Figure 45-1 Symbols that appear in the 2011 *Current Procedural Terminology (CPT)* code manual.

each providing a finer level of detail. The back of the manual contains an alphabetic index of procedures. The most common procedures performed in a given office are usually found on the charge slip and in the computer billing program. In the office itself, the provider usually checks off the codes for common procedures done during a patient visit and writes in the name of procedures not found on the charge slip. However, the patient may be billed from the medical office for services provided in another setting—for example, when a physician visits a patient in the hospital during morning rounds, when he or she examines a patient in the emergency room or a nursing home, and when he or she performs surgery in the hospital or an outpatient surgery setting. In most locations the office bills only for office services. If the office bills for labwork done by an outside reference lab, this must be indicated on the insurance form (see Chapter 46).

Category II Codes
Category II codes are optional codes that may be used to track performance. They are not reported to insurance carriers. The last character of these codes is the letter *F* instead

of a digit. Category II codes are found after the six main sections of the CPT. In addition, they are updated twice a year, and codes that have been added since publication of the most recent printed edition of the CPT can be found at the CPT website maintained by the AMA. Use of the code 1159F would mean that the medical record had been reviewed and a medication list was present.

Category III Codes
Category III codes are used to report services that represent emerging technology. They are temporary codes and can be used for up to 5 years. They consist of four digits followed by the letter *T*. These codes might be assigned to procedures (usually surgical procedures) that have not yet received U.S. Food and Drug Administration (FDA) approval. They are listed in their own section after the category II codes with an expiration date. Category III codes are updated twice a year and if available must be used instead of unlisted Category I codes. (Unlisted codes are used for procedures when no specific code can be found. They are found in the introduction to each section of the CPT manual.)

Appendices

Several appendices follow the Category III codes as indicated in the following list:

Appendix A—Modifiers

Appendix B—Additions, Deletions, Revisions

Appendix C—Clinical Examples for E/M Codes

Appendix D—Add-on Codes

Appendix E—Modifier -51 Exempt codes

Appendix F—Modifier -63 Exempt codes

Appendix G—Moderate Sedation codes

Appendix H—Alphabetical Clinical Topics Listing (removed and now only on the AMA website)

Appendix I—Genetic Testing Modifiers

Appendix J—Electrodiagnostic Medicine Listing of Sensory, Motor and Mixed Nerves

Appendix K—Product Pending FDA Approval

Appendix L—Vascular Families

Appendix M—Deleted CPT Codes

Appendix N—Resequenced CPT Codes

A **modifier** is an addition to a procedure code that indicates unusual circumstances related to the procedure, such as a more extensive procedure or two procedures performed in the same session. All modifiers are listed in Appendix A. The two-digit modifier can be added to the main code after a hyphen. The modifier can also be written as a separate five-digit code for electronic billing. The five-digit modifier always begins with 099 and ends with the two digits of the modifier (Table 45-1).

Appendix B is a summary of additions, deletions, and revisions from the previous year's manual. When the new manual is published, the medical assistant may not be able to find a code that has been used in the past. Appendix B provides a fast way to find out if the code has been deleted, changed, or included in another procedure.

Clinical examples of different codes are given in Appendix C. Reading these can be very helpful in learning how to decide what code to use, especially for E/M codes. The medical assistant should also become familiar with the other appendices in order to learn how to use them effectively.

Looking up CPT Codes in the Index

There are several steps in choosing a correct procedure code for a specific patient service. The first step in coding a procedure is to look up the procedure in the alphabetic index at the back of the CPT manual, but the code should not be recorded at this point. The medical assistant should never code directly from the index because it does not contain descriptions of the code and may result in use of an incorrect code.

It may be necessary to look up the procedure in several ways to locate the correct code. In the index, procedures may be located by looking under the name of the procedure, the anatomic location, and sometimes the diagnosis. The terms are arranged alphabetically with the main term in boldface type and modifying terms arranged below the main term. Each level of modifying term is indented further than the level above it. For example, the main term may be

Table 45-1 Selected CPT Modifiers Used in the Medical Office

(See the *Current Procedural Terminology* manual, Appendix A, for a complete list of modifiers.)

Modifier	Description
-21	Prolonged Evaluation and Management Services
-22	Increased Procedural Services (not used for E/M services)
-26	Professional Component
-32	Mandated Services
-47	Anesthesia by Surgeon (not including local anesthesia)
-50	Bilateral Procedure—This code is added to the second (bilateral) procedure performed at the same operation
-51	Multiple Procedures (performed at the same session)
-52	Reduced Services
-54	Surgical Care Only—This code is used when another physician provides preoperative and postoperative care
-55	Postoperative Management Only
-56	Preoperative Management Only
-57	Decision for Surgery (added to an E/M [Evaluation and Management] code when the physician makes the decision for surgery during an E/M visit)
-58	Staged or Related Procedure by the Same Physician during the Postoperative Session
-59	Distinct Procedural Service
-90	Reference (Outside) Laboratory
-91	Repeat Clinical Diagnostic Laboratory Test
-92	Alternative Laboratory Platform Testing
-99	Multiple Modifiers

an anatomic location, such as the foot. The first modifying term would identify either a condition, an anatomic location, or a procedure (such as Lesion, Nerve, or Repair). When a procedure is listed in the index (as the main term or any level of modifying term), it is followed by a code or range of codes (e.g., **Foot,** Nerve, Excision ...... 28055). Both main terms and modifying terms may point to a cross-reference using the word *See.* (See Figure 45-2.)

Several pieces of information may be significant when choosing the correct code for a procedure:

- Location
- Size of lesion or repair
- Method of performing the procedure, test, or surgery
- Number of minutes allotted for a treatment (e.g., acupuncture)
- Complexity of the procedure or service

Selecting a Specific CPT Code

After identifying a code or code range from the index, the medical assistant should read all relevant codes carefully in the main text. It may also be necessary to review the guidelines at the beginning of the appropriate section of the CPT manual to obtain additional information that can be helpful in choosing a code. The medical assistant should select the code that is the best match for the medical documentation

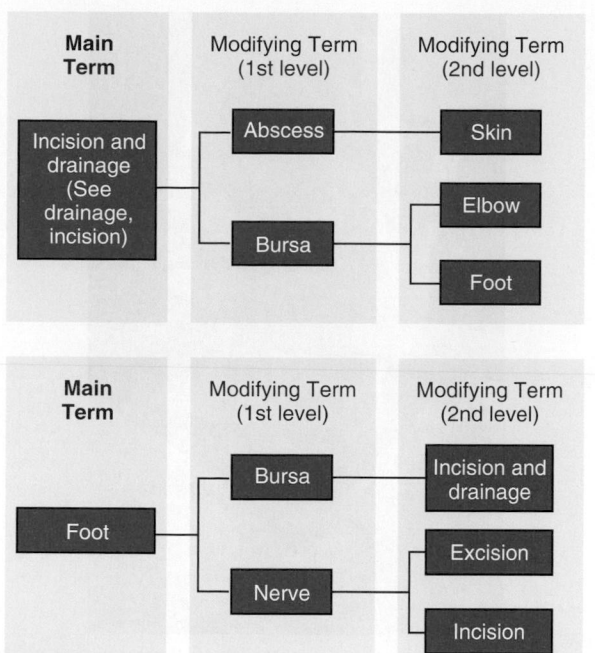

Figure 45-2 Examples of main terms and modifying terms in the index of the CPT manual when looking up the diagnosis *Incision and drainage of a bursa of the foot.*

and determine if it is necessary to use a modifier or an add-on code.

There are two types of CPT codes: stand-alone codes and indented codes. The stand-alone code contains a semicolon (e.g., 93000 Electrocardiogram, routine ECG with at least 12 leads; with interpretation and report). The indented code, which follows a stand-alone code or another indented code, provides only text to replace the words after the semicolon in the stand-alone code (e.g., 93005 [indent] tracing only, without interpretation and report). In the example given, the code 93000 would be used if the ECG tracing is made and the physician interprets the tracing in the same medical office. The code 93005 would be used if the ECG tracing is made in one office, but insurance should not be billed for the interpretation because it will be done by another physician and billed from another office (Procedure 45-1).

Evaluation and Management

The Evaluation and Management (E/M) section contains codes for office visits provided by primary care practitioners and specialists. E/M codes cover the service-oriented, rather than the procedure-oriented, parts of medical care. It is important to determine where the service was provided when selecting the correct E/M code.

Although procedures are fairly easy to define—for instance, incision and drainage of a cyst—the amount of service provided by a physician during an office visit is more difficult to describe. One physician may consider 20 minutes an appropriate amount of time for a visit, whereas another may consider 30 minutes the minimum amount of time to spend with a patient. One physician may focus strictly on the patient's presenting problem, whereas another may want to examine the patient more completely, especially if he or she has not been seen for several months.

The codes in the E/M section attempt to link reimbursement to the completeness of the examination and the amount of skill required to manage the patient's problems. Unfortunately, this may push the physician to limit the time spent with patients. If the patient does not have well defined, complex medical problems, the visit is reimbursed as uncomplicated, no matter how much time the visit took. For example, if a patient is in the office for a recheck of an ear infection, the visit would not usually take a significant amount of time. If the patient has several questions about methods other than antibiotics that could be used to treat ear infections, it will take more time for the physician to complete the examination, even though there is no additional medical problem or complication.

When determining the proper code for E/M services, the medical assistant must consider a number of factors.

1. For coding purposes, the patient is either an **established patient** (one who has been seen in the previous 3 years) or a **new patient** (one who has not had services performed by any provider in the medical office in the previous 3 years). There are separate groups of codes for each type of patient. New patients are expected to take longer to examine and are reimbursed at a higher rate. The patient is also either an **outpatient** (one who has not been admitted to a health care facility) or an **inpatient** (a patient who has been formally admitted to a health care facility). Although most services for patients who are inpatients are billed by the health care facility itself, physicians who are not employees of that facility bill for visits to the patient during a hospital admission, for inpatient consultations, for providing reports for some diagnostic tests performed at the hospital (such as cardiac stress tests), for critical care and intensive care services, as well as care for visits to patients in nursing homes.

2. There are separate groups of codes, depending on where the service is provided and whether the physician is the patient's primary care provider or a consultant. A medical service could have been provided in the office, in a nursing home, in a hospital to a patient who has been admitted, or in a hospital emergency department. The E/M section of the CPT manual is divided into several subsections, and it is important to select a code from the correct subsection, depending on the service that the physician provided and the location where the service was provided.

3. The level of service depends primarily on three key factors:
   • The extent of the medical history (number of body systems discussed)
   • The extent of the physical examination (number of body systems examined)
   • The complexity of medical decision making

Medical History

History taking consists of four levels: (1) problem focused, (2) expanded problem focused, (3) detailed, and (4) comprehensive.

- A problem-focused history is one that addresses the chief complaint, with a brief history of the illness or problem.
- An expanded problem-focused history addresses the chief complaint, a brief history of the present illness or problem, and a review of systems that have to do with the chief complaint.
- A detailed history addresses the chief complaint, an extended history of the present illness, and a review of body systems, including other systems beyond those related to the chief complaint. Family history is also reviewed as it relates to the present problem.
- A comprehensive history includes a chief complaint; an extended history of the present illness; a review of all body systems, especially those directly related to the present problem; and a complete family history.

Physical Examination

- A problem-focused examination is limited to the affected body system or organ.
- An expanded problem-focused examination is related to the affected body system, as well as other organs or systems that might be symptomatic. For example, the patient may be followed for angina (recurrent chest pain) and have a new complaint of calf pain when walking.
- A detailed examination includes the affected body systems or organs and other related systems or organs.
- A comprehensive examination is a multisystem examination, or a complete examination of one system.

Medical Decision Making

Medical decision making can be straightforward or have a low, moderate, or high level of complexity. If a patient has one problem, medical decision making is usually straightforward. When a patient has multiple problems, especially if they are causing severe or life-threatening symptoms, the decision-making process is more complex. For example, if a new patient has poorly controlled diabetes mellitus type 1, fever, and an increased white blood count, the decision-making process for the physician would be highly complex (Figure 45-3).

Secondary Factors

As secondary factors, the following may be considered when choosing an E/M code:

- Coordination of care
- Counseling
- The nature of the patient's problem
- The amount of time spent with the patient

Coordination of care refers to time spent arranging other services for the patient, such as home care or admission to a hospital or nursing home. Counseling includes discussions with the patient and/or family members reviewing the need for or results of diagnostic tests, discussing available

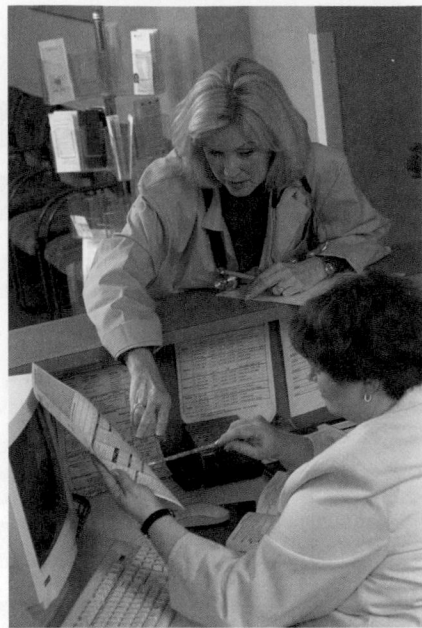

Figure 45-3 In the Evaluation and Management Section of the CPT manual, the type of decision making is one of the three key factors in selection of the correct level of service.

treatments and their risks and benefits, giving instructions, and so on. The nature of the patient's problem tends to determine the amount of service required and is usually found in the code description. For example, the description of code 99201 includes the following statement: "Usually the presenting problem(s) are self limited or minor." The amount of time spent is included in code descriptions as a guideline for code selection, but they are used for code selection only if more than 50% of the visit includes counseling the patient and/or family.

When coding for E/M services, it is vital to have documentation that supports the code chosen. Often the physician or other primary care provider checks the appropriate box on the charge slip at the time of the patient visit. Other times, the medical assistant may ask the physician about the level of service immediately after the visit (Figure 45-4). The medical assistant may also have to review the medical record when completing the insurance claim and decide which of the categories is supported by the physician's progress note. All of the key components must meet or exceed the stated level of care to qualify for a particular level of E/M service.

Anesthesia

Anesthesia is the administration of a drug that causes a total or partial loss of sensation. Anesthesia can be administered to provide analgesia (absence of pain) for a patient during a surgical procedure, wound closure, removal of a foreign body, childbirth, or a diagnostic test, including radiology, as well as for therapeutic radiology.

Anesthesia can be general, regional, or local. Local anesthesia by infiltration (the most common form of anesthesia

Type of Decision Making	Number of Diagnoses or Management Options	Amount of Complexity and/or Data to be Reviewed	Risk of Complications or Morbidity or Mortality
Straightforward	Minimal	Minimal or none	Minimal
Low complexity	Limited	Limited	Low
Moderate complexity	Multiple	Moderate	Moderate
High complexity	Extensive	Extensive	High

Figure 45-4 The medical assistant may need to question the physician about services provided to a patient.

used in the medical office) is included with the procedure and is not given a separate code. CPT codes for anesthesia are specified first by the anatomic region affected, then by the type of procedure. Anesthesia services are reimbursed based on a formula. Each anesthesia code is assigned a base unit value (B) which can be found in the Relative Value Guide published by the American Society of Anesthesiologists. The second component of the anesthesia formula is time (T), which is measured from the time the anesthesiologist first begins to manage a patient and ends when the patient is no longer under his or her care. Every 15-minute period is a unit. The final component is modifying units (M), which are assigned based on the patient's physical status as well as circumstances related to age. The total anesthesia units (B + T + M) are multiplied by a geographic factor to determine payment for anesthesia services.

The anesthesia section has two types of modifiers: standard modifiers and physical status modifiers. Standard modifiers are those used throughout the CPT code manual; physical status modifiers indicate the patient's condition at the time anesthesia was administered. Patient condition can influence the level of complexity of administering anesthesia in the proper dose over the proper time frame. The complete descriptions of these modifiers are found in the guidelines at the beginning of the anesthesia section of the CPT manual. Codes for conscious sedation (medication administered intravenously over a period of time to keep a patient calm without causing loss of consciousness) are found in the Medicine section.

Surgery

The surgery section is the largest section of the CPT manual. This section is organized by organ systems and within the systems by types of procedures.

Surgical procedures are coded as a surgical package. The term **surgical package** indicates that the code covers all routine services related to a surgery. The following areas are included in the surgical package and cannot be coded (or billed) separately:

- One evaluation and management visit that occurs after the decision for surgery has been made, either on the day before or the day of surgery
- Local or topical anesthesia or a digital nerve block
- Immediate postoperative care
- Writing orders for care after surgery
- Evaluating the patient in the recovery room
- Typical follow-up postoperative care

If complications occur during the surgery or during follow-up, treatment of the complications can be coded separately.

Radiology

The radiology section of the CPT manual includes radiology, nuclear medicine, diagnostic ultrasound, and radiation oncology. Radiology codes include both the technical component (creating the image) as well as the professional component (interpreting the image). If only one component is performed, this should be indicated by a modifier.

Most standard radiologic procedures are found in the diagnostic radiology subsection, including plain x-ray films, computed tomography (CT or CAT), magnetic resonance imaging (MRI), magnetic resonance angiography (MRA), and standard angiography. The codes for diagnostic radiology correspond to the anatomic site of the radiographic image, starting with the head and moving down. Some codes indicate a single view, whereas others indicate multiple views. The correct code may also indicate whether or not a contrast medium was used. In the outpatient setting, there is typically no additional charge for the physician's interpretation of the radiograph.

Pathology and Laboratory

The pathology and laboratory section of the CPT manual is organized by the type of tests performed, such as individual tests, panels, or assays. A **panel** is a group of laboratory tests, usually ordered together for diagnosis or screening, such as a cardiac panel (a group of tests ordered for a patient with cardiac symptoms). To use a panel code, each test in the panel must have been done. Additional or other tests are coded separately.

Different codes are used for laboratory tests performed by automated equipment and tests performed manually. When coding for a medical office, the medical assistant must be sure that patients are charged only for tests actually performed in the office (e.g., a dipstick urinalysis). If the medical assistant draws blood to be sent to an outside laboratory, the medical office charges the patient for the venipuncture (using the code 36415), but the laboratory bills separately for the diagnostic tests. The office does not charge separately for collecting urine and throat specimens if they are sent to an outside laboratory for processing.

Pathology testing, such as Pap tests and biopsies, is usually done by a special laboratory. The medical office charges for the visit or surgery during which the specimen is collected, but the laboratory usually bills for the actual specimen testing.

Medicine

The medicine section of the CPT manual gives the proper codes for noninvasive diagnostic and treatment services, many of which are performed in the offices of primary care physicians and specialists. (Invasive services, those that enter a body cavity, generally fall in the surgical section.) The medicine section is organized according to body system.

A number of highly specialized types of testing and treatment, ranging from electrocardiograms (ECGs) to ophthalmologic tests, are found in the medicine section. In addition, the medicine section contains the codes for immunizations and infusion therapies, including chemotherapy. Codes for procedures from this section that are performed frequently (e.g., ECGs in the office of an internist or cardiologist) are usually found on the charge slip and in the medical billing software. When a medical procedure is performed infrequently, the physician usually writes the name of the procedure on the charge slip, and the medical assistant may need to look up the code and enter it into the computer system for billing.

PROCEDURE 45-1   Performing CPT Coding

Outcome Perform CPT coding for procedures.

Equipment/Supplies

- Patient's medical record
- Charge slip
- CPT manual

1. **Procedural Step.** Find the name of the procedure to look up and information about the procedure (if necessary) using the patient's charge slip and/or medical record.
   Principle. The charge slip usually identifies the procedure(s) performed, but the medical record may be necessary to identify the appropriate level of service.
2. **Procedural Step.** For E/M services, identify if the patient is a new patient or an established patient.
   Principle. Different codes are used for new patients and established patients.
3. **Procedural Step.** For E/M services, identify if the patient was seen in the medical office or at another location, such as the hospital, emergency department, or nursing home.
   Principle. Different E/M codes are used depending on the location where the patient was seen. The coding and billing for visits provided by a physician to a hospitalized patient, nursing home resident, or patient in the emergency department are often done by staff at the physician's medical office.
4. **Procedural Step.** Using the index at the back of the manual, locate the section in which the category of codes will be found. You may need to look for the name of the procedure, the diagnosis, the type of patient, the location of service, or the location of the lesion.

Examples:
A. To locate an initial office visit for a new patient, look in the index under New Patient, Initial Office Visit (99201-99205) or under Evaluation and Management, Office and Other Outpatient (99201-99215).
B. To locate the code for a rapid strep test, look under *Streptococcus,* Group A, Direct Optical Observation (87880).

5. **Procedural Step.** Look in the manual at the code or range of codes to read the description and determine the correct code. Do not code from the index.
   Principle. You cannot be sure that you have identified the correct code without reading the description of the code. You may also find additional information in the section to help you code properly.
6. **Procedural Step.** If the service is unusual or does not seem to fit the description of the code completely, check the list of modifiers for the section of the manual to see if a modifier is necessary.

Example:
A patient has an abscess of the left upper arm, which required incision and drainage again today.
   1: In the index, you look up Abscess, Arm, Upper, Incision and Drainage. It refers you to codes 23930-23035.

Index*:

Abscess
(lines deleted)

Arm, Lower	25028
Excision	25145
Incision and Drainage	25035
Arm, Upper	
Incision and Drainage	23930-23935
Auditory Canal, External	69020

2: When you look at those codes, you see that these codes refer to deep abscesses.

Codes*:

Incision

(For incision and drainage procedures, superficial, see 10040-10160)

23030	Incision and drainage, upper arm or elbow area; deep abscess or hematoma
23931	bursa

3: You review the medical record and determine that the physician called the lesion a *subcutaneous abscess*.

4: For superficial abscesses, you are referred to codes 10040-10160. The code 10060 (incision and drainage of abscess: simple or single) appears to describe the procedure most accurately. Because the patient came for an office visit specifically for treatment of the abscess and no other E/M services were provided, you do not charge for a separate office visit.

Codes*:

Incision and Drainage

(For excision, see 11400, et seq)

10040	Acne surgery (leg, marsupialization, opening or removal of multiple milia, comedones, cysts, pustules)
10060	Incision and drainage of abscess (eg, carbuncle, suppurative hidradenitis, cutaneous or subcutaneous abscess, cyst, furuncle, or paronychial); simple or single
10061	complicated or multiple

7. Procedural Step. Enter the correct code(s) on the charge slip, on the encounter form, and if applicable in the patient's record in the computer so that it can be used for insurance billing.

Principle. Reimbursement is made by insurance companies based on the codes submitted. They must be accurate and reflect the service or procedure performed. In the example given earlier, the insurance company might refuse to pay for the service (as already provided) without the modifier, which indicates that it is in fact a repeat service of a procedure performed by another physician.

Putting It All into Practice

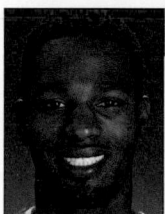

My name is John Grant, and I am a certified medical assistant. I work for a group of family practice physicians, and we have two offices. I am responsible for entering almost all of the information from the charge slips into the computer.

We have found that there is more consistency if one person is responsible for this task. Our physicians usually see patients in the office, but all of our physicians also visit their patients if they are hospitalized, visit patients in nursing homes, and sometimes see patients in the hospital emergency department in the evenings and on weekends. Each time a patient is seen in the office, a charge slip is filled out, and the physician checks beside the correct box for the type of visit. Our charge slips have the E/M codes on the slip so that we can distinguish between new and established patients, as well as levels of care provided. We also have all the codes for well visits and Medicare preventative services on the charge slip. When the physicians see patients in the hospital or in nursing homes, they fill out a log sheet we developed in the office so that we can be sure that we bill patients for all services and use the correct code for each service provided.

If the physician performs a procedure that is not on the charge slip, I look up the correct code and enter it into the computer system. In addition, I have to be sure that the correct place of service code is entered because insurance companies will reject a claim if the place of service does not match the service provided. For example, if I use the code 99281 for an emergency department visit, I have to be sure to use the place of service code 23 (emergency room—hospital).

I also look up diagnosis codes and enter them into the computer if necessary. The most common diagnosis codes are found in our computer system, but the physician often writes in a diagnosis that is not in the computer. The diagnosis has to correspond to the service, and sometimes the physician forgets to enter all of a patient's conditions on the charge slip. In those cases, I have to review the medical record to find the specific diagnosis that justifies a procedure. Coding is complicated, but in the long run it saves time to spend time making sure that the codes are entered correctly when the charges are entered. Otherwise, our insurance claims are rejected, and we spend a lot of time fixing mistakes and resubmitting claims. ■

What Would You Do? What Would You *Not* Do?

Case Study 1

When John is entering patient charges from the charge slips, he finds one charge slip on which the physician has checked the code for an expanded problem-focused office visit (99202) for a new patient named Peter Miller. John notices that the patient for whom he has a charge slip has other transactions in the computer from a previous visit about 12 months before the current visit. ■

HEALTHCARE COMMON PROCEDURE CODING SYSTEM LEVEL II CODES

HCPCS Level II codes use a five-digit alphanumeric coding system and designate specific services and equipment. Level II codes are used primarily for items and services that do not have Level I (CPT) codes. Examples of items with Level II codes include supplies, materials, specific medications, ambulance services, and some procedures. For example, if a patient is given a pair of metal underarm crutches after a cast is applied, the HCPCS code E0114 would be used to bill Medicare for the crutches. Note that the code begins with a letter that corresponds to the section of the Level II code manual. All codes are in the format of one letter followed by four digits, and they are arranged alphabetically by the first character and then numerically by the subsequent digits. Like CPT codes, they also have modifiers that should be used if necessary to clarify an individual code.

Level II codes are updated annually by the CMS. Most commercial insurance companies also accept Level II codes for covered items or services.

Looking up HCPCS Level II Codes

The process for locating accurate HCPCS Level II codes is almost the same as that for looking up CPT codes (Procedure 45-2). The medical assistant should first locate the item or service in the index at the back of the HCPCS manual. The index is in the form of main term followed by subterm(s). A single code or code range may be found in the index, but the medical assistant should always find the complete description in the list of codes before making a final selection. The codes consist of one letter followed by four numbers, and they are arranged alphabetically by the initial letter and then numerically by the four digits. Codes marked • are not valid for Medicare. They are used for other insurance carriers.

What Would You Do? What Would You *Not* Do?

Case Study 2

While entering charges for Joan Drysdale, a 72-year-old patient with Medicare insurance, John sees that the patient was charged for an intramuscular injection (90772) of methylprednisolone in addition to the office visit (99213). No other charges are listed on the charge slip. John needs to enter the charges and codes for this patient so that Medicare can be billed. ■

PROCEDURE 45-2 Performing HCPCS Coding

Outcome Perform HCPCS coding for services or equipment.

Equipment/Supplies

- Patient's medical record
- Charge slip
- HCPCS manual

1. **Procedural Step.** Refer to the charge slip or the patient's medical record to locate the service, supplies, or equipment requiring a HCPCS code.
   Principle. The charge slip usually identifies the procedure(s) performed, but the medical record may be necessary to identify more detail about the service, supplies, and so on.
2. **Procedural Step.** Using the index at the back of the manual, locate the code or range of codes. Look up medications in the Table of Drugs.
3. **Procedural Step.** Find the code or code range by locating first the initial letter (arranged alphabetically) and then the four-digit number (arranged numerically). Read the description and determine the correct code. Do not code from the index.
   Principle. You cannot be sure that you have identified the correct code without reading the description of the code. You may also find additional information in the section to help you code properly.
4. **Procedural Step.** Check to be sure that the code is valid for the patient's insurance.

Principle. Some HCPCS codes are valid for Medicaid or other insurance but not Medicare.
5. **Procedural Step.** Enter the correct code(s) on the charge slip, on the encounter form, and if applicable in the patient's record in the computer so that it can be used for insurance billing.
   Principle. Reimbursement is made by insurance companies on the basis of the codes submitted. They must be accurate and reflect the service or procedure performed.
   Example:
   1: To locate the code for an injection of diphenhydramine hydrochloride 25 mg, look up the drug in the index. (This medication may be given intramuscularly to treat an allergic reaction.) The code given for diphenhydramine hydrochloride is J1200.
   2: Look for the code in the list of codes first under J, then under 1200. The entry J1200 states that this code covers injections up to 50 mg. It would therefore be the correct code for this example.

DIAGNOSIS CODING

History of Diagnosis Coding

In addition to coding procedures, it is also necessary to code a patient's diagnosis or diagnoses. Diagnostic coding was originally developed to fulfill four purposes: track disease processes, classify the causes of death, collect data for medical research, and evaluate hospital service utilization.

In 1948 the World Health Organization (WHO) published the first edition of the *International Classification of Diseases,* which assigned numbers to specific diseases. This system was developed so that more accurate statistics could be collected about how often diseases and accidents occurred and were treated. The system proved to be useful for health care review and insurance claims processing.

WHO has revised the International Classification of Diseases several times since then. For insurance coding and review of medical records, a clinical modification tool was developed to better collect and compile data about specific diseases, conditions, and medical services for healthy individuals. The acronym for this coding system was ICD-9-CM, which stands for *International Classification of Diseases, Ninth Revision, Clinical Modification.* The ICD-9-CM became the system of choice for diagnostic coding after 1989. At that time Medicare began to require ICD-9 codes on all outpatient insurance claims forms. This soon became a requirement of all insurance companies.

The tenth edition (ICD-10) was published in 1993 by WHO. It has been used extensively in other parts of the world, but its acceptance in the United States has been delayed to October 1, 2014. This book will present both coding systems with greater emphasis on the ICD-10. For those who are accustomed to coding using the ICD-9-CM, it is important to note that there are five times more codes in the ICD-10. This allows for more precise coding of body part and patient encounter information. The ICD-9 coding system uses five alphanumeric characters with a decimal point after the third character. The only character that can be a letter is the first one. Compared with the ICD-9-CM, the ICD-10-CM includes several new features, such as the following:

- More extensive information related to ambulatory care and managed care encounters
- An expansion of injury codes
- New combination diagnosis and symptom codes to decrease the need for two codes
- An added sixth and seventh digit for some conditions
- Increased ability to locate and choose specific codes

In the ICD-10, for example, it is required for both diabetes mellitus and its complications to use a code that identifies the specific type or cause of the diabetes (type 1, type 2, due to drug or chemical, gestational, other, and so on). Conversion tables are available, but they are primarily useful for individuals who are already very familiar with the ICD-9.

It is necessary to use one or more diagnosis codes to have an insurance claim approved for reimbursement. If the proper ICD code(s) and coding format are not used, many insurance companies will reject a claim because the patient's diagnosis does not justify the procedures done for the patient. ICD coding is required by government-financed programs, such as Medicare and Medicaid, as well as most private insurance companies. The U.S. Department of Health and Human Services (HHS) is responsible for mandating accepted standards of electronic transmission and required code sets. As of January 1, 2012, the standard for transmission has been changed to Version 5010 which accommodates the longer ICD-10 codes.

ICD-9-CM MANUAL

The ICD-9-CM manual has three volumes. Volume 1 contains a tabular list of diseases, arranged numerically by disease classification. Volume 2 contains an alphabetic listing of diseases. Volumes 1 and 2 are used primarily in physicians' offices. In many handbooks, the index (Volume 2) is placed first and is followed by the tabular list of diseases (Volume 1). Volume 3, which has both a numeric tabular listing and an alphabetic listing of procedures, is primarily used in hospitals instead of the CPT manual. Volume III will be replaced by ICD-10-PCS.

Format of ICD-9-CM Codes

ICD-9-CM codes consist of three digits (from 001 to 999) that can be preceded by a letter and/or followed by a decimal point plus one or two additional digits. Digits after the decimal point make a given diagnosis more specific. They are arranged in numeric order. Following the numeric codes are codes that begin with certain letters.

Numeric Codes (001-999.9)

Numeric codes are arranged beginning with infectious diseases and followed by diseases or conditions related to individual body systems. For example, the first section of the tabular list (001-139) consists of infectious and parasitic diseases. The three-digit number for salmonella infections is 003, but this number cannot be used to code the disease. When coding a patient's diagnosis, the medical assistant should try to find a code with a decimal point followed by either one or two digits. Three-digit codes are less specific and, in most cases, not accepted. It is important to find the code that most exactly matches the diagnosis given by the physician. Zeros before the code and after the decimal point must always be included. If a code with two digits after the decimal is available, it should be selected.

In order to select the most specific and correct code, the medical assistant should not code from the index but always from the tabular list. As an example, assume that the physician lists the patient's diagnosis as *salmonella gastroenteritis.* If the medical assistant looks under *"Salmonella,"* the general code is given as 003.9. If the medical assistant looks in the tabular list, a more specific code (003.0) is easily located. In this case, the correct code could be found if the medical assistant looked in the index under *"Gastroenteritis, salmonella."*

Codes for Individuals Who Do Not Have a Disease or Injury

Codes that begin with the letter V (so-called V codes) follow the numeric codes. They identify factors influencing health status or an encounter with health services when there is no disease or injury, such as to receive an immunization. If a patient schedules an office visit because he or she has a family history of diabetes, the code V18.0 is used. The medical history alone justifies periodic examinations. V codes are used primarily for physical examinations, well-baby and well-child visits, and visits during pregnancy.

E codes cover external causes of injury or poisoning, such as injury due to collision of a motor vehicle with another motor vehicle. E codes are used in combination with other diagnosis codes to give more information about the cause of a medical problem. As an example, an open wound of the cheek without complications is given the code 873.41. In addition, an E code may be assigned to identify the cause of the wound (e.g., E 828.2, an accident to the rider of an animal, such as a horse riding accident). E codes facilitate the collection of statistics about causes and severity of injuries.

M codes describe **morphology** (structure and form) of neoplasms. A **neoplasm** is an abnormal growth or tumor. M codes, which are primarily used for statistical tracking, are included in Appendix A of the ICD-9-CM manual.

Using the Index (Volume 2)

The first step in coding a patient's diagnosis is to find the diagnosis in the alphabetic index. Some terms in the index may indicate that the diagnosis requires a fifth digit at the end of the code. Even though the categories of the fifth digit subclassification may be listed in the index, the medical assistant should never code directly from the index without looking up the code in the tabular list. The index does not contain the same detail as the tabular list of diseases.

The medical assistant must always keep in mind that insurance companies will be using the diagnosis code to pay for services. If the diagnosis codes are incorrect or incomplete, the insurance carrier may refuse to pay for the services provided. To find the diagnosis in the tabular list, the medical assistant may look under the main word of the patient's diagnosis. It is also possible to start from the anatomic location of the medical problem. A code must be identified for each diagnosis.

During the period when the physician is still trying to determine exactly what the patient's diagnosis is, symptoms may be listed on the charge sheet. These should be coded exactly as written. If the physician writes "rule out" or "r/O" with a diagnosis or condition, that condition may *not* be used for coding.

Examples

1. If the progress note describes the patient's problem as "recurrent right shoulder pain, rule out bursitis," the code can be located in the index under: pain, joint, shoulder (region) (719.41). If the medical assistant looks up shoulder, the following instruction is given: "see condition."

2. If the patient's diagnosis is given on the charge slip as diabetic neuropathy, the medical assistant can look in the index under diabetes (diabetic), neuropathy. The primary code is listed as 250.6 and 357.2 is listed in parentheses. The medical assistant should look up both codes as part of the process of selecting the correct code. The same information can also be located by looking in the index under neuropathy, diabetic. If a code cannot be used as a primary diagnosis, instructions are given to code the underlying disease first. When the medical assistant looks up the code 357.2, the code is listed as polyneuropathy in diabetes with instructions to code the underlying disease, diabetes mellitus, first. When the patient has the secondary condition (in this case polyneuropathy), it is important to include the code for diabetes because the code for polyneuropathy cannot be used independently.

Using the Tabular List (Volume 1)

Once a code or range of codes has been identified, the medical assistant should find the correct section and determine the best code to match the information on the patient's charge slip or in the medical record. It is important to look at the additional information given relating to the diagnosis.

In the tabular list, the medical assistant should always look for the most specific code possible, remembering that the code must be supported by the information in the medical record. A code labelled **NOS** is "not otherwise specified" and should be used when a more specific code cannot be identified. A code labelled **NEC** (which means "not elsewhere classifiable") should be used when the medical record indicates that more information is available but a more specific code cannot be found.

Selecting the Correct Fifth Digit

Certain codes require a fifth digit added after the subcategory code. Use of the fourth and fifth digits is not optional. If the diagnosis is diabetes mellitus, for example, a fifth digit is always required. The use of the fifth digit varies for each category where it is required, and it is necessary to review the instructions carefully before choosing the fifth digit.

When the tabular list is examined, it can be seen that the category for pain in a joint is 719.4, and a fifth digit is required. As noted earlier, the fifth digit is added as the second digit after the decimal point. The medical assistant should select the most specific digit from the table of possible fifth digits. For codes 719.4, the possible fifth digits are as follows:

0 site unspecified
1 shoulder region
2 upper arm

3 forearm
4 hand
5 pelvic region and thigh
6 lower leg
7 ankle and foot
8 other specified sites
9 multiple sites

The digits 0, 8, and 9 should only be used if one of the other digits does not match the diagnosis given by the physician. If the patient has pain in the left shoulder, the correct code would be 719.41.

ICD-10-CM MANUAL

The ICD-10-CM manual has two parts: the Index and the Tabular List. The Index is a list of diseases and conditions arranged in alphabetic order. The Tabular List is the section in which the actual codes are displayed, arranged in 21 chapters according to classification of the disease or condition or factors influencing health status or contact with health services. The ICD-9-CM had an additional volume, Volume 3, used to code hospital procedures. Volume 3 is replaced by the ICD-10-PCS (Procedure Coding System), which will not be discussed here because it is used for inpatient procedures only. CPT codes continue to be used to code outpatient procedures.

Format of ICD-10-CM Codes

The ICD-10-CM code begins with three characters followed by a decimal point. The first character is a letter, and the next two characters are usually digits. These first three characters show where the code occurs in the tabular list and stand for the basic condition. For example, Chapter 1 contains codes A00 to B99, which are infectious or parasitic diseases. There are 21 chapters, and most chapters contain the codes that begin with one letter of the alphabet. Chapters 3 to 14 are devoted to diseases or conditions of specific body systems. All the other chapters contain codes for types of diseases or conditions except the final chapter (Chapter 21), which contains codes for factors influencing health status. The codes from the last chapter are usually used for individuals who seek health screening or preventative care (see Table 45-2). Factors influencing health status include several reasons for an office visit besides illness, such as physical examinations, genetic carrier or genetic susceptibility, screening for various conditions, and contact with communicable diseases.

One to four characters (up to two more than for ICD-9) follow the decimal point. This allows for a total of up to seven characters in a valid code. Characters after the decimal point make a given diagnosis more specific. The first three characters after a decimal point may be digits or letters, and the final character (if needed) is a letter. A lower case x can be used as a place holder because each required digit or letter must be in the correct position (e.g., sixth character, seventh character) For example, the code for the initial encounter for a pathologic fracture in neoplastic disease in an unspecified site would be M84.50xA. The x is a placeholder for a sixth character that would indicate the site, which in this case is not specified. The seventh character, A, is required to indicate that the code refers to the initial visit.

Looking up Diagnosis Codes in the Alphabetic Index

When coding in the outpatient setting, the medical assistant should try to find the most specific code that matches each

Chapter	Codes	Diseases or Conditions
1	(A00-B99)	Certain Infectious and Parasitic Diseases
2	(C00-D49)	Neoplasms
3	(D50-D89)	Disease of the Blood and Blood-Forming Organs and Certain Disorders Involving the Immune Mechanism
4	(E00-E90)	Endocrine, Nutritional, and Metabolic Diseases
5	(F01-F99)	Mental and Behavioral Disorders
6	(G00-G99)	Diseases of Nervous System
7	(H00-H59)	Diseases of Eye and Adnexa
8	(H60-H95)	Diseases of Ear and Mastoid Process
9	(I00-I99)	Diseases of Circulatory System
10	(J00-J99)	Diseases of Respiratory System
11	(K00-K94)	Diseases of Digestive System
12	(L00-L99)	Diseases of Skin and Subcutaneous Tissue
13	(M00-M99)	Diseases of the Musculoskeletal System and Connective Tissue
14	(N00-N99)	Diseases of Genitourinary System
15	(O00-O99)	Pregnancy, Childbirth, and the Puerperium
16	(P00-P96)	Certain Conditions Originating in the Perinatal Period
17	(Q00-Q99)	Congenital Malformations, Deformations, and Chromosomal Abnormalities
18	(R00-R99)	Symptoms, Signs, and Abnormal Clinical and Laboratory Findings, Not Elsewhere Classified
19	(S00-T88)	Injury, Poisoning, and Certain Other Consequences of External Causes
20	(V01-Y99)	External Causes of Morbidity
21	(Z00-Z99)	Factors Influencing Health Status and Contact with Health Services

Table 45-2 Contents of the ICD-10-CM Manual

diagnosis given by the provider. The first-listed diagnosis describes the primary reason that the patient has sought care. This may be a disease or condition, if diagnostic testing has confirmed the diagnosis. It may be one or more symptoms, if a confirmed diagnosis is pending. It may also be a reason for seeking health care when the patient is not ill (such as a routine physical examination). In addition, the provider may list other diagnoses if the patient has complications or coexisting conditions, especially if they are the reason for procedures or diagnostic tests.

The first step is to locate the first-listed diagnosis in the alphabetic index. As an example, assume that the physician lists the patient's first diagnosis as *Salmonella gastroenteritis.* If the medical assistant looks under *Salmonella,* he or she is referred to *Infection, Salmonella* and the code listed is A02.9. If the medical assistant looks under *Gastroenteritis,* a subheading is found for *Salmonella* with the identical code. After locating the code in the index, the medical assistant should always follow up by reviewing the code in the tabular list in order to be sure that he or she has located the most specific code and has chosen a code with the required number of characters. It is not always possible to know from the index how many characters a specific code will require.

Codes for Individuals Who Do Not Have A Disease or Injury (Z01 to Z99)

Codes from Chapter 21 (Factors Influencing Health Status and Contact with Health Services) are used when the patient does not have a disease or injury and are referred to as *Z codes.* This code may be used as the first-listed diagnosis if the patient has sought health care to receive an immunization or for a physical examination. If the physician lists a diagnosis of family history of diabetes, the medical assistant would look up *History, family (of), diabetes mellitus* to find the code, Z83.3. Checking the tabular list would confirm that this is an acceptable first-listed or secondary diagnosis. The medical history alone justifies periodic examinations. It is important to note that even a code such as Z00.00 (Encounter for general adult medical examination without abnormal findings) is a diagnosis code and must be accompanied by a valid procedure code (CPT code) when billing the insurance company.

A Z code may also be used as a secondary code when a patient seeks care for a specific disease or condition. For example, a patient may seek care for an infection, but the care given may be influenced by the fact that the patient has a penicillin allergy that influences the care for the current condition. To code for the allergy, the medical assistant would look in the index under *History, personal allergy to, penicillin.*

External Cause Codes (V01 to Y99)

External cause codes cover external causes of injury or poisoning, such as injury resulting from collision of a motor vehicle with another motor vehicle. They facilitate the collection of statistics about causes and severity of injuries. These codes are used only in combination with other diagnosis codes to give more information about the cause of a medical problem. They are never the first-listed diagnosis. The External Cause Index is located before the Table of Drugs and Chemicals.

Using the Alphabetic Index

When looking up the diagnosis codes, the medical assistant must always keep in mind that insurance companies will be using the diagnosis code to pay for services. If the diagnosis codes are incorrect or incomplete, the insurance carrier may refuse to pay for the services provided.

To find the diagnosis in the index, the medical assistant may look under the main word of the patient's diagnosis. It is also possible to start from the anatomic location of the medical problem. The index is arranged with headings and subheadings. Each level of subheadings is also arranged alphabetically. In the examples that follow, a comma indicates that the next term is a subheading of the previous term.

During the period when the physician is still trying to determine exactly what the patient's diagnosis is, symptoms may be listed on the charge sheet. These should be coded exactly as written. If the physician writes "rule out (R/O)" with a diagnosis or condition, that condition may *not* be used for coding. If a patient has received ambulatory surgery, the medical assistant should look up the condition for which the surgery was done or the postoperative diagnosis, if it is different from the preoperative diagnosis.

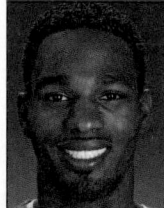

Memories *from* Externship

John Grant: My externship was performed in a large clinic where I spent some time in several departments. I was placed in the medical records department for 4 days, and I didn't understand why I needed to be there for such a long time. I was surprised to learn that not only was this department responsible for filing and taking care of the medical records, but they also did a considerable amount of coding. They asked me to look up diagnosis codes one day, and I spent all morning and part of the afternoon doing this. They gave me a stack of referral forms and told me to look up and write the diagnosis code on each form. If I couldn't find it or if I wasn't sure, I should put the form to one side so that someone could help me later. I was told to find the diagnosis in the index, and then look up the best code in the tabular list. I had had some practice in school, so this wasn't completely new to me. I have to admit that my pile of codes I was sure of was smaller than the pile I had questions about. I never realized that coding could be so complicated. There were some I couldn't find at all and others where I just couldn't decide what the best code was. For example, when the diagnosis was "unequal arm length due to old fracture" I found out that I should look up "Deformity, limb, unequal length, short site is …" in the index. I also found out that I would have to look at the medical record to identify the specific bone that had been previously fractured in order to select a specific code. This experience showed me that coding requires real attention to detail. ■

Examples

1. If the progress note describes the patient's problem as "recurrent right shoulder pain, rule out bursitis," the code can be located in the index under: *Pain(s), joint, shoulder* (M25.51-). The dash at the end of the code in the index indicates that at least one additional character is required (in this case to indicate if it is the right shoulder, left shoulder, or unspecified shoulder). If the medical assistant looks up *Shoulder* in the index, the following instruction is given: *see condition* (Figure 45-5).

2. If the patient's diagnosis is given on the charge slip as "diabetic neuropathy," the medical assistant should look in the index under *Neuropathy, diabetes*. The code range is listed as E09-E13 with .40. This means that types of diabetic neuropathy are listed under E09.40, E10.40, E11.40, and so on. It turns out that it is necessary to correlate the underlying type of diabetes (drug induced, type 1, type 2, or other) to the neuropathy. The medical assistant would find this information either in the medical record or by asking the physician. It is also possible to locate the code by looking in the index under *Diabetes, diabetic, with, neuropathy*, although the code given here refers specifically to type 2 diabetes mellitus.

Using the Tabular List

Once a code or range of codes has been identified, the medical assistant should find the correct section and determine the best code to match the information on the patient's charge slip or in the medical record. It is important to look at the additional information given relating to the diagnosis.

In the tabular list, the medical assistant should always look for the most specific code possible, remembering that the code must be supported by the information in the medical record. Parentheses are used in the index and tabular list to identify words that may be found in the diagnosis but are not required. When symbols indicate that codes require additional characters or cannot be used as a first-listed diagnosis, it is necessary to continue to look for a correct code. Codes may be identified as NOS or NEC as used in the ICD-9. A code that is identified by a symbol indicating that it is used for a complication or a comorbidity (additional disease or condition) should always follow another code related to the reason the patient has sought treatment (see Figure 45-5).

Instructional Notations

The word *Includes* may be used under a category and will identify additional names for conditions to the category or a description of conditions. For example, under the category code for *Mumps* (B26), the tabular list states, "Includes epidemic parotitis and infectious parotitis." The word *Excludes* identifies specific conditions that are not included in a category and usually points to an alternative code. *Excludes 1* means that the condition is not coded here, and the patient cannot have both the excluded condition and the condition listed above it. *Excludes 2* means that the condition is not included in this code, but the patient may have two conditions, the one included in the current code, as well as the condition using the correct code for the excluded condition. For example, in the category *Allergic contact dermatitis* (L23), the patient cannot have a diagnosis of contact dermatitis that does not specify allergy (Excludes 1), and conditions such as dermatitis caused by substances taken internally are not included (Excludes 2). (See Figure 45-6.)

More than one code may be required for a single disease or condition when a condition affects multiple body systems, is caused by or results from an underlying condition in another body system, and for late effects and complications. The instruction "Code first" instructs the coder to use another code first that will identify the cause or underlying condition. In the example of allergic contact dermatitis noted previously, an additional code that identifies the substance causing the allergic contact dermatitis should be used as the first code before the code for the dermatitis. There may also be an instruction to "Code also," which indicates that an additional code is required. In some cases, one code describes both the underlying condition and the manifestation and only one code is needed. For example,

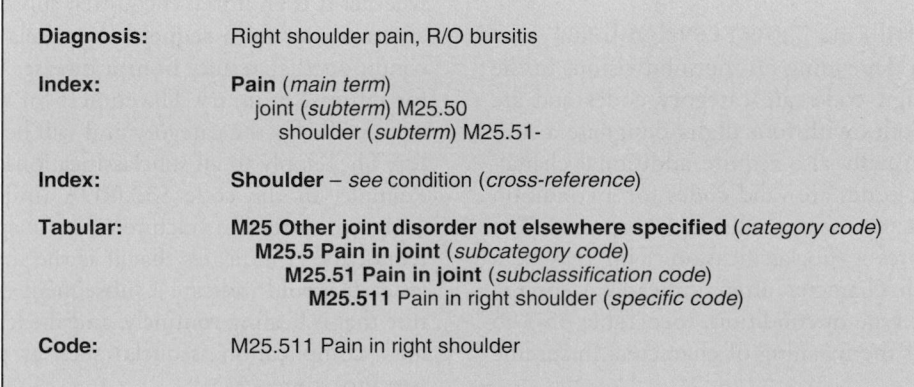

Diagnosis:	Right shoulder pain, R/O bursitis
Index:	**Pain** (*main term*)
	joint (*subterm*) M25.50
	shoulder (*subterm*) M25.51-
Index:	**Shoulder** – *see* condition (*cross-reference*)
Tabular:	**M25 Other joint disorder not elsewhere specified** (*category code*)
	M25.5 Pain in joint (*subcategory code*)
	M25.51 Pain in joint (*subclassification code*)
	M25.511 Pain in right shoulder (*specific code*)
Code:	M25.511 Pain in right shoulder

Figure 45-5 To code a diagnosis, look up the condition or location in the index, then find the most specific code in the tabular list.

● **L23 Allergic contact dermatitis**
   Code first (T36-T65), *to identify drug or substance*
   Excludes 1   allergy NOS (T78.40)
              contact dermatitis NOS (L25.9)
              dermatitis NOS (L30.9)
   Excludes 2   dermatitis due to substances taken
                 internally (L27.-)
              dermatitis of eyelid (H01.1-)
              diaper dermatitis (L22)
              eczema of external ear (H60.5-)
              irritant contact dermatitis (L24.-)
              perioral dermatitis (L71.0)
              radiation-related disorders of the skin and
                 subcutaneous tissue (L55-L59)
● **L23.0   Allergic contact dermatitis due to metals**
              Allergic contact dermatitis due to chromium
              Allergic contact dermatitis due to nickel
● **L23.1   Allergic contact dermatitis due to adhesives**
● **L23.2   Allergic contact dermatitis due to cosmetics**
● **L23.3   Allergic contact dermatitis due to drugs in contact
        with skin**
        Excludes 2   dermatitis due to ingested drugs and
                       medicaments (L27.0-L27.1)
● **L23.4   Allergic contact dermatitis due to dyes**

● Unacceptable first-listed diagnosois   ● Use additional character(s)
   Complication/comorbidity   Major C/C   Excludes 1   Excludes 2

Figure 45-6 A sample from the International Classification of Diseases, 10th Revision, Clinical Modification.

Table 45-3 Specificity of ICD-10 Codes			
Characters	Incomplete Code	Valid Code	Description
3	S22		Fracture of rib(s), sternum, and thoracic spine
4	S22.0		Fracture of thoracic vertebra
5	S22.01		Fracture of first thoracic vertebra
6	S22.010		Wedge compression fracture of first thoracic vertebra
7		S22.010A	Initial encounter for closed wedge compression fracture of first thoracic vertebra

a single code is sufficient for a sore throat cause by *Streptococcus* (J02.0 Streptococcal pharyngitis).

Selecting the Code with the Correct Level of Detail

Codes vary in length depending on the subdivisions in the tabular list. Three-digit codes are category codes and are rarely valid codes. Codes with four digits designate a subclassification. They usually also require additional characters. Some four-digit codes are valid codes for a condition whose location, cause, or other details are unspecified. The fifth character indicates a subclassification. This may be a body part. The sixth character often indicates a specific location or a specific type of condition. (See Table 45-3 to review an example of the meaning of characters in specific locations.)

Most codes are complete with five or six characters, but some require a seventh character (letter), usually to indicate whether it is an initial encounter, subsequent encounter, or an encounter for a **sequela.** A sequela (pl. *sequelae*) is any condition that results from a disease, injury, or treatment for a disease or injury. The choices for the seventh character are specific for the category and will be listed in the tabular list. They apply to all subclassifications of the category. For example, in the code S32.009A (initial encounter for a wedge compression fracture of an unspecified lumbar vertebra), the *A* indicates that it is the initial encounter. The letter *D* would indicate a subsequent encounter for a fracture that is healing routinely, and the letter *S* would be used for a complication (sequela) such as persistent back pain (see Procedure 45-3).

When medical codes are misused in order to obtain a higher level of reimbursement than is allowed, the process is called **upcoding**. Under Section 231 of the Health Insurance Portability and Accountability Act, nearly all federal health care programs can levy fines and penalties for failure to adhere to compliance with regulations for using correct codes on claims for reimbursements. A pattern or practice of upcoding can result in large fines, and ignorance of correct procedure is not considered a defense. Medicare analyzes claims to identify atypical billing and may follow up with a more detailed analysis when a pattern has been identified for a specific provider.

Some physician offices have contracted for independent review in order to identify coding and billing errors. After such a review, it may be found that in some cases codes do not reflect a high enough level of service, resulting in lower levels of reimbursement than are justified. An independent review can also discover cases in which the codes used on claims would result in charges that are higher than the level of service provided. Based on this information, the medical office can improve its coding procedures to maximize income without risking fines or other legal proceedings. ■

Case Study 3

When entering charges for Michael Drew, a 56-year-old patient, John sees that the physician has written the diagnosis "Diabetes Type 1." Just below the code, the physician has written "with diabetic polyneuropathy." John needs to enter the charges and codes into the computer so that this patient's insurance can be billed. John's office is using ICD-10 codes. ■

PROCEDURE 45-3 Performing ICD Coding

Outcome Perform ICD coding for a patient's diagnosis.

Equipment/Supplies

- Patient's medical record
- Charge slip
- Current ICD manual

1. **Procedural Step.** Refer to the patient's charge slip and/or medical record to identify the diagnosis. In the medical record, the physician may use the term "impression" or "diagnosis."

   Principle. The charge slip usually identifies the diagnosis, but the medical record may be necessary for additional information to select the correct code.

2. **Procedural Step.** Decide on the key word or phrase to look for the code in the alphabetic index of the most current ICD manual.

3. **Procedural Step.** Locate the key word and look for the body part or other distinguishing factors. Identify the possible code number(s).

4. **Procedural Step.** Locate the number(s) in the tabular list.

   Principle. You cannot be sure that you have identified the correct code without looking at the tabular list. You may also find additional information in the tabular list to help you code properly.

5. **Procedural Step.** Review the information given in the tabular list and select the most specific code that corresponds to the information on the charge slip and/or in the medical record. When there is a list of terminal characters (fifth digit for ICD-9-CM or seventh character for ICD-10-CM), select the character that makes the code as specific as possible.

   Principle. Reimbursement may be linked to selection of the correct code.

6. **Procedural Step.** Enter the correct code(s) on the charge slip, on the encounter form, and if necessary in the computer billing program so that it can be used for insurance billing.

   Principle. Reimbursement is made by insurance companies based on the codes submitted. Diagnosis codes must be accurate and justify the service provided.

   Example: Patient diagnosis is "precordial chest pain, possibly angina pectoris":

   1: To locate the code in the ICD-9-CM manual, first locate pain, then chest in the list of diseases (Volume 2). You will find entries similar to the following:

Index*:

Pain(s)

chest (central) 786.50
atypical 786.59
midsternal 786.51
musculoskeletal 786.59
noncardiac 786.59
substernal 786.51
wall (anterior) 786.52

Continued

2: Look up the code for central chest pain (786.50) in the tabular list (Volume 1).*

786.5 Chest pain
    786.50 Chest pain, unspecified
    786.51 Precordial pain
    786.52 Painful respiration
      Pain:
        anterior chest wall
        pleuritic
        pleurodynia
Excludes: *epidemic pleurodynia (074.1)*
    786.59 Other
        Discomfort in chest
        Pressure in chest
        Tightness in chest

The code 786.5 may be marked with a symbol that indicates a fifth digit is required (depending on the code manual). After reviewing all the codes in the category, it is clear that 786.51 *Precordial chest pain* corresponds best to the diagnosis given by the physician.

3: To locate the code in the ICD-10-CM manual, first locate pain, then chest, then precordial in the alphabetic index. Remember that terms preceded by "possibly" or "rule out" should not be coded. You will find entries similar to the following:

Index*:

Pain(s)
    chest (central) R07.9
      anterior wall R07.89
      atypical R07.89
      ischemic I20.9
      midsternal 798.51
      musculoskeletal R07.89
      non-cardiac R07.89
      on breathing R07.1
      pleurodynia R07.81
      precordial R07.2
      wall (anterior) R07.89

4: Look up the code for precordial pain (R.07.2) in the tabular list to validate that it is the most specific code.†

R07 Pain in throat and chest
    Excludes 1 epidemic myalgia (B33.0)
    Excludes 2 pain in breast (N64.4)
  R07.0 Pain in throat
      Excludes 1 chronic sore throat (J31.2)
        sore throat (acute) NOS (J02.1)
      Excludes 2 dysphagia (R13.1-)
        pain in neck
  R07.1 Chest pain on breathing
      Painful respiration
  R07.2 Precordial pain

*Buck C: *Saunders 2008 ICD-9-CM,* St. Louis, 2008, Saunders.
†Buck C: *Saunders 2011 ICD-10-CM,* St Louis, 2011, Saunders.

What Would You Do? What Would You *Not* Do? RESPONSES

Case Study 1
Page 1072

What Did John Do?
❑ Double-checked the medical record to find out if the charge slip was filled out for the correct Peter Miller and to find out if the patient had been seen before.
❑ Charged the patient correctly as an established patient if it turned out that he had been seen by any practitioner in the practice within the past 3 years.
❑ Filled out a new charge slip if it turned out from reviewing the medical record that Peter Miller was in fact a new patient with a different birth date and address.
❑ Checked with the physician to find out if he had checked the wrong box on the charge slip.

What Did John Not Do?
❑ Did not just assume that whatever box the physician checked was correct.
❑ Did not enter a charge for a new patient if the patient was in fact an established patient.
❑ Did not tell the physician to be more careful in the future when filling out the charge slip.

What Would You Do/What Would You Not Do?
Review John's response and place a checkmark next to the information you included in your response. List the additional information you included in your response.

_____
_____
_____
_____
_____

What Would You Do? What Would You *Not* Do? RESPONSES—cont'd

Case Study 2
Page 1072

What Did John Do?

❑ Entered the charges for the office visit and injection using the appropriate CPT codes in the computer.

❑ Looked up the Medicare code for methylprednisolone in the HCPCS Level II manual, where he noted that the correct code depends on the dose given.

❑ Checked the medical record to identify the dose of methylprednisolone given to the patient and selected the correct HCPCS code from that information.

What Did John Not Do?

❑ Did not assume that all the correct codes were found on the charge slip.

❑ Did not guess at the dose of methylprednisolone because he knew what dose the physician usually gave.

❑ Did not assume that he could save time by asking the physician what dose was given.

❑ Did not bother the physician with the details of this coding situation.

What Would You Do/What Would You Not Do?

Review John's response and place a checkmark next to the information you included in your response. List the additional information you included in your response.

_____
_____
_____
_____

Case Study 3
Page 1079

What Did John Do?

❑ Checked the ICD-10-CM manual to read all codes for diabetes mellitus and codes for diabetic polyneuropathy. He found a single code for type 1 diabetes with polyneuropathy. He used E10.42 Type 1 diabetes mellitus with polyneuropathy as the code. He selected (or entered) that code in the computer.

What Did John Not Do?

❑ Did not assume that two codes would be required because two codes were required when coding using the ICD-9-CM.

❑ Did not rely on his memory for the best code(s) for this condition.

❑ Did not bother the physician with the details related to this coding situation.

❑ Did not code from the alphabetic index of the ICD-10-CM manual.

What Would You Do/What Would You Not Do?

Review John's response and place a checkmark next to the information you included in your response. List the additional information you included in your response.

_____
_____
_____
_____
_____

↻ TERMINOLOGY REVIEW

Medical Term	Word Parts	Definition
Established patient		A patient who has been seen by one of the physicians in the practice within the past 3 years.
Inpatient		A patient who has been formally admitted to a health care facility.
Modifier		An addition to a *Current Procedural Terminology* code that indicates unusual circumstances related to the procedure, such as a more extensive procedure or two procedures performed in the same session.
Morphology	*morph-*: shape *-ology*: study of	The study of structure and form.
NEC		A diagnosis code that is not elsewhere classified. It is used when a more specific code for the condition is not available.
Neoplasm	*neo-*: new *plasma:* formation	Abnormal growth or tumor.

Continued

↻ TERMINOLOGY REVIEW—cont'd

Medical Term	Word Parts	Definition
New patient		For billing purposes, a patient who has not received services during the previous 3 years from a physician in a medical practice.
NOS		A diagnosis code that is not otherwise specified. It is used when there is not enough information given to select a more specific code.
Outpatient		A patient who has not been admitted to a health care facility.
Panel		A group of diagnostic tests done in one machine at the same time.
Sequela (pl. sequelae)	*sequi:* follow *-a:* noun ending	Any condition that results from a disease, injury, or treatment for a disease or injury.
Surgical package		Surgical services usually covered by a single procedure code that includes a preoperative visit, postoperative care, and local anesthesia (if applicable).
Upcoding		Using a code to obtain a higher level of reimbursement than is justified by medical procedures performed as documented in the medical record. This can result in serious fines and penalties.

≫ ON THE WEB

For information on CPT code information:

CPT—American Medical Association: www.ama-assn.org

CPT codes for CLIA Waived Laboratory Tests: www.cms.gov/Regulations-and-Guidelines/CLIA/downloads/waivedtbl.pdf

For information on ICD-9 codes:

ICD-9—National Center for Health Statistics: www.cdc.gov/nchs/icd/icd9cm.htm

For information on ICD-10 codes:

ICD-10—National Center for Health Statistics: www.cdc.gov/nchs/icd/icd10cm.htm#10updateICD-10

Centers for Medicare and Medicaid Services: www.cms.hhs.gov/ICD10/01_Overview.asp

Check out the Evolve site at http://evolve.elsevier.com/Bonewit/today/ to actively Prepare for your Certification, and to access additional interactive activities and exercises to help you study and prepare for success.

46

Medical Insurance

KEY TERMS

assignment of benefits
beneficiary
benefit
birthday rule
capitation
carrier
CHAMPVA
coinsurance
coordination of benefits
copayment
deductible
diagnosis-related groups (DRGs)
eligibility
explanation of benefits (EOB)
fee-for-service insurance

fiscal intermediary
formulary
group plan
guarantor
indemnity
insured
managed care
Medicaid
Medicare
nonparticipating provider (nonPAR)
participating provider (PAR)
preauthorization (PREE-awe-thur
  -i-zay-shun)
precertification (PREE-sur-ti-fi-kay-shun)
premium

primary care provider (PCP)
primary insurance
referral
reimbursement
resource-based relative value scale
  (RBRVS)
secondary insurance
self-referral
signature on file (SOF)
third-party payor
TRICARE
usual, customary, and reasonable (UCR)
utilization review
workers' compensation

INTRODUCTION TO HEALTH INSURANCE

The growth and change in the structure of health insurance has affected American health care since the end of World War II. When industrialized countries such as Canada and many countries in Western Europe were introducing government-provided health care, the United States was turning primarily to the private market to provide insurance coverage for Americans. This created the problem that many Americans could not afford health insurance. As health care costs continue to rise, so does the pressure to maintain high standards at a reasonable cost to both individuals and the government.

HISTORY OF HEALTH INSURANCE

Health insurance had its beginnings in accident insurance, which was first sold in the mid-1800s. In exchange for a monthly payment by a customer, the insurance company agreed to replace lost income resulting from an accident, and later resulting from a few specific illnesses, such as smallpox, diphtheria, typhoid, and scarlet fever.

In the 1930s a group of Dallas schoolteachers made an arrangement with Baylor Hospital to have any necessary hospital care provided in exchange for monthly premiums. This arrangement was the precursor to the Blue Cross and Blue Shield programs, which were incorporated as not-for-profit companies in each state. The amount of payment was based on the amount charged for the services provided. Other insurance companies began to offer health insurance using similar models. Labor unions began to negotiate for health insurance as an employee benefit that was not taxed as income in the same way as an increase in wages.

During World War II, Henry Kaiser created clinics in California to provide both inpatient and outpatient care for the workers in his shipyards. These clinics later opened themselves to other employers and individuals and became the Kaiser Permanente program. The employer paid a fixed amount per worker over a stated period of time for all necessary medical care. This method of payment is called **capitation,** and this type of health insurance is called a *prepaid health plan.* For many years Kaiser Permanente was the country's largest health maintenance organization (HMO). The philosophy behind the HMO movement was a belief that health care costs could be lowered if members were restricted to specific providers and facilities. Covered services also included preventive medical care in the hope of preventing conditions that would be expensive to treat. Over time, the HMO model broadened from one in which physicians were salaried employees and worked in a central facility to one in which HMOs contracted with private physicians in each community.

By the 1960s, many larger and even medium-sized businesses were providing company-paid health insurance benefits as a fringe benefit instead of increasing wages or salary. Health care costs began to increase faster than the general rate of inflation, with physicians beginning to earn large incomes. But certain groups of Americans—most notably the poor, elderly, and permanently disabled—were unable to obtain medical insurance through employment.

The federal government created two programs to try to close these large gaps in medical coverage. One was **Medicare,** the health insurance program for the elderly, disabled, and those with end-stage kidney disease. Medicare is paid for with federal taxes paid by employers and workers. The second government insurance program was **Medicaid,** the health insurance program for low-income individuals and families. The Medicaid program has different names in different states, and it is administered by each state. The federal government pays for the majority of required care and a smaller percentage of optional care, such as dental care, while the states pay for the rest. Each state sets its own criteria of eligibility for the Medicaid program.

Many senators, congresspersons, and physicians were against Medicare and Medicaid at the beginning, calling it "socialized medicine." But there were precedents for the government's involvement in paying for medical care. The Veterans Administration (VA) offered medical care for life for any man or woman who had seen active duty in the military, provided he or she wished to use the VA facilities. In addition, the Civilian Health and Medical Program of the Uniformed Services (CHAMPUS) program was developed to provide medical care at government expense for dependent spouses and children of active-duty military personnel. Today the former CHAMPUS program is called **TRICARE** (because there are three different plans). A companion program, the Civilian Health and Medical Program of the Department of Veterans Affairs **(CHAMPVA),** covers dependent spouses and children of military veterans with service-connected disabilities.

At the beginning of the twenty-first century, American society is still trying to resolve insurance issues. Low-wage workers often do not get health insurance through their employers or have insurance only for themselves and not their dependents. For more than 10 years the federal government has tried to pass legislation to expand insurance coverage to all or nearly all citizens, but the costs have made it difficult to gather enough support. The federal Patient Protection and Affordable Care Act, which became law in March 2010, attempts to define patients' rights and ensure that all Americans will have access to affordable, high-quality health care and preventative care. It remains to be seen whether this law can accomplish its mission, or even if it will survive efforts to challenge its legitimacy and/or constitutionality.

OBTAINING HEALTH INSURANCE

Individuals and families have basically three ways to obtain health insurance coverage: through a group plan, by purchasing an individual policy, or through one of the government plans described earlier.

Most **group plans** are available through an employer. A group plan is one insurance policy that covers a group of people. Larger employers generally have several different plans available. The employer pays a portion of the insurance costs. The amount paid by the employer for unionized workers tends to be greater than for workers not in a union.

Some small business owners can purchase insurance through group plans sponsored by a trade organization. Individuals sometimes have access to group plans through professional associations, or even college alumni associations. The self-employed can deduct a portion of their health insurance costs from their business income, as companies do.

As part of the process of gaining the right to sell health insurance in a particular state, most insurance plans are required to offer individual policies to individuals or families who are not covered under a group plan. An open-enrollment period usually occurs at least once per year for individuals to purchase coverage. Discussion has occurred at the federal level about allowing individuals or families who purchase their own insurance to claim a tax credit, or a larger tax deduction, for the cost.

Taxpayer-funded, or government, health insurance is usually provided as an entitlement when other conditions are met. For instance, when an individual reaches age 65, he or she is entitled to Medicare benefits if he or she has worked for at least 10 years in Medicare-covered employment. However, the individual must still file an application because the benefits do not begin automatically. An individual must meet other criteria for other government health insurance programs.

PAYING FOR HEALTH INSURANCE AND HEALTH CARE

The amount of money paid by the consumer to purchase health insurance is called the **premium.** This premium can be paid monthly, quarterly, semiannually, or annually. All or part of the premium may be paid by the person enrolled in the insurance plan or by the employer. In exchange for the payment of a premium, the insurance company or managed care plan agrees to provide payment for specific services provided by physicians, hospitals, laboratories, and other health care providers. Payment for a service covered by health insurance is called a **benefit,** and each individual covered by the health insurance plan is called a **beneficiary,** *enrollee,* or *member.* The **insured** is the individual who has the insurance, but the plan may also cover dependents of the insured including a spouse and children.

When the premium is paid by a person's employer, even if the employee is responsible for part of the cost, that premium is often paid with before-tax dollars. This means that the amount of the premium paid by the employer is not included in the amount of wages reported for the employee. The employee's portion may also be deducted before tax is calculated. In this case, the employee cannot use the payment for insurance as a tax deduction.

Another way to pay for health care using before-tax dollars is a medical savings account. This is a fund set up by the employer before tax is taken out of a person's earnings. The money in this fund can be used only for qualified health expenses, and it must be spent within a specified time frame. Money not used is lost to the employee.

Depending on the type of insurance policy, a patient may have to make certain payments for medical services. A **deductible** is an amount of money that must be paid for services provided to an individual or a family member in a group plan every calendar year before any insurance payments. After the deductible has been met, the patient may be required to pay a percentage of the allowed charge or a fixed fee every time service is received. If the patient is responsible for a specific percentage of the allowed charges (such as 20%), the patient portion is called **coinsurance.** An example of an insurance plan with coinsurance is Medicare Part B. If the patient is required to pay a fixed dollar amount every time he or she obtains medical services or fills a prescription, it is called a **copayment.** In some plans, the amount of the copayment is always the same, but often there are different amounts for different types of medical and/or pharmacy services.

FACTORS AFFECTING INSURANCE REIMBURSEMENT

Primary, Secondary, and Tertiary Insurance

If a person is covered by more than one insurance policy, the insurance to which the insurance claim is sent first is called the **primary insurance.** When the patient is the insured, that insurance is the primary insurance. Insurance held by another insured (such as a spouse) that provides additional insurance coverage would be **secondary insurance.** If a third type of insurance also covers the patient, that insurance would be tertiary insurance. As a general rule, private insurance must be billed before government insurance, and Medicaid is always the last insurance to be billed.

Coordination of Benefits

Some households have two working adults, both of whom are covered under separate employer health benefits. **Coordination of benefits** is a term for the rules insurance companies use to coordinate the payments for medical services so that no provider is paid more than 100% of the charge for any service provided.

If both members of a couple have insurance with coordination of benefits provisions, the following rules apply:

1. If the employee who holds the policy is the patient, his or her insurance is the primary insurance for any services obtained. The spouse's or partner's insurance becomes the secondary insurance and can be used to pay only for any portion of the charge not covered by the primary insurance. The deductible for the primary insurance may not be covered by the secondary insurance.

2. If a child is the patient, in most states the "birthday rule" applies. Under the **birthday rule,** the primary insurance for the child of parents who both have a family health plan is the insurance belonging to the working adult whose birthday comes first in the year. The insurance of the adult whose birthday is later is the secondary insurance.

3. When the patient is a child of divorced parents, the rules can get somewhat complicated. If a court has decreed that one parent is the "responsible party," that parent's policy provides the primary insurance. A responsible party ruling is often made in cases of joint custody, although the responsible party can also be a noncustodial parent. If no court ruling is in place, the custodial parent's policy is primary if the custodial parent has remarried. If there is no court ruling in place and the custodial parent has not remarried, the birthday rule remains in effect.

Coordination of benefits issues can be avoided if individuals in households with two working adults make modifications in their benefits. In order to reduce premium costs, some employers allow employees to take cash instead of health insurance if the family already has insurance. In cases where the company covers the complete cost for individual but not family coverage, only the husband or the wife needs to pay for family coverage. Of course, available plans should be compared for cost and benefits when deciding which policy to extend to family coverage.

4. If the patient is a Medicare recipient who also is covered by an employer's policy, the employer's policy is the primary insurance and Medicare is the secondary insurance. Patients with Medicare may also have supplemental insurance to cover what would normally be a patient responsibility. These plans, which are clearly defined as Medicare supplemental insurance, are considered secondary insurance.

Participating and Nonparticipating Providers

If the physician has a contract or agreement with a **third-party payor** (insurance **carrier** [company] or managed care organization), he or she is called a **participating provider (PAR).** One of the requirements is often that the physician accepts the insurance carrier's determination of the allowable fee and may not bill the patient for any additional amount that the insurance company did not allow. A **nonparticipating provider (nonPAR)** has no contractual agreement with the third-party payor and can bill the patient for the difference between the insurance payment and the amount billed. A PAR receives payment from the insurance carrier directly. A nonPAR must obtain payment from the patient (who receives **reimbursement** from the insurance carrier) unless the patient signs a form authorizing **assignment of benefits.** This term is used for the patient's request that the insurance carrier pay the provider directly. This authorization is usually part of the new patient information form.

Types of Reimbursement

Two basic types of insurance reimbursement exist: capitation and fee-for-service.

Under capitation, the primary care physician receives a monthly, quarterly, semiannual, or annual payment from the managed care insurance company. Specialists are usually not paid by capitation. The reimbursement per patient may vary depending on age and sex, but it does not depend on the amount of care the patient receives.

As discussed earlier, capitation moves some of the risk away from the managed care company and onto the primary care physician who treats the patient, and most physicians prefer other payment methods. In most circumstances, there will be enough healthy patients who cost the physician less to treat than the amount being paid by the company to make up for the few sick patients who cost more to treat.

Under **fee-for-service insurance,** the health care provider, including all physicians, is reimbursed for each treatment or procedure performed. In this case the only difference between traditional fee-for-service insurance and managed care is that managed care companies often negotiate a fee schedule that is lower than traditional indemnity plans.

In many instances, however, if the physician or other medical provider agrees to accept assignment of benefits, he or she cannot bill the patient for any portion of the charge not paid by the insurance company except the deductible and copayment or coinsurance.

TYPES OF INSURANCE

Several different types of health insurance are currently available. When learning about insurance, it is helpful to learn the characteristics of different types of insurance, although the medical assistant may also be responsible for finding out more specific information related to individual insurance plans.

Fee-for-Service Plans

Traditionally, private insurance plans provided payment, either to the physician or to the patient, for each medical service provided. These traditional plans are called *fee-for-service plans* or *indemnity plans.* The term **indemnity** means an obligation to compensate an individual for loss or damage. Until the late 1980s, fee-for-service plans dominated the health care industry. They were provided through private insurance companies and also through the Blue Cross and Blue Shield plans, which were established in each state as not-for-profit, quasi-governmental agencies. Since the late 1980s, the percentage of individuals covered under traditional fee-for-service plans has steadily decreased. Fee-for-service plans usually have a deductible, and the insurance pays for a percentage of the allowed charges (commonly 80%).

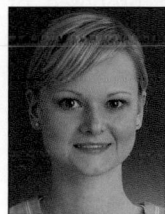

Putting It All into Practice

My name is Sandra O'Keefe, and I am a registered medical assistant. I work in the office of three dermatologists. With the advances in laser technology, there are many new procedures for removing spider veins, birthmarks, scars, hair, and tattoos. We also do Mohs micrographic surgery, a technique that removes skin cancers one layer at time with immediate tissue analysis. Using this technique the physicians can be sure that all malignant cells have been removed while taking a minimum of healthy tissue.

Billing in our office is somewhat complicated because many of the procedures are not covered by insurance. In general, insurance companies will pay for procedures that are medically necessary, like removal of skin cancers. They do not cover procedures that are strictly cosmetic, such as removal of spider veins (small varicose veins on the skin). Then there are some procedures that sometimes are covered by insurance and sometimes are not, such as the removal of birthmarks on the face.

When a procedure is medically necessary, we have to obtain preauthorization from the patient's insurance company, and sometimes we need to provide documentation for the insurance company to review before they give their approval. When a procedure is not covered, we have to be sure that the patient is willing to pay for it and knows how much it will cost. We can help arrange for the patient to obtain financing in order to pay for the procedure over a period of time.

Our physicians accept several different types of insurance including government plans, managed care plans, and traditional insurance plans. When patients are covered by managed care plans, we have to be sure that they have the proper referrals to cover each office visit, as well as the procedure. In some cases the insurance covers a consultation visit but the proposed treatment plan is not approved, and then the patients must decide about paying for any recommended procedure themselves. We do our best to complete all of the paperwork to obtain insurance coverage for our patients, but we are limited by the rules of each insurance company. ■

Case Study 1

Diane Bennett is a 35-year-old woman who has come to the office for treatment of a lesion on her neck. She has been referred from her primary care physician for up to three visits for consultation, diagnostic studies, and treatment. She is seen by one of the dermatologists in the practice, who recommends that the lesion be removed surgically in the office with a biopsy. During this visit the patient tells the physician that she has two other lesions she would like to have removed, one on her arm and one on her abdomen. The physician inspects the lesions and asks Sandra to contact the patient's managed care plan for authorization to treat the additional lesions. The patient says, "My physician gave me a referral to be treated by you. What's the problem? If these lesions need to be removed, I don't want any delay." ∎

The insurance company determines the allowed charge in two ways:

1. Through a fee schedule. A fee schedule says the insurance company will pay the specified percentage of a particular amount for a particular procedure. Any additional charges are the patient's responsibility.

2. Through service benefits, which define covered services but not the exact payments. Under service benefit plans, the insurance company will agree to pay the specified percentage of charges that are **usual, customary, and reasonable (UCR)** for the procedure and the state or region of the country in which it was performed. The usual fee is the amount that a physician usually charges or charges most often. The customary fee is the amount charged by physicians in the same specialty in the same geographic area (usually the 90th percentile amount of the charges of all physicians in the area. A reasonable fee meets the two criteria described earlier or is justifiable if there are special circumstances. Based on statistics kept by the insurance company, the fee actually charged by the physician is reviewed. The insurance company's payment is based on its own determination of what is UCR.

Under a traditional fee-for-service plan, a patient can make an appointment with any doctor, in any specialty, he or she wishes, and the insurance will pay the designated amount for the services. Some plans do have lists of approved providers for whom they pay 100% of charges and pay only a percentage of charges for other providers (similar to a preferred provider organization [PPO], discussed in more detail later in the chapter).

Managed Care Plans

Since the introduction of the Kaiser plan, HMOs have evolved into many forms. Both private insurance companies and government insurance plans offer HMOs, as well as other types of managed care plans. The various HMO models and their descendants, collectively, are known as **managed care.** This term is used in two ways: It describes the movement to control health care costs while improving preventive care and is a general term for insurance programs reimbursing care provided in this way. Managed care plans negotiate reimbursement amounts and limit patients to those providers and facilities with whom they have contracts.

Most insurance plans today involve some form of managed care. The patient's care is managed by the insurance plan in several ways:

1. Each patient chooses one physician as a **primary care provider (PCP),** a physician who provides most of the patient's care and also determines what other medical services the patient requires.

2. Care is usually restricted to specific providers, laboratories, and hospitals that have accepted the insurance plan's fee schedule or capitation payment plan.

3. The patient may or may not have access to providers and services outside the insurance plan. If there are tiers of providers, the patient must usually pay more for services obtained outside the plan. In addition, the patient may be subject to balance billing if he or she seeks service from a provider who is outside the managed care plan. This means that the patient must pay the difference between the amount allowed by insurance and the amount charged for services.

4. The insurance plan may require referrals from a PCP for services including consultations with specialists, therapy such as physical therapy or speech therapy, care outside of the medical office, and some diagnostic tests. The PCP functions as a "gatekeeper" to limit and approve access to specialty services. (The process of referrals is discussed later in this chapter.)

5. The insurance plan usually requires prior notification and/or **utilization review** (reviewing proposed or current care to determine medical necessity) before authorizing referral to specialists, certain procedures, therapy, surgery, and other types of care.

Health Maintenance Organization Models

In the original HMO concept, all medical care was provided for 1 year for a fixed premium, with no deductibles or coinsurance. The patient was responsible only for a fixed amount for each visit or prescription (copayment).

HMOs have always practiced preventive medicine, on the theory that much of the cost of medical care can be eliminated through routine care by PCPs. To reduce the cost of specialty care, PCPs including physicians, nurse practitioners, and physician assistants act as "gatekeepers," seeing patients first for nearly all illnesses and referring them to specialists only when necessary. The PCP is paid by capitation. HMOs are usually incorporated and regulated state by state. They are subject to regulation requiring more comprehensive quality assurance programs than other types of insurance. Medical record audits allow the HMO to check the records of any physician's patients to make sure the physician is not performing unnecessary procedures or ordering unnecessary tests.

Staff Model Health Maintenance Organization

The staff model HMO hires its physicians directly and pays them a salary for providing health care to members. The patient can receive care only at plan facilities. This type of plan was more common when the HMO movement first began and is rare today.

Network Health Maintenance Organization

The network model HMO contracts with various group practices for services to its members. Typically, the physicians also see patients who have other types of insurance. The HMO members must be referred to in-network providers if possible. Out-of-network coverage is allowed only in cases of emergency or urgent services.

Other Managed Care Models

Health care plans that are regulated by state and federal laws as insurance plans instead of HMOs may still maintain many features of managed care. Depending on the state, there may be separate regulatory agencies.

Preferred Provider Organization

A PPO provides coverage for in-network and out-of-network services to its members, but there is a financial incentive to use in-network services. These plans usually have deductibles and coinsurance. Patients may be required to pay a percentage of in-network costs, but they must usually pay a higher percentage of out-of-network costs.

Exclusive Provider Organization

An exclusive provider organization (EPO) is similar in structure and operation to a PPO, but its members must receive all health care services only within the network in order for them to be covered. Employers agree that the EPO is the only organization it will contract with for health services to employees. If a member receives health services outside the network (except for emergencies or when travelling out of the area), the cost will not be covered by insurance. In this way the EPO is similar to an HMO, but its legal structure is different because it is regulated as an insurance plan and not an HMO. The payment method is fee-for-service.

Independent Practice Association

The physicians of an independent practice association (IPA) work independently in the community but formally organize a physician association. They are paid from funds collected from subscribers of the health plan minus administrative costs, marketing and sales costs, and other overhead costs. IPAs often have a "hold back"—a portion of the agreed fee that is not paid to the physicians until after the end of the association's fiscal year, when the association determines if it has earned a profit or had financial losses. This way, the association requires member physicians to share some business risk.

Point-of-Service Plans

The point-of-service (POS) plan combines an in-network plan that is regulated as an HMO with an out-of-network plan that is regulated as an insurance plan. Members receive two certificates, one for an HMO for services provided by in-network providers and one for an indemnity carrier for out-of-network services. The POS plan functions as a combination of an HMO and a PPO. Members have a higher financial obligation when they seek out-of-network services. When they remain within the network, their only financial obligation is a copayment each time they seek service.

Government Plans

Medicare

Medicare is a federally funded plan administered by the Centers for Medicare and Medicaid Services (CMS). It pays for health care services for the following individuals:

- Individuals older than 65 who are eligible for Social Security
- Retired railroad employees and some retired federal employees
- Individuals who have been permanently disabled for 2 years
- Blind individuals
- Individuals with chronic renal disease who require dialysis or kidney transplant
- Kidney donors

The Medicare plan has several parts. Medicare Part A provides coverage of hospitalization services. Medicare Part B covers physician and other provider services. Together these two parts make up what is called the *Original Medicare Plan.* The patient's Medicare card identifies what type of coverage the patient has (Figure 46-1). Medicare was expanded to provide more choice in the types of available plans in 1997 (also known as *Part C*). Several Medicare Advantage Plans, including managed care plans and fee-for-service plans, replace the Original Medicare Plan if recipients choose them. Medicare Part D was passed in 2003 and

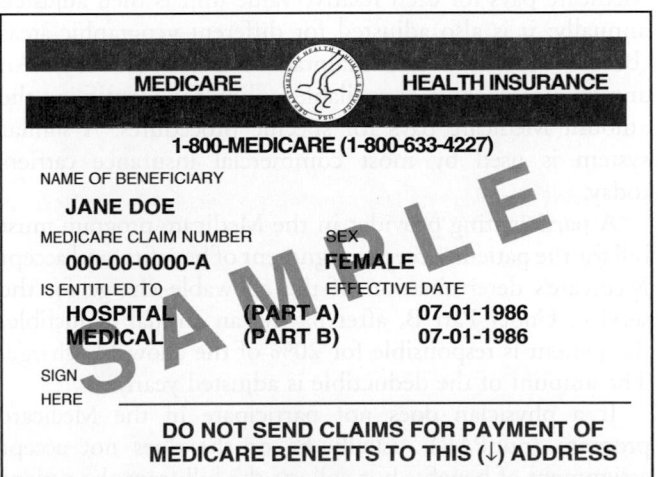

Figure 46-1 Identification card for Medicare.

went into effect in 2006. It adds a prescription drug benefit to the Original Medicare Plan and Medicare Advantage Plans that did not include this benefit. If the patient is enrolled in a Medicare Advantage plan, the physician must be a member physician of that plan in order for services to be covered.

Individuals aged 65 and older on Social Security, those younger than 65 but who collect Social Security disability benefits, and those who receive railroad retirement benefits are automatically enrolled in Medicare Part A. There is no premium for participation in Medicare Part A. The first day of each hospital admission is not paid by Medicare; this is the Part A deductible. Medicare Part A is funded through a tax paid by working individuals on all of their earned income.

Anyone eligible for Medicare Part A may also obtain Part B coverage. However, they must apply and pay a premium to obtain Medicare Part B or to enroll in one of the Medicare Advantage Plans. Former federal employees, who receive federal employee pensions rather than Social Security and are not covered by Medicare Part A, can purchase Medicare Part B coverage.

Medicare claims are handled by insurance companies that contract with CMS. A **fiscal intermediary** (insurance company that contracts to review and pay Medicare claims) processes claims in each state or group of states. The amount of payment for any service is standardized nationally.

Payment for hospitals for claims under Part A is based on **diagnosis-related groups (DRGs),** a system that classifies patients according to the diagnosis, treatment, and length of hospital stay. The patient is assigned a DRG based on the primary diagnosis, and the payment made by Medicare to a hospital is determined by the DRG rather than the length of time the patient remains in the hospital.

Since 1992, payments for services under Part B have been based on a **resource-based relative value scale (RBRVS)** developed by researchers at Harvard University. This system establishes relative value units for each procedure based on the amount of work involved, overhead expenses, and cost of malpractice insurance. The amount Medicare pays for each relative value unit is then adjusted annually; it is also adjusted for different geographic areas (because overhead and malpractice cost may vary). An annual fee schedule is available online for identifying the amount Medicare pays for specific procedures. A similar system is used by most commercial insurance carriers today.

A participating provider in the Medicare program must bill for the patient, accept assignment of benefits, and accept Medicare's determination of the allowable charge for the service. Under Part B, after paying an annual deductible, the patient is responsible for 20% of the allowable charge. The amount of the deductible is adjusted yearly.

If a physician does not participate in the Medicare program (nonPAR), usually he or she does not accept assignment of benefits but collects the bill from the patient up to a limiting charge (percent limit on fees above the fee-schedule amount) set by legislation.

Many patients purchase additional insurance (known as *Medicare supplemental* or *Medigap insurance*) that covers the annual deductible and 20% coinsurance for Part B, as well as the charge for the first day of a hospital stay (the deductible for Part A). Patients in most Medicare Advantage plans do not need supplemental insurance. Some patients may also be covered by employment plans after retirement. In this case, Medicare is the primary insurance and the Medigap or employment retiree plan is secondary. If a person continues to work after 65 and obtains insurance through employment, that insurance is the primary insurance for that individual and Medicare is the secondary insurance.

Medicaid

Medicaid, formally Title XIX (Title 19) of the 1965 amendments to the Social Security laws, provides for the federal government to give each state a grant to be used toward care of low-income residents. Along with the federal government's basic funding comes an obligation for the states to provide basic health care. States may add coverage for other care to their Medicaid laws but must pay for most of those costs, with the federal government paying a portion. The name of the Medicaid program as well as procedures for gaining access to it vary from state to state.

A patient's Medicaid eligibility must be checked at every office visit. In many states patients have a Medicaid card similar to a credit card with a magnetic stripe. The medical assistant uses a machine similar to a credit card reader to verify the patient's eligibility, as was discussed in Chapter 37.

Physicians may agree or decline to provide services to Medicaid patients. If they agree to treat Medicaid patients, physicians must agree to accept the state's payment for services, without billing patients for any difference between the state's payment and the actual charge.

Adults and children receiving basic welfare grants from a state are automatically eligible for Medicaid. Also, the children in many working households are eligible for Medicaid benefits if the parents' pay is low enough to put the family below the poverty line or if employee-provided medical insurance covers only the employed parent.

In addition to paying for medical services, Medicaid also covers the cost of long-term nursing home care for poor elderly and disabled individuals. Because nursing home care is so expensive, 20% of Medicaid beneficiaries—the elderly poor living in nursing homes—account for 70% to 80% of the cost of the Medicaid program.

Children's Health Insurance Program

The Children's Health Insurance Program (CHIP), established in 1997, is overseen by the CMS but managed by the individual states. The plan was expanded when President Obama signed the Children's Health Insurance Program Reauthorization Act in 2009. This program is administered and partially funded on a statewide basis. In some states eligible children are enrolled in the state's Medicaid plan. The medical assistant should familiarize himself or herself with the state requirements for this plan.

Insurance Plans for Dependents of Members of the Armed Services and Veterans

CHAMPUS was established by the federal government in 1966 to provide health benefits for the dependent spouses and children of active military personnel when receiving care from civilian physicians and health facilities. The name has been changed to TRICARE with the addition of managed care services because there are three plans available to members of the armed services: TRICARE Standard (formerly CHAMPUS), TRICARE Prime, and TRICARE Extra.

TRICARE Standard benefits are available to dependent spouses and children of active-duty military personnel, dependent spouses and children of military personnel who died while on active duty, and military retirees (and their dependents) who are not old enough to be eligible for Medicare. It is a standard fee-for-service plan.

TRICARE Prime is an HMO-type plan with optional participation. In addition to the services covered by TRICARE Standard, it includes preventive and primary care services.

TRICARE Extra allows an individual to seek care from a network provider on a visit-by-visit basis, receiving a discount on medical services provided and a lower copayment than when using TRICARE Standard.

In 1973 the federal government created CHAMPVA to provide both inpatient and outpatient medical benefits for the dependent spouses and children of veterans who have suffered total, permanent, service-connected disabilities and for surviving spouses and children of veterans who have died as a result of those service-connected disabilities. The nearest VA Medical Center determines eligibility and issues an identification card, but the CHAMPVA-covered patients are allowed to choose their own physicians and other medical service providers.

Workers' Compensation

Workers' compensation insurance covers lost wages and the cost of medical treatment for workers injured on the job or who fall ill as a result of workplace hazards or disease. Each state has its own workers' compensation program. The cost of workers' compensation insurance is paid by employers. The premium for a given employer depends on how many previous employees have made claims under workers' compensation.

Workers are required to make a prompt claim for workers' compensation coverage after an accident or the onset of an illness. In many states the employer and the insurance company issuing the policy have the right to choose the physician who treats the patient.

If a patient visits his or her regular primary care physician and says the illness or injury is workplace related, the medical assistant should check promptly with the employer to verify that the employee has made a report and that the care will be covered by the company's workers' compensation plan.

If a patient of the medical practice is seen for a workers' compensation case, separate medical and financial records should be established for that patient. Laws require that requests for medical records for compensation cases must contain only information associated with the work-related injury. If a workers' appeal board needs work-related injury records, it is important that no other medical information about the patient be released.

For a workers' compensation case, the physician must file a Physician's First Report of Injury. In most states this must be done within 72 hours of the patient's initial visit for a workplace injury. Four copies are prepared: one for the employer's compensation insurance carrier, one for the employer, one for the state compensation board, and one for the patient's medical record.

In addition to the report, the physician submits a statement of services to the insurance carrier. The physician must sign all forms because a stamped signature is not accepted for workers' compensation cases. As with most government programs, the physician must accept the payment provided as payment in full. The physician submits a report and a statement monthly until care is completed.

INSURANCE AND MANAGED CARE POLICIES AND PROCEDURES

Meeting Requirements for Insurance and Managed Care Plans

In order to obtain the maximum third-party reimbursement for services provided to patients, it is very important to be familiar with the requirements of each insurance carrier and HMO that provides insurance for the practice's patients. In addition, the same carrier may support more than one insurance plan. Each insurance plan works in its own way, and each one has a handbook for providers. This is available in hard copy and can also usually be accessed via the Internet and downloaded to the office network. The medical assistant should familiarize himself or herself with the various requirements of each particular insurance plan, including such things as whether a referral to a specialist must be in writing (hard copy or electronic) or can be given over the telephone. Each precertification and most referrals must be authorized by the HMO, and the authorization number should be noted on all of the certification or referral paperwork or electronic forms.

The medical assistant must also know which laboratory can do laboratory work for each plan and where patients can be referred for diagnostic follow-up. Most HMOs, for example, have contracts with a limited number of laboratories and/or medical facilities and will pay only for services provided by an approved facility (Procedure 46-1).

Because many patients have prescription drug benefits, the medical assistant should also learn the pharmacies that should be used for each plan and be sure that pharmacy information has been entered along with insurance plan information for each patient. The patient may have a separate pharmacy insurance card with specific information. This card should be copied for the patient file or scanned into the office computer system.

PROCEDURE 46-1 Applying Managed Care Policies and Procedures

Outcome Apply managed care policies and procedures.

Equipment/Supplies

- Managed care handbooks
- Managed care contract
- Username and password for managed care website

1. **Procedural Step.** Assemble information to review policies and procedures for a specific managed care organization, including hard copies of contracts and/or handbooks as well as information to log onto the organization's website.

2. **Procedural Step.** Sign into the managed care organization's website and/or use the contract and handbooks provided in hard copy to read about requirements for the managed care organization.

3. **Procedural Step.** Become familiar with any different plans offered by one organization, including covered services, covered hospitals, and covered laboratories, so that you can instruct patients and answer questions.
   Principle. Sometimes there are different plans whose benefits are different. The medical assistant should be able to answer patient questions.

4. **Procedural Step.** Become familiar with the preferred method to verify eligibility, notify the organization about proposed procedures or treatment, and obtain preauthorization or precertification.
   Principle. Each organization has its own requirements. Failure to meet the requirements of the managed care organization may result in denial of insurance benefits.

5. **Procedural Step.** Review all forms used by the managed care organization. Become familiar with electronic forms if that is the preferred method of submission. Download and print hard copies of any forms that will be submitted by mail, and make copies.
   Principle. Most managed care organizations prefer electronic submission of forms. The review process is faster, and authorized services can be viewed by other providers or hospitals.

6. **Procedural Step.** Repeat steps 1 to 5 for all managed care organizations with which the practice is affiliated.

7. **Procedural Step.** Make a note of the process for obtaining additional information if questions arise for each organization.

8. **Procedural Step.** Stay up to date and attend any training or information sessions provided by the various managed care organizations.
   Principle. Requirements change, so it is important to stay up to date with the latest information.

9. **Procedural Step.** Follow the guidelines for each managed care organization before providing services that require notification or authorization, when submitting insurance claims, and when answering patient questions about insurance.

Obtaining Preauthorization (Precertification)

Most insurance companies have a process for reviewing services such as surgery, treatment by a specialist, physical therapy, certain diagnostic tests, and so on. The services and specific requirements vary greatly and tend to be stricter for managed care plans. The first element of the process is often to verify **eligibility** status—that is, determine if the patient has health insurance coverage and will be able to receive health insurance benefits during the proposed time period. The patient's insurance card identifies telephone numbers, fax numbers, and usually a website where eligibility status can be verified (Figure 46-2). The second element is to verify insurance benefits—that is, determine if the patient's insurance covers the proposed service. The third element is to fulfill the insurance company's requirements for notifying the insurance company and obtaining authorization to provide the service.

Preauthorization (or prior authorization) and **precertification** are two terms used to indicate that the patient's health insurance company has verified that the service is covered by the patient's insurance policy and/or that the insurance company has reviewed the medical necessity for a service and agreed that a procedure is medically appropriate (utilization review). Different companies may use these terms in slightly different ways. In addition, some companies require formal notification of the intent to provide or receive service, either by the provider or the patient. The requirement may be for a telephone call or submission of an electronic or written form depending on the insurance company.

Preauthorization (precertification) is usually required for certain medical procedures, therapy (e.g., physical therapy, occupational therapy, speech therapy), certain diagnostic procedures, and consultations by a specialist physician, surgery, and hospitalization. Most insurance carriers prefer that requests for preauthorization (precertification) be submitted electronically using the insurance company's own website or an affiliate. The response is usually also provided electronically, usually with a form that can be printed and filed in a paper medical record or downloaded to an electronic medical record. Paper forms can be obtained for

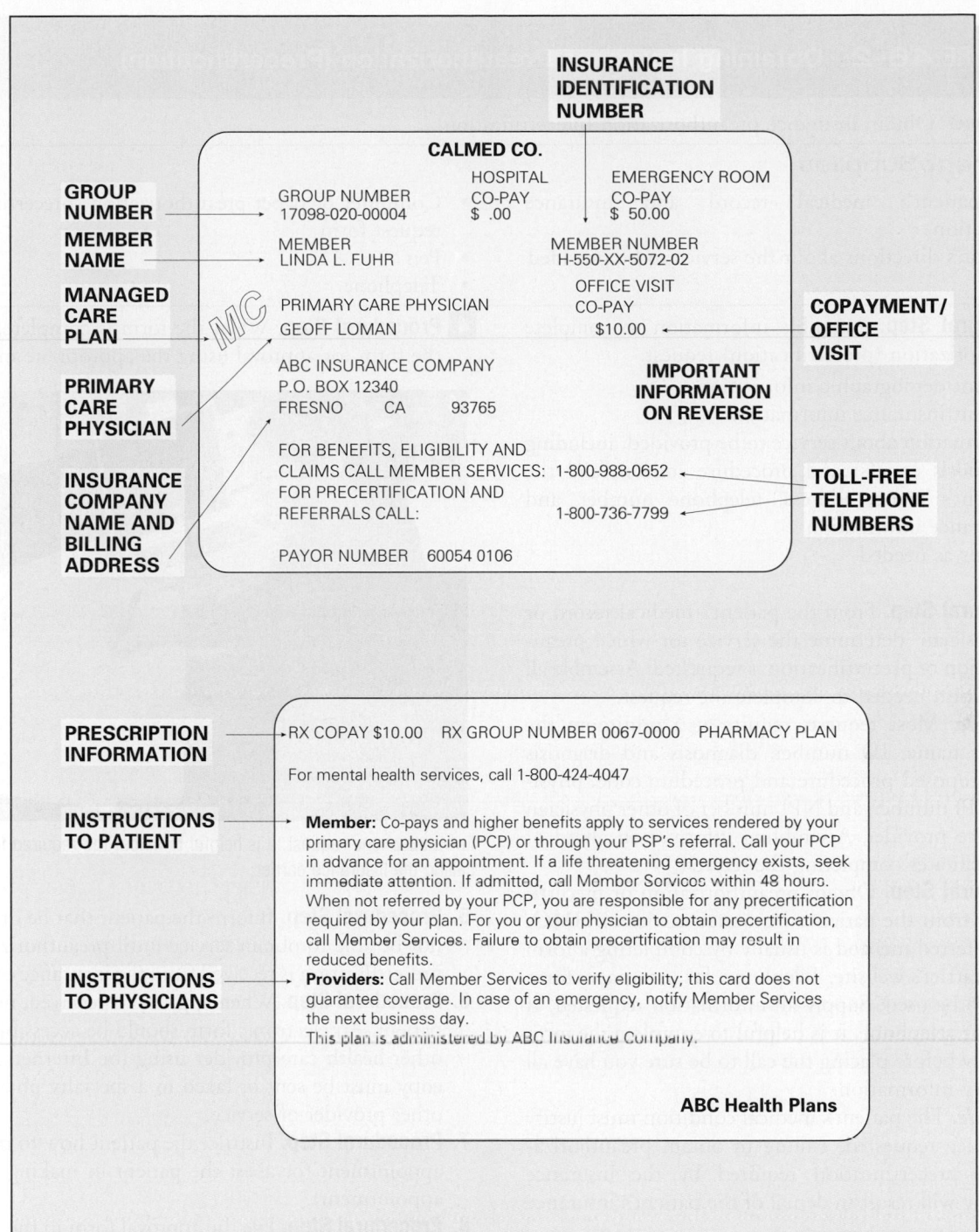

Figure 46-2 The patient's insurance card summarizes important information about the insurance plan.

fax or mail submission. Electronic requests can be approved more quickly.

The medical assistant should obtain the following information from the physician before initiating the request for preauthorization (precertification): a description of the service (e.g., number of visits to a specialist, type of therapy, surgery), the patient's diagnosis, any relevant information to justify the need for the service, and the proposed date of service (such as surgery or hospitalization). In addition, the medical assistant will need to provide the patient's

demographic and insurance information as well as the national provider identifier (NPI) numbers and contact information of the primary care physician, the physician who will perform the service, and the hospital or other health care facility where the patient will receive treatment (Procedure 46-2).

Referrals

A **referral** is the directing of a patient to a medical specialist by a primary care physician. (In managed care, a referral is

PROCEDURE **46-2**   Obtaining Insurance Preauthorization (Precertification)

Outcome Obtain insurance preauthorization (precertification).

Equipment/Supplies

- The patient's medical record and insurance information
- Physician's directions about the service to be provided
- Computer or paper preauthorization (precertification) request form
- Pen
- Telephone

---

1. **Procedural Step.** Assemble information to complete preauthorization (precertification) request:
   - Patient demographic information
   - Patient insurance information
   - Information about service to be provided, including diagnosis code(s) and procedure code(s), and the patient's name, address, telephone number, and insurance information
   - Forms as needed
   - Pen

2. **Procedural Step.** From the patient's medical record or the physician, determine the service for which preauthorization or precertification is requested. Assemble all information needed to complete the request.
   Principle. Most requests require at a minimum the patient's name, ID number, diagnosis and diagnosis code, proposed procedure and procedure code, physician's NPI number, and NPI number of other physician or service provider. Assembling information ahead of time facilitates completing the request.

3. **Procedural Step.** Obtain preauthorization or precertification from the patient's insurance carrier or HMO. The preferred method is usually by completing a form on the carrier's website. Telephone, fax, or a paper form may also be used. Supply all information requested. If using the telephone, it is helpful to complete the form manually before placing the call to be sure you have all necessary information.
   Principle. The patient's medical condition must justify the service requested. Failure to obtain preauthorization or precertification required by the insurance company will result in denial of the patient's insurance claim.

4. **Procedural Step.** When the form is complete, submit the form for approval using the appropriate method.

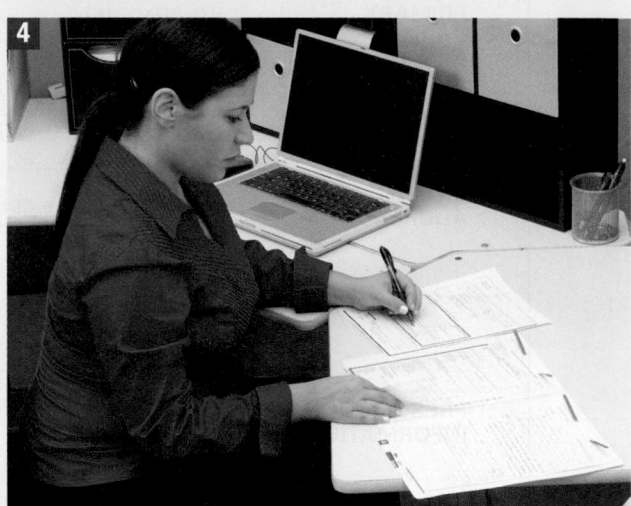

For a telephone request, it is helpful to fill out the required form before calling the insurance carrier.

5. **Procedural Step.** Inform the patient that he or she will not be able to obtain service until preauthorization or precertification is received from the insurance company.
6. **Procedural Step.** When approval is received, notify the patient. An electronic form should be accessible to any other health care provider using the Internet. A paper copy must be sent or faxed to a specialty physician or other provider of service.
7. **Procedural Step.** Instruct the patient how to make the appointment (or assist the patient in making the first appointment).
8. **Procedural Step.** File the approval form in the patient's medical record.

---

sometimes also used as the name for an authorization for a treatment, such as a referral for physical therapy). The PCP may be able to initiate a referral to a physician who participates in the patient's managed care plan without prior authorization, but usually a referral must be approved. This is consistent with the primary physician's role as "gatekeeper," or person responsible for deciding what care is medically necessary for the patient. For many managed care plans and for patients covered by Medicaid (government insurance for low-income patients), all care other than visits to the PCP must be approved. The process is basically the same as that for obtaining prior authorization, but a different form (electronic or paper) may be required. When the patient has a traditional fee-for-service insurance plan or if the patient has Medicare, authorization to see a specialist is not required. In this case, when a patient makes an appointment with a specialist, it is called a **self-referral.** This alerts the staff that no additional paperwork is required.

Formulary Exceptions

Insurance plans that include prescription drug benefits usually provide patients and providers with a list of preferred medications called a **formulary** (official list of covered medications to be used by network providers). This is an attempt to control costs by encouraging physicians to prescribe generic forms of a medication. Patients may have to pay either a larger copayment or the entire cost of prescription medications that are not approved by the insurance plan. If the physician wants to prescribe a medication that is not included in the insurance plan formulary, approval can be requested from the insurance plan using a form (electronic or paper) or by telephone. This approval will usually be granted only if formulary drugs have been tried and failed or caused an adverse outcome. The medical assistant might assist the physician with the paperwork or electronic documentation required.

INSURANCE CLAIM FORMS

The most commonly used insurance form in the medical office is the CMS-1500. This form began as the Health Insurance Claim Form, which was approved for use by the American Medical Association in 1975. It was gradually accepted by various insurance plans for payment of claims by those plans. In 1990 this form was revised and printed in red. It became the required form for Medicare claims in 1992. It is discussed in greater detail in the next section.

Another commonly used form is the UB-04 form, which is used by hospitals and other institutions to submit paper insurance claims.

The CMS-1500 Claim Form

Since the 1950s the Health Insurance Association of America has sought to have all medical insurance claims filed on a common form. After considerable work to develop a universal claim form, most insurance companies will accept the CMS-1500 form, either alone or as an attachment to the company's own form. This form was updated in 2005 to accept the NPI, a 10-digit identifier required for all health care providers that replaces all previous identification (ID) numbers (Figure 46-3). A claim form with minor revisions to accept ICD-10-CM diagnosis codes will be added.

Guidelines for Processing Insurance Claims

Because payment of a significant part of the bill for most patients is made by a third-party payor, it is important for the office to prepare and track insurance claims so that claims are processed in a timely manner without mistakes that will prevent or delay payment. This improves the cash flow for the office and avoids the need for the medical assistant to take extra time to correct errors. There are several general guidelines to facilitate the claim submission process.

1. Enter all patient and insurance information correctly into the computer, and be sure that insurance information is updated at each visit with an updated photocopy of the patient's insurance card.

2. Be sure there is a signature on file for each patient for whom an insurance claim is submitted.
3. Be aware of and follow requirements for all insurance companies related to verifying patient coverage, notifying before procedures, obtaining prior authorization, and using facilities such as laboratories, hospitals, and surgery centers as required by the insurance carrier.
4. Follow the correct procedure to transmit electronic information (which will be discussed later) or complete paper claims (when they are accepted) so that they can be read by automated equipment.
5. Proofread all claims for accuracy before submitting them. Numbers that are incorrect by one digit, missing information, and/or incorrect information can result in an automatic claim rejection. Be sure to submit additional information with a claim if it is required.
6. Submit claims or claim information promptly, and follow up to make sure that claims have been processed by the insurance carrier.
7. Follow up to correct and resubmit claims rejected for errors in a timely manner.

COMPLETING THE INSURANCE CLAIM FORM

In the medical office, the medical assistant usually prepares insurance claims using a computer billing program or submits claim information to an insurance billing clearinghouse. Since 2004, federal programs such as Medicare require electronic claim submission unless the office has been granted a waiver that allows submission of paper claims. Nevertheless, the medical assistant must know what information should be included so that each claim form can be reviewed before submission (Procedure 46-3).

Carrier Information

The name and address of the insurance company to which the claim will be sent is printed in the top section of the insurance claim form. For paper claims this address should be entered in uppercase letters without punctuation (except for the hyphen in the ZIP+4 code.)

Patient and Insured Information

Patient Information

The patient section contains the patient's basic demographic information. This includes the patient's name, address, date of birth, and sex. It also identifies whether the physician accepts assignment of benefits, which is authorized by the patient's signature. Instead of asking patients to sign every insurance claim, the phrase **signature on file** or the abbreviation **SOF** is often used to indicate that the office maintains a copy of the patient's signature authorizing submission of the claim and assignment of benefits.

1500

HEALTH INSURANCE CLAIM FORM

APPROVED BY NATIONAL UNIFORM CLAIM COMMITTEE 08/05

PICA
PICA

1. MEDICARE MEDICAID TRICARE CHAMPUS CHAMPVA GROUP HEALTH PLAN FECA BLK LUNG OTHER
   (Medicare #) (Medicaid #) (Sponsor's SSN) (Member ID#) (SSN or ID) (SSN) (ID)
   1a. INSURED'S I.D. NUMBER (For Program in Item 1)

2. PATIENT'S NAME (Last Name, First Name, Middle Initial)
3. PATIENT'S BIRTH DATE MM DD YY SEX M F
4. INSURED'S NAME (Last Name, First Name, Middle Initial)

5. PATIENT'S ADDRESS (No., Street)
6. PATIENT RELATIONSHIP TO INSURED Self Spouse Child Other
7. INSURED'S ADDRESS (No., Street)

CITY STATE
8. PATIENT STATUS Single Married Other
   Employed Full-Time Student Part-Time Student
CITY STATE

ZIP CODE TELEPHONE (Include Area Code) (   )
ZIP CODE TELEPHONE (Include Area Code) (   )

9. OTHER INSURED'S NAME (Last Name, First Name, Middle Initial)
10. IS PATIENT'S CONDITION RELATED TO:
11. INSURED'S POLICY GROUP OR FECA NUMBER

a. OTHER INSURED'S POLICY OR GROUP NUMBER
a. EMPLOYMENT? (Current or Previous) YES NO
a. INSURED'S DATE OF BIRTH MM DD YY SEX M F

b. OTHER INSURED'S DATE OF BIRTH MM DD YY SEX M F
b. AUTO ACCIDENT? YES NO PLACE (State)
b. EMPLOYER'S NAME OR SCHOOL NAME

c. EMPLOYER'S NAME OR SCHOOL NAME
c. OTHER ACCIDENT? YES NO
c. INSURANCE PLAN NAME OR PROGRAM NAME

d. INSURANCE PLAN NAME OR PROGRAM NAME
10d. RESERVED FOR LOCAL USE
d. IS THERE ANOTHER HEALTH BENEFIT PLAN? YES NO *If yes,* return to and complete item 9 a-d.

READ BACK OF FORM BEFORE COMPLETING & SIGNING THIS FORM.
12. PATIENT'S OR AUTHORIZED PERSON'S SIGNATURE I authorize the release of any medical or other information necessary to process this claim. I also request payment of government benefits either to myself or to the party who accepts assignment below.

SIGNED _____ DATE _____

13. INSURED'S OR AUTHORIZED PERSON'S SIGNATURE I authorize payment of medical benefits to the undersigned physician or supplier for services described below.

SIGNED _____

14. DATE OF CURRENT: MM DD YY ILLNESS (First symptom) OR INJURY (Accident) OR PREGNANCY(LMP)
15. IF PATIENT HAS HAD SAME OR SIMILAR ILLNESS. GIVE FIRST DATE MM DD YY
16. DATES PATIENT UNABLE TO WORK IN CURRENT OCCUPATION FROM MM DD YY TO MM DD YY

17. NAME OF REFERRING PROVIDER OR OTHER SOURCE
17a.
17b. NPI
18. HOSPITALIZATION DATES RELATED TO CURRENT SERVICES FROM MM DD YY TO MM DD YY

19. RESERVED FOR LOCAL USE
20. OUTSIDE LAB? YES NO $ CHARGES

21. DIAGNOSIS OR NATURE OF ILLNESS OR INJURY (Relate Items 1, 2, 3 or 4 to Item 24E by Line)
   1. ____ 3. ____
   2. ____ 4. ____
22. MEDICAID RESUBMISSION CODE ORIGINAL REF. NO.
23. PRIOR AUTHORIZATION NUMBER

24. A. DATE(S) OF SERVICE From MM DD YY To MM DD YY	B. PLACE OF SERVICE	C. EMG	D. PROCEDURES, SERVICES, OR SUPPLIES (Explain Unusual Circumstances) CPT/HCPCS MODIFIER	E. DIAGNOSIS POINTER	F. $ CHARGES	G. DAYS OR UNITS	H. EPSDT Family Plan	I. ID. QUAL.	J. RENDERING PROVIDER ID. #
1									NPI
2									NPI
3									NPI
4									NPI
5									NPI
6									NPI

25. FEDERAL TAX I.D. NUMBER SSN EIN
26. PATIENT'S ACCOUNT NO.
27. ACCEPT ASSIGNMENT? (For govt. claims, see back) YES NO
28. TOTAL CHARGE $
29. AMOUNT PAID $
30. BALANCE DUE $

31. SIGNATURE OF PHYSICIAN OR SUPPLIER INCLUDING DEGREES OR CREDENTIALS (I certify that the statements on the reverse apply to this bill and are made a part thereof.)

SIGNED _____ DATE _____

32. SERVICE FACILITY LOCATION INFORMATION
a. b.

33. BILLING PROVIDER INFO & PH # (   )
a. b.

790-0129 (08-05) (OCR) 1 PT.

CARRIER / PATIENT AND INSURED INFORMATION / PHYSICIAN OR SUPPLIER INFORMATION

NUCC Instruction Manual available at: www.nucc.org
APPROVED OMB-0938-0999 FORM CMS-1500 (08-05)

Figure 46-3 The CMS-1500 claim form (8/05 revision).

Outcome Complete or review a CMS-1500 insurance claim form.

Equipment/Supplies

- Patient information
- Patient account or ledger
- Copy of the patient's insurance card or computer patient information screen
- Insurance claim form
- Computer with medical billing program
- Printer

1. **Procedural Step.** Assemble information needed to prepare an insurance claim, including a claim form, information about the patient, the patient account or ledger, and a copy of the patient's insurance card or insurance information. Review the claim form guidelines for the specific insurance carrier.

2. **Procedural Step.** Enter (or review) information as required on the CMS-1500 form according to the following information. If paper claims will be submitted to be scanned by intelligent character recognition (ICR), use only capital letters and do not use commas, dollar signs, or other punctuation.

   Principle. Most insurance companies use ICR scanning to digitize information on paper claims, and the equipment works best when the guidelines outlined earlier have been followed.

3. **Procedural Step.** In the carrier section, enter or validate the name and address of the insurance company to which the claim will be sent using the following format:

   Line 1: Name of carrier
   Line 2: First line of address
   Line 3: Second line of address (if needed)
   Line 4: City [space] State [space] ZIP

   Example:

   3 line address:
   STANDARD HEALTH CARE
   1500 SUMMIT AVENUE
   WESTERN XY 45000

   4 line address:
   STANDARD HEALTH CARE
   SUITE 620
   1500 SUMMIT AVENUE
   WESTERN XY 45000

4. **Procedural Step.** Complete or review the patient and insured information on the claim form.

   Box 1—The type of insurance is indicated with an X. Only one box can be marked. Insurance obtained through employment is a Group Health Plan.

   Box 1a—The ID number of the individual who is insured as shown on the insurance card.

   Box 2—The patient's last name, first name, and middle initial (separated by spaces).

   Box 3—The patient's date of birth in the format MM DD YYYY and the patient's sex (M or F) marked with an X.

   Box 4—The name of the insured using the format last name, first name, middle initial (separated by spaces). If the patient and the insured are the same, this box does not have to be completed.

   Box 5—The patient's mailing address beginning with the street. Use the two-letter state code. Do not use commas, periods, or other punctuation in the address with the exception of the hyphen in a nine-digit ZIP code. Do not use a hyphen or space as a separator in the telephone number.

   Box 6—An X in the box that defines the patient's relationship to the insured (i.e., person whose name is on the insurance policy). The choices include self, spouse, child, and other.

   Box 7—The insured's mailing address beginning with the street. Use the two-letter state code. Do not use commas, periods, or other punctuation in the address with the exception of the hyphen in a nine-digit ZIP code. Do not use a hyphen or space as a separator in the telephone number. Complete this box if Box 4 is completed.

   Box 8—The boxes that best describe the patient's marital status and employment status are checked. If the patient has insurance through the employer, assume that he or she is employed. If the patient is a college student (older than 18), it may be important to determine if he or she is a full-time student. The choices include single, married, and other, and employed, full-time student, and part-time student.

   Box 9—If there is secondary insurance, the insured's name using the format described for Box 4.

   Box 9a-d—If there is secondary insurance, the subscriber policy (ID) or group number and subscriber date of birth, sex, employer, and insurance plan name.

   Box 10a-c—Information related to the cause of the patient's condition(s). The correct boxes are checked (yes or no) to answer the questions. If the patient's condition was caused by an automobile accident, the state where the accident occurred is identified using the correct two-letter code.

   Box 11—The insured's policy group or FECA number.

   Box 11a-d—If the patient is the insured, only box 11d must be completed. The insured's date of birth in the format MM DD YYYY and the insured's sex (M or F) marked with an X. The insured's employer and insurance plan name. An X is used in the correct box to indicate if there is additional insurance (yes or no). If "yes" is selected, Boxes 9a-d are filled out.

   Box 12—If the office has on file the patient's signature on a similar permission form, the initials "SOF" or the words "Signature on File" are placed in this box. Otherwise, the patient must sign and date the form.

Continued

4

1. MEDICARE ☐ (Medicare #) MEDICAID ☐ (Medicaid #) TRICARE CHAMPUS ☐ (Sponsor's SSN) CHAMPVA ☐ (Member ID#) GROUP HEALTH PLAN ☐ (SSN or ID) FECA BLK LUNG ☐ (SSN) OTHER ☐ (ID)	**1a.** INSURED'S I.D. NUMBER (For Program in Item 1)

2. PATIENT'S NAME (Last Name, First Name, Middle Initial)	**3.** PATIENT'S BIRTH DATE MM DD YY SEX M ☐ F ☐	**4.** INSURED'S NAME (Last Name, First Name, Middle Initial)
5. PATIENT'S ADDRESS (No., Street)	**6.** PATIENT RELATIONSHIP TO INSURED Self ☐ Spouse ☐ Child ☐ Other ☐	**7.** INSURED'S ADDRESS (No., Street)
CITY STATE	**8.** PATIENT STATUS Single ☐ Married ☐ Other ☐	CITY STATE
ZIP CODE TELEPHONE (Include Area Code) ( )	Employed ☐ Full-Time Student ☐ Part-Time Student ☐	ZIP CODE TELEPHONE (Include Area Code) ( )
9. OTHER INSURED'S NAME (Last Name, First Name, Middle Initial)	**10.** IS PATIENT'S CONDITION RELATED TO:	**11.** INSURED'S POLICY GROUP OR FECA NUMBER
a. OTHER INSURED'S POLICY OR GROUP NUMBER	**a.** EMPLOYMENT? (Current or Previous) ☐ YES ☐ NO	**a.** INSURED'S DATE OF BIRTH MM DD YY SEX M ☐ F ☐
b. OTHER INSURED'S DATE OF BIRTH MM DD YY SEX M ☐ F ☐	**b.** AUTO ACCIDENT? ☐ YES ☐ NO PLACE (State)	**b.** EMPLOYER'S NAME OR SCHOOL NAME
c. EMPLOYER'S NAME OR SCHOOL NAME	**c.** OTHER ACCIDENT? ☐ YES ☐ NO	**c.** INSURANCE PLAN NAME OR PROGRAM NAME
d. INSURANCE PLAN NAME OR PROGRAM NAME	**10d.** RESERVED FOR LOCAL USE	**d.** IS THERE ANOTHER HEALTH BENEFIT PLAN? ☐ YES ☐ NO *If yes,* return to and complete item 9 a-d.
READ BACK OF FORM BEFORE COMPLETING & SIGNING THIS FORM. **12.** PATIENT'S OR AUTHORIZED PERSON'S SIGNATURE I authorize the release of any medical or other information necessary to process this claim. I also request payment of government benefits either to myself or to the party who accepts assignment below. SIGNED _____ DATE _____		**13.** INSURED'S OR AUTHORIZED PERSON'S SIGNATURE I authorize payment of medical benefits to the undersigned physician or supplier for services described below. SIGNED _____

PATIENT AND INSURED INFORMATION

Patient and insurance information section.

Box 13—If the office has on file the patient's signature on a similar permission form, the initials "SOF" or the words "Signature on File" are placed in this box. Otherwise, the patient must sign and date the form.

5. **Procedural Step.** Complete the physician or supplier information using information from the patient charge slip.

Principle. If incomplete or incorrect information about primary and secondary insurance plans is given, the claim will be denied.

Boxes 14-16—Not usually required for Medicare, Medicaid, TRICARE, CHAMPVA, and most private insurance. If these boxes must be filled in, the dates are obtained from the patient's medical record and/or the physician.

Box 17—Name of the physician who referred the patient.

Box 17a—Blank.

Box 17b—The 10-digit NPI number of the referring physician.

Box 18—If the patient's claim is for a hospitalization, either a visit or surgery performed when the patient was hospitalized, and the dates of hospitalization. Otherwise, the box is left blank.

Box 19—Left blank unless instructed by a specific insurance carrier to use this box for information specific to that carrier.

Box 20—"No" is usually checked. If the office paid for outside laboratory services that are not itemized on one of the lines in Box 24, "yes" is checked. If "yes" is checked, enter the charges with a space between the dollars and cents. Only one outside service can be billed per claim form.

Box 21—The ICD code for up to four diagnoses. Use the most specific code possible according to the current diagnostic coding system (ICD-9-CM or ICD-10-CM). Leave a space for the period on the form.

Box 22—Left blank unless the claim is a Medicaid resubmission, when the code and original reference number are entered.

Box 23—Left blank unless a referral, preauthorization, or precertification number was assigned by the insurance company.

6. **Procedural Step.** Enter information in Box 24 on lines 1-6 for each procedure that is being billed to the insurance company. For more than six procedures, complete an additional CMS-1500 form.

Box 24A—The date service began under the "From" section in the format MM DD YYYY in the unshaded area. If the service occurred on 1 day only, the "To" section is left blank; otherwise, the date service ended.

Box 24B—The code for the place of service from Table 46-1.

Box 24C—This box is usually left blank. For some carriers, a "Y" is placed in this box if the service is an emergency service.

Box 24D—The CPT or HCPCS code and modifier(s) (if any) in the unshaded area.

Box 24E—The number(s) (from 1 to 4) that point to ICD-10-CM code(s) in Box 21 that justify the procedure. Only one digit can be used in this box for Medicare claims.

Box 24F—The charges in the unshaded area, leaving a space between the number of dollars and the number of cents instead of using a decimal point.

Box 24G—If charging for more than one of the same procedure (e.g., visits to a hospitalized patient on 3 consecutive days), the number of units of the procedure charged in the unshaded area. Otherwise, the number 1.

Box 24H—Left blank unless the patient is enrolled in the Medicaid program for early, periodic, screening, diagnosis, and service (EPSDT).

Box 24I—Blank.

Box 24 J—The 10-digit NPI number of the individual who provided service in the lower portion.

7. Procedural Step. Complete the remaining boxes on the CMS-1500 form.

Box 25—The tax ID number. If the Social Security number of an individual physician is used, box "SSN" is checked. If the employer ID number of a group practice is used, box "EIN" is checked.

Box 26—The patient account number. The box is left blank if there is no patient account number. Hyphens should not be used in this box.

Box 27—If the physician accepts assignment of benefits, an X is placed in the "yes" box. If assignment of benefits is not accepted, an X is placed in the "no" box.

Box 28—The total charges with a space between the number of dollars and the number of cents.

Box 29—The amount paid toward the covered charges, including any copayment. If the amount is zero, the box is left blank.

Box 30—The balance due, with a space between the number of dollars and the number of cents.

Box 31—SOF, Signature on File, or the physician's legal signature including credentials and the date.

Box 32—The name, address, city, state, and ZIP code of the facility where the services were provided without punctuation. If services were provided at the same address as the billing address, this box, as well as 32a and 32b, can be left blank.

Box 32a—The 10-digit NPI number of the service facility location.

Box 32b—For purchased diagnostic services (box 20) insert the supplier's PIN.

Box 33—The name, address, and telephone number of the physician group or supplier of services without punctuation. The telephone number is entered to the right of the title of the field without a hyphen. A hyphen is used in a nine-digit ZIP code after the fifth digit.

Box 33a—The 10-digit NPI number of the physician group or supplier of services.

Box 33b—Blank.

8. Procedural Step. Submit claim according to office policy. Copy a paper form before mailing, and keep the copy in an insurance claims file.

Provider and supplier section.

What Would You Do? What Would You *Not* Do?

Case Study 2

Daniel Litton is a 14-year-old new patient who has an appointment with one of the dermatologists in the office. He is brought to the office by his mother, who helps him fill out the new patient information form. In the section for insurance information, his mother indicates that he is covered by family insurance plans through both his father and his mother. His mother says, "I hope you will bill my insurance for him because I have better coverage for things like this." ■

Table 46-1 Place of Service Codes Used for Billing in the Medical Office

Code	Place of Service
11	Office
12	Home
21	Inpatient hospitalization
22	Outpatient hospitalization
23	Emergency room—hospital
24	Ambulatory surgical center
25	Birthing center
26	Military hospital or clinic
31	Skilled nursing facility
32	Nursing facility
33	Custodial care facility

From Hunt SA: *Saunders fundamentals of medical assisting,* St Louis, 2007, Saunders.

Subscriber and Insurance Information

The insurance information part of the insurance claim form includes the following information about the insured (sometimes called the *subscriber* or the *guarantor*): the name of the insured, address, and relationship to the patient. (It is important to create a computer record for the **guarantor,** the individual with financial responsibility and/or insurance, if he or she is not a patient. In addition, for employer-sponsored plans, the employer's name is listed. The insured has an ID number. In a family plan, other family members may use the same number as the insured, or each may be assigned a different number. For a group plan there is also a group number that is common to all members who obtain insurance from that employer or through that group.

If there is insurance in the name of a second party, this is also included on the claim form with the appropriate information about the insurance policy and ID (policy) and group numbers. On every claim form, information must be included to identify whether the claim relates to a work injury, auto accident, or other accident. This helps the insurance company identify which insurance is responsible for covering the claim.

Physician Information

The information about the medical service provided is entered in the lower half of the insurance claim form. In addition to information about the medical problem, the *International Classification of Diseases,* (ICD) code for each diagnosis (up to four) is listed. Each procedure must be linked to a primary diagnosis code to justify the procedure. On the lower lines, information about each procedure is given, including the date of service, place of service, pointer to the procedure code, charge for the service, number of units being billed, and NPI number for the provider of each service. See Table 46-1 for a list of codes commonly used for place of service when billing from the medical office. A revised claim form with minor changes to accommodate ICD-10 diagnosis codes will be used after June 2013.

SUBMITTING INSURANCE CLAIMS

Electronic Claims

Electronic submission speeds things up enormously. Submission is instantaneous, instead of taking a few days to move through the mail. The office may submit insurance claims directly to the insurance company or submit them to a clearinghouse that processes the data and submits the claim to the appropriate carrier. The procedure for submission depends on the computer software used by the office or clearinghouse. Insurance company personnel cannot make errors inputting the information into the company's computer system because the transmission is computer to computer.

Faster delivery and faster and more accurate processing means faster reimbursement. If electronic claim submission is coupled with electronic payment from the company to the practice's operating account, the entire turnaround time from submission to money in the bank can be days instead of weeks.

All parts of the Health Insurance Portability and Accountability Act of 1996 (HIPAA) affect insurance billing, but an important provision is the Transactions and Code Set Rule. This rule requires all health care providers to use American National Standards Institute (ANSI) technical content and format specifications for electronic transmissions. The electronic data interchange (EDI) Health Care Claim Transaction set 837P defines the format that must be used to submit health care claim billing information electronically by medical offices or to transmit this information between and within agencies involved in the reimbursement process. Because of the change from ICD-9 to ICD-10 diagnosis codes, the version of 837P has changed from ANSI version 4010A1 to ANSI version 5010 effective January 2012. This change as well as the change to ICD-10 codes affects the computer systems of almost all medical offices. Usually a new version of the office's electronic billing software incorporates the required changes.

Paper Claims

The CMS-1500 form is printed in red to facilitate optical scanning when paper forms are submitted. Although rarely used, paper claim forms can be purchased from medical office supply companies. For efficient processing, it is recommended to use all capital letters and no punctuation, to be sure that all information is within the required box, and to proofread for typographical errors that might cause the claim to be rejected. The medical assistant must be sure that the insurance company accepts paper claims. (Although there are some exceptions, in general, Medicare and Medicaid now require that all claims be submitted electronically.)

If the office submits claims by mail, the frequency of submission depends on the size of the office, the number of personnel devoted to processing claims, and the number of patients seen who are covered by any particular insurance plan. Submission is usually done daily or weekly.

TRACKING INSURANCE REIMBURSEMENT

Reimbursement is the payment received by the medical practice from the insurance company for the services performed.

Using a Claims Register

A record of every insurance claim filed should be kept using an insurance claims register. An insurance claims register can be kept either manually or on the computer (Figure 46-4).

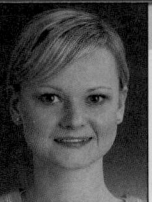

Memories *from* **Externship**

Sandra O'Keefe: My externship was done in the office of a single gynecologist in a medium-size city. Although the office had a computer billing program, we submitted most of the insurance claims on paper. After I had been at the office for several weeks, the office manager started having me fill out some insurance claim forms by hand. Then she would have me print the forms on the computer and compare my form with the computer-generated form. She said I needed to understand how to fill out the form myself, even if I didn't usually do it, so that I would know what kind of information should be in each box. At first I found it very confusing, but after a while I began to know what to look for. For example, an insurance company will deny a claim for a Pap test if the sex of the patient is given as male. I was always glad that I had some experience with insurance, although I don't think I realized how complex it really is until I actually began to work as a medical assistant. ■

What Would You Do? What Would You *Not* Do?

Case Study 3

Maria Santos, a 33-year-old woman, has been seen in the office for a physical examination. When reviewing insurance claims in the computer before submission, Sandra notices that the name of the insured on the claim for Maria Santos is Jose Santos, and his date of birth is the same as her date of birth. Sandra also notices that in box 8 there is an X beside the word "Employed." ■

The claims register includes the claim number (the number given to the claim as part of the office's tracking system); the patient's name and insurance group or policy number; the insurance company's name; the date and amount of the claim; a column for any follow-up actions taken (by mail or telephone); the date and amount of the paid claim; and any difference between the amount submitted and the amount paid.

The medical assistant should review the claims register on a regular basis to be sure that all claims have been paid and that the insurance company has not denied services that should be covered or paid less than it should for those services. If a pattern of rejected claims is seen, the medical

INSURANCE CLAIM REGISTER

BLACKBURN PRIMARY CARE ASSOCIATES, PC
1990 Turquoise Drive
Blackburn, WI 54937
608-459-8857

Claim number	Service	Insurance and ID and group no.	Date and amount of claim	Date and amount paid	Difference	Follow-up action

Figure 46-4 Insurance claims register.

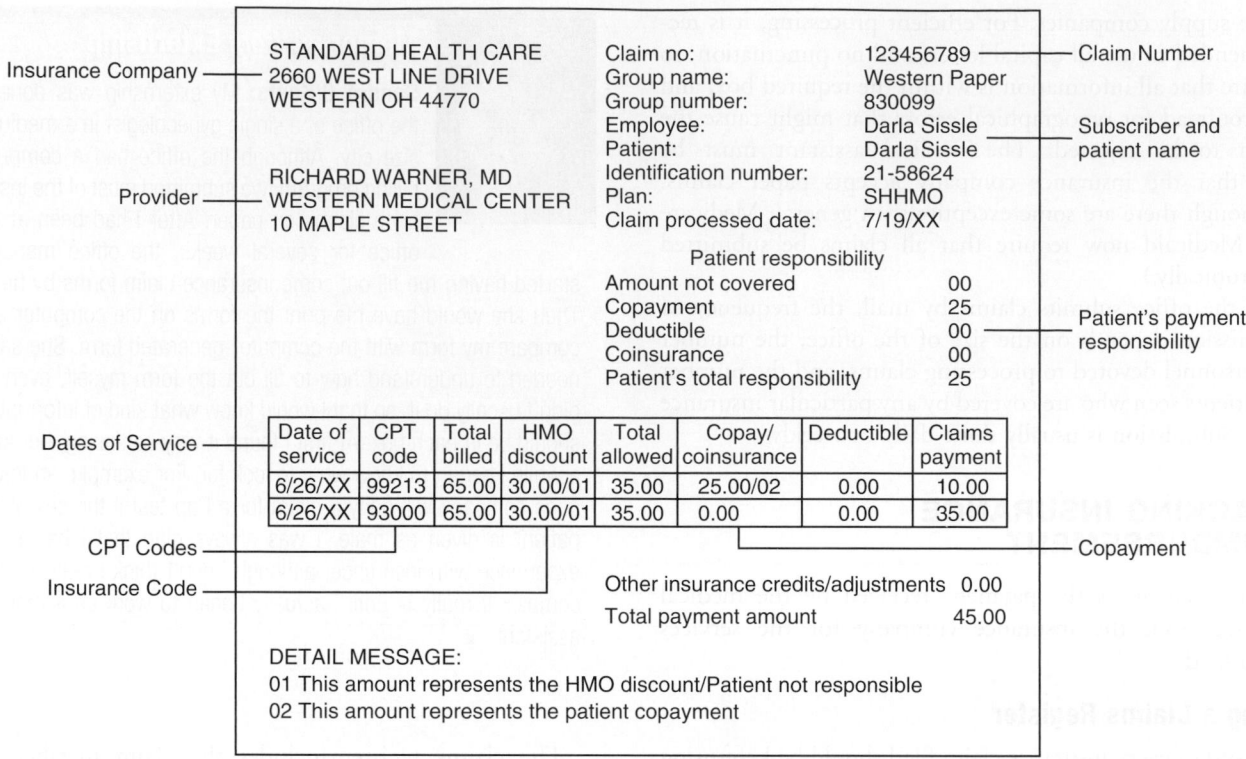

assistant should work together with other office staff to improve systems so that claims are not denied.

Explanation of Benefits Forms

After payment has been made by the insurance company to the physician, or if a claim is being denied, both the physician and the patient receive an **explanation of benefits (EOB)** form. Although each insurance carrier has its own form, the type of information contained on any EOB is similar, as shown in Figure 46-5. If the insurance company is denying the claim, the physician may also receive a remittance advice form, showing why the claim was disallowed.

Claims are usually denied for one of the following reasons: transposed names or numbers, incomplete information, incorrect or incomplete codes, or information that does not match codes or other information (Table 46-2). Claims may also be denied for late submission or late resubmission of a denied claim.

Follow-up and Resubmission of Claims

If a claim is denied, it should be resubmitted immediately, following any advice given by the company on the remittance advice form. Any questions about a denial should be discussed with a provider relations representative at the company.

If claims are not being paid or denied in a timely fashion, follow-up is in order. Follow-up can be made via letter or over the telephone. The claims log can be used to find all claims to any company that are becoming delinquent and to follow up with a call or letter.

Table 46-2 Common Errors on Insurance Claim Forms

Type of Error	Example
Transposing names or numbers	Reversing the name of the patient with the subscriber (guarantor)
	Reversing the primary insurance with the secondary insurance
	Transposing numbers in one of the identification numbers
Missing information	Missing signatures or signature stamps
	Missing or inaccurate physician national provider identifier number for each service, or not a physician registered with plan
	Required attachments missing (e.g., pathology report)
	Incomplete boxes
	No preapproval or preauthorization number
Inaccurate or incomplete codes	Inaccurate procedure or service codes (CPT or HCPCS)
	Missing modifier
Information does not match codes or other information	Diagnosis inconsistent with patient gender
	Diagnosis does not justify procedures performed
	Total amount of billing does not agree with services provided
	Place of service inconsistent with procedure code

Submitting claims for procedures that were not performed, coding for a higher level of care than can be justified by the medical record, and knowingly billing an insurance company for services to an uninsured individual are examples of insurance fraud. The medical assistant should be aware that fraud is a crime and can result in legal action against any individual involved. Individuals who have committed Medicare fraud may be excluded from participation in Medicare, Medicaid, or any other government health program. For the Medicare program alone, fraud and abuse cost taxpayers billions of dollars every year, even though the CMS encourages individuals to report any suspected Medicare fraud. The Red Flags Rule of 2009 (discussed in Chapter 37) describes the medical office's responsibility to make every attempt to detect identity theft so that insurance companies are not billed for services to uninsured individuals. ■

What Would You Do? What Would You *Not* Do? RESPONSES

Case Study 1
Page 1088

What Did Sandra Do?
❑ Explained to the patient that the original referral authorized treatment of only the lesion on the patient's neck, and the insurance company would not pay for other treatment without authorizing it.
❑ Explained that she would contact the insurance company and primary care physician and take care of any required paperwork.
❑ Promised to minimize delay as much as possible.
❑ Told the patient that she would be responsible for the cost of removal if proper authorization was not obtained from her insurance company.

What Did Sandra Not Do?
❑ Did not assume that the referral covered additional lesions not specifically mentioned on the referral form.
❑ Did not assure the patient that her insurance would automatically cover the cost of removing the additional lesions.
❑ Did not schedule the removal of the additional lesions until she had received insurance authorization or the patient promised to pay for the procedure.

What Would You Do/What Would You Not Do?
Review Sandra's response and place a checkmark next to the information you included in your response. List the additional information you included in your response.

_____
_____
_____
_____
_____

Case Study 2
Page 1100

What Did Sandra Do?
❑ Explained to Daniel's mother that there are rules governing coverage of children when both parents have insurance plans that cover their children.
❑ Asked Daniel's mother for her birth date and her husband's birth date.
❑ Explained to Daniel and his mother that usually children are covered by the insurance of the parent whose birth date comes first in the year.
❑ Asked Daniel's mother which insurance plan covered her children for their ordinary medical care.

What Did Sandra Not Do?
❑ Did not promise to send the insurance claim to the carrier the mother preferred unless it was the primary insurance carrier.
❑ Did not tell the mother not to worry because she would take care of it.
❑ Did not tell Daniel's mother that it was her responsibility to find out which insurance was the primary insurance.

What Would You Do/What Would You Not Do?
Review Sandra's response and place a checkmark next to the information you included in your response. List the additional information you included in your response.

_____
_____
_____
_____
_____

Continued

What Would You Do? What Would You *Not* Do? RESPONSES—cont'd

Case Study 3
Page 1101

What Did Sandra Do?
❑ Checked the new patient information form to be sure that the information about the insured's name and date of birth had been entered correctly because incorrect information could lead to denial of the insurance claim.
❑ Checked the new patient information form to be sure that the patient had listed an employer.

What Did Sandra Not Do?
❑ Did not assume that it was just a coincidence that the husband and wife had the same date of birth.

❑ Did not assume that a few errors on the insurance claim form would not matter.
❑ Did not assume that the information in the computer would always be correct.

What Would You Do/What Would You Not Do?
Review Sandra's response and place a checkmark next to the information you included in your response. List the additional information you included in your response.

_____
_____
_____
_____
_____

TERMINOLOGY REVIEW

Medical Term	Word Parts	Definition
Assignment of benefits		Authorization for insurance reimbursement to be made to the provider of health service rather than the insured individual.
Beneficiary		A person who can receive benefits under an insurance plan.
Benefit		Payment for a covered service under a health insurance plan.
Birthday rule		If both parents of a child have a family health plan, the insurance plan of the parent whose birthday comes earlier in the year is defined as the primary insurance plan covering the child. The insurance of the other parent becomes secondary insurance.
Capitation		A method of paying for insurance in which a fixed amount is paid to the provider per member for a specific time period regardless of the amount of care provided.
Carrier		An insurance company.
CHAMPVA		A government health insurance program that covers dependents of military veterans with service-connected disabilities.
Coinsurance		A percentage of the allowed charge for health services, which the patient is responsible for paying.
Coordination of benefits		Rules followed by insurance companies so that no claim is reimbursed at more than 100% of the charges.
Copayment		A fixed amount of money that the patient must pay for any health care service.
Deductible		An amount of money that an insured person must pay annually before health services are covered by the insurance plan.
Diagnosis-related group (DRG)		A system to determine Medicare reimbursement for a hospital stay on the basis of the patient's diagnosis.
Eligibility		Enrollment status related to a health insurance plan.
Explanation of benefits (EOB)		A statement issued by the insurance company explaining reimbursement for specific procedures.
Fee-for-service insurance		Insurance reimbursement that is directly related to the services provided and the amount charged by the provider.
Fiscal intermediary		An insurance company that contracts to review Medicare claims for the Centers for Medicare and Medicaid Services.
Formulary		An insurance carrier's official list of covered medications to be used by network providers.
Group plan		One insurance policy that covers a group of people.
Guarantor		A person with financial responsibility for a bill who may or may not also be a patient.
Indemnity		An obligation to provide compensation for loss or damage.

↻ TERMINOLOGY REVIEW—cont'd

Medical Term	Word Parts	Definition
Insured		The individual who has a specific insurance plan.
Managed care		A movement in health care based on reducing health care costs while providing high-quality care. The term may be used for the techniques used to reduce costs or for the companies that pay for the care provided.
Medicaid		The government insurance program for low-income individuals and families that is funded both by the federal government and by each individual state.
Medicare		The federal health insurance program that provides insurance coverage for the elderly, permanently disabled, and individuals with end-stage kidney disease.
Nonparticipating provider (nonPAR)		A physician who does not have any contract with a third-party payor.
Participating provider (PAR)		A physician who has a contractual agreement with a third-party payor.
Preauthorization		Verification from a patient's insurance company that a procedure is covered by the patient's insurance and/or agreement, after review, that the test or procedure is medically appropriate.
Precertification		Verification from a patient's insurance company that a procedure is covered by the patient's insurance and/or agreement, after review, that the test or procedure is medically appropriate.
Premium		An amount of money paid in a given period to purchase health insurance.
Primary care provider		The physician chosen by a patient to provide general medical care and also to determine and authorize additional medical services the patient may require.
Primary insurance		The insurance company that must be billed first for any individual.
Referral		The directing of a patient to a specialist physician by the primary care physician. Most managed care plans and some other insurance plans require the primary care physician to obtain prior authorization.
Reimbursement		The amount paid for a procedure by insurance.
Resource-based relative value scale (RBRVS)		A system to establish the Medicare fee schedule for Medicare Part B based on the service provided and the geographic location of the provider.
Secondary insurance		Insurance that an individual has in addition to primary insurance.
Self-referral		The process by which a patient makes an appointment with a specialist physician without requesting prior authorization from his or her primary care physician, usually because the patient's insurance plan does not require it.
Signature on file (SOF)		An indication on the insurance claim form that the signature of the patient is maintained by the medical office to authorize submission of insurance claims.
Third-party payor		Insurance carrier or managed care organization that pays health insurance claims.
TRICARE		A government insurance plan that provides medical care to spouses and dependents of individuals on active duty in the military. Formerly this program was called CHAMPUS.
Usual, customary, and reasonable (UCR)		A system for establishing the amount an insurance company will pay for a procedure. The reasonable charge is set by the insurance company on the basis of a physician's usual (most frequent) charge for the procedure and the customary charge of other physicians in the same geographic area.
Utilization review		Reviewing proposed or current care to determine medical necessity.
Workers' compensation		An insurance program that covers lost wages and health care costs of workers injured on the job or having work-related illnesses.

ON THE WEB

For information on the Centers for Medicare and Medicaid Services (Medicare, Medicaid, and CHIP):

Centers for Medicare and Medicaid Services: www.cms.gov

Medicare Coverage: www.cms.gov/center/PeopleWithMedicareCenter.asp

CMS-1500 Claim Form Fact Sheet: www.cms.gov/MLNProducts/downloads/form_cms-1500_fact_sheet.pdf

For information on CHAMPVA:

U.S. Department of Veterans Affairs: www.va.gov/hac/forbeneficiaries/champva/champva.asp

For information on CMS-1500 form—National Uniform Claim Committee:

National Uniform Claim Committee: www.nucc.org

For information on health care options and health care law:

U.S. Department of Health and Human Services: www.healthcare.gov

For information on TRICARE:

TRICARE Management Activity: www.tricare.mil

For information on U.S. Department of Labor—Office of Workers' Compensation Progams:

Office of Worker's Compensation Programs: www.dol.gov/owcp/owcpcomp.htm

---

 Check out the Evolve site at http://evolve.elsevier.com/Bonewit/today/ to actively Prepare for your Certification, and to access additional interactive activities and exercises to help you study and prepare for success.

47

Billing and Collections

INTRODUCTION TO BILLING

If patients have insurance, a bill is not usually sent to the patient until after the insurance company has paid its portion of the bill. If the patient is covered by a managed care policy, the copayment is usually collected at the time of the visit, and a bill may not be necessary. Often, however, the patient has a deductible and/or coinsurance, and a bill must be sent to the patient.

If a patient visit will not be covered by insurance, most physicians' offices request that payment be made at the time a medical service is provided. Medical offices usually also accept payment by credit card, which makes payment at the time of service possible and convenient for many patients. However, a number of patients still need to make arrangements to pay for their medical services over a period of time. In this case, the office must establish an account for the patient and send periodic bills. These bills are usually generated by computer software. Each bill is then placed in a window envelope and sent to the patient. Even if the patient's account is being paid by capitation, a billing record is usually kept for that patient, showing the amount of charges and payments.

The billing for physician offices that are affiliated with a hospital or large health group is usually done from a central location, and office employees are responsible only for posting charges. Patients and insurance companies make payments to the central office. Other offices may contract with an outside billing service. The medical assistant should understand the billing process, however, because efficient billing maximizes revenue for the medical practice.

BILLING CYCLE

Bills (also commonly called *statements*) can be sent to patients every 2 weeks, monthly, or at any regular period, such as once every 3 months (quarterly). The time between bills is called the *billing cycle*. A bill sent out at the end of a cycle will show the balance owed at the beginning of the cycle, any payments made during the billing cycle, any new charges for new services that occurred during the billing cycle, and the **balance due** (total amount owed) at the end of the cycle.

Patient accounts are often divided into equal parts, usually alphabetically. Each week a different section of the accounts receivable is billed. For instance, on the first week

of the month, patients with a last name beginning with the letters A to E may be billed; the second week, F to L; the third week, M to S; and the fourth week, T to Z. The same cycle is followed each month. Dividing the bills in this way makes more efficient use of staff time because billing is spread out over the month instead of being performed in only1 week of the month.

BILLING PROCESS

Bills can be produced manually using a word processing program and billing template, but in almost all medical offices they are produced using the medical office practice management program (Figure 47-1). If an outside billing service is used, the service can either send a paper record of all of the bills sent out at the end of each cycle or can transfer billing information from its computer to the office's computer, linking the information into the patient's financial record and the office's bookkeeping software.

At regular intervals, patient financial accounts should be examined and the accounts that must be billed should be processed. Billing insurance companies and billing patients are both straightforward transactions. However, the medical assistant should be aware of some special situations. A patient may have been treated for a final illness just before dying. In this case, any charges will have to be billed to the patient's estate. (Billing an estate is discussed in more detail at the end of this chapter.)

A patient may be a minor who sought treatment without his or her parent's knowledge. When minors are brought to a physician by a parent or guardian for treatment, the parent or guardian acknowledges that he or she is the responsible party for financial purposes. However, if a minor is treated without the parent's knowledge, the minor may be responsible for fees as well. Minors older than age 12 may give consent for certain kinds of treatment including treatment for sexually transmitted diseases (STDs), human immunodeficiency virus (HIV) testing, and treatment for drug or alcohol abuse. Because of confidentiality, the physician may not release information to the parent or guardian about the reason for the visit.

A patient may have a credit agreement with the practice, which allows the patient to pay bills off over time, along with interest on the balance due. This is important because in such situations, even though an outstanding balance may become old, it should not be considered delinquent and sent out of the office for collection (Procedure 47-1).

PROCEDURE 47-1 Processing Patient Bills

Outcome Process patient bills.

Equipment/Supplies

- Computer
- Patient accounts
- Window envelopes with two windows

- Statement template for word processing program (optional)
- Paper or statement forms

PROCEDURE 47-1 Processing Patient Bills—cont'd

1. **Procedural Step.** Locate patient accounts in the computer database.
2. **Procedural Step.** Identify patient accounts with an outstanding balance for which insurance payments have been made.
   Principle. Patients are usually not billed until insurance payments have been received.
3. **Procedural Step.** Create one or more patient bills manually using a statement template and word processing program, or compile outstanding bills using the computer program and view using *Print Preview.* Check all bills for completeness and accuracy.
   Principle. All bills must have the patient's name and address, previous activity for the account, and the amount due from the patient.
4. **Procedural Step.** Print patient statements using the office patient statement form. The statement form may

be printed with the bills from the computer program, or statement forms may be loaded in the printer.
5. **Procedural Step.** Make sure that statements have printed correctly.
6. **Procedural Step.** Fold statements so that the practice and the patient names and addresses will be visible through the windows in the envelopes.
   Principle. The practice purchases window envelopes with the windows positioned so that the return address of the practice shows through the upper window and the patient name and address show through the lower window.
7. **Procedural Step.** Insert statements in envelopes. Be sure that the names and addresses are visible.
8. **Procedural Step.** Place postage on envelopes and mail statements.

Putting It All Into Practice

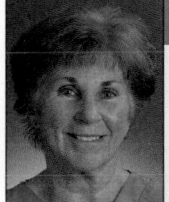

My name is Christa Wilson, and I have been working in the office of three physicians for the past 5 years. There are three medical assistants, and we all assist the physicians during office hours, but I am responsible for most of the billing. We use cycle billing in our office. The first week of the month we send out statements for patients whose last names begin with the letters A-F, the second week G-L, and so on. By the end of the month, every patient with an outstanding balance has received a statement, and we begin again. I am also responsible for posting payments received in the mail. Every month, we run an aging report, and I analyze it to see which accounts are overdue. Our computer program lets us add written

messages to the statements, but I add colored stickers for accounts that are older than 60 days because I think they are more likely to get the patient's attention. If there is a balance due from a patient after 90 days, I always follow up with a telephone call. When I first started making these calls, I used to get very nervous, but I have gotten accustomed to it now. I always try to stay calm and keep my cool. I have found that in most cases, there is a financial problem that makes it difficult for the individual or family to keep up with its debts. I try to work with our patients so that they pay something each month and remind them not to "forget" about their copayments. Eventually we do collect most of the money that is owed to us, and we feel that part of the reason is that we stay on top of our billing. ∎

BILLING PROBLEMS

Problems with Checks

From time to time the office may encounter a problem either with a check it has written or with one that has been written to the office by a patient.

Insufficient Funds in the Office Account

It is illegal to write a check for more than the amount of money in a bank account. However, this occasionally happens because of an arithmetic error in calculating the balance while writing checks or because of failure to reconcile a bank statement. If the office's account accidentally becomes overdrawn, the bank may refuse to honor any check written after the account is overdrawn. In this case the check will be returned to the person or company that deposited it marked NSF ("non-sufficient funds") in the

payer's account to cover the check. A check written on an account without adequate funds to cover it is called an **overdraft.**

It is a good practice to have overdraft protection for any office checking account. Although this protection may never be needed, it will prevent a check from bouncing in the event that the person who pays the bills in the medical office writes a check against an account without adequate funds to cover the check. In that case, funds will automatically be transferred from another office account, such as a savings account, and the bank will charge a small fee.

Stopping Payment

From time to time it may become necessary to ask the bank to stop payment on a check. A check might have been lost and a new check issued, or there may be a dispute between

PATIENT STATEMENT

WESTERN MEDICAL CENTER
109 RIVER STREET
WESTERN, OH 44770

Account # 1015
Date: 7/24/XX

DARLA SISSLE
10 MAPLE STREET
WESTERN, OH 44770

AMOUNT PAID

	Description	Charges	Credits	Balance
5/22/XX	Balance forward			$ 35.00
6/26/XX	Prob Focused OV	65.00		90.00
6/26/XX	EKG	65.00		165.00
6/26/XX	Patient payment - check		– 20.00	145.00
7/15/XX	Insurance payment		– 45.00	100.00
7/15/XX	Insurance adjustment		– 60.00	40.00

PLEASE PAY THIS AMOUNT $ 40.00

0 – 30 DAYS	**31 – 60 DAYS**	**61 – 90 DAYS**	**> 90 DAYS**	**> 120 DAYS**
5.00	35.00	0.00	0.00	0.00

Figure 47-1 A sample patient bill.

the practice and a vendor about a purchase or a previous payment. Banks charge a fee for stopping payment, so this practice should be used sparingly.

Insufficient Funds in a Patient Account

The bank may not honor a check deposited by the practice because a patient's account has insufficient funds. If a check is returned marked NSF, do not hesitate to call the patient and tell him or her of the problem. This may be the first of many checks that are being returned, and it is important for the person to find out why he or she is writing checks against insufficient funds. The bank usually charges fees both to the individual who wrote the check and to the medical office that tried to deposit the check. The amount of the NSF check must be added back to the balance owed by the patient as a positive adjustment that increases the amount owed. The fee charged by the bank is also added to the patient's balance, usually as a separate fee. As an example, assume that the patient paid a copayment of $20.00 at the time of the visit. The bank returned the check for insufficient funds and charged the medical office checking account a $15.00 fee. The medical assistant would charge the patient's account $35.00 to cover both the amount of the returned check and the additional fee charged by the bank. Most offices have a sign posted in the waiting room notifying patients of the additional charge for each returned check (Procedure 47-2).

Overpayments and Refunds

If the total of patient payments and insurance payments exceeds the allowed charge, it is called an *overpayment.* This might happen, for example, if a patient thought that he had not yet paid his annual deductible, when in fact he had. After all the payments have been posted, the balance on the account will be a negative number, or **credit balance,** indicating that the medical office owes money to the patient. Sometimes a small credit balance is left in place when a patient has a visit scheduled in the near future because new charges will be applied. Usually, however, the medical assistant will process a refund for the patient. The amount of the refund is posted to the patient's account, bringing the account balance to zero. The medical assistant sends a letter and a check to the patient with a brief explanation about the overpayment (Procedures 47-3 and 47-4).

PROCEDURE 47-2 Posting an NSF Check

Outcome Post a check returned for NSF.

Equipment/Supplies

- Computer
- Patient accounts
- Returned check

- Day sheet (optional)
- Calculator

1. **Procedural Step.** When the NSF check has been received, locate the patient account in the computer database. If using a day sheet, label the first open line with the name of the patient whose check was returned and enter the old balance in the *old balance* column.

2. **Procedural Step.** Create a new billing for the patient and post the returned check using the code for NSF check or "adjustment—charge" and entering the amount of the check. If using a day sheet, write "NSF check returned by bank" and the check number in the *professional service* column. Place the amount of the check in the *adjustment* column in parentheses to indicate that the amount is a debit adjustment (i.e., added to the patient's balance). Add the amount to the old balance and enter it in the *new balance* column.
   Principle. The amount of the returned check must be added to return the patient balance to the amount before the check was deducted.

3. **Procedural Step.** Post the amount charged by the bank as a charge using the code for a returned check fee. Record the total of the amount of the fee charged by the office for any returned check as a charge (fee). If recording on a day sheet, post the charge for the fee charged by the bank in the *fee* column. Add the amount

to the old balance and record in the *new balance* column.
   Principle. The bank fee is a new charge to the patient's account. Depending on office policy, the amount charged for the NSF check may be considered a fee or a debit adjustment.

4. **Procedural Step.** If using a computer program, be sure that the box indicating that insurance should be billed is *not* checked.
   Principle. Insurance is not responsible for the charge for a returned check.

5. **Procedural Step.** When totaling the columns of the day sheet at the end of the day, subtract any debit adjustment from the total of all credit adjustments.

6. **Procedural Step.** Notify the patient by telephone or letter that the check was returned and a fee has been charged. If sending a letter, enclose a patient statement with the letter showing the total amount of the returned check and the fee.
   Example: Darla Sissle's check for $15.00 was returned by the bank marked NSF. The bank also charged a fee of $15.00.

Charges:

Date	Procedure	Diag 1	Diag 2	Diag 3	Provider	POS	Units	Amount	Total
1/30/XX	99212	112.9			RW	11	1	55.00	55.00

Payments and adjustments:

Date	Pay/Adj Code	Paid By:	Description	Amount	Total
1/30/XX	Check	Darla Sissle	Patient Payment, Check	−15.00	40.00
2/4/XX	NSF		Check returned by bank	15.00	55.00
2/4/XX	FEE		Bank fee for NSF check	15.00	70.00

The NSF check and bank fee are posted to the patient's account.

What Would You Do? What Would You *Not* Do?

Case Study 1

The bank returns a check from a patient for NSF. The amount on the check is $25.00, and the bank includes a notice that the practice will be charged $15.00. Christa makes a telephone call to the patient, and she asks the patient to send the office a bank check or money order in the amount of $$40.00 The patient

becomes very upset. She says, "The bank will charge me the fee for the returned check, not you. All you have to do is send the check through again. There is money in the account now because I deposited my paycheck yesterday. You can't charge me a fee for this. You are just trying to make money out of this situation." ∎

PROCEDURE **47-3** Processing a Credit Balance

Outcome Process a credit balance.

Equipment/Supplies

- Computer
- Patient accounts
- Payment check(s)
- Day sheet
- Office policy manual
- Calculator

1. Procedural Step. When a payment has been made, locate the patient account in the computer. If using a day sheet, enter the patient's name on a new line and enter the previous balance in the *old balance* column.
Principle. Both insurance payments and patient payments must be entered in the correct patient account.

2. Procedural Step. Compare the amount of the payment against the total amount owed.
Principle. The total amount owed will be the balance due and charges for new services.

3. Procedural Step. Even if the payment is greater than the charges, post the payment to the computer system using the correct code (i.e., patient payment, check, insurance payment) and link to the visit for which the payment is made. If using a day sheet, post the payment on the line with the patient's name in the *payment* column.

4. Procedural Step. If an overpayment has occurred, note that the account balance in the computer is preceded by a minus sign. This means that the medical office owes the patient money. On the day sheet, subtract the amount of the payment from the patient's previous balance and record in the *new balance* column. Place a negative number in parentheses. When totaling the *new balance* column at the end of the day, subtract any negative number from the total instead of adding it.
Principle. A negative balance is indicated in accounting by enclosing it in parentheses. Care must be taken when totaling columns on a day sheet to subtract a negative number from the total.

5. Procedural Step. Take steps to clear the balance from the system according to your office policy. If the patient has another appointment scheduled, the negative balance may be carried for a short time. In most cases, a refund should be issued promptly (see Procedure 47-4).
Principle. Office policy guidelines indicate the proper management of a credit balance in a patient account.

PROCEDURE **47-4** Processing a Refund

Outcome Process a refund.

Equipment/Supplies

- Computer
- Patient accounts
- Payment check(s)
- Day sheet
- Office policy manual
- Calculator

1. Procedural Step. Locate the patient account in the computer. If using a day sheet, enter the patient's name on a new line and enter the amount of the credit balance in the *old balance* column.
Principle. All financial transactions must be entered in the correct patient account.

2. Procedural Step. Calculate the amount to be refunded (usually the amount of the negative balance).

3. Procedural Step. Create a new transaction for the patient in the computer account and choose "Refund" for the code. If using a day sheet, write "Refund for Overpayment" in the *professional service* column.

4. Procedural Step. Enter the amount of the refund in the "Amount" box of the transaction screen, and verify that the patient balance becomes zero. On the day sheet, record the amount of the refund in the *adjustment* column. Add this number to the patient's old balance (a negative number) so that the new balance becomes zero, and enter zero in the *new balance* column.
Example: The patient Edmund Hall paid $50.00 on his account followed by an insurance payment of $55.00, resulting in an overpayment of $15.00. A refund was issued for $15.00.

5. Procedural Step. Write a check for the refund amount including the date, amount in numbers, and amount in words on the line below. Leave the signature line blank.
Principle. The medical assistant is generally not authorized to sign checks for the medical office.

PROCEDURE 47-4 Processing a Refund—cont'd

6. **Procedural Step.** Record the check number, date, payee, and reason for the check on the check stub in the checkbook or in the check register.
7. **Procedural Step.** Subtract the amount of the check from the balance in the check register.
8. **Procedural Step.** Write a letter informing the patient of the refund, and prepare an envelope.

9. **Procedural Step.** Sign the letter and your title, or obtain the physician signature depending on office policy.
10. **Procedural Step.** Leave the check, letter, and envelope in the correct place to obtain an authorized signature on the check.

WESTERN MEDICAL CENTER
PATIENT ACCOUNT LEDGER
As of 4/19/20XX

Date	POS	Description	Procedure	Provider	Amount
EDMUND HALL					
Last Payment: −50.00 on 4/19/20XX					
3/21/20XX	11		99213	RW	65.00
3/21/20XX	11		88051	RW	25.00
3/30/20XX	11	Ins payment	INS	RW	−55.00
4/19/20XX	11	Patient payment	CHECK	RW	−50.00
4/19/20XX	11	Refund	REFUND	RW	15.00
Patient Total					0.00

Verify that the patient's account balance becomes zero.

ACCOUNT AGING

Account aging is the process of determining how long specific account balances have been outstanding.

Accounts Receivable Aging Records and Reports

An accounts receivable aging record should be created to identify accounts that are overdue. Accounts are aged in 30-day intervals. Figure 47-2 shows a sample accounts receivable aging record (see also Procedure 47-5).

Examining Accounts for Those Overdue

An account is considered overdue if it is not paid within 30 days of the date billed unless there is an outstanding credit

What Would You Do? What Would You *Not* Do?

Case Study 2
A patient calls the office to say that she has received her bill, and it does not show a payment of $10.00 that she made in cash at the time of the visit. The patient is upset, and she says, "I knew I shouldn't pay cash, because now I can't prove that I made that payment. I don't see why you can't keep accurate records." Christa asks the patient if she received a receipt for the cash payment. The patient says, "How do you expect me to remember that? This happened over a month ago." ■

PROCEDURE 47-5 Creating an Accounts Receivable Aging Record

Outcome Create and examine an accounts receivable aging record.

Equipment/Supplies
- Computer
- Patient accounts
- Accounts receivable aging record analysis form (optional)
- Office policy manual
- Pen

Continued

1. Procedural Step. Using the reports function of the computer billing program, create an aging report for patients and for insurance companies. It is also possible to create such a report manually using individual patient ledgers.

Principle. In a computerized billing system, the computer program can generate the report of all overdue accounts.

2. Procedural Step. Review the accounts on the report and mark the proposed action for each account according to your office policy.

Principle. Efforts to collect outstanding accounts should become increasingly more active as the account ages. Office policy may vary in respect to specific actions.

3. Procedural Step. Mark all accounts that are less than 31 days old "No Action Needed."

Principle. Accounts that are less than 31 days old are considered current.

4. Procedural Step. Mark bills with unpaid insurance claims that are older than 31 days "Follow up with insurance."

Principle. Patients usually do not pay on bills with outstanding insurance claims until they find out how much the insurance will pay. These bills, if overdue, need to be followed up with the insurance company.

5. Procedural Step. Mark accounts that are 31 to 60 days old, according to office policy. For example, a note may be attached to the statement saying, "Payment is now due." It may be possible to include payment notices in the computer program so that they print on the statement automatically if the account is overdue.

6. Procedural Step. Mark accounts that are 61 to 90 days old, according to office policy. For example, a note may be attached to the statement saying, "Payment of this bill is now overdue. Please pay the balance or contact the office."

7. Procedural Step. Mark accounts that are 91 to 120 days old, according to office policy. It may be office policy to place a telephone call to the patient at this point to discuss the account. Follow up with a letter confirming any agreement made.

8. Procedural Step. For accounts older than 120 days, review previous collection attempts. Unless there are known circumstances that warrant a delay in collection activity, send a collection letter stating that if payment is not received by a certain date the account will be given to a collection agency or pursued in small claims court (depending on the procedure used by the office to collect delinquent accounts).

Principle. After 120 days without activity, especially if the person owing money has been contacted by telephone and letter, it is unlikely that the bill will be paid without more aggressive collection measures.

9. Procedural Step. Record all action taken beside each account on the report.

Principle. This provides a written record of actions taken and results of telephone conversations.

10. Procedural Step. Write follow-up letters to document in writing any agreements made during telephone conversations. Attach a copy to the patient's medical record.

Principle. A written record of verbal communications regarding bills and payments provides evidence in case further legal action is necessary.

---

agreement. Accounts for which all the charges are from the previous billing period are considered current (0 to 30 days). Overdue accounts are categorized as 30 to 60 days, 60 to 90 days, and longer than 120 days.

An account with an outstanding balance after 120 days requires additional collection activity, such as sending the account out to a collection agency or writing a demand letter informing the account holder that a lawsuit will be brought if the account is not brought up to date. Most of the time, the balance of medical office accounts is small enough to permit legal action in small claims court. (Small claims court is discussed in more detail at the end of the chapter.)

COLLECTION ACTIVITIES

Many people who owe money have every intention of paying their bill but are unable to do so in the short term because of some emergency. As accounts age, it is appropriate to increase the forcefulness of any message to the patient

that the account is overdue. Patients should always be invited to call the office and make arrangements to pay over time if they have had a true emergency. Sometimes it is medical bills themselves that are piling up, especially in the case of a patient with a chronic illness who does not have adequate insurance.

Patients are also encouraged to discuss accounts for which insurance payment is expected but delayed. By working with the insurance company, the patient can more easily determine whose responsibility the bill is.

Past Due Accounts

Messages encouraging payment of the bill (often called **claim messages**) can be attached to bills or included in the billing envelope. Some computer programs will print a message on the bill itself.

A bill that is 60 days overdue should be accompanied by a claim message reminding the patient that the bill is overdue. Many offices use a series of messages that become more forceful as time passes without payment.

Enter credits in parentheses ( ) and subtract when totaling columns and P

ACCOUNTS RECEIVABLE AGING RECORD

Name		As of Date	Prepared by					Page of Page

NO.	ACCOUNT NAME	Insurance Information		Date of Last Payment	Current 1 to 30 days	31 to 60 days	61 to 90 days	91 to 120 days	121 days and over	TOTAL
		Date Claim Filed	Amount of Claim							
	Amounts brought forward									
1	Mary Smith			8/8/XX	120					120 -
2	John Payne			7/6/XX		250 -				250 -
3	Jack Desmonde			5/25/XX			500			500 -
4	Jill Jayne			4/2/XX		80 -				180 -
5										

A

Blackburn Primary Care Associates
Patient Aging

NAME	CURRENT 0 - 30	PAST 31 - 60	PAST 61 - 90	PAST 91 - 120	PAST over 120	Total Balance
Mary Smith Last Payment on 08/08/XX	$120.00					$120.00
John Payne Last Payment on 07/06/XX		$250.00				$250.00
Jack Desmonde Last Payment on 05/25/XX			$500.00			$500.00
Jill Jayne Last Payment on 04/02/XX		$80.00		$100.00		$180.00
Report Aging Totals Percent of Total Aging	$120.00 11.4%	$330.00 31.4%	$330.00 47.6%	$100.00 9.5%		$1,050.00 100.0%

B

Figure 47-2 Sample accounts receivable aging record: A, prepared by hand; B, prepared by computer.

Bills that are 90 days overdue should be followed up with a telephone call. By contacting patients directly, the medical assistant can determine why there has been no activity related to the account. The medical assistant must be careful to follow legal guidelines when discussing accounts with patients. The Fair Debt Collection Practices Act of 1966 identifies activities that are permitted and not permitted when contacting individuals who owe money. Most states also have debt collection laws with which the medical assistant should be familiar.

Collection Letters

Bills that are aged 120 days should either be accompanied by or followed up by a collection letter, such as the one shown in Figure 47-3. When writing a collection letter, the medical assistant should gather information related to the account before composing the letter. The recipient should be clearly informed about what action is expected, as well as the deadline for action. The letter should not threaten legal action or transfer to a collection agency unless the office is prepared to follow through.

Each medical office has its own policy about who should sign a collection letter. In many offices, the medical assistant signs the letters. In other offices there may be an office manager or billing specialist, or each physician may prefer to sign letters to his or her own patients (Procedure 47-6).

If the collection letter does not receive a response, another letter should be sent stating either that the account is now being turned over to a **collection agency** (a company that collects overdue bills for other companies) or that a lawsuit will be filed in small claims court if the account is not paid by a certain date. Some offices will continue to see patients with accounts in collection, but they usually require the patient to pay any current charges before the patient can be seen.

As in any case where it is important to have documentation that a letter was received, the letter should be sent Certified Mail, with a Return Receipt requested. If the patient is being asked to find a new provider, the letter should allow the patient at least 2 weeks to arrange alternate care.

Western Medical Center
107 River Street
Western, OH 44770

4/10/20XX

[Patient Address]

Dear [Patient Name],

Your account in this office is now more than 120 days overdue. We have made several previous attempts to set up a mutually agreeable payment schedule with you, but you have not followed through on your commitment. This will be your final notice. If you do not contact our office within 7 days of receipt of this letter, we will have no choice but to turn over this account to our collection agency. Please call us at (490) 220-1156 or send a check to pay the balance of your account if you wish to avoid collection activity.

Yours truly,

Richard Warner, MD

Richard Warner, MD

RW/mt

Figure 47-3 Sample collection letter.

Highlight on Guidelines for Telephone Collections

Things to Do

1. A creditor (person or company who is owed money) may contact the person who owes money by telephone during reasonable hours. The medical assistant should gather accurate information before placing the telephone call about an overdue account:
   a. Who owes the money?
   b. How much money is owed?
   c. How long has the money been owed?
   d. Is there any insurance claim pending?
   e. Has the insurance company processed the claim and/or made any payment?
2. A creditor may take measures to locate a person but may not divulge that he or she is trying to collect a bill to anyone other than the person who owes money. The medical assistant should ask to speak with the patient or the person responsible for the account when placing the call.
3. A creditor may not misrepresent himself or herself in order to trick the person who owes money into taking the call. After asking for the person responsible for the account, the medical assistant should identify himself or herself and the office or physician.
4. A creditor may not harass or intimidate a person who owes money. The medical assistant should speak calmly and professionally. The conversation should include a discussion of the different options for payment, including full payment, partial payment, and monthly installments. If possible, the medical assistant should obtain a verbal commitment for a date and amount of at least a first payment and/or a payment plan.
5. Although a verbal agreement is legally binding, a written agreement is easier to enforce if legal action becomes necessary. It is important to follow up any verbal agreement with a letter referring to the conversation and the agreement. If an arrangement was established for monthly payments, a truth-in-lending statement must be included, even if the patient will not pay interest.
6. Although it is not permitted to harass the patient, the medical assistant may contact him or her again if payments are not made as agreed. Often, the knowledge that attention is being paid to the account will encourage the patient to adhere to the repayment schedule.

Things Not to Do

1. A creditor should not call too early in the day or too late at night.
2. A creditor should not divulge to employers, neighbors, or other third parties that he or she is trying to collect a bill from the patient.
3. A creditor should not threaten.
4. A creditor should not end the conversation on vague terms.
5. A creditor should not call repeatedly. ■

Credit Agreements

Credit agreements are documents that allow patients to set up a schedule to pay off their bills as long as they make the specified monthly payments (Figure 47-4). If a patient decides independently to pay his or her bill in installments (i.e., without discussing it with the medical office), no credit agreement is necessary. If the office and patient make an agreement regarding installment payments, even if no interest is charged, the agreement must be in writing. An interest charge is often added to the balance due at the end of each billing cycle when a written agreement exists.

A credit agreement with a medical office is a type of revolving credit, like a department store or gasoline company charge card. As long as the monthly minimum is paid, the account is considered in good standing.

Truth in Lending Agreements

Because a credit agreement is a type of revolving credit, it falls under federal and state government fair lending practices. Therefore a truth in lending statement must be supplied to the patient when the agreement is made. **Truth in lending** refers to the legal requirement to disclose the terms of a loan to borrowers so that they can understand them.

This truth in lending statement includes facts about such things as the maximum amount the patient may charge to the account, the interest rate, how the interest is computed (e.g., average daily balance, or balance at the end of the billing period), and how the minimum monthly payment is computed (e.g., percentage of outstanding balance). Figure 47-4 shows a sample credit agreement.

Policy for Patients with Outstanding Balances

Most medical offices insist that a patient close out any current balance due before a credit agreement is written with that patient. If the practice has had trouble collecting bills from a patient in the past, it may write the credit agreement for a lower maximum balance. But the practice cannot charge a different interest rate or compute the minimum payment in a different way for different patients depending on past payment history.

Other Collection Techniques and Special Circumstances

Tracing "Skips"

Occasionally a bill is returned to the medical office from the post office with the notation "address unknown." This may be an innocent mistake—the result, perhaps, of an incorrect address on file or the patient's failure to notify the office after moving. On the other hand, it may be a deliberate attempt to "skip out" on the medical office's bill and the bills of other professionals and/or merchants.

A potential **"skip"** (account for which no billing information is available) should be followed up immediately.

Blackburn Primary Care Associates, PC
1990 Turquoise Drive
Blackburn, WI 54937
608-459-8857

Federal Truth in Lending Statement

Patient _____
Address _____

1. Fee for service of _____
2. Amount down _____
3. Amount financed _____
4. finance charge _____
5. total of payments 3 + 4 _____
6. number of payments _____
7. amount of each payment _____

Total no. of payments _____ payable over _____ monthly installments

In the amount of $_____. The first payment is due _____.

Date _____ Signed _____

Figure 47-4 Sample credit agreement.

The first step is to call the patient's phone number: It is very common to keep the same telephone number even if a person moves, or a person may have had the phone company use a "new number" message to forward calls. Because caller ID is a feature on many land lines and cell phones, a telephone call from a creditor may be ignored or the person answering the call may say that it is a wrong number.

If the patient cannot be contacted using the telephone number given at the office visit and if there is no new number listed, the next step is to call the patient's place of business and ask to speak with the individual. The medical assistant can try to get in touch with the person by contacting professional associations, unions, or other organizations with which the person is associated.

The medical assistant should never tell a third party that an individual owes money to the medical office and should not identify the employer; the medical assistant should say only that he or she wishes to speak with the person. Also, it is illegal to call a third party more than once in an attempt to trace a skip unless that person asks the medical assistant to call back. For example, the medical assistant may speak with a third party where the individual with an overdue account works, and that third party might ask the medical assistant to call back at the end of the day when he or she is not so busy.

Another way to attempt collection is to send a letter by Registered or Certified Mail, with a Return Receipt requested, to the individual at the old address. Even if the person did not ask the post office to forward all mail, he or she may have asked for certain types of mail to be forwarded. In this case, the letter should be placed in a plain envelope, with just the return street address and no office name. This minimizes the chances that the individual will refuse to accept the mail.

The medical office may also use one of several Internet resources to trace skips. These services usually charge a fee. The more information the office has about the individual, the more likely it is that the individual can be located.

If all of these efforts fail, the bill should be turned over to a collection agency used by the office as soon as possible. Most collection agencies handle far more "skips" than individual medical offices do and sometimes use other, more aggressive techniques. The sooner the collection agency receives the account, the better chance it has to collect the bill.

Sending Accounts to a Collection Agency

Collection agencies are in business specifically to collect accounts that have "aged out." This means that by the time a collection agency receives a delinquent account, the business such as a medical office has given the person who owes the money fair warning that the bill is overdue and that a professional collector is going to become involved.

Each state has specific laws under which collection agencies must work. These laws define when collection agency personnel can call, what they can say, and what other tactics they can use to collect the bill.

Collection agencies generally charge 20% to 40% of the amount they collect. They are not allowed to "cut a deal" with a patient and accept less than full payment unless the medical office has agreed to the arrangement for payment.

If a patient's account is in collection, usually the office has a policy not to see the patient unless any new charges are paid in full before the patient is seen by the physician. Other offices notify patients in writing that they will not be seen by any physician in the office until their outstanding balance has been collected.

When an account is turned over to a collection agency, the patient balance in the computer system is often adjusted to zero. The amount owed by the patient can still be seen clearly in the patient ledger, but the current balance is zero. This prevents bills to the patient from being generated, and the account no longer appears as overdue on account aging reports. The medical assistant should become familiar with the exact procedure used in his or her medical office. The medical office makes no further attempts at collection, and any payments received from the patient are sent directly to the collection agency. When a payment for the patient's account is received from a collection agency, it should be recorded on the daily ledger. In addition, it should be posted to the account for which it was collected. The patient's account balance, which is usually zero, is first increased (as a positive or debit adjustment) by the amount of the payment. Then the payment is posted as a payment, bringing the current account balance back to zero (Procedure 47-7).

PROCEDURE **47-6** Writing a Collection Letter

Outcome Write a collection letter.

Equipment/Supplies

- Accounts aging report
- Computer
- Patient accounts

- Letterhead stationery
- Envelope
- Printer

---

1. **Procedural Step.** After the accounts receivable aging record has been created, determine which accounts need a letter. In general, this will be the accounts that are 90 to 120 days old.

PROCEDURE 47-6 Writing a Collection Letter—cont'd

Principle. A letter is usually sent after reminders have been sent and a telephone call has been made to collect an outstanding account balance.

2. **Procedural Step.** Review each account for the amount due, how long it has been due, any previous activity, and special situations. If the account is due from the estate of a deceased patient or insurance, or if there is a known reason why delayed payment is acceptable, do not take action on the account.
Principle. There may be circumstances that justify the delay in payment.

3. **Procedural Step.** Otherwise, prepare a letter for each outstanding account. The letter should state clearly the amount of the outstanding balance, the date that the charges were incurred, the service provided, and the amount paid by insurance. It should also describe any previous conversations and/or agreements. The letter should clearly state that the outstanding balance is due and identify the date by which it is expected to be paid (usually in 10 days).
Principle. Even though the bill is overdue, the recipient of the letter is given a reasonable amount of time to respond to this letter.

4. **Procedural Step.** Enter the typed signature as indicated by office policy (the medical assistant, office manager, billing specialist, or physician). If you do not sign the letter yourself, place the name of the authorized individual on the written signature line and prepare a reference line using your own initials.
Principle. The letter should be signed by a person who is authorized by the medical practice to collect outstanding accounts.

5. **Procedural Step.** Prepare an envelope.

6. **Procedural Step.** Obtain the written signature on the letter.

7. **Procedural Step.** Place a copy of the letter in the patient's medical record. Place a notation that a letter was sent on the aging report and in the computer account if possible. You may also file a copy of the letter in a collection follow-up file.
Principle. Future activity to collect on the account should be based on a review of your current activity.

8. **Procedural Step.** Place the letter in the envelope and mail the letter.

PROCEDURE 47-7 Posting a Collection Agency Payment

Outcome Post a collection agency payment.

Equipment/Supplies

- Computer
- Patient accounts
- Payment check(s)
- Day sheet
- Office policy manual
- Calculator

1. **Procedural Step.** When a payment has been made from a collection agency, locate the patient account in the computer.
Principle. All financial transactions must be entered to the correct patient account.

2. **Procedural Step.** Be sure that the patient's balance was adjusted to zero at the time the account was sent to collection. On the day sheet, label the first open line with the name of the patient whose check was returned and enter zero in the *old balance* column.
Principle. It is standard procedure to write off the patient balance when an account is sent to collection. This decreases the total accounts receivable accounts by an amount that the medical office does not expect to be able to collect.

3. **Procedural Step.** Create a new transaction for the patient and select the code for reverse collection.

Enter the amount of the check and verify that the computer shows a positive patient balance after this entry.
Principle. The reverse collection code is used to increase the patient's balance before entering the payment.

4. **Procedural Step.** On the day sheet, enter the amount of the collection agency check in the *adjustment* column. The amount should be written in parentheses because it is a debit adjustment.
Principle. The patient balance, which has previously been adjusted to zero, must be increased to the amount of the collection agency check before posting the actual payment. In the computer, selecting the correct code automatically increases the patient balance. When using a day sheet, an adjustment must be added to the patient balance.

Continued

5. **Procedural Step.** When totaling the adjustment column of the day sheet, subtract the debit adjustment from the total of the credit adjustments.
6. **Procedural Step.** Enter the amount of the check in the *new balance* column. This figure is obtained by adding the adjustment to the previous balance of zero. If using a day sheet, on a new line enter "Collection Agency Payment" in the *professional service* column.
7. **Procedural Step.** In the computer, on a new line, select the code for collection agency payment and enter the amount of the collection agency check.
8. **Procedural Step.** Verify that the patient balance returns to zero in the computer account.
9. **Procedural Step.** On a new line of the day sheet, enter the patient's name and enter the amount of the collection agency check in the old balance column.

10. **Procedural Step.** Enter "Collection Agency Payment" in the *professional service* column of the day sheet.
11. **Procedural Step.** Enter the amount of the check in the *payment* column of the day sheet.
12. **Procedural Step.** Enter zero in the new balance column of the day sheet after subtracting the payment from the previous balance.
    Principle. After posting the collection agency payment, the patient's balance should again be zero.
    Example: The account of Robert Ricigliano, which was adjusted to zero when the account was turned over for collection, is increased to $25.00 using the code for reverse collection. Then a collection agency check for $25.00 is posted to the account leaving a zero balance.

Charges:									
Date	Procedure	Diag 1	Diag 2	Diag 3	Provider	POS	Units	Amount	Total
2/22/20XX	99212	I12.9			RW	11	1	55.00	55.00

Payments and adjustments:					
Date	Pay/Adj Code	Paid By:	Description	Amount	Total
2/22/20XX	WO		Send to collection	−55.00	0.00
4/18/20XX	REVERSE		Reverse collection	25.00	25.00
2/4/20XX	AGENCY	ABC Collection Agency	Collection agency payment	−25.00	0.00

There is a zero balance after posting the collection agency check.

Small Claims Court

Small claims courts exist in each state. They are special sessions of the local district court that deal only with civil lawsuits involving small amounts of money. Most small claims lawsuits involve disputes over payments. Each state has its own rules for the maximum claim that can be brought in small claims court. This maximum amount runs from about $1500 in some states to as much as $15,000 in others.

The question for a medical practice when choosing to use the court system is always whether it will sacrifice more in "good will" than it will gain in money if the collection is successful. Many offices bring suits in court only after a patient has left the practice without paying a bill in full. Furthermore, winning a judgment in small claims court is only the first step. The office must still collect the judgment.

Small claims courts are set up to reduce the legal fees for those seeking to collect relatively small amounts of money. Because there is no lawyer, the plaintiff (an individual or business) must represent himself or itself. The office manager or medical assistant might have to assume this duty if the office uses small claims court to try to collect on patient accounts. A collection agency cannot represent the office.

The clerk of the court has all of the documents necessary to file a small claim and can usually walk a first-time claimant through the process, explaining how to fill out the forms and which documentation to submit to back up the claim. Only the defendant can appeal a small claims court judgment; for the plaintiff, a negative judgment is final.

Billing an Estate

Patients do sometimes die without having paid their medical bills in full. In this instance the office will have to collect the balance due from the estate. Estates fall into an area of the law known as *probate*, and probate law is administered by a special section of the court system in each state.

It is not appropriate to send a bill to a deceased patient's estate immediately after the death while the family is grieving; however, the bill should be sent within 30 days. The bill should be sent to "The Estate of" the patient at the patient's address rather than to a family member or other individual unless that person has made a written promise to cover the deceased's medical costs.

If the deceased patient had a will, it usually has a provision that the costs of the patient's final illness be paid by the estate outside of the probate process. In such a case the bill will probably be paid promptly. The will should be filed within 30 days, and the clerk of the probate court should then be able to furnish you with the name of the executor or administrator (the person responsible for handling the estate's business dealings). An itemized final bill should then be sent to this individual by Certified Mail with a Return Receipt requested.

If the patient did not have a will, the medical practice's bill will be put in with other creditors' bills and paid only when payment is approved by the probate court and the administrator appointed by the court.

Bankruptcy

Bankruptcy laws are federal laws, meaning that they apply equally regardless of the state in which the bankrupt person lives. **Bankruptcy** is a means for an individual or business

to "get out from under" a crushing load of debt, either by reorganizing the debt or by liquidating assets and dividing the funds among all of the creditors.

Individuals file for personal bankruptcy under either Chapter 7 or Chapter 13 of the bankruptcy code.

A Chapter 7 bankruptcy is a liquidation of assets. Under such a bankruptcy, only secured creditors will be paid from the proceeds from the sale of any assets. If the bankrupt patient had a credit agreement, the medical office is a secured creditor. But if the office is merely trying to collect a bill, the office is an unsecured creditor and will not receive payment.

A Chapter 13 bankruptcy is an "Adjustment of Debts" bankruptcy. In such a bankruptcy, the debtor (patient) pays a particular amount determined by the bankruptcy court to the court-appointed trustee, who then distributes the money to creditors. The debtor, if he or she has a regular income, can be required to make payments from that income into the trustee account for 3 years, and the trustee makes payments to creditors under payment plans he or she works out.

During the period the debtor is under the jurisdiction of the bankruptcy court, no creditor may try to collect a debt outside the bankruptcy process. However, a medical office can demand payment in full for any additional service it provides to a patient from whom it is collecting old debts under a bankruptcy agreement.

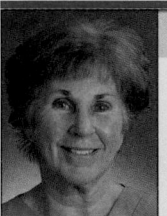

Memories *from* Externship

Christa Wilson: During my externship, I observed billing activities and I was allowed to assist in some ways. For example, I got a lot of practice at making sure that all bills printed correctly, checking each bill to make sure that there was an outstanding balance and that the insurance had already paid, and folding the bills to place them in window envelopes. The computer system used by the office where I did my externship printed the bills with an itemized statement of all activity on the account. The patient was expected to pay the balance on the bottom line of the statement. Sometimes patients called the office because they didn't understand what amount to pay. They usually spoke to the medical assistant at the office. I noticed that she was always polite and professional when she spoke to patients. The office also taught me how to post patient payments that were sent by check. I have to say I did not realize how important good billing practices are until my externship. I was grateful that I had experience at an office with a smooth-running system. ∎

What Would You Do? What Would You *Not* Do?

Case Study 3
On the day that Judith Mason is scheduled for an appointment, Christa notices that she has an outstanding balance of $58.00 from charges that were incurred 4 months ago. It is office policy that patients with a balance over 120 days are not seen until the balance has been paid. ∎

MEDICAL PRACTICE *and the* LAW

Several laws affect credit and collection activities.

Equal Credit Opportunity Act
The Equal Credit Opportunity Act is a federal law that prevents discrimination based on the following when offering credit:
- Sex, marital status, race, national origin, religion, age
- The fact that the applicant receives public assistance income
- The fact that the applicant has exercised rights under consumer credit laws

An applicant must be informed if credit is denied and has 60 days to request, in writing, the reason for denial of credit.

Fair Debt Collection Practices Act
The Fair Debt Collection Practices Act is a federal law that requires the fair treatment of debtors and prevents unfair debt collection measures, including harassment, false statements, and threats.
- The debt collector may not make frightening, verbally abusive, or threatening calls.
- The debt collector may not call before 8 AM or after 8 PM.
- The debt collector may not threaten action that cannot legally be taken or is not intended to be taken.

Continued

MEDICAL PRACTICE *and the* LAW—cont'd

Federal Truth in Lending Act

Installment agreements of more than four payments (or fewer if interest is charged) must be written. The Federal Truth in Lending Act is administered by the Federal Trade Commission. It requires creditors to provide applicants with a form disclosing in a clear and obvious way all finance charges and terms.

Fair Credit Reporting Act

The Fair Credit Reporting Act requires credit bureaus to supply correct and complete information to businesses to use in evaluating a person's application for credit, insurance, or employment.

Bankruptcy Abuse Prevention and Consumer Protection Act of 2005

The Bankruptcy Abuse Prevention and Consumer Protection Act of 2005 is a revision of federal bankruptcy laws that attempts to make it more difficult for individuals to file for bankruptcy under Chapter 7, by which most of the debts are forgiven by establishing a means test to determine if individuals are able to pay some of their debts. It also makes the process of filing for bankruptcy more difficult and expensive. Debtors are still able to file for bankruptcy under Chapter 13. ■

What Would You Do? What Would You *Not* Do? RESPONSES

Case Study 1
Page 1111

What Did Christa Do?

❏ Reassured the patient that the situation is upsetting, but it can happen sometimes.
❏ Explained that most banks charge both the account of the individual who writes a check against an account with insufficient funds, as well as the account where the check was deposited.
❏ Explained that the office had a policy of not sending a check through the bank a second time or accepting a personal check for payment after one check was returned.
❏ Suggested that the patient might want to consider overdraft protection.
❏ Explained politely that the office was only recovering its out-of-pocket expenses and was not, in fact, charging an additional fee.

What Did Christa Not Do?

❏ Did not get angry or raise her voice.
❏ Did not imply that the patient was trying to avoid payment or was a bad money manager.
❏ Did not make statements such as, "This better not happen again!" or "How do you expect us to pay our bills if our patients' checks bounce?"

What Would You Do/What Would You Not Do?

Review Christa's response and place a checkmark next to the information you included in your response. List the additional information you included in your response.

_____
_____
_____
_____
_____

Case Study 2
Page 1113

What Did Christa Do?

❏ Told the patient that she would check the receipt book, then went through the duplicate receipts of the day of the patient's visit.
❏ If a copy of the receipt for a cash payment was found, told the patient and entered the payment into the patient's account.
❏ If no copy of the receipt was found, explained to the patient that it is office policy to issue a receipt for any cash payment from a book where a duplicate is made automatically.
❏ If no copy of the receipt was found, suggested tactfully that the patient may not remember this specific visit, and perhaps she was unable to pay her copayment that day or forgot to pay it.
❏ If the patient continued to insist that she paid cash, offered to discuss the matter with the office manager or physician.

What Did Christa Not Do?

❏ Did not get angry at the patient or raise her voice.
❏ Did not say that unless the patient could show her a receipt, the office would automatically assume that she had not paid.
❏ Did not accuse the patient of trying to get out of paying the copayment.

What Would You Do/What Would You Not Do?

Review Christa's response and place a checkmark next to the information you included in your response. List the additional information you included in your response.

_____
_____
_____
_____
_____

What Would You Do? What Would You *Not* Do? RESPONSES—cont'd

Case Study 3
Page 1121

What Did Christa Do?
❑ Attempted to contact Ms. Mason by telephone to inform her of the office policy so that the patient could be prepared to settle her outstanding bill.
❑ If the patient could not be contacted before the appointment, took her to a private room when she arrived at the office to discuss her account.
❑ Strongly encouraged Ms. Mason to settle the account by check or credit card before she was seen by the physician.
❑ If Ms. Mason stated that she could not pay the balance on that day, left the final decision about whether she would be seen to the physician because the patient had not been informed of the office policy before coming to the office.

What Did Christa Not Do?
❑ Did not take the sole responsibility to tell the patient that if she did not pay, under no circumstances would she be seen by the physician.
❑ Did not raise her voice or get angry with Ms. Mason.
❑ Did not discuss Ms. Mason's financial matters where others could overhear the conversation.

What Would You Do/What Would You Not *Do?*
Review Christa's response and place a checkmark next to the information you included in your response. List the additional information you included in your response.

_____
_____
_____
_____

TERMINOLOGY REVIEW

Medical Term	Word Parts	Definition
Account aging		The process of finding out how long specific account balances have been outstanding.
Balance due		Total amount owed.
Bankruptcy		Legal process by which the debts of an individual or business are resolved if they cannot be paid.
Claim message		Messages encouraging payment of a bill, usually attached to or printed on the monthly statement.
Collection agency		A firm that is in the business of collecting overdue accounts.
Credit balance		A negative balance on a patient account (i.e., money is owed by the medical office), usually a result of an overpayment.
Overdraft		A check (or draft) that exceeds the amount of funds in a bank account.
Skip		Account for which no billing information is available.
Truth in lending		Legal requirement to disclose the terms of a loan in terms that the borrower can understand.

ON THE WEB

For information on the Federal Trade Commission:

Federal Trade Commission: www.ftc.gov

Check out the Evolve site at http://evolve.elsevier.com/Bonewit/today/ to actively Prepare for your Certification, and to access additional interactive activities and exercises to help you study and prepare for success.

The Medical Assistant as Office Manager

KEY TERMS

back order	net pay	salary
depreciation	per diem	service contract
gross pay	policy	Social Security tax (FICA)
inventory	procedure	vendor
invoice	reorder point	warranty
minutes	risk management	W-4

INTRODUCTION TO MEDICAL OFFICE MANAGEMENT

The medical assistant performs many tasks that promote the smooth running of the medical office. These tasks include maintaining the physical space, taking inventory, ordering supplies, monitoring programs such as risk management and employee safety programs, orienting new employees, and processing employee payroll. The responsibility for these management functions may be primarily that of the medical assistant in a small office, or primarily that of an office manager in a larger setting. Office management always provides the basis for effective patient care, and its importance cannot be overestimated.

MAINTAINING THE OFFICE

In many medical practices, a medical assistant assumes responsibility for maintaining the physical space of the medical office and performing general maintenance. Heavy cleaning and equipment repair are usually not performed by office staff, but rather by contractors. Thus the medical assistant may also be responsible for managing the relationship between the office and contractors or vendors of services, as well as medical, pharmaceutical, and office supply companies.

Administrative Area

When sitting at the front desk, the medical assistant must be able to effectively and efficiently answer two or three incoming calls, greet patients, and handle paperwork.

Depending on the size of the administrative area, supplies and equipment for correspondence and billing may be stored in this area, including stationery, envelopes, billing forms, and coding reference books. In addition to the telephone (discussed in detail in Chapter 39), the reception area usually contains a personal computer, which is usually linked to the office's computer network. Materials for creating new patient folders should also be at hand if a paper medical record system is used.

The administrative area needs to have enough room to perform the required activities without the patient files and other papers becoming mixed up, and it must also allow the medical assistant to maintain patient confidentiality (Figure 48-1).

Again, depending on the size of the office, business operations will either take place in the front office close to the reception area or in a separate area in the office. In the business office are the rest of the pieces of equipment necessary for administering the office, including the photocopy machine, fax machine, and postage meter or electronic mailing system. In small offices, an all-in-one printer-copier-fax may be used.

Patient billing records are available either in hard-copy files in the business office or on the computer. Charge slips, patient statements, and other documents are usually printed using a laser printer or ink jet printer.

The medical assistant should be familiar not only with the office equipment's operation, but also with the maintenance responsibilities, such as reloading paper and adding toner or printer cartridges. In addition, the medical assistant may need to follow the terms of any maintenance agreements when scheduling maintenance or repairs.

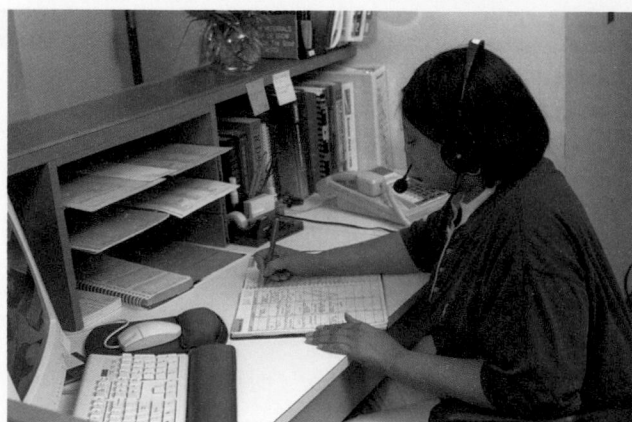

Figure 48-1 Well organized front office.

Offices should also have a paper shredder for disposing of confidential documents. Although medical records must be maintained indefinitely, old telephone logs, old payroll records, canceled checks more than 7 years old, and minutes of practice management meetings should all be shredded rather than simply thrown away in the wastebasket or in a wastepaper-recycling bin. Any documents with patient information that have been scanned into the electronic medical record should be shredded if they are not retained. Shredded paper can still be recycled, and there is no danger that sensitive personal or business information will be seen by anyone who should not have access to it.

Examination and Treatment Rooms

Each examination or treatment room also needs approximately 100 square feet of floor space to hold an examination or treatment table, cabinets and countertop, patient chair and physician stool, and a small surface for the physician to write on. The room should be laid out so that a physician and medical assistant can move freely about the room. Equipment and supplies should be within easy reach or stored in drawers or cabinets easy to reach.

Each examination or treatment room needs to have a sink, as well as soap and paper towel dispensers. Hand sanitizer may be in a wall-mounted or freestanding dispenser. The examination room must also contain a wall-mounted rigid container for the disposal of sharps, such as needles, scalpel blades, or other objects that might puncture a plastic bag. Biohazard wastebaskets with a biohazard plastic liner for materials that contain body fluids, such as blood, mucus, or pus, are located either in each examination room or in the hall. Containers for hazardous waste must be covered, except when adding waste. A foot pedal to open the cover facilitates use. The examination room usually contains an ordinary wastebasket for used paper towels and table paper.

For safety reasons, examination rooms should not contain syringes, needles, or medication samples. Cleaning materials and chemical solutions should never be stored under the counter in an examination room, especially if it is used for children.

Waiting Room

The waiting room makes a first impression on a new patient. It must be neat and welcoming. The waiting room needs two to four chairs for each physician in the office at one time, current magazines, and a table or magazine stand to hold them. If the practice sees children, some toys should be available in a separate play area. One person should be assigned to tidy up the waiting room a couple of times during the day.

A waiting room should have signs that inform patients about office policies. The signs depend on the policies of the individual office. Common signs include the following:

- No smoking
- Copayments are expected at the time of service (or some other language regarding the expectation of payment)
- The following credit cards are accepted (followed by names of credit cards)
- No eating or drinking
- A charge will be added for returned checks to cover any bank fees
- Patients will be charged for cancelled appointments unless at least 24-hour notice is given

Some offices have a display rack with health information brochures. Brochures are available from government agencies, public agencies, and many companies. With the approval of the physician(s), these brochures are often provided to help educate patients about health promotion and disease prevention.

Sometimes there is a television or DVD player in the waiting room. In some practices, health information videos are playing. Other practices have a radio tuned to an easy-listening station or a CD player with quiet pop or light classical music. The medical assistant may need to turn on this equipment at the beginning of the day.

Security Systems

A medical office maintains a number of different security systems.

First, if the office is entered from a corridor in an office building, the building owner or office condominium association most likely has an electronic security system for the building itself.

Second, regardless of whether the office is entered from a corridor or directly from the outside, the practice should maintain an electronic security system against break-ins to the office itself.

The office's security and safety alarm system is monitored by an alarm company and may or may not also be tied to the local police and fire departments. Whether or not the system is tied into the police and fire departments, the alarm company will call the practice's liaison to the company whenever the alarm goes off.

This designated person is often the practice administrator or "managing partner." However, two or three people are always listed as backups in case the liaison is not available.

Third, various places within the office require another layer of security. Medication cabinets—with all medications and prescription pads inside—should be locked, and a limited number of people should have keys to the medication cabinet lock. The laboratory, physicians' private offices, medical records cabinet or room, and business office are other areas that often have a lock and limited access.

If controlled substances are stored in the office, they should be "double-locked" (in a locked drawer within a locked cabinet). Two separate keys should open the two different locks.

ROUTINE MAINTENANCE

It is important to maintain the physical space of the medical office. Depending on the size of the office, many if not most routine maintenance activities are undertaken by staff. These include controlling the temperature, cleaning cabinets and drawers, changing lightbulbs and replacing batteries in battery-powered equipment, turning the security system on and off, making sure fire protection equipment is in working order, and performing some daily cleaning. In all activities, medical assistants and other staff must be sure to protect themselves and patients from hazards and injury. Good body mechanics should be used to move supplies and equipment and when cleaning, as well as when working with patients. The workplace should be arranged to minimize strain during all routine and maintenance activities.

Temperature and Ventilation

The reception area and examination rooms should be kept at a comfortable temperature. People who are ill are sensitive to cold and drafts. The reception and patient waiting areas and examination rooms should be about 70° to 72° F. The temperature in treatment rooms, the laboratory, and physicians' offices should be about 68° to 70° F. A room used for procedures or minor surgery can be kept a little cooler because the physician and medical assistant may be wearing gowns, masks, and hair covers.

Ventilation is also important. Keeping air circulating is important both to dissipate odors and to allow germs to escape from the office atmosphere.

General Cleaning

Larger offices may contract for cleaning services, or office cleaning may be included in the monthly rent, especially in buildings that are dedicated to medical offices. Contracted cleaning is usually done one or two times a week, so even if the major cleaning is contracted out, daily cleaning tasks still must be performed.

Daily cleaning includes tidying up all areas of the office—reception and waiting rooms, administrative space, physicians' offices, examination and treatment rooms, and the laboratory.

Sinks should all be toweled dry, and rest rooms should be checked to make sure ample toilet and facial tissue, soap,

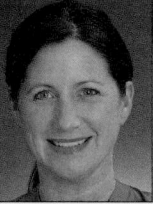

Putting It All Into Practice

My name is Kelsey Whitman, and I am a registered medical assistant. I usually work in one of the satellite offices of a large medical group that includes primary care providers and medical specialists. The office where I usually work was formerly a house. They are planning to close it next spring, tear it down, and build a modern office building. Even though there are some disadvantages to the current setting, it has a lot of charm. The waiting room and three small examination rooms are on the first floor with the physicians' office, and we use the rooms upstairs for storage, a break room, and meeting rooms. I have a small office upstairs, but I never have time to sit in it. Usually we have only one physician in the office. I work with one other medical assistant, but since I have been in the practice longer, I am responsible for making sure that everything runs smoothly. I have to go to the main office once a month for a staff meeting. The meetings are held once a month late on Wednesday afternoon. We discuss issues affecting all work areas. We have also been reviewing some of the procedures done by medical assistants to be sure that every medical assistant in every office does things the same way. The other medical assistant will be going out for maternity leave in a few weeks, and we have been interviewing for a replacement. After an initial screening interview, I have been asked to talk to three applicants, to give them a tour of our office, and to give my feedback about how they might fit into this setting. One of the applicants seemed like a real team player, and I hope they hire her. It is so important for everyone to be able to work well together. ∎

and paper towels are available. Any spills or puddles on the floor of the rest room should be mopped up using gloves as needed.

Waste containers and recycling containers should be checked daily and emptied as needed. Biohazard sharps containers should be checked daily and replaced when they are three-quarters full. The plastic liners of biohazard waste containers should be changed as needed. Contracted cleaning services will usually not empty biohazard waste containers because they contain regulated medical waste. The medical assistant must handle biohazard waste containers carefully to prevent an exposure incident. The OSHA Bloodborne Pathogen Standard outlines specific actions to take when handling regulated medical waste. These are outlined in Chapter 17.

If the office staff must do more intense cleaning, this should be done at least weekly. These tasks include mopping linoleum floors and vacuuming carpets, cleaning the glass at the reception area, polishing furniture and accessories, dusting, and thoroughly cleaning the rest rooms.

It is important to try to avoid a "medical smell" in the office. This is done by maintaining proper ventilation, as well as by cleaning up spills and accidents immediately, using light or unscented air fresheners in rest rooms and examination rooms, and keeping disinfectants and cleaning materials closed tightly when not in use and out of patients' reach.

Cleaning Cabinets and Drawers

Storage cabinets, drawers, and bookcases are cleaned less frequently, often on a day when the physician or some of the physicians in the practice are absent so that the room is not in use. After cleaning, the medical assistant should check labels on all items before putting them back on shelves. This is a good time to check for the expiration date on supplies and make a list of any items that need to be ordered or restocked from the general supply area to the cabinet. Outdated supplies must be disposed of properly (Figure 48-2).

What Would You Do? What Would You *Not* Do?

Case Study 1

Jean Highsmith has brought her 1-year-old twins, Scott and Lucy, to the medical office because they have been fussy and tugging at their ears. In the waiting room, she puts the twins on the floor to play with the toys while they are waiting. When Kelsey is able to take them to an examination room, she notices that the twins, who also have runny noses, have been chewing on some of the plastic toys in the waiting room. She notices that Mrs. Highsmith has left used tissues on one of the waiting room tables. After a few minutes in the examination room, Mrs. Highsmith comes to the door holding a child under each arm and tells Kelsey that Scott has thrown up a little on the examination room table. ■

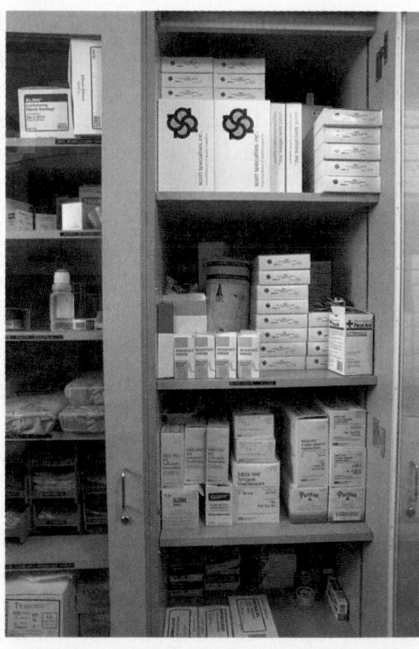

Figure 48-2 Well organized supply cabinet.

Miscellaneous Tasks

Among the miscellaneous tasks that have to be performed daily are rearranging the waiting room chairs and replacing magazines in their racks (as well as toys if toys are available); cleaning mirrors in the rest rooms and examination rooms; and cleaning the tops, fronts, and undersides of cabinets and paper towel dispensers. Toys must be cleaned and disinfected on a regular basis, because they can harbor microorganisms.

The medical assistant may be responsible for replacing lightbulbs in gooseneck lamps and other special lighting. Ceiling lighting is usually a responsibility of the maintenance staff employed by the building owner. If the space is owned by the practice, this may be a staff responsibility or may be covered by the cleaning or maintenance contract with an outside service.

PATIENT AND EMPLOYEE SAFETY

In addition to maintaining the physical environment of the medical office, it is also vital for all medical facilities to maintain a safe environment both for patients and for employees. This involves several measures.

1. Manage the environment to reduce hazards.
2. Train employees in general safety and to use correct methods and processes to prevent accident or injury.
3. Maintain equipment and perform regular safety inspections.
4. Create open lines of communication so that mistakes and accidents can be reported without fear of severe consequences.
5. Analyze all incidents including "near misses" to be sure that effective systems are in place. Constant awareness of potential hazards and a culture that expects each employee to respond to potentially unsafe conditions is one of the most effective tools for preventing accident or injury.

The following are general guidelines for workplace safety as recommended by the Occupational Safety and Health Administration (OSHA):

- Keep work areas, corridors, and hallways clear of obstacles.
- Exits should be accessible, clearly marked, and well lit. Be aware of state and/or local requirements for emergency lighting for exit signs.
- Keep floors dry, and clean up spills as soon as possible.
- Store waste in appropriate receptacles. Remove waste promptly and dispose of medical waste appropriately (see Chapter 17).
- Do not create high piles of materials that are likely to fall. Do not climb up on chairs or other unstable objects to retrieve objects stored on high shelves.
- Do not allow electrical cords to be present in areas where people walk.
- Do not leave drawers open.

Safe Work Practices

The office should have a safety plan, and all employees in the medical office should receive training so that they can carry out their duties correctly. The prevention of the spread of infection is always important. This is discussed in detail in Chapter 17. Equipment should always be checked for frayed electrical cords and used correctly to prevent injury. Hazardous chemicals should be handled and discarded safely as discussed in Chapter 18. Laboratory safety should be maintained according to guidelines in Chapter 29. There should be a plan to respond to spills of blood, body fluids, or chemicals. Areas that are restricted for safety reasons (such as the medical laboratory) should be clearly marked. Employees should report any unsafe condition to their supervisors. Protective equipment is provided by the employer and should always be used by each employee. Chapter 49 will discuss emergency and disaster response in detail.

Signs and Instructions

The office should post signs to instruct patients and employees as needed. As defined by OSHA, danger signs indicate that there is immediate danger and special precautions should be taken. These signs must be red on the upper panel with black lettering and a white background. They are more common in construction areas than the medical office. Caution signs warn against potential hazards. They should be predominantly yellow with either yellow lettering on a black background or black lettering on a yellow background. Caution signs should be used if potentially

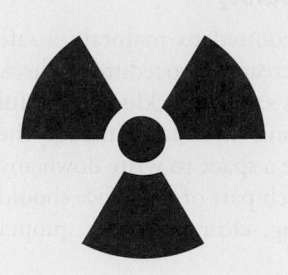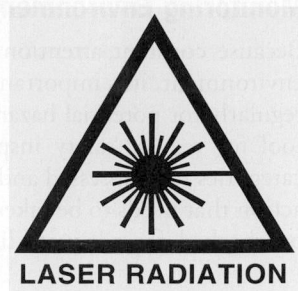

Figure 48-3 Examples of caution signs for radiation and laser radiation.

hazardous procedures are performed in the medical office such as x-ray examinations or laser treatments (Figure 48-3). Signs should designate areas where access is restricted. Safety instruction signs (if necessary for employees; e.g., at an eyewash station) should have an upper panel that is green with white lettering. Labels or color-coding should also be used for all biohazard boxes, biohazard waste, and flammable gases. Smoking should not be permitted in a physician's office, and signs advising patients and visitors that the office is a smoke-free environment should be clearly posted in the waiting area. Exits should be clearly marked, and an emergency evacuation map should be posted near the door to the waiting room. Exit signs should be white with red lettering not less than 6 inches high and ¾ inch wide. Lighted exit signs should be tested by shutting off the lights in the room; bulbs should be replaced if necessary.

Highlight on Ergonomics and Worker Safety

A typical working day in a medical office puts a lot of physical stress on personnel. Bending, lifting, reaching, squatting, having a telephone stuck in the crook of the neck, and repeatedly using a typing keyboard put stress on the body. The human body was not designed by nature to perform such activities so frequently.

Common causes for disabling workplace injury include the following:

- Overexertion injuries caused by excessive lifting, carrying, or pulling an object
- Falls either on the same level or from a higher to lower level
- Injuries caused by bending, tripping, slipping without falling, or attempting to avoid falling
- Repetitive strain injuries caused by performing a repetitive task in the same way over and over
- Being struck by or struck against an object

Ergonomics and Good Body Mechanics

The word *ergonomics* comes from the Greek root *ergon,* which means "work." Ergonomics is the study of maximizing work efficiency by adapting the work environment for optimal physical and mental function. For example, office seating should be designed to provide maximum support for the back, and computer keyboards

should be positioned to reduce repetitive motion injuries to the hands, wrists, and arms. But ergonomics does not have to be high tech; it can be as simple as placing a small footstool at the side of an examining table, not only so the patient can step up before sitting on the table, but also so the doctor, who stands and performs examinations for hours a day, can rest a foot there and take pressure off his or her lower back. Ergonomics can also affect selection of shelving and storage units to minimize strain when storing items or removing them from storage. In addition to adapting the environment, good body mechanics promote work efficiency and prevent injury. See the discussion in Chapter 22 of ways to use good body mechanics.

Preventing Falls

Most workplace injuries from falls occur in the service industry. Several measures can be implemented in the medical office to prevent personnel (as well as patients) from tripping and falling. Good lighting, preventing clutter in walkways, closing drawers, cleaning spills promptly, and emphasizing safety can reduce the likelihood of falls. Medical assistants should wear sturdy shoes and avoid walking too fast, carrying items that block vision, and failing to pay attention to their surroundings. ■

Monitoring Environmental Safety

Because constant attention is required to maintain a safe environment, it is important to create a procedure to check regularly for potential hazards. A safety checklist is a useful tool for regular safety inspections. It should include the categories to be assessed and have a space to write down any action that needs to be taken. Each part of the office should be checked for adequate lighting, clear walkways, proper storage of supplies, and removal of rubbish and biohazard waste. It is especially important to be sure that heavy boxes have not been stored in a high area where they could fall, that electrical cords are in good repair and do not cause a tripping hazard, and that spills have been attended to promptly. Storage of compressed gases, medications, and chemicals should be assessed according to office policies (Procedure 48-1).

PROCEDURE 48-1 Creating an Environmental Checklist and Performing a Safety Inspection

Outcome Perform and document a safety inspection after creating an environmental checklist.

Equipment/Supplies

- Area to be inspected
- Pen and paper (or computer and word processing file) to create an environmental checklist

1. **Procedural Step.** Create a checklist of types of hazards to be inspected for, including obstructed walkways and tripping hazards; electrical hazards; improperly stored boxes; inadequate lighting; wet floors; and improperly labeled and stored biohazards, medications, and chemicals.

2. **Procedural Step.** Moving from room to room in the designated area, first make a general inspection to be sure that floors are dry and all furniture and fixtures are in good repair. Then make a detailed inspection as required for each section on the checklist. If a problem is found, fix it if possible, but always note the problem on the checklist.

3. **Procedural Step.** Check for walkways that are wide enough for usual traffic without clutter. Be sure that there are no frayed carpets and no items that obstruct the walkway such as boxes, electrical cords, or debris. Be sure that there are no open drawers or cabinet doors.

4. **Procedural Step.** Check all electrical cords and plugs to ensure there is no fraying or malfunction. *Principle.* Frayed electrical cords are a potential fire hazard and can cause electrical shocks.

5. **Procedural Step.** Check all storage areas to be sure that the tops of cabinets are clear and that supplies have been stored without potential to fall and cause injury.

6. **Procedural Step.** Assess each light to be sure that all lightbulbs are in working order. Note any exceptions. Make a note if it seems that any area does not have adequate lighting.

7. **Procedural Step.** Depending on the type of area, be sure that all biohazards, chemicals, or other potentially hazardous materials are labeled correctly. Be sure that medication cabinets are locked. Be sure that chemicals are stored in secure areas away from patients.

8. **Procedural Step.** After completing the checklist, create a written plan to respond to any problems that you could not fix during the inspection.

MAINTAINING EQUIPMENT

Within the physical environment of the office there are many pieces of equipment, both for medical purposes and for business purposes. The medical assistant who manages the office is responsible for relationship management with the individuals or companies that sell and maintain the equipment, as well as with those who provide supplies for the equipment.

Inventory

An **inventory** is a detailed list of items in stock or in the possession of an individual or business. An equipment inventory lists each piece of equipment, the serial number, the date it was purchased, the length of the warranty, the name of the provider who services it, the manufacturer's suggested service schedule, and the last date of service. The office may also maintain a log validating maintenance and repair for larger pieces of equipment, such as computers and copiers.

An inventory is important for two reasons.

1. Tax consequence: Larger pieces of medical and office equipment are depreciated over 5 years, whereas smaller pieces of equipment and supplies can be fully deducted as an expense in the year in which they are purchased. (**Depreciation** is a name for the accounting methods used to account for the anticipated useful life of a piece of equipment and its loss of value over time.)

2. Theft or damage: In case of theft or damage, an inventory is necessary to make a complete report to the police and/or claim to the office's insurance company.

Operation manuals for the equipment can be stored centrally with the inventory list, or each manual can be stored with the piece of equipment for which it is used. Many pieces of equipment come with a plastic pouch on the side of the item or storage unit in which manuals and maintenance schedules can be kept.

Monitoring Equipment Function and Readiness for Use

The medical assistant should always be on the lookout for equipment problems, especially problems that could lead to a dangerous situation. All instruments should be checked when preparing them for sterilization. Before machines are used, the medical assistant should look for frayed wires, bent or damaged instruments, and machines that are not functioning properly.

Office machines should be dusted or wiped with a damp cloth regularly, following manufacturers' guidelines. Batteries, fluids, paper, toner, and other supplies should be replaced as needed. If there is a maintenance log for the piece of equipment (e.g., the autoclave log, copier log), the medical assistant should document any maintenance (Procedure 48-2).

The decision whether to repair or replace a piece of equipment will usually be made taking several factors into account:

- The age of the piece of equipment
- How expensive a new piece of equipment is
- The level of use the equipment gets
- Whether the manufacturer still produces parts for repair
- Whether any important features have been added to newer models of the equipment

If there is no service contract for the piece of equipment and the decision is made to repair it, a repair service must be located and a repair arranged. The manufacturer usually has a list of authorized repair services by region. In larger organizations, a purchase order is usually necessary for an equipment repair.

Emergency equipment must always be ready for use. This equipment must be checked at least monthly, and more often in many larger facilities. The contents of the emergency box or crash cart (discussed in detail in Chapter 35) should be checked for completeness by a designated person, who will initial a form to verify the presence of each item on the checklist.

Oxygen tanks are checked at the same time as emergency equipment. They should be sent to be refilled when the level falls to a predetermined level. Expiration dates of emergency medications are checked at the same time.

Service Contracts

Many pieces of medical office equipment are purchased with a service contract. A **service contract** is an agreement that provides for repair calls over a specific time period after the manufacturer's warranty has expired. A **warranty** is a promise by the manufacturer to repair or replace defective parts in an item during a specific time period. The service calls in a service contract may be free or have a specified charge, depending on the contract. Contracts usually call for larger pieces of equipment to be serviced at the physician's office. Smaller pieces of equipment often have a two-price contract: one price if the item is brought to a service center for repair and another price if repair is carried out on site.

Service Calls

Before calling in a service technician, the medical assistant should check the equipment thoroughly. A plug accidentally removed from a socket or a disconnected wire is often the cause of what seems like a machine breakdown.

If there is a service contract, all necessary routine maintenance should be performed in the office, or an appointment should be scheduled for a technician to perform it.

The medical assistant should keep a record of all service calls, the reason the call was made, the response, whether there was a service charge, and the suggested follow-up.

New Equipment Purchases

Although the physicians in the practice or the clinic administrator may be responsible for purchasing equipment, the medical assistant may be asked to help research options.

Manufacturers are glad to send information about the piece of equipment in question. Many companies now have websites that can be browsed to see product features and costs. Some sites even have video demonstrations. A demonstration can often be arranged.

Some practices look for used equipment or furniture. Companies that sell equipment from a number of manufacturers often have used equipment in inventory. Used equipment can also be found from physicians who are buying new equipment or retiring. Before purchasing a piece of used equipment, it is recommended to be sure that the manufacturer still supports the product (i.e., manufactures replacement parts so that it can be repaired).

The medical assistant may be asked to research the "lease versus buy" decision, whether to purchase the equipment or lease it over a period of time. Most medical and office equipment can be leased. Leasing and buying each have advantages and disadvantages, mostly in terms of tax treatment. The practice lawyer should be consulted on this decision. Laboratory equipment may be provided at a reduced cost or for a low monthly lease depending on the number of tests performed, so it is important to compare options among different companies.

When new equipment is received in the office, it is a good idea to note numbers of replacement parts, such as bulbs, batteries, and cartridges, and add them to the supply-ordering system.

PROCEDURE 48-2 **Performing Routine Maintenance of Equipment**

Outcome Perform equipment maintenance and document on equipment maintenance log.

Equipment/Supplies

- Piece of equipment to be maintained
- Cloth for dusting
- Maintenance log sheet

- Supplies necessary for the piece of equipment (e.g., paper, batteries, toner, fluids)

1. **Procedural Step.** Locate the piece of equipment to be checked.
2. **Procedural Step.** Check all electrical cords and plug to ensure there is no fraying or malfunction.
   Principle. Frayed electrical cords are a potential fire hazard and can cause electrical shocks.
3. **Procedural Step.** Check the piece of equipment for cracks, dents, or other damage; obvious impairment; or malfunction.
4. **Procedural Step.** Check any keyboard or keypad for cracks, faded numbers, or letters or other impairment.
5. **Procedural Step.** Dust or clean the outside or case of the piece of equipment according to manufacturer's directions.
   Principle. Dust can interfere with correct function of the machine.
6. **Procedural Step.** Check leads and other wires or other tubing.
7. **Procedural Step.** Check or change batteries, fluid, toner, or other essential components.

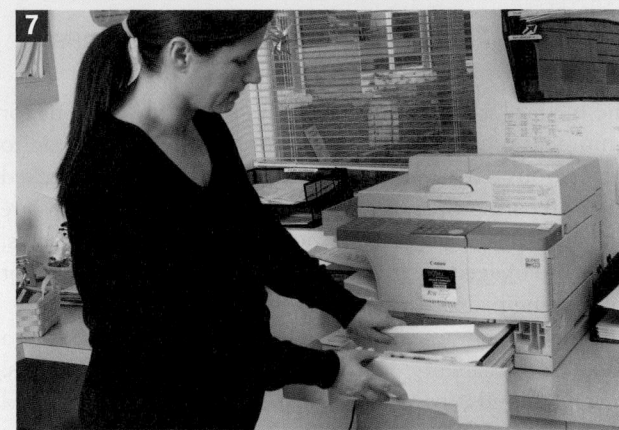
Add paper to the photocopier as needed.

8. **Procedural Step.** Schedule any required maintenance if appropriate.
9. **Procedural Step.** Fill out the equipment maintenance log.
   Example:

Equipment description:	BESTCOPY OFFICE PHOTOCOPIER		
Serial Number:	266XXX49500	Model Number:	6500AA

Date:	Action Taken/Comments:	Initials
5/26/XX	Machine checked, glass cleaned, toner added.	SH, CMA (AAMA)
5/30/XX	Streaks on copies, service call arranged. Technician cleaned drum.	SH, CMA (AAMA)
6/2/XX	Machine checked, glass cleaned.	SH, CMA (AAMA)

SUPPLIES

A busy medical office goes through an enormous amount of supplies—both clinical and administrative—in a month. Managing the purchase and stocking of supplies is another management task that often falls to a medical assistant.

The quantity of supplies that can be ordered at one time depends on the amount of storage space in the office. A practice can usually get a better price by ordering large amounts, but many offices are limited in the amount they can store. Sometimes it is possible to get extra storage space in the basement of the building where space is being rented.

Also, many physicians receive discounts on supplies by virtue of membership in some sort of a buying group or independent practice organization. Other practices are

beginning to move toward website-based purchasing of medical supplies, which may result in significant cost savings.

It is important to develop a good system of tracking supplies, usage, and storage capacity. In this way, reordering is not done too early when there is no room or too late when the practice may actually run out of important supplies.

When planning a new office or office move, it is important to plan for adequate supply-storage space.

Supply Inventory

A supply inventory is a listing of all the supplies regularly used in the office. This inventory can be kept in a notebook with a separate page for each supply, or it can be a set of cards—one for each supply item. Notebook pages or cards can be grouped either by the type of supply (e.g., surgical disposable, photocopier) or by the supplier. The inventory can also be kept on the computer. A list is printed when supplies are counted.

The information on the supply list should contain the following:

1. The item's name.
2. Any specific size used.
3. The usual supplier.
4. The cost per a standard quantity (e.g., $3.50 per 100) if known.
5. The **reorder point,** which is a number that identifies when the remaining quantity of the item is low enough that the item must be reordered. The reorder point is calculated by determining the number of

items used per day or week and the number of days or weeks it takes for an order to be received. For instance, if the office uses 100 pairs of gloves per day, there are 50 pairs in each box, and it takes 5 working days to receive a new order of gloves, the reorder point would be when fewer than 15 boxes (750 gloves) are in the supply room ($7\frac{1}{2}$ days' worth).

6. The quantity ordered each time.

Figure 48-4 shows a sample supply inventory. Information related to specific items is often maintained on cards or a sheet with the items ordered (Figure 48-5).

The card usually contains additional information about order dates and dates of receipt, initialed by the person who placed and/or received the order.

Most offices routinely order supplies on a monthly basis. Some supplies are routinely reordered each ordering

ITEM NAME	SUPPLIER	ITEM #	COST	REORDER AT	# TO ORDER
Bandages & Dressings					
nonsterile sponges 2" x 2"	H Medical	XY 2544	$3.50/pkg/200	5 pkg	10 pkg
nonsterile sponges 4" x 4"	H Medical	XY 7812	$8.25/pkg/200	5 pkg	10 pkg
sterile sponges 4" x 4"	H Medical	XY 5540	$22.00/box/00	2 box	5 box
non-sterile conforming bandage 2"	Winscott	49J265	$5.25/pkg/12	10 pkg	10 pkg
non-sterile conforming bandage 4"	Winscott	49J266	$8.62/pkg/12	10 pkg	10 pkg
paste bandage 4"	Winscott	57J381	$4.10 each	10	10
					10

Figure 48-4 Sample supply inventory.

ORDER (ITEM NAME) 3-ply Disposable Drape Sheets (white)7549 **ON ORDER**

ORDER QUANTITY _____ REORDER POINT ___100___

ORDER	QTY	REC'D	COST	PREPAID	ON ACCT	ORDER	QTY	REC'D	COST	PREPAID	ON ACCT
$^1/_{25}$	300	$^2/_{10}$	64.95	X							

INVENTORY COUNT

	JAN	FEB	MAR	APR	MAY	JUNE	JULY	AUG	SEPT	OCT	NOV	DEC
20 _00_	200											
20 _00_												

ORDER SOURCE

Patterson Office Supplies

201 Kenyon Road

Champaign, IL 61820

UNIT PRICE

100 - $23.95

300 - $64.95

Figure 48-5 Form for inventory control.

period, but others are ordered only on an "as needed" basis. For these items, the medical assistant may check the supply closet and generate a list of needed supplies. Computerized inventory record keeping can be maintained on a spreadsheet (Procedure 48-3).

Even if the office has been using the same supplier for a long time, it is a good practice to check other suppliers at least annually to see if a better relationship can be established. This might involve discounts for the volumes purchased, faster delivery, better prices overall, or availability of more products from another supplier than from the current supplier. If a new supplier has offered a better price,

the medical assistant should always give the current supplier the opportunity to "meet or beat" the current offer. An established relationship is a known quantity in terms of delivery reliability and overall quality of the relationship. When items are ordered repeatedly from the same supplier, the medical office is usually billed instead of having to pay in advance for the supplies.

When supplies are being stored in the main supply area, supplies with the expiration date closest to the current date should be placed at the front of the area so that they are used first. New supplies are stored behind the older supplies.

PROCEDURE 48-3 Taking a Supply or Equipment Inventory

Outcome Take a supply or equipment inventory.

Equipment/Supplies

- Inventory list
- Notebook or cards
- Items to inventory
- Pen

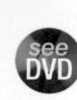

1. **Procedural Step.** Obtain a list of items in inventory—either on a written or computer-generated inventory list, inventory notebook, or box of inventory cards.
   Principle. The process of taking an inventory includes validating the presence or absence of a given set of items.

2. **Procedural Step.** Check each item in the inventory record against the items present in all areas of the medical office. For equipment, validate serial numbers. For supplies, consider the supplies on hand in examination rooms and storage areas, checking expiration dates and disposing of those that are expired.
   Principle. Expired items should be thrown away and not counted as part of the inventory. The point of taking inventory is to keep track of the number of items on hand that can be used.

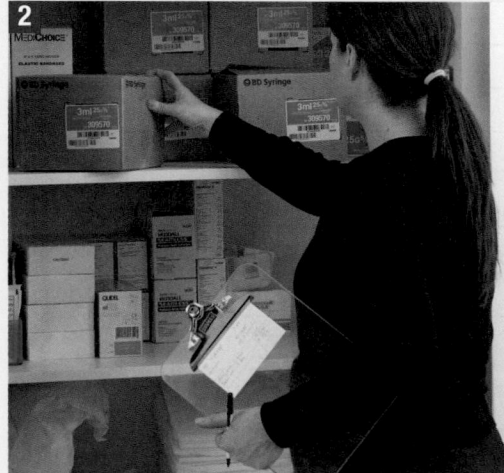

Check the quantity of supplies on hand.

3. **Procedural Step.** For an equipment inventory, make every effort to locate each piece of equipment on the list and validate that it is in working condition. Document if the item is missing or needs repair. For a supply inventory, check the quantity of supplies on hand against the quantity listed as the reorder point. If the quantity of items on hand is close to the reorder point, flag the item as one that needs to be reordered per the custom of your office.

4. **Procedural Step.** Check that the information on the inventory card or list is correct and complete. There should be a serial number for equipment and a description of the size, color, and price, as well as the usual supplier for supplies.
   Principle. You will need this information when replacing equipment or reordering supplies.

5. **Procedural Step.** Be sure that your storage space is tidy, that items can be found when needed, and that supplies are arranged so that those with the oldest expiration date are at the front of the storage shelf.
   Principle. Supplies are useless unless they can be found. Supplies with the oldest expiration date should be used first.

6. **Procedural Step.** Place inventory cards, computer printout sheet, or inventory book in the proper location for follow-up, including placing orders or updating computer information and storage until needed again.

Restocking

Moving supplies from the central supply area to the place where they will be used is called *restocking*. Examination rooms should be restocked once or twice daily. General supplies in administrative areas are usually restocked weekly. The photocopy and fax machines may need paper daily, depending on the volume of work done.

Ordering Supplies

A supply order is created by combining the list of supplies that are routinely ordered with the items that have been "flagged" using the inventory control system. When this list is complete, the supplier for each item must be identified and orders for that supplier created. Most offices will try to have one or two suppliers for clinical supplies and one or two for administrative supplies. Medications may be purchased from the same company as the one used for clinical supplies or from a pharmaceutical supplier.

Supplies are usually ordered in one of four ways: by telephone, by fax, by mail, or online (Figure 48-6). Even when using the telephone or computer, it is important to print or maintain a paper record of the transaction to reconcile against receipt of the supplies and for proper accounting. If ordering by fax, it is a good idea to make a follow-up phone call to make sure the fax has come through clearly and that the order-entry person at the supply house has no questions.

Fax or mail order purchases are submitted on a form listing the item, item number, amount, color, and so on. This form may be unique to the office or an order form supplied by the **vendor,** the company that sells the supplies or equipment. Some organizations may use a tracking number to reconcile receipt of supplies and payment of the invoice.

When the vendor cannot ship the item immediately, the item is said to be on **back order.** The order should be flagged to be sure it arrives when promised. A back-ordered item is usually not billed until it is shipped.

In some states, ordering of medications, needles, and sterile solutions requires an authorization from a physician

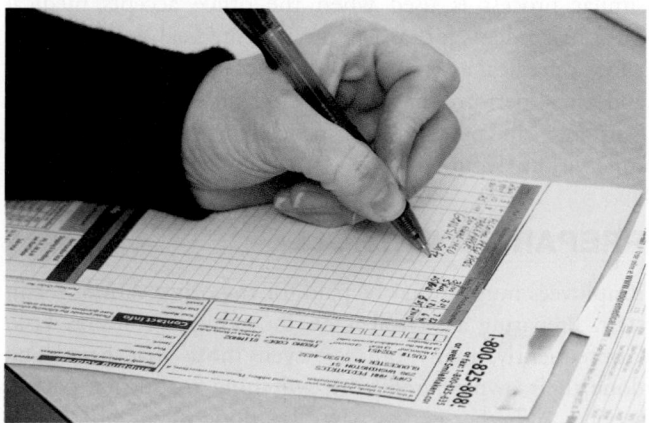

Figure 48-6 Supplies may be ordered using a catalog order form.

and a copy of the physician's state medical license for purchase. For purchase of controlled substances, such as narcotics, a physician authorization and a copy of the physician's federal Drug Enforcement Administration certificate is necessary.

What Would You Do? What Would You *Not* Do?

Case Study 2

Kelsey accepts a delivery of a large box of supplies from UPS at a time when the office is especially busy. She places the box in the supply room and continues with her work. Toward the end of the day, she realizes that she has not opened the delivery. She goes to the supply room and opens the outer box. Inside, there are boxes and packages of dressings, bandages, tape, tissues, gauze squares, and other items. Kelsey has an appointment, and she is anxious to finish up so that she can leave the office. ■

Receiving Supplies

Different suppliers ship their supplies in different ways, including using the U.S. Postal Service, large national package delivery companies such as United Parcel Service (UPS) or FedEx, and local courier services.

Most delivery services will ask for a signature to confirm that the delivery has been made. When supplies are received, they should immediately be brought to the storage room. At the first convenient opportunity, the packing slip should be inspected and reconciled with the order to make sure all items have been received or that items that are to be received in a separate delivery are noted on the packing slip. If the packing slip is incorrect, the missing items should be noted and the supplier notified.

The packing slip should be clipped to the order form. When all items have been received, the order form with all the packing slips attached should be marked "all items received" and placed in the accounts payable folder. If the order was not prepaid, the **invoice** (itemized bill for items that have not been prepaid) should arrive within a few days of delivery of the final items on the order.

Once the contents of a shipping box have been placed in storage, the box should be discarded. It is not recommended to keep boxes or cartons used for shipping because they may be dirty and can harbor insects or rodents.

CREATING AN ENVIRONMENT FOR TEAMWORK

Managing the medical office goes beyond the physical space, equipment, and supplies. It is also important to manage the people who work in the office. The medical assistant should help to establish an environment that supports teamwork, one in which people are willing to help one another out but are also willing to allow each individual to display her or his particular expertise. The medical assistant may help set the tone for teamwork by showing respect for each employee and his or her skills and pitching in to help orient new employees or anyone who needs a little assistance during an especially busy time.

Staff Meetings

In a busy office where each person is performing specialized tasks, regular staff meetings can also promote teamwork. These meetings should occur often enough—weekly or, at most, monthly—so that situations in need of correction can be dealt with quickly. The medical assistant may be responsible to schedule and/or lead these meetings.

The staff meeting should be used to share information or work through changes in office practice or procedures, discuss ways to improve patient satisfaction and office performance, and encourage staff to take advantage of opportunities to improve skills. Some skill improvement efforts can take place in the form of training sessions in the office on new equipment or computer systems. Others can be opportunities to attend off-site seminars and workshops.

In planning a meeting, a written agenda (list of specific items of business to be covered) assists in focusing the meeting and ensuring that all important business is considered in an organized way. One person should be assigned the task of taking **minutes** (a record of the meeting's proceedings).

Written minutes are valuable because they assist individuals who attended a meeting to follow up on suggestions and decisions. The agenda should be prepared in advance, but except for a large, formal meeting, it need not be circulated until the meeting begins. Minutes, however, should be circulated. They should be distributed as soon as possible after the meeting, although they are not usually formally approved until the beginning of the next meeting.

Orienting and Training Employees

A new employee will be required to provide documentation in order to be added to the office payroll. All employees must have a Social Security number and complete an I-9 (Employment Eligibility Verification) form before they can begin working. The medical assistant may be responsible for reviewing the Social Security card and/or documents that establish identity and eligibility to work in the United States. Information about obtaining or replacing a Social Security card or changing the name on a Social Security card is available from the Social Security Administration.

Before the end of the first withholding period, a new employee must fill out a W-4 form, which identifies the number of exemptions claimed for proper income tax withholding. This form is updated annually, and the current version can be obtained from the Internal Revenue Service (IRS) website. An employee can submit a new form any time that his or her status changes—for example, if the employee gets married or has a child. If the employee elects to claim fewer exemptions than he or she is legally entitled to, the medical office will withhold more money from the employee's paycheck. Individuals claim fewer exemptions

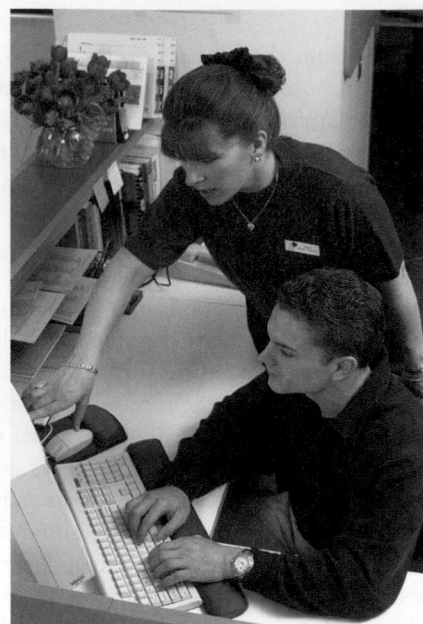

Figure 48-7 Medical assistants may need to help medical assisting students during their externship.

to be sure that adequate funds are withheld to cover their income tax liability.

A photocopy of any licenses or certificates should also be obtained from a new employee. All documents should be placed in the employee's personnel file.

Working with New Employees or Medical Assisting Students

The medical assistant may be asked to participate in the orientation and training of a new medical assistant. This usually involves explaining physician preferences and working with the new employee to be sure that he or she understands how all procedures should be performed. The office may have a checklist of skills or tasks that the new employee must demonstrate before being allowed to perform them without supervision. If a new employee is not familiar with a specific piece of equipment, such as the model of electrocardiograph or spirometer, the medical assistant may be responsible for training the new employee to use it. A similar process is used when the office accepts medical assisting students for externship. The medical assistant must allow a medical assisting student to observe each procedure and then perform it with supervision until the medical assistant can perform the procedure correctly without supervision (Figure 48-7).

PREPARING PAYROLL

Employees must always be paid, or the office cannot retain staff. Preparing a payroll is an increasingly complex task. Consequently, many offices—even those that have long done their own payroll—are switching to outside payroll services. Whether or not payroll is done in the office, files are kept on all employees.

Payroll records for individual employees include the following:

- Name, address, Social Security number, and occupation
- The employee's withholding allowance certificate **(W-4),** which is used to calculate the amount withheld for federal income taxes
- Dates of employment
- Record of hours worked, wages paid, annuity, and pensions
- Record of all payroll deductions

These records must be kept for at least 4 years and be available for review by the IRS.

Employees may fill out timecards to report the hours worked, or they may punch in and out using a time clock. Most medical assistants are paid an hourly rate. In this case the **gross pay,** the amount of money earned before any deductions, is calculated by multiplying the number of hours worked times the hourly rate. Some office employees may receive a **salary,** a fixed amount paid on a regular basis that does not depend on the number of hours worked. In this case the gross pay is the predetermined amount.

Deductions

Income Taxes

Employers are required to withhold federal income taxes based on the amount paid to an employee and the number of withholding allowances the employee claims. The IRS publication *Employer's Tax Guide* contains detailed information including tables to determine the amount to withhold.

Social Security and Medicare

Social Security tax (called *FICA* after the Federal Insurance Contributions Act) funds the national program of retirement benefits into which all workers pay 4.25% of the first $110,000 in income (for 2012). Employers still pay 6.2%. In addition, 1.45% of all employee wages are withheld for Medicare taxes, and the employer must pay an additional 1.45%.

State Taxes

Most states require employers to withhold state income tax based on the amount earned and the number of withholding allowances reported for the state (which may be different from the federal W-4 allowances).

Employer Obligations

The employer is required to deposit withheld income taxes, as well as employee and employer Social Security and Medicare taxes, following the schedule outlined in the IRS publication *Employer's Tax Guide.*

The employer is required to provide each employee with two copies of form W-2, the Wage and Tax Statement, by January 31. This form is used by the employee to complete his or her personal income tax forms. State income taxes are usually included on this form.

Unemployment Tax

Federal unemployment tax (FUTA) is paid by the employer on the first $7000.00 of income at a rate of 0.8% (for 2012). The money, which must be deposited quarterly, is used to pay unemployment compensation for workers who have lost their jobs. States also require employers to pay unemployment tax for their employees, and a few states also require employers to withhold an unemployment tax from their employees.

Preparing Payroll Checks

If the payroll is being done in the office, the individual who does the payroll must gather time sheets or timecards if they are used; calculate wages, taxes, and other deductions for each employee; prepare the checks; and record five items of information in the payroll record for each employee:

1. Total wages for the pay period (gross pay)
2. Federal, state, and (sometimes) local income taxes, as well as Social Security and Medicare taxes
3. Other deductions, such as health insurance, uncovered medical expenses, dependent care, and retirement savings
4. **Net pay,** or take-home pay (pay after deductions)
5. Gross pay, or total pay, from January 1 to the end of the pay period being recorded

Before wages are calculated, time sheets or timecards should be reviewed for accuracy. (If a time clock is used, the exact times of clocking in and clocking out are recorded.) If the payroll is being managed by a service outside the office, the supervising medical assistant is responsible only for collecting time sheets and transmitting to the payroll agency each employee's gross pay for the pay period.

MANAGING PHYSICIAN AND EMPLOYEE SCHEDULES

Physician Schedules

In addition to the medical office appointment schedule, physicians must be scheduled for other responsibilities related to patient care. In a group practice, one physician must always be on call (i.e., available to take telephone calls from patients and make arrangements so that urgent and emergency health care needs of patients will be met). Physicians in solo practice often collaborate with other physicians in their community to provide this service. The medical office usually develops a standard schedule, but individual physicians must be assigned to cover each on-call time period. After the schedule has been arranged, physicians usually must work with one another if they want to switch or change days.

If the medical practice has satellite offices, physicians must be assigned times to see patients in the main office and in the other offices. If possible, coverage must be coordinated so that there is at least one physician in the satellite office every day. A master schedule is usually created, but variations occur depending on time of year and circumstances. For example, sometimes satellite offices are closed during holiday or vacation periods.

In many practices the physicians make nursing home visits. In addition to scheduled blocks of time for these visits, there must also be a plan to provide urgent care if a nursing home resident becomes ill. Some physicians always see their own patients, and in other practices there is one physician who is responsible for nursing home patients on a given day.

Employee Schedules

Other staff members must also be scheduled to provide coverage in both the primary office and any satellite offices. Usually employees must submit requests in writing for days off, changes to the regular schedule, and vacation. Depending on the size of the office, the medical assistant or office manager may be responsible for creating the work schedule for staff other than the physicians. When one of the medical assistants or another staff member calls in sick, efforts must be made to find a replacement. The medical office often has contact with medical assistants or other employees who will work on a *per diem* basis; *per diem* is a Latin term meaning "per day" or "by the day." *Per diem* employees do not have a fixed schedule. They may be given a weekly schedule depending on office needs, and, in addition, they may be called in on a day when extra help is required. The office may also use an employment agency to obtain temporary employees, especially if one of the regular medical assistants is unable to work for an extended period of time.

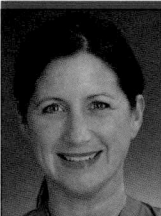

Memories *from* Externship

Kelsey Whitman: The office where I did my externship was in a physician office building next to the local hospital. It was a very clean, modern office, and I learned so much there. There were two physicians specializing in internal medicine. At the beginning of the day, we got everything ready for the patients. We made sure the waiting room was tidy, stocked every examination room, and turned on the CD player so that patients could listen to music. The office closed for an hour at noon, and after the morning patients had left, we checked the waiting room, picked up the magazines, and made sure there was no trash on the tables. In the afternoon, it was my job to go through the examination rooms and make sure that all items were restocked. While I was on my externship, one of the physicians went on vacation for a week, and we used that time to clean all the drawers and cabinets in the examination rooms. We took everything out and cleaned each area with soap and water. We found expired supplies at the back of the cabinets, and we had to discard them. It was a lot of work, but when we were done, everything seemed much better organized. Before my externship, I didn't realize the amount of work it is to keep everything looking neat and professional in a medical office. ∎

PROVIDING RESOURCES FOR STAFF AND PATIENTS

Office Policy and Procedure Manuals

Medical Office Policies

Effective management of the medical office requires activities to meet all legal requirements and to maintain a high standard of patient care. A guiding principle for management of the office is called a **policy.**

Often an organization formulates its own statements (written policies) to help it provide guidance to employees and adhere to laws or regulations. For example, a medical office might have written policies regarding sexual harassment, confidentiality, patient rights, and honest and ethical billing, to name just a few. Conditions of employment, including employee performance, attendance and punctuality, vacation time, sick time, paid time off, and employee evaluation are also included.

These are collected in a policy manual, which can easily be reviewed by employees and regulatory agencies. It is the responsibility of the manager to review existing policies and implement changes if necessary. A new employee might be required to review the policy manual and sign a statement to that effect.

If a policy needs to be reviewed, it is usually discussed in a staff meeting and a draft of the revision is circulated for review among office staff. Once there is consensus about the revision, the revised policy is accepted and the revised version is placed in all copies of the policy manual. The date of acceptance and/or revision should be clearly indicated on each policy. A new policy may be necessary, especially when new federal legislation is passed, such as the Health Insurance Portability and Accountability Act (HIPAA). A new policy is also written as a draft, circulated, discussed, and eventually accepted and added to the policy manual.

Written Procedures

In order to put policies into practice, an organization uses procedures. A **procedure** is a description of the steps to handle a specific situation or perform a certain task. Written procedure manuals are common in large organizations, but they can also benefit smaller medical offices, for several reasons. Procedures related to employment (such as requesting vacation days) are often included in the general policy manual.

Procedure manuals are excellent resources for new employees. They can also provide guidelines and information when a long-term employee suddenly becomes unavailable, either by changing jobs or becoming ill. They encourage office staff to reflect on the methods used to accomplish tasks and examine the reasons for specific actions. A procedure manual for laboratory tests is required under CLIA.

Regular review of procedures is necessary to be sure that they are up to date and conform to changes in legal regulations and/or improvements in technology. There may be separate procedure manuals for clinical procedures and administrative procedures.

Procedures that facilitate proper functioning of every area of the office should be available. New procedures should be written when they are missing or when new equipment or different supplies have changed how things are done. It is helpful to add photographs, especially of tray setups or supplies and equipment needed for special procedures. The medical assistant may oversee the job of setting the schedule to review or create procedures, obtaining written or verbal input from those who actually carry out the tasks, and finalizing the written procedures. Like policies, each procedure should be dated. Procedure manuals throughout the office should be kept up to date.

After the procedure manual has been created, all personnel, especially new staff members or those with questions, should be encouraged to use the procedure manual as a reference. It often seems easier to ask questions of co-workers with experience, but it increases independence and individual capability if staff is encouraged to refer to the written manual.

Locating Community Resources

The medical assistant can be helpful to patients by identifying community resources to meet patient health needs (Procedure 48-4). The medical office may keep a list of local organizations with telephone numbers or other contact information in the following areas:

- Support for alcoholism or addiction
- Support for caregivers of individuals with decreased mental or physical function
- Adult day care
- Visiting nurse and homemaker services
- Legal aid
- Local civic organizations including services for children, families, elders, and the homeless
- Local board of health
- Hospital-sponsored rehabilitation, weight control, smoking cessation programs
- Immunization clinics
- Cardiopulmonary resuscitation (CPR) and first aid training

National organizations focus on many diseases. Most will provide information, and some have local chapters or can refer patients to local organizations. The medical assistant can be helpful by assisting the patient to search the Internet for these organizations. Many hospitals also have extensive programs related to specific diseases or conditions, and the medical assistant should become familiar with those in his or her locality, especially those sponsored by the hospital with which the practice physicians are affiliated. The hospital newsletter is a good source of information on new programs for patients. See Appendix C on the Evolve site for the national contact information of some community resources.

PROCEDURE 48-4 Locating Community Resources

Outcome Locate appropriate community resources.

Equipment/Supplies

- Local telephone book
- Office list of community resources
- Computer
- Local hospital newsletter(s)
- Library access
- Local newspapers
- Pen
- Notepad

1. **Procedural Step.** Research local sources to identify community agencies with resources to assist patients. Potential sources of information include the library, local newspapers, local cable TV stations, local telephone books, local hospital newsletters, and the Internet.

   Principle. Familiarity with local agencies improves the medical assistant's ability to provide useful information about community resources to patients.

2. **Procedural Step.** As resources are identified, create a list including pertinent information about the resource: name, services available, address, telephone number, website address, contact name or information, and other useful information. The list may be created using pen and paper, but it should be transferred to a word processing file for ease of duplication.

3. **Procedural Step.** Once the document file has been substantially completed, group resources by subject and/or age group served. Alphabetize resources within each group.

   Principle. Arranging lists in alphabetic order facilitates finding specific information and avoids any impression of favoritism or recommending one agency more than another.

4. **Procedural Step.** When the list is complete, save and print copies as needed.

5. **Procedural Step.** Ask the office physicians to review and approve the list.

   Principle. Any referral made by a medical office should have the approval of the practice physicians.

6. **Procedural Step.** Update the list when information changes, when a new resource is identified, and on a periodic basis to be sure information is accurate.

7. **Procedural Step.** Use the list to make appropriate recommendations to patients either in response to patient questions or when instructed to by one of the office physicians.

RISK MANAGEMENT

Risk management is the process of assessing risk and putting in place policies and procedures that minimize it. Often, the focus of risk management activities is on avoiding lawsuits. Risk in a medical office comes in a number of forms.

Minimizing Risk of Injury or Illness

Physical risk involves the risk of injury or illness to employees, patients, and visitors. Business risk also exists: the risk of reduced patient visits because of poor "customer relations." Any medical office seeks to minimize these risks and prevent lawsuits that may result from injuries related to patient care or an accident in the office.

The medical assistant or office manager is often responsible for maintaining the risk management program, in close consultation with the physician or the managing partner among the physicians. In larger clinics or hospitals there may be a full-time risk manager, or risk management may be a part of the duties of one of the clinic's top administrators. Policies and procedures are designed by the physicians and the office's top administrator, who work closely with an attorney, an insurance professional, and a risk management professional. When a new policy is adopted, a copy is given to each employee covered by the policy. Policy and procedure manuals, once developed, should be accessible to all employees when questions arise.

Incident Reports

Whenever something happens in the office for which the office could be considered liable, an incident report should be filled out. An incident can be as simple as a staff member or patient tripping over a chair, or it could be as serious as a staff member sticking himself or herself with a needle that has just been used to give an injection.

The incident report should be initiated by the staff member who is injured or who is closest to the patient or visitor when he or she is injured. A supervisor should review the report before giving it to the individual who manages the risk management program.

Incident report forms vary widely but usually ask for the following information:
- Date and time that the incident occurred
- Name and identifying information of the individual(s) involved

- Address, building, and room number where the incident occurred
- Description of how the incident occurred and exactly what occurred
- Complete description of any injury or potential injury
- Name(s) and identifying information for any witnesses
- Name and contact information for the person in the organization to whom the incident was reported
- Date of receipt and follow-up by supervisor

Incident reports should always be filled out if a patient, employee, or visitor slips or falls, if a medication error is made, if blood is drawn from the wrong patient, if the number of surgical instruments counted after a procedure does not match the number counted before the procedure, or if an employee is stuck with a needle.

Any witnesses to the incident should be asked for their name, address, and phone number so that the office's insurance provider can call and investigate the incident further if necessary. The report should be dated and signed by the person filling it out. A physician and/or supervisor's signature also goes on the form, according to the office's policy for incident reports (Procedure 48-5).

Liability Coverage

Every office should have adequate insurance protection against liability, both professional liability (commonly called *malpractice*) and liability for any accident that might occur in the office.

Professional liability insurance covers a medical professional for patient claims that diagnostic procedures, tests, or treatments either caused an injury or failed to detect an existing medical condition that should have been detected using good medical practice.

Some physicians purchase insurance in their own name only and have professional staff members purchase their own professional liability policies. If this is the case, the medical assistant can purchase a professional liability policy through a professional organization, such as the American Association of Medical Assistants.

In other cases a practice purchases professional liability insurance for the entire staff. If this is the case, every professional staff member should be named on the policy.

The office should also have adequate insurance to cover property damage to the office because of fire, storm, or flooding (similar to homeowner's insurance). In addition, the practice should have adequate coverage against personal injury sustained on the office's property by a patient or employee. Many patients are ill and/or fragile, and a fall can occur at any time. The policy should cover any injury sustained on the property controlled by the practice. If the practice is in an office building, the public hallways are the responsibility of the landlord or medical office condominium association. If the office is in a freestanding building, the practice is responsible for any occurrences that happen on walkways, in the parking lot, or in other outdoor areas up to the public road or sidewalk.

Outcome Complete an incident report.

Equipment/Supplies

- Incident report form (such as OSHA Form 301)
- Pen
- Notes from witnesses to the incident

1. **Procedural Step.** Interview all witnesses to the incident, and make notes as needed to complete the incident report.
   Principle. The incident report is based on factual information, but individuals involved in the incident may not be available when the report is actually written.

2. **Procedural Step.** Obtain an incident report form and fill in information about the person (or persons) who are the main subject of the incident including name, date of birth, and address.

3. **Procedural Step.** Complete any information about health care provided including the names and identifying information for physicians or health care professionals who provided treatment.
   Principle. Risk management includes taking all possible steps to minimize an adverse result from an incident.

4. **Procedural Step.** Complete all information to describe the incident in detail including time, location (address, building, room number), what happened, and any injury or illness that resulted from the incident. Include the names and identifying information of any witnesses.
   Principle. Documentation of this information as soon as possible after the incident makes it easier to establish the facts about the incident at a later time.

5. **Procedural Step.** Include the name and contact information of the individual within the office to whom the incident was reported. The supervisor should add information about any follow-up that occurs at a later date. The supervisor should initiate any additional required reports to appropriate government agencies.
   Principle. Follow-up for an incident is a crucial step in effective risk management.

6. **Procedural Step.** Review the report with the subject of the incident if possible before signing the report and obtaining his or her signature, also if possible. Obtain a supervisor's signature as well.
   Principle. Signatures on an incident report indicate that parties involved have been informed of the contents of the report.

MEDICAL PRACTICE and the LAW

If an injury occurs in the medical office, it is usually necessary for the injured person to prove negligence in order to be compensated for the injury.

1. The medical office and its employees can be sued by patients and visitors to the office for accidental injuries that occur anywhere on the premises. Injury that is not a result of professional activity is covered by the office's general liability insurance policy. For example, if any individual other than an employee slips and falls on a wet floor in the office and is injured, the medical office would be legally liable.

2. A patient who is injured as a result of medical treatment might initiate a lawsuit for professional negligence (malpractice). For example, a patient might be accidentally burned from a hot pack that was too hot or left on too long. This type of lawsuit would be covered by professional liability insurance.

In a second category of injuries, liability is assumed and negligence does not have to occur.

1. Injury from defective equipment falls under the category of product liability. For example, a machine might suddenly create sparks and injure anyone near it. Provided that the office staff was using the equipment correctly and had maintained the equipment according to the manufacturer's directions, the manufacturer would be liable for any injury.

2. An injury to office employees while on the job is covered by mandatory workers' compensation insurance paid for by the employer. ■

What Would You Do? What Would You *Not* Do? RESPONSES

Case Study 1
Page 1128

What Did Kelsey Do?
❏ Put the twins in an examination room as soon as possible.
❏ Asked Mrs. Highsmith to place the used tissues in the wastebasket before taking the twins to the examination room. Then she provided hand sanitizer for Mrs. Highsmith.

❏ As soon as possible, put on disposable gloves and removed the plastic toys that the twins had had in their mouths so that they could be cleaned before other children played with them.
❏ When told that Scott Highsmith had thrown up a little, put on disposable gloves, used paper towels to absorb as much liquid as possible, and then promptly cleaned and disinfected the surrounding area.
❏ Reassured Mrs. Highsmith that children are ill sometimes and cleaning up is all in a day's work.

Continued

What Would You Do? What Would You *Not* Do? RESPONSES—cont'd

❑ Noted the color and amount of vomit so that she could inform the physician.

What Did Kelsey Not Do?

❑ Did not ask Mrs. Highsmith to prevent the twins from playing with any toys because they had colds.
❑ Did not tell other mothers in the waiting room that they might not want to let their children play with the toys until they could be disinfected.
❑ Did not wait to perform routine cleaning until the lunch break or after office hours.
❑ Did not tell another staff member or Mrs. Highsmith to clean up when Scott vomited.

What Would You Do/What Would You *Not* Do?

Review Kelsey's response and place a checkmark next to the information you included in your response. List the additional information you included in your response.

_____
_____
_____
_____
_____

Case Study 2
Page 1135

What Did Kelsey Do?

❑ Checked the number of each type of item against the packing slip to be sure the order was complete. Made a notation if any items were missing.
❑ Placed all the items in their assigned storage area, either that night or the next day. Placed newer items behind older items.
❑ When placing items into storage, checked items on the shelves to be sure that none of them had expired.
❑ If any items were missing or backordered, made a notation on the packing slip. Then she placed the packing slip in the accounts payable folder to indicate that the order had been received.
❑ Removed the shipping box to the designated area for trash.

What Did Kelsey Not Do?

❑ After opening the large box, did not leave the office before checking the packing slip. Another staff member might assume that the individual who opened the box had also checked the contents.
❑ Did not just stack the items on shelves in the storage room randomly because she was in a hurry.

❑ Did not discard the packing slip after checking the order.
❑ Did not keep the shipping box because it might be dirty or harbor pests.

What Would You Do/What Would You *Not* Do?

Review Kelsey's response and place a checkmark next to the information you included in your response. List the additional information you included in your response.

_____
_____
_____
_____
_____

Case Study 3
Page 1140

What Did Kelsey Do?

❑ Encouraged Ellen to reach out and find out if there were services that could help her mother.
❑ While Mrs. Brown was present, included her in the conversation.
❑ If speaking to Ellen privately was an option, offered understanding of how difficult it is to know what to do when a parent begins to be less able to function independently.
❑ Offered to help Ellen find resources for delivered meals or homemaking services in the community.
❑ Referred Ellen to local agencies that provide elder services.
❑ Offered to ask the physician if a referral to a visiting nurse would be appropriate.

What Did Kelsey Not Do?

❑ Did not exclude Mrs. Brown from the conversation or treat her like a child.
❑ Did not push Mrs. Brown or Ellen to accept her suggestions, but rather just offered information.
❑ Did not promise that the physician would make specific referrals.

What Would You Do/What Would You *Not* Do?

Review Kelsey's response and place a checkmark next to the information you included in your response. List the additional information you included in your response.

_____
_____
_____
_____
_____

TERMINOLOGY REVIEW

Medical Term	Word Parts	Definition
Back order		A term used for items ordered that cannot be shipped immediately, usually because they are out of stock.
Depreciation		Accounting methods to respond to the loss of value of a property or piece of equipment over time.
Gross pay		The total amount earned in a time period by an employee before any deductions.
Inventory		A detailed list of items in stock or in possession of an individual or business.
Invoice		An itemized bill for items whose cost has not been prepaid.
Minutes		A written record of the proceedings of a meeting.
Net pay		The actual amount of money paid directly to an employee after taxes and other deductions have been taken out.
Per diem		A term used for employees who do not have a fixed schedule but are scheduled by the day according to office needs.
Policy		A guiding principle for the management of a medical office or business.
Procedure		A list of the steps to handle a certain situation or perform a certain task.
Reorder point		A number on a supply inventory that indicates when a specific item should be reordered to be sure that the supply will not run out before the new order is received.
Risk management		The process of assessing risk and putting policies and procedures in place to minimize it.
Salary		A fixed amount of money paid on a regular basis that does not depend on the number of hours worked.
Service contract		An agreement that provides for service for a piece of equipment after the warranty expires.
Social Security tax (FICA)		A tax collected from employers and employees to fund the Social Security program, which provides benefits to retired workers.
Vendor		A company from whom supplies or equipment is purchased.
Warranty		A promise by the manufacturer to repair or replace defective parts in an item during a specific time period.
W-4		The form used to claim allowances for federal income tax reporting.

ON THE WEB

For information on U.S. government forms related to payroll and employment:

I-9 form (United States Citizen and Immigration Services): www.uscis.gov/files/form/i-9.pdf

Internal Revenue Service: www.irs.gov

  W-2 (Wage and Tax Statement)

  W-4 form (for employee withholding)

  Withholding tax tables

  Form 941 (employer's quarterly tax return)

  Form 940 (employer's annual federal unemployment [FUTA] tax return)

Social Security Administration: www.ssa.gov

  Obtain a Social Security number

  Apply for a replacement Social Security card

For information on worker safety:

OSHA Guide to Complicance for Medical and Dental Offices: www.osha.gov/Publications/osha3187.pdf

OSHA Small Business Handbook: www.osha.gov/Publications/smallbusiness/small-business.pdf

 Check out the Evolve site at http://evolve.elsevier.com/Bonewit/today/ to actively Prepare for your Certification, and to access additional interactive activities and exercises to help you study and prepare for success.

49

Emergency Protective Practices for the Medical Office

KEY TERMS

anxiety
evacuation plan
fire extinguisher

HAZMAT
man-made disaster
natural disaster

posttraumatic stress disorder (PTSD)
stress

INTRODUCTION TO DISASTER AND EMERGENCY PLANNING

Every healthcare facility faces the possibility that a disaster or serious emergency may cause damage and/or threaten its employees, patients, buildings and other assets with harm or inability to provide the usual services. All organizations must plan ahead to minimize the damage from any disaster or serious emergency and to facilitate recovery so that services can be restored as efficiently as possible.

TYPES OF SYSTEM-WIDE DISASTERS AND EMERGENCIES

Hazards are usually categorized as natural or man-made. A **natural disaster** results from a natural hazard (such as volcanoes, tornados, earthquakes, fires from lightning strikes, or hurricanes) that causes significant damage to the environment and leads to environmental, financial, and human losses. A **man-made disaster** refers to serious damage either directly or indirectly caused by intentional or negligent human actions or the failure of a man-made system (such as a fire, structural collapse, or terrorism).

Natural Disasters

Natural disasters may occur with or without warning. Earthquakes usually occur without warning, whereas hurricanes develop over a period of days, which allows for some preparation. In addition, the effect of natural disasters often seems random. Many communities must prepare when a hurricane or tornado is in the area because the exact track of the storm is difficult to predict. It is important for all employees of the medical office to be educated about immediate response to the types of natural disasters that tend to occur in their geographic area while still realizing that unusual events of great magnitude can also occur. The effect of serious natural disasters is felt far beyond the area that is affected. For example, Hurricane Katrina affected the entire United States, partly because of the shock that a disaster of such scope could even happen, partly because of the extensive relocation of people who lost their homes, and partly because of the massive relief effort, which included assistance from emergency workers and volunteers.

Man-made Disasters and Emergencies

As with natural events, the amount of threat or damage from man-made hazards can vary considerably; examples include a fire in a wastebasket that is quickly contained, a gunman threatening to injure all the employees of an office, a bomb threat, and a radiation incident that may involve an entire city or area. Man-made hazards include crime, many fires, terrorism, industrial hazards, structural collapse, power outage, radiation hazards, and chemical contamination. Municipal fire departments and police departments provide rapid assistance for fires, injury, and criminal activity, and the National Response Center of the Environmental

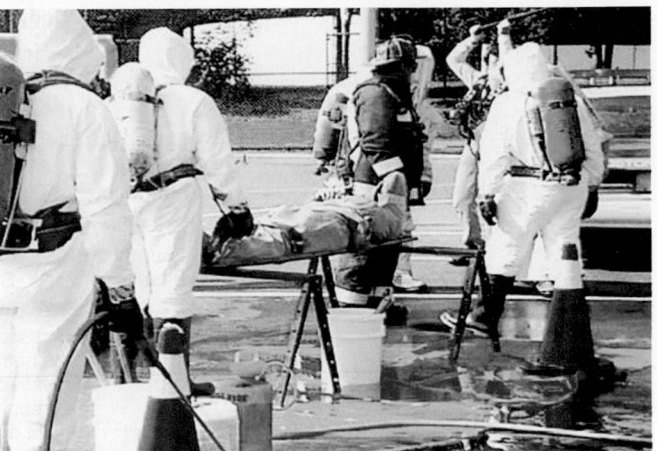

Figure 49-1 Teams responding to disasters involving hazardous materials (HAZMAT) must wear protective clothing and initiate decontamination of casualties.

Protection Agency responds to the release, or potential release, of oil, radioactive materials, or hazardous chemicals into the air, land, or water (Figure 49-1).

PSYCHOLOGICAL EFFECTS OF SERIOUS EMERGENCIES

Whenever an event occurs that causes or threatens to cause serious damage or interruption of the normal daily routine, individuals who are affected react positively and negatively to the loss of property or disruption of service. Positive reactions involve the triggering of resources, both internal and external, to meet the challenges. For example, when a serious flood threatens an area, both municipal and state employees and volunteers usually mobilize quickly to fill and place sandbags to minimize the anticipated damage. When physical and emotional resources are depleted, however, individuals react negatively. Disasters that tend to cause the most serious psychological effects include those with the following characteristics:

- Occur without warning
- Pose a serious threat to personal safety or have unknown health effects (such as the tsunami in Japan in 2011 or the damage from Hurricane Katrina)
- Have an uncertain duration (such as serious floods of major rivers)
- Result from malicious intent or human error
- Have symbolic significance (such as the 9/11 attacks)

The Stress Response

Stress is the body's response to threat or change. Hans Selye, an Austrian doctor who practiced in the middle of the twentieth century, described the body's reaction to stress as a four-part general adaptation syndrome (GAS), also known as the fight or flight response, which is shown in Figure 49-2. The four stages of the GAS are the alarm reaction, the stage of resistance, the recovery phase, and the stage of exhaustion.

Body Reaction When Stress Persists

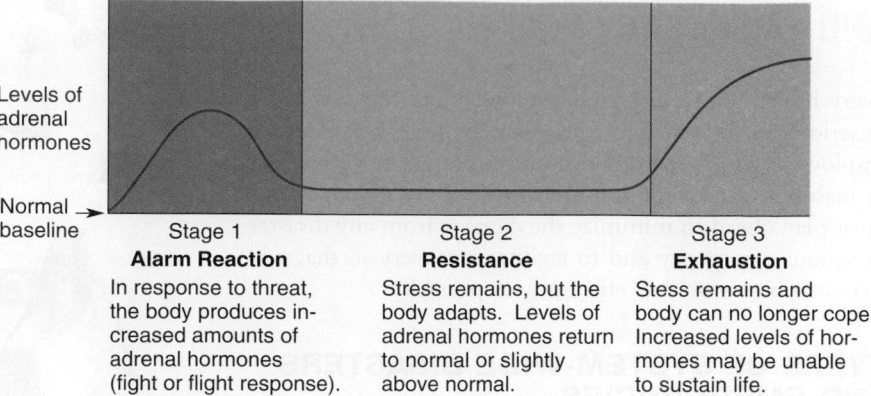

Levels of adrenal hormones

Normal baseline

Stage 1	Stage 2	Stage 3
Alarm Reaction	**Resistance**	**Exhaustion**
In response to threat, the body produces increased amounts of adrenal hormones (fight or flight response).	Stress remains, but the body adapts. Levels of adrenal hormones return to normal or slightly above normal.	Stess remains and body can no longer cope. Increased levels of hormones may be unable to sustain life.

Figure 49-2 Hans Selye's general adaptation syndrome (GAS).

Body Reaction When Stress is Removed

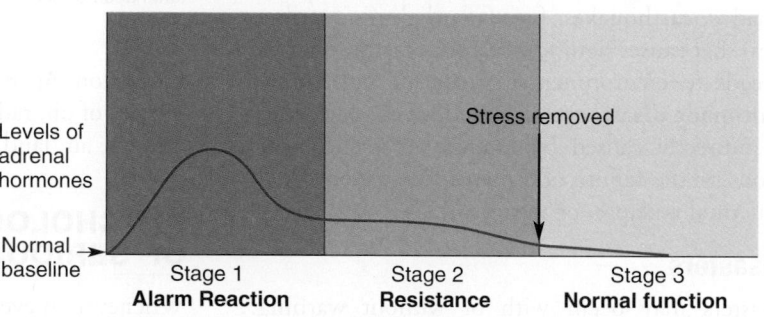

Levels of adrenal hormones

Normal baseline

Stress removed

Stage 1	Stage 2	Stage 3
Alarm Reaction	**Resistance**	**Normal function**

In the first stage, the alarm reaction, the body senses a stress and begins to react. Epinephrine is released from the adrenal medulla and stimulates the sympathetic nervous system. The pupils dilate, the heart beats faster, respirations become faster and deeper, and the blood pressure rises. The body prepares to fight or run away. The individual's attention becomes narrowly focused on the perceived threat or significant task. Some people experience the alarm reaction as energizing, whereas others quickly become extremely anxious.

In the second stage, the stage of resistance, the stress remains but the body adapts. This may occur within hours or days, depending on the circumstances. Levels of adrenal hormones may remain slightly high or drop back to normal. More energy is required to maintain the stage of resistance than the normal state.

After the stress has been removed, the body enters the recovery phase, and as the parasympathetic system begins to regain control, the body returns to its normal level of function.

If stress persists or is always present, it causes an increase in blood pressure, elevated glucose (blood sugar) level, increased metabolism, and increased pressure within the eye. This is why constant stress leads to fatigue, hunger, and headaches.

Eventually, in a person subjected to chronic stress, the body is unable to maintain the response, the immune system is compromised, and the person is more prone to a variety of illnesses.

Managing Anxiety

During the alarm reaction, anxiety is a normal part of the "fight or flight response." **Anxiety** is defined as a feeling of worry or uneasiness, often triggered by an event with an uncertain outcome. A person who is moderately to severely anxious is not able to notice details and think as clearly as in the normal state. Emergency procedures that have been learned and practiced help individuals to decide what to do without having to think through all possibilities. In addition, they tend to keep the anxiety level from rising because individuals feel more confident when they have a plan to respond to a threat.

Severe anxiety can be medically problematic. In an emergency situation it tends to immobilize an individual and stimulate anxiety in others. Symptoms of a full-blown anxiety attack include the following. An overly anxious person hyperventilates, has an extremely rapid heart rate, and becomes unresponsive. When there is an emergency, many people lose control of their emotions and cry or scream. The behavior can be minimized by giving the highly anxious person directions. It may be necessary to touch the person to gain his or her attention, and then directions should be given in short sentences, speaking a little more slowly than usual. Helping the person to breathe deeply will help reduce anxiety, but it is also important to direct the person exactly where to go if a dangerous area must be evacuated or if the person should take cover. Figure 49-3 shows the various stages of increasing anxiety.

If an emergency occurs while the medical assistant is at work, he or she should immediately focus on responding to

STAGES OF RISING ANXIETY

Panic

Severe state of psycholgic stess. Person unable to focus or cope. May focus on small details which are totally blown out of proportion.

Manifestations: incoherent speech, ineffective communication, sweating, rapid pulse and breathing, muscle tremors, increased muscle tension, elevated blood pressure.

Interventions: The panic state usually subsides fairly quickly because the body cannot sustain it. Interventions are the same for severe anxiety. It may be necessary to make transportation arrangements for the patient.

Severe anxiety

Painful level of anxiety produces loss of abstract thinking and consumes almost all of a person's energy. The person cannot notice what is going on even if it is pointed out.

Manifestations: crying, confused speech, dry mouth, sweating, rapid pulse and breathing, muscle tremors, increased muscle tension, elevated blood pressure

Interventions: Provide a quiet area for the person to regain control. A calm manner is reassuring. Encourage the patient to take slow deep breaths. Seek guidance from the physician if the patient is breathing faster than 22-24 breaths per minute.

Moderate anxiety

Attention is restricted to a particular task or problem rather than entire situation (called selective inattention). Still able to think fairly clearly but focuses on only one thing at a time.

Manifestations: sweating, rapid pulse and breathing, muscle tension and possible stomach pain, frequent urination and/or diarrhea

Interventions: A calm manner is reassuring. Acknowledge that the patient appears anxious. Focus on one thing at a time. Encourage the patient to take slow deep breaths.

Mild anxiety

Manifestations: The body functions well in this state. The person may feel a little nervous.

Figure 49-3 Stages of anxiety.

the immediate situation, implementing established procedures, and helping others. Deep breaths will help to control anxiety, which should be seen as a normal response. Even in disasters that have caused enormous amounts of physical damage, lives have been saved and injury has been minimized when people have been able to stay reasonably calm and follow procedures to stay as safe as possible.

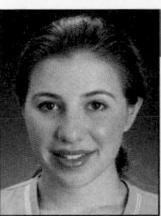

Putting It All into Practice

My name is Beth Ann Wilson, and I am a certified medical assistant. I have been assisting the office manager to update the equipment in our office that might be used in case of fire or natural disaster. We recently purchased an additional fire extinguisher for the staff break room, where we have a microwave and coffee maker. In addition, we have purchased an office disaster kit which has emergency supplies for 10 people for a few days including food, water, a flashlight, a radio, batteries, a first aid kit, and other supplies that might be useful in a building collapse. Of course we hope that we will never have to use these things. I was also one of the staff members from our office who participated recently as a "victim" in a mock disaster drill that was held for emergency personnel in our town. I pretended to be a victim with fractures of my arm and leg. I had never been in a situation where there were many people injured or been transported in an ambulance. The experience increased my understanding of the problems that emergency personnel face, and now I have a more personal understanding of how important it is to be prepared with training and equipment. ■

Posttraumatic Stress Disorder

After the initial phase of a disaster or serious emergency, in addition to a possible injury caused by the event, an individual may be in a state of shock as he or she adjusts to a changed situation. Depending on the individual and the damage to his or her health, property, and personal relationships, it is common to experience irritability, loss of appetite, self-blame, mood swings, physical symptoms such as headaches and stomach pain, nightmares and difficulty sleeping, fatigue, sadness, and depression. It is recommended to return to normal activities as soon as possible. Educational materials and/or grief crisis counseling are helpful as the person gradually adjusts and returns to a more normal state. In some cases, however, weeks or months after the catastrophic event, the individual begins to experience stronger symptoms of stress including flashbacks, memory disturbances, nightmares, severe irritability, severe depression, and impaired functioning. **Posttraumatic stress disorder (PTSD)** is the name given to the emotional disturbance that develops after a traumatic, catastrophic life disturbance when the disturbance lasts for at least a month. Individuals with possible PTSD should be referred for counseling, because this is one of the most effective treatments for this disorder.

FIRE SAFETY

Fire Hazards in the Workplace

Common fire hazards in the medical office include heating equipment that is poorly maintained or too close to flammable materials, overloaded electrical circuits, improper use of stoves or microwave ovens, and improper storage of oxygen, cleaning supplies, and other combustible materials. If the medical office processes its own laundry, poorly maintained washers and dryers can also cause fires, especially if the dryer is vented improperly or if the lint trap is not kept clean. Shipping boxes and other trash should be removed from the office as soon as possible to prevent the buildup of flammable material.

It is very important to avoid using damaged electrical cords, extension cords, and overloaded plug strips. The cords and plugs for all equipment should be inspected for fraying or cracking and replaced if damaged. Cords should not obstruct walkways, not only because they pose a tripping hazard but also because excessive pressure on a cord that is pulled sharply or stepped on may damage the cord and cause a fire. An extension cord may be used with supervision for a short period of time, but for long-term use a piece of equipment should always be plugged into a grounded outlet.

Fire Protection and Fire Safety Plan

Fire protection for an office building is the responsibility of the landlord or office condominium association (if the units are condominiums), but fire protection for the contents of the office is the responsibility of office staff.

Many states require sprinklers in commercial and office buildings. Some states that require sprinklers for larger office buildings do not require them for smaller offices, such as a physician's office that has been converted from a house.

In addition to the health hazards smoking presents, there are also potential fire hazards related to smoking. Smoking should not be permitted in a physician's office, and signs advising patients and visitors that the office is a smoke-free environment should be clearly posted in the waiting area.

Exits should be clearly marked, and an emergency evacuation map should be posted near the door to the waiting room. Lighted exit signs should be tested by shutting off the lights in the room; bulbs should be replaced if necessary.

In a large office or freestanding clinic, there may be fire doors at certain points in corridors. These doors are designed to contain any fire on one side of the door from going into another area of the building. Fire doors should never be propped open but should be allowed to shut to their naturally closed position. Fire alarm pull stations are frequently located in the building corridors. These alarms alert the entire building and also notify the fire department directly (Figure 49-4).

A **fire extinguisher** (a portable device that discharges foam or another material to extinguish a fire) should be positioned in each room near the exit, and they may also be located in the corridors of a large building. These fire extinguishers are important both for putting out small fires and for giving a person the ability to clear an exit path from a room that is on fire. There are many types of fire extinguishers, and many have a numeric rating that indicates how much fire they can handle. For the medical office, the extinguisher should be multipurpose and usually contains a dry chemical. Extinguishers are placed near the door so that the fire does not get between the person and the exit (Figure 49-5). There should always be a fire extinguisher within a 50-foot travel distance of flammable liquids that are stored in containers. Staff should be trained to use the fire extinguishers properly (Procedure 49-1).

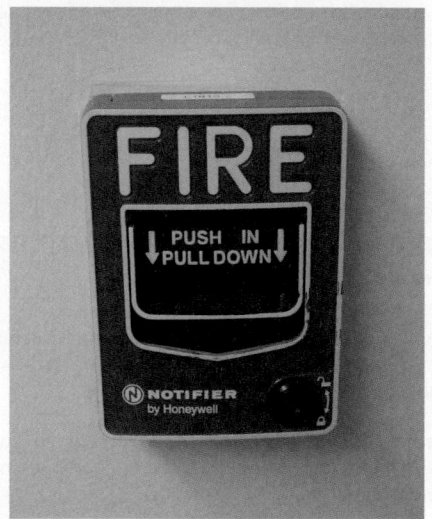

Figure 49-4 Fire alarm pull stations are commonly found in the corridors of an office building.

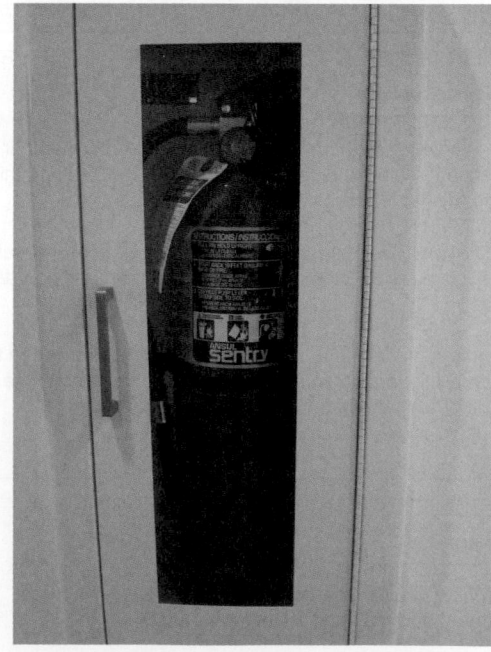

Figure 49-5 Fire extinguishers should be accessible for immediate use.

PROCEDURE 49-1   Demonstrating Proper Use of a Fire Extinguisher

Outcome Demonstrate proper use of a fire extinguisher.

Equipment/Supplies

- Portable office-size multipurpose (ABC) fire extinguisher

1. Procedural Step. Through role-playing (using a discharged fire extinguisher) or in an outdoor location using a new fire extinguisher, pull the safety pin from the handle of the fire extinguisher.
Principle. The fire extinguisher is prevented from discharging when the safety pin is in place.

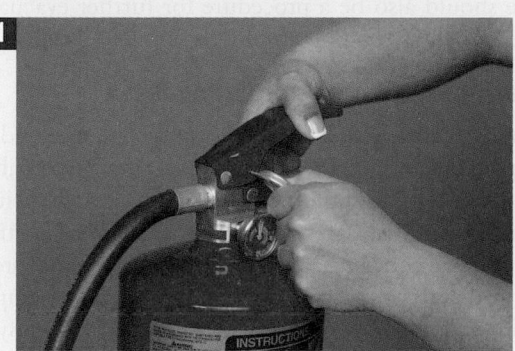
Remove the safety pin.

2. Procedural Step. Aim the nozzle or hose at the base of the fire.
Principle. It is more effective to apply the contents of a fire extinguisher directly to the burning area than to the upper flames.

3. Procedural Step. Stand at the recommended distance printed on the fire extinguisher and squeeze the

moveable top handle against the bottom handle until the extinguisher discharges.
Principle. Different fire extinguishers recommend use at different distances.

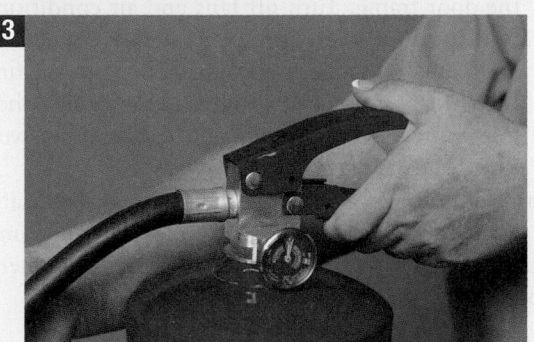
Slowly squeeze the movable top handle.

4. Procedural Step. Sweep the extinguisher from side to side until the flames are extinguished, gradually moving closer to the flames.

5. Procedural Step. Continue to watch the area to be sure that flames do not recur after having been extinguished.
Principle. Material that has been burning can remain hot enough so that flames reignite.

To use a fire extinguisher, the first step is to pull out the pin that keeps the extinguisher from discharging accidentally. Then the nozzle of the extinguisher should be aimed at the base of the fire (to prevent the fire from getting fuel). The handles should be squeezed slowly until the foam or other material is released. Finally the nozzle should sweep from side to side to cover all parts of the fire until the fire is out. The person can move toward the fire as it gets smaller. The acronym to remember these steps is PASS: Pull, Aim, Squeeze, Sweep.

Whenever possible, records should be stored in fire-resistant file cabinets. If the office uses a physical system to back up computer files (instead of a network or an Internet system), the backup drives should be stored in a fire-resistant file cabinet or fire-resistant box-type safe. It is always preferable to store a backup copy on the Internet or at another location.

Smoke detector laws vary by state, in terms of how many must be in an office and where they must be placed. In many buildings, smoke detectors are wired into the building's security and safety alarm system and are tied to the

sprinkler system. If the office has battery-operated smoke detectors, these should be tested monthly by pressing the test button. Batteries should be changed every 6 months, and the date should be noted on the detector.

Every medical office should have a fire safety plan, provide training to all employees, and perform regular fire drills as often as is required by local and/or state building codes.

What Would You Do? What Would You *Not* Do?

Case Study 1

Julie Manning, who is sitting in the waiting room, receives a telephone call, speaks on the telephone for a few minutes, and rushes to the front desk window. She tells Beth Ann that she has to leave immediately because she has just learned that there is a fire at her son's school. Julie speaks very quickly but her story seems disconnected. It is also clear that she is breathing very rapidly. ∎

Emergency Response

The acronym RACE is used to identify the steps in responding to a fire (RACE against fire).

Step 1: **Rescue** any person who is directly threatened by fire. Patient safety is always a first priority.

Step 2: **Activate** the emergency response system (or respond to the alarm of a smoke detector). This can be accomplished by using a fire pull alarm or using the telephone to call 911.

Step 3: **Confine** the fire by closing doors. If you hear a fire alarm, feel doors for heat. Do not open any door if it is warm or if you see smoke leaking out around the door frame. Turn off fans and air conditioners.

Step 4: **Extinguish** the fire or **Evacuate** the area. If the fire is small, use a fire extinguisher to put the fire out. If the fire cannot be extinguished, evacuate the area, following your fire safety plan to be sure that everyone leaves the area.

Large buildings may be designed so that only the affected areas evacuate during a fire, while employees remain in place in unaffected areas unless told to evacuate by emergency personnel.

EMERGENCY PREPAREDNESS IN THE MEDICAL OFFICE

Emergency Action Plan

A written emergency action plan is required by the Occupational Safety and Health Administration (OSHA) for almost all businesses. It must include several elements:

- A means of reporting fires and other emergencies
- Evacuation procedures and emergency escape routes
- Procedures for employees who remain if there are critical operations to be completed
- A way to account for all employees after evacuation
- Designation of rescue and medical duties
- Who to contact for additional information or clarification

Other elements that are recommended include a description of the alarm system to notify employees to evacuate, the site of an alternative communication center (if there is a fire or explosion), and a secure location to store originals or duplicate copies of essential records.

Evacuation Plan

The **evacuation plan** is an essential part of the emergency action plan in a medical office. It includes preplanned escape routes from the facility with diagrams posted in multiple locations. It identifies the conditions that would require evacuation of the area and the chain of command showing who can authorize an evacuation. Specific evacuation routes should be identified and marked on a floor plan, and these plans should be posted throughout the office. The floor plan should designate primary and secondary exits and remind individuals not to use elevators to reach an emergency exit (Figure 49-6).

The evacuation plan should also include information about evacuating individuals with disabilities, and the floor plan should indicate wheelchair accessible exits. Certain individuals may be designated to assist individuals who need extra assistance during evacuation. The duties of these individuals should be clearly defined. If necessary, some employees may be designated to stay behind briefly to operate fire extinguishers or shut down electrical equipment or special equipment that could be damaged if left operating. In high-rise buildings, the office evacuation plan should coordinate with the building evacuation plan.

Every plan should identify an assembly site for employees to meet after evacuation and the person designated to take a head count and account for all employees and all patients. There should also be a procedure for further evacuation if needed, such as sending employees home.

Orienting and Training Employees

When they are hired, all employees must be oriented to the emergency action plan and their specific responsibilities, and in most facilities they are required to review their training (especially fire safety training) annually. The training must include the fire hazards of the materials and processes used in the office, such as the use of oxygen. All employees should be trained in the evacuation plan, alarm systems, reporting procedures, types of potential emergencies, and the use of fire extinguishers. Employees who have special responsibility to assist in evacuation of other employees and patients are often called *fire wardens,* and they should be made aware of their responsibilities.

Fire Drills and Disaster Drills

Fire drills may be required at specific intervals depending on the municipal or state laws for the type of building and insurance requirements. Fire drills may be announced or unannounced. They remind the employees of a medical facility to review emergency escape routes and procedures to respond to a fire. One individual should coordinate the planning, implementation, and evaluation of the fire drill, including notification of the local fire department. This individual should also be responsible for keeping written records.

Disaster drills are usually more comprehensive than fire drills. Disaster drills often involve several community agencies, depending on the severity of the disaster scenario that will be simulated. Disaster drills are time-consuming, but they allow all participants to practice skills that would be needed in the event of a disaster. In addition, they allow organizations and communities to evaluate the effectiveness of their systems and identify potential weaknesses in the ability to respond to an actual disaster. An organization may also have drills to respond to a simulated environmental exposure disaster (Procedure 49-2). This term refers to exposure to pollutants or toxic substances. In a workplace, such exposure can be chronic, because of inadequate shielding or work practices. In addition, an acute incident can occur—for example, a gas leak, a radiation incident, or a spill of a hazardous substance.

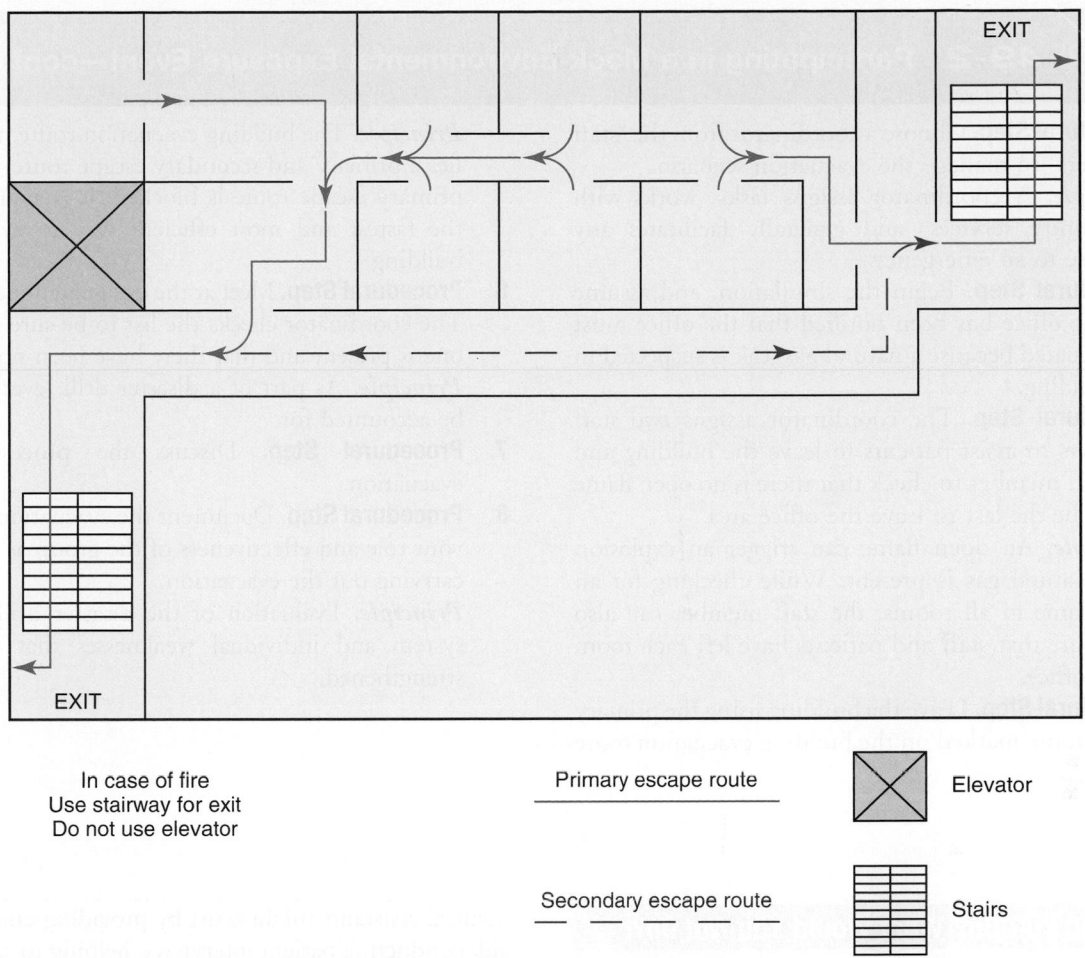

In case of fire
Use stairway for exit
Do not use elevator

Primary escape route

Elevator

Secondary escape route

Stairs

Figure 49-6 Evacuation floor plans should be posted in the medical office.

PROCEDURE **49-2** Participating in a Mock Environmental Exposure Event

Outcome Participate in a mock environmental exposure event.

Scenario: Role-play a scenario with your classmates. First review the directions, review your building evacuation route map, and make a list of all members of your group (the "employees" and "patients"). Designate a place to meet after evacuating the building.

In this scenario, the office manager of the medical office where your group works has been told to evacuate the office because a natural gas leak is suspected in the building. One member of your group should be chosen to coordinate the evacuation. He or she should assign two others to assist patients to leave the building and designate another member to be sure that there is no open flame in the office and be the last to leave the office. Carry out the evacuation, meet afterword, and account for everyone in your group. Discuss your process and document the steps in the evacuation.

Equipment/Supplies

- Scenario
- Evacuation plan

- Building evacuation route map
- Pen and paper

1. **Procedural Step.** Prepare for the disaster simulation by obtaining the building evacuation plan and floor map, reading the scenario, making a list of group members, assigning group members to be staff or patients, and designating a meeting place.

Principle. An evaluation plan includes all necessary details so that employees of a specific location know how to leave the location safely, know that they are responsible for patients, and can be accounted for after an evacuation.

PROCEDURE 49-2 Participating in a Mock Environmental Exposure Event—cont'd

2. **Procedural Step.** Choose a coordinator from the "staff members" to manage the evacuation scenario.
Principle. A coordinator assigns tasks, works with community services, and generally facilitates any response to an emergency.
3. **Procedural Step.** Begin the simulation, and assume that the office has been notified that the office must be evacuated because a natural gas leak is suspected in the building.
4. **Procedural Step.** The coordinator assigns two staff members to assist patients to leave the building and one staff member to check that there is no open flame and to be the last to leave the office area.
Principle. An open flame can trigger an explosion when natural gas is present. While checking for an open flame in all rooms, the staff member can also make sure that staff and patients have left each room in the office.
5. **Procedural Step.** Leave the building using the primary escape route marked on the building evacuation route map.

Principle. The building evacuation route map identifies a primary and secondary escape route. Unless the primary escape route is blocked, it is assumed to be the fastest and most efficient way to evacuate the building.
6. **Procedural Step.** Meet at the designated meeting area. The coordinator checks the list to be sure that everyone is present and that there have been no injuries.
Principle. As part of a disaster drill, everyone must be accounted for.
7. **Procedural Step.** Discuss the process of the evacuation.
8. **Procedural Step.** Document the evacuation including your role and effectiveness of the group as a whole in carrying out the evacuation.
Principle. Evaluation of the disaster drill identifies system and individual weaknesses that should be strengthened.

What Would You Do? What Would You Not Do?

Case Study 2
One afternoon, the office manager in the medical practice where Beth Ann works receives a telephone call from the building manager stating that the building must be evacuated because there is a smell of gas in the basement of the building. The office manager instructs Beth Ann to escort all the patients in the waiting room to the designated meeting place outside at the rear of the parking lot. There are three adults and two children in the waiting room, all able to walk. The office is on the fourth floor of an office building. When Beth Ann tells the patients that they will have to leave the building, one woman asks, "Can I just go to the rest room first?" ∎

Medical Assistant's Role

The medical assistant is an important team member in developing and implementing the emergency action plan for a health care setting and can also contribute to emergency preparedness in the community. He or she may make recommendations to supplement emergency equipment or facilities in the office, serve on a committee to review or revise the emergency plan, participate actively in all fire drills and disaster drills, and participate in the review of the effectiveness of any drill. In addition, the medical assistant must be prepared to provide emergency first aid or cardiopulmonary resuscitation (CPR), both in the workplace and in the community (see Chapter 35). In an actual disaster,

medical assistants might assist by providing emergency first aid, conducting patient interviews, helping to calm victims, documenting services provided, and performing phlebotomy or other procedures as directed.

COMMUNITY AND NATIONAL DISASTER PLANNING

Several very serious natural and man-made disasters have occurred since the 9/11 attack on the World Trade Centers, including Hurricane Katrina, major earthquakes and tsunamis, and other terrorist attacks and mass shootings. These have increased awareness of the need for all communities to increase preparedness and improve communication among different parts of the emergency response system. Community and state emergency preparedness plans involve coordination of all services including the emergency medical services (EMS) system, fire and police departments, the National Guard, the American Red Cross, and hospitals and other health care facilities (Figure 49-7). As the disaster unfolds, communication may be disrupted owing to electrical outages, damage to cell towers and television towers, and overloading of communication infrastructure. When a serious terror attack or disaster occurs, the governor of the affected state implements the state emergency plan and declares a disaster. If the state's resources are inadequate, the governor petitions the president to declare a major disaster. Federal assistance and resources then become available.

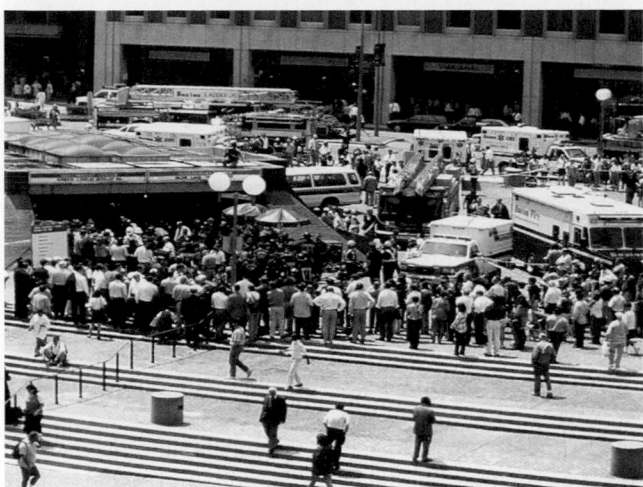

Figure 49-7 When multiple emergency units respond at a scene, it is important for the actions of police, fire, and emergency medical services (EMS) assets to be coordinated.

What Would You Do? What Would You *Not* Do?

Case Study 3

After a tornado that caused serious destruction in a neighboring town, Joanne Williams, a 32-year-old mother of two toddlers, asks Beth Ann how to prepare for a tornado. She tells Beth Ann that she lives in a fairly new house that doesn't have a basement. She says that she can't stop thinking about the images she saw on the television news, and she expresses fear that she might not be able to protect her children if a tornado were to strike her neighborhood. ∎

Community and National Organizations

The Federal Emergency Management Agency (FEMA), an agency of the Department of Homeland Security (DHS), is tasked with coordinating a response to any disaster that overwhelms the resources of state and local authorities. It also provides publications to assist with emergency preparedness planning for businesses and individuals. FEMA maintains 10 regional offices that work closely with the state agencies for emergency management in their region.

Citizen Corps is an agency coordinated by FEMA that coordinates volunteer activities to prevent crime and respond to emergencies. It was created to allow a means of service at the local level after the events of September 11, 2001. Citizen Corps Councils and various partners register with Citizen Corps. Many communities have established community groups of volunteers called Community Emergency Response Terms (CERTs). These groups may be community groups or affiliated in some other way (e.g., college, region). They receive disaster training to function as an extension of first responder services so that they can provide help in a disaster until professional services arrive.

A private agency that has a long history of disaster planning and relief is the American Red Cross. Local chapters provide assistance in disaster planning, and volunteers respond to fires and other emergencies. The Red Cross provides individuals and families a place to stay, food, and mental health services to help them meet their basic needs, recover from the disaster, and resume their normal activities.

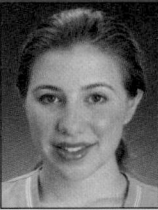

Memories *from* Externship

Beth Ann Wilson: The office where I did my externship was a clinic in a large city hospital. While I was there, I was allowed to attend a hands-on fire training session for hospital employees. We met at a training facility at the fire department where we saw two training films. One of them showed how to test a door for warmth and emphasized that a warm door or a door with smoke leaking around the edge should never be opened. In the film, a fireman did open the door, and we saw how the flames and smoke gushed out when the fire received the new supply of oxygen. Someone asked what you should do if you knew there was a patient in the room behind a warm door. The fireman answered that if possible, you should wait for a firefighter, who would be prepared to handle the flame and smoke. After the films, we were dressed in protective equipment and allowed to discharge fire extinguishers to put out small fires. Even though the fires were small, it was still a scary experience. I hope I never have to deal with a fire, even a small one, but I know that this experience helped to prepare me if it ever happens. ∎

Community Resources

The medical assistant should be aware of community resources for emergency preparedness (Procedure 49-3). The medical office may keep a list of local organizations with telephone numbers or other contact information in the following areas:

Emergency Management Services (911)

Poison Control Center

Telephone numbers of local hospitals

Telephone numbers of local and state health departments

Telephone number for the state HAZMAT response team (**HAZMAT** is an acronym constructed from "*haz*ardous *mat*erials." It refers to materials that pose a danger to health or the environment and require protective clothing for cleanup.)

The medical assistant should also be aware of community disaster plans and community organizations that might assist in a disaster. The website of the state emergency management agency often includes helpful articles related to the disasters that occur most frequently in that state. It is helpful to develop a list of useful resources for the medical office and update it regularly.

PROCEDURE 49-3 Maintaining a List of Community Resources for Emergency Preparedness

Outcome Maintain a list of community resources for emergency preparedness.

Equipment/Supplies

- Local telephone book
- Computer and Internet
- Telephone
- Pen and paper

1. **Procedural Step.** Prepare a list of community agencies for emergency response including EMS (911), the Poison Control Center, telephone numbers of local hospitals, telephone numbers of local and state health departments, and the telephone number for the state HAZMAT response team. This list should be posted by every telephone in a medical office.
   Principle. In an emergency situation, easy access to emergency telephone numbers saves time.
2. **Procedural Step.** Research and create a more detailed list of agencies to respond to a widespread disaster or emergency affecting the community. Locate telephone numbers and Web addresses of the local emergency management agency (LEMA) office, the local chapter of the American Red Cross, and any Citizen Corps council or Community Emergency Response Team (CERT) in your community. The list may be created using pen and paper, but it should be transferred to a word processing file for ease of duplication.
3. **Procedural Step.** Once the document file has been substantially completed, group resources by subject and/or age group served. Alphabetize resources within each group.
   Principle. Arranging lists in alphabetic order facilitates finding specific information and avoids any impression of favoritism or recommending one agency more than another.
4. **Procedural Step.** When the list is complete, save and print copies as needed.
5. **Procedural Step.** Update the list when information changes, when a new resource is identified, and on a periodic basis to be sure information is accurate.

MEDICAL PRACTICE and the LAW

A class-action lawsuit was filed against Tenet Healthcare Corporation and a subsidiary after Hurricane Katrina in 2011, claiming that deaths and injuries of several patients resulted from insufficiencies in Memorial Medical Center's backup electrical system and failed plans for patient care and evacuation. This lawsuit, brought on behalf of patients and visitors who were at the hospital during the hurricane, was eventually settled for $25 million. The problems experienced in New Orleans after Katrina stimulated nationwide reevaluation of institutional and community disaster plans. As this lawsuit demonstrates, medical facilities share in the responsibility to institute systematic policies and procedures to prepare as completely as possible for catastrophic conditions. ■

What Would You Do? What Would You *Not* Do? RESPONSES

Case Study 1
Page 1149

What Did Beth Ann Do?
- ❑ Told Mrs. Manning to stop and breathe and encouraged her to take several deep breaths.
- ❑ Recognized that Mrs. Manning was showing signs of severe anxiety, which would make it difficult for her to focus on driving safely.
- ❑ Said to Mrs. Manning that she seemed very upset by the news, reassured her that the fire department would respond promptly, and encouraged Mrs. Manning to sit down and relax for a minute until she collected herself.
- ❑ Asked Mrs. Manning if there was a family member or friend she could call to pick her up and drive her to her son's school.
- ❑ Listened attentively to Mrs. Manning's concerns.

What Did Beth Ann Not Do?
- ❑ Did not allow Mrs. Manning to leave and drive an automobile while in a state of severe anxiety.
- ❑ Did not tell Mrs. Manning to calm down because she was overreacting.
- ❑ Did not give Mrs. Manning a detailed explanation of the effects of anxiety.

What Would You Do/What Would You Not Do?
Review Beth Ann's response and place a checkmark next to the information you included in your response. List the additional information you included in your response.

_____

_____

_____

_____

_____

_____

Case Study 2
Page 1152

What Did Beth Ann Do?
- ❑ Spoke calmly but with authority when she requested that everyone in the waiting room come with her because it was necessary to evacuate the building.

What Would You Do? What Would You *Not* Do? RESPONSES—cont'd

❑ Instructed the woman who asked to use the rest room that she would have to wait because it was important to evacuate as quickly as possible.

❑ Allowed the patients to pick up their coats and personal items, but instructed them not to take time to put on coats or jackets.

❑ Looked at the posted sign containing evacuation routes, and led the patients along the nearest evacuation route using the stairs to reach the nearest emergency exit. Explained that this would leave the elevators available to any emergency personnel.

❑ Led the group to the designated meeting place and kept them there until all other staff arrived and everyone was accounted for.

What Did Beth Ann Not Do?

❑ Did not speak too quickly or in a high-pitched voice to avoid appearing upset. Did not guess about which evacuation route to use.

❑ Did not allow patients to spend unnecessary time making telephone calls, putting on coats or other clothing, or using the rest room.

❑ Did not allow patients to leave the parking lot area until everyone from the office had been accounted for.

What Would You Do/What Would You Not Do?

Review Beth Ann's response and place a checkmark next to the information you included in your response. List the additional information you included in your response.

_____
_____
_____
_____
_____

Case Study 3
Page 1153

What Did Beth Ann Do?

❑ Helped Mrs. Williams to find information about preparation for tornados.

❑ Asked questions to let Mrs. Williams express her fears and assess Mrs. Williams' anxiety level.

❑ Offered to ask the physician to recommend a counselor for Mrs. Williams to explore her feelings further.

❑ Reminded Mrs. Williams that serious disasters do happen, but they are not regular occurrences.

What Did Beth Ann Not Do?

❑ Did not say or imply that Mrs. Williams was overreacting or worrying for no reason.

❑ Did not push Mrs. Williams to accept her suggestions, but rather just offered information.

❑ Did not promise that the physician would make specific referrals.

What Would You Do/What Would You Not Do?

Review Beth Ann's response and place a checkmark next to the information you included in your response. List the additional information you included in your response.

_____
_____
_____
_____
_____
_____
_____

TERMINOLOGY REVIEW

Medical Term	Word Parts	Definition
Anxiety		A feeling of worry or uneasiness, often triggered by an event with an uncertain outcome.
Evacuation plan		A plan that includes escape routes for all locations in a building or other facility. Diagrams of these routes are posted in multiple locations.
Fire extinguisher		A portable device that discharges foam or another material to extinguish a fire.
HAZMAT		A word constructed from the beginnings of the two words "*haz*ardous *mat*erials." A material that poses a danger to health or the environment. It must be handled with protective equipment.
Man-made disaster		Serious damage either directly or indirectly caused by intentional or negligent human actions or the failure of a man-made system (such as some fires, structural collapse, or terrorism).
Natural disaster		Serious damage to the environment resulting from a natural hazard (such as volcanoes, earthquakes, or hurricanes) that leads to environmental, financial, and human losses.
Posttraumatic stress disorder (PTSD)		A psychiatric condition that develops months or years after a traumatic, catastrophic life experience.
Stress		The body's response to threat or change.

ON THE WEB

For Information on fire safety:

OSHA Fire Safety: www.osha.gov/SLTC/firesafety

U.S. Fire Administration: www.usfa.dhs.gov

For information on evacuation plans:

OSHA Evacuation Plans and Procedures: www.osha.gov/SLTC/etools/evacuation/eap.html

For information on emergency and disaster planning:

American Red Cross: www.americanredcross.org

CDC Emergency Preparedness: www.bt.cdc.gov/preparedness

Citizen Corps: www.citizencorps.gov

FEMA (Federal Emergency Management Agency): www.ready.gov

    Business emergency response plan: www.ready.gov/business/implementation/emergency

    Disaster help and resources: www.disasterassistance.gov

    State agencies: www.fema.gov/about/contact/statedr.shtm

Locate local emergency preparedness programs: www.citizencorps.gov/cc/searchCouncil.do?submitByZip

 Check out the Evolve site at http://evolve.elsevier.com/Bonewit/today/ to actively Prepare for your Certification, and to access additional interactive activities and exercises to help you study and prepare for success.

50

Obtaining Employment

INTRODUCTION TO OBTAINING EMPLOYMENT

After graduating from a medical assisting program, most medical assistants must begin the search for their first job. Sometimes the medical office where the graduate did a practicum (externship) asks the student to stay on as an employee. When this happens, it eases the transition from student to employed medical assistant. Because a student cannot count on this, it is important for the new graduate to see the process of learning how to seek employment as just another skill that must be mastered.

Finding a job involves more than simply answering a few newspaper advertisements or responding to one or two help-wanted notices on the school's career bulletin board. To find the right job, a medical assisting graduate needs to put time and effort into the job-hunting process.

SUCCESSFUL JOB SEARCH

Successful job hunting has two parts. The first is setting appropriate goals; the second is identifying potential employers where those goals might be met.

Setting Goals

Setting goals means identifying the ideal job for a medical assistant's current circumstances. The medical assistant should ask herself or himself the following questions:

- Do I want to work full-time or part-time?
- In what area of the country or region do I want to work?
- Do I want to work in a city? In the suburbs? In the country?
- What are my particular strengths and weaknesses?
- Am I interested in working in a particular medical specialty?
- Do I have a preference about the size of the organization where I would be happy?
- Do I want to specialize in either clinical or administrative duties, or do I want to do both?

Identifying Potential Employers

After a graduate has set goals, it is time to begin identifying potential employers. This is done by viewing online want ads and scanning newspaper ads to see what kinds of positions are being advertised and searching online or looking through the Yellow Pages to see what kinds of practices are in the community where the graduate wants to work. It is important to read carefully, because a graduate may be eligible for positions with different job titles. Many large organizations post job openings internally first. The graduate should ask family or friends who work in such institutions to keep an eye on the internal posting boards.

Larger institutions also often have personnel or human resource departments that keep files of potential employees to give to physicians or department administrators who need to fill a position. When an applicant fills out an application for such a facility, the application will stay on file for a period of time—usually 6 months or 1 year. After that, a new, updated application must be submitted.

During the job-hunting period, it is important to set aside some time each day to look for a job. The more opportunities a graduate explores, the better the possibility of not only finding a job but also finding the right job.

When looking for a job, it is important not to underestimate the importance of **networking,** contacting friends and acquaintances who may know of potential jobs. A personal network may include former instructors, contacts made during the medical assisting practicum, classmates, and even physicians the medical assistant knows or has worked with. It is important to develop a habit of maintaining professional contacts. Staying in touch, either through occasional telephone calls, e-mails, or meeting for coffee or lunch, provides opportunities to gain both support and information. A contact may call in the future when there is an opening at work or someone has asked for names of potential employees.

Potential employers may use the Internet to do research about job applicants, so when the job search begins, a graduate should use a Web browser and enter his or her own name, looking for both websites and images. Potential employers may look at public information on Facebook, Twitter, other social media sites, and blogs. The graduate should be sure that nothing appears that would prevent an employer from granting an interview. For example, a picture showing the graduate at a party, a comment criticizing the school the graduate attended, or even family photographs can create a negative impression. In addition, employers sometimes do credit checks, so it is recommended to review a personal credit history early in the job-hunting process and take steps to correct any errors.

TOOLS FOR A JOB SEARCH

Preparing a Résumé

The primary purpose of a résumé is to obtain an interview for an open position. A **résumé** is a summary of information about a person that describes education, work experience, and other information that employers may find pertinent in deciding whether or not to hire an individual.

A résumé is often important in making a first impression on a potential employer. It must be neat, professional, and informative. A paper résumé looks better if it is printed on high-quality paper. Employers, who often receive several résumés for one position, use the résumé to create a list of people with the desired training and/or experience to call in for personal interviews.

A résumé should describe a medical assistant's education, experience, and skills completely, but not in an exaggerated way. If possible, the résumé should be limited to one typewritten sheet. If the résumé is more than one page, the information that is especially pertinent to the job the medical assistant is applying for should appear on the first page. If a medical assistant is applying for many different types of positions, it may be desirable to have many variations of a résumé available, each one slanted toward the requirements of certain positions.

Personal information should not be included on a résumé. Information such as marital status, children, and hobbies does not relate to a medical assistant's credentials for a position. If personal information is included, the effect is most likely to be neutral or possibly negative, providing a reason not to grant an interview. For example, the employer may be afraid that a medical assistant with two or more children may need to be absent if the children become ill.

Résumé Styles

In general, there are three styles of résumés: chronologic, functional, and targeted.

A chronologic résumé contains a list of formal education, with degrees and certificates earned, followed by work experience (although work experience can come before education in this style). This is the most common type of résumé for applicants with limited work experience, or those who are seeking work similar to their present work.

A functional résumé categorizes experience according to skills or abilities, some of which may be a result of activities other than paid employment (e.g., volunteer work, unpaid work). A functional résumé is useful for an individual who wants to change from one type of work to a different type of work and wants to highlight how particular skills attained in one line of work can be helpful in the new position for which he or she is applying.

A targeted résumé organizes information about an individual who has targeted a particular job opportunity in such a way as to highlight the skills and work experiences being called for in the new employment. This type of résumé often begins with an employment objective that identifies the type of position the individual is seeking.

Information to Include

The basic pieces of information needed for a résumé are personal demographics, objective, education, experience, skills, credentials, and references. A number of computer programs are available for preparing résumés. If a computer program is used, the medical assistant should be sure to personalize the résumé. It is also helpful to use some sample résumés as guides (Figures 50-1, 50-2, and 50-3). Other samples may be available from the placement office of the graduate's college or medical assisting program, as well as résumé-writing books and websites.

Personal Demographics

Personal demographics include the name, address, telephone number, and e-mail address. This information is usually placed at the top of the résumé. The e-mail address should sound professional. If a graduate has been using an email address like "partyanimal@server.com" or if his or her personal e-mail has a link to Twitter or Facebook, he or she

should think about creating a new email account for the job search. The message on the cell phone and home phone should sound professional, without a child's voice or pet name. All identifying information should be large enough and in bold enough type to stand out.

Objective

The objective is a statement of the type of position the medical assistant is looking for. A medical assistant just graduating may be—even should be—flexible about the type of position being sought. If the objective is to obtain an entry-level position as a medical assistant, there may be better ways to use the limited space on a single-sheet résumé than stating this as an objective. This becomes a matter of personal preference.

A medical assistant with a more focused goal may wish to use a statement such as "To obtain a clinical medical assisting position in an office specializing in family practice or internal medicine." A specific objective reassures the potential employer that the candidate is interested in the position he or she is trying to fill, but it can limit the positions for which the candidate will be considered.

Education

The education section includes the institutions attended and degrees or certificates received. These should be arranged in chronologic order with the most recent first. At least one program should be listed with a degree, certificate, or diploma and the year it was received. Usually the high school diploma is included only if the candidate has no higher credential.

When identifying a school or program, the anticipated graduation date can be included if the résumé is prepared before the medical assistant graduates (e.g., A.S. in Medical Assisting, anticipated June 20XX). After graduation, the résumé should be revised before it is sent to other potential employers.

It is also appropriate to include the grade-point average (GPA) if it is above 3.0 and any honors or awards received from the educational institution, such as Dean's List.

Previous Experience

In the section on previous experience the following are included:

- The job title
- Years of employment
- Employer's name
- The town and state in which the work was performed

A new graduate may wish to present information about previous experience in two sections, titled *Related Experience* and *Other Experience.* The medical assisting practicum (externship) can be included under the heading *Related Experience,* but if the section is titled *Work Experience,* only paid employment should be included. Most employers do not like to see gaps in a work history, which might reflect jobs that the applicant does not wish to acknowledge. If the applicant has been a homemaker, it is recommended to

---

Susan Anderson
2314 May Avenue
Western, OH 44770
(490)111-1555
S.Anderson@anyserver.com

OBJECTIVE

To obtain an entry level position as a clinical medical assistant.

EDUCATION/CERTIFICATION

Associate in Science, Western Community College, Western, OH   June 2011

Major: Medical Assisting

GPA: 3.5

RELATED EXPERIENCE

Medical Assisting Externship (160 hours), Western Medical Associates,   2011
Western, OH

- Prepared patients for examination, took vital signs, patient history and chief complaint
- Performed diagnostic tests including throat cultures, rapid strep test, ECG's, dipstick urinalysis
- Answered telephones, filed, scheduled appointments and validated insurance coverage
- Entered patient information, patient charges and payments and insurance payments in the computer

Home Health Aide, Medical Home Care, Newtown, OH   2008-2011

OTHER EXPERIENCE

Cashier, Western Supermarket, Western, OH   2007

SPECIAL SKILLS

- Fluent in Spanish
- Keyboarding 45 wpm
- Microsoft Office, MediSoft, Practice Partner EMR

CERTIFICATIONS

Certified Medical Assistant: August 2011

BLS Healthcare Provider Level and First Aid April 2011

Figure 50-1 Chronologic résumé of a recent graduate.

include the years devoted to this under *Other Experience.* Any volunteer work can also be included.

For each position or type of experience, a short summary of responsibilities should be included. If the experience was in health care or medical assisting, more details should be included than for other jobs or experience. For example, more details should be included about specific responsibilities as a home health aide than as a cashier. Action verbs should be used in the description of previous experience (Figure 50-4). Any special achievements or projects should be included (e.g., setting up an electronic tickler file in a previous job as a secretary).

When preparing the descriptions of previous experience, the medical assistant should use one of two styles consistently. Either can be written in sentence form or as a list with bullets.

Describing Responsibilities Using Verbs in the Past Tense

Example in Sentence Form. Measured vital signs, prepared patients for examination, posted charges and payments, sent monthly bills, etc.

Example in Bullet Form

- Measured vital signs
- Prepared patients for examination
- Posted charges and payments
- Sent monthly bills

Describing Responsibilities Using Participle Form of the Verb

Example in Sentence Form. Responsible for measuring vital signs, preparing patients for examination, posting charges and payments, sending monthly bills.

Example in Bullet Form. Duties included:

Patricia A. Saychelles

26 Gillian Street
Western OH 44770
(490) 111-2728
saychelles@anyserver.com

OBJECTIVE

To obtain a challenging position as a medical assistant that will utilize my skills and training

EDUCATION

Certificate in Medical Assisting, Shamrock Institute, Western, OH   May 2011

SKILLS

- Developed clinical and medical assisting skills during classes and medical assisting externship at Western Medical Associates.
- Able to use computer programs including Microsoft Word, Microsoft Excel, MediSoft v. 16, Practice Partner EMR
- Managed, implemented and coordinated multiple activities and schedules for family members
- Able to plan events for large and small groups

COMMUNITY ACTIVITIES

- Chairperson of public library committee responsible for obtaining feedback from local community
- Volunteer for the DARE program at Western Middle School
- Secretary of the Western Women's League 2007-2009 responsible for secretarial duties, keeping the financial records and fund raising

CERTIFICATIONS

Registered Medical Assistant: August 2011
BLS Healthcare Provider Level and First Aid April 2011

EMPLOYMENT

Package Sorter United Parcel Service, Western, OH   2002-2003

Figure 50-2 Functional résumé of a woman who stayed home with children for several years before training as a medical assistant.

- Measuring vital signs
- Preparing patients for examination
- Posting charges and payments
- Sending monthly bills

Special Skills

The special skills section describes skills learned in an education program that may not be reflected in any direct experience, or that are usually not included in a medical assisting program. These may include computer skills with particular programs, ability to perform specific diagnostic tests, or knowledge of or fluency in a language other than English.

Activities and Other Credentials

In the section on activities and other credentials, the medical assistant may include certification as a CMA (AAMA) or RMA, memberships in professional organizations such as the American Association of Medical Assistants (AAMA) or the American Medical Technologists (AMT), and any other certifications or credentials including cardiopulmonary resuscitation (CPR) and/or first aid. Membership in community service organizations or disaster relief efforts may be included as well. Lists of unrelated activities, hobbies, and interests should not be included on a professional résumé.

References

Traditional résumés always included the following statement: References will be furnished on request. This statement is considered optional on a modern résumé because it is assumed to be the case. Actual references are not listed on the résumé because the goal is to be interviewed before the potential employer checks any references. After the interview, the medical assistant provides a list of references with contact information. Before using someone's name as

John Davidson
16 Carriage Way
Western, OH 44770
(490) 111-3235
airman@anyserver.com

OBJECTIVE

To obtain a position as a medical assistant or administrator in an emergency care setting with both clinical and management responsibilities.

SUMMARY

More than ten years of providing professional military and civilian health care, specializing in emergency treatment, supervision of personnel, physical examination, and health awareness training.

- Received qualifications from the U. S. Navy as Medical Assistant (MA), Nursing Assistant (NA), Emergency Medical Technician (EMT), Emergency Vehicle Operator (EVO) and Emergency Medical Dispatcher (EMD)
- Able to assist with and supervise personnel assisting with occupational, preventative, and emergent medical examinations, ECG's, and emergency procedures
- Able to facilitate hospital admission and maintain medical records
- Provided instruction in personal hygiene, preventative care and sanitary conditions

EMPLOYMENT

United States Navy

- *Hospital Corpsman First Class*, Naval Air Station, Harbor Bay, OH   2004-2011
- *Hospital Corpsman Second Class*, Naval Air Station, Seal Beach, CA   1999-2004

OTHER CREDENTIALS

Instructor: Emergency Medical Technician (EMT-B)

Instructor: American Heart Association BLS

Advanced Life Support (ACLS) provider

EDUCATION

Attended Western Community College from 1998-1999 taking general education courses and introductory health courses.

Figure 50-3 Targeted résumé of a man who received health care training in the Armed Services.

administer	distribute	process
analyze	document	proofread
arrange	establish	propose
assist	file	purchase
authorize	instruct	reconcile
balance	list	run
calculate	log	schedule
classify	mail	send
code	measure	set up
collect	monitor	sort
compose	order	stock
contact	organize	teach
coordinate	perform	write
copy	post	
develop	prepare	

Figure 50-4 Action verbs to use on a résumé.

a reference, the medical assistant should be sure to get that person's permission. It is also polite to call individuals whose names have been used so that they can be ready to receive a phone call or written request for a reference.

For references, a medical assistant who has recently graduated should choose a balance of instructors, practicum supervisor, other job supervisors, or co-workers from volunteer activities. It is not recommended to use friends or family for references. Sometimes the individual who will be used as a reference gives the medical assistant a letter that can be shown to a potential employer. More often, the potential employer contacts the individual given as a reference after interviewing the candidate.

Formatting the Résumé

The résumé should be formatted with at least 1-inch margins. It is important to lay out the résumé so that it looks balanced on the page with clear sections of information. After the résumé has been created, it should be proofread carefully. Spelling and grammar errors are unacceptable. A single spelling or grammar error may prevent a potential employer from offering an interview.

Often, the résumé is sent as an e-mail attachment or attached to an online job application. If the résumé will be sent through the mail, it should be a printed original, not a photocopy. It makes a good impression if a stationery-weight paper is used, which is slightly heavier than ordinary printer paper. Because medical assistants work in a fairly conservative segment of the job market, it is important to avoid using colored paper, unusual type fonts, or flashy formatting for the résumé.

Writing a Cover Letter

A **cover letter** is a letter sent with a résumé that explains briefly why the résumé is being sent. The cover letter clarifies whether the medical assistant is responding to an advertisement, has been referred by another individual, or is simply inquiring about possible job opportunities.

If sent through the mail, the cover letter should use the format for a business letter and should be printed on the same color paper as the résumé. If possible, the medical assistant should call the office to find out the name of the office manager or other individual responsible for hiring

medical assistants. If sent online with a résumé, the letter should be addressed to the human resources department.

The letter should begin with the reason for writing the letter and sending the résumé. This should be followed by a brief summary of the position being sought and the candidate's qualifications for filling that position. The final paragraph should be a request for an interview.

Each cover letter should be personalized because this is the first thing the potential employer will see. Of course, it should not contain any grammar or spelling errors. The reader should be referred to the résumé for details (Figure 50-5).

The medical assistant should keep a copy of all cover letters. The results (interview, second interview, job offer) can be written on the copy or on a separate log that keeps track of responses to all letters sent out.

Sending the Résumé

It is recommended to send résumés in 9×11-inch manila envelopes so that they do not need to be folded. If using a standard No. 10 business envelope, its color and weight should match the paper used for the résumé and cover letter if possible.

Increasingly, it is possible to respond to job openings using the Internet or to fax a résumé to an office. A cover letter is still recommended.

2314 May Avenue
Western, OH 44770
September 5, 20XX

Diane Wells, Practice Manager
Medical Practice Associates
525 Main Street
Western, OH 44770

Dear Ms. Wells:

I am sending you a copy of my resumé in response to your advertisement for a medical assistant in the Western Daily Item. As you will be able to see, I have recently completed an Associate's degree in Medical Assisting at Western Community College.

As part of our training, I was placed in an externship for 160 hours, and I was able to practice the skills that I learned in my training program. I have also passed the national certification exam in medical assisting given by the American Association of Medical Assistants.

I hope you will contact me at (490) 111-1555 to schedule an interview for this position. I am looking forward to hearing from you.

Sincerely,

Susan Anderson, CMA (AAMA)

Figure 50-5 Sample cover letter.

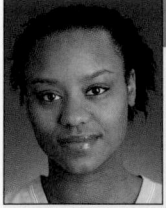
The advantage of a faxed or e-mailed résumé and cover letter is that the material arrives quickly, often within minutes of making a telephone inquiry. The disadvantage is that a fax or a printout of an e-mail does not look as crisp or professional as a mailed résumé and cover letter.

A few days after a mailed résumé should have arrived, a job applicant may call to see if the material did, indeed, arrive. At this time it is appropriate to ask if the person doing the hiring has an idea about the time frame in which a hiring decision will be made. However, a job applicant should not call again after that, to avoid appearing too aggressive.

Filling out an Employment Application

Most medical facilities require a completed job application in addition to a résumé. In large facilities, it may be necessary to complete the application before an interview is scheduled. In smaller offices, the application may be filled out at the time of the interview.

It is important to keep a list of information needed to fill out the job application. This includes the name and address of previous employers, dates of employment, names and telephone numbers of supervisors, as well as the names, addresses, and telephone numbers of references. Any letters of reference should be brought to the interview

so that the facility can make copies to attach them to the job application.

The medical assistant should answer all questions fully and truthfully on the application. If filling the application out by hand, the medical assistant should print legibly. All questions should be answered. It is not appropriate to refer the reader to the résumé. If a question does not apply, the medical assistant should write N/A or Not Applicable.

If the application asks for the reason for leaving a previous position, the medical assistant should avoid making any negative statements about the employer or supervisor. Common reasons for leaving are returning to school, relocation for a spouse's job, end of a temporary position, or exploration of new career options.

Some health care facilities may require applicants for medical assisting positions to take a keyboarding test or other skills test before an interview is granted.

Applying for Employment Using the Internet

The medical assistant may use an online employment website (e.g., Monster.com) to create a résumé, use that résumé to apply for open positions, and also post the résumé on the Web for potential employers to view it. The résumé that is created can be saved as a document file and used to apply for other positions. Many employers also advertise for medical assistants and accept applications using their own websites. When looking for employment, the medical assistant should visit the websites of potential employers, review job postings, and submit an application online if a suitable position is open. By networking with other students, instructors, and friends, the medical assistant can identify online resources that others have used successfully.

GETTING THE JOB

Interview Techniques

An employment interview provides a potential employer with an opportunity to assess a candidate's interpersonal and communication skills and preparation for a position in the medical setting. The interview also provides the medical assistant with a chance to assess the potential employer. The questions asked, the flow of the discussion, and the tour of the facility help the medical assistant decide whether the position fits appropriately with his or her work style and personality.

In order for a job to be offered, the medical assistant must do well in the interview. Often a candidate whose skills appear excellent on paper does not create a positive impression during the interview. The key for the employer is to find the person who seems to be the best fit for the position.

It is important for a medical assistant to accept any job interview offered, even if the position does not seem ideal. The more interviews a new graduate goes on, the more comfortable the job interview process becomes. It is not appropriate, however, to accept more job interviews after a position has been accepted.

Preparing for the Interview

Before the interview, the medical assistant should try to find out as much as possible about the practice or facility. Information can be obtained by talking to someone who works there or a patient of the office, if possible. The medical assistant should ask friends and other contacts if they know anyone with information about the potential employer.

Many medical offices have a website that describes the practice. The medical assistant should enter the name of the practice and/or physician(s) into a search engine. If the practice has a website, it will probably include the names of the physicians and other practitioners, the philosophy of the practice, and other background information. If the office is small, it may only be possible to locate telephone and address information. This may indicate that the office is not using as much modern technology as some other offices.

When the interview is arranged, the medical assistant should find out whether one person or a committee will conduct the interview, and if one person, the name and position of the individual.

The medical assistant should ask if there are any particular things that the interviewer(s) would like to know and if any background materials should be brought to the interview.

Appearance and Behavior

As always, a professional appearance is important. A female medical assistant should wear tailored, professional-looking clothing, such as a suit or blouse and skirt or dress slacks. Denim skirts, denim jeans, shorts, and mid-calf pants are not appropriate for an interview. Long hair should be worn pulled back and off the collar, as it would be when working as a medical assistant. It is recommended to avoid bulky jewelry, avoid false nails and visible piercings, and present a tailored appearance (Figure 50-6). For an interview the medical assistant should avoid sandals or athletic shoes and never wear flip-flops. A male medical assistant should wear a suit or dress slacks and sports coat or blazer, with a dress shirt and tie. Hair, including any facial hair, should be clean and neatly trimmed.

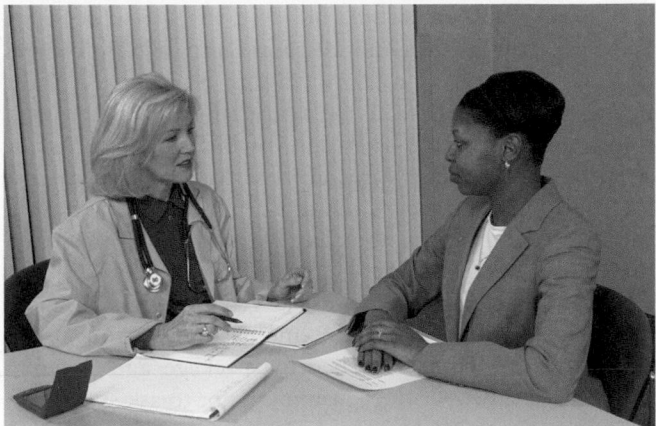

Figure 50-6 At a job interview, the medical assistant should look and act in a professional manner.

It is important to maintain good posture and look alert during the interview. The medical assistant should sit comfortably without slouching and avoid fidgeting or displaying nervous habits. At the same time, the medical assistant presents a better impression if he or she is relaxed and natural instead of reserved and stiff. The interviewer is looking for an individual who interacts well with patients and can make them feel at ease. If a job applicant smiles and makes conversation easily during an interview, it is likely that he or she will be comfortable with patients. A job applicant should never chew gum during an interview. Before the interview, the applicant should turn off his or her cell phone. It is useful to have a pen and notepad handy in order to make notes. It is also helpful to write down questions that might be encountered in future interviews, in order to practice answers before the next interview.

Questions That the Interviewer Should Not Ask

Interviewers are not supposed to ask questions that do not relate to the position, including marital status, number of children, and age (unless there is a legal age requirement as part of the job). If the interviewer asks a question about any of these things, the medical assistant should try to identify or respond to the underlying concern without directly refusing to answer the question.

Interviewer: "How many children do you have?"

Applicant: "Are you concerned about my ability to be dependable?"

What Would You Do? What Would You *Not* Do?

Case Study 2

When she was looking for a job, Deanna got lost on the way to an interview. The office was located about 30 minutes from her home. Deanna had allowed plenty of travel time, but she took the wrong turn off the highway and didn't realize it until she had gone almost 10 miles in the wrong direction. When she realized she was lost, she knew that backtracking would make her at least 15 minutes late. ■

Discussing Salary and Benefits

Specific salary is usually not discussed until a job is offered. But it is common for a salary range to be discussed. If the interviewer does not state the salary range, it is acceptable to ask about it as the interview is winding down. Asking about the salary range early in the interview may give the impression that money is the most important thing about the job. Failing to ask about a salary range may be interpreted as lack of interest.

It is also appropriate to ask a general question about benefits, such as how long an employee must work before becoming eligible for the benefits package and if health insurance is a benefit. It is customary not to ask specifically about vacation, sick days, and personal days until a job offer has been made.

When a position is offered, a discussion of salary and benefits helps the medical assistant make a decision about whether or not to accept the position. If the salary seems low or is less than the medical assistant currently earns, it is appropriate to ask about the specific time frame when performance will be reviewed and a raise will be possible.

Often, especially in larger facilities with rigid salary structures, a position is limited to a particular salary range. It is important to be sure that the salary is adequate to meet expenses before accepting the position. Usually an applicant can ask for 24 to 48 hours to consider a job offer.

Asking Questions

A good interviewer will ask a candidate at the end of the interview if he or she has any questions. The medical assistant may ask about who supervises the position, may ask the interviewer to clarify the job responsibilities, and/or may ask about the availability of training programs in-house or financial support for outside training or college courses. It is helpful to come to the interview with three or four written questions. If these were answered during the interview, the medical assistant can look over the list and say that it seems as though all his or her questions have been answered.

Determining the Timeline for Filling the Position

If the interviewer or lead interviewer in a committee does not state the employer's time frame for making a decision about filling the position, this is an important question to ask. Employers know that people must seek employment at many facilities, and most are willing to get back to applicants who have been interviewed within a few days.

Follow-up after an Interview

Although it may seem old-fashioned to write a written thank-you note after a job interview, most potential employers will be favorably impressed by this courtesy. It also provides an opportunity to include any additional information requested at the interview. See Figure 50-7 for a sample follow-up letter.

If the interviewer has not responded by the date expected, the medical assistant may telephone to ask if the position has been filled.

Highlight on Responding to Questions

Based on previous experience at interviews and suggestions from friends about their experiences, the medical assistant should try to prepare for questions the interviewer(s) will ask. Although it may seem awkward, it is helpful to practice answering sample interview questions out loud with friends, family, or a roommate. Several common interview questions and potential answers are presented in the following discussion.

1. What can I tell you about my organization?

   It is always important to have questions prepared. The medical assistant might ask about the history of the office or clinic and/or how long it has been in its present location. He or she should have found out how many physicians work there and what specialties are represented, but could ask how many medical assistants are employed.

2. What was your favorite subject in school?

   The answer is more powerful if it demonstrates enthusiasm and has some relation to the position being applied for. Math, English, science, computer courses, and medical assisting courses are good answers. If a job applicant says that poetry was her favorite subject, the interviewer may wonder if medical assisting is the applicant's real interest.

3. Why did you choose to study medical assisting?

People who choose this field are usually interested in health, like people, like a job where they can be active, and believe that preventive care and early diagnosis are important components of health. This question also gives the medical assistant an opportunity to demonstrate enthusiasm and caring.

4. What courses did you like least in school?

   It is better for the medical assistant to name one course and describe it as "difficult" or "challenging" (even if that does not directly respond to the question) instead of giving a long list of subjects that were boring. It is important to avoid looking like an individual who is uninterested in subjects that may relate to the job and also to avoid complaining or speaking negatively.

5. What campus activities did you participate in? What did you learn from them?

   The medical assistant can prepare by thinking of an interesting extracurricular activity he or she has participated in, even if there was not time to be a member of any club or organized activity in school. If the medical assistant worked for several hours while going to school, he or she might say so while identifying a hobby: "I worked as a cashier several hours a week in order to help pay for school, so I had to

Highlight on Responding to Questions—cont'd

leave school right after class. But I am working with a classmate to arrange for some of our graduates to get together monthly because I think that it would be too bad to lose contact with the friends I made in school."

6. Describe your responsibilities when you worked for XYZ Company.

   The medical assistant should identify his or her responsibilities, being sure to emphasize any special projects, promotions, or leadership roles. A medical assistant often has a part-time job while going to school, with some extra responsibility, such as opening or closing, training new employees, or rotating to different departments. If handling money was a job responsibility, it should be mentioned because it indicates reliability.

7. What types of problems have you encountered in your jobs? How did you handle them?

   The medical assistant should think of an example of a problem that might occur in a medical office, such as an angry or unsatisfied customer, telephones ringing off the hook, work backing up, and being overwhelmed at first. When discussing the problem, it is important to provide a realistic solution and explain how problem solving occurred.

8. What would your instructors or previous supervisors tell me about you if I were to call them?

   The medical assistant should identify his or her positive attributes and practice saying them calmly, even if it seems like bragging. "They would say that I work hard," "I am organized," "I catch on quickly," "I am good with people,"

and "I try hard to be accurate" are some examples. In an effective interview, the job applicant puts his or her best foot forward without exaggerating or distorting the truth.

9. What are some of your weaknesses or areas you need to work on?

   The medical assistant should think carefully about weaknesses that may be seen in some lights as positive, or weaknesses that everyone is subject to. Being a perfectionist, not liking to miss work for illness, and double-checking all work to be sure it is correct are examples of weaknesses that employers usually like. Being nervous in a new situation, becoming frustrated when there isn't enough time, and hating to see others sitting around when there is much work to do are traits common to many people. If a medical assistant is shy and reserved, this is a good opportunity to state that he or she is not always outgoing in new situations, but that it doesn't take very long to feel comfortable and open up more.

10. What are your long-term goals? or Where do you plan to be in 5 years?

   The prospective employer is trying to get a sense of how long the applicant plans to stay in the position if hired. In many areas, turnover of medical assistants is rapid, but an employer would like to be able to count on at least 2 years. If the medical assistant will be returning to school within 6 months, he or she should say so and identify whether part-time work would be possible at that time.

2314 May Avenue
Western, OH 44770
September 18, 20XX

Diane Wells, Practice Manager
Medical Practice Associates
525 Main Street
Western, OH 44770

Dear Ms. Wells:

I wanted to thank you for the opportunity to interview with you last week for the position of medical assistant. It is clear that your practice provides high quality care to patients. After meeting with you, I know that I would be glad for the opportunity to join your team.

I will wait to hear from you in about a week as we discussed. Please feel free to contact me at (490) 111-1555 or by email (S.Anderson@anyserver.com) if you have any questions. Thank you again for your time and consideration.

Sincerely,

Susan Anderson, CMA (AAMA)

Figure 50-7 Sample letter after an interview.

LIFELONG LEARNING

The field of health care is becoming more complex all the time. It is important for every member of the health care team to constantly improve his or her skills and stay up to date on new techniques in his or her field. To provide high-quality patient care, every member of the health care team must engage in lifelong learning.

Staying Current

Medical assistants must keep their skills current. This means keeping abreast of new techniques, as well as learning how to use the latest technology.

Administrative Skills

On the administrative side, computer software is constantly being updated. This includes operating systems and all programs used routinely in the medical office. Training to use updated versions of operating systems, word processing programs, or other general programs is often available online or through classes. If the office switches to an updated version of office management programs or an electronic medical record, the software company often provides training for office personnel.

Another area that requires constant updating relates to changes in coding and insurance claim submission. The medical assistant should read updates and attend classes as needed to keep skills current.

Clinical Skills

On the clinical side, it is important to learn to use new diagnostic or laboratory equipment. When a new piece of equipment is purchased, training should be arranged for all staff who will use it. The medical assistant must also stay current on new medications. Pharmaceutical representatives leave informational materials for the physician, and the medical assistant should make a point of reading this information.

Preparing for Increased Responsibility

The medical assistant may be trained to assist with special procedures. The medical assistant may be sent to an outside training program at office expense, or the physician or other staff member may provide the training. It is important to pay close attention during the training and take notes to be sure that all information is retained.

The medical assistant may also be given some responsibility to supervise other staff members. Classes or workshops in supervision, appraisal, conflict management, or other subjects may be helpful to ease this transition.

Avoiding Burnout

Burnout is a constant worry, especially for those in repetitive, high-stress jobs. **Burnout** is a term that has come to mean disillusionment with work and physical or emotional exhaustion. It is characterized by a loss of interest or enthusiasm and energy about work.

A person experiencing burnout may exhibit behavioral changes as well, including increased irritability, inability to empathize with patients, chronic fatigue, and poor relations with co-workers. Job burnout can be a precipitator for clinical depression and must be dealt with as a medical issue rather than a disciplinary problem.

Loss of enthusiasm at work may also result from factors outside the job. If an individual's life is out of balance, or if the individual is having problems with relationships within the family, he or she may not have the necessary energy to expend at work. This may appear as depression or burnout.

If a medical assistant arrives at the point where job burnout is a concern, it is important to take action. If possible, the medical assistant should reduce the hours of work, even if only for a 3- or 6-month period. Increased social activities, increased exercise, and focusing on physical and mental health can foster a more positive physical and emotional state. The medical assistant should try to find a hobby to help "decompress" from work.

Sometimes burnout is not recognized until the problems have progressed to such a degree that professional intervention is necessary. The individual with severe burnout may need counseling, therapy, or a job change; and if the individual has developed a substance abuse problem, he or she may even need inpatient rehabilitation. Many large facilities have in-house employee counseling.

What Would You Do? What Would You *Not* Do?

Case Study 3

After 6 months at the obstetrics and gynecology office where she was first hired, Deanna began to wish that she had more contact with other medical assistants to discuss job-related issues. The other medical assistants in her office seemed to be busy with their families, and they didn't socialize at all after work. Deanna wished that she knew more about new trends, new medications, and new technology. She had joined the American Association of Medical Assistants when she graduated, but there didn't seem to be an active chapter in her area. ∎

Professional Organizations and Peer Support

The AAMA and the AMT are professional organizations for medical assistants. Even if a medical assistant has not obtained certification, he or she can become a member of an active chapter of one of these organizations. Through local and national meetings and workshops, medical assistants are able to enter a network of peers with whom they can share and from whom they can learn. They can also obtain insurance at reasonable cost, professional journals, and other sources of information important to the profession.

For an annual membership fee, many benefits are available, including the following:

* Peer support
* Continuing education programs

- Legislative advocacy on issues important to medical assistants
- Publications and/or newsletters with information related to the profession of medical assisting

Legislation Affecting Medical Assistants

Professional organizations are able to advocate for pending state and federal legislation that may affect the medical assisting profession. Changes in legislation require actions by many people. In some states, issues for medical assistants arise from actions taken by other professionals to define legally who may perform certain procedures. As a result of such actions, medical assistants may not take radiographs in most states, and they may not be permitted to administer injections or draw blood, depending on the state.

A future task for the medical assisting profession will be to organize and help draft legislation giving medical assistants the right to perform in the workplace all skills for which they have been trained. This can best be accomplished by working with the national professional organizations and their state chapters.

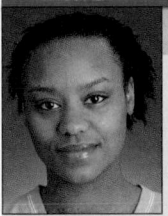

Memories *from* Externship

Deanna Taylor: The biggest difference between externship and employment is that it takes more effort to stay enthusiastic about showing up every day. When I was in the externship, everything was new. I was always excited to go because it seemed like there was a new experience every day. Now that I have been working for a few years, there are many days that seem very routine. There are new experiences, but I have to remind myself to notice them. One way that I have found to stay fresh and focused is to volunteer to be on committees to gather information or to plan the implementation of new equipment or new software. For example, we purchased three new meters for glucose testing a few months ago, and I volunteered to make a poster showing how to use the meters and to work with each staff member to make sure they were doing controls correctly. I also have been taking a general business course at night for the past month. I notice things at work that I never would have before, and I am now planning to take more courses in health administration or business administration. When I was in school, all I could think of was graduating and getting a job, but now that I am a medical assistant, I realize that my career is just beginning. I realize that I am personally responsible to find a way to keep my career rewarding and satisfying. ∎

Continuing Education Units

A **continuing education unit (CEU)** is a standard measure of qualified instruction as defined by a specific profession. Most health professions require a certain amount of continuing education for licensure or certification renewal. CEUs or contact hours of instruction are required for recertification as a CMA (AAMA) or RMA. The medical

assistant should keep a file with the paperwork acknowledging attendance at classes or workshops, together with the CEU credits or contact hours approved for them. With the constant change in the medical field, it is not merely important but necessary to keep skills up to date, attain new skills, and obtain new information about professional practices.

Medical assisting contact hours and CEUs can be obtained from education programs that have been approved by the particular certifying agency. These education programs may be given through the state and national organization, through other educational institutions, or through home or online study programs.

PLANNING FOR JOB ADVANCEMENT OR CAREER CHANGE

One of the best ways to avoid job burnout is to chart a course of career advancement.

Advancing to Management

If a medical assistant enjoys the administrative part of medical assisting, there are many opportunities to find a management position within the health care industry.

The larger the facility, the more the administrative and management tasks are broken into discrete parts, and the more management and administrative staff are in demand.

If a medical assistant is currently working in such a facility and would like to move up the management ladder, he or she should ask about the possibility of rotating through the various departments to gain experience in finance, billing, marketing, public relations, or any other department. If the medical assistant is working at a small facility or private practice, he or she should take the opportunity to learn about every job within the practice. This makes the medical assistant more versatile and more valuable as an employee. After gaining supervisory experience in a smaller facility, the medical assistant may wish to move to a larger facility.

Business courses or formal education in health administration is invaluable. A number of colleges have both bachelor's and master's degree programs in health care administration. A degree in public administration or business management would also be appropriate.

Upgrading Technical and Clinical Skills

In order to advance to a position of greater responsibility on the clinical side, it will probably be necessary to obtain more formal education. After a few years of experience, a medical assistant who wishes to remain in an outpatient setting might consider enrolling in a formal education program to become a physician's assistant, a registered nurse, a medical technologist, or an x-ray technologist.

The opportunities become broader if a medical assistant wishes to work in a hospital or rehabilitation center. The medical assistant should talk to various health professionals and explore several potential career options. Obtaining financial support for additional education may be a concern. The medical assistant must decide if financial support is available to pursue further education full-time. For most candidates, it will be necessary to continue working either part-time or full-time at their present positions. Many employers encourage education and pay all or part of an employee's education costs.

Transferring Skills

Over time, the medical assistant may have built up skills that would make it possible to find a position in a field such as computers, insurance, the pharmaceutical industry, or medical equipment sales. If a medical assistant develops a strong interest in one of these areas, he or she should develop contacts, gather information, and develop a strategy for making a lateral career move.

This discussion would also not be complete without a word about the enormous rewards that can come from teaching—transferring knowledge and abilities to others who would like to become medical assistants.

With a medical assisting degree or certificate, a certified medical assistant may be able to get some work teaching a specific class related to medical assisting skills. A medical assistant who is interested in teaching should speak to the director of the program where he or she trained about teaching opportunities.

In order to teach full-time, in addition to maintaining certification, the medical assistant should obtain a bachelor's degree and master's degree in a health care field, or in education. Depending on the financial resources available from a spouse or partner's income, family assistance, or scholarships and loans available, this may be as a part-time or full-time student.

MEDICAL PRACTICE and the LAW

Under the federal Equal Opportunity Employment laws, it is illegal for a company to discriminate in hiring practices on the basis of race, sex, religion, national origin, or age. Potential employers may ask questions related to job performance, but they should not ask any questions that might be interpreted as intent to discriminate. Some states also have legislation making it illegal to discriminate on the basis of sexual orientation. Under the Americans with Disabilities Act (ADA), employers must make "reasonable accommodations" to any individual with a physical or mental disability who is otherwise qualified to perform the tasks necessary in the job.

If a medical assistant believes that discrimination has occurred during the process of seeking employment or promotion, he or she should contact the U.S. Equal Employment Opportunity Commission (EEOC). A verbal contact must be made before a complaint can be filed. ■

What Would You Do? What Would You *Not* Do?   RESPONSES

Case Study 1
Page 1164

What Did Deanna Do?
- ❏ Reminded Andrea that employers usually consider work experience to include only paid positions.
- ❏ Pointed out tactfully that putting the practicum in the category of work experience might indicate unreliability or lack of knowledge to a potential employer.
- ❏ Advised Andrea to include the practicum in a section on the résumé called "Related Experience."
- ❏ Offered to look over Andrea's résumé to see if she could make other helpful suggestions.

What Did Deanna Not Do?
- ❏ Did not tell Andrea that she was being dishonest to put the practicum as work experience.
- ❏ Did not make a discouraging remark such as, "That won't help you get hired."

What Would You Do/What Would You Not Do?
Review Deanna's response and place a checkmark next to the information you included in your response. List the additional information you included in your response.

_____
_____
_____
_____
_____

Case Study 2
Page 1165

What Did Deanna Do?
- ❏ Made sure to take the name and telephone number of the person she was going to interview with.
- ❏ When Deanna realized that she was lost, she called the individual with whom she was scheduled to interview, explained

What Would You Do? What Would You *Not* Do? RESPONSES—cont'd

the situation, apologized, and asked if it would be better to come late or reschedule.
- ❏ At the same time Deanna asked for directions.
- ❏ Resolved always to get very clear directions before any other interview.

What Did Deanna Not Do?

- ❏ Did not show up 15 minutes late without making every effort to contact the individual with whom she was supposed to interview.
- ❏ Did not blame any individual for giving bad directions or failing to give directions.
- ❏ Did not act like being 15 minutes late was really not important.

What Would You Do/What Would You Not Do?

Review Deanna's response and place a checkmark next to the information you included in your response. List the additional information you included in your response.

_____
_____
_____
_____

Case Study 3
Page 1168

What Did Deanna Do?

- ❏ Found out where there were chapters of the AAMA in her state and made a point of attending a meeting. She also looked into attending the national meeting of the organization.

- ❏ Asked the practice manager if there were any continuing education programs at the local hospital that she could attend.
- ❏ Contacted graduates from her medical assisting program and arranged to get together with graduates with whom she had been friends when she was in school.
- ❏ Looked into the possibility of establishing a local chapter of the AAMA and tried to find one or two other medical assistants who might be interested in helping her.
- ❏ Looked at course offerings at the local community college to see if there were any courses or continuing education programs that she might be interested in attending.

What Did Deanna Not Do?

- ❏ Did not avoid taking responsibility to meet her own needs.
- ❏ Did not make excuses for putting off the process of seeking helpful contacts.
- ❏ Did not avoid reaching out to other medical assistants.

What Would You Do/What Would You Not Do?

Review Deanna's response and place a checkmark next to the information you included in your response. List the additional information you included in your response.

_____
_____
_____
_____

TERMINOLOGY REVIEW

Medical Term	Word Parts	Definition
Burnout		Disillusionment with work and physical or emotional exhaustion.
Continuing education unit (CEU)		A standard measure of qualified instruction or contact hours as defined by a specific profession.
Cover letter		A letter sent with one or more documents (such as a résumé) to provide an explanation.
Networking		Contacting acquaintances and their contacts who may know of potential jobs.
Résumé		A summary of information about a person that describes education, work experience, and other information related to an individual's suitability for employment.

ON THE WEB

For information about job discrimination:

U.S. Equal Employment Opportunity Commission (EEOC): www.eeoc.gov

For information on professional organizations:

American Association of Medical Assistants: www.aama-ntl.org

American Health Information Management Association: www.ahima.org

American Medical Technologists: http://www.americanmedtech.org/

American Society of Phlebotomy Technicians: www.aspt.org

For information on writing résumés and cover letters:

The OWL at Purdue University: owl.english.purdue.edu/owl/resource/719/01

Résumé Templates—Microsoft Office Online: office.microsoft.com/en-us/templates

Check out the Evolve site at http://evolve.elsevier.com/Bonewit/today/ to actively Prepare for your Certification, and to access additional interactive activities and exercises to help you study and prepare for success.

Glossary

ABA routing number A nine-digit number that identifies a bank; printed at the beginning of the magnetic ink character recognition line at the bottom of a check. It also appears in fractional form at the top right of the check under the check number.

Abandonment Failure to continue to provide medical care to a patient without proper notification.

Abortion The termination of a pregnancy before the fetus reaches the age of viability (20 weeks).

Abrasion A wound in which the outer layers of the skin are damaged; a scrape.

Abscess A collection of pus in a cavity surrounded by inflamed tissue.

Absorbable suture Suture material that is gradually digested and absorbed by the body.

Absorption The passage of digestive end products from the gastrointestinal tract into the blood or lymph.

Accommodation Mechanism that allows the eye to focus at various distances, primarily achieved by changing the curvature of the lens.

Account aging The process of finding out how long specific account balances have been outstanding.

Accounting Systematic recording and reporting of financial transactions.

Accounts payable The outstanding bills of a business, such as a medical office.

Accounts receivable Total amount owed to a business for goods and services.

Accreditation Credit or recognition for maintaining certain standards by a regional or national organization.

Accrual basis of accounting Accounting method in which income is entered at the time of sale or provision of service.

Acronym A word formed from the first letters in a name.

Act A bill or measure that has become law. Often refers to legislation with several parts.

Acting out Translating unconscious emotions into inappropriate behavior.

Action potential A nerve impulse; a rapid change in membrane potential that involves depolarization and repolarization.

Active listening Paying close attention to a speaker without thinking of anything else.

Active record The medical record of a patient who has been seen within a time frame specified by the office (usually 2 to 3 years).

Active transport Process that moves substances across or through a membrane and requires cellular energy.

Adenohypophysis Anterior portion of the pituitary gland; the gland that grows below the brain.

Adjustment A change to a patient account that is neither a charge nor a payment.

Adnexal Adjacent.

Adolescent An individual 12 to 18 years old.

Adventitious sounds Abnormal breath sounds.

Adverse reaction An unintended and undesirable effect produced by a drug.

Advocate A person who intercedes on another person's behalf.

Aerobe A microorganism that needs oxygen to live and grow.

Afebrile Without fever; the body temperature is normal.

Agglutination (as it pertains to blood) Clumping of blood cells.

Allergen A substance that is capable of causing an allergic reaction.

Allergy An abnormal hypersensitivity of the body to substances that are ordinarily harmless.

Alveoli Microscopic dilations of terminal bronchioles in the lungs, where diffusion of gases occurs; air sacs in the lungs.

Alveolus A thin-walled air sac of the lungs in which the exchange of oxygen and carbon dioxide takes place.

Ambulation Walking or moving from one place to another.

Ambulatory Able to walk as opposed to being confined to bed or a wheelchair.

Ambulatory care Medical care that is provided on an outpatient basis. The patient is able to come to the facility providing care and return home after receiving services.

Amenorrhea The absence or cessation of the menstrual period. Amenorrhea occurs normally before puberty, during pregnancy, and after menopause.

Amphiarthrosis A slightly movable joint; plural, *amphiarthroses.*

Amplitude Refers to amount, extent, size, abundance, or fullness.

Ampule A small sealed glass container that holds a single dose of medication.

Anaerobe A microorganism that grows best in the absence of oxygen.

Analyte A substance that is being identified or measured in a laboratory test.

Anaphylactic reaction A serious allergic reaction that requires immediate treatment.

Anatomic position Standard reference position for the body.

Anemia A condition in which there is a decrease in the erythrocytes or amount of hemoglobin in the blood.

Annotate To underline or highlight important words and phrases in correspondence.

Antagonist A muscle that has an action opposite to that of the prime mover.

Antecubital space The space located at the front of the elbow.

Antibody A substance that is capable of combining with an antigen, resulting in an antigen-antibody reaction.

Anticoagulant A substance that inhibits blood clotting.

Antigen A substance capable of stimulating the formation of antibodies.

Antipyretic An agent that reduces fever.

Antiseptic A substance that kills disease-producing microorganisms but not their spores. An antiseptic is usually applied to living tissue.

Anuria Failure of the kidneys to produce urine.

Anxiety A vague, unpleasant emotion of fear or dread often accompanied by restlessness or nervousness.

Aorta The major trunk of the arterial system of the body. The aorta arises from the upper surface of the left ventricle.

Apnea The temporary cessation of breathing.

Application software Software designed to accomplish a specific task (e.g., word processing); also called *application program* and *software program.*

Approximation The process of bringing two parts, such as tissue, together through the use of sutures or other means.

Arbitration A formal process by which the parties to a dispute agree to submit to the decision of a neutral party.

Arrector pili Muscle associated with hair follicles.

Artifact Additional electrical activity picked up by the electrocardiograph that interferes with the normal appearance of the ECG cycles.

Asepsis Free from infection or pathogens; the actions practiced to make and maintain an area or object free from infection or pathogens.

Assets In accounting, a combination of property owned and money owed to a business.

Assignment of benefits Authorization given by the patient to allow the insurance company to make payments directly to the health care provider instead of to the patient.

Assumption of risk A defense to a lawsuit that establishes the plaintiff assumed the risk of whatever caused the injury.

Astigmatism A refractive error that causes distorted and blurred vision for both near and far objects owing to a cornea that is oval.

Atherosclerosis Buildup of fibrous plaques of fatty deposits and cholesterol on the inner walls of an artery that causes narrowing, obstruction, and hardening of the artery.

Atrioventricular valve Valve between an atrium and a ventricle in the heart.

Attending physician The physician responsible for the care of a hospitalized patient.

Atypical Deviation from the normal.

Audiometer An instrument used to measure hearing acuity quantitatively for the various frequencies of sound waves.

Auscultation The process of listening to the sounds produced within the body to detect signs of disease.

Autoclave An apparatus for the sterilization of materials, using steam under pressure.

Autoimmune disease A condition in which the body's immune system produces antibodies that attack the body's own cells. The cause is unknown.

Autonomy Ability to make independent decisions without constraint or coercion from others.

Axilla The armpit.

Bacilli (sing. *bacillus*) Bacteria that have a rod shape.

Back order A term used for items ordered that cannot be shipped immediately, usually because they are out of stock.

Backup A duplicate copy of a program or data kept for reference in case the original is damaged, lost, or destroyed.

Balance due Total amount owed.

Bandage A strip of woven material used to wrap or cover a part of the body.

Bankruptcy Legal process by which the debts of an individual or business are resolved if they cannot be paid.

Barcode clear zone The area on the lower right corner of a card or letter that is left clear for the postal barcode to be printed.

Bariatrics The branch of medicine that deals with the treatment and control of obesity and diseases associated with obesity.

Baseline The flat horizontal line that separates the various waves of the ECG cycle.

Beneficence Acting in the best possible way; performing good deeds.

Beneficiary A person who can receive benefits under an insurance plan.

Benefit Payment for a covered service under a health insurance plan.

Bilirubinuria The presence of bilirubin in the urine.

Bill A law proposed by a legislative body.

Biopsy The surgical removal and examination of tissue from the living body. Biopsies are generally performed to determine whether a tumor is benign or malignant.

Birthday rule If both parents of a child have a family health plan, the insurance plan of the parent whose birthday comes earlier in the year is defined as the primary insurance plan covering the child. The insurance of the other parent becomes secondary insurance.

Bit The smallest unit of computer storage capacity.

Bladder catheterization The passing of a sterile catheter through the urethra and into the bladder to remove urine.

Blocked Term describing times in the appointment schedule when physicians are not available to see patients.

Blood antigen A protein present on the surface of red blood cells that determines a person's blood type.

Body language Communication that is expressed through facial expressions, body position, muscle activity, and other nonverbal means.

Body mechanics Use of the correct muscles to maintain proper balance, posture, and body alignment to accomplish a task safely and efficiently without undue strain on any muscle or joint.

Bookkeeping The process of recording financial transactions and keeping financial records.

Bounding pulse A pulse with an increased volume that feels very strong and full.

Bradycardia An abnormally slow heart rate (less than 60 beats per minute).

Bradypnea An abnormal decrease in the respiratory rate of less than 10 respirations per minute.

Brain stem The portion of the brain, between the diencephalon and spinal cord, that contains the midbrain, pons, and medulla oblongata.

Braxton Hicks contractions Intermittent and irregular painless uterine contractions that occur throughout pregnancy. They occur more frequently toward the end of pregnancy and are sometimes mistaken for true labor pains.

Broadband A method of transmitting electronic data that handles a wide range of frequencies.

Bronchial tree The bronchi and all their branches, which function as passageways between the trachea and the alveoli.

Buffy coat A thin, light-colored layer of white blood cells and platelets that lies between a top layer of plasma and a bottom layer of red blood cells when an anticoagulant has been added to a blood specimen.

Burn An injury to the tissues caused by exposure to thermal, chemical, electrical, or radioactive agents.

Burnout Disillusionment with work and physical or emotional exhaustion.

Byte A unit of computer storage capacity, usually eight bits. One byte is approximately equal to one character.

Calibration A mechanism to check the precision and accuracy of a test system, such as an automated analyzer, to determine if the system is providing accurate results. Calibration is typically performed using a calibration device, often called a *standard*.

Call-in times Blocks of time when a physician accepts telephone calls from patients.

Canthus The junction of the eyelids at either corner of the eye.

Capillary action The action that causes liquid to rise along a wick, a tube, or a gauze dressing.

Capitation A method of paying for insurance in which a fixed amount is paid to the provider per member for a specific time period regardless of the amount of care provided.

Cardiac cycle A complete heartbeat consisting of contraction and relaxation of both atria and both ventricles.

Carrier An insurance company.

Case law Law established by decisions of previous court cases.

Cash basis of accounting Accounting method in which income is entered when payment is received.

Cashier's check A check drawn on a bank instead of an individual account.

Celsius scale A temperature scale on which the freezing point of water is 0° and the boiling point of water is 100°; also called the *centigrade scale*.

Cerebellum Second largest part of the human brain, located posterior to the pons and medulla oblongata and involved in the coordination of muscular movements.

Cerebrum The largest and uppermost part of the human brain; concerned with consciousness, learning, memory, sensations, and voluntary movements.

Certificate of need A regulatory mechanism to ensure that new or expanded health care services will meet the needs of the community.

Certified check A check on an individual account that a bank assumes responsibility for, usually by withdrawing funds to cover the check from the checking account at the time the check is certified.

Cerumen Earwax.

Ceruminous gland A gland in the ear canal that produces cerumen or earwax.

Cervix The lower narrow end of the uterus that opens into the vagina.

CHAMPVA A government health insurance program that covers dependents of military veterans with service-connected disabilities.

Charge slip A form used to keep track of charges and payments at the time of a patient visit.

Charting The process of making written entries about a patient in the medical record.

Chemoreceptor A sensory receptor that detects the presence of chemicals; responsible for taste, smell, and monitoring the concentration of certain chemicals in body fluids.

Chemotherapy The use of chemicals to treat disease. Chemotherapy is most often used to refer to the treatment of cancer using antineoplastic medications.

Chondrocyte Cartilage cell.

Chronic Existing over a long period of time.

Chyme The semifluid mixture of food and gastric juice that leaves the stomach through the pyloric sphincter.

Cilia Slender, hairlike projections that constantly beat toward the outside to remove microorganisms from the body.

Civil law Law that regulates relationships and interactions among individuals and groups.

Claim message Messages encouraging payment of a bill, usually attached to or printed on the monthly statement.

Clinical diagnosis A tentative diagnosis of a patient's condition obtained through evaluation of the health history and the physical examination, without the benefit of laboratory or diagnostic tests.

Clinical messaging Communication among health professionals within the electronic medical record.

Cloning Producing genetically identical cells or individuals artificially.

Closed questions Questions that anticipate a yes/no or short answer.

Clustering Scheduling similar types of patients or examinations on the same day or part of the day.

Coagulation The process of blood clotting.

Cocci (sing. *coccus*) Bacteria that have a round shape.

Coinsurance A percentage of the allowed charge for health services, which the patient is responsible for paying.

Collagenous fibers Strong and flexible connective tissue fibers that contain the protein collagen.

Collate To assemble the pages of a document in numeric order.

Collection agency A firm that is in the business of collecting overdue accounts.

Colonoscope An endoscope that is specially designed for passage through the anus to permit visualization of the rectum and the entire length of the colon.

Colonoscopy The visualization of the rectum and the entire colon using a colonoscope

Colposcope A lighted instrument with a binocular magnifying lens used to examine the vagina and cervix.

Colposcopy Visual examination of the vagina and cervix using a colposcope (a lighted instrument with a magnifying lens).

Common law Unwritten body of law based on general custom.

Comparative negligence A defense to a lawsuit that establishes a percentage of responsibility for injury by the plaintiff.

Complimentary closing Words used as a polite ending to a letter just before the writer's signature.

Compress A soft, moist, absorbent cloth that is folded in several layers and applied to a part of the body in the local application of heat or cold.

Computer An electronic machine that has the ability to process data according to a program in order to produce a desired result.

Computer system All of the hardware and software components making up the computer.

Conduction The transfer of energy, such as heat, from one object to another by direct contact.

Conduction myofibers Cardiac muscle cells specialized for conducting action potentials to the myocardium; part of the conduction system of the heart; also called *Purkinje fibers*.

Consultation report A narrative report of an opinion about a patient's condition by a practitioner other than the attending physician.

Contagious Capable of being transmitted directly or indirectly from one person to another.

Contaminate To soil or to make impure. An aseptic object is contaminated when it touches something that is not clean.

Contingency A condition that must be met before a contract is binding.

Continuing education unit (CEU) A standard unit of measure for continuing education for professionals, defined as 10 contact hours of participation.

Contrast medium A substance used to make a particular structure visible on a radiograph.

Contributory negligence A defense to a lawsuit that establishes any responsibility for injury by the plaintiff.

Control A solution that is used to monitor a test system to ensure the reliability and accuracy of test results.

Controlled drug A drug that has restrictions placed on it by the federal government because of its potential for abuse.

Controlled substance A drug that has the potential for addiction or abuse.

Contusion An injury to the tissues under the skin that causes blood vessels to rupture, allowing blood to seep into the tissues; a bruise.

Convection The transfer of energy, such as heat, through air currents.

Conversion Changing from one system of measurement to another.

Coordination of benefits Rules followed by insurance companies so that no claim is reimbursed at more than 100% of the charges.

Copayment A fixed amount of money that the patient is responsible to pay at each visit.

Cover letter A letter sent with one or more documents (such as a résumé) to provide an explanation.

CPU (central processing unit) The "brain" of the computer housed in the main unit that interprets and executes the instructions that operate the computer. The CPU consists of the control unit and the ALU.

Crash cart A specially equipped cart for holding and transporting medications, equipment, and supplies needed for lifesaving procedures in an emergency.

Credit A posting that is subtracted from an account balance.

Credit balance A negative balance on a patient account (i.e., money is owed by the medical office), usually because of an overpayment.

Crepitus A grating sensation caused by fractured bone fragments rubbing against each other.

Crime An offense in violation of a law that prohibits or requires certain behavior.

Criminal law Law that regulates offenses against the public welfare.

Crisis A sudden falling of an elevated body temperature to normal.

Critical item An item that comes in contact with sterile tissue or the vascular system.

Cross-index To file under one unit and use a guide or card filed under another unit that refers to the primary filing location.

Cryosurgery The therapeutic use of freezing temperatures to destroy abnormal tissue.

Cubic centimeter The amount of space occupied by 1 milliliter (1 mL = 1 cc).

Culture The propagation of a mass of microorganisms in a laboratory culture medium.

Culture medium A mixture of nutrients on which microorganisms are grown in the laboratory.

Curative treatment Treatment that cures disease.

Cyanosis A bluish discoloration of the skin and mucous membranes.

Cytokinesis Division of the cell at the end of mitosis to form two separate daughter cells.

Cytology The science that deals with the study of cells, including their origin, structure, function, and pathology.

Data Raw, unorganized facts about subject matter presented to the computer for processing.

Data processing The changing of raw facts or data into usable information following a three-part sequence: input, processing, output.

Day sheet The record of daily transactions in the pegboard or "write-it-once system" and also in computer medical billing programs.

DEA number A registration number assigned to physicians by the Drug Enforcement Administration for prescribing or dispensing controlled drugs.

Debit A posting that is added to an account balance.

Decontamination The use of physical or chemical means to remove, inactivate, or destroy pathogens on a surface or item to the point where they are no longer capable of transmitting infectious particles; the surface or item is rendered safe for handling, use, or disposal.

Deductible An amount of money that an insured person must pay annually before health services are covered by the insurance plan.

Defendant The person or group against whom an action is brought in a court of law.

Denial Failure to acknowledge the reality of a situation.

Depreciation Accounting methods to respond to the loss of value of a property or piece of equipment over time.

Dermis Inner layer of the skin that contains the blood vessels, nerves, glands, and hair follicles.

Detergent An agent that cleanses by emulsifying dirt and oil.

Diagnosis The scientific method of determining and identifying a patient's condition.

Diagnosis-related group (DRG) A system to determine Medicare reimbursement for a hospital stay on the basis of the patient's diagnosis.

Diagnostic procedure A procedure performed to assist in the diagnosis, management, or treatment of a patient's condition.

Diapedesis The process by which white blood cells squeeze between the cells in a vessel wall to enter the tissue spaces outside the blood vessel.

Diaphysis The long straight shaft of a long bone.

Diarthrosis (pl. *diarthroses*) Freely movable joint characterized by a joint cavity; also called a *synovial joint*.

Diastole Relaxation phase of the cardiac cycle; opposite of systole.

Diastolic pressure The point of lesser pressure on the arterial wall, which is recorded during diastole.

Diencephalon Part of the brain between the cerebral hemispheres and the midbrain; includes the thalamus and hypothalamus.

Differential diagnosis A determination of which of two or more diseases with similar symptoms is producing a patient's symptoms.

Diffusion Movement of substances from a region of high concentration to a region of low concentration.

Digital image A picture stored in the computer in the form of pixels.

Dilation (of the cervix) The stretching of the external os from an opening a few millimeters wide to an opening large enough to allow the passage of an infant (approximately 10 cm).

Disbursements Money paid out.

Discharge summary report A brief summary of the significant events of a patient's hospitalization.

Disinfectant An agent used to destroy pathogenic microorganisms but not their spores. Disinfectants are usually applied to inanimate objects.

Dislocation An injury in which one end of a bone making up a joint is separated or displaced from its normal anatomic position.

Diuresis Secretion and passage of large amounts of urine.

Do not resuscitate (DNR) A medical order signed by a physician that relieves health care personnel from the obligation to resuscitate a patient who stops breathing or whose heart stops.

Documentation A written set of instructions accompanying an application program, designed to assist the user in understanding how to operate the program. Examples include the user manual, help screens, and reference cards.

Dose The quantity of a drug to be administered at one time.

Double booking Scheduling two patients for the same appointment time.

Drug A chemical used for the treatment, prevention, or diagnosis of disease.

Drug Enforcement Administration (DEA) The federal agency that enforces the Controlled Substances Act of 1970.

DSL (digital subscriber line) Technology that allows digital signals to be transmitted over telephone lines at high speed even if the telephone line is also being used for voice transmission.

Duplex To produce double-sided copies by storing images from both sides of the original in the memory of a photocopier.

Duty Commitment to act in a certain way.

Dysmenorrhea Pain associated with the menstrual period.

Dyspareunia Pain in the vagina or pelvis experienced by a woman during sexual intercourse.

Dysplasia The growth of abnormal cells. Dysplasia is a precancerous condition that may or may not develop into cancer.

Dyspnea Shortness of breath or difficulty in breathing.

Dysrhythmia An irregular heart rate or rhythm; also termed *arrhythmia.*

Dysuria Difficult or painful urination.

ECG cycle The graphic representation of a heartbeat.

Echocardiogram An ultrasound examination of the heart.

Ectocervix The part of the cervix that projects into the vagina and is lined with stratified squamous epithelium.

Edema The retention of fluid in the tissues, resulting in swelling.

Effacement The thinning and shortening of the cervical canal from its normal length of 1 to 2 cm to a structure with paper-thin edges in which there is no canal at all. Effacement occurs late in pregnancy, during labor, or both. The purpose of effacement along with dilation is to permit the passage of the infant into the birth canal.

Ego defense mechanism Unconscious mental process that offers psychological protection.

Elastic fibers Yellow connective tissue fibers that are not particularly strong but can be stretched and will return to their normal shape when released.

Electrocardiogram (ECG) The graphic representation of the electrical activity of the heart.

Electrocardiograph The instrument used to record the electrical activity of the heart.

Electrode A conductor of electricity, which is used to promote contact between the body and the electrocardiograph.

Electrolyte A chemical substance that promotes conduction of an electrical current.

Electronic health record (EHR) An individual patient's health record in digital format. Also called an *electronic medical record.*

Electronic medical record (EMR) A computerized record of the important health information regarding a patient including the care of that individual and the progress of the patient's condition. Also called an *electronic health record.*

E-mail The exchange of information from one computer to another using telecommunication.

Emancipated minor A person younger than the age of 18 with the rights of an adult including the ability to consent to medical care.

Embezzlement Fraudulent appropriation of funds or property of an employer or client.

Embryo The child in utero from the time of conception to the beginning of the first trimester.

Emergency medical services (EMS) system A network of community resources, equipment, and personnel that provides care to victims of injury or sudden illness.

Empathy Objective awareness and sensitivity to the feelings and emotions of others.

Empirically Learned from observation or experiment.

Encryption A process by which electronic information is changed into an unreadable form that requires the original encryption software to reverse the process.

Endocervix The mucous membrane lining the cervical canal.

Endocrine gland Gland that secretes its product directly into the blood; opposite of exocrine gland.

Endoscope An instrument that consists of a tube and an optical system that is used for direct visual inspection of organs or cavities.

Enema An injection of fluid into the rectum to aid in the elimination of feces from the colon.

Engagement The entrance of the fetal head or the presenting part into the pelvic inlet.

Enteral nutrition The delivery of nutrients through a tube inserted into the gastrointestinal tract.

Enunciation The act of speaking clearly and concisely.

Environmental exposure Employee's exposure to hazardous substances in the workplace.

Epidermis Outermost layer of the skin.

Epiphyseal plate The cartilaginous plate between the epiphysis and diaphysis of a bone; responsible for the lengthwise growth of a long bone.

Epiphysis The end of a long bone.

Erythema Reddening of the skin caused by dilation of superficial blood vessels in the skin.

Erythrocyte Red blood cell.

Erythropoiesis The process of red blood cell formation.

Erythropoietin A hormone released by the kidneys that stimulates red blood cell production.

Established patient A patient who has been receiving services from the same medical practice on a regular basis.

Etiquette Rules of socially acceptable behavior; manners.

Eupnea Normal respiration. The rate is 16 to 20 respirations per minute, the rhythm is even and regular, and the depth is normal.

Evacuated tube A closed glass or plastic tube that contains a premeasured vacuum.

Evacuation plan A plan that includes escape routes for all locations in a building or other facility. Diagrams of these routes are posted in multiple locations.

Exhalation The act of breathing out.

Exocrine gland Gland that secrets its product to a surface or cavity through ducts; opposite of endocrine gland.

Expected date of delivery (EDD) Projected birth date of an infant.

Explanation of benefits (EOB) A statement issued by an insurance company explaining reimbursement for specific procedures.

External os The opening of the cervical canal of the uterus into the vagina.

External respiration Exchange of gases between the lungs and the blood.

Externship or practicum A supervised work experience that is required in an educational program and usually unpaid.

Exudate A discharge produced by the body's tissues.

Fahrenheit scale A temperature scale on which the freezing point of water is 32° and the boiling point of water is 212°.

False negative A test result denoting that a condition is absent when it is actually present.

False positive A test result denoting that a condition is present when it is actually absent.

Familial Occurring in or affecting members of a family more frequently than would be expected by chance.

Fasting Abstaining from food or fluids (except water) for a specified amount of time before the collection of a specimen.

Fax Transmission of scanned, printed material by telephone. A short form of the word *facsimile*.

Febrile Pertaining to fever.

Fee-for-service A means of payment for health care in which reimbursement for each service provided is made in full or in part.

Fee-for-service insurance Insurance reimbursement that is directly related to the services provided and the amount charged by the provider.

Fee schedule List of charges (fees) for specific procedures that may be performed in a medical office.

Fee splitting The practice of sharing fees with colleagues, especially for making referrals.

Felony A serious crime punishable by death or imprisonment.

Fetal heart rate The number of times per minute the fetal heart beats.

Fetal heart tones The sounds of the heartbeat of the fetus heard through the mother's abdominal wall.

Fetus The child in utero from the third month after conception to birth; during the first 2 months of development, it is called an *embryo*.

Fever A body temperature that is above normal; synonym for *pyrexia*.

Fibroblast An immature cell from which connective tissue can develop.

Fidelity Faithfulness.

Filing system The way in which records are arranged. Common filing systems in the medical office include alphabetic, numeric, by subject, or chronologic.

Fire extinguisher A portable device that discharges foam or another material to extinguish a fire.

Firewall A system that protects a computer network from unauthorized access by users on its own network or another network, such as the Internet.

First aid The immediate care administered before complete medical care can be provided to an individual who is injured or suddenly becomes ill.

Fiscal intermediary An insurance company that contracts to review Medicare claims for the Centers for Medicare and Medicaid Services.

Fixed appointment scheduling An appointment scheduling method in which each patient is given a different, specific appointment time. Also called *stream scheduling, time-specified scheduling,* or *single booking.*

Flow rate The number of liters of oxygen per minute that come out of an oxygen delivery system.

Fluoroscope An instrument used to view internal organs and structures directly.

Fluoroscopy Examination of a patient by means of a fluoroscope.

Forceps A two-pronged instrument for grasping and squeezing.

Formulary An insurance carrier's official list of covered medications to be used by network providers.

Fracture Any break in a bone.

Fraud Intentional deception resulting in injury or loss.

Frenulum linguae The midline fold that connects the undersurface of the tongue with the floor of the mouth.

Frequency The condition of having to urinate often.

Full block style A letter format in which all parts of the letter are left justified.

Fundus The dome-shaped upper portion of the uterus between the fallopian tubes.

Furuncle A localized staphylococcal infection that originates deep within a hair follicle. Also known as a *boil.*

Gametes Sex cells: sperm and ova.

Gauge The diameter of the lumen of a needle used to administer medication.

Gene therapy Giving patients new genes or parts of genes to treat a disease or condition.

Genetic engineering Making, altering, or repairing genetic material.

Gestation The period of intrauterine development from conception to birth; the period of pregnancy. The average pregnancy lasts about 280 days, or 40 weeks, from the date of conception to childbirth.

Gestational age The age of the fetus between conception and birth.

Gigabyte (GB) A unit of computer storage capacity. One gigabyte is equal to a little more than 1 billion bytes or 1000 megabytes.

Glomerular capsule Double-layered epithelial cup that surrounds the glomerulus in a nephron; also called *Bowman's capsule.*

Glycogen The form in which carbohydrate is stored in the body.

Glycosuria The presence of glucose in the urine.

Glycosylation The process of glucose attaching to hemoglobin.

Gonads Primary reproductive organs; organs that produce the gametes: testes in the male and ovaries in the female.

Grammar The study of accepted rules used to create meaning in a language.

Gross pay The total amount earned in a time period by an employee before any deductions.

Group plan One insurance policy that covers a group of people.

Guarantor A person with financial responsibility for a bill who may or may not also be a patient.

Gynecology The branch of medicine that deals with the diseases of reproductive organs of women.

Hand hygiene The process of cleansing or sanitizing the hands.

Hard copy Printed output from a computer.

Hard disk A storage device consisting of one or more rigid, nonflexible platters coated with a magnetically sensitive material and encased in a permanently sealed, airtight container.

Hardware The physical devices making up a computer system (e.g., main computer unit, keyboard, monitor, printer).

Hazardous chemical Any chemical that presents a threat to the health and safety of an individual coming into contact with it.

Hazmat A word constructed from the beginnings of the two words "*haz*ardous *mat*erials."

HDL cholesterol A lipoprotein, consisting of protein and cholesterol, that removes excess cholesterol from the cells.

Health care proxy A legal document that names an agent to make decisions about a person's medical care if he or she becomes unable to make wishes known.

Health history report A collection of subjective data about a patient.

Health information exchange (HIE) The electronic exchange of healthcare-related data among different institutions.

Health insurance Purchase of protection for covered services related to health care.

Hematology The study of blood and blood-forming tissues.

Hematoma A swelling or mass of coagulated blood caused by a break in a blood vessel.

Hematopoiesis Blood cell production, which occurs in the red bone marrow; also called *hemopoiesis*.

Hematuria Blood present in the urine.

Hemoconcentration An increase in the concentration of the nonfilterable blood components in the blood vessels, such as red blood cells, enzymes, iron, and calcium, as a result of a decrease in the fluid content of the blood.

Hemocytoblast A stem cell in the bone marrow from which the blood cells arise.

Hemoglobin The protein- and iron-containing pigment of erythrocytes that transports oxygen in the body.

Hemoglobin A_{1c} Compound formed when glucose attaches or glycosylates to the protein in hemoglobin.

Hemolysis The breakdown of blood cells.

Hemophilia An inherited bleeding disorder caused by a deficiency of a clotting factor needed for proper coagulation of the blood.

Hemostasis The arrest of bleeding by natural or artificial means.

Hierarchy Classification according to rank or importance.

Histology Branch of microscopic anatomy that studies tissues.

Holistic Considering the whole; in medicine, considering the entire person when providing health care.

Home health care The provision of medical and nonmedical care in a patient's home or place of residence.

Homeostasis The state in which body systems are functioning normally and the internal environment of the body is in equilibrium; the body is in a healthy state.

Hormone A substance secreted by an endocrine gland.

Hospice An organization that manages care for dying patients (whose life expectancy is less than 6 months) including comfort, pain relief, and personal care. Services may be provided in the patient's home, a nursing home, or a special hospice facility.

Human anatomy Study of human body shape and structure and the relationships of its parts.

Human physiology Study of the functions of humans and their separate parts.

Hyperglycemia An abnormally high level of glucose in the blood.

Hyperopia Farsightedness.

Hyperpnea An abnormal increase in the rate and depth of respiration.

Hyperpyrexia An extremely high fever.

Hypertension High blood pressure.

Hyperventilation An abnormally fast and deep type of breathing, usually associated with acute anxiety conditions.

Hypoglycemia An abnormally low level of glucose in the blood.

Hypopnea An abnormal decrease in the rate and depth of respiration.

Hypotension Low blood pressure.

Hypothermia A life-threatening condition in which the temperature of the entire body falls to a dangerously low level.

Hypoxemia A decrease in the oxygen saturation of the blood. Hypoxemia may lead to hypoxia.

Hypoxia A reduction in the oxygen supply to the tissues of the body.

Immune globulin A blood product consisting of pooled human plasma containing antibodies.

Immunity The resistance of the body to the effects of a harmful agent, such as a pathogenic microorganism and its toxins.

Immunization (active, artificial) The process of becoming immune or of rendering an individual immune through the use of a vaccine or toxoid.

Impacted Wedged firmly together so as to be immovable.

In vivo Occurring in the living body or organism.

Inactive record The medical record of a patient who has not been seen within the past 2 to 3 years, or some other time frame specified by a given medical office.

Incision A clean cut caused by a cutting instrument.

Incubate In microbiology, the act of placing a culture in a chamber (incubator) that provides optimal growth requirements for the multiplication of the organisms, such as the proper temperature, humidity, and darkness.

Incubation period The interval of time between the invasion by a pathogenic microorganism and the appearance of first symptoms of the disease.

Indemnity An obligation to provide compensation for loss or damage.

Indexing units Pieces of information used to identify a correct filing location.

Induration An abnormally raised, hardened area of the skin with clearly defined margins.

Infant A child from birth to 12 months of age.

Infection The condition in which the body, or part of it, is invaded by a pathogen.

Infectious disease A disease caused by a pathogen that produces harmful effects on its host (also known as a *communicable disease*).

Infiltration The process by which a substance passes into and is deposited within the substance of a cell, tissue, or organ.

Inflammation A protective response of the body to trauma and the entrance of foreign matter. The purpose of inflammation is to destroy invading microorganisms and to remove damaged tissue debris from the area so that proper healing can occur.

Informed consent Consent given by a patient for a medical procedure after he or she has been informed of the nature of his or her condition and the purpose of the procedure, and has been given an explanation of risks involved with the procedure, alternative treatments or procedures available, the likely outcome of the procedure, and the risks involved with declining or delaying the procedure.

Infusion The administration of fluids, medications, or nutrients into a vein.

Inhalation The act of breathing in.

Inhalation administration The administration of medication by way of air or other vapor being drawn into the lungs.

Initiative The ability to begin or carry through on a plan of action independently.

Inoculate To introduce microorganisms into a culture medium for growth and multiplication.

Inpatient A patient who has been admitted to a hospital for at least one overnight stay.

Input 1. (noun) Data that have been entered into the computer. 2. (verb) The transfer of data to the computer for processing.

Input device A device for entering data into the computer (e.g., keyboard, mouse, scanner).

Inscription The part of a prescription that indicates the name of the drug and the drug dosage.

Insertion The end of a muscle that is attached to a relatively movable part; the end opposite the origin.

Inspection The process of observing a patient to detect signs of disease.

Instillation The dropping of a liquid into a body cavity.

Insufflate To blow a powder, vapor, or gas (e.g., air) into a body cavity.

Insured The individual who has a specific insurance plan.

Intercostal Between the ribs.

Internal respiration Exchange of gases between the blood and tissue cells.

Internet A global system of interconnected computer networks that use the Internet protocol (TCP/IP) to transmit and exchange data.

Interval The length of a wave or the length of a wave with a segment.

Intradermal injection Introduction of medication into the dermal layer of the skin.

Intramuscular injection Introduction of medication into the muscular layer of the body.

Intravenous (IV) therapy The administration of a liquid agent directly into a patient's vein, where it is distributed throughout the body by way of the circulatory system.

Inventory A detailed list of items in stock or in possession of an individual or business.

Invoice An itemized bill for items that have not been prepaid.

Irrigation The washing of a body canal with a flowing solution.

Ischemia Deficiency of blood in a body part.

Judgmental Describing one who makes judgments about what is good or bad based on personal opinion.

Juxtaglomerular apparatus Complex of modified cells in the afferent arteriole and the ascending limb and distal tubule in the kidney; helps regulate blood pressure by secreting renin; consists of the macula densa and juxtaglomerular cells.

Keratinization Process by which the cells of the epidermis become filled with keratin and move to the surface, where they are sloughed off.

Ketonuria The presence of ketone bodies in the urine.

Ketosis An accumulation of large amounts of ketone bodies in the tissues and body fluids.

Kilobyte (KB) A unit of computer storage capacity. One kilobyte is equal to 1024 bytes (characters).

Korotkoff sounds Sounds heard during the measurement of blood pressure that are used to determine the systolic and diastolic blood pressure readings.

Laboratory test The clinical analysis and study of materials, fluids, or tissues obtained from patients to assist in diagnosis and treatment of disease.

Laceration A wound in which the tissues are torn apart, leaving ragged and irregular edges.

Larceny Stealing another person's property or money without violence.

LDL cholesterol A lipoprotein, consisting of protein and cholesterol, that picks up cholesterol and delivers it to the cells.

Ledger A book, card, or computer account used to record financial transactions.

Left justified Format of a document in which the lines of type begin at the left margin.

Length (recumbent) The measurement from the vertex of the head to the heel of the foot in a supine position.

Letterhead A sheet of stationery preprinted with information about a business, including name, address, telephone number, and other information.

Leukocyte White blood cell.

Leukocytosis An abnormal increase in the number of white blood cells (greater than 11,000 per cubic millimeter of blood).

Leukopenia An abnormal decrease in the number of white blood cells (less than 4500 per cubic millimeter of blood).

Liabilities In accounting, the amount owed by a business to creditors.

Liability Legal responsibility.

License Official permission to perform an activity or practice a profession.

Licensure The process by which the state examines qualifications and gives permission to an individual or organization to engage in a profession or business.

Ligate To tie off and close a structure such as a severed blood vessel.

Lipoprotein A complex molecule consisting of protein and a lipid fraction such as cholesterol. Lipoproteins function in transporting lipids in the blood.

Litigation The process of taking a lawsuit through the courts.

Living will A legal document that specifies the kind of medical treatment a patient wants or does not want if he or she becomes incapacitated.

Load The articles that are being sterilized.

Local anesthetic A drug that produces a loss of feeling and an inability to perceive pain in only a specific part of the body.

Macrophage Large phagocytic connective tissue cell that functions in the immune response.

Main computer memory The part of the CPU that is responsible for temporarily storing information until it is needed for processing by the computer. Main memory in a microcomputer is known as *RAM.*

Mainboard The primary circuit board of the main computer unit, which allows all of the computer components to communicate with one another.

Malaise A vague sense of body discomfort, weakness, and fatigue that often marks the onset of a disease and continues through the course of the illness.

Malfeasance A crime or wrongdoing that is illegal or contrary to official obligation.

Malpractice Negligence by a professional.

Managed care A movement in health care based on reducing health care costs while providing high-quality care. The term may be used for the techniques used to reduce costs or for the companies that pay for the care provided.

Man-made disaster Serious damage either directly or indirectly caused by intentional or negligent human actions or the failure of a man-made system (such as a fire, structural collapse, or terrorism).

Manometer An instrument for measuring pressure.

Mast cell A connective tissue cell that produces heparin and histamine.

Material safety data sheet (MSDS) A sheet that provides information regarding a chemical, its hazards, and measures to take to prevent injury and illness when handling the chemical.

Matrix A rectangular or linear arrangement of numbers or information.

Mayo tray A broad, flat metal tray placed on a stand and used to hold sterile instruments and supplies when it has been covered with a sterile towel.

Mechanoreceptor A sensory receptor that responds to a bending or deformation of the cell; examples include receptors for touch, pressure, hearing, and equilibrium.

Mediation Negotiation by a third party to help two parties resolve a dispute.

Medicaid The government insurance program for low-income individuals and families that is funded both by the federal government and each individual state.

Medical asepsis Practices that are employed to reduce the number and hinder the transmission of pathogens.

Medical impressions Conclusions drawn by the physician from an interpretation of data. Other terms for impressions include provisional diagnosis and tentative diagnosis.

Medical practice management program A program that provides instructions to the computer for performing medical practice management procedures.

Medical record A written record of important information regarding a patient, including the care of that individual and the progress of the patient's condition.

Medical record format The way a medical record is organized. The two main types of medical record formats are the source-oriented record and the problem-oriented record.

Medical records management Activities related to the creation, management, use, and disposition of patient medical records.

Medicare The federal health insurance program that provides insurance coverage for the elderly, permanently disabled individuals, and individuals with end-stage kidney disease.

Megabyte (MB) A unit of computer storage capacity. One megabyte is equal to a little more than 1 million bytes or 1000 kilobytes.

Meiosis Type of nuclear division in which the number of chromosomes is reduced to one half the number found in a body cell; results in the formation of an egg or sperm.

Melanin A dark brown or black pigment found in parts of the body, especially skin and hair.

Melena The darkening of the stool caused by the presence of blood in an amount of 50 mL or greater.

Memo (memorandum) A form of communication within a company that is usually short and limited to one subject.

Meniscus The curved surface on a column of liquid in a tube.

Menopause The permanent cessation of menstruation, which usually occurs between the ages of 45 and 55.

Menorrhagia Excessive bleeding during a menstrual period, in the number of days or the amount of blood or both. Also called *dysfunctional uterine bleeding* (DUB).

Mensuration The process of measuring a patient.

Mesentery Extensions of peritoneum that are associated with the intestine.

Metabolism The total of all biochemical reactions that take place in the body; includes anabolism and catabolism.

Metered mail Mail for which the postage has been applied using a postage meter.

Metrorrhagia Bleeding between menstrual periods.

MICR line A line of numbers containing the ABA transit routing number and the account number that appears at the bottom left of a check. These numbers are read by a magnetic ink character recognition (MICR) system.

Microbiology The scientific study of microorganisms and their activities.

Microcomputer A small general purpose computer that relies on a tiny microprocessor chip to perform its processing functions.

Microorganism A microscopic plant or animal.

Micturition The act of voiding urine.

Minutes A written record of the proceedings of a meeting.

Misdemeanor A crime that is less serious than a felony; punishable by a fine or imprisonment for less than 1 year.

Misfeasance Performing a legal act in an improper way.

Mitosis Process by which the nucleus of a body cell divides to form two new cells, each identical to the parent cell.

Modified block style A format for business letters where the date line, complimentary close, and printed signature line are on a tab at the center or right justified and all other parts of the letter are left justified.

Modified wave scheduling An appointment system that has some fixed appointments and some appointment times during which patients are seen in order of arrival.

Modifier An addition to a *Current Procedural Terminology* code that indicates unusual circumstances related to the procedure, such as a more extensive procedure or two procedures performed in the same session.

Motor unit A single neuron and all the muscle fibers it stimulates.

Mucous membrane A membrane lining body passages or cavities that open to the outside.

Multigravida A woman who has been pregnant more than once.

Multipara A woman who has completed two or more pregnancies to the age of fetal viability regardless of whether they ended in live infants or stillbirths.

Myelin White, fatty substance that surrounds many nerve fibers.

Myopia Nearsightedness.

Nationwide Health Information Network (NHIN) A set of standards, services, and policies to facilitate national HIE (health information exchange).

Natural disaster Serious damage to the environment resulting from a natural hazard (such as volcanoes, earthquakes, or hurricanes) that leads to environmental, financial, and human losses.

NEC A diagnosis code that is not elsewhere classified. It is used when a more specific code for a condition is not available.

Needle biopsy A type of biopsy in which tissue from deep within the body is obtained by the insertion of a biopsy needle through the skin.

Negative feedback A mechanism of response in which a stimulus initiates reactions that reduce the stimulus.

Negligence Failure to act (or refrain from acting) as a reasonably prudent person would in similar circumstances.

Neoplasm Abnormal growth or tumor.

Nephron Functional unit of the kidney consisting of a renal corpuscle and a renal tubule.

Net pay The actual amount of money paid directly to an employee after taxes and other deductions have been taken out.

Networking Contacting acquaintances and their contacts who may know of potential jobs.

Neurilemma The layer of cells that surrounds a nerve fiber in the peripheral nervous system and, in some cases, produces myelin; also called *Schwann sheath*.

Neuroglia Supporting cells of nervous tissue; cells in nervous tissue that do not conduct impulses; nerve glue.

Neurohypophysis Posterior portion of pituitary gland; the gland that grows beneath the brain and contains axons of neurons.

Neuromuscular junction The area of communication between the axon terminal of a motor neuron and the sarcolemma of a muscle fiber; also called a *myoneural junction*.

Neuron Nerve cell, including its processes; conducting cell of nervous tissue.

Neurotransmitter A chemical substance that is released at the axon terminals to stimulate a muscle fiber contraction or an impulse in another neuron.

New patient For billing purposes, a patient who has not received services during the previous 3 years from any physician in a medical practice.

Nociceptor A sensory receptor that responds to tissue damage; pain receptor.

Nocturia Excessive (voluntary) urination during the night.

Nocturnal enuresis Inability of an individual to control urination at night during sleep (bedwetting).

Nonabsorbable suture Suture material that is not absorbed by the body and either remains permanently in the body tissue and becomes encapsulated by fibrous tissue or is removed.

Noncritical item An item that comes into contact with intact skin, but not with mucous membranes.

Nonfeasance Failing to perform an act that should have been performed, resulting in injury.

Nonintact skin Skin that has a break in the surface. It includes, but is not limited to, abrasions, cuts, hangnails, paper cuts, and burns.

Nonmalfeasance Ethical concept requiring that an action do no harm, or do less harm than good.

Nonparticipating provider (PAR) A physician who does not have any contract with a third-party payor.

Nonpathogen A microorganism that does not normally produce disease.

Nonverbal Describing communication that occurs without words, such as through body posture or facial expression.

Nonwaived test A complex laboratory test that does not meet the CLIA criteria for waiver and is subject to the CLIA regulations.

Normal flora Harmless, nonpathogenic microorganisms that normally reside in many parts of the body but do not cause disease.

Normal sinus rhythm Refers to an ECG that is within normal limits.

NOS A diagnosis code that is not otherwise specified. It is used when there is not enough information given to select a more specific code.

No-show A patient who does not keep a scheduled appointment.

Nullipara A woman who has not carried a pregnancy to the point of fetal viability (20 weeks of gestation).

Objective symptom A symptom that can be observed by an examiner.

Obstetrics The branch of medicine concerned with the care of women during pregnancy, childbirth, and the post-partal period.

Occult blood Blood in such a small amount that it is not detectable by the unaided eye.

Oliguria Decreased or scanty output of urine.

Oogenesis Process of meiosis in the female in which one ovum and three polar bodies are produced from one primary oocyte.

Open questions Questions that could have a variety of answers and encourage a personal response.

Operating system A type of system software that performs tasks required by the computer to operate itself.

Ophthalmoscope An instrument for examining the interior of the eye.

Opportunistic infection An infection that results from a defective immune system that cannot defend the body from pathogens normally found in the environment.

Optical disc A storage device consisting of a flat, round portable disk that stores data using laser technology.

Optical drive A device installed in a drive bay on the main computer unit that uses a laser to read an optical disc or write onto (burn) an optical disc.

Optimum growth temperature The temperature at which an organism grows best.

Oral Spoken; pertaining to the mouth.

Oral administration Administration of medication by mouth.

Origin The end of a muscle that is attached to a relatively immovable part; the end opposite the insertion.

Orthopnea The condition in which breathing is easier when an individual is in a sitting or standing position.

Osmosis Diffusion of water through a selectively permeable membrane.

Osteoblast Bone-forming cell; immature bone cell.

Osteochondritis Inflammation of bone and cartilage.

Osteoclast Cell that destroys, breaks down, or resorbs bone tissue.

Osteocyte Mature bone cell.

Osteomyelitis Inflammation of the bone or bone marrow as a result of bacterial infection.

Osteon Structural unit of bone; haversian system.

Otoscope An instrument for examining the external ear canal and tympanic membrane.

Outguide A cardboard or plastic card to insert in a file when a medical record is removed.

Outpatient A patient who has not been admitted to a health care facility.

Output 1. (noun) Information that has been generated by the computer. 2. (verb) The transfer of processed data back to the user.

Output device A device that transfers processed data to the user (e.g., computer monitor, printer).

Ovarian cycle Monthly cycle of events that occur in the ovary from puberty to menopause; occurs concurrently with the uterine cycle.

Ovarian follicle An oocyte surrounded by one or more layers of cells within the ovaries.

Overdraft A check (or draft) that exceeds the amount of funds in a bank account.

Oxygen therapy The administration of supplemental oxygen at concentrations greater than room air to treat or prevent hypoxemia.

Pager An electronic device that notifies the recipient to receive a message or return a telephone call.

Palliative treatment Therapy that reduces the effects of a disease or condition but does not remove the disease itself.

Palpation The process of feeling with the hands to detect signs of disease.

Panel A group of diagnostic tests done in one machine at the same time.

Paper-based patient record (PPR) A medical record in paper form.

Paraphrasing A restatement of the words of another, often to clarify meaning.

Parenteral Taken into the body through piercing of the skin barrier or mucous membranes, such as through needlesticks, human bites, cuts, and abrasions.

Participating provider (PAR) A physician who has a contractual agreement with a third-party payor.

Passive transport Process that moves substances across or through a membrane and does not require cellular energy.

Pathogen A disease-producing microorganism.

Patient An individual receiving medical care.

Patient self-scheduling The practice of allowing patients to have access to the computer scheduling program so that they can schedule their own appointments.

Payee The person to whom a check is made out.

PDA (personal digital assistant) A portable handheld computing device with access to various reference tools, such as a drug reference, calculator, and address book.

Peak flow rate The maximum volume of air that can be exhaled when the patient blows into a peak flow meter as forcefully and as rapidly as possible.

Pediatrician A physician who specializes in the care and development of children and the diagnosis and treatment of children's diseases.

Pediatrics The branch of medicine that deals with the care and development of children and the diagnosis and treatment of children's diseases.

Per diem Paid by the day; a term used in reference to employees who do not have a fixed schedule but are scheduled by the day according to office needs.

Percussion The process of tapping the body to detect signs of disease.

Percussion hammer An instrument with a rubber head, used for testing reflexes.

Perimenopause Before the onset of menopause, the phase during which the woman with regular periods changes to having irregular cycles and increased periods of amenorrhea.

Perinatal Relating to the period shortly before and after birth.

Perineum The external region between the vaginal orifice and the anus in a female and between the scrotum and the anus in a male.

Peristalsis Rhythmic contractions of the intestine that move food along the digestive tract.

Peroxidase As it pertains to the guaiac slide test, a substance that is able to transfer oxygen from hydrogen peroxide to oxidize guaiac, causing the guaiac to turn blue.

Petty cash A cash account kept in a business office to pay for incidentals, such as postage due and other small items.

pH The degree to which a solution is acidic or basic.

Phagocytosis Condition of cell eating; a form of endocytosis in which solid particles are taken into the cell.

Pharmacology The study of drugs.

Phlebotomist A health care professional trained in the collection of blood specimens.

Phlebotomy Incision of a vein for the removal of blood; the collection of blood.

Photoreceptor A sensory receptor that detects light; located in the retina of the eye.

Physical examination An assessment of each part of the patient's body to obtain objective data about the patient that assists the physician in determining the patient's state of health.

Physical examination report A report of the objective findings from the physician's assessment of each body system.

Physiologic Pertaining to body processes.

Pinocytosis Condition of cell drinking; a form of endocytosis in which fluid droplets are taken into the cell.

Pixels (picture elements) Dot locations on a computer screen that can be lit up as needed to display images.

Plaintiff The person or group that makes the complaint in a lawsuit.

Plasma The liquid part of the blood, consisting of a clear, yellowish fluid that makes up approximately 55% of the total blood volume.

Plicae circulars Circular folds in the mucosa and submucosa of the small intestine.

Poison Any substance that causes illness, injury, or death if it enters the body.

Policy A guiding principle for the management of a medical office or business.

Polycythemia A disorder in which there is an increase in the red blood cell mass.

Polyuria Increased output of urine.

Position The relation of the presenting part of the fetus to the maternal pelvis.

Postage meter A machine that automatically stamps a piece of mail with the correct postage.

Postal bar code A series of vertical bars of two lengths, which represent the delivery address of a piece of mail. The barcode facilitates automated sorting of mail.

Postexposure prophylaxis (PEP) Treatment administered to an individual after exposure to an infectious disease to prevent the disease.

Postoperative Occurring after a surgical operation.

Postpartum Occurring after childbirth.

Posttraumatic stress disorder (PTSD) A psychiatric condition that develops months or years after a traumatic, catastrophic life experience.

Preadmission testing (PAT) A series of diagnostic tests done before surgery to establish the patient's health status and identify any potential problems that may occur during surgery.

Preauthorization Verification from a patient's insurance company that a procedure is covered by the patient's insurance and agreement, after review, that the test or procedure is medically appropriate.

Precertification Verification from a patient's insurance company that a procedure is covered by the patient's insurance and agreement, after review, that the test or procedure is medically appropriate.

Preeclampsia A major complication of pregnancy, the cause of which is unknown, characterized by increasing hypertension, albuminuria, and edema. If this condition is neglected or is not treated properly, it may develop into eclampsia, which could cause maternal convulsions and coma. Preeclampsia generally occurs between the twentieth week of pregnancy and the end of the first week postpartum.

Premium An amount of money paid in a given period to purchase health insurance.

Prenatal Occurring before birth.

Preoperative Preceding a surgical operation.

Presbyopia A decrease in the elasticity of the lens that occurs with aging, resulting in a decreased ability to focus on close objects.

Preschool child A child 3 to 6 years old.

Prescription A physician's order authorizing the dispensing of a drug by a pharmacist.

Presentation Indication of the part of the fetus that is closest to the cervix and is delivered first. A cephalic presentation is a delivery in which the fetal head is presenting against the cervix. A breech presentation is a delivery in which the buttocks or feet are presented instead of the head.

Pressure point A site on the body where an artery lies close to the surface of the skin and can be compressed against an underlying bone to control bleeding.

Primary care provider The physician chosen by a patient to provide general medical care and also to determine and authorize additional medical services the patient may require.

Primary insurance The insurance company that must be billed first for any individual.

Prime mover The muscle that is mainly responsible for a particular body movement; also called *agonist.*

Primigravida A woman who is pregnant for the first time.

Primipara A woman who has carried a pregnancy to fetal viability (20 weeks of gestation) for the first time regardless of whether the infant was stillborn or alive at birth.

Printing speed The number of pages per minute (ppm) generated by a printer.

Privilege A special immunity that protects against legal liability.

Problem Any condition that requires further observation, diagnosis, management, or patient education.

Procedure A list of the steps to handle a certain situation or perform a certain task.

Processing The manipulation and reorganization of data according to the instructions in a program.

Product insert A printed document supplied by the manufacturer with a laboratory test product that contains information on the proper storage and use of the product.

Profile An array of laboratory tests for identifying a disease state or evaluating a particular organ or organ system.

Prognosis The probable course and outcome of a patient's condition and the patient's prospects for recovery.

Program A set of instructions, organized in a logical step-by-step sequence, that tells the computer how to perform a specific function.

Projection The act of experiencing one's own emotions as those of another.

Proof of posting A process of calculation to verify that calculations on a day sheet are internally consistent and all totals are correct.

Proofread To identify and correct errors in a document.

Proprioception The sense of body position and movements; responds to stimuli originating within an organism or muscle.

Proteinuria The presence of protein in the urine.

Prudent Using care or common sense.

Puerperium The period of time, usually 4 to 6 weeks after delivery, in which the uterus and the body systems are returning to normal.

Pulse oximeter A computerized device consisting of a probe and a monitor used to measure the oxygen saturation of arterial blood.

Pulse oximetry The use of a pulse oximeter to measure the oxygen saturation of arterial blood.

Pulse pressure The difference between the systolic and diastolic pressures.

Pulse rhythm The time interval between heartbeats.

Pulse volume The strength of the heartbeat.

Puncture A wound made by a sharp-pointed object piercing the skin.

Pyuria The presence of pus in the urine.

Qualitative test A test that indicates whether or not a substance is present in the specimen being tested and also provides an approximate indication of the amount of the substance present.

Quality control The application of methods to ensure that test results are reliable and valid and that errors are detected and eliminated.

Quantitative test A test that indicates the exact amount of a chemical substance that is present in the body, with the results being reported in measurable units.

Quickening The first movements of the fetus in utero as felt by the mother, which usually occur at 16 to 20 weeks of gestation and are felt consistently thereafter.

Radiation The transfer of energy, such as heat, in the form of waves.

Radiograph A permanent record of a picture of an internal body organ or structure produced on radiographic film.

Radiography The taking of permanent records (radiographs) of internal body organs and structures by passing x-rays through the body to act on a specially sensitized film.

Radiologist A physician who specializes in the diagnosis and treatment of disease using radiation and other imaging techniques.

Radiology The branch of medicine that deals with the use of radiation and other imaging techniques (such as ultrasound, CT scans, MRIs, and nuclear medicine) in the diagnosis and treatment of disease.

Radiolucent Describing a structure that permits the passage of x-rays.

Radiopaque Describing a structure that obstructs the passage of x-rays.

RAM (random-access memory) The main computer memory of a microcomputer, which is used to temporarily store items until needed by the computer for processing. Also known as *main computer memory.*

Reagent A substance that produces a reaction with a patient specimen that allows detection or measurement of the substance by the test system.

Reciprocity Automatic issuing of a license in one state to the holder of a license in another state.

Reconciling Making sure that two financial records agree, such as a bank statement and bank balance.

Reference range A certain established and acceptable parameter or reference range within which the laboratory test results of a healthy individual are expected to fall. (Also known as *reference value* and *reference interval.*)

Referral The directing of a patient to a specialist physician by the primary care physician. Most managed care plans and some other insurance plans require the primary care physician to obtain prior authorization.

Reflecting Expressing the meaning and emotion of another's words back to the person.

Refraction The deflection or bending of light rays by a lens.

Regulated medical waste (RMW) Medical waste that poses a threat to health and safety.

Reimbursement The amount paid for a procedure by insurance.

Renal threshold The concentration at which a substance in the blood that is not normally excreted by the kidneys begins to appear in the urine.

Renal tubule Tubular portion of the nephron that carries the filtrate away from the glomerular capsule; site where tubular reabsorption and secretion occur.

Reorder point A number on a supply inventory that indicates when a specific item should be reordered to be sure that the supply will not run out before the new order is received.

Reservoir host The organism that becomes infected by a pathogen and serves as a source of transfer of the pathogen to others.

Residency A program to provide training in a medical specialty to a physician who has finished medical school.

Resident flora Harmless, nonpathogenic microorganisms that normally reside on the skin and usually do not cause disease. Also known as *normal flora.*

Resistance The natural ability of an organism to remain unaffected by harmful substances in its environment.

Resolution The number of horizontal and vertical pixels in a display device, such as a computer screen.

Resource-based relative value scale (RBRVS) A system to establish the Medicare fee schedule for Medicare Part B based on the service provided and the geographic location of the provider.

Respiratory membrane Any surface in the lungs where diffusion occurs; consists of the layers that the gases must pass through to get into or out of the alveoli.

Respondeat superior A legal doctrine making an employer liable for the negligent acts of employees.

Résumé A summary of information about a person that describes education, work experience, and other information related to an individual's suitability for employment.

Retention The inability to empty the bladder. The urine is being produced normally but is not being voided.

Reverse chronologic order Arranging documents with the most recent document on top or in the front, which means that the oldest document is on the bottom or at the back of a section or file.

Right A claim that is expected to be honored.

Right justified Type that is aligned with the right margin of a document.

Risk factor Anything that increases an individual's chance of developing a disease. Some risk factors (e.g., smoking) can be avoided, but others (e.g., age and family history) cannot.

Risk management The process of assessing risk and putting policies and procedures in place to minimize it.

Router A wired or wireless device used to form or connect networks.

Routine test A laboratory test performed routinely on apparently healthy patients to assist in the early detection of disease.

Rugae Longitudinal folds in the mucosa of the stomach.

Salary A fixed amount of money paid on a regular basis that does not depend on the number of hours worked.

Saltatory conduction Process in which a nerve impulse travels along a myelinated nerve fiber by jumping from one node of Ranvier to the next.

Salutation The greeting that begins a letter.

Sanitization A process to remove organic matter from an article and to reduce the number of microorganisms to a safe level as determined by public health requirements.

SaO$_2$ (saturation of arterial oxygen) Abbreviation for the percentage of hemoglobin that is saturated with oxygen in arterial blood.

Scalpel A surgical knife used to divide tissues.

School-age child A child 6 to 12 years old.

Scissors A cutting instrument.

Sebaceous cyst A thin, closed sac or capsule that contains fatty secretions from a sebaceous gland.

Sebaceous gland An oil gland of the skin that produces sebum or body oil.

Secondary insurance Insurance that an individual has in addition to primary insurance.

Segment The portion of the ECG between two waves.

Seizure A sudden episode of involuntary muscular contractions and relaxation, often accompanied by changes in sensation, behavior, and level of consciousness.

Self-actualization The fulfillment of each individual's potential.

Self-referral Process by which a patient makes an appointment with a specialist physician without requesting prior authorization from his or her primary care physician, usually because the patient's insurance plan does not require it.

Semiblock style A letter format in which the date line, complimentary close, and printed signature line are on a tab at the center or right justified, all paragraphs are indented five to eight spaces, and the other parts of the letter are left justified.

Semicritical item An item that comes into contact with nonintact skin or intact mucous membranes.

Semilunar valve Valve between a ventricle of the heart and the vessel that carries blood away from the ventricle; also pertains to the valves in veins.

Sensory adaptation Phenomenon in which some receptors respond when a stimulus is first applied but decrease their response if the stimulus is maintained; receptor sensitivity decreases with prolonged stimulation.

Sequela (pl. *sequelae*) Any condition that results from a disease, injury, or treatment for a disease or injury.

Sequential-access memory Computer memory in which all stored data must be searched sequentially from beginning to end to locate the desired information.

Serum The clear, straw-colored part of the blood (plasma) that remains after the solid elements and the clotting factor fibrinogen have been separated out of it.

Server A large computer that stores data and manages tasks for other computers on a network.

Service contract An agreement that provides for service for a piece of equipment after the warranty expires.

Shock The failure of the cardiovascular system to deliver enough blood to all of the vital organs of the body.

Sigmoidoscope An endoscope that is specially designed for passage through the anus to permit visualization of the rectum and sigmoid colon.

Sigmoidoscopy The visual examination of the rectum and sigmoid colon using a sigmoidoscope.

Signatura The part of a prescription that indicates the information to print on the medication label.

Signature on file (SOF) An indication on the insurance claim form that the signature of the patient is maintained by the medical office to authorize submission of insurance claims.

Simplified letter style A letter format in which all elements are left justified. The greeting is replaced by a subject line in all capital letters. The complimentary close and typed signature are replaced by a typed signature in all capital letters.

Single booking An appointment scheduling method in which each patient is given a different, specific appointment time. Also called *stream scheduling* or *fixed appointment scheduling.*

Skip Account for which no billing information is available.

Smartphone A cell phone with computer capabilities.

Smear Material spread on a slide for microscopic examination.

Soak The direct immersion of a body part in water or a medicated solution.

SOAP format A method of organization for recording progress notes. The SOAP format includes the following

categories: subjective data, objective data, assessment, and plan.

Social Security tax (FICA) A tax collected from employers and employees to fund the Social Security program, which provides benefits to retired workers.

Software A general term for the programs or instructions that tell a computer what to do.

Sonogram The record obtained with ultrasonography.

Sorter A device that facilitates putting papers or records in alphabetic or numeric order.

Sound card A circuit board connected to the mainboard that converts computer audio output into electronic signals. The electronic signals are then sent to speakers, which convert them into sound.

Special keys Keys that issue commands to the computer to perform specific functions on the information displayed on the screen.

Specific gravity The weight of a substance compared with the weight of an equal volume of a substance known as the standard. In urinalysis, the *specific gravity* refers to the measurement of the amount of dissolved substances present in the urine compared with the same amount of distilled water.

Specimen A small sample or part taken from the body to show the nature of the whole.

Speculum An instrument for opening a body orifice or cavity for viewing.

Spermatogenesis Process of meiosis in the male in which four spermatids are produced from one primary spermatocyte.

Spermiogenesis Morphologic changes that transform a spermatid into a mature sperm.

Sphygmomanometer An instrument for measuring arterial blood pressure.

Spirilla (sing. *spirillum*) Bacteria that have a spiral or curved shape.

Spirometer An instrument for measuring air taken into and expelled from the lungs.

Spirometry Measurement of an individual's breathing capacity by means of a spirometer.

Splint Any device that immobilizes a body part.

SpO₂ (saturation of peripheral oxygen) Abbreviation for the percentage of hemoglobin that is saturated with oxygen in arterial blood as measured by a pulse oximeter.

Spore A hard, thick-walled capsule formed by some bacteria that contains only the essential parts of the protoplasm of the bacterial cell.

Sprain Trauma to a joint that causes injury to the ligaments.

Standard of care Level of appropriate care required of a health professional.

Statute of limitations A law limiting the time period for beginning a lawsuit.

Statutory law Law enacted by a legislative body.

Stem cells Cells that have the capacity to develop into various types of body tissue.

Sterile Free of all living microorganisms and bacterial spores.

Sterilization The process of destroying all forms of microbial life, including bacterial spores.

Stethoscope An instrument used for amplifying and hearing sounds produced by the body.

Storage capacity The maximum amount of information that a device can hold, measured in bytes.

Storage device A device that permanently stores information for later retrieval by a computer.

Strain A stretching or tearing of muscles or tendons caused by trauma.

Stream scheduling An appointment scheduling method in which each patient is given a different, specific appointment time. Also called *fixed appointment scheduling, time-specified scheduling,* or *single booking.*

Stress The body's response to threat or change.

Subcutaneous injection Introduction of medication beneath the skin, into the subcutaneous or fatty layer of the body.

Subcutaneous layer A sheet of areolar connective tissue and adipose tissue beneath the dermis of the skin; also called *hypodermis* or *superficial fascia.*

Subjective symptom A symptom that is felt by the patient but is not observable by an examiner.

Sublingual administration Administration of medication by placing it under the tongue, where it dissolves and is absorbed through the mucous membrane.

Subpoena A court order for a witness to appear and give testimony.

Subpoena *duces tecum* A court order to produce documents or records.

Subscription The part of the prescription that gives directions to the pharmacist and usually designates the number of doses to be dispensed.

Sudoriferous gland A gland in the skin that produces perspiration; also called *sweat gland.*

Summarizing Expressing the most important points of a conversation or written document.

Superbill An itemized charge slip usually also containing diagnosis codes and procedure codes required for insurance billing.

Supernatant The clear liquid that remains at the top after a precipitate settles.

Superscription The part of a prescription consisting of the symbol Rx (from the Latin word recipe, meaning "take").

Suppuration The process of pus formation.

Suprapubic aspiration The passing of a sterile needle through the abdominal wall into the bladder to remove urine.

Surfactant A substance, produced by certain cells in lung tissue, that reduces surface tension between fluid molecules that line the respiratory membrane and helps keep the alveolus from collapsing.

Surgery The branch of medicine that deals with operative and manual procedures for correction of deformities and defects, repair of injuries, and diagnosis and treatment of certain diseases.

Surgical asepsis Practices that keep objects and areas sterile or free from microorganisms.

Surgical package Surgical services usually covered by a single procedure code that includes a preoperative visit, postoperative care, and local anesthesia (if applicable).

Surname Last name or family name of an individual terminal digit filing.

Susceptible Easily affected; lacking resistance.

Sutures Material used to approximate tissues with surgical stitches.

Swaged needle A needle with suturing material permanently attached to its end.

Sympathy Feeling the same emotions as another.

Symptom Any change in the body or its functioning that indicates a disease might be present.

Symptomatic treatment Therapy for symptoms of a disease or condition that does not remove the disease itself.

Synapse The region of communication between two neurons.

Synarthrosis (pl. *synarthroses*) An immovable joint.

Synergist A muscle that assists a prime mover but is not capable of producing the movement by itself; two or more muscles work together to produce a movement.

System software A group of programs that control or maintain the operations of a computer.

Systole The phase in the cardiac cycle in which the ventricles contract, sending blood out of the heart and into the aorta and pulmonary aorta.

Systolic pressure The point of maximum pressure on the arterial walls, which is recorded during systole.

Tab A projection of a folder that extends beyond the top or side of the folder.

Tachycardia An abnormally fast heart rate (more than 100 beats per minute).

Tachypnea An abnormal increase in the respiratory rate of more than 20 respirations per minute.

Target tissue A tissue (cells) that responds to a particular hormone because it has receptor sites for that hormone.

Template A standard form to which additional information can be added as needed.

Terabyte (TB) A unit of computer storage. One terabyte is equivalent to a little more than a trillion bytes or 1000 gigabytes.

Terminal digit filing A chronologic filing system that uses the last number or number group as the first indexing unit.

Terminal phase The last stage of illness, usually used when death is expected to occur within 6 months.

Test system A setup that includes all of the test components required to perform a laboratory test such as testing devices, controls, and testing reagents.

Thermolabile Easily affected or changed by heat.

Thermoreceptor A sensory receptor that detects changes in temperature.

Thready pulse A pulse with a decreased volume that feels weak and thin.

Threshold stimulus Minimum level of stimulation that is required to start a nerve impulse or muscle contraction; also called *liminal stimulus.*

Thrombocyte One of the formed elements of the blood; functions in blood clotting; also called *platelet.*

Tickler file A chronologic file containing reminders of things to be done.

Time management Skills and techniques used to manage time in order to accomplish tasks and meet goals.

Time-specified scheduling An appointment scheduling method in which each patient is given a different, specific appointment time. Also called *stream scheduling, fixed appointment scheduling,* or *single booking.*

Tissue Group of similar cells specialized to perform a certain function.

Toddler A child 1 to 3 years old.

Topical administration Application of a drug to a particular spot, usually for a local action.

Tort An injury or wrong against a person or property that does not involve breach of contract.

Toxemia A condition that can occur in pregnant women that includes preeclampsia and eclampsia. If preeclampsia goes undiagnosed or is not satisfactorily controlled, it could develop into eclampsia, characterized by convulsions and coma.

Toxoid A toxin (a poisonous substance produced by a bacterium) that has been treated by heat or chemicals to destroy its harmful properties. It is administered to an individual to prevent an infectious disease by stimulating the production of antibodies in that individual.

Transcription The process of changing verbal dictation to typed or printed form.

Transfusion The administration of whole blood or blood products through the intravenous route.

Transient flora Microorganisms that reside on the superficial skin layers and are picked up in the course of daily activities. They are often pathogenic but can be removed easily from the skin by sanitizing the hands.

Triage The process of separating patients by the urgency of their need for care.

TRICARE A government insurance plan that provides medical care to spouses and dependents of individuals on active duty in the military. Formerly this program was called *CHAMPUS.*

Trimester Three months, or one third, of the gestational period of pregnancy.

Truth in lending Legal requirement to disclose the terms of a loan in terms that the borrower can understand.

Tympanic membrane A thin, semitransparent membrane between the external ear canal and the middle ear that receives and transmits sound waves. Also known as the *eardrum.*

Ultrasonography The use of high-frequency sound waves to produce an image of an organ or tissue.

Urgency The immediate need to urinate.

Urinalysis The physical, chemical, and microscopic analyses of urine.

Urinary incontinence The inability to retain urine.

URL The characters and/or words used to access a specific website or file on the World Wide Web.

User An individual using a computer.

Usual, customary, and reasonable (UCR) A system for establishing the amount an insurance company will pay for a procedure. The reasonable charge is set by the insurance company on the basis of a physician's usual (most frequent) charge for the procedure and the customary charge of other physicians in the same geographic area.

Uterine cycle Monthly cycle of events that occur in the uterus from puberty to menopause; also called the *menstrual cycle;* occurs concurrently with the ovarian cycle.

Utilization Review Assessing and reviewing medical services to determine whether they are appropriate, necessary, and of high quality.

Vaccine A suspension of attenuated (weakened) or killed microorganisms administered to an individual to prevent an infectious disease by stimulating the production of antibodies in that individual.

Vendor A company from which supplies or equipment is purchased.

Venipuncture Puncturing of a vein.

Venous reflux The backflow of blood (from an evacuated tube) into the patient's vein.

Venous stasis The temporary cessation or slowing of the venous blood flow.

Ventilation Movement of air into and out of the lungs; breathing.

Veracity Truthfulness.

Verbal Using words to communicate.

Vertex The top of the head.

Vial A closed glass container with a rubber stopper that holds medication.

Video card A circuit board connected to the mainboard that converts computer video output into electronic signals. The electronic signals are then sent to the monitor, where they are converted into text and images that can be viewed by the user.

Voicemail A method for delivery, storage, and retrieval of telephone messages that is built into the telephone system.

Void To empty the bladder.

Vulva The region of the external female genital organs.

W-4 The form used to claim allowances for federal income tax reporting.

Waived test A laboratory test that meets the CLIA criteria for being a simple procedure that is easy to perform and has a low risk of erroneous test results. Waived tests include tests that have been approved by the FDA for use by patients at home.

Warranty A promise by the manufacturer to repair or replace defective parts in an item during a specific time period.

Wave scheduling A method of scheduling appointments in which several patients are given the same appointment time and seen in the order in which they arrive.

Web browser A software program used to access the World Wide Web.

Webcam Small video camera attached to a computer that allows video to be transmitted on the Internet.

Wheal A tense, pale, raised area of the skin.

Wheezing A continuous, high-pitched whistling musical sound heard particularly during exhalation and sometimes during inhalation.

Workers' compensation An insurance program that covers lost wages and health care costs of workers injured on the job or who develop work-related illnesses.

World Wide Web A series of interlinked websites or files accessed via the Internet.

Wound A break in the continuity of an external or internal surface caused by physical means.

ZIP code A five-digit code that identifies the post office to which a given piece of mail is to be delivered.

ZIP+4 code A more detailed mailing code consisting of the original five-digit ZIP code followed by a hyphen and four additional digits. These digits identify a specific geographic segment within the delivery area.

Figure Credits

CHAPTER ONE

Figures 1-2, 1-3, and 1-6: From Hunt SA: *Saunders fundamentals of medical assisting,* St Louis, 2007, Saunders.

Figure 1-4: From Young-Adams AD, Proctor DB: *Kinn's the medical assistant,* ed 11, St Louis, 2011, Saunders.

Figure 1-5: Courtesy Gatterman MI: *Foundations of chiropractic: subluxation,* St Louis, 1995, Mosby.

Unnumbered Figures 1 and 2 in Highlight Box: Courtesy Blocker History of Medicine Collections, Moody Medical Library, University of Texas Medical Branch, Galveston, Tex.

Unnumbered Figures 3 and 4 in Highlight Box: Courtesy National Library of Medicine.

CHAPTER FOUR

Figures 4-1 and 4-4: From Hunt SA: *Saunders fundamentals of medical assisting,* St Louis, 2007, Saunders.

CHAPTER FIVE

Figures 5-1 through 5-28: From Applegate E: *The anatomy and physiology learning system,* ed 4, St Louis, 2011, Saunders.

CHAPTER SIX

Figure 6-1: From Applegate E: *The anatomy and physiology learning system,* ed 4, St Louis, 2011, Saunders.

CHAPTER SEVEN

Figures 7-1 through 7-4; 7-6 through 7-11; 7-17, and 7-18: From Applegate E: *The anatomy and physiology learning system,* ed 4, St Louis, 2011, Saunders.

Figures 7-5 and 7-12 through 7-16: Modified from Applegate E: *The anatomy and physiology learning system,* ed 4, St Louis, 2011, Saunders.

CHAPTER EIGHT

Figures 8-1 through 8-4: From Applegate E: *The anatomy and physiology learning system,* ed 4, St Louis, 2011, Saunders.

Figures 8-5 and 8-6: Modified from Applegate E: *The anatomy and physiology learning system,* ed 4, St Louis, 2011, Saunders.

CHAPTER NINE

Figures 9-1 through 9-8, 9-10, 9-12, and 9-13: From Applegate E: *The anatomy and physiology learning system,* ed 4, St Louis, 2011, Saunders.

Figures 9-9 and 9-11: Modified from Applegate E: *The anatomy and physiology learning system,* ed 4, St Louis, 2011, Saunders.

CHAPTER TEN

Figures 10-1 through 10-8: From Applegate E: *The anatomy and physiology learning system,* ed 4, St Louis, 2011, Saunders.

CHAPTER ELEVEN

Figures 11-1 through 11-3 and 11-5: From Applegate E: *The anatomy and physiology learning system,* ed 4, St Louis, 2011, Saunders.

Figure 11-4: From Applegate E: *The anatomy and physiology learning system,* ed 3, St Louis, 2006, Saunders.

CHAPTER TWELVE

Figures 12-1 through 12-15: From Applegate E: *The anatomy and physiology learning system,* ed 4, St Louis, 2011, Saunders.

CHAPTER THIRTEEN

Figures 13-1 and 13-4: From Applegate E: *The anatomy and physiology learning system,* ed 4, St Louis, 2011, Saunders.

Figures 13-2 and 13-3: Modified from Applegate E: *The anatomy and physiology learning system,* ed 4, St Louis, 2011, Saunders.

CHAPTER FOURTEEN

Figures 14-1 through 14-5; Figures 14-7 and 14-8: From Applegate E: *The anatomy and physiology learning system,* ed 4, St Louis, 2011, Saunders.

Figures 14-6 and 14-9: Modified from Applegate E: *The anatomy and physiology learning system,* ed 4, St Louis, 2011, Saunders.

CHAPTER FIFTEEN

Figures 15-1, 15-2, 15-4, and 15-6: From Applegate E: *The anatomy and physiology learning system,* ed 4, St Louis, 2011, Saunders.

Figures 15-3 and 15-5: Modified from Applegate E: *The anatomy and physiology learning system,* ed 4, St Louis, 2011, Saunders.

CHAPTER SIXTEEN

Figures 16-1 and 16-3 through 16-14: From Applegate E: *The anatomy and physiology learning system,* ed 4, St Louis, 2011, Saunders.

Figures 16-2: Modified from Applegate E: *The anatomy and physiology learning system,* ed 4, St Louis, 2011, Saunders.

CHAPTER SEVENTEEN

Figures 17-1, 17-2, and 17-4 through 17-14: From Bonewit-West K: *Clinical procedures for medical assistants,* ed 8, St Louis, 2011, Saunders.

Figure 17-3: From Goodman CC: *Pathology: implications for the physical therapist,* ed 3, St Louis, 2010, Saunders.

All Unnumbered Procedural Figures: From Bonewit-West K: *Clinical procedures for medical assistants,* ed 8, St Louis, 2011, Saunders.

Unnumbered Figure in Highlight Box: From Forbes CD: *Color atlas and text of clinical medicine,* ed 3, St Louis, 2003, Mosby.

CHAPTER EIGHTEEN

Figures 18-1 through 18-13: From Bonewit-West K: *Clinical procedures for medical assistants,* ed 8, St Louis, 2011, Saunders.

Figure 18-14: Courtesy of and modified from AMSCO/American Sterilizer Company, Erie, Pa.

Figure 18-15: Courtesy AMSCO/American Sterilizer Company, Erie, Pa.

All Unnumbered Charting Examples and Procedural Figures: From Bonewit-West K: *Clinical procedures for medical assistants,* ed 8, St Louis, 2011, Saunders.

CHAPTER NINETEEN

Figures 19-1 through 19-24: From Bonewit-West K: *Clinical procedures for medical assistants,* ed 8, St Louis, 2011, Saunders.

Figure 19-25: Robinson DS: *Essentials of dental assisting,* ed 4, St Louis, 2007, Saunders.

All Unnumbered Charting Examples and Procedural Figures: From Bonewit-West K: *Clinical procedures for medical assistants,* ed 8, St Louis, 2011, Saunders.

CHAPTER TWENTY

Figures 20-1, 20-3 through 20-5, and 20-7 through 20-12: From Bonewit-West K: *Clinical procedures for medical assistants,* ed 8, St Louis, 2011, Saunders.

Figure 20-2: From *Report of the Dietary Guidelines Advisory Committee on the dietary guidelines for Americans,* Washington, DC, 1995, U.S. Department of Health and Human Services.

Figure 20-6: From Applegate EJ: *The anatomy and physiology learning system,* ed 4, St Louis, 2011, Saunders.

All Unnumbered Charting Examples and Procedural Figures: From Bonewit-West K: *Clinical procedures for medical assistants,* ed 8, St Louis, 2011, Saunders.

CHAPTER TWENTY-ONE

Figures 21-1 through 21-5, 21-7, and 21-8: From Bonewit-West K: *Clinical procedures for medical assistants,* ed 8, St Louis, 2011, Saunders.

Figure 21-6: From Ishihara J: *Tests for color blindness,* Tokyo, 1920, Kanehara.

Figures 21-9 and 21-10: Courtesy GSI (Grayson-Stadler), Milford, NH.

Unnumbered Figure in Patient Teaching Box (Bacterial conjunctivitis): From Cuppett M, Walsh KM: *General medical conditions in the athlete,* St Louis, 2005, Mosby.

Unnumbered Figure in Patient Teaching Box (Chronic otitis media): From Damjanov I, Linder J: *Pathology: a color atlas,* St Louis, 1999, Mosby.

Unnumbered Figure in Patient Teaching Box (Serous otitis media): From Swartz MH: *Textbook of physical diagnosis,* ed 5, Philadelphia, 2006, Saunders.

All Unnumbered Charting Examples and Procedural Figures: From Bonewit-West K: *Clinical procedures for medical assistants,* ed 8, St Louis, 2011, Saunders.

CHAPTER TWENTY-TWO

Figure 22-1: From Wood LA, Rambo BJ: *Nursing skills for allied health services,* vol 2, Philadelphia, 1980, Saunders.

Figures 22-2 and 22-4: From Bonewit-West K: *Clinical procedures for medical assistants,* ed 8, St Louis, 2011, Saunders.

Figure 22-3: Courtesy 3M Health Care, St Paul, Minn.

All Unnumbered Charting Examples and Procedural Figures: From Bonewit-West K: *Clinical procedures for medical assistants,* ed 8, St Louis, 2011, Saunders.

CHAPTER TWENTY-THREE

Figures 23-1 through 23-6, 23-8, and 23-10 through 23-17: From Bonewit-West K: *Clinical procedures for medical assistants,* ed 8, St Louis, 2011, Saunders.

Figures 23-7 and 23-9: Modified from Mahon C, Manuselis G: *Textbook of diagnostic microbiology,* ed 3, St Louis, 2007, Saunders.

Unnumbered Figure in Box 23-1 (Embryo at approximately 9 weeks' gestation; Amniocentesis being performed under ultrasound guidance): From Greer IA, Cameron IT, Kitchener HC, Prentice A: *Mosby's color atlas and text of obstetrics and gynecology,* St Louis, 2001, Mosby.

Unnumbered Figures in Box 23-1 (Erect fetal penis; External female genitalia): From Callen P: *Ultrasonography in obstetrics and gynecology,* ed 4, Philadelphia, 2000, Saunders.

Unnumbered Figure in Box 23-1 (Twins): From Bonewit-West K: *Clinical procedures for medical assistants,* ed 8, St Louis, 2011, Saunders.

Unnumbered Figures in Box on Chlamydia and Gonorrhea Specimen Collection: From Bonewit-West K: *Clinical procedures for medical assistants,* ed 8, St Louis, 2011, Saunders.

All Unnumbered Charting Examples and Procedural Figures: From Bonewit-West K: *Clinical procedures for medical assistants,* ed 8, St Louis, 2011, Saunders.

CHAPTER TWENTY-FOUR

Figures 24-1 through 24-6, 24-8*B*, 24-9, 24-12, and 24-15 through 24-17: From Bonewit-West K: *Clinical procedures for medical assistants,* ed 8, St Louis, 2011, Saunders.

Figures 24-7, 24-8*A*, and 24-10: Courtesy Wyeth Laboratories, Philadelphia, Pa.

Figure 24-11: From Department of Health and Human Services, Centers for Disease Control and Prevention, United States, 2010.

Figure 24-13: Courtesy Centers for Disease Control and Prevention, Atlanta, Ga.

Figure 24-14: Modified from Immunization Action Coalition, St Paul, Minn.

All Unnumbered Charting Examples and Procedural Figures: From Bonewit-West K: *Clinical procedures for medical assistants,* ed 8, St Louis, 2011, Saunders.

CHAPTER TWENTY-FIVE

Figures 25-1, 25-2, 25-4 through 25-8, 25-10 through 25-16, 25-32 through 25-34, and 25-36: From

Bonewit-West K: *Clinical procedures for medical assistants,* ed 8, St Louis, 2011, Saunders.

Figure 25-3: Courtesy Elmed, Addison, Ill.

Figure 25-9: **A** modified from *Perspectives on sutures,* courtesy Davis & Geck, Danbury, Conn; **B** modified from Nealon TF Jr: *Fundamental skills in surgery,* ed 4, Philadelphia, 1994, Saunders.

Figure 25-17: Courtesy Diagnostic Pathology Associates, Columbus, Ohio.

Figure 25-18: From Weston, Lane, Morelli. In Sanders MJ: *Mosby's paramedic textbook,* ed 3, St Louis, 2007, Mosby.

Figure 25-19: From Nealon TF Jr: *Fundamental skills in surgery,* ed 4, Philadelphia, 1994, Saunders.

Figure 25-20: **A** from Braverman IM: *Skin signs of systemic disease,* ed 3, Philadelphia, 1998, Saunders. **B** from Nealon TF Jr: *Fundamental skills in surgery,* ed 4, Philadelphia, 1994, Saunders.

Figure 25-21: From LaFleur Brooks M: *Exploring medical language: a student-directed approach,* ed 7, St Louis, 2009, Mosby.

Figure 25-22: From White GM, Cox NH: *Diseases of the skin: a color atlas and text,* ed 2, St Louis, 2006, Mosby.

Figure 25-23: From Forbes CD: *Color atlas and text of clinical medicine,* ed 3, St Louis, 2003, Mosby.

Figure 25-24: From Goldman L: *Cecil medicine,* ed 23, Philadelphia, 2008, Saunders.

Figure 25-25: From Christensen BL: *Adult health nursing,* ed 5, St Louis, 2006, Mosby.

Figure 25-26: From Nealon TF Jr: *Fundamental skills in surgery,* ed 4, Philadelphia, 1994, Saunders.

Figure 25-27: From Seidel HM: *Mosby's guide to physical examination,* ed 6, St Louis, 2006, Mosby.

Figure 25-28: From Apgar BS, Brotzman GL, Spitzer M: *Colposcopy: principles and practice—an integrated textbook and atlas,* Philadelphia, 2002, Saunders.

Figure 25-29: From Damjanov I: *Pathology for the health-related professions,* ed 3, St Louis, 2006, Saunders.

Figure 25-30: Courtesy Elmed, Addison, Ill.

Figure 25-31: From Zakus S: *Clinical skills for medical assistants,* ed 4, Philadelphia, 2001, Saunders.

Figure 25-35: From Leake MJ: *A manual of simple nursing procedures,* Philadelphia, 1971, Saunders.

Unnumbered Figures in text (Suture insertion side table; Suture insertion sterile field; Sebaceous cyst removal sterile field): From Bonewit-West K: *Clinical procedures for medical assistants,* ed 8, St Louis, 2011, Saunders.

All Unnumbered Procedural Figures in Procedures 25-1 through 25-4: From Bonewit-West K: *Clinical procedures for medical assistants,* ed 8, St Louis, 2011, Saunders.

Unnumbered Figures in Procedure 25-5 (Steps 1 and 4): From Bonewit-West K: *Clinical procedures for medical assistants,* ed 8, St Louis, 2011, Saunders.

Unnumbered Figures in Procedure 25-5 (Step 6a and 6b): Modified from Nealon TF Jr: *Fundamental skills in surgery,* ed 4, Philadelphia, 1994, Saunders.

Unnumbered Figure in Procedure 25-5 (Step 6 [c]): Courtesy Ethicon, Somerville, NJ.

All Unnumbered Charting Examples and Procedural Figures: From Bonewit-West K: *Clinical procedures for medical assistants,* ed 8, St Louis, 2011, Saunders.

CHAPTER TWENTY-SIX

Figures 26-1 through 26-9, 26-11 through 26-17, 26-19 through 26-21, 26-24 and 26-25, and 26-27 and 26-28: From Bonewit-West K: *Clinical procedures for medical assistants,* ed 8, St Louis, 2011, Saunders.

Figure 26-10*A:* Becton-Dickinson Safety Glide Syringe.

Figure 26-10*B:* Monoject Safety Syringe.

Figure 26-10*C:* Vanish Point Syringe.

Figure 26-18: From Leahy JM, Kizilay PE: *Foundations of nursing practice: a nursing process approach,* Philadelphia, 1988, Saunders.

Figure 26-22: From Nairn R: *Immunology for medical students,* ed 2, Philadelphia, 2007, Mosby.

Figure 26-23: From Abbas AK: *Basic immunology: functions and disorders of the immune system,* ed 3, Philadelphia, 2004, Saunders.

Figure 26-26: From Shiland BJ: *Mastering healthcare terminology,* ed 3, St Louis, 2010, Mosby.

Figure 26-29: Copyright and courtesy Hollister-Stier, Spokane, Wash.

Figure 26-30: From Potter PA, Perry AG: *Basic nursing: essentials for practice,* ed 5, St Louis, 2002, Mosby.

Figure 26-31: Photo by Margaret Hartshorn. Courtesy of the Arizona Arthritis Center (www.arthritis.arizona.edu).

All Unnumbered Charting Examples and Procedural Figures: From Bonewit-West K: *Clinical procedures for medical assistants,* ed 8, St Louis, 2011, Saunders.

CHAPTER TWENTY-SEVEN

Figures 27-1 through 27-10, 27-12 through 27-16, 27-18 through 27-20, and 27-25: From Bonewit-West K: *Clinical procedures for medical assistants,* ed 8, St Louis, 2011, Saunders.

Figure 27-11 **D** From Long BW: *Radiography essentials for limited practice,* ed 3, St Louis, 2010, Saunders.

Figure 27-17: From Potter PA: *Basic nursing: essentials for practice,* ed 6, St Louis, 2007, Mosby.

Figure 27-21: **A** from Henry MC: *EMT prehospital care,* ed 4, St Louis, 2009, Mosby. **B** from Aehlert B: Paramedic practice today: above and beyond, 2-volume set, St Louis, 2009, Mosby.

Figure 27-22: From Perry AG: *Clinical nursing skills and techniques,* ed 7, St Louis, 2010, Saunders.

Figure 27-23: **A** from Sorrentino S: *Mosby's textbook for long-term care nursing assistants,* ed 5, St Louis, 2006, Mosby. **B** from Perry AG: *Clinical nursing skills and techniques,* ed 7, St Louis, 2010, Saunders.

Figure 27-24: **A** from Potter P: *Canadian fundamentals of nursing,* ed 4, Canada, 2010, Mosby. **B** and **C** from

Bonewit-West K: *Clinical procedures for medical assistants,* ed 8, St Louis, 2011, Saunders.

Unnumbered Figure in Highlight Box (Cardiac treadmill stress test): From deWit SC: *Medical-surgical nursing: concepts and practice,* St Louis, 2008, Saunders.

Unnumbered Figure in Highlight Box (Emphysema caused by smoking): From Little JW: *Dental management of the medically compromised patient,* ed 7, St Louis, 2008, Mosby. Courtesy R.N. McLay, J.H. Harrison, C.D. Fermin, H. Johnson, Tulane Gross Pathology Tutorial. Last modified July 15, 1997, Tulane University School of Medicine. Available at: http://www.som.tulane.edu/classware/pathology/medical_pathology/mcpath. Accessed August 22, 2006.

All Unnumbered Charting Examples and Procedural Figures: From Bonewit-West K: *Clinical procedures for medical assistants,* ed 8, St Louis, 2011, Saunders.

CHAPTER TWENTY-EIGHT

Figures 28-1 and 28-2, 28-4 through 28-6, 28-8, 28-9, and 28-11: From Bonewit-West K: *Clinical procedures for medical assistants,* ed 8, St Louis, 2011, Saunders.

Figure 28-3: From Lafleur Brooks M: *Exploring medical language: a student-directed approach,* ed 7, St Louis, 2009, Mosby.

Figure 28-7: From Lewis S: *Medical-surgical nursing,* ed 7, St Louis, 2007, Mosby.

Figure 28-10: From Meschan I: *Synopsis of radiologic anatomy with computed tomography,* Philadelphia, 1980, Saunders.

Figure 28-12: From Ballinger PW, Frank ED, eds: *Merrill's atlas of radiographic positions and radiologic procedures,* vol 2, ed 10, St Louis, 2003, Mosby.

Figure 28-13: From Prue L: *Atlas of mammographic positioning,* Philadelphia, 1994, Saunders.

Figures 28-14 and 28-15: From Meschan I: *Synopsis of radiologic anatomy with computed tomography,* Philadelphia, 1980, Saunders.

Figure 28-16: From Leonard PC: *Building a medical vocabulary: with Spanish translations,* ed 7, St Louis, 2009, Saunders.

Figure 28-17: From Tempkin BB: *Ultrasound scanning: principles and protocols,* ed 3, St Louis, 2009, Saunders.

Figure 28-18: From Kowalczyk N, Donnett K: *Integrated patient care for the imaging professional,* St Louis, 1996, Mosby.

Figure 28-19: From Snopek A: *Fundamentals of special radiographic procedures,* ed 4, Philadelphia, 1999, Saunders.

Figure 28-20: From Ballinger PW, Frank ED, eds: *Merrill's atlas of radiographic positions and radiologic procedures,* vol 3, ed 10, St Louis, 2003, Mosby.

Figure 28-21: From Donatelli RA: *Sports-specific rehabilitation,* St Louis, 2007, Churchill Livingstone.

Figure 28-22: Screenshot used by permission of MCKESSON Corporation. All rights reserved. Copyright MCKESSON Corporation, 2012. (From Buck CJ: *Electronic health record booster kit for the medical office,* St Louis, 2009, Saunders.)

Unnumbered Figure in Highlight Box (Colon cancer): From Forbes CD: *Color atlas and text of clinical medicine,* ed 3, Philadelphia, 2003, Mosby.

All Unnumbered Charting Examples and Procedural Figures: From Bonewit-West K: *Clinical procedures for medical assistants,* ed 8, St Louis, 2011, Saunders.

CHAPTER TWENTY-NINE

Figures 29-1 through 29-6, 29-8 through 29-24: From Bonewit-West K: *Clinical procedures for medical assistants,* ed 8, St Louis, 2011, Saunders.

Figure 29-7: Screenshot used by permission of MCKESSON Corporation. All rights reserved. Copyright MCKESSON Corporation, 2012. (From Buck CJ: *Electronic health record booster kit for the medical office,* St Louis, 2009, Saunders.)

CHAPTER THIRTY

Figures 30-1 through 30-6: From Bonewit-West K: *Clinical procedures for medical assistants,* ed 8, St Louis, 2011, Saunders.

Charting Example and Multistix Color Chart in Procedure 30-2: Modified and printed by permission of Siemens Medical Solutions Diagnostics, Tarrytown, NY.

All Other Unnumbered Charting Examples and Procedural Figures: From Bonewit-West K: *Clinical procedures for medical assistants,* ed 8, St Louis, 2011, Saunders.

CHAPTER THIRTY-ONE

Figures 31-1 through 31-26: From Bonewit-West K: *Clinical procedures for medical assistants,* ed 8, St Louis, 2011, Saunders.

All Unnumbered Charting Examples and Procedural Figures: From Bonewit-West K: *Clinical procedures for medical assistants,* ed 8, St Louis, 2011, Saunders.

CHAPTER THIRTY-TWO

Figures 32-1 through 32-4 and 32-6 through 32-8: From Bonewit-West K: *Clinical procedures for medical assistants,* ed 8, St Louis, 2011, Saunders.

Figure 32-5: From Custer RP: *An atlas of the blood and bone marrow,* ed 2, Philadelphia, 1974, Saunders.

Blood Smear slides in Procedure 32-2 (Step 4c): From Rodak BF: *Hematology: clinical principles and applications,* Philadelphia, 1995, Saunders.

All Other Unnumbered Charting Examples and Procedural Figures: From Bonewit-West K: *Clinical procedures for medical assistants,* ed 8, St Louis, 2011, Saunders.

CHAPTER THIRTY-THREE

Figures 33-1, 33-2, and 33-4 through 33-10: From Bonewit-West K: *Clinical procedures for medical assistants,* ed 8, St Louis, 2011, Saunders.

Figure 33-3: ATAC Lab System by Clinical Data, Inc.

Figures 33-11 and 33-13: From Garrels M, Oatis CS: *Laboratory testing for ambulatory settings,* ed 2, St Louis, 2011, Saunders.

Figure 33-12: Courtesy of and modified from Quidel Corporation, San Diego, Calif.

Unnumbered Figure in Patient Teaching Box on Diabetes: From Lewis S: *Medical-surgical nursing,* ed 7, St Louis, 2007, Mosby.

All Unnumbered Charting Examples and Procedural Figures: From Bonewit-West K: *Clinical procedures for medical assistants,* ed 8, St Louis, 2011, Saunders.

CHAPTER THIRTY-FOUR

Figure 34-1: From Fuerst R: *Frobisher and Fuerst's microbiology in health and disease,* ed 15, Philadelphia, 1983, Saunders.

Figures 34-2, 34-4, 34-5, 34-8: From Bonewit-West K: *Clinical procedures for medical assistants,* ed 8, St Louis, 2011, Saunders.

Figure 34-3: **A, B,** and **D** from Mahon CR, Manuselis G Jr: *Textbook of diagnostic microbiology,* ed 2, Philadelphia, 2000, Saunders; **C** courtesy Cathy Bissonette; **E** courtesy Dr. Andrew G. Smith.

Figure 34-6: Courtesy Quidel Corporation, San Diego, Calif.

Figure 34-7: From Mahon CR, Manuselis G Jr: *Textbook of diagnostic microbiology,* ed 2, Philadelphia, 2000, Saunders.

Figure 34-9: **A** courtesy Cathy Bissonette; **B** from Mahon CR, Manuselis G Jr: *Textbook of diagnostic microbiology,* ed 2, Philadelphia, 2000, Saunders.

All Unnumbered Charting Examples and Procedural Figures: From Bonewit-West K: *Clinical procedures for medical assistants,* ed 8, St Louis, 2011, Saunders.

CHAPTER THIRTY-FIVE

Figures 35-1 through 35-4, 35-6 through 35-9, 35-11, and 35-14 through 35-17: From Bonewit-West K: *Clinical procedures for medical assistants,* ed 8, St Louis, 2011, Saunders.

Figure 35-5: From Miller BF, Keane CB: *Encyclopedia and dictionary of medicine, nursing, and allied health,* ed 7, Philadelphia, 2003, Saunders.

Figure 35-10: From Connolly JF: *DePalma's the management of fractures and dislocations: an atlas,* Philadelphia, 1981, Saunders.

Figure 35-12: From Henry M, Stapleton E: *EMT prehospital care,* ed 2, Philadelphia, 1997, Saunders.

Figure 35-13: From Polaski AL, Tatro SE: *Luckmann's core principles and practice of medical-surgical nursing,* Philadelphia, 1996, Saunders.

CHAPTER THIRTY-SIX

Figure 36-1: Courtesy and modified from Colwell Systems, Champaign, Ill.

Figures 36-2, 36-6, 36-8, 36-9, 36-12 through 36-15, and 36-18 through 36-20: From Bonewit-West K: *Clinical procedures for medical assistants,* ed 8, St Louis, 2011, Saunders.

Figures 36-3, 36-5, 36-10, and 36-11: Modified from Diehl MO: *Medical transcription: techniques and procedures,* ed 6, St Louis, 2007, Saunders.

Figure 36-4: Form Number 3514. Courtesy Briggs, Des Moines.

Figure 36-7: Form Number 3507P. Courtesy Briggs, Des Moines.

Figure 36-16: Courtesy and modified from Miller Communications, Norwalk, Conn.

Figure 36-17: Form Number 653/2S. Courtesy Briggs, Des Moines.

All Unnumbered Charting Examples and Procedural Figures: From Bonewit-West K: *Clinical procedures for medical assistants,* ed 8, St Louis, 2011, Saunders.

CHAPTER THIRTY-SEVEN

Figure 37-1: From Klieger D: *Saunders textbook of medical assisting,* St Louis, 2005, Saunders.

Figure 37-3: Courtesy Bibbero Systems, Inc., Petaluma, Calif, (800) 242-2376; Fax (800) 242-9330; www.bibbero.com.

CHAPTER THIRTY-EIGHT

Figure 38-2: Courtesy Dell Computers, Round Rock, Tex.

Figure 38-11: Screenshot used by permission of MCKESSON Corporation. All rights reserved. Copyright MCKESSON Corporation, 2012.

Figures 38-13 and 38-14: Courtesy AltaPoint Data Systems, LLC.

CHAPTER THIRTY-NINE

Figure 39-3: From Young AP, Proctor DB: *Kinn's the medical assistant,* ed 11, St Louis, 2011, Saunders.

Unnumbered Figures in Procedure 39-2 (Step 4) and Procedure 39-3 (Step 7): From Hunt SA: *Saunders fundamentals of medical assisting,* St Louis, 2007, Saunders.

CHAPTER FORTY

Unnumbered Screenshot: Screenshot used by permission of MCKESSON Corporation. All Rights Reserved. Copyright MCKESSON Corporation, 2012.

CHAPTER FORTY-ONE

Figure 41-1: From Young AP, Proctor DB: *Kinn's the medical assistant,* ed 11, St Louis, 2011, Saunders.

Figure 41-2: Modified from Hunt SA: *Saunders fundamentals of medical assisting,* St Louis, 2007, Saunders.

Figures 41-3 and 41-4: Courtesy Bibbero Systems, Inc., Petaluma, Calif, (800) 242-2376; Fax (800) 242-9330; www.bibbero.com.

CHAPTER FORTY-TWO

Figure 42-6: From Diehl MO, Fordney, MT: *Medical typing and transcription: techniques and procedures,* ed 3, Philadelphia, 1991, Saunders.

Figure 42-7: From Hunt SA: *Saunders fundamentals of medical assisting,* St Louis, 2007, Saunders.

Figure 42-8: Courtesy Dell Corporation, Round Rock, Tex.

CHAPTER FORTY-THREE

Figures 43-2 and 43-6: Modified from Young AP, Proctor DB: *Kinn's the medical assistant,* ed 11, St Louis, 2011, Saunders.

Figure 43-3: From Young AP, Proctor DB: *Kinn's the medical assistant,* ed 11, St Louis, 2011, Saunders.

CHAPTER FORTY-FOUR

Figures 44-4 and 44-6: Courtesy Bibbero Systems, Inc., Petaluma, Calif, (800) 242-2376; Fax (800) 242-9330; www.bibbero.com.

Figures 44-5 and 44-8: From Hunt SA: *Saunders fundamentals of medical assisting,* St Louis, 2007, Saunders.

CHAPTER FORTY-FIVE

Figure 45-6: From Buck C: *Saunders 2011 ICD-10-CM,* St Louis, 2011, Saunders.

CHAPTER FORTY-SIX

Figure 46-2: From Fordney M: *Insurance handbook for the medical office,* ed 11, St Louis, 2010, Saunders.

Figure 46-4: From Hunt SA: *Saunders fundamentals of medical assisting,* St Louis, 2007, Saunders.

CHAPTER FORTY-SEVEN

Figures 47-2 and 47-4: From Hunt SA: *Saunders fundamentals of medical assisting,* St Louis, 2007, Saunders.

CHAPTER FORTY-EIGHT

Figure 48-4: From Hunt SA: *Saunders fundamentals of medical assisting,* St Louis, 2007, Saunders.

Figure 48-5: Courtesy Patterson Office Supplies, Champaign, Ill.

CHAPTER FORTY-NINE

Figures 49-1 and 49-7: From National Association of Emergency Medical Technicians: *PHTLS: Prehospital Trauma Life Support, Military Version,* ed 7, St Louis, 2011, Mosby.

Figures 49-2 and 49-3: From Hunt SA: *Saunders fundamentals of medical assisting,* St Louis, 2007, Saunders.

Unnumbered Photos from Procedure 49-1: From Sorrentino SA: *Mosby's textbook for long-term care nursing assistants,* ed 5, St Louis, 2007, Mosby.

CHAPTER FIFTY

Figure 50-4: Modified from Hunt SA: *Saunders fundamentals of medical assisting,* St Louis, 2007, Saunders.

Index

Page numbers followed by *f* indicate figures; *t*, tables; *b*, boxes.